Management of Common Musculoskeletal Disorders
Physical Therapy Principles and Methods

Management of Common Musculoskeletal Disorders
Physical Therapy Principles and Methods, Fourth Edition

Darlene Hertling, BS, RPT
Randolph M. Kessler, MD

With Contributors

LIPPINCOTT WILLIAMS & WILKINS
A **Wolters Kluwer** Company

Philadelphia • Baltimore • New York • London
Buenos Aires • Hong Kong • Sydney • Tokyo

Acquisitions Editor: Pam Lappies
Managing Editor: David Payne
Marketing Manager: Mary Martin
Project Editor: Paula Williams
Designer: Doug Smock
Artwork: Carolyn Kates, Kimberly Battista
Illustration Planning: Wayne Hubbel
Photography: Robert Riedlinger
Compositor: Circle Graphics
Printer: Courier-Kendallville

Copyright © 2006 Lippincott Williams & Wilkins

530 Walnut Street
Philadelphia, Pennsylvania 19106-3621 USA

351 West Camden Street
Baltimore, Maryland 21201-2436 USA

Printed in China

Library of Congress Cataloging-in-Publication Data

Hertling, Darlene.
    Management of common musculoskeletal disorders : physical therapy principles and methods / Darlene Hertling, Randolph M. Kessler ; with contributors.— 4th ed.
        p. ;   cm.
    Includes bibliographical references and index.
    ISBN-13: 978-0–7817–3626–8
    ISBN-10: 0–7817–3626–9 (alk. paper)
    1. Musculoskeletal system—Diseases—Physical therapy.   2. Musculoskeletal system—Diseases—Patients—Rehabilitation.
I. Kessler, Randolph M.   II. Title.
    [DNLM: 1. Bone Diseases—therapy.   2. Muscular Diseases—therapy.   3. Physical Therapy Techniques.   WE 140 H574m 2006]
RM700.H48   2006
616.7'062—dc22   2005022095

The publishers have made every effort to trace the copyright holders for borrowed material. If they have inadvertently overlooked any, they will be pleased to make the necessary arrangements at the first opportunity.

To purchase additional copies of this book, call our customer service department at **(800) 638-3030** or fax orders to **(301) 824-7390**. For other book services, including chapter reprints and large quantity sales, ask for the Special Sales department.

For all other calls originating outside of the United States, please call **(301) 714-2324**.

Visit Lippincott Williams & Wilkins on the Internet: http://www.lww.com. Lippincott Williams & Wilkins customer service representatives are available from 8:30 am to 6:00 pm, EST, Monday through Friday, for telephone access.

10 11 12 13
 6 7 8 9 10

To Max, Tess, Tera
Gunter, Sonja, and Dieter

Preface to the Fourth Edition

In 1983, Dr. Randolph Kessler and I published the first edition of *Management of Common Musculoskeletal Disorders: Physical Therapy Principles and Methods* to fill a void at that time in the rapidly expanding area of musculoskeletal medicine. The major focus of the first edition was on management of the extremity joints. The second edition in 1990 was extended to include the cervical and lumbar spine, and the third edition in 1996 was extended to embrace the thoracic spine, sacrum, and sacroiliac joint. All three editions were designed to bring together in one source the elements of anatomy, arthrology, biomechanics, and principles and methods of treatment clinically relevant to the study of spinal and extremity pain, in a form suitable for physical therapists and medical practitioners concerned with management of common musculoskeletal disorders. The present text continues and expands that tradition.

Modeled on the previous texts, this new edition draws on recent research developments in anatomy, biomechanics, and properties of dense connective tissue and wound healing. Moreover, the ambit of the text has now been extended to embrace soft tissue manipulations, functional exercises, stabilization techniques, and sensory motor and neuromuscular training.

ORGANIZATION AND NEW CONTENT FOR THIS EDITION

The edition is divided into three parts. Part I, "Basic Concepts and Techniques," has been expanded to include four new chapters on the properties of dense connective tissue, evaluation in somatic dysfunction, soft tissue manipulations, and functional exercises. Former chapters on wound healing, relaxation, and chronic pain management have been revised and expanded, capitalizing on recent research results on these topics.

In Part II, "Clinical Applications–Peripheral Joints," and Part III, "Clinical Applications–Spine," we deliberately avoid endorsing many contemporary theories about spinal and peripheral joint pain, because evidence for such endorsement is still lacking. However, the evaluation sections of these clinical chapters have been expanded to include an in-depth evaluation of the muscular system, embracing not only muscle strength and length but neuromuscular control and endurance. All these chapters have been expanded to cover ideas on sensory motor stimulation, neuromuscular training, stabilization techniques, and dynamic functional exercises. These chapters include insights from Butler, Cyriax, McKenzie, Edwards, Greenman, Grieve, Kaltenborn, Lewit, Janda, Jull, Maitland, Mulligan, McConnell, McGill, and others.

The final chapter, "Case Histories and Management Problems," provides the reader with a description of several case studies to integrate information learned in the relevant chapters and to present information across the lifespan.

PEDAGOGICAL FEATURES

The following features have been included as learning aids for the student:

- **Outlines.** As in the previous edition, detailed outlines are provided throughout the text to logically organize the content and make it easier to reference.
- **Boxes.** Special boxes, many of them illustrated, highlight techniques and other information.
- **Dynamic stabilization and functional exercises.** This special section, included at the end of many chapters, highlights new content on dynamic stabilization and functional exercise and is well illustrated.
- **New photos.** More than 600 new photos have been included in this edition.
- **Case studies.** A new chapter (Chapter 25) has been included that presents six case studies useful for applying the information covered in the text.

FINAL NOTE

My former co-author in the first edition, Randolph Kessler, MD, has become a recognized cardiovascular surgeon, which has restricted his availability for my recent editions. As I preface this new book, I continue to honor Dr. Kessler's major contributions to the first edition, and I shall endeavor to keep alive the spirit and tradition he championed in our earlier collaborative efforts.

Darlene Hertling
Seattle, Washington
2005

Preface to the Third Edition

In the decade that has elapsed since the first edition of Management of Common Musculoskeletal Disorders, a number of therapeutic advances have either been newly introduced or been made generally available. This book was conceived at a time when the lack of proper textbooks on impaired function and management of common musculoskeletal disorders was a major obstacle to teaching. Now there are numerous texts dealing with the teaching of soft tissue and joint mobilization, stabilization techniques, exercises, and so forth.

The third edition has again been expanded. Three entirely new chapters have been added. The techniques formerly described in the chapters on peripheral joint mobilization techniques and automobilization for the extremities have been absorbed into their respective peripheral joint chapters.

The book comprises three parts: Basic Concepts and Techniques, and Clinical Applications of the Peripheral Joints and the Spine. Part One, dealing with background material, is not meant to be a comprehensive discussion of the musculoskeletal system, which is well covered in other studies. A new Chapter 2, Properties of Dense Connective Tissue and Wound Healing, was authored by Larry Tillman and Neil Chasan. The overview of important concepts concerning connective tissue properties, behavior, injury, and repair is long overdue. The material vital for further discussion of a variety of topics is presented later in this text. We thank these authors for their work, cooperation, and patience.

Chapter 6, Introduction to Manual Therapy, includes a history of mobilization techniques (from the first edition) and a broad overview of manual therapy. This chapter addresses a number of new techniques that sometimes do not enjoy support in the literature but are being used by an ever-increasing number of therapists. It can be disastrous to confine one's interest to one area of specialty and to remain unaware of both the broader context of treatment and the possible alternatives.

The key chapter in this first section, from a clinical standpoint, is Chapter 5, Assessment of Musculoskeletal Disorders. A comprehensive system of patient evaluation is a crucial component of the clinician's overall approach to management. Ways to elicit subjective and objective data are presented, along with guides to the interpretation of findings.

Parts Two and Three encompass the clinical applications of the preceding materials as they relate to selected conditions affecting the peripheral joints and the spine. Each of the regional chapters in these sections is organized to include functional anatomy and biomechanics, specific regional evaluation, and common lesions and their management. Most of the chapters have been expanded, including Chapter 14, which formerly covered only the ankle and hindfoot and now includes the lower leg and forefoot. Chapters on the thoracic spine and the sacroiliac joint have been added for completeness.

Identification of the treatment most likely to succeed continues to improve, emphasizing either "hands on" procedures (Grieves 1986; Maitland 1987) or the "hands off" approach (McKenzie 1979; Holten 1984). Active mobility rather than passive mobility continues to be emphasized. Significant clinical contributions have been made by Robin McKenzie, a New Zealand physiotherapist of international renown who has expanded on an original contribution with his lateral shift treatment technique for patients with lumbar discogenic disorders, and by Brian Edwards of Australia, who has formalized combined movements in examination and treatment.

The works of Lewit, Fryett, Mitchell, Grieves, Janda and others have resulted in new methods of post-isometric relaxation techniques. Lewit (1985), having worked for about 30 years in the field of painful disorders stemming from impaired locomotor function, has observed that movement restrictions are not necessarily due to an articular lesion. Post-isometric relaxation techniques (which employ the patient's active participation during manual therapy techniques) are based on the prime importance of soft tissues, particularly the muscles, as opposed to the skeletal elements of joint structures, in producing various abnormal states of joint pain and movement limitations.

This book was originally written for the student in the advanced stages of training and for the practicing clinician. Originally it was directed toward physical therapists, but we soon recognized that its cross-sectional interest should be much broader. Patients with musculoskeletal disorders are likely to consult any one of a wide variety of practitioners. We trust that orthopaedists, osteopaths, physiatrists, rheumatologists, family practitioners, chiropractors, orthopaedic assistants, occupational therapists, physical therapy assistants, athletic trainers, massage therapists, orthopaedic nurses, and alternative somatic practitioners will also find it useful.

It is our hope that this third edition will continue to provide a foundation for designing creative and appropriate therapeutic programs. Occasionally we have chosen to introduce complex materials at a somewhat superficial level with the intent of exposing the reader to advanced concepts. Readers who wish to pursue topics in depth are encouraged to continue reading in the reference lists at the end of each chapter. Most of the techniques described here are widely accepted. No claim is made for original methods of treatment.

We thank the readers who have been so responsive to our efforts to develop a readable and comprehensive text on management of common musculoskeletal conditions and would like to encourage colleagues in the field to continue their dialogue with us. We acknowledge Professor Jo Ann McMillan, head of Physical Therapy, Rehabilitation Medicine, University of Washington Medical Center, for her support and continuous encouragement for the research and writing of this edition. Thanks are also due to various people—some students, some colleagues, patients, and a family member who allowed us to use them as pictorial models. Our thanks to the physical therapy students and the staff at the University of Washington for their contributions to the development of this edition: Laura Robinson, Jenny Cole, Anita Sterling, Beth Mortimer, Kelly Fitzgerald, and Robert Reif.

We particularly recognize the important role Elizabeth Kessler played in providing the art work as well as Bruce Terami in providing the photography. Finally, I am especially appreciative of the invaluable assistance and encouragement provided me by the following members of the editorial staff of Lippincott-Raven Publishers: Andrew Allen, Laura Dover, and Tom Gibbons.

Contributors

Mitchell G. Blakney, RPT
Practicing Physical Therapist
Gig Harbor, Washington

Neil Chason, PT, MMT
Practicing Physical Therapist
Bellevue, Washington

Joyce Engel-Knowles, PhD, OT
Occupational Therapy
University of Washington Medical Center
Seattle, Washington

June E. Hanks, PhD, PT
Department of Physical Therapy
University of Tennessee
Chattanooga, Tennessee

Karen E. Shrader DaSilva, RPT
Practicing Physical Therapist
Issaquah, Washington

Larry Tillman, PhD, PT
Department of Physical Therapy
University of Tennessee
Chattanooga, Tennessee

Reviewers

Jennifer Ellison, PhD, PT
Assistant Professor
Department of Physical Therapy
University of Texas Medical Branch
Galveston, Texas

Leslie Russek, PhD, PT, OCS
Associate Professor
Physical Therapy Department
Clarkson University
Potsdam, New York

Harvey Wallmann, PT, DPTSc, SCS, ATC, CSCS
Chair, Department of Physical Therapy
University of Nevada, Las Vegas
Las Vegas, Nevada

Reviewers

Jennifer Ellison, PhD, PT
Assistant Professor
Department of Physical Therapy
University of Texas Medical Branch
Galveston, Texas

Leslie Russek, PhD, PT, OCS
Associate Professor
Physical Therapy Department
Clarkson University
Potsdam, New York

Harvey Wallmann, PT, DPTSc, SCS, ATC, CSCS
Chair, Department of Physical Therapy
University of Nevada, Las Vegas
Las Vegas, Nevada

Acknowledgments

The writing of this fourth edition was an enormous undertaking, a task that could not have been accomplished without a supporting cast of friends, colleagues, and family. We acknowledge all the support provided by the editorial staff of Lippincott Williams & Wilkins. We wish to extend a special thanks to the managing editor, David Payne.

We are excited about the outstanding artwork and photographs that are included in this text. The art work was made possible by Carolyn Kates, Kimberly Battista, and Eliszabeth Kessler. The photographs were made possible by Robert Riedlinger and Bruce Terami. We would be remiss not to give thanks to the individuals who acted as models for this book: Sonja Atkinson, Joan Gelinus, Peggy Halwach, Andrew Headly, Harry Jackson, Diane Kamacho, Kali Kamacho, Christina Lee, Nancy Mitrano, Gae Naganuma Burton, Stacy Sherman, Frances Swain, Charles Tine, Kristi Trautmann, Scott Turnipseed, and Ann Yamanie.

Obviously, this new edition would not have been possible without contributing authors, who are listed by name in a separate section. Their willingness to share their expertise is immeasurably appreciated.

Contents

Basic Concepts and Techniques

I

Basic Concepts
and Techniques

Properties of Dense Connective Tissue

1

LARRY J. TILLMAN AND NEIL CHASAN

INTRODUCTION

Manual physical therapy has primary effects on dense connective tissue (DCT) structures. Through the application of scientific principles, the manual therapist can predict a level of success in the management of musculoskeletal problems. After the history taking and physical examination, the clinician should have some knowledge about the specific tissue(s) in a lesion. What happens next? By developing and implementing a treatment plan that is specific both to the tissue type(s) in a lesion and the state of wound healing (described in Chapter 2, Wound Healing: Injury and Repair of Dense Connective Tissue), the manual therapist can apply the "optimal stimulus for protein synthesis," which lends a high probability to success in the clinic.[11] Collagen has specific physical properties that can be taken advantage of during therapy. Furthermore, manual therapy joint articulation techniques (described in Chapter 3, Arthrology) have effects both on the mechanoreceptors and the DCT structures in which the receptors reside. For the reader to gain a full appreciation of soft tissue response to injury, a firm understanding of the physical properties of DCT and the biomechanical behavior of collagen is necessary.

FUNCTIONS, COMPOSITION, AND CLASSIFICATION OF DCT

DCT serves a variety of functions. Its most obvious function is to provide and maintain body structure. Additionally, DCT plays important roles in providing a defense and immunologic response to invading antigens. There is also an association between blood capillaries and DCT for the transport of nutrients and removal of metabolic wastes.[8,28]

By definition, DCT consists of an intricate extracellular matrix in contact with various cells and protein fibers. DCT structures differ considerably in appearance, consistency, and composition in different regions of the body according to the local functional requirements. These differences are related to the character of the extracellular matrix, the predominance of cell types, as well as the concentration, arrangement, and types of fibers. Table 1-1 summarizes the specific components of DCT.

DCT is classified by the degree of orientation in fibrous elements into irregular and regular types. The connective tissue sheaths of individual muscles (intermuscular septa) and synovial tendon sheaths are classified as **dense irregular connective tissue.** As the name implies, the connective tissue fibers are densely arranged, but in an irregular, more random fashion. In comparison, **dense regular connective tissue** includes those highly fibrous tissues with fibers regularly oriented to form either connective tissue sheets (such as aponeuroses and fasciae) or thicker bundles (such as ligaments or tendons). Other examples of dense regular connective tissue include the deep fascia of the lower extremity, the fascia lata of the thigh with its lateral iliotibial band, and crural fascia with its thickened retinacula.

Extracellular Matrix

The **extracellular matrix (ECM),** or ground substance, is an amorphous gel-like material occupying the interstitial space between the DCT cells and fibers. It is composed of a mixture of water and organic macromolecules interwoven with three major fiber-forming proteins—**elastin, reticulin,** and **collagen.** These macromolecules are secreted by **fibroblasts.**

Importantly, the ECM holds the connective tissue cells together and influences the development, shape, proliferation, migration, and metabolic functions of the cells that contact it.[1] The matrix has enormous water binding properties and acts as (1) a lubricant for movement of adjacent fibers

TABLE 1-1 COMPOSITION OF DENSE CONNECTIVE TISSUES

CELLS	FIBERS
Fibroblasts	Elastin
Chondroblasts	Collagen
Osteoblasts	
EXTRACELLULAR MATRIX	
Glycosaminoglycans	*Proteoglycans*
Hyaluronan	Hyaluronan (no protein core)
Chondroitin 4-sulfate	Aggrecan
Chondroitin 6-sulfate	Biglycan
Dermatan sulfate	Decorin
Heparan sulfate	Perlecan
Heparan	Syndecan
Keratan sulfate	Verican
Glycoproteins	*Tissue Fluid*
Fibromodulin	Water
Fibronectin	Electrolytes
Laminin	
Link protein	
Osteopontin	
Tenascin	
Thrombospondin	

and (3) **fibrous proteins.** The complex interaction among the ECM, cells, and fibers results in the formation of highly specialized connective tissue structures, such as basal lamina, bone, cartilage, ligaments, and tendons.

Glycosaminoglycans

Glycosaminoglycans (GAGs), also known as mucopolysaccharides, are a product of fibroblast metabolism. They are composed of repeating disaccharide units. One of the two sugar residues in the repeating disaccharide is always an amino acid, hence the name.[1] GAGs are highly negatively charged because of the presence of sulfate and/or carboxyl groups on many of the sugar residues. Enhanced by their high density of negative charges that attract osmotically active cations, GAGs are hydrophilic, attracting large amounts of water. Because of the porous and hydrated organization, GAGs allow rapid diffusion of water-soluble molecules and the migration of cells and cell processes. GAGs interact electrostatically with collagen fibers, binding them together, and thus contributing to their aggregation and strength.[3] The distinctive form in collagen fascicles is thought to be the result of the attachment of GAGs to the collagen fibers.[16,17,21]

Seven groups of GAGs have been identified by their sugar residues, the type of linkage between their residues, and the number and location of sulfate groups.[1,8] The particular type and distribution of GAGs in various tissues is demonstrated in Table 1-2. **Hyaluronan** or **hyaluronic acid (HA)** is common in cartilage and is thought to be responsible for cohesion within the collagen fibril, enabling the tissue to bear mechanical stresses without distortion.[4,23] HA exists as a very long carbohydrate chain of thousands of sugar residues, but it is not a typical GAG because it is not covalently linked to a protein core and none of the sugars is sulfated. HA has a special function supporting cell migration in DCT wound healing. Evidence suggests that increased local production of HA, which attracts water and therefore swells the matrix, may be one strategy used to facilitate cell migration during DCT repair.

over one another and (2) a source of nourishment for the fibroblasts.[7,12] The aqueous portion of the gel matrix permits the diffusion of nutrients and metabolites between the DCT cells and the blood.

The main components of ECM macromolecules that make up the matrix are (1) **glycosaminoglycans** (named **proteoglycans** when attached to a protein core), (2) **glycoproteins,**

TABLE 1-2 TYPE AND DISTRIBUTION OF GLYCOSAMINOGLYCANS

TYPE	DISTRIBUTION
Hyaluronan (HA)	Connective tissue, skin, cartilage, vitreous body, synovial fluid
Chondroitin 4-sulfate	Cartilage, bone, skin, arteries, cornea
Chondroitin 6-sulfate	Bone, skin, arteries, cornea
Dermatan sulfate	Dermis, tendon, ligament, cartilage, skin, blood vessels, heart valves
Heparan sulfate	Lung, arteries, cell surfaces
Heparan	Mast cells, skin, liver, lung
Keratan sulfate	Cartilage, intervertebral disc, cornea

Modified from Alberts B, Bray D, Lewis J, et al: Cell-cell adhesion and the extracellular matrix. In: Molecular Biology of the Cell. New York, Garland Publishing, 1983:703

This swelling pressure in the ECM temporarily protects the damaged structures by resisting compressive forces.[1]

Proteoglycans

Except for hyaluronan, GAGs covalently bind to protein chains in the ECM to form **proteoglycans (PGs).** PGs contain 90 to 95% carbohydrate by weight in the form of many long, unbranched GAG chains. They differ significantly in protein content, molecular size, and number and types of GAG chains per molecule. Each type of connective tissue, therefore, has unique PGs in various proportions. The role of PGs is to regulate collagen fibrillogenesis and accelerate polymerization of collagen monomers.[21] PGs are ordered in pattern, crossing the collagen fibrils at intervals of 67 nm, which is the same periodicity as that of the intrinsic cross-banding pattern of the collagen fibrils.[1]

Examples of true PGs include aggrecan, biglycan, decorin, perlecan, syndecan, and versican. These PGs have varied roles in the design and maintenance of DCT. Specific functions of PGs are to contribute to the mechanical stability of DCT by resisting compressive and tensional forces as well as to regulate cell growth, differentiation, and migration.[8] The

most understood PG is **aggrecan.** It is the predominant PG in articular cartilage and plays an important role in normal joint function. An example of the PG aggrecan is shown in Figure 1-1.

The percentage of PGs varies directly with the amount of stress or mechanical load placed on the DCT. For example, in tissues that resist tension, such as tendons and ligaments, PGs are in small concentrations (approximately 0.2% of dry weight). Articular cartilage, a tissue subjected to high compressive forces, has a relatively high percentage of PGs (approximately 8 to 10% of dry weight).[10]

CLINICAL CONSIDERATIONS

Extracellular viability depends on motion. GAGs and PGs have half-lives of 1.7 to 7 days, and motion is required for ECM production.[32] Early on, motion at the level of the DCT might imply gentle isometric contractions rather than gross osteokinematic movements. The forces generated by gentle isometric contractions are often sufficient to keep the DCT lubricated during the phase of recovery in which pain-induced splinting occurs. The absence of both weight bearing and movement can result in a large loss (up to 40%) of PGs in a

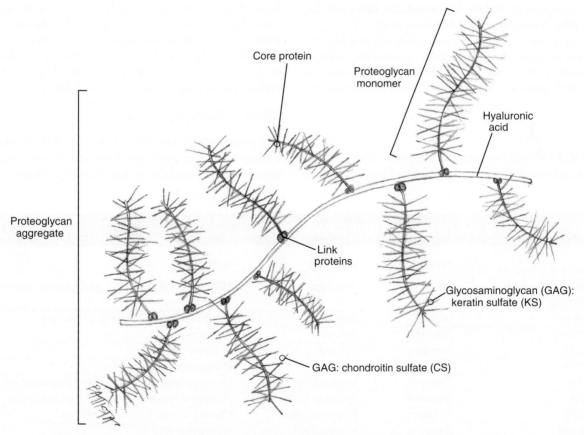

■ **FIG. 1-1.** Proteoglycan aggregate demonstrating several aggrecan monomers with keratan sulfate (KS) and chondroitin sulfate (CS) glycosaminoglycan side chains attached to the protein core.

short period (1 month).[15] Therefore, it is important to maintain some minimal level of joint motion during the early stages of DCT repair and healing.

Glycoproteins

Structural **glycoproteins** make up a small but significant proportion of the ECM. They are organic macromolecules containing a protein core to which small, complex, nonrepeating sequences of sugar molecules covalently attach. Glycoproteins usually contain only 1 to 6% carbohydrate by weight and thus are smaller than PGs.[1] Unlike PGs, the protein core predominates. Glycoproteins transport and exchange materials between DCT cells and their environment. Although they do not have a significant mechanical function in DCT, glycoproteins play an important role in the interaction between the cells and their adhesion to collagen. They are thought to enhance cell motility and stimulate cell proliferation.[8]

Two high molecular weight glycoproteins are widely distributed in the matrix of DCT. **Fibronectin** promotes cell adhesion of different soft tissue cells to each other as well as to collagen and other matrix substrates. It is composed of two disulfide-bonded subunits. **Laminin** is a major component of basal lamina. The basal lamina provides scaffolding along which regenerating cells can migrate following injury to epithelial, muscle, and nervous tissues.

Other glycoproteins include **fibromodulin, link protein, osteopontin, tenascin,** and **thrombospondin.** Examples of their varied functions include modulating cell attachments (fibronectin, tenascin, thrombospondin), controlling collagen fibril formation (fibromodulin), stabilizing PG aggregates in cartilage (link protein), and promoting tissue calcification (osteopontin).[8,13,14,30]

Cells

Cells of DCT fall into two general categories: those that are produced and remain locally (adipose cells, fibroblasts), and those cells that are produced elsewhere and are transient (leukocytes, macrophages, mast cells, plasma cells). Of the local cells, adipose cells store neutral fats for energy and heat production. Fibroblasts, and specialized osteoblasts in bone and chondroblasts in cartilage, are widely distributed in DCT. They are responsible for the production of protein fibers (collagen, elastin, reticulin) and the ECM (GAGs, PGs, glycoproteins) in the maintenance and repair of DCT.

Phagocytosis of foreign antigens is an important function of certain transient cells. Tissue macrophages are the first line of phagocytic defense during infection and inflammation. The next line of phagocytic activity comes from neutrophilic leukocytes, also known as polymorphonuclear leukocytes (PMNLs) or "polys" for short. These leukocytes migrate across the blood vessel wall to reach the bacteria. Monocytes are white blood cell macrophages that play a delayed role in phagocytosis, often following the tissue macrophages and PMNLs. Phagocytes will multiply in great numbers during the early stages of inflammation in an effort to control the spread of antigens and clean up the foreign debris.

Eosinophilic leukocytes release enzymes that destroy large parasites and help modulate allergic inflammatory reactions. Basophilic leukocytes are responsible for releasing histamine, a vasodilator, into the bloodstream in certain immune reactions. Mast cells, similar to basophils, release pharmacologically active substances, such as histamine, to produce an immediate hypersensitivity response to allergic reactions. Plasma cells, derived from activated B lymphocytes, produce antibodies and provide humoral immunity. T lymphocytes are responsible for cell-mediated immunity. A summary of DCT cells and their properties is found in Table 1-3.

Fibrous Proteins

The prominent protein fibers found in DCT are **elastin** and **collagen.** Elastin molecules form an extensive cross-linked network of fibers and sheets that can stretch and recoil, impart-

TABLE 1-3 CELLS OF DENSE CONNECTIVE TISSUES

CELL	TYPE	FUNCTION	ACTIVITY
Fibroblast, osteoblast, chondroblast	Local	Structural	ECM fiber and GAG, PG, glycoprotein synthesis
Adipose cell	Local	Storage	Fat stored for heat, energy production
Macrophage	Transient	Defense	Phagocytosis
Neutrophil	Transient	Defense	Phagocytosis
Monocyte	Transient	Defense	Phagocytosis
Eosinophil	Transient	Immunologic	Enzymes released during allergic/parasitic infections
Basophil	Transient	Pharmacologic	Histamine released during allergic reactions
Mast Cell	Transient	Pharmacologic	Histamine (and heparin) synthesis
Plasma cell	Transient	Immunologic	Humoral immunity
T lymphocyte	Transient	Immunologic	Cell-mediated immunity

ing compliance and elasticity to the matrix. Elastic fibers in tissues such as blood vessels, lung, and skin allow for reasonable deformation and repeated stretching without permanent damage. The quantity of elastin protein within DCT relates to the mechanical strain a particular structure undergoes and the amount of reversible deformation required. The amount of elastic fibers in skin decreases during the natural aging process. The depletion of elastin results in an observed loss of skin resilience.[6]

Collagen is a rope-like macromolecule that aggregates in long cable-like fibrils, resisting permanent stretching forces. It is the predominant fiber in DCT, making up one third of all protein in the human body. For example, a tendon is composed of 30% collagen, 65% water, 5% GAGs and glycoproteins. However, by dry weight, collagen makes up 99% of tendon.[28] It is important to study the physical and mechanical properties of collagen to understand fully the physical properties of DCT as a whole. The tension-resisting property of collagen is the principal means by which joint range of motion is limited, articular hyaline cartilage resists compression, striated skeletal muscle transmits forces, and tensile strength is imparted to bone.[8]

PHYSICAL PROPERTIES OF COLLAGEN

Reviewing collagen formation provides an appreciation of how collagen accounts for the viscosity of gelatinous structures, the toughness of deep fascia, and the tenacity of scar tissue adhesions. To understand the dynamics of scar tissue adhesions during wound healing, it is helpful to review the biochemistry and biomechanical behavior of collagen and its interaction with other macromolecules in the ECM.

Synthesis of Collagen

Collagen synthesis begins in the rough endoplasmic reticulum of connective tissue fibroblasts. In the intracellular endoplasmic reticulum, a repeating sequence of specific amino acids is assembled into long polypeptide chains of uniform length. The amino acid sequence of assembled peptide chains has a characteristic pattern of glycine-X-Y. Every third amino acid residue is glycine, and either proline or lysine amino acids are in the X-Y position on the peptide chain. Disruption of the glycine-X-Y amino acid sequence, such as occurs in osteogenesis imperfecta, leads to loss of the mechanical properties of collagen.[5] Three polypeptide chains attach in a right-handed triple helix formation to form the **procollagen** molecule. Because of the three-dimensional shape of each chain and the relative placement of radicals that react with each other through hydrophobic, hydrophilic, hydrogen, and covalent interactions, the chains fit together in specific configurations of fixed dimensions with uniform length and width (Fig. 1-2).[27] The procollagen molecule now has a rod-like structure of approximately 300 nm in length and 1.5 nm in diameter.

Once the procollagen molecule is extruded from the fibroblast into the interstitial space of the DCT matrix, cleavage at terminal sites of the molecule occurs and the nonhelical ends are removed. The slightly shortened molecule is now called **tropocollagen,** known as the basic building block of collagen. Five tropocollagen molecules rapidly aggregate in an overlapping array to form a collagen microfibril. Groups of microfibrils organize into the subfibril, and subfibrils combine to form fibrils. Assembly of the collagen fibril takes place as a complex interaction between the tropocollagen molecules, the fibroblast cell membrane surface, and the GAGs, PGs, and glycoproteins of the ECM. It is at the level of the collagen fibril that the characteristic periodicity or cross-banding observed in x-ray diffraction and electron microscopic studies is demonstrated (Fig. 1-3).[9] This periodicity is the result of the specific overlapping and stacking of the tropocollagen molecules within the larger units, emphasizing the highly structured molecular organization of collagen. The physical and mechanical properties of collagen, giving it the ability to withstand tensile loads, are governed directly by this hierarchy of organization.

Bundles of collagen fibrils combine to form connective tissue fascicles. It is at the level of the DCT fascicle that a tendon or ligament can first be tested mechanically. Whenever subjected to stress during formation, these fascicles form with a distinct waveform, know as **crimp.** Crimping occurs in all biologic collagenous tissues that undergo tension. The acute angle of crimping of collagen at this level of DCT development is 15 to 20° and is both predictable and measurable. The compliance of DCT is primarily, therefore, a function of removing the crimp or increasing the angle of crimping. In other words, when working within physiologic limits, collagen can be elongated temporarily with the straightening of the crimped DCT fascicles. However, as a result of the dimensions set by the molecular attachments, native collagen cannot shrink or be stretched with "permanent" elongation. Clinically speaking, any permanent elongation signifies tearing or denaturing of the collagenous structure with irreversible damage. Collagen fascicles combine to make up the gross structure of tendon, ligament, and joint capsule (Fig. 1-4).[19]

As presented, collagen is a complex structure. Nineteen types of collagen have been identified and categorized into six distinct classes based on the differences in their structure, location, and function.[2,20] Much of the biomechanical properties of DCT, however, have been studied on the fibril-forming collagens (Class 1), made up predominantly of collagen types I, II, and III (Table 1-4).[18] Tendons and ligaments are examples of those fibril-forming collagens whose primary function is to resist tensile forces. The larger structural, interstitial fibers of tendons and ligaments contain mostly type I collagen and, in smaller quantities, type II collagen. Articular cartilage, bone, dermis, and intervertebral disks are tissues that require resistance to applied tensile loads. Articular cartilage is typically composed of type II collagen, whereas bone, dermis, and fibrous cartilage (intervertebral disk) is type I. Type III collagen is found in expansible organs such as arteries, uterus, liver, spleen, kidney, and lungs and serves a structural support function.

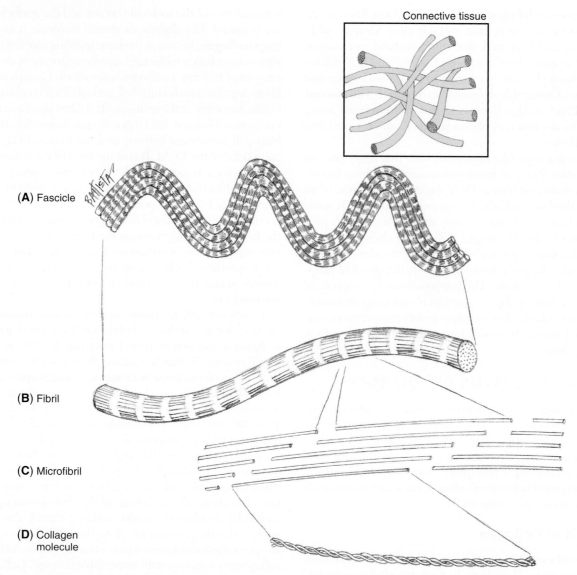

Connective tissue

(A) Fascicle

(B) Fibril

(C) Microfibril

(D) Collagen molecule

▪ **FIG. 1-2.** Collagen fibril formation. **(A)** Fibril with cross banding owing to overlapping tropocollagen units. **(B)** Extracellular stacking of tropocollagen molecules. **(C)** One tropocollagen molecule of fixed 300-nm dimension. **(D)** Right-handed triple helix.

CLINICAL CONSIDERATIONS

The collagen microfibril has been termed a "crystallite" structure because of the consistent spatial relationship of its molecules.[25] Collagen, therefore, is an organic crystal. The significance of these dimensions set by molecular attachments is that native collagen cannot shrink and cannot be stretched with permanent elongation, without denaturing or damaging the integrity of the soft tissue structure. The manual therapist must become comfortable working within the physiologic range of DCT if the treatment goal is not to tear or permanently damage a particular collagenous structure. One indication that the therapist is working outside the physiologic range, or "safe zone," is when the client complains of prolonged stiffness, pain, or both lasting longer than 1 hour after treatment.

Maturation Changes in Collagen

There are progressive changes in bonding as the collagen ages and matures. Once the tropocollagen molecules aggregate into microfibrils, gradual chemical changes occur resulting in the conversion of unstable hydrogen bonds into stable covalent bonds. New attachments are formed simultaneously with the organic molecules (GAGs) of the ground substance that result in additional stability. The end result is that the aging collagen becomes progressively rigid and strong. In addition to the increase in covalent bonding, two other factors thought to affect collagen strength during maturation include the continuous increase in size of the collagen fibers and the alignment of fibers along lines of stress.[24] Stress as a physical stimulus is a significant factor in the formation and maintenance of collagen in DCT.

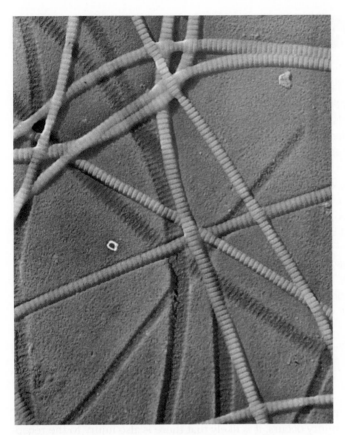

■ FIG. 1-3. Electron micrograph of metal-shadowed replica of collagen fibers from human skin, demonstrating cross-banding periodicity. (From de Duve C: A Guided Tour of the Living Cell, vol. 1. New York, Scientific American Library, WH Freeman, 1984:38, and Jerome Gross, Harvard Medical School, Boston, MA.)

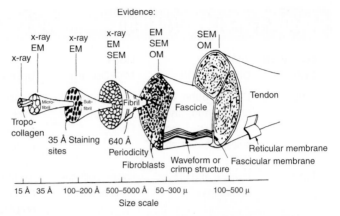

■ FIG. 1-4. Hierarchical organization of tendon. Note the cross-banding periodicity at the level of the collagen fibril and the specific crimp formation in the collagen fiber fascicle. *EM,* electron microscopy; *OM,* optical microscopy; *SEM,* scanning electron microscopy. (From Kastelic J, Galeski A, Baer, E: The multi-composite structure of tendon. Connect Tissue Res 6:21, 1978.) (Copyright 1978 from Connect Tissue Res 6:21 by J Kastelic. Reproduced by permission of Taylor and Francis Group, LLC, *http://www.taylorandfrancis.com.*)

Deprivation of physical stress results in actual quantitative loss of collagen fibers and progressive weakening of the DCT.

MECHANICAL PROPERTIES OF COLLAGEN

The mechanical behavior of tendon and other DCT can be studied by elongating collagen fibers to the point of rupture. The resulting changes in length and tension during stretch can be plotted to produce a **stress–strain curve. Stress** is the amount of load or tension per unit cross-sectional area placed on the specimen, whereas **strain** refers to the temporary elongation that occurs when stress is applied within physiologic limits.

Stress–Strain Curve

A stress–strain curve characteristic for tendon mechanically strained to the point of rupture includes five distinct regions as demonstrated in Figure 1-5.

1. Toe region. In the toe region, there is little increase in load with lengthening. This region represents a 1.2 to 2% strain, and occurs during loading for 1 hour or less. The load stays within the physiologic limit of the tissue. The crimp is tem-

porarily removed at the level of the DCT fascicle without permanently denaturing or damaging the tendon, thus allowing the therapist to remodel the connective tissue along lines of stress.
2. Linear region. In the linear region, increased elongation requires disproportionately larger amounts of stress. Microfailure of the tendon begins early in this region, plotted as a 2 to 6% strain. Clinically, the patient complains of tendon stiffness, a clue that treatment was slightly outside the physiologic range for working with collagenous tissues.
3. Region of progressive failure. In this region, the slope of the stress–strain curve begins to decrease, indicating microscopic disruption of sufficient amounts of DCT structure. The gross tendon, nonetheless, appears to be normal and intact. An observed decrease in the slope angle on the stress–strain curve is called **yield** and occurs around 6% strain.
4. Region of major failure. The slope of the stress–strain curve now flattens dramatically. Although the gross tendon is intact, there is visible narrowing at numerous points of shear and rupture. This narrowing at points of tear, demonstrated between 6 and 12% strain on the curve, is known as **necking.**
5. Region of complete rupture. The slope of the stress–strain curve falls off, indicating a total break in the gross tendon. Tendon failure occurs with 12 to 15% strain.

When a load is removed from a tendon before incomplete rupture, the tendon returns to its original starting length after a period of rest. The return of the temporarily elongated tendon to its original length is called **recovery.** Being a crystalline structure, collagen can be deformed temporarily by stress when working within physiologic limits, but with the removal of the load the collagen recovers to its original length.

TABLE 1-4 CLASS 1: FIBRIL-FORMING COLLAGENS

COLLAGEN TYPE	TISSUE DISTRIBUTION	LIGHT MICROSCOPY	ULTRASTRUCTURE	SITE OF SYNTHESIS	INTERACTIONS WITH GAGS	FUNCTION
Type I	Dermis, bone, tendon, dentin, fascias, sclera, organ capsules, intervertebral disk	Closely packed, thick, collagen fibers	Densely packed, thick fibrils with marked variation in diameter	Fibroblast, osteoblast, chondroblast, odontoblast	Intermediate level of interaction, especially with dermatan sulfate	Resistance to tension
Type II	Hyaline and elastic cartilages	Loose, collagenous network	No fibers; very thin fibrils embedded in abundant ECM	Chondroblasts	High level of interaction, mainly with chondroitin sulfates	Resistance to intermittent pressure
Type III	Smooth muscle, endoneurium, arteries, uterus, liver, spleen, kidney, lung	Loose network of thin reticular fibers	Loosely packed thin fibrils with uniform diameters	Smooth muscle, fibroblast, reticular cells, Schwann cells, hepatocytes	Intermediate level of interaction, mainly with heparin sulfate	Structural maintenance in expansible organs

Adapted with permission from Junqueira LC, Carneiro J, Long JA: Basic Histology, 6th ed. Los Altos, Lange Medical Publishers, 1968:92–104

CLINICAL CONSIDERATIONS

Manual therapy receptor techniques generally occur in the toe region of the stress–strain curve before any microtrauma. Type I, II, and III receptors are active in the beginning range, mid range, and end range of tension of the DCT structure in which they are located (Table 1-5).[33] Type IV receptors are stimulated once the DCT suffers irreversible damage, in the linear region. Trauma might bring the DCT into the region of progressive failure or the region of major failure. If DCT injury occurs, it is likely that there is also injury to the receptors typically residing within the traumatized structures. Early rehabilitation must therefore focus on joint proprioception.

Viscoelastic Properties of DCT

The viscoelastic properties of tendon and other DCT can be demonstrated when stress–strain studies plot the recovery of tendon following the removal of stress. Interrupted cyclical stress, in which a load is applied to and quickly removed from tendon, produces a stress–strain curve illustrated in Figure 1-6A. The tendon temporarily elongates (**compliance**) but quickly recovers to its original length (**elasticity**) with the removal of stress. The end result is an initial 1.5% strain with recovery. This example demonstrates the elastic behavior of DCT to cyclical (on/off) stress.[26]

When stress is applied to a tendon in a sustained fashion and recovery is allowed to occur, the constant (or uninterrupted cyclical) loading produces up to a 2.6% strain (Fig. 1-6B). This additional and gradual lengthening of the tendon with sustained stress is called **creep.** The phenomenon of creep describes the viscous or plastic behavior of tendon and DCT. The creep observed and plotted on a stress–strain curve responds to the physiologic removal of crimp at the level of the DCT fascicle, thereby temporarily elongating the DCT structure.

A tendon stressed 1% for 60 minutes recovers. It has been shown that all DCT creep found within physiologic limits and at 25°C is transitory.[29] In contrast, a 1% stress sustained over 1 hour results in irreversible damage to tendon structure and function. Creep in tendons, therefore, occurs at two levels: a

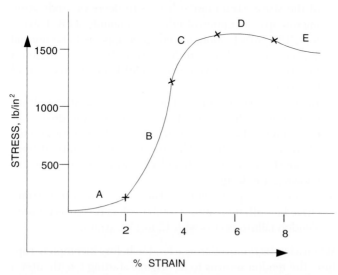

■ **FIG. 1-5.** Stress–strain curve for ruptured Achilles tendon in humans. Five distinct regions are (**A**) toe region, (**B**) linear region, (**C**) progressive failure region, (**D**) major failure region, and (**E**) complete rupture region.

TABLE 1-5 MECHANORECEPTORS OF THE DENSE CONNECTIVE TISSUES

RECEPTOR TYPE	WHERE ACTIVE	WHERE FOUND	ACTION/EFFECTS
Type I	Beginning and end range of tension	Superficial layers of joint capsules	Slow adapting, low threshold tension postural reflexogenic effects
Type II	Mid range of tension	Deep layers of joint capsules	Rapidly adapting, low threshold dynamic receptor
Type III	End range of tension	Intrinsic and extrinsic joint ligaments	Slow acting, high threshold dynamic mechanoreceptor
Type IV	Inactive normally; activated by noxious mechanical or chemical stimulation	Fibrous capsules, intrinsic and extrinsic ligaments, fat pads, and periosteum	Nonadapting, high threshold pain receptors

From Wyke B: The neurology of joints. Ann R Coll Surg Engl 41:25, 1967

temporary elongation that shows recovery when treatment is within physiologic limits, and a permanent elongation that progresses to irreversible damage and rupture.

CLINICAL CONSIDERATIONS

On occasion, the clinician might choose to perform a manipulation or stretching technique that results in permanent elongation or rupture of a DCT structure, such as with a small scar or capsular adhesion. In the event that the manual therapist performs a technique causing tearing of DCT, the injury caused by the technique should be managed as if it is an acute

trauma that will eventually result in fibrosis. Caution must be taken to prevent further adhesions requiring additional and aggressive care.

Rate of Stress on DCT

In addition to whether the applied stress to tendon is cyclical or sustained, the rate of stretch is also important.[26] Figure 1-7A illustrates that "slow" stretch allows creep to occur, and less force is required to provide more temporary elongation. In contrast, "fast" stretch (Fig. 1-7B) provides more resistance with the outcome of less elongation. With fast stretch, an

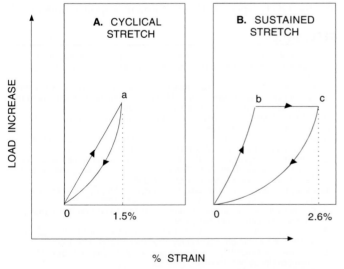

■ FIG. 1-6. Graphs illustrating the recovery of cyclical stretch (A) and sustained stretch (B). Increased strain occurs in a sustained stretch owing to the removal of crimp, indicated as b ▶ c. (Modified from Warren CG, Lehman JF, Koblanski JN: Elongation of rat tail tendon: Effect of load and temperature. Arch Phys Med Rehabil 52:466, 1971.)

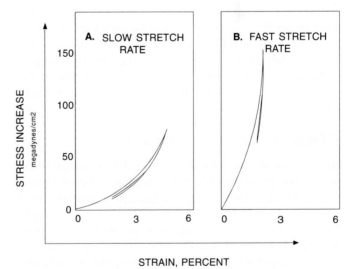

■ FIG. 1-7. Stress–strain data from extensor digitorum tendon. (A) Slow stretch rate. (B) Fast stretch rate. Slower rate of stretch produces greater strain with less stress. (Modified from Van Brocklin JD, Ellis DG: A study of mechanical behavior of toe extensor tendons under applied stress. Arch Phys Med Rehabil 46:371, 1965.)

increase of tendon resistance to stretch requires greater load to achieve elongation.[29] Although this higher stress might lead to more structural damage of the DCT, high-velocity techniques used to articulate joints benefit from the protection afforded the DCT by the increase in viscoelasticity with higher rates of stretch. In general, high-velocity techniques are performed at low amplitudes, which implies that the margin for error for the high-velocity thrust is greater at higher speed than for the same stretch applied at a slower rate. If such a technique were to be applied at high amplitudes, the likelihood that the DCT would be damaged is increased. Clinically, caution must be applied during the application of all techniques that stretch DCT so as to avoid permanent damage.

The physiologic limit of strain is only 1.5 to 2.6% with recovery.[25] With such a small, temporary strain, a therapist might ask what is the impetus to temporarily elongate tendon and other collagenous structures? Why bother to do it at all? The answer should be clearly understood. Stressing tendon within physiologic limits provides the effective and necessary stimulus for the remodeling of DCT. It has been demonstrated that collagen forms along lines of stress. Tension controls the direction of collagen fiber alignment and the formation of collagen into large fascicles. The manual therapist, therefore, can control how the newly synthesized collagen is laid down by providing the proper stimulus for remodeling. This concept is important to remember when dealing with scar tissue formation and wound healing.

CLINICAL CONSIDERATIONS

Rehabilitation of the musculoskeletal system requires that the patient exercise the injured joint(s). To stimulate the collagen structures appropriately with the "optimal stimulus for regeneration," the exercise must be dosed correctly. Early in the acute phase, the exercise dose must be sufficiently low so as to stress the collagen fibers without overloading them; as the fibers mature, the dose can be increased gradually. An important clinical consideration, therefore, is to think in terms of the collagen structures and the DCT in general when designing a rehabilitation program.

Effects of Temperature on DCT

Stress–strain studies have demonstrated that change in the viscoelastic properties of DCT is reversible below critical values of temperature, strain, and time. At strains between 1 and 4%, with temperatures up to 37°C, tendons recover to their original lengths following the removal of stress.[25] Temperatures between 37 and 45°C, however, do affect the viscoelastic properties of tendon. As the temperature increases, the ability of the collagenous structure to recover decreases. The risk factor for permanently damaging tendon and other DCT structures increases with higher temperatures. When a tendon is gradually heated at the critical temperature of 59 to 60°C, for example, it will undergo abrupt and irreversible shrinkage. This point of change is called the melt-

ing temperature, because the shrinkage reflects the melting or breaking of chemical bonds that maintain the structure of the collagenous fiber.

Additionally, increased temperature dramatically affects the rupture strain of tendons. Normally, tendons have rupture strains in the range of 8 to 14% at temperatures below 37°C. Below this temperature tendons can be strained repeatedly to 4% with no change in their stress–strain curves. However, tendon at 40°C has a rupture strain of only 3 to 4%.[25] This fact suggests that tendons are much more fragile when stressed at or above thermal transition temperatures. Using heat between 40 to 45°C requires a "working load" of one fourth that of the strain applied at 25°C if the goal is to work within the physiologic limits and not damage the DCT.[31]

CLINICAL CONSIDERATIONS

Working with heat, nonetheless, can have its advantages when the manual therapist carefully monitors the client's progress. The tendon becomes more ductile when heated; thus, there is faster creep in shorter periods with less strain applied. The rate of creep increases with increased temperatures, as reflected by the decreased time needed to achieve a 2.6% strain.[31] One recommended formula is to use 45°C with strains of less than 2.6% for short periods (less than 1 hour).[22] However, because the rupture load at 45°C is only one fourth of the value found when the tendon is tested at 25°C, the margin of error is minimal and extreme caution must be observed. When using a modality like ultrasound to achieve a temperature change in the DCT, the clinician must monitor for symptoms of periosteal pain that precedes the denaturing of collagen. Failure to adjust the dose immediately (by moving the ultrasound head away from the treatment area in this example) might permanently denature the DCT, especially if the treatment is applied under load.

REFERENCES

1. Alberts B, Bray D, Lewis J, et al: Cell-cell adhesion and the extracellular matrix. In: Molecular Biology of the Cell. New York, Garland Publishing, 1983:673–716
2. Bateman JF, Lamande SR, Ramshaw JAM: Collagen superfamily. In: Comper WE, ed: Extracellular Matrix, vol. 2: Molecular Components and Interactions. Amsterdam, Harwood Academic Publishers, 1996:22–67
3. Betch DF, Baer E: Structure and mechanical properties of rat tail tendon. Biorheology 17:83–94, 1980
4. Brody GS, Peng STJ, Landel RE: The etiology of hypertrophic scar contracture: Another view. Plast Reconstr Surg 67:673–684, 1977
5. Byres PH: Osteogenesis imperfecta. In: Royce PM, Steinmann BS, eds: Connective Tissue and Its Heritable Disorders: Molecular, Genetic, and Medical Aspects. New York, Wiley-Liss, 1993:317–350
6. Cleary EG: Skin. In: Comper WD, ed: Extracellular Matrix, vol. 1: Tissue Function. Amsterdam, Harwood Academic Publishers, 1996:77–109
7. Comper WD, ed: Extracellular Matrix, vol. 1: Tissue Function. Amsterdam, Harwood Academic Publishers, 1996.
8. Culav EM, Clark CH, Merrilees MJ: Connective tissues: Matrix composition and its relevance to physical therapy. Phys Ther 79:308–319, 1999
9. de Duve C: A Guided Tour of the Living Cell, vol. 1. New York, Scientific American Library, WH Freeman, 1984:38
10. Flint MH, Gillard GC, Merrilees MJ: Effects of local environmental factors on connective tissue organization and glycosaminoglycan synthesis. In: Parry DAD, Creamer LK, eds: Fibrous Proteins: Scientific, Industrial, and Medical Aspects. London, Academic Press, 1980:107–119
11. Grimsby O: Medical Exercise Training [Lecture]. Seattle, WA, Ola Grimsby Institute, March 1993
12. Harkness RD: Mechanical properties of connective tissues in relation to function. In: Parry DAD, Creamer LK, eds: Fibrous Proteins: Scientific, Industrial, and Medical Aspects. London, Academic Press, 1980:207–230

13. Heinegard D, Hascall VC: Aggregation of cartilage proteoglycans, III: Characteristics of the proteins isolated from trypsin digests of aggregates. J Biol Chem 249:4250–4256, 1974

14. Heinegard D, Oldberg A. Glycosylated matrix proteins. In: Royce PM, Steinmann B, eds: Connective Tissue and Its Heritable Disorders: Molecular, Genetic, and Medical Aspects. New York, Wiley-Liss, 1993:189–209

15. Hoiulbooke K, Vause K, Merrilees MJ: Effects of movement and weight-bearing on glycosaminoglycan content of sheep articular cartilage. Australian J Physiother 36:88–91, 1990

16. Hooley CJ, Cohen RE: A model for the creep behavior of tendon. Int J Biol Macromol 1:123–132, 1979

17. Hooley CJ, McCrum NG, Cohen RE: The viscoelastic deformation of tendon. J Biomech 13:521–528, 1980

18. Junqueira LC, Carneiro J, Long JA: Basic Histology, 6th ed. Los Altos, Lange Medical Publishers, 1968:92–104

19. Kastelic J, Galeski A, Baer E: The multicomposite structure of tendon. Conn Tissue Res 6:11–23, 1978

20. Kielty CM, Hopkinson I, Grant ME. Collagen: The collagen family, structure, assembly, and organization in the extracellular matrix. In: Royce PM, Steinmann BS, eds: Connective Tissue and Its Heritable Disorders: Molecular, Genetic, and Medical Aspects. New York, Wiley-Liss, 1993:103–147

21. Kirscher EM, Speer DP: Microvascular changes in Dupuytren's contracture. J Hand Surg 9A:58–62, 1984

22. Lehman JF, Masock AJ, Warren CG: Effect of therapeutic temperatures on tendon extensibility. Arch Phys Med Rehabil 50:481–483, 1970

23. Madden JW, De Vore G, Arem AJ: A rational postoperative management program for metacarpophalangeal joint implant arthroplasty. J Hand Surg 2:358–366, 1977

24. Madden JW, Peacock EE: Studies on the biology of collagen during wound healing: III. Dynamic metabolism of scar collagen and remodeling of dermal wounds. Ann Surg 174:511–520, 1971

25. Rigby BJ: The effect of mechanical extension upon the thermal stability of collagen. Biochem Biophys Acta 79:634–636, 1964

26. Rigby BJ, Hirai N, Spikes JD: The mechanical behavior of rat tendon. J Gen Physiol 43:265–283, 1959

27. Tagawa B, Prockop DJ, Guzman NA: Collagen diseases and biosynthesis of collagen. Hosp Pract 12:61–68, 1997

28. Tillman LJ, Cummings GS: Biological mechanisms of connective tissue mutability. In: Currier DP, Nelson RM, eds: Dynamics of Human Biologic Tissues. Philadelphia, FA Davis, 8:1–44, 1992

29. Van Brocklin JD, Ellis DG: A study of mechanical behavior of toe extensor tendons under applied stress. Arch Phys Med Rehabil 46:369–371, 1965

30. von der Mark K, Goodman S: Adhesive glycoproteins. In: Royce PM, Steinmann B, eds: Connective Tissue and Its Heritable Disorders: Molecular, Genetic, and Medical Aspects. New York, Wiley-Liss, 1993:211–236

31. Warren CG, Lehman JF, Koblanski JN: Elongation of rat tail tendon: Effect of load and temperature. Arch Phys Med Rehabil 52:465–484, 1971

32. Woo SL-Y, Mathews JV, Akeson WH, et al: Connective tissue response to immobility: Correlative study of biomechanical measurements of normal and immobilized rabbit knees. Arthritis Rheum 18:257–264, 1975

33. Wyke B: The neurology of joints. Ann R Coll Surg Engl 41:25–50, 1967

Wound Healing: Injury and Repair of Dense Connective Tissue

2

LARRY J. TILLMAN AND JUNE E. HANKS

- INTRODUCTION
- INFLAMMATORY PHASE
    - Acute Inflammation
    - Chronic Inflammation
- PROLIFERATIVE PHASE
    - Re-Epithelialization
    - Fibroplasia with Neovascularization
    - Wound Contraction
- REMODELING PHASE
    - Consolidation Stage
    - Maturation Stage
- EFFECTS OF STRESS ON SCAR REMODELING
    - Factors Impairing Wound Healing

INTRODUCTION

An injury can be defined as an interruption in the continuity of a tissue. Repair begins immediately following injury by attempting to reestablish that continuity. With the exception of teeth, all tissue within the body is capable of repairing injuries.[45,46] Generally, mammals do not regenerate tissue, they repair it with dense connective tissue (DCT) scarring. This quick process reduces the chances of infection. The prompt development of granulation tissue forecasts the repair of the interrupted DCT to produce a scar. It is important for the manual therapist to understand and apply basic biologic principles of inflammation, wound repair, and scar formation to predict the outcome of clinical wound management.

Wound injuries may occur as a result of surgery, trauma, or pressure. Surgical wounds heal by **primary intention** in which wound edges are drawn together to achieve closure. With primary intention healing, there is no major loss of tissue, the wound edges are smooth, and the wound is clean. Thus, wound healing by primary intention typically occurs quickly, with wound closure occurring in 3 to 7 days. **Delayed primary intention healing** is chosen when there is large tissue loss, when the wound is contaminated, and when closure by primary intention would put the patient at risk of infection. Typically, the wound is left open for several days and surgically closed at a later date when the risk of infection has decreased. **Secondary intention healing,** or healing by scar tissue formation, is the chosen method of healing when large amounts of tissue are lost, the wound margins are nonviable or cannot be approximated, or when the wound has a high bacterial bioburden.

The body produces a similar cellular response to tissue irritation, mechanical injury, surgical and other forms of trauma, and bacterial or viral invasion. In wound healing, this cellular response contributes to three broad phases of scar tissue formation: **inflammatory, proliferative,** and **remodeling phases.**[25]

INFLAMMATORY PHASE

Inflammation is a series of reactions by vascularized tissue in response to an injury. The purpose of the inflammatory reaction is to remove all foreign debris along with the dead and dying tissue, thereby reducing the likelihood of infection and providing an environment conducive to optimal wound healing. The inflammatory reaction attempts to control the effects of the injurious agent and return the tissue to a normal state. The inflammatory response and the process of repair are closely intertwined.

The inflammatory stage is traditionally studied by separating the tissue events into acute and chronic components. Acute inflammation is the immediate and early microvascular response to an injurious agent. The response is similar, with minor variations, in any particular tissue or body organ. Chronic inflammation is a longer-lasting response resulting from either an unresolved acute inflammatory process or a persistent injurious agent. The chronic response leads to a mostly DCT cell proliferation.

Acute Inflammation

Vascular and early cellular responses play a major role during the acute inflammatory phase. Depending on the size of the injury, this initial phase is of short duration (usually lasting only 24 to 48 hours; when extended, it is completed in 2 weeks). The clinical signs of **pain** (L. *dolor*), **heat** (L. *calor*), **redness** (L. *rubor*), **swelling** (L. *tumor*), and **loss of function** (L. *functio laesa*) relate directly to the sequence of acute hemodynamic changes. It is helpful to the manual therapist to correlate the signs of acute inflammation directly with the microscopic changes occurring in the injured tissues. Numerous chemical mediators of inflammation cause and respond to these microscopic changes.

VASCULAR RESPONSE

Initially, there is a neural reflex to cellular injury that causes transient vasoconstriction. This neurogenic response is quickly followed by a hyperemic response in which blood flows into the wound. Coagulation seals off the injured blood vessels and temporarily closes the wound space. Simultaneously, noninjured blood vessels in the vicinity of the wound dilate in response to various vasoactive chemicals released into the wound.[66] The duration of vasodilation depends on the chemical stimulus. The increased blood flow brings nutrients, oxygen, and phagocytic cells into the wound space.

Three interrelated plasma-derived systems stimulate and mediate the inflammatory response: the **kinin system,** the **complement system,** and the **clotting system.**[37] **Hageman factor XII,** a plasma protein, activates each of these three systems, releasing specific chemical mediators into the wound area. Hageman XII converts prekallikrein to kallikrein to start the release of kinins, stimulates plasmin interaction with complement proteins, and activates the coagulation proteins. Hageman factor XII becomes stimulated by surface-active agents, endotoxins, and contact with cartilage and basement membrane tissue.[18] The role Hageman factor XII plays in activating these systems is shown in Figure 2-1.

Kinins are plasma polypeptides found in the exudate. They contribute to the arteriolar dilation, increased venule permeability, contraction of smooth muscle, and increased pain sensation.[65] Once Hageman XII converts prekallikrein to kallikrein, kallikrein acts on high molecular weight kininogen (HMWK) to produce the final product bradykinin. **Bradykinin** participates in the early period of increased vascular permeability. The action of bradykinin is inactivated by the enzyme kininase.[12]

The complement system, known for its role in enhancing antibody–antigen immune complexes, also plays an important role in mediating inflammation. Complement plasma proteins affect vascular responses, leukocyte adhesion, and chemotaxis as well as enhance phagocytosis in inflammation.[65] In a sequential fashion, a series of nine plasma proteins (C1–C9), and their cleavage products, combine to form what is known as the complement cascade. Specific components of the complement cascade are important in the inflammatory phase of wound healing. Components of C3 and C5, for example, increase vascular permeability and cause vasodilation. C3 also assists in the process of phagocytosis by **opsonization.** Opsonization is the process by which bacterial antigens are coated with immunoglobulins that target the infectious agents for increased phagocytic destruction. Additionally, C5 is chemotaxic for neutrophils, eosinophils, basophils, and monocytes, attracting them to the injured site. The complement complex of C56789 attacks cell membranes causing lysis. Figure 2-2 demonstrates the complement cascade of events.

The complement cascade acts on DCT mast cells. Mast cells, located adjacent to the blood vessels, respond to specific complement proteins by releasing **histamine.** Histamine, a vasoactive amine also present in basophils and platelets, produces the initial, short-acting dilation of the noninjured arterioles and increases the vascular permeability of the venules. Histamine constricts the larger arteries. Allergic reactions, lytic enzymes, trauma, and heat can promote the release of histamine as well.

The release of these numerous chemical mediators causes vasodilation and an increased blood flow to the microvascu-

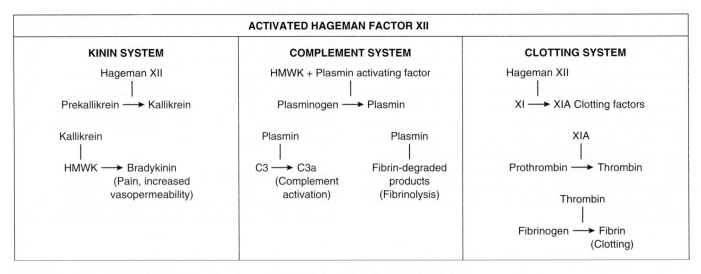

■ **FIG. 2-1.** Hageman factor XII activation. *HMWK,* high molecular weight kininogen.

COMPLEMENT CASCADE

1. Antigen-Antibody Complex → Activates C1 → Cleaves C4 and C2

2. C4 + C2 → C$\overline{42}$ Complex

3. C$\overline{42}$ → Cleaves C3a + C3b

4. C3a splits off *(increases vasopermeability)*

5. C3b *(opsonin for neutrophils, macrophages, and eosinophils)* + C$\overline{42}$ → C5a *(chemotactic for neutrophils and macrophages, increases vasopermeability, activates the lipoxygenase pathway of arachidonic acid metabolism)*

6. C5b + C6 + C7 → C$\overline{567}$ *(chemotactic for inflammatory cells)*

7. C$\overline{567}$ + C8 + C9 → C$\overline{56789}$ membrane attack complex *(lyses cell membranes, stimulates arachidonic acid metabolism)*

■ **FIG. 2-2.** Complement cascade. When the complement system is activated, proteolytic cleavage products are sequentially elaborated and significant inflammatory effects result.

lar beds. Heat and redness result as observed during the early hemodynamic changes. The dilated noninjured vessels initially release a **transudate,** composed mainly of water and electrolytes, from the blood into the connective tissue interstitium. Increased vascular permeability allows plasma proteins and a few white blood cells (WBCs) to escape into the wound area, and the serous transudate becomes a more viscous **exudate** (Fig. 2-3). The plasma proteins that leak into the tissues provide an osmotic gradient that brings more water into the wound area from the plasma. This exudation leads to the edematous swelling observed during the inflammatory phase.

The clotting system is also a series of plasma proteins. Hageman factor XII initiates clotting by converting prothrombin to thrombin (Fig. 2-1). Thrombin acts to convert fibrinogen to fibrin in the final step of the clotting cascade. Fibrinopeptides are formed during this conversion, which cause increased vascular permeability.[37] Fibrin plugs the capillaries and lymphatics around the wound to seal off the area, effectively preventing infection. Also, the water-binding properties of hyaluronic acid released from mast cells contribute to a "wound gel,"[10] which fills all space in the wound. During this process dermal fat is lost, leading to a thinning of the skin over the wound area.[29]

In addition to the plasma-derived protein systems, oxygenated **arachidonic acid (AA)** derivatives play a critical role in acute inflammation (Fig. 2-4). AA is a polyunsaturated fatty acid product of phospholipid breakdown in ruptured cell membranes that releases metabolites into the exudate. These products of AA metabolism are called **autocoids** and act as short-range local hormones. Three such groups of AA metabolites—**leukotrienes, prostaglandins,** and **thromboxanes**—can mediate virtually every step of acute inflammation.[37] Leukotrienes are a family of compounds that cause vasodilation and increased vascular constriction and permeability. Prostaglandins are longer-acting, local vasodilators that play a

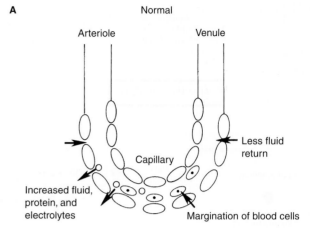

A   Normal

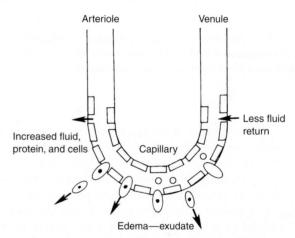

B   Edema—transudate

■ **FIG. 2-3.** Production of edema during inflammation. Initially a transudate consisting of water, electrolytes, and some plasma proteins is formed (**A**), followed by an exudate composed of increased plasma proteins and white blood cells (**B**). Daly TJ: The repair phase of wound healing—Re-epithelialization and contraction. In: Kloth LC, McCulloch JM, Feedar JA, eds: Wound Healing: Alternatives in Management, 2nd ed. Philadelphia, FA Davis, 1995.

role in pain transmission and fever production. Although unclear, increased fever might be the result of prostaglandins affecting the hypothalamus of the diencephalon, which in turn stimulates the sympathetic nervous system.[8] Nonsteroidal antiinflammatory drugs (NSAIDs) and corticosteroids inhibit the cyclooxygenase pathway biosynthesis of prostaglandins, thereby reducing the inflammatory reaction. Thromboxanes are involved in vasoconstriction and platelet aggregation. Synthesized by injured cell membranes, these chemical mediators prolong the edematous reaction of inflammation.

Other protein mediators of the acute inflammatory response include **lymphokines, neutrophil (polymorphonuclear [PMN]) products,** and **platelet activating factor (PAF).** Lymphokines are cytokines released from helper T lymphocytes. These vasoactive substances induce chemotaxis for

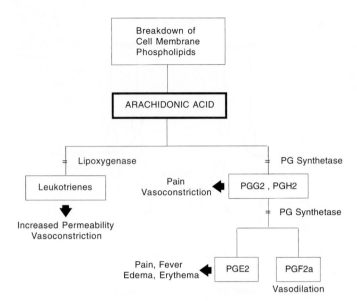

■ **FIG. 2-4.** Arachidonic acid metabolites in inflammation. Prostaglandin and leukotriene biosynthesis from the breakdown of cell membrane phospholipids.

PMNs and macrophages, in addition to their important role in immunologic reactions. Two lymphokines important in mediating inflammation are interleukin-1 (IL-1) and tumor necrosis factor (TNF). Proteins and proteases are released from the lysosomes of dying PMNs that can activate complement and kinin systems to stimulate vasodilation and enhance chemotaxis. PAF, released from mast cells and leukocytes, also increases vasopermeability and chemotaxis. A summary of the chemical mediators of acute inflammation is found in Table 2-1.

CLINICAL CONSIDERATIONS

During acute inflammation the vascular response almost always involves pain. Pain is produced by both the engorgement of tissue spaces from the swelling and resultant pressure, and by chemical irritation of pain-producing free nerve endings. Bradykinin, enhanced by prostaglandins, stimulates the nociceptor receptors in the skin. The increased pain causes the patient to guard the affected wound area, and loss of function results.

CELLULAR RESPONSE

The process of cell migration along a chemically mediated concentration gradient is called **chemotaxis.** Many of the chemical substances in the exudate are chemoattractants for WBCs. The arrival of leukocytes at the site of injury is a critical part of the inflammatory process because phagocytosis of cellular debris and foreign antigens is necessary to assure proper wound healing. Bacterial products, complement and fibrin fractions, histamine, and kinin components are chemotactic mediators of the WBC response that occurs during the inflammatory phase of wound healing.[7,22,50,55,66]

There is a cellular migration pattern into the inflamed tissue area. Tissue macrophages, also known as histiocytes, act as the first line of phagocytic defense against foreign antigens and bacterial debris. Macrophages are strongly chemoattractant for PMNs; therefore, WBC neutrophils are next in sequence to reach the inflamed tissue. With increased vascular permeability and escape of plasma proteins, the viscosity of the blood increases, causing sludging of red blood cells and increased frictional resistance to blood flow. During this process, short-lived PMNs follow a specific sequence of WBC events known as **margination, pavementing, emigration, chemotaxis,** and **phagocytosis.**

Initially the PMNs **marginate** to the inner walls of the capillaries and post-capillary venules; there they adhere to the walls, a process called **pavementing.** Next, these neutrophils **emigrate** through the permeable endothelial cells lining the vessels, into the surrounding interstitial space. They are then chemotactically drawn to the wound area where the bacteria are located. Blood monocytes, lymphocytes, eosinophils, and basophils all use this same pathway.[37] The primary goal of the PMNs is **phagocytosis** of bacterial products and other foreign antigens to prevent or eliminate infection in the wound. PMNs attach to and engulf the foreign particles, release proteolytic enzymes from lysosomal organelles, and it is hoped, degrade and digest the microorganisms. When large numbers of PMNs die and are lysed, the exudate forms pus and the wound is considered infected.

As the acute inflammatory phase progresses, the number of PMNs declines and DCT macrophages remain and predominate. Neutrophilic, bacterial, and complement fractions are chemoattractants for additional macrophages. These scavenger cells dispose of the remaining bacteria and necrotic tissue. Both neutrophils and macrophages function in a low oxygen, high acidotic environment. Hydrogen peroxide, ascorbic acid, and lactic acid are byproducts of phagocytosis.[67] Hydrogen peroxide controls anaerobic bacterial growth, while ascorbic and lactic acids further increase macrophage activity. This increased macrophage activity produces a more intense and prolonged inflammatory response.

Inflammation is necessary for tissue repair but it must subside for the progression of healing. Acute inflammation can completely resolve, heal by scarring, form abscesses, or progress into chronic inflammation. Host factors, wound size and location, persistent tissue trauma, and nutrition will influence outcomes.

MACROPHAGE SELECTIVE VERSUS NONSELECTIVE TISSUE DESTRUCTION

Macrophages attack and phagocytize bacteria and debris in a **selective** manner when the acutely inflamed area is not adversely disturbed through excessive movement or aggressive treatment. Through chemotaxis, mediators of inflammation attract the phagocytes to a confined, local area of injury. The macrophages clean up the foreign bacteria and debris, and the inflammatory response resolves in a timely fashion.

TABLE 2-1 CHEMICAL MEDIATORS OF ACUTE INFLAMMATION

CHEMICAL MEDIATOR	SOURCE	INCREASED ACTIVITY
VASOACTIVE AMINES		
Serotonin	Platelets	Vasopermeability
Histamine	Mast cells, platelets, basophils	Vasopermeability
PLASMA POLYPEPTIDES AND PROTEASES		
Kinins (bradykinin)	Plasma proteins	Vasopermeability, pain
Complement	Plasma proteins	
C3a		Vasopermeability
C5a		Vasopermeability, chemotaxis
Clotting cascade	Plasma proteins	Coagulation, fibrinolysis
ARACHIDONIC ACID DERIVATIVES		
Prostaglandins	Mast cells, cell membrane phospholipids, platelets	Vasodilation, pain, fever
Leukotrienes	Leukocytes, mast cells	Vasopermeability, chemotaxis
Thromboxanes	Platelets ?	Platelet aggregation, thrombosis
OTHER MEDIATORS		
Lysosomal proteases	Neutrophil, bacterial products	Vasopermeability, chemotaxis, cell damage
Platelet activating factor	Leukocytes, mast cells	Vasopermeability, chemotaxis
Cytokines (lymphokines)—IL-1, TNF	Lymphocytes, monocytes, macrophages	Vasopermeability, chemotaxis, fever
O_2-derived free radicals	Neutrophils, macrophages	Vasopermeability, cell damage

IL-1, interleukin-1; *TNF*, tumor necrosis factor.

With aggressive treatment or use of the acutely injured tissue, however, the macrophages participate in **nonselective** tissue destruction. Aggressive treatment of injured tissue leads to the release of additional chemical mediators, further stimulating the production of yet larger numbers of phagocytes. The result of this additional stimulation is that healthy tissue surrounding the injured area becomes destroyed by the macrophages in a nonspecific manner, which enlarges the initial area of injury, prolongs the inflammatory response, and retards wound healing. This type of nonselective tissue destruction, therefore, supports the concept of **rest** as an acceptable form of treatment during the acute phase of inflammation. However, the period of immobilization should be kept to a minimum.

Chronic Inflammation

Unlike acute inflammation, in which the emphasis is on hemodynamic activities, chronic inflammation follows a course leading mostly to a DCT cell proliferation. The differences between acute and chronic inflammation are highlighted in Table 2-2. Chronic inflammation lasts for months to years and results from either unresolved acute inflammation, repeated episodes of microtrauma, persistent chronic irritation, or hypersensitivity (immune) reactions. The chronically inflamed area is infiltrated with macrophages and monocytes. Macrophages

have the capacity to become metabolically active and secrete products that serve as mediators in chronic inflammation, thereby self-perpetuating the chronic response.[65] This macrophage self-perpetuation results in the infiltration of large numbers of activated fibroblasts that deposit increased amounts of collagen. Varying amounts of scar tissue form. With an increase in DCT cells and their products, the patient complains predominantly of stiffness with movement. Pain, the primary client complaint during acute inflammation, now becomes a secondary symptom in chronic inflammation.

The presence of a persistent irritant, local pressure (as in decubitus ulcers), poor oxygen supply, poor surgical closure, malnutrition, vitamin A and C deficiencies, radiation injury, or immunosuppression can prolong the chronic inflammatory phase. Wound healing and the prevention of infection are then adversely affected.[25] Assuming, however, that the phagocytes resolve the inflammatory response, the resultant clean wound bed is now ready for the rebuilding or fibroplastic phase of wound healing.

CLINICAL CONSIDERATIONS

The manual therapist must not allow treatment to become another chronic irritant that further enhances inflammation. Treatment is directed toward assisting the macrophages in their work through proper wound management to maintain a

TABLE 2-2 COMPARISON BETWEEN ACUTE AND CHRONIC INFLAMMATION

ACUTE INFLAMMATION	CHRONIC INFLAMMATION
Rapid response to injury	Slow response to injury
Dynamic vascular response	Proliferative DCT cellular response
Exudate production rich in fibrin	Collagen production leading to fibrosis
Typically produces a neutrophil and macrophage response	Macrophage, lymphocyte, plasma cell, and fibroblast response
Chemical mediators directed toward vascular permeability changes and release of exudate	Chemical mediators produced by cells recruiting macrophages and fibroblasts
Often results in resolution with some tissue destruction	Often results in significant tissue damage with fibrosis and scar formation
Throbbing pain	Stiffness with aching pain

clean, moist environment. Treatment also involves the implementation of the rest, ice, compression, elevation (RICE) regimen and proper positioning.[25] Additionally, the therapist can minimize some of these factors that prevent or prolong inflammation by application of receptor techniques for inhibition of pain and guarding, and introduction of carefully dosed, pain-free exercise for edema reduction.

PROLIFERATIVE PHASE

The proliferative phase of wound healing lasts approximately 3 weeks. This phase, also known as the granulation or fibroplastic phase, involves the DCT fibroblast that is primarily responsible for scar tissue formation by synthesizing new collagen and ground substance. Three major components occur simultaneously in this phase: **re-epithelialization, fibroplasia with neovascularization,** and **wound contraction.**

Re-Epithelialization

Within hours of an injury, superficial wounds initiate the re-epithelialization process in skin.[48,67] This process involves the re-establishment of the epidermis across the surface of the wound by mitotically active, basal cells of the uninjured epidermal margin. Epidermal growth factor is thought to stimulate the basal cell proliferation.[11] With a viable wound bed, these epithelial cells traverse the wound surface guided by matrix fibrin, fibronectin, and newly formed type IV collagen.[15,51]

Only 48 hours are required for approximated wound edges to re-epithelialize, well before fibroplasia begins.[9] The re-epithelialization of larger wounds takes longer; several weeks are required for the epithelial cells to differentiate into a functional, stratified epidermis firmly attached to the underlying dermis. The new epithelium forms deep to any scab, or eschar, to maintain contact with the vascular network.

CLINICAL CONSIDERATIONS

A clean, moist wound with ample blood supply will facilitate proper tissue repair and may reduce pain during healing. Although a scab acts as a temporary surface barrier against bacteria and foreign matter, in deeper wounds it impedes rapid re-epithelialization by retarding basal cell migration.[68] Scab formation of chronic wounds can be minimized by keeping the surface hydrated with various microenvironmental dressings.[26,54] Proper dressings create a wound environment that promotes an increased cell proliferation by retaining growth factors, proteins, and cytokines of wound exudate produced in response to injury and by promoting degradation of fibrin clots.[13,23,58] The appropriate dressing maintains adequate wound moisture and temperature and will protect the wound from contaminants and trauma. Although motion provides the ideal stimulus for collagen regeneration, repeated trauma to the wound surface through excessive skin stretching or multiple dressing changes may interfere with healing.

Fibroplasia with Neovascularization

Macrophages are not only essential to the inflammatory phase of wound healing, but are also necessary to direct the fibroblasts and angioblasts in the formation of new scar.[5] Macrophages release chemotactic substances, such as fibronectin, platelet-derived growth factor (GF), and other growth factors (epidermal GF, fibroblast GF, transforming GFs α, β),[19,27,33,36,60,61] which attract fibroblasts to the wound and play a role in adhesion of fibroblasts to the fibrin meshwork. Angioblasts contribute to the formation of new blood vessels at the wound edge.

In healthy tissue, fibroblasts are sparse and generally quiescent throughout the connective tissue matrix. After injury, fibroblasts are activated to migrate along the fibrin meshwork to the wound site as a result of the concentration gradients of chemical mediators, O_2, CO_2, lactic acid, and pH.[30] They proliferate and produce new collagen, elastin, GAGs, proteoglycans, and glycoproteins, which are utilized to reconstruct the connective tissue matrix.[46] The process of fibroblast migration and proliferation is called **fibroplasia.**

Healing will not be complete unless new, functioning capillaries develop to provide nourishment and oxygen to the injured tissue. Wound healing ends only when local hypoxia and lactic acid concentrations are reversed by the ingrowth of adequate circulation.[70] The process by which new blood vessels originate from pre-existing vessels at the wound margin and grow into the wound space is called **neovascularization** or **angiogenesis.** Within 24 hours and up to 5 days after an injury, as directed by macrophage-released chemotactic substances and ischemia,[54] patent blood vessels "sprout" cells called angioblasts into the wound space. When these cells contact each other, new capillary loops are formed. The increased vascular circulation to the new wound, together with immature collagen fibers, gives the surface of the wound a pink/red granular appearance; hence the term **granulation tissue.** The formation of granulation tissue is the hallmark of tissue healing during the proliferative phase.

The bulky scar at this stage is very fragile and easily disrupted.[39] The new collagen fibers are laid down randomly along strands of clot fibrin and initially are held together by weak hydrogen bonds. Immobilization is often prescribed to permit vascular regrowth and prevent microhemorrhages.[25] Use of gentle stretch to stress the scar will cause elongation of the scar by cell migration, but the application of excessive force will disrupt cell membranes, causing cellular death.[38] It is clinically important to note that edema may still be present in the newly formed granulation tissue, even after the inflammatory phase has ended. This edema is the result of plasma proteins leaking from the new capillaries into the extravascular space.[38]

CLINICAL CONSIDERATIONS

Open wounds progressing from the acute inflammatory to acute proliferative phase demonstrate increasing amounts of beefy red granulation tissue, with subsequent decrease in wound depth and size as epithelial cells migrate across the wound surface. The amount of serous or serosanguinous wound fluid will decrease as wound healing progresses. The periwound skin temperature, texture, and color will gradually return to normal.

A chronic wound that fails to progress appropriately through the proliferative phase will exhibit indications of poor blood supply, desiccation, infection, hypergranulation, or hypogranulation. Wound tissue may appear very pale or dark red and may have minimal exudate. In the case of infection, wound tissue may become bright red and wound fluid may become excessive, malodorous, viscous, and purulent. In some cases, granulation tissue may proliferate beyond the wound surface, resulting in the inhibition of epithelial cell migration. It is recommended that this hypergranulation tissue be disrupted by rubbing silver nitrate sticks or dry gauze across the wound surface or by trimming the hypergranulated tissue. An absence of the proliferation phase may result in hypogranulation of the wound bed, evidenced by a lack of change in wound depth, size, and surface area. Unless intrinsic and extrinsic conditions contributing to poor healing are addressed, wound closure is at risk.

Wound Contraction

Wound contraction is the mechanism by which the edges of a wound are centripetally drawn together because of forces generated within that wound. This normal healing process shrinks the defect, resulting in a smaller wound to be repaired by scar formation (Fig. 2-5). Although limited by how much each cell can contract, by the capacity of the extracellular fibers and ground substance to be compacted, and by the tension in surrounding tissues, this process is progressive. Wound contraction begins 4 days after injury and continues through day 21[49]; in other words, it lasts about as long as the fibroplasia. In certain circumstances, such as large burn scars, contraction remains active for longer periods, possibly owing to poor circulation associated with such scars.[31,64]

Wound contraction is predominantly mediated by cells called **myofibroblasts.**[38,43,46,69] Myofibroblasts are specialized fibroblasts containing muscle-like contractile proteins that enable them to extend and contract.[47] The myofibroblasts anchor to each other and to fibrillar structures in the extracellular matrix, so that the contraction of each cell is transmitted to the tissue as a whole. The interaction of the extracellular matrix and the cells of the granulation tissue form the wound contraction unit called the **fibronexus.** This unit is composed of the glycoprotein fibronectin, the contractile protein actin, the anchoring protein vinculum, and collagen types I and II. The actual process whereby the scar is made smaller can be compared to a ratchet where as collagen turnover occurs, the myofibroblasts reach out and contract the scar, and the new

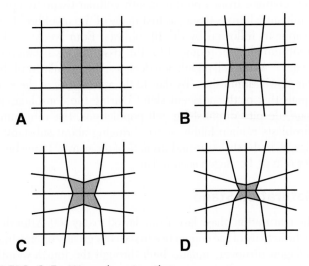

■ FIG. 2-5. Wound contraction.

collagen laid down occupies a smaller space, and so on.[6] The end result is a stable wound with a constant turnover of collagen as the matrix is remodeling. Large wounds contract 50% or one half their size at a rate of approximately 5 to 10% every 6 weeks or so. Linear, square, and rectangular wounds contract more rapidly than circular wounds.

CLINICAL CONSIDERATIONS

It is clinically important to distinguish between **wound contraction** and **scar contracture.** Wound contraction is a normal part of the healing process that reduces wound size, thereby decreasing the area needing to close by epithelialization. Scar contracture is the result of a contractile process occurring in a healed scar and often results in an undesirable fixed, rigid scar that causes cosmetic deformity and/or functional deficits, especially when occurring on the head, neck, hand, and joint surfaces. Scar contracture may be the result of wound contraction, adhesions, fibrosis, and other tissue damage.[2] Whereas wound contraction generally occurs in an incompletely epithelialized defect, scar contracture usually occurs in an epithelialized covered defect.[52,53] Range of motion and proper positioning are critical during scar formation to prevent functional impairment.

REMODELING PHASE

At the end of the fibroplastic stage, the myofibroblasts and fibroblasts start to leave the scar. At this point, the newly formed scar will undergo remodeling in an effort to strengthen the wound along appropriate lines of stress. By increasing the tensile strength of the scar, the ultimate goal of remodeling is the return of function. There are two distinct components of scar tissue remodeling, the **consolidation** and **maturation stages.**

Consolidation Stage

The consolidation stage lasts from day 21 to day 60. The scar typically stops increasing in size by day 21.[42] The tissue gradually changes from a predominantly cellular tissue to a predominantly fibrous tissue, as first many of the myofibroblasts disappear, followed by the fibroblasts. Four weeks is the minimum amount required for this tissue reorganization to occur.[1,26] As the cell population declines, the vascularity of the scar slowly diminishes. By day 42 the vascularity of the scar equals that of the adjacent skin.[1] During the consolidation stage, despite diminishing cell populations, the remaining fibroblasts remain highly active, bringing about substantial changes in the structure and strength of the scar.[1,28] Large bundles of type I collagen accumulate.

Maturation Stage

The maturation phase lasts from day 60 to day 360. After day 60 the activity of the connective tissue cells greatly diminishes. Collagen turnover remains high through the fourth month and then gradually tapers off.[3] Between 180 and 360 days, few cells are seen, and the tissue becomes tendon-like.[28,34] The changes in the scar during these last two stages occur very gradually as the scar, which starts out as an extremely cellular tissue, becomes predominantly fibrous by the end of the maturation stage. The bulk of the scar is formed by large and compact, type I collagen fibers. The fully mature scar is only about 3% cellular, and its vascularity is greatly reduced.[28,34] As immature scar is converted to mature scar, intracollagen molecular linkage changes from weak hydrogen bonding to strong covalent bonding, resulting in the gradual increase in scar strength.

EFFECTS OF STRESS ON SCAR REMODELING

Stress has a significant effect on scar remodeling, contributing to the shape, strength, and pliability of the scar.[28,34] The DCT cells, GAGs, proteoglycans, and collagen architecture are all affected by the direction and magnitude of mechanical stress applied to the scar.[34] Figure 2-6 illustrates the effect of stress on collagen formation. Collagen fibers are often randomly oriented in unstressed wounds yet aggregate in small, parallel bundles in wounds undergoing stress.

Fibroblasts, including their mitotic bundles, orient parallel to the lines of tension,[4] the long axis of the cells lying along stress lines. Mechanical forces, likewise, influence the metabolic activities of fibroblasts. It has been demonstrated that fibroblast tissue cultures subjected to a cyclic strain respond by increasing production of GAGs and proteoglycans after 24 hours.[57] Fibronectin, which anchors strands of myofibroblasts and provides a scaffold on which collagen fiber aggregation occurs, also lies parallel to the direction of wound contraction.[20] This model offers one explanation of how cellular orientation leads to collagen fiber orientation in the early development of DCT.[64]

Collagen fibers are laid down in response to lines of stress resulting from mechanical loads. Collagen under tension has different properties from collagen under compression, owing to the different distribution of piezo-electric charges on the collagen fibers. The physiologic loads of tension cause increased aggregation of collagen, whereas compression causes decreased fiber aggregation.[19] Collagen fibers laid down along stress lines involve the transduction of physical forces into electrochemical events at the molecular level.[64] As a result, the collagen fibers aggregate into small bundles oriented across the wound space, as dictated by the direction of stress.[21]

The magnitude and the duration of stress application also have an effect on collagen deposition, and in turn, on scar strength. If too much stress is applied to newly formed scar, the weakly bonded tissue pulls apart; it is not unusual for excessive strain to increase inflammation and decrease fibroplasia.[24] Several studies demonstrate the impact of overloading DCT structures.[56,59] Scar strength increases with not only the aggregation of collagen fibers along stress lines, but also with the increase of scar collagen volume and stable covalent bonding.[64,41]

The change in shape of scar tissue by remodeling is a slow process. Without the proper amount of stress stimulus, scar can take months to fill in a small space.[30] If remodeling is to occur, there must be a sufficient population of active con-

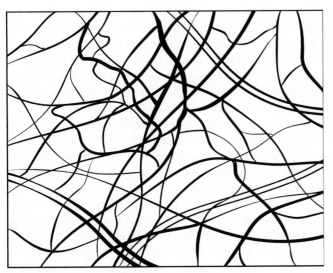
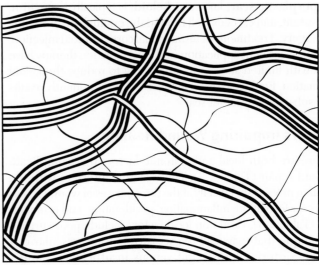

A Wound collagen, unstressed

B Wound collagen, stressed

■ **FIG. 2-6.** **(A)** Unstressed and **(B)** stressed wound collagen. In the wound subjected to stress, collagen reorganizes with larger, more parallel aligned fibers.

nective tissue cells to remodel the tissue, and the scar must be malleable enough for therapeutic stress to stimulate remodeling. Additionally, time governs the ability of scar to change shape. For example, a 4-week-old scar significantly remodels shorter to noncyclical strain, whereas a 14-week-old scar is unaffected by the remodeling.[41] This difference may be the result of the reduced number of DCT cells and stronger bonding in the maturing collagen architecture of the older scar.[64] Figure 2-7 summarizes the three overlapping phases of wound healing, to include a post-injury time scale of the events contributing to increased collagen accumulation, wound contraction, and scar strength.

CLINICAL CONSIDERATIONS

Scar has less innervation than normal skin, leading to decreased protective sensation and, in some persons, increased sensitivity to cold. Itching may occur as the scar matures to a deficiency of skin oils and the release of substances such as histamine in the wounded area. Nonperfumed lotions may be useful to decrease itching.

In normal healing, the pink maturing scar gradually blanches and conforms to the normal body contours. However, functional complications can result from contraction of the forming scar, especially when located over surfaces of joints. In cases of scar-impeded function, a surgical scar revision may be required. Small scars may be excised followed by primary wound closure. Larger scar excisions may require skin grafting for wound closure. Massage is useful in loosening adhesions between the scar and surrounding soft tissues. Slow, sustained elongation of the scar and adjacent tissue will promote function. Splints may be useful to maintain stretch on the scar and to counter scar contraction. The combination of heat application and stretching may increase collagen extensibility.

Some individuals have a genetically influenced imbalance between collagen synthesis and lysis, resulting in the formation of either hypertrophic or hyperplastic scars following wounding. A **hypertrophic scar,** associated with burns, appears as local areas of tissue overgrowth within the confines of the original wound that tends to soften and regress over time.

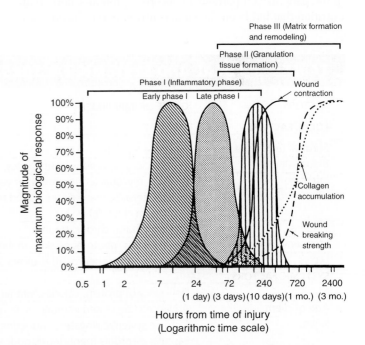

■ **FIG. 2-7.** The three overlapping phases of wound repair. Phase I, inflammation; phase II, granulation or fibroplastic; and phase III, remodeling. (Daly TJ: The repair phase of wound healing–Re-epithelialization and contraction. In: Kloth LC, McCulloch JM, Feedar JA, eds: Wound Healing: Alternatives in Management. New York, FA Davis, Holden and Publisher, 1990:15.)

Hyperplastic scar, known as **keloid,** is typically large, firm, persistent, and exceeds well beyond the original site of trauma or surgery. Treatments of intralesional corticosteroid injection, pressure garment application, and local radiation therapy have met with limited success in attempting to reduce the keloid formation. For keloid scars, surgical removal frequently results in a subsequently larger scar.

Factors Impairing Wound Healing

There are both local and systemic factors that complicate wound repair (Table 2-3). These factors interfere with the healing process specifically at the three phases of wound repair and scar formation: inflammation, proliferation, and remodeling (Table 2-4). Common local factors include poor surgical technique that may lead to excessive tension, vascular disorders (arteriosclerosis and venous insufficiency), infections caused by local microorganisms, locally administered medications (anesthetics, topical steroids, antibiotics, antineoplastic drugs, hemostatic agents), chronic trauma (chronic irritant, radiation), adverse wound microenvironment (dry/wet/semi-occlusive dressings), and development of ulcers (pressure, neuropathic).[14,16,32,40,44]

Systemic factors considered in the delay of wound healing include degree of malnutrition, patient age, pre-existing chronic illnesses, and systemic medications administered. Deficiencies of calories, proteins, vitamins (A and C), or trace metals (zinc and copper) all contribute to malnutrition of the patient.[35] Of particular concern is protein–calorie malnutrition that has been shown to contribute to reduced fibroblast proliferation, angiogenesis, and collagen synthesis. In the absence of adequate carbohydrate intake, body protein is used for energy.[63] Medications that may negatively affect wound repair include steroids, NSAIDs, and immunosuppressive agents. Steroids delay all phases of wound repair especially when taken at the time of wounding, thereby diminishing the inflammatory events and subsequent responses.[62] Additionally, decreased connective tissue strength and reduced blood flow to the wound have been associated with the use of NSAIDs.

Advanced aging has dramatic effects on wound healing. These aging effects include delayed wound contraction, decreased wound breaking strength, decreased epithelialization, attenuated metabolic response, delayed cellular migration and proliferation, decreased rate of wound capillary growth, delayed collagen remodeling, and increased rate of wound dehiscence. The state of general health is important to enhance optimal healing. Chronic debilitating illnesses, endocrine diseases, systemic vascular disorders, and various connective tissue diseases all retard wound closure. Corticosteroids, aspirin, heparin, Coumadin, penicillamine, nicotine, phenylbutazone, various NSAIDs, and antineoplastic agents all inhibit or arrest wound healing.[17] Tissues subjected to radiation therapy are at risk of breakdown and impaired healing. Ischemia induced by pressure over a bony prominence or by inadequate circulation may contribute to poor healing.

CLINICAL CONSIDERATIONS

If the more common factors complicating wound healing (e.g., infection, malnutrition, and problems indigenous to the

TABLE 2-3 LOCAL AND SYSTEMIC FACTORS IMPAIRING WOUND HEALING

FACTORS	CAUSE OF IMPAIRMENT
LOCAL FACTORS	
Surgical technique	Excessive tension
Blood supply	Atherosclerosis, venous insufficiency, tissue ischemia
Infection	Bacteria, mycobacterium, fungi, or yeast
Local medications	Topical steroids, many systemic and topical antibiotics, antineoplastic drugs, hemostatic agents (aluminum chloride)
Trauma	Foreign irritant, chronic trauma
Microenvironment	Dry dressings, photo-aged skin, radiation injury
Ulcers	Decubitus ulcers, neuropathic ulcers
SYSTEMIC FACTORS	
Nutrition	Deficiency of protein, calories, vitamins (A and C), trace metals (copper and zinc)
Age of client	Advanced (decreased immune system)
Illness	Chronic systemic illnesses, endocrine diseases (diabetes mellitus, Cushing's disease), systemic vascular disorders (periarteritis nodosa, vasculitis, granulomatosis, atherosclerosis), connective tissue disease
Systemic medications	Corticosteroids, aspirin, heparin, Coumadin, penicillamine, nicotine, phenylbutazone, other NSAIDs, antineoplastic agents

TABLE 2-4 CONDITIONS PROLONGING WOUND HEALING BY PHASES

INFLAMMATORY PHASE	PROLIFERATIVE PHASE	REMODELING PHASE
Magnitude of injury	Malnutrition (caloric, protein)	Vitamin A and C deficiency
Amount of tissue devitalization	Infection (bacteria, mycobacterium, fungi, yeast)	Mineral deficiency
Trauma (dehiscence, foreign matter)	Hypovolemia	Chronic steroid administration
Infection (bacteria, mycobacterium, fungi, yeast)	Chronic illness (diabetes mellitus, etc.)	Radiation treatment
Local topical steroids, NSAIDS	Trace metal deficiency (zinc, copper, magnesium)	
Vascular insufficiency	Chronic steroid administration, radiation treatment	

wound) are identified, the manual therapist must then explore other factors that might be contributing to the delayed healing process. Delayed wound closure and chronic wounds might involve (1) internal factors, such as those relating to the patient's general physical or mental health; (2) external factors, such as those relating to medical drug administration and treatments; or (3) iatrogenic factors, such as the way the therapist physically manages the wound. With delayed wound closure, all previous treatment regimens and modalities should be reviewed to ensure that no factor complicating the healing process has been overlooked.

REFERENCES

1. Akeson WH, Amiel D, Woo S L-Y: Immobility effects on synovial joints: The pathomechanics of joint contractures. Biorheology 17:95–110, 1980
2. Alvarez OM, et al: Wound healing. In: Fitzpatrick T, ed: Dermatology in General Medicine, 3rd ed. New York, McGraw-Hill, 1987:321–336
3. Amiel D, Akeson WH, Harwood FL, et al: Stress deprivation effect on metabolic turnover of the medial collateral ligament collagen. Clin Orthop 172:265–270, 1983
4. Arem AJ, Madden JW: Effects of stress on healing wounds: 1. Intermittent noncyclical tension. J Surg Res 20:93–102, 1976
5. Baur PS, Larson DL, Stacey TR: The observation of myofibroblasts in hypertrophic scars. Surg Gynecol Obstet 141:22–26, 1975
6. Baur PS, Parks DH: The myofibroblast anchoring strand—the fibronectin connection in wound healing and the possible loci of collagen fibril assembly. J Trauma 23:853–862, 1983
7. Bevilaquas MP, Pober JS, Wheeler ME, et al: Interleukin 1 acts on cultured human vascular endothelium to increase the adhesion of polymorphonuclear leucocytes, monocytes, and related leucocyte cell lines. J Clin Invest 76:2003–2011, 1984
8. Bryan J: Inflammation. In: Bullock BA, Henze RL, eds: Focus on Pathophysiology. Philadelphia, Lippincott Williams & Wilkins, 2000:260
9. Bryant WM: Wound Healing. Clinical Symposia. Philadelphia, CIBA 29(3), 1977
10. Cocke WM, White RR, Lynch DJ, et al: Wound Care. Ann Arbor, Books on Demand, 1986
11. Cohen S: The stimulation of epidermal proliferation by a specific protein (EGF). Dev Biol 12:394–407, 1965
12. Cotran RS, Kumar V, Collins T: Robbins Pathologic Basis of Disease, 6th ed. Philadelphia, Williams & Wilkins, 1999
13. Chen WYJ, Rogers AA, Lyndon MJ. Characterization of biologic properties of wound fluid collected during early states of wound healing. J Invest Dermatol 99(5):559–564, 1992
14. Chvapil M, et al: Local anesthetics and wound healing. J Surg Res 27:367, 1979
15. Clark RAF, et al: Fibronectin and fibrin provide a provisional matrix for epidermal cell migration during wound epithelialization. J Invest Dermatol 70:264–269, 1982
16. Corball M, et al: The interaction of vitamin A and corticosteroids on wound healing. Ir J Med Sci 154:306, 1994
17. Daly TJ: Contraction and re-epithelialization. In: Kloth LC, McCullough JM, Feedar JA, eds: Wound Healing Alternatives in Management, 2nd ed, Philadelphia, FA Davis, 1995
18. Fantone JC, Ward PA: Inflammation. In: Rubin E, Farber JL, eds: Pathology, 3rd ed. Philadelphia, Lippincott, 1999

19. Flint MH: The basis of the histological demonstration of tension in collagen. In: Longacre JJ, ed: The Ultrastructure of Collagen. Springfield, Charles C. Thomas, 1976:60–66
20. Frank C, Amiel D, Woo A L-Y, et al: Normal ligament properties and ligament healing. Clin Orthop 196:15–25, 1985
21. Forrester JC, Zederfeldt BH, Hayes TYL, et al: Tape closed and sutured wounds: A comparison by tensiometry and scanning electron microscopy. Br J Surg 57:729–737, 1970
22. Gamble JR, Harlan JM, Klebanoff SJ, et al: Stimulation of the adherence of neutrophils to umbilical vein endothelium by human recombinant tumor necrosis factor. Proc Natl Acad Sci USA 82:8667–8671, 1985
23. Garrett B, Barrett SB. Cellular communication and the action of growth factors during wound healing. J Wound Care 6(6):277–280, 1997
24. Goldstein WM, Barmada R: Early mobilization of rabbit medial collateral ligament repairs: Biologic and histologic study. Arch Phys Med Rehabil 65:239–242, 1984
25. Hardy MA: The biology of scar formation. Phys Ther 69(12):1014–1024, 1989
26. Hernandez-Jaurequi P, Esperabsa-Garcia C, Gonzales-Angulo A: Morphology of the connective tissue grown in response to implanted silicone rubber: A light and electron microscope study. Ann Plast Surg 75:631–637, 1974
27. Hinter J, et al: Expression of basement membrane zone antigens at the dermo-epibolic function in organ culture of human skin. J Invest Dermatol 74:200–205, 1980
28. Hooley CJ, Cohen RE: A model for the creep behavior of tendon. Int J Biol Macromol 1:123–132, 1979, and personal communication, 1981
29. Houck JC, Jacob RA: The chemistry of local dermal inflammation. J Invest Dermatol 36:451–456, 1961
30. Hunt TK, Banda MJ, Silver IA: Cell interactions in post-traumatic fibrosis. In: Fibrosis. Pitman, London (Ciba Foundation Symposium 114) 1985:128–149
31. Hunt TK, Van Winkle W: Wound Healing: Normal Repair–Fundamentals of Wound Management in Surgery. South Plainfield, Chirurgecom, 1976
32. Irwin TT: Wound Healing: Principles and Practice. London, Chapman & Hall, 1981:34.
33. Kariniemi A-L, et al: Cytoskeleton and pericellular matrix organization of pure adult human keratinocytes cultured from suction-blister roof epidermis. J Cell Sci 58:49–61, 1982
34. Kirscher CW, Speer DP: Microvascular changes in Dupuytren's contracture. J Hand Surg 9A:58–62, 1984
35. Kirsner RS, Bogensberger G: The normal healing process. In: Kloth LC, McCulloch JM, eds: Wound Healing Alternatives in Management, 3rd ed. Philadelphia, FA Davis, 2002
36. Kubo M, et al: Human keratinocytes synthesize, secrete, and deposit fibronectin in the pericellular matrix. J Invest Dermatol 82:580–586, 1984
37. Kumar V, Cotran RS, Robbins SL: Acute and chronic inflammation. In: Basic Pathology, 5th ed. Philadelphia, WB Saunders, 1992a:25–46
38. Kumar V, Cotran RS, Robbins SL: Wound healing: Repair, cell growth, regeneration, and wound healing. In: Basic Pathology, 5th ed. Philadelphia, WB Saunders, 1992b:47–60
39. Levenson SM, Grever EF, Crowley LV, et al: The healing of rat skin wounds. Ann Surg 161:293–308, 1965
40. Leyden JJ: Effect of bacteria on healing of superficial wounds. Clin Dermatol 2:81, 1984
41. Madden JW, DeVore G, Arem AJ: A rational postoperative management program for metacarpophalangeal joint implant arthroplasty. J Hand Surg 2:358–366, 1977
42. Madden JW, Peacock EE: Studies on the biology of collagen during wound healing: III. Dynamic metabolism of scar collagen and remodeling of dermal wounds. Ann Surg 174:511–520, 1971
43. Majno G, et al: Contraction of granulation tissue in vitro: Similarity to smooth muscle. Science 173:548–550, 1971

44. Marks JG, et al: Inhibition of wound healing by topical steroids. J Dermatol Surg Oncol 9:819, 1983

45. McMinn RMH: Tissue Repair. New York, Academic Press, 1989

46. Morgan CJ, Pledger WJ: Fibroblast proliferation. In: Cohen et al., eds: Wound Healing. Philadelphia, WB Saunders, 1992:63–75

47. Murray JC, Pollack SV, Pinnell SR: Keloids: A review. J Am Acad Dermatol 4:461–470, 1981

48. Odland G, Ross R: Human wound repair. I. Epidermal regeneration. J Cell Biol 39:135–151, 1968

49. Peacock EE, Van Winkle W: Structure, synthesis, and interaction of fibrous protein and matrix. In: Peacock EE, Van Winkle W, eds: Wound Repair. Philadelphia, WB Saunders, 1976:145–203

50. Pohlman TH, Stanness KA, Beatty PG, et al: An endothelial cell surface factor-s induced in vitro by lipopolysaccharide, interleukin 1, and tumor necrosis factor-alpha increases neutrophil adherence by a CDalpha18-dependent mechanism. J Immunol 136:4548–4553, 1986

51. Repesh LA, Fitzgerald TJ, Furcht LT: Fibronectin involvement in granulation tissue and wound healing in rabbits. J Histochem Cytochem 30:351–358, 1982

52. Rudolph R: Contraction and the control of contraction. World J Surg 4:279–287, 1980

53. Rudolph R, Van de Berg J, Ehrlich HP: Wound contraction and scar contracture. In: Cohen IK, et al., eds: Wound Healing. Philadelphia, WB Saunders, 1992:96–114

54. Ryan G, Majno G: Inflammation. Kalamazoo, Upjohn Company, 1977

55. Schliemer RP, Rutledge BK: Cultured human vascular endothelial cell surface acquires adhesiveness for neutrophils after stimulation with interleukin 1, endotoxin, and tumor-promoting phorbol diesters. J Immunol 136:649–654, 1986

56. Scully TJ, Besterman G: Stress fracture—A preventable training injury. Mil Med 147:285–287, 1982

57. Slack C, Flint MH, Thompson BM: The effect of tensional load on isolated embryonic chick tendons in organ culture. Connect Tissue Res 12:229–274, 1984

58. Slavin J. The role of cytokines in wound healing. J Pathol 178:5–10, 1996

59. Stacy RJ, Hungerford RL: A method to reduce work-related injuries during basic recruit training in the New Zealand army. Mil Med 149:318–320, 1984

60. Stanley JR, et al: Detection of basement membrane antigens during epidermal wound healing in pigs. J Invest Dermatol 77:240, 1981

61. Stenn KS, Madri JA, Roll FJ: Migrating epidermis produces AB2 collagen and requires continued collagen synthesis for movement. Nature 277:229–232, 1979

62. Stotts NA, Wipke-Tevis DD: Cofactors in impaired wound healing. In: Krasner DL, Sibbald RG, eds: Chronic Wound Care: A Clinical Source Book for Healthcare Professionals, 3rd ed. Wayne PA, HMP Communications 2001:271

63. Sussman C: Wound healing biology and chronic wound healing. In: Sussman C, Bates-Jensen BM, eds: Wound Care: A Collaborative Practice Manual for Physical Therapists and Nurses. Aspen Publishers, 1998:42

64. Tillman LJ, Cummings GS: Biological mechanisms of connective tissue mutability. In: Currier DP, Nelson RM, eds: Dynamics of Human Biologic Tissues, vol. 8. Philadelphia, FA Davis, 1992:1–44

65. Tortora GF, Funke BR, Case CL: Microbiology: An Introduction. Menlo Park, Addison Wesley Longman, 1998

66. Wahl LM, Wahl SM: Inflammation. In: Cohen et al., eds: Wound Healing. Philadelphia, WB Saunders, 1992:40–62

67. Werb A, Gordon S: Secretion of a specific collagenase by stimulated macrophages. J Exp Med 142:346–360, 1975

68. Winter GD: Formation of the scab and the rate of epithelialization of superficial wounds in the skin of the young, domestic pig. Nature 193:293, 1962

69. Wyke B: The neurology of joints. Ann R Coll Surg Engl 41:25, 1967

70. Yannas IV, Huang C: Fracture of tendon collagen. J Polymer Sci 10:577–584, 1972

Arthrology

DARLENE HERTLING AND RANDOLPH M. KESSLER

3

A complete study of human joints includes synchondroses, syndesmoses, symphyses, gomphoses, sutures, and synovial joints. Each of these classifications includes joints capable of movement. Movement definitely takes place at most syndesmoses, such as the distal tibiofibular joint. The symphysis pubis moves, especially during pregnancy. There is some movement of the teeth in their sockets (gomphoses). In fact, even the sutures of the skull are movable, at least through the third decade of life, and some investigators have claimed that they move spontaneously, with a rhythm independent of heart rate or respiratory rate.[20] Based on this claim, a few practitioners actually apply therapeutic mobilization to the sutures of the cranium.[20,44] However, for the sake of simplicity, and because the emphasis of clinical application is on joint mobilization techniques, the discussion in this chapter is restricted to the synovial joints, which are the most numerous and most freely movable of the various types of human joints.

The mutual influences of structure and function are emphasized because the two cannot be dealt with adequately or understood when considered independently. The traditional anatomic concept of synovial joints must be expanded to a physiologic concept; in addition to those structures that anatomically define a joint, those structures responsible for normal movement at the joint must also be included (Fig. 3-1). With this approach the synovial joint is considered the basic unit of the musculoskeletal system and used as a reference for discussing normal function and disorders of this system.

KINEMATICS

Classification of Joint Surfaces and Movements

The nature of movement at any joint is largely determined by the joint structure, especially the shapes of the joint surfaces. The traditional classification of synovial joints by structure includes the categories of spheroid, trochoid, condyloid, ginglymoid, ellipsoid, and planar joints.[58] It should be apparent even to someone with only a basic knowledge of human anatomy and kinesiology that this classification does not accurately define the shapes of joint surfaces or the movements that occur at each type of joint. The heads of the femur and humerus do not form true spheres or even parts of true spheres. A ginglymus, such as the humeroulnar joint, does not allow a true hinge motion on flexion and extension but rather a helical movement involving considerable rotation. The humeroradial joint, which is a trochoid joint, does not move about a single axis, or pivot, because the head of the radius is oval, having a longer diameter anteroposteriorly than mediolaterally. The interphalangeal joints, the carpometacarpal joint of the thumb, the humeroulnar joint, and the calcaneocuboid joints can be considered as sellar. However, the movements occurring at these joints vary greatly, as do the shapes of the joint surfaces. Therefore, although this classification of joint structure may serve a purpose for the anatomist, in itself it is not adequate for the clinician, such as the physical therapist, who must be concerned with the finer details of joint mechanics.

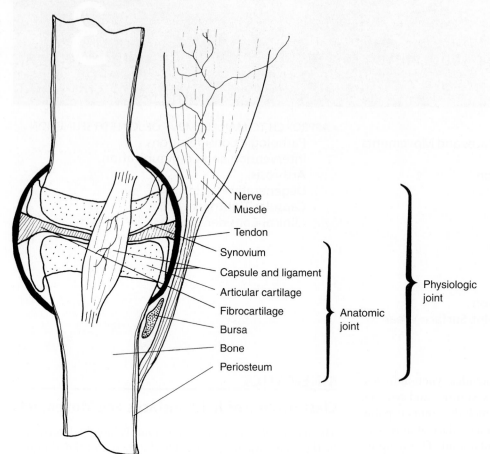

Nerve
Muscle
Tendon
Synovium
Capsule and ligament
Articular cartilage
Fibrocartilage
Bursa
Bone
Periosteum

Anatomic joint

Physiologic joint

▪ **FIG. 3-1.** Anatomic versus physiologic concept of the synovial joint.

A similar problem exists with classifying joint movement. The traditional classification of joint movement includes the following[58]:

Angular—Indicating an increase or decrease in the angle formed between two bones (e.g., flexion-extension at the elbow)

Circumduction—Movement of a bone circumscribing a cone (e.g., circumduction at the hip or shoulder)

Rotation—Movement occurring about the longitudinal axis of a bone (e.g., internal–external rotation at the shoulder)

Sliding—One bone slides over another with little or no appreciable rotation or angular movement (e.g., movement between carpals)

There are two problems with this classification system that make it inadequate for those clinicians concerned with joint mechanics. First, it describes movement occurring between bones but ignores movement occurring between joint surfaces. When movement is defined, what happens *at the joint* is often ignored. An analogy is to consider the movement of a door but to ignore the hinge. Second, angular movements almost never occur without some rotation; rotation nearly

always occurs with some angular movement; gliding usually involves angular and rotary movement, and so on. Again, the classification needs to be expanded to take into consideration the specifics of joint movement.

Movements occurring between bones must be defined in such a way that they can easily be related to movements occurring between respective joint surfaces. Therefore, it is helpful to define the **mechanical axis** of any joint as a line that passes through the moving bone, touching the center of the relatively stationary joint surface and lying perpendicular to it (Fig. 3-2). **Osteokinematic** movement (movement occurring between two bones) can now be defined according to the mechanical axis rather than according to the long axis of the moving bone, as has been done in the past.[30,58] By relating osteokinematic movement to **arthrokinematic** movement (movement occurring between joint surfaces), the movement of the mechanical axis of the moving bone relative to the stationary joint surface can be considered. In other words, one joint surface can be considered as stationary and its opposing joint surface as moving relative to it. This relative movement is defined according to the path traced by the line representing the mechanical axis of the joint on the stationary surface. The mechanical axis is determined at the starting point of a movement; once movement has begun, it maintains the same relationship to the moving bone while moving relative to the stationary bone.

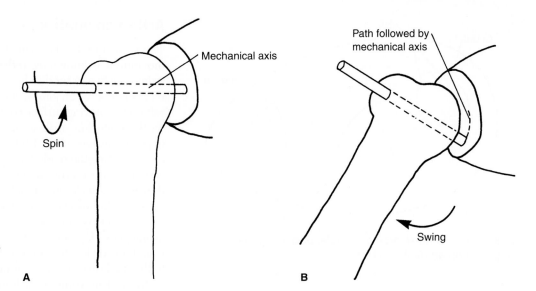

■ **FIG. 3-2.** Osteokinematic movements may be defined by the mechanical axis. These movements are **(A)** spin and **(B)** swing.

JOINT SURFACES

Before discussing types of movement, it is necessary to define the shapes of joint surfaces because they largely determine the types of movements that may occur at the joint. No joint surface resembles a true geometric form; joint surfaces are neither spheres, ovals, or ellipses, nor are they true parts of these. However, any joint surface can be thought of as being part of an ovoid surface, that is, resembling the surface of an egg (Fig. 3-3A). If a cross-section of an ovoid surface is examined, it is clear that the radius of the joint surface changes constantly, forming a cardioid curve (Fig. 3-4). A typical example is a sagittal section of a femoral condyle. Some joint surfaces, rather than representing part of a simple ovoid, might be considered a complex ovoid, or sellar, surface (Fig. 3-3B). A sellar surface is convex in one cross-sectional plane and concave in the plane perpendicular to it, although the surfaces of each of these cross-sections may be represented by a cardioid curve.

Referring again to a simple ovoid (Fig. 3-5), the shortest distance between any two points on the surface is termed a **chord,** and any other line of continuous concavity toward the chord is an **arc.** A three-sided figure made up of three chords is a **triangle.** A three-sided figure in which at least one side is formed by an arc is a **trigone.**

JOINT MOVEMENTS

Any movement in which the bone moves but the mechanical axis remains stationary is termed a **spin** (Fig. 3-2A). True spin of the humerus, then, would be a movement of flexion combined with some abduction, because the glenoid cavity faces slightly forward. The bone, during true spin, rotates about its mechanical axis. When the mechanical axis of the joint and the long axis of the moving bone coincide, such as at the metacarpophalangeal and the femorotibial joints, the spin is what is traditionally termed **rotation** at the joint. Where axes do not necessarily coincide, such as at the hip and shoulder, spin does not always occur when the joint "rotates." For example, spin occurs during internal and external rotation at the shoulder when the humerus is in 90° of abduction; the mechanical axis (defined according to the starting position of movement) coincides with the long axis of the humerus. However, internal and external rotations, performed with the

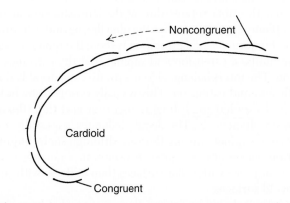

■ **FIG. 3-4.** A cardioid curve is representative of the cross-sectional shape of synovial joint surfaces. Because of the constantly changing radius, there is one position at which the radius of the opposing joint surface attains maximal congruency.

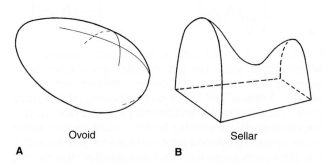

■ **FIG. 3-3.** Joint surfaces may be **(A)** ovoid or **(B)** sellar.

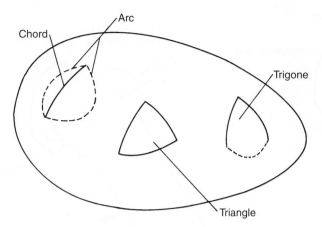

■ **FIG. 3-5.** Chord, arcs, a triangle, and a trigone are depicted on an ovoid surface.

arm to the side, do not involve spin at the joint surfaces; in this position, the mechanical axis does not coincide with the long axis of the humerus. A movement in which the mechanical axis follows the path of a chord is termed a **chordate,** or **pure,** swing. If the end of the mechanical axis traced the path of an arc during movement of the bone, the bone has undergone an **arcuate,** or **impure,** swing (Fig. 3-2*B*).

With flexion or abduction of the humerus, the movement is an impure swing. Pure swing of the humerus occurs during elevation in a plane somewhat midway between the planes of flexion and abduction (because the glenoid cavity faces approximately 40° forward). Also, internal and external rotation with the arm at the side is a movement of swing. An impure swing can be thought of as a pure swing with an element of spin, or rotation, about the mechanical axis. This element of rotation, which accompanies every impure swing, is termed **conjunct** rotation. Habitual movements at any joint are usually impure swings. It follows that most habitual movements, or those movements that occur most frequently at any joint, involve some conjunct rotation. It is well known, for example, that the tibia rotates during flexion-extension at the knee. If one carefully watches the ulna flexing and extending on the humerus, a similar rotation is seen; the ulna pronates at the limits of extension and supinates at the extremes of flexion. The interphalangeal joints rotate considerably during flexion and extension. This is easily observed by holding the extended small fingers together and then flexing them simultaneously. The distal phalanges, especially, can be seen to supinate during flexion. Although such conjunct rotation occurs at every joint, it occurs to a much greater degree at joints with sellar surfaces than at those with simple ovoid surfaces.

By now it should be evident that most of what have been traditionally considered "angular" movements are actually helical movements because of this element of conjunct rotation that accompanies them. This rotary component is an essential feature of normal joint mechanics.

Arthrokinematics

The study of what happens between joint surfaces on joint movement is known as **arthrokinematics.** When a bone swings relative to another bone, one of two types of movement may occur between joint surfaces.[30,58] If points at certain intervals on the moving surface contact points at the same intervals on the opposing surface, one surface is said to **roll** on the opposing surface (Fig. 3-6*A*). This is analogous to a tire on a car contacting the road surface as the car rolls down the street; various points on the tire contact various points on the road, the distance between contact points on the tire and road being the same. If, however, only one point on the moving joint surface contacts various points on the opposing surface, **slide** is taking place (Fig. 3-6*B*). This is analogous to a tire on a car that is skidding on ice; the tire is not turning but is moving relative to the road surface—it is sliding.

In most movements at human synovial joints, both slide and roll take place simultaneously. If only roll took place, the moving bone would tend to dislocate before much movement could occur; if only slide occurred, impingement of joint surfaces would prevent full movement (Fig. 3-7). Stated in another way, the moving bone must rotate about a particular center of motion (or centers of motion) for normal gliding to occur at the joint surfaces. If the bone should move about any other centroid of movement than what is normal for that joint,

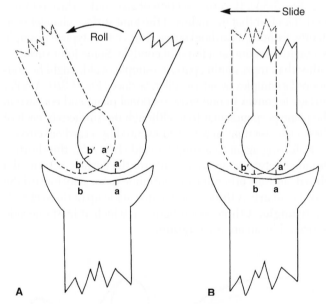

■ **FIG. 3-6.** Arthrokinematic movements showing **(A)** roll and **(B)** slide. The letters indicate points on the opposing joint surfaces that come in contact with one another. Points *a'* and *b'* are on the moving joint surface; points *a* and *b* are on the stationary joint surface. Note that during roll (A), points *a* and *b* contact various points on the opposing moving joint surface and that during slide (B), points *a* and *b* contact one point on the moving surface.

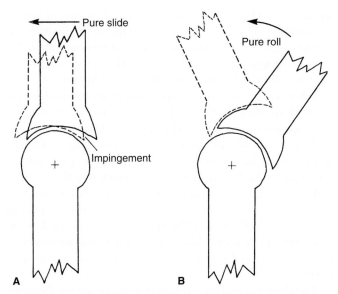

■ **FIG. 3-7.** Joint movements occurring in the absence of normal arthrokinematic movement cause (**A**) impingement or (**B**) dislocation.

abnormal movement will occur between joint surfaces. Conversely, if normal movement does not or cannot occur between joint surfaces, the moving bone cannot move about its normal centroid of movement. This will be discussed later, in the section on analysis of accessory joint motions. Clinically, a meniscus tear, which causes abnormal movement between joint surfaces, alters the normal centroid of movement at a joint.[15] This often results in abnormal stresses to the joint capsule, which are manifested as pain and muscle guarding. A tight joint capsule, which causes alteration in the normal centroid of movement, results in abnormal movement between joint surfaces, usually with premature cartilaginous compression before the movement is completed. Physiologically, the fact that slide and roll take place together allows for economy of

articular cartilage with respect to the size of the joint surface necessary for movement. It also prevents undue wearing of isolated points on joint surfaces, which would occur if, for example, only slide took place.

CONCAVE–CONVEX RULE

Obviously, roll always occurs in the same direction as the swing of the bone. However, the direction of joint slide can be determined only if the shapes of the joint surfaces are known. This is an important rule for anyone concerned with joint mechanics to know and will be referred to as the **concave–convex rule.** This rule states that if a concave surface moves on a convex surface, roll and slide must occur in the same direction; if a convex surface moves on a concave surface, roll and slide occur in opposite directions (Fig. 3-8). Therefore, if the tibia extends on the stationary femur, the tibia joint surfaces must roll forward and slide forward on the femoral condyles for full movement to take place. However, if the femur extends on the stationary tibia, the femoral condyles must roll forward but slide backward on the tibia. If the humerus is elevated, the humeral head rolls upward but must slide inferiorly. During external rotation, with the arm at the side (a movement of swing), the head of the humerus must slide forward, whereas during internal rotation it must slide backward.

Clinicians must apply these concepts in the approach to restoration of restricted joint motion. Traditionally, in attempts to restore joint movement clinicians have tended to work only on osteokinematic movements. For example, if flexion of the humerus is restricted, active or passive motion into flexion is used in an attempt to increase this movement. However, one must also consider that inferior slide of the head of the humerus on the glenoid cavity may be restricted as well. The manual therapist may use passive joint mobilization techniques to restore inferior slide to facilitate the restoration of upward swing of the humerus. Thus, by knowing the concave–convex rule, the therapist knows in which direction to apply joint slide mobilizations to increase any restricted swing of a bone.

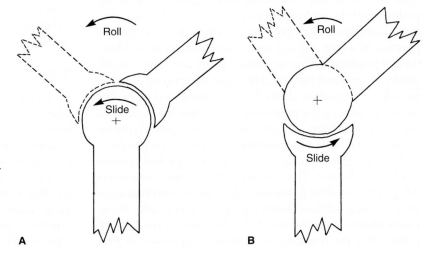

■ **FIG. 3-8.** Relationship between arthrokinematic movements and osteokinematic movements for the "concave–convex rule." (**A**) Concave surface moving on a convex surface. (**B**) Convex surface moving on a concave surface.

The type of joint surface motion that occurs with a spin of a bone about its mechanical axis is actually a form of slide. However, it should be apparent that while slide occurs in one direction at one half of the joint, it occurs in the opposite direction at the other half of the joint surface. This type of slide is referred to as **spin,** as is the osteokinematic movement it accompanies.

Biomechanical analysis demonstrates situations in which the concave–convex rule cannot be applied. These situations include movements at plane joints, movements for which the axis of rotation passes through the articulating surfaces, and movements at joints in which the concave side of the joint forms a deep socket.[28] Joints whose motions are largely dictated by the musculature and tension in the capsule (i.e., joints that are not track-bound), such as the glenohumeral joint, may be controlled more by the tension in the capsular tissue and musculature than by joint geometry.[22,23,36,46] However, the concave–convex rule is an excellent teaching tool for use with beginning students of manual therapy. This qualitative biomechanical analysis provides a methodical context from which to explain the application of the rule.[28]

CLOSE-PACKED POSITION

Separation of joint surfaces is termed **distraction;** approximation of opposing surfaces is **compression.** Whereas some bone movements are accompanied by a relative compression of joint surfaces, other movements involve distraction. By knowing the **close-packed position** of a joint, one can determine which movements involve compression and which involve distraction.

As mentioned, ovoid surfaces are irregular, in that in any one cross-sectional plane the ovoid surface is of constantly changing radius, defining a cardioid curve. If one imagines an opposing joint surface moving along this curve, it is clear that in most positions the two surfaces do not fit, or are noncongruent. However, one position exists in which the joint surfaces become relatively congruent because their contacting radii are approximately the same (Fig. 3-4). Thus, although synovial joint surfaces tend to be noncongruent, at least one position exists for each joint in which the surfaces become maximally congruent. This position is termed the close-packed position of a joint. At any joint, movement into the close-packed position involves an impure swing and so necessarily involves a conjunct rotation. The rotary component of movement into this position causes the joint capsule and major ligaments supporting the joint to twist, which in turn causes an approximation of joint surfaces. Once the close-packed position is reached, no further movement in that direction is possible.

Therefore, movement toward the close-packed position involves an element of compression, whereas movement out of this position involves distraction. MacConnaill and Basmajian point out that habitual movements at any joint involve movements directed into and out of the close-packed position.[30] It is likely that the resultant intermittent compression of joint surfaces has a bearing on nutrition and lubrication of articular cartilage. The squeezing out of synovial fluid with each compression phase facilitates exchange of nutrients and helps to maintain a lubricant film between surfaces (see sections on joint nutrition and lubrication later in this chapter).

Interestingly, moving the upper extremity in a reciprocating pattern, such that every joint is first moved simultaneously toward its close-packed position and then directly out of the close-packed position, resembles one of the basic patterns used by Knott and Voss in their proprioceptive neuromuscular facilitation techniques.[27] Considering the twisting and untwisting of the capsules and ligaments that occurs, and considering what is known of joint neurology with respect to joint-muscle reflexes (see the section on neurology later in this chapter), it seems likely that the facilitatory effect of the pattern may be related to joint position and muscle position.

The close-packed position also has important implications with respect to the pathomechanics of many injuries. For instance, many upper extremity injuries occur from falling on the outstretched hand; Colles' fracture at the wrist, supracondylar elbow fractures, posterior dislocation of the elbow, and anterior dislocation of the shoulder are but a few. This is not surprising if one realizes that falling on the outstretched hand, in such a way that the body rolls away from the arm on impact, throws every major upper extremity joint (except the metacarpophalangeal and acromioclavicular joints) into close-packing. As mentioned, once the close-packed position is reached, the joint becomes locked and no further movement is possible in that direction. If further force is added, a joint must dislocate, a bone must give, or both. The weak link tends to be determined by age; the child is likely to fracture the humerus above the elbow, the adolescent or teenager may dislocate the shoulder, and the middle-aged or elderly person invariably sustains a Colles' fracture. In general, most fractures and dislocations occur when a joint is in the close-packed position. Most capsular or ligamentous sprains occur when the joint is in a loose-packed position. This is simply because the tight fit of the adjoining bones in the close-packed position causes forces applied to the joint to be taken up by the bones rather than by the supporting structures; there is more "intrinsic stability" at the joint.

JOINT PLAY

In a loose-packed position, or in any position of the joint other than the close-packed position, the joint surfaces are incongruent. An obvious example is the knee joint in some position of flexion, although the menisci help to make up for the significant incongruence. In the loose-packed position, the capsule and major supporting ligaments remain relatively lax. This must be so in order to allow a normal range of movement. Thus, in most joint positions a joint has some "play" in it because joint surfaces do not fit tightly and because the capsule and ligaments remain somewhat lax.

This joint play is essential for normal joint function. First, the small spaces that exist because of joint incongruence are necessary to the hydrodynamic component of joint lubrication (see discussion later in this chapter). Second, because the joint surfaces are of varying radii, movement cannot occur around a rigid axis, and so the joint capsule must allow some play for full movement to occur. Related to this is the fact that if normal joint distraction (one form of joint play) is lost, then joint surfaces will become prematurely approximated when moving toward the close-packed position, and movement in this direction will therefore be restricted. Human synovial joints cannot be compared to a door hinge, except in a limited sense, because a door moves about a single axis at its hinge and requires little or no play. Third, most joint movements are helical, involving movement about more than one axis simultaneously. For this type of movement to occur, a certain amount of joint play must exist, unless the movement is track-bound, which is usually not the case. One may therefore presume that loss of joint play from some pathology, such as a tight joint capsule, will lead to alteration in joint function, usually involving restriction of motion or pain, or both. Mennell[41] uses the term **joint dysfunction** for loss of joint play. This term is useful in a general discussion of joint mechanics but in clinical use should be avoided in favor of terms that more precisely identify the responsible pathology, because there are many possible causes of loss of joint play.

CONJUNCT ROTATION

Conjunct rotation is the component of spin or rotation that accompanies any impure swing of a bone (Fig. 3-9). It is easily observed when the tibia extends on the femur, the distal phalanges of the fingers flex when held together, or the ulna flexes and extends on the humerus; such movements are helical. This rotation causes the joint capsule to twist when moving toward the close-packed position. At the shoulder, where a particularly large range of movement is possible, some rotation opposite the direction of normal conjunct rotation must occur at the later stages of movement. Thus, pure abduction in the frontal plane involves an impure swing with a medial conjunct rotation at the early phase, the first 90 to 120° of movement. This is because the glenoid cavity faces somewhat forward and the humerus on abduction swings out of the plane of the scapula. If this impure swing were left to continue, at full elevation the joint capsule would be completely twisted on itself. This, however, is impossible, because the twisting of the joint capsule would cause a premature approximation of joint surfaces before full elevation could be attained. To prevent this premature locking of the joint on abduction, the humerus must rotate laterally on its long axis during the final phase of movement, bringing the humeral head back toward the plane of the scapula. Similarly, sagittal flexion involves a lateral conjunct rotation but a medial longitudinal rotation during the final phase. This is best appreciated by observing it on a skeleton, noting the end position of the humerus on abduction or

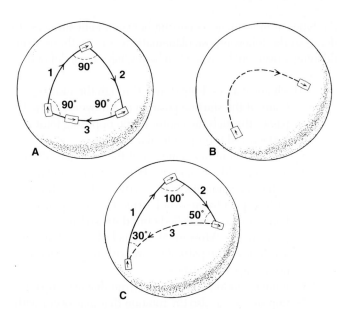

■ **FIG. 3-9.** Conjunct rotation occurring **(A)** with a succession of pure swings with return to the starting position (diadochokinetic movement), **(B)** with a single impure swing, and **(C)** with a completed cycle of pure and impure swings (also a diadochokinetic movement).

flexion without rotation and comparing it with elevation in the plane of the scapula, that is, about midway between flexion and abduction.

In addition to accompanying any impure swing, conjunct rotation may occur with a succession of swings, even if each of the swings is a pure swing. In a triangle drawn on a curved surface, such as an ovoid surface, the sum of the interior angles of the triangle may exceed 180° if the surface is convex, or the sum may be less than 180° if the surface is concave. During a succession of movements, in which the mechanical axis follows the path of a triangle or trigone, the amount of conjunct rotation that accompanies the completed cycle will be equal to the difference between the sum of the interior angles of the triangle or trigone and 180° (Fig. 3-9). This type of conjunct rotation can be visualized by moving the humerus through a succession of movements: starting with the arm at the side, elbow bent, fingers facing forward, flex the humerus 90°, abduct 90° horizontally, and then adduct 90°. The fingers are now directed laterally, indicating that the humerus, during this succession of movements, rotated outward 90°. The succession may only be carried out once or twice without derotating the humerus medially because of the twisting of the capsule that results from the lateral conjunct rotation.

Summary of Joint Function

The terminology of joint function has been expanded to accommodate the more specific features of joint kinematics, including the relationships between joint structure and function and the types of movements occurring between joint surfaces. In doing so the following osteokinematic terms, or those terms defining movement between two bones, have been defined:

Mechanical axis—Line drawn through the moving bone, at the starting position of a movement, that passes through the center of the opposing joint surface and is perpendicular to it

Spin–Movement of a bone about the mechanical axis

Pure swing—Movement of a bone in which an end of the mechanical axis traces the path of a chord with respect to the ovoid formed by the opposing joint surface; also called **chordate swing**

Impure swing—Movement in which the mechanical axis follows the path of an arc with respect to the opposing ovoid surface

Conjunct rotation—Element of spin that accompanies impure swing; also the rotation that may occur with a succession of swings

The following arthrokinematic terms, or those that define the types of movement occurring between joint surfaces, have also been defined:

Roll—Movement in which points at intervals on the moving joint surface contact points at the same intervals on the opposing surface

Slide—Movement in which a single contact point on the moving surface contacts various points on the opposing surface

Spin—Type of slide that accompanies spin of a bone; one half of the joint surface slides in one direction while the other half slides in the opposite direction (i.e., the moving joint surface rotates about some point on the opposing joint surface)

Distraction—Separation of joint surfaces

Compression—Approximation of joint surfaces; always occurs when moving toward the close-packed position

The close-packed position was defined for a joint in which the following three conditions exist:

1. The joint surfaces become maximally congruent.
2. The joint capsule and major ligaments become twisted, causing joint surfaces to approximate.
3. The joint becomes locked so that no further movement is possible in that direction.

Clinical Applications

TERMINOLOGY

A rationale for the approach to management of joint dysfunction, including the use of specific joint mobilization tech-

niques, can now be discussed based on the previous analysis of joint movement. However, some additional terms must first be presented. Unfortunately, a jargon has evolved relating to the clinical application of those concepts and is often the source of confusion because the terms are used inconsistently. Therefore, the most common and useful definitions of important terms are presented.

Accessory joint movements are simply those arthrokinematic movements that must occur for normal osteokinematic movement to take place. These include slides, rolls, distractions, compressions, or conjunct rotations. Consider the osteokinematic movement of the humerus moving from the resting position with the arm at the side to the close-packed position. The joint is convex-on-concave. The head of the humerus must roll in the same direction in which the bone swings. It must slide opposite this direction or somewhat inferiorly and inward. Because the close-packed position is being approached, the joint surfaces are becoming approximated. It is a movement of impure swing, so a conjunct rotation (in this case a lateral rotation) must occur. If any one of these accessory movements does not or cannot occur, then this particular swing of the humerus cannot be performed painlessly or harmlessly through the full range. If full osteokinematic movement does occur, it does so at the expense of the capsule or ligaments, which must be abnormally stretched, or of the articular cartilage, which must be abnormally compressed.

The term **component motions** can be used synonymously with **accessory movements.** For example, lateral rotation of the tibia is referred to as a component of knee extension. Likewise, spreading of the distal tibia and fibula is a component of dorsiflexion at the ankle. The clinician must be aware of the component motions necessary for each osteokinematic movement at a joint. Many of these are listed in Appendix.

Joint-play movements are those accessory movements that can be produced passively at a joint but cannot be isolated actively. They include distractions, compressions, slides, rolls, or spins at a joint in a particular position. Joint-play movements are used when applying specific mobilization techniques to restore accessory movements so that full and painless osteokinematic movement may be restored. For example, inferior glide occurs at the shoulder during active elevation. It can be performed passively, but in itself cannot be performed actively by voluntary muscle contraction; inferior glide is a joint-play movement at the glenohumeral joint.

Joint mobilization is a very general term that may be applied to any active or passive attempt to increase movement at a joint. In addition to traditional methods of increasing joint movement, such as active, passive, and active-assisted range-of-motion techniques, joint mobilization includes specific passive mobilization techniques. These techniques are aimed at restoring those component movements that permit pain-free or harmless osteokinematic movement. They are used especially to restore those joint-play movements that cannot be isolated actively.

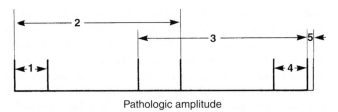

■ FIG. 3-10. Grades of joint-play movement.

Specific passive mobilization techniques are graded (Fig. 3-10). Grades 1 through 4 are often referred to as **articulation** techniques, which are passive rhythmic oscillations. Grade 5 is a **manipulation** technique that is a high-velocity, low-amplitude, passive thrust. These grades are relative to the pathologic amplitude of joint-play movement that exists at the joint and not to the normal amplitude that should exist. There are two main criteria for the selection of the particular grade to be used: (1) the degree of pain or protective muscle spasm during passive joint-play movement (irritability) and (2) the degree of restriction of joint-play movement. The greater the irritability, the lower the numeric grade of movement used. Pain and spasm must be avoided. Manipulation is used primarily when a very slight, minimally painful restriction exists. A third criterion of selection might apply here, namely the skill and experience of the operator, because manipulative maneuvers should only be attempted after articulation techniques have been mastered and after much practice. The terms of joint movement are shown in Figure 3-11.

Specific accessory joint motions that are limited may be restored by manual oscillations or thrusts. The primary goal of using specific joint mobilization techniques is restoration of normal, pain-free use of the joint. The emphasis is not on forcing a particular anatomic (osteokinematic) movement at a joint, as has been done in the past with traditional methods of mobilization; rather, it is on restoring normal joint mechanics to allow full, pain-free osteokinematic movement to occur. In this way, range of motion is restored to the joint with less risk of damaging the joint by compressing isolated portions of articular cartilage, and with less pain and muscle guarding from overstretching isolated capsuloligamentous structures, as may well occur if an osteokinematic movement is forced in the absence of necessary component movements. This is to say that specific passive mobilization, correctly applied, is a safer, more efficient, and less painful method of increasing range of motion at a joint. Mennell,[41] in his lectures, often uses the analogy of a door having lost movement because of a faulty hinge. Efforts to restore motion by pushing hard on the door are likely to result in further damage to the hinge. The logical method to remedy the situation is to direct one's attention to the hinge—to restore normal mechanics to the hinge, thereby restoring normal movement of the door.[41]

This discussion ignores the physiologic concept of the joint. This is done solely for the sake of simplicity. Obviously, when restoring normal joint mechanics is considered, attention must be given to the anatomic joint along with those structures responsible for active movement of the joint. For example, active abduction at the shoulder is often lost because of the absence of inferior glide. Relative to the anatomic joint, the joint-play movement of inferior glide may be limited. However, the problem may also be physiologic, in that inferior glide may not be occurring owing to weakness of the supraspinatus muscle. These are very different problems leading to similar results. The nature of the problem must be brought out by a thorough evaluation.

ANALYSIS OF ACCESSORY MOTIONS

Clinical Assessment. Many of the means of determining which accessory movements are components of specific osteokinematic movements have already been discussed. For instance, the direction of roll is always the same as that for the swing of the bone. If a convex surface moves on a concave surface, slide will occur in the direction opposite to the roll; if a concave surface moves on a convex surface, slide occurs in the same direction as the roll. Distraction occurs when moving out of the close-packed position; compression occurs when moving into the close-packed position. These components can all be determined for any joint moving in any direction. Some of the other component motions, as listed for each joint in the Appendix, must be memorized or deduced anatomically.

One way of assessing the state of a particular accessory movement (its amplitude and irritability) is clinically, by evaluating the joint-play movements. These examination maneuvers are essentially the same as the specific mobilization techniques. Rather than being performed as a graded, therapeutic technique, they are used to determine the amplitude of a joint-play movement and whether the movement causes pain or spasm. The amplitude of movement and possible restriction must be compared with the operator's concept of "normal" for that movement, at that joint, for that body type. This requires experience in evaluating normal as well as pathologic joints. Whenever possible, the pathologic joint must be compared with a healthy contralateral joint. The degree of irritability is determined by the patient's subjective response and by the presence of protective muscle spasm when performing the examination movement. (Refer to regional chapters for the joint-play techniques in Parts II and III.) Proficiency in clinically evaluating joint-play movements and correlating findings

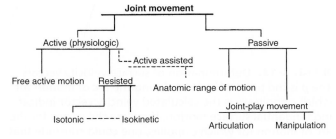

■ FIG. 3-11. Terms related to joint movement.

to knowledge of accessory movements at the joint, as well as other symptoms and signs presenting on examination, is essential to the effective application of joint mobilization techniques and management of musculoskeletal disorders.

Instant Center Analysis. The more scientific method of analyzing arthrokinematic movement has been described by Sammarco and coworkers.[51] This involves a determination of the centroid of movement, or instant center of movement, at various points throughout a joint movement. For any joint, the axis about which motion takes place changes constantly during a particular movement. This is because joint surfaces are irregular. The instant centers of motion can be plotted for a movement through the use of careful roentgenographic studies of a joint that record the relative position of the bones at various points throughout the movement. This is done by choosing two reference points on the moving bone; in Figure 3-12 the points lie on the central axis of the bone,

point *a* on the joint surface, point *b* 7 cm up on the shaft of the bone. A second roentgenogram taken after the bone has moved is superimposed over the original. In the new position, points *a'* and *b'* are determined along the central axis; *a'* is on the joint surface, *b'* is 7 cm up on the shaft. Now lines *aa'* and *bb'* are constructed, and perpendicular bisectors for each of these lines are drawn. The intersection of these bisectors is the instant center of motion, or the point of zero velocity, for this particular motion of the bone. Using this instant center of motion, point c, a velocity vector can be constructed showing the direction of surface motion that occurred for the particular movement. This is done by drawing a radius from the instant center to the point of contact between bones at the time for which the instant center was determined. In this case, the point of contact—the point at which the center axis of the bone crosses the joint surface—is called point p (Fig. 3-13). A perpendicular line drawn to this radius, at the joint surface, will indicate the direction of surface motion, with the arrow directed toward the movement of the bone.

After the instant center and surface-velocity vector are determined, an interpretation can be made. An instant center lying on the joint surface at the point of contact between the bones indicates that pure roll is taking place. An instant center lying far from the joint surface point of contact indicates that pure sliding is taking place. A velocity vector pointed away from the opposing (stationary) surface indicates a distraction

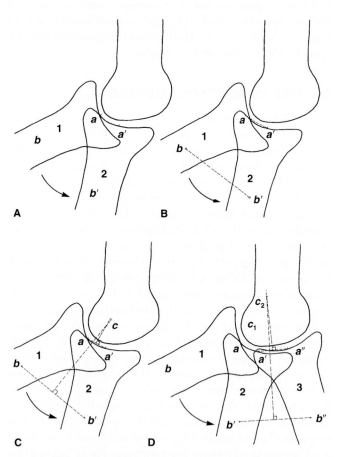

■ FIG. 3-12. Determination of instant centers of motion (c_1, c_2). **(A)** Two reference points on the moving bone are chosen; point *a* on the central axis of the joint surface and point *b*, 7 cm up the shaft of the bone (position *1*); the same points, *a'* and *b'*, are chosen in position *2*. **(B)** Lines *a-a'* and *b-b'* are constructed, and perpendicular bisections are drawn for these lines **(C, D)**. The intersection of the bisectors c_1 and c_2 are the instant centers of motion for movement from position *1* to *2* (C) and from position *2* to *3* (D).

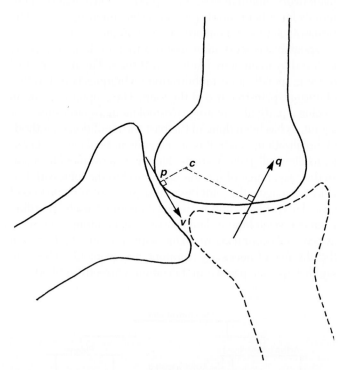

■ FIG. 3-13. Determination of surface velocity vectors. The *p* is the point of contact during the arc of motion for which *c* applies; *v* is the calculated velocity vector indicating tangential surface motion. If *q* were the vector for the arc of motion for which *c* applies, one could conclude that joint compression took place during this motion.

of the surfaces. A velocity vector aimed into the stationary surface indicates a compression of the surfaces. A velocity vector tangential to the joint surface suggests a smooth gliding motion is occurring.

The above analysis might seem somewhat complex at first but is actually quite simple. The difficult step is obtaining reliable roentgenograms that can be superimposed on each other. Plotting instant centers and surface velocity vectors for a particular movement throughout the range of motion can yield some very specific information about that motion. It reveals the relative amounts of roll and slide for various points throughout the range and how these values change during the complete motion: the closer the instant center comes to the point of contact, the more roll is taking place; the further it moves away, the more slide is occurring. Perhaps more importantly, it reveals possible abnormal compression or distraction of joint surfaces throughout the range (i.e., by comparison to what the operator considers "normal").

This type of scientific analysis of arthrokinematics is not practical for routine diagnostic purposes. However, it offers clinicians an opportunity to demonstrate the value of specific therapeutic interventions in improving abnormal joint mechanics. It has been used to show the value of certain surgeries (e.g., meniscectomy at the knee) in restoring normal joint mechanics.[15]

Because the information is obtained from roentgenograms, which are two-dimensional, arthrokinematic movements can be studied in only two dimensions. This analysis will not yield information concerning the amount of spin or conjunct rotation that is occurring.

NEUROLOGY

The neuroanatomy and, especially, the neurophysiology of joints are subjects not well covered in the current literature. Following the original works of Sherrington on neuromuscular physiology, a vast amount of information was collected concerning the role of muscle and tendon receptors in influencing posture, movement, muscle tone, and various reflex phenomena.[53] Little has been done until recently to identify specific joint receptors, and even less has been done to determine their clinical significance.[54,62] Because the subject of joint neurology is directly relevant to the management of common musculoskeletal disorders, an overview is presented here.

Innervation

Joints tend to receive innervation from two sources: (1) articular nerves that are branches of adjacent peripheral nerves and (2) branches from nerves that supply muscles controlling the joint. Each joint is usually supplied by several nerves, and their distributions tend to overlap considerably. In general, a particular aspect of a joint capsule is innervated by branches of the nerve supplying the muscle or muscles that would, when contracting, prevent overstretching of that part of the capsule.

One notable exception is the anteroinferior aspect of the glenohumeral capsule, which is innervated by a branch from the axillary nerve. The nerve fibers of an particular nerve are purely afferent, with the exception of small vasomotor efferents to the blood vessels. The fiber sizes range from large myelinated fibers to small myelinated and unmyelinated fibers.

Receptors

Joint receptors transmit information about the status of the joint to the central nervous system. The central nervous system interprets the information sent by the joint receptors and responds by coordinating muscle activity around the joint to meet joint mobility and stability requirements.[43,50] Joint receptors function to protect the joint from damage incurred by going into the pathologic range of motion. They are also partly responsible for determining the appropriate balance between synergistic and antagonistic muscular forces and for generating an image of body positioning and movement within the central nervous system. Four types of joint receptors have been identified, each serving a relatively specific role in the sensorimotor integration of joint function.[54,55,58,62]

Type I: Postural

Description—Encapsulated endings, similar to Ruffini corpuscle

Location—Numerous in the superficial joint capsule; usually found in clusters of six; located primarily in the neck, hip, and shoulder

Related fiber—Small (6 to 9 μm) myelinated (relatively slow conduction)

Stimulus—Changing mechanical stresses in the joint capsule; may be activated by the presence of positional faults; may be more active with traction techniques than with oscillations

Action—Slowly adapting (acts up to 1 minute following the initial stimulation), low threshold; mechanoreceptor

Function—Provides information concerning the static and dynamic position of the joint; is constantly firing; contributes to regulation of postural muscle tone; contributes to kinesthetic (movement) sense; senses direction and speed of movement; contributes to regulation of muscle tone during movement of the joint; produces increased tone in the muscle being stretched and relaxation in the muscle antagonistic to that being stretched; not active in mid–range-of-motion

Type II: Dynamic

Description—Thickly encapsulated, similar to pacinian corpuscle

Location—Sparse (relative to type I); found in joint capsule and ligaments (deeper layers and fat pads);

primarily located in the lumbar spine, hand, foot, and jaw

Related fiber—Medium (9 to 12 μm) myelinated

Stimulus—Sudden changes in joint motion; may be more active with oscillation techniques than with traction

Action—Rapidly adapting (acts for ½ second following each motion), low threshold; dynamic mechanoreceptor

Function—Fires only on quick changes in movement; provides information concerning acceleration and deceleration of joint movement; acts at initiation of movement as a "booster" to help overcome inertia of body parts; produces increased tone in the muscle being stretched and relaxation in the muscle antagonistic to the one being stretched when the joint is at end range, not active in mid–range-of-motion; inhibits pain

Type III: Inhibitive

Description—Thinly encapsulated, similar to Golgi end organ

Location—Primarily located in intrinsic and extrinsic joint ligaments, superficial layers of the capsule; in the lumbar spine not detected in the longitudinal posterior ligament, longitudinal anterior ligament, or iliolumbar ligament

Related fiber—Large (13 to 17 μm) myelinated (fast conduction)

Stimulus—Stretch at end range; more active with fast manipulation techniques

Action—Very slowly adapting (acts for several minutes following the initial stimulation), high threshold; dynamic mechanoreceptor

Function—Monitors direction of movement; has reflex effect on muscle tone to provide a "braking" mechanism against movement tending to overdisplace the joint (movement too fast or too far); inhibits muscle tone; responds to stretch at end of range

Type IV: Nociceptive

Description—Free nerve endings and plexus

Location—Located in most tissues: fibrous capsule, intrinsic and extrinsic ligaments, fat pads, periosteum (absent in articular cartilage, intra-articular fibrocartilage, and synovium)

Related fiber—Small (2 to 5 μm) myelinated and unmyelinated (2 μm) (slow conduction)

Stimulus—Significant mechanical deformation or tension; direct mechanical or chemical irritation

Action—Nonadapting, high threshold; pain receptors

Function—Inactive under normal conditions; active when related tissue is subject to significant deformation or other noxious mechanical or chemical stimulation; produces tonic muscle contraction

Clinical Considerations

It is apparent from the previous descriptions that stimulation of joint receptors contributes to sense of static position (type I), sense of speed of movement (type I), sense of change in speed of movement (type II), sense of direction of movement (types I and III), regulation of postural muscle tone (type I), regulation of muscle tone at the initiation of movement (type II), regulation of muscle tone during movement (coordination) (type II), and regulation of muscle tone during potentially harmful movements (type III). Of course, skin receptors, connective tissue receptors, and muscle receptors also contribute to many of these same functions. The following are some of the clinical problems that remain unresolved, or only partially resolved:

1. How important are these joint receptors, relative to muscle and skin receptors (e.g., in the regulation of muscle tone, posture, and movement)?
2. Are some of the persistent problems, such as chronic limp, residual incoordination, chronic instability ("giving way"), and chronic muscle atrophy, that are encountered in patients following some joint injuries the result of damage to these receptors?
3. How might treatment techniques, such as joint mobilization, neuromuscular facilitation, and inhibition, be refined to accommodate the functions of these joint receptors?

One particularly interesting study demonstrates a case in which malocclusion of dentures, causing abnormal afferent discharge from the temporomandibular joint capsules, resulted in an almost total reflex inhibition of the temporal muscles during active occlusion by the patient.[26] Restoration of normal joint mechanics, by remodeling of the dentures, restored normal muscular activity. A study by Wyke showed significant postural changes in a boy with apparent alteration of afferent impulses from the ankle capsule after injury to the lateral aspect of the capsule.[62] The postural deficit persisted despite an otherwise complete recovery, with restoration of normal strength and range of motion and with no residual pain. The boy's only complaint was that of occasional "giving way" of the ankle. Freeman advocates the use of coordination exercises on a balance board for patients with chronic ankle "instability" in the absence of demonstrable structural instability.[16] He reports good results with such a program, attributing such giving way at the ankle to alteration of normal joint afferent flow following injury to the joint, such as from an ankle sprain. Most physical therapists have encountered the common phenomenon of gross quadriceps atrophy following knee injury despite preventive efforts to maintain muscle function. Although there is little current literature on the subject, it seems reasonable to attribute this problem to reflex muscle inhibition by abnormal joint receptor stimulation.[9]

As far as techniques of treatment are concerned, it is interesting to relate what is known about the function of these joint receptors, and what is known of arthrokinematics, to techniques that have already evolved. Consider the diagonal pattern commonly used in proprioceptive neuromuscular facilitation techniques—moving the arm through flexion, abduction, external rotation to extension, adduction, and internal rotation. Part of the explanation of this pattern refers to moving from a position of maximum elongation and unspiraling of functionally related muscles to a position of spiraling and shortening of these same muscles.[57] In addition, this pattern involves moving all joints simultaneously from a close-packed to a loose-packed position. In doing so, the joint capsule of each joint moves from a position of maximum shortening and spiraling to a position of lengthening and unspiraling. Studies thus far on animals have indicated that maximum afferent stimulation occurs when approaching the close-packed position of a joint; this is to be expected since it is the position of maximum tightening of the capsule and ligaments in which the receptors lie. The techniques of proprioceptive neuromuscular facilitation evolved with primary consideration of the neurophysiology of muscles, using movement patterns that combine actions of functionally related muscles to bring about a mutual facilitation of each muscle in the chain. It is now suggested that these patterns also combine functionally related joint movements that add to the facilitative effect of the patterns on the muscles involved through joint receptor stimulation. It also seems probable that the joint receptors play a significant role in other techniques of facilitation, such as "quick stretch," that tend to stimulate the type II receptor.

It is important to consider the function of joint receptors when using joint mobilization or other treatment techniques involving joint movement. The effectiveness of efforts to increase movement at a joint will naturally be compromised by any muscle contraction tending to restrict joint movement. Emphasis, then, must be made on avoiding reflex muscle contractions that would tend to prevent or restrict a desired joint movement. For this reason—and for other obvious reasons—pain must be avoided during joint mobilization, because it is well known that pain at a joint tends to elicit a reflex muscle response to restrict movement at the joint. Sudden joint movement tends to stimulate firing of the type III receptors, which sets up a reflex muscle contraction to restrict further movement. Gradual initiation of movement tends to stimulate the type II receptor, which effects a small facilitative muscular response. Passive and active mobilization techniques are best performed rhythmically, without sudden changes in speed or direction of movement. A manipulation must be performed so quickly that it is completed before the reflex muscular response produced by stimulation of the type III receptor can act to interfere with the movement. Similarly, it must be performed through a very small amplitude to minimize the number of type III receptors stimulated.

With respect to the type IV pain receptors, it is worth emphasizing that articular cartilage, fibrocartilage (e.g., menisci), synovium, and compact bone are essentially aneural. This is well documented in anatomic studies and clinically.[25,54,62] In the anatomic joints the major pain-sensitive structures are the fibrous capsule, ligaments, and periosteum. This carries some important clinical implications. It suggests that pathologic conditions that might alter joint mechanics, such that the articular cartilage undergoes undue compression stress, may go unnoticed by the patient in the initial stages. In fact, the patient may note nothing until either joint mechanics are altered sufficiently to place an abnormal stress on the joint capsule or until the joint cartilage undergoes sufficient degeneration, causing a low-grade synovitis with resultant pressure on the capsule from effusion. This may explain why persons with "frozen shoulders" or osteoarthrosis of other joints often do not present to a physician until the disease has progressed considerably. It also suggests that clinicians must learn to examine routinely for subtle changes in joint mechanics rather than considering only gross range of motion, strength, and complaints of pain by the patient. Patients presenting with very early symptoms or signs of osteoarthrosis could enjoy complete arrest or reversal of the joint problem if properly managed, rather than resigning themselves to future joint replacement.

As is discussed in more detail in Chapter 6, Introduction to Manual Therapy, small oscillatory articulations may, in themselves, be useful in reducing pain at the joint being moved or at other joints derived from the same segment. The added proprioceptive input may inhibit the perception of pain through modulation at the substantia gelatinosa in the dorsal horn of the spinal cord.

JOINT NUTRITION

In addition to being aneural, articular cartilage is for the most part avascular. This is also true of intra-articular fibrocartilage. Because, in general, body tissues depend on blood supply for nutrition, these structures would seem to be at a disadvantage. It is generally believed that the articular margins do receive some nutrients from the highly vascularized synovium and periosteum adjacent to them.[18] The menisci at the knee also receive nutrients at their peripheral capsular attachments, and it is suggested that the deep layers of articular cartilage are fed by the blood supply to the subchondral bone. However, the problem of nutrition to the more superficial, centrally located portions of the articular cartilage and to the more centrally located parts of the intra-articular fibrocartilage remains. These cartilaginous areas are the primary articulating surfaces, not the more peripheral areas or deeper layers. It is generally agreed that nutrition to these regions occurs by diffusion and imbibition of synovial fluid. This is a unique situation because nutrients must cross at least two barriers to reach the chondrocytes embedded within the cartilage. First, they must pass from the capillary bed of the highly vascularized synovium.

Second, they must then diffuse through the superficial matrix layers of the cartilaginous surface, before reaching the cell wall of the chondrocyte. Thus, synovial fluid serves a major function as a source of nutrition for articular cartilage and intra-articular fibrocartilage.[18,32,33,35]

Intermittent compression and distraction of joint surfaces must occur for an adequate exchange of nutrients and waste products to take place. A joint that is immobilized undergoes atrophy of articular cartilage, just as a joint in which there is prolonged compression of joint surface undergoes similar atrophic changes.[2,12,13,60] The three primary mechanisms by which synovial joints undergo normal compression and distraction are the following: (1) weight bearing in lower extremity and spinal joints, (2) intermittent contraction of muscles crossing a joint, and (3) twisting and untwisting of the joint capsule as the joint moves toward and away from the close-packed position during habitual movements. With respect to the last mechanism, it is necessary to recall that as the joint approaches the close-packed position, its surfaces not only become compressed but also approach a position of maximal congruency. Thus, compression normally occurs in a position in which greater areas of the opposing joint surfaces are in contact. This ensures that relatively large portions of the joint surfaces undergo adequate exchange of nutrients. From a pathologic standpoint, a joint that has lost movement, such as from a tight joint capsule, does not receive a normal exchange of nutrients over the parts of the joint surfaces that no longer come into contact. This is especially true in the case of a tight joint capsule, since movements toward the close-packed position in which there is maximal joint surface contact are usually the movements that are most restricted.

Attritional changes in articular cartilage related to aging are observed in the relatively noncontacting portions of the joint surfaces.[4,38–40] Several reasons for this may be postulated. First, these are the areas of articular cartilage that undergo less deformation with use of the joint over time; as a result, the rate and degree of exchange of nutrient fluids are less in these areas. Also, with age there is a reduction of the chondroitin sulfate component of cartilaginous tissue. Because the fluid-binding capacity of articular cartilage is largely dependent on its chondroitin sulfate content, a decrease in this constituent might interfere with normal nutrition to the tissue. Furthermore, because loss of joint range of motion occurs with advancing age, the exchange of nutrients to portions of the articular cartilage is reduced.

Lubrication

In addition to serving as a nutritional source for articular cartilage, synovial fluid also acts as a lubricant to prevent undue wear of joint surfaces from friction.[11,37,61] In studying lubrication of human joints, however, not just the properties of synovial fluid and how they affect movement and friction between two surfaces are considered. In addition there are the shape and consistency of the joint surfaces as well as the types of movement that occur between joint surfaces. Many models have been proposed for human joint lubrication. Some of the earlier models tend to ignore many of the unique properties of human joints. The more recent models evolved with the sophistication of engineering principles, which are better able to deal with some of the complex factors involved in human joint lubrication. However, it is generally agreed that no one model of joint lubrication applies to all joints under all circumstances. The major mode of lubrication in a particular joint may change, depending on factors such as loading and speed of movement.

Synovial fluid has essentially the same composition as blood plasma, except for the addition of mucin. Mucin is mucopolysaccharide hyaluronic acid, which is a long-chain polymer. The viscous properties of synovial fluid are attributed to hyaluronic acid. The most important property to be considered in this respect is the **thixotropic** or non-newtonian quality of synovial fluid; the viscosity decreases with increased shear rate (increased speed of joint movement).

Models of Joint Lubrication

An analogy cannot accurately be drawn between a machine model of lubrication and the lubrication of synovial joints. One of the major reasons for this is that the physical properties of articular cartilage differ considerably from the physical properties of most machine components. Articular cartilage is porous and relatively spongelike in that it has the capacity to absorb and bind synovial fluid. Articular cartilage is also viscoelastic; the deformation rate is high on initial application of the load and levels off with time. When the load is removed, the initial "reformation" rate is high and decreases over time (Fig. 3-14). Although articular cartilage appears quite smooth and shiny microscopically, it is, in fact, relatively rough microscopically. Articular cartilage also has the tendency to adsorb large molecules, such as hyaluronic acid in synovial fluid, to its surface. The significance of this is discussed later in this section.

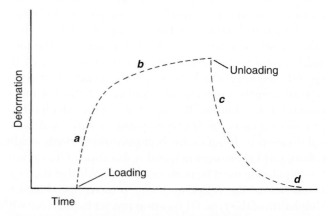

■ **FIG. 3-14.** Viscoelastic response of articular cartilage. Parts *a* and *c* of the curve are owing to elastic properties, whereas parts *b* and *d* show viscous behavior.

The early model of joint lubrication described a hydrodynamic, or fluid film, situation (Fig. 3-15).[27] In this case, synovial fluid fills in the wedges of space left by the joint surface incongruencies. On movement between surfaces the synovial fluid is attracted to the area of contact between the surfaces. This occurs because of (1) the pressure gradient produced by the movement and (2) the fact that relative movement tends to pull the viscous fluid in the direction of the moving surface. The result of this is the maintenance of a layer of fluids between joint surfaces during movement. Any friction occurring as a result of movement occurs within the fluid rather than between joint surfaces. This meets the requirements of a good lubrication system because it allows free movement and prevents wear to the joint surfaces. This system works well during movement; however, it would tend to fail under very slow velocity or under heavy loading. It would also fail under reciprocal motion, because it would not adapt well to changes in direction of motion, at which time the velocity of movement is zero. Because human joints often move slowly, under heavy loads, and reciprocally, by itself it seems an unsatisfactory model for human joint lubrication.

The hydrodynamic model, however, cannot be completely repudiated because the previous description does not consider the viscoelasticity of joint surfaces. This model can be modified to an elastohydrodynamic system (Fig. 3-15). Because of the nature of articular cartilage to deform, not all the energy of heavy loading goes to decreasing the thickness of the layer of film between the surfaces, thus increasing friction between the surfaces. Instead, deformation of the joint surfaces occurs, increasing the effective contact area between surfaces and thus reducing the effective compression stress (force per unit area) to the lubrication fluid. This allows the protective layer of fluid to remain at about the same thickness. Thus, the elastohydrodynamic model describes a system that withstands loading in the presence of movement. It fails to explain, however, the means of lubrication at the initiation of movement or at the period of relative zero velocity during reciprocating movements or during very heavy loading with very little movement.

This model of joint lubrication can be expanded by including the concepts of boundary lubrication and weeping lubrication.[37,48,56,61] With any materials undergoing relative shear between two surfaces, friction is the result of the irregularities of the surfaces; the greater the irregularities, the greater the friction. Effective lubrication must reduce this friction to a minimum, thus reducing wear of the surfaces to a minimum. In the case of boundary lubrication, the lubricant is adsorbed to the surface of the material, in effect, reducing the roughness of the surfaces by filling in the irregularities. Because articular cartilage is able to adsorb long-chain molecules of hyaluronic acid, these molecules are able to fill in the irregularities and to coat the surface. Any friction occurring as the result of shear movement occurs between molecules of the lubricant rather than between the joint surfaces themselves. This probably serves as an adjunct to the elastohydrodynamic system, especially in cases of extreme loading sufficient to decrease significantly the thickness of the layer of fluid maintained by the elastohydrodynamic model under lighter loads. It may also play a role at the initiation of movement or periods of zero velocity, since a layer of fluid would not be present because of its dependence on movement under an elastohydrodynamic system. The concept of weeping lubrication is actually an expansion of the elastohydrodynamic model. Because of the porosity and elastic qualities of articular cartilage, loading sufficient to cause a deformation of the articular surfaces also causes a "squeezing out" of the synovial fluid absorbed by the cartilage. The fluid that is squeezed out further serves to maintain a protective layer of lubricant between joint surfaces.

By the use of this "mixed lubrication" model, which combines elastohydrodynamic concepts with boundary lubrication concepts, the demands of human synovial joints are met.[11,47] The system allows movement, change in direction of movement, loading, and variations in congruencies of joint surfaces. It takes into consideration, at least in general terms, the properties of the lubricant (synovial fluid) and the surface materials. There is still considerable controversy over the relative importance of each of the lubrication models under various conditions, but most authors agree with the general concepts presented previously. Because it is still unknown how each model contributes to normal joint lubrication, very little investigation into the mutual effects of pathologic joint conditions and joint lubrication has taken place. A breakdown in some aspect of the lubrication system is likely to cause or add to the progression of joint disease, such as degenerative joint disease. On the other hand, certain joint diseases result in changes in structure and function of joint constituents. For instance, there is a loss of joint cartilage in degenerative joint disease and changes in synovial fluid viscosity in rheumatoid arthritis. It is probable that in such cases the disease will, in

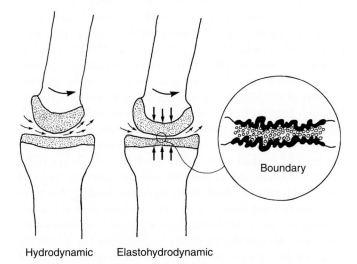

Hydrodynamic   Elastohydrodynamic

Boundary

■ **FIG. 3-15.** Hydrodynamic, elastohydrodynamic, and boundary models of joint lubrication.

turn, alter the function of the lubrication system, thus contributing to a progressive degenerative cycle.

Resolving Problems of Joint-Surface Wear

It has been emphasized that synovial joint surfaces are incongruent. Because of the incongruency that exists in most positions of movement, a relatively small contact area exists between joint surfaces. The wedges of space that surround this contact area are necessary for a hydrodynamic lubrication system to operate effectively; without these spaces the lubricant could not be drawn, or forced, between the contacting surfaces. One may wonder if such a small area of contact might increase the likelihood of wear between joint surfaces, since loading forces from weight-bearing and muscle contraction would be distributed over a small surface area, thus increasing the compressive stress to the joint. This would, in fact, be the case if the area of contact on one or both surfaces was consistently the same throughout habitual movements. In this respect the clinician might be concerned about joints that are relatively track-bound, such as the humeroulnar, patellofemoral, ankle mortise, and interphalangeal joints.

In each of these joints, movement tends to be restricted to one arc of movement that is determined almost entirely by the shapes of the joint surfaces. It would seem that during movement at these joints, the contacting area on one joint surface would consistently "follow a rut" on the opposing surface, increasing the likelihood of excessive wear in the rut or at the area of the surface contacting the rut. In these joints the problem of excessive wear is resolved in a number of ways. First, these joint surfaces are, relatively speaking, the most congruent in the body, so that forces are distributed over a somewhat larger area. Consider, for example, the close fit between the ulna and the trochlear surface of the humerus. Second, the contact area on each surface is constantly changing throughout an arc of movement. A change in contact areas occurs in one sense because a combination of roll and slide takes place between joint surfaces. In another sense, the contact area changes because contact alternates from the "bottom of the valley to the sides of the slopes" on one surface and correspondingly on the opposing surface. For instance, with the knee in full extension, the articular surface of the patella makes contact with the femur at a strip extending mediolaterally across the middle of the patellar surface. In flexion, however, only the medial and lateral margins of the patella make contact with the femoral condyles while the ridge in the middle of the patellar facets lies freely in the intercondylar notch.[21] A comparable situation occurs at the elbow, ankle, and finger joints throughout their respective movements. Note that at the ankle mortise, which undergoes intermittent heavy loading in habitual use, maximal loading (stance) takes place with the joint closer to its close-packed position, dorsiflexion. This is the position of maximal congruence and therefore the position in which the compressive force per unit area would tend to be smallest.

However, at joints such as the knee, a more complex situation exists. The knee is significantly incongruent compared with the joints discussed previously; it must be to allow some degree of rotation to occur independently of flexion or extension or in conjunction with them. The knee must also withstand heavier loading from weight bearing in a wide variety of positions. Thus, the knee is often required to undergo heavy loading in positions of flexion, in which the surfaces are very incongruent—a small area of contact withstands relatively large compressive forces. Thus, there might be concern that in a situation of heavy loading, relatively low velocity, and small contact area between surfaces, the lubrication system would not be sufficient to prevent excessive friction (shear) and wear between joint surfaces. This might very well be the case in a joint such as the knee that must undergo such conditions during normal daily activities, such as climbing stairs, squatting, and lifting. There might also be concern about the tendency for the femur to slip forward on the tibia under such conditions, again because of the incongruency of joint surfaces and the lack of intrinsic stability. Are the posterior cruciate, popliteus, and other intrinsic stabilizers sufficient to prevent this problem?

The knee, then, is a joint that must allow movement of spin between the tibia and the femur and swing between the tibia and femur because of the functional demands placed on it. For this to be possible, the joint surfaces must be sufficiently incongruent. However, because of this incongruence and because of normal heavy loading in a variety of positions, the knee appears susceptible to excessive shear forces between contacting joint surfaces during movement, excessive compressive forces between contacting surfaces on static loading, and intrinsic instability when loaded in flexion. It is probable that the intra-articular menisci serve to compensate for what would otherwise be unsatisfactory engineering at the knee joint—unsatisfactory in that the joint would not withstand the normal forces applied to it without giving way or undergoing premature wearing of joint surfaces.[29] Under heavy static loading, the menisci act to increase the effective load-bearing surface area at the joint, thus reducing the force per unit area. Being firmly attached to the joint capsule and tibia but mobile enough to conform to the shape of the articulating segments of the femoral condyles, they serve to increase the intrinsic stability of the joint by increasing the effective congruency between joint surfaces. During movement with heavy loading, they again act to increase the load-bearing surface area, but they also maintain a wedge-shaped interval surrounding the area of contact into which the lubricant fluid can be drawn.[29] Because the menisci are semicartilaginous, they can also absorb synovial fluid. With increased loading, fluid can be squeezed out from the menisci and the articular load-bearing surface, contributing to a weeping lubrication phenomenon. Also, as the menisci recede before the advancing condyles during movement, they can act to spread a layer of lubricant over the joint surfaces just before contact. This, incidentally, may also be a function of the rather large infrapatellar fat pad at the knee.[5] The menisci, because they are semimobile, allow the knee to act as though it were maximally congruent with respect to the requirements of lubrication and intrinsic stability, but to actually function as though it were very incongruent with respect to the types of movement that occur at the joint.

There is also considerable slide of the femoral condyles along the tibial surface during the complete range of flexion-extension. This feature also reduces the likelihood of excessive wear on the tibial surfaces by distributing the load-bearing surface over a larger area. The degree of slide could not occur normally without the extrinsic control provided by the cruciates, nor without the intrinsic stability provided by the menisci. This type of motion, in which the area of contact of a particular joint surface constantly changes with movement at the joint, is necessary to allow for the intermittent compression of articular cartilage essential to normal nutrition and lubrication. Loss of a constantly changing area of contact during use of a joint is likely to increase the probability of degeneration of articular cartilage by interfering with normal nutrition and normal lubrication, and by increasing the compressive forces over time per unit area per unit time. Unused areas of articular cartilage would not undergo necessary exchanges of nutrients; areas of cartilage in which loading occurs would eventually fail from fatigue (see section on arthrosis later in this chapter).

Fibrillation of articular cartilage in normal hip and shoulder joints occurs first in non-weight-bearing surfaces.[39] Also, a significant acceleration of degenerative changes occurs in weight-bearing animal joints in which a joint is immobilized but full use of the limb is allowed.[12] These are both examples of the effects on articular cartilage of the load-bearing contact area not being distributed over a large area of the opposing surfaces. This is perhaps a partial explanation for the frequency of degenerative arthritis occurring in human hip joints; a relatively small surface area is used for weight-bearing, while much of the articular cartilage receives little or no compression. As will be discussed later in the section on arthrosis, it also contributes to the explanation of how abnormal joint arthrokinematics may lead to joint pathology.

APPROACH TO MANAGEMENT OF JOINT DYSFUNCTION

The rationale for specific joint mobilization requires the restoration of normal joint play so that full, pain-free motion may occur at the joint. The term **joint dysfunction** is used by Mennell to indicate loss of normal joint play.[41] There are many explanations for the causes of joint dysfunction, some of which are specific for certain joints and some of which may be applied to all joints. In the spine, entrapment of "meniscoid inclusions" is postulated by some as a cause of joint dysfunction. Frankel et al.[15] and Sammarco et al.[51] have demonstrated through instant center analysis the presence of joint dysfunction at the knee from meniscus tears (confirmed later by surgery) and dysfunction in ankle joints that had been

classified as unstable, postfracture, or having degenerative disease. It has also been shown that joint dysfunction in "frozen shoulders" is often caused by adherence of the anteroinferior aspect of the joint capsule to the humeral head.[42] A loose body in a joint may be a cause of dysfunction, as may joint effusion causing some distention of the capsule. The list goes on, the point being that *there is no single cause of joint dysfunction.*

The use of specific mobilization is not indicated in all cases of dysfunction. For this reason, a thorough evaluation performed in an attempt to clarify the nature and extent of the lesion is a necessary step in the management of joint problems. Those cases in which a physical therapist must play a major role in treatment of joint dysfunction are those dysfunctions occurring as a result of isolated or generalized capsular tightness or adhesion. These typically follow traumatic sprains to the capsule or immobilization. In some cases, they occur for no apparent reason (e.g., "adhesive capsulitis" at the shoulder).

The traditional approach to management of patients presenting with loss of pain-free movement at a joint usually involves various modes of pain relief, active and passive measures to improve osteokinematic movement, and encouragement of normal use of the part. It should be clear that this approach is inadequate and perhaps dangerous. First, it ignores the basic problem, which is often loss of normal arthrokinematics. Second, it involves considerable forcing of osteokinematic movements in the absence of normal arthrokinematic movement, which may only occur at the expense of the articular cartilage. This is to say, the resiliency of the cartilage may allow a certain amount of osteokinematic movement to occur without the normal accompanying arthrokinematic movements. Frankel[14] describes the case of a boy who continued to use his knee in the absence of normal external rotation of the tibia on the femur during knee extension. One and a half years later, at surgery, dimpling of the articular cartilage of the medial femoral condyle was observable with the naked eye, presumably caused by continued abnormal compression of this portion of the articular surface from loss of normal arthrokinematic movement.

A more logical approach to the management of these patients emphasizes the restoration of joint play to allow free movement between bones. This can be achieved only by (1) evaluating to determine the nature and extent of the lesion, (2) deciding if joint mobilization is indicated based on the evaluation, (3) choosing the appropriate techniques based on the direction and extent of restrictions, and (4) skillfully applying techniques of specific mobilization. Efforts to relieve pain and reduce muscle guarding are, of course, important adjuncts to treatment but do not in themselves constitute a treatment program. Also, some movement should be encouraged in the cardinal planes, but only as normal kinematics are restored. To a certain extent, functional use of the part should be restricted through careful instructions to the patient until normal joint mechanics are restored. This approach minimizes the possible danger of undue stresses to the articular cartilage during attempts to restore movement. It also minimizes the possibility of discharging a patient who has relatively pain-free functional use of the joint but who may have some residual kinematic disturbance sufficient to cause cartilage fatigue over time and perhaps osteoarthrosis in later years.

Pathologic Considerations

A high percentage of the chronic musculoskeletal problems seen clinically are fatigue disorders. These are disorders in which abnormal stresses imposed on a structure over a prolonged period result in a tendency toward an increased rate of tissue breakdown. All tissues, including those with low metabolic activity such as articular cartilage, undergo a necessary process of repair to continuously replace the microdamage resulting from normal use. In bone, such microdamage involves fracturing of bony trabeculae, whereas in other connective tissues there is disruption of individual collagen fibers. As long as the rate of microtrauma does not exceed normal limits and the rate at which the tissue is able to repair itself is not compromised, the tissue remains "normal." The tendency to maintain an equilibrium against opposing, unbalancing factors is a homeostatic mechanism; a shift in the nature of one factor will cause a compensatory reaction by the body to correspondingly alter the other factor to maintain balance.

In general, the nature of the various pathologies affecting the musculoskeletal tissues can be considered according to this homeostatic model. The two factors that the body is attempting to balance are (1) the process of tissue breakdown and (2) the process of tissue production or repair. Thus, in discussing abnormal or pathologic situations, attention must be paid to the causes of and homeostatic responses to a tendency toward increased tissue breakdown and a decreased rate of breakdown. Factors that might disturb the body's ability to maintain an appropriate balance, such as those that might cause an abnormal degree of tissue production and those that might compromise the body's ability to produce enough tissue, must also be considered.

INCREASED RATE OF TISSUE BREAKDOWN

Increased tissue breakdown results when the frequency or magnitude of stresses to the part increases, when the capacity of the tissue to repair itself is reduced, or both. Under conditions of significantly increased stress over time, the body attempts to compensate by laying down more tissue to increase the capacity of the tissue to withstand the higher stress levels. The result is tissue hypertrophy. In well-vascularized tissues, this occurs in conjunction with a low-grade inflammatory process incited by the increased rate of tissue damage. A new equilibrium is reached in favor of a more massive structure, better able to withstand higher stress levels without failing. Typical examples include muscle hypertrophy in response to increased loading of a muscle over time; subchondral bony sclerosis in response to increased compressive forces over a joint; and fibrosis of a joint capsule receiving increased stresses from faulty joint movement over a prolonged period.

Such tissue hypertrophy, especially when affecting bone and capsuloligamentous structures, causes tissue to gain in strength at the expense of extensibility; the tissue becomes better able to withstand loads without undergoing gross failure but does not deform as readily when loaded. An increase in the ratio of collagen (mineralized collagen in the case of bone) to the remaining extracellular ground substance (mucopolysaccharide) reduces extensibility. This is believed to allow increased interfiber bond formation, with a subsequent reduced mobility, or gliding capacity, of individual elements. The added stiffness reduces the energy-attenuating capacity of the structure. Less of the energy of loading is attenuated as work, and more of the energy must be absorbed internally by the structure or attenuated by increased deformation of other structures that are in series with the hypertrophic tissues. Thus, with sclerosis of subchondral bone, the overlying articular cartilage is made to undergo greater strain per unit of load because of the reduced deformability of the subjacent bone. This is believed to be an important factor in the progressive degeneration of cartilage occurring with degenerative joint disease.[47] With fibrosis of tendon tissue, such as the extensor carpi radialis brevis origin at the elbow, the reduced extensibility of the tendon fibers results in greater strain to the tenoperiosteal junction of the tendon at the lateral humeral epicondyle. The ensuing inflammatory process is responsible for the symptoms and signs of the "tennis elbow" syndrome.

Although in such situations the hypertrophic structure is more massive and less likely to fail when loaded, the rate of microdamage may remain elevated. Although the stress to the structure tends to be reduced because of the increased cross-sectional area resulting from the hypertrophy, the internal energy within the structure may be increased because of the reduced extensibility. An increase in internal energy must be dissipated as heat or microfracturing of individual structural components. Clinically, a painful, low-grade inflammatory reaction may result from the added mechanical and thermal stimulation.

Thus, when a tissue hypertrophies in response to increased stress levels, the rate of microdamage tends to remain elevated—there is simply more tissue present to ensure that the structure, as a whole, does not fail. Pain may arise from the increased internal stresses on the involved tissue or from increased strain on connected tissues.

For any tissue there is a critical point past which the rate of breakdown may exceed the rate at which the tissue is able to repair or strengthen itself. Under normal metabolic conditions, this critical point is reached soonest in tissues with limited capacity for regeneration and repair. These are tissues that are poorly vascularized and have a low metabolic turnover. The typical example of such a tissue is articular cartilage. With increased compressive stress levels to a joint, the well-vascularized bone will tend to hypertrophy, while the cartilage degenerates. Even bone, however, can be stressed at a frequency or magnitude at which it can no longer repair itself fast enough to prevent progressive breakdown. A common clinical disorder in which this occurs is the stress fracture affecting athletes or other persons who habitually engage in high–stress-level activities.

REDUCED RATE OF TISSUE BREAKDOWN

Decreased stress levels on tissue over time will reduce the rate of breakdown. Thus, with relative inactivity the rate of microdamage is less and the body takes the opportunity to economize by reducing the rate of tissue production. The tissue no longer needs to be as strong because of the reduction in the everyday stresses it must withstand. The typical condition in which this occurs is disuse atrophy. When a part is immobilized, the bone becomes less dense, and capsules, ligaments, and muscles atrophy. The important clinical consideration in such situations is to increase gradually the stress levels on the tissue to promote strengthening of the structure by stimulating increased tissue production, but without causing the weakened structures to fail. This is especially true after healing of a structure such as bone or ligament; not only must new tissue be produced, but it must also mature. Maturation involves reorientation of major structural elements along the lines of stress that the structure will normally undergo. The process of maturation takes time, and the necessary stimulus is the judiciously applied loading of the part in ways that simulate the loads the part will need to withstand with normal use.

INCREASED RATE OF TISSUE PRODUCTION

The rate of tissue production increases in conjunction with any inflammatory process. The reparative phase that follows acute inflammation usually involves a proliferation of collagen tissue. This is especially true in certain virulent inflammatory processes associated with bacterial infections. Chronic, low-grade inflammation, such as that mentioned previously in conjunction with increased stress levels, is also accompanied by increased collagen production. Regardless of the cause, the result is a relatively fibrosed, less extensible structure. Loss of extensibility will be especially significant if the part is immobilized during the period of increased collagen production. The new collagen will not be laid down along the appropriate lines of stress, and abnormal interfiber cross-links develop that do not accommodate normal deformation. If, on the other hand, some movement of the part occurs during the period of increased collagen production, the loss of extensibility will not be so great. Appropriate orientation of the newly laid fibers is stimulated by the stresses imposed on the tissue by movement. Loss of extensibility in the immobilized part is owing to the increased density of the structure and the abnormal orientation of the structured elements. In the part in which some movement occurs, reduced extensibility is primarily a result of the change in density.

Clinically, a part that is strictly immobilized during an acute inflammatory process, such as that induced by surgery, trauma, infection, or rheumatoid arthritis, is likely to lose more movement. Further, this loss of movement is likely to be more persistent than in the case of a part in which some movement continues in the presence of a chronic, low-grade inflammation, such as degenerative joint disease.

Restoration of normal extensibility of the tissue requires (1) removing the stimulus of increased tissue production (e.g., stress, infection, trauma), (2) gradually stretching the structure to break down abnormal interfiber cross-links, and (3) restoring normal use of the part to induce normal orientation of structural elements.

REDUCED RATE OF TISSUE PRODUCTION AND REPAIR

Reduced rate of tissue production and repair occurs with reduced stress levels to the tissue, but it may also occur with some change in the metabolic status of the tissue. Examples of the latter include nutritional deficiencies, reduced vascularity, and abnormal hormone levels. When the cause is related to reduced stress levels, amelioration simply involves a gradual return to normal stress conditions. However, when the cause is metabolic, treatment is more complex and will vary with the type of disturbance. In these cases, stress levels must be reduced because the body is unable to keep up with the normal rate of tissue breakdown. Continued use of the part will result in fatigue failure of the involved tissues.

Typical examples of common musculoskeletal disorders that are related to such an alteration in the metabolic status of the involved tissues include the following:

Supraspinatus tendinitis at the shoulder—The tendon begins to fatigue from reduced vascularity in an area of the tendon close to its insertion. Occasionally the body attempts to compensate for its inability to produce new tendon tissue by laying down calculous deposits. These lesions often progress to complete tendon ruptures because the rate of breakdown continues to exceed the capacity of the tissue to repair itself.

Reflex sympathetic dystrophy—Generalized hypovascularity to a part, caused by increased sympathetic activity, results in atrophy of bone, nails, muscle, and skin—in short, all musculoskeletal components.

Senile and postmenopausal osteoporosis—Bone metabolism is compromised as a result of alteration in hormone levels and other age-related influences. The bone atrophy is most significant in cancellous bone, such as that of the vertebral bodies. Roentgenograms often show collapsed vertebrae, resulting from progressive trabecular buckling.

Age-related tissue changes—Aging, in itself, does not seem to result in changes in the collagen content of musculoskeletal tissues. However, with advancing age, the protein-polysaccharide (glycosaminoglycan) content of most somatic tissues is reduced. There is also an associated reduction in water content, since the protein-polysaccharide component of the tissue matrices is responsible for the fluid-binding capacity of the tissues. The result is a relative fibrosis of the involved tissues, because the ratio of collagen to ground substance is increased. It is postulated that the protein-polysaccharide ground substance normally acts as a lubricating spacer between collagen fibers. As its content is reduced, the collagen fibers approximate one another and form increased numbers of interfiber cross-links (intermolecular bonds), and the fibers no longer glide easily with respect to each other. Thus, the stiffness of the structure increases. Because of the increased stiffness, the tissue as a whole loses its deformability and therefore loses its ability to attenuate the energy of loading. With loading, more stress is imposed on individual structural elements and the rate of tissue breakdown subsequently increases. For many elderly persons this does not pose a problem because activity levels, and therefore stress levels, decrease with advancing age.

The reduced fluid-binding capacity of the tissue, associated with protein-polysaccharide depletion, may alter the nutritional status of the tissue. This is especially important in structures such as articular cartilage and intervertebral disks that depend on fluid inhibition for normal exchange of nutrients. Thus, the capacity of the tissue to repair itself is also reduced. This is a likely explanation for the degeneration of intervertebral disks and articular cartilage that occurs with advancing age.

Intervention and Communication

From a clinical standpoint, the clinician should be prepared to estimate the nature of a pathologic process according to this scheme. This is necessary to plan a treatment program specific for the type of pathologic process present. Awareness of the various ways the clinician can effectively intervene so as to appropriately alter the pathologic state is also important.

The terms used to refer to common musculoskeletal pathologies usually provide little information relating to the nature of the disorder. The same term may be applied to different conditions in which the cause and nature of the pathologic process are quite distinct. Tendinitis at the shoulder is an atrophic, degenerative condition resulting from reduced vascularity to an area of the rotator cuff tendons; tendinitis at the elbow is a hypertrophic, fibrotic condition often related to increased stress levels. Also, many terms, such as degenerative joint disease, refer to situations in which a number of tissues may be involved, and the nature of the changes affecting the involved tissues may differ. In the case of degenerative joint disease, for example, the subchondral bone and the joint capsule tend to hypertrophy while the articular cartilage atrophies and degenerates.

Therapeutically, there are many physical agents and procedures that may be used to influence various types of pathologic processes. Perhaps the most important form of intervention is well-planned instructions to the patient regarding the performance of specific activities. To give appropriate instructions the clinician must gear the patient's activity level to the nature of the disorder. This requires a knowledge of the response of tissues to various loading conditions under normal and abnormal circumstances. A careful examination must be carried out, including a biomechanical assessment. It also requires that the clinician be aware of the types of stresses imposed on a party by various activities. The patient must understand the instructions and be able and willing to follow them.

Arthrosis

When considering a diseased joint one usually thinks in terms of the physiologic changes that have occurred at the joint. There is much information concerning the histologic and biochemical changes in periarticular tissues, changes in hemodynamics, and synovial fluid changes that accompany some of the more common joint diseases.[3,7,31–34,38] Although mechanical changes also occur, these are usually not dealt with until advanced structural changes have resulted. The treatment then is usually surgical. The earlier, conservative treatment in joint disease typically involves measures to counter the physiologic changes taking place. This seems the logical approach in arthropathies in which the etiology is apparently some physiologic change and in which the primary joint changes are physiologic. Thus, in rheumatoid arthritis, gout, and spondylitis, the primary treatments are those aimed at controlling inflammation and metabolic disturbances. The mechanical changes in joint function are generally agreed to be secondary and often left to improve (or degenerate) along with the primary physiologic changes.

Although our knowledge of normal joint mechanics is becoming more sophisticated, little has been written concerning the mechanical changes that occur with, or possibly lead to, joint disease. It is well accepted, however, that joint disease may result from some mechanical disturbance. These cases are usually referred to as **secondary osteoarthritis,** in which some past joint trauma can be cited as a precipitating factor. This is distinguished by many researchers from **primary osteoarthritis,** in which several joints may be involved with no known causative factor. However, the pathologies of primary and secondary osteoarthritis are essentially identical, and because these disorders are for the most part noninflammatory, they are best referred to as **osteoarthroses.** As the probable etiologies of osteoarthroses are investigated, the more it appears that the classifications of primary and secondary are often arbitrary. Although it has been postulated by some that primary osteoarthrosis has a physiologic or metabolic etiology, it appears that in many cases it is owing to mechanical changes of much subtler onset than those causing secondary osteoarthrosis.[17,19,52]

It is generally agreed that changes in the articular cartilage trigger a cycle that leads to the progression of degenerative joint disease. Cartilage damage may occur after a single trau-matic incident, causing a tension or compression strain suffi-cient to interfere with the structural integrity of the cartilage. This is relatively rare and usually accompanies a fracture of the adjacent bone. More common is cartilage wearing from fatigue, or the cumulative effects of abnormal stresses, nei-ther of which is sufficient in itself to cause structural dam-age.[59] Cartilage may be susceptible to fatigue in part because it is aneural; any other musculoskeletal tissue is relatively immune to fatigue because protective reflex inhibition occurs with abnormal stress. This inhibitory response requires, of course, intact innervation. Cartilage is also susceptible to damage because it is avascular. It lacks the normal inflamma-tion and repair response that would replace damaged parts of the tissue. In fact, when cartilage is lacerated without involve-ment of the vascularized subchondral bone, a brief prolifera-tion of chondrocytes ensues but with no repair of the defect. If the lesion is sufficient to penetrate the subchondral bone, it immediately fills with blood and a clot is formed. This clot is invaded with new blood vessels that apparently bring in un-differentiated mesenchymal cells. These cells proceed to fill the defect with fibrocartilage (not hyaline cartilage).[10,24]

Hyaline cartilage partly makes up for the fact that it is aneural and avascular by its considerable ability to deform when loaded in compression. Much of the substance of artic-ular cartilage is a mucopolysaccharide ground substance, whose chief component is chondroitin sulfate. Chondroitin

sulfate is highly hydrophilic with the ability to bind large quan-tities of water. Cartilage is 70 to 80% water and depends on this water content for its resiliency—its ability to withstand com-pression stresses without structural damage. The energy of compressive loading is dissipated as cartilage undergoes strain, or deformation. This strain results in tension stresses that are absorbed by the collagen fibers embedded within the ground substance (Fig. 3-16). Thus, the extracellular carti-lage matrix normally withstands compression stresses through the mucopolysaccharide gel, and tension stresses through the collagen fibers. Interspersed throughout this matrix are the chondrocytes, or cartilage cells, that are responsible for production of the matrix components. Moreover, a con-siderable proportion of compressive forces is attenuated by the cancellous subchondral bone that, although stiffer than the articular cartilage, is thicker and has more volume for energy attenuation.[47]

Although cartilage was once believed to be inert metabol-ically, studies now indicate that turnover of cartilage does occur.[33] Chondrocytes apparently secrete some matrix material continuously to replace that lost by normal attrition. It has also been shown that in response to mild or moderate osteoarthro-sis in which cartilage degradation has increased, proliferation and metabolic activity of chondrocytes also increase. At least for a while the chondrocytes are able to keep pace with the disease. For some reason as yet unknown, this process shuts down in later stages of the disease. It is also poorly understood why

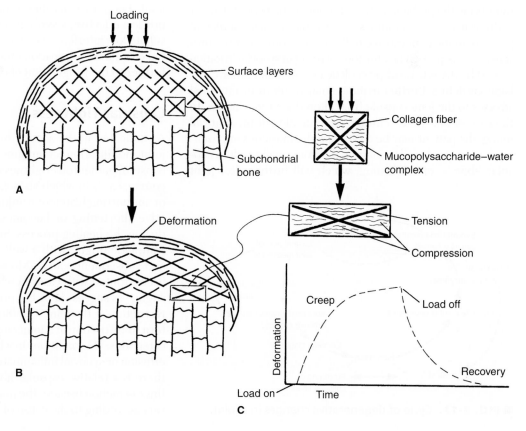

■ **FIG. 3-16.** **(A)** Compres-sive loading of articular car-tilage results in **(B)** tension stresses to the collagenous elements and compression stresses to the mucopoly-saccharide-water complex. **(C)** The total response is visco-elastic. The viscous creep with sustained loading is largely the result of a time-dependent squeezing out of fluid.

lacerations of cartilage do not undergo repair, whereas some repair does take place in the earlier stages of osteoarthrosis.

Degenerative Cycle

The initial changes that occur in the cartilage when abnormal stresses leading to acute damage or chronic fatigue are applied are (1) fibrillation, or fracturing of collagen fibers, and (2) depletion of ground substance, primarily a loss of chondroitin sulfate.[7,31,34,38–40,59] There remains some dispute over which change takes place first; however, it seems to be agreed that once initiated, a cycle of degeneration will follow. This cycle is countered up to a point by the proliferation of chondrocytes and the increased secretion of cartilage matrix by the chondrocytes. A cycle as shown in Figure 3-17 is likely to develop. Loss of chondroitin sulfate leaves the collagen fibers more susceptible to fracture; fracturing of these fibers causes a "softening" of the surface layers of the cartilage; the cartilage becomes less able to withstand stresses in this region, with the resultant death of local chondrocytes; and the death of chondrocytes is believed to allow the release of proteolytic enzymes that have a further degradative effect on chondroitin sulfate. The adjacent areas of cartilage, peripheral and deep to this damaged area, must now absorb increased stresses, so the process tends to spread. The chemical factor caused by destructive enzyme release adds to this spreading mechanical factor.[49]

Because of the absence of pain receptors in articular cartilage, considerable degeneration may take place before symptoms bring the problem to the attention of the patient. Pain or stiffness may not occur until synovial effusion causes sufficient pressure to the joint capsule to fire pain-sensitive or pressure-sensitive receptors. The effusion is a result of synovial irritation caused by the release of proteolytic enzymes and other cartilaginous debris. Further irritation may result from abnormal stresses to the joint capsule from altered joint mechanics. In the case of low-grade, chronic inflammation of the synovial lining, the patient may be aware of only transient symptoms. Such a low-grade inflammation, if chronic, will result in capsular fibrosis, or thickening, which will further alter joint

mechanics. Fibrosis of the joint capsule may be thought of as a relative increase in the collagen-mucopolysaccharide ratio. The result is that which occurs with any scarring process: reduced extensibility from loss of elasticity, gradual contracture, and adherence to adjacent tissues. The loss of capsular mobility often goes unnoticed by the patient until it causes limitation of motion sufficient to interfere with daily activities. In joints such as the shoulder, which in the inactive person may be used only through a small range of motion to perform daily activities, a rather significant limitation of movement may occur before the patient realizes that a problem exists. Such a lack of mobility of the joint capsule will, of course, contribute significantly to the cycle of degeneration shown in Figure 3-17 because of the resultant alteration of normal joint mechanics.

Other reactive joint tissue changes occur if the process is allowed to continue, including osteophyte formation, subchondral sclerosis, subchondral sclerosis, subchondral cyst formation, and eburnation of exposed bone. Subchondral bone changes are likely to lead to an alteration in the forces that must be absorbed by the articular cartilage, because normally subchondral bone takes up much of the force of compressive loading.[61] In fact, some researchers believe that subchondral bone changes, such as sclerotic changes owing to altered blood flow, are often the first changes to take place in the degenerative cycle.[7]

Changes in composition and structure of the articular surface, caused by fibrillation and chondroitin sulfate depletion, are also likely to compromise the lubrication system of the joint. Large irregularities gradually make boundary lubrication less effective; loss of cartilage resiliency from chondroitin sulfate loss interferes with weeping lubrication. These potential changes in lubrication efficiency also seem to contribute further to the progression of degeneration.

Capsular Tightness

As indicated in the section on clinical application, specific joint mobilization techniques are primarily used in cases of capsuloligamentous tightness or adherence. There are, of course, cases in which an isolated portion of a joint capsule or supporting ligament is injured and heals in a state of relative shortening or becomes adhered to adjacent tissues during the healing process. Such pathologies are usually of traumatic origin, with a well-defined mechanism of injury and subsequent course. More often, however, the therapist is confronted with cases in which the entire joint capsule is "tight," as suggested by the presence of a capsular pattern of restriction at the joint. Conditions that cause a capsular pattern of restriction at a joint can be classified into two general categories: (1) conditions in which there is considerable joint effusion or synovial inflammation and (2) conditions in which there is a relative capsular fibrosis. It is important to make this distinction because the implications for management will vary according to the cause of the restriction.

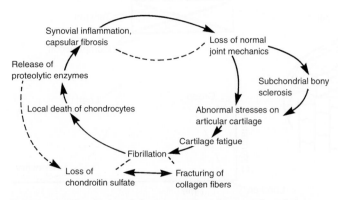

■ **FIG. 3-17.** Cycle of degenerative changes in a joint.

JOINT EFFUSION

Joint effusion causes a capsular pattern of restriction because of the distention of the joint capsule by the excessive intra-articular synovial fluid. Portions of the capsule that are normally lax to allow a certain range of movement become taut because of capsular distention. The joint tends to assume a position in which the joint cavity—the space enclosed by the joint capsule—is of maximum volume. The continuous pressure applied to the capsule by the joint fluid may effect abnormal firing of joint receptors, which results in an alteration in function of the muscles controlling the joint.[61] The rapid wasting of the quadriceps in the presence of knee joint effusion is believed to be a result of reflex muscle inhibition from abnormal receptor firing.[9] There may also be reflex facilitation of muscle activity, observed as muscle spasm or guarding, when the joint is moved. Those conditions that cause limited movement because of articular effusion may be classified broadly as inflammatory arthritis. These may, of course, include traumatic arthritis (in which some portion of the joint capsule is torn or stretched), rheumatoid arthritis (in which the synovial layer of the capsule is inflamed), infectious arthritis, gout, and others. In the acute stage of each of these conditions, the capsular restriction is primarily a result of the increased secretion of synovial fluid accompanying the acute stage of the inflammatory process, or it may result from reflex muscle guarding from abnormal firing of joint receptors. The cause of the restriction must be appreciated because, in such cases, clinicians do not wish to stretch the joint capsule to restore movement but rather to assist in the resolution of the acute inflammatory process.

RELATIVE CAPSULAR FIBROSIS

Relative capsular fibrosis most commonly accompanies one, or some combination, of the three following situations: (1) resolution of an acute articular inflammatory process; (2) a chronic, low-grade articular inflammatory process; and (3) immobilization of a joint.[2,12,13] The term **relative capsular fibrosis** has been used, up to this point, because histologically the capsular changes do not necessarily involve an increase in collagen content. It seems, instead, that inextensibility of capsular tissue may come about either from an increase in collagen content with respect to mucopolysaccharide content or from internal changes in the nature of the collagen tissue, such as changes in intermolecular cross-linking. The former might arise from an increased laying down of collagen, such as takes place during the repair phase of any inflammatory process.[1,8] It might also occur from a net loss of mucopolysaccharide content, with the total collagen content remaining constant. This typically occurs with prolonged immobilization of a joint.[12,45,60] One might consider the mucopolysaccharide content of connective tissue as serving as a lubricant for the collagen fibers; loss of the lubricant permits collagen fibers to approximate each other and to form abnormal interfiber cross-links. This inhibits their ability to glide against each other and thus reduces extensibility of the tissue.[1]

Clinically, it seems that conditions in which there is an actual increase in collagen content are more resistant to efforts to restore motion than are those cases of capsular restriction in which there is a net loss of mucopolysaccharide caused simply by immobilization. Also, inflammatory arthritis from infection resolves with a much greater degree of fibrosis (increase in collagen) than the capsular fibrosis that accompanies low-grade, noninfectious joint inflammation such as degenerative joint disease. Thus, the rate of improvement in range of motion might be expected to be more rapid in conditions at the top of the following list and slower when dealing with the capsular fibrosis that follows conditions near the bottom of this list:

> Simple immobilization
> Traumatic arthritis
> Degenerative arthrosis
> Rheumatoid arthritis
> Infectious arthritis

Several explanations are offered to account for the differences in rates of improvement noted above. First, relatively destructive processes, such as infectious arthritis or rheumatoid arthritis, might be met with a more vigorous repair response and, therefore, more collagen production during the resolution of the acute inflammatory process. Second, the period of immobilization, either prescribed or due to pain, is usually greater in acute inflammatory conditions, such as infectious or rheumatoid arthritis, than in relatively chronic conditions such as degenerative joint disease. The tendency, then, is for them to heal with less mobility. Third, during the mobilization period, the tissues may adapt more readily to increased mobility by laying down more mucopolysaccharide ground substance than they could by remodeling collagen. The maturation of the highly collagenous "scar tissue" is a longer, more involved process, involving reabsorption of excess collagen, realignment of collagen fiber orientation, and changes in the intermolecular cross-links within the collagen tissue.[1] In this way, capsular restriction from immobilization only, in which there is no increase in collagen content, is more easily resolved than conditions that lead to an actual increase in the collagen content of the joint capsules. It is clear from this discussion that the therapist must understand the nature of the pathologic process and its implications to set treatment goals accurately.

Clinical Considerations

Considering what is now known of the pathogenesis of osteoarthrosis, the accompanying biochemical responses, the pathologic tissue changes, and the clinical manifestations, some important conclusions and correlations are worth considering in the management of patients with arthrosis.

Subtle changes in joint kinematics, persisting over time, may cause abnormal stresses sufficient to result in gradual cartilage fatigue, which may, in turn, trigger a progression of changes leading to osteoarthrosis. Perhaps the most convincing evidence of this process is found in studies by Frankel and coworkers that show changes in the normal instant centers of motion in knee joints with minimal clinical signs or symptoms.[14,15] These changes suggested premature compression of joint surfaces accompanying knee extension. On careful clinical testing, loss of longitudinal external rotation of the tibia, with respect to the normal side, was found during extension on the involved side. Subsequent surgery revealed obvious "dimpling" of the cartilaginous joint surface, in the area of the cartilage compressed at full knee extension. In these cases internal derangement of the knee, although not sufficient to cause significant symptoms or signs, was responsible for altering normal knee mechanics enough to cause early cartilaginous changes, observable with the naked eye.

Up to a point in the progression of the disease, the cartilaginous destruction is repaired by increased proliferation and metabolic activity of chondrocytes, with laying down of new cartilage. The suggestion here is that osteoarthrosis is indeed somewhat reversible if managed correctly before severe progression has taken place. It is well known that osteotomy in the case of hip osteoarthrosis will cause the femoral head to become covered with fibrocartilage, with resultant restoration of the joint space on roentgenography. Studies suggest that it is partly a biologic phenomenon, perhaps from the hyperemia induced by the surgical procedure, as well as a mechanical phenomenon from the redistribution of stresses over the joint.[6]

If it is accepted that subtle changes in joint kinematics can lead to osteoarthrosis or, taken one step further, if this is the etiology in many of the cases that are considered primary or secondary osteoarthrosis, then evaluation techniques that can detect these changes are valuable. Instant center analysis is probably the best technique for detection of altered joint kinematics. However, because of the extra number of roentgenograms necessary, this technique is not practical for routine evaluation. In view of this, it seems that testing of joint-play movements is the most valuable technique clinically for detecting subtle joint changes that may be causing only minor signs or symptoms but may eventually lead to more serious joint changes in the form of osteoarthrosis. Joint-play techniques are important not only in evaluation of the patient presenting with obscure musculoskeletal complaints but also in evaluating the patient recovering from more serious trauma. Simply because a patient has regained full range of motion and strength does not guarantee that normal joint kinematics have been restored.

If osteoarthrosis may be caused by loss of normal joint mechanics, then primary treatments should be aimed at restoration of normal mechanics. This may entail surgery in cases such as meniscal tears and malalignment of bony structures. In cases of capsular tightness or capsular adhesion, treatment must consist of specific mobilization aimed at restoration of normal accessory movements at the joint. The approach to treatment of joint problems that appear to be mechanical should have a biomechanical basis. At present, treatment is too often "supportive" until obvious physiologic changes occur.

Current treatment tends to be directed at those physiologic changes, including various modalities for pain relief and pharmaceutical agents for controlling inflammation. Efforts to restore joint mechanics too often consist only of range-of-motion exercises and muscle strengthening, carried out without regard for the possible deleterious effects to the joint and without regard for abnormal reflex activity accompanying joint movement in the absence of normal arthrokinematics.

I believe that we, as clinicians, have yet to realize our full potential in the management of patients with mechanical joint disturbances. Knowledge of normal kinematics, ability to detect changes in joint mechanics through joint-play movements, and ability to restore normal component movements to a joint are necessary in successful management of patients with joint problems that are of a mechanical etiology or in which mechanical dysfunction is a prime factor.

REFERENCES

1. Akeson WH: An experimental study of joint stiffness. J Bone Joint Surg Am 43:1022–1034, 1961
2. Akeson WH, Amiel D, LaViolette D: The connective tissue response to immobility. Clin Orthop 51:183–197, 1967
3. Akeson WH, Woo SL, Amiel D: Biomechanical changes in periarticular connective tissues during contracture development in the immobilized rabbit knee. Connect Tissue Res 2:315–323, 1974
4. Barnett CH, Cochrane W, Palfray AJ: Age changes in articular cartilage of rabbits. Ann Rheum Dis 22:389–400, 1963
5. Barnett CH, Davies DV, MacConnaill MA: Synovial Joints: Their Structure and Function. Springfield, Charles C. Thomas, 1961
6. Bentley G: Articular cartilage studies and osteoarthrosis. Ann R Coll Surg Engl 57:86–100, 1975
7. Bollett AJ: Connective tissue polysaccharide metabolism and the pathogenesis of osteoarthritis. Adv Intern Med 13:33–60, 1967
8. Clayton ML, James SM, Abdulla M: Experimental investigations of ligamentous healing. Clin Orthop 61:146, 1968
9. de Andrade JR, Grant C, Dixon A: Joint distention and reflex muscle inhibition in the knee. J Bone Joint Surg Am 47:313–322, 1965
10. de Palma A, McKeever LD, Subin DK: Process of repair of articular cartilage demonstrated by histology and autoradiography with tritiated thymidine. Clin Orthop 48:229–242, 1966
11. Dowson D: Modes of lubrication in human joints. In: Lubrication and Wear in Living and Artificial Joints, vol. 181. London, Institute of Mechanical Engineers, 1967
12. Ely LW, Mensor MC: Studies on the immobilization of the normal joints. Surg Gynecol Obstet 57:212–215, 1963
13. Evans EB, Eggers GW, Butler JK, et al: Experimental immobilization and remobilization of rat knee joints. J Bone Joint Surg Am 42:737–758, 1960
14. Frankel VH: Biomechanics of the knee. In: Ingwersen O, ed: The Knee Joint. New York, Elsevier-Dutton, 1973
15. Frankel VH, Burstein AH, Brooks DB: Biomechanics of internal derangement of the knee: Pathomechanics as determined by analysis of the instant centers of motion. J Bone Joint Surg Am 53:945–962, 1971
16. Freeman MAR: Treatment of ruptures of the lateral ligament of the ankle. J Bone Joint Surg Br 47:661–668, 1965
17. Freeman MAR: The pathogenesis of primary osteoarthrosis. Mod Trends Orthop 6:40–90, 1972
18. Freeman MAR: Adult Articular Cartilage. London, Pitman & Sons, 1973
19. Freeman MAR: The fatigue of cartilage in the pathogenesis of osteoarthrosis. Acta Orthop Scand 46:323, 1975
20. Frymann VM: A study of the rhythmic motions of the living cranium. J Am Osteopath Assoc 70:928–945, 1971
21. Goodfellow J, Hungerford DS, Woods C: Patellofemoral joint mechanics and pathology: I and II. J Bone Joint Surg Br 58:287, 1976
22. Harryman DT, Sides JA, Clark JM, et al: Translation of the humeral head on the glenoid joint with passive glenohumeral motion. J Bone Joint Surg Am 72:1334–1343, 1990
23. Howell SM, Galinat BJ, Renzi AJ, et al: Normal and abnormal mechanics of the glenohumeral joint in the horizontal plane. J Bone Joint Surg Am 70:227–232, 1988
24. Johnell O, Telhag H: The effect of osteotomy and cartilage damage and mitotic activity: An experimental study in rabbits. Acta Orthop Scand 48:263–265, 1977
25. Kellgren JH: On the distribution of pain arising from deep somatic structures, with charts of segmental pain areas. Clin Sci 4:35, 1939

26. Klineberg IJ, Greenfield BE, Wyke B: Contribution to the reflex control of mastication from mechanoreceptors in the temporomandibular joint capsule. Dent Pract 21:73, 1970
27. Knott M, Voss D: Proprioceptive Neuromuscular Facilitation: Patterns and Techniques. New York, Harper & Row, 1968
28. Loubert PV: A qualitative biomechanical analysis of the concave–convex rule. Proceedings of the 5th International Conference of the International Federation of Orthopaedic Manipulative Therapists, Vail, Colorado, 1992:255–256
29. MacConnaill MA: The function of intra-articular fibrocartilage with special references to the knee and inferior radioulnar joints. J Anat 66:210–227, 1932
30. MacConnaill MA, Basmajian JV: Muscles and Movements: A Basis for Human Kinesiology. Baltimore, Williams & Wilkins, 1969
31. Mankin HJ: Biochemical and metabolic aspects of osteoarthritis. Orthop Clin North Am 2:19–31, 1971
32. Mankin HJ: The reaction of articular cartilage to injury and osteoarthrosis: I. N Engl J Med 291:1284, 1974
33. Mankin HJ: The reaction of articular cartilage to injury and osteoarthrosis: II. N Engl J Med 291:1335, 1974
34. Mankin HJ, Dorfman H, Lipiello L, et al: Biochemical and metabolic abnormalities in articular cartilage from osteoarthritic human hips. J Bone Joint Surg Am 53:523–537, 1971
35. Mankin HJ, Thrasher AZ, Hall D: Characteristics of articular cartilage from osteonecrotic femoral heads. J Bone Joint Surg Am 59:724–728, 1977
36. McClure PW, Flowers KR: Treatment of limited shoulder motions: A case study based on biomechanical considerations. Phys Ther 72:9229–9236, 1992
37. McCutcheon CW: Lubrication of joints. Br Med J 1:384–385, 1964
38. Meachim G: Articular cartilage lesions in osteoarthritis of the femoral head. J Pathol 107:199–210, 1972
39. Meachim G, Emergy IH: Cartilage fibrillation in shoulder and hip joints in Liverpool necropsies. J Anat 116:161–197, 1973
40. Meachim G, Emergy IH: Quantitative aspects of patellofemoral fibrillation in Liverpool necropsies. Ann Rheum Dis 33:39–47, 1974
41. Mennell J: Joint Pain. Boston, Little, Brown & Co, 1964
42. Nevaiser JS: Adhesive capsulitis of the shoulder: A study of pathologic findings in periarthritis of the shoulder. J Bone Joint Surg Am 27:211–222, 1945
43. Norkin CC, Levangie PK: Joint Structure and Function: A Comprehensive Analysis, 2nd ed. Philadelphia, FA Davis, 1992
44. Paris SV: Cranial manipulation. Fysioterapeuten 39:310, 1972
45. Peacock EE: Comparison of collagenous tissue surrounding normal and immobilized joints. Surg Forum 14:440, 1963
46. Poppen NK, Walker PS: Normal and abnormal motion of the shoulder joint. J Bone Joint Surg Am 58:195–201, 1976
47. Radin EL, Paul IL: Does cartilage compliance reduce skeletal impact loads? Arthritis Rheum 13:138, 1970
48. Radin EL, Paul IL: A consolidated concept of joint lubrication. J Bone Joint Surg Am 54:607–616, 1972
49. Roach JE, Tomblin W, Eyring EJ: Comparison of the effects of aspirin, steroids and sodium salicylate on articular cartilage. Clin Orthop 106:350–356, 1975
50. Rowinski MJ: Afferent neurobiology of the joint. In: Gould JA, Davies GJ, eds: Orthopaedic and Sports Physical Therapy, 2nd ed. St. Louis, CV Mosby, 1990
51. Sammarco GJ, Curstein AH, Frankel VH: Biomechanics of the ankle: A kinematic study. Orthop Clin North Am 4:75–95, 1973
52. Seileg AJ, Gerath M: An in vivo investigation of wear in animal joints. J Biomech 8:169–172, 1975
53. Sherrington C: The Integrative Action of the Nervous System. New Haven, Yale University Press, 1906
54. Skoglund S: Anatomic and physiologic studies of knee joint innervation in the cat. Acta Physiol Scand (Suppl) 124:1–100, 1956
55. Skolglund S: Joint receptors and kinaesthesis. In: Iggo A, ed: Handbook of Sensory Physiology, vol. II. Somatosensory System. New York, Springer-Verlag, 1973
56. Swanson SA: Lubrication of synovial joints. J Physiol 223:22, 1972
57. Voss D, Ionta MK, Myers BJ: Proprioceptive Neuromuscular Facilitation, 3rd ed. Philadelphia, Harper & Row, 1985
58. Warwick R, Williams P, eds: Gray's Anatomy, 36th ed. Philadelphia, WB Saunders, 1980
59. Weightman BO, Freeman MAR, Swanson SAV: Fatigue of articular cartilage. Nature 244:303–304, 1973
60. Woo SL, Matthews JV, Akeson WH, et al: Connective tissue response to immobility. Arthritis Rheum 18:257–264, 1975
61. Wright V, ed: Lubrication and Wear in Joints. Philadelphia, JB Lippincott, 1969
62. Wyke B: The neurology of joints. Ann R Coll Surg Engl 41:25–50, 1967

Chronic Pain Management in the Adult

JOYCE M. ENGEL

4

DEFINITION, INCIDENCE, AND COST OF CHRONIC NONMALIGNANT PAIN

The obligation to manage pain and relieve a patient's suffering is fundamental to healthcare. Cancer, traumatic injuries, and surgery result in millions of persons experiencing moderate to severe pain.[55] At least 50 million Americans live with chronic pain, and most are significantly disabled by it. The annual total financial cost (direct medical expenses, lost income, lost productivity, compensation payments, and legal fees) of all chronic pain syndromes is at least $100 billion.[1] Moreover, the cost of suffering cannot be estimated.

The International Association for the Study of Pain defines **pain** as "an unpleasant sensory and emotional experience associated with actual or potential tissue damage, or described in terms of such damage."[39] This definition conveys the multidimensional and subjective nature of pain.[54] Differentiating acute from chronic pain is essential for using the appropriate evaluation and intervention strategies. Acute pain and its associated physiologic, psychologic, and behavioral responses are almost invariably caused by tissue damage or irritating stimulation in relation to bodily insult or disease.[28] Chronic pain is described as a persistent pain that is not amenable to treatments based on specific remedies or to routine methods of pain control.[39] It does not serve a biologic purpose indicative of tissue damage or irritation. In chronic pain the body is unable to restore its physiologic functions to normal homeostatic levels.[34] Chronic pain often produces significant changes in mood (e.g., depression) and lifestyle.[21] Unrelieved pain may produce a decline in a person's routine activities and participation.[14]

Despite the magnitude of pain and suffering, chronic pain is often undertreated. The reasons for this include the low priority of providing consumers with pain relief in the healthcare system, lack of knowledge of pain interventions among healthcare professionals, and fear of opioid addiction among many healthcare professionals and the public.[1,7,21] Unfortunately, healthcare professionals often do not receive adequate education or training regarding appropriate evaluation and intervention for pain.[21,24]

COMMON CHRONIC PAIN SYNDROMES

Pain can be categorized by location or syndrome. In most persons with the complaints described below, usually the pain, not the underlying pathology, prevents them from achieving a productive and satisfying lifestyle.[5]

Low Back Pain

Most persons receiving physical therapy for pain complain of low back pain (LBP).[15] Approximately 3 to 7% of the population in Western industrialized countries experience chronic LBP. The impairment and disability associated with LBP often results in job absenteeism, loss of productive activity, and decreased participation.[58]

The most common causes of LBP are injury or stress resulting in musculoskeletal and neurologic disorders in the lumbosacral region (e.g., disk lesions, muscle spasm, sciatica). Pain may also result from infections, degenerative diseases, malignancies, and aging.[5] Poor posture may cause spinal disk degeneration and thus lead to LBP.[32] LBP tends to improve spontaneously over time.[60]

Headaches

Migraine and tension headaches are very common chronic pain complaints. Approximately 28 million Americans, roughly 18% of women and 6% of men, experience recurrent migraine headaches.[19] Experimental evidence supports the role of serotonin in migraine. Stress, attention, and mood (e.g., anxiety) affect these headaches. In contrast, tension headaches are generally considered to be muscular in origin. There is not sufficient evidence, however, for a specific pathophysiology.[3]

Myofascial Pain Syndrome

Myofascial pain syndrome (MPS) refers to a large group of muscle disorders characterized by highly sensitive trigger points within muscles or connective tissue. Myofascial pain is predominant and is perceived as a continual dull ache often located in the head, neck, shoulder, and low back areas. The trapezius muscle is one of the most commonly affected muscles. Myofascial pain may result from an acute strain caused by a sudden overload or overstretching of the muscle.[48]

Fibromyalgia

The prevalence of fibromyalgia ranges from 0.7 to 3.2% in the adult population. Fibromyalgia should not be confused with MPS. Although MPS and fibromyalgia may overlap clinically, they are two distinct pain syndromes. Skeletal muscles have been implicated as the cause of fibromyalgia, but no specific abnormalities have been identified. Abnormalities of the neuroendocrine system, autoimmune dysfunction, immune regulation, sleep disturbances, and cerebral blood flow difficulties have also been suggested.[22]

Chronic Pain Secondary to Physical Disability

Only recently has pain been investigated in persons who already have a physical disability. Chronic pain is a common problem following spinal cord injury (SCI). A recent community survey indicated 79% of adults with SCI reported a recurrent pain problem.[56] Pain may occur above, at, or below the level of injury in both complete and incomplete injuries. Neuropathic or central pain is the most frequent type of chronic pain in SCI and is believed to originate from abnormal processing of sensory input owing to damage to the central nervous system. Musculoskeletal pain complaints may result from a variety of factors, including wheelchair use.[11]

A typical consequence of amputation is phantom limb pain (PLP). As many as 85% of persons who undergo limb amputation will experience phantom limb pain. Residual limb pain ("stump pain") was reported by 72% of community-dwelling adults with lower limb amputations. Back pain has also been identified as a significant problem among many individuals with lower limb amputation.[11]

Adults with cerebral palsy frequently experience recurrent pain. Sixty-seven percent of a community sample reported chronic, bothersome pain. Low back and leg were identified as the most frequent sites. Pain has been associated with spasticity, scoliosis, and bony deformity resulting from spasticity.[11,45]

VIEWS OF PAIN

Because pain is viewed as being multidimensional and subjective, numerous theories and models exist to explain pain. Ideally, theories and models of pain transmission explain the range of pain phenomena.

Specificity Theory

The specificity theory was an initial attempt to explain the way the nervous system processes nociceptive (noxious stimuli) information. In 1894, Von Frey proposed that the sensation of pain resulted from a direct communication from specific pain receptors in the periphery to a central pain center in the brain. Physical characteristics of the pain stimulus (e.g., sharp quality) are transmitted from the pain receptors (free nerve endings) along specific peripheral nerve fibers (A-delta and C fibers) to the spinal cord. In the spinal cord, these impulses are conducted via the anterolateral spinothalamic tract to the brain (thalamus and higher centers), where they are then perceived as pain. Recently this theory has been criticized given current, observed clinical phenomena. The specificity theory assumes a direct relationship between stimulus intensity and perceived pain, yet the same stimulus may evoke varied responses in different individuals or even in the same individual under different conditions. In addition, interruptive surgical procedures like rhizotomy do not consistently eliminate pain despite interrupting this theoretical route of pain transmission.[54,4,12,44]

Pattern Theory

The pattern theory of pain transmission was proposed to address some of the limitations of the specificity theory. In 1894, Goldschneider suggested that it is not the direct stimulation of specific receptors, but the transmission of nerve impulse patterns coded at the periphery which causes the pain sensation. This theory proposes all nerve endings are alike, and the perception of pain is produced by intense stimulation of nonspecific receptors. The combination of direct stimulus added to other sensory inputs inform the central nervous system that pain is present. A key concept of this theory is the explanation it provides for phenomena such as phantom limb pain, in which the pain sensation continues to occur after the cessation of local stimulation. Several authors have criticized the pattern theory because it ignores evidence of receptor-fiber specialization such as the potential success of surgical procedures like cordotomy.[4,12,44]

Gate Control Theory

Melzack and Wall[38] offered a variation of the pattern and specificity theories to explain pain transmission. They suggested that skin receptors have specific physiologic properties by which they may transmit particular types and ranges of stimuli in the form of impulse patterns. According to this theory, pain is modulated by a "gating" mechanism located in the spinal cord that can increase or decrease the flow of nerve impulses to the brain. Afferent impulses can travel to the dorsal horn along large (A fiber) and small diameter (A-delta or C fiber) nerves associated with pain impulses. At the dorsal horn, these impulses encounter a gate thought to be substantia gelatinosa cells, This gate, which may be presynaptic or postsynaptic, can be closed, partially opened, or opened. When the gate is closed, pain impulses cannot proceed. When the gate is at least partially open, impulses stimulate T (transmission or trigger) cells in the dorsal horn which then ascend the spinal cord to the brain and pain perception results. Once the pain impulses are perceived, higher central nervous system structures (i.e., brainstem, thalamus, and cerebral cortex) can then modify pain by influencing T-cell activity. These structures can alter attention, memory, and affect, thereby contributing to an individual's unique pain perception.

Although the anatomic and physiologic bases of the gate remain controversial, this theory has been instrumental in furthering multidimensional pain evaluation and intervention. The gate control theory of pain implies psychology has much to offer in both understanding and treating pain. Motivational and cognitive processes thereby are examined in terms of their contribution to the pain experience.[12,44,50,53]

Loeser's Model

Loeser[32] proposed a biopsychosocial model of pain that suggests the phenomenon of pain can essentially be divided into four domains: nociception, pain, suffering, and pain behavior. **Nociception** is the detection of tissue damage by transducers in the skin and deeper structures and the central transmission of this information by A-delta and C fibers in the peripheral nerves. **Pain** thereby is the perception and interpretation of the nociceptive input by the highest parts of the brain. **Suffering** is the negative affective response to pain. It may be difficult to differentiate suffering from fear, anxiety, isolation, or depression. Lastly, **pain behavior** is what an individual says or does (e.g., taking medications) or does not say or do (e.g., job absenteeism), which leads others to believe that individual is suffering from noxious stimuli. Only pain behaviors are observable and measurable. Culture and environmental consequences influence pain behaviors. According to this model, one can experience or demonstrate some elements of the model in the absence of others. In chronic pain, pain behaviors and suffering often exist in the absence of nociception.[17,33,42,62]

ROLE OF THE PHYSICAL THERAPIST

Evaluation

The importance of adequate pain evaluation is being increasingly recognized in healthcare. Hospitals, outpatient clinics, home care agencies, nursing homes, and health plans accred-

ited by the Joint Commission on Accreditation of Health Care Organizations[27] require staff members to be competent in pain assessment. The American Pain Society (APS) has identified pain as the fifth vital sign. In addition, a goal of Healthy People 2010[41] is the promotion of the health of people with disabilities and the prevention of secondary conditions such as chronic pain. The inability to communicate verbally should not preclude pain assessment and treatment. Successful pain interventions are often predicated on accurate evaluation of the pain complaint.[42] Proper evaluation requires the use of valid and reliable instruments for determining the need for intervention and its effects.

PHYSICAL EXAMINATION

Traditionally, physical therapists have relied on clinical tests of impairment when evaluating the consumer. These tests, however, correlate poorly with self-reports of chronic pain and dysfunction. Standardized tests of range of motion and muscle strength lack sensitivity, specificity, and responsiveness. Complex and expensive isoinertial and isokinetic devices measure strength, range, and velocity of motion reliably, but the individual's performance can be affected greatly by factors such as fear of injury, motivation, and mood. In addition, use of these devices does not simulate activity performance and participation.[20]

FUNCTIONAL PERFORMANCE

Clinical improvement can be measured as improvements in activity performance and participation. The Brief Pain Inventory[9] is a reliable and valid instrument used to measure pain interference. Consumers rate on an ordinal scale how much their pain has interfered with general activity, mood, mobility, work, interpersonal relationships, sleep, enjoyment of life, self-care, and recreation.

PAIN INTENSITY

Because pain is a private experience that cannot be observed directly, assessment of the pain experience is frequently through self-reports. A reduction in pain intensity is typically the primary reason a consumer seeks services. Numerous measures exist to assess the severity of pain. The three most common measures are the verbal rating scale (VRS), the numerical rating scale (NRS), and the visual analog scale (VAS). The VRS consists of a list of adjectives ranging from no pain to extreme pain to describe different levels of pain. In contrast, the NRS requires consumers to rate their pain on a scale from 0 to 10 or 0 to 100, with the understanding that 0 is equal to "no pain" and the 10 or 100 is equal to the "most excruciating pain possible." Finally, the VAS consists of a 10-cm line for which the ends are labeled as the extremes (e.g., "no pain" to "pain as bad as it could be"). These rating scales are easy to administer and score, have good evidence for construct validity, are sensitive to treatment, and are used fairly reliably by consumers.[26,42]

PAIN BEHAVIORS

In accordance with Fordyce's seminal work[16] and Loeser's model of pain,[32] pain behaviors are to be considered in evaluation and intervention. For some individuals with severe disabilities pain behaviors are the only way to communicate pain. For others, pain behaviors can be explored within the context of functional analysis. Functional analysis can determine the degree to which pain behaviors are influenced by social and environmental variables.[42] Keefe et al.[29] suggested five options for assessing pain behavior: continuous observation, duration, frequency, time sampling (counting behavior at prespecified time intervals), and interval recording (observation broken into equal-length intervals). More in-depth information on pain behavior assessment and related treatment strategies can be found in Fordyce's publications.[16,33]

CULTURAL, FAMILIAL, AND SPIRITUAL INFLUENCES

Cultural, familial, and spiritual influences are other important factors to be considered in pain evaluation and intervention, especially when the pain etiology is unclear. Each culture, family, and religion has it own system of beliefs, attitudes, and values.[2] The individual therefore may be rewarded, ignored, or punished for having pain behaviors.[12]

Intervention

Pain interventions have changed dramatically over the years. The focus of treatment has shifted from dealing with impairments to emphasizing increasing function.[61] Healthcare consumers are no longer passive, and they expect practitioners to be accountable for provided services. A multidisciplinary team approach to chronic pain is common and includes the consumer as an active and educated participant.[24,46] The Commission on Accreditation of Rehabilitation Facilities (CARF) has identified pain management standards.[36] Other key team members in addition to the physical therapist are a physician and a psychologist or psychiatrist. An occupational therapist, vocational counselor, or dietician may also provide evaluation and intervention.[10] Chronic pain interventions strive to increase the consumer's activity performance and participation as well as reduce reliance on healthcare providers.

The data provided below are specific to the pain population identified for that intervention.

ACTIVE REHABILITATION PROGRAM

Physical therapy treatment goals may be achieved through physical restoration. An active rehabilitation program is not synonymous with exercise. In addition to prescribed exercises, an active rehabilitation program emphasizes behavioral strategies to help consumers better cope with and manage their pain.[18] The primary assumption of this intervention is that the major physical deficit is the "deconditioning syndrome," consequent to prolonged disuse of spinal joints and muscles. Physical therapy treatment therefore consists of individualized physical reconditioning exercises/activities based on objective quantification of physical functioning.[61] Treatment also needs to address long-term adaptations the body makes in its movement patterns and adaptations in connective tissue.[47] Ideally the physical therapist collaborates with the consumer in the development and implementation of the treatment program. Consumers should be informed that they might experience a slight increase in symptoms with the initiation of treatment and that increased pain with increased activity does not equal harm.[61]

THERAPEUTIC EXERCISE

Therapeutic exercise is a critical component of an active rehabilitation program. Exercise therapy is often prescribed for the relief of pain and improving function. Although rest may be beneficial for a few days after an acute injury, it is contraindicated for persons with chronic nonmalignant pain.[18,35] Prolonged rest and inactivity result in decreased mobility, reduced strength, lessened cardiopulmonary endurance, increased joint stiffness, and postural strain.[46,61] Wittink et al.[61] recommended that consumers be educated about the effects of deconditioning in addition to bodily changes occurring when an exercise program begins.

Evidence-based research supports active rehabilitation programs as the most effective means of achieving pain relief and reducing disability for persons with chronic LBP.[60] The recent Cochrane Review of exercise for LBP[51] indicated that exercises might be helpful for individuals to increase and tolerate routine activities of daily living, including work. It remains unclear, however, if any specific type of exercise (e.g., flexion or extension, strengthening) is superior. Success in an exercise program can make the difference between function and failure. Therefore, the physical therapist must assist the consumer in developing and implementing a daily exercise routine that is appropriate, structured, and meaningful.[61]

SOFT TISSUE MANIPULATION

Soft tissue manipulations can be directed at muscle, ligaments, and fascial layers to restore mobility and extensibility impacted by pain.[23] Information about soft tissue manipulation is provided in Chapter 8.

FELDENKRAIS METHOD

The Feldenkrais method is based on the premise that humans have a choice in developing habits of movement. In addition, mental and emotional activity are recognized as influencing human performance. The consumer is therefore invited to participate in intervention. Treatment consists of the physical therapist continually observing and then adapting stimuli to facilitate the consumer's exploration and development of adaptive skills to maximize function despite pain.[25] Further discussion of the Feldenkrais method is beyond the scope of this chapter.

QUOTA PROGRAMS

Increasing the consumer's activities and participation are the cornerstone of most chronic pain management programs. Intervention begins with a series of baseline trials in which the consumer is asked to perform a demonstrated exercise to tolerance. Tolerance is defined as the point at which an individual stops exercising because of pain or fatigue. Detailed pretreatment performances are documented. The physical therapist then establishes a quota for each prescribed mobility, strengthening, and/or cardiovascular endurance exercise/activity to be performed. Use of a quota system eliminates the linking of pain with function that often resulted in overdoing on "good days" and avoiding exercise on "bad days." Initial quotas are slightly lower than baseline trials (approximately 75% of average) and are increased by predetermined small increments (typically 10% every few days) regardless of how the consumer feels. Treatment also involves positively reinforcing (e.g., praising) the consumer's attempts and gains in functional performance. Resting before the quota is discouraged because it may reinforce pain behaviors.[16,30,61] A gradual increase in activity demands also decreases the likelihood of an exacerbation of pain.[61] Quota programs have been effective in increasing functional performance in persons with LBP.[17,18,31] Modalities (heat or cold) may be applied to prepare the consumer for therapeutic exercise or the initiation of activities.[12,20]

OPERANT TRAINING

Pain behaviors can be severely disabling. Vlaeyen et al.[59] used the operant principle of shaping (reinforcement of the small steps it takes to reach a goal) to increase sitting and standing tolerance in a consumer with chronic LBP after laminectomy. Each time a subgoal was achieved, a treatment team member provided social reinforcement. Treatment gains were generalized to a variety of settings and from an adjustable stool to a chair. Shaping principles were also successfully used to increase upper extremity use in adults with chronic pain and hysterical paralys.[8] A recent Cochrane Review indicated there is strong evidence that behavioral treatment of adults with chronic LBP resulted in small to moderate decreases in pain intensity and improved functional performance.[52]

MODALITIES

The use of modalities for persons with chronic pain complaints is disputed. Some practitioners advocate for only using self-management interventions (e.g., exercise, relaxation) because chronic pain cannot be "fixed."[61] Other practitioners do use modalities (e.g., heat therapy, transcutaneous electrical stimulation) and massage as an adjunct to other interventions.[15,47] Further discussion of modalities is beyond the scope of this chapter.

BODY MECHANICS AND POSTURAL INSTRUCTION

Instruction in and practice of proper body mechanics and postures that will not increase the risk of low back injury or strain are important for consumers experiencing both acute and chronic musculoskeletal pain as well as implications for primary prevention.[37] There is a lack of consensus in the literature, however, about specific lifting techniques.[49]

LUMBAR SUPPORTS

Lumbar supports may be used to reduce impairment and disability in persons with nonspecific LBP. Lumbar supports may also be used to prevent recurrences of LBP episodes. The Cochrane Review of lumbar supports for prevention and treatment of LBP indicated there is limited scientific evidence to advocate for the use of lumbar supports in pain relief.[58] There is some evidence that a lumbar support with a rigid insert in the back provides more overall improvement than a lumbar support without a rigid insert. In addition, there is conflicting evidence that consumers who use a lumbar support to return to work do so more quickly when compared with other interventions.[58] In some active rehabilitation programs consumers are weaned from lumbar supports as well as braces, canes, crutches, and pain medications.[61]

RELAXATION TRAINING

A variety of relaxation training strategies exist: autogenics; progressive, deep muscle relaxation; and guided imagery. Autogenics involves the silent repetition of phrases of self-directed formulas to describe the psychophysiologic aspects of relaxation (e.g., "My right arm is heavy"). The consumer passively concentrates on these phrases while assuming a reclined position, with eyes closed, in a quiet setting. The goal of this relaxation approach is to develop an association between a verbal cue (thought of relaxation) and a state of calmness. Progressive relaxation involves the systematic tensing of major musculoskeletal groups for a few seconds, passive focusing of attention on how the tensed muscle feels, and then release of the muscles and passive focusing on how relaxation feels. As the consumer learns to recognize the sensations of muscle tension, he or she can direct attention to inducing relaxation.

The rationale that underlies the analgesic effects of relaxation is that muscle tension results in pain. Muscle relaxation, therefore, will reduce or eliminate pain attributed to muscle tension. Guided imagery requires the consumer to develop a calm, peaceful image (e.g., a beautiful garden). He or she concentrates on that image for the duration of the pain or stress episode. The premise of this strategy is that an individual cannot concentrate on more than one thing at any given time. A strong image is needed to divert attention away from the pain complaint.[13,43] Relaxation training has been used successfully to relieve a variety of pain complaints, including headache, LBP, and myofascial pain.[57] In fact, the National Institutes of Health[40] concluded that, "The evidence is strong for the effectiveness of this class of techniques in reducing chronic pain in a variety of medical conditions." Additional details regarding relaxation training can be found in Chapter 9.

BIOFEEDBACK

Biofeedback refers to instrumentation used to provide consumers with immediate feedback of electronically monitored physiologic sites. This intervention assumes that a faulty body function causes pain, and that with feedback the consumer can learn to control the impairment.[57] Biofeedback does not do anything to the consumer; it merely facilitates learning body control. Biofeedback for pain control is typically done in conjunction with relaxation training. Skin temperature biofeedback to increase digital temperature in vascular pain complaints (e.g., migraine headaches) and electromyographic (EMG) biofeedback to decrease skeletal muscle pain (e.g., tension headaches) are standard treatments in multidisciplinary pain clinics. An evidence-based review by Turner and Chapman[57] revealed increased hand temperature resulted in decreased migraine headaches. Temperature changes, however, were not significantly correlated with symptom reduction. Therefore, other factors (e.g., suggestion, expectancy) may be responsible for the desired changes.[6]

Relapse Management

Consumers with chronic pain frequently experience an acute pain episode not related to their pain (nociception evident) or a significant exacerbation of their pain resulting from increased activity. Until the consumer has recovered from the acute incident, endurance (aerobic) conditioning exercises (e.g., walking, stationary biking, swimming) should be performed to help avoid dehabilitation from inactivity. An incremental, gradual increase in conditioning exercises can be implemented.[18]

CONCLUSION

Evaluation and treatment of individuals with chronic pain is complicated. Chronic pain is best managed by prevention.[46] Prevention reduces pain, suffering, healthcare costs, and the incidence of long-term disability. Physical therapists have a critical role in the prevention, evaluation, and treatment of persons with chronic pain.

REFERENCES

1. American Academy of Pain Medicine. FAQs. FAQs about pain [On-line]. Available at http://www.painmed.org/faqs/pain_faqs.html, 2001
2. Baptiste S: Chronic pain, activity and culture. Can J Occup Ther 55:179–184, 1988
3. Biber MP: Headache. In: Warfield CA, Fausett HJ, eds: Manual of Pain Management, 2nd ed. Philadelphia, Lippincott Williams & Wilkins, 2002:35–45
4. Bockrath M: Fundamentals. In: Carey KW, Forbes SL, Goldberg KE, et al., eds: Pain. Springhouse, Springhouse, 1985:6–24
5. Bonica JJ: General considerations of chronic pain. In: Bonica JJ, ed: The Management of Pain, 2nd ed. Philadelphia, Lea & Febiger, 1990:2–17
6. Boothy JL, Thorn BE, Stroud MW, et al: Coping with pain. In: Gatchel RJ, Turk DC, eds: Psychological Factors in Pain. New York, Guilford Press, 1999:343–359
7. Brownlee S, Schrof JM: The quality of mercy. U.S. News and World Report (March 17:55–57, 60–62, 65, 67, 1997
8. Cardenas DD, Larson J, Egan KJ: Hysterical paralysis in the upper extremity of chronic pain patients. Arch Phys Med Rehabil 67:190–193, 1986
9. Cleeland CS, Ryan KM: Pain assessment: Global use of the Brief Pain Inventory. Ann Acad Med 23:129–138, 1994
10. Commission on Accreditation of Rehabilitation Facilities: 2001 Medical Rehabilitation Standards Manual. Tucson, The Commission on Accreditation of Rehabilitation Facilities, 2001
11. Ehde DM, Jensen MP, Engel JM, et al: Chronic pain secondary to disability: A review. Clin J Pain. 2003, 19:3–17
12. Engel JM: Treatment for psychosocial components: Pain management. In: Neistadt ME, Crepeau EB, eds: Willard and Spackman's Occupational Therapy, 9th ed. Philadelphia, Lippincott, 1998:454–458
13. Engel JM: Pain management. In: Pedretti LW, Early ME, eds: Occupational Therapy: Practice Skills for Physical Dysfunction, 5th ed. St. Louis, Mosby, 2001:493–500
14. Engel JM: Pain management. In: Crepeau EB, Cohen E, Schell BA, eds: Willard and Spackman's Occupational Therapy, 10th ed. Philadelphia, Lippincott Williams & Wilkins, 2003:634–637
15. Fernando CK: Physical therapy and pain management. In: Weiner RS, ed: Pain Management: A Practical Guide for Clinicians, 6th ed. Boca Raton, CRC Press, 2002:739–747
16. Fordyce, WE: Behavioral Methods for Chronic Pain and Illness. St. Louis, CV Mosby, 1976
17. Fordyce WE: Contingency management. In: Bonica JJ, ed: The Management of Pain, 2nd ed. Philadelphia, Lea & Febiger, 1990:1702–1710
18. Fordyce WE, ed: Back Pain in the Workplace: Management of Disability in Nonspecific Conditions. Seattle, IASP Press, 1995:43–56
19. Gallagher RM: Primary headache disorders. In: Weiner RS, ed: Pain Management: A Practical Guide for Clinicians, 6th ed. Boca Raton, CRC Press, 2001:195–206
20. Harding VR, Simmonds MJ, Watson PJ: Physical therapy for chronic pain. Pain Clinical Updates, VI(3):1–4, Seattle, IASP Press, 1998
21. Hawthorn J, Redmond K: Pain: Causes and Management. Malden, Blackwell Science, 1998
22. Hernández-García JM: Fibromyalgia. In: Warfield CA, Fausett HJ, eds: Manual of Pain Management, 2nd ed. Philadelphia, Lippincott Williams & Wilkins, 2002:154–157
23. Hertling D, Kessler RM: Assessment of musculoskeletal disorders and concepts of management. In: Hertling D, Kessler RM, eds: Management of Common Musculoskeletal Disorders: Physical Therapy Principles and Methods, 3rd ed. Philadelphia, Lippincott-Raven, 1996:69–111
24. International Association for the Study of Pain ad hoc Subcommittee for Occupational Therapy/Physical Therapy Curriculum: Pain curriculum for students in occupational therapy or physical therapy. IASP Newslett Nov/Dec:3–8, 1994
25. Jackson-Wyatt O: Feldenkrais method and rehabilitation: A paradigm shift incorporating a perception of learning. In: Davis CM, ed: Complementary Therapies in Rehabilitation: Holistic Approaches for Prevention and Wellness. Thorofare, Slack, 1997:189–197
26. Jensen MP, Karoly P: Self-report scales and procedures for assessing pain in adults. In: Turk DC, Melzack R, eds: Handbook of Pain Assessment, 2nd ed. New York, Guilford Press, 1992:131–151
27. Joint Commission on Accreditation of Healthcare Organizations: Pain Standards for 2001. Oakbrook Terrace, Joint Commission on Accreditation of Healthcare Organizations, 2001
28. Katz ER, Varni JW, Jay SM: Behavioral assessment and management of pediatric pain. Prog Behav Mod 18:163–193, 1990
29. Keefe FJ, Williams DA, Smith SJ: Assessment of pain behaviors. In: Turk DC, Melzack R, eds: Handbook of Pain Assessment, 2nd ed. New York, Guilford Press, 2001:170–187
30. Linchitz RM, Capulong E, Battista DJ, et al: Physical modalities for pain management. In: Ashburn MA, Rice LJ, eds: The Management of Pain. New York, Churchill Livingstone, 1998:401–418
31. Lindstrom I, Ohlund C, Eek C, et al: The effect of graded activity on patients with subacute low back pain: A randomized prospective clinical study with an operant-conditioning behavioral approach. Phys Ther 27(4):279–293, 1992
32. Loeser JD: Concepts of pain. In: Stanton-Hicks M, Boas RA, eds: Chronic Low Back Pain. New York, Raven Press, 1982:145–148
33. Loeser JD, Fordyce WE: Chronic pain. In: Carr JE, Dengerink HA, eds. Behavioral Medicine in the Practice of Medicine. New York, Elsevier, 1983:331–345
34. Loeser JD, Melzack R: Pain: An overview. Lancet 353:1607–1609, 1999
35. Lynch MK, Kessler RM, Hertling D: Pain. In: Hertling D, Kessler RM, eds: Management of Common Musculoskeletal Disorders: Physical Therapy Principles and Methods, 3rd ed. Philadelphia, Lippincott Williams & Wilkins, 1996:50–68
36. MacDonell C: Accreditation of pain management programs. In: Ashburn MA, Rice LJ, eds: The Management of Pain. New York, Churchill Livingstone, 1998:227–234
37. McCauley M: The effects of body mechanics instruction on work performance among young workers. Am J Occup Ther 44:402–407, 1990
38. Melzack R, Wall, P: Pain mechanisms: A new theory. Science 50:971–979, 1965
39. Merskey H, Bogduk N, eds: Classification of Chronic Pain: Descriptions of Chronic Pain Syndromes and Definition of Pain Terms, 2nd ed. Seattle, IASP Press, 1994:210

40. National Institutes of Health: Integration of behavioral and relaxation approaches into the treatment of chronic pain and insomnia. NIH Technology Assessment Conference Statement, October 16, 1995, p. 9

41. Office of Disease Prevention and Health Promotion, Department of Health and Human Services: Healthy People 2010: Understanding and Improving Health (Stock No. 017-001-005550-9); retrieved July 15, 2001, from http://www.health.gov./healthypeople, 2001

42. Patterson DR, Jensen M, Engel-Knowles J: Pain and its influence on assistive technology use. In: Scherer MJ, ed: Assistive Technology: Matching Device and Consumer for Successful Rehabilitation. Washington, DC, American Psychological Association, 2002:59–76

43. Rice PL: Stress & Health, 2nd ed. Pacific Grove, Brooks/Cole Publishing, 1992

44. Schechter NL: Pain and pain control in children. Curr Probl Pediatr 15(5):3–67, 1985

45. Schwartz L, Engel JM, Jensen MP: Pain in persons with cerebral palsy. Arch Phys Med Rehabil 80(10):1243–1246, 1999

46. Scotece GG: Physical therapy and the management of pain. Orthop Phys Ther Clin North Am 4(4):541–554, 1995

47. Shillue KE. Physical therapy. In: Warfield CA, Fausett HJ, eds: Manual of Pain Management, 2nd ed. Philadelphia, Lippincott Williams & Wilkins, 2002:305–308

48. Sola AE, Bonica JJ: Myofascial pain syndromes. In: Bonica JJ, ed: The Management of Pain, 2nd ed. Philadelphia, Lea & Febiger, 1990:352–357

49. Strong J: Lifestyle management. In: Strong J, Unruh AM, Wright A, et al., eds: Pain: A Textbook for Therapists. New York, Churchill Livingstone, 2002:289–306

50. Suchdev PK: Pathophysiology of pain. In: Warfield CA, Fausett HJ, eds: Manual of Pain Management, 2nd ed. Philadelphia, Lippincott Williams & Wilkins, 2002:6–12

51. Tulder, MW van, Malmivaara A, Esmail R, et al: Exercise therapy for low back pain (Cochrane Review). In: The Cochrane Library, Issue 3. Oxford, Update Software, 2000

52. Tulder MW van, Ostelo RWJG, Vlaeyen JWS, et al: Behavioural treatment for chronic low back pain. In: The Cochrane Library, Issue 3. Oxford, Update Software, 2002

53. Turk DC, Genest M: Regulation of pain: The application of cognitive and behavioral techniques for prevention and remediation. In: Kendall PC, Hollon SD, eds: Cognitive-Behavioral Intervention: Theory, Research, and Procedures. New York, Academic Press, 1979:287–318

54. Turk DC, Meichenbaum D, Genest M: Pain and Behavioral Medicine. New York, Guilford 1983

55. Turk DC, Melzack R: The measurement of pain and the assessment of people experiencing pain. In: Turk DC, Melzack R, eds: Handbook of Pain Assessment. New York, Guilford Press, 1992:3–12

56. Turner JA, Cardenas DD, Warms CA, et al: Chronic pain associated with spinal cord injuries: A community survey. Arch Phys Med Rehabil 82(4):501–509, 2001

57. Turner JA, Chapman CR: Psychological interventions for chronic pain: A critical review. I. Relaxation training and biofeedback. Pain 12:23–46, 1982

58. Van Tulder MW, Jellema P, van Poppel MNM, et al: Lumbar supports for prevention and treatment of low back pain (Cochrane Review). In: The Cochrane Library, Issue 4. Oxford, Update Software, 2000.

59. Vlaeyen JWS, Groenman NH, Thomassen J, et al: A behavioural treatment for sitting and standing intolerance in a patient with chronic low back pain. Clin J Pain 5:233–237, 1989

60. Waddell G: A new clinical model for the treatment of low back pain. Spine 12:632–644, 1987

61. Wittink H, Michel TH, Cohen LJ, et al: Physical therapy treatment. In: Wittink H, Michel TH, eds: Chronic Pain Management for Physical Therapists. Boston, Butterworth-Heinemann, 1997:119–156

62. Wolff M, Wittink H, Michel TH: Chronic pain concepts and definitions. In: Wittink H, Michel TH, eds: Chronic Pain Management for Physical Therapists. Boston, Butterworth-Heinemann, 1997:1–26

Assessment of Musculoskeletal Disorders and Concepts of Management

DARLENE HERTLING AND RANDOLPH M. KESSLER

5

RATIONALE

A comprehensive examination is, without question, the most important step in the manual therapy practitioner's management of patients with common musculoskeletal disorders. The practitioner's role is to clarify the nature and extent of the lesion, to assess the extent of the resulting disability, and to record significant data to establish a basis against which progress can be judged. These activities must not be confused with or mistaken for the physician's diagnosis. The physician's diagnosis, in addition to clinical evaluation, often requires the use and interpretation of laboratory tests, roentgenograms, and other data employing skills and knowledge not included in most manual therapy practitioners' training. Diagnosis must differentiate a particular disease state from other possible causes of the symptoms and signs. The practitioner, in performing a clarifying examination, is not concerned with such differentiation but with collecting qualitative and quantitative data on the existing lesion.

A good manual therapy practitioner, however, is one who is trained in and acquainted with the global medical picture of organic and nonorganic causes of pain and who is clinically perceptive in quickly recognizing any potential danger ("red flag") signs and symptoms that would indicate the need to involve a medical practitioner. Patients need and appreciate early referral when appropriate. Important areas that demand surveillance and indicate the need for physician referral include metastatic disease, vertebrobasilar insufficiency, active infec-tion or inflammation (including rheumatoid arthritis), instability following trauma, and neurologic changes (such as spinal cord compression, cauda equina compression, and nerve root compression).

Diagnosis by a manual therapy practitioner means naming or labeling the movement dysfunction or problem that is the object of the therapy.[11,94] Diagnostic labeling is the result of the systematic analysis and grouping of the clinical manifestations of the patient.[5,28,51,91,94] Sahrmann[94] suggests the focus of such classification should be on the primary dysfunction identified in the evaluation. Jette[51] suggests that diagnostic categories should include physical impairment and functional disabilities based on the International Classification of Impairments, Disabilities, and Handicaps (ICIDH).[42] Both qualitative and quantitative data on the existing lesion are used to judge how best to apply certain treatment procedures and to assess their effectiveness.

Consider the case of a patient referred to a manual therapy practitioner with the diagnosis of "shoulder tendinitis." This is a condition easily managed by manual therapy over a relatively short period. However, for an effective program to be instituted, several features of the problem must be clarified. The clinician must determine which tendon is at fault to know where to direct treatment and at what site on the tendon the lesion exists. Assessment of the lesion's chronicity will influence the choice of treatment procedures and their application. It is important to know whether secondary problems such as stiffness or weakness exist; if so, they must be dealt with as well.

The practitioner must obtain information concerning the possible behavioral effects of the lesion. Are the conditions accompanying the problem reinforcing in any way to the patient's disease behaviors or is the patient "highly motivated?" Daily activities must be assessed not only to determine the existence of any functional deficit but also to judge whether any present activity will aggravate or prolong the condition. Generally, such information does not accompany the referral, but it is precisely this information that is required to institute an effective treatment program. The clinician must perform a thorough initial examination on every patient he or she treats.

As mentioned, information collected as part of the initial examination is used to set a baseline against which to judge progress and to assess the effectiveness of treatment. Therefore, the clinician not only must perform a complete initial examination but also must assess certain key signs before, during, and after each treatment session. In this way the clinician can determine whether, in fact, a particular procedure is effective and can quantitatively document the patient's progress. Progress must be judged on objective evidence. The patient's subjective report of the degree of pain must be considered but not dwelt on; in itself, it is not a valid measurement of progress. Instead, the clinician should be able to inform the patient as to whether the condition has improved. Treatment sessions should begin less often with, "Hello, Mrs. Jones. How is your back today?" but rather with, "Hello, Mrs. Jones. Let's take a look at your back to see how it's doing." This approach is possible only after complete initial examination and continued assessment of objective signs.

There are, of course, several approaches to patient examination.[17,37,56,57,73,74,77,78,80,81,105] Included in this group are Cyriax,[17] Kaltenborn,[56,57] Maitland,[73,74] McKenzie,[77,78] and Stoddard.[105] Their approaches are frequently used by practitioners of manual therapy to assess and treat muscle and joint problems. Regardless of which system is selected for assessment, the examiner must establish a sequential method to ensure that no crucial test or step is omitted; such an omission could prevent accurate interpretation. Perhaps no one has contributed more to systematization of soft tissue examination than James Cyriax.[17] His approach involves observation, subjective examination (patient history), objective examination (utilization of movements and special tests to elicit signs and symptoms of injury), palpation of soft tissues, and neurologic testing.[17]

One of the more common assessment recording methods used today is the problem-oriented medical records method, which uses SOAP notes.[61,69,120] SOAP stands for the four parts of the assessment—subjective (patient history), objective, assessment, and plan. Progress notes and the discharge summary should also follow the SOAP format and in combination with the initial examination, assessment, and treatment plan, they become the complete record for most patients. The assessment includes professional judgments about the sub-

jective and/or objective findings formulated into both long-term and short-term goals.

HISTORY

To help determine the nature and extent of the lesion and the resultant degree of disability, the clinician must gather data from the patient that cannot be determined by physical examination. These subjective findings are correlated with the findings of the physical examination.

In the case of common musculoskeletal disorders, the lesion is usually manifested primarily by pain. Some of the routine questions suggested here as part of every history are directed at obtaining a complete account of the history of the pain and the present status of the pain as perceived by the patient. However, the clinician must also inquire about other symptoms, such as paresthesias, feelings of weakness, feelings of instability, and autonomic disturbances. It is important to keep in mind that the patient's perception of pain and other symptoms offers valuable clues to the nature and extent of the lesion but does not alone serve as an indicator of progress. For that, the examiner must rely on assessment of objective signs and examination of the patient's functional status.

Determination of the degree of disability offers some data by which to judge progress legitimately. It also yields information concerning the nature and extent of the lesion. This is an important part of the history and is too often omitted. To determine the degree of disability the patient's "health-state" behaviors and activity level (occupation, recreation, and other activities of daily life) are assessed as well as the patient's "disease-state" behaviors and activity level. Documentation of the disease-state behaviors sets a baseline against which to judge progress; comparison with the patient's health-state behaviors may provide clues to the nature and extent of the problem. For example, the patient with a shoulder problem who has been able to comb her hair all her life but since the onset of the problem is unable to do so, lacks full, pain-free active elevation and external rotation. This is very suggestive of a capsular restriction. In this example there are some data to compare with the physical findings that may help determine the nature and extent of the lesion. One treatment goal will naturally be to restore the patient's ability to comb her hair. A criterion by which to judge progress has also been established. Consequently, when judging progress, the clinician must be less concerned with whether Mrs. Jones had shoulder pain that morning, its extent, or duration and be more concerned with whether Mrs. Jones was able to comb her hair.

Disability assessment and disease-state behavior assessment become especially important in evaluating patients with a chronic-pain state who have no physical findings or pain that is out of proportion to physical findings and in evaluating patients with a permanent functional deficit from some serious pathologic process. In the first situation, it is often necessary to change from a "medical model" (in which treatment is aimed at the lesion to change behavior) to an "operant model" (in which treatment is aimed at altering the consequences of the disease-state behaviors).[30–32] In the second situation, treatment is no longer directed at the primary lesion (e.g., a spinal cord lesion), but rather at improving residual function. There are some relatively common disorders in which pain complaints and functional disability are out of proportion to the extent of the pathologic process. Some of these abnormal pain states, such as reflex sympathetic dystrophy (see Chapter 13, Wrist and Hand Complex), have a physiologic basis. Other cases, such as those involving pending litigation, substantial monetary compensation, or welcomed time away from activities the patient finds undesirable, may have a psychosocial basis. The patient's pain or disability may promise rewards, which may in turn reinforce disease-state behaviors. It is essential that the presence of such abnormal behavior states be determined on examination. In these cases, treatment aimed primarily at some physical pathologic process may only serve to maintain the patient's disability. Primary emphasis must be placed on improved function by altering the consequences of the disabled state (Fig. 5-1).

Although this text emphasizes the assessment and treatment of the lesion itself, clinicians must not lose sight of the fact that they are treating patients and that the ultimate goal in any treatment program is rehabilitation of the patient. Even when treatment is aimed largely at the lesion, care must be taken not to reinforce the disease state or especially pain behavior. Similarly, clinicians must also be concerned with functional deficits associated with the disease state and see that they are resolved, when possible, along with the primary pathologic process. Thus, whether patient management is approached through a medical model or through an operant model, the primary goal is to restore health-state behaviors. When a well-defined lesion exists, and the consequences of the resulting disability appear to have a negative effect on the patient's attitude toward the disability, it can be reasonably expected that resolving the pathologic process will restore health-state behavior. However, when the consequences of disability are rewarding to the patient, treatment of the pathologic process may have little or no effect.

The specific inquiries during the initial history taking naturally vary according to the site of the lesion, the nature of the lesion, and other factors. Questions particularly important for specific anatomic regions are discussed in the respective chapters dealing with those regions. There are, however, certain routine inquiries that should be included in virtually every case.

The most efficient method of obtaining subjective information is to direct a list of specific, predetermined questions to the patient. However, this is not always the best method for eliciting certain important pieces of information, and it is certainly not the best method for developing the most effective patient–healthcare professional relationship. The direct-question approach is **close-ended;** it assumes that the relevant information will fall into predetermined categories, and it does not encourage consideration of factors outside these categories. It leads or directs the line of inquiry to specific categories. The patient often attempts to please the examiner by providing information related to these categories but not necessarily pertinent to the problem at hand.

A close-ended, direct-question method of interviewing creates a patient–manual therapy practitioner relationship in which the examiner assumes the authoritarian role of "healer" while the patient assumes a passive role. Within this relationship the patient need only provide the requested information, after which the examiner will perform the appropriate tests, decide what the problem is, and correct it. Such an approach favors the assumption that there is a specific pathologic process that the therapist will treat while the patient assumes a relatively passive role in the treatment program. This is consistent with a medical model of patient management and excludes from the outset the possibility of an operant disease state or an operant approach to management.

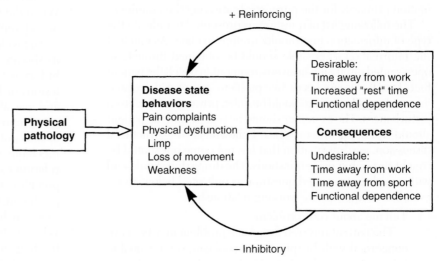

■ **FIG. 5-1.** Disability scheme.

Alternatively, a more **open-ended** approach guides the discussion but does not restrict information to certain categories. Furthermore, it allows the patient the freedom to relate what the patient feels is important in addition to what the examiner may feel is important. The open-ended patient interview is structured to be a discussion session rather than a question-and-answer period. The examiner structures the discussion carefully, however, to elicit the necessary information. In an open-ended interview, the examiner and patient discuss the patient's problem on a one-to-one basis. The examiner maintains a position as an expert in the field by virtue of the professional atmosphere in which the interview takes place. The patient is the expert with respect to the particular problem, being more familiar with it than anyone else. The interview serves as a forum in which the patient is encouraged to offer information and insight concerning the problem in return for advice and help in overcoming it. Both patient and examiner maintain distinct roles but remain equals. They establish an understanding that mutual cooperation and effort are required to execute an effective treatment program.

There are appropriate uses for both the open-ended and closed-ended approaches in history taking. In all situations, it is important to begin the interview open-endedly to establish an effective professional relationship and to get a feeling for the patient's problem. As the nature of the problem becomes more obvious, however, it is necessary to seek more detailed information by directing specific questions to the patient. However, even during a closed line of questioning, examiners must avoid asking leading questions that may elicit irrelevant or inaccurate information. For example, instead of asking, "Does the pain travel down the arm?" the examiner should ask, "Is the pain felt in any other parts?" Instead of, "Do you have a lot of pain in the morning?" one might ask, "When do you typically feel the pain?" The same is true when inquiring about disability. Rather than asking if a particular activity is painful or difficult, one should ask, "Which activities are particularly painful or difficult to perform?" In this way the patient is responsible for judging what information in a particular category is important and is less likely to provide information primarily for the purpose of satisfying the examiner.

The following list of questions is presented to indicate the type of information one should attempt to elicit. As much of the information as possible should be obtained through an open-ended discussion in an environment in which the patient feels free to discuss his or her problem and provide related information. The setting should be quiet, private, and free from disturbances. The examiner should be seated, and the patient should still be in street clothes. Following a well-structured discussion, any information that has not come out should be sought through specific questions. The discussion should end with a fairly open-ended question, as indicated below, to reestablish an appropriate working relationship.

1. Tell me about your problem.

   The patient referred for a back problem may be more concerned with his prostatic neoplasm; some valuable information may be elicited by letting the patient discuss freely whatever he feels is most important. On the other hand, the patient is likely to go on for as long as the examiner allows. One should be prepared to interrupt politely by saying, for example, "I'm beginning to get an idea of the nature of your problem. Now I would like to obtain some specific information pertaining to it." The patient, having been allowed the opportunity to talk freely, is assured that the examiner is interested in him as a person and has begun to involve him in the therapeutic process by listening to his opinion.

2. Where, exactly, is your pain?

   The patient is asked to indicate with one hand or one finger the primary area of pain and then any areas to which it might spread. It is important to determine whether in fact it does or does not spread.

   a. If the patient points to one small, localized area and claims that the pain does not spread from it, the lesion is probably not severe or it is relatively superficial, or both.

   b. If a diffuse area is indicated as the primary site, it suggests that the lesion is more severe or more deeply situated, or both.

   c. If the pain spreads, determine if it is confined to a segment. If so, determine if it follows a well-delineated pathway, as in dermatomic radiation, or if it is more diffuse, as in sclerotomic reference of pain. Well-delineated, radiating pain suggests pressure on a nerve root in which the A-delta fibers are irritated but still transmitting. Diffuse, segmental referred pain may have its origin in the viscera, a deep somatic structure, or a nerve root in which the large myelinated fibers are no longer conducting but the small C fibers are. Cyriax proposes that some structures such as the dura mater and viscera will refer pain extrasegmentally.[17]

   d. In general, reference of pain is favored by a strong stimulus (a severe lesion), a lesion of deep somatic structures or nerve tissues, and a lesion lying fairly proximally (because pain is more often referred distally than proximally).

3. When did the present pain arise? Was the onset gradual or sudden? Was an injury or unusual activity involved?

   An insidious onset unrelated to injury or unusual activity should always be viewed with suspicion, because this history is typical of a neoplasm. However, degenerative lesions or lesions caused by tissue fatigue are common and may also arise in this manner. If the patient blames some injury or activity, keep in mind that he or she may or may not be correct. The exact nature of the event or mechanism of injury should be determined so that correlation can be made to symptoms and signs for interpretation. Determining the direction and nature of forces producing the injury may give some clues as to which tissues may have been stressed.

4. What is the quality of the pain (sharp, dull, burning, tingling, aching, constant, boring, excruciating)? Has it changed at all in quality or intensity since its onset?

a. Sharp, well-localized pain suggests a superficial lesion.

b. Sharp, lancinating, shooting pain suggests a nerve lesion, usually at a nerve root, presumably affecting the A-delta fibers.

c. Tingling suggests stimulation of nerve tissue affecting A-alpha fibers. A segmental distribution suggests a nerve root; a peripheral nerve distribution implicates that nerve. Tingling in both hands, both feet, and all four extremities suggests spinal cord involvement or some other more serious pathologic process.

d. Dull, aching pain is typical of pain of deep somatic origin.

e. Excruciating pain, unrelenting pain, intolerable pain, and deep, boring pain all suggest a serious lesion.

f. Change in intensity of the pain may offer some clue as to the progression of the problem. This must be considered when treatment begins. If the patient's condition was getting worse before treatment and continues to worsen once treatment has begun, then the treatment has probably not been effective. However, it is probably not the cause of the worsening following initiation of treatment. On the other hand, if the patient's condition had been improving but stops getting better or gets worse once treatment has begun, the treatment is probably at fault.

g. Change in quality of the pain may offer many clues about the nature and extent of the lesion. Progression of nerve-root pressure, such as from a disk protrusion, typically leads to rather significant changes in symptoms (see Chapter 4, Chronic Pain Management in the Adult).

5. What aggravates the pain? What relieves it? Is it any better or worse in the morning or evening? When do you typically feel pain?

a. Pain not aggravated by activity or relieved by rest should be suspected as arising from some pathologic process other than a common musculoskeletal disorder. The exception is a disk problem that may be aggravated by sitting and relieved by getting up and walking.

b. Morning pain is suggestive of arthritis, especially the inflammatory varieties. Morning stiffness is suggestive of degenerative joint disease or chronic arthritis.

c. Pain that awakens the patient at night is typical of shoulder or hip problems that may be aggravated by lying on the affected side. Otherwise, a more serious problem should be suspected, particularly if the patient is kept awake and especially if the patient must get up and walk around.

d. Arthritis in weight-bearing joints leads to pain on fatigue (long walks, etc.) in its early stages. In later stages, the pain is felt when beginning a walk, somewhat relieved once going, and returns after walking too far.

6. Have you had this problem in the past? If so, how was it resolved? Did you seek help? Was there any treatment? Is the pain the same this time?

If the examiner should elicit a history of recurrence, the patient might be asked in depth about the first episode and the most recent episode, with an estimate of the number of intervening episodes. Recurrences are typical of spinal cord lesions, but many common extremity lesions such as ankle sprains, minor meniscus lesions or other internal derangements, minor degenerative joint problems, tendinitis, and frozen shoulder also may tend to recur.

By inquiring about previous management, some helpful information may be obtained for treatment planning. However, the patient's judgment of the effectiveness or value of previous treatment must not be weighed too heavily. If an injection helped before, for example, in the case of supraspinatus tendinitis, it does not necessarily follow that another injection is necessary or indicated. If treatment (perhaps inadequately instituted) was unsuccessful in the past, it should not be assumed that it will not be helpful on this occasion.

7. Are there any other symptoms that you have or have had that you associate with the problem, such as grinding, popping, giving way, numbness, tingling, weakness, dizziness, or nausea?

By concentrating on the patient's account of pain, the examiner may well overlook some other important symptoms. A wide variety of responses may be elicited with this question, each of which must be weighed carefully and considered. A patient's description of "numbness" is very often not true hypesthesia but is actually referred pain. In most cases, considerable weakness must be present before the patient can accurately perceive it as such, and very often what the patient describes as "weakness" is actually instability or giving way. Symptoms inconsistent with musculoskeletal dysfunction must be viewed with some suspicion and medical consultation sought for interpretation.

8. How has this problem affected your dressing, grooming, or other daily activities? Has it affected your ability to work at your job or around the house? Has it affected or altered your recreational activities? Is there anything that is difficult or impossible for you to do since the onset of this problem?

The patient's normal occupation and daily activity level is determined. The existence of a functional deficit often contributes to interpretation of the problem by considering the demands placed on various musculoskeletal structures in performing the task. Later, quantification of the deficit or residual function during physical examination will set a baseline against which to assess progress.

Any functional deficit must be correlated later with the apparent nature of the lesion, and any inconsistencies must be considered. In cases involving compensation or litigation, the disease state may be reinforced in such a way that a functional deficit is no longer the result of the problem but rather its cause.

9. What treatment are you having or have you had for the present problem? Are you taking any medications for this problem or for any other reason?

Here again, it may or may not be helpful to determine whether certain attempts at treatment have had any good or bad effects, especially treatments involving physical agents. The examiner must determine whether pain medications, anti-inflammatory agents, or muscle relaxants are being taken. Symptoms or signs may be masked accordingly. Certain medications may produce rather significant musculoskeletal changes (in addition to effects on other tissues and functions). Most important, perhaps, is the long-term use of corticosteroids, which produces osteoporosis; proximal muscle weakness; generalized tissue edema; thin, fragile skin; collagen tissue weakening; and increased pain threshold. These factors, of course, will affect findings on examination. More importantly, however, they must be considered when planning treatment.

10. How is your general health?

It is necessary to determine whether the patient has or has had any disease process or health problem that may have contributed to the present problem or that may influence the choice of treatment procedures.

11. Do you have any opinions of your own as to what the problem is?

Some useful information may be elicited concerning what the patient has learned from others, what his or her insight is into the problem, and so on. If nothing else, the patient can be reassured that the examiner is interested in the patient's opinions and that he or she is to be involved in the therapeutic program.

PHYSICAL EXAMINATION

A complete history performed by the experienced clinician will often be sufficient to determine the extent and nature of the lesion. Even so, the physical examination must not be excluded or cut short. Objective data are needed to facilitate or confirm the interpretation of subjective findings. It is equally important that every effort be made to quantify objective data to allow documentation of a baseline and, therefore, accurate assessment of progress.

Specific tests and measurements will vary, of course, depending on the area to be examined and to a certain extent on the information obtained from the history. This chapter presents a systematic approach that can be applied to any region to be evaluated; tests specific to particular regions are discussed in the chapters on those regions. This discussion will include general guidelines and statements meant to assist in interpretation of findings. The order of testing procedures presented here is for the sake of conceptual organization. Clinically, tests must be organized according to patient positioning. This point will be elaborated in the chapters on specific regions.

Having discussed the phenomenon of referred pain, it should be apparent that at times clinicians may be at a loss as

to which region should be singled out as the primary area to be examined. For example, elbow pain may have its origin locally or at the neck or shoulder, but surely it is not necessary that each of these areas be examined in depth. The physician's referral or the history, or both, will often implicate the involved area. However, this is not always the case. When such a difficulty arises, it is often helpful to perform a brief **scan examination.** This is done by asking the patient to actively move each joint within the suspected areas and by applying some passive overpressure to the extremes of each motion. If pain or dysfunction is noted at a particular area, it may be examined in depth. In general, every structure derived embryologically from the same segment must be considered as the segment or portion of a segment in which the patient indicates the pain exists.

The physical examination, briefly presented in this chapter, is described in detail in later chapters. The basic aims of the physical examination are (1) to reproduce the patient's symptoms and (2) to detect the level of dysfunction by provocation of the affected joint or tissues. The main components of the physical examination are as follows:

- Observation
- Inspection
- Selective tissue tension
  - Joint tests
    - Active movements
      - Passive movements
      - Passive physiologic movements
      - Joint play
    - Muscle tests
      - Muscle strength
      - Muscle control
      - Muscle length
      - Isometric muscle testing
      - Muscle bulk
  - Neuromuscular tests
  - Palpation
  - Provocation tests
  - Functional assessment
  - Special tests
  - Testing of related areas
  - Other investigations

Observation

The patient's general appearance and functional status can be observed when he or she walks in, during dressing activities, during the examination and treatment session, and as the patient leaves. If specific functional disabilities are related during the history, the examiner may ask the patient to attempt to perform the involved activity to assess the exact degree and nature of the disability.

The patient's general appearance and body build—slim, obese, muscular, emaciated, short, and tall—are noted and recorded. Obvious postural deviations and abnormalities in positioning of body parts are reported. It may well be that this informal observation is as informative as formal inspection, as the patient under such scrutiny may not adopt usual posture.

All functional abnormalities or deficits noted during the patient's visit are described as precisely as possible. These might typically include observations relating to gait, guarding of particular movements, use of compensatory or substitution movements, or use of certain aids or assistive devices.

Inspection

The inspection part of the examination entails a closer assessment of the patient's physical status. It is usually performed in conjunction with palpation, which is discussed later in this section. To avoid excluding crucial assessments, it is convenient and helpful to organize inspection of body parts according to the following three layers: bony structure and alignment, subcutaneous soft tissue, and skin.

BONY STRUCTURE AND ALIGNMENT

Inspection of the bony structure and alignment is a critical component of the biomechanical examination, especially when correlated with specific functional abnormalities such as gait deviances and altered range of motion. For example, a man with increased femoral antetorsion is likely to present with a loss of external rotation at the hip, but with respect to his structure, a decrease in average external rotation is normal. If a careful assessment of static alignment were not made, one might make the mistake of attempting to restore external rotation in this case. Similarly, a common gait abnormality seen clinically is increased pronation of the hindfoot during stance phase. This often occurs secondary to structural malalignments elsewhere in the lower limb, such as increased internal tibial torsion, increased femoral antetorsion, or adduction of the first metatarsal. The ultimate cause of the pronation can only be determined through a careful structural examination. Assessment of structural alignment is likewise of utmost importance following the healing of fractures. A person who has sustained a Colles' fracture invariably ends up with some residual angulation dorsally and radially; restoration of full wrist flexion and ulnar deviation should never be expected. Thus, structural assessment becomes important in planning treatment and in setting treatment goals.

The clinician observes posture by examining the anterior, lateral, and posterior views of the patient. Typical postural deviations, which will be observed, include the sway back posture (see Fig. 7-23) and handedness posture (see Fig. 7-26). Any asymmetry in posture from the normal should be corrected to determine its relevance to the patient's problem. If altering the posture changes the symptoms, this suggests that the posture is related to the problem; if the symptoms are not affected then the asymmetrical posture is probably not relevant to the patient's problem. Further details on examination of posture are found in Chapter 7, Myofascial Considera-

tions and Evaluation in Somatic Dysfunction, Kendall et al.,[58] Magee,[69] and other similar texts.

Assessment of a particular part in which some pathologic lesion may exist should often include structural assessment of biomechanically related parts. In the case of a patient with a low back disorder, the clinician should examine the alignment of the lower limbs and vice versa. The same is true for the cervical spine and upper limbs. Each part should be assessed with respect to frontal, sagittal, and transverse planes. Key bony landmarks are identified, and their relationships to fixed points of reference (e.g., the ground, wall, or a plumb-line) as well as their relationships to each other are determined. In judging whether malalignments exist, clinicians must often rely on their experience of what is normal and the comparison of the normal side in cases of unilateral problems. Malalignments should be documented through careful measurements when possible.

Specific assessments related to particular regions of the body are discussed in the chapters on those body regions. The following list includes some key bony landmarks that must often be identified when testing structural alignment and with which the clinician must become familiar:

- Navicular tubercles
- Talar heads
- Malleoli
- Fibular heads
- Patellar borders
- Adductor tubercles
- Greater trochanters
- Ischial tuberosities
- Posterior and anterior iliac spines
- Iliac crests
- Spinous processes
- Scapular borders
- Mastoid processes
- Clavicles
- Acromial processes
- Greater tubercles
- Olecranons
- Humeral epicondyles
- Radial and ulnar styloid processes
- Lister's tubercles
- Carpal bones

SUBCUTANEOUS SOFT TISSUES

The soft tissue is inspected and palpated for abnormalities. The examiner should look for swelling or increase in the size of an area, wasting or atrophy of the part, and alterations in the general contours of the region. When an increase in size is noted, an attempt should be made to distinguish the cause, whether generalized edema, articular effusion, muscle hypertrophy, or hypertrophic changes in other tissues. The area is examined for localized cysts, nodules, or ganglia. In the presence of wasting, the examiner should determine whether localized or generalized muscle atrophy exists or whether there is perhaps some loss of continuity of soft tissues.

Measurements should be taken to document carefully soft tissue changes and to use as baseline measurements. Volumetric measurements of small parts, such as fingers, hands, and feet, can be made by measuring the displacement of water in a tub. Swelling or wasting elsewhere in an extremity can often be documented with circumferential measurements using a tape measure.

SKIN AND NAILS

Local or generalized changes in the status of the skin are noted and recorded. These changes might include the following:

- Changes in color either from vascular changes accompanying inflammation (erythema) or vascular deficiency (pallor or cyanosis).
- Changes in texture and moisture. These commonly accompany reflex sympathetic dystrophy, in which the sympathetic activity of the part becomes altered. Increased activity results in hyperhidrosis; smooth, glossy skin; cyanosis; atrophy of skin; and splitting of the nails. Decreased sympathetic activity may result in pink, dry, scaly skin.
- Local scars, distinct blemishes, abnormal hair patterns, calluses, blisters, open wounds, and other localized skin abnormalities. When a scar exists, whether surgical or traumatic, the type of surgery or injury should be determined because it may have some bearing on the present problem. Blemishes such as large, brownish, pigmented areas (café au lait spots) and localized hairy regions often accompany underlying bony defects, such as spina bifida. Calluses develop with increased shear or compressive stresses; blisters occur with increased shear between the skin and subcutaneous tissue. When an open wound is observed, the clinician should determine whether it is of traumatic origin or of insidious origin, as often accompanies diabetes.

Local skin changes are described according to size and location. Size can be most precisely documented by outlining the borders of the defect on a piece of acetate, such as old x-ray film.

Selective Tissue Tension Tests

JOINT TESTS

Joint tests include active and passive physiologic movements of the joints and passive accessory movements underlying the symptoms and other relevant joints. Integrity tests to determine the stability of the joints are discussed in the relevant chapters. When properly interpreted, findings from these tests can yield very specific information relating to both the nature and extent of the pathologic process. The organization and interpretation of these tests is largely the work of Cyriax.[17]

I. Active Movements

These yield very general information, relating primarily to the patient's functional status. They provide information concerning the patient's general willingness and ability to use the part. They offer no true indication of the range of motion or strength of a part. If a patient is asked to lift an arm overhead and only lifts it to horizontally, it cannot be determined at that point whether the loss of function is owing to pain, weakness, or stiffness.

Therefore, active movement tests are used primarily to assess the patient's ability to perform common functional activities related to the part being evaluated. For lower quadrant and spinal regions, then, active movements should be performed while bearing weight. Upper quadrant parts should be moved in functional directions. At the shoulder, for example, internal and external rotation are performed by asking the patient to reach behind and to touch the back of the neck rather than rotating the humerus with the arm to the side.

The following should be noted and documented for the active movements tested:

A. The patient's account of the onset of, or increase in, pain associated with the movement, and at what point or points in the range of movement the pain occurs. The existence of a painful arc of movement is best detected on active, weight-bearing, or antigravity movements. A painful arc of movement, in which pain is felt throughout a small arc of movement in the midrange of motion, suggests an irritable structure being (1) pulled across a protuberance or (2) pinched between two structures. An example of the former is a nerve root pulled across a disk protrusion during straight-leg raises. An example of the latter is an inflamed supraspinatus tendon squeezed between the greater tubercle and the acromial arch during abduction of the arm.

B. The range of motion through which the patient is able to move the part. This should be measured by some easily reproducible method.

C. The presence of crepitus. This can usually be best detected on active movement, with the forces of weight bearing or muscle contraction maintaining compression of joint surfaces. Crepitus usually indicates roughening of joint surfaces or increased friction between a tendon and its sheath because of swelling or roughening of either the tendon or the sheath. Fine crepitus at a joint suggests early wearing of articular cartilage or tendinous problems, whereas coarser crepitus implies considerable cartilaginous degeneration. A creaking sound, not unlike that which a large tree makes when swaying in the wind, often occurs when bones articulate in the late stages of joint surface degeneration.

II. Passive Movements

A. Passive range of motion testing. The part is passively put through the major motions in the frontal, sagittal, and transverse planes that normally occur at the joint being moved. Very specific information concerning both the nature and extent of a disorder may be obtained by making the following assessments:

1. Range of movement. The examiner should determine whether movement is normal, restricted, or hyper-

TABLE 5-1 COMMON CAPSULAR PATTERNS FOR THE UPPER QUADRANT JOINTS

JOINT(S)	PROPORTIONAL LIMITATIONS
Temporomandibular	Limitation of mouth opening
Upper cervical spine (occiput–C2)	
OA joint	Forward bending more limited than backward bending
AA joint	Restriction with rotation
Lower cervical spine (C3–T2)	Limitation of all motions except flexion (sidebending = rotation > backward bending)
Sternoclavicular	Full elevation limited; pain at extreme range of motion
Acromioclavicular	Full elevation limited; pain at extreme range of motion
Glenohumeral	Greater limitation of external rotation, followed by abduction and internal rotation
Humeroulnar	Loss of flexion > extension
Humeroradial	Loss of flexion > extension
Forearm	Equally restricted in pronation and supination in presence of elbow restriction
Proximal radioulnar	Limitation; pronation = supination
Distal radioulnar	Limitation; pronation = supination
Wrist	Limitation; flexion = extension
Midcarpal	Limitation equal all directions
Trapeziometacarpal	Limitation abduction > extension
Carpometacarpals II–V	Equally restricted all directions
Upper extremity digits	Limitation flexion > extension

Adapted from references 17, 26, and 56.
OA, occipitoatlantal joint; *AA*, atlantoaxial joint.

---

mobile. The degree of any abnormal movements is measured carefully. If there is restriction of movement at a joint, the first determination that should be made is whether the restriction is in a capsular or noncapsular pattern. Tables 5-1 and 5-2 list the common capsular patterns present in the sequence of most to least restricted.

a. Capsular patterns of restriction indicate loss of mobility of the entire joint capsule from fibrosis, effusion, or inflammation. Differentiation can be

---

TABLE 5-2 COMMON CAPSULAR PATTERNS FOR THE LOWER QUADRANT JOINTS

JOINT(S)	PROPORTIONAL LIMITATIONS
Thoracic spine	Limitation of sidebending and rotation > loss of extension > flexion
Lumbar spine	Marked and equal limitation of sidebending and rotation; loss of extension > flexion
Sacroiliac, symphysis pubis, sacrococcygeal	Pain when joints are stressed
Hip	Limited flexion/internal rotation; some limitation of abduction; no or little limitation of adduction and external rotation
Tibiofemoral (knee)	Flexion grossly limited; slight limitation of extension
Tibiofibular	Pain when joint is stressed
Talocrural (ankle)	Loss of plantarflexion > dorsiflexion
Talocalcaneal (subtalar)	Increasing limitations of varus; joint fixed in valgus (inversion > eversion)
Midtarsal	Supination > pronation (limited dorsiflexion, plantar flexion, adduction, and medial rotation)
First metatarsal–phalangeal	Significant limitation of extension; slight limitation of flexion
Metatarsophalangeal (II–V)	Variable; tend toward flexion restrictions
Interphalangeal	Tend toward extension restrictions

Adapted from references 17, 23, 50, 57, and 69.

made by assessing the "end feel" at the extremes of movement (see following). Capsular restrictions typically accompany arthritis or degenerative joint disease (fibrosis, inflammation, or effusion) prolonged immobilization of a joint (fibrosis), or acute trauma to a joint (effusion).

Only joints that are controlled by muscles have a capsular pattern. Thus, joints such as the tibiofibular and sacroiliac do not exhibit a capsular pattern.

b. Noncapsular patterns of joint restrictions typically occur with intra-articular mechanical blockage or extra-articular lesions. Common causes include:

i. Isolated ligamentous or capsular adhesion. A common example of isolated ligamentous adhesion is that of adherence of the medial collateral ligament at the knee to the medial femoral condyle during healing of a sprain. This results in restriction of knee flexion to approximately 90°, with extension being of full range. Isolated anterior capsular tightness at the shoulder often occurs following an anterior dislocation, resulting in a disproportionate loss of external rotation.

ii. Internal derangements, such as displacement of pieces of torn menisci and cartilaginous loose bodies. These typically produce a mechanical block to movement in a noncapsular pattern. The most common example is a "bucket handle" medial meniscus tear, resulting in blockage of knee extension, with flexion remaining relatively free in the absence of significant effusion.

iii. Extra-articular tissue tightness, such as reduced lengthening of muscles from contracture (fibrosis) or myositis ossificans.

iv. Extra-articular inflammation or swellings, such as those accompanying acute bursitis and neoplasms.

2. **End feel** at extremes of painful or restricted movements. This is the quality of the resistance to movement that the examiner feels when coming to the end point of a particular movement. Some end feels may be normal or pathologic, depending on the movement they accompany at a particular joint and the point in the range of movement at which they are felt. Other end feels are strictly pathologic. The testing of end feel can be performed on both classic (osteokinematic) and accessory motions.

a. End feels that may be normal or pathologic include:

i. Capsular end feel. This is a firm, "leathery" feeling felt with a slight creep, for example, when forcing the normal shoulder into full external rotation. When felt in conjunction with a capsular pattern of restriction, and in the absence of significant inflammation or effusion, it indicates capsular fibrosis.

ii. Ligamentous end feel. This is a firm end feel with no give or creep. An example of normal ligamentous end feel is abduction of the extended knee.

iii. Bony end feel. This feels abrupt, as when moving the normal elbow into full extension. When accompanying a restriction of movement, it may suggest hypertrophic bony changes, such as those that occur with degenerative joint disease, or possible malunion of bony segments following healing of a fracture.

iv. Soft tissue approximation end feel. This is a soft end feel, as when fully flexing the normal elbow or knee. It may accompany joint restriction in the presence of significant muscular hypertrophy.

v. Muscular end feel. This more rubbery feel resembles what is felt at the extremes of straight-leg raising from tension on the hamstrings. It is less abrupt than a capsular end feel.

b. End feels that are strictly pathologic include:

i. Muscle-spasm end feel. Movement is stopped fairly abruptly, perhaps with some "rebound," owing to muscles contracting reflexively to prevent further movement. It usually accompanies pain felt at the point of restriction. When occurring with a capsular restriction, it indicates some degree of synovial inflammation of the portion of the joint capsule being stretched during the movement.

ii. Capsular (abnormal) end feel. The range of motion is obviously reduced, in a movement pattern characteristic for each joint. Some authors divide abnormal capsular end feel into **hard capsular end feel,** when the feel has a tight resistance to creep or thick quality to it, and **soft capsular end feel,** when it is similar to normal but is painful with induced muscle guarding. A hard end feel is seen in chronic inflammatory conditions. The soft capsular end feel is more often seen in acute inflammatory conditions, with stiffness occurring early in the range and increasing until the end range is reached. Maitland[72] calls this "resistance through range." Many authors also describe a boggy end feel that typically accompanies joint effusion in the absence of significant synovial inflammation.[13]

iii. Boggy end feel. This is a very soft, mushy end feel that typically accompanies joint effusion in the absence of significant synovial inflammation. It usually occurs together with a capsular pattern of restriction.

iv. Internal derangement end feel. This is often a pronounced, springy rebound at the end point of movement. It typically accompanies a noncapsular restriction from a mechanical block produced by a loose body or displaced meniscus.

v. Empty end feel. The examiner feels no restriction to movement, but movement is stopped at the insistence of the patient because of severe pain. This end feel is relatively rare except with acute bursitis at the shoulder or a few other painful extra-articular lesions such as neoplasms. The muscles do not contract to prevent movement because this would cause compression at the painful site and further pain.

c. Additional abnormal end feels described by Paris[87] include:

i. Adhesions and scarring with a sudden sharp arrest in one direction, commonly seen at the knee

ii. Bony block. This is a sudden hard stop short of normal range. Examples of abnormal bony blocks are callus formation, myositis ossificans, or fracture within a joint.

iii. Bony grate. The end feel is rough and grating as occurs in the presence of advanced chondromalacia.

iv. Pannus. This abnormal end feel is described as a soft, crunchy squelch. The exact nature is unknown but may include synovial infold or trapped fat pad.

v. Loose. Ligamentous laxity as seen in a ligamentous injury or rheumatoid arthritis.

The importance of the end feel is that it gives some indication of what is likely to be the most efficient treatment.

3. Another useful way to consider restricted motion is known as the barrier concept.[7,36,50] Barriers exist at the end of normal active range of motion, when the soft tissues about the joint have reached a degree of tension beyond which the person cannot voluntarily move. This is known as the **physiologic barrier.** Other barriers include:

a. Within the total range of motion there is a range of passive movement available that the examiner can introduce (Fig. 5-2A). The limits to this barrier have been described by some as the **elastic barrier.**[36] At this point all the tension has been taken up within the joint and its surrounding tissues.

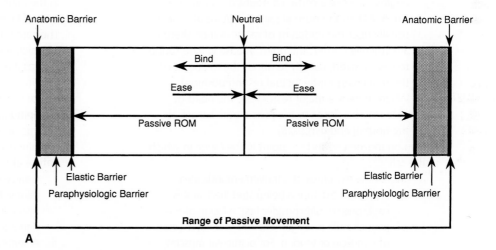

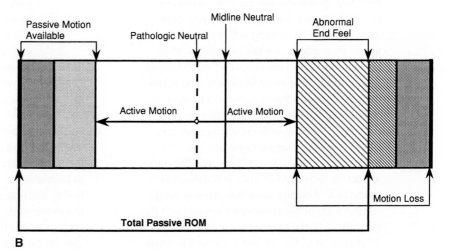

■ **FIG. 5-2.** Soft tissue tension development during examination procedures. **(A)** Normal mobility and associated barriers. **(B)** Dysfunction and associated restrictive barriers.

b. Passively, the joint may be taken beyond its elastic barrier to the **anatomic barrier.** Here the soft tissues are on maximum stretch, and going farther will either cause failure of the soft tissues or fracture. According to Sandoz[97] there is a small amount of potential space between the elastic barrier and anatomic barrier described as the **paraphysiologic space** (Fig. 5-2A). It is within this area that the high-velocity, low-amplitude thrust appears to generate the popping which is sometimes elicited from this maneuver.[36]

c. In a state of dysfunction, when motion is lost within the range, it can be described as a major or minor loss of mobility (Fig. 5-2B). The barrier, which prevents movement in the direction of motion lost, is defined as the **restrictive barrier.** The barrier may be described according to the abnormal end feel previously discussed.

d. The loose packed or resting position is often described as the **point of ease** (Fig. 5-2A).[36] Conversely, as one moves away from neutral or the point of maximum ease, in either direction, the soft tissue becomes more tense, where one begins to sense a certain amount of "bind" (see Fig. 5-2A). In the normal joint the point of ease is usually near the midpoint of range. When there is a restrictive barrier, the point of ease will be found to have moved, usually to about the midpoint of the remaining range (actual resting position). When there is a major restriction, the point of ease may be closer to the physiologic barrier at the normal end (Fig.5-2B).

4. Pain on movement and the point in the range in which it is felt.

a. Pain at the extremes of a movement indicates:

i. A painful structure is being stretched. In this case, one should consider first, a lesion of the joint capsule or a ligament and second, a lesion of a muscle or tendon. For biarticular muscles, the constant-length phenomenon can be used to differentiate the location. Otherwise one must correlate this finding with findings of isometric muscle tests (see below) to differentiate between capsuloligamentous and musculotendinous lesions. If the lesion lies in a muscle or tendon, resistance to the movement opposite the direction of the painful passive movement will be painful, whereas with capsuloligamentous lesions resisted movements are painless.

ii. A painful structure is being squeezed. This usually occurs with extra-articular lesions such as tendinitis and bursitis. An inflamed subdeltoid bursa is susceptible to impingement beneath the acromial arch; the trochanteric bursa is squeezed on abduction of the hip; the semimembranosus

bursa, when swollen, is squeezed on full knee flexion. With supraspinatus tendinitis, pain will be felt on elevation of the arm from squeezing of the involved part of the tendon between the greater tuberosity and the posterior rim of the glenoid cavity.

b. A painful arc may occur with passive movement tests. (See section on active movements for a discussion of its significance).

5. Joint sound on movement. When moving peripheral joints, the examiner will often feel or hear unusual joint sounds, which may indicate pathology.

a. Crepitus on movement. This is best detected by active movement testing but may be noted on passive movement as well. (See section on active movements for discussion.) A creaking, leathery (snowball) crepitus (soft tissue crepitus) is sometimes perceived in pathologies involving the tendons.[69] Soft tissue crepitus may be palpable in patients with degeneration of the rotator cuff and a bony crepitus will be evident in patients with osteoarthritis.

b. Clicks, such as the normal vacuum click, may be felt in the joint and are usually of no significance. In the normal knee, there is often a click on extension. They are particularly common in hypermobile joints in which the laxity of ligaments enables a bone to click as it moves in relation to its fellow bone.[16] Clicking is common in joints unsupported by muscles or when a loose body lies inside a joint.

c. Snapping may be heard or felt around joints as ligaments or tendons catch and then slip over a bony prominence. Less common causes of a pathologic nature are:

i. Coarse clunking types of noise accompanying joint subluxation or instability (e.g., rotatory instability of the knee owing to ligamentous damage or degenerative changes in the joint).[16]

ii. A semimembranosus bursa may snap as it jumps from one side of the tendon to the other, as the knee extends.[17]

iii. A trigger finger is often released into extension with a snap.[17]

d. Cracks may occur when traction is applied to a joint. Synovial fluid found in a joint cavity contains 15% gas, and the crack is thought to be caused by a bubble of gas collapsing.[17,112]

B. Passive joint-play movement tests (capsuloligamentous stress tests) are designed to stress various portions of the joint capsule and major ligaments to detect the presence of painful lesions affecting these structures or loss of continuity of these structures. (For the method of performing the movements and the various movements performed at each joint, see the mobilization techniques included in the specific joint chapters in Part II and Part III.)

Moving one of the articular surfaces of the joint in a direction that is either perpendicular or parallel to the joint (Fig. 5-3) assesses joint play. The treatment plane is at right angles to a line drawn from the axis of rotation to the center of the concave articulating surface and lies in the concave surface. Passively moving either bone in a direction perpendicular to the treatment plane constitutes a **traction** or distraction joint-play assessment, and moving either bone in a direction parallel to the treatment plane constitutes a **gliding** or oscillation joint-play assessment. Traction joint-play assessments directed along the axis of the long bone are called **long axis extension** or **distractions** to distinguish them from tractions administered perpendicular to the treatment plane.

Joint-play movement should be assessed in the loose (resting) position in which laxity of capsule and ligaments is greatest and there is the least bone contact (minimal congruency between the articular surfaces).[56] The greatest amount of joint play is available in the resting position that is usually considered in the midrange, or it may be just outside the range of pain and spasm (position of most comfort). If limitations in range of motion or pain prevent the examiner from placing the joint in the resting position, then the position most closely approximating the resting position should be used. This is called the actual resting position.[26] Examples of resting positions (loose packed) are shown in Table 5-3.

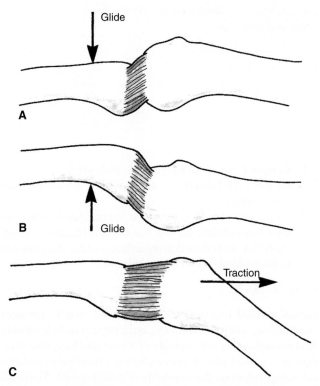

■ FIG. 5-3. (A, B) Glides and **(C)** traction. Traction is applied perpendicular, and glides are applied parallel to the treatment plane.

Joint-play assessment and treatment should not be performed or attempted in the maximal close-packed position (see Chapter 3, Arthrology). The close-packed configuration usually occurs at a position that is the extreme of the most habitual position of the joint, whereas the midrange of a joint movement will be closer to the loose-packed or resting position.[101] For example, the close-packed position for the wrist joint is full extension. The other extreme position of the joint that is less commonly assumed is also very congruent and is called the potential close-packed position.[3,68,117] Examples of the close-packed positions of most synovial joints are shown in Table 5-4.

If joint motion is to be avoided, the close-packed position can be used. For example, the spinal segments above and below a segment to be mobilized may be "locked" into a close-packed position in order to isolate the mobilizing force to a particular level. Generally speaking, rotation will cause a close-packed position.

Joint-play assessment entails determination of the type of resistance felt at the end of range of motion (end feel), the type of pain, and the amount of excursion present in a particular direction. Excursion is determined by comparing the joint with the same joint on the opposite side, assuming that it is not in dysfunction. Joint excursion is evaluated by performing either a glide or traction mobilization and by moving the bone up to and slightly through the first tissue stops. This corresponds to a grade 3 treatment glide or grade 2 to 3 treatment traction (see joint treatment techniques in Chapter 6, Introduction to Manual Therapy). The first tissue stop felt by the clinician corresponds with the end of the elastic phase and the beginning of the plastic phase on the stress–strain curve. Following this scheme one can assess:

1. The degree of mobility (amplitude). The possibilities include the following:
   a. Hypermobility, suggesting a loss of continuity (partial tear or complete rupture) of the structure being tested.
   b. Hypomobility, suggesting fibrosis, as from increased laying down of collagen in the presence of chronic stresses and low-grade inflammation, or suggesting adhesion to adjacent structures, as may occur during healing of a sprain. Hypomobility may be caused by protective muscle spasm, in which case some degree of inflammation of the structure or synovial lining is implied.
   c. Normal mobility, implying normal status of the structure being tested.
2. Presence of pain or muscle guarding (irritability) at extremes of movement. Pain on joint-play movement testing suggests the presence of a sprain or actual tear of the structure being stressed.
3. One must consider, then, six possible findings on joint-play movement testing and their probable interpretations:
   a. Normal mobility—painless. There is no lesion of the structure tested.
   b. Normal mobility—painful. There is a minor sprain of the structure tested.

TABLE 5-3 RESTING (LOOSE-PACKED) JOINT POSITIONS

JOINT(S)	POSITION
Vertebral	Midway between flexion and extension
Temporomandibular	Jaw slightly open (freeway space)
Sternoclavicular	Arm resting by side
Acromioclavicular	Arm resting by side
Glenohumeral	55–70° abduction; 30° horizontal adduction; neutral rotation
Elbow	
Humeroulnar	70° flexion and 10° supination
Humeroradial	Full extension and supination
Forearm	
Proximal radioulnar	70° flexion and 35° supination
Distal radioulnar	10° supination
Radio/ulnocarpal	Neutral with slight ulnar deviation
Hand	
Midcarpal	Neutral with slight flexion and ulnar deviation
Carpometacarpal (2 through 5)	Midway between flexion/extension, midflexion, and midextension
Trapeziometacarpal	Midway between flexion/extension and between abduction/adduction
Metacarpophalangeal	First MCP joint: slight flexion
	MCP joints 2–5: slight flexion with ulnar deviation
Interphalangeal	Proximal IP joints: 10° flexion
	Distal IP joints: 30° flexion
Hip	30° flexion, 30° abduction, and slight lateral rotation
Knee	25° flexion
Ankle/Foot	
Talocrural	Midinversion/eversion and 10° plantar flexion
Subtalar and midtarsal	Midway between extremes of range of motion with 10° plantar flexion
Tarsometatarsal	Midway between supination and pronation
Toes	
Metatarsophalangeal	Neutral (extension 10°)
Interphalangeal	Slight flexion

Adapted from references 26, 56, and 68.
MCP, metacarpophalangeal; *IP,* interphalangeal.

c. Hypomobility—painless. A contracture or adhesion involves the tested structure.

d. Hypomobility—painful. A more acute sprain of the structure may be accompanied by guarding. If the hypomobility is caused by muscle guarding, one cannot, at this point, know whether an actual tear or rupture exists.

e. Hypermobility—painless. A complete rupture of the structure is suggested; there are no longer intact fibers from which pain can be elicited.

f. Hypermobility—painful. A partial tear is present in which some fibers of the structure are still intact and being stressed.

4. Accessory movements are usually graded on a scale of 0 to 6, as listed in Table 5-5.[115] Such grading has the following treatment implications[26]:

a. Grades 0 and 6: Mobilization is not indicated. Surgery should be considered.

b. Grades 1 and 2: Mobilization is indicated.

c. Grade 3: Mobilization is not indicated to increase joint extensibility.

d. Grades 4 and 5: Mobilization is not indicated to increase joint extensibility. Taping, bracing, stabilization through exercises, and education regarding posture and positions to be avoided should be considered.

MUSCLE TESTS

Normal muscle function requires normal muscle strength, coordination, control, endurance, and length. A muscle must be short enough to provide stability of a joint and long enough to allow normal mobility. A muscle does not function in isolation and is dependent on the normality of its antagonist. There is a close relationship between agonist and antagonist muscles.

Muscle activation is associated with inhibition of its agonist so that overactivation of a muscle group as occurs in muscle

TABLE 5-4 CLOSE-PACKED POSITIONS OF THE JOINTS

JOINT(S)	POSITION
Vertebral	Maximal extension
Temporomandibular	Maximal retrusion (mouth closed with teeth clenched) or maximal anterior position (mouth maximally opened)
Glenohumeral	Maximum abduction and external rotation
Sternoclavicular	Arm maximally elevated
Acromioclavicular	Arm abducted 90°
Elbow	
Humeroulnar	Full extension and supination
Humeroradial	90° flexion, 5° supination
Forearm	
Proximal radioulnar	5° supination, full extension
Distal radioulnar	5° supination
Radiocarpal	Full extension with radial deviation
Hand	
Midcarpal	Full extension
Carpometacarpal	Full opposition
Trapeziometacarpal	Full opposition
Metacarpophalangeal	First MCP: full extension
Interphalangeal	Full extension
Hip	Ligamentous: full extension, abduction, and internal rotation
	Bony: 90° flexion, slight abduction, and slight external rotation
Knee	Full extension and external rotation
Ankle/Foot	
Talocrural	Full dorsiflexion
Subtalar	Full inversion
Midtarsal	Full supination
Tarsometatarsal	Full supination
Toes	
Metatarsophalangeal	Full extension
Interphalangeal	Full extension

Adapted from references 26, 56, and 68.
MCP, Metacarpophalangeal.

TABLE 5-5 GRADING ACCESSORY JOINT MOVEMENT

GRADE	JOINT STATUS
0	Ankylosed
1	Considerable hypomobility
2	Slight hypomobility
3	Normal
4	Slight hypermobility
5	Considerable hypermobility
6	Unstable

TABLE 5-6 FUNCTIONAL DIVISION OF MUSCLE GROUPS

MUSCLES PRONE TO TIGHTNESS (MAINLY POSTURAL [TONIC] FUNCTION)

Sternocleidomastoid	Hip flexor
Scalenes	Iliopsoas
Levator scapulae	Tensor fasciae latae
Pectoralis major (clavicular/sternal end)	Rectus femoris
Trapezius (upper part)	Lateral hip rotators
Flexors of the upper limb	Piriformis
Quadratus lumborum	Short hip adductors
Back extensors	Hamstrings
Erector spinae	Plantar flexors
Longissimus thoracis	Gastrocnemius
Rotatores	Soleus
Multifidus	Tibialis posterior

MUSCLES PRONE TO WEAKNESS (MAINLY DYNAMIC [PHASIC] FUNCTION)

Short cervical flexors	Rectus abdominus
Pectoralis major (abdominal part)	External/internal oblique
Trapezius (lower part)	Gluteus maximus
Rhomboids	Gluteus medius and minimus
Serratus anterior	Vastus medialis and lateralis
Subscapularis	Tibialis anterior
Extensors of upper limb	Peronei

Adapted from reference 45 and 54.

spasm, will be associated with inhibition of the antagonist group, which may then become weak. This situation produces what is known as imbalance (i.e., a disruption of the coordinated interplay of muscles).[88] Much of our current understanding of muscle imbalances and neuromotor training comes from the work of Janda,[43–49] Lewit,[66,67] Vasilyeva,[113,114] Kendall et al.,[58] Jull and Janda,[54] Sahrmann,[93–96] and Bookhout.[6] Janda[43–49] has observed that certain muscle groups respond to a dysfunction by tightening and shortening, while other muscle groups react by inhibition, atrophy, and weakness (Table 5-6). Until recently, evaluation of muscle function was concerned primarily with strength testing, with little attention paid to muscle tightness or resting muscle length. According to Janda's clinical experience, to try to strengthen a weakened muscle first is futile, because its shortened antagonist will inhibit it.[48] Muscle testing therefore involves examination of length and strength of both agonist and antagonist muscle groups.

The following tests are commonly used to assess muscle function: muscle length, muscle control, muscle strength, isometric muscle testing, and diagnostic muscle tests.

I. Muscle Length

    The purpose of assessment of muscle length (flexibility) is to determine whether the range of motion occurring at a joint is limited or excessive by the intrinsic joint structures or by the muscles crossing the joint. Muscle length is tested by the clinician stabilizing one end of the muscle and slowly and smoothly moving the body part to stretch the muscle (see Figs. 7-32 and 23-33). Muscle length testing allows the clinician to evaluate the tone of a muscle and to differentiate normal tone, hypertonicity, and tightness or adaptive shortening (see Chapter 8, Soft Tissue Manipulations). The following information should be noted:

    A. Tonal qualities and the presence of resistance through the range of movement and at the end of range of movement; the quality of resistance may identify whether neural tissue, joint, or muscle tissues are limiting.

    B. The quality of movement.

    C. The range of movement.

    D. Pain behavior (referred and local) through the range.

    E. Evidence of hypermobility suggesting excessive elongation of the myofascial system, looseness of joint capsular structures or laxity of supporting ligaments.

        Identification of a limitation or hypermobility of the joint resulting from muscular problems influences the treatment goals and success. The test position for assessment of muscle length is also a position for increasing the length or stretching the muscle. Reduced muscle length may occur with overuse, which causes the muscle initially to become short and strong, but later (over time) to become weak (owing to reduced nutrition).[88] This state is known as **stretch weakness.**[48]

II. Muscle Control

    The relative strength, endurance, and control of muscles are considered to be more important than the overall strength of muscle groups or a muscle.[54,55,95,122] Normal postural control involves the control of relative position of the body by skeletal muscles, with respect to gravity and to each other. Observing the activation, coordination, and recruitment patterns of synergistic muscles during active movements tests muscle control. Alterations in the optimal recruitment of synergistic muscles or over activity of certain muscles are often observed. For example, during shoulder elevation one may note excessive upper trapezius activity or early scapular elevation. Alterations in the optimal recruitment of synergistic muscles can cause action of the synergist to become more dominant than the action of other partici-

pating muscles.[96] The result is a movement that is in the direction of the dominant synergist. Although some active movements have been carried out (under joint test) there are other specific muscle tests which will be carried out here. Relative strength and control is assessed by observing the pattern of muscle recruitment, the quality of movement, monitoring the movement of the joints during active and passive motions, and by palpating muscle activity in various positions. For example, when assessing muscle control of the temporomandibular joint, the examiner can determine muscle hyperactivity by observation and indirectly by palpating the hyoid bone and suboccipital muscles (see Fig. 17-22).[65] Normally quick up and down movement of the hyoid should be felt with minimal contraction of the suboccipital muscles. With acquired anterior adult tongue thrust, a slow up and down movement of the hyoid bone is felt along with significant suboccipital muscle contraction. This excessive masticatory activity is though to be a factor in temporomandibular joint conditions.

III. Strength Test

    Strength tests are only a small part of the examination process and must be used with other information in the evaluation of muscle performance. Manual muscle testing is the most fundamental of all strength tests. Length-tension relationships, muscle imbalance, and positional weakness must be considered when choosing manual muscle test positions. Close attention to substitution patterns and testing in a variety of positions minimizes the chance of erroneous results. Muscle weakness, if elicited, may be caused by an upper motor neuron lesion, injury to a peripheral nerve, pathology at the neuromuscular junction, a nerve root lesion, or a lesion of the muscle, its tendons, or the bony insertions themselves. For the first three of theses causes the system of muscles testing grading may be used. For nerve root lesions, myotome testing is the method of choice (see below). Details of the system of muscle testing can be found in various texts including, Cole et al.,[14] Hislop and Montgomery,[40] Kendall et al.,[58] and Palmer and Epler.[86] Manual muscle testing often includes positional strength testing as advocated by Kendall et al.[58] and Sahrmann.[96]

    Positional strength testing is a specialized form of manual muscle testing that specifically tests the muscle in the short range to obtain information regarding the length-tension properties of the muscle. Positional strength testing is particularly useful in determining whether the muscle is weak because of general disuse or deconditioning, neurologic deficit, or muscle lengthening or strain. For example, if a muscle is lengthened, it tests weak in the short range but strong in a slightly more lengthened range. If a muscle is weak because of other causes, it tests weak throughout the range. Sahrmann[96] provides more information on positional strength testing.

IV. Isometric Muscle Testing

    These are tests designed to assess the status of musculotendinous tissue. With resisted isometric testing, the examiner is looking for problems of the contractile tissue, which consists of muscle, tendons, their attachments (e.g., bone), and the nervous tissue supplying the contractile tissue. In order to do so, ideally the clinician needs to stress the muscle and tendon that is to be tested without stressing other joint tissues. These tests are performed, then, as maximal isometric contractions, disallowing any movement of the joint. Realistically, in most cases other tissues are going to be squeezed or compressed by the contracting muscles, but this seldom poses a problem when the test is done correctly. A particular muscle and tendon are tested in the position that best isolates them, and in a position in which they are at an optimal length for maximal contraction (usually a midposition). Maximal stabilization is required to prevent substitution and to minimize joint movement.

When performing resisted isometric tests, one must determine whether the contraction is strong or weak and whether it is painful or painless. Weakness may be due to a neurologic deficit or to actual loss of continuity of muscle or tendon tissue; appropriate neurologic testing may be performed to determine which is the case. Few neurologic disorders result in isolated weakness of a single muscle. A painful contraction signifies the presence of some painful lesion involving the muscle or tendon tissues being tested. In the majority of cases the problem will be in the tendon, because muscle strains are rare except in sports-related injuries. Very often the patient feels the most pain as the contraction is released rather than during maximal contraction. When this occurs, it should be considered a positive test; the lengthening that occurs as a muscle relaxes apparently stresses the involved fibers sufficiently to cause more pain than does the shortening that occurs during contraction. Practically speaking, these resisted tests are often performed in conjunction with standard neuromuscular strength tests.

There are four possible findings on resisted movement tests:

A. Strong and painless—There is no lesion or neurologic deficit involving the muscle or tendon tested.

B. Strong and painful—A minor lesion of the tested tendon or muscle exists; usually the tendon is at fault. Occasionally auxiliary resisted tests must be performed to differentiate the involved structure from synergists.

C. Weak and painless.

1. There may be some interruption of the nerve supply to the muscle tested. The findings must be correlated with those of other muscle tests and neurologic tests.

2. There may be a complete rupture of tendon or muscle; there are no longer fibers intact from which pain can be elicited.

D. Weak and painful.

1. There may be a partial rupture of muscle or tendon in, which there are still some intact fibers that are being stressed. This may be the result of painful inhibition in association with some serious pathologic condition, such as a fracture or neoplasm or an acute inflammatory process.

V. Diagnostic Muscle Tests

These are particular tests that attempt to diagnose a muscle dysfunction. Examples include the shoulder drop arms test and the impingement syndrome test for involvement of the supraspinatus for rotator cuff tendinitis (see Fig. 11-31).

Neuromuscular Tests

If, at this point in the examination, one suspects that there may be a lesion interfering with neural conduction, the appropriate clinical tests should be performed in an attempt to detect loss of neurologic function. The common nerve lesions are extrinsic. Loss of conduction usually results from pressure on a nerve from some adjacent structure or structures. In the common nerve disorders, the pressure is usually minor or intermittent, or both, and usually involves a single nerve or segment. For this reason, the manifestations of the disorder are often quite subtle; findings on evaluation are largely subjective, and some objective signs may be detected only with more sophisticated electrotesting procedures.

When neurologic function is assessed clinically and a deficit is detected, the approximate site of the lesion can be estimated by correlating the extent of the deficit with peripheral nerve and segmental distributions. The effects of compression of the peripheral nervous system are as follows:

• Reduced sensory input
• Reduced motor impulses along the nerve
• Reflex changes
• Pain usually in the myotome or dermatome distribution
• Autonomic disturbance such as hyperesthesia, paraesthesia, or altered vasomotor tone

Sensory changes are caused by a lesion of the sensory nerves anywhere from the spinal nerve root to its terminal branches in the skin. The cutaneous nerve distribution and dermatome areas are shown in Figures 5-4 through 5-6. They do not correspond exactly to sclerotomes (Fig. 5-7). Recall

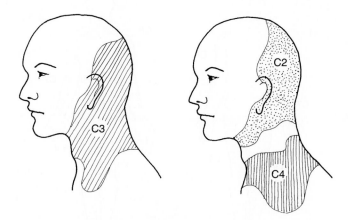

■ **FIG. 5-4.** Dermatomes of the head and neck. Note the three branches of the V cranial nerve (ophthalmic, maxillary, and mandibular divisions) supply the skin of the face, including that over the temporomandibular joint.

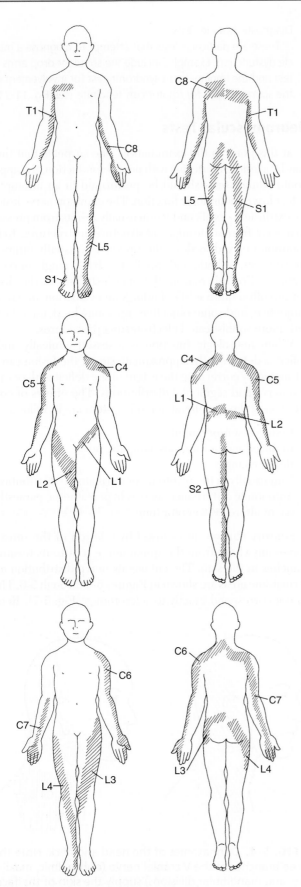

■ **FIG. 5-5.** Dermatomes of the body.

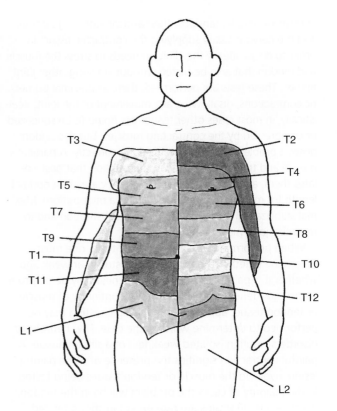

■ **FIG. 5-6.** Dermatomes of the trunk.

that a sclerotome comprises those deep somatic tissues (fascia, ligaments, capsules, and connective tissue) that are innervated by the same segmental spinal nerve. When a tissue of a particular sclerotome is irritated, the patient may perceive the resulting pain as arising from any or all of the tissues innervated by the same segmental nerve. This is a result of the lack of precision in central neural connection and is not related to abnormal impulses "spreading down a nerve." In other words, the "problem" is central, not peripheral, and there is nothing wrong with most of the area from which pain seems to arise. Furthermore, it crucial to realize that radiating pain does not necessarily imply nerve irritation.

Thus, patients with supraspinatus tendinitis often have pain referred down the lateral aspect of the arm and forearm to the wrist; disk protrusions may cause pain to radiate into limb without nerve-root pressure; and trochanteric bursitis is often mistaken for L5 nerve root irritation or is diagnosed as fascitis of the iliotibial band. Again, the clinical implications of referred pain cannot be overemphasized and must be appreciated by the clinician seeing patients with musculoskeletal disorders.

The terms **sclerotomic** and **dermatomic** are often used to distinguish between pain arising from deep somatic tissues and from the skin. Sclerotomic pain is typically deep, aching, and poorly localized, whereas dermatomic pain is sharp, sometimes shooting, and well localized. In most clinical setting, pain arising from the surface of the skin is not commonly encountered and therefore insignificant. However, a very important

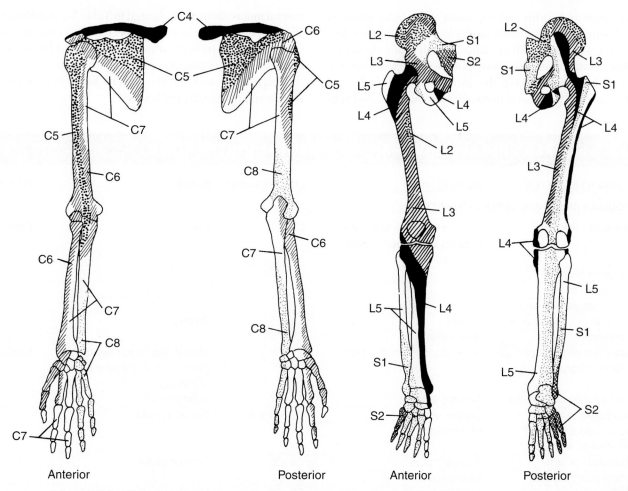

■ **FIG. 5-7.** Sclerotomes of the upper and lower limbs. (Reprinted with permission from Inman VT, Saunders JB: Referred pain from skeletal structures. J Nerv Ment Dis 99:660–667, 1944.)

source of both dermatomic and sclerotomic pain is direct irritation of a nerve pathway projecting afferent input from a particular area. This is properly referred to as **projected** (or radicular) pain, rather than **referred** (or spondylogenic pain), and the most common site of irritation is the nerve root. Thus, an intervertebral disk protrusion or bony osteophyte may directly excite nerve fibers subserving sensory or motor functions, producing symptoms or signs confined to the relevant dermatome, myotome, or sclerotome. The symptoms or signs will vary, depending on the fibers affected.

The largest myelinated nerve fibers are most sensitive to pressure, whereas small-diameter, unmyelinated fibers are lease sensitive. It is generally agreed that eventual dissociation of the quality of sensation is, in part, related to fiber size, and that sensation may arranged in order of decreasing fiber size as follows:

Vibration sense, proprioception—Large, myelinated (A-alpha) fiber
"Fast" (dermatomic) pain, temperature—Small, myelinated (A-delta) fiber
"Slow" (sclerotomic) pain—Unmyelinated (C) fiber

Touch and pressure travel over fibers spanning the entire range of diameters. Consistent with the above scheme is the clinical observation that patients presenting with nerve root irritation may complain of paresthesia (A-alpha stimulation); pain of a sharp, well-localized, dermatomic quality (A-delta irritation); or deep, aching, sclerotomic pain (C-fiber involvement). In any case, the sensation is perceived as arising from any or all of the tissues innervated by the involved nerve.

Differences in central projections between large-fiber afferent input and small-fiber input are responsible for observed differences in associated motor and sensory phenomena. Small-fiber afferent nerves transmitting sclerotomic and visceral pain follow a multisynaptic pathway with diffuse projections to areas such as the hypothalamus, limbic system, and reticular formation. These projections may mediate autonomic changes, such as changes in vasomotor tone, blood pressure, and sweat gland activity, which may accompany the pain experience. They may also be responsible for associated affective phenomena, such as depression, anxiety, fear, and anger. Sensory modalities transmitted over large fibers, such as dermatomic pain and non-noxious sensations, project largely to the thalamus and cortex and skip areas of the brain involved with affective and autonomic mediation. They are thus less likely to be associated with emotional or behavioral changes.

More central or serious lesions must be suspected when the extent of the deficit exceeds the distribution of a single segment or a single peripheral nerve. Peripheral nerve and segmental innervations are indicated in Table 5-7 and Figure 5-8. If a peripheral nerve lesion is suspected, the clinician may test the strength of individual muscles supplied by nerve (see above). Further details of peripheral nerve injuries are beyond the scope of this text, but they can be found in standard neurologic and orthopedic textbooks.

TABLE 5-7 PERIPHERAL NERVES AND SEGMENTAL INNERVATION

ACTION TO BE TESTED	MUSCLES	CORD SEGMENT	NERVES	PLEXUS
SHOULDER GIRDLE AND UPPER EXTREMITY				
Flexion of neck	Deep neck muscles (sternomastoid and trapezius also participate)	C1–C4	Cervical	Cervical
Extension of neck				
Rotation of neck				
Lateral bending of neck				
Elevation of upper thorax	Scaleni	C3–C5	Phrenic	
Inspiration	Diaphragm	C3–C5		
Adduction of arm from behind to front	Pectoralis major and minor	C5–C8 T1	Medial and lateral pectoral (from medial and lateral cords of plexus)	Brachial
Forward thrust of shoulder	Serratus anterior	C5–C7	Long thoracic	
Elevation of scapula	Levator scapulae	C5 (C3–C4)	Dorsal scapular	
Medial adduction and elevation of scapula	Rhomboids	C4–C5		
Abduction of arm	Supraspinatus	C4–C6	Suprascapular	
Lateral rotation of arm	Infraspinatus	C4–C6		
Medial rotation of arm	Latissimus dorsi, teres major, and subscapularis	C5–C8	Subscapular (from posterior cord of plexus)	
Adduction of arm front to back				
Abduction of arm	Deltoid	C5–C6	Axillary (from posterior cord of plexus)	Brachial
Lateral rotation of arm	Teres minor	C4–C5		
Flexion of forearm	Biceps brachii	C5–C6	Musculocutaneous (from lateral cord of plexus)	
Supination of forearm				
Adduction of arm	Coracobrachialis	C5–C7		
Flexion of forearm				
Flexion of forearm	Brachialis	C5–C6		Brachial
Ulnar flexion of hand	Flexor carpi ulnaris	C7–T1	Ulnar (from medial cord of plexus)	
Flexion of terminal phalanx of ring finger and little finger	Flexor digitorum profundus (ulnar portion)	C7–T1		
Flexion of hand				
Adduction of metacarpal of thumb	Adductor pollicis	C8–T1	Ulnar	Brachial
Abduction of little finger	Abductor digiti quinti	C8–T1		

TABLE 5-7 PERIPHERAL NERVES AND SEGMENTAL INNERVATION (Continued)

ACTION TO BE TESTED	MUSCLES	CORD SEGMENT	NERVES	PLEXUS
Opposition of little finger	Opponens digiti quinti	C7–T1		
Flexion of little finger	Flexor digiti quinti brevis	C7–T1		
Flexion of proximal phalanx; extension of two distal phalanges; adduction and abduction of fingers	Interossei	C8–T1		
Pronation of forearm	Pronator teres	C6–C7	Medial (C6, C7 from lateral cord of plexus; C8, T1 from medial cord of plexus)	Brachial
Radial flexion of hand	Flexor carpi radialis	C6–C7		
Flexion of hand	Palmaris longus	C7–T1		
Flexion of middle phalanx of index, middle, ring, little fingers	Flexor digitorum sublimis	C7–T1		
Flexion of hand				
Flexion of terminal phalanx of thumb	Flexor pollicis longus	C7–T1	Median	Brachial
Flexion of terminal phalanx of index finger, and middle finger	Flexor digitorum profundus (radial portion)	C7–T1		
Flexion of hand				
Abduction of metacarpal of thumb	Abductor pollicis brevis	C7–T1	Median	Brachial
Flexion of proximal phalanx of thumb	Flexor pollicis brevis	C7–T1		
Opposition of metacarpal of thumb	Opponens pollicis	C8–T1		
Flexion of proximal phalanx and extension of two distal phalanges of all fingers	Lumbricales (the two lateral) Lumbricales (the two medial)	C8–T1	Median Ulnar	Brachial
Extension of forearm	Triceps brachii and anconeus	C6–C8	Radial (from posterior cord of plexus)	Brachial
Flexion of forearm	Brachioradialis	C5–C6		
Radial extension of hand	Extensor carpi radialis	C6–C8		
Extension of phalanges of fingers	Extensor digitorum communis	C6–C8		
Extension of hand				
Extension of phalanges of little finger	Extensor digiti quinti proprius	C6–C8		
Extension of hand				
Ulnar extension of hand	Extensor carpi ulnaris	C6–C8	Radial	Brachial
Supination of forearm	Supinator	C5–C7		
Abduction of metacarpal of thumb	Abductor pollicis longus	C7–C8		
Radial extension of hand				
Extension of thumb	Extensor pollicis brevis and longus	C6–C8		

(continued)

TABLE 5-7 PERIPHERAL NERVES AND SEGMENTAL INNERVATION (Continued)

ACTION TO BE TESTED	MUSCLES	CORD SEGMENT	NERVES	PLEXUS
Radial extension of hand	Extensor indicis proprius	C6–C8		
Extension of index finger				
Extension of hand				
TRUNK AND THORAX				
Elevation of ribs	Thoracic, abdominal, and back		Thoracic and posterior lumbo-sacral branches	
Depression of ribs				
Depression of ribs				
Contraction of abdomen				
Anteroflexion of trunk				
Lateral flexion of trunk				
HIP GIRDLE AND LOWER EXTREMITY				
Flexion of hip	Iliopsoas	L1–L3	Femoral	Lumbar
Flexion of hip and eversion of thigh	Sartorius	L2–L3		
Extension of leg	Quadriceps femoris	L2–L4		
Adduction of thigh	Pectineus	L2–L3	Obturator	Lumbar
	Adductor longus	L2–L3		
	Adductor brevis	L2–L4		
	Adductor magnus	L3–L4		
	Gracilis	L2–L4		
Adduction of thigh	Obturator externus	L3–L4		
Lateral rotation of thigh				
Abduction of thigh	Gluteus medius and minimus	L4–S1	Superior gluteal	Sacral
Medial rotation of thigh				
Flexion of thigh	Tensor fasciae latae	L4–L5		
Lateral rotation of thigh	Piriformis	L5–S1		
Abduction of thigh	Gluteus maximus	L4–S2	Inferior gluteal	
Lateral rotation of thigh	Obturator internus	L5–S1	Muscular branches from sacral plexus	
	Gemelli	L4–S1		
	Quadratus femoris	L4–S1		
Flexion of leg (assist in extension of thigh)	Biceps femoris	L4–S2	Sciatic (trunk)	Sacral
	Semitendinosus	L4–S1		
	Semimembranosus	L4–S1		
Dorsiflexion of foot	Tibialis anterior	L4–L5	Deep peroneal	Sacral
Supination of foot				
Extension of toes II–V	Extensor digitorum longus	L4–S1		
Dorsiflexion of foot				
Extension of great toe	Extensor hallucis longus	L4–S1		
Dorsiflexion of foot				
Extension of great toe and the three medial toes	Extensor digitorum brevis	L4–S1		
Plantar flexion of foot in pronation	Peronei	L5–S1	Superficial peroneal	Sacral
Plantar flexion of foot in supination	Tibialis posterior and triceps surae	L5–S2	Tibial	Sacral

TABLE 5-7 PERIPHERAL NERVES AND SEGMENTAL INNERVATION (Continued)

ACTION TO BE TESTED	MUSCLES	CORD SEGMENT	NERVES	PLEXUS
Plantar flexion of foot in supination	Flexor digitorum longus	L5–S2		
Flexion of terminal phalanx of toes II–V				
Plantar flexion of foot in supination	Flexor hallucis longus	L5–S2		
Flexion of terminal phalanx of great toe				
Flexion of middle phalanx of toes II–V	Flexor digitorum brevis	L5–S1		
Flexion of proximal phalanx of great toe	Flexor hallucis brevis	L5–S2		
Spreading and closing of toes	Small muscles of foot	S1–S2		
Voluntary control of pelvic floor	Perineal and sphincters	S2–S4	Pudendal	Sacral

Adapted from Chusid JG: Correlative Neuroanatomy and Functional Neurology. Los Altos, CA, Lange Medical Publications, 1970.

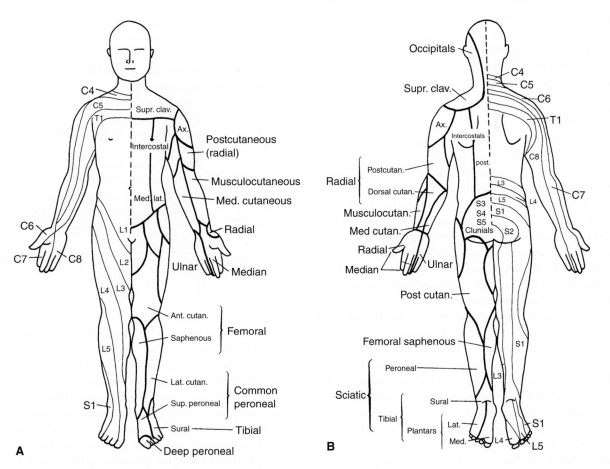

■ **FIG. 5-8.** **(A)** Segmental and **(B)** peripheral nerve distribution.

MYOTOME TESTING

Assessment of key myotomes is performed in any pathologic condition of nerve or muscle in which weakness is apparent or suspected. A finding of weakness during the upper-quadrant or lower-quadrant scan examination (see Chapter 21, Cervicothoracic-Upper Limb Scan Examination, and Chapter 24, Lumbosacral-Lower Limb Scan Examination) should alert the examiner that thorough muscle testing needs to be carried out on all the muscles innervated by that particular segmental nerve. Key segmental distributions, both myotomal and dermatomal, are listed in Table 5-8. These are the muscles and skin areas that are most likely to be affected by involvement of a particular segment. These are important to know because segmental deficits, such as those that occur with disk protrusions, are very common neural disorders seen clinically. Because of the overlapping of dermatomes and myotomes in the extremities, lesions involving a single segment—even when conduction is completely interrupted—result in only subtle deficits.

Myotome testing consists of carrying out an isometric contraction of a muscle group over a few seconds. The muscle is placed in the mid-position and the patient is asked to hold the position against the resistance of the examiner. Myotome testing is shown in Figures 5-9 and 5-10. The resistance is applied slowly to enable the patient to give the necessary resistance, and the amount of the force applied must be appropriate to the specific muscle group and to the patient. Myotomal testing is addressed throughout this text.

The tests described below may be used when performing clinical neurologic assessment

SENSORY TESTS

A pin, wisp of cotton, and tuning fork may be used to assess conduction along sensory pathways. Pressure on a nerve will usually result in loss of conduction along the large myelinated fibers first and the small unmyelinated fibers last. Therefore, minor deficits will often be manifested first by loss of vibration sense, with sensation to touch and noxious stimulation being reduced with more severe or long-lasting pressure.

The sensory examination is begun with a quick "scan" of skin sensation. To do this, the examiner runs his or her relaxed hands relatively firmly over the skin to be tested and asks the patient whether there are and differences (see Fig. 19-37). When performing detailed sensory tests for light touch (with a wisp of cotton or brush), a particular area on the normal side is tested and the patient is asked if the sensation is perceived. Then the involved side is retested and the patient is again asked if the sensation is felt. If sensation is intact on both sides, the patient is asked if it felt the same on both sides. This procedure is followed when testing each key segmental sensory area and each peripheral nerve distribution (Fig. 5-8). Sensory deficits and asymmetries in perception are noted.

Pain sensation can then be tested with a pin, pinwheel or other sharp object. Only light tapping should be used. The patient assesses the painful quality of the stimulus rather than

TABLE 5-8 KEY SEGMENTAL DISTRIBUTIONS (MYOTOMAL AND DERMATOMAL)

SEGMENTS	KEY MOVEMENTS TO TEST
C1	Upper cervical flexion
C2	Upper cervical extension
C3	Cervical side flexion
C4	Shoulder elevation, diaphragmatic function
C5	Shoulder abduction, external rotation
C6	Elbow flexion, wrist extension
C7	Elbow extension, wrist flexion
C8	Thumb extension
T1	Finger adduction
L2	Hip flexion
L3	Knee extension, hip flexion
L4	Ankle dorsiflexion, knee extension
L5	Extension of the big toe, ankle dorsiflexion
S1	Hip extension, contraction of buttock
S2	Toe standing, ankle plantar flexion
REFLEXES TO TEST	
Cranial nerve V	Jaw jerk[34,85]
C5, C6	Biceps, brachioradialis
(C7), C8	Triceps
(L3, L4)	Patellar tendon (quadriceps)
L5	Great toe jerk[37,108]
S1–S2	Achilles tendon
KEY SEGMENTAL SENSORY AREAS TO TEST (DISTAL PART OF SEGMENT)	
C6	Thumb and index finger, radial border of hand
C7	Middle three fingers
C8	Ring and small finger, ulnar border of hand
L2	Medial thigh
L3	Anteromedial, distal thigh
L4	Medial aspect of large toe
L5	Web space between large and second toes
S1	Below lateral malleolus, knee flexion
S2	Back of heel, knee flexion
S3–S4	Saddle, anal region

Others (e.g., upper cervical, thoracic, and lumbar) are less definite owing to overlapping.

the sensation of pressure or touch. The timing of the stimuli should be irregular so that the patient does not know when to expect the next pinprick or touch. Perception to pin prick may range from absence of awareness, through pressure sensation, hyperanalgesia with or without radiation, localization, and sensation of sharpness, to normal perception.[69]

Other sensations, which can be tested if abnormalities are found, are deep pressure, two-point discrimination, vibration sense, hot/cold sensation, proprioception, and stereognosis

Any abnormality of sensation is mapped out on a body chart. Positive finding must be re-examined at each attendance so

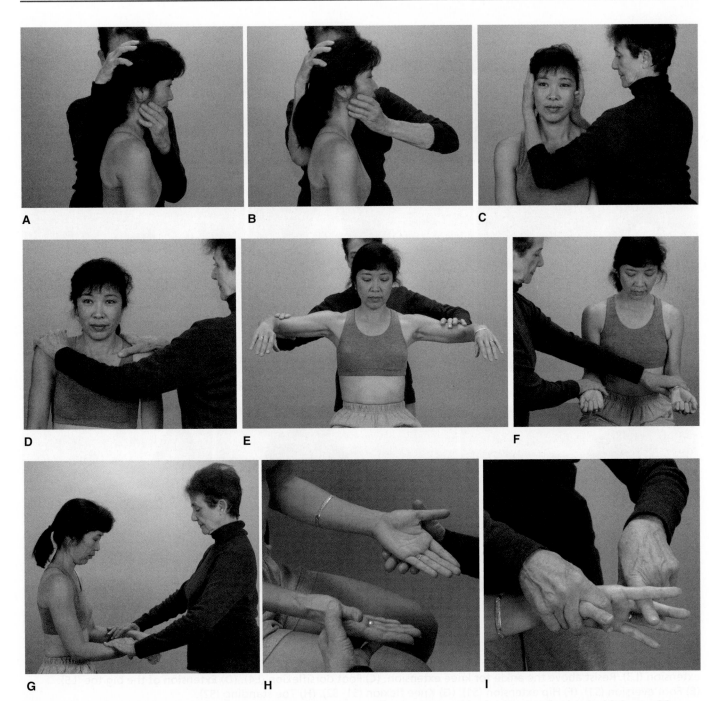

■ **FIG. 5-9.** Myotome testing for the cervical and upper thoracic nerve roots. The patient is asked to hold the position for at least 5 seconds so that the weakness can be noted. **(A)** Upper cervical flexion (C1). **(B)** Upper cervical extension (C2). **(C)** Cervical lateral flexion (C3). **(D)** Shoulder girdle elevation (C4). **(E)** Shoulder abduction (C5). **(F)** Elbow flexion (C6). **(G)** Elbow extension (C7). **(H)** Thumb extension (C6). **(I)** Finger adduction (T1).

that any progressive neurologic impairment can be identified and the necessary action taken.

DEEP TENDON REFLEXES

Lower motor neuron lesions, such as segmental or peripheral nerve disorders, may result in diminution of certain deeptendon reflexes, whereas more central, upper motor neuron lesions may cause hyperreflexia. The deep tendon reflexes are elicited by tapping the tendon a number of times. Incipient root involvement is missed if reflexes are tested once. Routine examinations should include tapping the tendon six successive times, to uncover the fading reflex response which indicates developing root signs.[37,73]

The commonly used deep tendon reflexes are the biceps, triceps, brachioradialis (see Fig. 11-24), patellar, and tendo-

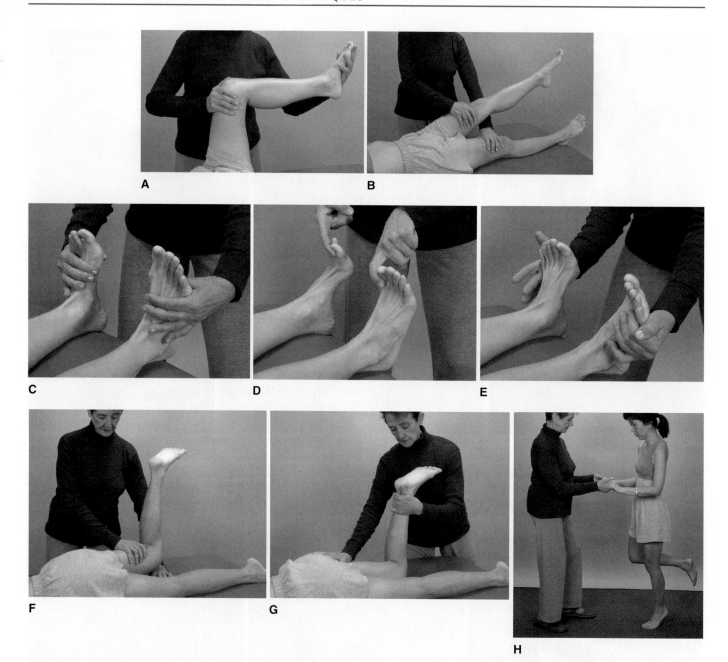

■ **FIG. 5-10.** Myotome testing for the lumbar and sacral nerve roots. **(A)** Hip flexion (L2). **(B)** Hip flexion and knee extension (L3). Resist above the ankle for knee extension. **(C)** Foot dorsiflexion (L4). **(D)** Extension of the big toe (L5). **(E)** Foot eversion (S1). **(F)** Hip extension (S1). **(G)** Knee flexion (S1- S2). **(H)** Toe standing (S2).

calcaneus (see Fig. 14-23). The jaw reflex (see Fig. 17-30) can be important to the neurologist in distinguishing cervical myelopathy (normal jaw reflex with exaggerated limb reflexes) from the possibility of an intracranial lesion.[37] If the reflex is absent or diminished, there may be pathology along the course of the fifth cranial nerve.

The important assessments to make when testing deep tendon reflexes are whether the responses at homologous tendons are symmetrical and whether any responses are clonic. The presence of hyporeflexia is difficult to judge, because some persons normally have reflexes that are difficult to elicit. In general, if it is equally difficult to elicit responses at corresponding tendons, no significance can be attributed. However, if upper extremity responses are difficult to elicit but lower extremity responses are strong, myelopathy or some other more serious pathologic process should be considered. The reflex response may be graded as follows:

Minus (−) or 0: absent
Minus (−) or 1: diminished

Plus (+) or 2: average
Plus (++) or 3: exaggerated
Plus (+++) or 4: clonus

Clonus is associated with exaggerated reflexes and is characterized by intermittent muscle contraction and relaxation produced by sustained stretching of a muscle. It is most commonly tested in the lower limb where the examiner sharply dorsiflexes the foot with the knee extended. An exaggerated reflex response suggests an upper motor lesion and if this is found, the plantar response should be tested. This involves stroking the lateral aspect of the foot and observing the movement of the toes. The normal response is for all the toes to plantarflex, while an abnormal response, confirming an upper motor neurone lesion consists of dorsiflexion of the great toe and downward fanning out of the remaining toes,[116] which is known as the extensor or Babinski response.

NEURAL EXTENSIBILITY TEST (MOBILITY OF THE NERVOUS SYSTEM)

Examination of the extensibility of the nervous system is examined by carrying out what are known as neurodynamic tests.[99] For more than 100 years,[22] the medical profession has used some of these tests; however, they have been more fully developed by several therapists.[9,27,73] Because neural tension (connective and conducting) can be a source of symptoms, tests of the neurodynamic often need to be included. Examples of tests of neurodynamics include the passive neck flexion, straight leg raise, prone knee bend, slump test (see Fig. 22-22), and upper limb tension tests, also known as brachial plexus tension tests (see Fig. 11-25 through 11-28).

The testing procedures follow the same format as those of joint movement. The resting symptoms are established before any testing movement and then the following information is noted:

- Range of movement
- Resistance through the range and at end range
- Duality of movement
- Pain behavior through the range

The clinician administering these tests should be skilled in the specialized features of sequencing the components of the test and understand what is considered normal or acceptable responses. Theoretical aspects of these tests and how the tests are performed can be found in Butler.[9]

Palpation

Palpation tests are usually conveniently performed at the same time as the inspection tests discussed previously. As in inspection, palpation tests should be organized according to layers, assessing the status of the skin, subcutaneous soft tissues, and bony structures (including tendon and ligament attachments). Significant findings are documented.

Palpation of all tissues associated with the area of symptoms discloses both physiologic and structural changes. The uninvolved side should be palpated first so that the patient has some idea of what to expect. The palpatory examination includes, but is not necessarily limited to, palpation of the myofascial structures in the form of layer palpation and palpation of the bony structures. The tissues that can be palpated include the skin, subcutaneous fascia, blood vessels, nerves, muscle sheaths, muscle bellies, musculotendinous junctions, tendons, deep fascia, ligaments, bones, and joint spaces.

For practical purposes, layer palpation may be categorized into superficial and deep palpation. Superficial palpatory examination includes assessment of tissue temperature and moisture as well as light touch to determine the extensibility and integrity of the superficial connective tissue.

SKIN

The examiner uses the back of the hand to initially discern variations in skin temperature and sweating between symptomatic and nonsymptomatic areas.

The movement of the skin over the underlying but superficial structures is checked next. Depending on the body part being tested, either the palm or the fingertips are used to detect restrictions. On broad body surfaces, the palm is firmly but lightly placed on the skin and then displaced in all directions to identify tension and resistance to gentle displacement.

More vigorous displacement in the form of skin rolling (if tolerated and indicated), skin gliding, skin distraction, and the pinch roll maneuver are often an important part of layer palpation; it gives additional information about the extensibility of the subcutaneous tissues and possible infiltration of the skin and subcutaneous tissue by cellulitis (see Figs. 7-40 through 7-43).[70,71] According to the minor intervertebral derangement theory of Maigne,[71] because of minor mechanical causes involving one or two apophyseal joints, the overlying skin is tender to pinching and rolling while the muscles are painful to palpation and feel cordlike. This is believed to be initiated by nociceptive activity in the posterior primary dermatome and myotome.

In general, the following should be noted:

- Tenderness. Minor pressure on a nerve supplying a particular area of skin may result in dysesthesia that may be perceived as a painful burning sensation to normally nonnoxious stimulation, such as light touch. A similar phenomenon may also occur in the presence of lesions involving other tissues innervated by the same segment. This is believed to be the result of summation of otherwise subthreshold afferent input to a segment of the spinal cord.
- Moisture and texture. Moisture and texture may be altered with changes in vascularity or changes in sympathetic activity to the part. In the presence of increased sympathetic activity, such as that which commonly occurs in the chronic stages of reflex sympathetic dystrophy, the skin will be abnormally moist and very smooth. With reduced sympathetic activity, sometimes preceding a reflex sympathetic dystrophy, the skin may be dry and scaly. Sudomotor stud-

ies have used an electrical skin resistance method for measuring sweat gland activity.[62-64]

- Temperature. Skin temperature will be elevated in the presence of an underlying inflammatory process or with reduced sympathetic activity.[1,21,41] A reduction in skin temperature may accompany vascular deficiency, increased sympathetic activity, or fibrofatty infiltration.[52] Thermocouples and infrared thermography are sometimes used for differential diagnosis of certain conditions.[83]
- Mobility. The skin should be moved relative to the underlying tissues to examine for the presence of skin adhesions. This is especially important following healing of surgical and other traumatic wounds.

SUBCUTANEOUS SOFT TISSUES

The soft tissues are palpated deep to the skin—fat, fascia, muscles, tendons, joint capsules and ligaments, nerves, and blood vessels. No more pressure than what is necessary is used. A common mistake is to press harder and harder in an attempt to distinguish deep structures. This only serves to desensitize the palpating fingertips and does not assist in determining the nature of the tissues being palpated.

The deep palpatory examination includes **compression,** which is palpation through layers of tissue perpendicular to the tissue, and shear. **Shear** is movement of the myofascial tissues between layers, moving parallel to the tissue.[10] Translational and longitudinal muscle play are effective assessment tools for assessing the mobility of a muscle or muscle group within the fascial sheath (see Figs. 7-45 and 7-46). Palpation may progress to probing, to grasping, or displacing muscle bellies and tendons. Resistance to displacement or stretch and crepitus or "catching" should be noted. It is most revealing to palpate the entire extent of a tendon sheath during contraction of its respective muscle. A characteristic vibration, as if the tendon needs lubrication, represents tenosynovitis.[115] Soft tissue palpation may offer information concerning the following:

- Tenderness. Tenderness of ligament, muscle, tendon, tendon sheath and nerve (including nerve tension points[9]) should be considered. Tenderness to deep palpation is a very unreliable finding. In itself it is never indicative of the site of a pathologic process because of the prevalence of referred tenderness with lesions of deep somatic tissues. The phenomenon is similar in all respects to that of referred pain. In many common lesions, the area of primary tenderness does not correspond well to the site of the lesion. Patients with low back disorders are often most tender in the buttock, those with supraspinatus tendinitis are most tender over the lateral brachial region, and persons with trochanteric bursitis are most tender over the lateral aspect of the thigh. These "trigger points," or referred areas of tenderness, are found in some area of the segment corresponding to the segment in which the lesion exists. Generally, tenderness associated with more super-

ficial lesions, such as medial ligament sprains at the knee, corresponds more closely with the site of the lesion than does tenderness occurring with more deeply situated pathologic processes.

- Edema and swelling. The size and location of localized soft tissue swellings are noted. Abnormal fluid accumulations should be differentiated as intra-articular or extra-articular. Articular effusion will be restricted to the confines of the joint capsule; pressure applied over one side of the joint may, therefore, cause increased distention observed over the opposite side. This type of **ballottement** test can be used with more superficial joints. Often articular effusion is distinguished by its characteristic distribution at a particular joint; these distributions are discussed in the chapters on specific regions. Extra-articular swelling may accompany acute inflammatory processes, such as abscesses and those following acute trauma, because of protein and plasma leaking from capillary walls. Generalized tissue edema may accompany vascular disorders, lymphatic obstructions, and electrolyte imbalances.
- Consistency, continuity, and mobility. Normal soft tissue is supple and easily moved against underlying tissue. Palpation for abnormalities such as indurated areas, loss of mobility, stringiness, doughiness, nodules, and gaps is done and results noted.
- Pulse. Palpating for the pulse of various major arteries can assist in assessing the status of blood supply to the part. Heart rate may also be determined.

BONY STRUCTURES

Bony structures also include ligaments and tendon attachments. When palpating bony structures, the following should be noted:

- Tenderness. As with deep, soft tissue tenderness, tenderness at various bony sites may be referred and is therefore often misleading. Lesions involving both ligaments and tendons commonly occur at the site where these structures join the periosteum. Typically, these are highly innervated regions and may be tender to palpation in the presence of tenoperiosteal or periosteoligamentous strains and sprains. Periosteal tenderness will also accompany specific bony lesions, such as stress fractures or other fractures.
- Enlargements. Bony hypertrophy often accompanies healing of a fracture and degenerative joint disease. In the latter, the bony changes will be noted at the joint margins in more superficial joints.
- Bony relationships. Structural malalignments, as discussed in the section on inspection, may be detected clinically by assessing the relationships, in the various planes of reference, of one bony structure to another. This is especially important following healing of fractures and in cases of vague, subtle, insidious disorders that may have a pathomechanical basis.

Provocation Tests

Provocation tests (auxiliary tests) are used only when no symptoms have been produced by full active movements and other selective tissue tension tests. Additional strategies may be required to reproduce symptoms.

Initial provocation tests may be undertaken in which gentle passive overpressure is applied at the end range of active or passive movement. Sometimes the symptoms are only at the end range, which the patient tends to avoid by moving just short of this point. Additional tests may include repeated active motions and repeated motions at various speeds and sustained pressures.

Should gentle overpressure, sustained pressure, or repeated motions fail to reproduce the pain, greater stress on the structures can be achieved by combined motions or by coupling movements in two or three directions (e.g., quadrant tests; see Chapter 22, Lumbar Spine). These tests have a considerable capacity to reproduce the patient's pain.

Special Tests

The administration of certain special tests, which pertain to the anatomy and pathologic condition of each peripheral joint or spinal region being examined, may be considered. These tests are structured to uncover a specific type of pathology, condition, or injury and are most helpful when previous portions of the examination have led the examiner to suspect the nature of the pathology or condition. These might include vacular tests, respiratory tests, tests for intermittent claudication, measurement for muscle bulk or edema, and tests of bony deformities or soft tissues (such as ligamentous laxity or meniscal tears in the knee). Other tests may include tests for malingering or nonorganic pain. These tests are discussed in the relevant chapters.

Examination of Related Areas

It is often necessary to test other related joints to determine if pain arises from these joints. For example, when assessing the lumbar spine, one may need to consider the sacroiliac or hip joint instead of, or in addition to, the spine. When examining the shoulder, one should consider lesion areas known to refer pain to it, including problems of the neck; for example, a herniated cervical disk may radiate pain to the shoulder or scapula, an elbow or distal humeral pathologies can radiate pain proximally (uncommon), and a myocardial infarction may radiate pain to the left shoulder. Shoulder symptoms may also be related to irritation of the diaphragm, which shares the same root innervation as the dermatome covering the shoulder's summit. A general physical examination including the chest may be necessary.

Functional Assessment

Functional assessment plays a very important role in the evaluation of the patient. It is different from the analysis of specific movement patterns of active, passive and isometric movements. Functional assessment may be as simple as observation of certain patient activities involving the joint or region being examined, or be more complex, such as a more detailed examination involving objective measurement of functional task performance. A number of functional tests are often part of the earlier observation section of the examination. Common functional tests carried out at this point for the lower quadrant include gait analysis, stair climbing, lifting, balance reach, single-leg squat excursions, and lunge distance. What the patient considers as an appropriate functional outcome and what the patient can or cannot do is extremely important in the choice of treatments that will be successful.

After any examination, the patient should always be warned of the possibilities of exacerbation of symptoms as a result of the assessment.

Other Investigations

Plain film radiography is the most common first-order diagnostic screening procedure in the evaluation of musculoskeletal diseases and dysfunction. X-ray films need not be taken routinely in all patients, and a particular radiologic lesion does not necessarily prove that it is the source of the patient's pain. They are often of most value in demonstrating that no abnormality is present in the bone or joints. At times, findings simply support a moderately firm clinical diagnosis; in others cases, however, the films may provide the only clue to a clinically obscure situation. If radiographs are available, they should be reviewed. If they are not available but the examiner believes they are needed, the examiner may request them before proceeding with treatment. The manual therapy practitioner must recognize the presence of skeletal conditions that contraindicate manual examination and treatment.

It is generally believed that procedural tests should be kept in reserve for chronic disorders, especially mechanical disorders, that remain undiagnosed and for situations in which surgical intervention is planned.[60] Depending on availability and merit, such tests include the following:

Computed tomography (CT)
Magnetic resonance imaging (MRI)
Myelography or radiculography
Discography
Bone scanning

RADIOGRAPHIC EXAMINATION

X-rays are the very short wavelength representatives on the spectrum of electromagnetic radiation. X-ray film, like photographic film, has a clear celluloid or plastic base coated with a silver bromide emulsion, which undergoes alterations in response to radiant energy. Chemical development then renders this visible as differential blackening and the resultant shadows or negatives are available for interpretation.

As the primary x-ray beam traverses a body part it will be absorbed to varying degrees depending on the density and volume of the tissue elements it encounters. High-density bone will absorb more x-rays than the adjacent soft tissues, leaving fewer photons available to expose the film, and the resultant image will have a white area of radiopacity. Fat and gas have lower x-ray absorption, permitting more film blackening or radiolucency.

In conventional x-ray films, the absorption densities of many musculoskeletal tissues—cartilage, tendon, and muscle—are identical. Fortunately, fat is often present along tissue planes and between muscle layers, providing visibility by virtue of its lower absorption density (Fig. 5-11). With experience, the examiner becomes able to detect on x-ray examination many important soft tissue changes such as effusion in joints, tendinous calcifications, ectopic bone in muscle, and tissue displaced by a tumor. Further, the studies enable the examiner to see fractures, dislocations, foreign bodies, and indication of bone loss (Figs. 5-12 and 5-13). For osteoporosis to be evident on film, approximately 30 to 35% of bone must be lost.

Basic proficiency in film interpretation is generally considered a clinical skill beyond the scope of manual therapy. However, a working knowledge of radiologic fundamentals and terminology greatly facilitates the study of the musculoskeletal system and provides access to pertinent information from the radiologist's report to form a more thorough history and physical evaluation of the patient.

The first step is to become familiar with the appearance of normal bones and tissues. They are characterized by clarity, contrast, and transparency of the structures as opposed to the haziness, indistinctness, and translucency associated with dis-

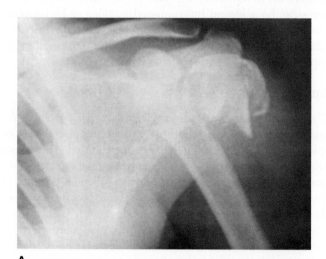

A

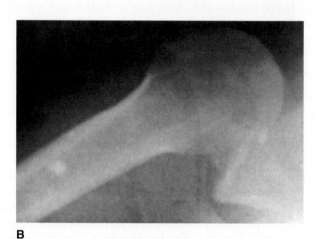

B

■ **FIG. 5-12.** **(A)** Roentgenogram of a fracture of the proximal humerus. **(B)** Axillary view of an anterior dislocation of the shoulder. A large defect (compression fracture) is present in the posterior position of the humeral head (Hill-Sack lesion). In both situations, the humeral head lies anterior to the glenoid cavity. (Reprinted with permission from D'Ambrosia RD: Musculoskeletal Disorders: Regional Examination and Differential Diagnosis, 2nd ed. Philadelphia, JB Lippincott, 1986.)

■ **FIG. 5-11.** Normal calcareous density, muscle density, and fat density. Fat pads help to outline tendons and articular cartilage at the knee. (Reprinted with permission from D'Ambrosia RD: Musculoskeletal Disorders: Regional Examination and Differential Diagnosis, 2nd ed. Philadelphia, JB Lippincott, 1986.)

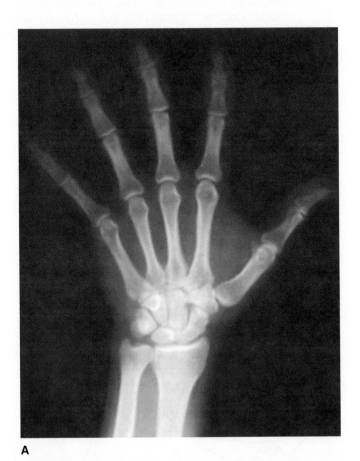

A

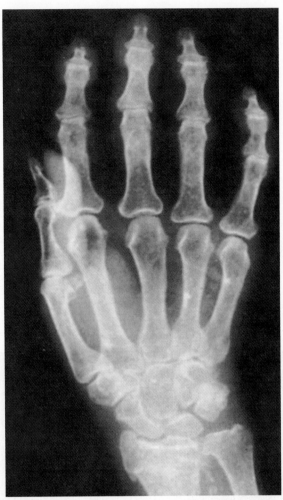

B

■ **FIG. 5-13.** **(A)** Radiograph shows normal shape of the bones of the wrist and hand. **(B)** Radiograph of a hand with senile osteoporosis shows a uniform loss of bone density with a thin, sharply defined cortex. A fracture of the distal radius is present. (A reprinted with permission from D'Ambrosia RD: Musculoskeletal Disorders: Regional Examination and Differential Diagnosis, 2nd ed. Philadelphia, JB Lippincott, 1986. B reprinted with permission from Greenfield GB: Radiology of Bone Disease, 4th ed. Philadelphia, JB Lippincott, 1986.)

eased tissue.[29] Evenness and regularity of outline, structure, and density further characterize healthy bone and tissue. Observation of bone films should include the following:

I. External Observations of Bone
   A. Bone shape. Each bone has its own characteristic shape and surface features (Fig. 5-13). The most frequently encountered example of a deviation from normal shape is a displaced fracture.[111]
   B. Bony surfaces. Cortical bone should be smooth, white, and intact, except for cortical roughening normally seen at the site of tendon attachments. Abnormalities of bone surfaces may include periosteal bone formation due to an underlying bone infection and focal erosions in rheumatoid arthritis.
II. Internal Structure of Bone

A. Diffuse changes. Less bone density than normal can be appreciated by comparing normal x-ray films with those that reflect disuse demineralization (see Fig. 5-13B).
B. Focal abnormalities. Slowly growing destructive bone lesions will modify the shape of surrounding bones and will often evoke a sclerotic reaction at the margin, which is evident by an increase in density (Fig. 5-13B). More radially growing lesions are characterized by poorly defined, permeative patterns of destruction.

Spinal radiographs are nearly always included to rule out fracture, dislocation, anomaly, or bone pathology. The radiographs are also used in biomechanical analysis to establish an initial course of treatment for patients. Radiographs of extremity skeletal structures may be included to rule out primary extremity pathologic processes.

Study of any skeletal region requires at least two views, preferably at right angles to each other (such as an anteroposterior [AP] and a lateral view). The patient's history and clinical evaluation are guides that help determine the different views that should be used. At times, modifications and supplementary techniques are required to pro-

vide precise diagnosis for effective therapy. For example, in the AP or frontal projection of the knee, it cannot be determined whether the patella is in front of, behind, or even within the femur (Fig. 5-14A, B). A lateral view will obviously localize the patella and give useful information about its configuration (Fig. 5-14C, D). However, if there

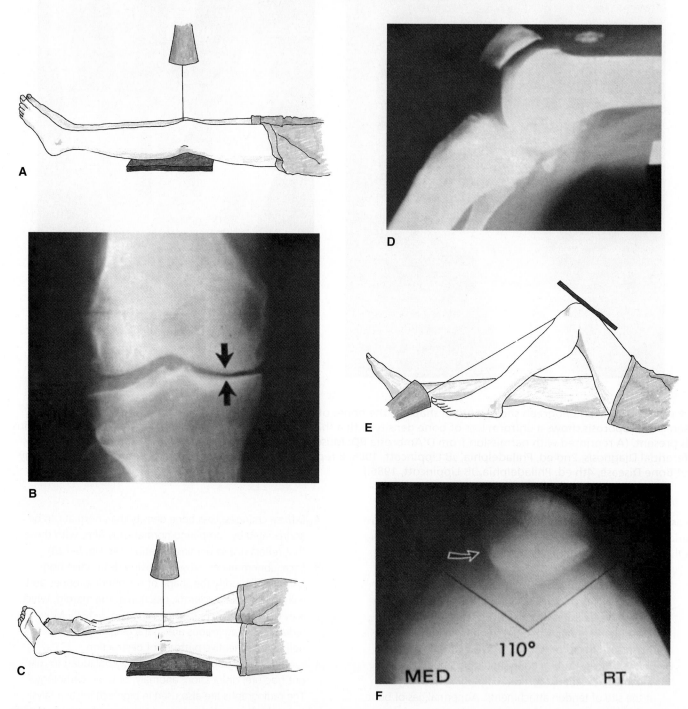

■ **FIG. 5-14.** Positioning and resulting radiographic appearance in standard projection for radiography of the knee. **(A, B)** Anteroposterior (AP) projection. **(C, D)** Lateral projection. **(E, F)** Tangential patellar (sunrise) view. (Reprinted with permission from D'Ambrosia RD: Musculoskeletal Disorders: Regional Examination and Differential Diagnosis, 2nd ed. Philadelphia, JB Lippincott, 1986.)

are really concerns about structural integrity of the patella itself, in order to rule out a fracture, a tangential or axial view of it would be necessary (Fig. 5-14*E, F*).[111]

III. Special Examination

Other supplementary techniques and modifications that may be required to provide precise diagnosis for effective therapy and often of particular interest to the manual therapist include:

A. Stress view. Although clinical tests for instability usually subjectively document that laxity is present, standard radiographs should be taken. They will indicate if the laxity is caused by an avulsion of the ligament with its bony attachment or by an epiphyseal separation. In order to determine whether the ligaments are intact after a joint injury, the joint may be x-rayed in a position that would normally tighten or stress the ligament in question; for example, by applying the appropriate varus–valgus or AP stress to a joint as a standard radiograph is taken. They have proved particularly useful for documenting instabilities at the ankle and epiphyseal injuries of the knee (Fig. 5-15).[59]

B. Dynamic studies. X-ray examinations in both still and cinematic format can be used to assess functional mobility as well as integrity of structure. Examples include cervical spine subluxations (Fig. 5-16) and upper limb motion at the wrist joint.

ARTHROGRAMS

Arthrography is the study of structures in an encapsulated joint using radiographic contrast media. Contrast medium is injected directly into the joint space, distending the capsule and outlining internal structures. When the clinical question is one of a torn meniscus (Fig. 5-17), focal erosion of articular cartilage or a non-opaque intramuscular fragment, arthrography is most informative. Arthrography has been commonly

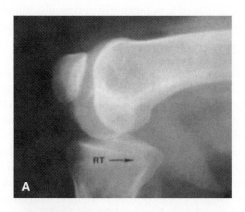

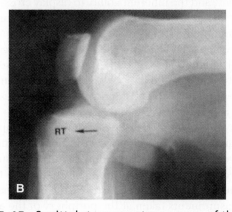

■ **FIG. 5-15.** Sagittal stress roentgenogram of the knee. **(A)** When a posterior drawer is done, the tibia has a normal relationship to the condyles. **(B)** With an anterior drawer, the tibia subluxes forward, suggesting anteromedial rotary instability. (Reprinted with permission from D'Ambrosia RD: Musculoskeletal Disorders: Regional Examination and Differential Diagnosis, 2nd ed. Philadelphia, JB Lippincott, 1986.)

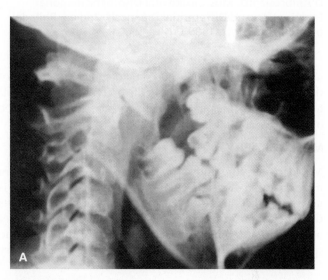

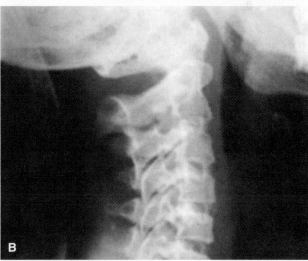

■ **FIG. 5-16.** Dynamic study of the cervical spine. **(A)** Flexion view shows significant anterior atlanto-axial subluxation. **(B)** Extension view shows normal atlanto-axial relationships. (Reprinted with permission from Greenfield GB: Radiology of Bone Disease, 4th ed. Philadelphia, JB Lippincott, 1986:856.)

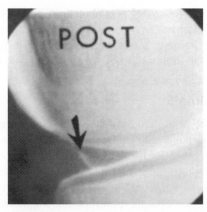

■ **FIG. 5-17.** Arthrogram shows a vertical tear (*arrow*) in the medial meniscus. (Reprinted with permission from D'Ambrosia RD: *Musculoskeletal Disorders: Regional Examination and Differential Diagnosis,* 2nd ed. Philadelphia, JB Lippincott, 1986.)

used in evaluating the knee and shoulder joint. Evaluation of the shoulder joint can determine the presence of rotator cuff tears (Fig. 5-18), bicipital tendinitis or tears, and the presence of adhesive capsulitis.

MYELOGRAPHY

Myelography is the study of spinal cord, nerve roots, and dura mater using radiographic contrast media. Myelography is now performed almost exclusively with water-soluble dyes through a spinal puncture. This technique is used to detect nerve root entrapment, spinal stenosis, and tumors of the spinal canal. Extradural techniques can yield supplementary

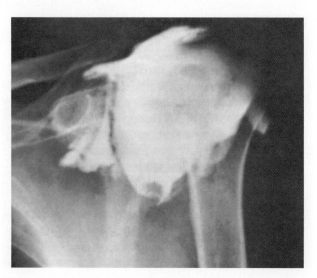

■ **FIG. 5-18.** Arthrogram of the shoulder in a patient with a rotator cuff tear. The dye can be seen leaking into the subdeltoid bursa through the tear. (Reprinted with permission from D'Ambrosia RD: *Musculoskeletal Disorders: Regional Examination and Differential Diagnosis,* 2nd ed. Philadelphia, JB Lippincott, 1986.)

information regarding the state of the disk. Indentation of the dural sac or filling defects indicates abnormality that needs explanation (see Fig. 22-4). Despite the decreased incidence of spinal headache and discomfort during this procedure, it is still significantly invasive and is usually reserved for chronic disorders that remain undiagnosed and unabated and in situations when surgical intervention is planned.[16,75] Plain films or CT may also be used to visualize more anatomic detail. When CT scanning is used in conjunction with myelography, the image is referred to as a CT myelogram.

DISCOGRAPHY

Discography involves the injection under x-ray control of a contrast medium (a water-soluble radiopaque dye) into the nucleus pulposus. Although rarely indicated, the technique can provide some useful information with respect to disk disease and the level of impingement (see Figs. 22-2A and 22-3A). The test interpretation depends on radiographic abnormalities of degeneration, identification of annular tears, epidural flow, or vertebral flow through vessels transiting the vertebral end-plate.[75]

Other contrast studies include angiography and arteriography (Fig. 5-19), used in evaluating hypervascular tumors, determining vascular anatomy,[8,106] and performing venography.

COMPUTED TOMOGRAPHY

CT uses a computerized display to recreate a three-dimensional image. Cuts of film are taken at specific levels of the body. Tomograms may be plain or computer-enhanced. In the latter case, they are referred to as CT scans or computer-assisted or enhanced tomography (CAT) scans.[69] CT has rapidly become the diagnostic procedure of choice for many conditions. Its diagnostic capabilities are based on tissue attenuation of a x-ray beam. Two features render it most useful for musculoskeletal radiology: greater tissue contrast resolution than conventional radiography, and the inherent ability to display cross-sectional anatomy.[35] The CT scan can also be contrast-enhanced (dye injected around the structure) to indicate tumor, bone, or soft tissue involvement. They are then referred to as computed tomoarthrograms (CTAs).[69] A CAT spinal scan is used to outline structural spinal problems involving both bone and soft tissues. These include spinal stenosis, vertebral diseases, disk prolapse, and abnormalities in the facet joint.

The process begins when a x-ray source rotates around the supine patient and x-rays penetrate the body from numerous angles. Detectors in the surrounding scanner measure tissue x-ray attenuation and transmit this information to the computer. The computer then reconstructs the body image using these measurements taken at the periphery of the axial slice of the body being scanned (Fig. 5-20).

NUCLEAR MAGNETIC RESONANCE AND MAGNETIC RESONANCE IMAGING

The nuclear magnetic resonance (NMR) scanner is one of the newest tools primarily devised to evaluate vertebral lesions. The development of surface coil technology in the mid-

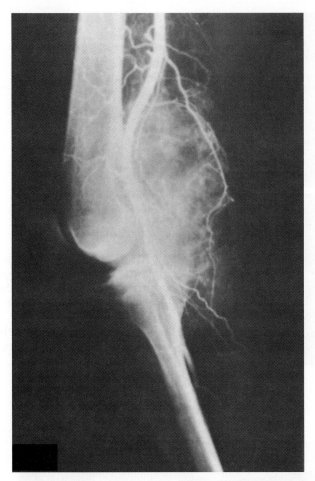

■ **FIG. 5-19.** Angiogram shows anterior displacement of the popliteal artery and a large soft tissue mass showing tumor vessels. (Reprinted with permission from Greenfield GB: Radiology of Bone Disease, 5th ed. Philadelphia, JB Lippincott, 1990.)

1980s[25] established MRI as a reasonable alternative to myelography and CT in the study of intervertebral disk disease.[2] This technique uses no ionizing radiation to visualize the structures being evaluated and can be used to obtain an image of bone and soft tissue (spinal cord and paravertebral masses). Recently, in orthopedic evaluation, the capabilities of MRI have expanded its role in examination of joints (Fig. 5-21). Excellent soft tissue and bone marrow contrast has led to the early detection of soft tissue and bone tumors.

BONE SCANS

Radioactive isotopes have been developed that will preferentially go to bone, showing increased uptake in portions of the skeleton which are hypervascular or which have an increased rate of bone mineral turnover (Fig. 5-22). Its major role is in identifying pathologic changes, especially infections, tumors, inflammatory diseases, or metabolic bone disease.[12,33,79] It is not specific in differential diagnosis of disease. It is, however, useful in locating a lesion that is symptomatic but not yet vis-

ible on roentgenograms. This procedure reveals metastases in 95% of cases.[100]

THERMOGRAPHY

Thermography is a noninvasive procedure that images the temperature distribution of the body surfaces. In contrast to radiography, CT, or myelography, which show only anatomic changes, thermography demonstrates functional changes in circulation consequent to damage to nerves, ligaments, muscles, or joints.[89,90,109,123] The procedure allows one to determine the degree of involvement of, for example, a limb in reflex sympathetic dystrophy or peripheral vascular disease. It also permits one to note the activity in stress fractures and diseases such as rheumatoid arthritis and to detect soft tissue tumors such as breast cancer.[15,125]

ULTRASONOGRAPHY

Other technologies such as ultrasound have been suggested as having potential for noninvasive measurement of spinal mobility.[76] High-frequency sound waves are reflected differently depending on the density of the reflecting tissues. They are received and used to form images of portions of the body. Ultrasonography is also ideally used for evaluating soft tissue masses in the extremities. It has been used in the knee and popliteal space to search for possible popliteal cysts or vascular aneurysms (Fig. 5-21*B*).[35]

ELECTRODIAGNOSTIC TESTING

The electromyogram (EMG) is the most commonly done of these tests and is extremely useful in evaluating nerve root denervation, muscular disease, and peripheral neuropathies. It is a helpful tool in the evaluation of herniated disk syndrome. Radicular pain with motor weakness (motor nerve involvement) is well evaluated by EMG.[38] It must be remembered, however, that it takes 21 days for the EMG to record denervation potentials.

Electromyography has been used for some time to analyze normal function and pathologic conditions in the spinal musculature. Two distinct patterns of EMG activity have clearly been identified in trunk movements: (1) trunk stabilization and (2) initiation of motion.[4,82] Different movements recruit muscles in different patterns of activity, but most spinal intrinsic musculature is involved in the initiation of most movement and maintenance of posture.[75]

Nerve conduction studies, measuring the velocity of an artificially induced signal through a peripheral nerve, may help to identify the existence and site of peripheral nerve root compression.[107] A current area of research is using somatosensory evoked potentials (SSEP) to assess the afferent system to identify lesions of nerves that fail to provoke motor involvement.

LABORATORY INVESTIGATIONS

Data derived from studies of blood and other material in the laboratory are peculiarly disappointing as diagnostic

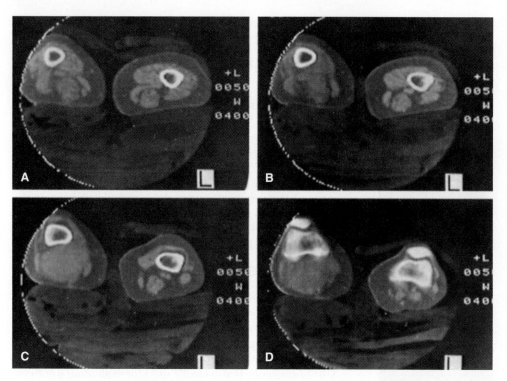

■ **FIG. 5-20.** (**A–D**) Computed tomography scans show a large soft tissue mass posterior to the left knee. (Reprinted with permission from Greenfield GB: Radiology of Bone Disease, 5th ed. Philadelphia, JB Lippincott, 1990.)

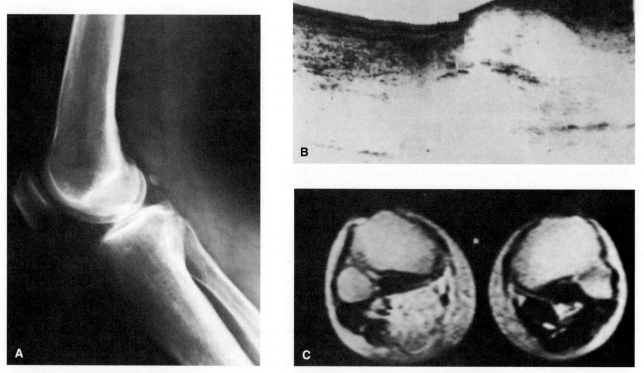

■ **FIG. 5-21.** Soft tissue mass in the popliteal region. (**A**) Lateral roentgenogram, (**B**) ultrasound scan, and (**C**) magnetic resonance imaging scan through the popliteal region show extent of the mass. (Reprinted with permission from D'Ambrosia RD: Musculoskeletal Disorders: Regional Examination and Differential Diagnosis, 2nd ed. Philadelphia, JB Lippincott, 1986.)

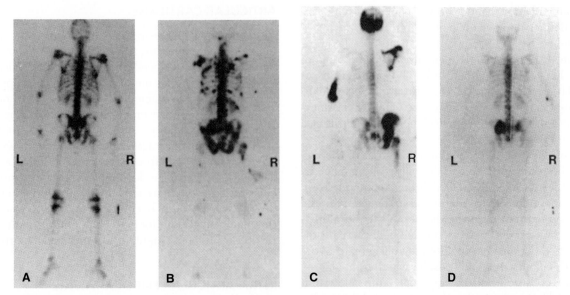

■ **FIG. 5-22.** Whole body bone scan. **(A)** Normal adolescent scan. **(B)** Abnormal bone scan showing foci of reactive bone formation consistent with metastatic disease of bone. **(C)** Abnormal bone scan showing patient with metastatic disease of bone. **(D)** Abnormal bone scan showing reactive bone formation secondary to bone tumor. (Reprinted with permission from Turek SL: Orthopaedics: Principles and Their Application, 4th ed. Philadelphia, JB Lippincott, 1984.)

aids in the search for the common causes of musculo-skeletal pain.[125] In the differential diagnosis of more serious pathologic conditions some studies may be invaluable. Bone marrow examination may be indicated for the diagnosis of generalized disorders, especially myeloma and tuberculosis.[104]

CLINICAL DECISION-MAKING AND DATA COLLECTION

Treatment Planning

Having completed all parts of the assessment, the examiner is now prepared to look at the pertinent subjective and objective facts, note the significant signs and symptoms to determine what is causing the patient's problems, and design a treatment regimen based on the findings. The re-evaluation process should be built into each treatment regimen. Quantified data obtained within the re-evaluation phase help to guide future decisions and to promote cost-effective treatment.

Clinical decision-making involves a series of interrelated steps that enable the manual therapy practitioner to plan an effective treatment compatible with the needs and goals of the patient and members of the healthcare team. Various systems and labels for describing the intellectual processes involved in clinical decision-making have been suggested: clinical reasoning,[53] clinical problem solving,[110] and clinical judgment.[20] The intellectual processes involved in clinical decision-making are not addressed in this chapter; rather, the purpose of this presentation is to offer a series of considerations to facilitate effective clinical problem solving. A varied spectrum of mod-

els to aid clinicians in their daily decisions has been developed.[11,23,24,39,53,84,92,98,118,119,121,124] Having several models may allow clinicians to identify which model works best with different types of patients.

Patients often present with a mixture of signs and symptoms that indicates overlapping problems. The novice may recognize the typical feature of an injury yet fail to exclude other potentially coexisting disorders that may share or predispose to the clinical presentation.[53] Only the examiner's knowledge, clinical experience, and diagnosis followed by trial treatment can conclusively delineate the problem. Diagnosis is one of the main decisional acts in clinical reasoning.[28]

Guides to Correlation and Interpretation

Correlation and interpretation of the examination findings is one of the most critical steps in clinical decision-making. This requires that the clinician give meaning and relevance to the data obtained during the examination.

The diagnostician must often make use of abstract relationships such as proximal–distal, deep–superficial, and gradual–sudden and not be centered purely on disjointed lists of signs and symptoms.[53] When faced with an atypical problem, the decision may be an educated guess; very few problems are textbook perfect. The precise diagnosis of patients with low back pain, for example, is unknown in 80 to 90% of patients.[103] Terms such as "disk disease" and "facet joint syndrome" in most instances are ambiguous because it is difficult to measure these phenomena or to define clearly their contribution to pain in a given patient.[18] Instead, terms such as "low back pain with referral into the leg," "low back pain without radiation," and "chronic pain syndrome" are more well-defined and unambiguous.

The Quebec Task Force on Spinal Disorders Classification System (QTFSD) clearly recognized this dilemma of diagnosis. They recommended only 11 classifications of activity-related spinal disorders.[102] DeRosa and Porterfield[18] have proposed a modified version of the QTFSD classification scheme most relevant to physical therapy diagnosis (see Table 22-1).

Judgments relating to the nature and extent of the disorder and the resultant degree of disability can be made by correlating the information obtained during a comprehensive initial patient examination. With respect to the nature of the problem, it is important to judge whether the disease state is a "medical" disorder or if perhaps operant behavior patterns have developed that may account for a significant part of the disability. The clinician should consider whether the degree of disability is consistent with the apparent nature and extent of the physical lesion or whether the patient is exhibiting disability behaviors that are out of proportion to clinical findings. If the latter is the case, the possibility that the disease state is being maintained by external consequences that have a reinforcing effect should be considered. It is essential that such determinations be made, because treatment directed at some physical pathologic process in the presence of an operant disease state will be futile and can further reinforce "learned" disability behaviors.

Nature of the Lesion

If it appears that some physical pathologic process is primarily responsible for the patient's disorder, the nature of the lesion should be estimated as precisely as possible. To do so, the information obtained on examination must be correlated with knowledge of anatomy, physiology, kinesiology, and pathology in order to identify the involved tissue or tissues. Some estimate should also be made concerning the extent to which these tissues are involved. A few common lesions make up the majority of disorders affecting each musculoskeletal tissue. For each of these lesions, there are also consistent key clinical findings. In developing judgments concerning the nature of common clinical disorders, it is helpful to be aware of the lesions common to each tissue and how they are manifested clinically. The following descriptions are meant to guide the clinician in this respect but are not meant to be all-inclusive.

BONE

Fractures are best identified in the physician's examination through the use of roentgenograms. When examining a patient following healing of a fracture, it is important to determine any malunion of bone on inspection of bone structure and alignment, as this may affect eventual functioning of the part. Dislocations are also best detected through the physician's interpretation of roentgenograms, although dislocations are often obvious on inspection.

ARTICULAR CARTILAGE

Degeneration from wearing due to fatigue is the most common lesion affecting this tissue. It causes roughening of the normally smooth surface layers of cartilage. Clinically this is manifested as crepitus on movements in which opposition of joint surfaces is maintained by weight bearing or other compressive forces. However, considerable degeneration must usually take place before crepitus is detected clinically.

A loose body is a fragment of articular cartilage that has broken away and lies free in the joint. This may occur in the late stages of cartilage degeneration or as a result of avascular necrosis of an area of subchondral bone (osteochondrosis). A loose body becomes symptomatic when it alters the mechanical functioning of the joint, usually causing a restriction of movement in a noncapsular pattern (joint block).

INTRA-ARTICULAR FIBROCARTILAGE

The common disorder affecting intra-articular fibrocartilaginous disks and menisci is tearing, usually from traumatic injury. Forces sufficient to tear a meniscus or disk in the limbs will usually also cause some strain on the joint capsule to which these structures attach. This causes synovial inflammation in the acute stage. Thus, movement is likely to be restricted in a capsular pattern.

Minor displacement of a torn fragment of fibrocartilage may simply result in "clicking" of the joint on specific movements. Lower extremity joints, namely the knee, may give way when a tag of a torn meniscus is caught between the articular surfaces, suddenly interfering with the normal mechanics of the joint.

A major displacement of a torn fragment may grossly interfere with normal mechanics and block joint movement in a noncapsular pattern. The classic example is a "bucket-handle" tear of a medial meniscus.

When the annular ring of a vertebral disk is torn, secondary neurologic symptoms or signs may result from bulging of the nucleus against adjacent nerve tissue.

JOINT CAPSULE

Fibrosis (see section on capsular tightness) typically occurs with prolonged immobilization of a joint, in association with a chronic, low-grade inflammatory process such as occurs with degenerative joint disease, and with resolution of acute inflammation of the synovium. Joint motion is limited in a capsular pattern, and there is a capsular end feel at the extremes of movement.

Synovial inflammation is commonly caused by rheumatoid arthritis, acute trauma to the joint, joint infection, and arthrotomy. Joint motion is limited in a capsular pattern. There is a painful muscle spasm end feel at the points of restriction of movements.

Inflammation of the synovium results in an increased production of synovial fluid, causing capsular distention and loss of the capsular laxity necessary for full movement. In the more superficial joints, the articular swelling can be observed and palpated. If the effusion persists after resolution of the synovial inflammation, motion will continue to be limited in a capsular fashion, with a boggy end feel to movement.

Patients with capsular pathology typically have some combination of fibrosis, synovial inflammation, and effusion. Therefore, end feels are not always distinct.

Forces sufficient to sprain a ligament usually cause some capsular disruption as well. Occasionally in traumatic injuries, a particular portion of a joint capsule is ruptured, such as the anterior capsule of the shoulder when the humerus dislocates anteriorly. Synovial inflammation and joint effusion usually follow capsular sprains.

In the case of a sprain, the joint-play movement that stresses the involved portion of the capsule will be of normal amplitude. In more severe sprains, the joint may be slightly hypermobile, with a painful muscle-guarding end feel.

LIGAMENTS

The history of a sprain invariably includes a traumatic onset. In the case of a mild sprain, the joint-play movement that stresses the ligament is of normal amplitude and is painful. More severe sprains (partial ruptures) will present as somewhat hypermobile and painful on the associated joint-play test. The synovial lining of the adjacent aspect of the joint capsule will often become inflamed, resulting in capsular effusion in the acute stage. There is usually tenderness over the site of the lesion.

The onset of a rupture is also usually traumatic. The associated joint-play movement test will be hypermobile and painless in the chronic stages. Even in the acute stage it is usually painless, because there are no fibers intact from which to elicit pain. If adjacent capsular tissue is also sprained, there may be some pain on stress testing in the acute stage. Capsular effusion often does not occur because fluid leaks through the defect. In the chronic stages the patient may give a history of instability. The joint gives way during activities that stress it in the direction that the ruptured ligament is supposed to check.

BURSAE

The common disorder of bursae is inflammation, secondary to chronic irritation, infection, gout, or, rarely, acute trauma. Movement of the nearby joint will cause pain or restriction of motion, or both, in a noncapsular pattern. There may be a painful arc of movement as well.

In acute bursitis, such as at the shoulder, the end feel to movement is often empty and painful; protective muscle spasm would only serve to squeeze the inflamed structure, increasing the pain. There is usually tenderness over the site of the lesion.

TENDONS

Tendinitis is a minor lesion of tendon tissue involving microscopic tearing and a chronic, low-grade inflammatory process.

In most cases it is degenerative; the lesion results from tissue fatigue rather than from acute injury. Because progression of the pathologic process will result in a partial tear (macroscopic) or rupture of the tendon, tendinitis should be considered on a continuum with more serious lesions.

The key clinical sign associated with tendinitis is a strong but painful resisted test of the involved musculotendinous structure. There may be pain at the extremes of the passive movement or movements that stretch the tendon. Seldom is there limitation of movement. There may be palpable tenderness at the site of the lesion or referred tenderness into the related segment, or both.

When the involved part of a tendon is that which passes through a sheath, two other terms are often used: tenosynovitis and tenovaginitis. **Tenosynovitis** is an inflammation of the synovial lining of a sheath resulting from friction of a roughened tendon gliding within the sheath. This will present similarly to tendinitis, but there is often pain on activity that produces movement of the tendon within the sheath. Thus, active movement in the direction or opposite the direction of pull of the tendon may be painful. In **tenovaginitis,** a tendon gliding within a swollen, thickened sheath causes pain. The classic example occurs with rheumatoid arthritis. The clinical signs are essentially the same as those for tenosynovitis. There may be palpable and visible swelling of the tendon sheath.

In the case of a partial tendon tear, actual loss of continuity of tendon tissue will cause weak and painful responses to the resisted test for the musculotendinous complex. The passive movement that stretches the tendon may be painful.

When the tendon has torn completely, the findings of the related resisted test will be weak and painless. In some cases, for example, rupture of the Achilles tendon, there may be a palpable gap at the site of the rupture.

MUSCLES

Muscle strains and ruptures are relatively rare. When they do occur they are invariably the result of acute trauma and are therefore most prevalent in sports medicine settings. Muscles, being well vascularized and resilient, do not commonly undergo fatigue degeneration as do tendons.

In the case of a strain, a minor tear of muscle fibers will result in a strong and painful finding on the resisted test that stresses the involved muscle. There may be pain on full passive stretch of the muscle and palpable tenderness. In the case of a rupture, the associated resisted test results will be weak and painless. A gap may be palpable, or occasionally visible, at the site of the defect.

NERVES

The common conditions affecting nerves are those in which some extrinsic source of pressure results in altered conduction along some or all of the nerve fibers—the so-called **entrapment syndromes.** The most common sites of pressure are the points of exit of the lower cervical and lower lumbar spinal nerves from the intervertebral foramina. Here pressure is usually from a protruding disk or projecting osteophyte. There are other common sites of pressure farther out in the periphery that affect the nerves to the extremities. Pressure tends to alter conduction first along the largest fibers and last along the smallest. Altered nerve conduction is usually manifested subjectively before any objective clinical evidence of neurologic dysfunction can be detected. In fact, in the case of the common entrapment syndromes, objective clinical findings are rare, and when present they are usually quite subtle. Often more sophisticated electrodiagnostic tests are required to objectively detect changes in nerve conduction.

The subjective complaints associated with common entrapment disorders can generally be classified as paresthesia (pins and needles), dysesthesia (altered sensation in response to some external stimulus), and pain. Although some patients may describe paresthesia and dysesthesia as painful, pain is usually not a primary complaint when there is pressure on a nerve farther out in the periphery rather than at the nerve-root level. Thus, patients with thoracic outlet syndrome, ulnar nerve palsy, and carpal tunnel syndrome, as well as those who have sat too long with the legs crossed, do not complain of pain but of a pins-and-needles sensation. Pain is a common complaint, however, in cases in which there is pressure on a nerve at nerve-root level. With initial pressure, when the larger, myelinated, "fast pain" fibers are stimulated, patients describe a sharp, shooting dermatomic quality of pain. With prolonged or increased pressure, when the larger fibers cease to conduct and the small, unmyelinated C fibers are stimulated, a dull, aching sclerotomic type of pain will be perceived.

Paresthesia, the primary subjective complaint with pressure farther out in the periphery, may occur with the onset of pressure or when the pressure is released, or both. For example, a person usually feels little or nothing when sitting with legs crossed, with pressure applied to the tibial or peroneal nerve. It is not until the person uncrosses the legs, releasing the pressure, that the pins-and-needles sensation of the foot being "asleep" is felt. A similar situation holds true for pressure on the lower cord of the brachial plexus from depression of the shoulder girdle; the patient invariably describes the onset of pins and needles in the early morning hours (1 or 2 AM) some time after the pressure is released. It seems that the interval between the release of pressure and the onset of paresthesia is in some way proportional to the length of time during which the pressure was applied. In other common nerve problems, the onset of symptoms occurs when the pressure is applied. For example, many patients with carpal tunnel syndrome describe paresthesia felt primarily during fine finger movements; the tension on the finger flexor tendons produces pressure on the median nerve sufficient to cause symptoms. Similarly, when a person sits or lies with pressure over the ulnar groove, pins and needles are usually felt in the ulnar side of the hand while the pressure is applied, and cease to be felt after the pressure is released.

As mentioned, more objective findings associated with common nerve-pressure disorders are usually very subtle when present. They are more common with nerve-root pressure from a disk protrusion than with more peripheral entrapment syndromes. The earliest evidence of decreased conduction will be related to those functions mediated by the largest myelinated fibers, because these fibers are most sensitive to pressure. Therefore, reduced vibration sense is often the earliest deficit detected by clinical testing. With increased or prolonged pressure, diminished deep-tendon reflexes may be noted, followed by reduced muscle strength. Finally, there is reduced sensation, first to light touch, then to noxious stimulation. Because of overlapping dermatomes and myotomes, and because each muscle and skin area typically receives innervation from more than one segment, even completely severing a nerve root will usually cause only a minor deficit.

Extent of the Lesion

When clinicians speak of acute and chronic lesions, it is often unclear whether they are referring to the length of time that the pathologic process has existed, the severity of the disorder, or the nature of the inflammatory process. There are relatively few consistent clinical findings related to either the duration or the severity of common musculoskeletal problems. However, there are certain symptoms and signs that are consistently present with acute inflammatory processes and others that are pathognomonic of lesions in which a more chronic inflammatory state exists. **Acute inflammation** is that stage or type of inflammatory process in which hyperemia, increased capillary permeability with protein and plasma leakage, and an influx of granulocytes and other defense cells takes place. **Chronic inflammation** is characterized by an attempt at repair, with increased numbers of fibrocytes and other "tissue-building" cells, and the presence of granulation tissue. An acute lesion is characterized by the following clinical findings:

1. Pain is relatively constant.
2. On passive range of motion of the related joint, there is a muscle spasm end feel or an empty end feel to movement.
3. Pain is likely to be referred over a relatively diffuse area of the related segment.
4. There may be a measurable increase in skin temperature over the site of the lesion.
5. There is often difficulty in falling asleep or difficulty in remaining asleep, or both.

In the presence of chronic lesions, the patient is likely to present with the following symptoms or signs:

1. Pain is increased by specific activities and relieved by rest.
2. On passive movement of the related joint, there is no muscle spasm or empty end feel.
3. Pain is likely to be felt over a relatively localized area, close to the site of the lesion, although often not directly over the site of the lesion.
4. There is little or no temperature elevation over the involved part.

5. Unless the lesion involves the shoulder or hip, there is little or no difficulty in sleeping.

Setting Goals and Priorities

Following the diagnosis, the clinician establishes short-term and long-term goals of treatment. Determining appropriate treatment goals assists the therapist in planning, prioritizing, and measuring the effectiveness of treatment. The goals are derived from the patient's symptom(s), signs, and diagnosis and from the patient's personal, vocational, and social goals. Involvement of the patient is critical in achieving patient compliance.[19] Information obtained from the patient should be integrated with the subjective and objective assessment data. A goal statement should be generated with the patient's full cooperation and understanding.

Long-term goals identify the functional behaviors to be attained by the patient by the end of the treatment program. Once long-term goals have been established, the next step is to determine the component skills that will be needed to attain these goals. Short-term goals identify the progressive functional levels to be attained by the patient at specific intervals within the projected period of treatment.[11] The clinician should determine the appropriate sequence of subskills and prioritize them accordingly. The patient advances through the sequence of short-term goals until he or she achieves the final end point of long-term goals. The goals and diagnosis direct treatment.

CONCEPTS OF MANAGEMENT

Only those procedures that may not be well understood or are new to most professional training programs are discussed in this section. It is assumed that the reader is familiar with many basic therapeutic procedures and modalities, such as therapeutic exercise, use of assistive devices, and electrotherapy. The application of these forms of treatment, in conjunction with traditional therapies, to specific pathologic processes affecting the various extremity regions is discussed in Parts II and III of this book.

Rehabilitation

The correlation and interpretation of findings from a comprehensive initial patient examination is the basis for developing a treatment plan. During the initial examination clinicians seek to elicit information that relates to the nature and extent of the pathologic process as well as to the degree of disability. The choice of therapeutic procedures depends on this information.

The primary considerations are the site of the lesion and the type of tissue involved. Once the nature of the lesion has been determined, there is often a tendency to direct treatment primarily at the site of the lesion, with the expectation that resolving the pathologic process will alleviate any resultant physical dysfunction and will in turn restore the patient to a normal health state.

There are many potential fallacies to this approach that make it unsuitable as a reliable treatment model. First, such an approach ignores the secondary effects that a lesion involving a particular structure may have on the normal functioning of other related structures. It calls for treatment of "anatomic structures" rather than "physiologic units." By considering the synovial joints as the basic physiologic—rather than anatomic—unit of the musculoskeletal system, one is better prepared to respect the interactions of the various components of this system under normal and abnormal conditions. This is essential because an alteration in one component of a functional unit often leads to dysfunction of other components of the same or neighboring units, which may act to maintain the primary pathologic condition, predispose to recurrence, or result in secondary disease. Thus, even in the case of relatively localized lesions, clinicians must respect such interactions and be prepared to deal with them therapeutically.

For example, a painful lesion of the supraspinatus tendon tends to result in reflex inhibition of the supraspinatus and other rotator cuff muscles. This will predispose to subacromial impingement from abnormal movement of the head of the humerus during elevation activities, which may further traumatize the supraspinatus tendon as well as the subdeltoid bursa. Also, muscles such as the deltoid and the trapezius may reflexively contract abnormally during movement of the arm, secondary to abnormal afferent input from the site of the lesion to the lower cervical segments. This may further interfere with normal joint mechanics at the shoulder as well as at the neck, to which the trapezius attaches. It is clear that effective treatment of this problem involves more than resolution of the pathologic process affecting the tendon. The rotator cuff muscles must, at some time, be strengthened; excessive elevation of the arm must be temporarily avoided; and relaxation of abnormally contracting muscles should be promoted. If one were to treat only the lesion of the tendon, it is likely that treatment would be ineffective or take much longer than necessary to be effective. Continued subacromial impingement would enhance the chance of recurrence. The patient would also be predisposed to the development of a coexistent cervical lesion from increased stresses to the neck owing to abnormal muscle activity.

Second, an approach in which treatment is aimed exclusively at some discrete pathologic process tends to ignore etiologic considerations. Temporary amelioration may ensue without true resolution of the problem. Unless underlying causes, such as biomechanical abnormalities, are recognized and dealt with, chronic recurrent problems can be expected. Thus, a patient with chondromalacia patellae resulting from abnormal foot pronation may temporarily do very well on a program of reduced activity and strengthening of the vastus medialis muscle. However, the patient is likely to experience similar problems with the resumption of normal activity levels unless the alignment of the foot and leg is corrected. Similarly, the patient with trochanteric bursitis caused by a tight iliotibial band usually responds well to ultrasound over the site of the lesion, but if extensibility of the iliotibial band is not increased, relief will be short lived. The clinician should implement the concept that prevention is the ultimate cure by attempting to identify etiologic factors and by employing appropriate measures to deal with them. This should be a major consideration in fatigue disorders that are chronic, because they tend to be self-resolving once the cause of the abnormal stresses is corrected (see the later outlined treatment of chronic disorders in this chapter).

Third, and most important, when treatment is directed only at a physical disorder, the psychosocial implications of the problem are not given due respect. Comprehensive rehabilitation requires restoration of an optimal level of function. Although a physical disorder may have been the original cause of physical dysfunction or other "disease behaviors" such as complaints of pain, there are often other factors that may serve to maintain or inhibit the disability behaviors. Such "motivational factors" may eventually assume a greater influence on the disability state than the original pathology (Fig. 5-1). These factors must be recognized because they often determine whether treatment is successful, whether an optimal level of function is restored, and whether disability behaviors (pain complaints, physical dysfunction, and functional dependence) are resolved. If being disabled carries excessively negative consequences for the patient, such as often occurs in sports medicine settings, these consequences will strongly inhibit the disability state. As a result, the patient often attempts to do more than is appropriate and imposes deleterious effects on the lesion. This may counteract any beneficial effects of other treatment procedures. On the other hand, if the patient stands to gain in some way from being disabled, such as time away from work, financial compensation, or welcomed dependence, the potential for gain may have a significant reinforcing effect on the disability state. The patient is not likely to improve despite otherwise effective treatment of the pathologic condition. In both of these situations, the psychosocial motivational influences are likely to have a greater effect on the disease state than the physical process itself. Unless these influences are dealt with, the patient cannot be truly rehabilitated. To estimate the relative influence of such factors, the clinician must determine whether the degree of disability is consistent with the symptoms and signs manifested by the disease. If there are inconsistencies, significant psychosocial influences affecting the nature of the disability state should be suspected.

Treatment of Patients with Physical Disorders

Although the principle of "treating the patient, not the disease" has become somewhat of a cliché, its application to patients with common musculoskeletal disorders is too often overlooked. The first consideration when devising a therapeutic program is how the patient's ability to function normally has been compromised. One must ask what conditions are responsible for the dysfunction and are these conditions reversible?

If they were reversible, what are the most appropriate means of intervening therapeutically so as to affect these conditions? If the conditions at fault appear irreversible, what can be done to optimize residual function? Finally, what can be done to prevent recurrences, secondary problems, and progression of the existing disorder? With such an approach, therapy is disability-oriented rather than pathology-oriented. The primary goal of management becomes restoration of an optimal level of functioning rather than simply resolution of some pathologic process. Resolution of a physical disorder does not necessarily lead to restoration of function, reduction in pain behavior, or other necessary signs of improvement.

In the case of many common musculoskeletal disorders, in which the degree of disability appears to be consistent with the nature and extent of the lesion, physical treatment will constitute a major component of the therapeutic program. When this is the case, clinicians must choose, among the various forms of intervention at their disposal, the procedures and modalities most appropriate for the management of the specific disorder. Treatment must be individualized for each patient and according to the nature and extent of the pathologic process. The tendency to incorporate "standardized" programs of exercises and other treatments, usually for the sake of efficiency, should be avoided. The controversies over and misconceptions about so many forms of treatment (e.g., massage, manipulation, traction, and certain exercises) stem largely from their having been advocated or misconstrued as panaceas for disorders affecting certain regions.

CLASSIFYING PATHOLOGIES: ACUTE VERSUS CHRONIC

As a preface to discussing specific types of treatments and their respective applications, some general concepts that are related to the overall approach to physical treatment are considered. As mentioned previously, approaches to treating a physical disorder should depend on its nature and extent. The two common terms used clinically to classify pathologic processes according to their nature and extent are acute and chronic. These terms should not be used to refer to the severity or duration of a disorder, since when used in these contexts they have little relationship to symptoms and signs. A patient with a relatively severe lesion such as a ligamentous rupture, for example, may present with much less pain and dysfunction than one whom has sustained a minor sprain. It is well known, even to those outside the healthcare professions, that a sprained ankle may be more painful and disabling shortly after injury than a fractured ankle. With respect to duration, disorders of fairly recent onset often present with subtle symptoms and signs when compared with certain long-standing problems. If a clinician has two patients, one with recent onset of aching in the shoulder but no gross loss of function and the other with long-standing severe pain and dysfunction, which condition is acute and which is chronic?

The terms **acute** and **chronic** have some significance when used to refer to the nature of the symptoms and signs with which a patient presents, as differentiated earlier in this chapter. This is because symptoms and signs reflect the nature of various disorders and, more specifically, they tend to reflect the nature of the inflammation or repair process that accompanies any physical lesion. Because these symptom–sign complexes do relate to the nature of pathologic processes, they are used here as a basis for a discussion of general approaches to management. The following scheme is based on the definitions of acute and chronic.

TREATMENT OF ACUTE AND CHRONIC DISORDERS

I. General Concepts
   A. Consider the nature and extent of the disorder, whether acute or chronic.
      1. These terms are sometimes used to refer to duration of the problem and not to symptoms and signs.
      2. They should be used to refer to the nature of the inflammatory process.
         a. Acute hyperemic phase
            i.   Pain is felt at rest and aggravated by activity.
            ii. Pain is felt over a relatively diffuse area and may be referred into any or all of the related segments (sclerotome).
            iii. Passive movement of related joints when limited is restricted by pain, muscle guarding, or both.
            iv. Skin temperature over the site of the lesion is often elevated.
         b. Chronic/reparative phase
            i.   There is no pain at rest and pain is felt only with specific activities.
            ii. Pain is felt over a fairly localized area, close to the site of the lesion (often not directly over the site of the lesion, however).
            iii. Movement of related joints, when limited, is restricted by soft tissue tightness; pain is felt only at the extremes of movement or through a small arc of movement.
      3. The terms are not useful in describing the severity of the lesion. For example, a patient with a complete rupture of a ligament may present with less pain, less disability, and fewer cardinal inflammatory signs than a person with only a partial tear of a ligament.
   B. Assess, control, and monitor the patient's functional status.
      1. Assess the degree of disability from findings of the history and physical examination. Compare disease (injury) status with health (normal) status, and compare with other symptoms and signs.
         a. Is the degree of disability consistent with the apparent nature and extent of the disorder? This yields important information relating to the patient's motivational status and is a major consideration in treatment planning.
            i.   The well-motivated patient is one for whom the consequences of injury (disability) are punishing. For example, they imply time away from desirable situations or possibility of financial loss. It can be presumed that resolution of the disease will lead to resolution of the disability state. A medical approach to treatment is appropriate.
            ii. The poorly motivated patient is one for whom the consequences of disability are reinforcing. For example, they offer time away from undesirable situations or the possibility of financial gain. It cannot be presumed that treatment of the disease will result in resolution of the disability state. Rehabilitation must include attempts to alter the consequences to disability. An operant approach must be incorporated into the treatment program.
         b. Record and use information as baselines by which to judge progress.
      2. Control functional status (see below under techniques of management).
         a. Inappropriate activities must be restricted to prevent prolongation or recurrence of the disorder.
         b. Appropriate activities must be resumed as the pathologic process resolves. This is the *ultimate goal* of management.
      3. Monitor functional status to judge improvement. The patient is not rehabilitated until an optimal level of function is restored, regardless of the state of the lesion.

II. Treatment of Acute Inflammatory Disorders (Traumatic)
    The primary goal is to promote progression to a chronic state while minimizing dysfunction.
    A. Physiologic intervention to control the acute inflammatory response:
       1. Ice—To reduce blood flow.
       2. Compression—To prevent and reduce swelling.
       3. Elevation—To prevent and reduce swelling and hyperemia.
       4. Relaxation—To reduce pain and muscle spasm.
    B. Avoidance and prevention of continued trauma and irritation by reducing loading of the part.
       1. Braces, slings, splints, assistive devices, strapping.
          a. Lower extremity—Crutches or canes to reduce forces of weight bearing; splints, braces, or strapping to reduce forces of movement.
          b. Upper extremity—Slings to reduce forces of gravity and, therefore, postural muscle tone; splints, braces, or strapping to reduce the forces imposed by movement.
          c. Spine—Passive support with collar or corset if indicated.
       2. Control of activities causing undesirable loading of the part. This requires careful, well-understood instructions to the patient.
    C. Maintaining optimal levels of function and preventing unnecessary dysfunction.

1. Isometric resistive exercises to maintain muscle function while avoiding undesirable movement of the part.
2. In acute nuclear prolapse, isometric activities (e.g., pelvic tilt exercises, straining, and Valsalva maneuvers) must be avoided.
3. With respect to the spine:
   a. Rest is interspersed with periods of controlled activity.
   b. Positions that increase intradiskal pressure should be avoided (e.g., acute disk protrusions).
4. Gentle active or passive movement (when appropriate according to the nature of the disorder) to avoid pain and muscle guarding.

III. Treatment of Chronic Disorders
A. Causative factors. The majority of disorders seen in most clinical settings have two primary causes:
1. Abnormal modeling of tissue during resolution of an acute disorder. The following are examples:
   a. Malunion of fractures resulting in a change in the direction or magnitude of forces acting on the part during use (increased stress).
   b. Abnormalities in collagen maturation or production (scarring, fibrosis, adhesions). An excess amount of collagen may be produced, and that which is produced may not be oriented along the normal lines of stress. Abnormal collagen cross-links are formed, and the tissue may adhere to adjacent structures. The net result is reduced extensibility and therefore reduced capacity to attenuate energy by deforming when stressed.
2. Fatigue response of tissues. There are two types of response:
   a. Tissue breakdown. The rate of attrition exceeds the rate of repair (e.g., stress fractures and cartilage degeneration). The tissue becomes "weaker" and begins to yield under loading conditions. It occurs with mild to moderately increased stress levels in tissues with low regenerative capacity (e.g., articular cartilage), with higher stress levels in other tissues (e.g., tendon, bone), and under conditions of altered tissue metabolism (e.g., hypovascularity).
   b. Tissue hypertrophy (e.g., fibrosis and sclerosis) occurs with mild to moderately increased stress levels in tissues with good regenerative/repair capacity, acting over a prolonged period. Tissue becomes stiffer, with reduced energy attenuation capacity. Individual fibers or trabeculae begin to yield under loading conditions, resulting in low-grade inflammation, pain, increased tissue production, and so on.
B. Treatment planning.
1. Reduce magnitude of loading (control of activities).
   a. Reduce magnitude of loading (control of activities).
   b. Reduce magnitude of stresses by altering direction or magnitude of forces acting on the part through control of activities, use of protective/assistive devices, and use of orthotic devices to control position of the part.

c. Increase surface area of loading (e.g., foot orthosis).
d. Provide for external energy attenuation (e.g., pads, helmets, and cushioned heels).
2. Increase energy-attenuating capacity of the part.
   a. Increase compensatory muscle strength/activity with strengthening exercises; increase neuromuscular facilitative (afferent) input (e.g., taping, coordination training).
   b. Increase tissue extensibility (ability to deform without loss of structural integrity):
      i. Active stretching.
      ii. Passive stretching, using passive range-of-motion stretching for musculotendinous tightness and specific joint mobilization for capsuloligamentous tightness.
      iii. Use of ultrasound in conjunction with stretch.
      iv. Use of transverse friction massage to increase interfiber mobility and to prevent or reduce fibrous adhesion without longitudinally stressing the tissue.
      v. Soft tissue manipulations directed at muscle, ligaments, and fascial layers to restore mobility and extensibility.
   c. Promote increase in structural integrity of the part (increased "strength"). This requires tissue hypertrophy, without loss of extensibility from overproduction of immature collagenous tissue, and so on, and maturation of collagen fiber orientation along normal lines of stress and development of appropriate cross-links.

   The necessary stimulus is stress to the part. This means gradual, controlled return to participation in high–stress-level activities (training).
3. Resumption of optimal activity levels and prevention of recurrence. Judgments are based on the following:
   a. Clinical evidence of having accomplished above objectives.
   b. Awareness of the nature of stresses imposed by various activities and an estimate of the capacity of the part to withstand those stresses. This requires biomechanical assessment and analysis and familiarity with research related to biomechanical properties of musculoskeletal tissues under various conditions of loading and healing.
   c. Extrinsic "motivational" factors—the consequences of disability for the patient.

Patients with true chronic pain syndrome should not be treated with the emphasis on pain modulation. Whereas acute pain bears a relatively straightforward relationship to peripheral stimulus, nociception, and tissue damage, chronic pain disability becomes increasingly dissociated from the original physical basis and there may be little if any evidence of any remaining nociceptive stimulus. Emphasis should be placed on functional restoration, which uses sports medicine principles. This approach emphasizes the recognition, through objective quantitative assessment of physical function, of the loss of physical capacity that accompanies disuse (termed the **deconditioning syndrome**).[76] The focus should be on augmenting function and on increasing physical activity, mobility, strength, endurance, and cardiovascular improvement.

Evaluation of the Treatment Program

The last step is ongoing and involves continuous re-evaluation of the patient and efficacy of treatment. Recognition of the original problems that have been solved and those that need further attention must be made. New short-term goals should be established and appropriate procedures selected. In determining and implementing revised goals and related treatment and criteria, the clinician is again at the problem-solving stage of determining and administering treatment. When long-term goals are reached or are close to being reached, discharge planning and plan for follow-up care (when indicated) are initiated. The overall success of the treatment plan is dependent on the therapist's clinical decision-making skills and on engaging the patient's cooperation and motivation.[84]

REFERENCES

1. Agarwal A, Lloyd KN, Dovey P: The dermography of the spine and sacroiliac joints in spondylitis. Rheum Phys Med 10:349–355, 1970
2. Aprill C: Radiologic imaging techniques of the spine. In: Hochschuler SH, Cotler HB, Guyer RD, eds: Rehabilitation of the Spine. St. Louis, CV Mosby, 1993:79–111
3. Barnett C, Davies D, MacConaill MA: Synovial Joints: Their Structure and Mechanics. Springfield, IL, Charles C. Thomas, 1961
4. Basmajian J: Muscles Alive: Their Functions Revealed by Electromyography, 4th ed. Baltimore, Williams & Wilkins, 1978
5. Behr D, Katz, Krebs D: Diagnosis enhances, not impedes boundaries of physical therapy practice. Orthop Sports Phys Ther 13:218–219, 1991
6. Bookhout MR: Examination and treatment of muscle imbalances. In: Bourdillon JF, Day EA, Bookhout MR, eds: Spinal Manipulation, 5th ed. Oxford, Butterworth-Heinenmann, 1992:313–333
7. Bourdillon JG, Day EA, Bookhout MR: Examination: General considerations. In: Bourdillon JG, Day EA, Bookhout MR, eds: Spinal Manipulation, 5th ed. Oxford, Butterworth-Heinemann, 1992:46–80
8. Bowers TA, Murray JA: Bone metastases from renal carcinoma: The preoperative use of transcatheter arterial occlusion. J Bone Joint Surg Am 64:749–754, 1982
9. Butler DS: Mobilisation of the Nervous System. Melbourne, Churchill Livingstone, 1991
10. Cantu RI, Grodin AJ: Myofascial Manipulation: Theory and Clinical Application. Gaithersburg, Aspen, 1992
11. Catlin PA: Elements of problem solving. In: Greenfield BH, ed: Rehabilitation of the Knee: A Problem-Solving Approach. Philadelphia, FA Davis, 1993:66–84
12. Citrin DL, Bessent RG, Greig WR: A comparison of the sensitivity and accuracy of the Tc-99 phosphate bone scan and skeletal radiographs in the diagnosis of bone metastases. Clin Radiol 28:107–117, 1977
13. Clarkson HM, Gilewich GD: Assessment: Joint Range of Motion and Manual Muscle Strength. Baltimore, Williams & Wilkins, 1989
14. Cole JH, Furness AL, Twomey LT: Muscles in Action, An Approach to Manual Muscle Testing. Edinburg, Churchill Livingstone, 1996
15. Colodney AK, Raj P: Reflex Sympathetic Dystrophy. In: Hochschuler SH, Cotler HB, Guyer RD, eds: Rehabilitation of the Spine: Science and Practice. St. Louis, CV Mosby, 1993:509–532
16. Corrigan B, Maitland GD: Examination. In: Corrigan B, Maitland GD, eds: Practical Orthopaedic Medicine. London, Butterworth, 1985:9–17
17. Cyriax JH: Textbook of Orthopaedic Medicine, vol. 1. Diagnosis of Soft Tissue Lesions, 8th ed. London, Bailliere Tindall, 1982
18. DeRosa CP, Porterfield JA: A physical therapy model for treatment of low back pain. Phys Ther 72:261–269, 1992
19. DiMatteo M, DiNicola D: Achieving Patient Compliance. New York, Pergamon Press, 1982
20. Downie J, Elstein AS, eds: Professional Judgement: A Reader in Clinical Decision Making. New York, Cambridge University Press, 1988

21. Duensing F, Becker P, Rittmeyer K: Thermographic findings in lumbar disc protrusions. Arch Psychiatr Nervevenkr 217:53–70, 1973
22. Dyke P: Lumbar nerve root: The enigmatic eponyms. Spine 9:3–6, 1984
23. Dyrek DA: Assessment and treatment planning strategies for musculoskeletal deficits. In: O'Sullivan SB, Schmitz TJ, eds: Physical Rehabilitation and Assessment and Treatment, 3rd ed. Philadelphia, FA Davis, 1994:61–82
24. Echternach JL, Rothstein JM: Hypothesis-oriented algorithms. Phys Ther 69:559–564, 1989
25. Edelman R, Schoukimas G, Stark D, et al: High resolution surface coil imaging of lumbar disc disease. Am J Radiol 144:1123–1129, 1985
26. Edmond SL: Manipulations and Mobilization: Extremity and Spinal Techniques. St. Louis, CV Mosby, 1993
27. Elvey RL: Brachial plexus tension tests and the pathoanatomical origin of arm pain. In: Glasgow EF, Twomey LT, Scull ER, et al., eds: Aspects of Manipulative Therapy. Melbourne, Churchill Livingstone, 1980:105–110
28. Feinstein AR: Clinical Judgement. Malabar, Robert E. Kreiger, 1967
29. Ferguson AB, D'Ambrosia RD: Roentgenogram Interpretation. In: D'Ambrosia RD, ed: Musculoskeletal Disorders: Regional Examination and Differential Diagnosis, 2nd ed. Philadelphia, JB Lippincott, 1986:21–58
30. Fordyce WE: Behavioral Methods for Chronic Pain and Illness. St. Louis, CV Mosby, 1976
31. Fordyce WE: Evaluating and managing chronic pain. Geriatrics 33:59–62, 1978
32. Fordyce WE, Fowler RS, Lehmann JF, et al: Operant conditioning in the treatment of chronic clinical pain. Arch Phys Med Rehabil 54:399–408, 1973
33. Galasko CSB: The significance of occult skeletal metastases, detected by skeletal scintigraphy, in patients with otherwise apparent "early" mammary carcinoma. Br J Surg 67:694–696, 1975
34. Goldie IF, Reichman S: The biomechanical influence of traction on cervical spine. Scand J Rehab Med 9:31–34, 1977
35. Greenfield GB: Analytical approach to bone radiology. In: Greenfield GB, ed: Radiology of Bone Disease, 4th ed. Philadelphia, JB Lippincott, 1986:1–30
36. Greenman PE: Barrier concepts in structural diagnosis. In: Greenfield GB, ed: Principles of Manual Therapy, 2nd ed. Baltimore, Williams & Wilkins, 1996:39–44
37. Grieve GP: Mobilisation of the Spine: Notes on Examination, Assessment and Clinical Method, 5th ed. Edinburgh, Churchill Livingstone, 1991
38. Handel J, Selby D: Spinal instability. In: Hochschuler SH, Cotler HB, Guyer RD, eds: Rehabilitation of the Spine: Science and Practice. St. Louis, CV Mosby, 1993:153–166
39. Harris BA, Dyrek DA: A model of orthopaedic dysfunction for clinical decision making in physical therapy. Phys Ther 69:548–553, 1989
40. Hislop HJ, Montgomery J: Daniel's and Worthingham's Muscle Testing: Techniques of Manual Examination, 6th ed. Philadelphia, WB Saunders, 1995
41. Huskisson EC, Berry H, Browett J, et al: Measurement of inflammation. Ann Rheum Dis 32:99–102, 1973
42. International Classification of Impairments, Disabilities, and Handicaps. Geneva, Switzerland, World Health Organization, 1980
43. Janda V: Muscles, central nervous motor regulation and back problems. In: Korr I, ed: The Neurobiologic Mechanisms in Manipulative Therapy. New York, Plenum Press, 1978:27–41
44. Janda V: Muscles as a pathogenic factor in back pain. In: The Treatment of Patients. Proceedings of the 4th International Federation of Orthopaedic Manipulative Therapists, Christchurch, New Zealand, 1980
45. Janda V: Muscle Function Testing. London, Butterworth, 1983
46. Janda V: Muscle weakness and inhibition (pseudoparesis) in back pain syndromes. In: Grieve GP, ed: Modern Manual Therapy of the Vertebral Column. Edinburg, Churchill Livingstone, 1986:197–201
47. Janda V: Muscles and cervicogenic pain syndromes. In: Grant R, ed: Physical Therapy of the Cervical and Thoracic Spine, New York, Churchill Livingstone, 1988
48. Janda V: Muscle strength in relation to muscle length, pain and muscle imbalance. In: Harms-Rindahl K, ed: Muscle Strength. New York, Churchill Livingstone, 1993:83–105
49. Janda V: Evaluation of muscular imbalance. In: Liebenson C, ed: Rehabilitation of the Spine. Philadelphia, Lippincott, Williams & Wilkins, 1996:97–112
50. Jensen GM: Musculoskeletal analysis. In: Scully RM, Barnes MR, eds: Physical Therapy. Philadelphia, JB Lippincott, 1989:326–339
51. Jette AM: Diagnosis and classification by physical therapist: A special communication. Phys Ther 69:967–969, 1989
52. Jones C: Physical aspects of thermography in relation to clinical techniques. Bibl Radio 6:1–8, 1975
53. Jones MA: Clinical reasoning in manual therapy. Phys Ther 72:875–884, 1992
54. Jull GA, Janda V: Muscles and motor control in low back pain. In: Twoney LT, Taylor JR, eds: Physical Therapy of the Low Back. New York, Churchill Livingstone, 1987:253–278
55. Jull GA, Richardson CA: Rehabilitation of active stabilization of the lumbar spine. In: Twoney LT, Taylor JR, eds: Physical Therapy of the Lumbar Spine, 2nd ed. New York, Churchill Livingstone, 1994:251–283
56. Kaltenborn FM: Mobilization of the Extremities, 3rd ed. Oslo, Olaf Norlis Bokhandel Universitetsgaten, 1980
57. Kaltenborn FM: The Spine: Basic Evaluation and Mobilization Techniques, 2nd ed. Oslo, Olaf Norlis Bokhandel Universitetsgaten, 1993

58. Kendall FP, McCreary EK, Provance PG: Muscle Testing and Function. 4th ed. Baltimore, Williams & Wilkins, 1993

59. Keene JS: Ligament and muscle-tendon-unit injuries. In: Gould JA, Davies GJ, eds: Orthopaedic and Sports Physical Therapy. St. Louis, CV Mosby, 1985:135–165

60. Kenna C, Murtagh J: Back Pain and Spinal Manipulation. Sydney, Butterworth, 1989:1–34

61. Kettenbach G: Writing SOAP Notes. Philadelphia, FA Davis, 1990

62. Korr IM, Thomas PE, Wright HM: Patterns of electrical skin resistance in man. Acta Neuroveget 17:77–96, 1958

63. Korr IM, Wright HM, Chase JA: Cutaneous patterns of sympathetic activity in clinical abnormalities of the musculoskeletal system. Acta Neuroveget 4:589–606, 1962

64. Korr IM, Wright HM, Thomas PE: Effect of experimental myofascial insults on cutaneous patterns of sympathetic activity in man. Acta Neuroveget 23:329–355, 1962

65. Kraus SL: Physical therapy management of TMD. In: Kraus SL, ed: Temporomandibular Disorders, 2nd ed. Edinburgh, Churchill Livingstone, 1994:161–216

66. Lewitt K: Manipulative Therapy in Rehabilitation of the Locomotor System. Oxford, Butterworth-Heinemann, 1991

67. Lewitt K: Role of manipulation in spinal rehabilitation. In: Liebenson C, ed: Rehabilitation of the Spine. Philadelphia, Lippincott, Williams and Wilkins, 1996

68. MacConaill MA, Basmajian JV: Muscles and Movement. Hunting, Robert E. Krieger, 1977:13–44

69. Magee DJ: Principles and concepts. In: Magee DJ, ed: Orthopedic Physical Assessment, 3rd ed. Philadelphia, WB Saunders, 1997:1–52

70. Maigne R: Manipulation of the spine. In: Basmajian JV, ed: Manipulation, Traction and Massage. Baltimore, Williams & Wilkins, 1986:71–96

71. Maigne R: Orthopedic Medicine: A New Approach to Vertebral Manipulations. Springfield, Charles C. Thomas, 1972

72. Maitland GD: Palpation examination of the posterior cervical spine: The ideal, average and abnormal. Aust J Physiother 28:3–11, 1982

73. Maitland GD: Vertebral Manipulation, 5th ed. Boston, Butterworth, 1986

74. Maitland GD: Peripheral Manipulation, 3rd ed. London, Butterworth-Heinemann, 1991

75. Mayer TG, Gatchel RJ: Quantitative lumbar spine assessment to address the deconditioning syndrome. In: Mayer TG, Gatchel RJ, eds: Functional Restoration for Spinal Disorders: The Sports Medicine Approach. Philadelphia, Lea & Febiger, 1988:115–138

76. Mayer TG, Gatchel RJ: The role of the physical therapist: Active sports medicine, not passive modalities. In: Mayer TG, Gatchel RJ, eds: Functional Restoration for Spinal Disorders: The Sports Medicine Approach. Philadelphia, Lea & Febiger, 1988:218–240

77. McKenzie RA: The Lumbar Spine: Mechanical Diagnosis and Therapy. Waikanae, New Zealand, Spinal Publications, 1981

78. McKenzie RA: The Cervical and Thoracic Spine: Mechanical Diagnosis and Therapy. Waikanae, New Zealand, Spinal Publications, 1990

79. McNeil BJ: Value of bone scanning in neoplastic disease. Semin Nucl Med 4:277, 1984

80. Mennell JM: Back Pain: Diagnosis and Treatment Using Manipulative Techniques. Boston, Little, Brown, & Co., 1960

81. Mitchell FL Jr, Moran PS, Pruzzo NA: An Evaluation and Treatment Manual of Osteopathic Muscle Energy Procedures. Valley Park, MO, Mitchell, Moran, and Pruzzo Associates, 1979

82. Morris J, Benner G, Lucas D: An electromyographic study of the intrinsic muscles of the back in man. J Anat 196:509–520, 1962

83. Nyberg R: Clinical assessment of the low back: Active movement and palpation testing. In: Basmajian JV, Nyberg R, eds: Rational Manual Therapies. Baltimore, Williams & Wilkins, 1993:97–140

84. O'Sullivan SB: Clinical decision making: Planning effective treatments. In: O'Sullivan SB, Schmitz TJ, eds: Physical Rehabilitation Assessment and Treatment. 3rd ed. Philadelphia, FA Davis, 1994:1–8

85. Ongerboer DE, Visser BW, Goor C: Jaw reflexes and masseter electromyograms in mesencephalic and pontine lesions: An electrodiagnostic study. J Neurol Neurosurg Psychiatry 39:90–92, 1976

86. Palmer ML, Epler ME: Fundamentals of Musculoskeletal Assessment Techniques, 2nd ed. Philadelphia, Lippincott, Williams & Wilkins, 1998

87. Paris CP: End feel testing: Interrater reliability of end feel testing—Elbow flexion and extension. Proceedings of the 5th International Conference of the International Federation of Orthopaedic Manipulative Therapists, Vail, CO, 1992:103–105

88. Petty NJ, Moore AP: Neuromusculoskeletal Examination and Assessment. Edinburgh, Churchill Livingstone, 1998

89. Pochazesky R, Wexler CE, Meyers PH, et al: Liquid crystal thermography of the spine and extremities. J Neurosurg 56:386–395, 1982

90. Pochazesky R: Thermography in skeletal and soft tissue trauma. In: Taveras J, Ferrucci J, eds: Radiology. Philadelphia, JB Lippincott, 1987

91. Rose SJ: Physical therapy diagnosis: Role and function. Phys Ther 69:535–537, 1989

92. Rothstein JM, Echternach JL: Hypothesis-oriented algorithm for clinicians: A method for evaluation and treatment planning. Phys Ther 66:1388–1394, 1986

93. Sahrmann SA: A program for correction muscular imbalances. Clin Man Phys Ther 3:21–28, 1983

94. Sahrmann SA: Diagnosis by the physical therapist: A prerequisite for treatment. Phys Ther 68:1703–1706, 1988

95. Sahrmann SA: Diagnosis and treatment of muscle imbalances and associated regional pain. Continuing Education Course. Seattle, WA, 1993

96. Sahrmann SA: Diagnosis and Treatment of Movement Impairment Syndromes, St. Louis, Mosby, 2002

97. Sandoz R: Some physical mechanisms and effects of spinal adjustments. Ann Swiss Chiro Assoc 6:91–141, 1976

98. Schenkman M, Butler RB: A model for multi-system evaluation, interpretation and treatment of individuals with neurologic dysfunction. Phys Ther 69:538–547, 1989

99. Shaddock M: Neurodynamic. Physiotherapy 81:9–16, 1995

100. Sim FH: Diagnosis and Management of Metastatic Bone Disease: Multi-disciplinary Approach. New York, Raven Press, 1988

101. Simons A, Trossman P: Biomechanical assessment in clinical practice. In: Abreu BC, ed: Physical Disabilities Manual. New York, Raven Press, 1981:41–56

102. Spitzer WO: Quebec task force on spinal disorders: Scientific approach to the assessment and management of activity-related spinal disorders. Spine 12:S1–S58, 1987

103. Spratt KF, Lehmann TR, Weinstein JN, et al: A new approach to the low-back physical examination. Spine 15:96–102, 1990

104. Stahl DC, Jacobs B: The diagnosis of obscure lesions of the skeleton. JAMA 201: 229–231, 1967

105. Stoddard A: Manual of Osteopathic Practice. London, Hutchinson & Co., 1969

106. Sunndaresan N, Galicich JH, Lane JM, et al: Surgical treatment of spinal metastases in kidney disease. J Clin Oncol 4:1851–1856, 1985

107. Taylor RG, Fowler WM Jr: Electrodiagnosis of musculoskeletal disorders. In: D'Ambrosia RD, ed: Musculoskeletal Disorders: Regional Examination and Differential Diagnosis, 2nd ed. Philadelphia, JB Lippincott, 1986:59–94

108. Taylor TKF, Weinir M: Great-toe extensor reflexes in the diagnosis of lumbar disk disorders. Br Med J 2:487–489, 1969

109. Thomas PS, Zauder HL: Thermography. In: Raji PP, ed: The Practical Management of Pain. St. Louis, Mosby-Year Book, 1986

110. Thomas-Edding D: Clinical problem solving in physical therapy and its implications for curriculum development. Proceedings of the Tenth International Congress of the World Confederation for Physical Therapy. Sydney, New South Wales, Australia, 1987:100–104

111. Troupin RH: Radiologic evaluation of the musculoskeletal system. In: Rosse C, Clawson DK, eds: The Musculoskeletal System in Health and Disease. Philadelphia, Harper and Row, 1980:103–118

112. Unsworth A, Doverson D, Wright V: Cracking joints: A bioengineering study of cavitation in the metacarpophalangeal joint. Ann Rheum Dis 30:348–358, 1971

113. Vasilyeva LF, Kogan OG: Manual diagnosis and manual therapy of atypical motor patterns. Presented at the 10th International Congress of the Federation Internationale de Medicine Manuelle (FIMM), Brussels, September 1992

114. Vasilyeva LF, Lewitt K: Diagnosis of muscular dysfunction by dysfunction. In: Liebenson C, ed: Rehabilitation of the Spine. Philadelphia, Lippincott, Williams & Wilkins, 1996:113–142

115. Wadsworth CT: Manual Examination and Treatment of the Spine and Extremities. Baltimore, Williams & Wilkins, 1988:12–27

116. Walton Lord: Essentials of Neurology, 6th ed. Edinburgh, Churchill Livingstone, 1989

117. Warwick R, Williams P, eds: Gray's Anatomy, 35th ed. Philadelphia, WB Saunders, 1973

118. Watt NT: Decision analysis: A tool for improving physical therapy practice and education. In: Wolf SL, ed: Clinical Decision Making in Physical Therapy. Philadelphia, FA Davis, 1985:7–23

119. Watt NT: Clinical decision analysis. Phys Ther 69:569–576, 1989

120. Weed L: Medical records that guide and teach: Part I. N Engl J Med 278:593–600, 1968

121. Weed LL, Zinny NJ: The problem-oriented system, problem-knowledge coupling, and clinical decision making. Phys Ther 69:565–568, 1989

122. White SG, Sahrmann SA: Movement system balance approach to management of the musculoskeletal pain. In: Grant R, ed: Clinics in Physical Therapy of the Cervical and Thoracic Spine, 2nd ed. Edinburg, Churchill Livingstone, 1994:339

123. Wilson P: Sympathetically maintained pain. In: Stanton-Hicks M, ed: Sympathetic Pain. Boston, Kluwer, 1989

124. Zinny NJ, Tandy CJ: Problem-knowledge coupling: A tool for physical therapy clinical practice. Phys Ther 69:155–161, 1989

125. Zohn DA, Mennell J: Ancillary aids in diagnosis. In: Zohn DA, Mennell J, eds: Musculoskeletal Pain: Diagnosis and Physical Treatment. Boston, Little, Brown & Co., 1976:65–88

RECOMMENDED READINGS

Physical Examination
American Academy of Orthopaedic Surgeons: Joint Motion, Method of Measuring and Recording, 3rd ed. New York, Churchill Livingstone, 1990

Akeson WH, Amiel D, LaViolette D, et al: The connective tissue response to immobility: An accelerated aging response? Exp Gerontol 3:289–300, 1968

Basmajian JV, Nyberg R, eds: Rational Manual Therapies. Baltimore, Williams & Wilkins, 1993

Boissonault WG: Examination in Physical Therapy Practice, 2nd ed. New York, Churchill Livingstone, 1995

Bourdillon JF, Day EA, Bookhout MR: Spinal Manipulation, 5th ed. Oxford, Butterworh-Heinemann, 1992

Brownstein B, Bronner S: Evaluation, Treatment and Outcomes: Functional Movement in Orthopaedic and Sports Physical Therapy. New York, Churchill Livingston, 1995

Butler DS: Mobilization of the Nervous System. Melbourne, Churchill Livingstone, 1991

Cantu R, Grodin AJ: Myofascial Manipulation: Theory and Clinical Application, 2nd ed. Gaithersburg, Aspen, 2001

Clayton ML, James SM, Abdulla M: Experimental investigations of ligamentous healing. Clin Orthop 61:146, 1968

Corrigan B, Maitland GD: Practical Orthopaedic Medicine. Boston, Butterworth, 1985

Cyriax J: Textbook of Orthopaedic Medicine, vol. I. The Diagnosis of Soft Tissue Lesions, 8th ed. London, Bailliere-Tindall, 1982

Cyriax JH, Cyriax PJ: Illustrated Manual of Orthopaedic Medicine, 11th ed. London, Butterworth, 1984

Dvorak J, Dvorak V: Manual Medicine: Diagnostics, 2nd ed. New York, Thieme Medical, 1990

Dvorak J, Dvorak V, Tritschler T: Manual Medicine: Therapy. New York, Thieme Medical, 1988

Edmond SL: Manipulation & Mobilization: Extremity and Spinal Techniques. St. Louis, Mosby-Year Book, 1993

Edwards BC: Manual of Combined Movements: Their Use in the Examinations and Treatment of Musculoskeletal Vertebral Column Disorders. Oxford, Butterworth-Heinemann, 1999

Fordyce WE: Behavioral Methods for Chronic Pain and Illness. St. Louis, CV Mosby, 1976

Fordyce WE, Fowler RS, Lehmann JF, et al: Operant conditioning in the treatment of chronic clinical pain. Arch Phys Med Rehabil 54:399–408, 1973

Frankel VH: Recent advances in the biomechanics of sport injuries. Acta Orthop Scand 46:484–497, 1975

Gradosar IA: Fracture stabilization and healing. In: Gould JA, Davies GL, eds: Orthopaedic and Sports Physical Therapy. St. Louis, CV Mosby, 1990

Goodman CC, Synder K: Differential Diagnosis in Physical Therapy, 2nd ed. Philadelphia, WB Saunders, 1995

Greenman PE: Principles of Manual Therapy, 2nd ed. Baltimore, Williams & Wilkins, 1996

Grieve G: Modern Manual Therapy of the Vertebral Column. Edinburgh, Churchill Livingstone, 1986

Grieve G: Common Vertebral Joint Problems, 2nd ed. Edinburgh, Churchill Livingstone, 1988

Hammer WI: Functional Soft Tissue Examination and Treatment by Manual Methods: The Extremities. Gaithersburg, Aspen, 1991

Hartley A: Practical Joint Assessment: A Sports Medicine Manual. St. Louis, Mosby–Year Book, 1990

Hettinga DL: Inflammatory response of synovial joint structures. In: Gould JA, Davies GL, eds: Orthopaedic and Sports Physical Therapy. St. Louis, CV Mosby, 1990

Hoppenfeld S: Physical Examination of the Spine and Extremities. New York, Appleton-Century-Crofts, 1976

Kaltenborn FM: The Spine: Basic Evaluation and Mobilization Techniques, 2nd ed. Oslo, Olaf Norlis Bokhandel, 1993

Keene JS: Ligament and muscle-tendon unit injuries. In: Gould JA, Davies GL, eds: Orthopaedic and Sports Physical Therapy. St. Louis, CV Mosby, 1990

Kenna C, Murtagh J: Back Pain & Spinal Manipulation: A Practical Guide. Sydney, Butterworth, 1989

Kennedy JD, Hawkins RJ, Willis RB, et al: Tension studies in human knee ligaments. J Bone Joint Surg Am 58:350–355, 1976

Knight K: The effects of hypothermia on inflammation and swelling. Athlet Train 11:1, 1976

Lehmann JF, DeLateur BJ, Stonebridge JB, et al: Therapeutic temperature distribution produce by ultrasound as modified by dosage and volume of tissue exposed. Arch Phys Med Rehabil 48:662–666, 1967

Lehmann JF, Warren CF: Therapeutic heat and cold. Clin Orthop 99:207–245, 1974

Lewit K: Manipulative Therapy in Rehabilitation of the Locomotor System, 2nd ed. Oxford, Butterworth-Heinemann, 1991

Lieberson C: Rehabilitation of the Spine. Philadelphia, Lippincott, Williams & Wilkins, 1996

Magee DJ: Orthopedic Physical Assessment, 3rd ed. Philadelphia, WB Saunders, 1997

Maitland GD: Musculoskeletal Examination and Recording Guide, 3rd ed. Adelaide, Lauderdale Press, 1981

Maitland GD: Vertebral Manipulation, 5th ed. London, Butterworth, 1986

Maitland GD: Peripheral Manipulation, 3rd ed. London, Butterworth-Heinemann, 1991

Mannheimer JS, Lampe GN: Clinical Transcutaneous Electrical Nerve Stimulation. Philadelphia, FA Davis, 1984

McRae R: Clinical Orthopaedic Examination, 2nd ed. Edinburgh, Churchill Livingstone, 1983

Murtagh J, Kenna C: Back Pain and Spinal Manipulation: A Practical Guide, 2nd ed. Oxford, Butterworth-Heinemann, 1997

Norkin CC, Levangie PK: Joint Structure and Function, 2nd ed. Philadelphia, FA Davis, 1992

Noyes FR, Edward SG: The strength of the anterior cruciate ligament in humans and rhesus monkeys. J Bone Joint Surg Am 58:1074–1082, 1976

Noyes FR, Grood ES, Nussbaum NS, et al: Effects of intra-articular corticosteroids on ligament properties. Clin Orthop 123:197–209, 1977

Noyes FR, Torvik DJ, Hyde WB, et al: Biomechanics of ligament failure: An analysis of immobilization, exercise and reconditioning effects in primates. J Bone Joint Surg Am 56:1406–1418, 1974

Palmar L, Epler ME: Fundamentals of Musculoskeletal Assessment Techniques, 2nd ed. Philadelphia, Lippincott Williams & Wilkins, 1998

Petty NJ, Moore AP: Neuromusculoskeletal Examination and Assessment: A Handbook for Therapists. Edinburg, Churchill Livingstone, 1998

Radin EL, Paul IL: A comparison of the dynamic force transmitting properties of subchondral bone and articular cartilage. J Bone Joint Surg Am 52:444–456, 1970

Sahrmann SA: Diagnosis and Treatment of Movement Impairment Syndromes. St. Louis, Mosby, 2002

Starkey C: Evaluation of Orthopedic and Athletic Injuries. Philadelphia, FA Davis, 1996

Warren CG, Lehmann JF, Koflanski JN: Heat and stretch procedures: An evaluation using rat tail tendons. Arch Phys Med Rehabil 57:122–126, 1976

White AA, Panjabi MM: Clinical Biomechanics of the Spine, 2nd ed. Philadelphia, JB Lippincott, 1990

Clinical Decision-Making and Data Collection

Boissonault WG, ed: Examination in Physical Therapy Practice: Screening for Medical Disease. New York, Churchill Livingstone, 1991

Feinstein A: Scientific methodology in clinical medicine, Part I: Introduction, principles and concepts. Ann Intern Med 61:564–579, 1964

Feinstein A: Scientific methodology in clinical medicine, Part IV: Acquisition of clinical data. Ann Intern Med 61:1162–1193, 1964

Feinstein A: An additional basic science for clinical medicine, Part IV: The development of clinometrics. Ann Inter Med 99:843–848, 1983

Payton O, Nelson C, Ozer M: Patient Participation in Program Planning: A Manual for Therapists. Philadelphia, FA Davis, 1990

Stith JS, Sahrmann SA, Dixon KK, et al: Curriculum to prepare diagnosticians in physical therapy. Phys Ther 9:46–53,1995

Weinstein M, Fineberg H: Clinical Decision Analysis. Philadelphia, WB Saunders, 1980

Wolf S: Clinical Decision Making in Physical Therapy. Philadelphia, FA Davis, 1985

Introduction to Manual Therapy

6

DARLENE HERTLING AND RANDOLPH M. KESSLER

HISTORY OF JOINT MOBILIZATION TECHNIQUES

Although specific mobilization techniques were introduced in physical therapy curricula in the United States in the 1980s, their use in the management of patients with musculoskeletal disorders is certainly not new. It seems somewhat odd that physical therapists have been slow in adopting joint mobilization techniques. After all, therapists have been delegated the duty of passive movement for years, and joint mobilization is simply a form of passive movement.

Some time in the past this important method of treatment was lost from medical practice and is just beginning to emerge again. The explanation for its disappearance probably lies in the fact that early users of mobilization techniques based their value on purely empirical evidence of their effectiveness; there was no scientific basis for their use. Later, specific joint mobilization was practiced only by more esoteric "professions" that claimed beneficial effects on all disease processes, usually from manipulations of the spine. This tended to further alienate orthodox medical practitioners, with the result that the use of any and all forms of joint mobilization, other than movement in the cardinal planes, became taboo. The approach to the management of many joint conditions is still largely influenced by the teachings of the early orthopedic surgeons, who advocated strict rest in the management of all joint conditions. Although scientific proof of the effectiveness of specific joint mobilization is still largely lacking, our expanded knowledge of joint kinematics at least provides a scientific basis for its use. It is becoming evident that to treat mechanical joint dysfunctions effectively and safely, a knowledge of joint kinematics and skill in joint examination and mobilization techniques are required.

Early Practitioners

The use of specific mobilization techniques did not arise with the emergence of osteopathy and chiropractic. Some of the earliest recorded accounts of the use of joint manipulation and spinal traction are from Hippocrates, a physician in the fourth century, BCE. In fact, Hippocrates proposed refinements in some of the techniques used in his time. For example, one traction technique required that the patient be tied to a ladder and dropped 30 feet, upside down, to the ground. Hippocrates suggested that ropes be tied to the ladder so that two people could shake it up and down, thus affecting an "intermittent" traction. Hippocrates also developed many of the methods of reducing dislocations that are still in use today. Accounts of the use of manipulation by Cato, Galen, and other physicians during the time of the Roman Empire also exist.[24]

Little is known of the practice of joint manipulation during the disintegration of the Roman Empire and the beginning of the Middle Ages. During this time most hospitals were attached to monasteries, and treatment was carried out by members of the religious orders. Friar Moulton, of the order of St. Augustine, wrote *The Complete Bonesetter*. The text, which was revised by John Turner in 1656, suggests that manipulation was practiced in medical settings throughout the Middle Ages and early Renaissance. With the reign of Henry VIII in England and the subsequent dissolution of the monasteries, medicine lost its previous "mystic" influences and became the practice of "art and science."

The English orthopedic surgeons of the late 1700s and early 1800s, such as John Hunter and John Hilton, advocated strict rest in the early management of joint trauma.[62] This view was emphasized by Hugh Owen Thomas in the late 1800s. For two centuries this influence prevailed, and joint manipulation remained in the hands of "bonesetters." Bonesetting was practiced by lay people, and the art was passed down over the centuries within bonesetters' families. The bonesetters had no basis for the use of their manipulations other than past experience. The successful bonesetters were those who remembered details of cases in which ill effects had resulted and avoided making the same mistakes again. Bonesetters tended to guard their techniques, keeping them secret among family members. A few bonesetters, because of their success, became quite famous. One such bonesetter, a Mrs. Mapp, was called on to treat nobility and royalty.

BONESETTERS VERSUS PHYSICIANS

During this period there was extreme rivalry and animosity between physicians and bonesetters. Physicians were well aware of disastrous effects that bonesetting had at times on tuberculous joints or other serious pathologies. It is interesting that Thomas, who was particularly outspoken against bonesetters, was the son and grandson of bonesetters. Thomas, who gave his name to the **Thomas splint,** was the originator of many of the orthopedic principles concerning immobilization of fractures and joint injuries still adhered to today. It goes without saying that medical opinion of joint manipulation has changed very little since his time.

Despite medical opinion, Sir James Paget, a famous surgeon and contemporary of Thomas in England, recognized the value of judiciously applied bonesetting techniques. His lecture entitled "Cases that Bonesetters Cure," which appeared in the *British Medical Journal* in 1867, spoke of the rivalry between bonesetters and physicians. He described types of lesions for which manipulation may be of value and advised that physicians "imitate what is good and avoid what is bad in the practice of bonesetters." Unfortunately, the medical profession at the time, and for years to come, ignored this advice.

The first medical book on manipulation since Friar Moulton's work was published in the 1870s. It was written by Dr. Wharton Hood, whose father, Dr. Peter Hood, treated a bonesetter, a Mr. Hutton, for a serious illness. Dr. Hood did not charge Hutton since he was aware of Hutton's free services to many poor people. In repayment, however, Hutton offered to teach Hood all he knew of bonesetting. The elder Hood was too busy to accept the offer, but his son Wharton did. In his paper on the subject, published in *Lancet* in 1871, Hood describes Hutton's techniques of spinal and peripheral manipulation.[93] He lists the conditions that Hutton was willing to treat as primarily postimmobilization stiffness, displaced cartilage and tendons, carpal and tarsal subluxations, and ganglionic swellings; he also states that Hutton avoided working on acutely inflamed joints. Hutton usually applied heat before manipulating, especially to the larger joints. Hood describes Hutton's manipulations as being very precise as to the direction and amplitude of motion. They were always of a high-velocity thrust. The illustrated descriptions of some of the common manipulations used by Hutton show them to be essentially identical to the manipulations used by manual

therapists and even some orthopedists and physiatrists today. Hutton admitted to knowing nothing of anatomy and felt that in all of his cases a bone was "out." Of his techniques he says that forced pushing and pulling are useless; "the twist is the thing."

OSTEOPATHY AND CHIROPRACTIC

Meanwhile in the United States, Dr. Andrew Taylor Still was practicing medicine in Kansas.[251] It happened that Still's children contracted meningitis and all three died. Still, being frustrated and angered by the failure of current medical practices to save his children, set out to find a solution. For a time he spent his days studying the anatomy of exhumed Indian remains, paying special attention to the relationships among bones, nerves, and arteries. In 1874, through a "divine revelation," Still claimed he had discovered the cause of all bodily disease. His "law of the artery" claimed that all disease processes were a direct result of interference with blood flow through arteries that carried vital nutrients to a part. If normal blood flow to the part could be restored, then the body's natural substances would resolve the disease process. In 1892, Still founded the first school of osteopathy in Kirksville, Missouri, offering a 20-month course. By 1916 the osteopathic course was extended to 3 years, and by 1920 the United States Congress granted equal rights to osteopaths and MDs.[186] In the early 1900s, the osteopathic profession gradually became aware that some of Still's original proposals were incorrect. Over the years they incorporated traditional medical thought with the practice of joint manipulation. Especially during the past decade, osteopathic schools have de-emphasized the practice of manipulation and have attained essentially the same standards as medical schools. Osteopaths now qualify for residency programs in all medical and surgical fields.

In 1895 a grocer named D. D. Palmer, who had been a patient of Still, founded the Palmer College of Chiropractics in Davenport, Iowa. No prior education was required, and one of the first graduates was Palmer's 12-year-old son, B. J. Chiropractic theory evolved around the "law of the nerve," which stated that "vital life forces" could be cut off from any body part by small vertebral subluxations placing pressure on nerves. Since this could cause disease in the part to which the nerve ran, most, if not all, disease could be prevented or cured by maintaining proper spinal alignment through manipulation. Chiropractic was a "drugless" remedy that often supplemented manipulative treatment with various herbs, vitamins, and so forth. The chiropractic profession was fraught with internal turmoil from the outset.[226] (B. J. apparently grew up hating his father and later bought him out. When the father died, he stipulated that B. J. was not to attend his funeral.) Unlike osteopaths, most chiropractors adhered to their original concept, the law of the nerve, although the profession has always been divided into two or more schools of thought. They have received bitter opposition from the medical profession, which views them as charlatans and quacks. Today there remains some division in chiropractic philosophy. The "straights" continue to follow the law of the nerve, claiming to treat most disease by manipulating the spine or other body parts. The "mixers" tend to accept the limitations of this practice and use local application of ultrasound, massage, exercises, and so on to supplement their manipulative treatment. It is significant that because of a strong lobbying force and the realization by chiropractors that to survive professional standards and education must be upgraded, chiropractors are rapidly gaining acceptance by governing bodies, the public, and even some physicians. It will be interesting to see if the profession of physical therapy keeps abreast of this trend.

Current Schools of Thought

Despite efforts by Paget and Hood to emphasize the value of bonesetting techniques, manipulation was not readopted as a method of treatment by medical doctors until the late 20th century. The earliest physicians to practice manipulation were English. Books on the subject were published by A. G. Timbrell Fisher, an orthopedic surgeon, in 1925, and by James Mennell in 1939.[62,164] Mennell was a doctor of physical medicine at St. Thomas' Hospital. Both he and Fisher often performed their manipulations with the patient anesthetized. In 1934 Mixter and Barr published an article in the *New England Journal of Medicine,* and T. Marlin published *Manipulative Treatment for the Medical Practitioner.*[150,153,171,180] These works have had a powerful effect on medical thought, stimulating much interest and leading to a series of excellent publications since then. Later in the century books advocating manipulative treatment were published by Alan Stoddard and James Cyriax.[38,230] Cyriax was to succeed Mennell at St. Thomas' Hospital. Cyriax advocated manipulations performed without anesthesia. Most of allopathic medicine's knowledge of manipulations can be traced to Mennell and Cyriax; the former made contributions in the field of synovial joints, the latter in the area of the intervertebral disk. Cyriax's examination approach is considered superb and contains a wealth of medical logic.

Currently, a school of thought that has attracted some attention (especially in Europe) is being led by Robert Maigne, who has postulated the "concept of painless and opposite motion."[146] This concept states that a manipulative maneuver should be administered in the direction opposite to the movement that is restricted and causing pain. Maigne, like Cyriax, has worked hard to focus medical attention on manipulative therapy as an effective modality in the relief of pain.

The driving force behind a school of thought that has flourished in Scandinavia is F. M. Kaltenborn.[113] Under his leadership, a systematic postgraduate education program that requires passage of practical and written examinations leads to certification in the specialty of manual therapy. The philosophy behind Kaltenborn's technique is a fusion of what he has considered the best in chiropractic, osteopathy, and physical medicine. He uses Cyriax's methods to evaluate the patient and employs mainly specific osteopathic techniques for treatment. Disk degeneration and facet joint pathologies are the two main spinal pathologies that the Scandinavians theorize are amenable to physical therapy.

Maitland, an Australian physical therapist whose approach is currently being taught in Australia, has a nonpathologic orientation to the treatment of all joints.[35,147] His techniques are fairly similar to the "articulatory" techniques used by osteopaths, involving oscillatory movements performed on a chosen joint. To increase movement of a restricted joint, movement is induced within the patient's available range of movement tolerance. He distinguishes between mobilizations and manipulations but puts heavy emphasis on mobilization. A meticulous examination is essential to this method because examination provides the guideline to treatment.

A prominent figure in the United States has been Dr. John Mennell, the son of the late James Mennell, who came to practice in the United States. His work on the spine and extremities has been described in several publications and is particularly well known in the United States. He has made a significant contribution to a better understanding of joint pain and its treatment by placing stress on the function of small involuntary movements within a joint. He refers to these small movements as **joint play;** a disturbance of these movements is termed **joint dysfunction.** He states that full, painless, voluntary range of motion is not possible without restoration of all joint-play motions.[164,165]

In spite of their efforts, Mennell, Cyriax, Stoddard, and Maigne remain among the very few medical physicians to practice joint manipulation. As a result, manipulative treatment was not—and still is not—available to most patients seeking help from the medical profession. The original reasons for avoiding the practice of manipulation stemmed from the teachings of Hilton, Thomas, and Hunter, and the occasional disasters that occurred at the hands of bonesetters and other manipulators. Today many more medical physicians accept the value of judiciously applied manipulative treatment. However, to be effective, this treatment requires considerable evaluative and therapeutic management, and most physicians simply do not have the time to learn or practice manipulative technique.

Role of the Physical Therapist

Physical therapists are the logical practitioners to assume the responsibility for manipulative treatment. They work closely with physicians, who are capable of ruling out serious pathology. They tend to develop close and ongoing rapport with patients because the nature of their work requires close patient contact. They are taught to evaluate and treat by use of the hands. The advantages of the physician–physical therapist team in orthopedic manual therapy are perhaps best described by Cyriax: "Between them they have every facility: informed selection of cases, a wide range of different types of treatment, alternative approaches when it is clear that manual methods cannot avail."[39]

The United States, which has lagged far behind other countries in the development of orthopedic manual therapy, is gradually catching up. Thanks to the efforts of Mennell and Stanley Paris, a therapist originally from New Zealand, American therapists have at least had the opportunity to take postgraduate courses and to gain some competency in manual therapy and the management of orthopedic patients. It is hoped that the formation of the Orthopaedic Section of the American Physical Therapy Association in 1974 and increased education will improve this situation. Graduate courses in the physical therapy schools, clinically oriented long-term courses, postgraduate apprenticeships, and orthopedic specialization in master's and doctorate degree programs are developing.

Currently, the techniques therapists use to restore accessory movement are termed **articulations** or **joint mobilizations** and **manipulations.** Generally, manipulation means passive movement of any kind. Many therapists prefer to use the term articulation to denote a passive movement directed at the joint without any high-velocity thrust and within the range of the joint. Articulations or joint mobilizations are passive movements performed at a speed slow enough that the client can stop the movement. The technique may be applied with a sustained stretch or oscillatory motion: a gentle, coaxing, repetitive, rhythmic movement of a joint that can be resisted by the patient. The technique is intended to decrease pain or increase mobility. Unlike manipulation, it can be performed over a wide range and thus involve a series of movements referred to as **stages** (grades of movement). The techniques may use physiologic movements or accessory movements.

Manipulation, in this context, would then denote only passive movement involving a high-velocity, small-amplitude thrust that proceeds quickly enough that the relaxed patient cannot prevent its occurrence. The motion is performed at the end of the pathologic limit of the joint and is intended to alter positional relationships, to stimulate joint receptors, and to snap adhesions.[187] **Pathologic limit** means the end of available range of motion when there is restriction. Thus, the speed of the technique, not necessarily the degree of force, differentiates the two categories of passive movement. Joint manipulation is sometimes referred to as **thrust manipulation** or more recently, in osteopathic manual medicine, as **mobilization with impulse.**[218]

The basic spinal and peripheral joint mobilization techniques presented in this book are only part of the larger scope of manual therapy. Manual therapy is concerned with the establishment of the normal structural integrity of the body and, to achieve this end, uses a variety of methods. The following is an overview of the practice of manual therapy.

HYPOMOBILITY TREATMENT

The term **hypomobility** denotes a decrease in the range of motion in an extremity joint or a spinal segment. In hypomobility there is a subjective stiffness and often pain, particularly when the joint is forcibly moved. Such restrictions often force adjacent joints to become hypermobile to compensate and enable a full range of movement to take place in the area.

Treatment methods directed at hypomobility are classified in four groups.

1. Soft tissue therapies other than joint corrections to normalize activity status, restore extensibility, reduce pain, and relieve abnormal tension in muscles, ligaments, capsules, and fascia.
2. Neural tissue mobilization to increase mobility of dura mater, nerve roots, and peripheral nerves.
3. Techniques of joint mobilization or articulation for the normalization of mobility and position. With hypomobility, the goal of treatment is to mobilize the restricted joint or spinal segment.
4. Other methods that have as their aim the improvement or restoration of normal body mechanics, such as relaxation training, correction of posture, exercise, and activities that help to maintain the improved normal mechanics, soft tissue length and mobility, and joint mobility.

All these methods fall within the broader aspect of the manual therapy approach.

Soft Tissue Therapies

Soft tissue therapies involve manual contacts, pressures, or movements primarily to myofascial tissues. Soft tissue work may be classified into four categories: massage, soft tissue mobilizations or manipulations, acupressure, and stretching techniques ("active" relaxation of muscles, such as proprioceptive neuromuscular facilitation [PNF] and muscle energy techniques, as well as "passive" stretching of shortened muscles and associated connective tissues). **Soft tissue mobilization** is simply defined as the manual manipulation of soft tissues administered for the purpose of producing effects on the nervous, muscular, fascial, lymphatic, and circulatory systems.[263]

CLASSIC MASSAGE

Classic massage includes the traditional massage techniques that are often taught in the physical therapy curriculum and will not be covered here. The techniques consist of three generally used strokes: effleurage or stroking, pétrissage or kneading, and friction. With the exception of tapotement and friction massage, slowly applied sustained pressure is recommended for decreasing soft tissue tone and for improving soft tissue extensibility (see Chapter 8, Soft Tissue Manipulations).

FRICTION MASSAGE

A particular method of friction massage (transverse frictions) was discussed in the 1940s by Mennell[163] and was clinically described later as Cyriax's deep massage and manipulation.[39] Although not yet demonstrated by adequately controlled histologic studies, friction massage represents an excellent empirical method of healing that has stood the test of time for the treatment of pathology caused by chronic overuse soft tissue syndromes (see Chapter 8, Soft Tissue Manipulations).[247]

SOFT TISSUE MANIPULATIONS

Soft tissue manipulations have undoubtedly been performed since the beginning of time and have evolved into a variety of formats.[8–11,30,32,76,81,105,135,140,146,149,174,202,236] Soft tissue manipulations (including myofascial manipulations and stretching and release treatment methods), as in joint mobilizations, may be used to restore mechanical function of the soft tissue, especially its elasticity and mobility relative to other tissues or tissue layers, to exert a therapeutic effect on the autonomic nervous system by decreasing reflexive holding patterns (connective tissue massage)[13,32,43,47,69,123,184,236] or to change abnormal movement patterns through movement, posture, and body awareness.[10,30]

Mechanical approaches differ from autonomic approaches in that they seek to make mechanical or histologic changes in the myofascial structures.[10,30] **Myofascial manipulations** have been defined as the forceful passive movement of the musculofascial elements through their restrictive direction(s), beginning with the most superficial layers and progressing in depth while taking into account their relationship to the joints concerned.[30] According to Lewit,[140] the technique is characteristically uniform, which distinguishes it from difference between classical massage and myofascial-release types of soft tissue manipulations or mobilizations is that massage ignores the barrier-and-release phenomenon and with its moderate to rapid movements fails to achieve myofascial release. In the movement of shifting or stretching, one first takes up the slack (engages a barrier), after which a release occurs. Release is hypothesized as following reflex neural efferent inhibition and biomechanical hysteresis within the tissues.[76] The resistant barrier may be engaged directly or the tissue may be stretched in a direction away from the barrier in an indirect fashion. There are many combinations, and different authors and teachers of myofascial manipulations show similarities and differences.[10,30,76,81,149,217]

Substantial research has been performed by Akeson, Amiel, Woo, and others to determine the biomechanical characteristics of normal and immobilized connective tissues.[2–7,261] Because the literature is currently inconsistent and available research does not clearly explain how connective tissue is changed with soft tissue mobilization, practitioners must rely on clinical experience until further research is published.[42,73,81,234,235]

ACUPRESSURE

Acupressure is a method of point massage to acupuncture points or along meridians for the purpose of analgesia. It acts particularly on reflex changes in the soft tissue. Typically, fingertip pressure is used over a finite acupuncture point of highly discernible tenderness according to anatomy or traditional acupuncture, trigger points, or spontaneously tender points (Ah Shi points).[21,83,140,160,205,242] Pressure may also be applied by the thumbs, knuckles, palms, elbows, or even the feet for specific techniques. The stimulus applied may be either deep pressure on trigger points or Ah Shi points that are in muscle, circular or transverse frictions over acupuncture points, or kneading or palm pressure along the course of the meridian. Different systems suggest sustaining pressure from 3 to 90 seconds when a number of points are treated; however, one point can be treated as long as 3 to 4 minutes.[204] It has been found most effective to sustain pressure for as long as it takes to feel a softening of the tissue.[15] Although acupuncture and the various methods of acupuncture point stimulation have gained some acceptance in Western medicine, the theoretical basis for the effects of this type of treatment are viewed with a degree of skepticism. Research into the effects has tied it to the endogenous opiate system.[177]

TRIGGER POINT THERAPY

Trigger point therapy gained prominence as an important modality in treating myofascial pain in the 1960s. Although it had been a recognized type of therapy for many years, it was brought to the forefront by Janet Travell, John Mennell, and David Simons, who supplied much of the needed neurophysiologic information, and trigger point therapy became an accepted therapeutic modality. A **trigger point** is best described as an area of hypersensitivity in a muscle from which impulses travel to the central nervous system, giving rise to referred pain.[243]

Myofascial pain syndrome (MPS) is defined by Travell and Simons as "localized musculoskeletal pain originating from a hyperirritable spot or trigger point with a taut band of skeletal muscle or muscle fascia."[243] Involved muscles may present with a stretch length limitation (muscle tightness) and a local twitch response on palpation.[224,260,264] Physical treatments reported in the literature include transcutaneous nerve stimulation,[71,161] deep massage,[39,224] myofascial manipulations,[10,30,81,149] acupressure or isometric pressure,[21,149] reflex inhibition following minimal or maximal isometric contraction (muscle energy or post-isometric relaxation),[140,160,161,204] laser therapy,[221,228,229,250] ultrasonography,[21,22] trigger point injection or anesthetic blocks,[15,61,64,65,82,161,183] dry needling,[21,83,250] massage with an ice cube, and intense cold and stretching techniques using vapocoolant spray.[15,86,88,89,97,204,220,225,227,241–244] Travell and Simons[243] have stated that "stretch is the action, spray is the distraction." They believe that the cooling effect of the vapocoolant spray blocks pain and reflex muscle spasm, which occurs when a muscle with a trigger point is stretched, thus allowing greater elongation and passive range of motion. A multifaceted approach is needed along with myofascial stretching, exercise, and corrective posture activities.[89,149,154,203]

MUSCLE ENERGY (POST-ISOMETRIC RELAXATION)

Muscle energy is a form of manipulative treatment using active muscle contraction at varying intensities from a precisely controlled position in a specific direction against a counterforce. The origin of muscle energy is credited to Fred Mitchell, Sr., an osteopathic physician, who described the technique in the 1950s. His work has been documented by Mitchell

Jr. and associates.[169,170] Its other term, **post-isometric relaxation,** indicates the patient's active participation by muscular contraction and inspiration or expiration during manual treatment techniques.[17,53,70,75,80,126,127,140,141,169,170] These techniques rest on the prime importance of soft tissues, particularly muscles, in producing various, moderately abnormal states of joint pain and movement limitation.

Muscle energy techniques may be used to decrease pain, stretch tight muscles and fascia, reduce muscle tonus, improve local circulation, strengthen weak musculature, and mobilize joint restrictions.[70] This method uses muscle contraction by the patient followed by relaxation and stretch of an antagonist or agonist. It is essentially a mobilization technique using muscular facilitation and inhibition.[141] Moderate to maximal contractions are used to stretch muscles and their fascia while minimal to moderate contractions are used for joint mobilizations.

Lewit[141] has found that muscle energy techniques are as advantageous for muscle relaxation as they are for joint mobilization, if there is muscle spasm and particularly if there are active trigger points. Lewit recommends the following procedure. The muscle is first brought into a position in which it attains its maximum length without stretching, taking up the slack in the same way as in joint mobilization. In this position, the patient is asked to resist with a minimum of force (isometrically) and to breathe in. This resistance is held for about 10 seconds, after which the patient is told to "let go." With patient relaxation, a greater range is usually obtained. The slack is taken up and the procedure repeated three to five times. If relaxation proves to be unsatisfactory, the isometric phase may be lengthened to as much as half a minute. Wherever possible, the force of gravity is used, as described by Zbojan,[265] for isometric resistance and for relaxation. This method is comparable with the "spray and stretch" method of Travell[240,243,244] but places greater emphasis on relaxation.

THERAPEUTIC MUSCLE STRETCHING

Therapeutic muscle stretching (specific muscle stretching performed, instructed, or supervised by a manual therapy practitioner in a patient with dysfunctions of the musculoskeletal system) has been promoted by Bookhout,[16] Janda,[98] Muhlemann and Cimino, [175] Saal, [210] and Evjenth and Hamberg.[53] The latter investigators have developed highly specific techniques for stretching individual muscles that minimize the risk of injuring the surrounding tissue. Relaxation of incoming neural input is essential for lengthening a contractile unit.[80] This relaxation is best accomplished by a stretch that occurs slowly and evenly and is accompanied by gentle contraction of the antagonist muscle.[126] **Proprioceptive neuromuscular facilitation techniques** (PNF) are methods of promoting or hastening the response of the neuromuscular system through the stimulus of proprioceptors.[127] PNF is used in the approach of Evjenth and Hamberg. This approach as well as muscle energy is used to bring about relaxation of the antagonist muscle group according to the laws of reciprocal innervation proposed by Sherrington.[80,222] Primary objectives of PNF are also to develop trunk or proximal stability and control as well as to coordinate mobility patterns.

Performing stretching exercises both before and after an exercise period has been demonstrated to result in increased flexibility gains.[172] The ideal length of time for an individual to hold an isolated stretch is probably 15 to 30 seconds.[211] Continuation of the stretch for a period longer than this will not generate any greater flexibility gains, except in the case of pathologic contracture.[131,210,211]

RELAXATION EXERCISES

Relaxation exercises are of particular value in patients with musculoskeletal pain associated with psychogenic or tension states (see Chapter 9, Relaxation and Related Techniques). For example, tension headaches and muscular pain in the region of the cervical spine are often associated with prolonged muscle tension. Relaxation refers to a conscious effort to relieve tension in muscles. These exercises are usually based on the technique described by Jacobson[96] in which minimal contraction of each muscle is followed by a period of maximum relaxation. In addition, as a muscle is contracting, its corresponding antagonistic muscle is inhibited (Sherrington's law of reciprocal innervation).[80,222] Conscious thought can also be used to affect tension in muscle. This has been demonstrated in biofeedback, transcendental meditation, and autogenic training (see Chapter 9, Relaxation and Related Techniques).[144,145,219,248]

Neural Tissue Mobilization

Nerve tension tests of the lower limb have been incorporated into mobilization techniques for some time.[147] Both straight leg raising and the slump test position used in testing of the lumbar spine can be used as a treatment mobilization.[27,147] These methods can be applied when the symptoms or signs indicate pain is arising from the nerve root or its associated investments. Straight leg raising is an example of a direct method of mobilization of the nervous system. It is not considered a method of choice when the limitation is muscular and it should not be used, according to Maitland,[147] until other techniques that do not move the nerve root so much have been found ineffective.

The incorporation of the upper limb tension test (ULTT) into clinical practice was introduced by Robert Elvey (see Chapter 11, Shoulder and Shoulder Girdle).[50–52] According to Maitland,[147] the ULTT is a most important evaluation tool and should be used by all physical therapists, even at the undergraduate level. The utilization of the ULTT as a treatment technique is just beginning to be developed and there is much more to be learned and many combinations of movements to be explored.[27,52,118] It can be used as an effective treatment technique for both chronic and acute cervical pain and shoulder pain.

When indicated by the examination, Butler[27] gives three related ways of approaching a tension component related to the patient's disorder.

1. Direct mobilization of the nervous system via tension tests and palpation techniques
2. Treatment via interfacing and related tissue such as joints, muscles, and fascia
3. Indirect treatment such as postural advice

Introduction to Joint Mobilization Techniques

GENERAL RULES

The following rules and considerations should guide the therapist when performing joint mobilization techniques.

I. The patient must be relaxed. This requires that the patient is draped properly, that room temperature is comfortable, and that there are no distracting noises. Joints, other than the joint to be mobilized, must be at rest and well supported.

    The operator's handholds must be firm but comfortable. He or she must remove watches, jewelry, and so forth and be sure that buttons and belt buckles are not in contact with the patient.

II. The operator must be relaxed. This requires good body mechanics, especially with regard to the spine. The operator should attempt to create a situation in which his or her body and the part to be treated "act as one." This requires close body contact between the operator and patient for optimal control and mobilization.

III. Pain must be monitored. Therapy must not move into or through the point of pain. The operator must be able to determine the difference between the discomfort of soft tissue stretch, which is at times desirable, and the pain and muscle guarding that are a signal to ease up lest damage be done.

    The advanced manual therapist at times will move into or through the point of pain, but only in highly selective circumstances. These techniques are not to be taught, nor are they expected to be learned in a basic level course.

IV. Position of the patient must be correct. The following criteria must be satisfied:
    A. The joint under treatment is accessible and the full range of movement remains unrestricted.
    B. The movement can be localized to the exact area required.

V. The operator should use good body mechanics. The mobilizing force should be as close to the operator's center of gravity as possible. The force ideally should be directed with gravity assistance, especially when treating larger joints.

VI. When performing an assessment mobilization, the joint should be tested in the resting position if the patient is capable of attaining that position. If not, the joint should be tested in the actual resting (present neutral or loose-packed position) position. Maximum joint traction and joint play are available in that position. In some cases, the position to use is the one in which the joint is least painful.

VII. Each technique is both an evaluative technique and a treatment technique; therefore, the clinician continually evaluates during treatment. Formal assessments also should be made before and after treatment.

VIII. In Peripheral Joints:
    A. The direction of movement during treatment is either perpendicular or parallel to the treatment plane. **Treatment plane** is described by Kaltenborn[113] as a plane perpendicular to a line running from the axis of rotation to the middle of the concave articular surface. The plane is the concave partner, so its position is determined by the position of the concave bone.
        1. Gliding mobilizations are applied parallel to the treatment plane (see Fig. 5-3).
        2. Gliding mobilizations are usually performed in the direction in which the mobility test has shown that gliding is actually restricted (direct technique).
        3. If the mobility test in the desired direction produces pain, gliding mobilization in the other direction should be used (indirect technique).[146] Other indications for the indirect method include joints that are hypermobile or that have little movement (amphiarthrosis).[113]
        4. Joint traction or distraction techniques are applied perpendicular to the treatment plane.[113] The entire bone is moved so that the joint surfaces are separated (see Fig. 5-3).
    B. Treatment force in gliding techniques is applied as close to the opposite joint surface as possible. The larger the contact surface is, the more comfortable the procedure will be.
    C. One hand will usually stabilize while the other hand performs the movement. At times the plinth, the patient's body weight, and so on, are used for external stabilization. This allows both hands to assist in the movement. The therapist uses the hand or a belt to fix or stabilize the joint partner against a firm support. The fixation is maintained close to the joint surface without causing pain. The mobilizing hand grips the joint structure to be moved as close to the joint space as possible.
    D. The grip must be firm, yet painless and reassuring, while simultaneously allowing the fingertips to be free to palpate the tissues under treatment.
    E. The operator must consider the following:
        1. Velocity of movement. Slow stretching for large capsular restrictions; faster oscillations for minor restrictions.
        2. Amplitude of Movement. Graded according to pain, guarding, and degree of restriction.
    F. Accessory joint movement is compared with the opposite side (extremity), if necessary, to determine presence or degree of restriction.
    G. One movement is performed at a time, at one joint at a time.

IX. In Spinal Joints:
    A. In the sitting position it is essential that the patient is kept "in balance" so the occiput is in line with the coccyx, thus keeping the apex above the base.
    B. The direction of mobilization is determined by the results obtained from provocation tests. Mobilization initially is in that direction in which the pain and nociceptive reaction are diminished.
    C. Traction may be used to improve pain (levels I–II) before applying the specific mobilization technique.
X. Each Technique Can Be Used As:
    A. An examination procedure, by taking up the slack only, to determine the existing range of accessory movement and the presence or absence of pain.
    B. A therapeutic technique in which a high-velocity, small-amplitude thrust or graded oscillations are applied to regain accessory joint movement and relieve pain.
XI. Reassessment. This should be done at the beginning of each treatment session and during the treatment session. A selection of a few important "markers" for assessment enables a quick estimate of progress to be made without repeatedly going through the whole examination procedure.

INDICATIONS

Joint mobilization techniques are indicated in cases of joint dysfunction owing to restriction of accessory joint motion causing pain or restriction of motion during normal physiologic movement. However, as discussed in Chapter 3, Arthrology, there may be numerous causes of loss of accessory joint movement. The most common of these include capsuloligamentous tightening or adherence; internal derangement, as from a cartilaginous loose body or meniscus displacement; reflex muscle guarding; and bony blockage, as from hypertrophic degenerative changes. From this it should be clear that the proper indication for using specific mobilization techniques is loss of accessory joint motion (joint-play movement) secondary to capsular or ligamentous tightness or adherence. Other causes of joint dysfunction are relative contraindications. Refer to the section on capsular tightness in Chapter 4, Chronic Pain Management in the Adult.

CONTRAINDICATIONS

I. Absolute
    A. Any undiagnosed lesion
    B. Joint ankylosis
    C. The close-packed position (close-packed positions produce too much compression force on the articular surfaces)
    D. In the spine:
        1. Malignancy involving the vertebral column
        2. Cauda equina lesions producing disturbance of bladder or bowel function if the lumbar spine is being treated
        3. Where the integrity of ligaments may be affected by the use of steroids, traumatized upper cervical ligaments, Down's syndrome, and rheumatoid collagen

necrosis of the vertebral ligaments, particularly if the cervical spine is involved and being treated
        4. Any indication of vertebrobasilar insufficiency in the cervical spine if the cervical spine is being treated
        5. Active inflammatory and infective arthritis
II. Relative
    A. Joint effusion from trauma or disease
    B. Arthrosis (e.g., degenerative joint disease) if acute or if causing a bony block to movement to be restored
    C. Rheumatoid arthritis
    D. Metabolic bone disease, such as osteoporosis, Paget's disease, and tuberculosis
    E. Internal derangement
    F. General debilitation (e.g., influenza, chronic disease)
    G. Hypermobility. Patients with hypermobility may benefit from gentle joint-play techniques if kept within the limits of motion. Patients with potential necrosis of the ligaments or capsule should not be mobilized.
    H. Joints that have yet to ossify. The epithelium is very sensitive in babies owing to the rich blood supply; therefore, in children younger than 18 to 24 months of age, the authors work with mobility via muscle elongation and movement.
    I. Total joint replacements. The mechanism of the replacement is self-limiting, and therefore mobilizations may be inappropriate.
    J. In the spine:
        1. Pregnancy, if the lumbar spine or pelvis is being treated
        2. Spinal cord involvement or suspected aneurysm in the area being treated
        3. Spondylolisthesis or severe scoliosis in the area being treated
        4. Where there are symptoms derived from severe radicular involvement

Peripheral Joint Mobilization Techniques

GRADING OF MOVEMENT

Gaining a feel for the appropriate rate, rhythm, and intensity of movement is perhaps the most difficult aspect of learning to administer specific joint mobilization. Generally, rate, rhythm, and intensity must be adjusted according to how the patient presents—whether acute or chronic—and according to the response of the patient to the technique. When significant pain or muscle spasm is elicited, the rate of movement must be adjusted, or the intensity reduced, or both.

The type of movement performed ultimately depends on the immediate effect desired. In the majority of cases, these techniques are used to provide relief of pain and muscle guarding, to stretch a tight joint capsule or ligament, and rarely to reduce an intra-articular derangement that may be blocking movement.

MANUAL TRACTION[113,114]

Traction mobilizations are performed at a right angle to the treatment plane. Treatments are graded according to the amount of excursion imparted to the joint. The distance a joint is passively moved into its total range is its amplitude or grade of mobilization. Traction treatment mobilizations are graded as follows (Fig. 6-1):

Grade 1: Traction mobilization is applied by slowly distracting the joint surfaces, then slowly releasing until the joint returns to the starting position. There is little joint separation. Traction grade 1 may be used with all gliding tests and mobilization techniques.

Grade 2: Slow, larger amplitude movement perpendicular to the joint surface is applied, taking up the slack of the joint and the surrounding tissues.

Grade 3: Slow, even larger amplitude movement perpendicular to the joint surface is applied, stretching the tissues crossing the joint.

Grades 1 and 2 are used for pain reduction, whereas grade 3 is used to reduce pain and increase periarticular extensibility.

Other forms of manual traction include oscillatory, inhibitory, progressive, adjustive, and positional traction (see Figs. 19-59 and 22-48). Positional traction may also be applied mechanically. A manual adjustive traction employs a high-velocity thrust.[186]

Kaltenborn[112] advocates the use of **three-dimensional traction,** which describes traction to a joint, which has been positioned with respect to the three cardinal planes. For example, a painful joint may be positioned in a pain-free position with a certain amount of abduction, flexion, and rotation before traction is applied to alleviate the pain.

Gliding Mobilizations. Two systems of grading dosages for gliding mobilizations are commonly used: graded oscillation techniques and sustained joint-play techniques.[113–115,148] However, a number of mobilization methods may be considered, such as progressive stretch, continuous stretch, muscle energy techniques, functional techniques, and counterstrain.[19,94,109,182]

I. Sustained Translational Joint-Play or Stretch Techniques[113–115]
   A. Grade 1: Small-amplitude glide is applied parallel to the joint surface and does not take the joint up to the first tissue stop (at the beginning of range); used to reduce pain.

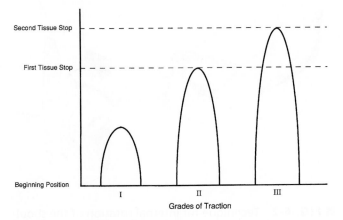

■ **FIG. 6-1.** Grades of traction.

B. Grade 2: The bone is moved parallel to the joint surface until the slack is taken up and the tissues surrounding the joint are tightened; used to decrease pain.
C. Grade 3: The bone is moved parallel to the joint surface with an amplitude large enough to place a stretch on the joint capsule and on surrounding periarticular structures.

   Traction is always the first procedure. Gliding mobilization is then performed in the direction in which the mobility test has shown that the gliding is actually restricted (direct technique). For restricted joints, apply a minimum of a 6-second stretch force, followed by partial release (to grade 1 or 2), then repeat at 3- to 4-second intervals. When applying stretching techniques, move the bony partner through the available range of motion first (until resistance is felt), and then apply the stretch force against the resistance.

II. Graded Oscillation Techniques (see Fig. 3-10)[148]
   Glides are graded along a scale of 1 to 5 as follows:
   A. Grade 1: Slow, small-amplitude oscillation parallel to the joint surface at the beginning of range; used to reduce pain.
   B. Grade 2: Slow, large-amplitude oscillation parallel to the joint surface within the free range; used to reduce pain (does not move into resistance or limit of range).
   C. Grade 3: Slow, large-amplitude oscillation parallel to the joint surface from middle to end of range; used to increase mobility (reaches the limit of range or takes the joint through the first tissue stop).
   D. Grade 4: Slow, small-amplitude oscillation parallel to the joint surface at the limit (end) of range; used to increase mobility.
   E. Grade 5: Fast, small-amplitude, high-velocity, non-oscillatory movement parallel to the joint surface beyond the pathologic limitation of range (through the first tissue stop), also called a thrust manipulation. Grade V is used when resistance limits movement, in the absence of pain.
      Some indications for a thrust manipulation (Grade V) of the peripheral joints may include:[36]
      1. Replacement of a joint dislocation (e.g., a subluxed cuboid, a dislocated shoulder, or in a child with a pulled elbow).
      2. Reduction of an internal derangement of a joint in which a torn meniscus (knee) or loose body (elbow) produces blocking of movements.
      3. Stretching or breaking down adhesions. In chronic adhesive capsulitis of the shoulder, thrust manipulation may be used to break down periarticular adhesions and increase joint mobility.

The oscillatory treatment movements (grades I–III) may be smooth and regular or performed with an irregular rhythm in an attempt to trick muscles when large-amplitude treatment movements are hindered by tension.[36] The oscillatory movements are usually used in one or two methods, either (1) as small- or large-amplitude movements, at a rate of two or three per second, applied anywhere within the range, or (2) combined with sustained stretch as small-amplitude oscillations applied at the limit of the joint range. One may vary the speed of oscillations for different effects such as low-amplitude, high-speed to inhibit pain, or slow speed to relax muscle guarding.[147] If gliding in the restricted direction is too painful, gliding mobilization can be started in the painless direction.

The only consistency between the dosages of the two gliding methods is with grade 1, in which no tension is placed on the joint capsule or surrounding tissue.[124] The choice of using oscillatory or sustained techniques depends on the patient response. When dealing with pain management or high tone, oscillatory techniques are recommended. When dealing with loss of joint play and decreased functional range, sustained techniques are recommended. Traction, grade 1, is used with all gliding tests and gliding mobilizations.

TECHNIQUES FOR THE RELIEF OF PAIN AND MUSCLE GUARDING

Relief of pain and muscle guarding is desirable in relatively acute conditions, as a treatment in and of itself, and in chronic conditions to prepare for more vigorous stretching. The techniques in acute conditions are performed to increase proprioceptive input to the spinal cord so as to inhibit ongoing nociceptive input to anterior horn cells and central receiving areas. They are what Maitland refers to as grades I and II techniques.[147] Movement is performed at the beginning or midpoint of the available joint-play amplitude, avoiding tension to joint capsules and ligaments. A rhythmic oscillation of the joint is produced at a rate of perhaps two to three cycles per second.

In the case of acute joint conditions, these may constitute the only passive mobilization techniques used until the acute manifestations subside. In more chronic cases, these techniques should be used at the initiation of a treatment session, between stretching techniques, and at the end of a session in order to promote relaxation of muscles controlling the joint. Chronically, they are used on a continuum with stretching techniques, gradually increasing in intensity as the patient relaxes.

Stretching Techniques. Because clinicians use these techniques primarily in cases of capsular tightness or adherence, the ultimate goal is to apply an intermittent stretch to the particular aspect of the capsule that is to be mobilized. In doing so, the clinician must move the joint up to the limit of the pathologic amplitude of a particular joint-play movement and attempt to increase the amplitude of movement. These techniques must be applied rhythmically—no abrupt changes in speed or direction—to prevent reflex contractions of muscles about the joint that might occur from overfiring of joint receptors. They must also be applied slowly in order to allow for the viscous nature—resistance to quick change in length—of connective tissue. The slack that is taken up in the joint-play movement is not released as the movement is performed. In effect, one is applying a prolonged stretch with superim-

posed rhythmic oscillations of small amplitude. The rationale is twofold. A prolonged stretch is the safest, most effective means of increasing the extensibility of collagenous tissue. In addition, rhythmic oscillations reduce the amount of discomfort and facilitate maximal relaxation during the procedure, presumably by increasing large-fiber input to the "gate."

Stops. When stretching at the limits of a particular osteokinematic movement in the presence of a tight capsule, it is usually helpful to provide a rigid "stop" against which the oscillation is made. It is best for the practitioner to arrange one of his or her body parts (e.g., thigh, forearm, or trunk) as a stop. In this way the stop is easily moved to allow progressively increased range of movement. Such a stop also gives the patient an indication of exactly how far the therapist is going to move the part during a particular series of oscillations. This will reduce anticipatory muscle guarding to a minimum. If a greater range of movement is desired, the patient is informed where the stop will be made. The therapist rearranges the stop so as to allow a small increase in motion, and the oscillations are resumed. Such a technique seems to be most effective if the patient's body part is brought up rather firmly against the stop with each oscillation. For example, when mobilizing the shoulder, the therapist's thigh is brought up on the plinth to act as a stop for internal (Fig. 6-2) or external rotation (Fig. 6-3).

SPINE

There are some specific technical points to be mentioned with respect to the spine. For instance, because it is not possible to move a single segment actively, passive movement represents, as it were, joint play. Because of this relative difficulty in moving single joints, both specific and nonspecific techniques will be described in the spinal chapters. In the practice of spinal mobilization therapy there are scores of techniques available to the manual therapy practitioners. Most of the techniques

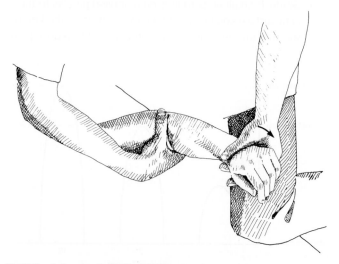

■ **FIG. 6-2.** Technique for internal rotation of the shoulder joint (arm close to 90° abduction) using a stop.

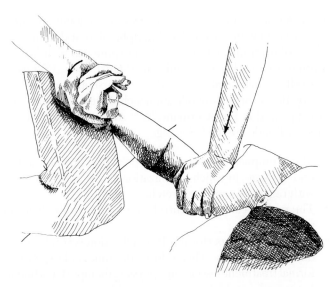

■ **FIG. 6-3.** Technique for external rotation of the shoulder joint (posterior glide, arm close to 90° of abduction) with a stop.

employed by practitioners have either osteopathic or chiropractic components, although some occasionally make use of Cyriax's and Mennell's techniques.[180] Mobilization can be performed in a physiologic direction (namely, rotation, extension, lateral flexion, or flexion) or in a nonphysiologic direction (e.g., longitudinal traction or anterior-directed posterior-anterior gliding). In practice, rotation, posterior gliding, and traction techniques are mainly employed.[117] Spinal mobilization techniques can be classified under the headings of indirect mobilizations, direct mobilizations, specific mobilizations, nonspecific manipulations, oscillatory techniques, progressive loading, and manipulative thrusts.[180] Although there are many mobilization techniques, it is necessary to become proficient with only a few.

Indirect Mobilizations. When using these techniques the operator uses the limbs or pelvic or shoulder girdle as natural levers to influence the spinal column or sacroiliac joint.[180] For example, when a patient is sidelying with the operator applying pressure on the pelvis and the shoulder in opposite directions, the resulting force can cause rotation of the lumbar spine (see Fig. 22-41). Contract–relax or muscle energy techniques may be used to facilitate maximum range of motion or to correct an anterior sacroiliac dysfunction (see Fig. 22-46). The leg is used as a lever.

Direct Mobilizations. Direct mobilizations involve direct manual pressure on the vertebrae in order to influence the intervertebral joints under treatment. These techniques are sometimes described as pressure techniques. The maneuvers are essentially those of chiropractors.[180] They are executed with the heel or ulnar border of the hand; more exactly, it is the pisiform, which constitutes the point of pressure, which is either applied at the level of the transverse process or the spinal process (see Fig. 22-34).

Specific Mobilizations. There are specific mobilization techniques intended to influence only one joint at a time. This is achieved in several ways.

Positioning of the Area of Spine Under Treatment. When treating the lumbar spine, the operator should position the lumbar spine in extension when mobilization of the upper lumbar intervertebral joints is desired, and with a flexed spine for the lower lumbar intervertebral joints (see Figs. 22-33 and 22-37).

Locking. One way of achieving a specific effect is to apply "locking" techniques. To make such a technique specific, the clinician must try to lock all segments except for the one to be mobilized. The principle of locking consists of bringing the segments that are not to be moved into an extreme position, under a certain degree of tension. The mechanism is either tension of ligaments or opposition of bony structures (facet locking).

Ligamentous locking is achieved by moving the joint to the limit of joint range possible and utilizing the resulting capsular tension to lock the joint. The therapist locks the spinal segment by placing it in a movement pattern that constrains movement. When using ligamentous tension locking for localization, it is often desirable to use manual contact to achieve some degree of specificity. For example, a vertebra may be fixed by direct manual contact in a least one direction (e.g., fixation of a spinous process from the side prevents rotation in the opposite direction).

Facet locking is achieved mainly by a careful combination of movement patterns (noncoupled or coupled) that constrains such movement as sidebending and rotation, making use of bony opposition. The therapist positions the patient just short of complete fixation so that a small range of movement is possible in the joint in question but less in the adjacent joints above and below. Usually segments cranial to the treated segment are locked. In some instances, locking may be used both cranial to and caudal to the spinal segment. An in-depth discussion of spinal joint locking is presented by Evjenth and Hamberg.[53] To achieve the maximum specific effect, a combination of leverage and locking techniques with direct contact and fixation is commonly used.

Leverage of Movement (Long-Lever Techniques). This is another way to achieve specificity. For example, for treatment of the lower lumbar intervertebral joints, mobilization can be effected by rotating the pelvis or legs on a relatively fixed trunk up to the segment to be mobilized (see Figs. 22-39 and 22-40). Following this principle, the trunk can be rotated on a relatively fixed spine for the treatment of the thoracic spine (see Fig. 20-48).

Nonspecific Manipulations. There are also nonspecific techniques that can be useful in mobilizing larger sections of the spinal column, such as traction along the long axis of the spine. Whereas traction along the long axis of the spine (see Fig. 22-43) acts on the intervertebral disk, distraction of the apophyseal joints is provided by rotation and side flexion around that same axis (see Fig. 22-48). Other types of nonspecific methods are represented by soft-tissue mobilization, general spinal manipulations, and noncontact manipulations.[87] Nonspecific manipulations are techniques whereby the manipulative force falls on more than one joint. Most of Cyriax's techniques fall under this category in which massive traction is applied to the area of the spine under treatment simultaneously with the manipulative thrust.[38–40] A potential complication of nonspecific techniques (traction and nonspecific manipulations) is the possibility of increasing motion in an unstable joint that was not detected during the evaluation.

Oscillatory Techniques. A variety of oscillatory techniques have evolved. However, more than anyone else, Maitland has successfully developed an excellent system for the application of oscillatory techniques.[147,148] As with the peripheral joints, the operator is guided by the signs and symptoms that the patient brings into the treatment situation. The operator oscillates into the patient's pain but not beyond it. An important feature of these techniques is that the patient is the controller of the treatment, thereby minimizing the possibility of harm. Another component of these techniques is rhythm. The more rhythmic the oscillations, the more tolerable and pleasant the treatment will be for the patient and the more effective.[180] Any diagnostic label is de-emphasized, while the amount of movement in the joint becomes the subject of treatment. This purpose is very much facilitated if the joint is positioned somewhere in mid range in order to move the joint in a chosen direction. (see above for grading of these techniques)

Progressive Loading. Progressive loading mobilization involves a successive series of short-amplitude, spring-type pressures.[188] Pressure is imparted at progressive increments of the range on a 1 to 4 scale, as are graded oscillations. The pressures used are transmitted at different ranges; however, the amplitude of each pressure is the same.[181,182] Grades 1 to 3 occur within the available active range of motion. Grade 4 goes beyond the restrictive barrier and into the passive motion barrier.

Manipulative Thrusts. A manipulative thrust (grade V) involves a high-velocity, small-amplitude thrust beyond the pathologic limits of range (through the first tissue stop). Only properly trained and experienced clinicians should apply manipulative thrusts of the spine owing to the skill and judgment necessary to their safe and effective practice. Most therapists have found that they can achieve the same effects by prudent application of other methods of spinal mobilization techniques. The great hallmark of mobilization is its relative safety.

Self-Mobilization Techniques of the Spine. Traditionally, home programs have included exercise regimens dealing in a general way with the affected region rather than with the specific segment involved. Many of these home programs for joint dysfunction have, for the most part, stressed active or passive motions that are often poorly controlled by the patient, thus leading to further pain and joint stiffness.[45,195] The logical and most effective approach in the management of capsular restriction is increasing the extensibility through techniques applied directly to the joint. This has led

to the development of special exercises for the joints and muscles involved with vertebral and peripheral joint dysfunction. Self-mobilization techniques of the spine are well known through the works of Kaltenborn,[112] Gustavsen,[84,85] Fisk,[63] Buswell,[25,26] and Lewit.[139,140] In 1975, the first of a series of articles by Rohde on self-mobilization techniques of the extremities appeared in East Germany.[198–201] Among the advantages cited by Rohde are the following:

- Major emphasis is placed on a pain-free position at the end of range, in which mobilization can be most effective with regard to capsular stretch.
- The patient can often control pain more readily than can the therapist.
- The patient can perform self-mobilization several times a day independently. This reduces the time and expense of formal treatment sessions in a physical therapy department.
- Increased range of motion is possible without excessive force.
- The techniques are simple, easy to apply, and are not time consuming.

Furthermore, it is probable that the oscillatory nature and repetitive motion working within the painful limits reduces pain by increasing proprioceptive input.[31,162] When pain is present, joint irritability is carefully monitored and patients are advised to observe pain behavior and to discontinue the movement if there is an increase in peripheral pain. Self-mobilization must be gentle, slow, and as specific as possible.

In general, self-mobilization is indicated in subacute or chronic painful conditions of the joints, which have resulted in a capsular pattern of restriction and for which restoration of range of motion appears possible. The basic rules and indications are essentially the same as for other mobilization techniques. Precise clinical diagnosis and indication are mandatory. For restricted movement, the patient is advised to gradually work into the painful range in order to stretch tight structures. A particularly effective variation in peripheral joint mobilization is the use of hold–relax techniques applied directly before a specific self-mobilization. All exercises are further enhanced by purposeful breathing.[26] An active altered posture is recommended for all spinal patients.[156,157,191,245]

Self-mobilization exercises are aimed at self-treatment, making the patient the most active member of the rehabilitation team. Selected examples of specific exercise for the relief of pain and increased mobility are described in subsequent chapters.

MUSCLE ENERGY AND FUNCTIONAL TECHNIQUES

Muscle energy is an extremely valuable technique for correcting positional faults or joint hypomobility, because the technique combines methods to increase extensibility of periarticular tissue with methods to restore a length–tension relationship to the muscles controlling joint motion. The techniques of muscle energy are discussed in a previous section regarding soft tissue mobilization techniques. When muscle energy is used for joint restrictions, the joint is placed in a specific position to facilitate optimal contraction of a particular muscle or muscle group. Isometric muscle contraction against counterpressure provided by the clinician causes the muscle to pull on the bony attachment that is not being stabilized, thus moving one bone in relation to its articulating counterpart. Most isometric contractions are held for 3 to 7 seconds, and techniques are repeated approximately three to five times before reassessment. When isometrics are used for joint mobilization, maximal contractions are not desirable since they tighten, or freeze, the joints.[140] Moderate contractions are much more appropriate for joint mobilization.

An important consideration in this approach is the particular type of three-dimensional movement posture that will best localize the effect to a particular vertebral segment or rib joint. Localization of the force is more important than intensity of force. What is especially welcome about these methods is that they are alternatives to manipulative procedures.[17]

To understand the principles and applications of muscle energy techniques and functional techniques (two forms of post-isometric relaxation techniques), one must be familiar with the concepts of segmental facilitation proposed by Korr and with the work of Patterson and Sherrington on spinal reflexes.[128,129,189,222] According to Korr,[128] when the gamma motoneuron discharge to the muscle spindle is excessive, less external stretch is required to fire the primary annulospiral endings, which reflexly fire the extrafusal muscle fiber via the alpha motoneuron. The exaggerated spindle responses are provoked by motions, which tend to lengthen the facilitated muscle and therefore create a restrictive spinal fault. The aim of both muscle energy and functional techniques is to restore the normal neurophysiology of the segment.

Harold Hoover, an osteopathic physician, originated the functional method.[19,20,94,106,136] The aim of functional techniques is to reduce the exaggerated spindle response from the facilitated segmental muscles and thus restore normal joint mobility.[20,137] Like combined movements[48,49] and strain and counterstrain,[108,109,134] functional techniques utilize combinations of movements to find the most pain-free starting position, and superimpose on this starting position gentle, repetitive motions or sustained holding.[20,137] The goal of these approaches is to obtain an antalgic starting position, with subsequent reduction in the input from depolarized nociceptors.[136]

STRAIN–COUNTERSTRAIN TECHNIQUE[41,44,77,108,109,134,182]

Strain and counterstrain became popular in the 1970s and the number of practitioners is increasing. The technique was devised by Lawrence Jones, an osteopathic practitioner. It is considered an indirect manipulative technique of extreme gentleness for the treatment of somatic dysfunctions. In *Strain and Counterstrain*, Jones offers two definitions of the technique.[109]

1. "Relieving spinal or other joint pain by passively putting the joint into its position of greatest comfort."
2. "Relieving pain by reduction and arrest of the continuing inappropriate proprioceptor activity." To accomplish this, the muscle that contains the malfunctioning muscle spindle is significantly shortened by applying mild strain to its antagonist.

The position of injury is one of strain, which places some muscles in a shortened state and other muscles in a lengthened state. The rationale for strain and counterstrain is based on a neurologic model first proposed by Dr. Irvin Korr in 1975.[129,130] According to Korr's muscle spindle theory for neuromuscular disorder, the gamma motor neuron activity to the intrafusal fibers of the shortened muscles is turned up instead of decreased. The resultant tension in the intrafusal mechanism of the shortened muscles causes excitation of the central nervous system, stimulation of the alpha motor neurons, and the maintenance of extrafusal fiber contraction.

Diagnosis in this method is made by the presence of a specific tender point that overlies the muscle. The tender points may be related to myofascial trigger points and acupuncture points.[44] The treatment technique is positional. According to Jones, positioning the joint in the exact opposite position to the one that produces the pain will relieve the pain and dysfunction. There are two important aspects of this treatment procedure:[134]

1. Using the tender point as a monitor, the operator is guided into a position of comfort that reduces aberrant afferent flow and returns the muscle to "easy neutral."
2. The position of comfort is held for 90 seconds, the amount of time required for the proprioceptive firing to decrease in frequency and amplitude, and then it is returned to neutral slowly after the positional release.

Strain and counterstrain is considered a gentle, nontraumatic type of mobilization technique especially effective when irregular neuromuscular activities have maintained and perpetuated abnormal mechanical stress to tissue in both acute and chronic conditions. Strain and counterstrain can make a significant contribution when integrated with other manual medicine techniques (i.e., joint mobilization, muscle energy, myofascial release).[134] Although there is limited research data in this area to support the model, the observation of practitioners points to a neural basis through a principle of afferent reduction of abnormal mechanoreceptor and nociceptor stimulation.[77]

HYPERMOBILITY TREATMENT

The term **hypermobility** denotes an increase in the range of motion in an extremity joint or a spinal segment. One can differentiate between minor hypermobility without pain, hypermobility with pain, and complete instability that is considered to be pathologic.[85] Pain may be caused by continued postural imbalances, continued motor performance abnormalities, or delayed stretch pain (tendon pain resulting from overstretching of one or several tendons). According to Gustavsen,[85] this type of tendon pain appears a few seconds after bringing the joint to its barrier and decreases very slowly when the joint is carried to a more normal position.

The two basic types of hypermobility include systematically acquired hypermobility (general constitutional type) and local hypermobility of a peripheral joint or spinal segment. Hypermobility is not a pathologic motion state of a joint but rather one end of the normal mobility spectrum.[72] Hypermobility may be generalized to both spinal and peripheral joints, or it may be a feature of spinal joints alone, peripheral alone, or isolated to one spinal segment. Symptomatic hypermobility occurs when musculoskeletal signs and symptoms may be ascribed to the presence of hypermobility.[46,68] An unstable joint is one with increased range of movement in one (or more) directions in which there is insufficient soft tissue control, be it ligamentous, disk, muscular, or all three.[72]

Many definitions of spinal instability exist without any real consensus.[44,56,66,68,78–80,95,120–122,176,188,190,193,211] One consideration is the difference between functional (clinical instability) and mechanical instability. Whereas **mechanical instability** is described as consisting of a measurable abnormal translation of joint opening that is the direct result of disruption of one or more of the mechanical stabilizers of the joint, **functional instability** (which can occur in the absence of measurable mechanical instability) is manifested by instability of the joint under load.[194] In most cases, functional instability is caused by muscular or proprioceptive deficit.

Spinal segment hypermobility may be the result of compensation seen with acquired motion restrictions or congenital motion restrictions. Junctional areas (i.e., C4–5, lumbosacral junction and thoracolumbar junction) of the spinal column tend to become especially hypermobile.[237] Hypermobility in the C4–5 segment is often accompanied by hypomobility in segments C2 and C3 and the cervicothoracic junction as well.[85] Muscular dysfunction is usually present with shortened upper deep neck muscles and weakened long neck and prevertebral muscles. Hypermobility of L4, L5, and S1 is often caused by inappropriate motor activities.[85] Typically these individuals have forgotten how to control their lumbar spine in a position of stability when carrying out activities of daily living. Management of segmental instability should include pain reduction methods. Pain may be caused by continued postural imbalance, continued motor performance abnormalities, or delayed stretch pain. Passive mobilization (grades 1 and 2, posterior–anterior pressures) of the affected segment within its range is particularly effective.[85] Stabilizing and controlling procedures (collars, corsets, taping) when the spinal area is very painful or very unstable, or both, may be helpful.[116,168,176,212,213,216,252,258] These procedures should be temporary while the exercise program is developed.

Regional Exercises

LUMBAR AND THORACIC SPINE

Therapeutic exercises that improve muscle strength, endurance, coordination, and control should be started as soon as possible. Isometric, gravitational exercises, and other forms of exercise should be considered.[78–80,119,166,188] If the spinal extensors (thoracic and lumbar spine) are weak, exercises to strengthen them should avoid inner range hyperextension movements. The starting position should be arranged so that the resisted movement occurs in mid range and the excursion ceases when normal postural length of the muscle is reached.[80] A potent cause of aggravation of low back pain, due to hypermobility, is that of forced extension in the starting position of lying prone. Rotational exercises have been effective in patients who do not respond to other treatments.[192] By increasing muscle control and strength, postural backache and locking will be reduced.

The learning of physiologically correct movement patterns and postural advice is vital and should include avoidance of positions and exercises that lead to strain on joints, such as hyperextension. Exercises need to be selected with care, since those which stress extreme joint positions are liable to exacerbate the condition. In general, one should start with many repetitions at low speed with minimal resistance performed at middle or beginning range. Progression of exercises should focus on increased (isometric) contractions in the inner range of motion and finally on submaximal resistance in any range except the outer range. The purpose is not so much to develop strength but endurance and technique (physiologically correct movement patterns).

Swimming is considered excellent for the lumbar and thoracic spine, because there is little back movement and strong muscle work including co-contractions.[72] Balance exercises using a wobble board, Tumble Form, or Feldenkrais foam roll in standing, sitting, and lying positions are used to improve muscular "speed" reactions and balance reactions. The patient's balance may be challenged also with the use of the Swiss gymnastic ball.[132,138]

The emphasis of long-term management involves the avoidance of excessive load, sustained activities, and especially end-of-range postures.

CERVICAL SPINE

Training follows similar lines as for the thoracic and lumbar spine. Patients will usually benefit from postural retraining of the entire spine. Lumbar exercises offer a properly aligned base of support for the thoracic spine, whereas the position of the thoracic cage is the key to postural control of the balanced cervical spine.[232] As with the thoracic and lumbar spine, the learning of physiologically correct movement patterns, use of relief postures, ergonomic advice, and increased postural awareness are vital to bring about dynamic changes in the musculoskeletal system. Longstanding compulsive patterns need to be modified or removed from the nervous system.[152] Imposing traditional exercise movements on changed or faulty postures and movement patterns will often only perpetuate the existing condition.[60] There are several very effective methods and techniques in current use to facilitate body awareness and movement including the Feldenkrais method,[57-60,151] the Alexander technique,[11,33,67,107] Aston Patterning,[8,9,143,167] ideokinetic facilitation and related body alignment techniques,[233,239] and Kein-Vogelbach's functional kinetics.[125]

There are many methods of strengthening the paravertebral muscles of the neck including proprioceptive facilitation and simple self-administered resistance by hand pressure.[1,25,28,29,185,197,214,215,266] Exercises for the cervical, upper through mid-thoracic and shoulder girdle region are functionally interrelated and need to be addressed. Exercises should not be given arbitrarily as a group but should be judiciously chosen for the treatment program.

Localized Active Stabilization Techniques (Segmental Strengthening)

Patients with spinal dysfunction need to learn to actively stabilize hypermobile spinal areas. This requires strong and well-functioning muscles. The small extensor and rotator muscles close to the hypermobile joint must become strong enough to be able to fixate a hypermobile segment. Strengthening the segmental musculature is achieved by the principle of stimulating the small but important muscle groups to work isometrically in maintaining the orientation in space of a single segment.[80] Clear evidence exists that degenerative joint conditions are accompanied by changes in the relative population of "fast" and "slow" fibers in the segmental musculature (e.g., multifidus).[110] The deeper intersegmental and polysegmental muscles, particularly the multifidi, are primarily stabilizers controlling posture and assisting in fine adjustments and segmental movement.[12,90,121,249] The multifidi are also believed to protect the facet capsule from being impinged during movement because of its attachment to the joint capsule.[14]

DIRECT METHOD

These stabilization techniques involve direct manual pressure on the spinous process of the hypermobile segment. The thumb pads may be applied to the side of the spinous process in a lateral or oblique direction (lateral technique) or over the spinous process in a posteroanterior direction (sagittal technique) to recruit the small rotators or extensors (see Figs. 22-62C and 22-63A). Moderate but sustained pressure is applied to the bony point while the patient is instructed not to allow the vertebra to be displaced. With encouragement and practice the patient is able to localize the muscular effort. Progression is made by increasing the pressure, both in intensity and duration. Positioning is usually with the spine in a resting position. One can also use ligamentous or facet locking and positioning out of the resting position to influence localization. Progression can also be increased by using an antigravity position (see Fig. 19-63).

INDIRECT METHOD

When using indirect techniques the operator uses the limbs, sacrum, or head to influence the small muscles along the spinal column. For example, when treating the lumbar spine with the patient in a prone position, one hand of the operator is placed on the lumbar region immediately above the segment(s) concerned while moderate but increasing and sustained pressure is applied to the sacrum with the other hand (see Fig. 22-62C).

Self-Stabilization Exercises

At home, another person can be taught to give resistance, or pressure can be self-administered by the patient (see Figs. 19-61, 19-62, 22-62B,C, 22-63A,B). Indirect methods use specific starting positions so that the painful and hypermobile segment does not move during these exercises. Stabilization programs in which the extremities are involved may require a special exercise program to train the muscles so that they can develop the required stabilizing effect (see therapeutic exercises, following). Exercises should emphasize diagonal motion to strengthen the small muscles around the spine.[85]

THERAPEUTIC EXERCISES

Therapeutic exercises have been widely recommended to help prevent the development of spinal and peripheral pathology, to decrease pain, and to increase function. The benefits of exercise extend beyond the obvious improvement in muscle performance to include positive effects on the cardiovascular system, bone and connective tissue. Exercise may have a positive effect on the strength, integrity and organization of collagen that is found in all types of connective tissue.[7,37,55,133,178,238,246] Although disuse and inactivity cause atrophy and weakening of connective tissues such as tendons and ligaments, physical training can increase the maximum tensile strength and the amount of energy absorbed before failure.[231,262] Physical activity returns damaged tendons and ligaments to normal tensile strength faster than complete bed rest.[238]

Numerous types of exercises are recognized as necessary to prevent, restore, or maintain a healthy and functional musculoskeletal system: strength training, power training, flexibility training, balance and agility training, endurance training, aerobic training, speed training and neuromuscular control training. Much of our present-day understanding of muscle imbalances and neuromuscular control training comes from the work of Bookhout,[16] Janda,[99-102] Jull and Janda,[111] Lewit,[140] Kendall et al.,[116] and Sahrmann.[212,213] Janda has observed that certain muscle groups respond to dysfunction by tightening and shortening, while other muscle groups react by inhibition, atrophy, and weakness (see Table 5-6).

Therapeutic exercises should be directed by someone who understands the rehabilitation process, the concept of soft tissue healing, the demands of the sports or activities on the musculoskeletal system, the musculoskeletal deficits of the individual, and the principles of sound exercise program design, including appropriate frequency and dosage, intensity, duration of the exercises, and the concepts of specificity, recovery, and gradual progression. The first and immediate reason following injury for rehabilitation is to resolve the clinical symptoms and signs that exist. Criteria for advancement include pain control, adequate tissue healing, near-normal ROM and tolerance for strengthening. In the recovery stage of functional rehabilitation, when tissue healing is complete or nearly complete (see Chapter 2, Wound Healing: Injury and Repair of Dense Connective Tissue), treatment emphasis shifts from resolution of clinical signs to restoration of function. The remodeling tissue can now be appropriately loaded to regain local flexibility, proprioception and strength.

In the past 20 years, both clinicians and patients have shown increasing support for the concepts of self-treatment.[155–159] Training programs such as medical exercise training (MET),[91,92,223] medical training therapy (MTT),[84,85] functional exercise, (see Chapter 10, Functional Exercise)[34,74] aerobic training,[18,153,173,179,259] back and neck schools,[54,56,142,232,253–257] sensory motor stimulation[23,103,104] and dynamic stabilization programs (particularly for the lumbar spine),[153,173,185,196,206–209,211,214,215,232,256] have increased our knowledge of how to carry out a patient-oriented training program to provide optimal stimulation of the functional qualities of muscle strength, flexibility, endurance, coordination, and cardiovascular fitness for retraining and improving function.

REFERENCES

1. Adler SS, Beckers D, Buck M: The neck. In: Adler SS, Beckers D, Buck M, eds: PNF in Practice: An Illustrated Guide. Berlin, Springer-Verlag, 1993:141–151
2. Akeson WH, Amiel D: The connective tissue response to immobility: A study of the chondroitin 4 and 6 sulfate and dermatan sulfate changes in periarticular connective of control and immobilized knees of the dog. Clin Orthop 51:190–197, 1967
3. Akeson WH, Amiel D: Immobility effects of synovial joints: The pathomechanics of joint contracture. Biorheology 17:95–110, 1980
4. Akeson WH, Amiel D, LaViolette D: The connective tissue response to immobility: An accelerated aging response? Exp Gerontol 3:289–301, 1968
5. Akeson WH, Amiel D, Mechanic GL, et al: Collagen cross-linking alteration to joint contractures: Changes in the reducible cross-linking in periarticular connective tissue collagen after nine weeks of immobilization. Connect Tissue Res 5:15–19, 1977
6. Akeson WH, Woo SL-Y, Amiel D, et al: The connective tissue response to immobilization: Biomechanical changes in periarticular connective tissue of the rabbit knee. Clin Orthop 93:356–362, 1973
7. Akeson WH, Woo SL-Y, Amiel D et al. The chemical basis of tissue repair: The biology of ligaments. In: Hunter LY, Funk FJ, eds: Rehabilitation of the Injured Knee. St. Louis, CV Mosby, 1984:93–148
8. Aston J: Movement Dynamics, I. Continuing Education Course. Seattle, WA, Aston Training Center, 1990
9. Aston J: Movement Dynamics, II. Continuing Education Course. Incline Village, NV, Aston Training Center, 1992
10. Bajelis D: Hellerwork: The ultimate. Int J Altern Complement Med 12:26–39, 1994
11. Barlow W: The Alexander Technique. New York, Warner Books 1973
12. Basmajian JV: Muscles Alive: Their Functions Revealed by Electromyography. Baltimore, Williams & Wilkins, 1978
13. Bischof I, Elminger G: Connective tissue massage. In: Licht S, ed: Massage, Manipulation & Traction. Baltimore, Waverly, 1963:57–85
14. Bogduk N, Twomey LT: Clinical Anatomy of the Lumbar Spine. New York, Churchill Livingstone, 1987
15. Bonica JJ: Management of myofascial pain syndromes in general practice. JAMA 164:732–738, 1957
16. Bookhout MR: Examination and treatment of muscle imbalances. In: Bourdillon JF, Day EA, Bookhout MR, eds: Spinal Manipulation, 5th ed. Oxford, Butterworth-Heinemann, 1992:313–333
17. Bourdillon J, Day EA, Bookhout MR: Spinal Manipulation, 5th ed. Oxford, Butterworth-Heinemann, 1992
18. Bower KD: The role of exercises in the management of low back pain. In: Grieve GP, ed: Modern Manual Therapy of the Vertebral Column. Edinburgh, Churchill Livingstone, 1986:839–848
19. Bowles CH: A functional orientation for technique. Yearbook of the Academy of Applied Osteopathy. 1955:177–191
20. Bowles CH: Functional technique: A modern perspective. J Am Osteopath Assoc 80:326–331, 1981
21. Bradley JA: Acupuncture, acupressure, and trigger point therapy. In: Peat M, ed: Current Physical Therapy. Toronto, BC Decker, 1988:228–234
22. Brown BR: Diagnosis and therapy of common myofascial syndromes. JAMA 239:646–648, 1978
23. Bullock-Saxton JE, Janda V, Bullock MI: Reflex activation of gluteal muscles in walking: An approach to restoration of muscle function for patients with low back pain. Spine 18:704–708, 1993
24. Burke GL: Backache from Occiput to Coccyx. Vancouver, MacDonald, 1964
25. Buswell JS: A manual of home exercises for the spinal column. Auckland, Pelorus Press, 1977
26. Buswell JS: Exercises in the treatment of vertebral dysfunction. In: Grieve G, ed: Modern Manual Therapy of the Vertebral Column. Edinburgh, Churchill Livingstone, 1986:834–838
27. Butler DS: Mobilisation of the Nervous System. Melbourne, Churchill Livingstone, 1991
28. Cailliet R: Soft Tissue Pain and Disability, 3rd ed. Philadelphia, FA Davis, 1996
29. Cailliet R: Subluxations of the cervical spine: The whiplash syndromes. In: Cailliet R, ed: Neck and Arm Pain, 2nd ed. Philadelphia, FA Davis, 1991:81–121
30. Cantu RI, Grodin AJ: Myofascial Manipulation: Theory and Clinical Application. Gaithersburg, Aspen, 1992
31. Casey KL, Melzack R: Neural mechanism of pain: A conceptual model. In: Way EL, ed: New Concepts in Pain and Its Clinical Management. Philadelphia, FA Davis, 1967
32. Chaitow L: Modern Neuromuscular Techniques. New York, Churchill Livingstone, 1996
33. Chaplan D: Back Trouble: A New Approach to Prevention and Recovery. Gainesville, Triad, 1987
34. Chason NP, Kane DM: Functional training for low back patient. Orthop Phys Ther Clin North Am 8:451–477, 1999
35. Cookson JC, Kent BE: Orthopedic manual therapy—An overview. Phys Ther 59:136–146, 1979
36. Corrigan B, Maitland GD: Practical Orthopaedic Medicine. London, Butterworth, 1985
37. Curwin S, Standish W: Tendinitis: Its Etiology and Treatment. Lexington, Collamore, 1984:1–67
38. Cyriax J: Textbook of Orthopaedic Medicine, vol. 1. Diagnosis of Soft Tissue Lesions, 8th ed. London, Balliere Tindall, 1982
39. Cyriax J, Coldham M: Textbook of Orthopaedic Medicine, vol. 2. Treatment by Manipulation, Massage and Injection, 11th ed. London, Balliere Tindall, 1984
40. Cyriax JH, Cyriax PJ: Illustrated Manual of Orthopaedic Medicine. London, Butterworth, 1983
41. D'Ambrogio KJ: Positional Release Therapy: Assessment & Treatment of Musculoskeletal Dysfunction. St. Louis, Mosby, 1997
42. Danneskiold-Samsoe B, Christiansen E, Anderson RB: Myofascial pain and the role of myoglobin. Scand J Rheumatol 15:174–178, 1986
43. Dicke E, Schliack H, Wolff A: A Manual of Reflexive Therapy of the Connective Tissue. Scarsdale, Simon, 1978
44. DiGiovanna EL: Counterstrain. In: DiGiovanna EL, Schiowitz S, eds: An Osteopathic Approach to Diagnosis and Treatment. Philadelphia, JB Lippincott, 1991:85–87
45. Dontigny RL: Passive shoulder exercises. J Phys Ther 50:1707–1709, 1970
46. Dupuis PR, Young-Hing K, Cassidy JD, et al: Radiologic diagnosis of degenerative lumbar spinal instability. Spine 10:662–676, 1985
47. Ebner M: Connective Tissue Manipulations. Malbar, Robert E. Kreiger, 1985
48. Edwards BC: Combined movements in the lumbar spine: Examination and significance. Aust J Physiother 25:147–152, 1979
49. Edwards BC: Combined movements in the lumbar spine: Examination and treatment. In: Grieve GP, ed: Modern Manual Therapy of the Vertebral Column. Edinburgh, Churchill Livingstone, 1986:561–566
50. Elvey RL: Brachial plexus tension tests and the pathoanatomical origin of arm pain. Proceedings of the Multidisciplinary International Conference of Manipulative Therapy, Melbourne, Australia, 1979:105–111
51. Elvey RL: Brachial plexus tension test and the pathoanatomical origin of arm pain. In: Idczack RM, ed: Aspects of Manipulative Therapy. Carlton, Australia, Lincoln Institute of Health Sciences, 1981

52. Elvey RL: Treatment of arm pain associated with abnormal brachial plexus tension. Aust J Physiother 32:225–230, 1986
53. Evjenth O, Hamberg J: Muscle Stretching in Manual Therapy: A Clinical Manual, vol. 1. The Extremities: Vol. 2. The Spinal Column and the TMJ. Alfta, Sweden, Alfta Rehab Forlag, 1984
54. Fahrni WH: Back school back then: A personal history. In: White AH, Anderson R, eds: Conservative Care of Low Back Pain. Baltimore, Williams & Wilkins, 1991:37–38
55. Falkel JE, Cipriani DY: Physiological principles of resistance training and rehabilitation. In: Zwachazewski JE, Magee DJ, Quillen WS, eds: Athletic Injuries and Rehabilitation. Philadelphia, WB Saunders, 1996
56. Farfan HF, Gracovetsky S: The nature of instability of the spine. Spine 9:714–719, 1984
57. Feldenkrais M: Awareness through movement. New York, Schocken Book, 1979
58. Feldenkrais M: The master moves. Cupertino, CA, Meta Publications, 1984
59. Feldenkrais M: Potent self. Cambridge, Harper & Row, 1985
60. Feldenkrais M: Bodily expressions. Somatics 4:52–59, 1988
61. Fine PG, Milano R, Hare BD: The effects of myofascial trigger point injections are naloxone reversible. Pain 32:15–20, 1988
62. Fisher AGT: Treatment by Manipulation, 5th ed. New York, Paul B. Hoeber, 1948
63. Fisk JW: The Painful Neck and Back: Diagnosis, Manipulation, Exercise, Prevention. Springfield, Charles C. Thomas, 1977:154–205
64. Frost A: Diclofenac versus lidocaine as injection therapy in myofascial pain. Scand J Rheumatol 15:2153–2156, 1986
65. Frost A, Jessen B, Siggaard-Andersen J: A control, double-blind comparison of mepivacaine injection versus saline injection for myofascial pain. Lancet 8:499–500, 1980
66. Frymoyer JW, Krag M: Spinal stability and instability: Definitions, classifications and general principles of management. In: Dunsker S, Schmidek H, Frymoyer J, et al., eds: The Unstable Spine. Orlando, Grune & Stratton, 1986:1–16
67. Gelb M: An Introduction to the Alexander Technique: Body Learning. New York, Henry Holt and Co., 1981
68. Gertzbein SD, Seligman J, Holtby R, et al: Centrode patterns and segmental instability in degenerative disc disease. Spine 10:257–261, 1985
69. Gifford J, Gifford L: Connective tissue massage. In: Wells PE, Frampton V, Bowsher D, eds: Pain Management in Physical Therapy. Norwalk, Appleton & Lange, 1988:218–238
70. Goodridge JP: Muscle energy technique: Definition, explanation, methods of procedure. J Am Osteopath Assoc 81:249–254, 1981
71. Graff-Radford SB, Reeves JL, Baker RL, et al: Effects of transcutaneous electrical nerve stimulation on myofascial pain and trigger point sensitivity. Pain 37:1–5, 1989
72. Grant ER: Lumbar sagittal mobility in hypermobile individuals and professional dancers. In: Grieve GP, ed: Modern Manual Therapy of the Vertebral Column. Edinburgh, Churchill Livingstone, 1986:405–415
73. Gratz CM: Biomechanical studies of fibrous tissues applied to facial surgery. Arch Surg 34:461–495, 1937
74. Gray G: Lower Extremity Functional Profile. Adrian, MI, Wynn Marketing, 1995
75. Greenman PE: Principles of muscle energy techniques. In: Greenman PE, ed: Principles of Manual Medicine, 2nd ed. Baltimore, Williams & Wilkins, 1996:93–98
76. Greenman PE: Principles of myofascial release technique. In: Greenman PE, ed: Principles of Manual Medicine, 2nd ed. Baltimore, Williams & Wilkins, 1996:145–158
77. Greenman PE: Osteopathic manipulation of the lumbar spine and pelvis. In: White AH, Anderson R, eds: Conservative Care of Low Back Pain. Baltimore, Williams & Wilkins, 1991:200–215
78. Grieve G: Lumbar instability. Physiotherapy 68:2–9, 1982
79. Grieve G: Lumbar instability. In: Grieve G, ed: Modern Manual Therapy of the Vertebral Column. Edinburgh, Churchill Livingstone, 1986:416–441
80. Grieve GP: Mobilisation of the Spine: Notes on Examination, Assessment and Clinical Method, 5th ed. Edinburgh, Churchill Livingstone, 1991
81. Grodin AJ, Cantu RI: Soft tissue mobilization. In: Basmajian JV, Nyberg R, eds: Rational Manual Therapies. Baltimore, Williams & Wilkins, 1993:199–241
82. Grosshandler S, Burney R: The myofascial syndrome. NC Med J 40:562–565, 1979
83. Gunn CC, Ditchburn FG, King MH, et al: Acupuncture loci: A proposal for their classification according to known neural structures. Am J Chin Med 4:183–195, 1976
84. Gustavsen R: Fra aktiv avspenning til trening. Oslo, Norlis, 1977
85. Gustavsen R, Streeck R: Training Therapy: Prophylaxis and Rehabilitation. New York, Thieme Medical, 1993
86. Halkovich LR, Personius WJ, Claman HP, et al: Effect of Fluori-Methane spray on passive hip flexion. Phys Ther 61:185–188, 1981
87. Harris JD: History and development of manipulation and mobilization. In: Basmajian JV, Nyberg R, eds: Rational Manual Therapies. Baltimore, Williams & Wilkins, 1993:7–20
88. Hey LR, Helewa A: The effects of stretch and spray on women with myofascial pain syndrome: A pilot study [abstract]. Physiother Can 44:4, 1992

89. Hey LR, Helewa A: Myofascial pain syndrome: A critical review of the literature. Physiother Can 46:28–36, 1994
90. Hollinshead WH: Functional Anatomy of the Limbs and Back. Philadelphia, WB Saunders, 1976
91. Holten O: Medical Training Therapy. Continuing Education Course. Salt Lake City, Holten Institut for Medisinsk Treningsterapi, 1984
92. Holten O: Norwegian medical exercise therapy. Proceedings of the 5th International Conference of the International Federation of Orthopaedic Manipulative Therapists, Vail, Colorado, 1992:58–61
93. Hood W: On so-called bone-setting: Its nature and results. Lancet 7:344–349, 1871
94. Hoover HW: Functional technique. Yearbook of the Academy of Applied Osteopathy. 1958:47–51
95. Ito M, Tadano S, Kaneda K: A biomechanical definition of spinal segmental instability taking personal and disc level differences into account. Spine 18:2295–2304, 1993
96. Jacobson E: Progressive Relaxation, 4th ed. Chicago, University of Chicago Press, 1962
97. Jaeger B, Reeves JL: Quantification of changes in myofascial trigger point sensitivity with the pressure algometer following passive stretch. Pain 27:203–210, 1986
98. Janda V: Die Bedeutung der musklaren fehlhatung als pathogenetisher Faktor vertebragener Storungen. Arch Phys Ther 20:113–116, 1968
99. Janda V: Muscles, central nervous motor regulation and back problems. In: Korr I, ed: The Neurobiologic Mechanisms in Manipulative Therapy. New York, Plenum Press, 1978:27–41
100. Janda V: Muscles as a pathogenic factor in back pain. In: The Treatment of Patients. Proceedings of the 4th International Conference of the International Federation of Orthopaedic Manipulative Therapists, Christchurch, New Zealand, 1980:1–23
101. Janda V: Muscle Function Testing. London, Butterworth, 1983
102. Janda V: Muscles and cervicogenic pain syndromes. In: Grant R, ed: Physical Therapy of the Cervical and Thoracic Spine. New York, Churchill Livingstone, 1988:153–166
103. Janda V, Vavrova M: Sensory Motor Stimulation: A Video. Presented by JE Bullock-Saxton. Brisbane, Australia Body Control System, 1990
104. Janda V, Vavrova M: Sensory motor stimulation. In: Liebenson C, ed: Rehabilitation of the Spine: A Practitioner's Manual. Philadelphia, Lippincott, Williams & Wilkins, 1996:319–328
105. Johnson G: Soft tissue mobilizations. In: Donatelli R, Wooden MJ, eds: Orthopaedic Physical Therapy, 3rd ed. New York, Churchill Livingstone, 2001:578–617
106. Johnston WL: Functional technique. In: Basmajian JV, Nyberg R, eds: Rational Manual Therapies. Baltimore, Williams & Wilkins, 1993:335–346
107. Jones F: Body awareness. New York, Schocken Books, 1979
108. Jones LH: Spontaneous release by positioning. Doctor Osteopathy 4:109, 1964
109. Jones LH, Kusunose R, Goering DO: Strain and Counterstrain. Boise, ID, Jones Strain-Counterstrain, 1996
110. Jowett RL, Fidler MW: Histochemical changes in the multifidus in mechanical derangements of the spine. Orthop Clin North Am 6:145–161, 1975
111. Jull GA, Janda V: Muscles and motor control in low back pain. In: Twomey LT, Taylor JR, eds: Physical Therapy of the Low Back. New York, Churchill Livingstone, 1987:253–278
112. Kaltenborn FM: Extremity Mobilizations. Vail, Institute of Graduate Health Sciences, 1975
113. Kaltenborn FM: Manual Therapy for the Extremity Joints, 3rd ed. Oslo, Olaf Norlis Bokhandel, 1980
114. Kaltenborn FM: The Spine: Basic Evaluation and Mobilization Techniques, 2nd ed. Oslo, Olaf Norlis Bokhandel, 1993
115. Kaltenborn FM, Evejenth O: Manual Mobilization of the Extremity Joints, vol. II: Advanced Treatment Techniques. Oslo, Olaf Norlis Bokhandel, 1986
116. Kendall FP, McCreary EK, Provance PG: Muscles: Testing and Function, 4th ed. Baltimore, Williams & Wilkins, 1993
117. Kenna C, Murtagh J: Back Pain and Spinal Manipulation. Sydney, Butterworth, 1989
118. Kenneally M, Rubenach H, Elvey R: The upper limb tension test: The SLR test of the arm. In: Grant R, ed: Physical Therapy of the Cervical and Thoracic Spine. New York, Churchill Livingstone, 1988:167–197
119. Kennedy B: An Australian programme for management of back problems. Physiotherapy 66:108–111, 1980
120. Kirkaldy-Willis WH: Presidential symposium on instability of the lumbar spine: Introduction. Spine 10:25, 1985
121. Kirkaldy-Willis WH, Burton CV: Managing Low Back Pain, 3rd ed. New York, Churchill Livingstone, 1993
122. Kirkaldy-Willis WH, Farfan WH: Instability of the lumbar spine. Clin Orthop 165:110–123, 1982
123. Kisler CD, Taslitz N: Connective tissue massage: influence of the introductory treatment on autonomic functions. Phys Ther 48:107–119, 1968
124. Kisner C, Colby LA: Therapeutic Exercise: Foundations and Techniques, 2nd ed. Philadelphia, FA Davis, 1990
125. Klein-Vogelbach S: Therapeutic Exercises in Functional Kinetics: Analysis and Instruction of Individually Adaptive Exercises. Berlin, Springer-Verlag, 1991

126. Knott M, Voss DE: Proprioceptive Neuromuscular Facilitation: Patterns and Techniques. New York, Hoeber-Harper Books, 1956
127. Knott M, Voss D: Proprioceptive Neuromuscular Facilitation, 2nd ed. New York, Harper and Row, 1968
128. Korr IM: Proprioceptors and somatic dysfunction. J Am Osteopath Assoc 74:638–650, 1975
129. Korr IM: The facilitated segment: A factor in injury to the body framework. In: The Collected Papers of Irvin M Korr. Newark, OH, American Academy of Osteopathy, 1979
130. Korr IM: The neural basis of the osteopathic lesion. In: The Collected Papers of Irvin M Korr. Newark, OH, American Academy of Osteopathy, 1979
131. Kottke F, Pauley D, Ptak R: The rationale for prolonged stretching for correction of shortening of connective tissue. Arch Phys Med Rehab 47:345–352, 1966
132. Kucera M: Exercise on the Gymball. Stuttgart, Gustav Fischer Verlag, 1993
133. Kuist M, Jarvinen M: Clinical histochemical and biomechanical features in repair of muscle and tendon injuries. Int J Sports Med 3:12–14, 1982
134. Kusunose RS: Strain and counterstrain. In: Basmajian JV, Nyberg R, eds: Rational Manual Therapies. Baltimore, Williams & Wilkins, 1993:323–333
135. LaFreniere JG: LaFreniere Body Techniques: A Therapeutic Approach by Physical Therapy. Chicago, Year Book Medical Publishers, 1984
136. Lamb DW: A review of manual therapy for spinal pain with reference to the lumbar spine. In: Grieve GP, ed: Modern Manual Therapy of the Vertebral Column. Edinburgh, Churchill Livingstone, 1986:605–621
137. Lee D: Principles and practice of muscle energy and functional techniques. In: Grieve, ed: Modern Manual Therapy of the Vertebral Column. Edinburgh, Churchill Livingstone, 1986:640–655
138. Lester MN: Spinal stabilization and compliance utilizing the therapeutic ball. Proceedings of the 5th International Conference of the International Federation of Orthopaedic Manipulative Therapists, Vail, Colorado, 1992:159
139. Lewit K: Manuelle Therapie (im Rahmen der artlichen Rehabilitation). Leipzig, JA Barth, 1973
140. Lewit K: Manipulative Therapy in Rehabilitation of the Locomotor System, 2nd ed. Oxford, Butterworth-Heinemann Ltd, 1991
141. Lewit K, Simons DG: Myofascial pain: Relief by post-isometric relaxation. Arch Phys Med Rehabil 64:452–456, 1984
142. Liston CB: Back schools and ergonomics. In: Twomey LT, Taylor JR, eds: Physical Therapy of the Low Back. New York, Churchill Livingstone, 1987:279–301
143. Low J: The modern body therapies: A first hand look at leading bodywork therapies, part four. Aston Patterning. Massage Mag 16:48–56, 1988
144. Luthe W, ed: Autogenic Therapy, vol. 1–6. New York, Grune & Stratton, 1969–1972
145. Maharishi MY: The Science of Being and Art of Living. London, International SRM Publications, 1966
146. Maigne R: Orthopedic Medicine. Springfield, Charles C. Thomas, 1972
147. Maitland GD: Vertebral Manipulations, 5th ed. London, Butterworth, 1986
148. Maitland GD: Peripheral Manipulations, 3rd ed. London, Butterworth-Heinemann, 1991
149. Manheim CJ: The Myofascial Release Manual. Thorofare, Slack, 2001
150. Marlin T: Manipulative Treatment for the General Practitioner. London, Edward Arnold & Co., 1934
151. Masters R, Houston J: Listening to the Body: The Psychophysical Way to Health and Awareness. New York, Delta Books, 1978
152. May P: Exercise and training for spinal patients: Movement awareness and stabilization training. In: Basmajian JV, Nyberg R, eds: Rational Manual Therapies. Baltimore, Williams & Wilkins, 1993:347–359
153. Mayer TG, Gatchel RJ: Functional Restoration for Spinal Disorders: The Sports Medicine Approach. Philadelphia, Lea & Febiger, 1988
154. McCain GA: Role of physical fitness training in fibrositis/fibromyalgia syndrome. Am J Med 81(Suppl 3A):73–77, 1986
155. McKenzie RA: The Lumbar Spine. Waikanae, New Zealand, Spinal Publications, 1980
156. McKenzie RA: Treat Your Own Back. Waikanae, New Zealand, Spinal Publications, 1981
157. McKenzie RA: Care of the Neck. Waikanae, New Zealand, Spinal Publications, 1983
158. McKenzie RA: Mechanical diagnosis and theory for low back pain: Toward a better understanding. In: Twomey LT, Taylor JR, eds: Physical Therapy of the Low Back. New York, Churchill Livingstone, 1987:157–174
159. McKenzie RA: The Cervical and Thoracic Spine: Mechanical Diagnosis and Therapy. Waikanae, New Zealand, Spinal Publications, 1990
160. Melzack R: Prolonged relief of pain by brief intense transcutaneous somatic stimulation. Pain 1:357–373, 1975
161. Melzack R, Stillwell DM, Fox EJ: Trigger points and acupuncture points for pain: Correlations and implications. Pain 3:3–23, 1977
162. Melzack R, Wall PD: Pain mechanisms: A new theory. Science 150:971–979, 1965
163. Mennell JB: Physical Treatment by Movement, Manipulation and Massage, 5th ed. Philadelphia, Blakiston, 1947
164. Mennell JB: The Science and Art of Joint Manipulation. London, J & A Churchill, 1949
165. Mennell J McM: Joint Pain. Boston, Little, Brown & Co., 1964
166. Milanowska K: Conservative treatment. In: Weistein JN, Wiesel SW, eds: The Lumbar Spine. Philadelphia, WB Saunders, 1990:500–515
167. Miller B: Alternative somatic therapies. In: White A, Anderson R, eds: Conservative Care of Low Back Pain. Baltimore, Williams & Wilkins, 1991:120–133
168. Million R, Nilson KH, Jayson MV, et al: Evaluation of low back pain and assessment of lumbar corsets with and without back supports. Ann Rheum Dis 40:449–454, 1981
169. Mitchell FL Jr: Elements of muscle energy technique. In: Basmajian JV, Nyberg R, eds: Rational Manual Therapies. Baltimore, Williams & Wilkins, 1993:285–321
170. Mitchell FL Jr, Moran PS, Pruzzo NA: An evaluation and treatment manual of osteopathic muscle energy procedures. Valley Park, MO, Mitchell, Moran, and Pruzzo, 1979
171. Mixter WJ, Barr JS: Rupture of the intervertebral disc with involvement of the spinal canal. N Engl J Med 211:210–215, 1934
172. Moller M, Oberg B, Gilquist J: Stretching exercise and soccer: Effect of stretching on range of motion in the lower extremity in connection with soccer training. Int J Sports Med 6:50–52, 1985
173. Morgan D: Concepts in functional training and postural stabilization for the low-back-injured. Top Acute Care Trauma Rehabil 2(4):8–17, 1988
174. Mottice M, Goldberg D, Benner EK, et al: Soft Tissue Mobilization Techniques. Monroe Falls, OH, JEMD Publications, 1986
175. Muhlemann D, Cimino JA: Therapeutic muscle stretching. In: Hammer WI, ed: Functional Soft Tissue Examination and Treatment by Manual Methods. Gaithersburg, Aspen, 1991
176. Nachemson A: Lumbar spine instability: A critical update and symposium summary. Spine 10:290–291, 1985
177. Nicholson GG, Clendaniel RA: Manual techniques. In: Scully RM, Barnes MR, eds: Physical Therapy. Philadelphia, JB Lippincott, 1989:926–985
178. Noyes FR, Trovik PJ, Hyde WB: Biomechanics of ligament failure: An analysis of immobilization, exercise and deconditioning effects in primates. J Bone Joint Surg Am 56:1406–1418,1974
179. Nutter P: Aerobic exercise in the treatment and prevention of low back pain. Occup Med 3:137–145, 1988
180. Nwuga VC: Techniques of spinal manipulation. In: Nwuga VC, ed: Manipulation of the Spine. Baltimore, Williams & Wilkins, 1976:47–81
181. Nyberg R: Clinical decision making in orthopaedic physical therapy: The low back. In: Wolf SL, ed: Clinical Decision Making in Physical Therapy. Philadelphia, FA Davis, 1985:255–293
182. Nyberg R: Manipulation: Definition, types, application. In: Basmajian JV, Nyberg R, eds: Rational Manual Therapies. Baltimore, Williams & Wilkins, 1993:21–48
183. Pace JB: Commonly overlooked pain syndromes responsive to simple therapy. Postgrad Med 58:107–113, 1975
184. Palastanga N: Connective tissue massage. In: Grieve G, ed: Modern Manual Therapy of the Vertebral Column. Edinburgh, Churchill Livingstone, 1986:827–833
185. Pardy W: Exercise and training for spinal patients: Strength training. In: Basmajian JV, Nyberg R, eds: Rational Manual Therapies. Baltimore, Williams & Wilkins, 1993:387–425
186. Paris S: The Spinal Lesion. Christchurch, New Zealand, Pegasus Press, 1965
187. Paris S: Mobilization of the spine. Phys Ther 59:988–995, 1979
188. Paris S: Physical signs of instability. Spine 10:277–279, 1985
189. Patterson MM: A model mechanism for spinal segmental facilitation. J Am Osteopath Assoc 76:121–131, 1976
190. Pettman E: Hypermobility/instability. Proceedings of the Fifth International Conference of the International Federation of Orthopaedic Manipulative Therapists, Vail, Colorado, 1992:40–41
191. Pickering SG: Exercises for the Autonomic Nervous System. Springfield, Charles C. Thomas, 1981
192. Polermo F, Panjabi MM: Role of trunk rotation endurance exercise in failed back treatment. Arch Phys Med Rehabil 67:620, 1986
193. Pope M, Punjabi M: Biomechanical definitions of spinal instability. Spine 10:255–256, 1985
194. Porter-Hoke A: Lumbar instability: Manual therapy evaluation and management. Continuing Education Course. Seattle, WA, 1993
195. Robins V: Should patients with hemiplegia wear a sling? J Phys Ther 49:1029, 1970
196. Robinson R: The new back school prescription: Stabilization training, Part I. Spine: State of the Art Reviews 5(3):341–355, 1991
197. Rocabado M, Iglarsh ZN: Physical modalities and manual techniques used in the treatment of maxillofacial pain. In: Rocabado M, Iglarsh ZN, eds: Musculoskeletal Approach to Maxillofacial Pain. Philadelphia, JB Lippincott, 1991:174–193
198. Rohde J: Die automobilisation der extremitatengelenke (I). Zeitschrift fur physiotherapie. 27:57, 1975
199. Rohde J: Die automobilisation der extremitatengelenke (II). Zeitschrift fur physiotherapie. 28:51, 1976
200. Rohde J: Die automobilisation der extremitatengelenke (III). Zeitschrift fur physiotherapie. 28:121, 1976
201. Rohde J: Die automobilisation der extremitatengelenke (IV). Zietschrift fur physiotherapie. 28:427, 1976

202. Rolf I: Rolfing: The Integration of Human Structures. Santa Monica, Dennis-Landman, 1977
203. Rosomoff HL, Fishbain DA, Goldberg M, et al: Physical findings in patients with chronic intractable benign pain of the neck and/or back. Pain 37:279–287, 1989
204. Rubin D: Myofascial trigger point syndromes: An approach to management. Arch Phys Med Rehabil 62:107–110, 1981
205. Rumsey J: Guidelines for acupuncture massage—Neck pain. Sports Med, Bull APTA 4:8–9, 1977
206. Saal JA: Rehabilitation of sports-related lumbar spine injuries. Phys Med Rehabil State of the Art Reviews 1:613–638, 1987
207. Saal JA: Dynamic muscular stabilization in the nonoperative treatment of lumbar pain syndromes. Orthop Rev 19:691–700, 1990
208. Saal JA: The new back school prescription: Stabilization training, Part II. Spine: State of the Art Reviews 5(3):357–366, 1991
209. Saal JA, Saal JS: Nonoperative treatment of herniated lumbar intervertebral disk with radiculopathy: An outcome study. Spine 14:431–437, 1989
210. Saal JS: Flexibility training. In: Saal JS, ed: Rehabilitation of Sports Injuries. Philadelphia, Hanley & Belfus, 1987
211. Saal JS, Saal JA: Strength training and flexibility. In: White AH, Anderson R, eds: Conservative Care of Low Back Pain. Baltimore, Williams & Wilkins, 1991:65–77
212. Sahrmann S: A program for correction of muscular imbalance and mechanical imbalance. Clin Manage PT 3:21–28, 1983
213. Sahrmann S: Diagnosis and Treatment of Movement Impairment Syndromes. St. Loius, Mosby, 2002.
214. Saliba VL, Johnson GS: Lumbar protective mechanisms. In: White AH, Anderson R, eds: Conservative Care of Low Back Pain. Baltimore, Williams & Wilkins, 1991:112–119
215. Saliba VL, Johnson GS, Wardlaw CF: Proprioceptive Neuromuscular facilitation. In: Basmajian JV, Nyberg R, eds: Rational Manual Therapies. Baltimore, Williams & Wilkins, 1993:243–284
216. Saunders DH: Spinal orthotics. In: Saunders DH, ed: Evaluation, Treatment and Prevention of Musculoskeletal Disorders. Minneapolis, Viking, 1985:285–296
217. Scariati PD: Myofascial release concepts. In: DiGiovanna EL, Schiowitz S, eds: An Osteopathic Approach to Diagnosis and Treatment. Philadelphia, JB Lippincott, 1991:363–368
218. Schneider W, Dvorak J, Dvorak V, et al: Manual Medicine Therapy. New York, Thieme Medical, 1988
219. Schultz JH, Luthe W: Autogenic Training: A Psychophysiologic Approach in Psychotherapy. New York, Grune & Stratton, 1959
220. Schwartz RG, Gall NG, Grant AE: Abdominal pain in quadriparesis: Myofascial syndrome as unsuspected cause. Arch Phys Med Rehabil 65:44–46, 1984
221. Scudds RA, Ewart NK, Trachsel L: The treatment of myofascial trigger points with Helim-Neon and Gallium-Arsenide LASER: A blinded, crossover trial [abstract]. Pain Suppl 5:768, 1990
222. Sherrington C: The Integrative Action of the Nervous System. New Haven, Yale University Press, 1961
223. Sihvonen T, Hanninen G, Kankkunin P, et al: The relief of static work loading to shoulder musculature [abstract]. Scand J Rheum (Suppl) 60:51, 1986
224. Simons DG: Fibrositis/fibromyalgia: A form of myofascial trigger points? Am J Med 81:93–98, 1986
225. Skootsky SA, Jaeger B, Oye RK: Prevalence of myofascial pain in general internal medicine practice. Western J Med 151:157–160, 1989
226. Smith RL: At Your Own Risk: The Case Against Chiropractics. New York, Trident Press, 1969
227. Snow CJ, Aves Wood R, Dowhopoluk V, et al: Randomized controlled clinical trial of stretch and spray for relief of back and neck myofascial pain [abstract]. Physiother Can 44:8, 1992
228. Snyder-Mackler L, Barry AJ, Perkins AL, et al: Effects of helium-neon laser irradiation on skin resistance and pain in patients with trigger points in the neck or back. Phys Ther 69:336–341, 1989
229. Snyder-Mackler L, Bork C, Bourbon B, et al: Effect of helium-neon laser on musculoskeletal trigger points. Phys Ther 66:1087–1090, 1986
230. Stoddard A: Manual of Osteopathic Technique. London, Hutchinson, 1978
231. Stone MH: Implications for connective tissue and bone alterations resulting form resistance exercise training. Med Sci Sports Exerc 20:S162–S168, 1988
232. Sweeney T: Neck school: Cervicothoracic stabilization training. Occup Med: State of the Art Reviews 7:43–54, 1992
233. Sweigard L: Human Movement Potential: Its Ideokinetic Facilitation. New York, Harper and Row, 1974
234. Tabery JC, Tabery C, Tardieu C, et al: Physiologic and structural changes in the cat's soleus muscle due to immobilization at different lengths in plaster casts. Am J Physiol 224:231–244, 1972
235. Tabery JC, Tardieu C: Experimental rapid sarcomere loss with concomitant hypoextensibility. Muscle Nerve May/June:198–203, 1981
236. Tappan FM: The bindegewebsmassage system. In: Tappan FM, ed: Healing Massage Techniques, 2nd ed. Norwalk, CT, Appleton Lange, 1988
237. Tilscher H: Die Rehabilitation von wirbelsaulengestorten. Schriftenreihe Manuelle Medizin. Heidlberg, Verlag fur Medizin, 1975
238. Tipton CM, Matthes RD, Maynard JA et al: The influence of physical activity on ligaments and tendons. Med Sci Sports Exerc 7:165–175, 1975
239. Todd ME: The Thinking Body. New York, Dance Horizons, 1937
240. Travell J: Myofascial trigger points: Clinical view. In: Bonica JJ, Albe-Fessard A, eds: Advances in Pain Research and Therapy, vol. 1. New York, Raven Press, 1976:919–926
241. Travell J: Identification of myofascial trigger point syndromes: A case of atypical facial neuralgia. Arch Phys Med Rehabil 62:100–106, 1981
242. Travell J, Rinzler SH: Myofascial genesis of pain. Post Grad Med 11:425–434, 1952
243. Travell JG, Simons DG: Myofascial Pain and Dysfunction: The Trigger Point Manual, vol. 1. Baltimore, Williams & Wilkins, 1983
244. Travell JG, Simons DG: Myofascial Pain and Dysfunction: The Trigger Point Manual, vol. 2. Baltimore, Williams & Wilkins, 1992
245. Tucker WE: Home Treatment and Posture. London, E & S Livingstone, 1969
246. Vailas AC, Tipton CM, Matthes RC et al: Physical activity and its influence on the repair process of medial collateral ligaments. Connect Tissue Res 9:25–31,1981
247. Walker JM: Deep transverse friction in ligamentous healing. J Orthop Sports Phys Ther 6:89–94, 1984
248. Wallace RK: Physiological effects of transcendental meditation. Science 167:1751–1754, 1970
249. Warwick R, Williams PL, eds: Gray's Anatomy, 35th British ed. Philadelphia, WB Saunders, 1973
250. Waylonis GW, Wilke S, O'Toole D, et al: Chronic myofascial pain: Management by low-output helium-neon laser therapy. Arch Phys Med Rehabil 69:1017–1020, 1988
251. Webster, GV: Concerning Osteopathy. Norwood, Plimpton, 1921
252. Wells PE: Manipulative procedures. In: Wells PE, Frampton V, Bower D, eds: Pain Management in Physical Therapy. Norwald, Appleton & Lange, 1988:181–217
253. White AA, Punjabi MM: Clinical Biomechanics of the Spine. Philadelphia, JB Lippincott, 1990:106–115
254. White AH: Back School and Other Conservative Approaches to Low Back Pain. St. Louis, CV Mosby, 1983
255. White AH: Back school: State of the art. In: Weinstein JN, Wiesel SW, eds: The Lumbar Spine. Philadelphia, WB Saunders, 1990
256. White AH: Stabilization of the lumbar spine. In: White AH, Anderson R, eds: Conservative Care of the Low Back. Baltimore, Williams & Wilkins, 1991:106–111
257. White AH, ed: Back school. Spine: State of the Art Reviews, 5(3):325–506, 1991
258. Willner S: Effect of a rigid brace on back pain. Acta Orthop Scand 56:40–42, 1985
259. Wolf LB: Exercise and training for spinal patients: Aerobic exercise. In: Basmajian JV, Nyberg R, eds: Rational Manual Therapies. Baltimore, Williams & Wilkins, 1993:425–440
260. Wolfe F: Fibrositis, fibromyalgia and musculoskeletal disease: The current status of the fibrositis syndrome. Arch Phys Med Rehabil 69:527–531, 1988
261. Woo S, Matthews JV, Akeson WH, et al: Connective tissue response to immobility. Arthritis Rheum 18:257–264, 1975
262. Woo SLY, Ritter MA, Amiel D et al: The biomechanical and biochemical properties of swine tendon–Long term effects of exercise on the digital extensors. Connect Tiss Res 7:177–183, 1980
263. Wood EC, Becker PD: Beard's Massage, 3rd ed. Philadelphia, WB Saunders, 1981
264. Yunus MB, Kalyan-Raman UP, Kalyan-Raman K: Primary fibromyalgia syndrome and myofascial pain syndrome: Clinical features and muscle pathology. Arch Phys Med Rehabil 69:451–454, 1988
265. Zbojan L: Antigravitá_cna relaxacia, jej podstata a pou_ztie. (Gravity induced relaxation, its principles and practical application). Praktick'y Leka 68:147, 1988
266. Zohn DA, Mennell J McM: Musculoskeletal pain conditions. In: Zohn DA, Mennell JM, eds: Musculoskeletal Pain: Diagnosis and Physical Treatment. Boston, Little, Brown and Co., 1976:171–198

Myofascial Considerations and Evaluation in Somatic Dysfunction

DARLENE HERTLING

7

- ▪ MYOFASCIAL CONSIDERATION IN SOMATIC DYSFUNCTION
    - Connective Tissue
    - Myofascial Tissue
    - Dysfunction
- ▪ POSTURAL MUSCULOFASCIAL SYSTEMS
    - Cranial and Cervical Fascial System
    - Myofascial System of the Shoulder Girdle
    - Myofascial System of the Lumbo-Pelvic-Hip Complex

- ▪ MYOFASCIAL INTEGRATION AND DYSFUNCTION
    - Muscle Imbalance Syndromes
    - Types of Muscle Dysfunctions
- ▪ SKIN AND SUBCUTANEOUS SOFT TISSUE DYSFUNCTION
- ▪ EVALUATION OF SOFT TISSUE DYSFUNCTION
    - Evaluation of Posture and Movement Patterns
    - Selective Tissue Tension Tests
    - Palpatory Evaluation

The term soft tissue manipulation can be used to encompass all manual methods that address tissue other than bone and includes massage[16,40,53,54,56,132,185,264] myofascial manipulation,[11,35,101,176,177,230] stretching,[2,14,23,36,62,71–73,121,142,146,148,151,197,214,215,234,236,237,257,261,264,271,272] postisometric relaxation (muscle energy),[24,42,59,88,96,159,160,195,246,279] strain–counter strain (positional release),[43,57,96,133,134,154,278] and neural tissue treatment.[29,30,68–70,106,107,143,174,250,257] These methods can all be used as effective measures to detect and to help normalize soft tissue dysfunction. When treating any musculoskeletal dysfunction, a comprehensive approach must be considered. Any one technique used to the exclusion of another will not address the totality of the problem when joint, myofascial, and neuromuscular components are present. The techniques and concepts reviewed here are typically used in conjunction with therapeutic exercise, joint articulations, and functional carry-over ensuring comprehensive management of dysfunction.

Current therapies used to control wound contracture in traumatized tissue involve biomechanical control of collagen production of myofibroblastic activity and physical means.[232] Physical measures imposed to prevent contractures include static splinting, which is presumed to counter the tactile property of the fibroblast, and range of motion exercises, which are performed to orient new collagen fibers that proliferate during wound healing.[7] Mechanical forces utilized in these methods to elongate restrictive tissues include low-load applications maintained for extended periods.[242]

Soft tissue manipulations have been described as a system of manual techniques using low-load, long-duration forces applied in approximation, traction, and torsional vectors to improve mobility between underlying and adjacent connective tissue layer throughout the body to restore normal intratissue

and intertissue mobility of the fascial system.[194,263] It is often defined as "the forceful passive movement of the muscle-fascial system element thorough its restrictive direction beginning with the superficial layers and progressing into depth while taking into accord the relationship of the joints concerned."[35] Soft tissue manipulation differs from most approaches to massage in that it usually places fascia and muscle in an elongated rather than a relaxed or shortened position. This achieves multiple therapeutic outcomes, including surface exposure of the tissue to be treated, elongation of connective tissue, and change in the resting length of muscle.[84] Soft tissue manipulations therefore simultaneously incorporate the principles of massage, joint articulations, and therapeutic exercise. Whether one chooses to perform soft tissue or joint articulation techniques to improve mobility, the tissue being affected (joint capsule, ligament, tendon, muscle, or fascia) are all forms of connective tissue.

MYOFASCIAL CONSIDERATIONS IN SOMATIC DYSFUNCTION

Striated muscle, along with its organizing areolar and dense connective tissue, forms a functionally inseparable composite termed **myofascia.** Myofascial structures are those tissues that are either musculoskeletal or connective tissue in makeup and origin. The interrelationship between these tissues and the mechanical dysfunction that can be directly linked to their aberrant function demands the closest attention.

Connective Tissue

The largest component of the human body, connective tissue, chiefly comprises ligaments and tendons as well as aponeuroses, fascia, synovial membranes, joint capsules, and intrinsic elements of muscle (dense and loose irregular).[108,277] Connective tissue are organized into three types based on fiber density and arrangement: dense regular, dense irregular, and loose irregular. Dense regular connective tissue, which is characterized by a high proportion of collagen fibers to ground substance and a uniplanar or linear fiber orientation, provides tensile strength required by ligaments and tendons (see Fig. 1-4).[108,116,277] Characteristics allow for high tensile strength and low extensibility. Dense regular connective tissue has poor vascularity; therefore, healing time is significantly increased after trauma.

Dense irregular connective tissue is found in fascial sheaths, aponeuroses, dermis of the skin, capsules, and periosteum. Irregular connective tissue is recognized by its multidirectional fiber orientation, which provides necessary strength, in all directions. Because of its structure it is able to limit forces in a three-dimensional manner.[47]

Loose irregular connective tissue is found in the superficial and deep fascia as well endomysium, nerve, and muscle sheaths and the supportive structure of the lymph system. A sparse, multidirectional framework of collagen and elastin (Fig. 7-1) generally characterizes it. Because of sparse concentrations of collagen in this type of tissue, loose irregular connective tissue is the most elastic and typically has the greatest potential for change when manipulated by external forces such as myofascial techniques.[35,47,48,100,101,108,277]

Myofascial Tissue

The majority of loose connective tissue (see above) is fascia. The mechanical role of fascia is reflected in its composition: a small number of randomly oriented fibers embedded within a watery ground substance. The ground substance is the gel-like supporting substance for metabolic transport and reduces friction between fibers. Fascia is an elastocollagenous tissue that exists in variable dense areolar and seromembranous forms depending on its local functional specialization. Continuous throughout the entire body, the fascial system interconnects with tendons, aponeuroses, ligaments, capsules, peripheral nerves, and intrinsic elements of muscle.[5] Because the fascia comprises a single structure, the implications for body-wide repercussion of distortions in that structure are clear. This abundant material separates and surrounds structures, serves as a packing material that lies between areas of more specialized tissue (such as muscles), and facilitates movement between adjacent structures. It also plays a major role in inflammation and repair because it is vascular and contains cells vital to the repair process. Its several functions include the following:

- Providing origins and insertions for muscles
- Serving as an elastic sheath for muscles
- Forming specialized retaining bands (retinacula and fibrous sheaths for tendons)
- Providing pathways for the passage of vessels and nerves, surrounding these structures as neurovascular sheaths (the central nervous system [CNS] is surrounded by fascial tissue [dura mater])
- Allowing sliding or gliding of one structure on another
- Assisting in stabilization and permitting motion initiated by muscular activity (acts as a harness that converts energy generated by the sarcomeres)

Fascia is more or less continuous over the entire body but it is commonly named according to regions. For example, the pectoral fascia invests the pectoralis major and continues to the latissimus dorsi and floor of the axilla.[82] Fascia is usually continuous with specialized elements such as ligaments and tendons. Specialized mechanoreceptors and proprioceptors are within these specialized elements of the fascia that report information to the spinal cord and brain on body position and movement, both normal and abnormal.[96] Proprioceptive endings are numerous in aponeuroses and retinacula.[82] This abundance suggests that these structures have a kinesthetic and a mechanical function. Bands of fascia may also act as tendon. An extreme instance is that of the fascia lata of the thigh, whose iliotibial band is in fact the principle tendon of insertion for the gluteus maximus and the tensor fascia latae muscles (Fig. 7-2).[89]

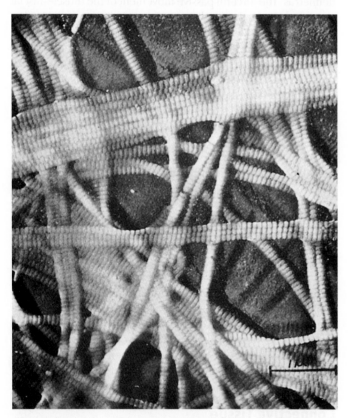

■ **FIG. 7-1.** Prepared micrograph of loose irregular connective tissue showing both multidirectionality and low-density connective tissue fibers. (Reprinted with permission from Copenhaver WM, Bunge RB, Bunge MB: Bailey's Textbook of Histology. Baltimore, Williams & Wilkins, 1975:117.)

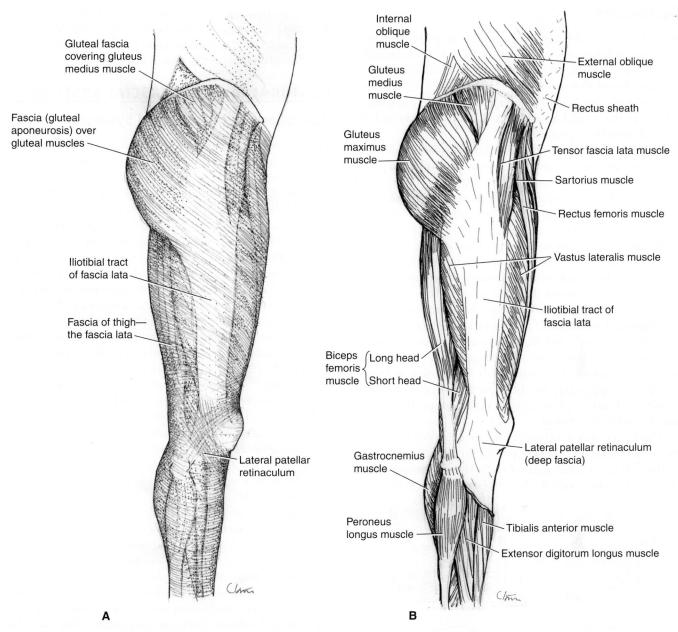

■ **FIG. 7-2.** Lateral thigh. **(A)** Superficial fascia. **(B)** The fascia lata and iliotibial tract. The fascia lata becomes particularly strong laterally where it is reinforced by tendon fibers derived from the insertions of the tensor fasciae latae and gluteus maximus muscles; below it blends with the retinacula of the knee and helps form the fibrous capsule at the knee joint.

Cathie[39] regards the following properties of fascia as being important to therapeutic consideration:

1. It is richly endowed with nerve endings.
2. It has outstanding properties of contractility and elasticity.
3. It gives extensive muscular attachment.
4. It supports and stabilizes, thus enhancing the postural balance of the body.
5. It is vitally involved in all aspects of motion.
6. It aids in circulatory economy, especially of venous and lymphatic fluids.
7. Fascia is a major arena of inflammatory processes.
8. Fluids and infectious processes often travel along fascia planes.
9. Fascial changes precede many chronic degenerative diseases
10. Fascial changes predispose toward chronic tissue congestion.
11. Such chronic passive congestion precedes the formation of fibrous tissue that increases hydrogen ion concentration of articulator and periarticular structures.
12. Fascial specializations produce definite stress bands.
13. Sudden stress (trauma) on fascial tissue will often result in burning pain.

Dysfunction

In dysfunction (inflammation, adhesion, or postural stress), the tissue develops intermolecular cross-linking of the collagen fibers, in which the fibers adhere to each other with a resultant loss of glide or mobility (Fig. 7-3).[1,4,191,216,286] Ground substance also becomes more dense or viscous, which interferes with the normal removal of catabolic products and the relay of anabolic requirements.

Dysfunctional tension also compromises venous and lymph return, because normal myofascial activity provides the pump for lymphatic and venous return in the limbs. Freedom of movement of the nerves and vessels may also be impaired by entrapments in the areas where they must pierce through sleeves of dense fascia.

Balance is the term given to the ideal state in which soft tissue tension has free and appropriate movement in three dimensions. In dysfunction, the balance system is disturbed by (multiple) tissue restrictions that interfere with the normal alignment and mobility of individual body areas as a whole. Malalignment, immobility, and inappropriate movement patterns reinforce and exacerbate tissue restrictions. Abnormal tension of fascia may have several causes: faulty muscular activity, alterations in the position or relationship of bones, change in the position of the viscera, or the use of an unnatural position.[39] It accompanies altered vertebral mechanics that may be sudden or gradual.

The degree of dysfunction varies depending on factors such as general health and nutrition, posture, and movement habits. Cathie refers to certain areas of the body as "postural" fascia because they are among the first to show changes in the pres-

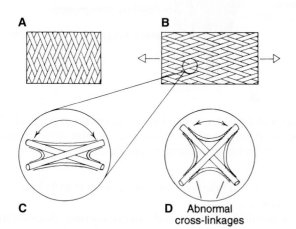

■ **FIG. 7-3.** Collagen fiber orientation and alignment. **(A)** Normal collagen fiber orientation in a relaxed state. **(B)** Extended fiber alignment. **(C)** Magnified area of unrestricted fiber gliding when extended. **(D)** Abnormal cross-linkages limiting fiber gliding and tissue extensibility. (Reprinted with permission from Henry JA: Manual therapy of the shoulder. In: Kelly JM, Clark WA, eds: Orthopedic Therapy of the Shoulder. Philadelphia, JB Lippincott, 1995:290.)

ence of postural defects. They include the (1) cervical and cranial fascia, (2) thoracolumbar fascia, and (3) iliotibial band of the fascial lata and gluteus maximus (Fig. 7-2) which assist in stabilization and permit motion initiated by muscular activity.

POSTURAL MUSCULOFASCIAL SYSTEMS

Cranial and Cervical Fascial System

The support of the weight of the shoulder girdle depends on the fascia and suspensory muscles of the head and neck and their support of the scapulae and clavicles through their joining to the sternum and ultimately through the ribs to the spine. Each rib hangs at a particular vertebral level, and its weight with that of the soft tissue attachments is supported by the vertebrae with which it attaches. The sternum gives support, through the cartilages of the ribs, to the entire rib cage and supports the upright position of the skull. The skeletal muscles of the head and neck must be very strong to balance and move the head on its platform the atlas-axis mechanisms. This necessitates many guy wires that are amply supplied on all sides by fascia, muscles, and tendons running from the ribs, sternum, scapulae, and clavicle to the head and reinforced by side ties between the ribs and cervical vertebrae (see Figs. 7-22, 17-18, 19-9, 19-10).[269] The spine affords the head a secure upright support through its opposing curves and its powerful muscles and ligaments. If the occipital condyles rest evenly on the surface of the atlas, a balanced relationship of the atlas and other cervical vertebrae follows, facilitating muscular freedom. This in turn favors the adjustment of the rest of the spine to its load because in the erect position, the head furnishes the cue for the balance of the entire body.[269]

Fascia plays an important role in directing the force of muscle contraction through the weight-bearing tissues such as the articular cartilage of the apophyseal joints and vertebral body-intervertebral disk interface. As in the limbs and other parts of the body, the principle muscle masses, the main nerves and blood vessels of the neck and viscera are contained within fascial coverings composed of connective tissue organized in well-defined sheets and membranes (Fig. 7-4). The cervical fascia "affords that slipperiness which enables structures to move and pass over one another without difficulty, as in swallowing, and allowing twisting of the neck without it creaking like a manila rope—a looseness, moreover, that provides the easiest pathways for vessels and nerves to reach their destination."[282] The deep fascia of the neck is generally described as comprising three layers: investing, pretracheal, and prevertebral (Fig. 7-5).

INVESTING CERVICAL FASCIA

The thick, tough investing layer of the cervical fascia (Figs. 7-4 and 7-5) encloses or forms a collar around the neck, surrounding all the structures of the neck except the platysma. The investing layer is attached superiorly to the nuchal line of the occiput, the mastoid process, the zygomatic arch, the liga-

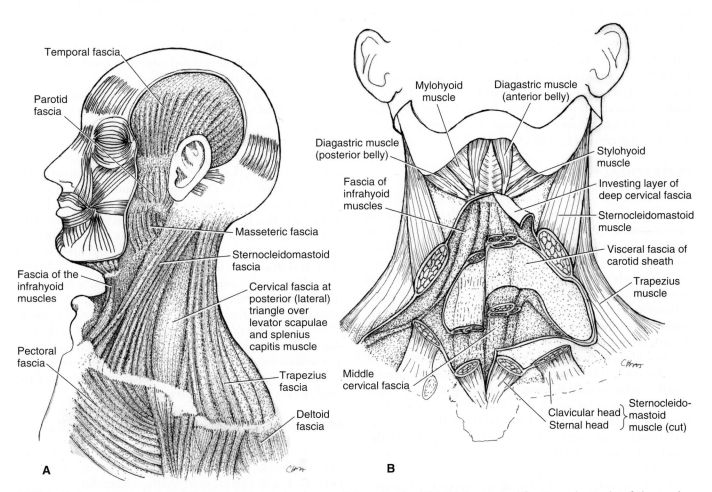

■ **FIG. 7-4.** Head and neck. **(A)** External investing layer of deep fascia. **(B)** Middle cervical fascia and muscle of the neck (anterior view).

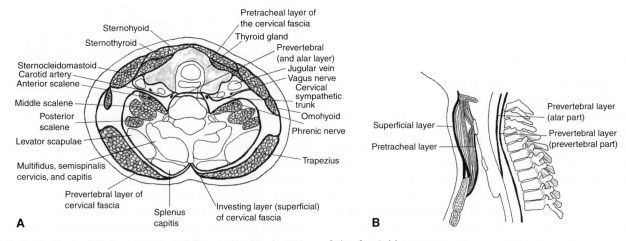

■ **FIG. 7-5.** Neck. **(A)** Cross-section. **(B)** Longitudinal section of the fascial layers.

mentum nuchae, and the spinous processes of the cervical vertebrae.[196,288] Beyond these lines of bony attachment, the layer continues into the face as the parotid and masseteric fasciae, investing the masseter and parotid glands. Inferiorly, the investing layer is attached to the manubrium of the sternum, the clavicle, and the acromion and spine of the scapula. From these bony attachments, it is carried beyond into continuity with the pectoral and deltoid fascia (Fig. 7-4A). It splits into two sheets to enclose the sternocleidomastoid and trapezius muscle but exists as a single sheet over the anterior and posterior cervical triangles.[288]

PRETRACHEAL FASCIA

Underneath the investing fascia lies the middle cervical aponeurosis or pretracheal fascia into which the infrahyoid musculature is embedded (Fig. 7-5). It unsheathes both the superficial and deep layers of the infrahyoid muscles and thus possesses superficial, mid, and deep septi. Superiorly each septum attaches to the hyoid bone. Inferiorly all three fascial divisions attach to the sternum. Laterally, the fascia attaches to the clavicle, first rib, subclavius muscles, and bony and firm landmarks of the thoracic inlet.[12] It comes in contact with the deep or prevertebral layer of the cervical fasciae. It surrounds the thyroid gland, the air and food passages, and is connected with the connective tissue sheath around the neurovascular bundle (common carotid artery, internal jugular vein, vagus nerve) as the carotid sheath (Fig. 7-4B).[218] The pretracheal layer extends in a craniocaudal direction from the hyoid bone to the manubrium sterni and the clavicles. Cranially from the hyoid bone, the pretracheal layer fuses with the superficial layer of the cervical fascia.

According to Barrel,[12] this fascial system has two essential functions: circulatory and muscular. From a muscle standpoint, it supports the infrahyoids in an optimal orientation. This structure is affected by all traumas to the cervical spine or thorax and by cardiac or pleuropulmonary disorders.[12] Because of its vascular connection, it is often involved in circulatory problems of the cervicothoracic junction.

PREVERTEBRAL FASCIA

The prevertebral fascia is firmly adherent to the anterior aspect of the cervical vertebrae and the clavicle (Fig. 7-5). It proceeds medially to attach to the transverse processes of the cervical vertebrae and covers all the cervical nerve roots, the muscles anteriorly (scaleni), and continues laterally and posteriorly to cover the paraspinal cervical muscles. The fascia on the deep aspect of the scalene muscles spreads over the cupula (dome) of pleura, reinforcing it and giving it superior support. This is known clinically as **suprapleural membrane** (Sibson's fascia).[288] The prevertebral layer is continuous with the thoracolumbar fascia. In front of the subclavian artery, it is prolonged laterally as the axillary sheath, which invests the brachial plexus in addition to the vessels. The fascia does not ensheathe the subclavian or axillary veins and

therefore cannot cause venous congestion. However, with all the other nerves and vessels so ensheathed, it is apparent that constriction of theses vital structures is possible.[31,32] Because nerves of the sympathetic outflow (from the stellate ganglia) penetrate this fascia, fibrous constriction can entrap or irritate the sympathetic nerves and cause symptoms attributable to sympathetic nerve stimulation.[32]

The investing layer of cervical fascia encloses all except the most superficial structures of the neck, but within it are other compartments. The prevertebral layer forms a complete enclosure for a compartment containing the cervical vertebrae and their associated longitudinal musculature, vessels, and nerves (Fig. 7-5). The contents of the neck (the larynx, pharynx, esophagus, trachea, and thyroid gland) with the parathyroid glands lie between the pretracheal and prevertebral layers and are invested by the cervical visceral fasciae. In front of the bodies of the cervical vertebrae, an additional layer (the alar fascia) is found between the pretracheal and prevertebral layer. It is attached to the transverse processes (Fig. 7-5B).[82]

In the posture causing scapulocostal syndrome symptoms, the depressed scapula places strain on the fascia and the scapular musculatures.[70] Obliteration of the radial pulse, as observed in Adson's maneuver, can be attributed to the tension of the cervical fascia on rotation of the head and neck. Traction on the lower trunk of the brachial plexus may well cause pain and numbness in the ulnar distribution of the hand, which is common in this syndrome.

Myofascial System of the Shoulder Girdle

Officially, the shoulder girdle is composed of the humerus, scapula, clavicle, and the sternum. However, considering the extensive kinesiology involved and the relationship of shoulder girdle movement, the rib cage, spine, head, and pelvic girdle complex should be considered as essential parts of motion (see below). The shoulder girdle is surrounded by its own fascia to permit free movement of the muscles against each other. Particularly strong fasciae are the pectoral fascia, axillary fascia, clavipectoral, and suspensory ligaments (Cooper's ligaments) (Fig. 7-6).[196,218] The pectoral fascia encloses the pectoralis major muscle and continues to the latissimus dorsi where it divides into two layer that ensheathes the latissimus dorsi and are attached behind to the spine of the thoracic vertebrae.[82]

The deeper clavipectoral fascia surrounds the subclavius, the pectoralis minor, and partly extends over the coracobrachialis muscle (Fig. 7-6).[218] The connection of the clavipectoral fascia with the clavicle supports and suspends the floor of the axilla (composed of axillary fascia and skin).[196] The suspensory ligaments, fibrous bands of the axillary fascia, attach behind the lateral border of the pectoralis major and ensheathe the pectoralis minor. By its traction effect the suspensory ligaments produce the hollow of the arm when the arm is abducted and supports the breasts.

The muscular fasciae of the scapular region are continuous with one another. The fascia of the infraspinatus and teres minor is continuous with the teres major and after

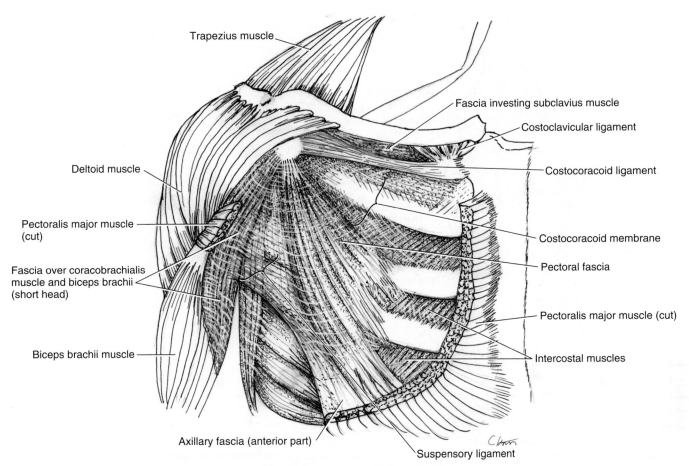

Trapezius muscle

Deltoid muscle

Pectoralis major muscle (cut)

Fascia over coracobrachialis muscle and biceps brachii (short head)

Biceps brachii muscle

Axillary fascia (anterior part)

Fascia investing subclavius muscle

Costoclavicular ligament

Costocoracoid ligament

Costocoracoid membrane

Pectoral fascia

Pectoralis major muscle (cut)

Intercostal muscles

Suspensory ligament

■ **FIG. 7-6.** Fascia of the anterior shoulder girdle. Pectoral, clavipectoral, axillary (anterior part) fasciae, and the suspensory ligament of the axilla.

attachment to the border of the scapula, with the fascia of the subscapularis.[288]

SHOULDER GIRDLE MYOLOGY AND MYOFASCIAL MOBILITY

Muscles of the axial skeleton (trunk) that are considered muscle of the shoulder region include the trapezius, latissimus dorsi, pectoralis major, levator scapulae (Fig 7-7), rhomboid minor, rhomboid major (see Fig. 7-12B), and pectoralis minor (Fig. 7-7C).[222] This group of extrinsic muscles of the shoulder functions to stabilize and move the shoulder girdle. Two of these muscles cross the shoulder joint and thus move the humerus. Overall these muscles move and stabilize the scapula and thus provide maximal mobility of the hand while providing a firm base on which the arm, forearm, and hand function.[222] With the exception of the trapezius, the small branches of the brachial plexus innervate them.

Trapezius and Levator Scapulae (Fig. 7-7A). The intimate relationship between the trapezius and the investing fascia is not often appreciated: the deep surface of the investing fascia serves an attachment for much of the trapezius muscle tissue.[220] The upper trapezius, upper serratus ante-

rior, levator scapulae, and the associated fascia support the shoulder girdle against the downward pull of gravity (Fig. 7-7). The upper trapezius and upper serratus anterior muscles form one segment of a force couple that drives the scapula in elevation of the arm.[206] The lower trapezius (Fig. 7-7A) and lower serratus anterior muscle (Fig 7-7B) form the second segment to the force couple. These muscles often suffer postural strain or acute strain. The upper trapezius has a tendency to develop tightness, whereas the middle and lower trapezius tend to develop inhibitory weakness.[128] A depressed scapular position lengthens the upper fibers of the trapezius muscle and produces a lateral translation and compression force on the cervical spine leading to hypermobility in various planes, depending on the angle of pull.[144]

The connective tissue matrix in this region is an important factor in tissue resilience. In dysfunction there is often fascial clumping generally occurring close to bony insertions.[247] These areas of fascial clumping are often tight as well as tender to palpation and are often difficult to influence toward renewed movement. Some common examples are the attachment of the trapezius as it crosses the scapula below the scapular spine and insertion of the levator scapulae at the upper medial border of the scapula.[247]

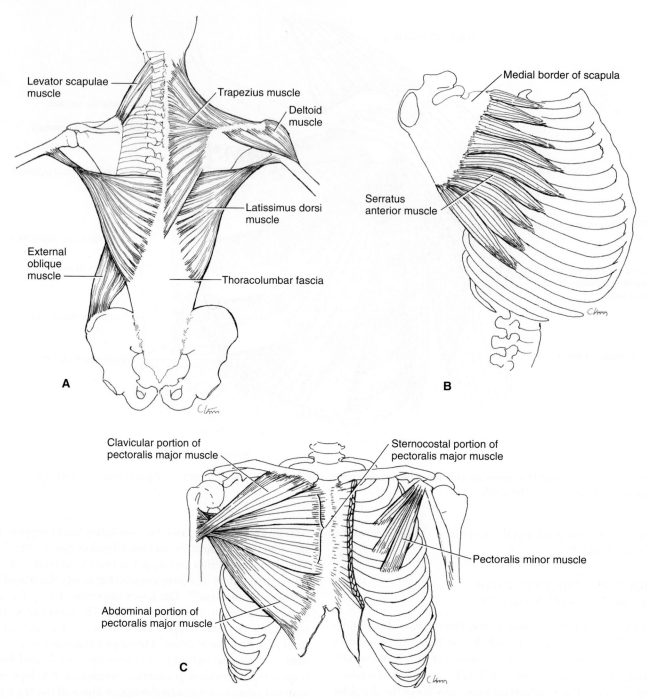

■ FIG. 7-7. Muscle of the axial skeleton considered muscle of the shoulder region. **(A)** Trapezius, latissimus dorsi, levator scapulae. **(B)** Serratus anterior. **(C)** Pectoralis major and pectoralis minor.

The levator scapulae (Fig. 7-7A) acts in concert with the trapezius in shrugging the shoulder. It elevates the scapula and acts along with the rhomboids to help retract the scapula. When its insertion is fixed, it acts unilaterally to provide sidebending and rotation of the neck. According to Porterfield and DeRosa,[220] it is optimally aligned to direct posterior shear forces to the vertebrae of the cervical spine. In this regard, its function might be compared with those of the deep erector spinae of the low back. A forward-head posture increases the anterior shear force, and this posture obligates the levator scapulae to maintain a continuous contractile state to dynamically minimize this force. This muscle often develops strain, especially at the point of insertion. It tends to develop tightness with time.[128]

Both the upper trapezius and levator scapulae have broad insertions into the cervical spine. Alterations in the shoulder girdle resting position and function change the length of these muscles, affecting both the shoulder girdle and cervical spine. For example, in a faulty posture with forward head with posterior cranial rotation and kyphosis, the cervical spine is in extension and the upper trapezius and levator muscles are in a shortened position.

Rhomboid Muscles. The rhomboids (see Fig. 7-12*B*) retract the scapula during movement of the upper limb and rotate the scapula to depress the glenoid cavity. They are used when forcibly lowering the raised upper limbs (e.g., when driving a stake into the ground).[196] Another important action of the rhomboids is deceleration of the scapula during protraction movements of the scapula (as in throwing).[220] These muscles can suffer postural strain or acute strain and tend to develop weakness with time.[128] In the scapular elevation-downward rotation syndrome, described by Sahrmann,[235] they tend to be short along with the levator scapula and upper trapezius.

Pectoral Muscles (Fig 7-7C). The fascial sheath enclosing the pectoralis major is attached at its origin to the clavicle and sternum.[196] It leaves the lateral border of the pectoralis major to form the axillary fascia in the floor of the axilla. Its broad origin includes the manubrium, adjacent ribs and/or cartilage, and the deep fascia of the abdominal wall (see below).

The main action of the pectoralis major is that of a strong adductor and medial rotator of the humerus. When the arm is flexed, the sternocostal head raises the ribs during forced expiration.[196] The sternocostal and abdominal portions, together with the latissimus dorsi, are primary depressors of the shoulder girdle complex.[206,222] In climbing, when the arms are fixed, this muscle draws the body upward. It also assists the deltoid in glenohumeral flexion and aids in throwing, pushing, and shoveling.[82] The pectoralis major (and minor) are both prone to tightness.[128,236] Pectoral tension can be associated with lack of mobility in the midthoracic region.

The pectoralis minor is surrounded by the clavipectoral fascia that runs from the clavicle to the axillary fascia inferiorly (Fig 7-6). The primary action of the pectoralis minor is to protract the scapula. It also participates in a force couple with the levator scapula and rhomboids to provide downward rotation of the scapula, there by tilting its glenoid cavity inferiorly.[51,196] A contracted pectoralis minor tilts the scapula anteriorly pulling the shoulder girdle down and forward. With attachment of the pectoralis minor on the coracoid process, tightness of this muscle depresses the coracoid anteriorly causing pressure and impingement on the cords of the brachial plexus and the axillary, blood vessels that lie between the coracoid and rib cage.[142] Loss of correct posture of the shoulder girdle with tightness of the pectorals, the levator scapula, and neck musculature is significant because scapular protraction approximates the clavicle to the first rib. Change in the position of the scapula can result in compression of the neurovascular bundle and narrowing of the thoracic outlet (see Chapter 11, The Shoulder and Shoulder Girdle).[220,238] The resulting forward-head, round-shoulder posture, also results in humeral internal rotation, which narrows the subacromial space and predisposes the suprahumeral tissues to impingement (see Chapter 11, Shoulder and Shoulder Girdle; Chapter 17, Temporomandibular Joint and Stomatognathic System; and Chapter 19, Cervical Spine).

Myofascial System of the Lumbo-Pelvic-Hip Complex

One of the best examples of the intricacies of the neuromuscular mechanism is the lumbar-pelvic-hip complex, which requires an integration of the muscles and fascia of the lumbar spine, abdomen, pelvic girdle, and hips. The lumbar-pelvic-hip complex has been called the "hub" for both weight bearing and functional kinetic chain movement.[27,221] The role of the myofascial and skeletal tissues in this region is to absorb forces, initiate and control movement, and transfer forces to the surrounding tissues from either ground reaction forces transmitted superiorly at heel strike or upper extremity trunk forces transmitted inferiorly. Muscles such as the middle trapezius and latissimus dorsi acting over the shoulder girdle influence the lumbopelvic hip mechanics (Fig. 7-7A). The lumbar-pelvic-hip complex stability and mobility are dependent on several musculofascial systems: the thoracolumbar fascia, abdominal fascia, fascia of the thigh (fascia lata), and transversalis fascial systems.

THORACOLUMBAR FASCIAL SYSTEM

The thoracolumbar (lumbodorsal) fascia has a tensile strength of nearly 2,000 pounds per square inch and serves as one of the most important noncontractile structures of the spine.[75]

Traditionally, the thoracolumbar fascia has been ascribed not only as fascia but the fused aponeuroses of several muscles with no other function then to invest the muscles of the back and to provide attachment for the internal oblique and transverse abdominus (Fig. 7-8).[246] However, recent studies in the significance of its biomechanical role in the stability of the lumbar spine have created considerable interest in its function (particularly in lifting and forward bending) and its anatomy.[18,20,74,91–93,274]

The thoracolumbar fascia consists of three layers of fascia (anterior, middle, and posterior) with both skeletal and muscular attachments (Fig. 7-8B).[18,221] The thin anterior layer is derived from and envelops the quadratus lumborum and continues medially to attach to the lumbar transverse processes. The middle layer, which lies behind the quadratus lumborum and attaches to the transverse processes, contributes to the lateral raphe and becomes the aponeuroses of the transverse abdominis and internal oblique (Fig. 7-9). The thick posterior layer of the thoracolumbar fascia, which can be used for load transfer, is of special interest because of multiple connections. At the sacral region it fuses with the underlying erector spinae aponeuroses and blends with fibers of the gluteal muscles (Figs. 7-10 and 7-11).

Anatomically, the posterior layer covers the back muscles from the sacral region through the thoracic region as far

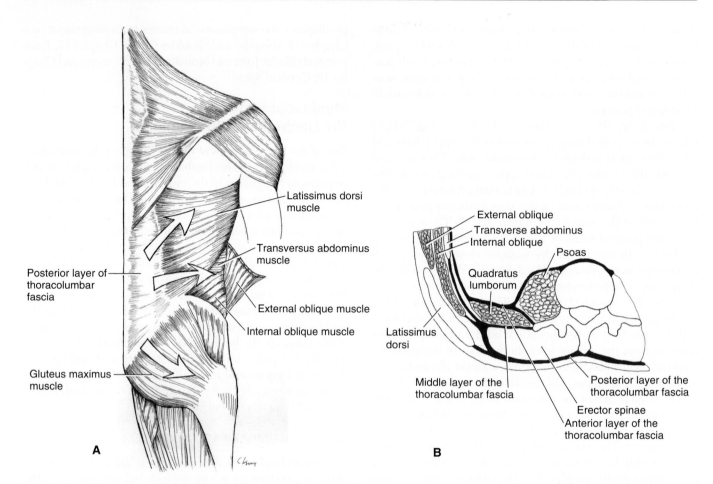

■ **FIG. 7-8.** Thoracolumbar fascia. **(A)** Posterior view. Note how various muscles act to exert tension on this structure. **(B)** Cross-section showing the anterior, middle, and posterior layers.

splenius muscle and ligamentum nuchae of the cervical spine (Fig. 7-12). In the lower thoracic and lumbar regions this fascia is much thicker than the rest of the spinal area, because it represents not only fascial tissue but also the fused aponeuroses of several muscles. It functions in many respects as a ligament, because it invests epaxial muscles that course along the spinous processes and is reinforced by the aponeurotic origin of the latissimus dorsicranially and by the attachment of the erector spinae (epaxial paravertebral) mass caudally into the sacrum and sacral ligaments. At the level of L4–L5 and the sacrum, strong connections exist between the superficial and deep lamina. The transverse abdominal and internal oblique muscles are indirectly attached to the thoracolumbar fascia through a dense raphe formed by fusion of the middle layer of the thoracolumbar fascia and both laminae of the posterior layer (Figs. 7-9 through 7-11).[19] This "lateral raphe" is localized lateral to the erector spinae and cranial to the iliac crest.

At the sacral levels, the superficial lamina is continuous with the fascia of the gluteus maximus (Fig. 7-11): the fibers of the superficial lamina fuse with those of the deep lamina. Because the fibers of the deep lamina are continuous with the sacrotuberous ligament (Fig. 7-10), an indirect link exists

between this ligament and the superficial lamina.[274] Vleeming et al.[274] applied traction to a variety of muscles to study the displacement of the posterior layer. They found that the superficial lamina is tensed by contraction of muscles, such as the latissimus dorsi, gluteus maximus, and erector spinae muscles, and the deep lamina by contraction of the biceps femoris. These findings and others suggest the anatomic structures normally described as hip, pelvis, and leg muscles interact with so-called arm and spinal muscles via the thoracolumbar fascia.[274] This allows for effective load transfer between spine, pelvis, and legs—an integrated system. It is suggested that the gluteus maximus muscle and contralateral latissimus are functionally coupled, especially during rotation of the trunk, and the combined action of theses muscles assists in rotating the trunk while simultaneously stabilizing the lower lumbar spine and sacroiliac joints.

Because the thoracolumbar fascia encloses a space on each side of the spine, contraction of the erector spinae muscle mass (with consequent increase in transverse muscle area) tends to tighten the thoracolumbar fascia greatly. It functions as part of an active mechanism for pulling the vertebrae posteriorly and controlling shear and flexion during lifting. On full flexion, as

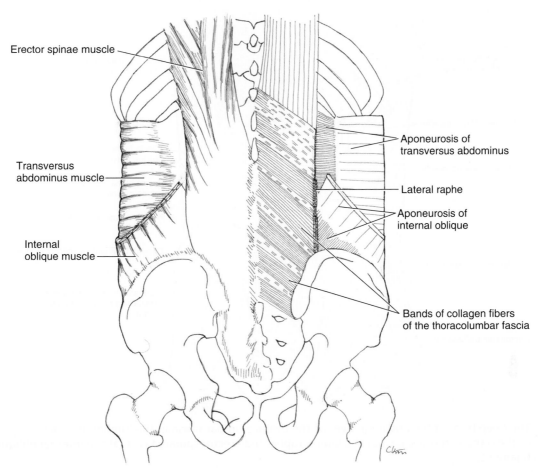

Erector spinae muscle

Transversus
abdominus muscle

Internal
oblique muscle

Aponeurosis of
transversus abdominus

Lateral raphe

Aponeurosis of
internal oblique

Bands of collagen fibers
of the thoracolumbar fascia

■ **FIG. 7-9.** Middle layer of the posterior layer of the thoracolumbar fascia (right) showing its bands of collagen fibers passing from transverse processes to the midline of the lateral raphe, posterior superior iliac spine, and the aponeurosis of the transverse abdominus and internal oblique.

the muscles become electrically silent, the thoracolumbar fascia becomes the major force against further flexion.[165] On extension from a fully flexed position, the gluteus maximus and hamstrings act in concert with the thoracolumbar fascia to initiate extension.[90] With increased activity of these muscles, the fascia serves to increase their efficiency.[93] It also serves as a protective ligament against excessive flexion, and as the muscle mass contracts, the increased diameter of the muscle exerts a wedging effect on the aponeurosis. This is believed to relieve some of the shear load on the articular facet joints and disks in flexion-extension movements of the spine.[76]

The thoracolumbar fascia contains free nerve endings and two types of mechanoreceptors: Ruffini's and Vater-Pacini corpuscles. The presence of these nerve endings supports the hypothesis that the thoracolumbar fascia may play a neuro-sensory role in lumbar spine pain mechanism.[262]

It has been further demonstrated on the basis of dissections and histologic observations that the muscles of the abdomen have the potential to stabilize the vertebral column through the action of the thoracolumbar fascia. This can be brought about, according to Tesh and associates,[268] by

(1) the intrinsic nature of the fascia without direct involvement of the vertebral ligaments, (2) muscle contraction modifying longitudinal ligament tension by the thoracolumbar fascia, or (3) a combination of both mechanisms.

ABDOMINAL FASCIAL SYSTEM: MUSCULATURE AND THE RELATED FASCIAL SYSTEM

The abdominal fascial system, having broad attachments to the ribs, pelvic girdle and thoracolumbar fascia provides support for the viscera, act as prime movers for spinal motion and act as postural muscles (Fig. 7-13). Abdominal muscles include the rectus abdominus, internal and external obliques, and transverse abdominus (Fig. 7-13A). The rectus abdominus parallels the superficial erector spinae in that it is primarily responsible for producing large trunk movements, in this case forward flexion, and it has an important overall postural role in preserving lumbar lordosis. The rectus abdominis muscle is surrounded by its own fascial layer (the rectus sheath) formed by the individual aponeurotic contributions of the transverse abdominis and the oblique muscles as they converge toward

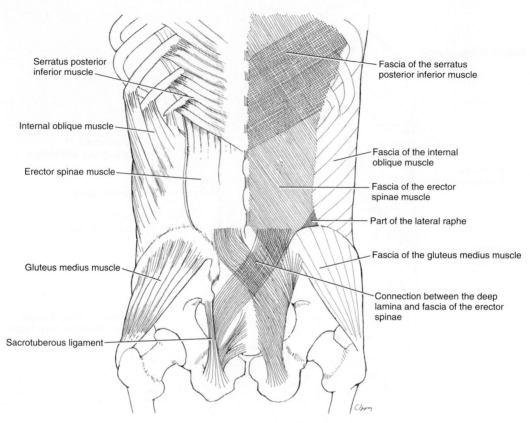

Serratus posterior inferior muscle

Internal oblique muscle

Erector spinae muscle

Gluteus medius muscle

Sacrotuberous ligament

Fascia of the serratus posterior inferior muscle

Fascia of the internal oblique muscle

Fascia of the erector spinae muscle

Part of the lateral raphe

Fascia of the gluteus medius muscle

Connection between the deep lamina and fascia of the erector spinae

■ **FIG. 7-10.** The deep layer of the posterior layer of the thoracolumbar fascia in the lumbar and sacral region showing its connection to the gluteal muscles, part of the lateral raphe, the erector spinae, fascia of the internal oblique, and the sacrotuberous ligament.

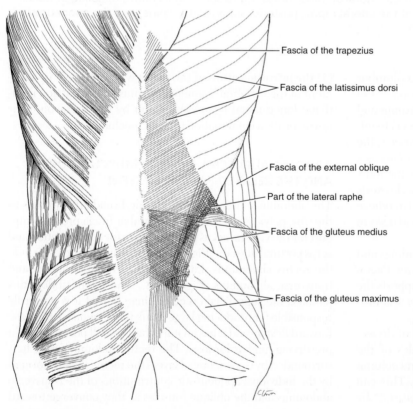

Fascia of the trapezius

Fascia of the latissimus dorsi

Fascia of the external oblique

Part of the lateral raphe

Fascia of the gluteus medius

Fascia of the gluteus maximus

■ **FIG. 7-11.** Superficial lamina of the posterior layer of thoracolumbar fascia which is continuous with the aponeurosis of latissimus dorsi and fascia of the gluteus maximus, fascia of the gluteus medius, part of the fascia of the external oblique, and the trapezius muscle.

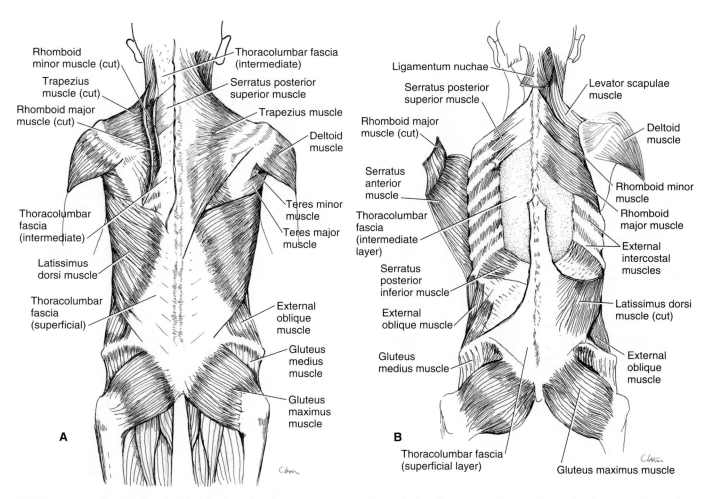

■ FIG. 7-12. Thoracolumbar fascia showing its entire extent through the thoracic region as far as the fascia nuchae of the cervical spine. **(A)** Superficial layer. **(B)** Intermediate layer.

the linea alba (Fig. 7-13A, D). Below the umbilicus, all three lateral abdominals pass aponeurotic expansions anterior to the rectus abdominis (Fig. 7-13A). According to Porterfield,[221] a possible explanation for such an arrangement might be that below the umbilicus the added aponeuroses anterior to the rectus offers additional connective tissue support to counter anterior shear stress of the lumbar spine and abdominal viscera in this region.

The investiture of the internal oblique and transverse abdominus into the thoracolumbar fascia and the fiber orientation of both the external and internal oblique contribute to sagittal control of the pelvis, and the transverse and frontal stabilizers of the trunk to accommodate upper and lower extremity motions.[27] The transversus abdominus, oblique abdominals, and their investing fascia have gained considerable notoriety as important stabilizers of the spine.[136–138,226,227,283] The transverse abdominus is the first muscle to be recruited during small amplitude, rapid trunk movements and when limb movements are initiated.[50,117] It inserts anteriorly in the rectus sheath (Fig. 7-13C). The transverse abdominus is the only muscle to demonstrate significant activity with isometric trunk

extension and is the muscle most consistently related to changes in abdominal pressure for increased spinal stability.[208] The internal oblique and transverse abdominus are the only muscles to have both anterior trunk and spinal connections.[208]

The abdominal wall muscles work synergistically with the scapula retractors, diaphragm, and pelvic floor muscles to align the abdomen and thorax as well as the relationship of the scapula to the thorax.[220] Weakness of the abdominal muscles results in the sternum and chest being carried more caudally and may contribute to the rounded shoulder posture. A comprehensive treatment approach for the forward-head, rounded shoulder posture therefore should include scapular retractor strengthening, anterior shoulder girdle lengthening, scapulothoracic postural positioning, and abdominal wall training.

FASCIA LATA AND RELATED MUSCULATURE

Another fascial system that is significant for posture is the fascia lata, which unsheathes all the muscles of the thigh and covers the gluteal region (Fig. 7-2). The iliotibial tract, a band of fascia, acts as the principle tendon for insertion of the

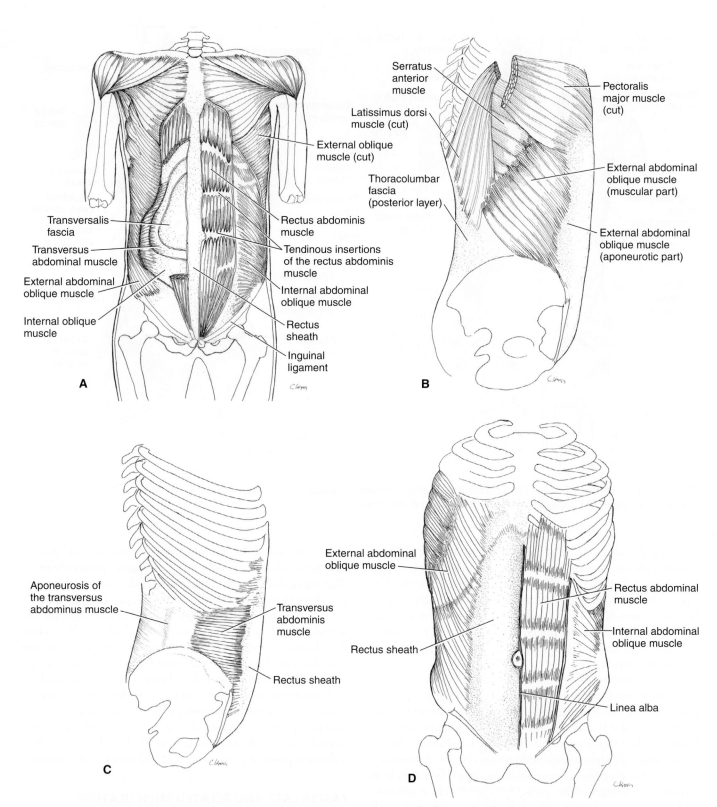

■ **FIG. 7-13.** Abdominals. **(A)** Abdominal wall from the front. On the left, a section of each muscle has been removed to reveal deep muscles and fascia. **(B)** Lateral view of the external oblique muscle. **(C)** Lateral view of the transversus abdominal muscle and aponeurosis. **(D)** Anterior view of the internal and external abdominal oblique muscles.

gluteus maximus and the tensor fascia latae muscle. The fascia lata (fascia of the thigh) begins at the coccyx and sacrum and extends forward along the entire length of the crest of the ilium. It also attaches to the inguinal and sacrotuberous ligaments. Inward extension from its deep surface forms the lateral and medial intermuscular septae of the thigh.[82]

The fascia lata also blends with the aponeurotic insertions of the vastus medialis and lateralis to form the lateral and medial retinacula of the patella (Figs. 7-2 and 7-14A). The part of the fascia overlying the vastus lateralis forms the iliotibial tract.[82] Findings from cadaver studies performed by Terry et al.[267] indicate that the iliotibial tract at the knee separates into two functional components, the iliopatellar band and the iliotibial tract (Fig. 7-14B). The iliopatellar band anatomically connects the anterior aspect of the iliotibial tract and femur to the patella. The iliotibial tract is a multilayered structure consisting of deep capsuloligamentous, middle, superficial, and aponeurotic layers.[94] The iliotibial tract inserts at the tibial tubercle of Gerdy. The iliotibial tract attachments include the lateral intermuscular septum, the lateral femoral condyle, the lateral capsular ligament, the biceps femoris tendon, and the fibula.[223] The iliotibial tract is pulled posteriorly by the

biceps femoris tendon throughout knee flexion. Because of its angle of insertion, the iliotibial tract is a knee extensor from 0 to 30° of extension and a knee flexor when the knee is flexed 30° or more.[179] The tensor fascia lata, acting through the band, is also a weak external rotator of the tibia relative to the femur (see Chapter 15, Knee).

The fascia lata also blends with the aponeurotic insertions of the vastus medialis and lateralis to form the medial and lateral patellofemoral retinacula of the patella. Static stability of the knee is provided by the osseous structures, the capsule of the knee joint, and patellofemoral retinaculum. Henry[113] describes thickening of the lateral retinaculum, which contributes to lateral tilt and possible lateral subluxation of the patella in cases of hypomobility (see Chapter 15, Knee). Hypermobility of the medial structures of the knee, including the medial patellar retinaculum, from trauma or congenital maldevelopment can also increase the likelihood of lateral patella instability or abnormal patellar tracking.[113]

The gluteus maximus and tensor fasciae latae are inserted into the tract and with the tract and septus, form a continuous, strong musculoskeletal apparatus that is important in locomotion and maintaining posture (Fig. 7-2). The fascia is dynami-

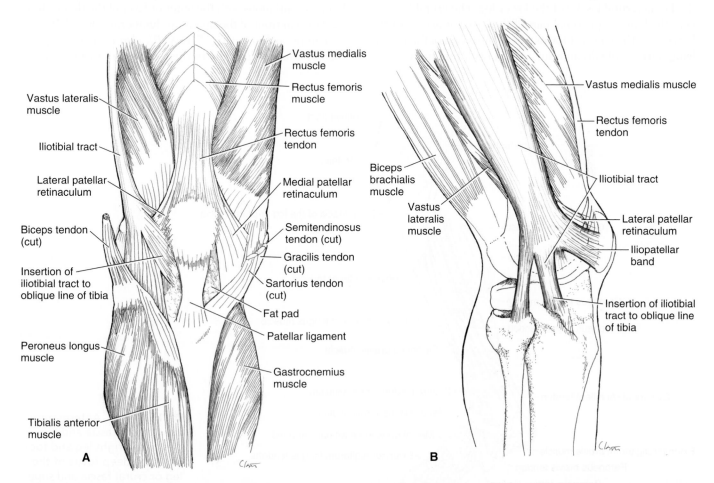

■ **FIG. 7-14.** Knee joint. **(A)** Anterior and **(B)** lateral views showing the iliotibial tract, quadriceps femoris muscles, and soft tissue attachments to the knee. The attachment of the biceps brachii tendons to the head of fibula has been removed.

ni on-

TRANSVERSALIS FASCIA SYSTEM: MUSCULATURE AND RELATED FASCIA SYSTEMS

Another important lumbo-pelvic-hip fascial system is the transversalis fascia (Figs. 7-13A and 7-16). This fascia is the internal investing layer that lines the entire abdominal wall. It covers the deep surface of the transversalis muscle and its aponeurosis. Each part of the transversalis is named according to the structures on which it lies, hence the names diaphragmatic fascia on the thoracoabdominal diaphragm (Fig. 7-17). the psoas fascia on the psoas, the iliac fascia on the iliacus (Fig. 7-16A), and the pelvic fascia in the pelvis.[196] The transversalis fascia is continuous with the anterior layer of the thoracolumbar fascia in front of the quadratus lumborum (Fig. 7-16B).

The psoas fascia (Fig. 7-16A, B), also termed the psoas sheath, attaches laterally to the transverse processes of the

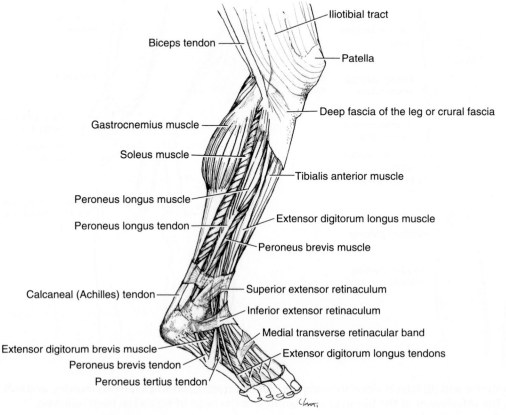

■ **FIG. 7-15.** Anterolateral view of the fascia and muscles of the right leg and foot. Note the deep fascia of the leg or crural fascia and superior and inferior retinaculum of the foot and ankle.

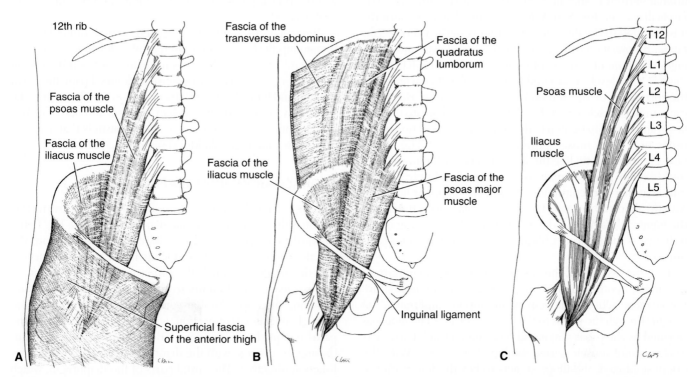

■ **FIG. 7-16.** Psoas and iliacus. **(A)** Anterior view of the fascia of the psoas, iliacus, and proximal thigh. **(B)** Fascia of the psoas, iliacus, and its relationship to the transversus abdominus and quadratus lumborum. **(C)** The psoas and iliacus muscles.

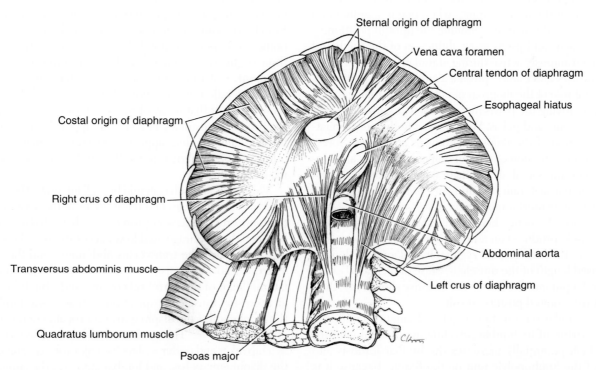

■ **FIG. 7-17.** Thoracoabdominal diaphragm. The abdominal surface is showing its relationship to the quadratus lumborum and psoas.

lumbar vertebrae and medially to the lumbar vertebrae. The fascia iliaca (see Fig. 8-16A, B) covers the iliacus. Superiorly, it is attached to the iliac crest, together with the transversalis fascia. Below, it contributes to the femoral sheath and to the inguinal ligament and is continuous with the fascia lata of the thigh.[82] It is closely associated with the pelvic fascia and with the formation of the femoral canal and femoral ring. The psoas minor muscle inserts by a long strap tendon into the iliac fascia and serves to tighten it, thus integrating the action of the psoas and iliacus muscles through its course.[269] The iliacus fascia is aponeurotic like the heavy fasciae of the muscles of the shoulder girdle (similarity in pectoral and pelvic girdle musculature) and continues deep in the inguinal ligament with the iliopsoas tendon. The iliacus fascia is also attached to the inguinal ligament and participates with it in giving origin to fibers of the internal oblique and transversus abdominus muscles.[281]

Like the fascia lata, this fascial system plays an important part in the coordination of the pelvis and thigh musculature for balanced action in movement and support and transfer of weight through the pelvis to the legs and feet.[269] The iliopsoas (formed by the psoas major and psoas minor) and iliacus acts as a one-joint muscle across the hip (Fig. 7-16C). With the origin stabilized, the iliopsoas acts to flex the femur on the trunk. With the insertion stabilized, the muscle acts bilaterally to flex a stable trunk over the femurs as in a sit-up. With the femur fixed, the iliopsoas, acting unilaterally produces ipsilateral flexion of the lumbar spine with rotation contralaterally. Acting bilaterally it increases lumbar lordosis (assists in extension of the lumbar spine) when one is standing and plays a significant role in maintaining the upright position.[271] Both the iliacus and psoas assist abduction of the thigh and may be continuously active during ambulation.

Grocovetsky and Faran[92] present a model that hypothesizes a significant role of the iliopsoas of not only controlling lordosis but also driving the pelvis in gait through its attachment at the lumbar spine and pelvis. With respect to the pelvis, bilateral contraction of the iliopsoas produces an anterior force, causing anterior motion of the innominate as well as an anterior force on the sacral ala. Unilateral contraction causes an anterior force ipsilaterally, resulting in anterior rotation of the innominate and anterior movement of the sacrum.

Under closed kinetic chain conditions, contraction of the iliacus muscle produces an anterior torsion of the ilium and extension of the lumbosacral zygapophyseal joint. If there is a decreased length of the muscle because of increased efferent neural input into the muscle, or adaptive shortening, then an anteriorly rotated position results.

Under similar circumstances (closed kinetic chain), the psoas by virtue of its lumbar attachment is one of anterior shear which potentially increases the lumbar lordosis and flexion of the lumbopelvic unit on the femur. Because it is strategically placed, it has numerous control functions related to the lumbar spine motions, and altered contraction patterns or shortness of the muscle may jeopardize the biomechan-

ical relationship between the facet joint and the intervertebral disks.[221]

Being a postural muscle, it tightens with dysfunction, producing hip flexion and increased lumbar lordosis. According to Lewit,[159] the psoas behaves in many ways as if it were an internal organ. Psoas spasms cause abdominal pain, flexion of the hip, and typical antalgic (stooped) posture. Tension in the psoas may be secondary to kidney disease, and one of its frequent clinical manifestations when in spasm is that it reproduces the pain of gallbladder disease.[42]

THORACOABDOMINAL DIAPHRAGM

Another clinically important contractile structure in this region is the thoracoabdominal diaphragm (Fig. 7-17). In the forward-head, protracted shoulder, slumped position, the anterior elements collapse, reducing diaphragmatic excursion. The diaphragm, although the primary muscle of inspiration, has extensive attachments to the musculoskeletal system, including the upper lumbar vertebra, the lower six ribs, and through myofascial connections with the lower extremities, the psoas and quadratus lumborum. Both the psoas and quadratus through this merge with the diaphragm influence respiratory function directly.[42] The costal parts of the diaphragm, which forms the right and left "domes," arise from the lower six costal cartilages and lower four ribs, They interdigitate with the transversus abdominus at their costal attachments (Fig. 7-17). The lumbar part arises from two aponeurotic arches. The lateral arch envelops the quadratus lumborum, and the medial arch envelops the psoas major muscle. The lumbar part also arises from two tendinous crura (legs) that take their origin from the bodies and intervertebral disks of the first two (left crura) or three (right crura) lumbar vertebrae and anterior longitudinal ligament.[255] Although formal studies have not been completed, detailed examination of the crura and their attachments suggest that many of the tendinous fibers of the crura are prolonged caudally beyond the upper three lumbar vertebrae. These tendons appear to constitute much of what has otherwise been interpreted as the lumbar anterior longitudinal ligament.[18]

The thorax and pelvis should be well integrated by use of the lumbar-pelvic muscles and the muscles of the abdominal wall to stand erect. Balancing forces involve a balanced action between the diaphragm and lower accessory muscle of breathing, particularly the transversus abdominis, and the psoas.[269] The quadratus lumborum, which is normally thought of as a lateral flexor of the vertebral column and a hip hiker, is also an accessory muscle of expiration.[206] It acts as a stabilizer for the diaphragm as the diaphragm eccentrically contracts during phonation.[13,82,180,244] The quadratus lumborum seldom functions as a hip hiker and perhaps plays its major role as a stabilizer for the diaphragm, pelvis, and lumbar spine (in the frontal, horizontal, and sagittal planes) working with such structures as the thoracolumbar fascia, psoas major, hip muscles, deep portion of erector spinae, and the iliolumbar ligament.[221]

The diaphragm, in addition to being the chief muscle of respiration, is used during weight lifting, giving additional support to the vertebral column through increased intra-abdominal support, and is an important muscle in abdominal straining during micturition, defecation, and parturition.[196] According to Richardson et al.,[226] the diaphragm and muscles of the pelvic floor are activated in synergy with the transverse abdominus and lumbar multifidus during the action of drawing in the abdominal wall. This coactivation of the transversus abdominus and muscles of the pelvic floor and diaphragm is likely to act to maintain the intra-abdominal pressure at a critical level, thus allowing cocontraction of the transversus abdominus to affect spinal support.

The diaphragm is situated in close proximity of the abdominal organs whose nerve supply often communicates with that of this major respiratory muscle. The phrenic nerve, which is the sole motor nerve supply to the diaphragm, is mainly derived from the 4th cervical nerve, with contributions from the 3rd and 5th nerves. Thus irritation of inflamed pleura, by diaphragmatic movement during respiration, may produce shoulder symptoms and chest pain.

PELVIC DIAPHRAGM, ENDOPELVIC FASCIA, AND MUSCLE OF THE PELVIC FLOOR

Endopelvic Fascia. The endopelvic fascia is a segment of the great lining fascia of the abdominal cavity; it is continuous with the transversalis, lumbar, iliacus, and subdiaphragmatic fasciae.[163] The endopelvic fascia is a lining made of a mesh of smooth muscle fibers, ligaments, nerves, blood vessels, and connective tissue; it supports and covers the bladder, the uterus in females, and inner organs such as the intestine.[37,38] Some of the ligaments of the endopelvic fascia connect to the lumbar spine and symphysis pubis. Although endopelvic fascia cannot be exercised, training the pelvic floor muscles of the second layer (pelvic diaphragm) can improve back pain by support of the bladder and uterus (in females) from below and can decrease the strain on the ligaments.[37]

In the true pelvis, the endopelvic lining fascia is divided into the parietal fascia, the fascia of the outlet diaphragm, and the visceral pelvic fascia.

The parietal fascia (piriformis and obturator fascia) covers the piriformis and the obturator internus muscle (Fig. 7-18A). It also attaches to the ligaments and bones of the pelvic outlet and is continuous superiorly with the iliopsoas fascia and transversalis fascia.[163]

The fascia of the pelvic outlet diaphragm covers the superior surfaces of levator and coccygeus (Fig. 7-18B), deep transverse perineal muscle, and sphincter of the membranous urethra (and sphincter vaginae in the female).

The visceral fascia is derived from the superior layer of the fascia of the levator and urogenital diaphragm (Fig. 7-18C) and is reflected from the muscle complexes onto the various pelvic viscera, blending with their outer muscular coats and forming their muscular sheaths.

Muscle of the Pelvic Floor. The most common terminology used in reference to the pelvic floor is "levator ani" or "the pelvic diaphragm complex."[275] The pelvic floor complex consists of the visceral pelvic fascia and pelvic diaphragm as well as the urogenital anal triangles with superficial and deep genital muscles. The pelvic diaphragm is responsible for most of the function or dysfunction of this area. This layer is divided into the coccygeus muscle and the levator ani muscles. Dysfunction of the musculature of the pelvic floor commonly referred to as the levator ani group can play a significant role in the mechanics of the pelvic ring when there is hypertonus, denervation, or trauma to the levator ani.[22] When dysfunction is unilateral, potential muscle imbalances exist, which can cause asymmetric pull on one side of the coccyx, on the pubis, or on one of the ilia.

The levator ani group is composed of two morphologically distinct sections, the pubococcygeus and the iliococcygeus (Fig. 7-18C). The function of the levator ani group is to compress the vagina, urethra, and rectum for continence and support the pelvic viscera.[17,61] In doing so it must counteract gravitational and intra-abdominal forces. The strength of the levator ani is considered the primary factor in the maintenance of normal anatomic relationships of the pelvic viscera with ligamentous forces when pelvic floor muscle support is diminished.[58,241]

The coccygeus muscle (Fig. 7-18A–C) originates on the spine of the ischium and inserts on the anterior portion of the coccyx. It flexes the coccyx, assists in support of pelvic viscera, and stabilizes the sacroiliac joint. It also has powerful leverage for rotating the joint, and abnormal tension of the coccygeus muscle could easily hold the sacroiliac joint in a displaced position.[271] Ventral coccygeal tenderness is often associated with a blocked sacroiliac joint.[160]

The pelvic floor diaphragm muscles are approximately 70% slow-twitch muscle fiber (type 1) and 30% fast-twitch muscle fiber (type 2).[248] A complete exercise program must train both types of fibers. The pelvic floor muscles have the sensation of proprioception and deep pressure through the pudendal nerve. They respond to quick stretch and have extensive fascia throughout the muscle layers. The pelvic floor muscles support the viscera and in doing so must counteract gravitational and intra-abdominal forces.

In conclusion, anatomic structures normally described as the abdominal wall, hip, pelvic, and leg muscles interact with so-called arm and leg muscles via the thoracolumbar fascia. This allows for effective load transfer between spine, pelvis, legs and arms—an integrated system.[274] In both the sagittal and transverse planes, the tensile forces of the muscles attached to and contained within the thoracolumbar fascia provide important passive control of trunk motions. Because of the distance of the contractile portion of the latissimus dorsi, it has the largest moment arm on the fascia.[25] Positions of the humerus will further affect the length of this moment arm as will the amount of anterior pelvic tilt. Increased tensile muscle forces will have a net effect of tightening the thoracolumbar fascia and increasing its rigidity in stabilizing function.[25]

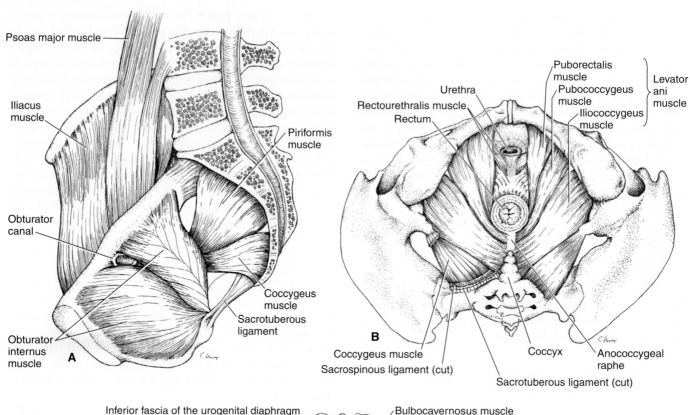

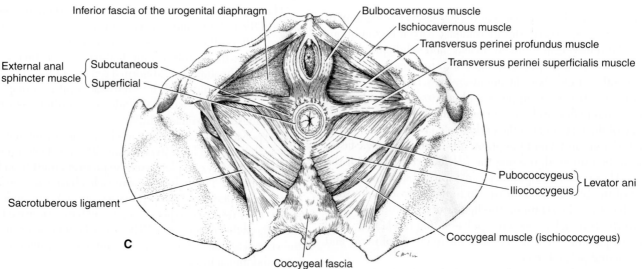

■ FIG. 7-18. Pelvic musculature. **(A)** Right medial view. **(B)** The male pelvic diaphragm (from below). **(C)** The female pelvic diaphragm (from below).

MYOFASCIAL INTEGRATION AND DYSFUNCTION

Skeletal muscle is structurally and functionally integrated by fascia on both a macroscopic and a microscopic level. The description **myofascial** is quite accurate because skeletal muscle, for all practical purposes, does not exist without fascia.

Skeletal muscle (which is the focus here) consists of two basic components: the muscle fibers (the contractile component) and connective tissue (the noncontractile compo-

nent). The structural unit of skeletal muscle is virtually sheathed in fascia. The muscle interior, the sarcomere muscle cells, are arranged linearly in tubes of elastic fascia, the endomysium. The contractile units are organized into fascicles or bundles by fibroelastic fascia, the perimysium, which is continuous with the epimysium, or outer layers of deep investing fascia that wraps the entire muscle.[89] Muscle is also functionally categorized by biochemistry, circulation, metabolism, and in fiber type based on speed of contraction or relaxation.

All skeletal muscles have a mixture of both fiber types, although in most there is a predominance of one or the other. The following fiber type classification is currently widely used.[83] There are those that contract slowly (slow twitch or slow red fibers) which are classified as Type I. These have very low stores of energy-supplying glycogen but carry high concentrations of myoglobulin and mitochondria. These fibers fatigue slowly and are mainly involved in postural or stabilizing tasks.

Type IIa fibers (also called fast twitch/oxidative or fast red fibers) are intermediate fibers that have a faster contraction time than Type I fibers while remaining moderately fatigue resistant with high concentrations of mitochondria and myoglobulin. Type IIb muscle fibers (also called fast twitch glycolytic or fast white fibers), which have a faster contraction time, are less fatigue resistant and depend more on glycolytic sources of energy, with low levels of mitochondria and myoglobulin. Finally, Type IIm fibers (superfast fibers) are found mainly in jaw muscles and depend on a unique myosin structure which, along with a high glycogen content, differentiates it from the other Type II fibers.[231]

The implications of the effects of prolonged stress on these different muscle fiber types cannot be stressed too strongly. Long-term stress involving Type I fibers indicates that they will shorten, whereas Type II fibers, undergoing similar stress, will weaken without shortening over their whole length (although they may develop shortened areas within the muscle).[42]

Muscles can also be classified as those that maintain postures, the so-called static muscles, and those that provide movement, the so-called phasic muscles. Muscles can perform both functions but usually one will predominate. Among the more important postural muscles that become hypertonic in response to dysfunction are the following (see Table 5-6):

- Sternocleidomastoid (Fig. 7-4), pectoralis major (clavicular and sternal end) (Fig. 7-7C), upper trapezius, latissimus dorsi, levator scapulae (Fig. 7-7A) in the upper trunk, and flexors of the upper limbs
- Iliopsoas, quadratus lumborum (Fig. 7-16), tensor fascia lata (Fig. 7-2), rectus femoris (Fig. 7-19), adductors (pectineus, adductor longus, gracilis, and adductor magnus) (Fig. 7-20), hamstrings (Fig. 7-21), and lumbar erector spinae in the lower half of the body (Fig. 7-10)

Dynamic phasic muscles, which respond by inhibition, hypotonicity, and weakness, include:

- Scaleni muscles (Fig. 7-22). (start out as phasic but may end up as postural muscles)[41]

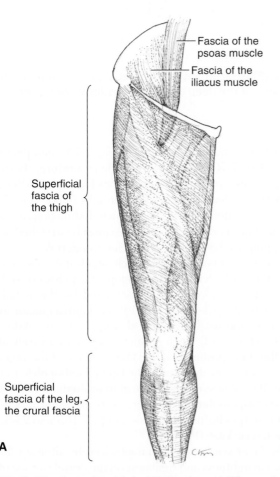
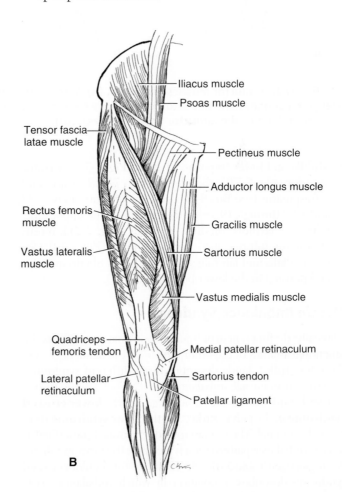

■ **FIG. 7-19.** Anterior thigh. **(A)** Fascia and **(B)** muscles.

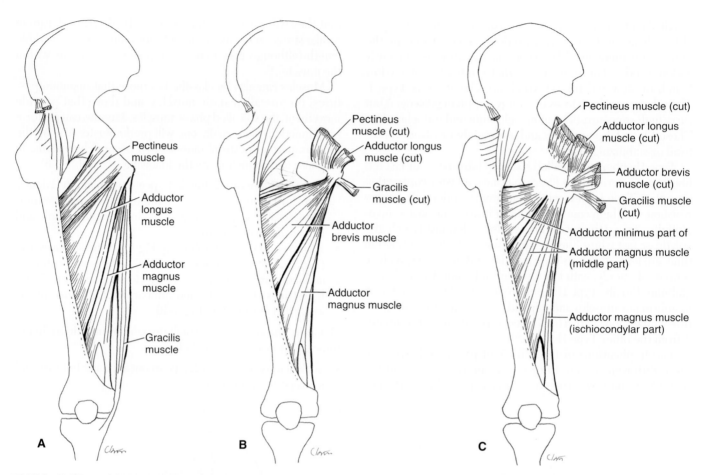

■ **FIG. 7-20.** Adductor muscles of the hip. **(A)** Superficial adductors. **(B)** Attachment of the deep adductor muscles. The overlying pectineus and adductor longus have been cut. **(C)** Attachment of the deep adductor muscles showing the adductor minimus (the adductor brevis has been cut).

- Middle and lower trapezius, deltoid (Fig. 7-7A), serratus anterior (Fig. 7-7B), rhomboids (Fig. 7-12B), supra and infraspinatus (see Box 8-1), deep neck flexors (Figs. 7-22 and 19-9 through 19-10) and extensors of the upper limb
- Gluteus maximus, medius, minimus (Fig. 7-21), rectus abdominis, internal and external obliques (Fig. 7-13), vastus medialis and lateralis (Fig. 7-19), and tibialis anterior and peronei in the lower body (Fig. 7-15)

Muscle Imbalance Syndromes

Clinically, dysfunction in or injury to one area often affects the functional abilities of the other area (e.g., the head, neck, and shoulder girdle). Janda describes three different syndromes resulting from muscle imbalance.[124,127,136] They are the **upper crossed syndrome** in the shoulder girdle, the **lower crossed syndrome** in the pelvic girdle, and the **layer syndrome** from caudad to cranial. The upper crossed syndrome is described as muscle imbalance pattern seen typically in the head and shoulder region (see Table 5-6).[122,127] The upper or shoulder crossed syndrome describes a situation in which imbalance exists between the weak lower stabilizers of the scapula and deep neck flexors (Figs. 7-22 and 19-10) and the tight and shortened

upper trapezius, levator scapulae (Fig. 7-7A), and pectoralis group (Fig. 7-7C). With a forward head posture, shortened suboccipitals (see Fig. 19-8), sternocleidomastoid (Figs. 7-4 and 19-9), scalene (Fig. 7-22), pectoralis minor (Fig. 7-7C) muscles are often present. When such dysfunctions are present, the shortened muscles and fascia must be stretched before the training of the weakened muscles is undertaken.

Another common region in which muscle imbalance is more evident or in which it starts to develop is the pelvic crossed syndrome. This syndrome is characterized by the imbalance between tight hip flexors (Fig. 7-16), and lumbar erector spinae (Fig. 7-9), and weakened gluteal (Fig. 7-21) and abdominal muscles (Fig. 7-13). Such an imbalance can adversely affect both the static posture and dynamic function of the region.[136] An imbalance can also exist in the lateral lumbopelvic musculature. If weakness occurs in the gluteus medius (Fig. 7-21) it can be compensated for by overactivity and tightness in the ipsilateral quadratus lumborum (Figs. 7-16B and 23-8) and tensor fasciae latae (Fig. 7-2).[136]

The layer syndrome is characterized by alternate bands of muscle tightness and weakness on the dorsal surface of the body beginning from below upward.[122,136] It is usually characterized by tightness of the gastrocsoleus muscles (Fig. 7-15),

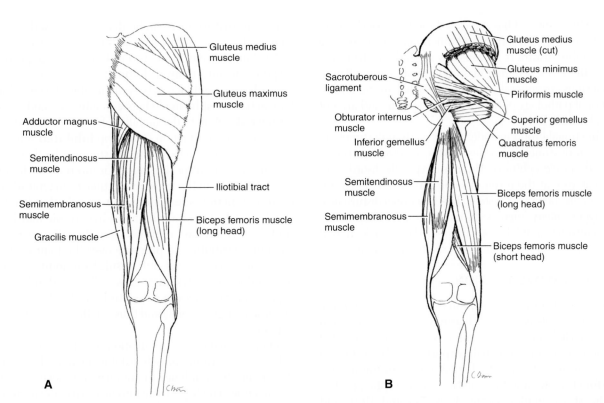

■ **FIG. 7-21.** Muscles of the hip and thigh. Posterior view showing **(A)** hamstring and gluteals and **(B)** piriformis and external rotators.

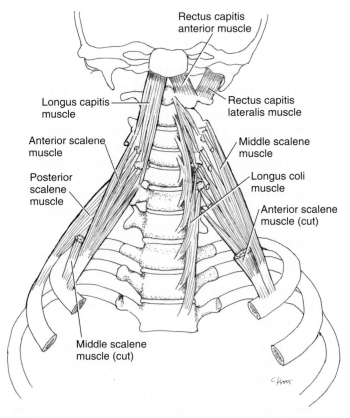

■ **FIG. 7-22.** Scalene and prevertebral muscles (longus colli, rectus capitis, and longus capitis).

hamstrings (Fig. 7-21), lower thoracic and upper cervical erector spinae (see Fig. 18-17), upper trapezius, and levator scapulae (Fig. 7-7). Weakness of the glutei (Fig. 7-21) and lower erector spinae (Fig. 7-9), rhomboids (Fig. 7-12), and lower trapezii is usually present (Fig. 7-7). Another feature of the layer syndrome is "banding" in the erector spinae musculature. With close observation, the examiner can identify sequential areas of hypertonicity and inhibition in various groups of the erector spinae group (Fig. 7-10).

According to Janda's clinical experience, to try to strengthen a weakened muscle first is futile, because its shortened antagonist will inhibit it.[122,136] Attention in the exercise program should be directed initially toward normalizing the length of the myofascial system. Having assessed that a muscle is tight, the clinician must further differentiate whether the muscle is in spasm or whether structural changes, including shortening of connective tissue, have occurred. Such an assessment will direct the clinician to the treatment technique(s) that should be used to achieve normal muscle length. Until recently, evaluation of muscle function was concerned primarily with strength testing, with little attention paid to myofascial tightness and resting muscle length.

Types of Muscle Dysfunctions

Many types of muscle dysfunction have been described in the literature. Examination and treatment will vary depending on the type of dysfunction. Janda[126] delineated seven types of muscle dysfunction and has separated the types of dysfunction into two groups: structural and functional. The structural group contains disorders of muscles caused by structural lesions in the CNS resulting in spasticity or rigidity. These types of lesions are generally not the types that are significant in functional pathology of the locomotor system and are not included here.[164,254,290,291]

The functional group includes limbic system dysfunction, interneuron dysfunction, reflex spasm, myofascial trigger points, and muscle tightness. These are typically disorders of muscle that arise as the result of some sort of functional disturbance in the locomotor system. The functional disturbance may be hypertonicity (increase in muscle tone) or hypotonicity (also referred to as inhibition), in which there is a decreased readiness for the nervous system to activate the muscle.[201]

LIMBIC SYSTEM DYSFUNCTION

The **limbic system** is the functional link between mental activity, and muscle activity.[104] There is a direct connection between the thalamic and the limbic system that is involved in the memory of previous pain experience. According to Janda,[126] muscles affected by hypertonicity in limbic system dysfunction include those in the cervical spine, particularly the sternocleidomastoid (Figs. 7-4 and 19-9) and posterior cervical muscles including the trapezius (Figs. 7-7 and 19-7). Muscle involved in the lower quadrant include the lumbar spine muscles, particularly the erector spinae (Fig. 7-10) and muscles of the pelvic floor (Fig. 7-18). Palpation will reveal a distinct area of tenderness over the involved muscles with a gradual transition from tender areas to nontender areas. Generalized hypertonicity is the most common finding although specific trigger points may be identified within the muscle.[200,201]

INTERNEURON DYSFUNCTION

Interneuron muscle dysfunction is altered tone caused primarily by joint dysfunction. There is a population of cervical mechanoreceptors in the zygapophyseal joints that is relatively small in number that is believed to have an influence on the activity of the gamma motor neurons that innervate the muscle spindles.[182,183] These are consistent in type to those arranged into the classification scheme proposed by Wyke[289] (see Chapter 3, Arthrology). In addition there are a great number of nociceptor afferents in the joint capsules that also influence gamma motor neuron activity.[45,86,182,183,187,292]

When a joint becomes dysfunctional, a decrease in the activation of the mechanoreceptors as well as an increase in the activation of the nociceptors in the joint capsule may develop. This alteration in balance of activity between the afferent in the activity of the two joint afferent systems allows for the transmission of nociceptive impulses relatively unchecked.[192,249] Because of the influence to these two afferent systems on the gamma motor neuron system, an alteration in the sensitivity of the muscle spindle may occur leading to disturbance in

tone. This disturbance can be that of decreased[6,114,260,292] or increased[77,132] tone depending on the muscle involved.

Certain muscles tend to easily become hypertonic in response to interneuron dysfunction (see above) whereas others have a tendency to become inhibited (see Table 5-6). Distinction must be made between inhibited and weak. The term **weak** refers to the inability of a muscle to provide sufficient torque production. The term **inhibited** refers to the inability of a muscle to respond to stimuli—be they be external, in the form of perturbation, or internal, in the form of central order—in the appropriate time or magnitude to perform its function adequately.[201] A muscle that is inhibited may be weak and a muscle that is hypertonic may be weak. Both hypertonic and inhibited muscle will cause an alteration of distribution of pressure over the joint(s) that they cross and thus may not only result from joint dysfunction, but produce joint dysfunction as well.[126] Both inhibited and hypertonic muscles are susceptible to the development of myofascial trigger points and thus can themselves be a source of pain.[123]

On examination (see evaluation of soft tissue dysfunction below), a hypertonic muscle exhibits increased resistance to stretch and the tendency to dominate on movement pattern examination. The hypertonic muscle is typically shortened but may be of normal resting length so that resting length is not necessarily a reliable indicator of hypertonicity. Muscle tone should be determined by assessment of function involving observation of movement patterns (quality of coordinated muscle activity), active-assistive, passive movements, and palpation as well as muscle length and accessory muscle lengthening (see evaluation of soft tissue dysfunction below).

REFLEX SPASM (INVOLUNTARY GUARDING, CHEMICAL MUSCLE HOLDING, AND VOLUNTARY GUARDING)

Much confusion exists regarding the term reflex spasm or **spasm.** Clinicians are inclined to use the term spasm to describe any change in muscle behavior; however, the term becomes too broad and it fails to identify the numerous entities that might be contributing. True spasm is defined as an "uncontrolled involuntary jerking of muscle."[60] Greenstein[97] defines spasm as an involuntary contraction of muscle that may involve the whole muscle or part of a muscle. It can be caused by injury to a muscle or by a biochemical imbalance (hypercalcemia, hyperkalemia, or other electrolyte imbalances). There is no cerebral cortex involvement.[97] Paris[215] describes the following forms of muscle dysfunction that help to clarify the type of muscle dysfunction often described as muscle spasm.

1. Involuntary guarding. This is the most common of the hypertonic muscle states found in the spine, usually involving the multifidus group, and will invariably coexist with most underlying joint dysfunction.[215] The resultant hypertonicity (present in standing and sitting) will invariably disappear in lying if the patient is adequately supported. This

is thought to be a protective mechanism to "splint" the injured tissue and protect it from further injury. Involuntary guarding (reflex spasm) can occur, as a result of intense nociception arising from virtually any tissue, but is especially common when the pain-generating tissue is the intervertebral disk.[201] Involuntary guarding (often referred to as reflex spasm) related to nociception from the intervertebral disk was demonstrated in an animal model by Indahl et al.,[119] who stimulated the annular fibers of the disk in pigs. They demonstrated a reactive increase in resting EMG activity in the multifidus and longissimus muscles at the stimulated segment.

2. Chemical muscle holding. When muscles have been overused, such as the leg muscles in hiking, the muscles will ache and feel doughy and tender to touch. In the spine this may result from overuse, but is more commonly the result of sustained involuntary guarding described above.[215]

3. Voluntary guarding. The patient may voluntarily hold the affected part fixed with voluntary muscle guarding owing to the fear of creating more pain.

MYOFASCIAL TRIGGER POINTS

Myofascial pain syndrome with the presence of myofascial trigger points is a specific form of somatic dysfunction with subjective pain, objective weakness, and autonomic and vascular-lymphatic characteristic[152] (see Chapter 6, Introduction to Manual Therapy and Chapter 17, Temporomandibular Joint and Stomatognathic System). According to Korr,[149] a **trigger point** is a localized area of somatic dysfunction that behaves in a facilitated manner. For example, it will amplify and be affected by any form of stress imposed on the individual whether this is physical, chemical, or emotional. Trigger point develops when there occurs a localized shortening of a fascicle of muscle fibers in which a group of sarcomeres remain in a state of contracture rather than returning to their normal resting length.[252] This contracture can be palpated as an indurated "taut band" that is painful on compression and may give rise to characteristic referred pain (target area), tenderness, and autonomic phenomena.[270] It may produce a jump sign and when stroked (transverse) will cause an involuntary jump sign. Muscles housing trigger points can frequently be identified as being unable to achieve their normal resting length using standard muscle evaluation procedures.[123] Recent research has demonstrated that there is spontaneous EMG activity in the nidus of the trigger point that is not present in the rest of the taut band or the other fascicles within the muscle.[118,253]

It is believed that a trigger point can develop in a muscle when the muscle is subject to direct trauma, acute strain, sustained tension, gravitational strain pathophysiology, overwork, hormonal or nutritional inadequacies, or joint dysfunction leading to dysafferentation and interneuron dysfunction.[152,245] **Dysafferentation** is an expression used when alteration in the balance between the two afferent systems has occurred when a joint becomes dysfunctional (see above).[249]

Myofascial dysfunction is capable of initiating and maintaining pain syndromes (myofascial pain syndrome), systemic dysfunction, and instability. The most prominent manifestations of gravitational pathophysiology are altered postural alignment and recurrent somatic dysfunction.[153] Although the dysfunction induced by gravitational stress and strain is muscle specific, general patterns are characteristic.[120,124,139,153,270,271] Travell and Simons[270,271] definitively describe and map individual myofascial trigger points but also consistently report associated trigger point patterns in myostatic units. The myostatic unit, a complex of muscles sharing the same functional responsibilities or stress, is at increased risk of myofascial dysfunction. Travell and Simons' myofascial trigger points and treatment techniques are described in detail in several texts.[252,270–272]

MUSCLE TIGHTNESS

Muscles undergo adaptive shortening and remodeling if maintained in a shortened position.[157,161] Adaptive shortening or lengthening of a muscle and its connective tissue is a slow, nonpathologic process occurring in response to the range of motion being utilized in the related joints. With shortening, the connective tissue elements of a muscle are in a continuously shortened state and the muscle has increased reactivity to both central and peripheral stimuli.[126] Because of the involvement of connective tissue contracture, muscle tightness is distinguished from hypertonicity related to interneuron dysfunction in that it is shortened in its resting state.[201] A muscle affected by muscle tightness also tends to provide greater resistance to lengthening than does one with hypertonicity caused by interneuron dysfunction, because not only do the contractile elements provide increased resistance, the noncontractile elements do as well. As with interneuron dysfunction, certain muscles tend to become tight (or hypertonic) easily and certain muscles tend to become inhibited easily (see Table 5-6).

A muscle that is tight will have a tendency to dominate the movement patterns in which it is involved and provide increased resistance to stretch. It will have the tendency to inhibit its antagonist, causing those muscles to tend to be left out of the movement patterns in which they are supposed to be involved. Reasons for muscle shortening have been discussed extensively. Overuse, poor posture, lack of exercise or stretching, and reflex mechanisms are all considered contributing factors.

SKIN AND SUBCUTANEOUS SOFT TISSUE DYSFUNCTION

When joint or muscle dysfunction occurs, reflex changes can take place in the skin and subcutaneous tissue that can become their own locus of aberrant afferent input to the CNS, leading to pain and other reflex changes.[160] The most common of these is the **hyperalgesic skin zone (HSZ).**[160,199]

The HSZ is an area of skin that develops increased sensitivity so that stimuli that are normally innocuous become painful. It occurs as a result of dysfunction in another part of the locomotor system and is frequently found in an area that is dermatomally or sclerotomally related to the area of dysfunction.[115,158] The mechanism by which HSZ and other skin and subcutaneous dysfunctions occur is unknown. However, Korr et al.[150] found that myofascial insults induced either by injection of hypertonic saline or from specific postural stresses produced lowered electrical skin resistance in areas remote from the stimulation and represented autonomic responses.

The area of skin affected by HSZ exhibits increased tension, manifested clinically as an increased resistance to stretch.[160] Increased resistance is also known to occur in skin overlying the spine, correlating to levels of joint dysfunction.[168–173,266] Skin can also lose normal mobility secondary to trauma, scar tissue formation, and immobility. With the loss of this mobility the underlying structures can be impeded in their functional capacity and normal coordinated movement patterns of the kinetic chain altered. The skin is continuous with the deep fascia and underlying structures through the attachment of the superficial fascia to the basement membrane of the dermis.[108]

EVALUATION OF SOFT TISSUE DYSFUNCTION

A general approach to the assessment of the musculoskeletal system is discussed in Chapter 5, Assessment of Musculoskeletal Disorders and Concepts of Management, Chapter 21, Cervicothoracic–Upper Limb Scan Examination, and Chapter 24, Lumbosacral–Lower Limb Scan Examination. However, there are additional concepts and techniques specific to the evaluation of the myofascial system. The aspects of myofascial evaluation considered in this chapter are the evaluation of postural and movement patterns, functional testing (active and passive movement analysis), and palpation. The myofascial aspects of this evaluation are stressed. This assessment represents only one aspect of the total evaluation, and the results should always be correlated with other findings to assess accurately the functional (or dysfunctional) state of the spine and or limbs.

Evaluation of Posture and Movement Patterns

The examination of posture and movement patterns allow the examiner to assess the locomotor system in a global way to identify chains of disturbance that can have an impact on the myofascial and skeletal system as a whole and can help identify localized dysfunction. The locomotor system works as a functional whole and all movements occur as a result of a chain of muscle activity, with each muscle involved serving its own particular role in carrying out smooth, efficient, and stable movement patterns.[28]

The examination of posture and movement patterns should occur in the subacute or chronic states only. In the acute stage, alteration of posture and movement is adaptive and there is nothing to be gained by performing these examination procedures. The subacute or chronic stage, however, is the time

to evaluate for the presence of significant dysfunctions that have the potential to perpetuate the patient's pain or dysfunction. This is also the time to look for chain reactions that may be present. These key links may require treatment. Dysfunction in the locomotor system most often occurs in chains, as a result of the alteration of neurologic programs such as gait, prehension, and breathing.[201] It is essential that the examiner be able to identify the key link(s) in the chain (i.e., the joint, muscle, skin, fascial, or programmatic dysfunction that is most responsible for the perpetuation of the chain).

STATIC POSTURAL ANALYSIS

Through careful observation, the postural, bony structure and soft tissue components are analyzed for patterns of dysfunction. Because soft tissue dysfunction results in postural change, the postural assessment should be very detailed. Although lack of symmetry is not necessarily indicative of myofascial dysfunction (because asymmetry tends to be the norm in the human body), myofascial dysfunction is often reflected in structural asymmetry.[9,35,110,287] Taking into account the natural asymmetric state of each individual, **efficient posture** can be defined as the balanced three-dimensional alignment that provides for optimal functional capacity, shock absorption, and weight attenuation.[132] It is the position the body assumes in preparation for the next movement; it is not necessarily a static position. Common postural faults include:

- The proximal or shoulder crossed syndrome (see Chapter 8) in which there is elevation and protraction of the shoulders, abduction (winging) and rotation of the scapulae, and forward head posture.[128]
- The pelvic or distal crossed syndrome (see below) in which there is an anteriorly rotated pelvis, an increased lumbar lordosis, and slight flexion of the hips.[129,136]
- The kyphosis-lordosis posture.[141,142] This type of posture is shown in Figure 7-23 and is more or less equivalent to the proximal and distal crossed syndromes. The anterior longitudinal ligament will be lengthened, the posterior disk space narrowed, and the facet joint approximated with accompanying dural compression and synovial irritation.[207]
- The flat back posture.[141,142] The flat back posture (Fig. 7-24) is characterized by flexion of the upper part of the thoracic spine, reduction in the lumbosacral angle, and posterior tilting of the pelvis. The lordosis is lost and an extension dysfunction is present. This is thought to be caused by elongated and weak hip flexors and short strong hamstrings. Sahrmann[236] considers the lumbar paraspinals to be long as well.
- The sway back posture.[141,142] The sway back posture (Fig. 7-25) is one in which the whole pelvis is shifted anteriorly and the hips are forced into extension. It is characterized by a forward head posture, increased flexion and posterior displacement of the upper trunk, flexion of the lumbar spine, and posterior pelvic tilt. The iliofemoral ligaments are stretched, as are the anterior longitudinal ligament of

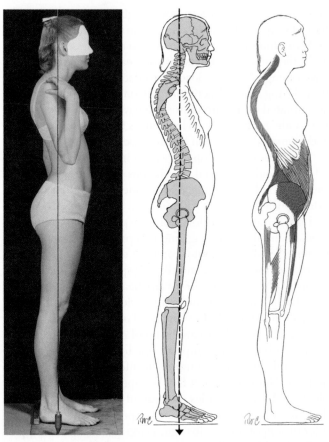

■ **FIG. 7-23.** Kyphosis-lordosis posture. Short and strong: neck extensors, hip flexors, lumbar erector spinae (strong, may be short). Elongated and weak: neck flexors, upper back erector spinae, external oblique. Hamstrings (elongated, may be weak). (Reprinted with permission from Kendall HO, McCreary EK, Provance PT: Muscle Testing and Function, 4th ed. Baltimore, Williams & Wilkins, 1993:84)

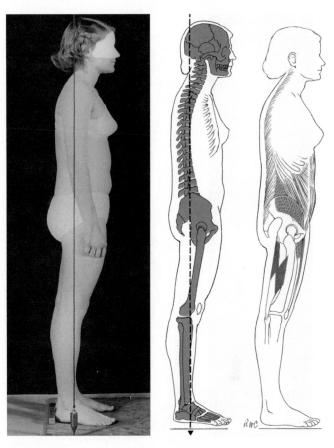

■ **FIG. 7-24.** Flat back posture. Short and strong: hamstrings. Elongated and weak: one-joint hip flexors. (Reprinted with permission from Kendall HO, McCreary EK, Provance PT: Muscle Testing and Function, 4th ed. Baltimore, Williams & Wilkins, 1993:87.)

the lower spine and the posterior longitudinal ligament of the upper lumbar and thoracic spine.[207] If the posture is asymmetrical and weight bearing is taken onto only one leg, the iliotibial band is also tightened on the straight leg side.

- The handedness posture.[141,142] The right-handedness posture (Fig. 7-26) is characterized as a low right shoulder, adducted scapulae with scapular depression, a thoracolumbar curve convex to the left, lateral pelvic tilt, right hip joint adducted with medial rotation, and left hip joint abducted with some pronation of the right foot. There is the appearance of a longer right leg. The left tensor fascia latae is usually strong and there maybe tightness of the iliotibial band.
- Layer syndrome.[124,136] Like the crossed syndromes (see above), the layer syndrome is often described as a muscle imbalance syndrome. The layer syndrome involves generalized deconditioning and extensive muscle imbalances throughout the body. Alternating layers of tight and weak

muscle groups with disturbance of several movement patterns are found. Overactivity is found in the hamstrings, thoracolumbar erector spinae, scapular elevators, and deep neck extensors with weakness in the gluteals and lower scapular fixators, abdominals (rectus abdominis and transversus abdominis), and deep neck flexors. Clinical consequences include poor trunk stabilization, joint hypomobility especially in transitional regions, symptom chronicity, and potential for poor clinical outcome.[44]

Clinical examination of the pelvic posture in standing and sitting, palpable assessment of paired anatomic landmarks, and comparison of leg length (in standing) can be completed quite quickly. In both standing and sitting, assessment (in all planes) of total body alignment as well as segmental alignment of each body part should be noted and described. One should generally assess the overall body type, contour, and balance of the patient's posture. Changes in attitude (deformity), contour (swelling, muscle wasting, and guarding), color (alterations in circulation or inflammation), and skin appear-

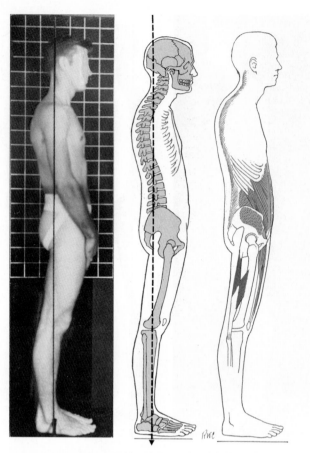

■ **FIG. 7-25.** Sway back posture. Short and strong: hamstrings, upper fibers of internal oblique. Strong but not short: lumbar paraspinal muscles. Elongated and weak: hip flexors, external obliques, upper back extensors, and neck flexors. (Reprinted with permission from Kendall HO, McCreary EK, Provance PT: Muscle Testing and Function, 4th ed. Baltimore, Williams & Wilkins, 1993:85.)

ance should be noted, taking into account general body build and age.

Integrating the myofascial system into the postural evaluation, the entire body should be viewed globally for fascial plane restrictions, because fascial planes can be restricted over large areas of the body.[35] Much information can be gained in the diagnosis of muscular dysfunction by inspection. Hyperactivity and shortening results in visible hypertonus. Change in body shape and contour are so specific and relevant that often it is possible by mere inspection to identify the single muscle involved, movement affected, and related joint dysfunction.[125,160,273] Diagnosis of muscular dysfunction by inspection has proven to be most informative and is illustrated and described in great detail by Vasilyeva and Lewit.[273]

An important objective assessment of vertical alignment of the spine is the vertical compression test (see Fig. 20-4 and Chapter 20, Thoracic Spine).[35,67,132,155,239] The concept behind compressive testing is to test the amount of "spring" that the spine has when a direct compression is imparted.[35] It provides

kinesthetic feedback as to how weight is transferred to the base of support, the compliance of the structural components, and symptoms produced from habitual postures.[35,132,239] Generally the spines of patients with decreased curvatures will not have enough "spring," leading to decreased shock attenuation during normal activities.[35] Conversely, patients with accentuated spinal curvatures will have an increased springiness, indicating increased lever arms for the effect of gravity and increased stresses on the myofascial system.

The three-dimensional position in space of each skeletal part should be noted. Deviations from the norm can be expressed in biomechanical terms such as rotations (flexion-extension, left and right rotations, left and right sidebending) and translations (anterior-posterior positioning), left-right, medial-lateral positioning, and compressed-distracted positioning.[280,281] For example, common deviations noted in the position of the cranium and cervical spine are anterior translation of the head (i.e., forward head), cervical extension (usually in the upper and midcervical joints), and lateral translation (lateral shift) of the head on the neck.

In addition to the relationship of each skeletal part with the whole-body base of support (the feet in standing, and the pelvis and thighs in sitting) each inferior part provides an individual base of support for the superior part.[194] For example, the rib cage provides the base of support for the shoulder girdle. In the forward shoulder posture with inadequate inferior support of the rib cage, a large portion of the support of the shoulder girdle must come from the suspensory muscles of the cervical spine (i.e., rhomboids, levator scapulae, and trapezius [Fig. 7-7]) leading to dysfunction.

Another useful way of viewing the body is with a spatial perspective in mind.[9,194] The examiner notes the three-dimensional structural components of the skeletal and soft tissue systems (i.e., its length, depth, and width).[9] In the efficient state, each individual has an inherent proportional balance between length, width, and depth of his or her structural components.[9,39,147] Dysfunction often diminishes and restricts functional capacity and weight distribution. Because muscle overactivity involves a process of shortening, the resulting decrease in span can be detected readily by comparative differences in the dimensions of a body region. For example, cervical muscles that are in a chronic state of cocontraction will often pull the neck into a shortened position. Thus, the dimension that is diminished is length. Tight pectoral muscles will pull the shoulder girdle into protraction causing an anterior narrowing of the shoulder girdle. In this instance, the decreased dimension is width. In sacral sitting, the pelvis is displaced posteriorly in relationship to the upper body, in a way that creates excess tension in the back muscle. In this instance the decreased dimension is depth. Noting these alterations in body dimension can be a useful guide in identifying myofascial restriction and directing treatment.[194] Keep in mind that the body is a kinetic chain and that postural malalignment in any part of the body causes postural malalignment throughout the body.

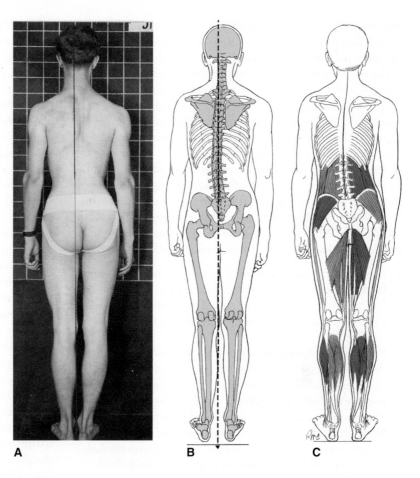

■ **FIG. 7-26.** Handedness posture. Short and strong: right lateral trunk muscles, left hip abductors, right hip adductors, left peroneus longus and brevis, right tibialis posterior, right flexor hallucis longus, right flexor digitorum longus, left tensor fascia latae may be weak. Elongated and weak: left lateral trunk muscles, right hip abductors, left hip adductors, right peroneus longus and brevis, left tibialis posterior, left flexors hallucis longus, left flexor digitorum longus. Right tensor fascia latae may be weak. (Reprinted with permission from Kendall HO, McCreary EK, Provance PT: Muscle Testing and Function, 4th ed. Baltimore, Williams & Wilkins, 1993:89.)

A   **B**   **C**

It is an instructive habit, during this stage of the clinical examination, to include a general palpation of the relevant muscles groups in different postures for muscular state, palpable asymmetry, postural guarding, and alterations in muscle tone. As clinical experience mounts, the examiner progressively gains a familiarity with how postural changes normally modify the tonus of the major muscle groups of each region.[99]

DYNAMIC POSTURAL ANALYSIS

As with the bony structural examination (see Chapter 5, Assessment of Musculoskeletal Disorders and Concepts of Management), all cardinal planes of spinal movement including forward bending, sidebending, and rotation should be observed. Combined movements (see Chapter 22, Lumbar Spine) should also be observed, because daily movements and resulting dysfunction occur in multiple planes. This is especially important when dealing with the myofascial system because it is multidirectional.[35]

Combined spinal movements are also designed to position spinal joints under maximum stress by opening or closing one side of the intervertebral segment.[26,63–65] In evaluating active spinal motion from a myofascial standpoint, the examiner should look first regionally and then segmentally. Regional observation will reveal myofascial abnormalities; segmental observation reveals more specific joint abnormalities and localized myofascial restrictions.

When examining movement patterns, it is important that the patterns are representative of basic stereotyped patterns.[201] Basic patterns include gait, getting up from a recumbent or sitting position, stability responses, respiration, and others. These patterns are programed in the CNS, and the programs call for specific muscles to become activated to specific magnitudes at specific points during the carrying out of each pattern. Faulty movement patterns typically result from alteration of the function of one or more of the muscles that are involved in the pattern.[201] For example, if the sternocleidomastoid and/or the suboccipital muscles become hypertonic as the result of dysfunction owing to trauma, misuse, or other causes, they may tend to dominate the movement patterns in which they are involved. Muscles that are inhibited, such as the middle and lower trapezius, may be activated to a lesser degree. When evaluating a typical stereotyped pattern such as asking the patient to get up from sitting to standing, the normal pattern would be for the patient to lead with the posterosuperior aspect of the head. If the sternocleidomastoid and suboccipitals are dominating, however, the patient will lead with the chin.

Dynamic postural screening is important in most musculoskeletal dysfunctions. The job of the clinician is to identify any abnormalities of movement. Rarely will joint pathology be linked directly to postural deviations. For example, rarely will shoulder pathology be linked directly to postural deviations of the upper quarter; however, shoulder rehabilitation must address postural changes as it relates to dysfunction. These postural deviations lead to shortening and tightening of certain muscle groups and lengthening of other muscle groups.[10] Through the course of time this leads to ultimate weakness, neuromuscular dysfunction, and pain.

Pain-related postural problems are most often caused by mechanical stresses that exceed the supporting capabilities of the tissues resulting in tissue breakdown. If this continues without adequate healing, overuse syndromes with inflammation and pain will affect function without any apparent injury. Pain syndromes related to poor posture include the following:[146]

1. Postural fault and the postural pain syndrome. A **postural fault** is a posture that deviates from normal alignment but has no structural limitations, but if the postural habit continues, strength and flexibility imbalance will eventually develop.
2. **Postural dysfunction** differs from the postural pain syndrome in that adaptive shortening of soft tissues and muscle weakness is involved. The cause may be the result of contracture and adhesions formed during the healing of tissues after trauma or surgery or prolonged poor postural habits. Strength and flexibility imbalances may predispose the area to injury or overuse syndromes that a normal musculoskeletal system could sustain (see overuse syndromes below).

STATIC POSTURAL EVALUATION IN STANDING AND SITTING: SAGITTAL PLANE

The clinician should relate head, neck, and trunk posture and note any increased or decreased curvatures (see Fig. 7-23 through 7-25). Relating an imaginary plumb line to what should be the apex of the thoracic curve, determine if this plumb line also touches the occiput and buttocks. The distance from this plumb line to the apex of the lumbar lordosis is approximately 5 cm in normal adult sagittal plane posture and approximately 6 cm to the apex of the cervical lordosis.[279] The individual should be observed from both sides.

Typical postural dysfunction includes the forward head posture (see Chapter 17, Temporomandibular Joint and Stomatognathic System). This common postural defect increases the gravitational forces on the head and may lead to hyperextension of the head on the neck (posterior cranial rotation), flexion of the neck over the thorax, and posterior migration of the mandible (see Fig. 17-19).[228,229] Myofascially, there is lengthening and weakening of the anterior cervical soft tissue and hyoid muscles, hypertrophy of the masticatory muscles, and hypertonicity of the suboccipital musculature which maintain the occiput in an extended position. In the upper thoracic area, the facets are in a forward bent position, with the posterior myofascial structures being placed on stretch. The myofascial structures of the anterior chest wall are held in a shortened

position. The shoulder complex is held in a protracted position with the tendency for the head of the humerus to be displaced anteriorly (protrudes in front of the acromion).[235] The lumbar spine can be either hyperlordotic or hypolordotic. If hypolordotic, muscle findings include short external obliques combined with a short rectus abdominis.[235] This combination causes thoracic kyphosis, a depressed chest, and narrow infrasternal angle (less than 90°). The anterior thorax is held in a shortened position, diaphragmatic breathing is compromised, and the accessory muscles of respiration are facilitated. Posteriorly, there is flattening of the lumbar spine with a posterior pelvic tilt resulting in stretching of the posterior structures, and hypermobility and atrophy of the lumbar paraspinals. This can be critical when rotation stress is placed on vertebral segments.

According to Sahrmann,[235] short external obliques (with normal length rectus), with narrowing of the infrasternal angle, also pulls the thoracolumbar fascia taut. The taut thoracolumbar fascia pulls the lumbar spine into a long lordosis and can contribute to muscle atrophy of the lumbar paraspinal muscles. The spine is supported by passive tension of the taut thoracolumbar fascia rather than muscular support.

If hyperlordotic, all the abdominals tend to be long with the pelvis tilted anteriorly (Fig. 7-23). Abdominal weakness results in the sternum and chest being carried more caudally, which accentuates a rounded-shoulder posture.[220] When addressing a rounded-shoulder posture commonly attributed to the lengthening or weakness of the scapular retractors, one should also address the role that the abdominal wall muscles play. The abdominal wall muscles work synergistically with the scapular retractors, diaphragm, and pelvic floor muscles to align the abdomen and thorax. Also, apparent excessive lumbar lordosis may be an indication of dysfunction of the lumbosacral junction (hypomobility) and the sacroiliac joint rather than excessive lumbar extension.[279] There may be a component of anterior shearing of the lumbar vertebrae contributing to this apparent excessive lordosis.

DYNAMIC POSTURAL EVALUATION: SAGITTAL PLANE

Dynamic spinal motions should be compared with the static postural evaluation. The application of Fryette's[78] third law (see Appendix) explains how static postural dysfunction affects dynamic movement. Fryette noted that when movement is taken up on any one plane, the potential for movement in other planes is reduced. For example, with typical postural dysfunction of lumbar hyperflexion, there is likely to be full flexion but lumbar extension range will be limited. Similarly, the static forward head posture owing to flexed vertebrae is likely to present with full flexion but limited cervical extension.[279]

Trunk Flexion (Forward Bending) During Standing and Sitting. Physiologic movements of the cervical, thoracic, and lumbar spine should be assessed through full ranges of flexion. The quality, timing, movement pattern, and symmetry of motion are observed in standing (Fig. 7-27) and sit-

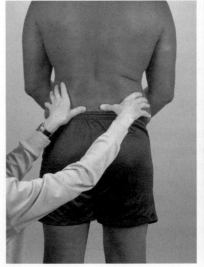 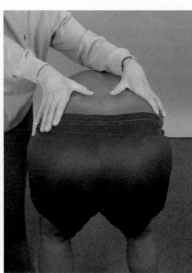

■ **FIG. 7-27.** Standing flexion test. **(A)** Starting position with feet approximately 4 inches apart. **(B)** End position.

A   **B**

ting (Fig. 7-28). Comparison of findings in seated flexion with those of standing flexion tests evaluates the behavior of the vertebral complex without the influence of the lower extremities. The movement pattern should start with the posterosuperior aspect of the head. Assessment is made of the lumbopelvic rhythm (basic neuromuscular activity) as the forces of forward bending proceed from the cervical spine down into the pelvis.[33,91] Trunk rotation or sidebending should not occur, and if present will require further specific mobility testing. This test is very sensitive to dysfunction in the articulations of the bony pelvis (see Chapter 23, Sacroiliac Joint and Lumbar–Pelvic–Hip Complex) and fasciae of the trunk and lower extremities. Views from the side, from behind, and in front of the patient will frequently demonstrate pelvic rotation alterations, flattening of one paravertebral mass, verte-

bral rotation, maintenance of a rigid lumbar mass, and lateral trunk deviation to one side.[99] Loss of movement in a particular region of the spine is most often the result of either true myofascial tightness, protective muscle guarding, or both.[219] Normal limiting factors include tension in the posterior longitudinal, supraspinous, and interspinous ligaments; the ligamentum flavum; and the spinal extensor muscles. If the body deviates to the right or left while forward bending, it may indicate that the body is moving around a disk fragment in the joint or spasm caused by disk herniation. Interruption of a smooth pelvic rotation can also imply tight hamstrings, hip dysfunction, or sacroiliac dysfunction.

With nonstructural scoliosis, the observed scoliotic curve in standing will disappear on forward flexion; with structural scoliosis it will remain (see Fig. 20-8).

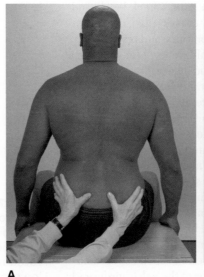 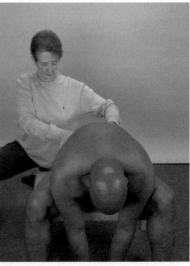

■ **FIG. 7-28.** Seated flexion test. **(A)** Starting with knees apart and feet flat on the floor. **(B)** End position.

A   **B**

Trunk Extension (Backward Bending). As the patient extends, the lumbothoracic curve should curve back in a smooth, even manner. The examiner should again look for the preferred movement pattern and apparent areas of tightness or angulations when the movement is performed. Many patients with back pain backward bend by simply hyperextending the hips (a protective guarding mechanism).[221] The anterior fascial planes of the trunk should be observed for myofascial restrictions. Motion is often limited by a tight rectus abdominus. With multisegmental capsular restriction, the range will be limited because of premature close packing of the facet joints. In the presence of any inflammation, a painful arch or painless end feel may accompany spinal motion. Backward bending should be repeated with the arms elevated overhead to assess mobility of the thorax and for actual backward bending of the vertebrosternal and vertebrochondral regions (see Fig. 20-15).[155]

STATIC POSTURAL EVALUATION: CORONAL PLANE

Comparing right and left discrepancies of anatomic landmarks and restrictions of the myofascial system assesses coronal plane postural dysfunction. From the front, relate the head, neck, and trunk to an imaginary perpendicular or a "grid" background. Note the horizontal level of the eyes, position of the chin and neck, contour and symmetry of the clavicular joints, shoulder joints, subclavicular hollows, chest deformities, waist angle, high point of the iliac crests, anterior superior iliac spines, level of pubic bones, and any lower limb discrepancies.

From behind the client's unstructured stance is noted. In this habitual stance the patient may be compensating for a number of postural asymmetries.[255] Next observe the posture in structured stance with the client standing with the feet hip width apart and perpendicular to a line to detect a number of postural asymmetries (Fig. 7-29). Check the contour of the posterior cervical musculature, trapezius, latissimus dorsi, sacrospinous muscles, and posterior fascial planes for restrictions. Note bulk and muscle symmetry, especially of the medial scapular region. Check levels and attitude of scapulae, horizontal body curves (ribs), deviations of spinous processes, back muscle contours, and resting tone. The right and left gluteal folds should be level (in standing) as well as the posterior iliac spines and iliac crests. If in standing, the iliac crest is elevated on the right side compared with the left, there is a pelvic obliquity (lateral pelvic tilt) indicating limitation in lumbar range of motion (Fig. 7-30).[279] Right elevation indicates that the lumbar spine is sidebent to the right, and there will be limitation in left lumbar sidebending. Muscle findings may reveal a unilaterally taut quadratus lumborum resulting in the limb appearing to be shorter on that side with S curve functional scoliosis of the spine.[271] Other findings may include an actual leg length discrepancy, a tight ipsilateral hip abductor muscle, a tight contralateral hip adductor, and weakness of the contralateral hip abductor muscles.[213]

Comparison of findings of sitting flexion with those of standing flexion helps to assess the behavior of the pelvic girdle and

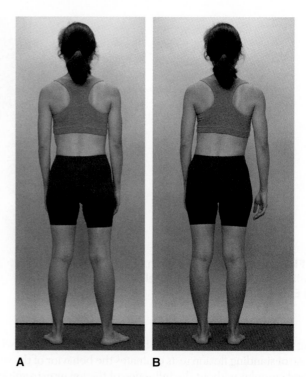

■ **FIG. 7-29.** Postural evaluation (coronal plane). **(A)** Structured and **(B)** unstructured stance.

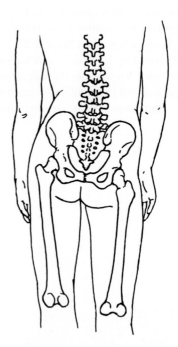

■ **FIG. 7-30.** Lateral pelvic tilt (coronal plane) showing lateral tilt of the pelvis (pelvic obliquity) with associated relative abduction and adduction of the legs. (Reprinted with permission from Palmer ML, Epler M: Clinical Assessment Procedures in Physical Therapy, 2nd ed. Philadelphia, Lippincott Williams & Wilkins, 1998:67.)

vertebral complex without the influence of the lower extremities as the patient is sitting on the ischial tuberosities. Unleveling of the iliac crest (when seated) is suggestive of inequality in the size of the left and right innominates (hemipelvis)[96,271,272] or unilateral muscle atrophy of the gluteal muscles

DYNAMIC POSTURAL EVALUATION: CORONAL PLANE

The patient actively sidebends to the left and right as far as possible without bending forward (Fig. 7-31). Observation is made of the symmetry of range and the induced spinal symmetrical C curve. Straightening of segments of the induced curve are highly suggestive of significant vertebral motion segment dysfunction which will require further specific mobility testing to determine its cause. In the anterior view, check for any discrepancies of bony landmarks suggesting pelvic obliquity (see above).

Observation (in standing) is also made of any pelvic shifts to the right and left during sidebending and whether loading of the lower extremities appear symmetric. The fascial planes on the contralateral side can be evaluated for restrictions. Soft tissues that may limit motion include the following:[111]

- Latissimus dorsi, quadratus lumborum, deep spinal muscles, lateral fibers of the external and internal obliques muscles
- Thoracolumbar fascia
- Capsular facet ligaments
- Iliolumbar and iliofemoral ligaments
- Intertransverse ligaments

Active lateral shifts (sidegliding) motions are performed. Watch for unilateral restrictions or blocking. Movement is restricted in the opposite direction when a patient has a lateral shift of the thoracic lumbar spine.

STATIC POSTURAL EVALUATION: TRANSVERSE PLANE

Transverse plan postural dysfunction represents rotation dysfunction of the limbs (see Chapter 15, Knee) and spine. Faulty myofascial rotatory dysfunction of the head and neck may be owing to tightness of the sternocleidomastoid, upper trapezius, scalene, and intrinsic rotator muscles on one side and elongation of the contralateral rotator muscles.[213] There is associated compression and rotation of the vertebrae.

Normal soft tissue limiting factors of thoracic and lumbar spinal rotation include tension in the costovertebral ligaments and annulus fibrosus of the intervertebral disks, tensions in the ipsilateral external oblique and contralateral internal obliques, and opposition of the articular facets.[45] Muscle findings with pelvic rotation (medial pelvic rotation) and ipsilateral lumbar rotation include tightness of medial rotators, hip flexor muscles, and iliotibial band on the rotated side.

In conjunction with pelvic rotation in the transverse plane, the position of the lower limbs may be altered in the transverse plane by torsion of the femoral neck (antetorsion-retrotorsion), femoral shaft (see Fig. 14-3) or tibial shaft. Retrotorsion (patellae angle in) with compensated internal tibial torsion may reveal tightness of the lateral hip rotators and weakness of the medial rotators.[213] Antetorsion (patellae angle out) with compensated external tibial torsion (see Fig. 14-3) and external tibial torsion (compensated) may exhibit weakness of the lateral rotators and tightness of the iliotibial band.[213]

Locally, spinal rotatory dysfunction can be assessed via the posterior prominence of the paravertebral soft tissues and transverse processes by observation and palpation. With the patient sitting or standing the examiner palpates the posterior aspects of the transverse processes and the paravertebral structures, using the thumbs or dorsum of the fingers of both

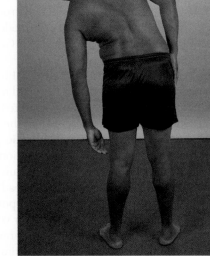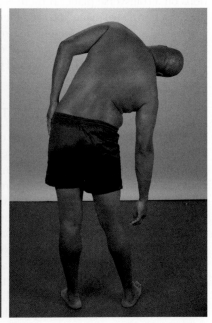

■ **FIG. 7-31.** Active movements of the trunk. **(A)** Side flexion left and **(B)** side flexion right. Observation is made of symmetry of range, the induced spinal curve, any straightening of segments of the induced curve, symmetry of pelvic shift left and right, and whether loading of the lower extremities appears symmetric.   **A**   **B**

hands. The total spine and sacral segments can be evaluated in this way for transverse rotatory plane postural asymmetry.[96,156,279] If the left transverse processes of several spinal segments are more prominent dorsally, this represents a rotation dysfunction of the vertebrae to the left of these segments with limitation to the right of those segments. Positional tests can also be performed in hyperflexion and hyperextension.

Shoulder girdle transverse plane dysfunction can be evaluated in a similar fashion.[279] Forward shoulders (scapulae abducted) are commonly associated with shortened serratus anterior, pectoralis minor and upper trapezius.[142] Muscles in a lengthened position include the middle and lower trapezius. Based on Fryette's third law, if the right shoulder girdle is more protracted, there will be limitation in right shoulder girdle retraction and horizontal adduction.[78]

DYNAMIC POSTURAL EVALUATION: TRANSVERSE PLANE (AXIAL ROTATION)

With the patient standing or sitting, he or she is instructed to rotate the head and trunk to either side (see Fig. 20-16). The ability of the trunk to produce a smooth regional spinal S curve is noted. A lack of movement or a kink in the spinal curve requires further specific mobility testing to determine the cause. It is helpful to repeat axial rotation passively through the client's shoulders, sensing the range, quality of movement, and end feel (see Fig. 20-17). Over pressure may help pinpoint the location of restriction or pain. Limitation of range of motion and/or pain on the side that is opposite the direction of rotation suggests a muscle strain (or restriction, usually of the obliques or thoracolumbar fascia).[111] Limitation and/or pain on the same side as the rotation suggests a disk or facet lesion.

Findings should be correlated with static postural deviations on a transverse plane. If there is a static postural deviation on a transverse plane, the examiner can anticipate finding a physiologic limitation of motion in rotation to the opposite side. With dysfunction, the opposite deep rotators, internal oblique, and thoracolumbar fascia and the external oblique on the same side will limit movement.

COMBINED SPINAL MOVEMENT TESTING

Virtually all natural movements are coupled or combined. Hence, examination of the neuromusculoskeletal system will elicit the most precise and fullest clinical information when combined movements are added to cardinal plane movements (see Chapter 22, Lumbar Spine). Examination techniques enhance the precision of clinical findings, allow recognition of regular and irregular patterns of response, and can be used to assess further the flexibility of the myofascial system. Functional movements combined with spinal flexion help assess the flexibility of the myofascial system on the contralateral posterior side, whereas those patterns combined with spinal extension are most useful in assessing the flexibility of the anterior fascial planes for restriction. With the patient in sitting and/or

standing, he or she may be instructed in the following combined spinal movements:

1. Combined lateral flexion in forward flexion (see Fig. 22-9)
2. Combined forward flexion and rotation (see Fig. 22-10)
3. Combined lateral flexion in extension (see Fig. 22-11)
4. Combined extension and rotation to one side and then the other (see Fig. 22-12)

Many other combinations of two or three movement patterns and varying sequencing of movements allow for more detailed assessment of the spinal joints and the myofascial system.

STATIC AND DYNAMIC POSTURE EVALUATION OF THE LIMBS

The upper and lower limbs can be evaluated for both static and dynamic postural dysfunction on the sagittal, coronal, and transverse planes. Specific assessment of the limbs is discussed in the chapters on those body regions.

OTHER POSTURES

Non–weight-bearing positions (particularly the supine position) in which the effects of gravity have been eliminated and positions on the hands and knees add yet another dimension in the assessment of static and dynamic posture and associated dysfunction of the myofascial and articular systems. Supine posture is often a better barometer of the patient's posture than standing. In standing the patient adapts to postures that are comfortable, thus compensating for areas of restriction and minimizing pain. In the infant and the nonambulatory adult, these positions may be the only postures available for assessment.

The assessment of posture should include both static and dynamic postural analysis. When we speak of normal posture, remember that it is theoretical and represents the most efficient use of energy. The "relative normal" is function that represents the most economic performance of an individual's own body.[66] Static postural analysis is a present-status comparison to a theoretic construct known as the ideal or standard posture model. Specific models of static posture as theorized by Arnhiem,[8] Cailliet,[33,34] Giallonardo,[85] Kendall,[141,142] Kisner,[146] Magee,[166] McKinnis,[181] McMorris,[184] Mensendieck,[189,190] Norkin,[206] Palmer,[213] Phelps,[217] Sahrmann,[237] Williams and Worthingham,[284] and many others differ in details and rationale. It is important to be familiar with the wealth of information presented in these works.

Dynamic posture is defined as the result of the coordinated functioning of proximal and distal neuromuscular strategies to attain a goal or task.[224] Dynamic postural analysis includes head and trunk control, balance and equilibrium in various support postures, active and passive range of motion, capacity for voluntary control, and strength.[181] Dynamic posture in different sporting positions might include, for example, lifting positions in weight training, lower limb kinematics in runners, and upper limb mechanics in throwing athletes.

Much of the effort of earlier times that was devoted to the study of static posture is now directed to research and evaluation concerning dynamic posture. Dynamic posture in different sporting and functional activities may be assessed using video playback.

Selective Tissue Tension Tests

Selective tissue tension tests involve active, active-assistive, passive, and resisted movements as well as muscle length, accessory lengthening (traction), and joint play (gliding and translatory motions).

ACTIVE AND ACTIVE-ASSISTIVE MOTIONS

Active motions demonstrate the patient's willingness to do the movement, the joint range of motion possible, and the ability or muscle power to do the movement. It allows the examiner to look globally at the patient with regard to coordination and to the quality of movement related to certain basic stereotyped activities. It also allows the detection of important localized areas of dysfunction (key links) that may require treatment. Usually the examiner judges available active movement and determines the pattern or quality of the movement, movement of associated joints or substitutions, the presence of pain, and the cause of limitation if present.

Active-assistive motions with the patient in a functional weight-bearing position are particularly valuable.[194] The examiner gently moves the body part a few degrees in each direction with light, gentle, slow movements, noting the patient's responsiveness to the movement (i.e., how readily, easily, and willingly the patient moves). Turning the head, for example, with the patient in sitting, may elicit the patient's responsiveness to the movement by the patient actively going along with the movement and perhaps involving the participatory action of the upper trunk. This induced motion has the quality of a passive motion because it is manually initiated by the examiner, but it also has the quality of active motion because the patient actively goes along with the movement and does not totally remain passive. The feel of resistance to this movement is noted and can be described as initiation feel (early range).[95] If the amplitude of motion progresses further (into midrange), a through-range feel can be appreciated.[233] Active and active-assistive assessment to resistance motion offers information that differs from the more commonly assessed end feel (end range).[194]

PASSIVE MOVEMENTS

Passive movements are used to detect lesions in inert structures, because the latter are subject to stretch when the joint is moved passively. Inert structures are tested by measuring the range of motion and/or the degree of pain. Thus, moving the joint passively through as full a range as possible selectively stretches the inert structures. Concurrently, the examiner notes the amount of range obtained in each direction, the amount of pain caused by the movement, and finally what the movement felt like at the end of range (end feel). End feel, at extremes of restricted or painful movement, is the quality of resistance to movement that the examiner feels when coming to the end point of a particular movement. End feel may be normal depending on the on the movement accompany it at a particular joint and the point in the range of movement at which it is felt. Other end feels may be abnormal or pathologic. Types of normal and abnormal end feel are discussed in Chapter 5, Assessment of Musculoskeletal Disorders and Concepts of Management.

Assessment of passive motion also assists in the determination of muscle flexibility and reveals subjective information about the responsiveness of muscles to stretch stimulus. Care must be taken to differentiate between structural limitation of range of motion, soft tissue shortening, bony changes, and hypertonicity. When tone is normal the limb moves easily and the examiner is able to alter the direction and speed without feeling abnormal resistance. **Muscle tone** is defined as the resistance of muscle to passive elongation or stretch.[212] Resistance may be owing to physical inertia, intrinsic mechanical-elastic stiffness of muscle and connective tissues, and reflex muscle contraction (tonic stretch reflexes).[140] Hypertonic limbs generally feel stiff and resistance to movement while flaccid limbs feel heavy and unresponsive. A qualitative determination of the degree of tone should be made. In cases of localized or unilateral dysfunction, comparison to the unaffected limb is helpful.

Passive testing is also a key test for tension-related conditions, because it may be impossible to do a pure passive motion and the patient will actually assist you in moving the part. Although assistance is the most prevalent sign with passive movements, tense patients may actually resist movement.

FLEXIBILITY (MUSCLE LENGTH TESTING)

One of the most important methods by which individual muscle function is evaluated is through the use of muscle length tests. Shortening of various muscle groups, especially hip and two-joint muscles, can contribute to or occur in response to a variety of postural joint dysfunctions. For example, hamstring tightness may contribute to flattening of the lumbar spine with a posterior pelvic tilt, restriction of knee extension when the hip is flexed, or restriction of hip flexion when the knee is extended.[142] Unilateral hamstring tightness is frequently associated with posterior rotated ilia.[255]

Muscle length tests allow the clinician to evaluate the tone of a muscle and to differentiate normal tone, hypertonicity, and tightness or adaptive shortening. This is done by lengthening the muscle to the point at which the barrier is engaged and assessing the degree of length that is attained, as well as the amount of resistance that the muscle provides when the clinician attempts to lengthen it beyond the barrier. The most reliable clue to dysfunction caused by muscle shortening is an altered end feel.[55] Normally, a soft-elastic end feel is typically felt when limitation of movement is owing to approximation or elongation of muscle tissue. When this soft-elastic end feel is felt in a position which allows less movement than normal, muscle shortening is a likely cause.

One can assess the length of individual muscles or groups of muscles via well-documented muscle length tests[62,71–73,123,142,236,271,272] involving various combinations of physiologic movements. It should be remembered that a large number of muscles are biarticular and have complex muscle fiber arrangement (multiangular as opposed to pure parallel). Emphasis should be placed on arcuate pathways with respect to fiber orientation rather than cardinal plane of motion both in assessment and therapeutic myofascial stretching techniques. Examples of assessment of hamstrings spasm and contracture

in cardinal planes include the straight leg raising test (see Fig. 14-8) and the popliteal angle (90°/90° hamstring assessment for knee flexion contractures [see Fig. 15-27]).[3,52,166,198,213,243] Length testing and stretching maybe carried out for the biceps femoris, medial and lateral (Fig. 7-32A–C). The following method of arcuate assessment of muscle length and myofascial stretching for the hamstrings may be used for selective elongation of the medial hamstrings, lateral hamstrings, and biceps femoris with respect to muscle fiber orientation (Fig. 7-32D).[162,271]

Because one muscle can have one or several function at one or several joints, muscle shortening can cause a variety of effects. Shortened muscles with more than one function at

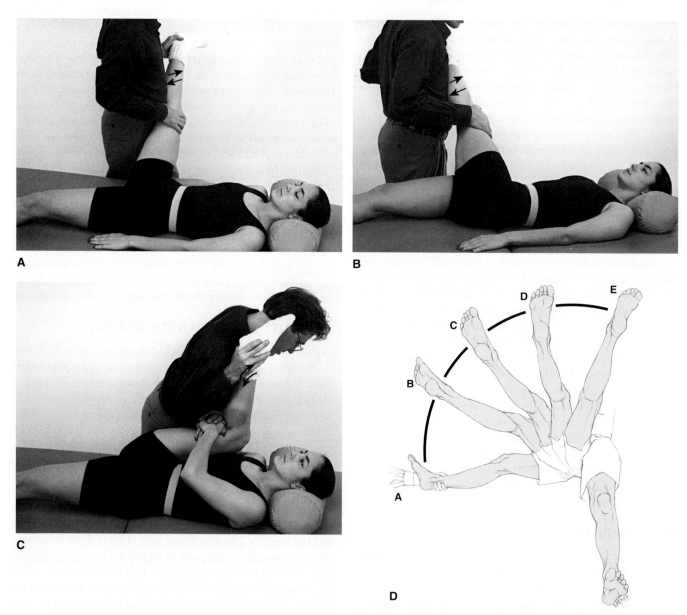

■ **FIG. 7-32.** Hamstrings myofascial length testing and stretching. **(A)** Medial hamstrings. **(B)** Lateral hamstrings. **(C)** Biceps femoris. **(D)** A full arcuate pathway. Postisometric techniques can be used for treatment. (Reprinted with permission from Liebenson C: Rehabilitation of the Spine: A Practical Manual. Lippincott Williams & Wilkins, 1996:259.)

a single joint can restrict range of motion at a single joint in all directions that oppose the directions of their contractile force. Shortened muscles with one or more functions at two or more joints (multiarticular) can restrict range of motion in all directions that oppose the directions of their contractile force at any or all of the joints that are moved by these muscles.[109] For example, a shortened rectus femoris, which functions as a knee extensor and hip flexor with the pelvis fixed (and a pelvic extensor with the femur and leg flexed), will not allow full knee flexion if the hip is fully extended or full hip extension if the knee is flexed (see Fig. 23-33). Tightness of the rectus femoris is also associated with hyperlordosis of the lumbar spine.

Associated muscle of the trunk and lower limbs usually checked for muscle length include the spinal muscles, latissimus dorsi, quadratus lumborum, rectus abdominus, lateral abdominals, internal and external obliques (Fig. 7-33), hip flexors, rectus femoris, tensor fascia latae, hip adductors and rotators, gluteals, hamstrings, and gastrocsoleus.

Muscles length testing of the cervical spine and shoulder girdle includes the pectoral muscles, shoulder rotators, teres minor, the upper trapezius and scalene muscles (Fig. 7-34), suboccipital muscles (Fig. 7-35), sternocleidomastoid (Fig. 7-36), and levator scapulae (Fig. 7-37). The clinician should evaluate muscle tension, contour, as well as range of motion and end feel barrier.

Typically, prolonged alterations can result in muscle length changes. The time a muscle spends in the shortened range and the amount muscle is contracted in the shortened range determine whether it becomes shortened.[285] Adaptive shortening or lengthening of a muscle and its connective tissue is a slow, nonpathologic process occurring in response to the range of motion being used in the related joints. Continuous functioning in a shortened range can reduce the mechanical stimulation necessary for tissue maintenance, resulting in functional adaptation and sarcomere depletion.[112] Certain muscles show a greater propensity for adaptive shortening. These are considered in more detail earlier in this chapter.

ACCESSORY LENGTHENING

One can also assess the accessory lengthening ability (or extensibility) of soft tissues (including muscle, fascia, and neuromuscular elements) by applying a light tensile load, sustaining it, and noting the resulting distribution of tensile deformation.[112,176,177,194] During arm traction or arm pull techniques (through an arcuate pathway), restrictions are perceived as remote "tethering" (i.e., the tissue will fail to elongate in proportion to adjacent tissue) (Fig. 7-38).[94] Restrictions can be perceived along the linear extent of the entire upper quarter as well as in the cross section of the upper limb and forequarter.[194] Stiffer elastic barriers are felt with myostatic contracture, and a hard end feel is usually indicative of bony approximation (i.e., acromioclavicular approximation).[112] Lower limb traction (i.e., leg pulling) of the lower quadrant and trunk can be evaluated and treated as well (Fig. 7-39).

Additional selective tissue tension assessment procedures such as joint play, muscle strength, muscle control and coordination of muscle during active movements are discussed in detail under the respective chapters on the limbs and spinal joints as well as in Chapter 5, Assessment of Musculoskeletal Disorders and Concepts of Management.

Palpatory Evaluation

In this book, many aspects of the palpatory part of the examination are described in Chapter 5, Assessment of Musculoskeletal Disorders and Concepts of Management and chapters in Parts II and III on clinical application. Having completed an evaluation of posture (see above) the examiner has already gained an appreciation of tension patterns in weight-bearing postures throughout the body which can be correlated with the observation of alignment and selective tissue tension tests and muscle length testing (see above).

Palpation seeks to identify various tissue abnormalities, such as undue tissue tenderness, soft tissue thickening, bony abnormalities, and generalized or discrete muscle spasm, as

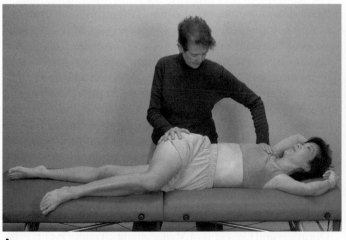
A

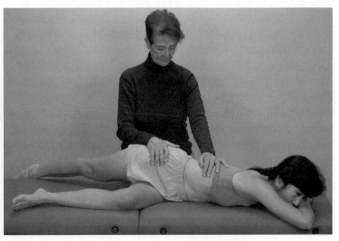
B

■ **FIG. 7-33.** Myofascial length test of the (**A**) external and (**B**) internal oblique abdominal muscles.

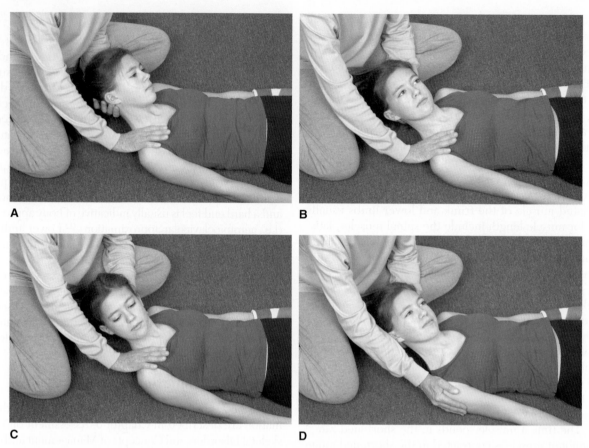

■ FIG. 7-34. Myofascial length testing and stretching of the scalene and upper trapezius muscles. With the patient supine, one hand stabilizes the proximal shoulder girdle while the other assists in sidebending the head away from the involved muscle. Three positions of the head and cervical spine are required to lengthen the scalene. **(A)** To lengthen the posterior scalene, the face is turned away from the involved muscle. **(B)** To lengthen the middle scalene, the face looks forward. **(C)** To lengthen the anterior scalene the face is turned toward the involved muscle. **(D)** To lengthen the upper trapezius, stabilize the shoulder while introducing sidebending and slight rotation to the opposite side. All these length tests can be used as stretching techniques.

well as attempts to reproduce the patient's symptoms. When palpating, the examiner is also interested the presence of swelling, tenderness, crepitus, and alterations in skin temperature.[49] Increased warmth indicates the presence of increased metabolic activity caused by inflammation or hemarthrosis. Alterations in skin temperature (hot or cold) accompanied by sweating and a clammy feeling may indicate sympathetic involvement. Skin temperature can be tested with the back of the hand. Soft tissue crepitus may be palpable in degenerative lesions (e.g., rotator cuff degeneration). Palpation is also used for assessment of abnormal soft tissue or bony masses, vascular pulses, and lymph nodes. Palpable lymph nodes may suggest the presence of infections or neoplasms.

PALPATION FOR TENDERNESS

Tenderness must be differentiated from hyperesthesia of the skin from pinching, compression, or rolling friction (superfi-

cial tenderness) and hyperalgesia of the underlying muscle, ligaments, or tendons that occurs when the skin is pressed against soft tissue or bone (deep tenderness).[258,259,265] Certain areas of the body are always somewhat tender to palpation because of their anatomic location and therefore can be misleading as to the source of pain. Tissues lying directly over or against bone, the heel cord, and upper trapezius are prime examples.[178] The first rib, clavicle, and midthoracic spinous processes are usually tender in young females.[99] Such tenderness existing without other objective signs is unreliable.[99] Normal ligaments and capsules are never tender to palpation.

Palpation should also include palpation for tender acupuncture points, motor points, trigger points, and tender points of fibromyalgia (see Chapter 5, Assessment of Musculoskeletal Disorders and Concepts of Management). Tender points existing in muscles of the anterior and posterior rami of one root may signify the segmental level of spinal involvement.[178]

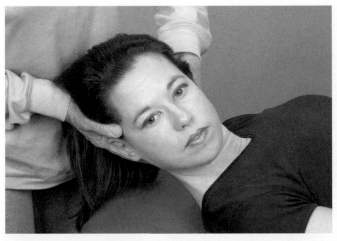

■ **FIG. 7-35.** Myofascial length testing of the suboccipital muscles and testing for restricted movement of the atlantoaxial articulation. Position the patient's head in full flexion to take up all the slack in the lower cervical spine and localize motion to upper cervical spine. Apply rotation movement to each side. Restriction to one side could indicate myofascial tightness and/or atlantoaxial articulation joint restriction. This same position can be used for treatment using muscle energy or postisometric relaxation techniques.

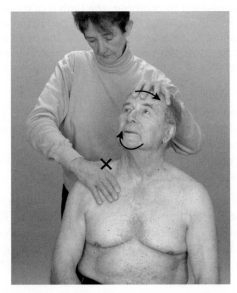

■ **FIG. 7-36.** Myofascial length testing of the sternocleidomastoid. Fixate the shoulder with one hand and at the same time palpate the clavicular and sternal muscle insertion of the sternocleidomastoid. Using the other hand, introduce first maximum upper cervical spine flexion of the head and then maximal sidebending to the opposite side, with subsequent minimal rotation to the same side. During this maneuver, the examiner evaluates the tension of the muscle insertion.

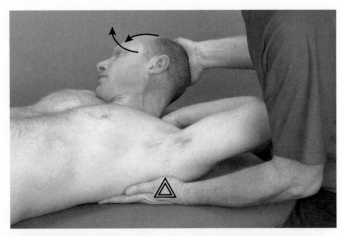

■ **FIG. 7-37.** Myofascial length testing of the levator scapulae. The arm of the supine patient is maximally elevated at the shoulder with the elbow supported against the examiner's abdomen. The stabilizing hand fixates the superior aspect of the scapula while the other hand introduces flexion and rotation of the head in the opposite direction. With this maneuver the examiner evaluates whether pain is introduced as well as assesses range of motion and palpatory changes.

PALPATION OF PERIPHERAL ARTERIAL PULSES

Palpation of peripheral arterial pulses may reveal important information regarding the status of the cardiovascular system. When assessing the abdomen, especially before doing soft tissue mobilization for the abdominal region, the examiner should palpate for the presence of an aortic aneurysm.[21] Also palpate for abdominal aortic aneurysm in back patients, particularly men in the sixth or seventh decade of life who present with a deep, boring pain in the midlumbar region.[87] On occasion, an abdominal aortic aneurysm can cause severe back pain. Most aortic aneurysms occur caudal to the renal artery. A palpable pulse greater than 2 to 3 inches wide should raise suspicion of the presence of aneurysm. Prompt medical attention is imperative because rupture can result in death.

PALPATION OF THE NERVOUS SYSTEM

Palpation of the nervous system is a new idea to many examiners; however, the peripheral nervous system is readily available to palpation and much valuable information can be gleaned.[29,30] Normal nerves, where accessible, should feel firm and round. One should be able to move the nerve from side to side easily. Transverse range of movement will be lessened if the nerve is under tension. In addition to determining if the nerve is under tension, palpation may evoke local pain from irritated and/or scarred connective tissue sheaths or from mechanosensitive sites of abnormal impulse generation.[29,30]

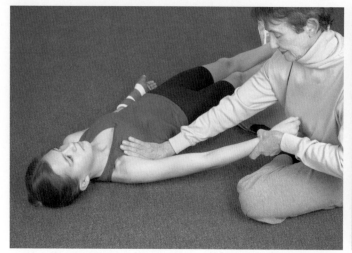

A

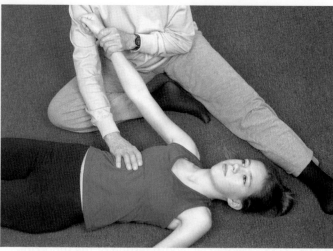

B

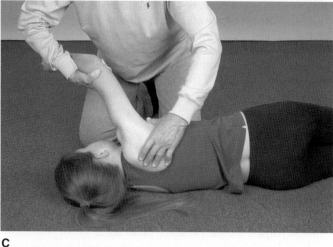

C

■ **FIG. 7-38.** Accessory myofascial lengthening or arm traction. Starting in anatomical neutral (**A**) light traction is introduced (enough to take out the slack in the fascial sleeve). (**B**) The arm is gradually abducted with some twisting in the direction of external rotation. (**C**) As traction is maintained throughout, the limb is gradually taken through its full available range of circumduction assessing and engaging the elastic barrier. Allow the head of the humerus to rotate with physiologic motion. The induced relaxation should dictate the pace of passive motion.

In the clinical context of upper quadrant pain syndromes, the most relevant and commonly palpated nerves include[29,30,68,70,107]:

1. Greater occipital nerve as it exit the fascia at the base of the skull
2. Spinal nerves as they exit from the gutters of the transverse processes of C4–C6
3. Upper and middle trunks of the brachial plexus
4. Neurovascular bundle of the brachial plexus underlying the tendon of the pectoralis minor
5. Neurovascular bundle in the axilla incorporating the axillary artery and vein together the median, radial and ulnar nerves
6. Median, radial, ulnar, axillary, dorsal scapular, and suprascapular nerves

In the lower quadrant, the following neural structures are commonly examined[29,107]:

1. Sciatic nerve in the gluteal region
2. Ventral rami in the belly of the psoas
3. Femoral nerve in the inguinal region
4. Common peroneal nerve (fibular head), deep peroneal (lateral to the extensor hallux longus muscle), and superficial peroneal (dorsum of foot)
5. Tibial nerve centrally, posteriorly at the knee joint, and at the posterior tarsal tunnel

Palpation may turn into a local massage treatment or friction treatment.[29] Oscillatory pressures can be placed on the nerve or the surrounding fascia can be frictioned and released. Methods for assessment and treatment exist, and appropriate texts should be consulted for details of these.[29,68,70,106]

PALPATION FOR SOFT TISSUE MOBILITY, CONSISTENCY, AND CONTINUITY

The palpatory examination for mobility, consistency, and continuity reveals additional information that may be correlated to previous findings. Palpation for abnormalities such as loss of mobility, nodules, and gaps should be noted. Palpation involves careful assessment of the following structures by feel: subcutaneous tissue, fat, fascia, crepitus masses, muscles tendons and bursa, the joints and their surrounding tis-

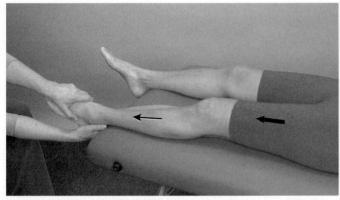

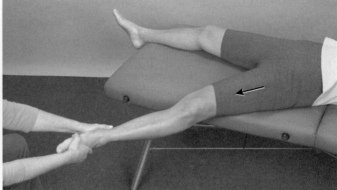

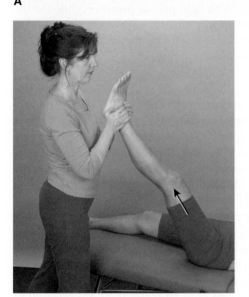

■ **FIG. 7-39.** Accessory myofascial lengthening or lower limb traction. **(A)** Starting in anatomical neutral (grasp the foot with one hand, the heel with the other hand), introduce enough traction to take out the slack in the fascial sleeve. **(B)** As gentle traction is maintained throughout, slowly move the lower limb into abduction and external rotation. **(C)** When possible, take the limb through its full available range of circumduction, allowing the head of the trochanter to rotate with the physiologic motion and the pelvis to protract.

sue (capsules and ligaments), and if indicated vascular pulses, lymph nodes, and the nerves. With educated hands, mobility and qualities such as softness, hardness, shape, texture, size, depth, thickness, and position can be detected and discriminated. Palpation is used to find asymmetry of position or structure, changes in tissue texture, mobility and quality of motion, and the type of soft tissue end feel. The goal of palpatory diagnosis is to identify and define areas of somatic dysfunction.[96] **Somatic dysfunction** is the impaired or altered function of related components of the somatic (body framework) system: skeletal, arthrodial, myofascial structures, and related vascular, lymphatic, and neural elements.[145] Once such an area of dysfunction is defined, the goal of manual therapy is to improve the mobility of tissues (joint, muscle, ligament, fascia, fluid) and to restore normal physiologic motion as much as possible.

LAYER PALPATION OF THE MYOFASCIAL STRUCTURES

Layer palpation is a systematic method of assessing the mobility and condition of the myofascial structures, starting from the most superficial structures and progressing to the deepest. Skin mobility, scar tissue palpation for restriction, and deeper tissue mobility are assessed by skillful loading of the myofascial system by the examiner who monitors the quality and quantity of deformation that results. Restrictions may be palpated in the passive inability of the skin or other superficial tissues to glide over deeper structures, or in the loss of passive lateral gliding of the tissue being assessed. At times, restrictions may be observed in puckering or gathering in of the tissues and in color changes of the skin as tension is applied.

It is generally agreed that the pads of the fingers are the most sensitive portions of the hand available for palpatory diagnosis.[41] Depending on the body part or structure being examined, the thumb, finger pads, or palm(s) may be used to detect restrictions. On broad surfaces, such as the trunk the entire palmar surface may be place on the skin and then pushed in all directions to feel for freedom of movement or lack of it.

The examiner stresses the tissue by loading the structures with both compressive forces and shear forces. Compression implies applying a force perpendicular to the tissue surface, where shear forces are applied by a force parallel or oblique direction to the tissue being assessed.[35,96] Tissue characteristics have been well described in the literature and include tissue extensibility, recoil, end feel, and independent play.[40,41,59,130,160,176,177]

1. Extensibility and recoil. Tissue extensibility is the ability of the tissues to elongate to an optimal range and still have a springy end feel. Recoil is evaluated by how the tissue returns to its normal resting length. In dysfunction specific restrictive points and the direction of greatest restriction or barrier should be identified.

2. Tissue end feel is the quality of tension felt when tissue is manually deformed through direct pressure to the limit of its physiologic or accessory range.[55] Normal myofascial tissues and skin have a springy end feel; ligaments feel firm with little give or creep; capsules feel firm with a slight creep. Tissues in a state of dysfunction may have a variety of abnormal end feels. Muscle may exhibit an abnormal elastic resistance or hard end feel; in hypertonicity a feeling of firmness or turgor; in hypotonicity a feeling of decrease in normal tone or no tone. Skin, in the presence of hyperalgesia, presents with less spring and slack is taken up sooner. In ligamentous laxity there may be a loose end feel. In the presence of adhesions or scarring there is a sudden sharp arrest.

3. Independent play. According to Johnson,[131] one can think of all soft tissue normal states as having independent accessory mobility in relationship to surrounding structures. The degree and extent of mobility varies from one structure to another. In a healthy state this may be described as normal play. In a dysfunctional state there is reduced play between adjoining tissues. In myofascial tissues this is termed restricted muscle play. Dysfunctional tissues can be further evaluated by conducting palpation during passive and active movements.

METHODS OF SOFT TISSUE EVALUATION: PALPATION

Superficial Palpation (Skin and Fascial Planes Assessment). Superficial palpations are targeted at the skin and superficial connective tissue. Palpatory examination includes the assessment of tissue temperature, moisture, texture, and mobility. Various techniques are available for assessing and treating mobility of the subcutaneous tissues. These include skin gliding, skin rolling, and "skin distraction" or stretching method advocated by Lewit.[160]

In skin gliding (Fig. 7-40), the soft tissues are first examined for mobility by placing the finger pads in light contact with the skin and then gliding the tissues alternately in all directions (Fig. 7-40A). Normally the skin and superficial fascia should possess multidirectional extensibility and glide freely over the underlying muscle. Assess the mobility and end feel. Note the direction of any restrictions. On broad surfaces, such as the back, the entire palmar surface may be used (Fig. 7-40B). With light palmar pressure, glide the tissues in all directions. Once superficial restrictions in the skin and subcutaneous tissue are found they can be released by number of soft tissue manipulations (i.e., "J" stroking, skin distraction, and skin rolling).

In skin rolling, the skin and subcutaneous tissues are rolled over the deep structures (Fig. 7-41). Using the thumbs and usually the first two fingers of each hand, the thumbs move slowly along the surface of the skin while the fingers gather up the skin in front of the thumbs causing a wave of skin and subcutaneous tissue to roll onward in advance of the thumbs. One should start in an area with minimal restriction and gradually roll into adjacent areas of restriction. Normally, the dermis and hypodermis should lift readily off the deeper fascia. Skin rolling assessment that detects tightness and tenderness is a valuable tool in identifying levels of somatic dysfunction.[96] When used as a technique, as the restrictions are felt, greater force can be used to lift and pull the skin upward, forward and backward until all restrictions are released.[176] Skin rolling is used to restore mobility, reduce pain and to stimulate circulation and lymph drainage.[41,112]

The pinch and roll maneuver may be used to reveal involvement of the dermatome of the nerve in minor derangement of the spine.[172,259] According to Maigne,[167,168,170,172] spinal lesions are often accompanied by some changes in tissues supplied by

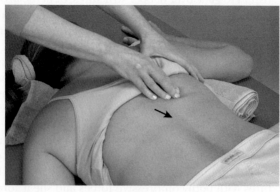 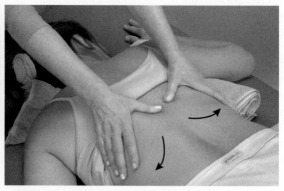

A   **B**

■ **FIG. 7-40.** Skin gliding showing **(A)** digital contact and **(B)** open palmar contact for evaluation of the superficial tissues.

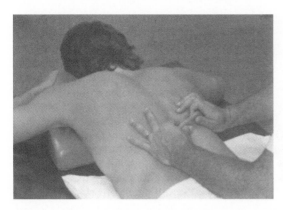

■ **FIG. 7-41.** Skin rolling of the skin and subcutaneous tissues over the deep structures. (Reprinted with permission from Henry JA: Manual therapy of the shoulder. In: Kelly JM, Clark WA, eds: Orthopedic Therapy of the Shoulder. Philadelphia, JB Lippincott, 1995:300.)

the corresponding posterior and anterior primary rami of the spinal nerve. To carry out this maneuver, a cutaneous fold of skin is pinched and rolled between the thumb and index finger (Fig. 7-42). When involved and compared to adjacent and opposite areas it appears thickened, grainy, and very sensitive. These changes frequently are localized to the cutaneous area overlying the joint abnormality.[259] The superficial tender-

ness found in all or part of the dermatome is most probably of neurotropic origin and is owing to nerve root damage[172] or mediated via preganglionic efferent neurons sharing in the heightened activity of a facilitated cord segments.[259] It should be recalled that the cutaneous territory of the posterior rami at the thoracic and lumbar levels is usually located at four levels or more below the level of exit. For example, the skin in the area of the iliac crest and of the lateral fossa is innervated by posterior rami T11, T12, L1, and L2 (see Fig. 20-7).[172]

Gunn and Milbrandt[102,103] have described early and subtle signs in cervical and low back pain. Skin, connective tissue and muscle may share in sensory disorders that may be caused by irritation of autonomic neurons, and these detectable changes may be confusing in their atypical and unexpected distribution more to a vasal rather than a neural topography. They are described to early and reversible neuropathy, rather than late and severe denervation. There is a gradual fibrosis of the subcutaneous tissue, and overlying skin tends to be fissured and prone to heavy folds producing a "peau d' orange" effect (previously described by Stoddard[259]) when squeezed together. There is pitting edema to small localized pressure ("matchstick test") and this last longer than in normal skin.

The technique of skin distraction[160] may be used either for assessment or for therapy. Any area of the skin may be assessed with fingertips (both index) placed close together resting on the tissue to be tested (Fig. 7-43). By separating the fingers the

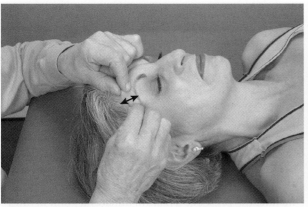

A

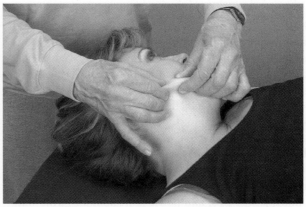

B

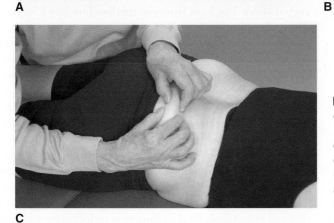

C

■ **FIG. 7-42.** Pinch-roll maneuver used to demonstrate areas of subcutaneous tenderness illustrating a painful (**A**) eyebrow pinch roll, indicating possible irritation of the anterior branch of C2–C3 found in headaches of cervical origin, (**B**) mandible pinch roll, indicating irritation of the anterior branch of C2 and C3, and (**C**) gluteal pinch roll, suggesting irritation of spinal nerves T12, L1–L2.[172]

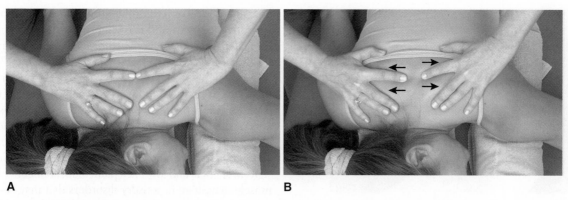

■ FIG. 7-43. Skin distraction. **(A)** Starting position. Fingertips of both hands are placed close together, resting on the tissue to be stretched. **(B)** By separating the fingers, the skin is stretched by simply taking out the slack in the skin. This is compared in several directions, noting the end feel.

skin is stretched and extensibility assessed. A minimum of force is used to take out the slack in the skin. The end position and the degree of "springing" in the tissue are noted. This is compared in several directions over the area to be examined. When used therapeutically, end position of resistance is held for approximately 10 seconds or longer until resistance is felt to ease and the normal physiologic degree of springing is noted. Larger areas are contacted by using the ulnar borders of the hands. The arms are crossed over each other. Stretching is introduced by separation of the hands.

Deep Palpation. Deep palpation examination includes the assessment of the deep fascia (parallel layers of collagen fibers), ligaments, joint capsule, myofascial unit, tendon, and peritoneum. Deep palpatory methods include compressions and shear. Shear is movement of the tissues between layers perpendicular to the tissues. The identification of depth is achieved via the angle of inclination the palpatory digit or hand contact assumes. The more horizontal the contact, the more superficial the tissue palpation. Changing the angle of inclination to a more vertical orientation allows for greater depth of penetration.

Palpation for Soft Tissue Mobility Around Bony Prominence. Evaluation of soft tissue mobility along bony contours as they insert and anchor into the periosteum of the spine, limbs joints, ribs, and pelvic and shoulder girdle may provide valuable information about the overall condition of the multiple layers of soft tissues that attach to bony contours.[67,131,177,202,247] Assessment of these restrictions is easily done with digital palpation using one or both hands. The initial stroke is carried out at a superficial level, with subsequent strokes performed at deeper levels. Restrictive barriers are noted as attention is given to the direction and depth of the tissue barrier evaluated.

Common sites of soft tissue restrictions associated with the spinal dysfunction are the paravertebral musculature between the spinous processes (see pinch and roll evaluation above), posterior arch, and transverse processes. Restricted barriers, increased tone, tenderness of the erector spinae motor points, and underlying trigger points of the deeper paraspinal muscu-

lature can be identified.[178] Other sites in the thoracic and lumbar region include the pad created by the latissimus dorsi at the lumbosacral junction, the interaction between the trapezius and latissimus dorsi at the lumbothoracic hinge, and along the iliac crest.[247] Various muscular and fascial attachments along the iliac crest are also vulnerable to myofascial restrictions. Movement restrictions in forward bending, sidebending, and also backward bending can occur here.[35]

In the cervical region the attachment of the occipital muscles and the levator scapulae to the base of the occiput and the upper four cervical vertebrae are frequently involved.[247] A forward head posture accentuates the anterior shear force at the cervical spine, and this posture necessitates the levator scapulae to maintain a continuous contractile state to minimize this force.[220] The distal attachment of the levator scapulae is commonly associated with palpable induration and a taut band that causes excessive tension. Tension in the levator scapulae is a common cause of neck stiffness. The diagnoses of scapulocostal syndrome,[31,32,193,211] levator scapulae syndrome,[186] and stiff neck syndrome[256,272] are terms commonly applied to muscular symptoms of persistent pain between the shoulder blades. Pain in this region is often sequela of radiculitis of cervical diskogenic disease.[46] Other signs of cervical involvement include the presence a painful unilateral point in the T5 or T6 region about 1 or 2 cm from the median line (see Chapter 20, Thoracic Spine).[172]

Other common areas of bony contour abnormalities and fascial clumping that patients complain about in this region are the trapezius as it crosses the tip of the shoulder (acromion) and as it crosses the scapula below the scapular spine.[247] Anteriorly, common sites of bony contour abnormality include the inferior border of the clavicle; the sternum, sternal manubrial and costochondral junction and the inferior borders of the costochondral arch.[67] Both anteriorly and posteriorly structural rib dysfunctions commonly appear with positional alterations as well as myofascial restrictions of the intercostal muscles.[67] The intercostal soft tissues become restricted from either traditional musculoskeletal dysfunction or following pulmonary

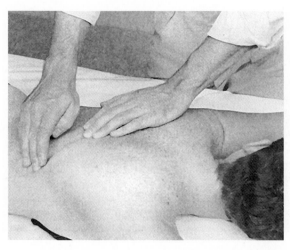

■ **FIG. 7-44.** Evaluation and treatment of bony edges of the ribs and intercostal muscles. Either supine or prone positions maybe used, depending on which aspect of the rib cage is being evaluated (or treated). Digital contact is used pushing laterally along the intercostal space. This stroke maybe repeated several times at each tissue depth so the borders of the ribs and the intercostal mobility can be assessed (or treated). (Reprinted with permission from Scully RM, Barnes MR: Physical Therapy. Philadelphia, JB Lippincott, 1989:966.)

problems.[202] Soft tissue mobilization techniques are an effective method of restoring costal mobility. Examination and treatment of the intercostal tissues is performed with either the distal phalanx of the first, second, or third digit (Fig. 7-44).[202]

Muscle Mobility and Tone. Muscle tone has been used by clinicians to refer to a variety of conditions or states.

Attempts to define and clearly measure quantity of tone have met with little success. Muscle tone is used here to describe tissue firmness to the touch with respect to the resting tonus of adjacent and contralateral myofascial structures. Muscle tone is a function of the natural fullness (turgor) of the muscular and fibrous tissue and of the response of the nervous system to stimuli.[98] Normal muscle has a particular turgor or firmness to it when palpated. Muscle tone, in state of increased tone, feels harder, denser, and may be painful. Atrophied or diseased muscles may feel pasty, or soft and boggy.

Muscle tissue mobility is used to identify restriction within and between the muscles themselves: the assessment of muscle play. **Muscle play** is describe as the quality of accessory mobility of a muscle in relationship to the surrounding structures, which allows for full functional excursion during muscle contraction.[130] Muscle play also includes the ability of the muscle cell bundles to slide in relationship to each other, which allows for full active and passive functional excursion of that muscle. Muscle play or accessory myofascial mobility is related to the amount of intrinsic mobility of a muscle and its related noncontractile elements demonstrated in relationship to their surrounding osseous myofascial, articular, and visceral structures.[67,130] Abnormal muscle play is characterized by a lack of elasticity and by resistance to deformation when outside pressure it applied. The ability to shear muscles freely from their adjacent and underlying structures as well as the ability to move in an uninterrupted fashion through the separate muscle groups is evaluated by perpendicular (transverse deformation) to the muscle fibers or parallel (longitudinal) along the borders of the muscle belly obtaining a parallel separation.

1. Evaluation of transverse (perpendicular) muscle play (Fig. 7-45). Starting at the most superficial level, pressure

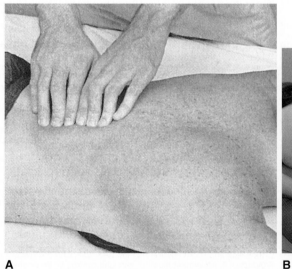

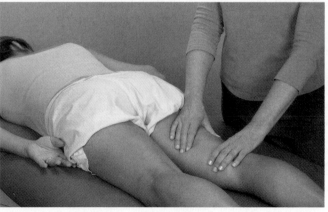

A   B

■ **FIG. 7-45.** Evaluation and treatment of transverse (perpendicular) muscle play of the **(A)** erector spinae and **(B)** the hamstrings muscles. (A Reprinted with permission from Scully RM, Barnes MR: Physical Therapy. Philadelphia, JB Lippincott, 1989:968.)

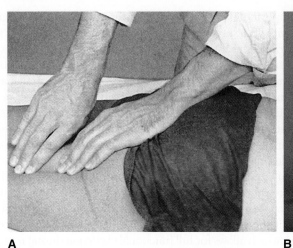
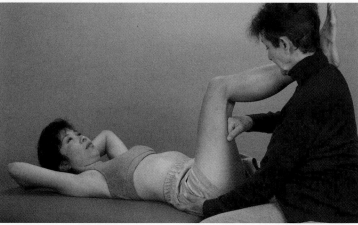

A   B

■ **FIG. 7-46.** Evaluation and treatment of longitudinal (parallel) muscle play of the (**A**) low back and (**B**) the hamstring muscles. (A Reprinted with permission from Scully RM, Barnes MR: Physical Therapy. Philadelphia, JB Lippincott, 1989:968.)

is applied to gently deform the muscle tissue by pressing the contact point against the border of the muscle. When the end range or barrier is reached, the pressure on the tissue is released. As this process is repeated along the length of the muscle the end-feel of the tissue is noted. Restrictions are noted for its site, depth, direction, and degree of restriction. When used as a treatment technique, transverse muscle play may be used to mobilize the fascial sheath surround the muscle to provide more space for it to contract and to reduce adhesions between muscle fibers.

2. Evaluation of longitudinal (parallel) muscle play (Fig. 7-46). Starting with light pressure to examine the superficial tissue, finger pressure is applied along the border of the muscle belly, deforming it until the end range is attained and then allowing the edge of the muscle to pass back beneath the contact point(s). Pressure is gradually increased on subsequent strokes to examine the deep layers. Restrictions are noted as with the previous evaluation technique. When use as a treatment technique, the purpose of this approach is to mobilize the muscle in preparation for more aggressive stretching.

Muscles may be restricted in a longitudinal, transverse (medial-lateral) or in a diagonal direction.[35] By identifying and treating the dysfunction in the appropriate plane, specific restrictions may be released and the flexibility of the muscle increased before lengthening or stretching.

REFERENCES

1. Akeson WH, Amiel D, Woo SLY: Immobility effects on synovial joint: The pathomechanic of joint contracture. Biorheology 17:95–110, 1980
2. Alter MJ: Science of Stretching. Champaign, IL, Human Kinetics, 1988
3. American Orthopaedic Association: Manual of Orthopaedic Surgery. Chicago, American Orthopaedic Association, 1972
4. Amiel D, Frey C, Woo SLY, et al: Value of hyaluronic acid in the prevention of contracture formation. Clin Orthop 196:306–311, 1985
5. Anderson JE: Gray's Atlas of Anatomy, 8th ed. Baltimore, Williams & Wilkins, 1985
6. Aniss AM, Gandevia SC, Milne RH: Changes in perceived heaviness and motor commands produced by cutaneous reflexes in man. J Physiol 397:113–126, 1988
7. Arem AJ, Madden JW: Effects of stress on healing wounds: Noncyclical tension. J Surg Res 20:93–102, 1976
8. Arnheim D, Auxter D, Crowe WC: Principles and Methods of Adapted Physical Education. St. Louis, CV Mosby, 1969
9. Aston J: Movement dynamics II: Continuing Education Course. Incline Village, NV, Aston Training Center, 1990
10. Ayub E, Glasheen-Wray M, Kraus S: Head posture: A case study of the effects on the rest position of the mandible. J Orthop Sports Phys Ther 5:179–185, 1995
11. Bajelis D: The ultimate in myofascial release. J Altern Complement Med 12:26–30, 1994
12. Barral J-P: Urogenital Manipulation. Seattle, Eastland Press, 1993
13. Basmajian JV, DeLuca CJ: Muscles Alive, 5th ed. Baltimore, Williams & Wilkins, 1993
14. Beaulieu JE: Stretching for All Sports. Pasadena, Athletic Press, 1980
15. Beckman M, Craig R, Lehman RC: Rehabilitation of patellofemoral dysfunction in the athlete. Clin Sports Med 8:841–860, 1989
16. Benjamin PJ: Massage therapy in the 1940's and the College of Swedish Massage in Chicago. Massage Ther J 32:56–62, 1993
17. Benson JT, ed: Female Pelvic Floor Disorders. New York, North Medical Books, 1992
18. Bogduk N: Clinical Anatomy of the Lumbar Spine and Sacrum. New York, Churchill Livingstone, 1997
19. Bogduk N, Macintosh J: Applied anatomy of the thoracolumbar fascia. Spine 9:164–170, 1984
20. Bogduk N, Windsor M, Inglis A: The innervation of the cervical intervertebral discs. Spine 13:2–8, 1988
21. Boissonnault WG: Examination in Physical Therapy Practice: Screening for Medical Disease, 2nd ed. New York, Churchill Livingstone, 1995
22. Bookhout MM, Boissonnault JS: Musculoskeletal dysfunction in the female pelvis. Orthop Phys Ther Clin North Am 5:23–45, 1996
23. Bookhout MR: Examination and treatment of muscle imbalances. In: Bourdillon JF, Day EA, Bookhout MR, eds: Spinal Manipulation, 5th ed. Oxford, Butterworth Heinemann, 1992:313–333
24. Bourdillon JF, Day EA, Bookhout MR, eds: Spinal Manipulation, 5th ed. Oxford, Butterworth Heinemann, 1992
25. Bronner S: Functional rehabilitation of the spine: The lumbopelvis as a key point of control. In: Brownstein B, Bronner S, eds: Evaluation Treatment and Outcomes in Orthopedic and Sports Physical Therapy. New York, Churchill Livingstone, 1995:141–190
26. Brown L: An introduction to the treatment and examination of the spine by combined movements. Physiotherapy 74:347–353, 1988
27. Brownstein B: Evaluation, Treatment and Outcomes: Functional Movement in Orthopaedic and Sports Physical Therapy. New York, Churchill Livingstone, 1997
28. Brownstein B: Movement biomechanics and control. In: Brownstein B, Bonner S, eds: Evaluation Treatment and Outcomes: Functional Movement in Orthopaedic and Sports Physical Therapy. New York, Churchill Livingstone, 1997:1–42
29. Butler D: Mobilisation of the Nervous System. Melbourne, Churchill Livingstone, 1991

30. Butler D: Commentary: Adverse mechanical tension in the nervous system: A model for assessment and treatment. In: Maher C, ed: Adverse Neural Tension Revisited. Melbourne, Australian Physiotherapy Association, 1998:33–35
31. Caillet R: Neck and Arm Pain, 3rd ed. Philadelphia, FA Davis, 1991:69
32. Caillet R: Shoulder Pain. Philadelphia, FA Davis, 1991
33. Caillet R: Low Back Pain, 5th ed. Philadelphia, FA Davis, 1995
34. Caillet R: Soft Tissue Pain and Disability, 3rd ed. Philadelphia, FA Davis, 1996
35. Cantu R, Grodin A: Myofascial Manipulation. Gaithersburg, Aspen, 1992
36. Carriere B: The Swiss Ball: Theory, Basic Exercises and Clinical Application. Berlin, Springer-Verlag, 1998
37. Carriere B: Fitness for the Pelvic Floor. New York, Thieme, 2002
38. Carriere B, Felix L: In consideration of proportions. Clin Man 4:93, 1993
39. Cathie A: Considerations of fascia and its relation to disease of the musculoskeletal system. Yearbook of the American Academy of Osteopathy, 1974
40. Chaitow L: Soft tissue manipulation. Rochester, VT, Healing Arts Press, 1980
41. Chaitow L: Modern Neuromuscular Techniques. New York, Churchill Livingstone, 1996
42. Chaitow L: Muscle Energy Techniques. New York, Churchill Livingstone, 1996
43. Chaitow L: Positional Release Techniques. New York, Churchill Livingstone, 1996
44. Chapman SA, DeFranca CL: Rehabilitation of low back pain. In: Cox JM, ed: Low Back Pain: Mechanism, Diagnosis, and Treatment. 6th ed. Baltimore, Williams & Wilkins, 1999:653–678
45. Clarkson HM, Gilewich GB: Musculoskeletal Assessment: Joint Range of Motion and Manual Muscle Strength. Baltimore, Williams & Wilkins, 1989
46. Cloward RB: Cervical diskography: A contribution to the etiology and mechanism of neck, shoulder, and arm pain. Ann Surg 150:229, 1947
47. Cobb DS, Cantu R: Myofascial treatment. In: Donatelli R, eds: Physical Therapy of the Shoulder, 3rd ed. New York, Churchill Livingstone, 1997
48. Copenhaver WM, Bunge RP, Runge R, et al: Bailey's Textbook of Histology. Baltimore, Williams & Wilkins, 1975
49. Corrigan B, Maitland GD: Practical Orthopaedic Medicine. London, Butterworth, 1983
50. Cresswell A, Gundstrom A, Thorstensson A: Observation on intra-abdominal pressure and patterns of abdominal intramuscular activity in man. J Acta Physiol Scand 144:409–418, 1992
51. Cropper JR: Regional anatomy and biomechanics. In: Flynn TW, ed: The Thoracic Spine and Rib Cage: Musculoskeletal Evaluation and Treatment. Boston, Butterworth-Heinemann, 1996:3–29
52. Cusick BD: Progressive Casting and Splinting for Lower Extremity Deformities in Children with Neuromotor Dysfunction. Tucson, Therapy Skill Builders, 1990
53. Cyriax J: Clinical application of massage. In: Licht S, ed: Massage, Manipulation and Traction. New Haven, Elizabeth Licht, 1960:122–139
54. Cyriax J: Deep massage. Physiotherapy 63:60–61, 1977
55. Cyriax J: Textbook of Orthopaedic Medicine: Diagnosis of Soft Tissue Lesions, vol. I, 8th ed. London, Bailliere Tindall, 1982
56. Cyriax J, Coldham M: Textbook of Orthopaedic Medicine, vol. I. 11th ed. London, Bailliere Tindall, 1984
57. D'Ambrogio KJ, Roth GB: Positional Release Therapy: Assessment & Treatment of Musculoskeletal Dysfunction. St. Louis, Mosby, 1997
58. DeLancey J: Anatomy of genital support. In: Benson JT, ed: Female Pelvic Floor Disorders, Investigation and Management. New York, WW Norton, 1992
59. DiGiovanna EL, Schiowitz: An Osteopathic Approach to Diagnosis and Treatment. Philadelphia, JB Lippincott, 1991
60. Dorland's Illustrated Medical Dictionary, 27th ed. Philadelphia, WB Saunders, 1985:130
61. Dunbar A: Physical therapy management of uterine prolapse. J Obstet Gynecol Phys Ther 17:3–11, 1993
62. Dvorak J, Dvorak V: Manual Medicine: Diagnostic. New York, Thieme Medical, 1990
63. Edward BC: Combined movements of the lumbar spine: Examination and significance. Aus J Physiother 25:147–152, 1979
64. Edward BC: Combined movements in the lumbar spine: Their use in examination and treatment. In: Grieve GP, ed: Modern Manual Therapy of the Vertebral Column. New York, 1986:561–566
65. Edward BC: Clinical assessment: The use of combined movements in assessment and treatment. In: Twomey LT, Taylor JR, ed: Physiotherapy of the Low Back. New York, Churchill Livingstone, 1987:175–198
66. Einhorn AR, Mandras M, Sawyer M, et al: Evaluation and treatment of the shoulder. In: Brownstein B, Bronner S, eds: Evaluation, Treatment, and Outcomes: Functional Movement in Orthopedic and Sports Physical Therapy. New York, Churchill Livingstone, 1995:89–139
67. Ellis JJ, Johnson GS: Myofascial considerations in somatic dysfunction of the thorax. In: Flynn TW: The Thoracic Spine and Rib Cage: Musculoskeletal Evaluation and Treatment. Boston, Butterworth-Heinemann, 1996:211–262
68. Elvey R: Treatment of arm pain associated with abnormal brachial plexus tension. Aust J Physiother 32:225–230, 1986
69. Elvey R: Commentary: Treatment of pain associated with abnormal brachial plexus tension. In: Maher C, ed: Adverse neural tension revisited. Melbourne, Australian Physiotherapy Association, 1998:13–17
70. Elvey R, Hall T: Neural tissue evaluation and treatment. In: Donatelli R, ed: Physical Therapy of the Shoulder, 3rd ed. New York, Churchill Livingstone, 1997:132–152
71. Evjenth O, Hamberg J: Muscle Stretching in Manual Therapy: A Clinical Manual, vol. I: The Extremities. Sweden, Alfta Rehab Forlag, 1984
72. Evjenth O, Hamberg J: Muscle Stretching in Manual Therapy: A Clinical Manual, vol. II: The Spinal Column and the TMJ Joint. Sweden, Alfta Rehab Forlag, 1984
73. Evjenth O, Hamberg J: Autostretching. Sweden, Alfta Rehab Forlag, 1997
74. Fairbank JCT, O'Brien JP: The Abdominal Cavity and Thoracolumbar Fascia as Stabilizer of the Lumbar Spine in Patients with Low Back Pain, vol. 2. Engineering Aspects of the Spine. New York, Mechanical Engineering, 1980:83–88
75. Farfan HF: Mechanical Disorders of the Lumbar Spine. Philadelphia, Lea & Febiger, 1973
76. Farfan HF: Muscular mechanism of the lumbar spine and the position of power and efficiency. Orthrop Clin North Am 6:135–144, 1975
77. Fredin Y, Elert J, Britchgi N, et al: A decreased ability to relax between repetitive muscle contractions in patients with chronic symptoms after whiplash trauma to the neck. J Musculoskel Pain 5:55–70, 1997
78. Fryette HH: Principles of Osteopathic Technique. Carmel, American Academy of Osteopathy, 1954
79. Fulkerson JP: Awareness of the retinaculum in evaluating patellofemoral pain. Am J Sports Med 10:147–149, 1982
80. Fulkerson JP: The etiology of patellofemoral pain in young patients: A protective study. Clin Orthop 179:129–133, 1983
81. Fulkerson JP, Hungerford D: Disorders of the Patellofemoral Joint. Baltimore, Williams & Wilkins, 1990
82. Gardner E: Muscular system. In: Gardner E, Gray DJ, O'Rahilly R, eds: Anatomy: A Regional Study of Human Structure, 4th ed. Philadelphia, WB Saunders, 1978
83. Gauthier GF: Skeletal muscle fiber types. In: Engel AG, Banker BQ, eds: Myology. New York: McGraw-Hill, 1986:225–284
84. Geiringer SR, Kincaid CB, Rechtien JJ: Traction, Manipulations, and Massage. In: Delisa JA, ed: Rehabilitation Medicine: Principles and Practice. Philadelphia, JB Lippincott, 1988
85. Giallonardo LM: Posture. In: Sgarlat Meyer R, ed: Saunders Manual of Physical Therapy. Philadelphia, WB Saunders, 1995:1087–1103
86. Giles LGF, Harvey AR: Immunohistochemical demonstration of nociceptors in the capsule and synovial folds of human zygapophyseal joints. Br J Rheumatol 26:362–364, 1987
87. Goodman CC, Synder TE: Differential Diagnosis in Physical Therapy, 2nd ed. Philadelphia, WB Saunders, 1995
88. Goodridge JP: Muscle energy technique: Definition, explanation, methods of procedure. J Am Osteopath Assoc 81:249–254, 1981
89. Goss CM: Gray's Anatomy, 29th ed. Philadelphia, Lea & Febiger, 1973
90. Gould JA: The spine. In: Gould JA, Davies GJ, eds: Orthopedics and Sports Physical Therapy, 2nd ed. St. Louis, CV Mosby, 1985:518–549
91. Gracovetsky S: The Spinal Engine. Springer-Verlag, New York, 1988
92. Gracovetsky S, Farfan HF: The optimum spine. Spine 11:543–573, 1986
93. Gracovetsky S, Farfan HF, Lamy C: The mechanism of the lumbar spine. Spine 6:249–262, 1981
94. Greenfield BH, ed: Rehabilitation of the Knee: A Problem Solving Approach. Philadelphia, FA Davis, 1993
95. Greenman PE, ed: Concepts and Mechanisms of Neuromuscular Function. New York, Springer-Verlag, 1984
96. Greenman PE: Principles of Manual Therapy, 2nd ed. Baltimore, Williams & Wilkins, 1996
97. Greenstein GM: Clinical Assessment of Neuromuscular Disorders. St. Louis, Mosby, 1997
98. Gregor RJ: The structure and function of skeletal muscle. In: Rasch PJ, ed: Kinesiology and Applied Anatomy, 7th ed. Philadelphia, Lea & Febiger, 1989:32–47
99. Grieve GP: Mobilization of the Spine. A Primary Handbook of Clinical Method, 5th ed. Edinburgh, Churchill Livingstone, 1991
100. Grodin A, Cantu R: Myofascial Manipulation: Theory and Clinical Management. Berry, VA, Forum Medicum, 1989
101. Grodin A, Cantu R: Soft tissue mobilization. In: Basmajian JV, Nyberg R, eds: Principles of Manual Therapy. Baltimore, Williams & Wilkins, 1993:199–221
102. Gunn CC, Milbrandt WE: Tenderness at motor points: An aid in diagnosis of pain in the shoulder referred from the cervical spine. J Am Osteopath Assoc 77:196–175, 212–219, 1977
103. Gunn CC, Milbrandt WE: Early and subtle sings in low back pain. Spine 3:267–282, 1978
104. Guyton AC: Textbook of Medical Physiology, 7th ed. Philadelphia, Lea & Febiger, 1989
105. Hall CM, Brody LT: Therapeutic Exercise: Moving Toward Function. Philadelphia, Lippincott Williams & Wilkins, 1998
106. Hall TM, Elvey RL: Evaluation and treatment of neural tissue pain disorders. In: Donatelli RA, Wooden MJ, eds: Orthopaedic Physical Therapy, 3rd ed; New York, Churchill Livingstone, 2001:618–639
107. Hall TM, Zusman M, Elvey RL: Adverse mechanical tension in the nervous system? Analysis of straight leg raise. Man Ther 3:140–146, 1998
108. Ham A, Cormack D: Histology. Philadelphia, Lippincott, 1979
109. Hammer WI: Functional Soft Tissue Examination and Treatment by Manual Methods: The Extremities. Gaithersburg, Aspen, 1994
110. Hanlon WH: Taproots: Underlying Principles of Milton Erickson's Therapy and Hypnosis. New York, WW Norton, 1987
111. Hartley A: Practical Joint Assessment: Lower Quadrant, 2nd ed. St. Louis, Mosby, 1995

112. Henry JA: Manual therapy of the shoulder. In: Kelly MJ, Clark WA, eds: Orthopedic Therapy of the Shoulder. Philadelphia, JB Lippincott, 1995:285–336

113. Henry JH: The patellofemoral joint. In: Nicholas JA, Hershmann EB, eds: The Lower Extremity and Spine in Sports Medicine. St. Louis, CV Mosby, 1986:1013–1054

114. Hides JA, Stokes MJ, Saide M, et al: Evidence of lumbar multifidus muscle wasting ipsilateral to symptoms in patients with acute/subacute low back pain. Spine 19:21–27, 1994

115. Hochaday JM, Whitty WM: Patterns of referred pain in the normal subject. Brain 90:481–496, 1967

116. Hollinshead WH: Functional Anatomy of the Limbs and Back: A Textbook for Students of the Locomotor Apparatus. Philadelphia, Saunders, 1976

117. Hodges P, Richardson C: Contraction of the transversus abdominus invariably precedes upper limb movement. Exp Brain Res 114:362–370, 1997

118. Hubbard DR, Berkoff GM: Myofascial trigger points show spontaneous EMG activity. Spine 18:1803–1807, 1993

119. Indahl A, Kaigle AM, Reikeras O, et al: Interaction between the porcine lumbar intervertebral disk, zygapophyseal joints and paraspinal muscles. Spine 22:2834–2840, 1997

120. Institute for Gravitational Strain Pathology. The Jungmann Concept and Technique of Antigravity Leverage, 2nd ed. (revised). Rangeley, Maine Printing Exchange, 1992

121. Janda V: Die bedeutung der muskularen fehlhaltung als pathogenetischer faktor vertebraler stoerungen. Arch Phys Ther 20:113–116, 1968

122. Janda V: Muscles, central nervous motor regulation and back problems. In: Korr I, ed: The Neurobiologic Mechanism in Manipulative Therapy, New York, Plenum Press, 1978:27

123. Janda V: Muscle Function Testing. London, Butterworths, 1983

124. Janda V: Muscle weakness and inhibition (pseudoparesis) in back pain syndromes. In: Grieve GP, ed: Modern Manual Therapy of the Vertebral Column. Edinburg, Churchill Livingstone, 1986

125. Janda V: Differential diagnosis of muscle tone in respect of inhibitory techniques. In: Patterson JK, Burn L, eds: Back Pain, an International Review. Boston, Kluwer, Drodrecht, 1990

126. Janda V: Muscle spasm–A proposed procedure for differential diagnosis. Man Med 6:136–139, 1991

127. Janda V: Muscle strength in relation to muscle length: pain and muscle imbalance. In: Harms-Rindahl K, ed: Muscle Strength. New York, Churchill Livingstone, 1993

128. Janda V: Muscle and motor control in cervicogenic disorders: Assessment and management. In: Grant R, ed: Physical Therapy for Cervical and Thoracic Spine, 2nd ed. Edinburgh, Churchill Livingstone, 1994:195–216

129. Janda V: Evaluation of muscular imbalance. In: Liebensen C, ed: Rehabilitation of the Spine: A Practitioner's Manual. Baltimore, Williams & Wilkins, 1996:97–112

130. Johnson GS: Soft tissue mobilization. In: Donatelli R, Wooden MJ, eds: Orthopaedic Physical Therapy, 2nd ed. New York, Churchill Livingstone 1994: 697–756.

131. Johnson GS: Soft tissue mobilization. In: Donatelli R, Wooden MJ, eds: Orthopaedic Physical Therapy, 3rd ed. New York, Churchill Livingstone, 2001:150–156

132. Johansson H, Sojka P: Pathophysiological mechanisms involved in genesis and spread of muscular tension in occupational muscle pain and in chronic musculoskeletal pain syndromes: A hypothesis. Med Hypotheses 35:196–303, 1990

133. Jones LH: Strain and Counterstrain. Newark, OH, American Academy of Osteopathy, 1981

134. Jones LH, Kudunose R, Goering E: Jones Strain-Counterstrain. Boise, Jones Strain-Counterstrain, 1995

135. Jones SL, Bates BT, Osternig LR: Injuries to runners. Am J Sports Med 6:40–50, 1978

136. Jull GA, Janda V: Muscles and motor control in low back pain. In: Twomey LT, Taylor JR, eds: Physical Therapy of the Low Back. New York, Churchill Livingstone, 1987:253–278

137. Jull G, Richardson C: Rehabilitation of active stabilization of the lumbar spine. In: Twomey L, Taylor JR, eds: Physical Therapy of the Low Back, 2nd ed. New York, Churchill Livingstone, 1994:251–274

138. Jull G, Richardson C, Toppenberg R, et al: Towards a measurement of active muscle control for lumbar stabilization. Aust J Physiother 36:6–11, 1990

139. Jungmann M, McClure CW: Backaches, postural decline, aging and gravity-strain. Proceedings of the New York Academy of General Practice, New York City, October 17, 1963

140. Katz R, Rymer Z: Spastic hypertonia: Mechanisms and measurement. Arch Phys Med Rehabil 70:144–155, 1989

141. Kendall HO, Kendall FP, Boynton DA: Posture and Pain. Huntington, NY, Robert E. Kreiger, 1970

142. Kendall HO, McCreary EK, Provance PT: Muscles Testing and Function, 4th ed. Baltimore, Williams & Wilkins, 1993.

143. Kenneally M, Rubenach H, Elvey R: The upper limb tension test: The SLR test of the arm. In: Grant R, ed: Physical Therapy of the Cervical and Thoracic Spine. Edinburgh, Churchill Livingstone, 1998:167–194

144. Kennedy CN: The cervical spine. In: Hall CM, Thein Brody L, eds: Therapeutic Exercise: Moving Toward Function. Philadelphia, Lippincott Williams & Wilkins, 1998:525–548

145. Kimberly PE, ed: Somatic Dysfunction: Principles of Manipulative Treatment and Procedures. Kirksville, MO, Kirksville College of Osteopathic Medicine, 1980

146. Kisner C, Colby LA: Therapeutic Exercise: Foundations and Techniques, 3rd ed. Philadelphia, FA Davis, 1996

147. Klein-Vogelback S: Functional kinetics: Observing, Analyzing and Teaching Human Movement. Berlin, Springer-Verlag, 1990

148. Knott M, Voss DE: Proprioceptive Neuromuscular Facilitation. New York, Hoeber, 1968

149. Korr I: Spinal cord as organizer of the disease process. 1976 Yearbook of the Academy of Applied Osteopathy, 1977

150. Korr IM, Wright HM, Thomas PE: Effects of experimental myofascial insults on cutaneous patterns of sympathetic activity in man. Neurol Transm 23:330–355, 1962

151. Kraftsow G: Yoga for Wellness. Healing with Timeless Teachings of Viniyoga. New York, Penguin Books, 1999

152. Kuchera ML: Tavell's myofascial trigger points. In: Ward R, ed: Foundations for Osteopathic Medicine. Baltimore, Williams & Wilkins, 1997

153. Kuchera ML: Treatment of gravitational strain pathophysiology. In: Vleeming A, Mooney V, Dorman T, et al., eds: Movement, Stability & Low Back Pain: The Essential Role of the Pelvis. New York, Churchill Livingstone, 1997

154. Kusunose R: Strain and counterstrain. In: Basmajian JV, Nyberg R, eds: Rational Manual Therapy. Baltimore, Williams & Wilkins, 1993:323–333

155. Lee D: Manual Therapy for the Thorax. British Columbia, Delta, 1994

156. Lee D, Walsh CM: A Workbook of Manual Therapy Techniques for the Vertebral Column and Pelvic Girdle. Delta, BC, Nascent Publishing, 1991

157. Lentill G, Hetherington T, Eagan J, et al: The use of thermal agents to influence the effectiveness of a low-load prolonged stretch. J Orthop Sports Phys Ther 5:200–207, 1992

158. Lewis T, Kellgren JH: Observation related to referred pain, visceromotor reflexes and other associated phenomena. Clin Sci 4:47–71, 1939

159. Lewit K: Manipulative Therapy in Rehabilitation of the Motor System. London, Butterworth, 1985

160. Lewit K: Manipulative Therapy in Rehabilitation of the Motor System, 2nd ed. London, Butterworth, 1991

161. Lieber RL: Skeletal muscle structure and function. Baltimore, Williams & Wilkins, 1992

162. Lieberson C, ed: Rehabilitation of the Spine: A Practical Manual. Philadelphia, Williams & Wilkins, 1996

163. Linder HH: Clinical Anatomy. Norwalk, Appleton & Lange, 1989

164. Ludlow CL, Naunton RF, Sedory SE, et al: Effects of botulism toxin injections on speech in adductor spasmodic dysphonia. Neurology 38:1220–1225, 1988

165. MacConaill MA, Basmajian JV: Muscles and Movement. Baltimore, Williams & Wilkins, 1969

166. Magee DJ: Orthopedic Physical Assessment, 3rd ed. Philadelphia, WB Saunders, 1997

167. Maigne R: Orthopaedic Medicine. Springfield, Charles C. Thomas, 1972

168. Maigne R: La semeiolgie clinique des derangements intervertebraus mineurs. Ann Med Physique 15:275–292, 1972

169. Maigne R: Fondamenos fisiopatologicos de la manipulacion vertebral. Rehaiblitacion 4:427–422, 1976

170. Maigne R: Orthopedic Medicine: A New Approach to Vertebral Manipulations. Springfield, Charles C. Thomas, 1976

171. Maigne R: Dolleurs d'origine vertebrale et traitements par manipulations (les derangements intervertebraux mineurs), 3rd ed. Paris, Expansion Scientifique, 1978

172. Maigne R: Manipulations of the spine. In: Rogoff JB, ed: Manipulation, Traction and Massage. Baltimore, Williams & Wilkins, 1980:59–120

173. Maigne R, Le Corre F: Sur l'origine cervicale de certaines dorsalgies rebeles et benignes. Ann Med Phys 1:1–18, 1964

174. Maitland G: Vertebral Manipulations, 5th ed. London, Butterworths, 1986

175. Mangine R, Heckman T: The knee. In: Sanders B, ed: Sports Physical Therapy. Norwalk, Appleton & Lange, 1990:423–450

176. Manheim CJ: Myofascial Release Manual, 2nd ed. Thorofare, Slack, 1994

177. Manheim CJ: Myofascial Release Manual, 3rd ed. Thorofare, Slack, 2001

178. Mannheimer JS, Lampe GN: Clinical Transcutaneous Electrical Nerve Stimulation, Philadelphia, FA Davis, 1984

179. Marshall JL, Girgis FG, Zelko RR: The biceps femoris tendon and its functional significance. AM J Bone Joint Surg 54:1444–1450, 1972

180. Massery M: Respiratory rehabilitation secondary to neurological deficits: Understanding the deficits. In: Frownfelter DL, ed: Chest Physical Therapy and Pulmonary Rehabilitation, 2nd ed. Chicago, New Book, 1987:499–528

181. McKinnis DL: The posture-movement dynamic. In: Richardson JK, Iglarsh ZA, eds: Clinical Orthopedic Physical Therapy. Philadelphia, WB Saunders, 1994

182. McLain RF: Mechanoreceptor endings in human facet joints. Spine 19:495–501, 1994

183. McLain RF: Mechanoreceptor endings of the cervical, thoracic and lumbar spine. Iowa Orthop J 15:145–155, 1995

184. McMorris RO: Faulty posture. Pediatr Clin North Am 8:213–224, 1961

185. Meagher J: Sports massage. Barrytown, Station Hill Press, 1990
186. Menachem A, Kaplan O, Dekel S: Levator scapulae syndrome: An anatomic clinical study. Bull Hosp Joint Dis 53:21–24, 1993
187. Mendel T, Wink CS, Zinny ML: Neural elements in human intervertebral discs. Spine 17:132–135, 1992
188. Mennell JB: Physical Treatment by Movement, Manipulation, and Massage, 5th ed. Philadelphia, Blakiston, 1947
189. Mensendieck B: It's Up to You. New York, JJ Little & Ives, 1931
190. Mensendieck B: Mensendieck System of Functional Exercises. Portland ME, Shorthwork, Anthoesen Press, 1937
191. Meyer K: Mucopolysaccharides and connective tissue. Verth Dtsch Ges Rheumatol Suppl 2:5–9, 1972
192. Meyer RA, Campbell JN, Raja SN: Peripheral neural mechanisms of nociception. In: Wall P, Melzack R, eds: The Textbook of Pain, 3rd ed. New York, Churchill Livingstone, 1997:13–44
193. Micheli AA, Eisenberg J: Scapulocostal syndrome. Arch Phys Med Rehabil 49:383–387, 1968
194. Miller B: Manual therapy treatment of myofascial pain and dysfunction. In: Rachlin ES, ed: Myofascial Pain and Fibromyalgia. St. Louis, CV Mosby, 1994:415–454
195. Mitchell FL Jr, Moran PS, Pruzzo NA: An Evaluation and Treatment Manual of Osteopathic Muscle Energy Procedures. Valley Park, MO, Mitchell, Moran, and Pruzzo, 1979
196. Moore KL: Clinically Oriented Anatomy, 3rd ed. Baltimore, Williams & Wilkins, 1992
197. Muhlemann D, Cimino JA: Therapeutic muscle stretching. In: Hammer WI, ed: Functional Soft Tissue Examination and Treatment by Manual Methods. Gaithersburg, Aspen, 1991
198. Mundale MO, Hislop HJ, Rabideau RJ, et al: Evaluation of extension of the hip. Arch Phys Med Rehabil 37:75–80, 1956
199. Murry DR: Hyperalgesic skin zones: A case report. Chiro Tech 4:124–127, 1992
200. Murry DR: The seven types of hypertonicity of muscle. J Myofasc Ther 1:33–36, 1995
201. Murry DR: Conservative Management of Cervical Spine Syndromes. New York, McGraw–Hill, 2000
202. Nicholson GG, Clendaniel RA: Manual techniques. In: Scully RM, Barnes MR, eds: Physical Therapy, Philadelphia, JB Lippincott, 1989:926–985
203. Noble CA: Iliotibial band friction syndrome in runners. Br J Sports Med 8:232–234, 1980
204. Noble HB, Hajek HR, Porter M: The iliotibial band friction syndrome. Br J Sportsmed 10:67–74, 1982
205. Noble HB, Hajek HR, Porter M: Diagnosis and treatment of iliotibial band tightness in runners. Phys Sports Med 10:67–74, 1982
206. Norkin CC, Levangie PK: Joint Structure & Function: A Comprehensive Analysis, 2nd ed. Philadelphia, FA Davis, 1992
207. Norris C: Sports Injuries: Diagnosis and Management for Physiotherapists. Oxford, Butterworth-Heinemann, 1993
208. Norris C: Spinal stabilization. 3. Stabilization mechanism of the lumbar spine. Phys Ther 81:72–79, 1995
209. Nyberg GF: Pelvic girdle. In: Payton OD, ed: Manual of Physical Therapy. New York, Churchill Livingstone, 1989:363–382
210. O'Neill DR, Micheli LJ, Warner JP: Patellofemoral stress: A prospective analysis of exercise treatment in adolescents and adults. Am J Sports Med 20:151–156,1992
211. Ormandy L: Scapulocostal syndrome. VA Med Q 121:105–108, 1994
212. O'Sullivan SB: Motor control assessment. In: O'Sullivan SB, Schmitz TJ, eds: Physical Rehabilitation: Assessment and Treatment, 3rd ed. Philadelphia, FA Davis, 1994:111–131
213. Palmar ML, Epler M: Clinical Assessment Procedures in Physical Therapy, 2nd ed. Philadelphia, JB Lippincott, 1998
214. Paris SV: Clinical decision making: Orthopaedic physical therapy. In: Wolf SL, ed: Clinical Decision Making in Physical Therapy. Philadelphia, FA Davis, 1985:215–254
215. Paris SV: Differential diagnosis of lumbar and pelvic pain. In: Vleeming A, Mooney V, Snijders CJ, et al.: Movement Stability and Low Back Pain: The Essential Role of the Pelvis. New York, Churchill Livingstone, 1997
216. Peacock E, VanWinkel W: Wound Repair, 2nd ed. Philadelphia, WB Saunders, 1976
217. Phelps, WM, Kiphuth RJ, Goff CW: The Diagnosis and Treatment of Postural Defects, 2nd ed. Springfield, Charles C. Thomas, 1956
218. Platzer W: Color Atlas and Textbook of Human Anatomy, vol. 1: Locomotor System. Stuttgart, Georg Thieme, 1978
219. Porterfield JA: The SIJ. In: Gould J, ed: Orthopaedic and Sports Physical Therapy. St. Louis, CV Mosby, 1985
220. Porterfield JA, DeRosa C: Mechanical Neck Pain: Perspective in Functional Anatomy. Philadelphia, WB Saunders, 1995
221. Porterfield JA, DeRosa C: Mechanical Low Back Pain. Perspectives in Functional Anatomy, 2nd ed. Philadelphia, WB Saunders, 1998
222. Pratt NE: Clinical Musculoskeletal Anatomy. Philadelphia, JB Lippincott, 1991
223. Puniello MS: Iliotibial band tightness and medial patellar glide in patients with patellofemoral dysfunction. J Orthop Sports Phys Ther 17:144–148. 1993
224. Reed ES: Changing theories of postural development. In: Woollacott MH, Shumway-Cook A, eds: Development of Posture and Gait Analysis Across the Life Span. Columbia, University of South Carolina Press, 1989
225. Renne JW: The iliotibial band friction syndrome: J Bone Joint Surg Am 57:1110–1111, 1975
226. Richardson C, Jull G, Hodges P, et al: Therapeutic Exercise for Spinal Segmental Stabilization in Low Back Pain: Scientific Basis and Clinical Approach. Edinburgh, Churchill Livingstone, 1999
227. Richardson C, Toppenberg R, Jull G: An initial evaluation of eight abdominal exercises for their ability to provide stabilization for the lumbar spine. Aust J Physiother 36:6–11, 1990
228. Rocobado M: Biomechanical relationship of the cranial cervical and hyoid region. J Craniomandib Pract 1:61–66, 1983
229. Rocabado M, Iglarsh ZA: Musculoskeletal Approach to Maxillo-Facial Pain. Philadelphia, JB Lippincott, 1991
230. Rolf IP: Rolfing: The Integration of Human Structures, Santa Monica, Denis–Landman, 1977
231. Rowlerson A, Pope B, et al: A novel myosin present in cat jaw closing muscles. J Muscle Res Cell Motil 2:415–438, 1981
232. Rudolph R: Contraction and control of contraction. World J Surg 4:279–287, 1980
233. Rywerant Y: Feldenkrais Method. San Francisco, Harper & Row, 1983
234. Saal JS: Flexibility training. In: Saal JS, ed: Rehabilitation of Sports Injuries. Philadelphia, Hanley & Belfus, 1987
235. Sahrmann S: Diagnosis and Treatment of Muscle Imbalances and Associated Regional Pain Syndromes. Course notes, St. Louis, Washington University, 1992
236. Sahrmann SA: Diagnosis and Treatment of Movement Impairment Syndromes. Course outline. St. Louis, Washington University, 1998
237. Sahrmann SA: Diagnosis and Treatment of Movement Impairment Syndromes. St. Louis, Mosby, 2001
238. Saidoff DC, McDonough AL: Critical Pathways in Therapeutic Intervention: Upper Extremity. St. Louis, Mosby, 1997
239. Saliba VI, Johnson GS: Lumbar protective mechanism. In: White AH, Anderson R, eds: Conservative Care of Low Back Pain. Baltimore, Williams & Wilkins, 1991:112–119
240. Sanders B, ed: Sports Physical Therapy. Norwalk, Appleton & Lange, 1990
241. Santiesteban AJ: Electromyographic and dynamometric characteristics of female pelvic floor musculature. Phys Ther 68:344–350, 1988
242. Sapega A, Quedenfeld T, Moyer R, et al: Biophysical factors in range of motion exercise. Phys Sports Med 9:57–65, 1981
243. Saudek CE: The hip. In: Gould JA, ed: Orthopedic and Sports Physical Therapy. St. Louis, CV Mosby, 1990
244. Schafer RC: Clinical Biomechanics: Musculoskeletal Actions and Reactions. Baltimore, Williams & Wilkins, 1983
245. Schneider MJ: Principles of Manual Trigger Point Therapy. Self-published, 1994
246. Schneider W, Dvorak J, Dvorak V, et al: Manual Medicine Therapy. New York, Thieme Medical, 1988
247. Schultz RL, Feitis R: The Endless Web: Fascial Anatomy and Physical Reality. Berkeley, North Atlantic Books 1996
248. Schussler B, Laycock J, Nortin P, et al., eds: Pelvic Floor Re-Education Principle and Practice. New York, Springer-Verlag, 1994
249. Seaman DR, Winterstein JF: Dysafferentation: A novel term to describe the neuropathophysiological effects of joint complex dysfunction. A look at likely mechanism of symptom generation. J Manipulative Physiol Ther 21:267–280, 1998
250. Shacklock M: Neurodynamics. Physiotherapy 1:9–16, 1995
251. Shacklock M: Case study: Positive upper limb tension test in a case of surgically proven neuropathy: Analysis and validity. Man Ther 1:154–161, 1996
252. Simons DG: Myofascial pain syndrome due to trigger points. In: Goodgold J, ed: Rehabilitation Medicine. St. Louis, Mosby, 1988
253. Simons DG: Hong CY, Simons LS: Prevalence of spontaneous electrical activity at trigger spots and at control sites in rabbit skeletal muscle. J Musculoskel Pain 3:35–48, 1995
254. Simons DG, Mense S: Understanding and measurement of muscle tone as related to clinical muscle pain. Pain 75:1–18, 1998
255. Smith SS: Musculoskeletal analysis: The lumbar spine and lumbopelvic region. In: Scully RM, Barnes MR, eds: Physical Therapy. Philadelphia, JB Lippincott, 1989:438–464
256. Sola AE, Williams RL: Myofascial pain syndromes. Neurol 6:91–95, 1956
257. Spring H, Illi U, Kunz HR, et al: Stretching and Strengthening Exercises. New York, Thieme Medical, 1991
258. Stoddard A: Manual of Osteopathic Technique. London, Hutchinson. 1978
259. Stoddard A: Manual of Osteopathic Practice. London, Hutchinson, 1978
260. Stokes M, Young A: The contribution of reflex inhibition to arthrogenous muscle weakness. Clin Sci 67:7–14, 1989
261. Sullivan PE, Markos PD: Clinical Decision-Making in Therapeutic Exercise. Norwalk, Appleton & Lange, 1994
262. Suseki K, Takahashi Y, Takahashi K et al: Innervation of the lumbar facet joints: Origins and functions. Spine 22(5): 477–485, 1997
263. Sutton GS, Bartel MR: Soft-tissue mobilization techniques for the hand. J Hand Ther 7:185–192, 1994

264. Tappan FM, Benjamin PR: Tappan's Handbook of Healing Massage Techniques: Classic, Holistic, and Emerging Methods. Stamford, Appleton & Lange, 1998
265. Tarsy JM: Pain Syndromes and Their Treatment. Springfield, Charles C. Thomas, 1953
266. Taylor T, Tole G, Vernon H: Skin rolling technique as an indicator of spinal dysfunction. Chiro Assoc 34:82–86, 1990
267. Terry GC, Hughston JC, Norwood LA: The anatomy of the iliopatellar band and the iliotibial tract. Am J Sports Med 14:39–45, 1986
268. Tesh JH, Evans J, Shawdunn J, et al: The mechanical interaction between the thoracolumbar fascia and the connective tissue of the posterior spine. In: Buerger AA, Greenman PE, eds: Empirical Approach to the Validation of Spinal Manipulation. Springfield, Charles C. Thomas, 1985
269. Todd ME: The Thinking Body, Brooklyn, Dance Horizons, 1979
270. Travell JG, Simons DG: Myofascial Pain and Dysfunction: The Trigger Point Manual. Baltimore, Williams & Wilkins, 1983
271. Travell JG, Simons DG: Myofascial Pain and Dysfunction: The Lower Extremities, vol. 2. Baltimore, Williams & Wilkins, 1992
272. Travell JG, Simons DG, Simons LS: Myofascial Pain and Dysfunction: The Trigger Point Manual, vol. 1: Upper Half of the Body, 2nd ed. Baltimore, Williams & Wilkins, 1999
273. Vasilyeva LF, Lewit K: Diagnosis of muscular dysfunction by inspection. In: Liebenson C, ed: Rehabilitation of the Spine. Philadelphia, Lippincott Williams & Wilkins, 1996
274. Vleeming A, Pool-Goudzwaard AL, Stoeckkhart R, et al: The posterior layer of the thoracolumbar fascia: Its function in load transfer from spine to legs. Spine 20:753–758, 1995
275. Wallace KA: Pelvic floor muscle dysfunction and its behavioral treatment. In: Agostini R, ed: Medical and Orthopedic Issues of Active and Athletic Women. Philadelphia, Hanely & Belfus, 1994:200–212
276. Walters PM, Millis MB: Hip and pelvic injuries in the young athlete. Clin Sports Med 7:513–526, 1988
277. Warwick R, Williams PL, eds: Gray's Anatomy 37th ed. Edinburgh, Churchill Livingstone, 1989
278. Weisel S: Manual Therapy with Muscle Energy Technique: For the Pelvis, Sacrum, Cervical, Thoracic & Lumbar Spine. East Hamstead, NH Northeast Seminars, 1994
279. Weiselfish S: Developmental Manual Therapy for Physical Rehabilitation for the Neurologic Patient: A Learner's Manual. East Hamstead, NH Northeast Seminars, 1994
280. White AA, Panjabi MM: Clinical Biomechanics of the Spine, 2nd ed., Philadelphia, JB Lippincott, 1990
281. White SS: Musculoskeletal analysis: The lumbar spine and lumbopelvic region. In: Scully RM, Barnes MR, eds: Physical Therapy. Philadelphia, JB Lippincott, 1984:438–464
282. Whitnall SE: The Study of Anatomy, 4th ed. London, Arnold, 1939
283. Wilke I-IJ, Wolf S, Clase LE, et al: Stability increase of the lumbar spine with different muscle groups: A biomechanical in vitro study. Spine 20:192–198,1995
284. Williams M, Worthingham C: Therapeutic Exercise for Body Alignment and Function, 2nd ed. Philadelphia, WB Saunders, 1977
285. Williams PE, Goldspink G: Changes in sarcomere length and physiological properties in immobilized muscle. J Anat 127:459–468, 1978
286. Woo SLY, Gomez MA, Woo YK, et al: II. Mechanical properties of tendon and ligaments. The relationship of immobilization and exercise on tissue remodeling. Biorheology 19:397–408, 1982
287. Wood J: Aston-Patterning: Recognizing individuality: A whole person approach. Massage & Bodywork, Winter:80–82, 1997
288. Woodburne RT: Essentials of Human Anatomy, 4th ed. London, Oxford University Press, 1969
289. Wyke B: Neurology of the cervical spinal joints. J Physiother 65:73–76, 1979
290. Young RR, Wiegner AW: Spasticity. Clin Orthop 219:50–62, 1987
291. Young A, Stokes M, Iles JF: Effect of joint pathology on muscle. Clin Orthop Rel Res 219:21–27, 1987
292. Zoppi M, Chrubasik S: Neural control of joint pain. Rheum Pain Feb:2–8, 1997
293. Zoten DJ, Clancy WG, Keene JS: A new operative approach to snapping hip and refractory trochanteric bursitis in athletes. Am J Sports Med 14:201–204, 1986

SYSTEMS OF SOFT TISSUE MANIPULATIONS

Over the past two decades interest in soft tissue manipulations procedures has dramatically increased.[6,7,10,11,65,69,70,83,97,122,172,216,277,278,302,311,343,425,429–432,448,488] From a historical perspective many of the current soft tissue approaches used by clinicians have been adapted from traditional orthopedic massage,[91–95,190,297–301] osteopathic methods,[69–73,108,151,308,411,412] physical therapy,[20,106,244,291,429–432] massage and muscular therapy,[23–29,499] massage of acupuncture and trigger points,[1,5,12,18,44,48,68,70,71,133,137,147,170,173,176,187,255,265,275,276,277–279,282,283,289,294–296,318–320,332,336,342,348,349,386–388,393–396,430,431,436–440,450–453,455,470,475,489] and specialized systems developed by Dicke (connective tissue massage),[32,49,106,115–118,143,145,191–193,352] Rolf (structural integration or Rolfing),[83–85,343,361–363,382,433] Inghram (foot reflexology),[27,28,44,62,134,188,204,234,238,262,333,335,370,430,431] Hellar (Hellarwork movement),[10,11,177] Aston (Aston patterning)[6,7,67,306,307] Trager (Trager Approach),[221,259,413,448,473,486,487] Vodder (manual lymph drainage),[234,240–242,431,432,488] and others. Types of soft tissue manipulations or mobilizations, considered myofascial in nature, are difficult to pinpoint but basically there are three types: autonomic approaches, mechanical approaches, and movement approaches. Many approaches use a combination of the above.

Autonomic Approaches

The autonomic approaches attempt to exert their effect mainly through the skin and superficial connective tissue.[65,106,115–118]

CLASSIC MASSAGE

Because massage and soft tissue manipulations are interchangeable in concept, the available research on massage's effect on the body needs to be considered. Massage can be defined broadly as the manipulation of the soft tissues, performed with the hands for the purpose of producing a direct or indirect effect on the autonomic, somatic, and central nervous systems; on muscle and connective tissues; and on psychologic states.[179] The therapeutic effects are felt to result in relaxation (local and general), pain relief, increased range of joint and limb motion, stimulation of blood and lymph circulation, and facilitation of healing.[101] Details of the methods, effects, and indications for massage in its various forms have been described in the literature, and only a few general indications and methods are addressed below.[16,72,101,107,131,132,183,184,195,205,264,297,423,429–432]

Stroking and Effleurage. Effleurage is considered synonymous with the term stroking. Effleurage will vary in pressure from slight to firm, which allows tissues to be treated at different levels. Effleurage may be applied firmly and deeply with the greatest possible area of hand contact, to relieve fluid congestion of a body part, but is more often employed as a method of inducing relaxation. Deep effleurage, to the level of the outer layer of investing fascia, can be used to gently elongate and stretch fascia. Both superficial effleurage and deep effleurage may be used as an evaluation tool. Superficial effleurage gives initial information about the skin and superficial muscle groups. Alterations in contour, texture, tone, skin sensitivity, temperature, and elasticity are readily assessed. Deep effleurage stroking and special variations of this stroke, such as skin rolling (see Fig. 7-41) and skin dragging, are useful for identifying specific localized changes in skin, superficial fascia, and specific muscles or segments of muscles both superficial and deep.

Kneading and Petrissage. Kneading and pétrissage are not dissimilar, in that both techniques are directed at improving the tissue–fluid exchange and vascularity (when muscle congestion and hypertonicity are present) and normalizing texture of subcutaneous and deep soft tissue. The various manipulations all have the quality of alternate traction, picking up and relaxing movement of a localized mass of tissue held between one or two hands. In extremely small areas it can be performed by two fingers, or a finger and thumb. Many variations exist in these techniques and methods may be combined with stretching or with inhibitory pressures. Greater effect is produced on the sensory receptor system with the muscle and fascia, which can participate in reflex reduction of neuromuscular hypertonicity and neuromodulation of nociceptor activity than effleurage.[179] (Henry)

INHIBITORY PRESSURES

Muscle tone can be addressed with a wide array of techniques designed to reduce hypertonicity. Hold-relax or contract-relax at minimal levels of activation can be used to eliminate excessive muscle tonus that the patient is often unaware of using owing to sensorimotor amnesia phenomena described by Hanna.[171] Methods of treating localized regions of increased muscle activity (spasms) include perpendicular strumming techniques and sustained pressures. The probable underlying therapeutic mechanism of sustained pressure is by Golgi tendon organ stimulation with resulting reduction of neuromuscular sensitivity to pressure and stretch. Sustained pressure applied into the muscle belly can also produce neuromuscular relaxation, probably by altering the mechanical tension in the gamma spindle loop, which is not accompanied by dynamic change in muscle position or length.[179]

Sustained Pressures. Sustained pressures involve the application of direct pressure to discrete areas of local soft tissue dysfunction, such as tendons, the muscle belly, and origins or insertions of a muscle, for 1 minute or more in a "make and break" manner to reduce hypertonic contraction or for its reflex effect.[73] Sustained pressures works well over broad flat tendons adjacent to or over the osseous junction (e.g., the trapezius and splenius capitis), or muscles such as the psoas major or pectoralis major. Initially, to obtain an environment of comfort, respective tissues are placed on slack by altering the surrounding tissue by positioning and/or by using one hand to place the tissue on slack (Fig. 8-1). Treatment with tissues on slack or the shortened range is followed by treatment in the resting position (neutral) and finally in the lengthened range.[122]

Inhibition can be done effectively in most areas of the lumbar and thoracic spine by using sustained pressure of the fingertips, the palmar surfaces of both thumbs (Fig. 8-2), or the heels of the hands over an area of muscle involvement.[272,411,412] The body part used to apply the sustained pressures will vary depending on the size and depth of the area to be treated. Small superficial regions can be treated with the pad of the thumb or finger whereas deeper and slightly larger regions may require the use of all the knuckles or the elbow (Fig. 8-3). When applied to tendon, sustained pressure is applied with the fingertips directly perpendicular to and into the tendon. Muscle is placed on enough tension to engage the first barrier without additional stretch or the amount of pressure just less than that, which will further increase muscle contraction. As the operator maintains constant pressure (for 60 to 120 seconds), softening of the tissue can be felt indicating neuromuscular relaxation. With relaxation of the muscle, the therapist can apply the pressure at a deeper level by allowing the contact surface to sink through the relaxed muscle.

These techniques can be enhanced by having the patient perform deliberate slow deep breathing with emphasis on long exhalations and with imagery or visualization. The basic technique can be applied with various modifications to increase its

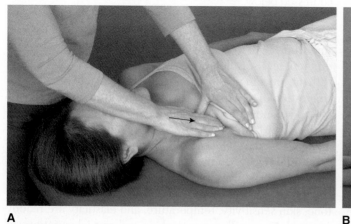
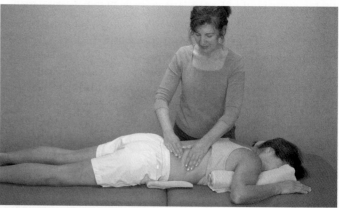

A   **B**

■ **FIG. 8-1.** Sustained pressure of the superficial connective tissue (fascia and underlying tissue) placed on slack with the assisting hand. **(A)** Clavipectoral and **(B)** thoracolumbar fascia.

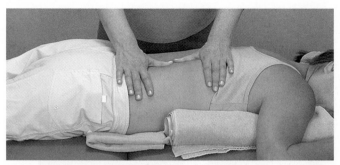

■ **FIG. 8-2.** Sustained pressures using the palmar surface of both thumbs to produce a slow traction of the paravertebral muscles. At end range (barrier) the pressure is released for a while and repeated. This maneuver should be quite rhythmic and continuous without losing contact even during the period of relaxation.

effectiveness. Some options include sustained pressure with oscillation of adjacent body parts and sustained pressure with localized muscle contraction.[232]

One particularly effective application of this technique is in the treatment of the psoas muscle. In many conditions of acute low back pain, sciatic cases, sacroiliac dysfunction, as well as postural dysfunctions, such as significant lumbar lordotic and scoliotic conditions, the iliopsoas is found to be involved with increased tone, limited extensibility, and loss of muscle play.[8,9,72,154,210,298]

Tests for psoas tightness include the Thomas test (see Fig. 14-19) and Michele's test.[303,446] Patients with acute muscle spasm cannot assume these positions. According to Chaitow,[72] x-ray diagnosis is the only sure method to determine psoas contracture. Asymmetric psoas weakness often suggests L1–L3 radiculopathy.[9]

Therapeutic treatment often is directed at the muscle belly. With the patient's abdominal muscles relaxed, the practitioner gently presses posteriorly until the anterior surface of the psoas is contacted (lateral to the fourth to fifth lumbar vertebrae). The psoas can be identified while palpating the muscle belly while the patient gently flexes the ipsilateral hip. While palpating along the muscle, regions of increased muscle activity or tenderness will be noted. Both psoas motor points are tender in psoas dysfunction/insufficiency syndrome (PDIS).[9]

These regions can be effectively treated with sustained pressure techniques following the guideline mentioned previously (Fig. 8-4). Sustained pressure techniques may be effectively combined with gentle active contraction of the muscle or passive leg movement. Following treatment, the psoas muscle should be less painful to palpation and it should display a greater resting length. If PDIS is present and etiologic, following psoas stretch there is a significant increase in range of forward bending.[9] Muscle lengthening, muscle energy, and positional release techniques are also effective methods of treatment. Appropriate texts should be consulted for details of these techniques.

Transverse Strumming. Transverse strumming is a technique used for evaluation and treatment of increased muscle contraction and the loss of muscle play. Transverse strumming employs either specific contacts such as the thumbs, a knuckle, or general contact such as the distal phalanges of the fingers (Fig. 8-5) or the elbow. The technique is applied through repeated rhythmic deformation of the muscle belly. When perpendicular strumming is used in the treatment of involuntary muscle activity, increased tone, or spasms, the strumming is conducted along the muscle belly until the activity is decreased. The frequency and amplitude of the strumming should be large enough so that the rest of the

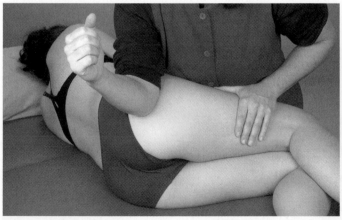

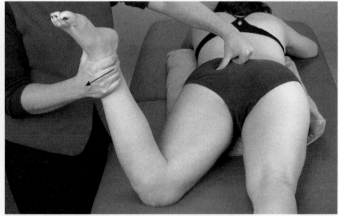

A   **B**

■ **FIG. 8-3.** Sustained pressures using the elbow (olecranon) or palmar surface of the thumb to apply firm pressure with slow circulatory movements concentrated on the area of restriction. **(A)** Elbow pressure to the piriformis. **(B)** Thumb pressure to the piriformis muscle. The stabilizing hand grasps the ankle and internally rotates the hip. Both hands may also work in a pumping motion to massage the piriformis muscle.

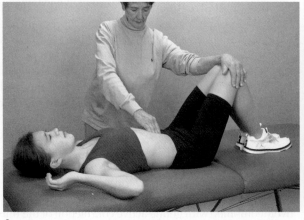

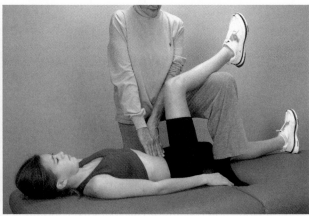

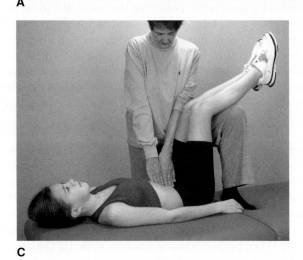

■ **FIG. 8-4.** Sustained pressure to the psoas muscle, with the patient in supine with the (**A**) hips and knees flexed (feet supported on table), (**B**) one leg supported by the operator, or (**C**) both legs supported by the operator.

patient's body oscillates during the treatment thus providing the inherent relaxation qualities of oscillatory motions.[135,216,323]

When used as a treatment technique for loss of muscle play, this technique can be performed either unilaterally or bilaterally. The bilateral technique requires that contact be made on both borders of the muscle belly.[323] The tissues are deformed by the thumbs in one direction and by the fingers in the opposite direction (Fig. 8-6A). It is important to maintain a consistent rhythm with this technique. Although strumming can be used to treat muscle condition, play, and tone simultaneously, subtle variations in how it is performed usually shift the emphasis from one to the other. Strumming can be performed

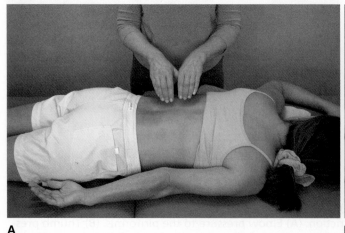

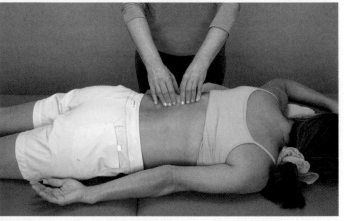

■ **FIG. 8-5.** Perpendicular strumming to the erector spinae. (**A**) Hand position. (**B**) Technique.

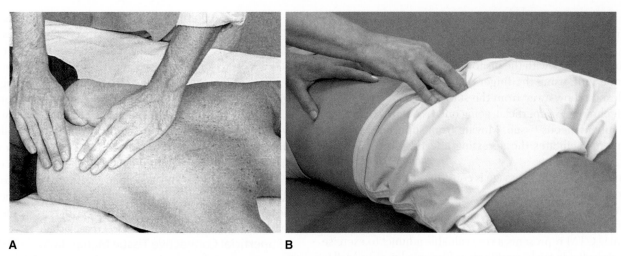

A   **B**

■ **FIG. 8-6.** Myofascial strum release techniques. **(A)** Bilateral strum technique using fingertips and thumbs on both borders of the muscle (erector spinae). **(B)** Small-amplitude parallel or perpendicular strumming to gluteal muscle. (Part A reprinted with permission from Scully RM, Barnes MR: Physical Therapy. Philadelphia, Lippincott, 1989:971.)

softly, as a hypostimulation technique, to mainly reduce tone or it can be performed more vigorously, as a hyperstimulation technique, to produce an irritating response accompanied by reactive production of neuroanalgesic substance.[122] When performed in this manner, both muscle condition and muscle play is affected more. This form of strumming is used as a very deep release (often painful) technique by gradually increasing transverse or longitudinal pressures applied to the restricted muscle site.[277,278] A back and forth scrubbing motion is then used to break loose the deep myofascial restriction applied with a knuckle, elbow, or fingertips. The hand may be cupped and held in a claw-like position as a "windshield wiper motions" are performed with deep pressure parallel or perpendicular to the muscle fiber (Fig. 8-6B).[277,278] These more forceful types of strumming can be used around the knee to release a tight medial retinaculum when abnormal patellar tracking is present, along the erector spinae to break up long standing hypomobility of one or more vertebral segments, and along bony attachments (i.e., ischial tuberosity) to release restricted connective tissue.[277,278]

All the massage techniques and inhibitor methods of evaluation above may be used for their mechanical effect.

CONNECTIVE TISSUE MANIPULATIONS

Connective tissue manipulation (CTM) is one of many systems of soft tissue manipulations that uses reflex effects diagnostically and therapeutically.[32,49,71,101,106,115–118,143,145,191–193,239,429–431] CTM was developed in the 1920s and early 1930s by German physiotherapist Elizabeth Dicke. CTM involves special stroking maneuvers that use short, hooking, and pulling strokes to restore extensibility in the skin and free gliding mobility between the dermis and underlying fascia promoting remodeling of collagen. Strokes can be applied directly in the direction of restriction with short excursion through the plane of the der-

mis. According to Ebner,[118] the palpable reflex tissue changes utilized in diagnosis and treatment in CTM methodology can take any of the following forms:

• Drawn-in bands of tissue
• Flattened areas of tissue
• Elevated areas giving the impression of localized swelling
• Muscle atrophy or hypertrophy
• Osseous deformity of the spinal column

It is suggested that the method's effectiveness is based on the cutaneovisceral reflex, knowledge of which has helped, in part, to explain and lead to the development of many successful therapeutic procedures directed at apparent deeper tissue dysfunction.[72,411,412,451] CTM emphasizes autonomic nervous system reflex interaction of the integumentary system with visceral and organic dysfunction. Treatment of these conditions is thought to be facilitated by correcting superficial connective-tissue changes sustained by sympathetic influences. CTM techniques in this text are only considered for its usefulness in the treatment of localized soft tissue changes manifested as a component of somatic dysfunction. It is most often used when the patient shows signs of being autonomically facilitated or extremely sensitive. For a patient with such symptoms starting with a deep touch is counterproductive.

There are principally three kinds of strokes: (1) pulling, (2) pull and hook on, and (3) widening.[32] Each stroke is performed with the tips of the third and fourth finger of either hand. There are many different ways to perform the strokes depending upon the part of the body for which treatment is desired. The proper stroke in CTM is always a pull on the tissue, never a push. The proper pull requires a well-controlled motion arising in the shoulder and transmitted to the tissues through the arm, hand and fingers. It may be partially steep, flat, or steep. An example described by Cantu and Grodin[65] for the lumbar spine is an excellent means of offering an entryway into deep techniques by quieting the autonomic system. One hand is placed on the patient to stabilize the subcutaneous tissue. The treatment hand uses a flat hand pulling approach, with the pisiform being the axis of motion. A gentle pull, using the finger pads is executed by moving the flexed elbow away from the stabilizing hand (Fig. 8-7). This technique is superficial, going only as deep as the superficial subcutaneous tissue. Moving from superficial to deep treatment facilitates the accessing and treating of deeper myofascial elements.

Connective tissue massage is considered the most important reflex zone massage known.[239] By stimulating the nerve endings of the autonomic nervous system one is offered an entryway into deeper techniques by quieting the autonomic system.[65] CTM represents a very valuable adjunct to exercise and pain relief in such conditions as fibromyalgia[49] and reflex sympathetic dystrophy.[130] It has been widely used to treat signs and symptoms of circulation disorders, respiratory conditions and connective tissue disorders.[101]

Mechanical Approaches: Myofascial Manipulations

Mechanical approaches differ from autonomic approaches in that they primarily seek to make histologic or mechanical changes in the myofascial structures. Many of the autonomic approaches discussed above can be used as mechanical approaches (i.e., transverse strumming techniques).

SKIN AND SUPERFICIAL FASCIA MANIPULATIONS

Examination of the skin and superficial fascia includes evaluation of the mobility of these tissues over the underlying structures (see Chapter 7). Superficial restrictions detected during the palpation examination (e.g., subcutaneous restriction detected during skin rolling) must be treated initially otherwise the treatment of deeper tissues will be painful and inefficient. Treatment of theses superficial restrictions may

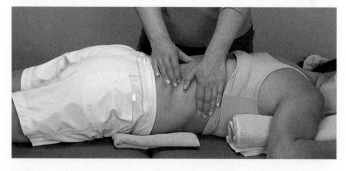

■ **FIG. 8-7.** Connective tissue manipulations showing a superficial hook on type stroke used as an autonomic or reflexive technique. The stroke consists of a tangential pull on the skin and subcutaneous tissues away from the underlying fascia.

be done in several different ways depending upon the severity of the restrictions. The following are a few examples.

J-Stroking[277,278]**.** J-Stroking is similar to CTM, with definite lines of stroking. It is used as a treatment technique for a specific area identified as being restricted and not throughout a generalized area as in CTM. This technique is performed by taking up the slack with the non mobilizing hand which stretches and stabilizes the area around which the mobilizing hand carries out firm "J"-like strokes across the area of restriction with the second and third fingers held against each other for support (Fig. 8-8). The technique is designed with a torque at the end of the motion to twist and work into the restriction. The technique is repeated several times, with reassessment of the tissue mobility performed between each trail.

Superficial Connective Tissue Manipulation[65,122,216,323]**.** The purpose of these techniques is elongation of the superficial connective tissue involving sustained application of low-load force in the superficial plane utilizing a pushing or pulling pressures upon the restriction. Because the subcutaneous tissue is multidirectional in fiber orientation, restrictions may be in any direction and must be determined by examination. Techniques are applied by using one hand or part thereof to apply pressure on the restriction while the other hand assists to facilitate a release. A wide variety of options may be used to apply pressure from one or two digits to the entire palmar surface of the hand. The slack is taken up and held at the motion barrier with one hand until it releases allowing soft tissue deformation to occur. The assisting hand can facilitate a release by placing the skin on slack (Fig. 8-1) or placing the tissue in a position of increased tension by altering the surrounding tissue by proximal stabilization, traction, or lengthening the tissue in the opposite direction (Fig. 8-9).

Other methods of releasing superficial restrictions are considered extension of the examination and include "skin rolling" (see Fig. 7-41), Lewit's[253] skin distraction method (see Fig. 7-43), and skin gliding or fascial glide (see Fig. 7-40).

SOFT TISSUE MANIPULATIONS AROUND BONY PROMINENCES

Common sites for restricted connective tissue is at their attachment to bone. Owing to the extensive attachment of soft issues to bony contours, evaluation of each layer provides valuable information related to overall condition of the soft tissues of the trunk and limbs (see Chapter 5, Assessment of Musculoskeletal Disorders and Concepts of Management). Common sites for restriction of the trunk and pelvic girdle include the rib cage, iliac crest, ischial tuberosity, greater trochanter, and the spinous processes. An example of a general technique to treat and assess restrictions of greater magnitude is soft tissue mobilization of the erector spine group and myofascial tissues of the lumbar, thoracic, and to a certain extent the cervical spine muscles. A bony contour technique is directed along the groove between the spinous processes of the patient in a sitting or quadruped position (Fig. 8-10).[65,122,323] One advantage to this

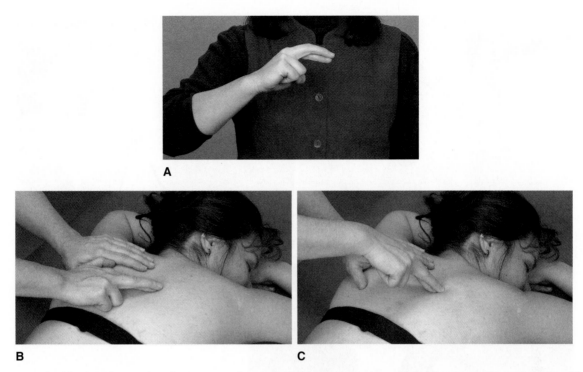

■ FIG. 8-8. J-Stroking. A focused technique used to release skin restrictions and adhesions. (**A**) J-stroke hand position. (**B**) Superficial J-stroke. (**C**) Deep J-stroke.

technique is that the patient can actively participate rather than remain passive. As discussed earlier, soft tissue and joint mobilization have a unique relationship in that either the soft tissues or the joint may be contributing to hypomobility. Passive segmental mobility of a joint may change dramatically after releasing the soft tissue.

To treat these soft tissue limitations, the therapist can use sustained pressure techniques similar to those for the treatment of the skin and superficial connective tissues. Typically digital contact is used and the tissue is treated by moving the fingers parallel along the edges of the bone by placing them on stretch, by shortening the tissues around the site of restric-

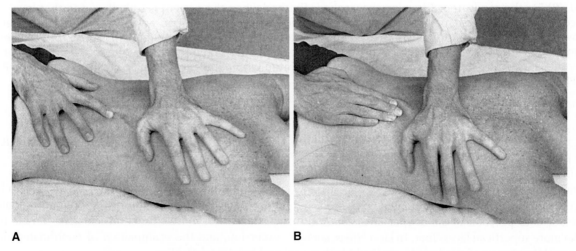

■ FIG. 8-9. Soft tissue mobilization of superficial connective tissue by placing the tissue under tension by (**A**) taking up all the slack in the direction of the restriction while the opposing hand stabilizes or tractions the skin in the direction opposite the restriction, or if the restriction is severe (**B**) using a unlocking spiral technique in a clockwise or counterclockwise direction depending on the direction of greatest restriction. The area is reassessed, and the examination or technique proceeds. (Reprinted with permission from Scully RM, Barnes MR: Physical Therapy. Philadelphia, Lippincott, 1989:963.)

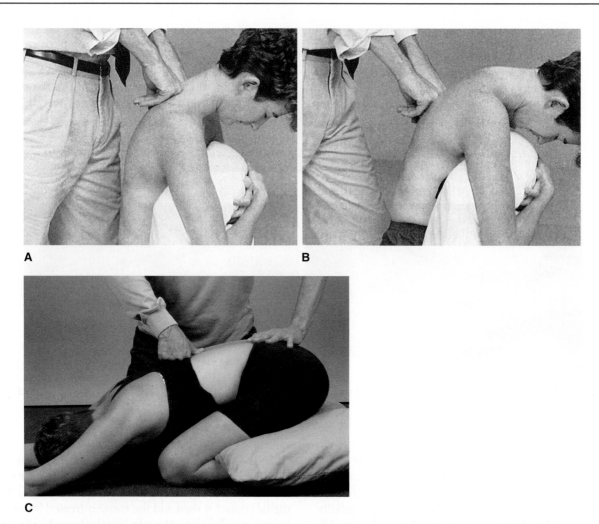

■ **FIG. 8-10.** General treatment technique and examination of the paraspinal musculature. **(A)** Starting in sitting, slight pressures are applied anteriorly and inferiorly (with dorsal surface of the proximal phalanges, elbow, forearm, or reinforced thumb) as the patient is instructed to flex forward slowly to the level of the therapist's hands. If a localized restriction is found, the patient is asked to stop the movement and a sustained pressure is applied until the restriction is released. **(B)** For the cervicothoracic spine the stroke is finished when the patient is fully flexed to that level. **(C)** For the thoracolumbar spine this same technique may be applied starting in quadriped while instructing the patient to slowly move backward to sit on the heels. Bilateral or unilateral stroked maybe applied with active forward bending, sidebending, and rotation. It is important that the therapist and patient time this technique so the patient does not flex below the level of the therapist's hands. (Part A, B reprinted with permission from Scully RM, Barnes MR: Physical Therapy. Philadelphia, Lippincott, 1989:970.)

tion, or by using a spiraling technique. Superimposed on the sustained pressure technique, greater or less tension can be created by applying clockwise or counterclockwise rotatory motions to the tissue. The clinician must concentrate on the layer of tissue that is being examined or treated. A common error is to proceed to the deeper layers without clearing the more superficial layers first. In large areas, such as the iliac crest, treatment of restrictions (particularly those of greater depth) may be performed with the forearm or even the elbow (Fig. 8-11). Myofascial restrictions along the iliac crest are especially prevalent in lumbosacral dysfunction and fibromyalgia.[65]

MUSCLE TISSUE EVALUATION AND MANIPULATION

The next aspect of the treatment and examination scheme is to identify restrictions within and between muscles themselves. Evaluation of the myofascial structures should include assessment of muscle tone, muscle play, muscle functional excursion, and the examination of coordinated movement and functional abilities.

Direct myofascial or soft tissue manipulation of muscle tissue imparts firm mechanical force in the direction of restriction for the purpose of breaking up abnormal cross-linkage, loosening the connective tissue weave, and restoring indepen-

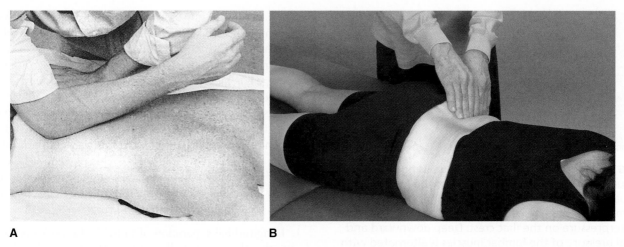

A   **B**

■ **FIG. 8-11.** Treatment and evaluation of soft tissue restrictions along the iliac crest using **(A)** an elbow or **(B)** reinforced hand. The entire expanse of the ilium should be mobilized or at least palpated for restrictions. (Part A reprinted with permission from Scully RM, Barnes MR: Physical Therapy. Philadelphia, Lippincott, 1989:967).

dent mobility to muscle and fascial compartments.[179] Treatment of muscular restrictions may be done either with specific or general, direct or indirect techniques. Specific techniques usually involve lateral stretching, linear stretching, deep pressure, bending techniques, traction, and/or separation of muscle origin and insertion.

Transverse Muscle Play or Perpendicular (Lateral) Stretching Techniques. Perpendicular stretching employs a force at right angles to the long axis of the muscle.[151] Various parts of the hands, fingers, and thumb pads are used to employ a slow rhythmical (oscillatory) or sustained stretch over the involved area. One or both hands may be used to mobilize the soft tissues. Often one hand is used to stabilize or apply a counterforce as the opposing hand mobilizes. One variation is the 'S' contact technique described by Lewit.[253] The hands are positioned in such a way as to allow thumb or hand pressure to be applied across the fibers of the involved muscle or soft tissue area so that the contacts are traveling in opposite directions to each other (Fig. 8-12). As pressure is applied simultaneously, the tissue between the two contacts will progressively have the slack removed and be placed on stretch until a release occurs. Other variations include the following.

1. Decontractions employing counterpressure.[271–273] Decontractions are performed with one hand applying a slow, steady, uninterrupted stretch over the involved site while the opposing hand applies a counterforce by stabilizing a body part or moving a body part in the opposite direction to progressively take up the slack. For example, as deep pressure is applied downward and laterally on the lumbar muscle, a counterforce can be applied by lifting the patient's ilium in the opposite direction (Fig. 8-13).

2. Bending technique.[65,82,179,297] In this technique the fibers of the involved muscle or soft tissues are stretched in a

manner similar to that whereby the hands are attempting to snap a twig (Fig. 8-14). Repetitive lifts and release cycles are applied, taking up all the transverse slack so as to produce simultaneous bending and shearing force in the involved tissue. The thumbs function as a fulcrum as the pronating wrists move into ulnar deviation away from each other. Manipulation in this manner is thought to break up cross-fiber restrictions.[179] Areas typically treated by this method include the thigh adductors, tensor fascia lata (iliotibial band), and the pectoralis mass (including the deep clavipectoral fascia and the suspensory ligament of the axilla) (Fig. 8-14).

3. Transverse (perpendicular) sustained or oscillatory stretching technique.[323] The clinician applies enough pressure to localize the treatment at the desired tissue depth. The

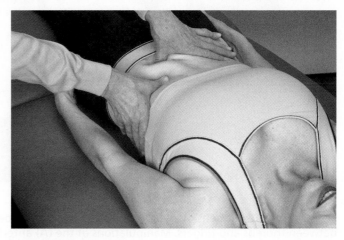

■ **FIG. 8-12.** Perpendicular (lateral stretch) S myofascial pressure release.

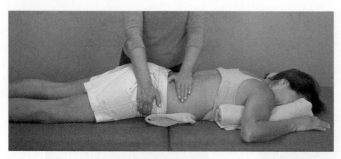

■ FIG. 8-13. Decontraction technique using counter pressure to the myofascial structures of the lumbar spine. Manual stretch and soft tissue manipulation of the mass of lumbar muscles and connective tissue are applied with counterpressure on the iliac crest. Deep downward and lateral pressure of the lumbar muscles is alternated with counter pressure on the iliac crest. Alternate deep pressure is applied slowly and rhythmically.[272]

clinician repeatedly deforms the muscle to the point of tension in the direction of restriction (end-range deformation) (see Fig. 7-45). Gentle oscillatory (at rate of several cycles per second) or sustained pressures can applied.

Transverse (perpendicular) pressures can be performed in a firm manner on a fixed site of muscle or tendon to facilitate tissue analgesia and healing (see Cyriax's transverse friction massage below) or in an oscillatory fashion such as strumming (Fig. 8-6).

Longitudinal Muscle Play or Parallel Stretching. Force applied in the direction of the long axis of the muscle is generally called longitudinal, parallel, or linear stretch-

ing.[151,179,277] Any muscle or muscle group that allows the placement of two hands or even two fingers can be relieved of myofascial restrictions. For small areas only one or two fingers or thumb are needed. For a large muscle group better leverage is achieved by crossing the arms and using the entire surface of both hands (Fig. 8-15). Both hands apply slowly increasing pressures proximal to the attachment of the muscle(s) to be stretched in the direction of the muscle fibers. Just enough pressure is applied to stretch the superficial skin, fascia, and underlying muscle(s). This position is held until the soft tissue is felt to relax. Longitudinal stretching continues by taking up the slack created by the release. Variations of this technique include the following:

1. Longitudinal separation of individual muscles or fascicle within the muscle bellies (Fig. 8-16).[179] Stretch is directed from origin to insertion by drawing or pushing along the myofascial structure. By applying each pass progressively deeper, the tissues are spread apart, helping to restore dimensional mobility, free space, and muscle play. Parallel separation techniques can be performed along the muscle belly or in a similar fashion along the bony attachment of muscle (see above). These linear strokes may be applied with the lateral edge of the finger (Fig. 8-16A), an individual knuckle, or even the elbow along fascial clefts and muscle borders obtaining a parallel separation of the muscle from adjacent soft tissues. Gross stretch of the diagonal fibers may be enhanced by providing additional passive stretch via positioning the patient's leg or arm in flexion and extension (Fig. 8-16B).[278]

2. Longitudinal stretch of the trunk. Typically this soft tissue stretching technique employs the use of both forearms and hands to stretch or elongate the myofascial structures. This technique is typically used on lumbar

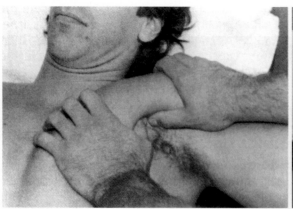

A

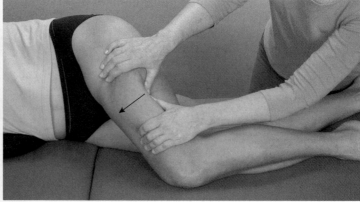

B

■ FIG. 8-14. Treatment of myofascial restrictions using a bending or "twig snapping" approach by grasping the tissues between thumbs and fingers. Manipulations of the **(A)** anterior pectoral fascia and **(B)** iliotibial band. The movement can be sustained or oscillatory. (Part A reprinted with permission from Kelley MJ, Clark WA: Orthopedic Therapy of the Shoulder. Philadelphia, Lippincott, 1995:301.)

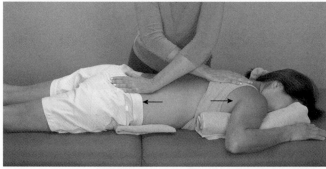

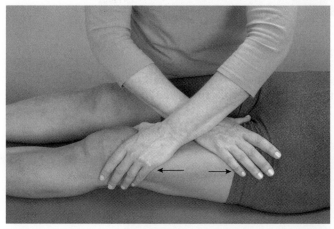

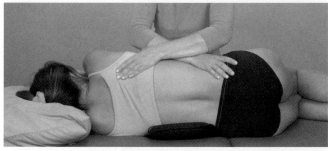

■ **FIG. 8-15.** Longitudinal myofascial stretching using a cross-arm technique showing stretching of (**A**) the myofascial planes of the back, (**B**) the quadriceps, and (**C**) the quadratus lumborum in sidelying.

spine with forearms or hands on the sacrum and lower thoracic spine (Fig. 8-17C).[244] Stretch is performed with forearms and hands in opposite directions to extend muscles and spinal joints that are restricted and tight. Alternatively, one arm may stabilize as the other stretches. Greater stretch can be further achieved by increasing trunk motions (i.e., spinal flexion over a ball, 8-17A,B) or using the weight of the lower limbs to apply traction (Fig. 8-17C). These techniques are both evaluative and therapeutic and

serve as useful techniques in preparation for joint mobilization. When used directly over the spine, they serve as a manual spinal traction technique.

3. Upper quadrant. Elongation of a muscle at functional end range can be achieved via arm or leg traction while anchoring the proximal attachment of the myofascial structure to be treated. This can also be reversed by maintaining the limb near end range while further elongation is achieved with the proximal hand stretching or mobilizing the proximal attachment in the opposite direction (Fig. 8-18). By using three planar diagonals of movement, maximum twisting and untwisting of the muscles and joint capsules can be facilitated. For example, the proprioceptive neuromuscular pattern (PNF) flexion–abduction–external rotation (D2F) of the upper limb allows for maximum twisting of the glenohumeral joint capsule (approaching the closed-packed position) as the muscles are untwisting. This is in keeping with normal coordinated patterns of motion, which are diagonal in direction with spiral components.

4. Lower quadrant. In the lower limb near end range of a muscle can be achieved using a closed-kinetic chain (Fig. 8-19) or limb traction, leaving both hands free to apply end-range soft tissue mobilization directly to the involved tissue. (Fig. 8-20). Stationary longitudinal pressures may be applied to the restricted myofascial structures around a joint, guiding it in the proper direction, and improving "tracking of movement" as the patient performs active physiologic movements.[307,363]

Longitudinal techniques may consist of long, continuous strokes or short, interrupted strokes designed to improve muscle play. Techniques can be facilitated with active participation of the patient and three planar movements.[65,323]

ARM AND LEG TRACTION TECHNIQUES (ARM AND LEG PULL)[39,179,277]

These techniques are used to enhance mobility of the limbs and trunk by releasing regional fascia, thereby affecting restrictions not addressed fully by specific muscle stretching. They are effective in the treatment of myofascial pain and other mechanism of pseudomyostatic contracture and following immobilization.[179,277,278]

The mechanism of release here is felt to be both mechanical and neuromuscular. The introduction of twisting and shearing forces combined with traction loads the fascia in an attempt to break up mechanical restrictions and change the viscosity of the ground substance. Sustained traction activates the Golgi tendon organs (GTO) situated in the muscle tendons and in the intermuscular septum producing neuromuscular relaxation.[179]

The "release" phenomenon is performed slowly and in stages with great emphasis on the attentiveness regarding what the clinician is feeling. Throughout the technique the clinician should stay within the available pain-free range, remembering

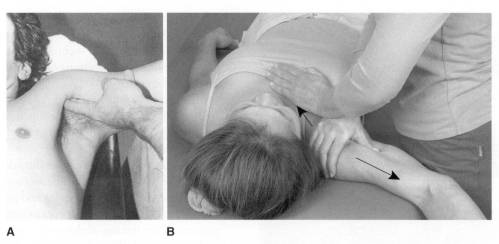

A B

■ **FIG. 8-16.** Pectoralis major. **(A)** Longitudinal myofascial separation technique of the sternal portion of the pectoralis major (muscles on slack, initially) and **(B)** gross manual stretch of the diagonal fibers allowing gravity and the position of the patient's arm to provide additional stretch. Provide the patient with additional feedback on the necessary angle at the shoulder to target restricted diagonal fibers. (Part A reprinted with permission from Kelley MJ, Clark WA: Orthopedic Therapy of the Shoulder. Philadelphia, Lippincott, 1995:302.)

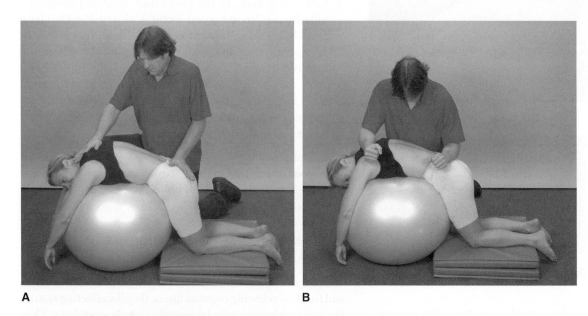

A B

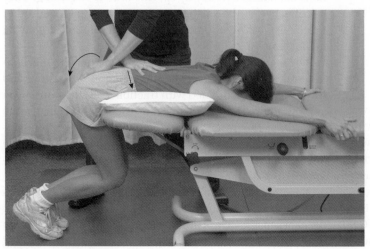

C

■ **FIG. 8-17.** Longitudinal or diagonal stretch to the thoracolumbar spine using **(A)** the hands to stretch in the opposite directions or **(B)** using both forearms or one forearm or hand to stabilize as the other elongates the tissue. Further stretch can be achieved by positioning the spine in increased flexion (e.g., over a ball) or **(C)** using the lower limbs to apply traction (e.g., legs over the edge of a table).

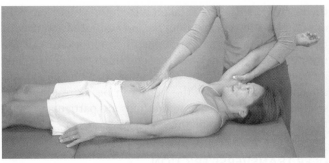
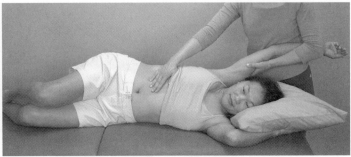

A   **B**

■ **FIG. 8-18.** Anterolateral fascial elongation to the superficial fascial sheaths of the anterior thorax. **(A)** As the arm is tractioned into elevation (various patterns and degrees of flexion and abduction), a traction force is applied in the direction of the umbilicus in supine or **(B)** sidelying.

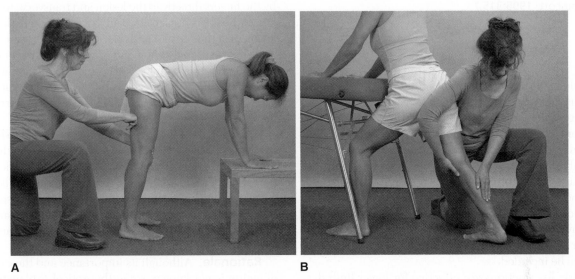

A   **B**

■ **FIG. 8-19.** Longitudinal soft tissue stretch technique of the **(A)** hamstrings and **(B)** the gastrocnemius using a closed-kinetic chain to place the tissues on further stretch.

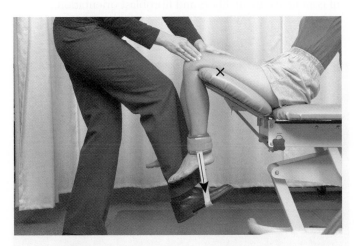

■ **FIG. 8-20.** Longitudinal soft tissue stretch technique of the quadriceps, retinaculum, and insertion of the iliotibial band employing limb traction with either passive or active motion of the knee. This method of limb traction (with a belt) can also be used effectively during joint articulations of the knee.

that this type of release is not purely mechanical. It is not the amount of the force that creates the release; rather, it is the low load over time. Gentle increases in traction may be applied until an end feel has been reached, indicating that the limb is stretched as far as it can be in that position at that time.[277,278] Elapsed time is typically in the range of 2 minutes to obtain maximum benefit.[179] Active exercise, flexibility, mobilization, and function rehabilitation are recommended to help reestablish neuromuscular communication. Arm traction can be used with patients who experience upper limb dysfunction and it is also an excellent treatment of cervical and thoracic dysfunction (see Figs. 7-38 and 7-39).

A modification of the arm traction technique is a glenohumeral joint capsular twist that localizes the forces to the capsule by moving the hand grips proximally on the humerus (Fig. 8-21).[179] Twisting and stretching are introduced in an attempt to increase the extensibility of the capsule and break up any adhesions. This technique has been found to be particularly useful in the management of adhesive capsulitis or frozen shoulder.[179] Increase in collagen fiber density and

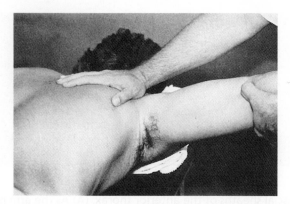

■ FIG. 8-21. Capsular twist technique of the gleno-humeral joint. (Reprinted with permission from Kelley MJ, Clark WA: Orthopedic Therapy of the Shoulder. Philadelphia, Lippincott, 1995:315.)

interfiber cross-links can involve the full depth or extent of the capsule resulting in significant multidirectional motion restrictions.[89,93,103,321,322,334] The synovial reaction gives rise to the formation of adhesions, mainly located in the axillary folds and anatomical neck of the humerus,[93,103] which will limit shoulder motion particularly during glenohumeral abduction and lateral rotation. Capsular stretching procedures and specific joint articulation procedures are indicated to restore joint play and normal arthrokinematics (see Chapter 11, Shoulder and Shoulder Girdle). Scapular stabilization, biofeedback, and postural awareness, emphasizing control of the rhomboids and lower trapezius, and strengthening of the rotator cuff should also be included.

Likewise, leg tractions are effective for lower limb dysfunction, pelvic girdle, and lumbar spine dysfunction. For example, the hip adductor can be lengthened indirectly by applying light traction to the whole leg (see Fig. 7.39). As

the leg relaxes, the leg is taken into the next barrier. Various combinations of rotation, flexion and extension may be used to influence the various adductor muscles. All the muscle groups of the pelvis, hip, and thigh can be stretched indirectly in this fashion. When more than one clinician is available large areas of the body can be more efficiently stretched (Fig. 8-22). These methods are particularly helpful for the trunk musculature.[277]

DEEP TRANSVERSE FRICTION MASSAGE[75,91,101,145,167,168,334,337,464,494]

A particularly important massage technique in the management of many musculoskeletal disorders is deep transverse friction massage. Deep transverse massage implies massage applied by the fingers directly to the lesion and transverse to the direction of the fibers in a localized area of tendon, muscle, fascia, or ligament at the site of scar tissue, adhesions, or pain. For many years before steroids where introduced, it was the only alternative to infiltration with local anaesthetics.[95] Friction is usually slower in effect than injections but leads to a physically more fundamental resolution, resulting in less reoccurrence and more permanent cure.[334]

A major part of the role of friction massage is to help identify areas of dysfunction and also offer help in the differential diagnosis Friction strokes provide localized specific information about certain connective tissue structures. The compliance and adherence of connective tissue can be assessed. The fascial compartments, sheaths of muscle, joint capsules (especially around superficial joints), tendon sheaths, and related structures can be identified and evaluated.

Rationale. Although its importance and the exact mode of action is not known, some theoretical explanations have been put forward. Friction has a local anti-inflammatory and pain-diminishing effect and also results in better alignment of connective tissue fibers and fibroblast orientation.

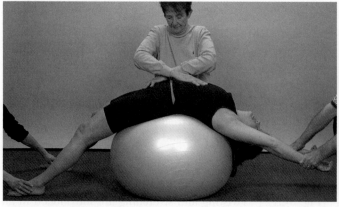

A

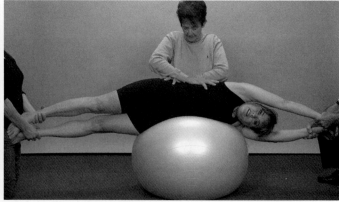

B

■ FIG. 8-22. Three-person arm and leg traction with focused stretching on **(A)** the rectus abdominis and **(B)** the quadratus lumborum.

Relief of Pain. This massage technique temporarily reduces pain by activating the "gate" mechanism[145] and according to Cyriax[95] increases destruction of Lewis' substance P, thought to be the principal chemomediator of pain impulses from the periphery to the central nervous system.[498] An appropriate dose of friction massage can result in a sustained period of posttraumatic analgesia through the depletion of subtonic P in the locally sensory neuron.

Movement imparted through friction results in stimulation of the mechanoreceptors that transmit impulses along large-fiber afferent pathways to the spinal cord. They serve to decrease nociceptor transmission to higher pain centers. It appears that as the patient responds to friction massage, on subsequent treatments the time for anesthesia to occur lessens. The temporary relief at the end of a treatment session of friction massage permits other treatments.

Prevention and Breaking Up Adhesions. Friction massage for conditions of the soft tissues, usually muscles, ligaments, tendons, and tendon sheaths, for the prevention and treatment of inflammatory scar tissue has been used and recommended by numerous authors.[75,91,95,100,142,158,167,168,200,210,297,334,337,464] Friction has an effect on connective tissue in that it prevents and/or ruptures abnormal cross-links and adhesions.[268,334,464,485] It involves applying deep massage directly to the site of the lesion in a direction perpendicular to the normal orientation of fibrous elements. This maintains mobility of the structure with respect to adjacent tissues and probably helps to promote increased interfiber mobility of the structure itself without longitudinally stressing it. Friction massage increases myotendinous scar pliability and facilitates normal collagen fiber orientation as they are produced. Kessler[231] likens this effect to the effect of rolling your hand over an unorganized pile of toothpicks; eventually the toothpicks will all become oriented perpendicular to the direction in which the hand moves.

Transverse frictions also assists fibroblast orientation.[334] In the early stage of fibroblast proliferation when cross-links are absent or still weak, friction must be very light and given only over a short period so as to cause only minimal discomfort. In later stages, if strong cross-links have formed, intense friction is needed to break these down.[75,268,464,485]

In some pathologic cases, such as rotator cuff tendinitis, in which the etiology may be related to nutritional deficit arising from hypovascularity, the hyperemia induced by the deep friction massage may also contribute to the healing process. Another purpose of deep friction massage is to provide deep pressure over myofascial trigger points to produce a reflex effect.[277,347] Friction over a trigger point may create exquisite pain and elicit a "jump sign" with referred pain in a specific pattern. After a trigger point is reduced, friction may be used to eliminate the taut fascia that can be the promoter of the trigger point.[167]

Indications

Diagnostic. Diagnostically, friction anesthesia may help to define the exact site of the lesion or source of pain in problems related to muscle, tendinous or ligamentous lesions. Numbing an area of pain that was previously sensitive on isometric testing (muscles or tendons) and is much less sensitive after friction on postisometric testing affirms that one is dealing with the probable source of pain. Friction anesthesia can also help to distinguish between a partial and a complete tear of a tendon.[167] For example, in a suspected tear of a rotator cuff tendon of the shoulder limited by pain and weakness, if motion significantly improves after the application of friction anesthesia, this may be evidence that a partial tear rather than a complete tear exists.

Therapy. Deep transverse friction can be used after an injury and for mechanical overuse in ligamentous, tendinous, and muscular structures. It is primarily indicated for chronic conditions of soft tissues arising from abnormal modeling of fibrous elements in response to fatigue stresses or accompanying resolution of an acute inflammatory disorder. The intent is to restore or maintain mobility of the structure with respect to adjacent tissues and to increase the extensibility of the structure under normal loading conditions. The approach is to allow for increased energy-attenuating capacity of the part with reduced strain to individual structural elements.

Tendons. Most mechanical tendinitis and tenosynovitis can be treated by deep friction massage. In tendinitis of tendons without a sheath, a painful scar in the tendon body or at the periosteal insertion may follow repetitive overuse or sudden strain.[334] Friction massage is applied directly over the site of the lesion with minimal tensile tension in tendons. In tenosynovitis occurring with a sheath, roughening of the gliding surfaces of both the tendons and the sheath gives rise to pain and sometimes crepitus suggesting roughening of the gliding surfaces. For maximal efficacy, the tendon with its sheath must be put under tension during massage so that the tendon forms an immobile base against which the tendon is moved. It would appear that massage, by manual rolling of the tendon sheath to and fro against the tendon, serves to smooth off the gliding surfaces.[91] During the treatment of tendinitis, tenovaginitis, or tenosynovitis, the patient must avoid all activity that provokes pain. Typical types of tendinitis treated by friction massage include:

- Supraspinatus or infraspinatus (shoulder) (tendinitis) (Box 8-1, Figs. *A–C*).
- Subscapularis (tendinitis) (Fig. 8-23)
- Infraspinatus (tendinitis) (Box 8-1, Fig. *D*)
- Biceps tendon at the bicipital groove (bicipital tendinitis) (Box 8-1, Fig. *E*; also see Fig. 11-19)
- Tennis elbow (medial and lateral tendinitis) (Box 8-1, Fig. *F*)
- De Quervain's (wrist)(tenovaginitis of the abductor pollicis longus and extensor pollicis brevis) (Fig. 8-24).

BOX 8-1	USE OF FRICTION MASSAGE IN SOME COMMON UPPER LIMB TENDINITIS

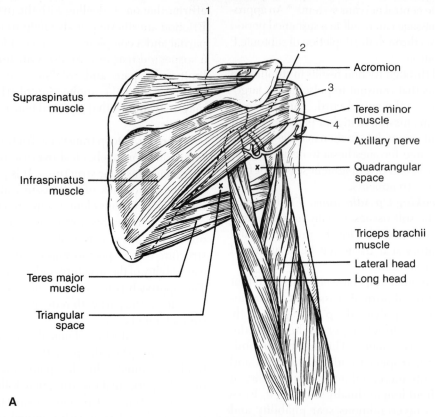

A

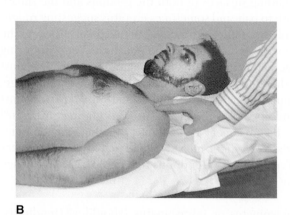

B

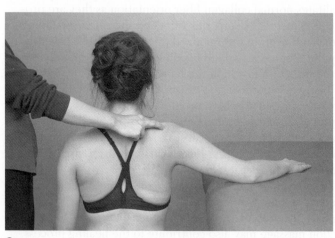

C

(**A**) Posterior view of the intrinsic muscles of the shoulder and lesions of the supraspinatus. *1*, musculotendinous insertion; *2*, dentoperiosteal insertion. Infraspinatus: *3*, body of tendon; *4*, dentoperiosteal insertion.

(**B**) Deep friction to the superficial and deep periosteal junction of the supraspinatus (the arm may be resting at the side or positioned in internal rotation allowing the tendon to be brought into a more sagittal position just below the anterior acromion).

(**C**) Deep friction to the musculotendinous lesion of the supraspinatus (the shoulder should be in a rested position of 90° of abduction).

Box 8-1. continued

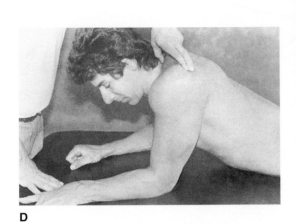

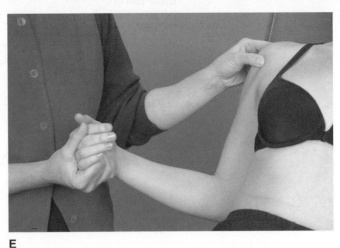

D

E

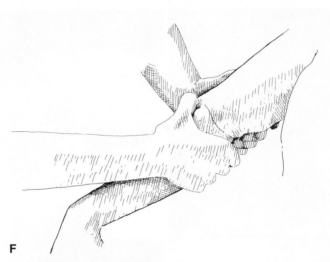

F

D) Deep friction to the infraspinatus. The most tender area, either the tendon body or the insertion into the greater tuberosity, is frictioned.

(E) Deep friction to the to the long head of the biceps (lesions in the sulcus). Friction is applied by rotating the patient's arm, allowing the tendon to glide under the thumb. Pronation-supination movements of the therapist's contralateral arm have the same effect. The active moment is on supination.

(F) Deep friction to the extensor carpi radialis tendon at the lateral humeral epicondyle.

(Part A reprinted with permission from Pratt NE: Clinical Musculoskeletal Anatomy. Philadelphia, JB Lippincott, 1991:82. Parts B and D Reprinted with permission from Kelley MJ, Clark WA: Orthopedic Therapy of the Shoulder. Philadelphia, Lippincott, 1995:304.)

- Wrist extensors: extensor carpi radialis longus and/or brevis and extensor carpi ulnaris tendinitis (Fig. 8-25; also see Fig. 13-33)
- Wrist flexor: flexor carpi radialis and flexor carpi ulnaris tendinitis (Fig. 8-26; also see Fig. 13-34)
- Patellar tendinitis and quadriceps expansion (knee) (Box 8-2, Figs. *B* and *C*; also see Fig. 7-14)
- Achilles tendinitis (Box 8-2, Fig. *F*).

- Peroneal tendinitis (ankle or foot) (Box 8-2, Fig. *G*; also see Fig. 7-15)

Boxes 8-1 and 8-2 depict the locations where friction massage should be applied in tendinitis of the upper and lower limb. Following friction massage, tendons should only be exercised (i.e., passively stretched) if there is minimal discomfort and no pain. Later in the healing phase, active

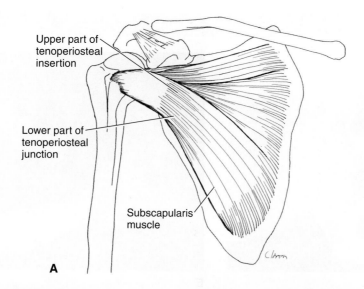

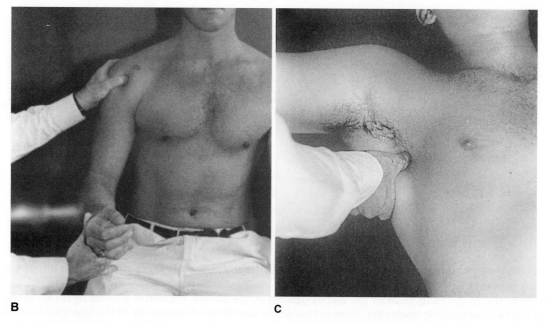

■ **FIG. 8-23.** **(A)** Subscapularis muscle as seen from the front. Friction may be necessary **(B)** at the most tender level of the bony lesser tuberosity (tenoperiosteal junction) and **(C)** muscle belly (lateral aspect). (Part B, C reprinted with permission from Kelley MJ, Clark WA: Orthopedic Therapy of the Shoulder. Philadelphia, Lippincott, 1995:265–266.)

and passive full range of motion (ROM) and a strengthening programs (isometric, isotonic, isokinetic, and Isoflex exercise) are introduced.

Ligaments. Most ligaments link two bones together while permitting movement at the joint they span. This mobility has to be maintained after a recent sprain or must be restored if posttraumatic adhesions have already been allowed to consolidate themselves. In recent ligamentous sprains, gentle transverse frictions are used to encourage mobile scar formation. Passive and free active movement or light resisted exercises are begun within the limits of pain to maintain normal gliding of the ligament over adjacent bone. In the

lower limb instruction in a pain free gait follows as well as exercises for the adjacent joints.

After significant pain-free range of movement is obtained, the rehabilitation program progresses to include more vigorous activities, to increase mobility, and to introduce strength training. In chronic conditions, forceful manipulation may be necessary for reducing the restricting adhesions. In such cases the friction thins out and numbs the ligament at the point of fibrous adherence, thus facilitating movement. Some ligamentous lesions that are only curable by friction and are never forced by manipulations include the posterior carpal ligaments at the wrist (Box 8-3, Fig. *B*), the coro-

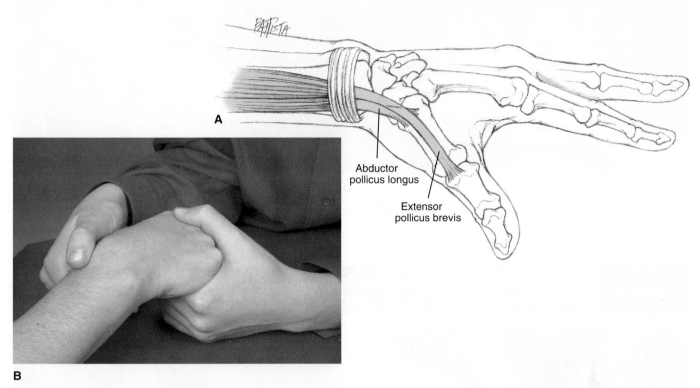

A

B

■ **FIG. 8-24.** **(A)** Extensor pollicis brevis (upper tendon) and abductor pollicis longus (lower tendon) and their common sheath. **(B)** Friction may be necessary at their shared sheath (de Quervain's) or where the muscles pass over the wrist extensors (intersection syndrome).

nary ligament at the knee (Box 8-3, Fig. *D:* also see Fig. 15-7), and the tibiotalar ligaments (anterior and posterior) (Fig. 8-27).[334]

Other subacute or chronic ligamentous sprains treated effectively with friction massage include (Box 8-3) the following:

- Acromioclavicular ligament (Box 8-3, Fig. *A;* also see Fig. 11-4)
- Medial collateral ligament (knee) (Box 8-3, Fig. *C;* also see Fig. 15-8)
- Lateral ankle ligaments: calcaneofibular, calcaneocuboid, and tibiofibular ligaments (see Fig. 16-14)

(text continues on page 200)

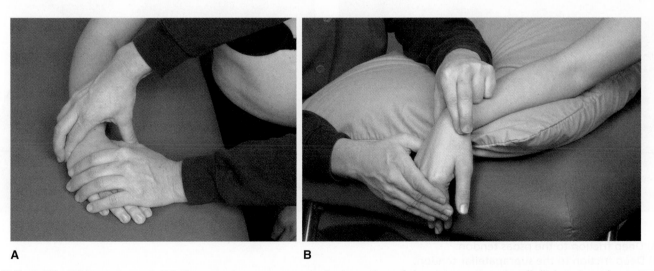

A   **B**

■ **FIG. 8-25.** Wrist extensors. Friction may be necessary at the insertion of the extensor carpi radialis brevis and extensor carpi radialis longus **(A)** or the extensor carpi ulnaris **(B)**. The wrist is treated in flexion if a sheath is involved.

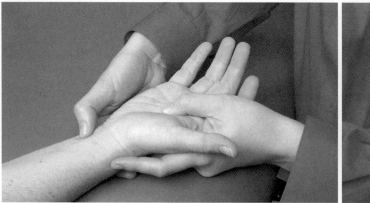
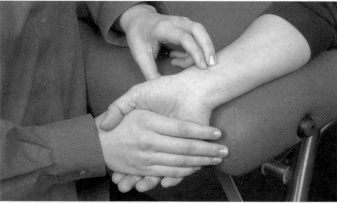

A   **B**

■ **FIG. 8-26.** Wrist flexors. Friction may be necessary near the insertions of the flexor carpi ulnaris (**A**), the flexor carpi radialis (**B**), or tendons of the finger flexors.

BOX 8-2	**USE OF FRICTION MASSAGE IN SOME COMMON LOWER LIMB TENDINITIS LESIONS**

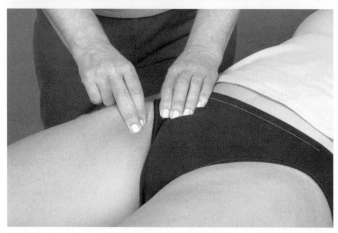
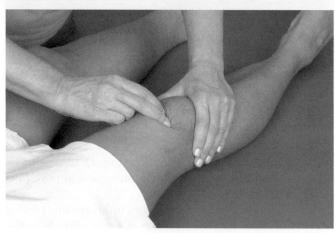

A   **B**

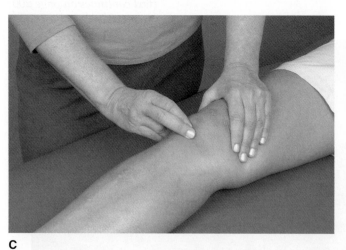
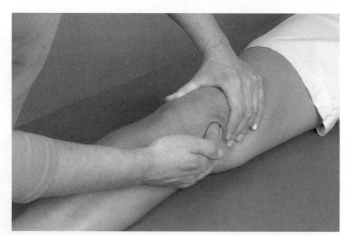

C   **D**

(**A**) Deep friction to the psoas tendon.
(**B**) Deep friction to the suprapatellar tendon.
(**C**) Deep friction to the infrapatellar tendon.
(**D**) Deep friction to the quadriceps expansion.

Box 8-2. continued

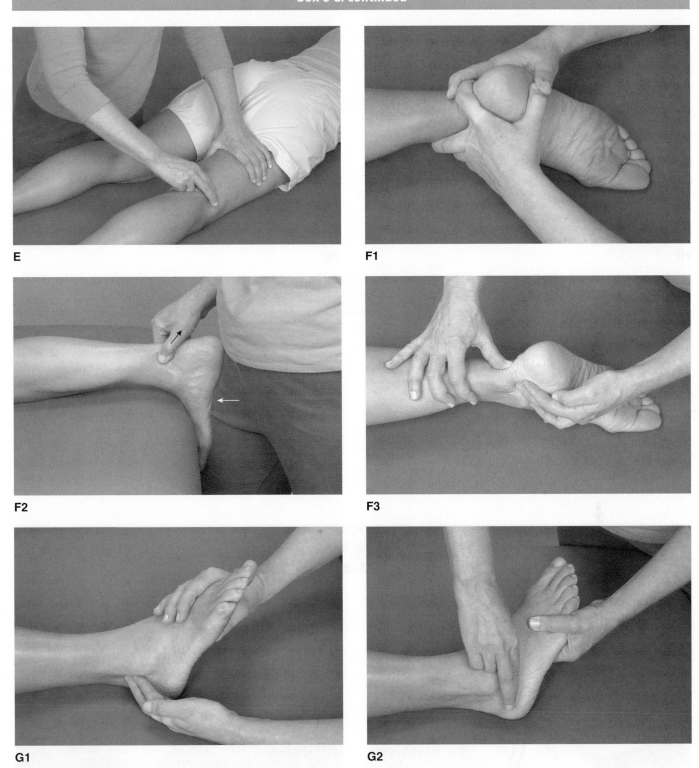

E

F1

F2

F3

G1

G2

(**E**) Deep friction to the biceps tendon.
(**F**) Deep friction to the (*1*) Achilles tendon to the insertion, (*2*) medial and lateral aspect, and
(*3*) anterior aspect of the tendon.
(**G**) Deep friction to the peroneal tendons (*1*) under the malleolus and (*2*) level with the malleolus (peroneal tendinitis).

(*continued*)

Box 8-2. continued

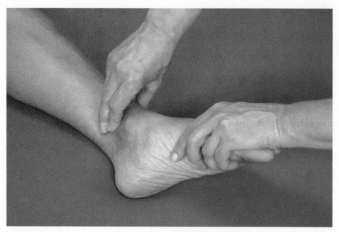

H1

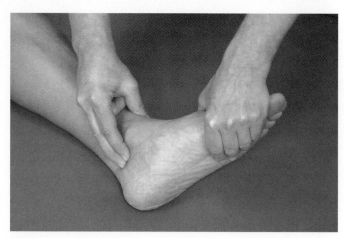

H2

(H) Deep friction to the (*1*) upper part of the tibialis posterior muscle and (*2*) to the tendon and muscle (overuse tendinitis) This muscle is usually involved in anterior shin splints at its musculotendinous area.

- Affected ligaments of the coccyx (Fig. 8-28; also see Box 8-3, Fig. *E*)[15,95,334]

In recent ligamentous sprains, local swelling is removed as much as possible by effleurage. It is followed by friction massage of short duration (approximately 1 minute) for the first 2 days.[334] As pain diminishes the intensity and time are increased. From the third day, friction is followed by pas-sive and active movements within the limits of pain to maintain normal gliding over adjacent bones.

Muscle Bellies. The main function of striated muscle is to contract. As muscles contract, their fibers broaden and separate. Full mobility a toward broadening out must be maintained or restored in muscles that have been the site of a minor rupture, contusion, major strain, or of repeated overuse (myosynovitis).[91,334] Loss in mobility toward broad-

BOX 8-3 | **EXAMPLES OF THE USE OF FRICTION MASSAGE TO SOME COMMON LIGAMENTOUS SPRAINS**

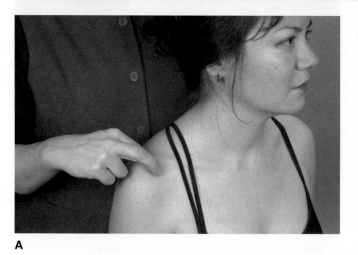

A

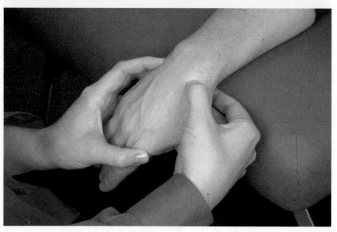

B

(A) Deep friction to the superficial acromioclavicular ligament in sprains without displacement.
(B) Deep friction to the dorsal carpal ligaments at the wrist.

Box 8-3. continued

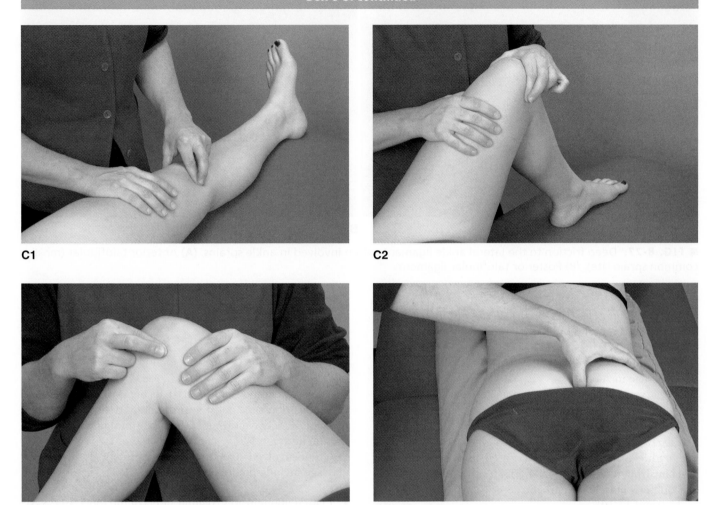

C1

C2

D

E

(C) Deep friction to the medial collateral ligament (*1*) in extension and (*2*) in flexion. A sprain of this ligament should be frictioned at the most tender site during maximum allowable flexion and extension.
(D) Deep friction to the meniscotibial (coronary) ligament. The knee is flexed and the tibia externally rotated to expose the medial side of the knee.
(E) Deep friction to the affected ligaments of the coccyx (posterior sacrococcyx ligament, the intercoccygeal ligaments) and the origin of the gluteus maximus (see Fig. 8-28).

ening owing to abnormal cross-links between fasciculi can be mobilized by transverse frictions that mobilize the longitudinal muscle fibers without pulling on the tear (in the early stage) or break down (in the chronic stage) abnormal cross-links. To stretch out a muscle does not widen the distance between muscle fibers; on the contrary, during stretching they lie more closely together. Deep transverse friction passively restores mobility to muscles in the same way that joint mobilizations frees a joint. Friction massage is always given with the muscle fully relaxed or in a shortened position.

In recent minor tears, friction is followed by active contraction with the muscle in a position of maximum relax-

ation. In long-standing cases the friction is followed by normal use of the muscles. During the treatment period all activities or movement that bring on pain should be avoided. Friction can be used for all muscle bellies. According to Ombregt et al.,[334] the following muscles can only be treated effectively by frictions:

- Subclavius (see Fig. 7-6)
- Brachialis (see Fig. 12-12)
- Supinator (see Fig. 12-14)
- Adductor of the thumb (Fig. 8-29)
- Oblique muscles of the abdomen (see Fig. 7-13)

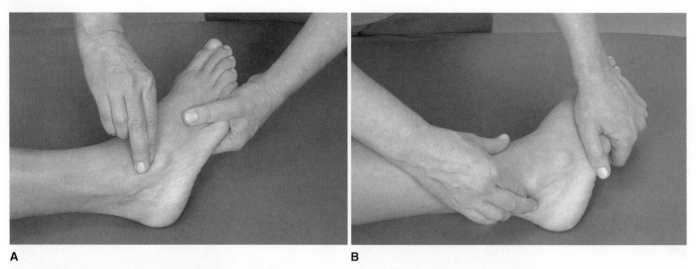

A | **B**

■ **FIG. 8-27.** Deep friction to the lateral ankle ligaments often involved in ankle sprains. **(A)** Anterior talofibular (most common sprain site). **(B)** Posterior talofibular ligament.

- Intercostal muscles (Fig. 8-30; also see Fig. 7-6)
- Interosseus muscles of the foot and hand

Other musculature that can be treated effectively by friction massage include:

- Occipital insertions of semispinalis or splenius capitis muscles (posttraumatic lesions) (Box 8-4, Fig. *A;* also see Fig. 19-7)
- Quadriceps muscles (Box 8-4, Fig. *B;* also see Fig. 7-14)
- Hamstring muscles (Box 8-4, Fig. *C;* also see Fig. 7-21)
- Popliteus muscle (strain) (Box 8-4, Fig. *D,* also see Figs. 15-9 and 15-10)

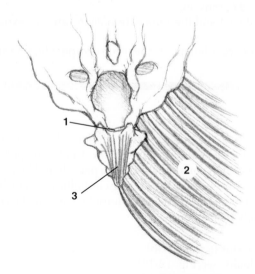

■ **FIG. 8-28.** The coccyx (*1*) showing its articulation with the sacrum, the insertion of the gluteus maximus (*2*), and the superficial fibers of the sacrococcygeal ligament (*3*).

- Tibialis anterior (myosynovitis) (Box 8-4, Fig. *E;* also see Fig 7-15)
- Tibialis posterior (see Box 8-2, Fig. *H1*)
- Gastrocnemius (tennis leg) (see Fig. 7-15)

Musculotendinous junctions that contain both muscle and tendinous fibers are most appropriately treated by friction massage.[334] Active movements in minor muscular tears follow friction massage.

Other involved structures treated effectively by friction massage include the following:

- Plantar aponeuroses (plantar fascia of the foot) (Fig. 8-31; also see Fig. 16-22)
- Plicae around the knee joint (Fig. 8-32; also see Fig. 15-42),
- Superficial joint capsules such as the cervical facet joints (complicating osteoarthritis), (see Figs. 19-1 and 19-2),
- Temporomandibular joint (see Box 8-6, Fig. *C* and Figs. 17-5 through 17-8),
- Acromioclavicular joint (see Box 8-3, Fig. *A,* and Fig. 11-4),
- Trapezium–first metacarpal joint capsule (Fig. 8-33; also see Fig. 13-8).

Contraindications. Contraindications are similar to those of other massage techniques and include the following[91,179,334]:

1. Bacterial and rheumatoid-type tendinitis, tenosynovitis, and tenovaginitis
2. Calcification and ossification of soft tissues
3. Disorders of nerve structures, for example carpal tunnel syndrome.
4. Skin problems such as psoriasis, ulcers or blisters
5. Hematoma
6. Acute bursitis

Hammer[168] found friction massage clinically effective in management of chronic bursitis of both the hip and the shoul-

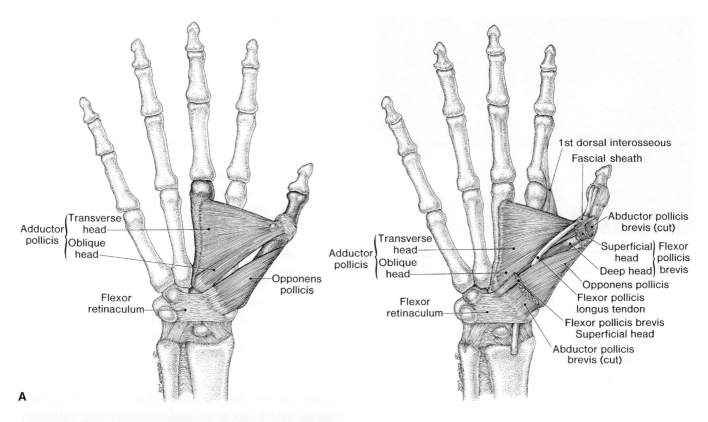

Adductor pollicis { Transverse head / Oblique head

Opponens pollicis

Flexor retinaculum

A

1st dorsal interosseous

Fascial sheath

Abductor pollicis brevis (cut)

Adductor pollicis { Transverse head / Oblique head

Superficial head } Flexor pollicis brevis
Deep head }

Opponens pollicis

Flexor pollicis longus tendon

Flexor pollicis brevis Superficial head

Abductor pollicis brevis (cut)

Flexor retinaculum

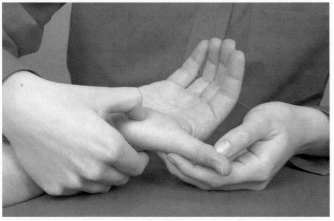

B

■ **FIG. 8-29.** **(A)** Opponens pollicis and adductor pollicis muscles. Lesions of the adductor pollicis may follow an abduction sprain of the thumb. The origin of the oblique portion of the adductor pollicis muscle at the palmar aspect of the base of the second or third metacarpal is most commonly affected.[334] **(B)** Treatment consists of a few sessions of deep transverse frictions. (A: Reprinted with permission from Simons DG, Travell LS, Simons LS: Travell & Simons' Myofascial Pain & Dysfunction: The Trigger Point Manual, vol. 1, 2nd ed. Baltimore, Williams & Wilkins, 1999:778.)

der. It appears that the adhesions in chronic bursal problems that are related to pre-existing tendinitis are positively affected by friction massage in the breakdown of bursal scar tissue. The bursae are believed to be secondarily involved.[45,261,379,426,457]

Technique. Therapeutically, friction massage is aimed directly at the site of the lesion. To this end a correct diagnosis must be achieved. The part should be well exposed and supported so as to reduce postural muscle tone. It should be positioned so that the site of the lesions is easily accessible to the fingertips. The structure to be treated is usually put in a position of neutral tension (e.g., tendons and ligaments) while muscles are best manipulated in a relaxed position, thus avoiding excessive damage to the muscle cells. If adherence

between a tendon and its sheath is suspected, then the tendon should be kept taut to stabilize it while the sheath is exposed. The patient's skin and the clinician's finger must move as one, so that the deep layers of the skin move over the affected fibers. Therefore, no lubricant is used.

The clinician should be seated, if possible with the elbow supported to reduce muscle tension of more proximal parts. When employing transverse friction, the thumb, heel of the hand, or the index finger supported by the middle finger or the middle finger with two adjacent fingers supporting it provide a strong treatment unit in the application of concentrated, repetitive stroking. Stroking is directed perpendicular to the fiber orientation of the structure being evaluated or

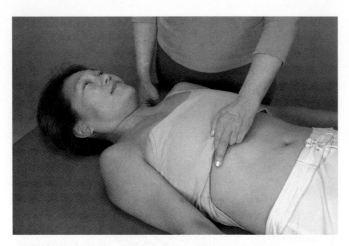

■ **FIG. 8-30.** Deep friction to an intercostal muscle. Sprained intercostal muscles are usually the result of direct injury to the chest.

treated. The superficial tissues are moved over the underlying structures by keeping the hand or fingers in firm contact with the skin. Friction massage begins with the initial gentle transverse movements that gradually bear more deeply into the tissue and continue for 5 to 15 minutes. With the exception of muscle, most soft tissue structures are treated with to-and-fro movements provided by the use of the flexor muscles or by pronation/supination of the forearm. A pinch grip is the normal technique used for a muscle belly with the pinch provided between the thumb and other fingers (Box 8-4, Figs. *B* and *C*). The practitioner grasps the involved area with the flexed fingers of one or both hand and pulls the contracted muscle belly. Contact is held without sliding the fingers as attempts are made to broaden the muscle.

Friction massage is followed by active movement in minor muscular tears, by passive movement in ligamentous tears, and by the avoidance of painful activity in tendinous lesions until full resolution has been achieved. It is vital that deep friction be performed only at the site of the lesion. The effect is so local that unless the finger is applied to the exact site and friction given in the right direction, relief cannot be expected.

An initial dose of 2 to 3 minutes is adequate to assess the response to treatment. Analgesic benefits can be achieved from this brief application in many cases.[179] Chronic conditions may require a minimum of 10 minutes or more over 6 to 10 sessions. Most overuse conditions respond within 2 weeks to 2 months.[167]

Friction massage is used to restore mobility between otherwise freely moving structures and to render adhesions less capable of acting as a source of mechanical restriction and irritation. It is designed to increase mobility and the deformation of soft tissue. Movement may enhance the arrangement of newly synthesized collagen fibers to align so as to permit the restoration of physiologic mobility and pliability specific to the tissue in which the process of healing is taking place.[95]

MODIFICATION OF SCAR TISSUE

Scar tissue adhesions can develop from callous formation following a fracture or from soft tissue trauma. The trauma could be from a specific injury, a laceration, or surgical incision. Scar tissue mechanics differ somewhat from normal connective tissue. Normal connective tissue is mature and stable, with limited pliability. Mature scar tissue is often reverts to an inactive nonpliable status. The scar becomes inextensible and nondynamic.

Scar tissue formation occurs in four distinct phases: (1) the inflammatory phase, (2) the granulation phase, (3) the fibroplastic stage, and (4) the maturation phase (see Chapter 2, Wound Healing: Injury and Repair of Dense Connective Tissue).[89,90] The final phase of scar tissue formation is the maturation phase. At this point maximal stress can be placed on the tissue without risk of tissue failure. Because collagen syntheses is still accelerated, significant remodeling can take place when appropriate mobilizations are performed.[65] If scar tissue is left unchecked, the collagen fibers can cross-link and the tissue can shrink significantly.

Soft tissue mobilization techniques are useful in loosening adhesions between the scar and surrounding tissues. Slow, sustained elongation of the scar and adjacent tissue will help promote function. Splints (serial or dynamic) may be useful to maintain stretch on the scar and to counter scar contraction. The combination of soft tissue mobilization, joint mobilization techniques in the presence of capsuloligamentous tightness or adherence, heat applications (ultrasound may increase collagen extensibility), stretching, and PROM are important aspects of treatment. The prevention of scar tissue adhesion following surgery is of great importance. Following back surgery, for example, the introduction of passive straight leg raising is often recommended. This can be done with the use of slings and pulleys or the help of nurses and relatives. Once the surgical site has stabilized, gentle active ROM exercises may be started. Mobilization of the nervous system should be considered to limit postlaminectomy scarring in any of the intraneural or extraneural tissue.[61] During the acute postsurgical phase, depending on the type of surgery, prone knee bend and SLR can be introduced in a limited, gentle, and nonprovocative way. As the patient's recovery progresses, treatment of the nervous system is usually still necessary and may be carried out in sitting via cervical and thoracic flexion. The patient can also flex and extend the knee with the body in a partial slumped position (slump test position) (see Fig. 22-22).

Scar tissue is assessed by appreciating and observing:

1. The stage of healing and reactivity.
2. Intrinsic mobility of the scar (in all planes).
3. Influence of scar tissue on muscle recruitment and osteokinematic motion patterns of related articular segments.
4. Dissociation from adjacent and underlying structures.

Any scar should be examined for tender spots on deep palpation. With increased resistance (adhesions) there may be a

BOX 8-4   EXAMPLES OF MUSCULATURE THAT CAN BE TREATED EFFECTIVELY BY FRICTION MASSAGE

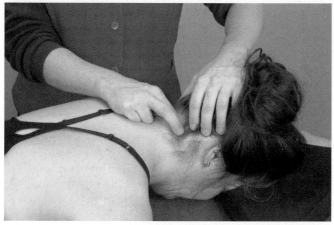

A

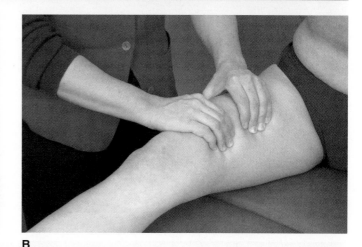

B

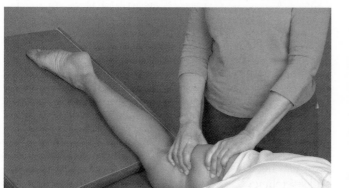

C

D

(A) Deep friction to the occipital insertion of semispinalis and/or splenius capitis muscle (posttraumatic lesions). Pressure is imparted upward and forward, thus catching the muscle against the bone.

(B) Deep friction to the quadriceps belly (posttraumatic lesion). The quadriceps are placed in a resting position (knee extended and hip flexed). The thumbs are used as a fulcrum as flexion of the fingers draws the tissues upward (the skin must move with the fingers). After friction, isometric contractions are done over 5 to 10 minutes.

(C) Deep friction to the hamstring belly (muscle strain). The technique is similar to the one used in quadriceps lesions. The patient lies prone, with the hip extended and the knee passively flexed to 90° to produce complete relaxation of the muscle's belly. Using the thumbs as a fulcrum an extension movement at the wrists moves the flexed fingers upward. After friction, isometric contractions are done.

(D) Deep friction to the popliteus (muscle or tendon strain). The patient adopts a prone position with the knee slightly bent. One thumb reinforced by the other is placed on the affected area. Deep friction is given by a supination of both arms.

(continued)

Box 8-4. continued

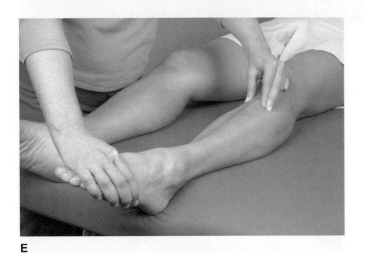

(E) Deep friction to the tibialis anterior (myosynovitis). With the foot in full plantar flexion and eversion (to stretch the muscle), the thumb is placed on the medial aspect and the fingers on the lesion. The thumb is used as a fixed point as the fingers apply transverse friction over the muscle.

hyperalgesic skin zone around the scar, best detected by skin stretching.[253]

Superficial Release. Superficial restrictions can be released easily by superficial techniques such as J-stroking (Fig. 8-8), perpendicular "skin gliding" (see Fig. 7-40), or skin rolling techniques (see Fig. 7-41). When employing skin rolling techniques, as the restrictions are felt, slightly greater force can be used to lift and pull the skin upward and backward until all the restrictions are released. The S pressure release technique (Fig. 8-12) can be applied to the subcutaneous tissue, to active scars

with tender points and surrounded by an hyperalgesic skin zones (HSZ).[72,253] Subcutaneous scar tissue can be loosened by careful and persistent transverse friction (see above) or circular friction massage (see below).[20,430]

Deep Release. Scar tissue releases epitomize the concept of the myofascial onions metaphor.[277,278] The layer-by-layer approach allows a complete release of the superficial scar and its deeper layers. Over time, once the initial superficial scar tissue release is completed, another layer of the surrounding layer of the scar tissue and restriction of the surrounding layer can be released using local scar tissue manipulations and stretching.

Using this concept, circular frictions may be performed with the whole or proximal part of the palm or with the palmar surface of the distal phalanx (Box 8-5, Fig. A). Circular friction massage is applied in the direction (clockwise or counterclockwise) which will produce tension on the involved scar and there by stretch and loosen it. One or both hands may be used.

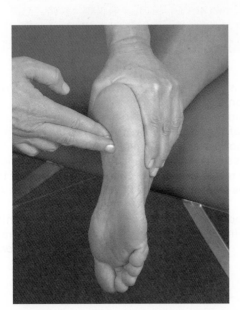

■ **FIG. 8-31.** Deep friction to the insertion of the plantar fascia on the calcaneus. When frictions are applied to the aponeuroses of the foot (plantar fascia of the foot), a rubber-tipped T bar may be necessary because of the density of the tissue.

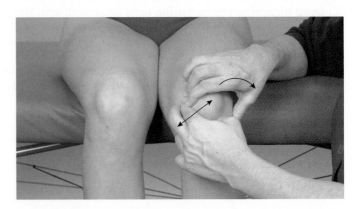

■ **FIG. 8-32.** Deep friction to the medial patellar plica (plica syndrome)

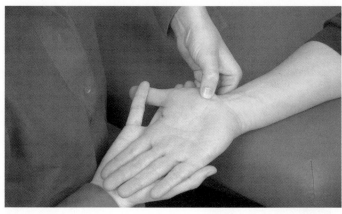
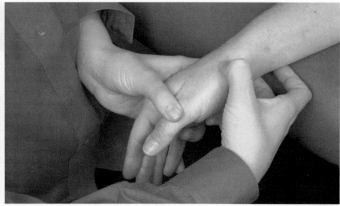

A   B

■ **FIG. 8-33.** Deep friction to the anterior (**A**) and anterolateral capsule (**B**) of the trapezium–first metacarpal joint.

1. Two thumbs may work closely together, alternating clockwise or counterclockwise movements (Box 8-5, Fig. *B*).
2. One thumb may give support or stabilize as the opposing thumb or fingers work against it as the friction movement is performed.
3. Over a large flat surface one palm does the friction movement reinforced by the other hand.

Transverse or circular friction manipulations may be performed with a rubber glove or a piece of Dyson material to assist in softening the scar and increasing the extensibility.

The use of non–water-based lubricants such as cocoa butter or lanolin rich lotions are often recommended to soften the skin and maintain tissue mobility.[291,430]

Other forms of deep releases include:

1. Pinching and lifting techniques of the scar tissue away from the body (Box 8-5, Fig. *C*). The scar is gathered in a pincer grip with the thumbs and fingers and lifted directly and slowly upward from the body. Once a full stretch away from the body is completed, maintain the vertical traction and move the tissue in all planes to determine the areas of restrictions. Once the direction(s) of the barrier is determined, change the angle of stretch in response to feedback. Hold, wait for the release, and stretch again. Repeat the stretch until a soft end feel is reached.
2. Stretching techniques of deeply indented scar tissue (Box 8-5, Fig. *D*). Scar tissue can be stretched in a similar manner as a muscle is stretched. Depending on the barrier the scar tissue may be stretched in a longitudinal, horizontal, or diagonal direction. When used on large surfaces both hands are used. The hands may stretch in the opposite direction or one hand may stabilize while the other hand mobilizes. Sometimes it is advantageous to use an indirect technique in which the opposing hand feed the tissue into the mobilizing hand.

Skin rolling (see Fig. 7-41) is a good final technique to verify that all restrictions have been released.

Scar tissue is a common and frequently ignored source of myofascial pain either locally or at a distance. The exact mechanism is not known, but it is possible that it may be owing to neuroma formation, which causes an aberrant input into the central nervous system, or it may be owing to a restriction of glide of the layers of fascia.[48] Scar desensitization should be initiated gently and can be performed in many ways. These methods include manual self-massage, deep soft tissue manipulations, S contact technique, trigger point release and injections, the use of vibrators, acupuncture (local anesthesia), and rubbing the skin with different textures such as a towel.[48,253,277,278,281,451,452] Scar tissue can be stimulated by either therapeutic laser or by "peppering" the scar with an acupuncture needle.[48] With hand involvement, gripping of different textured particles by the patient has been found to be a useful desensitization technique. Gripping is not only beneficial for scar site desensitization but the encouragement of active wrist extension with finger flexion.[281]

Scar tissue massage and/or desensitization techniques become an important component of the home program and the patient is advised to perform these activities several times per day. As the patient progresses through the various stages of wound healing, his or her response to treatment is constantly assessed and treatment is modified or advanced.

MUSCLE LENGTHENING AND INHIBITION TECHNIQUES

Several types of muscular dysfunction were discussed in Chapter 7, Myofascial Considerations and Evaluation in Somatic Dysfunction. Specific treatment approaches that are designed to address these unique characteristics for improvement in function will vary since each type of muscle dysfunction is manifested differently and has different neurophysiologic characteristics.

| BOX 8-5 | SOFT TISSUE MANIPULATIONS USED IN THE TREATMENT OF SCAR TISSUE |

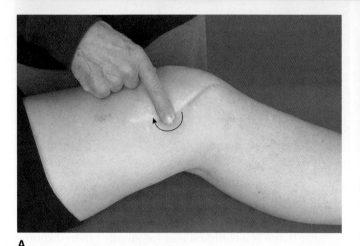

A

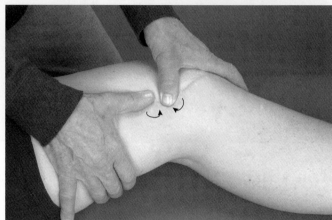

B

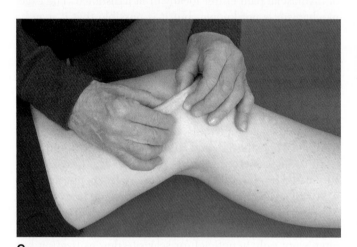

C

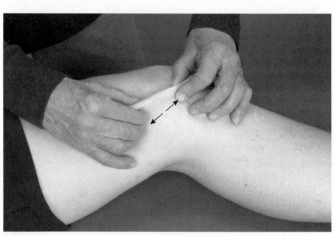

D

(A) Clockwise or counterclockwise circular frictions with one finger. The angle and direction is changed in response to feedback. When the scar adhesion is placed on maximum stretch, feedback will guide the therapist to increase the vertical pressure until an end feel is reached.
(B) Circular friction with two thumbs working closely together or one thumb stabilizes while the opposing thumb or fingers work against it.
(C) Vertical lifting and rolling technique.
(D) Stretching technique

Limbic System Dysfunction

The **limbic system** is the functional link between mental activity, particularly as related to emotions, and muscle activity (see Chapter 7). The muscles affected in limbic system dysfunction include those in the cervical spine, particularly the posterior cervical muscles, the sternocleidomastoid and the upper trapezius, the lumbar muscles, particularly the erector spinae, and the muscles of the pelvic floor.[212] The involved muscles are predisposed to developing myofascial trigger points and

are thus capable of creating referred pain syndromes, particularly headache and low back pain.[317]

Treatment for limbic system dysfunction involves some form of relaxation training if lasting relief of pain is to be expected (see Chapter 9, Relaxation and Related Techniques). This can take the form of biofeedback, progressive relaxation, autogenic training and other forms of psychophysiologic relaxation techniques including meditation.[225,317] Meditation, in particular can be a powerful tool in treatment of patients with chronic cervical and lumbar syndromes. It has been demonstrated that it is possible to reduce the sensitivity of the stretch reflex and muscle tone, via conscious effort.[125,490-492]

In addition to relaxation training the muscles can be treated with soft tissue manipulations, muscle re-education, postisometric relaxation, and positional release to reduce tone or ischemic compression for any trigger points that may be present.

Interneuron Dysfunction

Interneuron dysfunction is alteration of muscle tone that results from joint or muscle dysfunction.[212,316] Hypertonicity related to interneuron dysfunction can be detected by muscle length testing. The treatment of choice for joint dysfunction is joint articulations (see Chapter 6, Introduction to Manual Therapy) which often resolves the muscle dysfunction. Changes in muscle activity have been demonstrated following manipulation.[153,162,185,186,442] Joint manipulation may not always be sufficient to resolve the hypertonicity of the muscle. This is particularly true when hypertonicity is well established as a result of plastic range that has taken place in the neuromuscular system.[317] Soft tissue manipulation and postisometric relaxation techniques (applied directly to the involved muscles to produce normalization of muscle tone) are usually necessary.

Postisometric relaxation (muscle energy) techniques (see Chapter 6, Introduction to Manual Therapy) are very effective in producing muscular relaxation. They can also be used to treat muscular spasms, trigger points and even referred pain.[253] Postisometric relaxation can also be used to influence joint position and mobility (see Figs. 17-32, 8-43, 8-49, 8-65, and 8-66). The principles applied in postisometric techniques are similar to those of PNF techniques employed to release tight myofascia and to reeducate neuromuscular function and joint control (see Chapter 6).

Reflex Spasm

The obvious treatment for reflex spasm is rapid reduction of nociception. The principle of effective management includes patient education, controlling the inflammatory responses, treating the pain-producing structures and promoting healing through controlled movements and reduced stresses. Joint mobilization or manipulations can relieve reflex spasm related to spinal injury.[203]

Myofascial Trigger Points Management

Knowledge of trigger points and skill in deactivating them are felt to be essential to relieve myofascial pain. It is important however to be able to differentially diagnose myofascial from articular sources of pain. It is not possible to differentiate between joint and muscle sources on the basis of the location of the pain. Both muscle and joints can cause local or referred pain. If an active trigger point is found (taut band, twitch response, positive jump sign, referred pain to target area), the following approach is recommended.[257,451]

1. Assess for muscle imbalances
2. Assess for joint dysfunction
3. Identify work or lifestyle factors
4. Aim treatment at remediating joint dysfunction and restoring muscle balance
5. If treatment fails and corticalization of pain and fibromyalgia have been ruled out consider methods to deactivate the active trigger point.

Trigger points may be deactivated by a variety of non-manual methods including cryotherapy, saline injections, dry needling, anesthetics, transcutaneous nerve stimulation and acupuncture (see Chapter 6, Introduction to Manual Therapy and Chapter 17 Temporomandibular Joint). Manual methods found to be effective in deactivating trigger points include deep stroking massage (stripping), vibrations, percussive strokes, acupressure, deep friction at the trigger point, ischemic compression, and use of integrated neuromuscular inhibition technique.[48,72,278,432,452] No one technique has emerged which is superior to the others. Myofascial stretching, strain–counterstrain (positional release), postisometric relaxation, or functional techniques are usually part of a multifaceted approach to trigger point treatment.[72,317] The preferred type of stretching in this sequence is to activate the fibers involved using isometric contractions (PNF) or postisometric relaxation techniques.[72]

The application of ischemic compression, advocated by Travell and Simons,[451] involves applying direct compression to the trigger point. Trigger points are released manually by carefully graded increasing pressure using one finger, several fingers, the knuckle, or elbow with enough pressure to elicit the referred pain pattern without causing significant pain. With this method, the pressure is held until the referred pain disappears for approximately 1 minute. One application is made to each TP using this technique. A knowledge of trigger points and their radiation patterns will help the practitioner understand complicated pain complaints. Both volumes of *Myofascial Pain and Dysfunction* by Travell and Simons[452,453] describe the primary trigger points and their radiation patterns. In treating trigger points, the method of chilling the offending muscle while holding it on stretch to achieve this end, was advocated by Travell and Simons. In recent publications, Travell and Simons have moved towards Lewit's viewpoint, using postisometric relaxation as a starting point before stretching the offending muscles.[452,453]

Another method of ischemic compression developed by Nimmo[79] follows similar guidelines (as above) but the pressure is held for only 5 to 7 seconds, after which finger pressure is quickly withdrawn, another trigger point found, and the same technique used. After several trigger points are treated in this way (compression held for 5 to 7 seconds with a quick release), the clinician returns to the first trigger point and again treats it in the same manner, with repeated applications to each of the treated trigger points. Each trigger point is treated three times.

The variations of applying manual ischemic compression are unlimited. A particular approach that this author has found to be highly effective is that advocated by Manheim[277,278] in which trigger point releases follow the same pattern as other myofascial releases. The initial pressure takes up the available slack in the surrounding tissue in a downward or inward direction. As the trigger point gradually relaxes, the pressure is increased to take up additional slack. Following the initial release, the inherent tissue motion will draws the finger(s) farther down into the trigger point in a spiral fashion. Feedback from the patient directs the treatment. When no further releases occur, pressure is slowly released. Manheim[277,278] provides detailed information on this method.

No matter what technique or combinations of techniques are used, the basic goal of treatment remains the same. Local pain relief is necessary to allow restoration of normal movement. Normal movement can be restored through a number of techniques including mobilization of stiff joints, soft tissue manipulations, stretching of tight myofascial structures, and strengthening of weakened muscles groups. Normal movement must be maintained through postural alignment and relaxation. Positions and movements that cause prolonged misalignment of body parts should be avoided.

THERAPEUTIC MUSCLE STRETCHING

Therapeutic muscle stretching (see Chapter 6: Introduction to Manual Therapy), specific muscle stretching instructed by a practitioner in patients with dysfunction of the musculoskeletal system, has been promoted by numerous authors.[2,3,19,22,42,114,126,127,207,230,245,247,314,338,339,372,373,406,432,452,453,503] Stretching is considered important because it is believed to provide many physical benefits, including improved flexibility,[46,164,399] injury prevention,[399,403] improved muscle or athletic performance,[484,495] improved running economy,[146,403] promotion of healing, and possibly decreased onset of muscle soreness.[59,105]

Three common methods of stretching are generally used in the attempt to elongate the muscle tendon unit and the periarticular connective tissue. These methods are manual or mechanically applied passive stretch (static stretch) (Fig. 8-34), active inhibition through the use of various proprioceptive neuromuscular techniques (PNF), and self-stretch.[22,77,95,224,233,235,236,245,285,338,339,391,392,422,454]

The rationale for various forms of muscle stretching such as static stretch (SS),[52,104,233,236,339,378,408,462,471,472,501–503] static stretch with yoga poses,[30,52,86,87,159,237,246,249,350,351,365,435,445] self-stretch,[3,52,112,128,151,161,163,233,247,383,456] postisometric relaxation,[252,253] muscle energy,[47,148,150,155,308,477] contract–relax (CR) (synonymously called hold–relax),[80,126–128,285,345,369,422,428,460,462] and contract–relax–antagonist–contract (CRAC),[81,480] hold relax with agonist contraction (HR-AC),[80,123,126,127,309,462] and agonist contraction (AC)[13,77,80,126,127] techniques have been well documented. Numerous researchers have compared various stretching techniques to determine which technique is most effective for increasing ROM.[197,369,399,467,482]

Passive and Static Stretch

Static stretching is a method of stretching in which a stationary position is held for a period during which specific joints are locked into a position that places the muscles and connective tissues at their greatest length.[502] Passive stretch may be applied either manually or by sustained mechanical stretch (Fig. 8-34; also see Fig. 12-29).

MANUALLY APPLIED STATIC STRETCH

Manually applied stretching is usually applied for 15 to 30 seconds. Continuation of the stretch for a period longer than this will generally not generate any greater flexibility gains.[13,270,367,368,460] It has, however been demonstrated that 60-second stretching can yield a greater rate of improve-

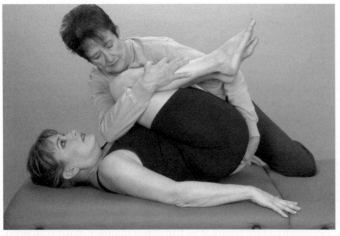
A

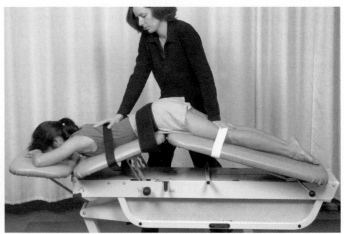
B

■ **FIG. 8-34.** Manual **(A)** and **(B)** mechanical stretch of the myofascia of the lumbar spine by positioning.

ment in knee extension ROM then similar regimens of 15- or 30-second stretches in elderly people.[129] The advantages of manual static stretching when compared to ballistic stretching (quick stretch imposed upon the muscles and connective tissue structures) are (1) energy requirements are lower, (2) there is little danger of exceeding the extensibility of the tissues involved, and (3) muscle soreness is less likely and may be relieved.[105] Static stretching also has the advantages of minimizing any impact of the Ia and II spindle afferent fiber stimulation and maximizing the impact of Golgi tendon organ, thereby decreasing the contractile elements of resistance to deformation.[501] A low-intensity maintained stretch that is applied gradually is also less likely to facilitate the stretch reflex and increase tension in the muscle being lengthened.[140,144]

MECHANICAL STATIC STRETCH

When muscle contracture has been present for some time or when the patient is too large, a mechanical assist is useful. A low-intensity external force is applied to shortened tissues over a prolonged period with mechanical equipment. The stretch force may be applied through positioning of the patient (Fig. 8-34B), with dynamic splints or serial casts, with weighted traction and pulley systems, or with weights (5 to 15 lb or 5 to 10% of body weight)(see Fig. 12-29).

When using mechanical sustained stretch, the muscle will resist; therefore, the mechanical stretch is usually applied for at least 15 minutes. Duration of 20 minutes or longer seems to be more effective, and the possible reason is that the stretch reflex of muscle has been fatigued.[40,338,378] Low-intensity stretch (5- to 12-lb stretch force applied 1 hour per day) has been shown to be significantly more effective than manual passive stretching over a 4-week period in patients with long-standing bilateral knee flexion contractures.[258]

Sustained, low-intensity stretch can also be accomplished with dynamic splints such as the Dynasplint.[181] This type of splint is applied for 8 to 10 hours. Units are available for the elbow, wrist, knee, and ankle. Dynamic wrist and hand splints have self-adjusting resilient or elastic components such as wire, rubber bands, or springs that create mobilizing force on a segment, resulting in passive or passive-assisted motion of a joint or successive joints.[384]

Plastic changes in noncontractile and contractile tissue may be the basis of "permanent" or long-term improvement in flexibility when using this type of prolonged stretching.[40,90]

PNF Stretch

Various authors and studies have concluded that PNF stretching techniques are effective in increasing flexibility. There is no consensus regarding which is the single best technique.[81,263,280,285,309,345,346,369,428,462,467,504] CRAC stretching as been shown to be significantly better than CR stretching ($P <$ 0.05).[81,480] CR was significantly better than HR ($P < 0.05$) and CR and HR was demonstrated to be significantly better than static or ballistic stretching ($P < 0.05$).[263,345,369,428,467] These

techniques seek to capitalize on the use of the neurophysiologic concept of stretch activation and to facilitate the GTO to inhibit the muscle in which it lies or the principle of reciprocal inhibition.[462] Prestretch conditioning through active or passive movements (e.g., active repetitive eccentric contractions or passive oscillations) may loosen actin-myosin bonds and increase stretching effectiveness.[202]

Self-Stretch

Self-stretch is a type of flexibility exercise that clients carry out themselves. Self-stretch may be passive or active, depending on whether the muscles actively participate in promoting the stretch. In passive self-stretch the muscles are relaxed while they are stretched. The force to stretch them come either from the muscles on the opposite side of the joint involved, using body weight, or from an external force (or restraint) or from a combination of these forces. Another method of passive self-stretch of the limbs is by moving the body or trunk in relationship to the stabilized extremity (see Figs. 11-63 through 11-70). This type of self-ROM or self-stretch affords an excellent stretch of the myofascial system, minimizes incorrect movements by the patient, and allows a greater degree of pain-free movement.[111,156]

In active self-stretch, the muscles are alternately contracted and relaxed as the stretch progresses. Using PNF techniques, such as successive contract-then-relax cycle, enables further gains in the lengthening to be attained under control. Because the muscles stretched are actively involved, active stretching tends to be more comfortable than passive stretching.

Most self-stretch exercises may be done actively or passively or may contain both active and passive phases. These stretching techniques require careful instructions and communication with the client to ensure that neither over stretching nor excessive resistance produces muscle injury. Immature collagen cannot tolerate excessive stress and strain. In general, active stretching is preferable, because if affords greater control of the stretch and therefore minimizes the risk of uncontrolled overstretching.[161] Self-stretch enable clients to independently maintain or increase ROM gained in treatment sessions.

In summary, ROM may be limited as a result of contractures, adhesions, and scar tissue formation, leading to shortening of muscles, connective tissue, and skin. The overall goal of the various types of stretching described above is to regain normal ROM of joints and mobility of the soft tissues that surround the joints; to increase the ability of the muscle to lengthen through the necessary ROM in the most efficient manner. PNF forms of stretching, although potentially the most effective, requires time and expertise. Emphasis should be placed on arcuate pathways with respect to the myofascial system and fiber orientation rather than cardinal planes of motion (see Fig. 7-32D). When there is muscle weakness and opposing tissue tightness, tight muscles must be elongated before weak muscles can be strengthened effectively.[208,210] A shortened and tight muscle appears to be over activated in various movement patterns, and this activation may be so intense that it makes strengthening exercise of the weakened muscle impossible due to the reflex inhibition.[208,210]

Manual Stretch and Soft Tissue Manipulations

While the soft tissue or stretching techniques is intended to affect specific muscles or muscle groups of muscles, they are essentially regional techniques. Soft tissue techniques often involve stretching connective and muscle tissue in an abnormal state that generally crosses joints, which prohibit normal painless joint ROM. For example, the sacrospinalis muscle group (quadratus lumborum and erector spinae) and connective tissue (thoracolumbar fasciae) in an abnormal state (e.g., spasm, acute lumbago, tightness, and ultimately some degree of fibrosis) may need unilateral stretching and mobilization as well as the more intrinsic joint structures. This may be achieved in part by the use of localized stretching and soft tissue manipulation (including orthodox massage) and by using methods which also have a considerable effect on the more intrinsic joint structures (Fig. 8-35, Fig. 8-36, Fig. 8-37).[126,127,155,272,411,427]

Many soft tissue spinal stretching techniques have similarly have appeared under the guise of manual traction techniques (Fig. 8-34A) because the division between stretching and traction is largely notational. Nevertheless, stretching generally refers to soft tissues, which have length, whereas traction generally indicates concern with immediate peri-articular and intra-articular structures.[154] Similarly, a unilateral soft tissue stretch to a given segmental level of the spine is also asymmetrical traction for the associated intrinsic vertebral joint structures. Many nonspecific joint mobilization techniques are also considered soft tissue stretching techniques (see Figs. 22-25 through 22-30).

CAPSULAR STRETCH

Hip Joint

One should also consider stretching of restrictive joint capsules. In the early stages of osteoarthrosis, stretching of the joint capsule is often the treatment of choice. The decision to use stretching depends largely on the clinical findings. For example, in osteoarthritis of the hip, early arthrosis with a slight capsular pattern and a more or less elastic end feel usually respond quite well to such treatment.[334] The result to be expected is not a marked increase in range but a decrease in pain. Used in the early stage, years of relief can often be obtained.[334] Ombregt and associates recommend stretching the joint capsule in three directions: flexion (Fig. 8-39), internal rotation (Fig. 8-40), and extension (Fig. 8-41) for 5 to 10 minutes each. Self-mobilization techniques can be carried out at home (see Figs. 14-35 and 14-36). Rocking-chair therapy is an excellent form of sensory stimulation for relieving pain that should also be considered.[93,497] Following the early stages a more vigorous and comprehensive program should be considered (see Chapter 14, Hip).

Many patients, particularly those with significant medial femoral torsion, may require stretching of the anterior joint structures to increase their available lateral rotation and to help the gluteals muscles work in the inner range. Patient-assisted stretch of the anterior structures can be carried out effectively in the figure-of-four position (Fig. 8-42).[152] The patient is instructed to push along the length of the thigh to try to flatten the pelvis against the treatment table (see Fig. 8-42A). When this can be achieved, glutei (gluteus medius muscle in the inner range) facilitation techniques can be started. The patient is instructed to keep the pelvis on the

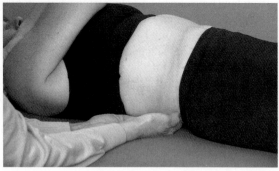 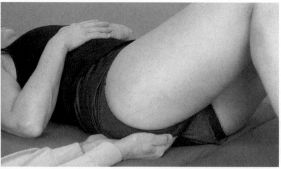

A   **B**

■ **FIG. 8-35.** Manual stretch and soft tissue manipulation of **(A)** mass of lumbar muscles (erector spinae and quadratus lumborum) and connective tissue. The region is distracted on the ipsilateral side with the tips of the fingers applied against the spinous processes and lateral borders of the sacrum. While using this leverage formed by the wrist and forearm, pressure is also applied upward with the fingers. This combined pressure-distraction is maintained for some time, then released to be applied again. This maneuver has a very sedative effect in acute low back problems. **(B)** It is also an effective technique in mobilizing the connective tissue along the borders of the sacrum before attempting to mobilize the sacrum out of various positions of dysfunction.[272]

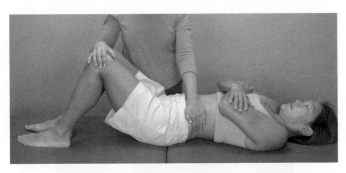

■ **FIG. 8-36.** Manual stretch and soft tissue manipulation of the lumbar mass with counter pressure of the legs. Slow and very rhythmic transverse pull on the mass of lumbar muscles is applied toward the therapist as the knees are pushed away. This maneuver should be applied slowly and rhythmically.[272]

table while lifting the knee of the laterally rotated leg off the table (see Fig. 8-42*B*). Because training is specific to limb position, it is essential that gluteus medius is mainly trained in weight bearing (see Fig. 14-39).

Shoulder Joint

In the later stages of shoulder adhesive capsulitis, aggressive self-stretching of the capsule (see Fig. 11-62) and surrounding musculature can be used effectively. Aggressive capsular stretching is started when the patient has attained flexibility of at least 90° abduction and the end feel is firm with a painless end point. Patients are instructed in either a high-load, short-duration stretch (10 seconds) or low-load, long-duration stretch (40 seconds or longer). An effective indirect method

of facilitating extensibility of the glenohumeral joint capsule is a modification of the arm traction technique employing a capsular twist (Fig. 8-21).[179]

COMMON MYOFASCIAL LESIONS AND THEIR MANAGEMENT

Craniomandibular Dysfunction

There is an intimate relationship between the head and neck as well as surrounding joint and soft tissue structures.[357,358] Trauma as well as occlusal and postural abnormalities (see forward head posture below) and/or dysfunction affecting one structure frequently result in problems at an adjacent region.

The upper quarter and the stomatognathic system includes the cranium, mandible, temporomandibular joint (TMJ), dentition, upper and lower cervical spine, cervicothoracic junction, upper thoracic spine, first and second ribs, sternum, and shoulder girdle. Each of these are connected via soft tissue comprising muscles, ligaments, fascia, and tendons as well as interrelated neural innervation, circulation, and lymphatic systems. Because one of the main symptoms of craniomandibular disorders is myofascial tenderness, the status of the cervicovertebral region and head posture is likely to be affected in a patient suffering from such disorders.

Comprehensive treatment of the temporomandibular and craniocervical disorders can be broken down into four areas: modalities, mobilization, exercise (neuromuscular re-education, facilitory exercises), and patient education (see Chapter 17, Temporomandibular Joint and Stomatognathic System). Effective soft tissue manipulations techniques include deep pressure joint massage, transverse friction massage to the capsule (Box 8-6, Fig. *C*, as well as the myofascial system),

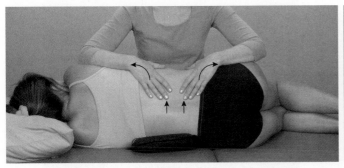

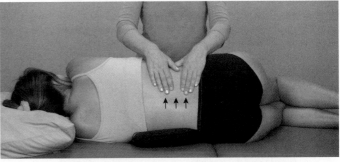

A   B

■ **FIG. 8-37.** Manual stretch and soft tissue manipulation of the mass of erector spinae, thoracolumbar fascia, and quadratus lumborum muscles. **(A)** The myofascial structures are placed in some degree of stretch (by using a roll under the lumbar spine and flexing the patient's bottom leg). The therapist applies outward pressure with both forearms. **(B)** Alternatively, the therapist may apply transverse soft tissue stretch with the myofascial tissues on stretch. Further stretch can be achieved by flexing both legs towards the chest and the therapist's using his or her thighs to push the patient's knees further into lumbar flexion to the desired degree of stretch. Alternating pressure on the knees varies the tension on the myofascial structures. Rhythmic motion against the knees, counterbalanced by the pulling action to the hands, is an effective way of releasing the connective tissue and sacrospinal muscles.[441,442]

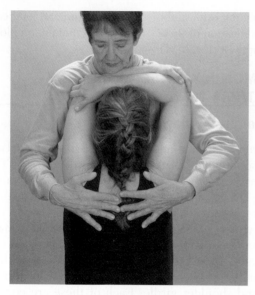

■ **FIG. 8-38.** Manual stretch of the upper thoracic spine and the pectoral soft tissue. A walk stand posture is used with the patient's arms supported on the operator's chest while rhythmically leaning backward.

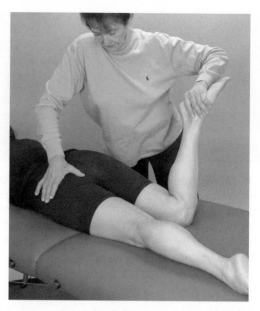

■ **FIG. 8-40.** Capsular stretch—hip internal rotation. The hip is moved into medial rotation until the opposite ilium is lifted off the table. At this point the operators applies pressure to the opposite ilium downward toward the plinth. When the thigh of the affected side is firmly in the rotated position, this downward pressure will increase the outward stress on the affected hip.

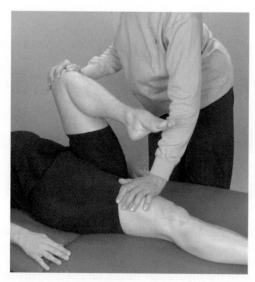

■ **FIG. 8-39.** Capsular stretch—hip flexion. This position is maintained for as long as the patient can comfortably tolerate it (e.g., for 1 minute). The degree of force applied is determined by the ratio of pain to end feel.

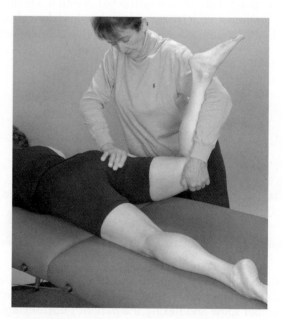

■ **FIG. 8-41.** Capsular stretch–hip extension. By sidebending the body, the operator pulls the patient's thigh upward while the pelvis is pushed down forcefully. Pain and the end feel determine the degree and duration of force used.

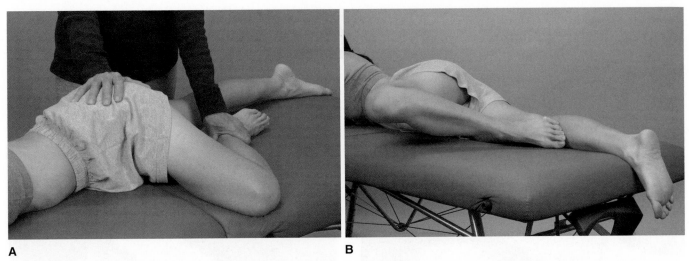

A   **B**

■ **FIG. 8-42.** Anterior stretch of the capsule and other soft tissue structures of the hip region. **(A)** Patient-assisted stretch in the figure-of-four position. The patient is instructed to push along the length of the thigh to try to flatten the anterior superior iliac spine onto the treatment table. **(B)** Facilitation of the gluteus medius occurs when the patient elevates the knee while trying to maintain the pelvis on the table.

gentle kneading or stroking techniques intraorally to inhibit pain (to the insertion of the temporalis, medial, and lateral pterygoid musculature) (see Figs. 17-23*B*, 17-24, 17-25*B*, and 17-26), connective tissue massage, myofascial manipulations or release, postisometric relaxation techniques (see Fig. 17-32), strain–counterstrain (Box 8-6, Fig. *E*), stretching, and craniosacral therapy.[75,96,113,126–128,273,278,334,358,453] Exercise is critical to maintain the gained extensibility of the soft tissues.[358] The major muscles of mastication which can be treated effectively by soft tissue manipulations include the following:

1. Masseter
2. Temporalis
3. Medial pterygoid
4. Lateral pterygoid

Pain originating from these muscles is present in the great majority of TMJ patients. Soft tissue manipulations and stretching have been found to be particularly helpful to release the temporal masseter complex and pterygoid musculature. Box 8-6 provides a number of examples of soft tissue manipulations and stretching techniques for these primary muscles of mastication.

Because of the intimate relationship between the upper cervical spine and the TMJ,[113] soft tissue release techniques can be applied to cervical spine musculature and upper cervical joints. Figures 8-43 and Box 8-7, show generalized releases that aid in balancing asymmetries of the maladjusted musculature and joints. These techniques bring freedom to the restricted infrahyoid, anterior deep cervical (longus colli, longus capitis), and ligamentous support structures.[113] Also released are the superficial skin, the fascia, the platysma, the sternocleidomastoid belly, and the anterior division of the scaleni. Lateral cervical releases (Box 8-7, Fig. *C*) are effective in releasing the

sternocleidomastoid, anterolateral ligamentous support structures, and anterior and medial portions of the scalenes that are important in balancing the cranium. Shortening or spasms of the scalenes may inhibit the movement cephalad in the kinetic chain.[357] Box 8-7 provides a number of examples of soft tissue manipulations and stretching techniques of the upper cervical spine, prevertebral and anterior muscles of the neck, and the suboccipital muscles (also see Figs. 7-34, 8-43 through 8-46, 8-52, and 8-53).

Proximal or Shoulder Girdle Crossed Syndrome and the Forward Head Posture

The proximal crossed syndrome has been described earlier (see Chapter 7, Muscle Imbalance Syndromes).[207,208,210–214,223] This pattern of muscle imbalance produces typical changes in posture and motion. In standing, elevation and protraction of the shoulders are evident as well as counterclockwise rotation and abduction of the shoulder blades and a forward head posture (FHP) (see Fig. 17-19). This altered posture is likely to stress the cervicothoracic and cervicocranial junctions.[215]

Muscle findings in the FHP typically reveal shortening of the suboccipital muscles and compression forces on the trigeminocervical complex and vertebral artery. Other findings include the following:

• Imbalance between the sternocleidomastoid, levator scapula, and trapezius which tighten and shorten. An altered direction of the axis of the glenoid fossa will develop resulting in the humerus needing to be stabilized by additional levator scapula and upper trapezius activity, with additional activity of the supraspinatus as well.[75]
• Imbalances of the supra and infra hyoid muscles. The suprahyoids tend to shorten and develop increased tension

| BOX 8-6 | EXAMPLES OF SOFT TISSUE MANIPULATIONS AND STRETCHING TECHNIQUES FOR THE PRIMARY MUSCLES OF MASTICATION AND TMJ CAPSULE |

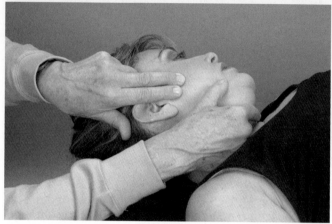

A

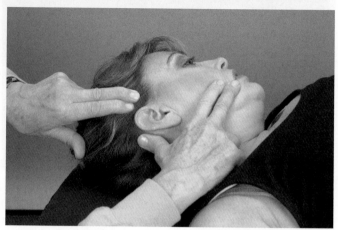

B

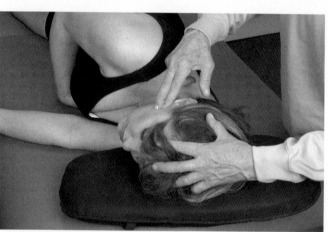

C

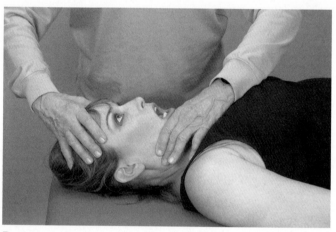

D

(A) Masseter release. Stretch of small muscles can be performed using one or two fingers or a thumb. Stretch a small segment of the muscle to take up the slack. Hold and wait for a release and stretch again. Repeat this sequence until an end feel is reached. Move to another area of involved muscle and repeat the sequence again.

(B) Temporalis and masseter complex release. A modification of the technique shown in A simultaneously incorporating the masseter and temporalis. This technique is valuable for patients who have temporal headaches and for treating patients who chronically clench.

(C) Deep friction to TMJ joint capsule. The reinforced index finger applies transverse frictions to the capsule.

(D) Postisometric relaxation of the masseter, medial pterygoid, and the temporalis. The patient is instructed to breathe out after the slack has been taken up and then open the mouth wide and take a deep breath. During the relaxation phase passive deviation of the mandible may be introduced to selectively stretch the muscles in question.

Box 8-6. continued

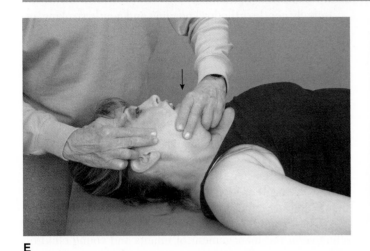

E

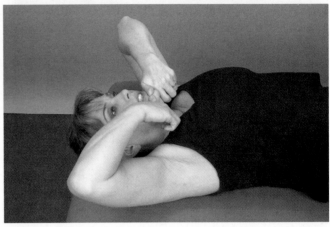

F

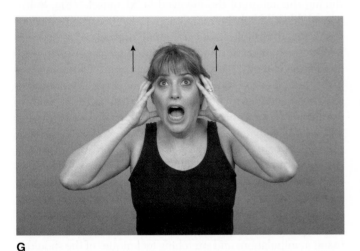

G

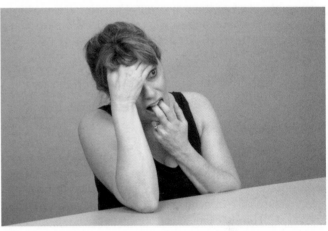

H

(E) Strain–counterstrain of the masseter. Treatment involves pushing the slightly open mandible toward the side of the deviation. The tender point is usually found near the front of the ascending ramus of the mandible.

(F) Self-stretch of lateral pterygoid. The same as postisometric relaxation of the masseter (part E) except the patient uses her own thumbs.

(G) Self-stretch of temporalis. The jaw elevator muscles are elongated by opening the mouth to a comfortable position. The patient presses firmly in the upward direction just above the temples with her fingers, stretching the temporalis muscle while taking a long full breath to facilitate relaxation.

(H) Self-stretch (using postisometric relaxation) of the masseter, medial pterygoid, and the temporalis muscle. The patient sits with the propping hand on her forehead; the fingers of the other hand are on the lower incisors. After opening her mouth to take up the slack, she breathes out; during inhalation she opens her mouth as wide as possible.

while there is lengthening of the infrahyoid. The muscle of mastication and the digastric are also frequently involved (see Chapter 17, Temporomandibular Joint and Stomatognathic System, and Figs. 17-31 and 17-32). Shortening of all the shoulder girdle internal rotators, including the latissimus dorsi, subscapularis, pectoralis, and teres major occurs.

- Respiration shows increased activity of the accessory muscles with decreased utilization of diaphragmatic breathing. There is a decreased ability for the lower rib cage to expand, leading to an upper respiratory sequence of breathing.

- Scalene shortness can be assumed if there is any indication of upper chest breathing. Typically there is elevation of the first and second ribs.

The suboccipital muscles (rectus capitis posterior major and minor, obliquus capitis inferior and superior) help provide and control movements of nodding, rotation, and sidebending. They are a common source of headache and are shortened in the FHP with a posterior rotated cranium. It is often helpful to deactivate the trigger points or tender points (of fibromyal-

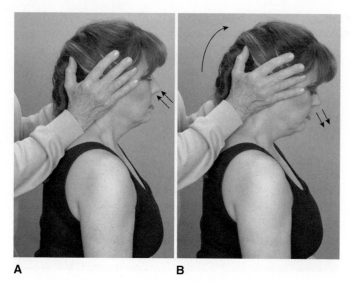

A   **B**

■ **FIG. 8-43.** Postisometric release of the suboccipital muscles. **(A)** The operator flexes the patient's head to take up the slack in the suboccipital muscles; then, while the patient looks up and slowly takes a deep breath, the operator gently resists the patient's tendency to extend. **(B)** The patient then slowly exhales fully, looks down, and allows the head to flex while the operator exerts upward traction at the occiput and takes up the slack that develops.

gia) along the occiput region before stretching or release of the suboccipital muscles by augmented postisometric release or positional release (Fig. 8-43).[253,453] Often occipitoatlantal (OA), alantoaxial (AA), and C2 on C3 joint dysfunction coexist and must all be checked and treated.

There is no absolute test for shortness of the sternocleidomastoid (SCM) (see Fig. 7-36), but observation of posture (FHP) and palpation of the degree of induration, fibrosis, and trigger point activity can all alert to probable shortness of the SCM.[74,215] The authors have found that soft tissue manipulations of the SCM are often more effective in increasing its extensibility than are traditional stretching methods and places less stress on the cervical joints.[33] Traditionally, to stretch the SCM, the head and neck must be put into an extreme of rotation and lateral flexion, which can be uncomfortable and can also be damaging to the joints and smaller muscles. This is particularly true in the acceleration injury (acute whiplash). The most common injuries in acceleration injuries found in a study by McNab[269] were complete and partial tears of the SCM muscle followed by complete tears of the longus colli and complete and partial tears of the anterior longitudinal ligament. The SCM muscles will often be overshortened and very strong. Any strengthening program that increased the strength of the SCM or anterior neck musculature will contribute to muscle imbalance. The most effective method for the longus colli and multifidi is to restore normal resting length (slight lordosis) of the cervical spine[357,358] and to retrain

these muscles for deep segmental muscle control and support rather than strength training.[222]

Initially gentle orthodox kneading and gentle stroking are quite effective in decreasing tone of the SCM. Release the SCM by gently squeezing the muscle between your thumb and flexed index finger and unwind the muscle laterally (Fig. 8-44). Transverse stroking may be used along the muscle belly where trigger points, tender areas, and areas of hypertonicity are encountered. In more chronic conditions, after releasing the muscle edges and bony insertions (Fig. 8-45), vigorous forms of soft tissue manipulations may be carried out as well as muscle energy techniques. The SCM and upper trapezius (which are synergistic) can be tested and treated quite effectively together.[151] The resistive force is to the patient's shoulder girdle rather than the head and neck.

We have found strain–counterstrain techniques to be quite effective in the management of infants and young children with acute torticollis. Treatment is a simple matter of reproducing the action of the involved SCM muscle (Fig. 8-46). The child will likely be more cooperative because treatment is more comfortable than traditional methods of stretching. Follow-up facilitation techniques and treatment for neck elongation and postural control are important. Ultimately, we want the infant to establish full range of cervical motion and dynamic head control in relationship to full body motion.

The shoulder girdle muscles that often require stretching and soft tissue manipulation are the levator scapula (Fig. 8-47), upper trapezius (Fig. 8-48), and rhomboids (Fig. 8-49). Although the rhomboids usually tend to develop weakness, in the scapular elevation-downward rotation syndrome described by Sahrmann,[371] they tend to be short along with the upper trapezius and levator scapulae. Soft tissue attachments along the scapulae are frequently restricted. Some methods of soft tissue manipulations and stretching techniques of the shoulder girdle complex are depicted in Box 8-8. A number of techniques, which are shown in Figures 11-53 and 11-54, are also considered scapulothoracic articulations.[155]

In the FHP, the anterior elements collapse, reducing diaphragmatic excursion and expansion of the lower rib cage. For patients to perform postural reeducation techniques successfully and elongate the thoracic area, the contracted area of the anterior trunk must be supple and mobile. Release of the intercostals (Fig. 8-50)[155,273,278,323,453] and diaphragm (Fig. 8-51)[65,161,334] may be indicated. Sprained intercostal muscles and lesions of the diaphragm (peripheral costal insertion) respond very well to a few session of deep transverse friction.[334]

Although the scalene muscles have been classified in the past as accessory muscles of respiration, they serve as primary muscles of inhalation.[453] The assessment for muscle length of the scaleni muscles can be used as an effective method for lengthening these muscles (see Fig. 7-34A–C). Soft tissue manipulations (Fig. 8-52),[414,415,421] muscle energy manipulative techniques,[151,308] and strain–counterstrain (positional release) therapy are useful.[96,219,220] Such techniques are augmented greatly with self-stretch by the patient (Fig. 8-53).

BOX 8-7 | **EXAMPLES OF SOFT TISSUE MANIPULATIONS AND STRETCH TECHNIQUES OF THE NECK; PREVERTEBRAL, ANTERIOR, AND SUBOCCIPITAL MUSCLES**

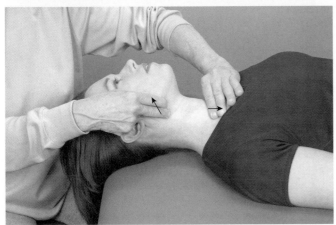

A

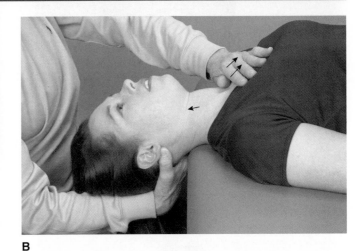

B

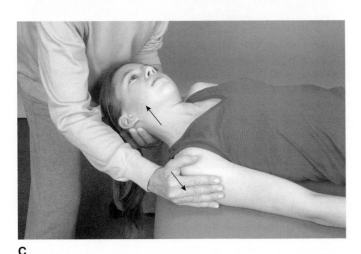

C

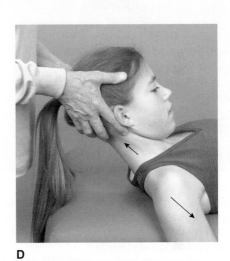

D

(**A**) Infrahyoid release. Using the fingertips, contact is made at the proximal and distal end of the infrahyoid. Gently take up the slack and wait for a release. Repeat this sequence until an end feel is reached. This technique may be used to decrease spasms in the overstretched infrahyoid musculature seen in postcervical whiplash patients.
(**B**) Anterior cervical release (longus colli and capitis, sternocleidomastoid, and ligamentous support structures).
(**C**) Lateral cervical release. The scalenes, sternocleidomastoid, and anterior and lateral support structures are released using this technique.
(**D**) Posterior cervical release. This technique is used to release the trapezius, levator scapulae, splenius capitis, and semispinalis capitis.

(continued)

Box 8-7. continued

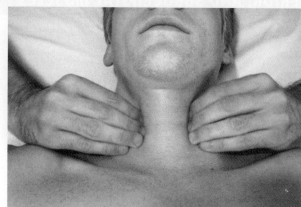

E

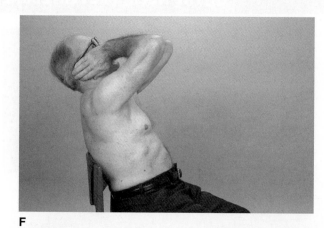

F

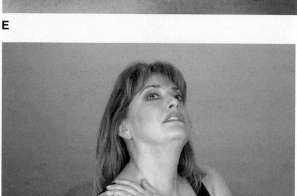

G

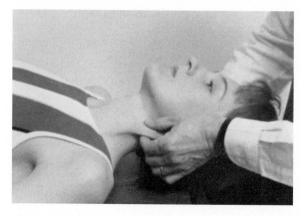

H

(E) Fingertip release of the prevertebral muscles (longus coli, longus capitis). Gently place the fingers of both hands length-wise along the borders of the trachea. Slowly and lightly slide the fingers medial under the trachea toward the anterior bodies of the cervical vertebrae. Moving the fingers of one hand at a time along the prevertebral muscles, feel for knots and taut bands. Work each side individually.
(F) Self-stretch of anterior neck muscles. PNF or postisometric relaxation may be used to facilitate muscle relaxation.
(G) Self-stretch of the sternocleidomastoid.
(H) Self-stretch of the suboccipital muscles. PNF or postisometric relaxation may be used to facilitate muscle relaxation.
(Part E reprinted with permission from Scheumann DW: The Balanced Body: A Guide to Deep Tissue and Neuromuscular Therapy, 2nd ed. Baltimore: Lippincott Williams & Wilkins, 2002:212.)

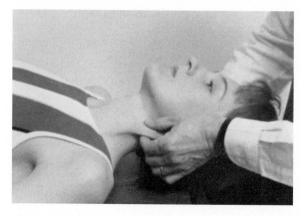

■ **FIG. 8-44.** Massage of muscle belly of the sternocleidomastoid.

In the final stage of restoring full range to the movement of shoulder girdle complex, soft tissue stretch of the gleno-humeral joint capsule (see Figs. 8-21 and 11-62) and the muscles that blend into the capsule (supra and infraspinatus) may be necessary (Figs. 8-54 and 8-55). Additional considerations include treatment of the soft tissues of the clavicular area (Fig. 8-56), upper thoracic spine (Fig. 8-57), and as joint articulations of the associated joints (see Chapter 11, Shoulder and Shoulder Girdle).[65,109]

The osseous components of the "functional shoulder girdle" include the following:

- Upper thoracic vertebrae
- First and second rib
- Manubrium

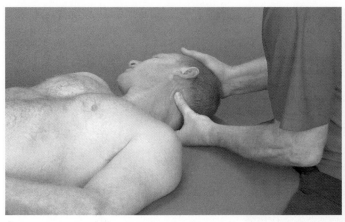
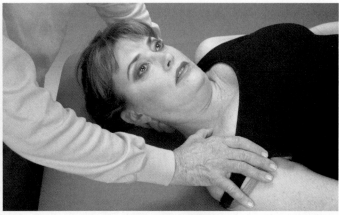

A   **B**

■ **FIG. 8-45.** Clearing the bony attachments of the sternocleidomastoid. **(A)** Clear the bony attachment of the sternoclei-domastoid (SCM) by placing the thumb posterior to the SCM tendon at the mastoid process and displacing the tendon anteriorly while simultaneously pressing into the mastoid process. Use static pressure or transverse friction. **(B)** Release of the bony insertions of the SCM. Medial to lateral friction may be used on the sternal and clavicular attachment.

- Scapula
- Clavicle
- Humerus

The spine must be stable for this complex to functional adequately. To achieve full arm elevation, the upper thoracic vertebrae must be able to extend, rotate, and sidebend to the ipsilateral side, and the bodies of the first and second ribs must be able to descend and move posteriorly with vertebral rotation.[228] The manubriosternal joint, costomanubrial joint, and sternoclavicular joint must permit the manubrium to sidebend and rotate to the ipsilateral side. While the upper thoracic vertebrae must be able to extend, rotate and sidebend to the ipsilateral side, the lower thoracic must be able to sidebend away from the side of motion. For full elevation (180°) exaggeration of the lumbar lordosis becomes necessary and is achieved by the action of the spinal muscles.

In FHP it is essential to release most components of the shoulder girdle and associated fascial connections. Correcting abnormal lumbopelvic mechanics and strengthening posterior shoulder girdle muscles will help maintain the areas of release and improvement of posture that has been achieved. It is imperative that these procedures are augmented with functional carryover as well as stretching and strengthening exercises by the patient.

Upper Limb Nerve Compression and Pain Syndromes

Some of the more common upper limb nerve compression disorders and pain syndromes that lend themselves to the application of nerve and soft tissue manipulations as well as stretching include syndromes of the thoracic outlet, cubital tunnel, radial tunnel, posterior interosseous nerve, pronator, and carpal tunnel. Soft tissue tightness secondary to healed fractures, burns, Dupuytren's disease, reflex sympathetic dystrophy, peripheral nerve injury, and tendinitis almost always exhibits improvement with use of these procedures (see "Stiff Hand" in Chapter 13, Wrist and Hand Complex). De Quervain's and extensor indicis tendinitis of the hand and lateral and medial epicondylitis of the elbow are conditions that respond well to friction massage (see above) and deep fascial releases.[398,405]

Soft tissue manipulations and deep fascial releases are generally thought of in relationship to large muscle groups of the body. However, these methods can also be adapted successfully for use in a hand clinic in addition to postsurgical and post plastic surgery cases. The effects of trauma or inflammation of

■ **FIG. 8-46.** Strain–counterstrain technique for congenital torticollis (sternocleidomastoid). Treatment includes sidebending toward and rotation slightly away from the tender point (2 to 3 cm lateral to the medial end of the clavicle and origin of the sternocleidomastoid). The weight of the head is supported by the operator's hand.[220]

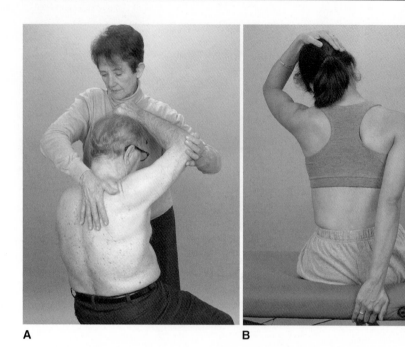

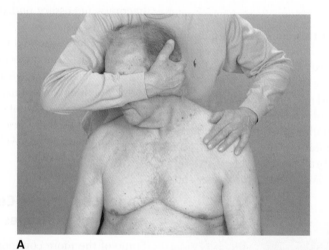

■ **FIG. 8-47.** (**A**) Manual and (**B**) self-stretch of the levator scapula. For self-stretching, fixation of the scapula can be achieved by gripping the chair seat behind the hip while bowing the head into flexion, side flexion, and rotation away from the affected side.

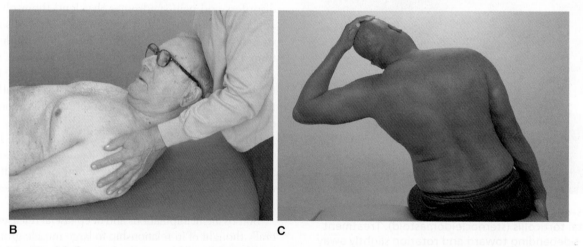

■ **FIG. 8-48.** Stretch for the upper trapezius. (**A**) Postisometric stretch with cervical spine traction. (**B**) Manual stretch in conjunction with sternocleidomastoid. (**C**) Self-stretch in conjunction with sternocleidomastoid.

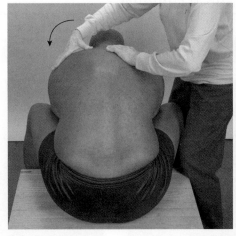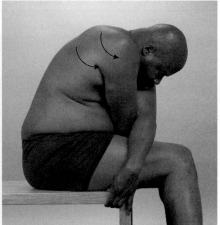

■ **FIG. 8-49.** (**A**) Postisometric stretch for the left rhomboids. The operator slightly resists scapular adduction as the patient slowly breathes in and looks upward to the left. The patient then looks downward while breathing out and relaxing fully. As the muscle releases, the operator's hand follows the movement of the scapula, taking up the slack into abduction. (**B**) Self-stretch (gravity assisted).

A   **B**

BOX 8-8	SOFT TISSUE MANIPULATIONS, SELF-STRETCH, AND MANUAL STRETCH TECHNIQUES OF THE SHOULDER GIRDLE COMPLEX

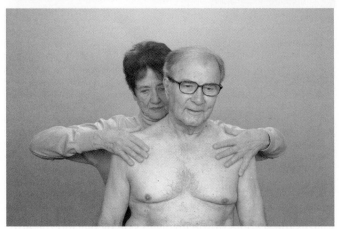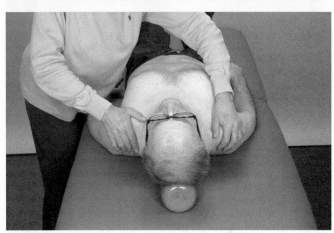

A   **B**

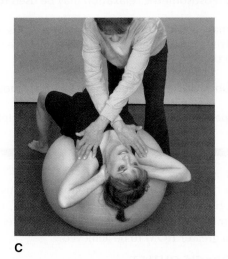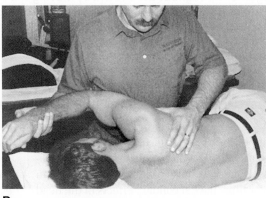

C   **D**

(**A**) Expanding the upper chest. Unilateral or bilateral pectoral anterior fascial stretch.
(**B**) Manual and self-stretch of the pectoralis minor over a roll positioned under the thoracic spine.
(**C**) Manual and self-stretch of the pectoralis major over a ball.
(**D**) Manual stretch of the lateral border of the scapula: latissimus dorsi, teres minor, and major.

Box 8-8. continued

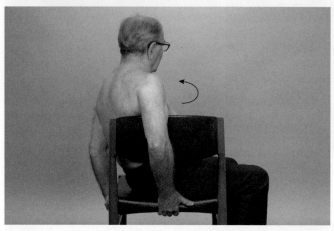
E

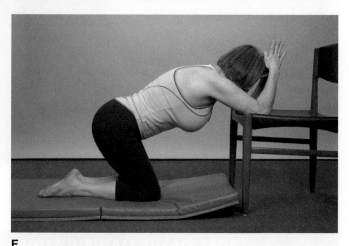
F

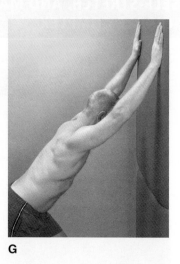
G

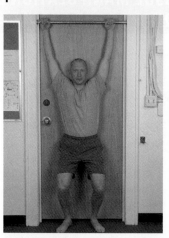
H

(E) Self-stretch of the serratus anterior in sitting. The patient stabilizes the scapula of the involved side by placing the arm behind their back and, after exhaling slowly, turns the thorax away. Postisometric relaxation may be used to facilitate muscle relaxation.
(F) Self-stretch of the latissimus dorsi in kneeling. To promote external rotation of the shoulders the hands and elbows should be held together throughout the stretch. By moving the pelvis into a posterior tilt, a more selective stretch is placed on the latissimus dorsi as the patient attempts to sit back on the heels.
(G) Self-stretch of the latissimus dorsi and teres major in standing
(H) Wall hanging stretch for the latissimus dorsi, teres major, and subclavius. Wall hanging is one of the most effective ways to stretch the muscle of the shoulder girdle.
(Part D reprinted with permission from Kelley MJ, Clark WA: Orthopedic Therapy of the Shoulder. Philadelphia, Lippincott, 1995:310.)

the fascia of the upper limb can result in a binding down of the three-dimensional web of fascia leading to abnormal pressure on blood vessels, nerves, muscles, and bones. This can create pain and, over time, have secondary effects in the head and neck area as well as the thorax.

When modifying soft tissue manipulations for the upper limb, the main concern is to exert a lighter pressure, as the areas to be treated are smaller and more cutaneous. Strumming or transverse friction pressure should not cause undue

pain or discomfort such as numbness or tingling. Combing soft tissue manipulations with joint ROM, muscle energy, contract–relax, or postisometric relaxation techniques allows even greater ROM to be achieved.

THORACIC OUTLET SYNDROME[88,119,189,124,229,366,374,377,414,415,421,453,468,479,493,506]

Thoracic outlet syndrome may involve structural restrictions of the first rib or the muscular or fascial compression

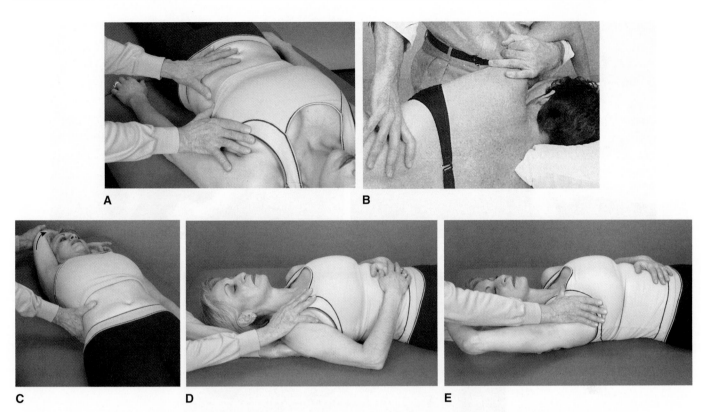

■ FIG. 8-50. Manual stretch for the intercostals and ribs. **(A)** Gross stretch using both thumbs placed parallel to each other on the superior and inferior borders of the ribs. Stretch in the directions of the tightest fibers by pushing the ribs apart. **(B)** Gross stretch for the lower intercostals in sidelying. **(C)** Gross stretch for the lower intercostals in supine. **(D)** Gross stretch for the upper intercostals, using one hand posteriorly to apply pressure in a cephalad direction and one anteriorly over the affected ribs to apply caudal pressure. **(E)** Alternate stretch of the upper intercostals with the arm positioned in elevation. Rib elevation is resisted when the patient inhales and then assisted when the patient exhales. (Part B reprinted with permission from Scully RM, Barnes MR: Physical Therapy. Philadelphia, Lippincott, 1989:971.)

of vascular and neurologic branches as they exit the spine and descend laterally to the upper limb. Clinically, what is seen is often a painful region in the upper back with associated stiffness in the upper trapezius. The scalene and brachial plexus are reactive to palpation. There may also be a positive Tinel sign over the supraclavicular area at the insertion of the anterior scalene muscle.[189,366,377,493] Cervical ROM is usually limited and patterns of weakness and tightness are common in this area (see Chapters 19, Cervical Spine, and 20, Thoracic Spine). In evaluating and developing an effective program treatment program it is necessary to think of thoracic outlet syndrome as multifactorial rather than having a single cause.[119,453,506]

Treatment approach for the thoracic outlet syndrome is based on evaluative findings. If the problem is identified early, then muscle wasting, weakness, and inhibition are less likely, but the painful condition may still remain. Systematically looking at myofascial restrictions, joint dysfunction, muscle imbalances, and upper limb tension tests is most useful in the assessment and management of these cases. Upper limb tension tests to evaluate and treat abnormal

neural dynamics in the brachial plexus are most valuable (see Fig. 11-25 and Chapter 11, Shoulder and Shoulder Girdle).[61,114,468]

Stretching and soft tissue manipulations of the scalenes (see Figs. 7-34, 8-52, and 8-53), upper trapezius (see Fig. 8-48C), pectorals (see Box 8-8), pretracheal fasciae (middle cervical aponeurosis) (Fig. 8-58), and other involved tissues should be considered.[14] The general rule is to stretch the antagonist before strengthening the agonist. These muscles groups should be addressed before strengthening exercises performed for the middle and lower trapezius and serratus anterior which are generally inhibited. Initially, emphasis is placed on high repetition and low resistance exercise.[417] Otherwise, excess shortening of the muscles will lead to recurrence or reactivation of pain and trigger points. Joint mobilization of the first and second ribs, lower cervical, upper thoracic spine, and clavicle joints may be necessary. Posture correction is critical because of the intimate relationship between the neurovascular structures and the shoulder girdle. Stabilization of the lumbopelvic region may be necessary. Work, sleep postures, and leisure activities should be modified as needed to decrease pressure on these structures.

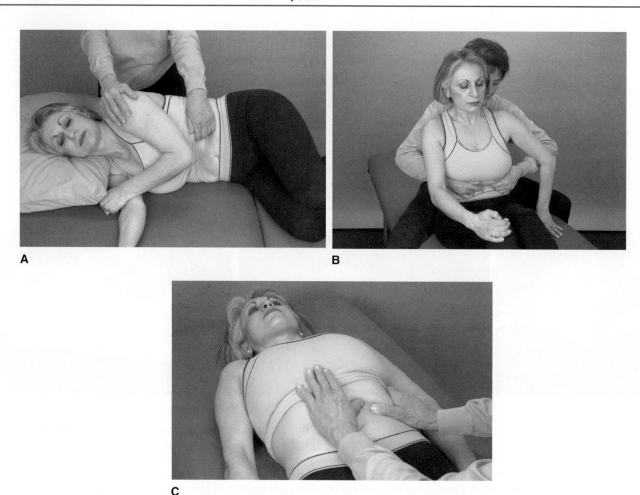

■ **FIG. 8-51.** Respiratory diaphragm bony contour and soft tissue mobilization **(A)** in sidelying with the hip and knees flexed (shorten position), **(B)** in sitting in a slump position (attempt a more erect position to allow lengthening) and **(C)** in a supine lengthened position.

NEUROPATHIES AROUND THE ELBOW AND WRIST

Cubital Tunnel Syndrome. Cubital tunnel syndrome (see Fig. 12-13) is considered the second most common entrapment neuropathy in the arm, second to carpal tunnel syndrome (see Chapter 12, Elbow and Forearm).[136] Entrapment or irritation of the ulnar nerve at the elbow is associated with compression under the flexor carpi ulnaris. The flexor digitorum (profundus or superficialis), pronator teres, and flexor carpi radialis may also be involved.[139,421] Soft tissue manipulations are clearly indicated and therapeutic. Stretching exercises should focus on extrinsic flexor and extensor muscles along with ulnar–nerve-innervated intrinsic muscles. Nerve gliding techniques may be appropriate for patient with intermittent symptoms (Fig. 8-59).[61] Precipitating or aggravating postures or movements that compress the ulnar nerve should be avoided. Some patients can be helped by the use of a night splint for several months.[389]

Radial Tunnel Syndrome. Radial tunnel syndrome (arising from adverse mechanical neural tension) and posterior interosseous nerve syndrome (implying irritation of injury of the radial nerve as it passes through the supinator or arcade of Frohse [(see Fig. 12-14B)] along the posterolateral proximal forearm) are a fairly common diagnoses.[61,260,265,266,340,341,360,374,404] Several clinicians have observed similarities between radial tunnel syndrome and lateral epicondylitis, complicating the diagnosis.[99,340,404] Frequently patients with radial tunnel syndrome have undergone unsuccessful treatment for lateral epicondylitis. Tennis elbow straps may increase symptoms because of the increased compression.[52] Ischemic compression and soft tissue manipulations effectively treat trigger points or taut bands identified in these muscles of the forearm.[421,453] The supinator responds well to postisometric relaxation (Fig. 8-60) and is also valuable as a self-treatment at home.[254,453] Additional treatment consists of radial nerve gliding, therapeutic exercises, and stretching to restore full extrinsic wrist extensors and flexor muscle length. Other considerations include the use of wrist cock-up splints, activity modification, and surgery. Postoperatively, scar and pain management as well as strengthening and stretching programs are used.

Pronator Syndrome. Pronator syndrome (see Fig. 12-15) refers to compression of the median nerve (1) by the pronator

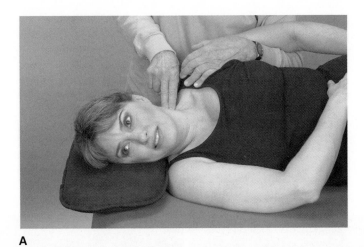

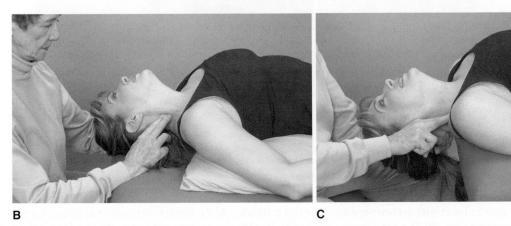

■ **FIG. 8-52.** Soft tissue mobilization of the scalene muscles **(A)** sidelying, **(B)** supine with a pillow under the thorax to increase cervical extension, and **(C)** supine with head and the shoulders extended over the edge of the table (head supported by operator's knees).

teres muscle as the median nerve passes through the heads of that muscle, (2) to a lesser extent by a fibrous band near the origin of the deep flexor muscles, known as the lacertus fibrosis and flexor digitorum superficialis arcade,[21] and (3) even less commonly by the ligament of Struthers, an anomalous structure found in 1% of the population.[405] The syndrome commonly occurs in patients whose job requires repetitive pronation–supination. Pronator syndrome may be characterized by pain in the forearm on resistance to pronation and flexion of the long and ring finger flexor digitorum superficialis. Tinel's sign may be present at the site of compression.

Treatment includes soft tissue manipulations and stretching to both pronator and supinator muscles. Muscle energy is an effective technique, gradually increasing the supination.[421] Another approach involves direct pressure to the pronator, enhanced by gradually increasing the supination or combining it with muscle energy (Fig. 8-61).[226,308,340,421]

CARPAL TUNNEL SYNDROME

Carpal tunnel syndrome (CTS) at the wrist is the most common peripheral compression neuropathy of the upper limb.[374,463]

CTS commonly affects middle-aged women between 40 and 60 years of age, a characteristic suggestive of a hormonal aberration as a cause in the development of this disorder.[359] Often these patients, present with the double crush phenomena described by Upton and McComas.[458] Both ulnar nerve neuropathy and carpal tunnel may be involved in the double-crush syndrome.[124] A **double-crush syndrome** is a condition in which a nerve may be compressed at more than one site. Nonsurgical treatment or treatments are described in Chapter 13, Wrist and Hand Complex. Soft tissue manipulations described by Sucher have been found to be extremely effective,[416,418–421] as have tendon-gliding[447] and nerve-gliding exercises (Fig. 8-62).[61,199,447]

Tendon-gliding exercises[374,476] are used to facilitate isolated excursion of each of the two flexor tendons to each finger passing through the tunnel. Each exercise is initiated from a position of full finger and wrist extension. The patient then completes a hook-fist position to obtain maximum differential gliding of the profundus, a straight fist to obtain maximum flexor digitorum superficialis excursion, and a full fist to maximize full excursion of the tendons through the carpal tunnel (Fig. 8-63).

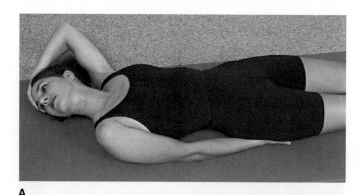

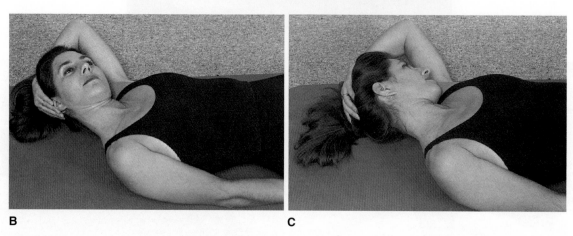

■ FIG. 8-53. Self-stretch for the scalene muscles. Each of the three major scalene muscles is stretched in the supine position with the hand on the side to be stretched anchored under the buttock. **(A)** To stretch the scalenus posterior the face is turned away from the involved side. **(B)** The face looks forward to stretch the scalenus medius. **(C)** The face is turned toward the involved muscle to stretch the scalenus anterior. These stretches can also be done in sitting with the hand on the side to be stretched secured under the seat as each position is assumed and the patient leans his or her trunk away from the involved side. (Reprinted with permission from Liebenson C: Rehabilitation of the Spine: A Practical Manual. Philadelphia, Lippincott Williams & Wilkins, 1996:280.)

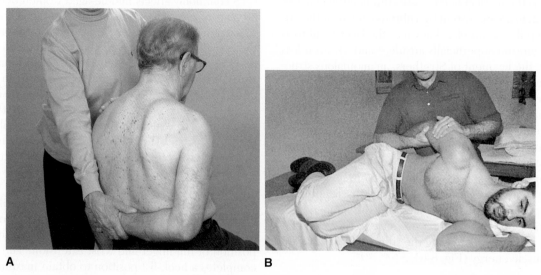

■ FIG. 8-54. Manual stretch for the supraspinatus. **(A)** Optimum position. **(B)** Combined with lateral glide, arm at the side. Snapping and clicking sounds may occur around the shoulder joint because of tautness of the supraspinatus fibers interfering with normal glide of the humeral head.[453] (Part B reprinted with permission from Kelley MJ, Clark WA: Orthopedic Therapy of the Shoulder. Philadelphia, Lippincott, 1995:310.)

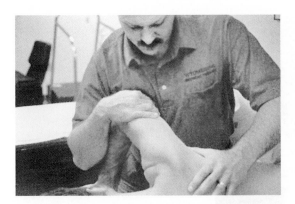

■ **FIG. 8-55.** Manual stretch for the infraspinatus and teres minor. Restriction in simultaneous internal rotation and adduction of the shoulder is often present. (Reprinted with permission from Kelley MJ, Clark WA: Orthopedic Therapy of the Shoulder. Philadelphia, Lippincott, 1995:310.)

The most currently documented manipulative techniques for CTS, described by Sucher,[415,416,421] have emphasized three components employing (1) transverse extension or opening of the canal using a three-point opening maneuver, (2) transverse extension and pulling the thumb into radial abduction and extension, and (3) finally stretching the carpal region directly by extending the wrist and digits (Fig. 8-64). This manual approach to treatment is complemented with a regimen of self-stretching several times daily.[421] Muscle energy[151,308] to the abductor pollicis brevis can be applied to further increase the stretch to the carpal ligament.

Gentle mobilization of the pisiform, with the wrist in flexion (carpal tunnel on slack), is often effective as is myofascial manipulation of the entire forearm. Posture correction and activities of daily living modification are indicated. Performing repetitive wrist flexion–extension exercise motions, certain wrist and hand postures, and repetitive wrist flexion–extension

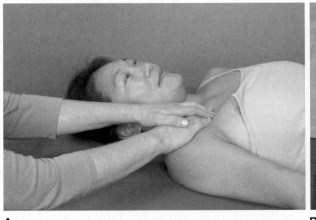
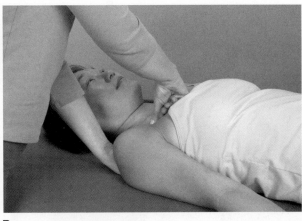

A   **B**

■ **FIG. 8-56.** Release of the clavicular area. **(A)** Deep anterior technique applied with reinforced hands. The stroke is applied through the fingertips from medial to lateral. **(B)** Deep anterior technique applied through the reinforced thumb from medial to lateral.

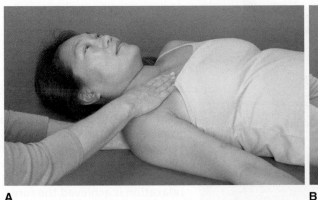
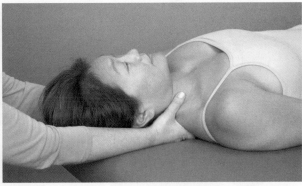

A   **B**

■ **FIG. 8-57.** Release for the upper thoracic. **(A)** Unilateral anterior-posterior technique progressing medially to laterally pulling the hands toward the glenohumeral joint. **(B)** Bilateral technique. Gentle cephalad-caudad oscillations with deep pressure are applied on the upper thoracic paravertebral musculature.

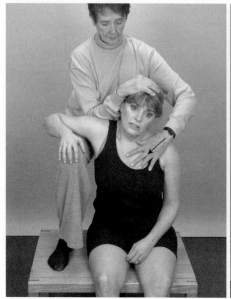

A

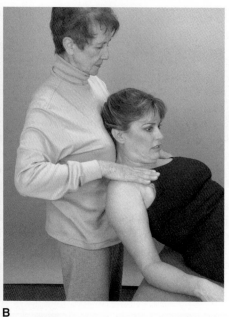

B

■ **FIG. 8-58.** Soft tissue manipulation of the pretracheal (middle cervical aponeurosis). **(A)** Seated position. **(B)** Supine position.

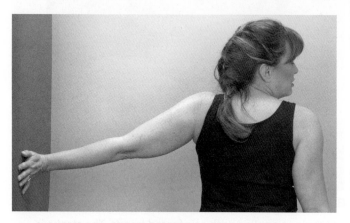

■ **FIG. 8-59.** Ulnar nerve gliding stretch, with wrist extension, forearm supination, and elbow extension.

motions (such as pinching and gripping) should be avoided. It is imperative to evaluate the work environment and to make suggestions for modification.

Upper limb releases of the radial nerve and scars resulting from carpal tunnel or De Quervain's disease surgery respond well to soft tissue manipulations and scar tissue release (see above). The therapist should initiate scar desensitization when the surgical incision is closed.[281] Methods include soft tissue manipulations, self-massage, or the use of a mini-vibrator. The patient massages the scar by applying firm pressure to mobilize the scar over subcutaneous tissues. Massage is usually performed in a circular motion three or more times daily for 10 minutes. As therapy progresses, various densities of pressure stents may be applied to compress the scar. Lightweight foam may be upgraded to a denser foam or to molded Otofoam

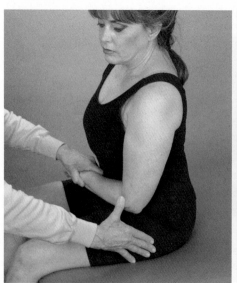

A

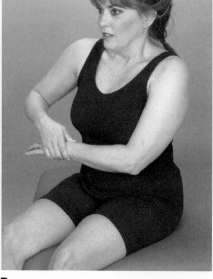

B

■ **FIG. 8-60.** Supinator. **(A)** Post-isometric relaxation examination and treatment. The forearm is pronated to take up all the slack. The patient supinates with minimal force with resistance from the operator several times followed by relaxation. When relaxation is achieved the forearm is pronated until all the slack has been taken up. **(B)** Self-treatment. The patient performs the same movements with her opposite hand as did the operator.

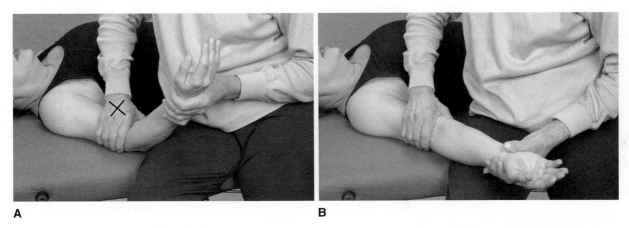

■ **FIG. 8-61.** Muscle energy technique for the pronator teres. (**A**) Starting position. (**B**) Final position.

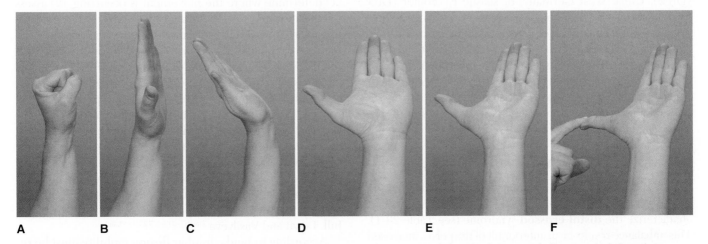

■ **FIG. 8-62.** Nerve gliding exercise for mobilization of the median nerve. (**A**) Wrist in neutral, fingers and thumb in flexion. (**B**) Wrist in neutral, fingers and thumb extended. (**C**) Thumb in neutral, wrist and fingers extended. (**D**) Wrist, fingers, and thumb extended. (**E**) Same as position D, with forearm in supination. (**F**) Same as position as E, with other thumb gently stretching thumb.

■ **FIG. 8-63.** Tendon gliding exercises for the tendons passing through the carpal tunnel. (**A**) Starting position with full finger extension. (**B**) Ten repetitions of the hook fist, (**C**), straight fist, (**D**) and full fist are performed to maximize differential tendon gliding and full excursion of the tendons through the carpal tunnel.[476]

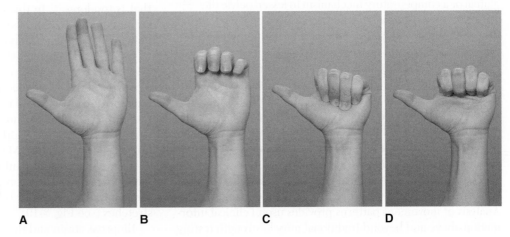

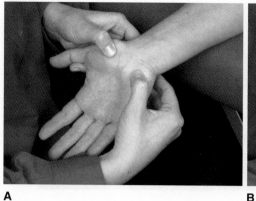
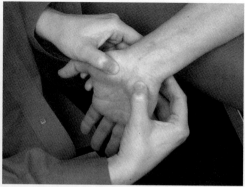

A   **B**

■ **FIG. 8-64.** Manipulation in carpal tunnel syndrome. **(A)** Thumb pressure is applied along the attachment edges of the carpal ligament at the medial and lateral borders of the carpal bones. At the same time the patient's thumb is pulled into radial abduction with extension. **(B)** Same as (A) except the patient's wrist and digits are hyperextended, further opening and extending the canal.[421]

(Dreze, Unna, West Germany) or silastic Elastomer (Dow Corning, Midland, MI) stent. These pressure pads may be held in place with Coban wrap or a compression stockinette. The patient should be advised to wear the pliable foam stents when performing activities and exercise and to incorporate the pads into the resting phase when the hand is relatively less mobile.[199] The desensitization process is initiated slightly irritating but tolerable; as tolerance increases, more noxious stimuli are introduced.[17,281,474]

Pelvic or Distal Crossed Syndrome

Tightness of the hip flexors and spinal extensors, and inhibition of and weakness of the gluteals and abdominal muscles,[215,223] characterize the **distal crossed** syndrome (see Table 23-1). This imbalance results in an anterior tilt of the pelvis, increased flexion of the hips, and compensatory hyperlordosis. This can result in changes in posture in other parts of the body: increase thoracic kyphosis and increase in cervical lordosis. The hamstrings are frequently found to be tight in this syndrome as well. This may be a functional compensation for the inhibited gluteal or a compensatory mechanism to lessen pelvic tilt.[252,253] Decreased hip extension during gait is often observed. Other postural muscles around the hip and back that may shorten include the piriformis and hip adductors.

Imbalance can also exist in the lateral trunk musculature. Gluteus medius weakness is usually compensated for by tightness and over activity in the ipsilateral quadratus lumborum and tensor fasciae latae.[223] Clinical consequences of the lower crossed syndrome include increased thoracolumbar facet and sacroiliac joint strain, altered hip mechanics, and overstress of the lumbosacral junction.[76,210,215,223]

These muscle imbalance in general are identified by posture inspection, gait evaluation, and movement assessment. Analysis of movement patterns provides useful clinical information above and beyond traditional muscle strength testing procedures. This assessment of kinesiopathology is diagnostic for muscular imbalances and provides information that guides therapeutic and rehabilitation decisions.[210,215,223] Three main objectives emerge when analyzing a particular movement:

(1) determine where the movement is occurring, (2) assess the quality of the movement, and (3) assess the range or quantity of the movement. For example, in assessing trunk curl, the rectus abdominus is the primary mover in trunk flexion with the iliopsoas acting as a powerful synergist.[215,355,367,481] As the patient is asked to sit up, lumbosacral hyperextension indicates poor stability, overactive erector spinae and poor abdominal control. Abdominal protrusion is correlated with lack of transversus abdominus and multifidi co-contraction.[330,356] Shaking of the body during the movement indicates poor abdominal recruitment. Lifting the feet off the table demonstrates iliopsoas hyperactivity. For more details of this method of analysis of movement patterns and in depth diagnosis of muscular dysfunction by postural inspection see the works of Janda, Jull, Lewit and Vasilyeva.[209,211–213,223,252–254,459]

According to Janda, lumbar flexion mobility must be regained first, after which treatment proceeds to strengthen the abdominal muscles. Stretching needs to be completed frequently throughout the day, such as four times per day.[13] Conversely, Sahrmann teaches that the most effective way of lengthening a short muscle is by working its antagonist that is too long.[165] In this example, do not stretch first, but strengthen the lengthened lower abdominals. This strengthening will lengthen the short lumbar paraspinals.

Box 8-9 illustrates self-stretches for muscles prone to tightness of the trunk and lower quadrant (mainly postural muscles) found in the pelvic or distal crossed syndrome. The lateral trunk muscles and rotators (e.g., erector spinae, quadratus lumborum), piriformis, iliotibial band and tensor fasciae latae, hamstrings, hip short adductors, iliopsoas, and rectus femoris are illustrated. Many patients' collagen properties will not allow a significant change in length to occur from stretching alone. Therefore, it is recommended that soft tissue manipulations be performed and added while the patient stretches (see Fig. 8-19).

Iliopsoas strain and the snapping iliopsoas syndrome are rather common sports-related injuries that may also result in hip flexor tightness. The snapping iliopsoas syndrome is due to snapping of the tendon over the iliopectineal eminence.

(text continues on page 238)

BOX 8-9	SELF-STRETCH OF MYOFASCIAL STRUCTURES OF THE TRUNK AND LOWER QUADRANT

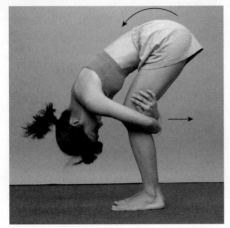

A1

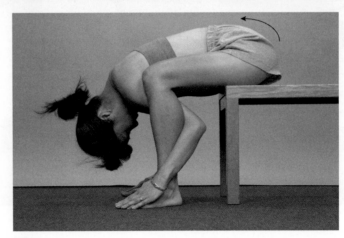

A2

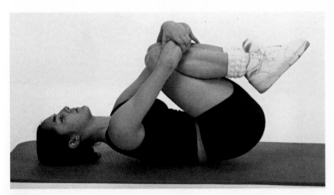

A3

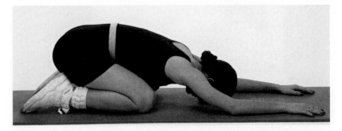

A4

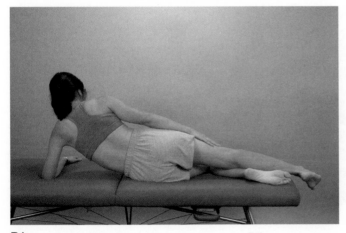

B1

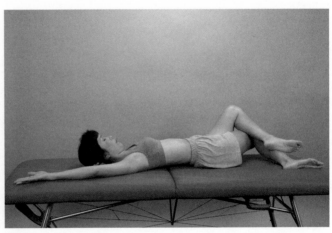

B2

(A) Self-stretch of the erector spinae of the lumbar and thoracic spine and myofascial structures of the low back (latissimus dorsi and thoracolumbar fascia). (*1*) Self-stretch in standing, (*2*) sitting, (*3*) supine, and (*4*) heels on buttock. **(B)** Self-stretch of the quadratus lumborum. (*1*) Sidelying. (*2*) Supine with a twist.

(*continued*)

Box 8-9. continued

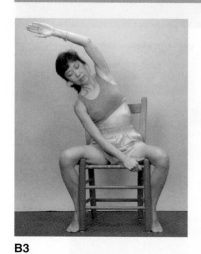

B3

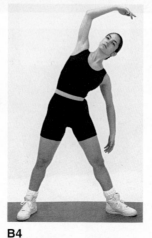

B4

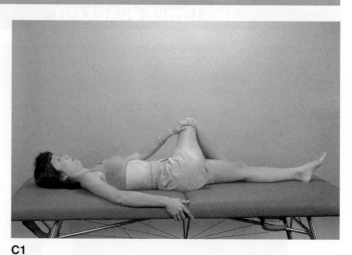

C1

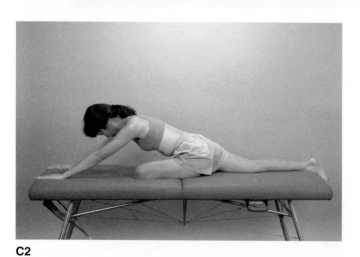

C2

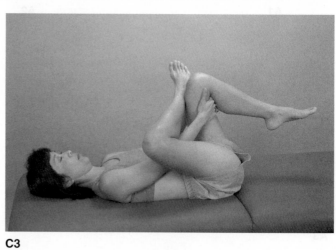

C3

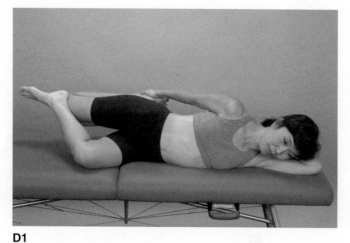

D1

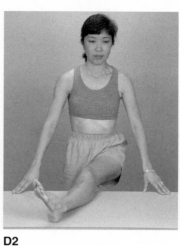

D2

(B) *(3)* Sitting. *(4)* Standing. **(C)** Self-stretch for the piriformis and hip external rotators. *(1)* Supine with a twist. *(2)* Semi-prone. *(3)* Supine with hips flexed. **(D)** Self-stretch for the iliotibial band, tensor fascia latae, and its associated lateral structures. *(1)* Sidelying taking up the slack with hand behind back and using the weight of the opposite foot to apply a stretch. *(2)* Horizontally adducting with hip internal rotation of the hip.

Box 8-9. continued

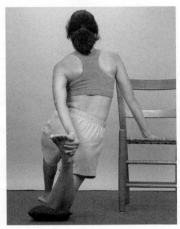

D3

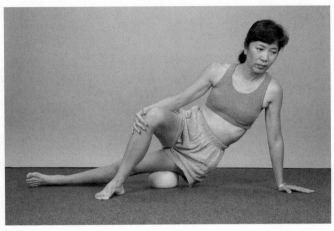

D4

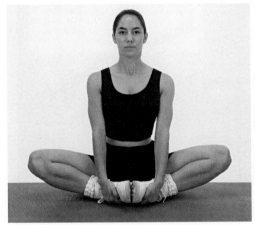

E1

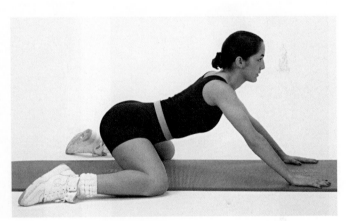

E2

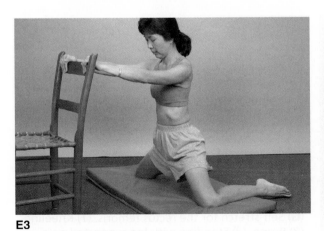

E3

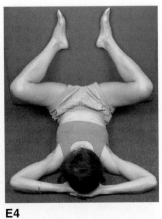

E4

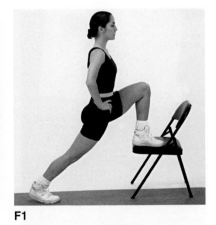

F1

(D) (*3*) Kneeling with crossed legs; shift right hip outward and forward and drop the left hip. (*4*) Rolling on a ball to stretch target areas selectively. **(E)** Self-stretch for the short adductors. (*1*) Sitting. (*2*) Quadriped. (*3*) Kneeling with weight bearing on the knee. (*4*) Supine with the legs supported by a wall. **(F)** Self-stretch for the iliopsoas. (*1*) Standing.

(*continued*)

Box 8-9. continued

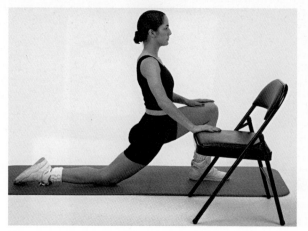

F2

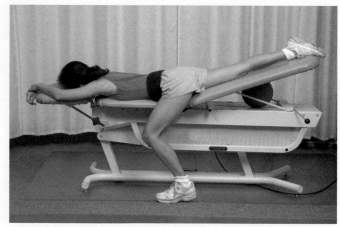

F3

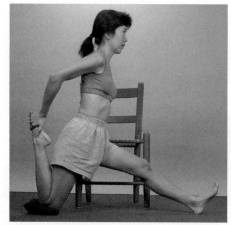

G1

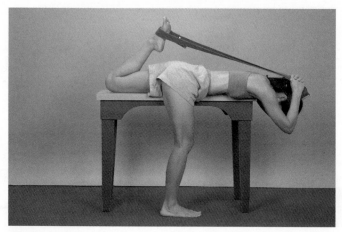

G2

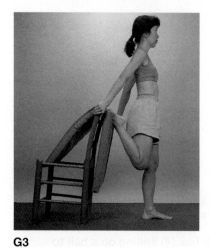

G3

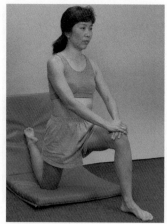

G4

(F) (*2*) Kneeling. (*3*) Prone with leg elevated.
(G) Self-stretch for the rectus femoris. (*1*) Kneeling.
(*2*) Prone. (*3*) Standing with leg supported on a
chair. (*4*) Kneeling with leg supported on a wall.

Box 8-9. continued

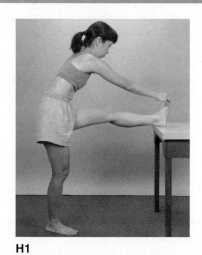

H1

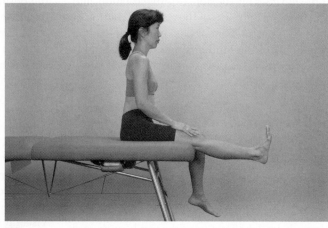

H2

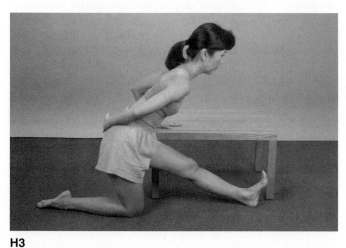

H3

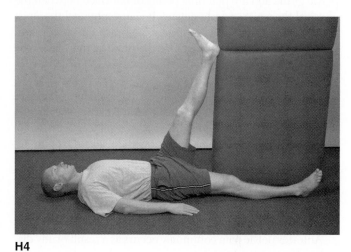

H4

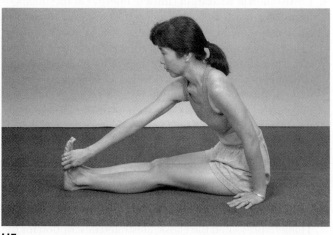

H5

(**H**) Self-stretch for the hamstrings. (*1*) Standing with leg supported on a chair or table. (*2*) Sitting (patient should avoid backward pelvic rock). (*3*) Kneeling. (*4*) Supine with leg supported on a wall. (*5*) Sitting.
(Parts A3–4, B4, C2–3, E1–2, F1–2 reprinted with permission from Liebenson C: Rehabilitation of the Spine: A Practical Manual. Philadelphia, Lippincott Williams & Wilkins, 1996:260–272.)

Snapping of the iliopsoas can be painful as a result of a secondary bursitis that may develop following repetitive friction to the bursa as the hip goes into flexion, external rotation, and full extension.[293] Bilateral tightness of the vertebral portion of the iliopsoas may result in an increased compression load on the posterior elements of the lumbar spine. Bilateral tightness (contraction of the psoas) causes excessive backward bending of the lumbar spine.

Pelvic Floor Disorders (See Chaper 7 and Fig. 7-18)

Back, pelvic, hip, and abdominal pain are common symptoms associated with urogenital diseases and frequently encountered by family medicine and primary care practitioners of obstetrics/gynecology. Symptoms in these areas also frequently arise from musculoskeletal dysfunction of the trunk, spine, and pelvic girdle and are potential points of interface between the physical therapist and physicians. Because physical therapist may be the first healthcare professional responsible for adequate screening, it is important for the physical therapist to be aware of obstetric and gynecologic concepts and make appropriate referrals.

In general, orthopedic causes of pelvic pain in women are easily recognized by the physical therapist. Posterior pelvic pain originating in the lumbosacral, sacroiliac, coccydynial, and sacrococcygeal regions present with localized pain in the lower lumbar spine and over the sacrum often radiating over the sacroiliac ligaments and referred into the posterior thigh and buttock.[218] Coccydynial and sacrococcygeal pain are very common presentations in women often associated with a fall on the buttock or following childbirth.[15]

Anterior pelvic pain commonly occurs as a result of any disorder affecting the hip joint; pregnancy with separation of the symphysis pubis; local injury to the insertion of the adductor muscles, rectus femoris, or rectus abdominus; femoral neuralgia; and psoas abscess.[218]

The myofascial component of pelvic floor pain has been a focus of recent attention in the field of physical therapy. When the muscular floor sags or sustains a muscle tear during childbirth, pelvic floor weakness results in pelvic laxity and disrupts the functioning and positioning of the pelvic organs. Chronic back, pelvic, and leg pain, urinary incontinence, and organ prolapse may accompany pelvic floor weakness. Severe pain in the pelvic region of women with fibromyalgia is not uncommon.[218]

Detailed management of pelvic floor disorders is beyond the scope of this chapter and the reader is referred to the current literature.[4,31,34–38,41,55,57,63,66,112,169,182,198,217,248,313,324,380,390,409,410,466,478] Postgraduate study is recommended in directly treating pelvic floor muscles. A major focus of treating this area is on strengthening the pelvic floor muscles and reducing pain and altered tone. Pain and altered tone impairments may be caused by lumbopelvic joint mobility impairment, tonic holding patterns of the pelvic floor muscles, abdominal adhesions, adhered scars in the trunk, and perineum and hip balance impairment. It is often difficult to pinpoint the origin of pain in the lower pelvic region. Muscle spasm and trigger points are a common cause of pain in the perineum, groin, and coccyx areas. Travell and Simons[452] describe referred pain patterns from trigger points in the adductors, pelvic floor muscles, obturator internus, and piriformis. Treatment of pelvic floor muscle spasm includes manual soft tissue manipulations of pelvic floor muscles vaginally, rectally (see Thiele's massage below), or externally around the coccyx and ischial tuberosities and sacrum (Fig. 8-28 and Box 8-3, Fig. *E*).

Spasms of the pelvic floor muscles are often related to sacroiliac, sacrococcygeal, pubic symphysis, and lumbar joint mobility impairments. These impairments may be primary or secondary and include hypomobility or hypermobility. Mobility restrictions of scar tissue and connective tissue in the perineum and groin can also affect pelvic floor function greatly. Visceral adhesions may cause sacroiliac joint mobility impairments, especially if unilateral adhesions from organ to sacrum are severe.[15] Specialized therapists and osteopathic practitioners use visceral mobilization techniques to manipulate organs and abdominal fascial tissue. Soft tissue mobilization of abdominal adhesions and organs can enhance organ function and help in maintaining normal mobility in the pelvic joints. A number of soft tissue manipulations may be considered in the management of pelvic floor disorders including:

1. Scar tissue manipulations and friction massage externally and internally.
2. Friction massage for irritation of the coccygeal fibers of the gluteus maximus muscle and contusions and sprains of the intercoccygeal ligaments and sacrococcygeal joint (see Figs. 8-28, 18-19; also see Box 8-3, Fig. *E*).[334]
3. Strain and counterstrain techniques (see Fig. 23-63) for sacral and coccygeal tender points (levator ani, pubococcygeus, sacrotuberous, and sacrospinous ligaments).[95]
4. Postisometric relaxation (muscle energy) in the management of a tender coccyx owing to increased tension in the levator ani and gluteus maximus (a frequent cause of pain).[253] If postisometric relaxation treatment of the levator ani and gluteus maximus fails (Fig. 8-65), the cause is usually tension in the piriformis, which can be treated with postisometric relaxation (Fig. 8-66) and sustained pressures (see Fig. 8-3). Treatment of the gluteus maximus (Fig. 8-65*B*) and piriformis can also be administered as a self-treatment.
5. Stretching techniques of the levator ani as part of the massage procedure.[452]
6. Thiele's massage, which as been found effective in patients with coccygodynia and low back pain.[452]

Thiele[443] presented the classic illustrated description for the examination and treatment by massage of the surfaces of the coccygeus and levator ani muscles and the sacrococcygeal ligament via the rectum. The patient is positioned in sidelying for both examination and treatment. The clinician, using a gloved hand and vaginal gel, inserts the full length of the index finger into the rectum. When performing the massage technique,

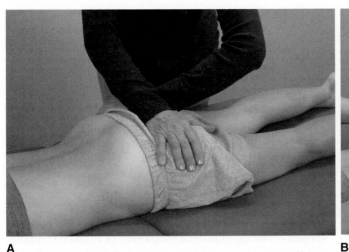 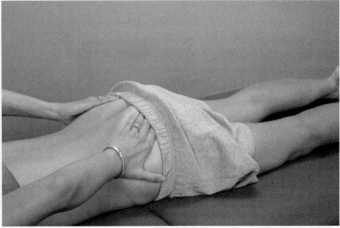

A   **B**

■ **FIG. 8-65.** (A) Examination and postisometric relaxation treatment of the gluteus maximus. Using crossed arms, the hands are placed on each buttock at the level of the anus. The patient is instructed to press the buttock together with little force and to maintain it for 10 seconds and then release. This is repeated three to five times. As the gluteus maximus contracts and relaxes so does the levator, and palpation of the coccyx is usually painless. **(B)** This technique can also be used as self-treatment.

the index finger sweeps from side to side massaging lengthwise the muscle fibers of the coccygeus and levator ani muscle (10 to 15 times) on each side of the pelvis. Sustained pressure is applied to the sacrococcygeal ligament. The massage usually lasts 5 minutes. If the patient does not improve after the first four to six treatments another consultation

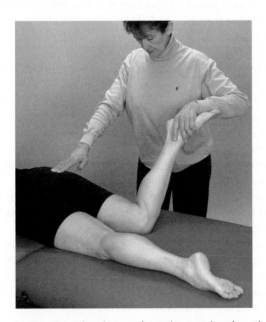

■ **FIG. 8-66.** Examination and postisometric relaxation treatment of tension of the piriformis. The leg is rotated outward at the hip to take up the slack. The patients is requested to give slight counter pressure (which is resisted for approximately 10 seconds) and then told to let go. During relaxation internal rotation at the hip is increased. This is repeated three to five times.

should be considered. This author has found this technique to be very useful before manipulation of the coccyx (see Chapter 23, Sacroiliac Joint and Lumbar–Pelvic–Hip Complex).

For the patient with involvement of the pelvic floor muscles, the clinician should identify and if possible correct any articular dysfunction's of the lumbosacral region, sacroiliac joints, and sacrococcygeal articulations. General strengthening of the pelvic floor muscles is essential. The clinician should be able to develop an effective exercise program for both slow-twitch and fast-twitch contractions as well as exercises for the unstable pelvic girdle, lumbar spine, and hips. Use of the pelvic floor muscle is one of the most effective methods of achieving contraction of the transversus abdominus to contribute to stabilization of the spine.[355] Exercises to tone the peritoneum and sphincters should be carried out several times per day.[15] Additional considerations include patient education, biofeedback, and postural awareness.

Overuse Syndromes of the Lower Quadrant

Overuse syndromes, repetitive strain injury, and cumulative trauma disorders,[206] are used to describe the repetitive nature of precipitating events. Overuse syndromes resulting in muscle strain occurs along a continuum from acute macrotraumatic injury to chronic microtraumatic overuse injuries. Acute traumatic injuries occur when a muscle is rapidly overloaded or overstretched, and the tension generated exceeds the tensile capacity of the musculotendinous unit.[274] Many injuries do not result from a single traumatic injury but most occur insidiously, resulting from overuse of various musculoskeletal tissues. Typically these overuse injuries result from repetitive subtraumatic forces. Breakdown of microscopic tissue occurs faster than the tissue can heal or repair itself. Repetitive microtrauma overload over time result in structural weakness or fatigue breakdown of connective tissue with collagen fiber cross-link breakdown and inflammation, muscle strain, ligament failure, tendinitis, tendon rupture, and stress fracture.[121]

Overuse injuries of the lower quadrant affect different anatomic sites and tissues. A survey by Clement conducted in 1981 of 1,819 runners indicated the most common anatomic areas affected were the knee (41.7%), lower leg (27.9%), foot (18.1), hip (5%), lumbar spine (3.7%), and upper leg (3.6%).[78] Specific syndromes included patellofemoral joint pain syndrome (patellar dysfunction) (25.8%), tibia stress syndrome (medial tibial stress syndrome) (13.2%), Achilles tendinitis (6%), plantar fasciitis (4.7%), patellar tendinitis (4.5%), iliotibial friction band syndrome (iliotibial band syndrome) (4.3%), (see Chapters 14–16 for details of these common lesions), metatarsal fractures (3.2%), and tibial fractures (2.6%) Based on this survey and others,[120,206] the most common overuse injuries affect the knee, lower leg, ankle, foot, upper leg, hip, and pelvis.

These common syndromes occur most often in individuals (both young and old) participating in sports activities.[344,402] Like young adults, older people are participating in sport activities in larger numbers than ever before at all levels of competition.[483] Older athletes may be more prone to overuse injuries than younger athletes.[284] Several factors may contribute to this predisposition. First, they are less flexible than younger athletes.[141,284,400,465] Second, muscle mass is reduced.[156] Third, most have at least some arthritic changes in the weight-bearing joints.[141] Degenerative changes in articular cartilage,[56,315] tendon,[175,227] bone,[60,286] and muscle reduce the force-generating and absorbing capacity of the musculoskeletal system. Changes in reaction time,[251] proprioception, strength, and vision all place the older athlete at risk of injury in sports that require movement such as skiing and tennis.

Injuries secondary to recurrent microtrauma are also becoming increasingly common in the pediatric population.[50,304] Overuse syndromes account for the majority of sports medicine problem in children and adolescents.[407] Although many sports injuries in children are similar to those found in adults, two major differences have been identified.[292,305]

1. Trauma to a joint may cause fracture of epiphyseal growth plate instead of a ligamentous injury.
2. Stress injuries related to differential growth or strength of musculoskeletal structures.[292,305]
   A. Decrease in flexibility as growth occurs.
   B. Imbalance of muscle strength around individual joints.
   C. Length changes in the musculotendinous system and the skeletal system do not occur concurrently.

The classic example of an overuse or overstress syndrome in children and young adults is that of the Little League elbow (see Chapter 12, Elbow and Forearm). Others include stress fractures, sprains and strains, tendinitis, impingement of the rotator cuff, patellofemoral joint pain syndrome, involvement of the extensor mechanism of the knee, Osgood–Schlatter's

disease, and problems related to abnormal foot pronation (see Chapter 11, Shoulder and Shoulder Girdle; Chapter 15, Knee; and Chapter 16, Lower Leg, Ankle, and Foot).

In rehabilitating overuse syndromes, stresses placed on the healing tissues should not exceed the tissue's readiness to accept these forces. Motion must be full, unrestricted, and pain free. During the chronic inflammation phase, proper management must involve selective reduction of abnormal stresses. The approach used must be in accordance of findings on evaluation, including information relating to the patient's present and former activity level. In developing a program of management, it must be kept in mind that the tissue pathology resulting in the painful condition may be owing to normal stresses occurring at too great a frequency, to abnormal high stresses occurring at normal frequency, or to some combination thereof. In general management of overuse syndromes involves measures to either reduce either the frequency or the magnitude of stresses, or both. General treatment goals and plan of care during the chronic inflammation phase and return to function phase may consist of the following:

1. Chronic inflammation and the reduction of pain should be managed by judicious use of cryotherapy, compression (constant or intermittent), elevation, and rest. Rest and protection of the part (i.e., cessation of athletic activities; protection via taping, lift, or pad; and very limited barefoot walking) are necessary to promote healing initially.
2. Patient education and counseling on biomechanics to eliminate irritating factors. Integration of specific structural or biomechanical components that may relieve symptoms, including the choice of shoes or custom biomechanical orthoses.
3. Soft tissue techniques and friction massage as indicated for increased tissue length and elasticity and to develop a strong, mobile scar.
4. Joint mobilization as indicated to restore joint mobility.
5. Develop a balance in length and strength of muscle. Correct cause of faulty muscle and joint mechanics with appropriate graded stretching and strengthening exercises.
6. Cardiovascular exercises as appropriate for improved metabolism and increased endurance.
7. Develop support in related regions via awareness training and stabilization exercises. Include neuromuscular, balance, and proprioceptive re-education.
8. Progressive gait training for stance stability and control of excessive pronation as indicated. Step progression to hopping and jumping as tolerated (plyometrics goal for the young athlete). Such activities should be gauged as symptoms allow.

ITB FASCITIS (INFLAMMATION OF THE FASCIAL BAND) AND TENSOR FASCIAE LATA (TFL) OR ILIOTIBIAL OVERUSE SYNDROME

The ITB is commonly involved in overuse syndromes (see Chapter 7, Myofascial Systems of the Lumbo-Pelvic-Hip

Complex), lower kinetic chain problems, the sacroiliac joint, lumbar–pelvic–hip complex, knee, foot, and ankle dysfunction.[54,63,65,71,72,95,109,110,166,174,230,233,257,297,301,329,334,372,373,376,441,446,461] Many diffuse "referred pain" syndromes in the lower limb, lumbar spine, and pelvic girdle can be traced to iliotibial dysfunction.

The ITB is an important lateral stabilizer and helps to maintain posture during gait. Tightness often affects a person's ability to shift weight over the base of support (because of lateral tightness) and to perform lateral motions.[298] Often there is associated postural dysfunction of an anterior pelvic tilt posture (kyphosis-lordosis posture) with lower limb compensation including medial rotation of the femur, genu valgum, lateral tibial torsion, pes planus and hallux valgus, flat back posture, or handedness posture (see Figs. 7-23 and 7-26).[230,273] According to Sahrmann,[372,373] overuse of the TFL rather than gluteus maximus leads to lateral knee pain from ITB tension or medial rotation of the femur with medial knee stresses from increased bowstring effect. Overuse of the two-joint hip flexors (TFL, sartorius, and rectus femoris) may cause knee pain or faulty hip mechanics from overuse of these muscles.

Low Back and Sacroiliac Dysfunction. Limited mobility of the ITB is probably a major contributor to quadratus myofascial disorders, lumbar spine immobility, and pain.[257,298] ITB fasciitis, seen in elderly patients when it is severe enough, is often wrongly diagnosed as unilateral spinal stenosis.[372] When contracted or pathologically tight, the ITB is often misdiagnosed as sciatica or a sacroiliac problem.[72] The signs of a tight ITB are those of subluxation, usually backward rotation of one sacroiliac joint.

Snapping Hip Syndrome. When the band becomes singularly taut over the hip region (often with inflexibility of the gluteal muscles as well), the symptoms of a "snapping hip" and generalized aching in the thigh may develop. Sprain of the ITB, described by Cyriax,[94] occurs primarily in dancers and athletes, causing symptoms similar to trochanteric bursitis. On examination, the snap may be reproduced, by flexing and extending the hip in adduction, revealing the cause to be the iliotibial tract moving over the greater trochanter.[324,364] Cyriax[94] listed four characteristics. The first is pain on the involved side with side flexion toward the painless side (which increases if the patient crosses the legs before bending sideways) while other lumbar spine movements are free. Other characteristics are pain on passive adduction of the hip, no pain on any other passive motion, and no pain on resisted abduction of the hip. Palpation reveals a painful spot around the greater trochanter.

Clicks, pops, and snaps around the hip are most often associated with the tensor fascia lata tendon passing over the greater trochanter or the iliopsoas tendon snapping over the anterior hip.[375,505] Renstrom[354] describes two types of hip snaps. The first type he describes occurs laterally from either a thickened posterior border of the iliotibial band or anterior border of the gluteus maximus moving over the greater trochanter often producing secondary bursitis. The second type is described as a more medial problem, which results from the iliopsoas tendon passing over the iliopectineal eminence.

ITB Tendinitis or ITB Friction Syndrome. Because of the attachments of the ITB to the lateral retinaculum and to the patella, the ITB has a significant effect on the patellar position and patellar pain, especially when it is excessively tight. ITB tendinitis or ITB friction syndrome presents itself with pain along the lateral side of the knee proximal to Gerdy's tubercle or over the prominence of the lateral femoral condyle. The ITB has two components at the lateral knee: the iliopatellar band and the iliotibial tract (see Fig. 7-14B). The iliopatellar band reinforces the lateral retinaculum, participates, and adds stability to the lateral capsule of the knee. The ITB friction syndrome is caused by friction between the lateral femoral condyle and iliotibial band while flexing and extending the knee. It is most common in varus knee alignment and often present in clients with a rigid cavus (non–shock-absorbing) foot because stress is transferred to the lateral side of the knee. It usually occurs in long distance runners who run 20 to 40 miles per week and have recently changes their running training habits (i.e., speed, terrain, footwear, running surface, or distance).[174] Climbing stairs or running on an incline aggravates the pain. This condition is aggravated on the downhill side when running on a sidehill.[446] Frequently there is localized effusion and occasionally palpable crepitus over the femoral condyle on repeated flexion and extension of the knee. Most patients with this problem will also have a positive Ober's test and Noble's compression test the majority of the time (see Chapter 14, Hip).

Foot Problems related to ITB Dysfunction. The cause of pain in the foot may be found in the iliotibial band, which, if it is pathologically tight, causes eversion at the ankle and external rotation of the foot.[301] Clinical studies have shown pes cavus–related ITB friction syndrome (see above) can take up to twice as long to resolve as pronation-related patellofemoral problems.[424] According to Mennell,[301] Achilles tendon insufficiency is associated with an accentuation of the drop of the foot at rest, resulting in the course of time, in shortening of the plantar fascia and myostatic contractures of the intrinsic muscles of the foot. This in turn results in impairment of foot joint function. Plantar fasciitis has a component in Ober's syndrome, a chronic condition of the plantar fascia. Achilles tendon insufficiency is often not only associated with a taut iliotibial bands, but chronic lumbosacral and sacroiliac joint problems as well.

Stretched TFL and ITB. Although the condition of pain associated with a contracted TFL/ITB is more common, there are instances of a strain and stretch of the TFL/ITB. This commonly occurs in unilateral TFL/ITB tightness on the high side (usually opposite to the tight side) of the pelvis as occurs in handedness postures (see Fig. 7-26).[230] When the leg is in a position of postural adduction, there is continuous tension of the abductors and ITB of the thigh and pelvis on that side. The TFL/ITB can also be stretched by a fall sideways or by a sideways thrust in which the pelvis moves laterally on a fixed pelvis. Symptoms of pain may be quite acute. Pain is referred to the lateral knee via the fascia lata. For strained TFL/ITB due to continuous tension or a fall, taping techniques to

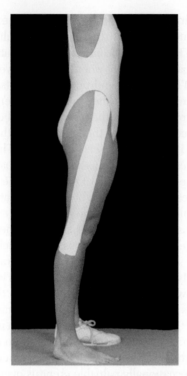

■ FIG. 8-67. Unloading the tensor fasciae lata/iliotibial band with lateral longitudinal taping using a technique developed by Florence Kendall.[230] (Reprinted with permission from Kendall HO, McCreary EK, Provence PT: Muscle Testing and Function, 4th ed. Baltimore: Williams & Wilkins, 1993:363.)

unload the ITB used in such a way that limits adduction have been quite successful (Fig. 8-67).[166,230] See the works of Hall and Kendall et al. for more information.[166,230]

Specific Evaluation and Differential Diagnosis

I. Subjective Complaints
   A. When overuse syndrome is a contributing factor, there will be a characteristic history of gradual onset of pain that may be accentuated by excessive running, excessive pronation or supination, or prolonged sitting with the hip too flexed.
   B. With TFL and ITB shortening referred pain/or burning is generally along the lateral aspect of the thigh to the knee or may extend upward over the buttock and involve the gluteal fascia (ITB fasciitis).[257,371] Pain eases slightly with movement but worsens after walking and with fatigue. Often pain is felt as the leg is brought forward through the swing phase.[326] Pain may wake the patient at night. Pain occurs primarily on the involved limb.
   C. ITB friction syndrome pain is typically of an aching type in the lateral knee. This can be sharp at a certain level of activity (e.g., at specific mileage threshold in runners).[446] Iliotibial knee pain may refer proximally or distally. Climbing stairs or running on inclines aggravates pain.

D. The patient may report numbness along the peroneal distribution (lateral calf).[230]

II. Key Objective Findings
   A. There may be some predisposing structural factors such as excessive pronation or supination, tibial varum, or the coxa varum-genu valgum combination, genu varus, medial femoral torsion, lateral tibial rotation, pes planus, or a rigid cavus foot.
   B. Observation may also reveal a groove present in the iliotibial band and lateral deviation of the patella. Unilateral tightness of the iliotibial band is associated with a lateral pelvic tilt low on the side of tightness.[230]
   C. Palpation may reveal a painful tender point over the greater trochanter (snapping hip syndrome). Trigger points may be found superior or in the midportion of the muscle. Palpation in ITB fasciitis may reveal nodules along the band and tenderness.
   D. The patient can usually point to a specific spot on the lateral aspect of the knee in ITB friction syndrome. There may be some swelling and occasionally thickening of the tissue in this area. There may be palpable crepitus on repeated flexion and extension of the knee.
   E. Key tests (ITB fasciitis). Hip flexion, abduction and medial rotation (TFL manual muscle test) may test painful. The Ober test reveals shortness of the TFL/ITB, and further stretch may elicit pain.[166] Positional weakness of the synergistic muscles of the gluteus maximus, iliopsoas and quadriceps is present.
   F. Key tests (ITB friction syndrome). Ober's test (see Fig. 14-20) and Noble's Compression Test (see Fig. 14-24) will be positive. Palpation of the femoral condyle reproduces the patient's pain.
   G. Associated findings may revel excessive medial rotation relative to lateral rotation hip ROM, antalgic gait, or positive Trendelenburg sign; excessive medial rotation or limited hip extension in gait[310]; hip antetorsion and joint dysfunction; and sacroiliac and patellofemoral joint.
   H. Other TFL/ITB overuse syndromes include trochanteric bursitis (see Chapter 14, Hip), extensor mechanism disorders (see Chapter 15, Knee), and faulty movement patterns at the hip and tibiofemoral joints. Sahrmann[373] provides more information on faulty movement patterns.[373]

Treatment of Iliotibial Overuse Syndromes. Treatment of this area becomes important in a variety of problems (see above), even if the patient has no conscious awareness of pain in the area of the ITB. Treatment of ITB syndromes should address all contributing factors (i.e., forefoot instability [excessive pronation], prolonged sitting with hip too flexed, compensation to a weak gluteus medius, lateral pelvic shift, and repetitive strain from running). Symptomatic relief measures such as iontophoresis, ice, ultrasound, rest, and position can help control pain and inflammation. Patients should avoid activities or postures that increase mechanical stress on the ITB (e.g., repetitive strain from running, prolonged sitting with the hip too flexed).[257] The patient should avoid standing in medial rotation and hip adduction with a high iliac crest, and hip adduction during sitting.[371]

Friction massage (Fig. 8-68), manually applied stretch (Fig. 8-69), and self-stretching (Box 8-9, Fig. *D*) help lengthen the ITB and TFL.[325,326,334] Self-stretching should be performed on a regular basis (once or twice a day) to prevent recurrence of viscoelastic stiffness or elevated neuromuscular tension.

Soft tissue manipulations may employ focused stretch, a direct approach, to the ITB as advocated by Mennell.[297,299,301] This technique actually addresses three distinct areas: (1) the anterior ITB and the groove between the quadriceps, (2) the posterior fibers of the ITB and the groove between the hamstrings, and (3) the ITB over the greater trochanter. The patient lies in the sidelying position with the leg to be treated uppermost. Both legs should comfortably flexed at the hip and knee with upper leg resting in front of the lower one.

1. Focused stretching used to stretch the anterior fibers of the band distal to the greater trochanter uses a bending or "twig snapping" technique (Fig. 8-14*B*). The fingers of both hands are laid over the anterior fibers of the band, starting at the knee. The thumbs are used as a fulcrum and placed against the edge of the posterior band. The movement is exactly that which corresponds to an attempt to snap a twig across: the thumbs are driven up against the posterior edge of the band, while the fingers of the two hands are separated from one another by twisting both hands into ulnar deviation in a controlled manner. The main force is transmitted through the thumbs. It is recommended to start stretching at the knee and work slowly up to the greater trochanter.

2. Focused stretching of the posterior band is achieved in a push-pull manner. The heels of the hands (the wrists being fully extended) are placed against the posterior aspect of the band. While the heel of one-hand pushes forward, the other hand pulls backward against the fibers, but without any alteration in the position of the fingers and the wrist (Fig. 8-70). The movement is then reversed Pressure is exerted perpendicular to the long axis of the femur. The whole length of the band can be treated in this way

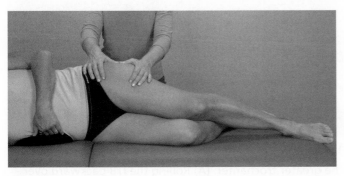

■ FIG. 8-68. Deep frictions to a lesion of the iliotibial band.

3. The region overlying the trochanter is treated by rolling it backwards and forward over the bony prominence (Fig. 8-71).[297] The fascia is first moved posteriorly by using the thumbs to press downward and backward (see Fig. 8-71A). The roll is attempting to take the band posteriorly over the trochanter. To press the back of the band forward and down toward the ilium at the same time, the middle fingertips (or the ulnar border of a reinforced fist) roll the band over the greater trochanter (see Fig.8-71B). Downward pressure in both of these techniques is through the weight of the operator. When the band is tight, as the tissue is rolled backward, the heel of the foot on the treated side should rise from the table.

Mennell's method of treating the fascial tissues above the greater trochanter and the TFL is the use of gentle kneading massage and effleurage.[299]

Other methods of focused stretch to the ITB below the trochanter include longitudinal stretch of the posterior band and hamstring, the anterior band and the quadriceps and along the band itself (Fig. 8-72). Focused stretch to the belly of the TFL may employ the forearm, one or more fingers or more of both hands as well as the palmar surface of the thumb. A small involved section of the TFL may be mobilized by taking up the slack (one hand stabilizes or tractions the tissue as the opposing hand stretches in the opposite direction) and elongating the involved tissues. The stretch is held while waiting for a release. When no further stretch is available another section is mobilized until all involved portions of the TFL have been released.

Soft tissue manipulation and stretching of other musculature of the lower quadrant (when tightness is present) should also be considered as well as joint mobilization/stabilization as indicated by the ongoing evaluation (see manual stretch [Fig. 8-73] and self-stretch to the gluteal musculature and external rotators [Fig. 8-74] as well as the quadratus lumborum [Box 8-9, Fig. *B*]). A number of joints in the lower quadrant, including the sacroiliac and lumbar spine, may be involved. As the patient progresses, include strengthening of the gluteus medius and other underused synergists. Instruct patients to recruit gluteus medius versus TFL in single leg stance (see Fig. 14-39). One may actually need to strengthen TFL/ITB if the condition is chronic.[371]

Patients should gradually return to a normal routine. Runners with ITB friction syndrome should avoid excessive side-hill running (see above) and all patients should avoid excessive use of stairs. One may also want to do patellofemoral taping to stretch the lateral retinaculum (see Figs. 15-39–15-41).[152,287] Patients need to wear shoes with good shock absorbency and should attempt to run on a softer surface. Carefully designed orthotic devises may help.

PIRIFORMIS MUSCLE SYNDROMES: SHORT AND LONG PIRIFORMIS SYNDROMES

The piriformis muscle as been implicated as a potential source of sciatic symptoms causing buttock and hamstring pain.[138,500]

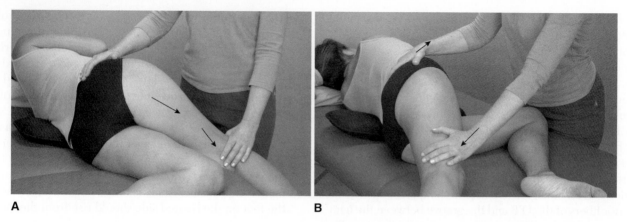

■ **FIG. 8-69.** Manual stretch of the tensor fasciae lata. **(A)** In sidelying with hip flexion. **(B)** In sidelying with hip extension. Postisometric relaxation and muscle energy may be used with both techniques.

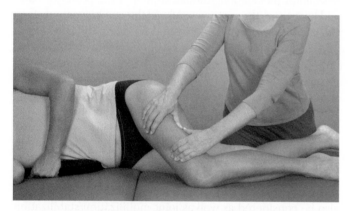

■ **FIG. 8-70.** Focused stretch of the iliotibial band of the posterior band along its length achieved in a push-pull manner; while pushing forward with the heel of one hand, the other hands pulls the tissue backward.

In sports medicine practice, in which chronic hamstring pain is a common diagnostic problem, this syndrome is often put forward as a possible cause of these symptoms.[258] Most often the piriformis syndrome is described as being associated with a contracted piriformis (short piriformis syndrome). However it is the opinion of Kendall et al.[230] and others that the piriformis is often associated with a stretched piriformis (long piriformis syndrome).[166,230,373]

The piriformis, the obturator internus, the superior and inferior gemelli, the quadratus femoris, and the obturator externus muscles are designated as the short external rotators of the femur (see Figs. 7-18*A* and 7-21*B*). Although, according to Hollinshead,[194] the piriformis muscle usually is designated as the key to arrangement of the nerves and vessels in the buttock. Whether the piriformis muscle is the cause of the compression has not been established. It is possible that the obturator internus/gemelli complex is an alternative

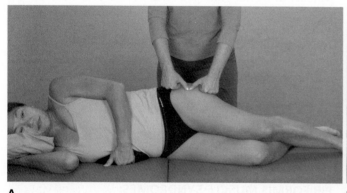
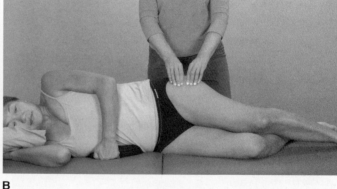

■ **FIG. 8-71.** Focused stretch of the iliotibial band (ITB) over the greater trochanter. **(A)** Rolling the ITB backward over the greater trochanter through pressure exerted through the thumbs. **(B)** Rolling the ITB forward over the over the greater trochanter with pressure exerted through the fingertips.[297]

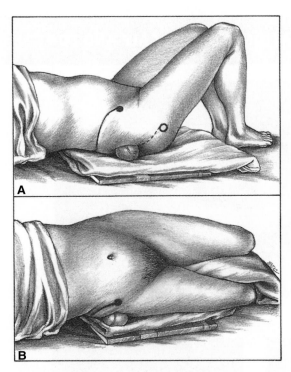

■ FIG. 8-78. **(A)** Self-ischemic compression therapy using a tennis ball place over the TP of the gluteus medius and gluteus minimus. **(B)** Pressure in applied by rolling the body weight onto the ball. (Reprinted with permission from DG Simons, LS Travell, LS Simons: Travell & Simons' Myofascial Pain & Dysfunction: The Trigger Point Manual, vol. 2. Baltimore, Williams & Wilkins, 1999:164.)

evident that, because causes of gluteus medius pain and spasm are often from other structures, correct and specific diagnosis is paramount. A common movement imbalance in neuromusculoskeletal pathology (e.g., nerve root, peripheral nerve) is between weak gluteal muscles with hyperactive hip flexors, and hyperactive lumbar erectores spinae with weak abdominal muscles. Soft tissue manipulations of the gluteus medius are often used to facilitate treatment of the gluteus medius syndrome by directly neutralizing muscle hypertonicity. The gluteus medius is a powerful hip abductor. The posterior portion of the gluteus medius primary role is to provide stabilization of the hip and control the femoral head in the acetabulum.[149]

The patient with gluteal tendinitis presents with pain that is usually well localized over the greater aspect of the greater trochanter but may refer to the posterior lateral aspect of the thigh. This overuse lesion tends to occur in two group of patients: those involved in sporting activities that involve extensive running, and in middle-aged, usually female, and often overweight patients with associated degenerative changes in the lower lumbar spine. Pain is usually brought on by hip movements, especially stair climbing and walking. Pain is reproduced by stretching, contracting the gluteus medius tendon, or on resisted contraction of the muscle. Calcification in the tendon or bursa may be found on radiographs in up to 20% of cases.[82]

Treatment. Treatment of gluteal tendinitis consists of rest from activities that produce this condition. Physical methods of treatment include ice or heat, stretching of the tendon, soft tissue manipulations (see above), and deep friction massage. Joint mobilization techniques may be effective (see Chapter 14, Hip) and are continued if the pain-free range improves.[82] Exercises are contraindicated in the early stages.

Balancing of the hip musculature is an important aspect of treatment in the many conditions involving the gluteus medius (e.g., neuromuscular pathology, muscle strain, altered-length tension relationships, pain, general weakness because of disuse, and subacute stages of gluteal tendinitis). Often there is faulty recruitment (incoordination) of the tensor fascia latae and gluteus medius during hip abduction.[253,373] When palpating these muscles to see whether both contract during active abduction, outward rotation and hip flexion may indicate that the gluteus medius is contracting too little, too late, or not at all.[253] One should also watch for undesirable contraction of the quadratus lumborum during manual muscle testing.

Overuse syndromes of the lower limb are discussed in the chapters on knee, lower leg, ankle, and foot (see extensor mechanism disorders, Chapter 15, Knee, and overuse syndromes of the leg and problems related to abnormal foot pronation, Chapter 16, Lower Leg, Ankle, and Foot). Box 8-10 provides examples of soft tissue manipulations and stretching techniques for common overuse syndromes of the leg and foot (e.g., compartment syndromes, plantar fasciitis). Also see the following soft tissue manipulation and stretching techniques for the lower limbs in Figs. 7-32, 7-39, 7-46B, 8-6, 8-19, 8-20, 8-27, 8-31, 8-32, 8-40–8-42, 8-68, and 8-78.

Common overuse syndromes of the upper limbs include impingement syndrome (rotator cuff pathology), biceps tendinitis, elbow tendinitis (lateral and medial epicondylitis), posterior impingement of the elbow (triceps tendinitis), compression neuropathies and compartment syndromes of the forearm, CTS (see above). De Quervain's syndrome and a variety of overuse syndromes at the wrist (extensor carpi ulnaris and radialis tendinitis, flexor carpi ulnaris and radialis tendinitis, as well as pisotriquetral and intersection syndrome–cross-over tendinitis) and hand may be encountered. These syndromes are particularly prevalent in the athletic world in sports such as baseball pitching, swimming, tennis, golfing, rowing, strength training, and racket sports (e.g., squash, badminton); work-related cumulative trauma disorders; and in spinal cord injury survivors.

In the recovery stage of overuse syndromes, treatment shifts from resolution of clinical signs and symptoms to restoration of function. When tissue healing is complete or nearly complete, the tissue can be appropriately loaded to facilitate remodeling and to regain local flexibility, proprioception, and strength. Also, other tissue subjected to chronic overload prior to injury and/or as the result of injury itself is treated. Secondary biomechanical deficits in flexibility, strength, and balance at sites other than the overuse syndrome or injury itself should be addressed. While some manual therapy for

(text continues on page 252)

BOX 8-10   EXAMPLES SOFT TISSUE MANIPULATIONS FOR THE CALF AND FOOT

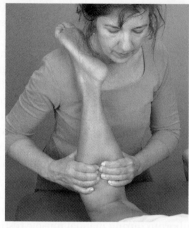

A1

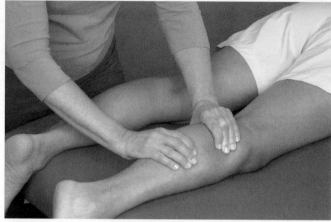

A2

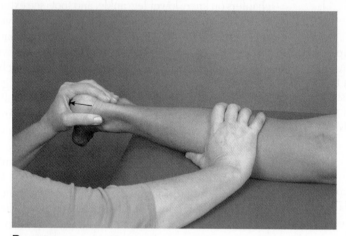

B

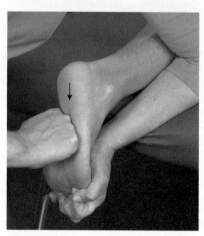

C1

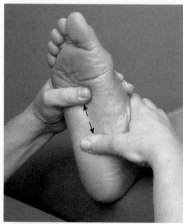

C2

(**A**) Manual techniques of the calf. (*1*) Lateral expansion with the knee in various degrees of flexion. (*2*) Bending or twig technique with the knee extended.
(**B**) Manual release of the tissue around the malleolus by spreading the myofascial structures in a lateral direction and by applying sustained traction to the calcaneus.
(**C**) Manual elongation of the plantar fascia. (*1*) Elongation with a knuckle sweep. (*2*) Stretching in conjunction with dorsiflexion.

Box 8-10. continued

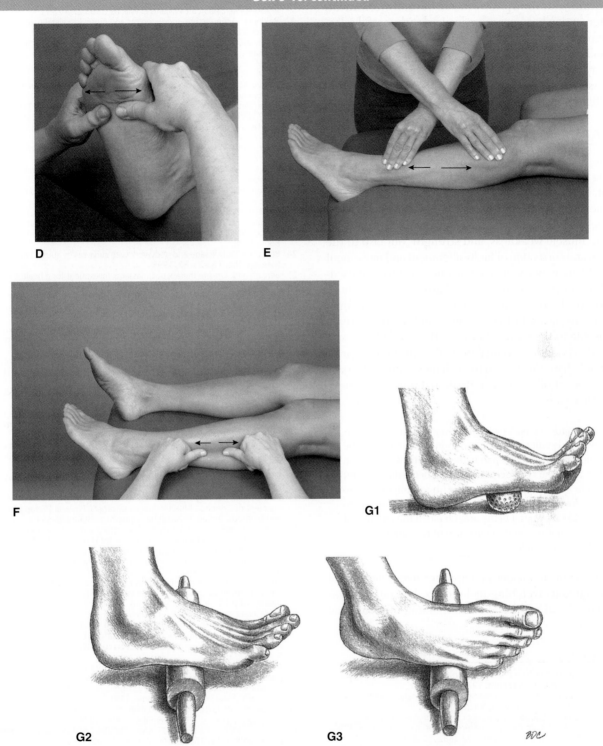

D

E

F

G1

G2

G3

BDC

(**D**) Widening of the planter fascia of the foot by lengthening the tissue in a lateral direction.
(**E**) Gross focused stretching of the anterior tibialis (anterior compartment).
(**F**) Focus stretch of the peroneals (lateral compartment).
(**G**) Self-stretch of the plantar fascia of the foot using (*1*) a golf ball or (*2*) a rolling pin. (Reprinted with permission from Simons DG, Travell LS, Simons LS: Travell & Simons' Myofascial Pain & Dysfunction: The Trigger Point Manual, vol. 2. Baltimore, Williams & Wilkins, 1999:518.)

myofascial and articular mobilization may continue, treatment emphasis shifts away from passive modalities and medications. Active intervention becomes more focused with careful selection of exercise treatment (i.e., limb position, joint angle, limb velocity and type of contraction). Criteria for advancement in the recovery stage or rehabilitation include complete pain control and tissue healing with essentially full painless ROM and good flexibility.

SUMMARY

Soft tissue manipulations are flexibly adapted according to presenting signs and symptoms; as these change, so should treatment. Before treatment, assessment of joint restrictions, relative shortness of postural muscles, and the myofascial system is necessary. Attention should be paid not only to myofascial length, muscle weakness, and strength, but also to the observation and correction of faulty alignment and movement patterns, which can perpetuate recurrent and chronic musculoskeletal dysfunction. Myofascial and articular dysfunctions typically coexist to some extent. Each component of dysfunction requires its own set of examination and treatment techniques specific to the tissue. As to whether the joint or soft tissues need to be addressed first, the truly well-rounded practitioner should have the tools to treat all these parts of the system. The concept of connective tissue tightness is not new. Mennell[299] has said:

"It is very remarkable how widespread may be the symptoms caused by unduly taut fascial planes. Though it is true that the fascial bands play a principle part in the mobility of the human body, they are often conducive to binding between two joint surfaces. For obvious reasons it is of the utmost importance to restore the lost mobility in the joints, before attempting to stretch the fascial planes. On the other hand, if the mobility of these planes is not restored, recurrence of the binding of the joints is almost inevitable."

This chapter is by no means a comprehensive treatment of all myofascial and stretching techniques, but rather gives the clinician a solid and basic understanding of myofascial manipulation.

REFERENCES

1. Academy of Traditional Chinese Medicine: An Outline of Chinese Acupuncture. Peking, Foreign Language Press, 1975
2. Alter MJ: Science of Stretching. Champaign, Human Kinetics, 1988
3. Anderson B: Stretching. Bolinas, CA, Shelter, 1985
4. Appell RA, Bourcier AP, Torre FL: Pelvic Floor Dysfunction—Investigations and Conservative Treatment. Rome, Cassa Editrice Scientifica Internazionale, 1999
5. Armstrong ME: Acupuncture. Am J Nurs 72:1582–1588, 1972
6. Aston J: Aston Bodyworks II. Continuing Education Course. Seattle, WA, The Aston Training Center, 1996
7. Aston J, Pollock JP: Integrating Aston concepts into a massage therapy practice. Massage March/April, 1996
8. Bachrach RM: The relationship of low back pain to psoas insufficiency. J Orthop Med 13:34–40, 1991
9. Bachrach RM: Psoas dysfunction/insufficiency, sacroiliac dysfunction and low back pain. In: Vleeming A, Mooney V, Dorman T, et al., eds: Movement, Stability and Low Back Pain. New York, Churchill Livingstone, 1997
10. Bajelis D: The ultimate in myofascial release. J Altern Complement Med 12:26–30, 1994
11. Bajelis D, Bell S, Haller J, et al: Alternative movement-related therapies. In: Hall CM, Thein Brody L, eds: Therapeutic Exercise: Moving Toward Function. Philadelphia, Lippincott Williams & Wilkins, 1998:274–285
12. Baldry PE: Acupuncture, trigger points and musculoskeletal pain. London, Churchill Livingstone, 1993
13. Bandy WD, Irion JM: The effect of time of static stretch on the flexibility of the hamstring muscles. Phys Ther 74:845–852, 1994
14. Barral J-P: The Thorax. Seattle, Eastland, 1991
15. Barral J-P: Urogenital Manipulation. Seattle, Eastland, 1993
16. Batavia M: Contraindications for therapeutic massage: Do sources agree? J Bodywork Move Ther 8:48–57, 2003
17. Baxter-Petralia P, Penny V: Cumulative trauma. In: Stanley BG, Tribuzi SM, eds: Concepts in Hand Rehabilitation, Philadelphia, FA Davis, 1992:419–445
18. Beal NW: Acupuncture and related treatment modalities. Part I: Theoretical background. J Nurse Midwife 37:254–259, 1992
19. Beam J, Delany W, Haynes W, et al: The stretching debate. J Bodywork Move Ther 7:80–96, 2003
20. Beard G, Wood EC: Massage Principles and Techniques. Philadelphia, WB Saunders, 1964
21. Beaton LE, Anson BJ: The relation of the median nerve to the pronator teres muscle. Anat Rec 75:23–28, 1939
22. Beaulieu JE: Stretching for All Sports. Pasadena, Athletic Press, 1980
23. Benjamin BE: Are You Tense? The Benjamin System of Muscular Therapy: Tension Relief through Deep Massage and Body Care. New York, Pantheon Book, 1978
24. Benjamin BE: Massage and bodywork with survivors of abuse. Part I. Massage Ther J 34:23–32, 1995
25. Benjamin PJ: On-site therapeutic massage: Investment for a healthy business. Information brochure. Rockford, IL, Hemingway Publications, 1994
26. Benjamin PJ: The California revival: Massage therapy in the 1970–80's. Presentation at the AMTA National Education Conference in Los Angeles, CA, June 1996
27. Benjamin PJ, Eunice D: Ingham and the development of foot reflexology in the United States. Part one: The early years to 1946. Massage Ther J Spring:38–44, 1989
28. Benjamin PJ, Eunice D: Ingham and the development of foot reflexology in the United States: Part two: On the road 1946–1974. Massage Ther J 32:56–62, 1989
29. Benjamin PJ, Limp SP: Understanding Sports Massage. Champaign, Human Kinetics, 1996
30. Benson H, Stuart EM: The Wellness Book: The Comprehensive Guide to Maintaining Health and Treating Stress-Related Illness. New York, Simon & Schuster, 1992
31. Berghams LC, Hendricks HJ, Bo K, et al: Conservative treatment of stress urinary incontinence. A systematic review of randomized clinical trials. Br J Urol 82:181–191, 1998
32. Bischoff I, Elminger G: Connective tissue massage. In: Licht S, ed: Massage, Manipulation and Traction, Baltimore, Waverly Press, 1963
33. Blakney MG, Hertling D: The cervical spine. In :Hertling D, Kessler RM: Management of Common Musculoskeletal Disorders, Physical Therapy Principles and Methods, 3rd ed. Philadelphia, Lippincott, 1996:528–559
34. Bo K: Pelvic floor muscle exercise for the treatment of stress urinary incontinence. An exercise physiology perspective. Int Urogynecol J 6:282–291, 1996
35. Bo K: Single blind, randomized controlled trial of pelvic floor exercises, electrical stimulation, vaginal cones, and no treatment in management in genuine stress incontinence in women. BMJ 318:487–493, 1999
36. Bo K, Hagen RH, Kvarstein B, et al: Pelvic floor muscle exercise for the treatment of female stress urinary incontinence. III: Effects of two different degrees of pelvic floor muscle exercise. Neurourol Urodyn 9:489–502, 1990
37. Bo K, Kvaarstein B, Hagen R, et al: Pelvic floor muscle exercise for the treatment of female stress urinary incontinence. II. Validity of vaginal pressure measurements of pelvic floor muscle strength and the necessity of supplementary methods for control of correction contraction. Neurourol Urodyn 9:470–487, 1990
38. Bo K, Talseth T: Long term effect of pelvic floor muscle exercise five years after cessation of organized training. Obstet Gynecol 87:261–265, 1996
39. Boehme R: Myofascial Release and its Application to Neuro-Developmental Treatment. Milwaukee, Regi Boehme, 1991
40. Bohannon RW: Effect of repeated eight-minute muscle loading on the angle of straight leg raising. Phys Ther 64:491–496, 1984
41. Bookhout MM, Boissonnault JS: Musculoskeletal dysfunction in the female pelvis. Orthop Phys Ther Clin North Am 5:23–45, 1996
42. Bookhout MR: Examination and treatment of muscle imbalances. In: Bourdillon JF, Day EA, Bookhout MR, eds: Spinal Manipulation, 5th ed. Oxford, Butterworth-Heinemann, 1992:313–333
43. Booth B: Shiatsu. Nurs Times 89:38–40, 1993
44. Booth B: Reflexology. Nurs Times 90:38–40, 1994
45. Booth RE, Marvel JP: Differential diagnosis of shoulder pain. Orthop Clin North Am 6:353–379, 1975
46. Borms J, VanRoy P, Santen JP, et al: Optimal duration of static stretching exercises for improvement of coxa-femoral flexibility. J Sports Sci 5:39–47, 1987
47. Bourdillon JF, Day EA, Bookhout MR, eds: Spinal Manipulation, 5th ed. Oxford, Butterworth- Heinemann, 1992

48. Bradley JA: Acupuncture, and trigger point therapy. In: Peat M, ed: Current Physical Therapy. Toronto, BC Decker, 1988:228–234
49. Brattberg G: Connective tissue massage in the treatment of fibromyalgia. Eur J Pain 3:235–244, 1999
50. Brenneman SK, Stanger M, Bertoti: Age-related considerations: Pediatrics. In: Sgarlat R, Meyer R, eds: Saunders Manual of Physical Therapy Practice. Philadelphia, WB Saunders, 1995:1229–1283
51. Brownstein B: Movement biomechanics and control. In: Brownstein B, Bronner S, eds: Evaluation Treatment and Outcomes: Functional Movement in Orthopaedic and Sports Physical Therapy, New York, Churchill Livingstone, 1997
52. Brody L: Mobility impairment. In: Hall CM, Brody L, eds: Therapeutic Exercise: Moving Toward Function. Philadelphia, Lippincott, Williams & Wilkins, 1998:87–111
53. Brody L: Pain. In: Hall CM, Brody L, eds: Therapeutic Exercise: Moving Toward Function. Philadelphia, Lippincott Williams & Wilkins, 1998:145–164
54. Brownstein B, Bronner S: Evaluation, Treatment, and Outcomes. Functional Movement in Orthopedic and Sports Medicine Physical Therapy. New York, Churchill Livingstone, 1995:1–42
55. Brubaker L, Benson JT, Bent A, et al: Transvaginal electrical stimulation for female urinary incontinence. Am J Obstet Gynecol 177:536–540, 1997
56. Buckwalter JA, Kuettner KE, Thonar EJ-M: Age related changes in articular cartilage proteoglycans: electron microscopic studies. J Orthop Res 3:215, 1985
57. Burgio KI, Goode PS, Locher JL: Behavioral training with and without biofeedback in the treatment of urge incontinence in older women: A randomized control trial. JAMA 288:2293–2299, 2001
58. Buckwalter JA, Woo SL-L, Goldberg VM, et al: Current concepts review: Soft tissue aging and musculoskeletal function. J Bone Joint Surg Am 75:1533–1548, 1993
59. Buroker KC, Schwane JA: Does postexercise static stretching alleviate delayed muscle soreness? Phys Sportsmed 17:65–83, 1989
60. Burstein AH, Reilly DT, Martens M: Aging of bone tissue: Mechanical properties. J Bone Joint Surg Am 58:82–86, 1976
61. Butler DS, Slater H: Neural injury in the thoracic spine: A conceptual basis for manual therapy. In: Grant R, ed: Physical Therapy of the Cervical and Thoracic Spine. New York, Churchill Livingstone, 1994:313–338
62. Byer DC: Better Health with Foot Reflexology. St. Petersburg, Ingham, 1991
63. Calais-Germain B: Female Pelvis Anatomy and Exercise. Seattle, Eastland, 2003
64. Canavan PK: Rehabilitation in Sports Medicine: A Comprehensive Guide. Stanford, Appleton & Lange, 1998
65. Cantu R, Grodin A: Myofascial Manipulation. Gaithersburg, Aspen, 1992
66. Carriere B: Fitness for the Pelvic Floor. Stuttgart, Thieme, 2002
67. Centeno K: An exclusive interview with Judith Aston. Massage Bodywork Spring:53–58, 1996
68. Chaitow L: The Acupuncture Treatment of Pain. Rochester, VT, Healing Arts Press, 1991
69. Chaitow L: Soft-tissue manipulation. Rochester, VT, Healing Arts Press, 1980
70. Chaitow L: Soft-tissue Manipulation: A Practitioner's Guide to the Diagnosis and Treatment of Soft-Tissue Dysfunction and Reflex Activity. Rochester, VT, Healing Arts Press, 1987
71. Chaitow L: Modern Neuromuscular Techniques. New York, Churchill Livingstone, 1996
72. Chaitow L: Muscle Energy Techniques. New York, Churchill Livingstone, 1996
73. Chaitow L: Positional Release Techniques. New York, Churchill Livingstone, 1996
74. Chaitow L: Cranial Manipulation, Theory and Practice: Osseous and Soft Tissue Approaches. Edinburgh, Churchill Livingstone, 1999
75. Chamberlain GJ: Cyriax's friction massage: A review. J Orthop Sports Phys Ther 4:16–22, 1982
76. Chapman SA, DeFranca CL: Rehabilitation of low back pain. In: Cox JM, ed: Low Back Pain: Mechanism, Diagnosis, and Treatment, 6th ed. Baltimore, Williams & Wilkins, 1999:653–678
77. Cherry D: Review of physical therapy alternatives for reducing muscle contracture. Phys Ther 60:877–881, 1980
78. Clement DB: A survey of overuse running injuries. Phys Sports Med 9:47–58, 1981
79. Cohen JH, Schneider MJ: Receptor-tonus technique: An overview. Chiro Tech 2:13–16, 1990
80. Condon SM, Hutton RS: Soleus muscle electromyographic activity and ankle dorsiflexion range of motion during four stretching procedures. Phys Ther 67:24–30, 1987
81. Cornelius W, Jackson A: The effects of cryotherapy and PNF on hip extensor flexibility. Athlet Train 19:183–184:1984
82. Corrigan B, Maitland GD: Practical Orthopaedic Medicine. London, Butterworth, 1983
83. Cottingham JT: Healing Through Touch: A History and Review of the Physiological Evidence. Boulder, Rolf Institute, 1985
84. Cottingham JT, Porges SW, Lyon T: Effect of soft tissue mobilization (Rolfing pelvic lift) on parasympathetic tone in two age groups. Phys Ther 68:352–356, 1988

85. Cottingham JT, Porges SW, Richmond K: Shifts in pelvic inclination angle and parasympathetic tone produced by Rolfing soft tissue manipulation Phys Ther 68:1364–1370, 1988
86. Couch J, Weaver N: Runner's World: Yoga Book: Stretching and Strengthening Exercises for Runner and Other Athletes, 2nd ed. Mountain View, CA, Runner's World Books, 1982
87. Crisswell E: How Yoga Works–An Introduction to Somatic Yoga. Phoenix, Freeperson Press, 1989
88. Cuetter AC, Bartoszek DM: The thoracic outlet syndrome: Controversies, overdiagnosis, and recommendations for management. Muscle Nerve 12:410–419, 1989
89. Cummings CG, Crutchfield CC, Barnes BM: Orthopedic physical therapy series, vol. 1: Soft tissue changes in contractures. Atlanta, Stokesville, 1983
90. Cummings GS, Tillman LJ: Remodeling of dense connective tissue in normal adult tissues. In: Currier DP, Nelson RM, eds: Dynamics of Human Biologic Tissues. Philadelphia, FA Davis, 1992
91. Cyriax J: Clinical applications of massage. In: Licht S, ed: Massage, Manipulation and Traction. New Haven, Elizabeth Licht Publishers, 1960:122–139
92. Cyriax J: Deep massage. Physiotherapy 63:60–61, 1977
93. Cyriax J: Textbook of Orthopaedic Medicine: Diagnosis of Soft Tissue Lesions, vol. I, 8th ed. London, Bailliere Tindall, 1982
94. Cyriax JH, Cyriax PJ: Illustrated Manual of Orthopaedic Medicine. London, Butterworth, 1983
95. Cyriax J, Coldham M: Textbook of Orthopaedic Medicine, vol. II. 11th ed. London, Balliere Tindall, 1984
96. D'Ambrogio KJ, Roth GB: Positional Release Therapy: Assessment & Treatment of Musculoskeletal Dysfunction, St. Louis, Mosby, 1997
97. Davidson CJ, Ganion LR, Gehlsen GM, et al: Rat tendon morphologic and functional changes resulting from soft tissue mobilization. Med Sci Sports Exerc 29:313–319, 1997
98. Davis DG: Manipulation of the lower extremity. In: Subotnick SI, ed: Sports Medicine of the Lower Extremity, 2nd ed. New York, Churchill Livingstone, 1999:443–453
99. Dawson DM, Hallett M, Millender LH: Radial nerve entrapment. In: Entrapment Neuropathies. Boston, Little Brown, 1983:141–168
100. de Bruijn R: Deep transverse friction: Its analgesic effect. Int J Sports Med 5(Suppl):35–36, 1984
101. De Domenico G, Wood EC: Beard's Massage, 4th ed. Philadelphia, WB Saunders, 1997
102. DePalma AF: Surgery of the Shoulder. JB Lippincott, Philadelphia, 1983
103. DePalma B: Rehabilitation of the groin, hip and thigh. In: Prentice WE, Voight MI, eds: Techniques in Musculoskeletal Rehabilitation. New York, McGraw, 2001:509–540
104. DeVries HA: Evaluation of static stretching procedures for improvement of flexibility. Res Q 3:222–229, 1962
105. DeVries HA: Physiological effects of an exercise training regimen upon men aged 52 to 88. J Gerontol Biol Sci Med Sci 25:325–336, 1970
106. Dicke E, Schliack H, Wolff A: A Manual of Reflexive Therapy of the Connective Tissue "Bindegewebsmassage." Stuttgart, Germany, Sidney S. Simon, 1978
107. Diego MA, Field T, Hernandez-Reif M, et al: HIV adolescents show improved immune function following massage therapy. J Neurosci 106:35–45, 2001
108. DiGiovanna EL, Schiowitz S: An Osteopathic Approach to Diagnosis and Treatment. Philadelphia, JB Lippincott, 1991
109. Donatelli RA, Wolf SL: The Biomechanics of the Foot and Ankle. Philadelphia, FA Davis, 1990
110. Donatelli RA, Wooden MJ: Orthopaedic Physical Therapy, 3rd ed. New York, Churchill Livingstone, 2001
111. Dontigny RL: Passive shoulder exercises. J Phys Ther 50:1707–1709, 1970
112. Dumoulin C, Seaborne DE, Quirion-DeGirardi C, et al: Pelvic-floor rehabilitation, Part 2: Pelvic floor reeducation with interferential currents and exercise in the treatment of genuine stress incontinence in postpartum women–cohort study. Phys Ther 75:1075–1081, 1995
113. Dunn J: Physical therapy. In: Kaplan AS, Assel LA, eds: Temporomandibular Disorders. Philadelphia, WB Saunders, 1991:455–500
114. Dvorak J, Dovrak V: Manual Medicine: Diagnostic. New York, Thieme Medical, 1990
115. Ebner M: Connective tissue massage. S Afr J Physiother 21:4–7, 1965
116. Ebner M: Connective tissue massage: Therapeutic application. N Z J Physiother 3:18–22, 1968
117. Ebner M: Connective tissue massage: Physiother JCSP 64:208–210, 1978
118. Ebner M: Connective Tissue Manipulation: Theory and Therapeutic Application, 2nd ed. Malabar, Robert E. Krieger, 1985
119. Edgelow PI: Neurovascular consequences of cumulative trauma disorders affecting the thoracic outlet: A patient centered treatment approach. In: Donatelli RA, ed: Physical Therapy of the Shoulder, 3rd ed. New York, Churchill Livingstone, 1997:153–178
120. Eggold JF: Orthotics in prevention of runner's overuse injuries. Phys Sports Med 9:125–131, 1981
121. Elliot B, Achland T: Biomechanical effects of fatigue on 10,000 meter running techniques. Res Quart Ex Sports 52:160–166, 1981

122. Ellis JJ, Johnson GS: Myofascial considerations in somatic dysfunction of the thorax. In: Flynn TW, ed: The Thoracic Spine and Rib Cage: Musculoskeletal Evaluation and Treatment. Boston, Butterworth-Heinemann, 1996:211–262

123. Etnyre BR, Abraham LD: H-reflex changes during static stretching and two variations of proprioceptive neuromuscular facilitation techniques. Electroencephalogr Clin Neurophysiol 63:174–179, 1986

124. Eurroll R, Hurst L: The relationship of the thoracic outlet syndrome and carpal tunnel syndrome. Clin Orthop 164:149–153, 1982

125. Evatt ML, Wolf SL, Segal RL: Modification of human spinal stretch reflexes: Preliminary studies. Neurosci Lett 105:278:299–304, 1989

126. Evjenth O, Hamberg J: Muscle Stretching in Manual Therapy: A Clinical Manual, vol. 1: The Extremities. Alfta, Sweden, Alfta Rehab Forlag, 1984

127. Evjenth O, Hamberg J: Muscle Stretching in Manual Therapy: A Clinical Manual, vol. 2: The Spinal Column and the TM Joint. Alfta, Sweden, Alfta Rehab Forlag, 1984

128. Evjenth O, Hamberg J: Autostretching. Sweden, Alfta Rehab Forlag, 1997

129. Feland JB, Myrer JW, Schulthies SS, et al: The effect of duration of stretching of the hamstring muscle group for increasing range of motion in people 65 years or older. Phys Ther 81:1110–1117, 2001

130. Fialka V, Sadil V, Ernst E: Reflex sympathetic dystrophy (RSD)—A century of investigation and still a mystery. Eur J Phys Med Rehab 2:26–28, 1991

131. Field T, Delage J, Hernandez-Reif: Movement and massage therapy reduce fibromyalgia pain. J Bodywork Move Ther 7:49–52, 2003

132. Field T, Diego M, Cullen C, et al: Fibromyalgia pain and subtonic P decreases and sleep improves after massage therapy. J Clin Rheumatol 8:72–76, 2002

133. Fischer AA: Documentation of myofascial trigger points. Arch Phys Med Rehabil 69:286–291, 1988

134. Fitzgerald WH, Bower EF: Zone Therapy. Columbus, IW Long, 1917

135. Flynn TW: The Thoracic Spine and Rib Cage: Musculoskeletal Evaluation and Treatment. Boston, Butterworth-Heinemann, 1996

136. Foberg CR, Weiss AP, Akelmann E: Cubital tunnel syndrome. Part I: Presentation and diagnosis. Orthop Rev 23:136–144, 1994

137. Fox EJ, Melzack R: Transcutaneous electrical stimulation and acupuncture: Comparison of treatment for low back pain. Pain 2:141–148, 1976

138. Freiburg A, Vinkle T: Sciatica and sacro-iliac joint. J Bone Joint Surg 16:126–136, 1934

139. Gabel GT, Morrey BF: Operative treatment of medial epicondylitis: Influence of concomitant ulnar neuropathy at the elbow. J Bone Joint Surg Am 77:1065–1069, 1995

140. Gajdosik RL: Effects of static stretching on the maximal length and resistance to passive stretch of short hamstring muscles J Orthop Sports Phys Ther 14:250–255, 1991

141. Gambert SR: Rheumatologic problems in the elderly. In: Gambert SR, Benson DM, Gupta KL, eds: Handbook of Geriatrics. New York, Plenum, 1987:95–120

142. Gerstein JW: Effect of ultrasound on tendon extensibility. Am J Phys Med 34:662, 1955

143. Gifford J, Gifford L: Connective tissue massage. In: Wells BE, Frampton V, Bowsher D, eds: Pain Management in Physical Therapy. Norwalk, Appleton & Lange, 1988

144. Gillette TM, Holland JGJ, Williams JV, et al: Relationship of body core temperature and warm-up to knee range of motion. J Orthop Sports Phys Ther 13:126–131, 1991

145. Goats GC, Kerr K: Connective tissue massage. Br J Sports Med 25:131–133, 1991

146. Godges JJ, MacRae H, Longdon C, et al: The effects of two stretching procedures on hip range of motion and gait economy. J Orthop Phys Ther 10:350–357, 1989

147. Goldenberg DL: Treatment of fibromyalgia syndrome. Rheum Dis Clin North Am 15:61–71, 1989

148. Goodridge JP: Muscle energy technique: Definition, explanation, methods of procedure. J Am Osteopath Assoc 81:249–254, 1981

149. Gottschalk F, Kourosh S, Leveau B: The functional anatomy of tensor fascia latae and gluteus medius and minimus. J Anat 166:179–189, 1989

150. Greenman PE, ed: Concepts and Mechanisms of Neuromuscular Function. New York, Springer-Verlag, 1984

151. Greenman PE: Principles of Manual Therapy, 3rd ed. Baltimore, Williams & Wilkins, 2003

152. Grelsamer RP, Mc Connell J: The Patella: A Team Approach, Gaithersburg, Apsen, 1998

153. Grice AS: Muscle tonus changes following manipulations. J Can Chiro Assoc 18:29–31, 1974

154. Grieve GP: Common Vertebral Joint Problems, 2nd ed. Edinburgh, Churchill Livingstone, 1988.

155. Grieve GP: Mobilization of the Spine: A Primary Handbook of Clinical Method, 5th ed. Edinburgh, Churchill Livingstone, 1991

156. Grimby G, Danneskiold-Samsoe B, Hvid K: Morphology and enzymatic capacity in arm and leg muscles in 78–81 year old men and women. Acta Physiol Scand 115:125–134, 1982

157. Grimsby O: Fundamentals of Manual Therapy: A Course Workbook. Everett, WA, Sorlandets Institute, 1985

158. Gross MT: Chronic tendinitis: Pathomechanics of injury, factors affecting the healing response, and treatment. J Orthop Sports Phys Ther 16:248–261, 1992

159. Gudmestad J: Ease on back. Yoga J 153:94–101, 2000

160. Guidotti TL: Occupational repetitive strain injury. Am Fam Physician 45:585–592, 1992

161. Gunnari H, Evjenth O, Brady MM: Sequence Exercise: The Sensible Approach to All-Round Fitness. Oslo, Dreyers Forlag, 1984

162. Gumimaraes ACS: Reflex responses associated with manipulative treatments on the thoracic spine: A pilot study. J Manipulative Physiol Ther 18:233–236, 1995

163. Gustavsen R, Streeck R: Training Therapy: Prophylaxis and Rehabilitation. New York, Thieme, 1993

164. Halbertsman JPK, Van Bolhuis AI, Goeken LNH: Sport stretching: Effect on passive muscle stiffness of short hamstrings. Arch Phys Med Rehabil 77:688–692, 1996

165. Hall CM: Diagnosis and Treatment of Movement System Imbalances with Musculoskeletal Pain as taught by Shirley Sahrmann. Continuing Education Course, Seattle, WA, 1993

166. Hall CM: The hip. In: Hall CM, Brody LT, eds: Therapeutic Exercise: Moving Toward Function. Philadelphia, Lippincott Williams & Wilkins, 1998:387–436

167. Hammer WI: Friction Massage. In: Hammer WI, ed: Functional Soft Tissue Examination and Treatment by Manual Methods: The Extremities. Gaithersburg, Aspen, 1991:235–249

168. Hammer WI: The use of transverse massage in the management of chronic bursitis of the hip and shoulder. J Manipulative Ther 16:107–111, 1993

169. Hampton E: The relationship between pelvic floor and abdominal musculature: Clinical recommendations for rehabilitation based on emerging literature. J Section Women's Health 27:22–25, 2003

170. Han JS: The neurochemical basis of pain relief by acupuncture: A collection of papers 1973–1987. Beijing, Chinese Medical Science & Technology Press, 1987

171. Hanna T: Somatics: Reawakening the Mind's Control of Movement, Flexibility and Health, 4th ed. Reading, MA, Addison–Wesley, 1991

172. Hanten WP, Chandler SD: Effects of myofascial release leg pull and sagittal plane isometric contract-relax techniques on passive straight-leg raise angle. J Orthop Sports Phys Ther 20:138–144, 1994

173. Hare ML: Shiatsu acupressure in nursing practice. Holistic Nurs Pract 2:68–74, 1988

174. Hartley A: Practical Joint Assessment: Lower Quadrant, 2nd ed. St. Louis, Mosby 1995

175. Hattrup SJ: Rotator cuff repair: Relevance of patient age. J Shoulder Elbow Surg 4:95–100, 1995

176. He L: Involvement of endogenous opiod peptides in acupuncture analgesia. Pain 31:91–121, 1987

177. Hellar J, Jenkin WA: Bodywise. Berkeley, Wingbo, 1991

178. Hendrickson, T: Massage for Orthopedic Conditions. Philadelphia, Lippincott Williams & Wilkins, 2003

179. Henry JA: Manual therapy of the shoulder. In: Kelly MJ, Clark WA, eds: Orthopedic Therapy of the Shoulder. Philadelphia, JB Lippincott, 1995:285–336

180. Henry JH: The patellofemoral joint. In: Nicholas JA, Hershman EB, eds: The Lower Extremity and Spine in Sports Medicine. St. Louis, CV Mosby 1986:1013–1054

181. Hepburn G: Case studies: Contracture and stiff joint management with dynasplint. J Orthop Sports Phys Ther 8:498–504, 1987

182. Herman H: Urogenital dysfunction. In: Wilder E, ed: Clinics in Physical Therapy, vol. 20, Obstetric and Gynecologic Physical Therapy, New York, Churchill Livingstone, 1988

183. Hernandez-Reif M, Field T, Krasnegor J, et al: Lower back pain is reduced and range of motion increased after massage therapy. Int J Neurosci 106:1–15, 2000

184. Hernandez-Reif M, Field T, Largie C, et al: Parkinson's disease symptoms are differentially affected by massage therapy vs. relaxation: A pilot study, J Bodywork Move Ther 6:177–182, 2002

185. Herzog W: Mechanical and physiological responses to spinal manipulative treatments. J Neuromusculoskel Sys 3:1–9, 1995

186. Herzog W, Conway PJ, Zgang YZ, et al: Reflex response associated with manipulative treatment of the thoracic spine. J Neuromusculoskel Sys 2:124–130, 1994

187. Hey LR, Helewa A: Myofascial pain syndrome: A critical review of the literature. Physiother Can 46:28–36, 1994

188. Hillman J: Zone therapy. Nursing 3:225–227, 1986

189. Hirsch LF, Thanki A: The thoracic outlet syndrome. Postgrad Med 77: 197–207, 1985

190. Hoffa A: Technik der Massage, 14th ed. Stuttgart, Ferdinand Ernke, 1978

191. Holey EA: Connective tissue zones: An introduction. Physiother JCSP 8:366–368, 1995

192. Holey EA: Connective tissue manipulation-toward a scientific rationale. Physiother JCSP 81:730–739,1995

193. Holey EA, Watson M: Inter-rater reliability of connective tissue zones recognition. Physiother JCSP 81:369–372, 1995

194. Hollinshead WH. Functional Anatomy of the Limbs and Back. A Text for Students of the Locomotor Apparatus. Philadelphia, Saunders, 1976

195. Hollis M: Practical Exercise Therapy, 2nd ed. Oxford, Blackwell Scientific, 1982

196. Hollis M: Massage for Therapists. Oxford, Blackwell. 1987
197. Hortobagyi T, Faludi J, Tihanyi J, et al: Effects of intense "stretching"—Flexibility training on the mechanical profile of the knee extensors and on the range of motion of the hip joint. Int J Sports Med 6:317–321, 1985
198. Howard FM, Perry CP, Carter JE, et al: Pelvic Pain: Diagnosis & Management. Philadelphia, Lippincott, Williams & Wilkins, 2000
199. Hunter JM, Schneider LH, Mackin EJ, et al., eds: Rehabilitation of the Hand: Surgery and Therapy, 3rd ed. St. Louis, Mosby 1990
200. Hunter SC, Poole RM: The chronically inflamed tendon. Clin Sports Med 5:371–388,1987
201. Hurwitz S, Ernst GP, Yi S: The foot and ankle. In: Canavan PK, ed: Rehabilitation in Sports Medicine: A Comprehensive Guide. Stamford, Appleton & Lange, 1998:325–382
202. Hutton RS: Neuromuscular basis of stretching exercises. In: Kormi PV, ed: Strength and Power in Sports. Boston, Blackwell Scientific, 1992:29–38
203. Indahl A, Kaigle AM, Reikeras O, et al: Interaction between the porcine lumbar intervertebral disc, zygopophyseal joints and paraspinal muscles. Spine 22:2834–2840, 1997
204. Ingham ED: Stories the Feet Can Tell [revised as Stories the Feet Have Told Through Reflexology]. St, Petersburg, Ingham, 1984
205. Ironson G, Field T, Scafidi F, et al: Massage therapy is associated with enhancement of the immune system's cytotoxic capacity. Int J Neurosci 84:204–217, 1996
206. James SL, Bates BR, Ostering LR: Injuries to runners. Am J Sports Med 6:40–50, 1978
207. Janda V: Die Bedeutung der musklaren Fehlhatung als pathogenetisher Faktor vertebagener Storungen. Arch Phys Ther 20:113–116, 1968
208. Janda V: Muscles, central nervous motor regulation and back problems. In: Korr I, ed: The Neurobiologic Mechanism in Manipulative Therapy. New York, Plenum Press, 1978:27
209. Janda V: Muscle Function Testing. London, Butterworths, 1983
210. Janda V: Muscle weakness and inhibition (pseudoparesis) in back pain syndromes. In: Grieve GP, ed: Modern Manual Therapy of the Vertebral Column. Edinburgh, Churchill Livingstone, 1986
211. Janda V: Differential diagnosis of muscle tone in respect of inhibitory techniques. In: Patterson JK, Burn L, eds: Back Pain, an International Review. Boston, Kluwer Drodrecht, 1990
212. Janda V: Muscle spasm—A proposed procedure for differential diagnosis. Man Med 6:136–139, 1991
213. Janda V: Muscle strength in relation to muscle length; pain and muscle imbalance. In: Harms-Rindahl, ed: Muscle Strength. New York, Churchill Livingstone, 1993
214. Janda V: Muscle and motor control in cervicogenic disorders: Assessment and management. In: Grant R, ed: Physical Therapy of the Cervical and Thoracic Spine, 2nd ed. Edinburgh, Churchill Livingstone, 1994:195
215. Janda V: Evaluation of muscular imbalance. In: Liebensen C, ed: Rehabilitation of the Spine: A Practitioner's Manual. Baltimore, Williams & Wilkins, 1996:97–112
216. Johnson GS: Soft tissue mobilization. In: Donatelli R, Wooden MJ, eds: Orthopaedic Physical Therapy, 3rd ed. New York, Churchill Livingstone, 2001:578–617
217. Johnson VY: How the principles of exercise physiology influence pelvic floor muscle. J Wound Ostomy Cont Nurs 28:150–155, 2001
218. Jones DG: Orthopedic causes of pelvic pain. In: Rocker I, ed: Pelvic Pain in Women: Diagnosis and Management. New York, Springer-Verlag, 1990:150–156
219. Jones LH: Strain and Counterstrain. Newark, American Academy of Osteopathy, 1981
220. Jones LH, Kudunose R, Goering E: Jones Strain-Counterstrain. Boise, Jones Strain-Counterstrain, 1995
221. Juhan D: An Introduction to Trager Psychophysical Integration and Mentastics Movement Education. Mill Valley, CA. The Trager Institute, 1989
222. Jull GA: The physiotherapy management of cervicogenic headaches: Non traumatic and traumatic models of neck pain. Cervical Spine and Whiplash Research Unit, Department of Physiotherapy, University of Queensland, Australia, Seattle, WA, January 2001
223. Jull GA, Janda V: Muscles and motor control in low back pain. In: Twomey LT, Taylor JR, eds: Physical Therapy of the Low Back. New York, Churchill Livingstone, 1987:253–278
224. Kabat H: Studies on neuromuscular dysfunction: XII: New concepts and techniques of neuromuscular re-education for paralysis. Permanente Found Med Bull 8:21–143, 1950
225. Kabat-Zinn J, Lipworth L, Burney R: The clinical use of mindful meditation for self regulation of chronic pain. J Behav Med 8:163–190, 1985
226. Kaner JJ: Entrapment neuropathies. Osteopath Ann 9:13–20, 1981
227. Kannus P, Jozsa L: Histopathological changes preceding spontaneous rupture in tendon. J Bone Joint Surg Am 73:1507–1525, 1991
228. Kapandji IA: The Physiology of the Joints. Edinburgh, Churchill Livingstone, 1970
229. Karas SE: Thoracic Outlet Syndrome. Clin Sports Med 9:297–310, 1990
230. Kendall FP, Mc Creary EK, Provance PT: Muscles Testing and Function, 4th ed. Baltimore, Williams & Wilkins, 1993
231. Kessler RM: Friction massage. In: Kessler RM, Hertling D, eds: Management of Common Musculoskeletal Disorders: Physical Therapy Principles and Methods. Philadelphia, Harper & Row, 1983:192–201
232. Kirkadly-Willis WH: Managing Low Back Pain, 2nd ed. New York, Churchill Livingstone, 1988
233. Kisner C, Colby LA: Therapeutic Exercise: Foundations and Techniques, 3rd ed. Philadelphia, FA Davis, 1996
234. Knaster M: Discovering the body's wisdom. New York, Bantam Books, 1996
235. Knott M, Voss DE: Proprioceptive Neuromuscular Facilitation. New York, Hoeber, 1968
236. Kottke FJ, Pauley DL, Park KA: The rationale for prolonged stretching for correction of shortening of connective tissue. Arch Phys Med Rehabil 47:345–352, 1966
237. Kraftsow G: Yoga for Wellness. Healing with the Timeless Teachings of Viniyoga. New York, Penguin Books, 1999
238. Kunz K, Kunz B: The Complete Guide to Foot Reflexology. Englewood Cliffs, NJ: Prentice-Hall, 1982
239. Kuprain W: Massage. 2nd ed. Philadelphia, WB Saunders, 1995
240. Kurz W, Wittlinger G, Litmanovitch YI, et al: Effect of manual lymph drainage massage on urinary excretion of neurohormones and minerals in chronic lymphodema. Angiology 29:64–72, 1978
241. Kurz I: Introduction to Vodder's manual lymphatic drainage. Vol 2, Therapy 1. Heidelberg: Haug Publishers, 1986
242. Kurz I: Introduction to Vodder's manual lymphatic drainage. Vol 3, Therapy 2. Heidelberg, Haug Publishers, 1990
243. Kusunose R: Strain and counterstrain. In: Basmajian JV, Nyberg R, eds: Rational Manual Therapy. Baltimore, Williams & Wilkins, 1993:323–333
244. La Freniere JG: La Freniere Body Techniques: A Therapeutic Approach by Physical Therapy. Chicago, Year Book, 1984
245. Lardner R: Stretching and flexibility: its importance in rehabilitation. J Bodywork Move Ther 5:254–263, 2001
246. Laster J: Untying the knot: Yoga as physical therapy. In: Davis CM, ed: Complementary Therapies in Rehabilitation. Holistic Approaches for Prevention and Wellness. Thorofare, Slack, 1997:125–132
247. Laughlin K: Overcome Neck & Back Pain. New York, Fireside, 1995
248. Laycock J, Haslam J: Therapeutic Management of Incontinence and Pelvic Pain Organic Disorders. London, Springer-Verlag, 2002
249. Lazater J: Relax and Renew: Restful Yoga for Stressful Times. Berkeley, Rodmell, 1995
250. Lenz FA, Gracely RH, Zirh AT, et al: The sensory-limbic model of pain memory: Connections from the thalamus to the limbic system mediate the learned component of the affective dimension of pain. Pain Forum 6:22–31, 1997
251. Lewis RD, Brown RMM: Influence muscle activation dynamics on reaction time in elderly. Eur J Appl Physiol 69:344–349, 1994
252. Lewit K: Manipulative Therapy in Rehabilitation of the Motor System. London, Butterworth, 1985
253. Lewit K: Manipulative Therapy in Rehabilitation of the Motor System, 2nd ed. Oxford, Butterworth-Heinemann, 1991
254. Lewit K, Simons DG: Myofascial pain: Relief by postisometric relaxation. Arch J Phys Med 65:452–456, 1984
255. Lidell L: The Book of Massage. The Complete Step-by-Step Guide to Eastern and Western Techniques. London, Ebury Press, 1984
256. Liederbach M: Movement and function in dance. In: Brownstein B, Bronner S, eds: Evaluation, Treatment and Outcomes: Functional Movement in Orthopaedic and Sports Physical Therapy. New York, Churchill Livingstone, 1995:253–310
257. Liebenson C, ed: Rehabilitation of the Spine: A Practical Manual, Philadelphia, Lippincott, Williams & Wilkins, 1996
258. Light KE, Nuzik S, Personius W, et al: A low-load prolonged stretch vs. high brief stretch in treating knee contractures. Phys Ther 64:330–333, 1984
259. Liskin J: Moving Medicine: The Life and Work of Milton Trager. Barrytown, NY, Talman, 1996
260. Lister GD, Belsole RB, Kleinert HE: The radial tunnel syndrome. J Hand Surg 4:52–60, 1979
261. Little H: Tronchanteric bursitis: A common clinical problem. Orthop Clin North Am 120:456–458, 1979
262. Lockett J: Reflexology—A nursing tool? Aust Nurses J 22:14–15, 1992
263. Louden KL, Bollier CE, Allison KA, et al: Effects of two stretching methods on the flexibility and retention of flexibility at the ankle joint in runners. Phys Ther 65:698, 1985
264. Lovas JM, Ashley RC, Raison RL, et al: The effects of massage therapy on the human immune response in healthy adults. J Bodywork Move Ther 6:143–150, 2002
265. Lundberg T, Nordemar R, Ottson D: Pain alleviation by vibratory stimulation. Pain 20:25–44, 1984
266. Lunborg G, Dahlin LB: Pathophysiology of nerve compression. Nerve Compression Syndromes. In: Szabo RM, ed: Thorofare, Slack, 1989
267. MacConaill MA, Basmajian JV: Muscles and Movement. Baltimore, Williams and Wilkins, 1969
268. MacGregor M: Manual treatment of the knee. Physiotherapy 57:207–211, 1971

269. MacNab I: Acceleration injuries of the cervical spine. J Bone Joint Surg Am 46:1797–1799, 1964

270. Madding SW, Wong JG, Hallum A, et al: Effects of duration of passive stretching on hip abduction range of motion. J Orthop Sports Phys Ther 8:409–416, 1987

271. Maigne R: La semeiologie clinique des derangements intervertebraus mineurs. Ann Med Physoque 15:275–292, 1972

272. Maigne R: Orthopedic Medicine: A New Approach to Vertebral Manipulations. Springfield, Charles C. Thomas, 1976

273. Maigne R: Manipulation of the spine. In: Rogoff JB, ed: Manipulation, Traction and Massage. Baltimore, William & Wilkins, 1980:59–120

274. Malone TR, Garrett E, Zachazewski JE: Muscle: Deformation, injury and repair. In: Zachazewski JE, Magee DJ, Quillen WS, eds: Athletic: Injuries and Rehabilitation. Philadelphia, WB Saunders, 1996

275. Man P, Chen C: Acupuncture anesthesia—A new theory and clinical study. Curr Ther Res 14:390–394, 1972

276. Mance D, McConnell B, Ryan PA, et al: Myofascial pain syndrome. J Am Podiatr Med Assoc 76:328–331, 1986

277. Manheim CJ: Myofascial Release Manual, 2nd ed. Thorofare, Slack, 1994

278. Manheim CJ: Myofascial Release Manual, 3rd ed. Thorofare, Slack, 2001

279. Mann F: Acupuncture: The ancient Chinese art of healing and how it works scientifically. New York, Random House, 1973

280. Markos PD: Ipsilateral and contralateral effects of proprioceptive neuromuscular facilitation techniques on hip motion and electromyographic activity. Phys Ther 59:1366–1373, 1979

281. Maser BM, Clark CM, Giraid D: Carpal tunnel syndrome: Postoperative management. In: Maxey L, Magnusson J, eds: Rehabilitation for the Postsurgical Orthopedic Patient. St. Louis, Mosby, 2001:101–119

282. Masunaga S: Keiraku to Shiatsu. Yokosuka, Ido-No-Nihonsha, 1983

283. Masunga S. Ohashi W: Zen Shiatsu: Tokyo, Japan Publications, 1977

284. Matheson GO, MacIntryre JG, Tauton JE, et al: Musculoskeletal injuries associated with physical activity in older adults. Med Sci Sports Exerc 21: 379–385, 1989

285. McAtee RE: An overview of facilitated stretching. J Bodywork Move Ther 6:47–54, 2002

286. McCalden RW, McGeough JA, Barker MB, et al: Age-related changes in the tensile properties of cortical bone. J Bone Joint Surg Am 75:1193–1205, 1993

287. McConnell J: The management of chondromalacia patellae: A long-term solution. Aus J Physiol 2:215–223, 1986

288. McCrory P, Bell S: Nerve entrapment syndromes as a cause of pain in the hip, groin and buttock. Sport Med 27:261–274, 1999

289. McGarey WA: Acupuncture and Body Energies. Phoenix, Gabriel Press, 1974

290. McMillan M: Massage and Therapeutic Exercise. Philadelphia, WB Saunders, 1921

291. McMillan M: Massage and Therapeutic Exercise, 2nd ed. Philadelphia, WB Saunders, 1925

292. McPoil TG: Considerations in management of pediatrics and adolescent sports injuries. In: Touch Topics in Pediatric, Lesson 3, Department of Education. A PTA, Alexandria, VA, American Physical Therapy Association, 1990

293. Meese M, Black K: The hip and pelvis. Athletic injuries of the hip and pelvis. In Canavan PK: Rehabilitation in Sports Medicine. A Comprehensive Guide. Stamford, Appleton & Lange, 1998:257–267

294. Melzack R: Myofascial trigger points: Relation to acupuncture and mechanisms of pain. Arch Phys Med Rehab 62:114–117, 1985

295. Melzack R: Hyperstimulation analgesia. Clin Anaesthesiol 3:81–82, 1985

296. Melzack R, Stillwell D, Fox E: Trigger points and acupuncture points for pain: Correlation and implications. Pain 3:3–23, 1977

297. Mennell JB: Physical Treatment by Movement, Manipulation, and Massage, 5th ed. Philadelphia, Blakiston, 1947

298. Mennell JB: The Science and Art of Manipulation, vol. 2. London, Churchill, 1952

299. Mennell J McM: Back Pain. Boston, Little Brown and Co., 1960

300. Mennell J McM: Joint Pain. Boston, Little, Brown and Co., 1964

301. Mennell J McM: Foot Pain. Boston, Little, Brown and Co., 1969

302. Mettler PR: The Mettler Release Technique. A new manual treatment. Phys Ther Today 17(1):33–42, 1994

303. Michele A: Iliopsoas. Springfield, Charles C. Thomas, 1962

304. Micheli LG: Overuse injuries in children's sports: The growth factor. Orthop Clin North Am 142:337–360, 1983

305. Micheli LG, Smith AD: Sports injuries in children. Curr Prob Pediatr 12:4–54, 1982

306. Miller B: Alternative somatic therapies. In: White AH, Anderson R, eds: Conservative Care of Low Back Pain. Baltimore, Williams & Wilkins, 1991:120–136

307. Miller B: Manual therapy treatment of myofascial pain and dysfunction. In: Rachlin ES, ed: Myofascial Pain and Fibromyalgia. St. Louis, CV Mosby, 1994: 415–454

308. Mitchell FL Jr., Moran PS, Pruzzo NA: An Evaluation and Treatment Manual of Osteopathic Muscle Energy Procedures. Valley Park, MO, Mitchell, Moran, and Pruzzo, 1979

309. Moore MA, Hutton RS: Electromyographic investigation of muscle stretching. Med Sci Sports Exerci 12:322–324, 1980

310. Moore MO, Hislop HJ, Rabideau RJ, et al: Evaluation of extension of the hip. Arch Phys Med Rehabil 37:75–80, 1956

311. Motice M, Goldberg D, Benner EK, et al: Soft Tissue Mobilization Techniques. Munroe Falls, OH, JEMD Publications, 1986

312. Morkved S, Bo K: Effect of postpartum pelvic floor muscle training in prevention and treatment of urinary incontinence. BJOG 107:1022–1028, 2000

313. Morkved S, Bo K, Schei B, et al: Pelvic floor muscle training during pregnancy to prevent urinary incontinence: A single–blind randomized controlled trial. Obstet Gynecol 101:313–319, 2003

314. Muhlemann D, Cimino JA: Therapeutic muscle stretching. In: Hammer WI, ed: Functional Soft Tissue Examination and Treatment by Manual Methods. Gaithersburg, Aspen, 1991

315. Murrata H, Ikuta Y, Murkami T: An anatomic investigation of the elbow joint, with special reference to aging of articular cartilage. J Shoulder Elbow Surg 2:175–181, 1993

316. Murry DR: The seven types of hypertonicity of muscle. J Myofasc Ther 1:33–36, 1995

317. Murry DR: Conservative Management of Cervical Spine Syndromes. New York, McGraw-Hill, 2000

318. Namikoshi T: Japanese Finger-Pressure, Shiatsu. Tokyo, Japan Publications, 1969

319. Namikoshi T: Shiatsu. San Francisco, Japan Publications, 1969

320. Namikoshi T: The Complete Book of Shiatsu Therapy. Tokyo, Japanese Publications, 1981

321. Neviaser R: Adhesive capsulitis. Orthop Clin North Am 18:439–443, 1987

322. Neviaser R, Neviaser T: The frozen shoulder: Diagnosis and management. Clin Orthop Rel Res 223:59–64, 1987

323. Nicholson GG, Clendaniel RA: Manual techniques. In: Scully RM, Barnes MR, eds: Physical Therapy. Philadelphia, JB Lippincott, 1989:926–985

324. Nitsch W: Chronic pelvic pain in women: Etiology and intervention—A review of the literature and its implications for physical therapists. J Section Women's Health 25:7–12, 2001

325. Noble HB, Hajek HR, Porter M: The iliotibial band friction syndrome. Br J Sportsmed 10:67–74, 1982

326. Noble HB, Hajek HR, Porter M: Diagnosis and treatment of iliotibial band tightness in runners. Phys Sport Med 10:67–74, 1982

327. Nordin M, Frankel VH: Basic Biomechanics of the Musculoskeletal System. Philadelphia, Lea & Feiger, 1989

328. Norman L, Cowan T: Feet First: A Guide to Reflexology. Englewood Cliffs, Simon & Schuster, 1988

329. Norris C: Sports Injuries: Diagnosis and Management for Physiotherapists. Oxford, Butterworth-Heinemann, 1993

330. Norris C: Spinal stabilization. 3. Stabilization mechanism of the lumbar spine. Phys Ther 81:72–79, 1995

331. Nyberg GF: Pelvic girdle. In: Payton OD, ed: Manual of Physical Therapy. New York, Churchill Livingstone, 1989: 363–382

332. Ohashii W: Do-it-yourself Shiatsu, New York, EP Dutton, 1976

333. Oleson T, Flocco W: Randomized controlled study of premenstrual symptoms treated with ear, hand, and foot reflexology. Obstet Gynecol 82:906–911, 1993

334. Ombregt L, Bisschop P, ter Veer HJ, et al: A System of Orthopaedic Medicine. London, WB Saunders, 1995

335. Omura Y: Accurate localization of organ representation areas on the feet & hands using the bi-digital O-ring test resonance phenomenon: Its clinical implication in diagnosis and treatment—Part I: Acupuncture Electro Ther Res Int J 19:153–190, 1994

336. Ortego NE: Acupressure: An alternative approach to mental health counseling through bodymind awareness. Nurse Pract Forum 5:72–76, 1994

337. Palastanga N: The use of transverse frictions in soft tissue lesions. In: Grieve GP, ed: Modern Manual Therapy of the Vertebral Column. New York, Churchill Livingstone, 1986: 819–826

338. Paris SV: Clinical decision making: Orthopaedic physical therapy. In: Wolf SL, ed: Clinical Decision Making in Physical Therapy. Philadelphia, FA Davis, 1985: 215–254

339. Paris SV: Differential diagnosis of lumbar and pelvic pain. In: Vleeming A, Mooney V, Snijders CJ, et al., eds: Movement, Stability, and Low Back Pain: The Essential Role of the Pelvis. New York, Churchill Livingstone, 1997: 319–330

340. Pecina MM, Krmpotic J, Markiewitz AD: Tunnel Syndromes. Boca Raton, CRC Press, 1991

341. Peimer CA, Wheeler DR: Radial tunnel syndrome/posterior interosseus nerve compression. In: Szabo RM, ed: Nerve Compression Syndromes. Englewood, CO, American Society for Hand Surgery, 1994

342. Peppard A: Trigger-point massage therapy. Phys Sports Med 1:59–162, 1983

343. Perry J, Jones MH, Thomas L: Functional evaluation of Rolfing in cerebral palsy. Dev Med Child Neurol 23:717–729, 1981

344. Plona, Browstein B: Function in older individuals–Orthopaedic geriatrics. In: Browstein B, Bonner S, eds: Evaluation, Treatment and Outcomes: Functional Movement in Orthopaedic and Sports Physical Therapy. New York, Churchill Livingston, 1995: 311–349

345. Prentice WE: A comparison of static stretching and PNF stretching for improving hip joint flexibility. Athlet Train 18:56–59, 1983

346. Prentice WE: Therapeutic Modalities in Sports Medicine, 3rd ed. St. Louis, Mosby, 1994
347. Prentice WE: Therapeutic Modalities for Allied Health Professionals. New York, McGraw-Hill, 1998
348. Prudden B: Pain Erasure: The Bonnie Prudden Way. New York, M Evans, 1980
349. Prudden B: Myotherapy: Bonne Prudden's Complete Guide to Pain-Free Living. New York, Ballantine Books, 1984
350. Pullig Schatz, M: Back Care Basic. A Doctor's Gentle Yoga Program for Back and Neck Pain Relief. Berkeley, Rodmell, 1992
351. Raju PS, Madhavi S, Prasad KV, et al: Comparison of effects of yoga & physical exercise in athletes. Indian J Med Res 100:81–86, 1994
352. Reed B, Held J: Effects of sequential connective tissue massage on autonomic nervous system of middle-aged and elderly adults. Phys Ther 68:1231–1234, 1988
353. Reed ES: Changing theories of postural development. In: Woollacott MH, Shumway-Cook A, eds: Development of Posture and Gait Analysis Across the Life Span. University of South Carolina Press, Columbia, SC, 1989:3
354. Renstrom P: Tendon and muscle injuries in the groin area. Clin Sports Med 11:815–831, 1992
355. Richardson C, Jull G, Hodges P, et al: Therapeutic Exercise for Spinal Segmental Stabilization in Low Back Pain: Scientific Basis and Clinical Approach. Edinburgh, Churchill Livingstone, 1999
356. Richardson C, Toppenberg R, Jull G: An initial evaluation of eight abdominal exercises for their ability to provide stabilisation for the lumbar spine. Aust J Physiother 36:6–11, 1990
357. Rocobado M: Biomechanical relationship of the cranial cervical, and hyoid region. J Craniomandib Prac 1:61–66, 1983
358. Rocabado M, Iglarsh ZA: Musculoskeletal Approach to Maxillo-facial Pain, Philadelphia, JB Lippincott, 1991
359. Rodman GP, Schumacher HR: Primer on the Rheumatic Diseases, 8th ed. Atlanta, Arthritis Foundation, 1983
360. Roles NC, Mausley RH: Radial tunnel syndrome, resistant tennis elbow as a nerve entrapment. J Bone Joint Surg. 54(B):499–508, 1972
361. Rolf IP: Structural Integration: A contribution to the understanding of stress. Confinia Psychiatrica 16(2): 60–79, 1973
362. Rolf IP: Rolfing and physical reality. Rochester, VT, Healing Arts Press, 1990
363. Rolf IP: Rolfing: The Integration of Human Structures. New York, Harper and Row, 1997
364. Romero JA: The hip and pelvis. In: Sanders B, ed: Sports Physical Therapy. Norwalk, Appleton & Lange, 1990:397–421
365. Ross R: Yoga and neurological illness. In: Weintraub M, ed: Alternative Medicine in Neurological Illness. Philadelphia, WB Saunders, 2001
366. Roos DB, Owens JC: Thoracic outlet syndrome. Arch Surg 93:71–74, 1966
367. Saal JS: Flexibility training. In: Saal JS, ed: Rehabilitation of Sports Injuries. Philadelphia, Hanley & Belfus, 1987
368. Saal J, Saal J: Non-operative treatment of herniated lumbar intervertebral disk herniated lumbar intervertebral disk herniations with radiculopathy. Spine 14:431–437, 1989
369. Sady SP, Wortmann M, Blake D: Flexibility training: Ballistic, static or proprioceptive neuromuscular facilitation. Arch Phys Med Rehabil 63:261–263, 1982
370. Sahai ICM: Reflexology—Its place in modern health-care. Prof Nurse 8:722–725, 1993
371. Sahrmann S: A program for identification and correction of muscular and mechanical imbalance: principles and methods. Clin Man 3:23–28, 1983
372. Sahrmann SA: Diagnosis and Treatment of Movement Impairment Syndromes. Course outline. St. Louis, MO: Washington University, 1998
373. Sahrmann SA: Diagnosis and Treatment of Movement Impairment Syndromes. St. Louis, Mosby 2001
374. Saidoff DC, McDonough AL: Critical Pathways in Therapeutic Intervention: Upper Extremity. St. Louis, Mosby, 1997
375. Sammarco G: The dancer's hip. Clin Sports Med 2:485–498, 1983
376. Sanders B, ed: Sports Physical Therapy. Norwalk, Appleton & Lange, 1990
377. Sanders J, Hung CE: Thoracic Outlet Syndrome. Philadelphia, JB Lippincott, 1991
378. Sapega A, Quedenfeld T, Moyer R et al: Biophysical factors in range of motion exercise. Phys Sports Med 9:57–65, 1981
379. Schapira D, Nahir M, Scharf Y: Trochanteric bursitis: A common clinical problem. Arch Phys Med Rehabil 67:815–817, 1986
380. Scheufele L: Pelvic floor muscle exercise and the postpartum female: A review of the current literature. J Section Women's Health:27:29–36, 2003
381. Scheumann, DW: The Balanced Body: A Guide to Deep Tissue and Neuromuscular Therapy, 2nd ed. Philadelphia, Lippincott Williams & Wilkins, 2002
382. Schleip R: The golgi tendon reflex arc as a new explanation of the effect of Rolfing. Rolf Lines 17:18–20, 1989
383. Schneider W, Dvorak J, Dvorak V, et al: Manual Medicine Therapy. New York, Thieme, 1988
384. Schultz-Johnson, K: Splinting: A problem solving approach. In: Stanley BG, Tribuzi SM, eds: Concepts in Hand Rehabilitation. Philadelphia, FA Davis, 1992: 239–271
385. Schussler B, Laycock J, Nortin P, et al., eds: Pelvic Floor Reeducation Principles and Practice. New York, Springer-Verlag, 1994
386. Serizawa K: Massage, the Oriental Method. Tokyo, Japanese Publications, 1972

387. Serizawa K: Effective Tsubo Therapy. Tokyo, Japanese Publications, 1984
388. Serizawa K: Tsubo, Vital Points for Oriental Therapy, Tokyo, Japanese Publications, 1984
389. Seror P: Treatment of ulnar nerve palsy at the elbow with a night splint. J Bone Joint Surg Br 75:322–327, 1993
390. Shelly B: The pelvic floor. In: Hall CM, Brody LT, eds: Therapeutic Exercise: Moving Toward Function. Baltimore, Lippincott Williams & Wilkins, 1999: 253–386
391. Sherrington CS: On plastic tonus and proprioceptive reflexes. Q J Exp Physiol 2:109–156, 1909
392. Sherrington CS: The Integrative Action of the Nervous System. New Haven, Yale University Press, 1920
393. Simons DG: Myofascial pain syndromes due to trigger points: Treatment and single-muscle syndromes. Manual Med 1:72–77, 1985
394. Simons DG: Myofascial pain syndrome due to trigger points. In: Goodgold J, ed: Rehabilitation Medicine. St. Louis, MO, Mosby, 1988
395. Simons DG: Travell JG: Myofascial pain syndromes. In: Wall PD, Melzack R, eds: Textbook of Pain, 2nd ed. Edinburgh, Churchill Livingstone, 1989:368–385
396. Simons DG, Hong CY, Simons LS: Prevalence of spontaneous electrical activity at trigger spots and at control sites in rabbit skeletal muscle. J Musculoskel Pain 3:35–48, 1995
397. Simons DG, Mense S: Understanding and measurement of muscle tone as related to clinical muscle pain. Pain 75:1–18, 1998
398. Sisco M: Adaptation of myofascial release techniques in a hand and plastic surgery clinic. Phys Ther Forum 6(48):1–4, 1987
399. Smith CA: The warm-up procedure: To stretch or not to stretch. A brief review. J Orthop Sports Med Phys Ther 19:12–17, 1994
400. Smith JR, Walker JM: Knee and elbow range of motion in healthy older individuals. Phys Occup Ther Geriatr 2:31–38, 1983
401. Smith LK, Weiss EL, Lehmkuhl LD: Brunnstrom's Clinical Kinesiology, 5th ed. Philadelphia, FA Davis, 1996
402. Snyder-Mackler L, Knarr JF: The older athlete. In: Guccione A, ed: Geriatric Physical Therapy. St. Louis, Mosby, 1993:403–411
403. Spense AP: Biology of Human Aging. Engelwood Cliffs, Prentice-Hall, 1989
404. Spinner M, The radial nerve. In Injuries to the Major Branches of Peripheral Nerves of the Forearm, 2nd ed. Philadelphia, WB Saunders, 1978: 79–157
405. Spinner M, Spencer PS: Nerve compression lesions of he upper extremity: A clinical and experimental review, Clin Orthop Rel Res 104:46–67, 1974
406. Spring H, Illi U, Kunz HR, et al: Stretching and Strengthening Exercises, New York, Thieme, 1991
407. Staheli LT: Fundamentals of Pediatric Orthopedic. Philadelphia, Lippincott-Raven, 1992
408. Starring DT, Grossman, Nicholson GG, et al: Comparison of cyclic and sustained passive stretching using a mechanical devise to increase resting length of hamstring muscles. Phys Ther 68:314–320, 1988
409. Steege JF: Office management of chronic pelvic pain. Clin Obstet Gynecol 40:554–563, 1997
410. Steege JF, Metzger DA, Levy BS: Chronic Pelvic Pain: An Integrated Approach. Philadelphia, WB Saunders, 1998
411. Stoddard A: Manual of Osteopathic Technique. London, Hutchinson, 1978
412. Stoddard A: Manual of Osteopathic Practice. London, Hutchinson, 1978
413. Stone AR: The Trager approach. In: Davis CM, ed: Complementary Therapies in Rehabilitation: Holistic Approaches for Prevention and Wellness. Thorofare, Slack, 1997: 199–216
414. Sucher BM: Thoracic outlet syndrome. A myofascial variant: Part 1. Pathology and diagnosis. J Am Osteopath Assoc 90:686–704, 1990
415. Sucher BM: Thoracic outlet syndrome—A myofascial variant: Part 2. Treatment. J Am Osteopath Assoc 90–810–823,1990
416. Sucher BM: Myofascial release of carpal tunnel syndrome J Am Osteopath Assoc 93:92–101, 1993
417. Sucher BM: Thoracic outlet syndrome—A myofascial variant. Part 3. Structural and postural considerations. J Am Osteopath Assoc 93:334–345, 1993
418. Sucher BM: Myofascial manipulative release of carpal tunnel syndrome. Documentation with magnetic resonance imaging. J Am Osteopath Assoc 93:1273–1278, 1993
419. Sucher BM: Palpatory diagnosis and manipulative management of carpal tunnel syndrome. J Am Osteopath Assoc 94:647–663, 1994
420. Sucher BM: Palpatory diagnosis and manipulative management of carpal tunnel syndrome: Part 2. "Double crush" and thoracic outlet syndrome. J Am Osteopath Assoc 95:471–479, 1995
421. Sucher BM, Glassman JH: Upper extremity syndromes. Man Med 7(4):787–810, 1996
422. Sullivan PE, Markos PD: Clinical Decision-Making in Therapeutic Exercise. Norwalk, Appleton & Lange, 1994
423. Sunshine W, Field T, Quintino O, et al: Fibromyalgia benefits from massage therapy and transcutaneous electrical stimulation. J Clin Rheumatol 2:18–222, 1996
424. Sutker AV, Jackson DW, Pagliano JW: Iliotibial band syndrome in distance runners. Phys Sportsmed 9:69–73, 1981
425. Sutton GS, Bartel MR: Soft-tissue mobilization techniques for the hand. J Hand Ther 7:185–192, 1994

426. Swezey RL: Pseudo-radiculopathy in subacute trochanteric bursitis of sub-gluteal maximus bursa. Arch Phys Med Rehabil 57:387–390, 1976

427. Sydenham RW: Manual therapy techniques for the thoracolumbar spine. In: Donatelli RA, Wooden MJ, eds: Orthopaedic Physical Therapy. New York, Churchill Livingstone, 2001:335–365

428. Tanigawa MC: Comparison of the hold-relax procedure and passive mobilization for increasing muscle length. Phys Ther 52:725–735, 1972

429. Tappan FM: Massage. In: Wall PD, Melzack R, eds: Textbook of Pain. Edinburgh, Churchill Livingstone, 1984: 735–740

430. Tappan FM: Healing Massage Techniques, Holistic, Classic, and Emerging Methods. Norwalk, Appleton & Lange, 1988

431. Tappan FM, Benjamin PR: Tappan's Handbook of Healing Massage Techniques: Classic, Holistic, and Emerging Methods. Stamford, Appleton & Lange, 1998

432. Tappan FM, Benjamin PR: Joint movements. In: Tappan FM, Benjamin PR, eds: Tappan's Handbook of Healing Massage Techniques: Classic, Holistic, and Emerging Methods. Stamford, Appleton & Lange, 1998:107–132

433. Tavrazich J: Rolfing, Hellerwork, and soma. In: Davis C, ed: Complementary Therapies in Rehabilitation: Holistic Approaches for Prevention and Wellness, Thorofare, Slack, 1997:69–80

434. Taylor MJ: Yoga therapeutics in neurologic physical therapy: Application to a patient with Parkinson's disease. Neurol Rep 25:55–62, 2001

435. Taylor MJ, Majmundar M: Incorporating yoga therapeutic into orthopedic physical therapy. Ortho Phys Ther Clin North Am 9:341–360, 2000

436. Teeguarden IM: Acupressure Way of Health: Jin Shin Do. New York, Tokyo, Japan Publications, 1978

437. Teeguarden IM: Jin Shin Do Handbook, 2nd ed. Felton, CA. Jin Shin Do Foundation, 1981

438. Teeguarden IM: Acupressure in the Classroom. East West J 15:22, 1985

439. Teeguarden IM: Joy of Feeling: Bodymind Acupressure. New York/Tokyo: Japan Publications, 1987

440. Teeguarden IM: A Complete Guide to Acupressure. New York/Tokyo, Japan Publications, 1996

441. Terry GC, Hughston JC, Norwood LA: The anatomy of the iliopatellar band and the iliotibial tract. Am J Sports Med 14:39–45, 1986

442. Thabe H: Electomyography as a tool to document findings and therapeutic results associated with somatic dysfunction in the upper cervical spinal joints and sacroiliac joints. Man Med 2:53–58, 1986

443. Thiele GH: Coccygodynia: Cause and treatment. Dis Colon Rectum 6:422–463, 1963

444. Thomas HO: Diseases of Hip, Knee, and Ankle Joints with Their Deformities Treated by New and Efficient Means, 2nd ed. Liverpool, Dobb 1976

445. Tobias M, Stewart M: Stretch and Relax, London, Dorling Kindesley, 1985

446. Tomberlin JP, Saunders HD: Evaluation, Treatment and Prevention of Musculoskeletal Disorders, vol. 2. Extremities, 3rd ed. Chaska, MN, The Saunders Group, 1994

447. Totten P, Hunter J: Therapeutic techniques to enhance nerve gliding in thoracic outlet syndrome and carpal tunnel syndrome. Hand Clin 7:505–520, 1991

448. Trager M Guadagno C: Trager Mentastics: Movement As A Way to Agelessness. Barrytown, NY, Station Hill, 1987

449. Travell J, Rinzler GH: Relief of cardiac pain by local block of somatic trigger area. Pro Soc Exp Biol Med 63:480–487, 1946

450. Travell J, Rinzler GH: The myofascial genesis of pain. Postgrad Med 11:425–434, 1952

451. Travell JG, Simons DG: Myofascial Pain and Dysfunction: The Trigger Point Manual. Baltimore, Williams & Wilkins, 1983

452. Travell JG, Simons DG: Myofascial Pain and Dysfunction: The Lower Extremities, vol. 2. Baltimore, Williams & Wilkins, 1992

453. Travell JG, Simons DG, Simons LS: Myofascial Pain and Dysfunction: The Trigger Point Manual: Vol. 1: Upper Half of the Body, 2nd ed. Baltimore, Williams & Wilkins, 1999

454. Trombly CA: Occupational Therapy for Physical Dysfunction, 2nd ed. Baltimore, Williams & Wilkins, 1983

455. Tsay RC: Textbook of Chinese Acupuncture Medicine. General Introduction to Acupuncture, vol. 1. Wappinger Falls, NY: Association of Chinese Medicine and East-West Medical Center, 1974

456. Tyne PJ, Mitchell M: Total Stretching. Chicago, Contemporary Books, 1983

457. Uhthoff HK, Sarkar K, Hammond DI: The subacromial bursa: A clinicopathological study of the shoulder. In: Bateman JE, Welch RP, eds: Surgery of the Shoulder. St. Louis, CV Mosby, 1984: 121–125

458. Upton A, McComas A: The double crush in nerve entrapment syndrome. Lancet 2:359–362, 1973

459. Vasilyeva LF, Lewit K: Diagnosis of muscular dysfunction by inspection. In: Liebenson C, ed: Rehabilitation of the Spine, Philadelphia, Lippincott Williams & Wilkins, 1996

460. Vesco JJ: Principles of stretching. In: Torg JS, Welsch RP, Shepard RJ, eds: Current Therapy in Sports Medicine, vol. 2. Toronto, BC Decker, 1990

461. Vleeming A, Pool-Goudzwaard AL, Stoeckkhart R, et al: The posterior layer of the thoracolumbar fascia: its function in load transfer from spine to legs. Spine 20:753–758, 1995

462. Voss DE, Ionta MK, Myer GJ: Proprioceptive Neuromuscular Fascilitation Patterns and Techniques, 3rd ed. Philadelphia, Harper & Row, 1985

463. Wadsworth C: The wrist and hand. In: Malone TR, McPoil T, Nitz AJ, eds: Orthopedic and Sports Physical Therapy, 3rd ed. St. Louis, CV Mosby, 1997

464. Walker H: Deep transverse frictions in ligament healing. J Orthop Sports Phys Ther 6:89–94, 1984

465. Walker JM, Sue D, Miles Elkousy N, et al: Active mobility of the extremities in older subjects. Phys Ther 64:919–923, 1984

466. Wallace K: Female pelvic floor functions, dysfunctions and behavior approaches to treatment. Clinics in Sports Medicine 13: 459–481, 1994

467. Wallen D, Ekblom B, Grahn R, et al: Improvement of muscle flexibility: a comparison between two techniques. Am J Sports Med 13:263–268, 1985

468. Walsh MT: Therapist management of thoracic outlet syndrome. J Hand Ther 9:131–144; 1994

469. Walsh MT: Hand therapists are you prepared? Rehab Manag 9:49–53,1996

470. Wanning T: Healing and the mind/body arts. Am Assoc Occup Health Nurses 41:349–351, 1993

471. Warren CG, Lehmann JF, Koblanski JN: Elongation of rat tail tendon: Effect of load and temperature. Arch Phys Med Rehabil 52:465–471, 1971

472. Warren CG, Lehmann JF, Koblanski JN: Heat and stretch procedures: An evaluation using rat tail tendon. Arch Phys Med Rehabil 57:122–126, 1976

473. Watrous I. The Trager approach: An effective tool for physical therapy. Phys Ther Forum 72:22–25,1992

474. Waylett-Rendall J: Desensitization of traumatized hand. In: Hunter JM, Mackin EJ, Callahan AD, eds: Rehabilitation of the Hand: Surgery and Therapy, 4th ed. St. Louis, Mosby, 1995

475. Weaver MT: Acupressure: An overview of theory and application. Nurse Practitioner 10:38–42, 1985

476. Wehbe M: Tendon gliding exercises. Am J Occup Ther 41:164–167, 1987

477. Weiselfish S: Manual Therapy with Muscle Energy Technique: for the Pelvis, Sacrum, Cervical, Thoracic & Lumbar Spine. East Hampstead, NH Northeast Seminars, 1994

478. Weiss JM: Pelvic floor myofascial trigger points: Manual therapy for interstitial cystitis and urgency-frequency syndrome J Uroloy 166:2226–2231, 2001

479. Whitenack SH, Hunter JM, Jaeger SH, et al: Thoracic outlet syndrome complex: Diagnosis and treatment. In: Hunter JM, Schneider LH, Mackin EJ, et al., eds: Rehabilitation of the Hand: Surgery; and Therapy, 3rd ed. St. Louis, Mosby, 1990

480. Wiktorsson-Moller M, Obergt B, Ekstrand J et al: Effects of warming up, massage, and stretching on range of motion and muscle strength in the lower extremities. Am J Sports Med 11:249–252, 1983

481. Wilder D, Aleksiev A, Magnussin M, et al: Muscular response to sudden load. Spine 21:2628–2639, 1996

482. Williford HN, Smith JF: A comparison of proprioceptive neuromuscular facilitation and static stretching techniques. Am Corr Ther J 39:30–33, 1985

483. Wilmore JH: The aging of bone and muscle. Clin Sports Med. 10:231–244, 1991

484. Wilson GJ, Elliot BC, Wood BA: Stretch shorten cycle performance enhancement through flexibility training. Med Sci Sports Exerc 24:116–123, 1992

485. Winter B: Transverse frictions. S Afr J Physiother 24:5–7, 1968

486. Witt P: Trager psychophysical integration: A method to improve chest mobility of patients with chronic lung disease. Phys Ther 66:214–217, 1986

487. Witt P, Parr C: Effectiveness of Trager psychophysical integration in promoting trunk mobility in a child with cerebral palsy: A case report. Phys Occup Ther Pediatr 8:75–94, 1988

488. Wittinger H, Wittinger G: Introduction to Dr. Vodder's manual lymphatic drainage, vol. 1. Heidelberg, Haug, 1982

489. Wolfe F: Fibrositis, fibromyalgia and musculo-skeletal disease: The current status of fibrositis syndrome. Arch Phys Med Rehab 69:527–531, 1988

490. Wolpaw JR: Reflexes capable of change: Models for the study of memory. Fed Proc 42:2146, 1982

491. Wolpaw JR: Adaptive plasticity in the primate spinal stretch reflex: reversal and redevelopment. Brain Res 278:299–304, 1983

492. Wolpaw JR, O'Keefe JA: Adaptive plasticity in the primate spinal stretch reflex: Evidence for two-phase process. J Neurosci 4:2718–27–24, 1984

493. Wood VE, Twito R, Verska JM: Thoracic outlet syndrome. The results of first rib resection in 100 patients. Orthop Clin North Am 19:131–146, 1988

494. Woodman R, Pare L: Evaluation and treatment of soft tissue lesions of the ankle and forefoot using Cyriax approach. Phys Ther 62:1114–1147, 1982

495. Worrell TW, Smith TL, Winegardner JW: Effect of hamstring stretching on hamstring muscle performance. J Orthop Sports Phys Ther 20:154–159, 1994

496. Wyke B: Neurology of the cervical spinal joints. Physiother 65:73–76, 1979

497. Wyke B: Articular neurology and manipulative therapy. In: Idezak RM, ed: Aspects of Manipulative Therapy. Carlton, Victoria, Australia, Lincoln Institute of Health Sciences, 1980

498. Yamashita T, Cavanaugh J, Cuneyt Ozaktay A, et al: Effect of substance P on mechanosensitive units of tissues around and in the lumbar facet joints. J Orthop Res 11:205–214, 1993

499. Yates J: A physicians guide to therapeutic massage: Its physiological effects and their application to treatment. Vancouver BC, Canada, Massage Therapists Association of British Columbia, 1990

500. Yeoman W: The relationship of arthritis of the sacro-iliac joint to sciatica. Lancet ii:1119–1122, 1928

501. Zachazewski JE, Reischl SR: Flexibility for the runner: Specific program considerations. Top Acute Care Trauma Rehabil 1:9–27, 1986
502. Zachazewski JE: Flexibiity for sports. In: Saunders B, ed: Sports Physical Therapy. Norwalk, Appleton & Lange, 1990:201–238
503. Zakas A, Galazoulas C, Grammatikopoulou G, et al: Effect of stretching exercise during strength training in prepubertal, pubertal and adolescent boys. J Bodywork Move Ther 6:170–176, 2002
504. Zebas CJ, Rivera ML: Retention of flexibility in selected joints after cessation of a stretching exercise program. In: Dotson CO, Humphrey JH, eds: Exercise Physiology: Current Selected Research. New York, AMS Press, 1985
505. Zolten DJ, Clancy WG, Keene JS: A new operative approach to snapping hip and refractory trohanteric bursitis in athletes. Am J Sports Med 14:201–204, 1986
506. Zuniga L: Management of thoracic dysfunction. In Canavan PK: Rehabilitation in Sports Medicine: A Comprehensive Guide, Stamford, Appleton & Lange, 1997: 93–108

RECOMMENDED READINGS

Bogdux N: Clinical Anatomy of the Lumbar Spine and Sacrum. New York, Churchill Livingstone, 1997
Butler D: Mobilization of the Nervous System, Melbourne, Churchill Livingstone, 1991
Cantu R, Grodin A: Myofascial Manipulation. Gaithersburg, Aspen, 1992
Chaitow L: Modern Neuromuscular Techniques. New York, Churchill Livingstone, 1996
Manheim CJ: Myofascial Release Manual, 3rd ed. Thorofare, Slack, 2001
Myers TW: Anatomy Trains: Myofascial Meridians For Manual and Movement Therapist. Edinburgh, Churchill Livingstone, 2001
Ombregt L, Bisschop P, ter Veer HJ, et al: A System of Orthopaedic Medicine, London WB Saunders, 1995
Schultz L, Feitis R: The Endless Web. Berkeley CA, North Atlantic Books, 1996

RECOMMENDED READINGS

Relaxation and Related Techniques

9

JOYCE M. ENGEL

INTRODUCTION

Relaxation training is no longer perceived as alternative or complementary medicine. It is now recognized as a viable intervention for the reduction of anxiety and stress, distraction from pain, alleviation of skeletal muscle tension, reduction of fatigue, sleep hygiene, enhancement of pain relief measures, and improvement of muscle control.[4,17,18,28] This chapter defines stress, describes theories of stress, identifies the benefits of relaxation training, states how the healthcare practitioner can assist consumers in how to use relaxation techniques, and effectively outlines methods of relaxation induction.

DEFINITIONS OF STRESS

Pressure. Tension. Strain. These are common terms people use when talking about stress. These terms all have a negative connotation. When defining stress, however, we are simply referring to change. Selye[23] proposed that stress could be divided into two categories: distress and eustress. Distress is damaging or unpleasant stress. In contrast, eustress is uplifting and pleasurable. Eustress can heighten awareness, increase mental alertness, and improve cognitive and behavioral performance.[21]

Cannon[6] also introduced terminology for stress. Cannon proposed the idea of homeostasis, the tendency of an organism to maintain a stable internal environment. He also investigated the fight-or-flight response as a mechanism of emergency preparedness.[21]

THEORIES OF STRESS

Selye's View

Stress is a common condition for humans. Selye[23] may be the most influential pioneer in the field of stress theory and research. His work popularized the concept of stress and its relationship to illness. Selye stated all organisms have an innate drive for equilibrium. Homeostasis is the process that maintains this internal balance. Selye described the general adaptation syndrome (GAS) as the body's generalized attempt to defend itself against stressors (noxious agents such as germs or excess work demands). This stress response is nonspecific. It consists of three stages, beginning with the alarm reaction. Not everyone experiences all three stages. During the alarm stage the body's defenses against a stressor are activated. An immediate reaction of the sympathetic division of the autonomic nervous system occurs. Body systems are activated to increase strength in preparation for "fight or flight." Adrenaline (epinephrine) is released, heart rate and blood pressure elevate, respiration increases, blood is diverted from the internal organs to the skeletal muscles, the gastrointestinal system slows, and sweat glands are activated. Cortisol is released as a natural defense for the body by reducing swelling from injury that might occur.[5,21]

The second phase of GAS is the stage of resistance. Adaptation to the stressor occurs during this stage. The span of this stage is dependent on the severity and duration of the stressor as well as the adaptive capacity of the organism. Although the individual appears normal on the outside, the body's internal functioning is not stable. Continuing stress results in constant neurologic and hormonal (e.g., cortisol) changes. Seyle hypothesized that prolonged activation of this stage causes diseases of adaptation (e.g., hypertension, cardiovascular disease, peptic ulcers). He further hypothesized that resistance to stress causes changes in the immune system, making infection more likely. Chronic stress may also increase vulnerability to disease and compromise recovery.[5,21]

The third and final stage of GAS is exhaustion. The organism can no longer defend itself. The parasympathetic division of the autonomic nervous system becomes activated and functions at a low level. When the reserve of adaptive energy is depleted, death may occur.[5,21]

Mason's View

Selye's work has been criticized because of its lack of addressing cognitive and psychosocial factors critical to understanding human stress. Mason proposed an alternate view of stress. He challenged Selye's belief that stress is a nonspecific response. Mason also proposed that emotional stress was an underlying mechanism. He suggested this emotional reaction creates the illusion of a generalized response to stress.[5]

Lazarus' View

In contrast to Selye and Mason, Lazarus proposed that cognitive variables that affect the interpretation of stressful events (perceptions) are more important than the events themselves. This perception includes potential threats, challenges, and one's abilities to cope with these stressors. The individual's appraisal of the situation is paramount. Stress is simply the consequence of appraisal. Lazarus and his colleagues pioneered stress assessment scales that measure daily hassles and uplifts (positive experiences).[5,13,15]

PHYSIOLOGIC, COGNITIVE, EMOTIONAL, AND BEHAVIORAL INDICATORS OF RELAXATION

Relaxation can counteract the above-described responses to stress. Relaxation affects physiology, cognition, emotion, and behavior. A summary of the key indicators of relaxation is provided in Table 9-1.

ROLE OF THE HEALTHCARE PRACTITIONER

The healthcare practitioner is in an ideal position to teach bodily relaxation. Practitioners can teach consumers how to recognize stress and learn relaxation strategies. As described below, there are many techniques available for inducing relaxation. Progressive muscle relaxation and autogenic training are the relaxation techniques most often used by U.S. physical therapists.[15] Personal preference for relaxation strategies should be addressed. Written relaxation protocols facilitate home practice. This home practice is essential for skill acquisition. Eventually, a few deep breaths or a key relaxation phrase may induce deep relaxation.

Relaxation Strategies

Relaxation can be induced in a variety of ways. Relaxation strategies use many of the same concepts to achieve the desired effect. The first similarity is the use of a repetitive verbal, visual, or physical stimulus. A second similarity is the use of a passive attitude. Distracting thoughts are ignored and attention redirected to the relaxation technique. Third, a prescribed protocol is used. A fourth commonality is the use of a comfortable posture that minimizes muscular work (e.g., semireclined position). A fifth

TABLE 9-1 PHYSIOLOGIC, COGNITIVE, EMOTIONAL, AND BEHAVIORAL INDICATORS OF RELAXATION

PHYSIOLOGIC	COGNITIVE	EMOTIONAL	BEHAVIORAL
Reduced muscle tension	Slowed neural impulses to the brain; change from beta consciousness to alpha consciousness	Feelings of well-being	Little or no movement
Vasodilatation with increased temperature in extremities	Improved memory	Sense of comfort, peacefulness, and tranquility	Eye closure
Lowered heart and respiratory rates	Increased concentration; decreased distractibility	Content not to do anything temporarily	Lack of facial expression
Decreased blood pressure	Enhanced creativity		Jaws drop
Constricted pupils	Positive attitude		Head drops or slightly tilts to side
Decreased perspiration			Palms open with fingers curled
Decreased oxygen consumption and elimination of carbon dioxide			
Slowed metabolic rate			
Lowered serum levels of epinephrine and norepinephrine			
Cortisol released			

Adapted from Townsend MC: Relaxation therapy. In: Psychiatric Mental Health Nursing: Concepts of Care, 3rd ed. Philadelphia, FA Davis, 2000:186.

shared feature is the use of a quiet environment. Finally, the participant needs to assume responsibility for participation in treatment.[10,20] Relaxation techniques often serve as an adjunct to medical treatment or are used to prevent health problems.

ABDOMINAL BREATHING

Our breathing rate reflects the emotional or physical demands on ourselves at any given time. For example, we may pant after running a long distance. We may briefly hold our breath when startled. Because breathing leads directly to the autonomic nervous system, its potential for inducing relaxation is increased.[22] Breathing is the simplest means to inducing relaxation. In addition, most breathing exercises can be done anywhere, thereby allowing for generalization of the relaxation skill. Rhythmic breathing for the purpose of healing can be traced back to ancient Egyptians, Hebrews, and Tibetans. The learning sequence begins with (1) awareness of breathing pattern, (2) inhalation, and (3) slow exhalation. Breathing awareness focuses on chest and abdominal movements that accompany respiration. Breathing in a stressed individual is characterized by rapid, mostly upper costal movement and typically involves contraction of the shoulder girdle muscles. Relaxation is associated with a reduced breathing rate. Abdominal breathing emphasizes the downward expansion of the chest. The participant begins abdominal breathing exercises by assuming a comfortable position (e.g., semi-reclined seating with eyes closed and arms and legs uncrossed) and quietly resting. Breathing then proceeds at the natural rate for that person. Air is let in through the nose and gently exhaled. Artificially deep breathing is avoided so as to not induce hyperventilation.[22] A sample abdominal breathing exercise is provided in Table 9-2.

TABLE 9-2 ABDOMINAL BREATHING EXERCISE

Assume a comfortable body position

Place one hand across your abdomen and the other hand across your chest

Pay attention to your breathing pattern without attempting to alter it

Scan your body for any tension indicators

Take a comfortable breath in through the nose, hold it, and gently exhale through pursed lips

Feel your abdomen gently rise and fall while your chest is relatively still

Continue breathing in this manner, taking about twice the time to exhale as to inhale

Practice for 5–10 minutes

Once mastered, only a few deep breaths are necessary to become more relaxed.

PROGRESSIVE MUSCLE RELAXATION

Jacobson introduced progressive muscle relaxation in the early 1900s. Jacobson proposed that muscle tension is required for task completion. Many persons, however, use excess tension that results in complaints such as muscle spasm, pain, and fatigue. Stressors were also believed to trigger muscle tension. Progressive muscle relaxation involves teaching the participant to systematically contract and relax the major skeletal muscle groups.[11,19] This intervention emphasizes the participant learning to differentiate muscle tension and relaxation so that with one's first awareness of tension, muscle relaxation should begin (Table 9-3). The learning sequence is (1) focusing attention on the muscle group, (2) systematic tensing and relaxing

TABLE 9-3 ABBREVIATED PROGRESSIVE MUSCLE RELAXATION EXERCISE

Assume a comfortable body position, gently close your eyes, and listen to yourself breathe

Breathe in r-e-l-a-x-a-t-i-o-n and exhale t-e-n-s-i-o-n

Allow your body to be supported

Feel your body sink

Scan your body for tension indicators

Feel the tension leaving your body as you become more relaxed and comfortable

Inhale and begin by tightening your arms by making fists

Study the tension

Now exhale, relax, and feel all the tension leaving your arms

Next inhale and tighten your legs by pointing your toes

Now exhale and let your legs go limp with relaxation

Inhale and draw your abdominal muscles in, making the abdomen "hard"

Release your breath and relax

Inhale up into your chest

Hold your breath as you tighten your pectorals

Exhale, relax, and feel the tension leave your body

Inhale and tense your shoulders and back by shrugging

Breathe out as you let your shoulders and back relax

Inhale and gently bring your chin toward your chest, hold it, and exhale as you relax

Breathe in and tense your face by squinting and your lips

Exhale and let your face relax

Allow the relaxation to spread throughout your body

Be aware of how much more relaxed and comfortable you feel

As you return to your normal level of awareness, concentrate on bringing back with you these feelings of comfort and relaxation

Gently open your eyes and stretch

of muscle groups to verbal cues, (3) systematic relaxing of muscle groups to verbal cues, and (4) relaxing muscle groups by suggestion.[12,20] Playing soft background music may facilitate relaxation. Bernstein and Borkovec[2] introduced an abbreviated version of progressive relaxation. Progressive relaxation is contraindicated for persons with upper motor neuron lesions and spasticity, hypertension, or cardiac disease.[12] Physician authorization should be obtained for using progressive muscle relaxation with persons having severe back injuries, recent muscle strains, or fractures because moderate strain is placed on bones and muscles with this intervention.[21] Research findings support the use of progressive muscle relaxation in the treatment of tension headaches.[2]

AUTOGENIC TRAINING

Autogenic training developed out of the hypnosis work of Schultz in the 1930s. Autogenic training involves the silent repetition of phrases about the ideal psychophysiologic state (Table 9-4). Autogenics strives toward a restoration of homeostasis. This approach uses autosuggestion (self-produced) to induce sensations of physical heaviness and warmth to achieve muscle relaxation and vasodilatation. The learning sequence is (1) scanning the mind and body for tension indicators, (2) using correct body posture (e.g., seated with back support), (3) reducing external stimuli, (4) passively concentrating on internal physical and mental states, and (5) following verbal cues for heaviness and warmth of the extremities, a calm heart beat, paced respiration, abdominal warmth, and a cool forehead.[27] The phrases of relaxation are repeated to emphasize their effect and to draw the participant's attention away from external stimuli.[22] Visualization is an integral part of advanced autogenics.[21] Autogenic training has been effective in treating persons with tension headache,[16] asthma,[25] and substance abuse.[9] Autogenic training has also been used for coping and wellness and in the treatment of persons with cardiac arrhythmias, hypertension, musculoskeletal disorders, neurologic disorders (e.g., Parkinsonism), and phobias. Autogenics is not recommended for persons who are agitated or actively psychotic.[12] Participants should be monitored to learn if any of the suggestions are aversive (e.g., feelings of heaviness).[22]

GUIDED IMAGERY

Guided imagery is the purposeful use of images/imagination to reduce the body's response to stress. Imagery may also be used to distract one's attention away from intrusive thoughts. The participant selects the relaxing environment (e.g., sunny beach, floating on a cloud). The same image should be used throughout that relaxation session.[24] Guided imagery has been helpful in reducing anxiety.[26]

MEDITATION

Relaxation, with an emphasis on peacefulness, is one goal of meditation. Meditation involves focusing attention on a rhythmic, repetitive word, phrase, or sensation while maintaining a passive attitude.[19] The learning sequence is (1) scanning for muscle tension, (2) paying attention to position, (3) performing a winding-down procedure, (4) concentrating on an everyday stimulus (concentration on the breath, a repeated phrase, or visual object), and (5) returning to routine daily activities. Meditation has been demonstrated to reduce hypertension.[24] It is contraindicated for persons experiencing acute psychosis.[22]

RELAXATION RESPONSE

After studying transcendental meditation and major religions, Benson[19] surmised four elements were necessary to produce therapeutic benefits: (1) a quiet environment, (2) a comfortable position, (3) a mental device, and (4) a passive attitude. These key elements form the relaxation response. Benson emphasizes a mental device to free the mind from external stimuli. The relaxation response is synonymous with parasympathetic nervous activity.[22] He recommends relaxation practice twice daily for 10 to 20 minutes. Benson's research advocates the use of the relaxation response for reducing hypertension.

TABLE 9-4 AUTOGENIC TRAINING EXERCISE
Assume a comfortable body position, gently close your eyes, and listen to yourself breathe
Breathe in r-e-l-a-x-a-t-i-o-n and exhale t-e-n-s-i-o-n
Allow your body to be supported
Feel your body sink as you become more relaxed
Scan your body for tension indicators
Feel the tension leaving your body as you become more relaxed and comfortable
Repeat the following phrases silently to yourself as you feel your body becoming more relaxed and comfortable
My arms and legs are heavy
My arms and legs are warm
My heartbeat is calm and regular
My body breathes itself
My center is warm
My forehead is cool
My mind is at peace
Allow the relaxation to proceed on its own
As you return to your normal level of awareness, concentrate on bringing back with you these feelings of comfort and relaxation
Gently open your eyes and stretch

Biofeedback

Biofeedback refers to instrumentation used to provide participants with feedback of electronically monitored physiologic events (e.g., muscle activity, skin surface temperature). This intervention assumes that a faulty body function is responsible for the participant's complaint of discomfort and that the impairment can be controlled when the participant is provided with immediate feedback.[2] Both autogenic training and progressive relaxation are used in conjunction with biofeedback. The learning sequence is (1) skin surface sensors are placed to monitor the desired body function (e.g., skeletal muscle activity), (2) instruction that a signal from the equipment (e.g., blinking light) monitors ongoing physiologic changes, (3) practice of relaxation or voluntary control to modify physiology, and (4) concentration on what the participant did to obtain the desired signal that is indicative of autonomic function. Skin temperature feedback to increase digital temperature in vascular conditions (e.g., migraine headaches) and electromyographic feedback to lessen muscle tension complaints (e.g., low back pain) are standard treatments in interdisciplinary pain clinics. Several studies[2] have reported that finger warming resulted in reduced migraine headaches. Temperature changes, however, were not significantly correlated with symptom reduction. It has therefore been suggested that other factors (e.g., changes in cognition) might be responsible for the desired changes.[1] Special training is required to become a biofeedback practitioner.

Massage

Massage can induce muscle relaxation. The contrast method of relaxation teaches the participant the difference between muscle contraction and relaxation. The participant contracts groups of muscles for 3 to 5 seconds and then focuses on relaxation. It is believed that muscle relaxation is increased following a strong contraction. The induction method uses a variety of strokes (e.g., centrifugal) and pressures to bring about relaxation.[3] Heat or cold are typically used before massage.[15] The reader is referred to the work of De Domenico and Wood[7] for a review of the massage literature and massage techniques.

Yoga

Yoga prescribes a lifestyle that requires rigorous physical and mental exercises. Ethical teachings emphasize restraint of antisocial and selfish behaviors with an emphasis on positive conduct. The learning sequence involves (1) specific postures (asanas), (2) breathing rituals (pranayamas), (3) withdrawal of the senses (pratyahara), (4) meditation, (5) contemplation, and (6) isolation. Yoga intends to recondition the mind to release creative energy and free the individual from unconscious impulses. The stretching and asanas involved in yoga are often relaxing.[7,21]

Physical Exercise

Exercise yields not only physical benefits but also enhances psychological well-being and ability to manage stress, thereby providing relaxation. Clinical populations have reported reduced fatigue, tension, insomnia, aggression, and depression in addition to increased self-esteem with regular exercise. The engagement in physical activity, whether aerobic or nonaerobic, appears to improve stress control.[22]

EVALUATION OF RELAXATION EFFECTIVENESS

Evidence of relaxation is made through observing the participant for indicators of relaxation as outlined in Table 9-1. Self-reports of relaxation are also beneficial. Relaxation reports can be assessed using an 11-point scale with 0 equal to "complete relaxation" and 10 equal to "tense as I can be." Table 9-5 is a sample relaxation monitoring sheet.

CONCLUSION

Chronic stress can activate physiologic arousal that may have many adverse effects. Relaxation may counter the stress response. The criteria of successful intervention are the sensation of relaxation and lack of distress that the participant experiences. Biofeedback instrumentation may be used to validate physiologic responses. Daily relaxation rehearsal is recommended, because stress reduction is temporary and symptomatic. If relaxation practice is haphazard, the techniques become less efficacious over time.

TABLE 9-5 RELAXATION MONITORING SHEET

SESSION	DATE	RELAXATION TECHNIQUE USED	OBSERVABLE INDICATORS OF RELAXATION	SELF-REPORTS OF RELAXATION
1				
2				
3				

REFERENCES

1. Benson H: The Relaxation Response. New York, Avon Books, 1975
2. Bernstein DA, Borkovec TD: Progressive Relaxation Training: A Manual for the Helping Professions. Champaign, Research Press, 1973
3. Boothby JL, Thorn BE, Stroud MW, et al: Coping with pain. In: Gatchel RJ, Turk DC, eds: Psychological Factors in Pain. New York, Guilford, 1999:343–359
4. Bottomley JM: Biofeedback: Connecting the body & mind. In: Davis CM, ed: Complementary Therapies in Rehabilitation: Holistic Approaches for Prevention and Wellness. Thorofare, Slack, 1997:101–123
5. Brannon L, Feist J: Health Psychology: An Introduction to Behavior and Health, 2nd ed. Belmont, Wadsworth, 1992
6. Cannon WB: The Wisdom of the Body. New York, Norton, 1932
7. De Domenico G, Wood EC: Beard's Massage, 4th ed. Philadelphia, WB Saunders, 1997
8. Giles GM, Neistadt ME: Treatment for psychosocial components: Stress management. In: Neistadt ME, Crepeau EB, eds: Willard & Spackman's Occupational Therapy, 9th ed. Philadelphia, Lippincott, 1988:458–463
9. Henry M, DeRivera JLG, Gonzales-Martin IJ, et al: Improvement of respiratory function in chronic asthmatic patients with autogenic therapy. J Psychosom Res 37:265–270, 1993
10. Hertling D, Jones D: Relaxation and related techniques. In: Hertling D, Kessler RM, eds: Management of Common Musculoskeletal Disorders, 3rd ed. Philadelphia, Lippincott Williams & Wilkins, 1996:140–162
11. Jacobson E: Progressive Relaxation. Chicago, University of Chicago Press, 1938
12. Jacobson E: You Must Relax, 5th ed. New York, McGraw-Hill, 1978
13. King JV: A holistic technique to lower anxiety: Relaxation with guided imagery. J Holistic Nurs 6:16–20, 1988
14. Lasater J: Untying the knot: Yoga as physical therapy. In: Davis CM, ed: Complementary Therapies in Rehabilitation: Holistic Approaches for Prevention and Wellness. Thorofare, Slack, 1997:125–131
15. Lazarus RS: Evolution of a model of stress, coping, and discrete emotions. In: Rice VH, ed: Handbook of Stress, Coping, and Health: Implications for Nursing Research, Theory, and Practice. Thousand Oaks, Sage, 2000:195–222
16. Luthe W: Autogenic Training. New York, Grune & Stratton, 1965
17. McCaffery M: Nursing Management of the Patient with Pain. Philadelphia, JB Lippincott, 1979
18. National Institutes of Health Technology Assessment Panel on Integration of Behavioral and Relaxation Approaches into the Treatment of Chronic Pain Conditions: Integration of behavioral and relaxation approaches into the treatment of chronic pain and insomnia. JAMA 276:313–318, 1996
19. Payne RA: Relaxation Techniques: A Practical Handbook for the Health Care Professional, 2nd ed. New York, Churchill Livingstone, 2000
20. Pelletier KR: Holistic Medicine: From Stress to Optimum Health. New York, Delacorte, 1979
21. Rice PL: Stress & Health, 2nd ed. Pacific Grove, Brooks/Cole, 1992
22. Rosch PJ, Hendler NH: Stress management. In: Taylor RB, Ureda JR, Denham JW, eds: Health Promotion: Principles and Clinical Applications. Norwalk, Appleton-Century-Crofts, 1982:339–371
23. Selye H: The Stress of Life, revised ed. New York, McGraw-Hill, 1976
24. Sharp C, Hurford DP, Allison J, et al: Facilitation of internal locus of control in adolescent alcoholics through a brief biofeedback-assisted autogenic relaxation training procedure. J Subst Abuse Treat 14:55–60, 1997
25. Spinhoven P, Corry A, Linssen G, et al: Autogenic training and self-hypnosis in the control of tension headache. Gen Hosp Psychiatry 14:408–415, 1992
26. Townsend MC: Relaxation therapy. In: Psychiatric Mental Health Nursing: Concepts of Care, 3rd ed. Philadelphia, FA Davis, 2000:177–186
27. Turner JA, Chapman CR: Psychological interventions for chronic pain: A critical review. I. Relaxation training and biofeedback. Pain 12:1–21, 1982
28. Turner JA, Romano JM: Cognitive-behavioral therapy. In: Bonica JJ, ed: The Management of Pain, 2nd ed. Philadelphia, Lea & Febiger, 1990: 1711–1721

RECOMMENDED READINGS

Reid GJ, McGrath PJ: Psychological treatment for migraine. Biomed Pharmacother 50:58–63, 1996
Turner JA, Chapman CR: Psychological intervention for chronic pain: a critical review. 1. Relaxation training and biofeedback. Pain 12:1–21, 1982

Functional Exercise

NEIL CHASAN

INTRODUCTION

"The term 'function' is used in orthopedics to describe the complex combination of multiple systems (musculoskeletal, CNS, sensory, motor, visual, vestibular) and their interactions."[3] Various authors have attempted to define functional exercise. Gray defined function by coining the term **mostability,** a synergistic combination of motion and stability. He goes on to define mostability as "the ability to functionally take advantage of just the right amount of motion at just the right joint in just the right plane in just the right direction at just the right time."[8] Additionally, no one has done a better job of defining functional exercise and testing than Gray with Team Reaction in the book *The Lower Extremity Functional Profile.*[7,9]

Our objective as therapists is ultimately to restore function, thus enabling normal participation in activities of daily living, including work and athletics. As therapists, we often spend much time on minutia. However, with the advent of managed healthcare in the 1990s, there has been a significant limitation in the number of visits that are allowed or reimbursed. These restrictions on care are a function of actuarial data and have resulted in therapists having to be both accountable and effective during increasingly limited contact with patients. In addition, home exercise compliance is a problem, as reported by numerous authors.[1,2,9,10,13,17,18,19] A cursory overview of the obesity data in the United States implies lack of participation in any exercise program whatsoever. The resulting dilemma—fewer visits and poor compliance with home exercise programs—requires an innovative solution. Because we have fewer visits to work with, we need to teach our patients effective methods to judge their own progress and to self-monitor. Empowering people will enhance participation, improving the effectiveness of home exercise programs. If one were to examine the activities of patients once they left the clinical environment, one would not be surprised to learn that they typically performed normal activities of daily living. It is from this point of view that functional exercise begins to make sense as a strategy for guiding rehabilitation. If an exercise program were more aligned to the daily life of each patient, the opportunity for increased compliance would be enhanced. After all, our muscles and joints work together to complete even the most mundane task.

LOWER EXTREMITY FUNCTIONAL PROFILE

The **Lower Extremity Functional Profile** is a great place to start because the profile is really an assessment tool that allows us to establish a firm starting point based on objective measurement. Further, the profile can be prescriptive as well and also allows the clinician to track actual functional progress objectively. This sort of objectivity is necessary in charting and will, in the end, be the tool that differentiates physical therapists from personal trainers in the minds of insurance providers.

As a point of interest, functional exercise should be differentiated from closed chain exercise. Although many of the lower extremity functional exercises are closed chain activities, the idea is to match the exercise to the function. If the job is throwing, as in the rehabilitation of an athlete, then the exercise program must include functional elements of throwing. Naturally, this will include various ankle, knee, hip, and trunk closed chain activities as well as open chain shoulder, elbow, and wrist activities. It would be more accurate to consider function in the context of the "Kinetic Link" described by Kibler[12] as well as Ellenbecker and Davis[5] as a series of sequentially activated body segments. The kinetic link explores the idea that motion begins proximally and proceeds to distal segments. Distal segments can be, and often are, open chain segments (as in the kicking foot or the throwing hand).

Functional testing depends on the definition of the components of function and on a set of tools to measure these components accurately, inexpensively, and repeatedly with accuracy. Further, clinicians should be able to communicate with each other referencing such tests in a common language so that the tests can be duplicated. Any clinician should be able to measure function easily. "Functional testing must determine an individual's threshold of function."[9] Functional testing must be "objective, specific, and meaningful."[9] When practiced in this fashion, functional testing provides a starting point for rehabilitation and quantifiable tools for measuring progress toward function. As Gray puts it, "The value of a battery of tests lies within the features of those tests. *The Lower Extremity Functional Profile* features specific qualities that prove its benefit to specifically determine functional thresholds and functional profiles. *The Lower Extremity Functional Profile* provides the need to objectify measurements of function, communicate function, direct rehabilitative and conditioning efforts, document efficacy and prove credibility."[9]

In a functional rehabilitation environment, the role of pronation and supination is important to understand. We think of pronation and supination as motions related to and associated with the foot. Usually, pronation and supination are motions thought to be associated with the subtalar joint. In a functional paradigm, however, motion in the subtalar joint is transmitted to the knee via the tibia and from the knee to the hip via the femur. Therefore, pronation that begins at heel strike becomes pronation at the knee, visible to the eye as flexion, internal rotation and genu valgus (abduction). At the hip, one sees pronation as internal rotation flexion and adduction. The transmission of pronation carries on up through the pelvis and trunk as the **pronation response**[7] resolves.

In the context of a gravitational environment, one can think of pronation as the way the musculoskeletal system deals with the absorption of energy. With each joint and all the muscles that cross the joint involved in the absorption of energy we can say that pronation is the absorption of energy of the entire functional chain. Excessive or prolonged subtalar pronation will cause increased frontal plane valgus stress to the knee, resulting in increased tibial internal rotation, knee flexion, and femoral internal rotation.[4,14,20]

In contrast, supination begins as the foot moves from being a mobile adaptor to being a rigid lever, on up through the subtalar joint, the ankle, the knee, the hip, and up through the spine as the power needed to accelerate away from the ground overcoming gravity is generated in initiating and producing movement. Supination is illustrated as motion of the calcaneus from eversion to inversion. Then motion occurs at the ankle, from dorsiflexion to plantar flexion, and then from knee flexion and valgus to extension and varus. The hip then moves from flexion and internal rotation to extension and external rotation. The pelvis rotates and the spine extends. Effectively propulsion. Gray refers to propulsion as the "**supination response.**"[7] He goes on to describe pronation as "giving in to gravity to accommodate and absorb load," where muscle activity is primarily in the form of eccentric loading to decelerate motion while supination, on the other hand, typically overcomes gravity to propel with muscle actions that are concentric to accelerate loads.[11]

In a functional rehabilitation environment, transformation from pronation to supination and vice-versa is key. The timing of change, the latency, the quality of motion, and the range of motion as well as the power able to be generated by the subject are all issues to focus on in the clinic. Plane dominance is also relevant and must be addressed by the clinician. Specific adaptation to imposed demand (the SAID principle) should govern the functional progression of the rehabilitation process. Nociceptive mechanoreceptors generally report and respond to weight-bearing postures more specifically. As such, weight-bearing exercise that simulates or even exceeds the expected postrehabilitation demand will further prepare the tissues for the loads to come (Box 10-1).

To help the reader contemplate the possibilities, following are several clinically useful functional exercises. One could prescribe the identical exercise for two completely separate conditions. For example, an anterior medial balance and reach exercise (Fig. 10-1) is an excellent exercise in the rehabilitation of an injured ankle or an injured knee. The exercise causes loaded dorsiflexion at the ankle of the weight-bearing foot as well as flexion and abduction of the loaded knee. Muscularly, the exercise challenges the muscles that decelerate dorsiflexion with bent knee (soleus, tibialis posterior, flexor digitorum, and others) as well as the muscles which decelerate knee flexion and abduction under load (quadriceps, sartorius, gluteus medius, and others). The clinician could also prescribe two completely different exercises for the identical condition. This decision may depend on the environment in which the patient spends his or her time, the demands expected to be placed on the tissues following recovery, or any other set of variables. The point is that the clinician must prescribe the right exercise to be completed in the right way to the right dose. This is what makes for a successful clinician.

The prescribed exercise could be used to challenge proprioception, range of motion, strength, or endurance. Which variable is controlled (time, speed, repetitions, range of motion, load) changes the purpose of the exercise completely. As a result, the idea is not to define functional exercise protocols. Rather, various functional exercises must be examined from the point of view of the specific functional deficit of the individual patient. The emphasis on one joint or another is going to be dictated by their specific dysfunction. The identical exercise for knee pain and hip pain would be dosed differently and directed differently depending on the functional quality for which the clinician was searching. For that reason, there is no discussion on dose for a particular exercise beyond the following. As a general rule, it does not make sense to exercise in a manner that increases pain. It does not make sense to exercise in a manner that promotes substitution or accommodation. Quality of movement is important. How much weight should a person use? The clinician must adjust

BOX 10-1   TERMINOLOGY FROM THE LOWER EXTREMITY FUNCTIONAL PROFILE

Planes of motion: Sagittal, transverse, and frontal planes

Triplanar motion: Motion that crosses all three planes

Pronation: Generally implies collapsing under the force of gravity

Supination: Generally implies accelerating against the force of gravity

Vector: The direction of motion

Joints of motion: Simply, the joints involved in the motion named

Range of motion: Dependent on the tests chosen, direction of the tests, and the manipulation of other variables

Loading: Intrinsic or extrinsic loading of various types specifically varied to change movement reactions and requirements

Speed and time: These variables can be considered for each test

Control: Various types, directions, and amounts of control can be introduced to increase or decrease difficulty, or increase safety

Feedback: Another testing variable that is left to the examiner to introduce to improve the quality of testing

Balance: Measures the time an individual can maintain his or her balance on one foot; balance is challenged by various head, arm, and leg positions or movements

Peripheral balance: Balance reach tests measure the distance individuals can reach with their arms or the opposite leg to challenge their ability to stand on one leg

Excursion: Measures the amount of motion that can be controlled at a specific joint within a specific plane while in a unilateral stance

Lunge: Lunge tests measures the distance an individual can lunge along various test vectors; the lunge leg does most of the work

Step-up: Step-up tests measure the height of the step an individual is able to take, with an emphasis on the leg on the step and inhibition of the ground leg

Step down: As in the step up, but the step down is tested with a successful return to the start position

Jump: Jump tests measure the distance an individual can jump along a specific vector by taking off of one leg and executing a successful two-leg landing

Hop: Hop tests measure the distance an individual can hop along a specific vector by taking off of one leg and executing a successful same-leg, one-leg landing

---

the dosage (i.e., the weight, speed of motion, range of motion, number of repetitions, and other variables) to make patients successful in their efforts. Success is defined as the ability of the patient to perform the task safely and correctly without cognition. In this manner, the patient happily progresses toward full functional restoration. In addition, consideration must be given to regularly modifying the exercise prescription to progress the patient along the **functional spectrum.** In other words, it makes sense to move from simple tasks to complex exercises, from one plane of motion to triplanar motion, and from easy challenges to difficult challenges.

A patient might well tolerate activities in the transverse plane but avoid stresses in the frontal plane. It is the duty of the clinician to find a way to stimulate the patient by stressing the frontal plane, in this example, at a low enough dose so as to avoid or eliminate the avoidance behavior. This might take form with the verbal directive, "Reach for this target here," or it might take the form of a biomechanical solution, for example, changing the surface orientation by placing a wedge under the medial surface of the foot. Clinical expertise in directing functional exercise programs implies that the clinician will recognize when a patient is performing the exercise in a manner that is inconsistent with optimal function and make appropriate changes to the dose by adjusting or tweaking one or more variables to get the desired result. Gray calls this clinical skill "tweakology."[8] He suggests that it is best to provide an instruction or correction that is not associated with the desired movement (e.g., if you wish to have the knee move across the foot into an abducted position of the knee during loaded flexion, changing the direction of the reaching foot to a more medial target will often cause the loaded knee to acquire more abduction as the hip adducts without asking the patient to "abduct the knee" as he or she bends the loaded leg). These functional puzzles are an exciting application of a physical therapist's knowledge base. A clinician should be able to explain to another clinician why he or she is having a patient perform a particular task in a particular way from an anatomic point of view. In other words, a prescribed exercise should be designed to elicit a specific functional response that will aid the recovery toward full function.

An argument can be made that when one exercises functionally, the improvement seen is secondary to proprioceptive learning. The mechanoreceptors, which are housed in dense connective tissue structures, all function best in a weight-bearing position. There is a significant amount of motor learning that can be enhanced by varying the proprioceptive environment. Altering the surface to make balance more difficult increases the difficulty of the exercises disproportionately. This is easily accomplished by having the patient stand on a foam pad or some other soft surface. A good rule in the clinic is to introduce a balance challenge when thinking about the next progression.

Muscle function during various activities generally falls into one of two categories. Pronation is usually associated

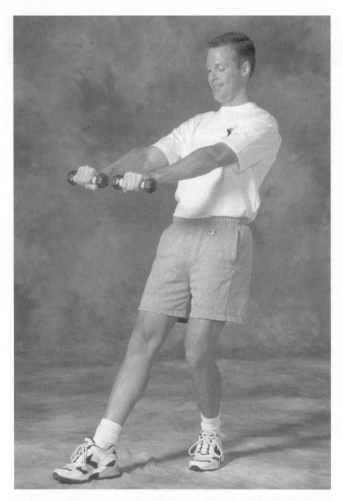

■ FIG. 10-1. Anterior medial balance and reach, hands at waist height. (Photograph by Norm Hirsom Photography.)

with eccentric contractions, and supination is usually associated with concentric contractions. During function, without thought, we pronate (reduce loads) and supinate (produce loads) causing our muscles to shift between eccentric and concentric contractions frequently.[6] Thinking about function, it seems that the key "moment of truth," so to speak, is the point of transition between the two. As a muscle decelerates momentum reducing the load (eccentrically) it must begin to accelerate producing a load in an alternative direction (concentrically). Large two-joint muscles can therefore undergo both of these functions simultaneously in different planes of motion. Transformation is key to restoring function. To train transformation, the patient must decelerate momentum by focusing on eccentric loading and unloading activities. Further, eccentric training excites the muscle spindle leading to improved coordination of motion. Proprioception is a key component of this process.

Much has been said about momentum as a deleterious concern during weight training. Examination of function

demonstrates that momentum is a natural part of everyday life. Training using free weights as an amplifier of momentum helps prepare a body for action against everyday loads. Naturally, using free weights as opposed to machines implies that the functional restrictions that exercise machines place on movement are eliminated. As such, the clinician must be vigilant to ensure that the patient is exercising safely. Although one might encourage the patient to "work as quickly as possible," it is important to monitor the quality of movement and the range of movement and to ensure that no substitutions are used to overcome weakness, fatigue or pain. Keep in mind that increasing the speed of movement effectively increases the load that the patient must decelerate and accelerate.

One element of functional exercise worthy of consideration is the idea of "integrated" versus "isolated" movement patterns. Whereas most machine-based exercises isolate a particular motion at a particular joint effectively training a muscle in one plane, functional exercises tend to be multiplanar or triplanar, since true functional movement occurs in a triplanar fashion.[3] Thus, while the clinician might be emphasizing a particular muscle in a given exercise, the triplanar exercise can be set up by the clinician to isolate the muscle being trained into a normal integrated functional movement pattern. Along with this is the idea that the way to proceed clinically is proximal to distal, or core to periphery. Motion patterns have been described by Putnam as "proximal to distal sequencing."[15] Stability, therefore, is generated by the core muscles, and as such, a functional exercise model should begin with core strengthening. This strategy provides the stability needed to progress a patient towards full function without reaching or being affected by artificial barriers to progress.

EXERCISE PROGRESSIONS

In general, patient progress during rehabilitation occurs along the following lines[6]:

- From simple movements to complex movements.
- From easy to more difficult movements and movement patterns.
- Execution of the activities is important, and it is best to begin with correct execution. After which, as the form is mastered, the patient can begin to increase the number of repetitions and eventually increase the intensity of the exercises.
- Finally, exercises that mimic the patients' specific functional goals are necessary. This is why soccer players need to finally perform exercises that mimic the demands of play on the soccer field, and injured workers need to be able to demonstrate the critical demands of their jobs before returning to work.

Home exercise programs must be established in a manner that eliminates barriers to participation. Simple exercises that are **home-workable** are best. Retesting a patient against the initial data gathered will encourage and perhaps ensure compliance.

In the final analysis, applying and implementing a functional exercise strategy in a physical therapy clinic will broaden the arsenal of tools that clinicians have at their disposal. Combining functional exercise with manual therapy and various other exercise models will augment the rehabilitative potential of the patient.[3] Restoring a functional lifestyle is the goal of our patients, and we should do all we can to facilitate their goals (Fig. 10-2).

Plane Emphasis

It is possible to make the plane of motion the emphasis of the exercise program. Although all muscles essentially function in a triplanar fashion, it is possible to focus the dominant motion in one plane or another, or even to combine two planes over the third. For example, each of the exercises shown in figures 10-5, 10-6, and 10-7, emphasize a different plane.

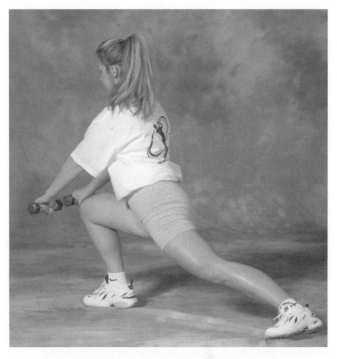

■ **FIG. 10-3.** Posterior lateral rotation lunge, hands reaching to knee height. (Photograph by Norm Hirsom Photography.)

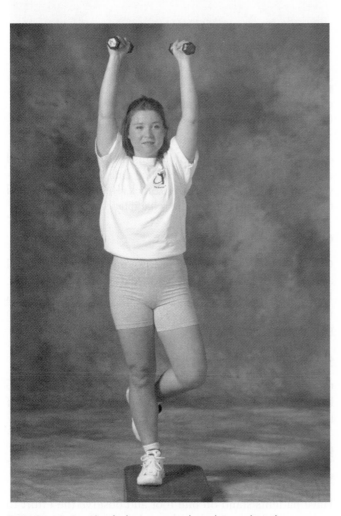

■ **FIG. 10-2.** Single leg stance, hands overhead. (Photograph by Norm Hirsom Photography.)

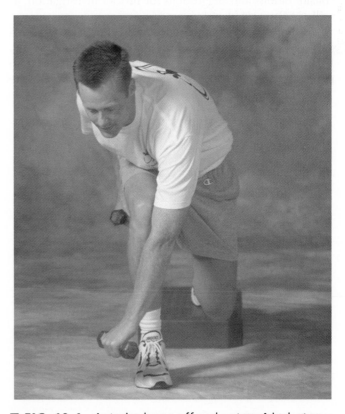

■ **FIG. 10-4.** Anterior lunge off and onto a 4-inch step. Opposite hand reaches across the foot at ankle height. (Photograph by Norm Hirsom Photography.)

Sagittal Plane Exercise: Anterior Lunge

Frontal Plane Exercise: Lateral Slides

Transverse Plane Exercise: Trunk Rotation

TESTING FOR FUNCTION[7]

Functional testing is a component of a physical therapy evaluation. Once the "serious stuff" is ruled out through proper screening tests, a series of functional tests are necessary to make a "functional diagnosis" of the dysfunction present. The objective clinician must differentiate between an "attractor-well" for example versus "accommodation" secondary to pain. It is important to assess the level of function to define an appropriate starting point for a rehabilitative exercise program. The tools used during a functional assessment are commonly found in the clinic. These include a goniometer, a stop watch, a tape measure, and steps of various sizes. It is also helpful to use a compass on the floor or a mat that is so printed. Defining the parameters of testing is important so that there is good interrater and intrarater reliability in the data gathered.

Establishing a starting point for rehabilitation begins with an evaluation. In the case of functional assessment, one must begin with the basics. As an example, the lower extremity evaluation is developed, with the progression of functional considerations and suggestions for further investigation, as well as treatment planning.

The functional spectrum, as defined by Gray, allows the progressive increase in intensity, load, and demand to be assessed. In this section, the idea is developed to allow the clinician to move the evaluation along quickly while gathering appropriate

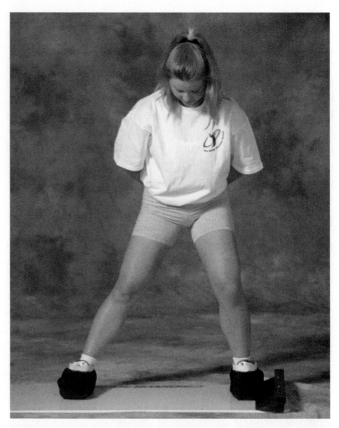

■ **FIG. 10-6.** The slide board is a functional exercise that challenges the lower extremities in the frontal plane. (Photograph by Norm Hirsom Photography.)

data—in effect, the significant signs that can be monitored accurately and efficiently. Recording data using naming conventions already discussed allows quick retests to be conducted to monitor progress during the rehabilitation process.

Gait

Observe gait first. Look for plane dominance at the feet and ankles, the knee and hip, the pelvis and spine, and the trunk. Begin by noting the gait deviations from normal (such as a medial heel whip, excessive calcaneal eversion, or excessive pelvic sway) and record those.

Structure and Alignment

Observe the patient standing in front of you. Look at bony landmarks to evaluate their symmetry and alignment. Note if the patients is favoring one leg or the other.

LOWER EXTREMITY FUNCTIONAL PROFILE

Static Balance (Box 10-2)

Have patients stand on one foot and observe the effort to maintain balance. Look at how they recover, noting the strategy used to maintain single leg stance. If they are com-

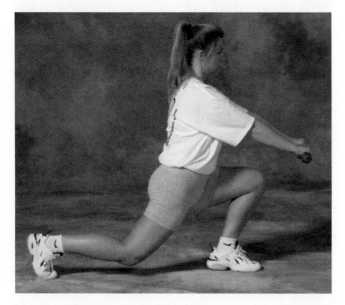

■ **FIG. 10-5.** The anterior lunge with hands reaching at waist height is a sagittal-plane–dominant exercise. (Photograph by Norm Hirsom Photography.)

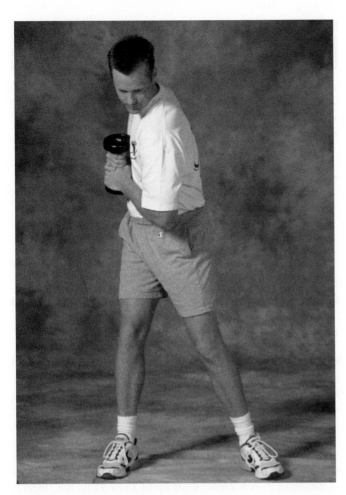

■ **FIG. 10-7.** The trunk rotation exercise is a transverse-plane–dominant exercise that challenges the rotators of the spine and hip in the transverse plane. (Photograph by Norm Hirsom Photography.)

BOX 10-2	STATIC BALANCE CHALLENGES

- Time: 30 seconds
- Head movement
  - Rotation
  - Sidebending
  - Back bending
- Visual challenges
  - Eyes closed
  - One eye closed
  - Open and close eyes
  - Open and close eyes alternately
  - Blink rapidly
- Head positions
  - Side bent
  - Rotated
  - Extended
- Arm/leg movement; swing arms/legs in various planes
  - Frontal
  - Sagittal
  - Transverse
- Surface challenges
  - Stable
  - Unstable

Peripheral Dynamic Balance (Box 10-3)

Using either the arms (hands) or the other leg (foot) have patients reach out in various planes along a given vector without transferring their weight. Have them demonstrate (this is the important part) an ability to return to the starting point without losing balance or having to cheat (use another joint strategy) to return to the starting position safely. For example, in a sagittal plane balance and reach, the instruction might be, "Stand on your left foot, reach as far out in front of you along this line using your right foot, toe touch, and return to standing." The patient might try to maintain a straight leg and use the hip to achieve the motion. Being interested in their knee, you might offer them the following corrected instruction, "Do it again, but this time try to keep your shoulders back as you reach out with your right foot." This instruction would have the impact of shifting the motion dominance from the hip to the knee. You would measure the shortest distance, the space between their left toe and the point of contact of their right foot, and record it in centimeters or inches. Then you would have them repeat the task using their opposite foot and compare the result to the other side. Gray suggests that you have the subject repeat a single test several times, each being a slightly longer reach than the preceding reach until their maximum reach is established.[8] Observing a significant difference in distance reached, or if they were only able to execute the motion using a strategy that kept the demand off the knee and loaded the hip instead, you might conclude that they have a sagittal plane peripheral balance deficit in the left

fortable and clearly able to balance (30 seconds is a good indicator that they are), introduce a balance challenge to test the plane in which they showed a little trouble. If you are unsure, introduce multiple challenges to tease out the plane of weakness. For example, you might have the patient swing the arms or legs from side to side to increase frontal plane forces. If patients maintain balance comfortably for 30 seconds, perhaps have them tilt the head to one side or the other to challenge them by altering their cervical spine receptor and visual receptor inputs. Static balance often gives you clues about the real underlying deficits. After a few minutes, you should have an idea about what you will likely find as you increase the load and demand on the tissues.

Excursion

Using a goniometer, measure both loaded and unloaded range of motion. Compare one side to the other, noting the significant findings.

knee. You would repeat the test with a frontal plane balance and reach, and a transverse plane balance and reach. Note the plane of weakness and record the appropriate data. Figure 10-8 illustrates a typical balance and reach test.

Load/Unload (Lunging) (Box 10-4)

The next level of loading involves pronation and supination under load, or lunging. Once again, have the patient work along a particular vector allowing you to identify the specific plane of motion. You might offer the following instruction, "Take a big step with your left leg along this line, touch the ground with both hands in front of your foot, and return to standing. Do it three times, each time trying to go just a bit further each time, so on the third try, you are stepping as far as you can safely." Once again, monitor the movement strategy. Make sure you are seeing similar strategies for each leg, and in this case, in which you are evaluating a left knee problem, make sure patients do not pull themselves back to standing with their right leg when they step onto their left leg. If they do, note that they do, and try to offer a suggestion to correct the strategy to really evaluate the loading deficit. You might say something like, "Try taking a smaller step so you don't have to rely on your right leg to get back." Measure the shortest distance between their left and right foot, note their movement strategy, and repeat for the other two planes. You might find that they can safely manage a sagittal/frontal plane along a 45° vector, but not a frontal plane lunge along a 90° vector. Make a note of this and the hand position reached during the test and move on to the next test (Fig. 10-5).

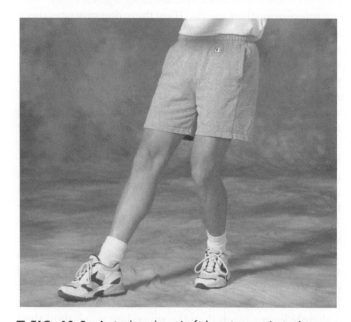

■ **FIG. 10-8.** Anterior view. Left leg stance. Anterior-lateral balance and reach rest. Measure the shortest distance between the toe of the left foot and the heel of the right foot. The patient needs to be able to reach and get back to upright stance safely. (Photograph by Norm Hirsom Photography.)

- Time
- Repetitions per unit time
- Repetitions
- Plane
  - Sagittal, transverse, frontal
  - Vectors between planes
- Hand positions
  - Hands at side
  - Reach at ankle height
  - Reach at knee height
  - Reach at waist height
  - Reach at shoulder height
  - Reach overhead
- Use of weight in hands

Step Up/Step Down (Box 10-5)

Once you have established the tolerances of pronation and supination from static balance to lunging in all three planes, the next level of testing is loading while changing elevation. Using steps of various heights, we can simply increase or decrease the load as we modify our evaluation to suit the particular patient in question. A set of steps of various heights allows the examiner to quickly move the patient from one step to the next as the investigation continues. Typically, a clinic might have steps in 2-inch or 4-inch increments up to 18 or 24 inches. Placed side by side, the patient can simply move from the lower steps to the higher, while the examiner evaluates movement patterns and strategies. Pain is a natural stopping point, but substitutions are common on steps. A knee patient will often use a hip-dominant strategy rather than a knee-dominant strategy, and this shows up on step up and step down testing more often

BOX 10-4 **LUNGE CHALLENGES**

- Time
- Repetitions per unit time
- Repetitions
- Plane
  - Sagittal, transverse, frontal
  - Vectors between planes
- Hand positions
  - Hands at side
  - Reach at ankle height
  - Reach at knee height
  - Reach at waist height
  - Reach at shoulder height
  - Reach overhead
- Use of weight in hands

than not. The instruction to the patient would be something like, "Face the step, and step up with the right, then down with the left back to your starting position." This instruction would examine the quality of motion and the movement strategy for a right leg step up and a right leg step down in the sagittal plane. An anterior right leg step down, in contrast, would require that the left leg lead the right leg as it would if one were descending stairs. Naming the tests is important because the examiner will likely want to retest weaknesses after a time. The same instruction, but with a slight variation, would change the test to a frontal plane test. "Stand with the step to your right and step up onto the step using your right leg. Then step down using your left leg to lead. Return to the starting position." To make the test a transverse plane test, the instruction must be modified: "Stand facing away from the step at a 45° angle. Step up onto the step using your right leg. Rotate 135° to the right as you do, so you finish facing to the right. Then step down with your left leg, finishing the way you started." Remember that functional testing tests the leg doing the work.

It is not uncommon to need "more gravity" to tease out an expected dysfunction.[8] For example, in the event that you are examining a very muscular man, simple step up and step down tests (even onto and off a 24-inch step) are insufficient loads to incriminate a particular tissue or plane of motion. In situations such as this, one might consider having the subject hold additional weight, as much as 25 pounds in each hand, to increase the load. If the net effect of the increased load is to cause the patient to modify the movement strategy sufficiently, one can draw the conclusion that the step up (or down) plus 50 pounds of load was sufficient to incriminate a particular tissue or plane of motion. It is important to record such modifications to the test procedure in your records so you can repeat the test in the future. Figure 10-9 demonstrates step up-step down on a 4" step as an exercise.

Jumping (Box 10-6)

Assuming that the preceding tests revealed only minor deficits of function one side to the other, the next level of intensity is jumping. A jump is defined as taking off on one foot and landing on two feet. The instruction is to, "Stand on your right foot. Jump as far as you can along this line (straight ahead), and land

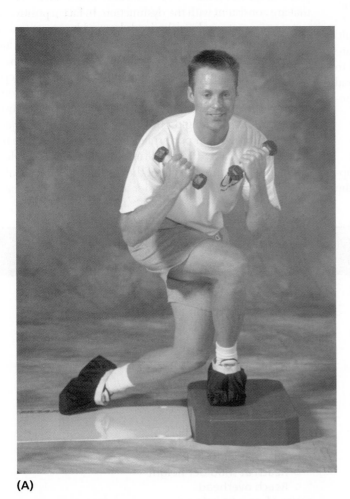

(A)

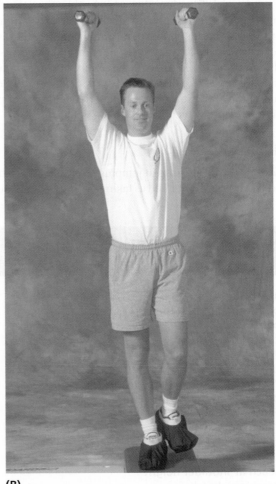

(B)

■ **FIG. 10-9.** Anterior view. Right leg anterior medial step up. **(A)** Starting position. **(B)** Finish position. (Photograph by Norm Hirsom Photography.)

BOX 10-5	STEP-UP CHALLENGES

- Time
- Repetitions per unit time
- Repetitions
- Step height
- Plane
  - Sagittal, transverse, frontal
  - Vectors between planes
- Hand positions
  - Hands at side
  - Reach at ankle height
  - Reach at knee height
  - Reach at waist height
  - Reach at shoulder height
  - Reach overhead
- Use of weight in hands

---

on two feet. You must stick the landing. Repeat the jump three times, each time jumping a bit further than the time before." The testing clinician will then ask the patient to repeat the test on the opposite side and compare the result. Often, deficits that show up during lunging and step tests are invisible in jumping because of the ability of the patient to substitute. In cases like that, having the patient use additional weights, adding repetitions, making the demand time dependent and so on are ways to tease out the deficit.

Hopping (Box 10-7)

Deficits that do not show up in jumping often show up in hopping tests. Hopping is defined as taking off and landing on the

same foot. Having the patient hop three successive times, stick the last landing, allows a cumulative deficit to appear. A small difference between legs on one hop often looks substantially larger when compared after three hops. Hopping to the side is named from the point of view of the leg doing the work. For example, the instruction, "Stand on your right leg and hop to the right three times," would be called a right lateral hop. It is also possible to test the frontal plane in the other direction. The instruction, "Stand on your right foot and hop three times to the left," would be named a right medial hop. Adding rotation to jumping and hopping allows the examiner to test the ability of the patient to supination and pronation forces in the transverse plane as well. The nomenclature for naming transverse plane jumps and hops is similar to that for naming frontal plane jumps and hops. A right lateral rotational hop would be a hop in which the subject stood on their right leg, hopped to the right while rotating in mid air, and landed on the same leg facing a given rotation away from the starting position.

Assessment and Exercise Planning

Armed with the information gathered during the assessment phase of the examination, the clinician can introduce exercises that are consistent with the dysfunction. In fact, a positive dosing strategy is to reduce the load demand by a nominal percentage and ask the patient to repeat the test to the reduced load point as an exercise, completing so many repetitions in a given time. One might ask the patient to complete 20 repetitions in 30 seconds, performing a balance and reach exercise to a point at 80% of the maximum shown during the testing procedure. By working on the limited activity, the subject is likely to improve their performance incrementally. If the therapist asks the patient to perform several exercises, each one originating as a direct result of the testing procedure, patient compliance is likely to be higher and good outcomes can be

---

BOX 10-6	JUMPING CHALLENGES

- Time
- Repetitions per unit time
- Repetitions
- Distance
- Plane
  - Sagittal, transverse, frontal
  - Vectors between planes
- Hand positions during jumping
  - Touch the floor
  - Reach at ankle height
  - Reach at knee height
  - Reach at waist height
  - Reach at shoulder height
  - Reach overhead
- Use of weight in hands

BOX 10-7	HOPPING CHALLENGES

- Time
- Repetitions per unit time
- Repetitions
- Distance
- Plane
  - Sagittal, transverse, frontal
  - Vectors between planes
- Hand positions during jumping
  - Touch the floor
  - Reach at ankle height
  - Reach at knee height
  - Reach at waist height
  - Reach at shoulder height
  - Reach overhead
- Use of weight in hands

expected. Gray coined the expression "causative-cure," implying that the patient must do the task that caused the injury (dosed correctly, that is dosed low enough to avoid further injury) to optimally provide the best stimulus for repair of both the tissue in dysfunction and the neurology supporting the coordination of the joint or muscles in question.[8] It is this idea that the clinician can employ to design the optimal exercise program for the particular dysfunction and also the reason why specific exercise protocols are irrelevant. Armed with this strategy, the therapist might develop an exercise plan that might include only a few of the thousands of permutations of several exercises available.

Specific parameters of testing can include modifications of range of motion, repetitions, time, repetitions per unit of time, additional load (weight), modification of surfaces (toward more unstable or stable surfaces), and removal or addition of other sources of neurologic input (e.g., closing the eyes). Whichever modification the clinician makes to the test procedure, it is important to include the notation in the record so that the test is reproducible.

Follow up of patients who have been tested in this manner is easy if the clinician has properly recorded the test and the deficit. Patients are often very eager to show the clinician the progress that they have made because they see the value of such exercises to their well-being. Retesting is much more efficient than initial testing, because during retesting only the injured extremity needs to be tested and only the specific limitation needs to be rechecked. In fact, it takes just a few minutes to quickly retest a patient each visit, allowing the clinician to make an educated and accurate decision with respect to progressing the patient along the functional spectrum toward full function.

Ultimately, the exercise program must look like the tasks patients expect their rehabilitated selves to perform. In the end, if, for example, the activity goal is unrestricted participation in competitive soccer, the exercises must look like the demands on the field of competition. This should include high intensity action lasting 20 seconds or less as well as jumping, backward running, and numerous changes of direction during sprinting activities.[6] If the demands related to returning to work in a material handling environment include 30 lifts per minute of a 20-pound box from floor to overhead, then the exercise program must finally include box lifting from floor to overhead on a timed basis. In either case, this is not where the rehabilitation would begin, but it should be where it ends.

The functional examination procedure described in the *Lower Extremity Functional Profile* is one flavor of testing that the clinician uses to be able to accurately answer the question that every patient asks: "When can I play [or work] again?" As physical therapists, we are catering to the patient, the physician, and the insurance carrier. Everybody want answers to the posed question that suite them. To answer suitably for all three, we need to use an array of tools to get valid answers and ensure the best result we can as efficiently and economically as possible. Functional testing and exercise strategies broaden our arsenal of tools to this end dramatically.

REFERENCES

1. Blampied P: Why don't patients do their home exercise program. J Orthop Sports Phys Ther 25(2):101–102, 1977
2. Cain RE: Effect of instruction on perceived physical ability and exercise adherence. Percept Mot Skills 82:494, 1996
3. Chasan N, Kane M: Functional training for the low back patient. Orthop Phys Ther Clin North Am 8(4):1059–1056, 1999
4. Donatelli RA, ed: The Biomechanics of the Foot and Ankle. Philadelphia, FA Davis, 1990:32
5. Ellenbecker T, Davies GJ: Closed kinetic chain exercise. Human Kinetics, 2001
6. Gambetta V: The Gambetta method. Vern Gambetta Publisher, 1998:9–16
7. Gray G: Lower Extremity Functional Profile. Wynn Marketing, 1995
8. Gray G: Chain Reaction Festival. personal communication, 1996
9. Gray G: Functional kinetic chain rehabilitation: Overuse and inflammatory conditions and their management . . . a strategy of oxymorons. Sports Med Update 24–30, 1995
10. Roush SE, Sonstroem RJ: Development of the physical therapy outpatient satisfaction survey (POPTS). Phys Ther 79(2):159–170, 1999
11. Jenkins W, Bronner S, Mangine R: Functional evaluation and treatment of the lower extremity. In: Functional Movement in Orthopedics and Sports Physical Therapy. New York, Churchill Livingstone, 1995:194
12. Kibler WB: The role of the scapula in the overhead throwing motion. Contemp Orthop 22:535–532, 1991
13. Mayo NE: Patient compliance: Practical implications for physical therapists. Phys Ther 58(9):1083–1090, 1978
14. McCulloch MU, Brunt D, Linden DV: The effect of foot orthotics and gait velocity on lower limb kinematics and temporal events of stance. J Orthop Phys Ther 17:2–10, 1993
15. Putnam CA: Sequential motions of the body segments in striking and throwing skills: Descriptions and explanations. J Biomech 26 Suppl 1:125–135, 1993
16. Root ML, Orien WP, Weed JH: Normal function of the foot. In: Clinical Biomechanics. Los Angeles, Clinical Biomedics Corp., 1971
17. Sluijs EM, Kok GJ, Van der Zee J: Correlates of exercise compliance in physical therapy. Phys Ther 73(11):771–786, 1993
18. Sluijs EM, Knibbe JJ: Patient compliance with exercise: Different theoretical approaches to short term and long-term compliance. Patient Educ Counsel 17:191–204, 1991
19. Sluijs EM: A checklist to assess patient education in physical therapy practice: Development and reliability. Phys Ther 71(8):561–568, 1991
20. Tiberio D: The effect of excessive sub talar pronation on patellofemoral mechanics: A theoretical model. J Ortho Sports Phys Ther 9:160–165, 1987
21. White SA, Corce RV, Loureiro EM, et al: Effects of frequency and duration of exercise sessions on physical activity levels and adherence. Percept Mot Skills 73,172–174, 1991

Clinical Applications— Peripheral Joints

PART II

Shoulder and Shoulder Girdle

11

DARLENE HERTLING AND RANDOLPH M. KESSLER

REVIEW OF FUNCTIONAL ANATOMY

Osseous Structures

The osseous components of the functional shoulder girdle include the upper thoracic vertebrae, the first and second ribs, the manubrium, the scapula, the clavicle, and the humerus (Fig. 11-1). For this complex to function adequately, the spine must be stable. To achieve full arm elevation, the upper thoracic vertebrae must be able to extend, rotate, and sidebend to the ipsilateral side, and the bodies of the first and second ribs must be able to descend and move posteriorly (with vertebral rotation). The manubriosternal, costomanubrial, and sternoclavicular joints must permit the manubrium to sidebend and rotate to the ipsilateral side.

The acromioclavicular and sternoclavicular joints provide the mobility of the scapulothoracic mechanism. Movement of the glenohumeral joint provides between 90° (active) and 120° (passive) elevation. For full elevation of the arm, scapular rotation, clavicular elevation, and thoracic extension must accompany humeral elevation. During ipsilateral elevation the upper thoracic vertebrae must be able to extend, rotate, and sidebend to the ipsilateral side, while the lower thoracic vertebrae must sidebend away from the side of motion. For full vertical eleva-

tion, exaggeration of lumbar lordosis becomes necessary and is achieved by the action of the spinal muscles.[120]

Although the joints act interdependently and in concert, we must discuss their structure and movement individually to understand their functions and significance.

Glenohumeral Joint

The humeral head, in the anatomic position, faces medially, slightly posteriorly, and superiorly. The head forms almost half a sphere, with an angular value of about 150°. It forms an angle of about 45° with the humeral shaft (Fig. 11-2).

The glenoid cavity faces laterally, forward, and superiorly. It has an angular value of only 75°. This incongruity between the humeral head and the glenoid cavity is partially compensated for by the fibrous or fibrocartilaginous glenoid labrum, which serves to deepen the glenoid cavity. The glenoid is pear-shaped—narrow superiorly and wider inferiorly.

Acromioclavicular Joint

The clavicle is S-shaped, the lateral third being concave anteriorly (Fig. 11-3A). This provides for extra motion during elevation of the arm (see Biomechanics below). The articular

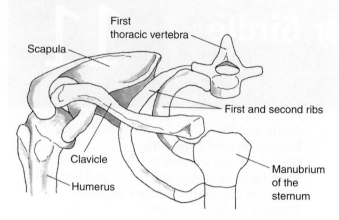

■ **FIG. 11-1.** Osseous components of the functional shoulder girdle.

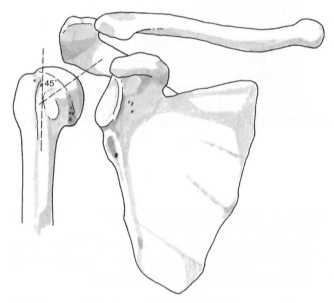

■ **FIG. 11-2.** Anterior view of the relationship of the bones of the glenohumeral joint.

surface of the clavicle is convex. The concave articular surface of the acromion process faces medially and somewhat antero-superiorly. This joint is oriented in such a way that a strong compression force tends to cause the clavicle to override the acromion. This is what occurs in an acromioclavicular separation, usually caused by a fall on the tip of the acromion.

Sternoclavicular Joint

The sternal end of the clavicle is somewhat bulbous. It is convex in the frontal plane and has a slight concavity antero-posteriorly. It articulates with the upper lateral edge of the manubrium, as well as with the superior surface of the medial aspect of the cartilage of the first rib. It tends to extend above the superior surface of the manubrium by as much as half its width.

Scapulothoracic Mechanism

The scapulothoracic joint complex or mechanism (Fig. 11-4) is not a true anatomic joint, because it has none of the usual joint characteristics. Movements are inescapably associated with the sternoclavicular and acromioclavicular joints. These two anatomic joints and the functional thoracic joint form a closed kinetic chain in which movement in one joint invariably causes motion in the other.

The scapula, viewed from above at rest, makes an angle of about 30° with the frontal plane (Fig. 11-3A). It makes an angle of about 60° with the clavicle, viewed from above.

The medial portion of the scapular spine usually lies level with the T3 spinous process, whereas the inferior angle lies level with the T7 or T8 spinous process. The medial border lies about 6 cm lateral to the thoracic spinous processes.

Ligaments

Glenohumeral Joint

The articular capsule of the glenohumeral joint (Fig. 11-4) is quite thin and lax, with redundant folds situated anteroinferi-orly when the arm is at rest. This allows a full range of eleva-tion. Because of the laxity of the joint capsule, the head of the humerus can be distracted laterally about 2 cm in the cadaver, with the arm in a position of slight abduction. With the arm at the side, the superior joint capsule remains taut, whereas the rest of the capsule assumes a forward and medial twist. The tendons of the supraspinatus, infraspinatus, teres minor, and subscapularis blend with the fibers of the joint capsule.

The glenohumeral ligaments provide some reinforcement to the capsule anteriorly, helping to check external rotation. The middle glenohumeral ligament limits lateral rotation up to 90° abduction and is an important anterior stabilizer of the shoulder joint.[134] The inferior glenohumeral ligament is the thickest of the glenohumeral structures and attaches to the anterior, inferior, and posterior margins of the glenoid labrum.[215,248] It strengthens the capsule anteriorly and inferi-orly, helping to prevent anterior subluxation and dislocation.[226]

The coracohumeral ligament strengthens the superior cap-sule and is important in maintaining the glenohumeral rela-tionship. Largely the superior capsule and the coracohumeral ligament counteract the downward pull of gravity on the arm. From the root of the coracoid process, the coracohumeral ligament extends to the greater and lesser tubercles of the humerus beneath the supraspinatus tendon. The ligament blends with the rotator cuff and fills in the space between the subscapularis and the supraspinatus muscles.[189] Tension develops mainly in the anterior band during extension and in the posterior band during flexion. The anterior band, running somewhat anteriorly to the vertical axis about which rotation occurs, checks external rotation and perhaps extension. The tension in the posterior band is thought to be a factor in assist-ing the glenohumeral ligament in medial rotation of the shoul-der during flexion.[24,185]

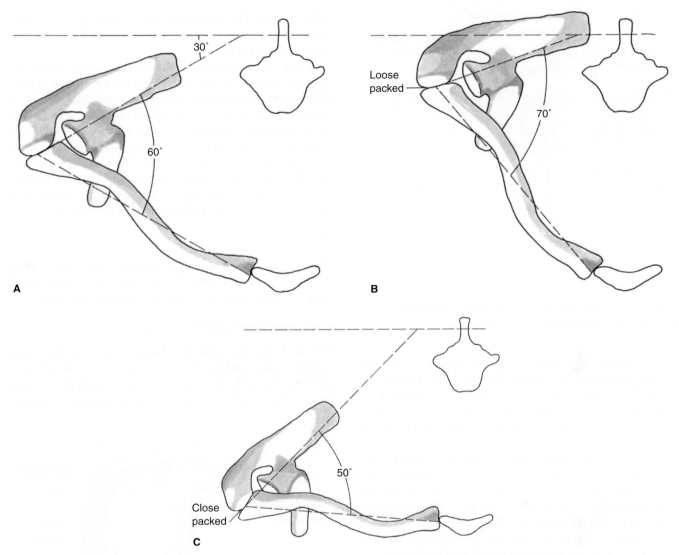

■ **FIG. 11-3.** Acromioclavicular, sternoclavicular, and scapulothoracic articulations shown at rest (**A**), in retraction (**B**), and in protraction (**C**).

The transverse humeral ligament traverses the intertubercular (bicipital) groove, acting as a retinaculum for the tendon of the long head of the biceps.

Acromioclavicular Joint

The major ligaments of the acromioclavicular joint (Fig. 11-4) are the superior and inferior acromioclavicular ligaments and the coracoclavicular ligaments. The superior and inferior ligaments offer some protection to the joint and help prevent overriding of the clavicle on the acromion. Although situated away from the joint, the coracoclavicular ligaments are of the most importance in providing acromioclavicular joint stability.

The trapezoid ligament lies almost horizontally in the frontal plane and is positioned in such a way that it can check overriding, or lateral, movement of the clavicle on the acromion.

It also helps prevent excessive narrowing of the angle between the acromion and clavicle (viewed from above), as occurs with protraction.

The conoid ligament is oriented vertically, medial to the trapezoid ligament, and is twisted on itself. It primarily checks superior movement of the clavicle on the acromion; it also prevents excessive widening of the scapuloclavicular angle. As the arm is abducted, the scapula rotates in such a way that the inferior angle swings laterally and superiorly. This movement increases the distance between the clavicle and the coracoid process, pulling the conoid ligament taut. This tightening causes posterior or external (backward axial) rotation of the clavicle, bringing the acromioclavicular joint back into apposition (because of the S shape of the clavicle). It is necessary for full elevation of the arm (see Biomechanics below).

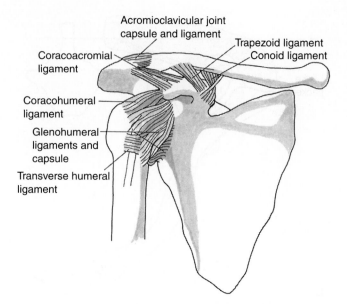

■ **FIG. 11-4.** Anterior view of the ligaments of the glenohumeral and acromioclavicular joints.

These ligaments suspend the scapula from the clavicle and transmit the force of the superior fibers of the trapezius to the scapula.[53] Anteriorly, the space between the ligaments is filled with fat and frequently a bursa. In up to 30% of subjects the bony components may be opposed closely and may form a coracoclavicular joint.[53,269]

The coracoacromial ligament, the acromion, and the coracoid process form an important protective arch over the glenohumeral joint (Fig. 11-4).[164] The arch forms a secondary restraining socket for the humeral head, preventing dislocation of the humeral head superiorly. This arch can be the site of impingement on the greater tubercle, supraspinatus tendon, or subdeltoid bursa in cases of abnormal joint mechanics.

Sternoclavicular Joint

The relatively lax sternoclavicular joint capsule is reinforced anteriorly by the anterior sternoclavicular ligament, posteriorly by the posterior sternoclavicular ligaments, and superiorly by the interclavicular ligament (Fig. 11-5). The costoclavicular ligament lies just lateral to the joint. Its anterior fibers run superiorly and laterally and check elevation and lateral movement

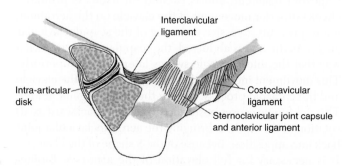

■ **FIG. 11-5.** Sternoclavicular joint.

of the clavicle. The posterior fibers run superiorly and medially from the first rib and check elevation and medial movement of the clavicle.

An intra-articular disk is attached above to the clavicle and below to the first costal cartilage and the sternum. It is especially important in helping to prevent medial dislocation of the clavicle, which can occur with a fall on the outstretched arm or on the point of the shoulder. Invariably the clavicle will break or the acromioclavicular joint will dislocate before the sternoclavicular joint dislocates medially. This is true despite the fact that the medial sloping of the joint surfaces and the superior overlap of the clavicle on the sternum would seem to make the joint susceptible to medial dislocation.

Bursae

There are usually considered to be eight or nine bursae about the shoulder joint. Practically speaking, only two are worth considering here, because of their clinical significance.

Subacromial or Subdeltoid Bursa

The subacromial or subdeltoid bursa extends over the supraspinatus tendon and distal muscle belly beneath the acromion and deltoid muscle. At times it extends beneath the coracoid process (Fig. 11-6A). It is attached above to the acromial arch

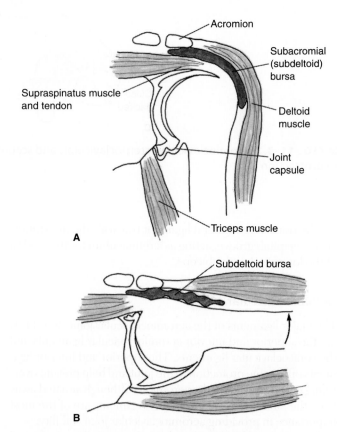

■ **FIG. 11-6.** **(A)** Subacromial (subdeltoid) bursa. **(B)** As the humerus elevates, the bursal tissue gathers beneath the acromion.

and below to the rotator cuff tendons and greater tubercle. It does not normally communicate with the joint capsule but may in the case of a rotator cuff tear. This is seen on arthrography as dye leaking over the top of the supraspinatus tendon. The bursa is susceptible to impingement beneath the acromial arch, especially if it is inflamed and swollen (Fig. 11-6B). Inflammation of the bursa is often attributed to rupture of a supraspinatus calcium deposit superiorly into the underside of the bursa.

Subscapular Bursa

The subscapular bursa overlies the anterior joint capsule and lies beneath the subscapularis muscle. It communicates with the joint capsule and fills with dye on arthrography. Articular effusion may be manifested clinically by an anterior swelling, caused by distension of the bursa (Fig. 11-7).

Vascular Anatomy of Rotator Cuff Tendons

The tendons of the rotator cuff include the supraspinatus, infraspinatus, teres minor, and subscapularis. As implied by the term *rotator cuff,* they are not discrete tendons but blend to form a continuous cuff surrounding the posterior, superior, and anterior aspects of the humeral head. The fibers of the tendinous cuff attach to the articular capsule of the glenohumeral joint by blending with it. This allows the cuff to provide dynamic stabilization of the joint.

The rotator cuff is a frequent site of lesions—usually of a degenerative nature—in response to fatigue stresses. Lesions usually affect the supraspinatus and to a lesser extent the infraspinatus portions of the cuff. Because such degeneration often occurs with normal activity levels, the nutritional status of this frequently involved area of the cuff is of particular interest. Most fatigue or degenerative lesions occur either from increased stress levels or from a nutritional deficit.

The primary blood supply to the rotator cuff tendons is derived from six arteries, three of which contribute in virtually all persons and three of which are sometimes absent (Fig. 11-8).[174] The posterior humeral circumflex and the suprascapular arteries are usually present; they supply primarily the infraspinatus and teres minor areas of the cuff. The subscapularis is supplied by the anterior humeral circumflex artery, which is usually present; the thoracoacromial artery, which is occasionally absent; and the suprahumeral and subscapular arteries, which are often absent. The supraspinatus region receives its supply primarily from the thoracoacromial artery, which as mentioned is not always present. This artery anastomoses with the two circumflex arteries, which also contribute some to the supraspinatus region.

The most significant feature of the blood supply to the rotator cuff is that the supraspinatus and to a lesser extent the infraspinatus regions of the cuff are often considerably hypovascular with respect to the rest of the tendinous cuff. This has been confirmed by injection studies as well as by histologic sections. Rothman and Parke[208] found that regardless of age, the supraspinatus region was hypovascular in 63% of 72 specimens, and that the infraspinatus region was hypovascular in 37%. When the infraspinatus was undervascularized, so was the supraspinatus. Hypovascularity was demonstrated in the subscapularis region in only 7% of the specimens.

Clinically, the relative incidence of tendinitis in these tendons correlates well with the above relative incidences of hypovascularity. Also, the incidence of shoulder tendinitis tends to increase with advancing age, which is consistent with the findings that tendon hypovascularity in general progresses with age.[174]

It has been proposed that the hypovascularity in the supraspinatus region is at least partly the result of pressure applied to the underside of the tendon by the superior aspect of the humeral head as the tendon passes around and over its insertion on the greater tubercle of the humerus.[153]

BIOMECHANICS

Joint Stabilization

As mentioned above, the glenohumeral joint capsule is relatively lax. This is somewhat unusual, because most joints rely primarily on their capsules and ligaments to maintain proper orientation of joint surfaces during movement and in response to external forces. The shoulder joint capsule does provide some stabilization of the joint when the arm is at the side, and it does help guide movement of the joint. At the shoulder, however, the muscles also play an essential role in these functions. The shoulder, then, relies on active and passive stabilizing components to maintain joint integrity. This is necessary at the glenohumeral joint because the incongruent bony constituents confer little intrinsic stability, such as that present at the hip joint.

When the arm hangs freely to the side, the superior joint capsule and coracohumeral ligament are normally taut, and

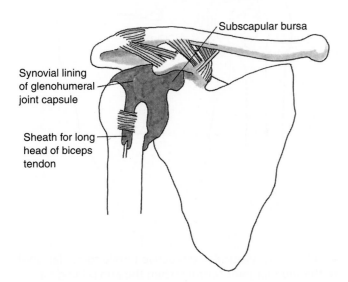

Subscapular bursa

Synovial lining
of glenohumeral
joint capsule

Sheath for long
head of biceps
tendon

■ **FIG. 11-7.** Subscapular bursa.

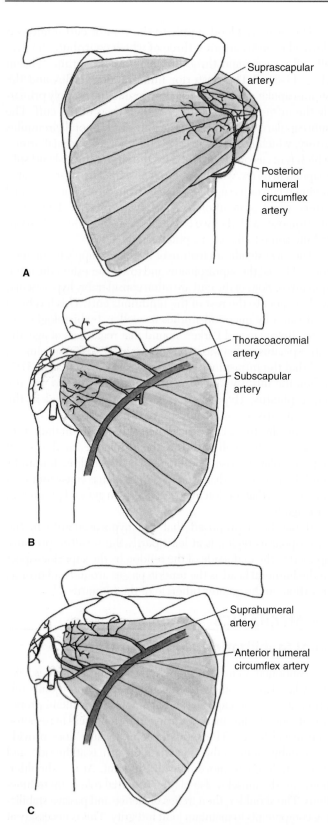

A — Suprascapular artery; Posterior humeral circumflex artery

B — Thoracoacromial artery; Subscapular artery

C — Suprahumeral artery; Anterior humeral circumflex artery

■ **FIG. 11-8.** Vascular supply of the rotator cuff muscles: posterior view (**A**), anterior view showing the thoracoacromial and subscapular arteries (**B**), and anterior view showing the suprahumeral and anterior humeral circumflex arteries (**C**).

the plane of the glenoid cavity faces somewhat upward. A vertical force produced by the weight of the hanging arm is met by a reactive tensile force to the superior joint capsule. The result of these two forces is a force that tends to pull the head of the humerus in against the upward-facing glenoid cavity (Fig. 11-9). In this way the tightness of the superior joint capsule and the orientation of the glenoid stabilize the humerus when the arm hangs freely at the side. Little or no muscle contraction by the deltoid or the rotator cuff muscles is necessary to prevent inferior subluxation of the humerus, even when some weight is held in the hanging hand.[15,16]

Once the arm is elevated from the side in any plane, tension is lost in the superior joint capsule so that it can no longer contribute to the maintenance of joint integrity (Fig. 11-10). Now the rotator cuff muscles, supraspinatus, subscapularis, and teres minor must contract to hold the humerus in a proper orientation with respect to the glenoid cavity during arm movement (Fig. 11-11). In this way, the rotator cuff tendons, which blend with the joint capsule, provide for stabilization of the glenohumeral joint when the arm is held away from the side.[15–17,53,108]

Clinically there are some common conditions in which these normal stabilizing mechanisms are compromised. The two common causes are alterations in the normal structural alignment of the bony constituents of the shoulder girdle, and rotator cuff muscle weakness. In a person with a thoracic kyphosis, the scapula follows the contour of the thorax and assumes a downward rotated position; the glenoid cavity no longer faces upward. Also, in this position the freely hanging

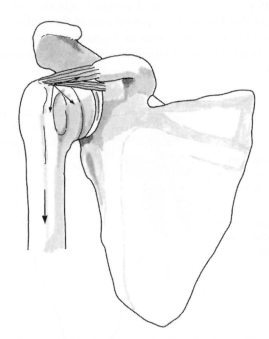

■ **FIG. 11-9.** Vertical and reactive tensile forces (arrows) to the superior joint capsule when the arm is hanging freely at the side.

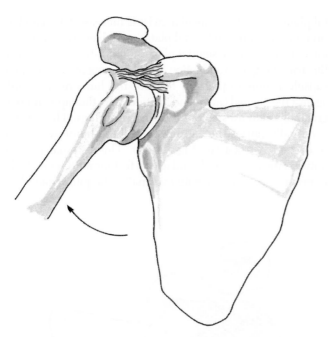

■ **FIG. 11-10.** During elevation of the arm, tension is lost in the superior joint capsule.

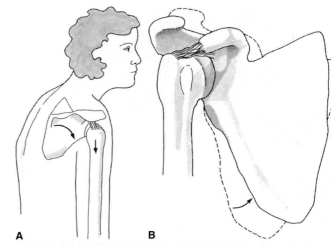

■ **FIG. 11-12.** In a person with thoracic kyphosis, the scapula assumes a downward, rotated position so that the glenoid fossa no longer faces upward (**A**), and the freely hanging humerus assumes a position of relative abduction with loss of tension in the superior joint capsule (**B**).

humerus assumes a position of relative abduction with respect to the scapula, and tension is lost in the superior joint capsule (Fig. 11-12). In this situation, the rotator cuff muscles must contract to maintain joint integrity with the arm at the side, thus preventing inferior subluxation of the humerus. Therefore, the person with a thoracic kyphotic deformity must main-

tain increased tone in the rotator cuff muscles to compensate for the loss of capsular stabilization. Thoracic kyphosis may be an etiologic factor in some cases of frozen shoulder. The increased tone of the rotator cuff muscles results in increased tensile stresses to the joint capsule, with which the rotator cuff tendons blend (Fig. 11-13). The increased stress to the capsule stimulates an increase in collagen production, which leads to a gradual loss of extensibility of the capsule—in other words, capsular fibrosis.

In the patient with shoulder girdle muscle paresis, a similar situation may exist; the weakness of the scapular muscles allows the scapula to assume a downward rotated position on the chest wall (Fig. 11-14A). The common condition in which this occurs is hemiplegia after a stroke. In these patients, rotator cuff muscle activity may also be reduced, and the arm is predisposed to inferior subluxation because of the loss of active and passive stabilizing components (Fig. 11-14B).

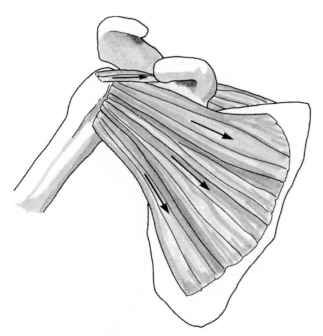

■ **FIG. 11-11.** Rotator cuff muscles contract to hold the humerus in proper orientation with respect to the glenoid during movement of the arm.

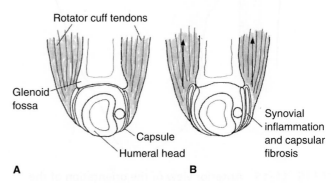

Rotator cuff tendons

Glenoid fossa

Capsule

Humeral head

Synovial inflammation and capsular fibrosis

A   **B**

■ **FIG. 11-13.** Transverse section of the glenohumeral joint depicting normal (**A**) and increased (**B**) cuff tension.

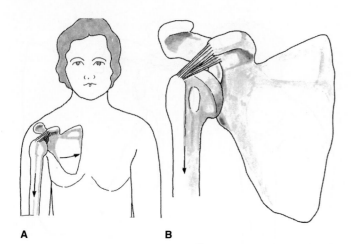

■ FIG. 11-14. In the person with shoulder girdle muscle paresis, the scapula assumes a downward, rotated position on the chest wall (**A**), and reduced rotator cuff tension predisposes to inferior subluxation (**B**).

Influence of Glenohumeral Joint Capsule on Movement

The orientation and configuration of the shoulder joint capsule play a major role in determining the degree and type of movement that occur at the joint. When the arm hangs freely to the side, the fibers of the joint capsule are oriented in a forward and medial twist (Fig. 11-15).[116] Because the plane of the scapula is oriented midway between the frontal and sagittal planes,[134,198] this capsular twist is increased with abduction (elevation in the frontal plane) and decreased with flexion (elevation in the sagittal plane; Fig. 11-16).[134,198] Thus, as the arm swings into abduction, the increasing twist in the joint capsule begins to pull the head of the humerus in tightly against the glenoid cavity, and the tension in the capsular fibers gradually increases as the twisting continues. The tension eventually causes the capsule to pull the humerus around into external rotation (Fig. 11-17). This external rotation untwists the joint capsule and allows further movement. If the humerus were not to rotate externally, the joint would lock

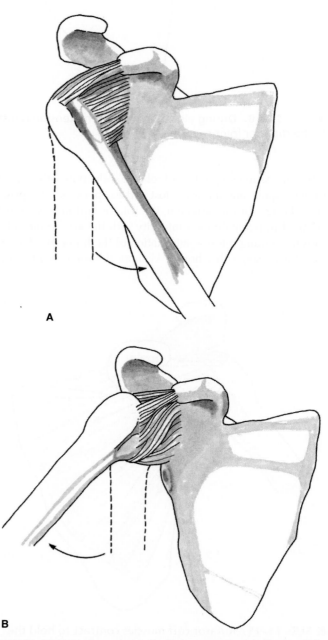

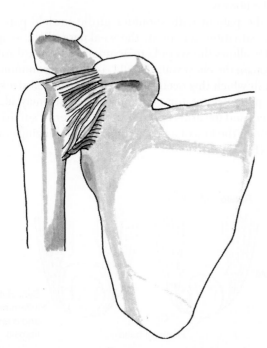

■ FIG. 11-15. Anterior view of the orientation of the fibers of the joint capsule when the arm hangs freely at the side.

■ FIG. 11-16. Capsular twist is decreased with flexion (**A**) and increased with abduction (**B**).

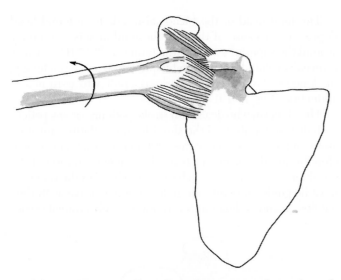

■ **FIG. 11-17.** Capsular pull results in external rotation of the humerus and "untwisting" of the capsule during abduction.

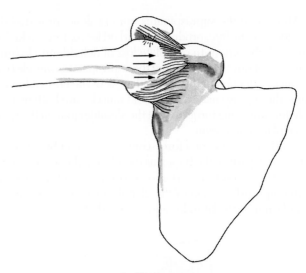

■ **FIG. 11-18.** Locking of the joint and impingement of the greater tubercle results if lateral humeral rotation does not occur during abduction.

at the midrange of abduction from the combined effects of abnormal compression of joint surfaces and excessive tension on the capsular fibers. The external rotation that occurs also causes the greater tubercle to clear the coracoacromial arch during abduction.[46,108,148] In this way, the external rotation of the humerus that takes place during abduction is a passive phenomenon, occurring as a result of the twisted configuration of the glenohumeral joint capsule, combined with the fact that abduction involves movement out of the plane of the scapula in a direction that tends to increase the twist. If lateral rotation does not occur, full movement is restricted because the joint locks and the greater tubercle impinges on the acromial arch (Fig. 11-18).

A common condition in which external rotation of the humerus becomes restricted is frozen shoulder. With capsular fibrosis at the shoulder, the anterior joint capsule becomes especially tight. The capsule adheres to the anterior aspect of the humeral head, whereas the redundant folds of the capsule situated anteroinferiorly adhere to one another.[170] In the presence of capsular tightness at the shoulder, abduction is restricted by locking and impingement; this movement should not be forced until external rotation is gained.

Muscular Force-Couple

The rotator cuff muscles act with the deltoid muscle in a force-couple mechanism during elevation to guide the humerus in its movement on the glenoid cavity.[55,108,148,201,207] The force of elevation, together with active inward and downward pull of the short rotator muscles, establishes the muscle force-couple necessary for limb elevation. When the arm is by the side, the direction of the deltoid muscle force is upward and outward with respect to the humerus, whereas the force of the infraspinatus, teres minor, and subscapularis is inward and down-

ward. The force of the deltoid muscle, acting below the center of rotation, is opposite that of the force of the three rotator muscles applied above the center of rotation and produces a powerful force-couple.[20]

Some anatomists consider the primary function of the supraspinatus muscle to be only the initiation of abduction, thus necessitating contraction of the rotator cuff muscle for the arm to be swung from the side. However, Howell and associates have observed that in the shoulder with a paralyzed supraspinatus muscle, the deltoid can initiate and generate a significant torque from 0° to 30° elevation in the plane of the scapula.[106]

For the glenohumeral joint to be stable and functional within its range, the muscles must generate sufficient force throughout the entire range. The deltoid is well suited in two ways to fulfill this need. First, the muscle fibers are in a multipennate arrangement.[96] Functionally, this means there is less change in length of each fiber while providing maximal force during contraction. For a muscle to be powerful, it must develop maximal tension over the range as quickly as possible. This is accomplished better in a multipennate arrangement. Therefore, multipennate muscles are more powerful than muscles with parallel fibers. The second reason why the deltoid is well designed to provide stability to the glenohumeral joint is related to its attachments. Arising from the scapular spine, acromial arch, and clavicle, the deltoid has a broad base and a large muscle mass. More importantly, the origins can be raised during humeral elevation. This scapular rotation decreases the range over which the deltoid must contract during humeral elevation, which in turn increases muscle power throughout the entire range. The combination of the multipennate design and movable origin is of considerable functional advantage for the deltoid and glenohumeral joints.[52]

Absence of the supraspinatus muscle alone, provided the shoulder is pain-free, produces a marked loss of force in higher ranges of abduction. In complete loss of deltoid muscle function, the rotator cuff (including the supraspinatus muscle) can produce abduction of the arm with 50% of the normal force.[20] Thus, the supraspinatus and deltoid muscles are both responsible for producing torque about the shoulder joint in the functional planes of motion.

Another example of a force-couple is the combined action of the three parts of the trapezius muscle and the serratus anterior.[151] The serratus acts as a force-couple with the trapezius during upward rotation of the glenoid fossa by tr°acking the scapula anteriorly, laterally, and superiorly.[46]

The long head of the biceps also aids in humeral head depression because of the way the tendon acts as a pulley around the superior aspect of the humerus.[108,148] If the arm is externally rotated so that the bicipital groove faces laterally, the long head of the biceps works as a pulley to assist in arm abduction (Fig. 11-19).

The clinician who deals with stroke patients, or any patient with diffuse paralysis of the shoulder musculature, must be aware of the importance of the rotator cuff muscles in guiding glenohumeral movement. If passive range of motion of the shoulder is performed in such cases, the head of the humerus must be guided into inferior glide (depression) passively during flexion and abduction. If it is not, the subacromial tissues

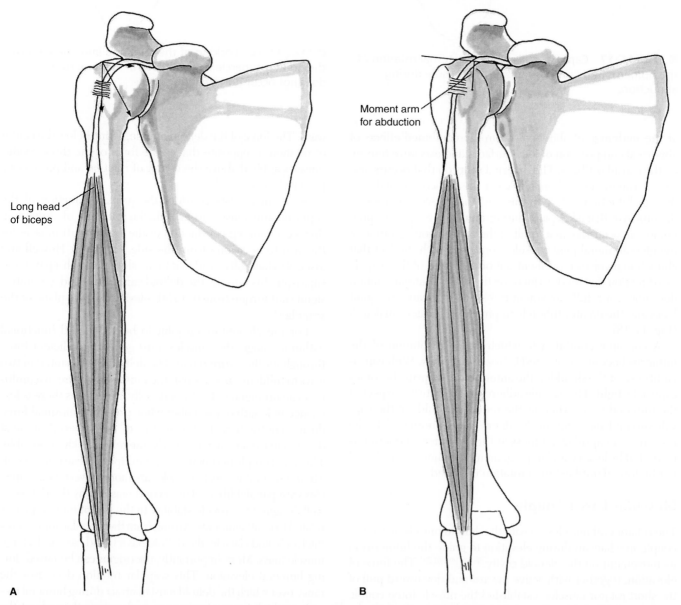

Long head of biceps

Moment arm for abduction

A

B

■ **FIG. 11-19.** Long head of the biceps acts in the muscular force-couple to create vertical and reactive tensile forces (**A**) and moment arm during humeral elevation (**B**). The increasing medial twist is a result of medial conjunct rotation from movement of the humerus around the medial axis as defined at the beginning of movement. This occurs because abduction is an impure swing in which the humerus moves out of the plane of the scapula.

may be subjected to repeated trauma. This may explain the onset of shoulder pain in many of these patients as sensation to the shoulder returns. It also emphasizes that "routine" range of motion must be performed by a skilled professional.[169]

Analysis of Shoulder Abduction

When we consider function at the shoulder, we must be concerned with the contribution of several joints in addition to the glenohumeral articulation. These include the acromioclavicular joint, the sternoclavicular joint, the articulation between the scapula and the thorax, the joints of the lower cervical and upper thoracic spine, and the articulation between the coracoacromial arch and the subacromial tissues. An analysis of the function of each of these structures during abduction of the arm emphasizes the importance of a normal interplay between the components of the shoulder complex.

During the first 15 to 30° abduction, much of the movement occurs at the glenohumeral joint, although this varies among people.[76,108,146] During this early phase, the muscles controlling the scapula contract to stabilize the scapula against the chest wall, preparing it for subsequent movement. Because the glenohumeral joint capsule is twisted forward and medially at the starting position, and because abduction is a movement of the humerus out of the plane of the scapula, the medial twist of the capsule begins to increase as abduction proceeds.[116]°

Beginning at 15 to 30° abduction, the scapula begins to move to contribute to arm elevation. In doing so, it moves forward, elevates, and rotates upward on the chest wall. Much of this movement of the scapula can occur because of movement at the sternoclavicular joint; the clavicle protracts about 30°, elevates about 30°, and rotates backward around its long axis about 50°.[56,108,178] The acromioclavicular joint contributes much less to scapular movement because its planar joint surfaces do not allow much angular movement. The scapula rotates some at the acromioclavicular joint at the beginning of scapular movement. Viewed from above, the angle between the scapula and clavicle narrows as the scapula slides around and forward on the chest wall (Fig. 11-3C). The rotation that the scapula undergoes in the frontal plane, with respect to the clavicle, causes the conoid ligament to tighten. Because this ligament attaches to the backside of the clavicle, as it pulls tight, it pulls the clavicle into a backward axial rotation. As the angle between the scapula and clavicle narrows (as viewed from above), the joint close-packs quite early. However, because the clavicle rotates axially and because it is S-shaped, the joint surfaces maintain a more constant relationship than they would otherwise. Furthermore, less movement is required of the acromioclavicular joint because of this axial rotation and the shape of the clavicle (Fig. 11-20). Thus, of the roughly 60° that scapular movement contributes to arm

---

° The increasing medial twist is a result of medial conjunct rotation from movement of the humerus around the medial axis as defined at the beginning of movement. This occurs because abduction is an impure swing in which the humerus moves out of the plane of the scapula.

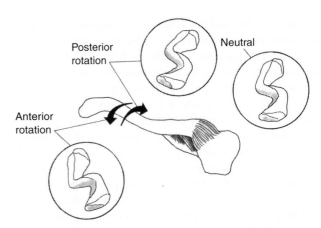

■ **FIG. 11-20.** Clavicular rotation in the sagittal plane, as viewed from the proximal end of the clavicle and the frontal plane.

elevation, about 30° occurs at the sternoclavicular joint, and the rest occurs from the combined effects of clavicular rotation, which causes the clavicular joint surface to face upward, and the movement that occurs at the acromioclavicular joint.

From 15 to 30° abduction, the humerus continues to elevate with respect to the scapula through a total of 90 to 110°.[19,76,108,148] The humerus contributes about 10° of movement for every 5° contributed by scapular motion. As the humerus elevates, the greater tubercle begins to approximate the coracoacromial arch, and the capsular fibers continue to twist medially. Once a certain amount of tension develops in the joint capsule, the capsule pulls the humerus around into a lateral axial rotation, causing the greater tubercle to be directed behind and beneath the acromion. As this occurs, the subdeltoid bursal tissue is gathered proximally beneath the acromion (Fig. 11-6). If the bursa is distended, or if the tubercle rides too high or does not rotate laterally, subacromial impingement will occur, with either loss of movement or chronic trauma to the subacromial tissues, or both.

The combined glenohumeral and scapular movements contribute about 160° to the full range of abduction. The remaining movement occurs as a result of movement at the lower cervical and upper thoracic spines. If both arms are raised simultaneously, extension occurs at these regions. In unilateral abduction, the spine bends away from the side of arm movement. The contribution of spinal movement to the full 180° elevation of the arm is often overlooked. The person with a fixed spinal deformity, such as a thoracic kyphosis, cannot be expected to demonstrate full elevation of the arm.

EVALUATION OF SHOULDER

A general approach to the evaluation of soft tissue lesions is discussed in Chapter 5, Assessment of Musculoskeletal Disorders and Concepts of Management. However, there are additional concepts and techniques specific to evaluation of the shoulder region.

The shoulder and the arm are common sites of referred pain from other areas, such as the myocardium, cervical region, and diaphragm. Usually the history will suggest the origin of pain. If not, a scan examination consisting of active motion of the neck and all major upper extremity joints, with passive overpressure at the extremes of each motion, may be useful in reproducing the pain and suggesting the site of the lesion. In discussing examination of the shoulder itself, we assume that the physician's examination, the history, or the scan examination has localized the lesion to the shoulder region. The clinician's in-depth examination clarifies the nature and extent of the lesion so that treatment modalities may be safely and effectively applied; it also establishes a baseline for judging progress.

I. History
   A. Specific questions for shoulder lesions:
      1. Does the pain ever spread to below the elbow?
      2. Can the patient lie on the shoulder at night?
      3. Can the patient use the arm to comb his or her hair?
      4. Can the patient reach into a hip pocket or fasten a bra behind her?
      5. Can the patient eat comfortably with the arm?
      6. Does it hurt to put on or remove a shirt or jacket?
      7. Is it difficult to perform activities that require reaching above shoulder level?
   B. Site of pain. Except in acromioclavicular joint sprains, pain is seldom felt at the shoulder itself but rather over the lateral brachial region. It may spread to all or any part of the limb innervated by that spinal segment, from which the glenohumeral joint structures are primarily derived, usually the C5 segment or, in the case of acromioclavicular problems, the C4 sclerotome (see Fig. 5-7).
   C. Nature of pain. Common lesions at the shoulder tend to be aggravated by use and relieved by rest. Patients with capsular lesions give a history of painful limitation, especially with movements into external rotation and abduction. Patients with noncapsular lesions often present with painful "twinges" during various functions, such as donning a jacket or reaching above shoulder level. In acute bursitis, which is relatively rare, the pain may become quite intense and is often felt even at rest.
   D. Onset of pain. Except in athletic settings, a history of trauma does not accompany most common shoulder lesions. More often the onset is insidious, as in tendinitis or capsular tightening. In these, the onset is very gradual, whereas in acute bursitis, the patient notes a rapid buildup of pain for 12 to 72 hours.
   E. General health. The final set of subjective questions should consider the patient's general health, in particular disorders of the cardiac and visceral organs that may cause pain to be referred to the shoulder region (e.g., diaphragmatic irritation, cardiac ischemia, gallbladder problems, pancreatic disease).[26] Ask questions during the history taking regarding cardiac problems,

diaphragm or respiratory dysfunction, and chest or upper abdominal problems (liver, gallbladder, pancreas, spleen). Has the patient experienced symptoms of spinal cord compression, which are bilateral tingling in the hands or feet or disturbance of gait?
      1. During the physical examination, observe for normal respiratory movements and function. Diaphragm, lung, or respiratory problems can refer pain along the C4 and C5 nerve root. Also observe for chest or abdominal scars from a laparotomy, cholecystectomy, or previous heart surgery.
      2. Obtain information routinely regarding weight loss, drug therapy, neurologic symptoms, and dizziness. Dizziness is relevant when there are symptoms of pain, discomfort, or altered sensation emanating from the cervical spine where vertebral insufficiency may be provoked. Further questions about dizziness and testing for vertebrobasilar insufficiency are described more fully in Chapter 19, Cervical Spine.

II. Physical Examination
   A. Observation
      1. Posture of upper quadrant in standing position, noting the posture of the shoulder, shoulder girdle, head and neck, thoracic spine, and soft tissue contours around the region
         a. Does the patient hold the arm close to the side or across the chest?
         b. Does the patient tend to support the arm?
      2. Function, particularly dressing, and general willingness to use the arm
      3. Observation of the patient's attitude and feelings
   B. Inspection
      1. Structure. Observe the patient in a relaxed standing position for:
         a. Upper spinal curvatures
         b. Shoulder heights
         c. Bony relationships—acromioclavicular joint, acromion-to-greater-tubercle distance, sternoclavicular joint
         d. Position of scapulae. Note any winging of the scapula. Winging may be due to pseudowinging[75] (e.g., asymmetry of the bony anatomy, as in scoliosis), generalized neuropathy or neuropathy of the long thoracic nerve,[33,75,81,85,156,218,227] muscle injury or muscle disease[143] (e.g., muscular dystrophy), or voluntary winging.[227] This phenomenon, commonly seen in swimmers, is normal.[227] The most common cause of scapular winging is trauma or overuse injury of the long thoracic nerve.
         e. Rotary position of the humerus hanging freely at the side, as judged by the orientation of the epicondyles and antecubital space.
         f. Step deformities over the shoulder. Such a deformity may be caused by an acromioclavicular deformity, with the distal end of the clavicle lying

superior to the acromion process. Flattening of the normally round deltoid may indicate an anterior dislocation of the glenohumeral joint or atrophy of the deltoid muscle. If deformity appears when traction is applied to the arm, it may be secondary to multidirectional instability, leading to inferior subluxation. This deformity is referred to as *sulcus sign* (See Fig. 11-39).[155,178]

A specific abnormal posture relevant to the shoulder region is the shoulder crossed syndrome[111] where there is elevation and protraction of the shoulders, winging of the scapulae, and a forward head posture, which has been described in Chapter 7, Myofascial Considerations and Evaluation in Somatic Dysfunction. Other abnormal postures are also described in Chapter 7.

2. Soft tissues. With the patient sitting, observe for:
   a. Atrophy—especially over the shoulder girdles
   b. Swelling
      i. Anteriorly for joint effusion
      ii. Laterally for bursal swelling
      iii. Entire limb for edema, as from reflex sympathetic dystrophy
   c. General contours—note asymmetries
3. Skin (entire extremity and shoulder girdle)
   a. Color
   b. Moisture
   c. Texture
   d. Scars and blemishes
C. Cervical screening
   1. AROM
   2. PROM
   3. Quadrant compression tests
D. Functional movements. The shoulder complex plays an integral role in activities of daily living (ADL), sometimes acting as part of a closed kinetic chain and sometimes acting as part of an open kinetic chain. Usually three functional movements are used to predict the patient's ability to perform ADLs. Active functional movements concurrently test joint mobility, muscle strength, and willingness to move. The three functional movements are:
   1. Hands behind neck. Combined glenohumeral elevation, external rotation, and scapular rotation into the middle phase of elevation are required to complete this movement. This may affect a number of ADLs such as grooming, and activities overhead such as throwing and manipulating objects overhead.
   2. Hands to opposite shoulder. Combined glenohumeral flexion and horizontal adduction are required to complete this movement. This may affect a number of ADLs such as washing the opposite shoulder, manipulating objects across the body, and many sport maneuvers such as a golf swing or baseball pitch.
   3. Hands behind back. Combined glenohumeral extension, adduction and internal rotation, and scapular

distraction are required to complete this movement. Limitation of this movement may affect many ADLs such as tucking in a shirt behind the back, perineal care, fastening bra, or reaching the back pockets.

Other common functional testing of the shoulder and ADLs include eating, putting something on a shelf, and dressing. Other assessments may include activities associated with work or recreation. Often a numerical scale is used.
E. Joint tests. Selective tissue tension tests

Joint tests include active and passive physiologic movements and passive joint-play movements. Integrity tests for instability completes the joint tests and are described in the common lesions section on instability. For both active and passive physiologic joint movements, the examiner should note the following:
   • Range of motion
   • Quality of movement
   • Behavior of pain through the range of motion
   • Type of end feel and resistance through the range
   • Any provocation of spasm
1. Active physiologic movements with passive overpressure (sitting or standing)
   a. Observation
      i. Routine active movements of the shoulder girdle—protraction, retraction, elevation, circumduction, and depression
      ii. Detailed examination with applied passive overpressure at the limits of each active shoulder movement
   • Flexion and extension (observe the scapulohumeral rhythm posteriorly)
   • Abduction (determine whether a painful arc exists)
   • Horizontal adduction and abduction
   • Lateral rotation (arm at side with forearm at 90° flexion) and hand behind the neck
   • Medial rotation with back of hand moving up between scapulae
      iii. Note these factors:
   • Willingness to move
   • Limited range and what appears to limit it
   • Quality of movement
   • Nature of end feel
   • Presence of crepitus
   • Presence and nature of pain
   • Presence of a painful arc
      iv. For further information about active range of motion, the following can be carried out:
   • The movement can be repeated several times.
   • The speed of movement can be altered.
   • Two or more physiologic movements can be performed together.
   • Compression or distraction to the glenohumeral, acromioclavicular, and scapulohumeral joints can be added.

2. Passive movements (supine)
   a. Perform
      i. Flexion and extension
      ii. Internal/external rotation (with elbow bent and arm at 45° abduction)
      iii. Abduction (note painful arc)
      iv. Horizontal adduction
   b. Record
      i. Range of motion
      ii. Pain
      iii. End feel
      iv. Crepitus
      v. The response of symptoms to the active and passive movement to help determine whether the structure at fault is noncontractile (articular) or contractile (extra-articular).
      vi. Whether a capsular or noncapsular pattern is present. The capsular pattern for the glenohumeral joint is limitation of lateral rotation, abduction, and medial rotation.

3. Joint-play movements
   a. Glenohumeral joint (passive joint-play movements). Tests may be performed either in sitting or supine position. For most of the tests, the open-packed position (resting position) should be used (55 to 70° abduction; 30° horizontal abduction).
      i. Inferior glide (sitting; see Fig. 11-45*A*)
      ii. Inferior glide (supine; see Fig. 11-44*F*)
      iii. Lateral glide (distraction) with the arm at side (see Fig. 11-48*B*)
      iv. Posterior glide (supine; see Fig. 11-46*A*)
      v. Anterior glide (prone; see Fig. 11-47*B*)
   b. Glenohumeral joint play with active movement. These sustained mobilizations carried out with active movements are a development from Kaltenborn's[118] work and have been devised and fully described by Mulligan.[170] It is proposed that the mobilization with movement affects and corrects a bony positional fault, which produces abnormal tracking of the articular surfaces during movement.[72,170,192] An increase in range and no pain or reduced pain are positive examination findings.
      i. Mobilization with movement for glenohumeral abduction (Fig. 11-21). The patient sits with the arm at the side. The examiner applies an anteroposterior glide to the head of the humerus during active glenohumeral abduction.[192]
      ii. Mobilization with movement for glenohumeral medial rotation (Fig. 11-22). The patient sits with the hand behind the back. The examiner stabilizes the scapula while applying an inferior glide (longitudinal caudal glide) to the humerus at the same time the

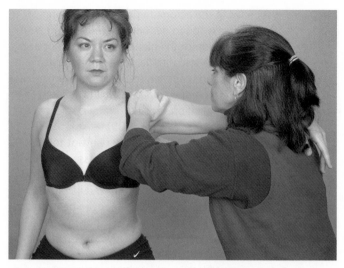

■ **FIG. 11-21.** Mobilization with movement for glenohumeral abduction.

patient actively rotates the glenohumeral joint medially.[192]
   c. Compare to other arm and record
      i. Amplitude of joint play (normal, restricted, hypermobile)
      ii. Presence of pain or muscle guarding
   d. Passive joint-play movements may need to include tests for the cervical and upper thoracic spine and the following related joints:
      i. Sternoclavicular joint (see Fig. 11-50*A–D*)
      ii. Acromioclavicular joint (see Fig. 11-51*A–C*)
      iii. Scapulothoracic mechanism (see Fig. 11-54*A,B*)

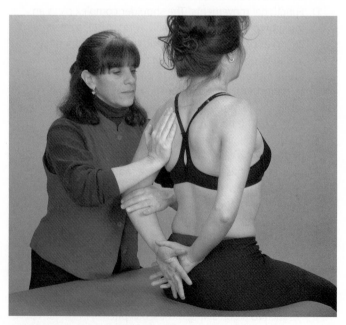

■ **FIG. 11-22.** Mobilization with movement for glenohumeral medial rotation.

Other joints apart from the glenohumeral and scapular girdle that may need to be examined to prove or disprove their relevance to the patient's condition include the cervical spine, thoracic spine, elbow joint, wrist, and hand. These joints can be tested fully (see relevant chapters), or if they are not suspected of being a source of symptoms then the relevant clearing test can be used (see Chapter 21, Cervicothoracic–Upper Limb Scan Examination). In addition one should consider evaluation of the kinematic chain as well.[130] The hip and knees should be assessed for any incompletely resolved injury. Lumbar flexibility, both in flexion and lateral bending, should be measured, lumbar lordosis should be checked, and trunk musculature strength should be evaluated (see below). Finally, the thoracic spine should be evaluated for kyphosis or scoliosis. Both of these conditions can alter overhead activities and may also disrupt normal scapulothoracic motion.

F. Muscle tests

Muscle tests include examining muscle strength, control, length, isometric contraction, and muscle and specific diagnostic tests. When testing for muscle lesions, it is more appropriate to test for resisted isometric movement first to determine which movements are painful, then perform individual muscle test.

1. Resisted isometric movements (supine)
   a. Strong isometric contractions with the arm close to the side (material in parentheses indicates tendons most commonly involved if test is positive)
      i. Internal rotation (subscapularis)
      ii. External rotation with arm close to side (infraspinatus)
      iii. External rotation with arm at 75° abduction (teres minor)
      iv. Abduction with arm close to side (supraspinatus)
      v. Elbow flexion (long head of biceps)
      vi. Forearm supination (biceps)
      vii. Others as necessary for differentiation of the status of the musculotendinous tissue
   b. Record whether strong or weak, painful or painless
2. Muscle strength. When indicated, strength should be estimated by means of standard manual muscle tests as described by Cole et al.,[47] Hislop and Montgomery,[102] Kendall et al.,[125] and Palmer and Epler[186] to determine exactly which muscle is at fault. This often includes positional strength testing as advocated by Kendall et al.[125] and Sahrmann[211,212] (see Chapter 5, Assessment of Musculoskeletal Disorders and Concepts of Management).
   a. Test of shoulder girdle elevation, depression, protraction, and retraction plus the shoulder joint flexors, extensors, abductors, adductors, and medial and lateral rotators should be included, as well as the elbow flexors and extensors.
   b. Neck musculature should be checked for whether there is any suggestion of neck pathology or stiffness. Greater detail may be required to test the strength of individual muscles, in particular those muscles prone to become weak, i.e., the deep neck flexors.[111]
   c. Evaluation of the trunk musculature strength should be evaluated as part of the kinematic chain of the shoulder and shoulder girdle.
3. Muscle control. Relative strength is assessed indirectly by observing posture and the quality of active movement, noting any changes in the muscle recruitment patterns, and by palpating muscle activity in various positions. Muscle imbalances around the scapula have been described by a number of workers[111,117,130,188,212] and can be assessed by observation of upper limb movements. For example:
   a. Performing a slow push-up from prone position. The clinician can observe for any excessive or abnormal movement of the scapula. Muscle weakness may cause winging of the scapula or the scapula to rotate and glide laterally or to move superiorly.[111]
   b. Analyzing shoulder abduction performed slowly with the elbow flexed. Observe the quality of movement of the scapula and shoulder joint. Note abnormal, insufficient, or excessive movements such as insufficient scapular adduction or excessive humeral medial rotation or anterior glide. Humeral anterior glide and pain may be more evident during shoulder rotation in the frontal plane versus the scapular plane.[212]
   c. Synchronous motions. Of particular benefit in visual assessment is the observation of synchrony of motion.[130,188] *Synchronous motions* refer to identical movements of the shoulder girdle complex bilaterally. It is best observed by having the client simultaneously and sequentially abduct to 90°, horizontally extend, and externally rotate the shoulders while seated. Smooth symmetrical motion in both ascending and descending phase should be observed. Asymmetry, which is usually noted in the descending phase, suggests weakness in the scapula force-couple. By observing the client from behind, one can notice asynchrony in such areas as (1) elevation of one shoulder above the other, indicating use of the upper trapezius to assist in abduction; (2) muscle fasciculations, indicating local muscular weakness; (3) oscillating movements of the scapula, indicating the inability

to fixate the scapula; and (4) excessive lateral rotation of the scapula during external rotation, indicating a tight anterior capsule, which limits external rotation.

Scapular stabilizer control and strength may be assessed by prone (see above) push-ups or wall push-ups, and "lateral" slide measurements (Fig. 11-23). These tests measure the ability of the scapular muscles to stabilize the thoracic wall in response to imposed load.[130]

4. Muscle length. Test the length of individual muscles, in particular those muscles prone to become short: the glenohumeral lateral rotators, teres major, the scalene (see Fig. 7-34), levator scapula (see Fig. 7-36), sternocleidomastoid (see Fig. 7–37), the pectoralis major and minor, upper trapezius, and latissimus dorsi (rhomboids; Box 11-1).[12,63,110,125,212,246]

5. Muscle bulk. Measure the circumference of the muscle bulk (if indicated) with a tape measure and compare left with right.

G. Neuromuscular tests. These tests may be performed if neurologic involvement is suspected, such as after anterior humeral dislocation or accompanying a cervical nerve root impingement (see Chapter 5, Assessment of Musculoskeletal Disorders and Concepts of Management). Included might be:

1. Dermatomes or peripheral nerves (see Tables 5-7, 5-8). Light touch and pain sensation of the upper limb are tested. A knowledge of the cutaneous distribution of nerve roots (dermatomes) and peripheral nerves enables the clinician to distinguish the sensory loss caused by a root lesion from that caused by a peripheral nerve lesion.

2. Myotomes or peripheral nerves. Cervical and upper thoracic myotome testing is shown in Figure 5-9. A working knowledge of the muscular distribution of nerve roots (myotomes) and peripheral nerves (see Fig. 5-8, Tables 5-7, 5-8) enables the examiner to distinguish the motor loss caused by a root lesion from that caused by a peripheral nerve root.

3. Reflex testing. The following deep tendon reflexes are tested:
   • C5–C6: biceps (Fig. 11-24*A*)
   • C7: triceps (Fig. 11-24*B*)

4. Neural tension tests (also known as the brachial tension test and upper limb tension tests).[35,36,67–71,86,119,126,157] Tests of neural tension proposed for the upper limb, upper limb tension tests (ULTTs), have been developed much more recently than those for the lower limb and trunk. Elvey[67] and the Western Australia Institute of Technology are continuing this valuable work. ULTTs are recommended for all patients with symptoms in the arm, head, neck, and thoracic spine.[35,36,157] Because methods of testing for movement of the cervical nerve roots or their sleeves are not yet clearcut and continue to be developed and

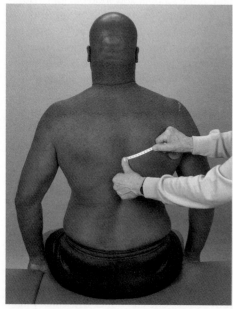 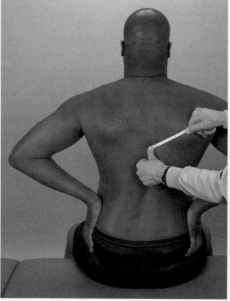 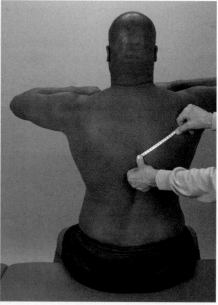

A   **B**   **C**

▪ **FIGURE 11-23.** Lateral slide measurements: Measurements are taken from the inferior tips of the scapula to the nearest spinous process. **(A)** Position 1, with arms in the anatomic rest position. **(B)** Position 2, with hands on hips (thumbs pointing posteriorly). **(C)** Position 3, with arms abducted to 80 to 90° and maximum glenohumeral internal rotation. This position places maximum load on the scapular stabilizers.

BOX 11-1   **MUSCLE LENGTH TESTS OF THE SHOULDER GIRDLE**

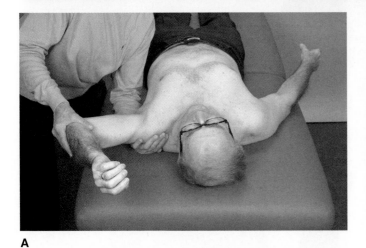

A

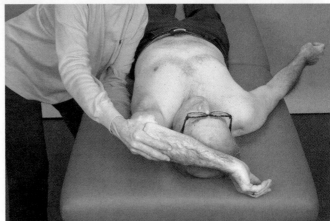

B

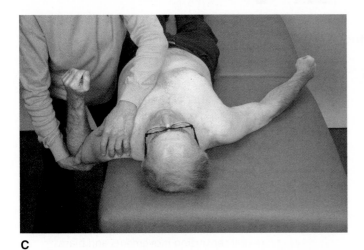

C

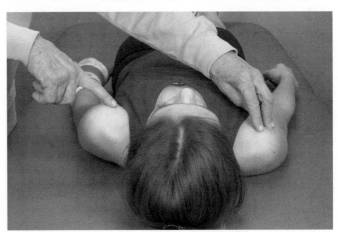

D

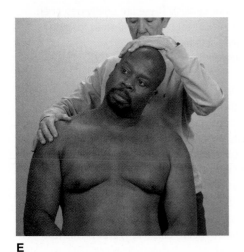

E

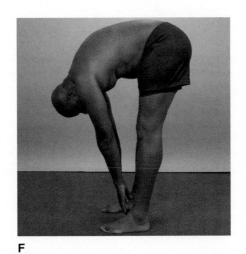

F

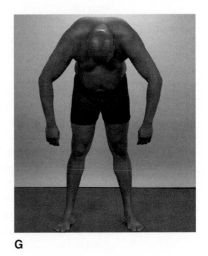

G

Muscle length tests of the shoulder girdle. Pectoralis major5: (**A**) Sternal portion of pectoralis major; normal range is 30° past midline. (**B**) Costal portion of pectoralis major; normal range allows the humerus to be 20–30° away from the ear. (**C**) Clavicular portion of pectoralis major; full range is 30° below midline. (**D**) Pectoralis minor: right, normal length; left, short, shoulder held forward. (**E**) Upper trapezius: normal range of motion is 35–40°. Latissimus dorsi and rhomboids (major and minor): (**F**) arms held back (latissimus dorsi tight) and (**G**) shoulder blades pulled together (rhomboids tight).

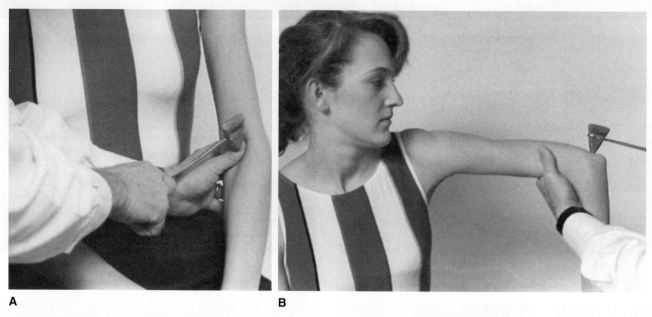

A   **B**

■ **FIG. 11-24.** Tests for upper limb reflexes: biceps **(A)** and triceps **(B)**.

modified, the reader should refer to the most current literature. The base test (ULTT 1) based on Elvey's original work[68] has been described by Hall and Elvey,[93] Butler,[35,36] and Kenneally and associates.[126] One variation of this test is described below.

a. ULTT 1. Neural provocation test biased to the median nerve trunk (base test).

   i.   The patient lies supine, with the examiner facing the patient. The examiner's inner hand maintains constant depressive force over the top of the shoulder girdle with a light and sensitive grasp. With the elbow flexed, the arm is passively abducted (about 110°) and externally rotated at the glenohumeral joint and supported by the operator's thigh (Fig. 11-25A).

   ii. While continuing to stabilize the shoulder girdle, the elbow is carefully extended and the forearm supinated. In an asymptomatic person the elbow can be fully extended (Fig. 11-25B).

   iii. Active wrist extension is added depending on the degree of irritability. If indicated, passive overpressure is applied first to wrist extension and then to finger extension (Fig. 11-25C,D). Normal response to this position is a stretch sensation over the anterior shoulder and over the cubital fossa and may be accompanied by slight or definite tingling in the lateral three digits.[86]

   iv. To impart maximal tension to the neural tissues, in nonirritable conditions contralateral and ipsilateral active cervical side flexion are added while maintaining shoulder girdle depression (Fig. 11-25E).

Symptoms and symptom changes must be identified after each step. This is regarded as the base test of the median nerve.[35] Additional motions that may be added to the base test include cervical rotation, cervical flexion, bilateral straight leg raising (SLR), and the combination of cervical flexion with double SLR.[91] ULTTs can be directed at any nerve. Butler[35,36] and others[86,119,157] have written extensively on this subject and have encouraged clinicians to use neural sensitizing movements and biases toward particular nerve trunks (median, radial, and ulnar nerves). These are briefly described below. Each test begins by testing the non-involved side first.

b. ULTT 2. Median nerve bias (Fig. 11-26). This test involves:

   i.   Shoulder girdle depression with approximately 10° shoulder joint abduction elbow extension

   ii. Lateral rotation of whole arm

   iii. Wrist, finger, and thumb extension
        If symptoms are minimal or no symptoms appear, cervical side flexion may be added (sensitizing test). The desensitizing test is cervical side flexion toward the symptomatic side or release of shoulder girdle depression.

c. ULTT 3. Radial nerve bias (Fig. 11-27). This test involves:

   i.   Shoulder girdle depression and abduction (10°)

   ii. Elbow extension

   iii. Medial rotation of the whole arm

   iv. Wrist flexion and lunar deviation

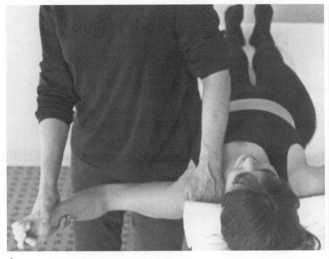

A

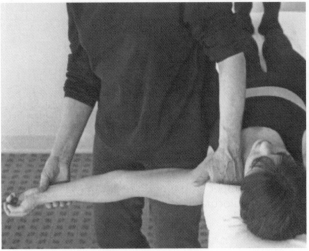

B

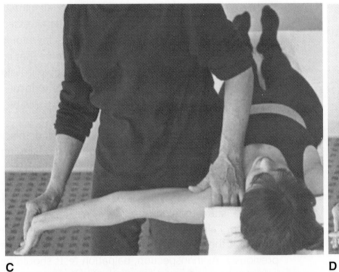

C

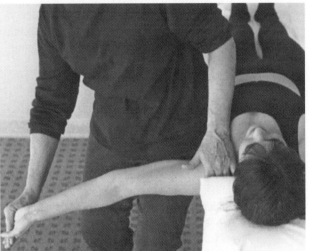

D

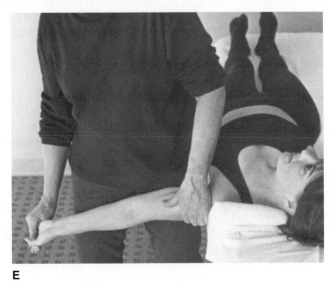

E

■ **FIG. 11-25.** Upper limb tension tests (ULTT) 1: Median nerve bias (anterior interosseus nerve C5, C6, C7). With the arm abducted and in about 10° of extension, the arm is supported, on the examiner's thigh, in external rotation (**A**), the elbow is extended and supinated (**B**), the wrist is extended (**C**), and the fingers are extended (**D**). (**E**) Cervical side flexion may be added.

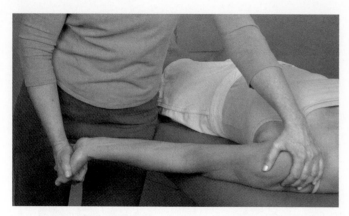

■ **FIG. 11-26.** Upper limb tension test (ULTT) 2: Median nerve bias (musculocutaneous, axillary nerve).

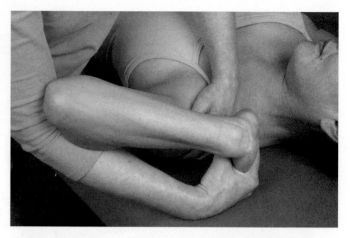

■ **FIG. 11-28.** Upper limb tension test (ULTT) 4: Ulnar nerve bias.

    v. Finger and thumb flexion
        The sensitizing test is cervical side flexion away from the symptomatic side or shoulder abduction. The desensitizing test is cervical side flexion toward the symptomatic side or release of shoulder depression.
  d. Ulnar nerve bias (Fig. 11-28). This test involves:
    i. Wrist extension and radial deviation
    ii. Finger and thumb extension
    iii. Pronation or supination (pronation more sensitive) of the forearm
    iv. Elbow flexion
    v. Shoulder girdle depression
    vi. Shoulder lateral rotation
    vii. Shoulder abduction (hand to ear)
        The sensitizing test is cervical side flexion away from the symptomatic side and cervical side flexion toward the symptomatic side to desensitize.

Before neural mobility testing, all joints moved during the tests should be assessed for mobility and symptoms. Muscles should not be placed in stretched positions that could confound the findings. When nerve irritation is present, the patient's response to local palpation or pressure on the nerve will be exaggerated.[119]

Additional tests for the ULTT include placing the other arm in a ULTT position and adding in either the SLR or slump test.

Note: When abnormal tension signs are present, treatment should be aimed at the neural tissue rather than capsular or muscle tissue.

H. Palpation. Palpation tests are usually conveniently performed at the same time as the inspection tests discussed previously. As in inspection, palpation tests should be organized according to layers, assessing the status of the skin, subcutaneous soft tissues, and bony structures. For further details see Chapter 5, Assessment of Musculoskeletal Disorders and Concepts of Management.
  1. Skin
    a. Temperature over joint regions and entire extremity
    b. Moisture and texture, especially distally
    c. Mobility of skin over subcutaneous tissues
    d. Tenderness, especially if neurologic involvement is suspected
    e. Texture
  2. Soft tissues
    a. Consistency, tone, and mobility of the shoulder girdle and brachial region
    b. Swelling. Joint effusion may be palpable anteriorly; bursal effusion may be noted laterally.
    c. Tenderness. Referred tenderness over the lateral brachial region accompanies most common shoulder lesions. Do not be misled.

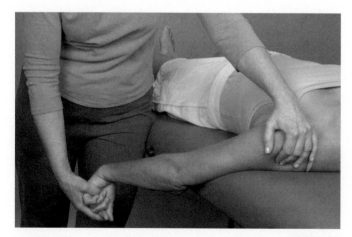

■ **FIG. 11-27.** Upper limb tension test (ULTT) 3: Radial nerve bias.

3. Bones and soft tissue attachments
   a. Bony relationships
      i. Acromioclavicular joint
      ii. Sternoclavicular joint
      iii. Acromion-to-greater-tubercle distance
   b. Tenderness
      i. Tenoperiosteal junctions of the supraspinatus, infraspinatus, subscapularis, teres minor, and biceps
      ii. Acromioclavicular joint
      iii. Sternoclavicular joint
   c. Bony contours

I. Special tests. Only those special tests that the examiner feels have relevance should be performed. If the patient's signs, symptoms, or dysfunction have not been reproduced, additional tests may include:

1. Locking test.[48,158] The patient lies supine with the arm initially at the side of the body. The examiner's forearm is used to stabilize the lateral border of the scapula, and the clavicle is stabilized by placing the supinated hand under the shoulder and over the trapezius to prevent shoulder girdle elevation (Fig. 11-29). With the other hand, the operator flexes the patient's elbow and extends the humerus on the glenohumeral joint with slight internal rotation. The humerus is abducted until it reaches a position where it becomes locked and further movement is impossible, resulting in compression against the inferior surface of the acromion. Normally this maneuver is painless. In some shoulder abnormalities the locking position may not be obtainable and may be painful.

2. Quadrant test.[48,158] The locking position is obtained as described above. The arm is carried forward by first relaxing the pressure on the abducted arm so that it can be moved anteriorly from the coronal plane. The small arc of movement that can be felt

during this anterior and rotation movement is known as the *quadrant position.* The humeral head is now unlocked; the arm and forearm are rotated externally and then brought up toward full flexion to a vertical position over the subject's head (Fig. 11-30), producing stress on the anteroinferior joint capsule. The degree and site of pain should be observed.

Overpressure is applied to the arm, moving it backward, which increases the stress on the joint capsule and compresses the acromioclavicular joint. The range of this movement in the sagittal plane should be noted. Patients with joint laxity demonstrate a pronounced forward movement of the humeral head into the anterosuperior portion of the axilla.

3. Supraspinatus tests
   a. Abduction in the coronal plane is accomplished mainly by the middle portion of the deltoid muscle and the supraspinatus. The patient's arms are abducted to 90° with neutral rotation, and resistance is applied to abduction bilaterally. With the arms abducted to 90°, the forearm maximally rotated, and the arms positioned 30° forward of the coronal plane or in the plane of the scapula, resistance is again given while the examiner looks for weakness or pain, reflecting a positive test result. A positive result may indicate neuropathy of the suprascapular C5 nerve or a possible tear of the supraspinatus.
   b. Drop-arm test.[167] The drop-arm test is used as an adjunctive test in the assessment of a rotator cuff tear, specifically of the supraspinatus. The examiner abducts the arm to 90° and asks the patient to slowly lower the arm from the abducted posi-

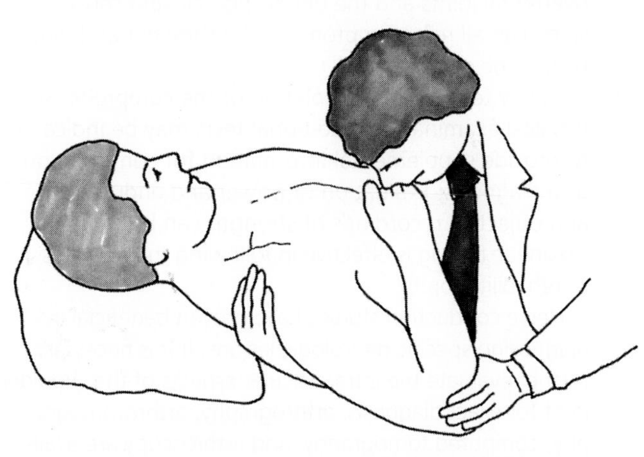

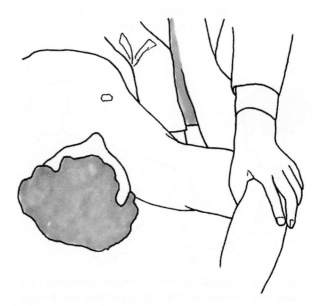

■ **FIG. 11-29.** Locking position of the shoulder causing compression of the subacromial physiologic joint.

■ **FIG. 11-30.** Quadrant position of the shoulder.

tion back to the side in the same arc of movement. A positive result is confirmed if the patient cannot return the arm to the side slowly or has severe pain when attempting to do so.

4. Impingement syndrome test. An impingement test is positive when pain is elicited by internal rotation of the humerus in the forward flexed position (horizontal adduction). The examiner flexes the arm (elbow flexed, forearm pronated) passively (Fig. 11-31). This maneuver tends to drive the greater tubercle under the acromial arch. The significant structures involved are the supraspinatus and the biceps tendon.[37]

5. Test for bicipital tendinitis. Stretching or contracting (isometrically) the biceps tendon may reproduce the patient's pain. Several tests have been devised to reveal involvement of the biceps muscle or tendon and the integrity of the transverse humeral ligament; these include the Yergason test, Lippman test, Ludington test, Booth and Marve transverse humeral ligament test, and the Speed's test.[19,99,145,149,268] There are, however, no data as to the sensitivity or specificity of any of these tests on patients with shoulder pain. The most important question when performing provocative tests on any part of the musculoskeletal system is "Does this maneuver specifically reproduce the patient's pain?"

   Speed's test is considered one of the more reliable tests.[155] The Speed's test or Hawkins and Kennedy's test is a resistive test.[99] The examiner palpates the biceps tendon while resisting shoulder flexion (with the patient's elbow extended and forearm supinated; Fig. 11-32). The test may also be performed by flexing the patient's arm forward to 90° and then asking the patient to resist an eccentric movement into extension.[155] Tenderness or pain in the bicipital groove is a positive finding that may suggest bicipital tendinitis.

6. Tests for thoracic outlet syndrome. Because thoracic outlet syndrome includes pain in the shoulder, spe-

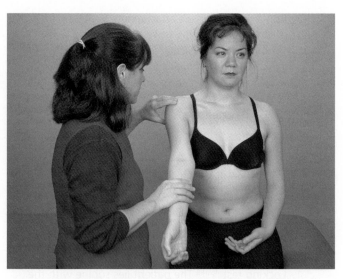

■ **FIG. 11-32.** Speed's test (biceps or straight-arm test). Tenderness in the bicipital groove when shoulder forward flexion is resisted (with forearm supination and elbow joint extension) indicates bicipital tendinitis.

cific tests should be used to rule it out; these include the Adson's maneuver, Allen test, provocative elevation test, and cervical rotation lateral flexion tests (CRLF; Box 11-2).[2,6,97,106,147,225,270] All of these maneuvers are provocative movements and postures that attempt to reproduce pain, paresthesia, a change in a radial pulse, or a supraclavicular bruit. The reliability of these tests have never been established, and it is now apparent that positive findings occur in many normal people who have no arm symptoms whatsoever.[213,231] Nevertheless, judgment of the clinical significance of a positive result may be made when one considers the speed of onset and the severity of symptoms during examination.[252]

J. Miscellaneous. Because the shoulder and upper extremity articulate with the thorax and spine, they function as a kinetic chain. Involvement of costosternal and costovertebral joints and the upper thoracic and cervical spine can all refer symptoms to the shoulder and may need to be checked.

K. Ancillary tests. After completion of the comprehensive physical examination, additional tests may be indicated to provide supplemental information for confirmation of a diagnosis. Evaluation of power and endurance and objective recordings of strength can be valuable. Isokinetic testing is effective in following the progress of rehabilitation.[263]

   Nerve conduction studies have proven beneficial in diagnosing specific neurologic lesions. If it is necessary to further evaluate the intra-articular aspects of the shoulder joint for exact diagnosis, arthrography, arthrotomography, computed tomography, and arthroscopy are available. Shoulder arthrography has been valuable for evaluating rotator cuff pathology.[46]

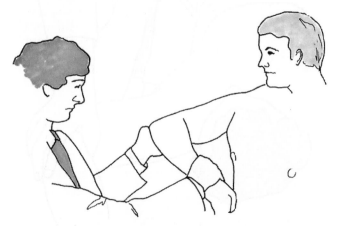

■ **FIG. 11-31.** Shoulder impingement syndrome test of possible involvement of the supraspinatus and biceps tendon.

BOX 11-2   PROVOCATION TESTS IMPLICATING THORACIC OUTLET SYNDROME

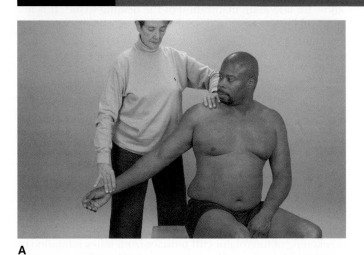

A

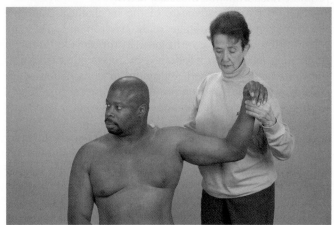

B

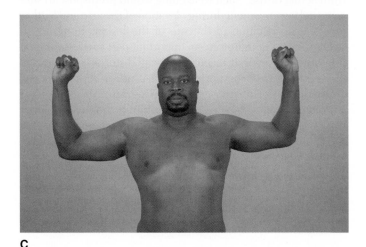

C

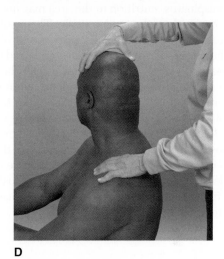

D

(A) Adson's maneuver, using abduction, extension, external rotation in association with a deep breath, and head extension and turning to the same side to elicit symptoms. This maneuver decreases the interscalene space and increases any existing compression of the subclavian and lower components (C8 and T1) of the brachial plexus against the first rib. **(B)** Allen test. Adson's maneuver but with the head turned toward the opposite side. Both the Adson's maneuver and Allen test assess vascular structures primarily and have a high incidence of false findings. **(C)** Provocative elevation test. The patient elevates both arms and opens and closes the hands 15 times. Fatigue, cramping, or tingling indicates a positive test for thoracic outlet syndrome. **(D)** Cervical rotation lateral flexion test. To complete this maneuver, the head is rotated toward the suspected side of dysfunction. The head is then bent toward the chest in a gentle fashion to assess the influence of the first rib as associated with thoracic outlet dysfunction.

COMMON LESIONS

Rotator Cuff Pathology

Rotator cuff disease involves a spectrum of pathology including tendinitis, subacromial bursitis, impingement syndrome, and partial and full-thickness tears. Overuse is an important factor in most cases. Partial tears are usually seen in young individuals, with total tears typically seen in adults older than 40 years of age.[8] In older adults, chronic tears can lead to

cuff thinning, degeneration, and finally, total rupture of the supraspinatus tendon.

Impingement Syndrome

The impingement symptom complex primarily involves the coracoacromial arch intruding on the rotator cuff, subacromial bursa, or biceps tendon.[37] There are three theories regarding the factors involved in the development of impingement syndrome: the mechanical-anatomic theory; the vascular compromise theory; and a theory proposed by Perry,[190] which implicates kinesiologic factors that limit scapular rotation or promote uncoordinated muscular activity.

Neer,[173] a strong advocate of the mechanical-anatomic theory, recognizes three stages of the syndrome: (1) a benign, self-limiting, overuse syndrome, (2) the development of thickening and fibrosis followed by repeated episodes of the first stage, and (3) development of bony changes, including spurs and eburnation of the humeral tuberosity, leading to possible complications such as rotator cuff tears (Fig. 11-33).

Tendinitis at the shoulder is common. It occurs in young active persons as well as in older persons, and about equally in men and women. In the case of a younger person it may be caused by activities such as tennis, racquetball, or baseball, which increase the stress levels to the rotator cuff tendons. In the older person it is more likely to be a degenerative lesion. Because of the relatively poor blood supply near the insertion of the supraspinatus, nutrition to the area may not meet the metabolic demands of the tendon tissue. The resultant focal cell death sets up an inflammatory response, probably as a result of the release of irritating enzymes and dead tissue acting as a foreign body.[56,153] The body may react by laying down scar tissue or calcific deposits. Such calcific deposits may be visible on radiographs; however, they are often seen in the absence of symptoms, and conversely, they are not always present in known cases of tendinitis. Superficial migration of these deposits with rupture into the underside of the subdeltoid bursa is thought to be a major cause of acute bursitis at the shoulder.[154] Because of the poor blood supply to the region, adequate repair may not occur, and the lesion may develop into an actual tear in the tendon.

The degenerative lesions tend to be persistent, with little likelihood of spontaneous resolution. The combined effects of poor blood flow and continued stress to the tendon do not allow for adequate maturation of the healing tissue. It is not unusual for a patient to describe a history of several years of constant or intermittent problems with the shoulder. This by no means should suggest that such patients cannot be helped, as they do respond well, and often dramatically, to the program outlined below.

Transverse friction massage is an essential component of the treatment program in chronic cases (see Box 8-1). The beneficial effects of friction massage in such cases are not well understood. However, it is proposed that an increase in the mobility of the developing, or developed, scar tissue occurs without stressing the tendon longitudinally (see Chapter 8, Soft Tissue Manipulations). This prevents the healing tissue from being continually torn again during daily activities.

A factor that may contribute to chronicity and recurrence is weakening of the rotator cuff muscles from reflex inhibition or from actual disuse. Such weakening would predispose to subacromial impingement during elevation of the arm and further mechanical irritation to the site of the lesion. Rotator cuff strengthening is, therefore, an important part of the treatment program. However, if recent or repeated steroid injections to the tendon have been performed, it is necessary to proceed gradually with the strengthening program. Although local steroids do relieve the pain by inhibiting the inflammatory response, they have an antianabolic effect on connective tissue, which may result in structural weakening of the injected tendon.[235]

The differential diagnosis of shoulder pain has been well documented in other publications, and specific conditions afflicting athletes have also been reported.[9,23,91,99,128,188,221]

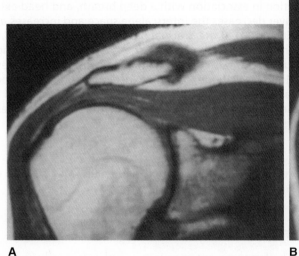
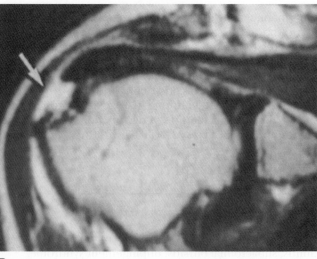

A   B

■ **FIGURE 11-33.** Magnetic resonance images of normal shoulder rotator cuff (**A**) and a complete rotator cuff tear (**B**; arrow). (Reprinted with permission from Esch JC, Baker CL: Arthroscopic Surgery: The Shoulder and Elbow. Philadelphia, JB Lippincott, 1993:31.)

According to Cahill,[37] the four types of pathologic processes most often neglected are glenohumeral instability, primary acromioclavicular lesions, groove syndrome, and quadrilateral space syndrome. Of these conditions, glenohumeral instability is the one most frequently confused with impingement syndromes. Treatment for impingement syndrome will not benefit the patient with instability.

I. History
   A. Site of pain. Lateral brachial region, possibly referred below to the elbow in the C5 or C6 sclerotome
   B. Nature of pain. Sharp twinges felt on various movements, such as abduction, putting on jacket, or reaching above shoulder level
   C. Onset of pain. Usually gradual with no known trauma. May be related to occupational or recreational overuse. May have been present for many months, or even years.
II. Physical Examination
   A. Observation
      1. Postural assessment. Observe the patient's posture, body type, and ability to move freely. Note postural deviations (i.e., forward head, rounded shoulders, flattening of thoracic spine).
      2. Shoulder girdle asymmetry
      3. Ability to achieve a more balanced postural position
      4. Biomechanical screening
         a. Antalgic movement patterns with dressing activities
         b. Functional use of upper extremity during gait
         c. Scapulohumeral rhythm
   B. Inspection
      1. Usually negative
      2. Some atrophy may be noted if chronic
   C. Cervical screening
      1. AROM
      2. PROM
      3. Overpressure
      4. Quadrant compression test
   D. Upper limb functional ROM
   E. Shoulder girdle mobility
      1. Active movements. Relatively full range of motion. Often a painful arc is present at midrange of abduction. There is usually slight limitation and pain at full elevation caused by pinching of the lesion between the greater tubercle and the posterior rim of the gleaned cavity.
      2. Passive movements
         a. Essentially full range of motion
         b. Pain at full elevation, but full range of motion is usually present
         c. May be a painful arc on rotation and abduction
         d. May be pain on stretch of the involved tendon (e.g., on full internal rotation in the case of supraspinatus or infraspinatus tendinitis)
      3. Resisted movements. The key test:
         a. Maximal isometric contraction of the relevant muscle will reproduce the pain.
         b. In the case of simple tendinitis, the contraction will be fairly strong; if an actual tear exists, it will be weak.
         c. The supraspinatus is the most commonly involved tendon.
         d. Others (biceps, subscapularis, teres minor) are rarely involved.
         e. Supraspinatus isolation ("empty can" position)
            i. Shoulder is internally rotated, thumb pointed to floor
            ii. Abduct the arm to 90° maintaining a position 30° anterior to the midfrontal position (scaption)
   F. Palpation
      1. Tenderness, usually over the involved tendon near its insertion. Soft tissue crepitus may be palpable in patients with degeneration of the rotator cuff and a bony crepitus in patients with osteoarthritis.[48]
         a. The supraspinatus tendon insertion may be easily palpated as the examiner stands behind the patient and places two fingers of one hand over the greater tuberosity.[48] With the other hand the examiner grasps the forearm above the elbow and passively rotates the arm medially and laterally, while also applying long-axis extension caudally. The normal tendon insertion can be felt to move as a firm cord under the examiner's fingers. At times a gap may be felt if the tendon is disrupted.
         b. The infraspinatus is best palpated near its insertion just below the acromion process and posterior border of the deltoid while the arm is held with the glenohumeral joint at 90° of forward flexion.[48]
         c. The tendinous insertion of the subscapularis may be palpated over the lesser tuberosity just medial to the tendon of the long head of the biceps.
         d. Usually referred tenderness over the lateral brachial region. *Do not be misled.*
   G. Special tests
      1. Supraspinatus tests (see above)
         a. Abduction in the coronal plane
         b. Drop-arm test
      2. Impingement syndrome test
   H. Muscle tests
      1. Muscle strength
      2. Muscle control
      3. Muscle length
   I. Neurologic tests
      1. Integrity of the nervous system
      2. Mobility of the nervous system
III. Management. The presence or absence of a calcific deposit, as demonstrated by radiographs, should not affect the treatment plan.
   A. Ultrasound
      1. Resolution of inflammatory exudates
      2. Increased blood flow to assist the healing process

3. May provide some pain relief, although persistent pain is usually not a problem
B. Friction massage. A key component of the treatment program
   1. Mobile scar formed
   2. The hyperemia induced by the massage may enhance blood flow to the area to assist the healing response.
C. Instruction in appropriate use of the arm
   1. Strict avoidance of activities that may cause impingement or tension stress at the site of involvement while painless scar forms
   2. Gradual return to normal use as healing progresses
   3. Restrengthening of involved muscles and other measures to restore normal joint mechanics

GENERAL GUIDELINES

In most cases of tendinitis at the shoulder, perhaps the only dispensable component of the above program is the use of ultrasound. In our experience, failure to institute any of the remaining measures appropriately increases the likelihood that treatment will be unsuccessful or that the patient will suffer a recurrence. The younger person whose primary complaint is pain during recreational activities such as baseball or racquetball must be advised that temporary abstinence from certain activities is an essential remedial measure. However, restricting activities to "resting" the part is usually not sufficient in itself to effect a resolution of the pathology, although the reduction in pain experienced may often suggest this. Usually, resumption of activities will be accompanied by a recurrence of the previous symptoms, because simply resting the part does not ensure the development of a mature, mobile cicatrix. This is also true for the older person, who may experience pain during normal daily activities. Although appropriate control of activities is necessary for resolution of the problem, it alone is usually inadequate. The use of friction massage (see Box 8-1), passive range of motion (PROM), and, perhaps more importantly, restrengthening exercises should not be excluded.

The therapist must, through a complete history, become aware of the patient's habitual daily activities. This is important because the patient often engages in activities that may contribute to the problem without actually realizing it. Such "fatigue" disorders typically result from the accumulation of otherwise asymptomatic stresses. Activities that particularly must be avoided are those involving repetitive elevation of the arm to shoulder level or above.

The importance of strengthening exercises can be appreciated by understanding the key role the muscles play in the normal functioning of the shoulder joint. As mentioned earlier, the supraspinatus is largely responsible for maintaining adequate depression of the humeral head during abduction. In the presence of a weak supraspinatus, the head of the humerus will tend to ride high in the glenoid during elevation of the arm because of the disproportionate contraction

of the deltoid. This would predispose to impingement of the greater tubercle, along with its tendinous attachments, against the coracoacromial arch. Thus, in cases of tendinitis there is a tendency toward muscle atrophy from reflex inhibition or disuse, and this is often a factor in prolonging the pathologic process.

The muscles of the rotator cuff are tonic and therefore highly dependent on adequate blood supply and oxygen tension. The key to rotator cuff rehabilitation is to provide a pain-free environment for revascularization of the tendons of the rotator cuff. Motion and strengthening exercises that are pain-free stimulate collagen synthesis and collagen fiber organization and neuromodulate pain.[3,261,266]

Remedial strengthening exercises are best performed with the arm close to the side to prevent the possibility of impingement and reflex inhibition during the exercises.

During the early stages of rehabilitation, isometric exercises may be performed with the shoulder in a neutral position after warm-up. *Warm-up* is an increase in body heat by active muscle use for the purposes of lowering soft tissue viscosity and enhancing body chemical and metabolic functions, to protect and prepare the body for more aggressive physical activity.[19,140] General central muscular body activity (e.g., calisthenics or riding a stationary bicycle) or local exercises (e.g., saw or pendulum exercises) may be used.[23,51] Active muscle activity is likely to be more productive than passive means of heating, because passive heating does not enhance the metabolic and cardiac factors, which are also important.[176]

The position of the shoulder can be altered in several ways to enhance the isometric strengthening of appropriate muscle groups at different angles and lengths in the pain-free range.[77] If pain from joint compression occurs, the use of manual resistance and slight traction to the joint as resistance is given is helpful. Ice is frequently used to reduce postexercise soreness, but the value of ice alone has been questioned on the basis of experimental data.[267]

A particularly useful rehabilitation approach is that proposed by Grimsby,[88] in addition to the regimen for progression of resistive exercises and repetition patterned after Holten's 1-RM (100% resistance maximum) pyramid (Fig. 11-34).[90,103] The initial goal is to facilitate tendon revascularization through isolation and reinforcement of high-repetition, nonresistive tonic cuff musculature activity.[88] The concept of unloading is an integral part of this treatment program. During acute inflammation, the weight of the arm alone is enough to aggravate pain.[223] Techniques for performing unweighted axial humeral rotation are initiated, progressing from 50 to 100 repetitions a day of simple pain-free, active internal and external rotation to three sets of 100 repetitions a day. An overhead pulley with forearm support may be used to unweight the limb (Fig. 11-35). Cumulative total repetitions should be 5,000 to 6,000. Abduction, followed by forward flexion, begins gradually in an unweighted environment. Axial rotation is again stressed in varying degrees of abduction and forward flexion. Once satisfactory increases in flexion and abduction have been

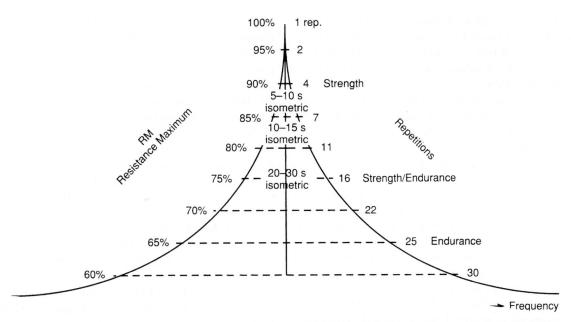

■ **FIG. 11-34.** The Odvar Holten pyramid diagram. (Reprinted with permission from Skyhar MJ, Simmons TC: Rehabilitation of the shoulder. In: Nickel LV, Botte MJ, eds: Orthopaedic Rehabilitation. New York, Churchill Livingstone, 1992:758.)

gained with the arm unweighted, active motions are started in a pain-free environment without irritating the involved muscle(s). This regimen allows the therapist to assess and treat any stage of muscle rehabilitation objectively. Rehabilitation of the scapular stabilizers begins simultaneously with that of the rotator cuff. Finally, sport-specific exercises may begin.

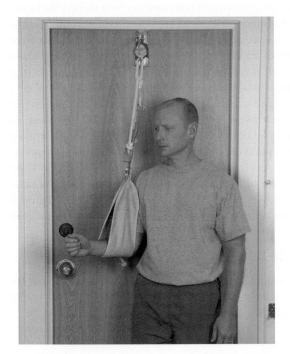

■ **FIG. 11-35.** Technique for performing unweighted axial humeral rotation.

This is a brief overview of this approach. The reader should refer to the works of Holten,[103] Grimsby,[88] and Gustavsen[90] to adequately plan such a treatment program.

As range of motion improves and healing progresses, the patient is graduated to isotonic exercises for the rotator cuff muscles with manual resistance, free weights, or elastic tension cord resistance (Isoflex exercises). Isoflex exercises are convenient, particularly for home programs, and effective, and they allow unlimited arcs of motion with both concentric and eccentric muscle training.[60,78,176]

To strengthen the supraspinatus, the patient should stand with the arm at the side and rotate the shoulder internally to pronate the forearm (see Fig. 11-80). Then, moving the arm in a diagonal direction of abduction, the patient should aim to achieve 90° abduction at 30 to 40° in front of the coronal position. This position aligns the muscle parallel to arm movement (in the plane of the scapula); in this position the electromyographic output of the supraspinatus is greatest.[115]

A strong rotator cuff assists in depression of the scapula and the humeral head in the glenoid during overhead activities.[127] It is therefore important to attain a strong rotator cuff before initiating shoulder elevation above 90°. Range of motion can be increased gradually as long as impingement is avoided.

From a functional standpoint, strengthening of the deltoid (particularly the anterior portion) is also important.[29,159] According to Matsen and colleagues,[160] the initial premise that the supraspinatus muscle is the primary depressor and is necessary for full shoulder elevation is incorrect. It primarily functions along with the other rotator cuff muscles as a head concavity compressor and stabilizer. *Concavity compression* is a stabilizing mechanism in which compression of the convex humeral head into the concave glenoid fossa stabilizes it against translating forces.[160] Even patients with massive tears of the supraspinatus can still fully elevate their arms. The deltoid plays the major role in elevation of the arm with active flexion and abduction in these conditions.[29,108,191]

Two other exercises important in the prevention of impingement are shoulder shrugs and push-ups with the arm abducted to 90° (see Fig. 11-76).[30] These exercises strengthen the upper trapezius and serratus anterior, providing normal scapular rotation and thus allowing the acromion to elevate without contracting the rotator cuff.

Shoulder elevation above 90° should be initiated with a D1F (flexion–adduction–external rotation; see Fig. 11-83) proprioceptive neuromuscular (PNF) pattern before advancing to a D2F (flexion–abduction–external rotation) pattern (see Fig. 11-84).[229] Rotator cuff dysfunction may result in both reduced humeral depression and external rotation.[18,32,40] Neer[172] has reported that the functional arc of shoulder elevation is not lateral, as previously thought, but forward. This results in the suprahumeral structures being impinged against the anterior part of the acromion when the humerus is internally rather than externally rotated.

The advanced phase of rehabilitation concentrates on the progressive return to normal function. In general, the patient continues self-stretching of the rotator cuff and inferior capsule as normal strength and endurance return. During this phase, exercises may be performed on an exercise machine (e.g., Nautilus, Universal). Free weights should be used until the patient can safely transfer to the exercise machines for resistive exercise.[30] Pool therapy can be effective for power and endurance training using PNF patterns with hand paddles facilitated by the isokinetic resistance of water,[76] and can also restore range of motion.[50,264]

Closed-chain exercises popular with the lower extremity[187,220] are useful in providing joint approximation forces that promote a cocontraction about the joint and provide joint stability.[45,58,183,230,253] Closed-chain training enhances static stability by facilitating compression of the glenohumeral capsule and stimulating joint receptors to provide static control. Traditional closed-chain exercises provide an external fixed motion apparatus or use the patient's body as the external resistance (i.e., basic push-offs [see Fig. 11-71] and push-ups [see Figs. 11-75A, 11-76A]), but the nontraditional closed-chain exercises advocated by Cipriani,[45] Dickhoff-Hoffman,[58] and Wilk[253] include the use of a dynamically fixed distal segment (e.g., dynamic push-ups on a Profitter [Fitter International, Calgary, Alberta, Canada] balance board or ball(s) [see Fig 11-76B], hand gait on a treadmill, and hand stair climber), requiring the shoulder girdle complex to function not only with great stability but also with great mobility (see dynamic stabilization techniques at the end of this chapter).

Although plyometric activity is primarily used for lower-limb training, it has an important place in training the upper limb.[78,177,242,256] Various types of throwing drills and catching activities are examples (see Fig. 11-89). Plyometrics are pri-

marily used in late-stage rehabilitation and functional pre-competitive testing after the injury of an athlete.

Total body fitness should be initiated no later than the early part of the advanced stage of rehabilitation. This program should consist of exercises to develop cardiovascular fitness, leg strength, and endurance.[165] This is especially important for athletes who engage in sports that predominantly use the muscles of the upper extremity but also require strong lower extremities. It is important to maintain the central cardiovascular system by general aerobic conditioning. A specific aerobic exercise to enhance the endurance of the upper extremity muscle group consists of sitting behind a stationary bike and pedaling with the hands.

Rehabilitation after surgical repair of the rotator cuff is lengthy and is characterized by slow progress. The surgical techniques are beyond the scope of this text but are well documented in the literature.[19,55,131,169,221,249] Rehabilitation requires an average of 12 to 14 months for an athlete to return to his or her level of activity before the injury.[48] General mobilization to restore accessory motion should be initiated after immobilization. Caudal glides of the humeral head should be emphasized to increase the available space between the acromion and humerus. A program of general shoulder strengthening, capsular stretching, and specific rotator cuff strengthening exercises should be continued as long as the patient uses the shoulder to any great degree in activities of daily living and sports.[30]

Many injuries of the shoulder can be classified as overuse problems resulting from repetitive stresses, with minimal abnormalities.[226] Abnormalities that represent deficits in strength, flexibility, or technique are often easily remedied through appropriate intervention by a skilled therapist.

The successful use of friction massage requires precision with respect to the site of application and the intensity or depth of application (see Chapter 8, Soft Tissue Manipulations). If it is impractical for the patient to be seen regularly for treatment, consider instructing a family member in the technique of application or instructing the patient in self-administration. However, application by a skilled, experienced practitioner is preferred to ensure that the appropriate technique is used and to monitor and document results accurately. As athletic activities or activities involving repetitive elevation of the arm are resumed, instructing the patient in self-administered friction massage before engaging in the particular function may be an important preventive measure.

Acute Bursitis

Acute bursitis is relatively rare and is thought to occur secondary to calcific tendinitis, in which the deposit migrates superficially into the floor of the subdeltoid bursa.[168]

I. History
   A. Site of pain. Lateral brachial region, possibly referred distally

B. Nature of pain. Intense, constant, dull, sometimes throbbing pain. The patient may present with the arm in a sling, or supporting the arm at the elbow with the uninvolved hand. During this acute period, very little relief is found in any position. All movements are reported to be painful.

C. Onset of pain. History may suggest a chronic tendinitis. The acute pain, however, usually arises during a period of 12 to 72 hours, with a gradual buildup of pain during this period.

II. Physical Examination

A. Active movements. Marked restriction in all planes with evidence of severe pain on attempts to elevate the arm

B. Passive movements. Restricted by pain in a noncapsular pattern with an "empty" end feel; no resistance is felt to movement, but the patient insists that movement be ceased because of intense pain. Rotation with the arm at the side may be fairly free, but abduction past 60° or flexion past 90° is usually not permitted because of complaints of severe pain.

C. Resisted movements. There may be some hesitation to perform a maximal contraction, with perhaps some pain on resisted abduction caused by squeezing of the inflamed bursa. When carefully tested, however, most contractions are strong and painless.

D. Palpation. Possibly some warmth and swelling of the region overlying the subdeltoid bursa; usually considerable tenderness in this area.

E. Inspection. Often unremarkable; possibly some visible swelling laterally at the side of the bursa

III. Management

A. Early stages

1. Resolution of the acute inflammatory process
   - Ice or superficial heat
   - Support of the arm with a sling to reduce postural tone in the muscles adjacent to the bursa, thereby relieving pressure to the inflamed area

2. Manual therapy
   - Soft tissue techniques to the shoulder girdle complex
   - Maintain range of motion. Gentle active-assisted exercises such as wand and pendulum exercises
   - Joint mobilization
   - Mobilization techniques as patient presentation dictates to cervical and thoracic spine and sternoclavicular, acromioclavicular, and scapulothoracic joints
   - Grades I–II glenohumeral joint mobilization to inhibit pain

3. Exercise and home program
   - Active assistive or AROM in pain-free range
   - Rest
   - Cryotherapy
   - Perform in pain-free ROM with low load, high repetitive format, inhibiting deltoid cocontraction to decrease excessive subacromial compression

B. Chronic stage. With the above measures, it is rare for the condition to remain acute for longer than a few days. The absence of pain at rest and localization of pain to the lateral brachial region characterize resolution of the acute stage. The patient can actively elevate the arm to at least 90° flexion or abduction.

1. Resolution of chronic inflammatory process. Bursitis at the shoulder and of the trochanteric bursa are, in our experience, the two conditions in which the use of ultrasound to provide relief of symptoms, in the presence of a subacute or chronic inflammation, will often have an unequivocally beneficial effect. The increased blood flow induced by the local heat apparently aids in a more rapid resolution of inflammatory irritants and debris.

   Unlike tendinitis or frozen shoulder, acute bursitis at the shoulder tends to be self-limiting during a period of several weeks. With appropriate therapy few patients have significant pain or disability 2 weeks after the onset of acute symptoms. However, because calcific rotator cuff tendinitis is often a preexisting condition, it is important as the acute phase of the bursitis resolves to test for the presence of tendinitis, the clinical signs of which may be obscured by the acute symptoms of bursitis. If tendinitis does exist, appropriate treatment measures should be instituted (see previous discussion on tendinitis).

2. Restoration of full range of motion, joint play, and strength
   a. Instruction in home range of motion procedures
   b. Specific joint mobilization (automobilization or passive movements) if warranted
   c. Instruction in home strengthening exercises

Bicipital Brachii Tendinitis

The most common cause of bicipital tendinitis actually results as a secondary involvement of the biceps after primary impingement or tearing of the rotator cuff.[213] Bicipital tendinitis may also be related to shoulder laxity, instability, or traction overload tendinitis.[260] The long head of the biceps acts as a humeral stabilizer as well as a decelerator of elbow extension. When there is increased translation of the humeral head with activity, more stress is placed on the biceps and ligamentous structures.

Injury to the biceps brachii often occurs from repetitive overuse during rapid overhead movements involving shoulder abduction and external rotation and excessive elbow flexion and supination activities, such as those performed by pitchers, racquet sports players, and swimmers. Possible causes of discomfort observed with ultrasound include subluxating biceps tendon, synovitis or effusion of the bicipital groove, cysts of the tendon, and mineralization of the transverse ligament.[265] The problems most frequently seen in this injury are anterior shoulder pain and chronic degenerative changes similar to those of the rotator cuff because of its long intra-articular course.[202]

Bicipital tendinitis may also be associated with a partial subluxation of the tendon or laxity of the transverse humeral ligament. Chronic irritation of the biceps tendon for a prolonged period, repeated corticosteroid injections, or a traumatic injury may cause rupture of the tendon and distal retraction of the muscle mass with a diagnostic lump in the forearm. Rupture occasionally occurs distally where the tendon attaches to the bicipital tuberosity on the radius with proximal retraction of the muscle mass. Distal ruptures occur in patients primarily older than 30 years of age.[94] Surgical intervention is usually required.

I. History
   A. Usually significant history of tendinitis (previous injection therapy) cuff disease, or impingement syndrome.
   B. Nature of pain. Vague pain and snapping in the region of the anterior shoulder joint, proximal humerus and tendon
   C. Subluxation or dislocation. Sensation of popping or catching during arm rotation.
   D. Rupture. Usually dramatic injury associated with a snap or pop
II. Physical Examination
   A. Active movements. Pain with shoulder internal and external rotation. In internal rotation, the pain stays medial; in external rotation, the pain is located in the midline or just lateral to the groove.[8] The possibility of a painful arc elicited with the palm facing upward at approximately 80° maybe present.[98,224]
   B. Cervical screening and upper limb functional ROM.
   C. Passive movements. There may be pain with passive stretching of the biceps in shoulder hyperextension with elbow extension and forearm pronation.[74]
   D. Resistive movements and special tests. Increase pain with resistance of shoulder flexion. The results of Yergason's test is positive. The test is performed by having the patient supinate the forearm against resistance; in so doing, pain is produced in the bicipital groove. Speed's test (Fig. 11-32; biceps or straight arm test) will also increase pain. If profound weakness is found on resisted supination, a severe second-degree or third-degree (rupture) strain of the distal biceps should be suspected.[22]
   E. Palpation. Pain in the bicipital groove. Tenderness and crepitus over the bicipital groove; the findings move laterally with external rotation or medially with internal rotation; anterior cubital fossa (distal rupture).
   F. Inspection
      1. Ecchymosis
      2. Palpable visible gap in muscle belly (complete rupture)
      3. "Popeye" deformity in proximal long head ruptures (distal movement of the muscle mass)
III. Management. Surgery for subluxation or dislocation: repair of the transverse humeral ligament. Rupture: tenodesis for all distal and proximal ruptures in younger, more athletic patients. In the absence of a rupture consider the following:

A. Initial: Ice, rest, and anti-inflammatory medications. Rest of approximately a week may be needed followed by gradual progression back to activity.
B. Friction massage to the long head of the biceps (see Box 8-1). This lesion responds well to deep friction.
C. Restrengthening the internal and external rotators while avoiding horizontal abduction. Shoulder elevation and elbow curls with the shoulder elevated with emphasis on the eccentric phase.[49]
D. Counterforce bracing to proximal biceps belly
E. Other measures to restore joint mechanics and maintain adequate flexibility

Glenohumeral Instability

Instabilities may be caused by either static or dynamic factors. Dynamic factors occur primarily as a result of rotator cuff weakness; static factors include damage to the anterior capsule, glenohumeral ligament, and glenoid labrum. Several classifications of glenohumeral instabilities are described in the literature. The degree of instability (subluxation or dislocation), the nature (voluntary or involuntary), and the chronicity are all important parameters that must be addressed in the rehabilitation program.[159–161] Shoulder instabilities may be classified as traumatic, atraumatic, or acquired. Matsen and associates[159,161] have provided useful acronyms for this classification. *T*raumatic patients exhibit *u*nilateral or *u*nidirectional instabilities, caused by a *B*ankark lesion, and usually require *s*urgery to stabilize the shoulder joint (TUBS). The second type of patient is the *a*traumatic, *m*ultidirectional unstable patient, usually *b*ilaterally involved, in whom *r*ehabilitation is the first line of defense; if conservative treatment fails, then an *i*nferior capsular shift procedure is performed, which tightens the inferior capsule and the rotator *i*nterval (AMBRII).

Burkhead and Rockwood[34] reported only 15% good to excellent results with conservative treatment in patients with traumatic shoulder dislocations. The success rate was 85% with the atraumatic patient.

I. History. The aim is to ascertain the degree (subluxation, dislocation), direction (anterior, posterior), and onset (traumatic, atraumatic, overuse). Considering the two main groups of instability patients (see above) allows us to better appreciate the variations in symptomatic presentation. The AMBRII patient presents with no history of trauma and describes symptoms brought on by certain arm positions or activities. The TUBS patient describes a significant injury causing a dislocation requiring reduction and often subsequent recurrent dislocations. With a subluxation, the patient may describe a feeling of the shoulder "slipping out of the joint" momentarily but going back into place spontaneously. Apprehension is a common feature in patients with recurrent dislocations or subluxation. It is important to determine the nature of the onset of the instability. In traumatic recurrent instability, the shoulder usually displaces anteriorly and rarely posteriorly; in the atraumatic group, multidirectional and posterior displacements are more common.[97]

A. The traumatic patient is asked to reenact the mechanism of injury to help clarify the body position and the stress placed on the involved tissue. This helps to determine the damaged structure and injury mechanism. The AMBRII patient is asked to demonstrate the positions in which the shoulder feels unstable. Anterior instability is usually associated with the externally rotated and abducted arm position. Posterior instability is manifested with the arm in flexion, internal rotation, and adduction. Inferior laxity is usually noted with axial downward traction on the arm, manifested by a sulcus sign.

B. Patients are asked routinely whether they can dislocate the shoulder voluntarily; determine whether voluntary instability is the predominant problem or whether it is just a minor facet of the shoulder going out involuntarily. The patient with atraumatic voluntary instability has no history of injury but can remember since childhood the ability to slip one or both shoulders out of place with minimal discomfort.[161] A general appreciation of ligamentous laxity can be observed with bilateral extension of the elbow and thumb to forearm.[21]

II. Physical Examination

A. Observation. In the sagittal view, note any anterior displacement of the humeral head. No more than a third of the head of the humerus should be in front of the acromion. Sahrmann's three-finger test may be used.[211] The examiner places the thumb over the head of the humerus anteriorly, the index finger over the acromioclavicular joint, and the ring finger on the posterior aspect of the scapular spine, and notes the relationship of the head of the humerus to the acromion. From the anterior view, note any step deformities suggesting an acromioclavicular dislocation. If the deformity appears when traction is applied to the arm, it may be caused by multidirectional instability (sulcus sign).[79,161]

B. Cervical screening and upper limb functional ROM

C. Joint-play movements are considered key tests for the assessment of instabilities. The amplitude of joint play (hypermobility) and the presence of pain and muscle guarding are noted and compared with the other arm (see Figs. 11-44D, 11-45A, 11-46A, 11-46B).

D. Tests for instability. Static instability may be assessed clinically by the anterior and posterior drawer test.[79] Anterior and posterior instability is initially tested with the patient sitting with the forearm resting in the lap and the shoulder relaxed. The examiner grasps the proximal humerus and gently presses the humeral head toward the scapula to center it in the glenoid, ensuring a neutral starting position (Fig. 11-36A). The head is first pushed forward to determine the amount of anterior displacement possible (Fig. 11-36B). The normal shoulder reaches a firm end feel with no pain, apprehension, or clunking. The humerus is returned to the neutral position and then pulled posteriorly to determine the amount of posterior translation relative to the scapula. According to Matsen and associates,[161] the normal shoulder allows posterior translation up to about half of the humeral head diameter. Increased posterior and anterior translation suggests multidirectional instability. A more rigorous test (fulcrum test) is to position the

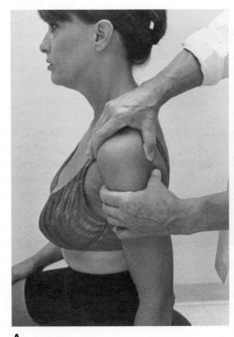
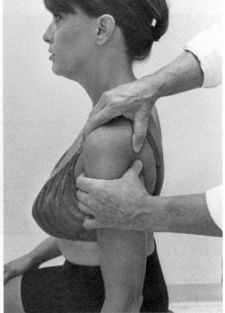

■ **FIG. 11-36.** Anterior-posterior drawer test: starting position (**A**) and end position (**B**).

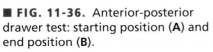

A   **B**

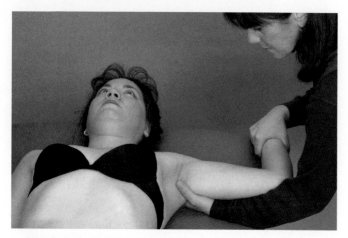

■ **FIG. 11-37.** Fulcrum test. With the shoulder in 90° abduction, the examiner adds lateral rotation and extension. This test is considered positive—indicating instability—if the patient becomes apprehensive.

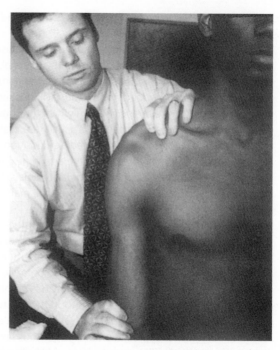

■ **FIG. 11-39.** Sulcus test. The examiner applies a longitudinal caudad force to the humerus. A positive test is indicated if the patient's pain is reproduced or a sulcus appears distal to the acromion, suggesting inferior instability of the shoulder. (Reprinted with permission from Kelly MJ, Clark WA: Orthopedic Therapy of the Shoulder. Philadelphia, JB Lippincott, 1995:253.)

patient in the supine position, with the injured shoulder over the edge of the table (Fig. 11-37). The arm is abducted to 90° and externally rotated, and from this position the examiner applies an anterior or posterior force.[161]

Numerous other tests are available to assess multidirectional instability,[203,209] anterior instability,[56,79,99,139,161,200,203,210,245] posterior instability (Fig. 11-38),[51,161,179] and inferior instability (Fig. 11-39).[79,161] The drawer test, however, has the advantage of eliciting evidence of capsular laxity without threatening the patient with dislocation. Clinical laxity testing has

shown that in a few subjects, the magnitude of translation for shoulders with atraumatic instability is essentially the same as that of normal shoulders or shoulders with traumatic instability.[160] Therefore, pay particular attention to the patient's response during the test and determine whether the test duplicates his or her symptoms.

E. Muscle tests should include strength, muscle control (a key muscle test), and resisted isometrics.

III. Management. The strength of the rotator cuff muscles is probably the single most important consideration.[177,228] Whether management is nonoperative or rehabilitative after surgery, strengthening exercises of the rotator cuff (see above) and scapular stabilizing muscles are critical to optimal outcome. According the Sutter,[230] conservative management should be based on immediate motion and strengthening. Several investigators have documented that the incidence of recurrent instability is not affected by the length of glenohumeral immobilization.[65,105,210] The scapulothoracic joint should be strengthened by exercising the muscles that control scapular rotation: the levator scapulae and the rhomboids (rowing), the serratus anterior (push-ups), the latissimus dorsi (pull-downs), and the trapezius (shrugging).[177]

Recurrent multidirectional, inferior, and involuntary instability is common in the AMBRII syndrome. Vigorous

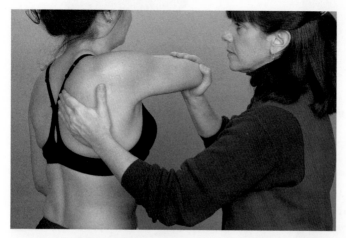

■ **FIG. 11-38.** Jerk test. With the shoulder abducted to 90° and medially rotated, the examiner applies a longitudinal cephalad force to the humerus and moves the arm into horizontal flexion. A positive test is indicated if there is a sudden jerk as the arm is moved into horizontal flexion and as it returns to the start position.

rotator cuff strengthening can ameliorate the effects of generalized capsular instability. The goals of instability rehabilitation are to strengthen specific muscle groups and more importantly to increase their sensitivity to stretch. Grimsby's three-stage program is particularly useful.[88,223]

A. Stage 1 begins with low-speed, high-repetition minimum resistance in the beginning and middle range of motion. This stage is meant to increase muscle endurance and circulation, avoiding overexertion.

B. Stage 2 involves increasing resistance and adding isometrics in the inner ranges of motion. This is designed to increase strength and sensitivity to stretch.

C. Stage 3 continues to increase resistance (usually 80% 1-RM) and adds isometrics through a full but not maximal range of motion.

Multidirectional instability requires comprehensive rotator cuff rehabilitation. When treating anterior instability, rehabilitation should concentrate on the internal rotators and adductors (pectorals, subscapularis, latissimus dorsi, anterior deltoid).[223] The external rotators and teres minor and major are emphasized for posterior instability.

The treatment program should also include exercises to enhance neuromuscular control (comprehensive stability and force-couple control), closed-chain (weight-bearing) exercises to facilitate cocontraction, and PNF diagonal patterns with or without the use of equipment and shoulder stabilization programs (see below).[10] Flexibility training and soft tissue (see Chapter 8, Soft Tissue Manipulations) and joint mobilization are included as necessary. Specificity regarding concentric or eccentric muscle function, aerobic or anaerobic energy pathways, and velocity of movement should be addressed in the final aspects of the program.

Scapular Impairment: Dyskinesis and Instability

The importance of the scapula as the base of support for the glenohumeral joint is well documented.[124,166,184,194–197,222,254] The scapular stabilizing muscles place the scapula in a position for optimal glenohumeral function and provide a stable base of support. Faulty scapular alignment and dyskinesis contribute to a variety of syndromes affecting the upper quadrant and trunk (cervical, thoracic and lumbar spine, and pelvic girdle). Upper quadrant diagnoses may include the following:

• Neural entrapment syndromes in the region of the shoulder girdle contributing to distal upper limb neuropathies
• Shoulder impingement syndromes
• Glenohumeral instability or hypermobility
• Cervical strain
• Muscle strains (i.e., middle and lower trapezius strain)
• General weakness from disuse because of muscle imbalances (i.e., upper trapezius dominance) or deconditioning[109]
• Altered length–tension relationships

• A variety of scapular syndromes described by Sahrmann (i.e., scapular downward rotation syndrome, scapular abduction syndrome, and scapular winging syndrome)[212]
• Adhesive capsulitis (see below)
• Thoracic outlet syndrome (see below)

Scapular faulty alignment and dyskinesis is very common in shoulder injuries. Very rarely is there direct nerve involvement. The most common cause of scapular dyskinesis is muscle inhibition secondary to some other pain syndrome such as glenohumeral disorder (rotator cuff, labrum, instability; see above).[130] Treatment of the underlying problem relieves inhibition and allows the patient to enter a scapular and shoulder functional stability program (see below). This may be done in coordination with treatment protocols for the underlying disorder.

I. History. Onset and progression will likely fall into one of two major categories: macrotrauma (i.e., paralysis of the serratus anterior after direct trauma to the long thoracic nerve) or microtrauma. The most common is microtrauma resulting from repetitive stress to the tissues, characterized by an insidious onset of symptoms. When microtrauma is suspected, the clinician must identify the patient's daily activities and postures to determine both intrinsic and extrinsic factors that may contribute to the problem.

A. Intrinsic factors. Physical characteristics that predispose the individual to microtrauma such as malalignment, anatomic variations, age, flexibility, endurance, and muscle strength and length.[7,130,135] Examples might include strength deficits of the rotator cuff or a muscle length deficit of the scapula. In the downward rotation scapular syndrome, described by Sahrmann,[212] one may find shortness of the deltoid and supraspinatus, resulting from excessive length of the upper trapezius muscle or shortness or stiffness of the levator scapulae.

B. Extrinsic factors. Result of external conditions under which an activity is performed that predisposes an individual to microtrauma injuries, such as training errors (e.g., duration, intensity, and progression) and environmental conditions. Usually high-velocity repetitive microtrauma (shot putting, back-scratching position during tennis serve) on a background of excessive shoulder motion is a precipitating factor.[94]

C. Nature of pain. Acute after nerve or muscle injury; chronic if secondary to other glenohumeral disorder. Dull ache or pain in the shoulder girdle; usually asymptomatic. There may be increased pain with contralateral head tilting or ipsilateral arm elevation.[94]

II. Physical Examination

A. Observation. May have normal resting alignment. There may be evidence of forward head, rounded shoulders, scapular depression, downward rotation, scapular winging, or tilting with hypertrophy of certain scapulohumeral muscles groups. A slouched thoracic posture diminishes shoulder abduction force and range of motion along with diminishing posterior scapular tilt.[123]

B. Cervical screening and upper limb functional ROM

C. Active movements. May reveal clunking (a sensation of the shoulder slipping out of the socket), snapping, or crepitus with arm elevation, possible winging when the arm is brought into the elevated position; emphasized when the patient pushes against a wall with arms extended or with sitting push-ups.

D. Passive movements. As with AROM, the examiner must be alert for motions of the involved side that only appear to have full mobility because of excessive motion at adjacent joints. For example, when the inferior capsule of the glenohumeral is restricted, the patient may substitute excessive extension of the trunk or excessive lateral rotation of the scapula.

E. Key tests. Include muscle tests for muscle length, strength, muscle control, dyskinesis, isometric resistive tests, joint-play movements, and tests for instability.

F. Test for instability. Include those for the glenohumeral joint (i.e., may have increased accessory glide at the glenohumeral joint in any direction), functional tests for scapular winging (see above), and test for scapular stability.[129] The lateral slide test evaluates the function of the muscles that stabilize or externally rotate the scapula (serratus anterior, rhomboids major and minor, upper trapezius and lower trapezius). A measurement is taken from the inferior angle of the scapula to the nearest thoracic segment in three different glenohumeral positions (Fig. 11-23).[129] A difference of 1 cm or greater in the second and third position is associated with microtrauma of the shoulder.

G. Special test. Tests to be considered include those associated with thoracic outlet syndrome, glenohumeral impingement, and scapulothoracic bursitis. Scapulothoracic bursitis is common in sports requiring repetitive shoulder motion (e.g., swimming, throwing, racquet sports).[94]

III. Management. Management follows a similar line as for glenohumeral instability. Addressing biomechanics and limiting the patient to reasonable volume of activity is the first step in managing these problems. Emphasis is placed on resolving the underlying disorders that commonly accompany scapular instability (see above).

A. Acute phase (when present). Initially, emphasis is placed on resolving the symptoms of pain, swelling, or mechanical derangement. Medications, ultrasound or other modalities, and relative rest are commonly used in the acute phase.

B. Recovery phase. After the acute symptoms have been resolved, entry into the recovery phase will be implemented. The protocols for glenohumeral or scapular instability are basically the same at this point, differing only by whatever tissue overloads or biomechanical deficits are found on the ongoing evaluation. The primary focus is regaining trunk and scapular control. The significance of the scapular rotators is frequently and

erroneously overlooked.[184,197] The rehabilitation program (see shoulder and functional scapular stabilization) at the end of this chapter places considerable emphasis on retaining the scapular muscles. Other considerations include the following:

1. Reeducation of postural habits. Determination of involved muscle groups, likely to have shortened or weakened, will be noted on the examination. Prescribed postural activities will address issues that are often related to months or even years of poor posturing and positioning. Effectiveness is achieved through education and patient compliance.

2. Scapular taping techniques applied with the individual in a corrected resting thoracic and scapular posture. These techniques can provide cutaneous feedback to maintain correct posture via increased skin tension (Fig. 11-40) and improve the resting alignment of the related joints and length–tension properties of the shared musculature between the scapula and other regions of the upper quadrant.[92,104,122,237]

C. Functional phase. Shoulder and scapular stabilization program (see Dynamic Stabilization and Functional Exercise section). The focus on this phase is to:

1. Increase power and endurance of the upper limb complex

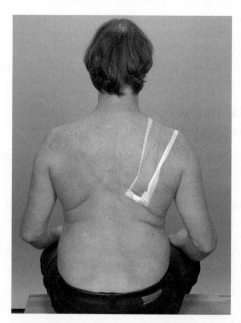

■ **FIG. 11-40.** Example of scapular taping technique to facilitate correct posture and scapular position (in this case to produce scapular posterior tilt and slight retraction). Tape originates over the anterior shoulder (acromion) and is applied diagonally across the back and ends just lateral to the spinous processes of T6–T12. The strips of tape follow the line of pull of the lower and middle trapezius.

2. Increase neuromuscular control in multiple planes of motion
3. Prepare for return to normal activity
D. Return to normal activity. The final phase of any rehabilitation treatment plan must prepare the patient for activity that will be performed. This phase must be especially designed for the individual patient.

Adhesive Capsulitis—Frozen Shoulder

Capsular tightening at the shoulder, another common disorder, is usually referred to as *frozen shoulder* or *adhesive capsulitis*. In most patients seen by physical therapists, no specific cause can be determined for the stiffening. It affects women more often than men, and middle-aged and older persons more often than younger persons. Some so-called idiopathic cases of frozen shoulder probably result from an alteration in scapulohumeral alignment, as occurs with thoracic kyphosis. This is consistent with the fact that women are more frequently affected, because women are also more predisposed to developing thoracic kyphosis than men are. Some believe that this problem is a progression of rotator cuff lesions, in which the inflammatory or degenerative process spreads to include the entire joint capsule, resulting in capsular fibrosis.[56,154,168] This may be true in some cases, but there are two major contradictions to this proposal: rotator cuff tendinitis affects men and women fairly equally, whereas frozen shoulder is much more common in women; and persons with a frozen shoulder rarely present with coexistent tendinitis, as evidenced by the absence of pain on resisted movement.

It is commonly thought that these patients stop using the arm because for some reason it is painful, and motion is therefore lost from disuse. In our experience, this is rarely true; instead, the loss of motion is responsible for the pain. The patient continues to use the arm until the restriction of motion progresses to the extent that it interferes with daily activities. Not until this point is reached does the patient feel much pain or become aware of a problem with the arm. The woman first notices that it is difficult to comb her hair and fasten a bra. She may also be awakened at night when rolling onto the affected side. The man notes difficulty reaching into the hip pocket and combing his hair, and may be similarly awakened at night. Because much shoulder motion can be lost before interfering with daily activities in this age group, these patients invariably do not seek medical help until the shoulder has lost about 90° abduction, 60° flexion, 60° external rotation, and 45° internal rotation. In fact, it is rare for a patient to present with significantly more or significantly less than this amount of movement.

Of course, some cases of capsular tightening at the shoulder are associated with particular disease states or conditions. Conditions that might result in capsular tightness at the glenohumeral joint include:

Degenerative joint disease. This is rare at the shoulder and, if present, is relatively asymptomatic.

Rheumatoid arthritis. The smaller joints of the hand and feet are usually affected first.

Immobilization. For example, after fracture of the arm, forearm, or wrist, or dislocation of the shoulder[100]

Reflex sympathetic dystrophy (see Chapter 13, Wrist and Hand Complex). This condition may occur after certain visceral disorders such as a myocardial infarction, or it may occur after trauma, such as a Colles' fracture. Capsular stiffening of the joints of the hand, wrist, and shoulder is a common component of this syndrome. A frozen shoulder occurring in conjunction with a reflex sympathetic dystrophy is usually more refractory to treatment, probably because of the abnormal pain state that tends to accompany the disorder.

I. History
A. Site of pain. Lateral brachial region, possibly referred distally into the C5 or C6 segment
B. Nature of pain. Varying from a constant dull ache to pain felt only on activities involving movement into the restricted ranges. The patient is often awakened at night when rolling onto the painful shoulder.
C. Onset of pain. Very gradual. May be related to minor trauma, immobilization, chest surgery, or myocardial infarction. More commonly, no cause can be cited.
II. Physical Examination
A. Active movements. Limitation of motion in a capsular pattern: little glenohumeral movement on abduction, much difficulty and substitution getting the hand behind the neck. Usually there is some limitation when flexing the arm or trying to put the hand behind the back.
B. Passive movements. Limitation in a capsular pattern: external rotation is markedly restricted, abduction is moderately restricted, flexion and internal rotation are somewhat limited.
   1. May be limited by pain with a muscle guarding end feel (acute)
   2. May be limited by stiffness with a capsular end feel (chronic)
C. Joint play. Restrictions of most joint-play movements, especially inferior glide
D. Resisted isometric movements. Strong and painless, unless a tendinitis also is present
E. Palpation. Often referred tenderness over the lateral brachial region. There is often a feeling of increased muscle tone, with induration over the lateral brachial region.
F. Inspection. Often negative. Observe for a surgical scar.
III. Acute vs. Chronic
A. Acute
   1. Pain radiates to below the elbow.
   2. The patient is awakened by pain at night.
   3. On passive movement, limitation is caused by pain and muscle guarding, rather than stiffness per se.

B. Chronic
   1. Pain is localized to the lateral brachial region.
   2. The patient is not awakened by pain at night.
   3. On passive movement, limitation is caused by capsular stiffness, and pain is felt only when the capsule is stretched.
C. Subacute. Some combination of the above findings
IV. Management
   A. Acute stage
      1. Relief of pain and muscle guarding to allow early, gentle mobilization
         a. Ice or superficial heat
         b. Grade I or II joint-play oscillations
      2. Maintenance of existing range of motion and efforts to gently begin increasing range of motion
         a. Grade I or II joint-play mobilization. At this stage it is often best to perform these with the patient lying prone and the arm hanging freely at the side of the plinth (see Fig. 11-44A–C). Inferior glide is particularly comfortable for most patients and is usually most helpful in relieving muscle spasm. This is an important movement to perform because the spasm, which is usually present in the acute stage, causes the humerus to assume a superior position in the glenoid cavity, further interfering with normal joint mechanics.
         b. Initiation of active assisted range of motion exercises at home, such as automobilization techniques and wand and pendulum exercises.
      3. Instruction in isometric strengthening exercises, especially for the rotator cuff muscles. The movements associated with isotonic exercises will usually cause pain and reflex inhibition, thus reducing their effectiveness.
      4. Prevention of excessive kyphosis and shoulder girdle protraction. When appropriate, provide instruction in postural awareness for the upper trunk and shoulder girdles such that the patient learns to differentiate proprioceptively between a kyphotic, protracted posture and a relatively upright, retracted position. A system of regular "postural checks" should be incorporated into the patient's daily activities.
      5. Gradual progression of the above program as the condition becomes more chronic (see below)
   B. Chronic stage. Increase the extensibility of the joint capsule, with special attention to the anteroinferior aspect of the capsule.
      1. Ultrasound preceding or accompanying stretching procedures
      2. Specific joint mobilizations, with emphasis on the anteroinferior capsular stretch

General Guidelines

When using specific joint mobilization techniques in the presence of a chronically tight joint, the primary objective is to stretch the joint capsule. To do so, the more vigorous grade IV techniques must be used. It is usually best, however, to start with grade I or II oscillations in preparation for more intensive stretching. The lower grades of oscillations promote reduced muscle spasm and pain, probably by increasing large fiber sensory input. Perhaps the best technique to use when beginning glenohumeral mobilization is the *inferior glide* with the arm to the side (see Fig. 11-44D–F); this technique, especially, seems to induce relaxation. These are also good techniques for relieving the cramping sensation a patient may feel during more vigorous movements.

Before or during capsular stretching procedures, ultrasound can be used to help increase the extensibility of the tissue. For example, perform the anteroinferior capsular stretch while an assistant directs ultrasound to the anteroinferior aspect of the joint. Specific joint mobilization techniques are most effective when used in conjunction with the motions they are intended to restore, such as inferior glide performed simultaneously with abduction or flexion, posterior capsular stretch with internal rotation, and anterior capsular stretch with external rotation (see the section on Self Capsular Stretches). Passive stretching can also be combined with appropriate accessory movements (e.g., flexion with inferior glide or abduction with inferior glide).

Instruct the patient in home range of motion exercises. These are necessary to maintain gains made in treatment and to help increase movement. A major goal of the treatment program is to promote independence in mobilization procedures. Once about 120° abduction, 140° flexion, and 60° external rotation are achieved, many patients continue to make satisfactory improvement in range of motion by continuing on a supervised home exercise program. From the outset, though, it is difficult for most patients to make substantial gains in range of motion with home exercises alone; skillfully applied passive movement will significantly accelerate improvement in the early phases of treatment. This is probably because in the relatively acute stage, the reflex muscle spasm that accompanies active movement of the joint prevents patients from exerting an effective stretch to the joint capsule—they simply fight against their own muscles. The therapist skilled in the use of passive joint mobilization procedures can localize the stretch to specific portions of the joint capsule and carefully graduate the intensity of the stretch to avoid eliciting protective muscle contraction. Also, the therapist can combine joint-play movements with certain movements of the arm to reduce cartilaginous or bony impingement at the extremes of movement. For example, when moving the arm into abduction, the therapist can passively move the head of the humerus inferiorly to prevent impingement of the greater tubercle against the acromial arch, which would tend to occur from the loss of external rotation and from a loss of inferior glide of the joint. By doing so, muscle spasm is reduced and a more effective stretch to the inferior capsule is effected. In fact, until significant gains in external rotation are made, patients should not be instructed to stretch into abduction on their own:

attempts to do so may traumatize the subacromial tissues more than stretching the inferior aspect of the joint capsule.

The primary goal of treatment is to restore painless functional range of movement; regaining full movement of the arm is not always realistic. This is especially true for persons with some degree of increased thoracic kyphosis, because full elevation of the arm involves extension of the upper thoracic spine. For these patients "normal" elevation is usually about 150° to 160°. Range of motion of the uninvolved shoulder should serve as a guide for setting treatment goals.

In more acute cases of frozen shoulder, the patient's major complaint is often the inability to get a good night's sleep: each time he or she rolls onto the involved side, he or she is awakened by pain. The resultant fatigue adds to the patient's general debilitation. Fortunately, with appropriate management this is usually the first aspect of the problem to resolve. In fact, subjective improvement, in the form of significant reduction in night pain, will usually precede any evidence of objective improvement, such as increased range of motion. In our experience, one or two sessions of gentle joint-play oscillations, especially into inferior glide, preceded by superficial heat or ice, are often enough to alleviate nocturnal symptoms. This leads us to speculate whether the night pain may be related more to the fact that the joint is compressed in a position in which the humerus is held into a cephalad malalignment by muscle spasm, rather than being the result of compression of an inflamed joint capsule. At any rate, relaxation of the associated muscle spasm seems to be one of the more important measures in reducing pain in the acute phase.

In the chronic stage, pain is primarily the result of repeated tensile stresses to the tight joint capsule during daily activities. Treatment is directed primarily at increasing range of motion, although some restriction of activities may be warranted. For the most part, however, in the chronic stage, encourage the patient to use the arm as much as tolerable to minimize habitual disuse, which can be a factor in perpetuating the disorder.

Some authors claim that adhesive capsulitis is a self-limiting disorder, and that spontaneous resolution can be expected in about 12 months.[169,174,235] This has not been consistent with our clinical experience. Even if it were true, this should not be a reason for failing to institute active treatment, because with appropriate therapy satisfactory results can be expected within no longer than 3 to 4 months. The only common exception is when a frozen shoulder is part of a sympathetic reflex dystrophy. These cases are often refractory to conservative management and may require supplementary measures such as sympathetic blocks or manipulation under anesthesia.

Although in most cases of frozen shoulder the prognosis for functional recovery is good, the time frame of recovery is rarely linear. Improvement tends to be characterized by spurts and plateaus. Both the therapist and patient should realize this to avoid undue frustration during periods of limited progress.

Thoracic Outlet Syndrome

The thoracic outlet syndrome (TOS) complex refers to a series of neurovascular syndromes in the shoulder region. Today TOS is recognized as an entrapment compression vasculopathy of the subclavian vessels but more commonly involving the lower trunk or medial cord of the brachial plexus at four common sites.[213,219] The four common sites include (Fig. 11-41):

1. The sternocostovertebral space. Pancoast tumors present at this locale.
2. The scalene triangle is narrower in many patients with TOS resulting in emergence of the neurovascular bundle from the apex of that triangle.[205] This may cause excessive rubbing of the neurovascular bundle against the adjacent structures. Nerve adhesions to muscle may occur at this site.
3. The costoclavicular space contains all the structures of the scalene triangle and the subclavian vein.
4. The coracopectoral space contains the inferior trunk of the brachial plexus.

Because many anatomic structures can impair free passage, TOS has previously been termed scalene anticus syndrome, cervicodorsal outlet syndrome, hyperabduction syndrome, cervical rib syndrome, clavicocostal syndrome, subcoracoid pectoralis minor syndrome, hyperabduction syndrome, quadrilateral space syndrome (located over the posterior scapular and subdeltoid region), and droopy shoul-

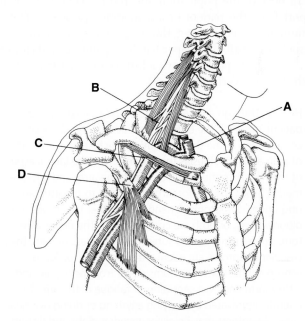

■ **FIG. 11-41.** The four sections of the thoracic outlet. **(A)** Sternoclavicular space. **(B)** The scalene triangle. **(C)** The costoclavicular space. **(D)** The coracopectoral space. (Reprinted with permission from Kelly MJ, Clark WA: Orthopedic Therapy of the Shoulder. Philadelphia, JB Lippincott. 1995:145.)

der syndrome.[38,39,41,213,252] Obstruction may be caused by a number of abnormalities, including degenerative joint or bony disorders (the presence of a cervical rib, malunion of old clavicular fractures, the presence of a cervical rib, pseudarthrosis of the clavicle, and exostosis of the first rib), fascial fusions of muscles, fibromuscular bands, vascular abnormalities, spasms of the scaleni or pectoralis minor. According to McNair and Maitland[162] and Maitland,[157] the syndrome is a product of the combined anomalies of soft tissues and bony boundaries of the outlet; hence treatment must address both conditions. It is necessary to think of TOS as multifactorial rather than having a single cause as the basis for evaluating and developing an effective treatment program.[64,234,246] Often patients with TOS are suffering from additional secondary system complaints including myofascial trigger points, primary or secondary glenohumeral joint pathologies, cervical pathologies, or more distal peripheral neuropathies.[246]

Risk factors in the development of TOS include congenital structural anomalies, traumatic structural alterations in the size of the thoracic outlet (i.e., fractures of the clavicle), and postural alteration in the size of the thoracic outlet.[252] Scapular ptosis has been identified as a significant factor in the production of symptoms of TOS.[138,232] Disuse of the shoulder because of pain or immobilization from any cause may result in atrophy of the trapezius, levator scapulae, and rhomboids. This in turn will result in ptosis of the scapula.[232] Other theories presented by authors regarding the cause of TOS related to soft tissues include shortening of the pectoralis minor, shortening of the scaleni, and muscle hypertrophy.[217]

In 60% of the population affected by TOS, there is no report from the patient of any inciting episode.[138] TOS is commonly seen in racquet, throwing, and aquatic sports, and in such occupations as paper handing, painting, and carpentry.[121,150] Thirty percent have a history of repetitive activity with the arm overhead.[94]

I. History. Through a detailed history and evaluation of a patient's activity, the clinician can identify the cause of compression in the thoracic outlet. The history is often that of pain and paresthesias that extend from the lateral aspect of the neck into the shoulder, down the arm, and into the medial aspect of the forearm and hand to the little and ring finger. Symptoms depend on whether the nerves, the blood vessels, or both are compromised. The nerve symptoms are paresthesia and subjective weakness or pain; the vascular symptoms are edema, discoloration, pallor, or venous congestion. Symptoms range from neck pain and diffuse arm pain to a sensation of fatigue in the arm, frequently aggravated by carrying anything or doing overhead work. Symptoms may be experienced at night and disturb sleep. There may be referred pain to the ipsilateral breast or chest. In axonopathic TOS, there is objective weakness and wasting of the median and ulnar nerve distribution of the hand and forearm.[39] Sensory impairment is usually of the ulnar distribution. Pain tends to be in the dermatomal dis-

tribution. Differentiation should be made between TOS symptoms that most commonly affect the C8 and T1 nerve roots and cervical radicular syndromes that usually affect C5, C6, and C7.

II. Physical Examination

A. Observation. Observation is an essential part of the examination; one must look for unequal shoulder height and protective positioning of the upper quarter to reduce stress on the vascular and neural structures. The examiner should also look for forward head posture, particularly for prominence in the cervical thoracic junction.[64] There may be edema in the supraclavicular fossa or extremity. The hand may be cool to touch, and there may be signs of reflex sympathetic dystrophy (RSD). Scars on the palms and elbows may be seen because of previous unsuccessful carpal tunnel and cubital tunnel releases.[252]

The breathing pattern is always paradoxic, with the scalene muscle active on inspiration from the initiation of inspiration throughout the full expiratory phase.[64] The patients often have difficulty breathing with the diaphragm.

B. Upper quadrant screening. Cervical spine range of motion, the Spurling's test (Fig. 19-38), and the vertebral artery test should be performed. Myotomal scanning for muscle strength and reflex testing are also performed (see Chapter 5, Assessment of Musculoskeletal Disorders and Concepts of Management). Careful sensory evaluation should be carried out to investigate (1) dermatomal distribution to rule out cervical root involvement; (2) sensory disturbances related to brachial plexus and its divisions; and (3) peripheral nerve distribution to rule out possible local peripheral nerve entrapment neuropathies.[246]

C. Myofascial length testing. The deltoid fascia and pectoralis minor and scaleni (see Fig. 7-34) should be examined.

D. Joint-play movements. The first and second rib joints and the apophyseal joints, especially in the lower cervical spine and upper thoracic spine, must be examined. The acromioclavicular, glenohumeral, and possibly the elbow and wrist joints need to be examined, particularly if a double or multiple crush syndrome is evident.[152,238]

E. Palpation. Palpate the upper quadrant for myofascial trigger points and peripheral nerves to determine irritability and relationship to the patient symptomatology. In patients with neurogenic TOS there may be pain with direct palpation over the scalene muscles and also on the brachial plexus.[64] There may also be a positive Tinel sign over the supraclavicular area at the insertion of the scalene muscle.[101,206,214,262] Tenderness in the region of the subclavius muscle is also common. The supraclavicular fossa should be palpated for fibromuscular bands, percussed for brachial plexus irritability, and auscultated for vascular bruits that appear by placing the upper limb in the position of vascular compression.[62]

F. Neural tension tests. According to Butler,[35] all tension tests should be performed (see above). Tension tests on the opposite arm and a slump test, both in long sitting and in sitting, are suggested to look for any spinal canal components of adverse tension. When examining the upper limb tension test, it is essential to examine the initial barrier or point at which involuntary muscle guarding comes into play.

G. Traditional objective tests for TOS. Several authors[14,39,71,94,157,162,193] have outlined test procedures to help differentiate the most likely offending soft tissue or bony structure. Although it is beyond the scope of this text to describe all the tests needed to diagnosis TOS, the Wright's test, Adson's maneuver, Allen test, provocative elevation test, and cervical rotation lateral flexion test (CRLF; Box 11-2) are often included in differential diagnosis of TOS.

The problem with many of these traditional tests is that when pulse obliteration is used as the critical sign, the tests have shown too many false-positive results to be reliable, because the majority of asymptomatic individuals have pulse changes with the maneuvers.[73,80] Reproduction of the patient's symptoms is a more reliable sign of TOS.

H. Special studies. Diagnosis of vascular TOS is made by duplex scanning (i.e., ultrasound combined with Doppler velocity waveforms), angiography, or venography. Electrodiagnostic tests can reveal chronic, severe lower trunk brachial plexopathy.

III. Management. Muscle strengthening, postural reeducation of the neck and shoulder girdle, and mobilization of the whole shoulder complex remains the cornerstone of conservative management of the complex problems of TOS. Therapeutic exercises should be used to correct physiologic impairments linked to posture and movement impairments such as force-generating capacity or length–tension properties of underused synergists or antagonists such as the lower trapezius to offset short pectoralis minor or the upper trapezius to alleviate a depressed scapula. The suspensory muscles—middle and upper trapezius, levator scapulae, and sternocleidomastoid—the thoracic outlet "openers," generally need to be strengthened.

Muscle lengthening and soft tissue mobilizations such as improving the length of the scaleni, subclavius, pectoralis major and minor—the thoracic outlet "closers"—should be instituted to increase the space of the thoracic outlet (see Chapter 8, Soft Tissue Manipulations). Proper breathing should also be reviewed with the patient. The scalene muscles act as accessory breathing muscles, and improper breathing techniques can lead to tightening of these muscles.

A. Stage 1. It is imperative that those activities, positions, and treatments that exacerbate and relieve the patient's symptoms be identified. Careful positioning of the upper limb such that the brachial plexus is neither compressed nor stretched should be emphasized. This rest position is with the scapula in abduction and elevated and the shoulder internally rotated (that is the hand is placed on the contralateral shoulder). The resting position in sitting can be achieved with the forearm supported on a table and in sleeping by a modified fetal position (with the arms supported by pillows) or in supine with a pillow to support the arm on the patient's stomach. The use of modalities such as heat, cold, ultrasound, electrical stimulation, laser, and electroacupuncture have been used in providing temporary pain relief.[13] Other considerations include taping the scapula in elevation or the use of a figure-of-eight strap to pull the shoulders back out of the forward round-shoulder posture.[92,213] Relaxation exercises to relax the upper thorax and diaphragmatic breathing should be emphasized throughout the program.

B. Stage 2. The protocol should include joint mobilization (grades I–IV) and soft tissue mobilization of acromioclavicular, sternoclavicular, and scapulothoracic joints, first and second ribs, and cervical–upper thoracic spine as indicated; deep stretching and soft tissue manipulations of the clavipectoral fascia, pectoral muscles, scaleni, and other tight structures in the upper limb. Peripheral nerve mobilization (see above) and brachial plexus gliding as described by Totten and Hunter[233] may be instituted (Fig. 11-42).

C. Stage 3. The treatment program involves conditioning and strengthening of those muscles necessary to maintain postural correction. Maintenance of the patient's ability to tolerate adverse neural tension with activities of daily living (ADL) and functional and occupational activities are also addressed. Restoration of functional range of motion and increased aerobic capacity become important as well as educating patients about posture and levels of activity that they can tolerate during stages 2 and 3.

Acromioclavicular Joint Sprains and Degeneration

The most common conditions affecting the acromioclavicular (AC) joint are sprains and degeneration.

INJURIES

The AC joint is exposed to a high level of stress because it is the main articulation suspending the upper limb from the trunk. This predisposes that joint to chronic injury, especially in situations with repetitive high demands. Injuries to the AC joint are among the most commonly occurring problems in the athletic population.[141,236] AC joint separations are commonly classified into six types (Fig. 11-43). Clinical evaluation involves determination of the stability of the AC joint using stress x-ray, if the extent of the injury is not otherwise apparent.

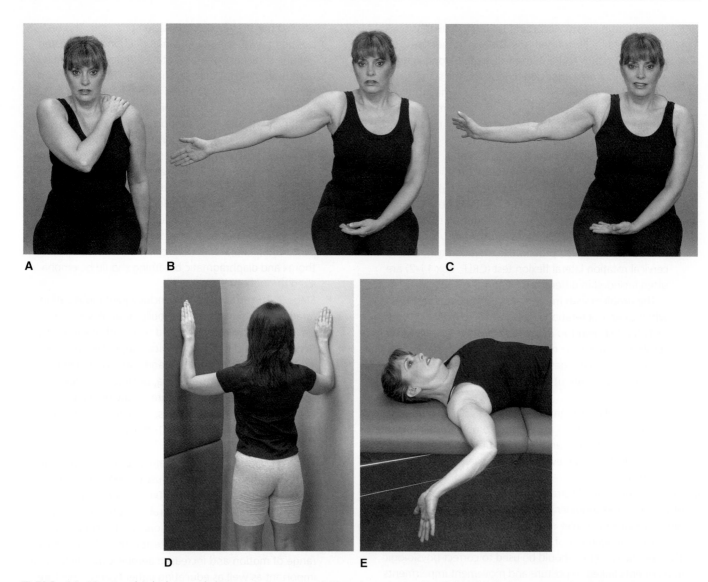

■ **FIG. 11-42.** Brachial plexus gliding exercises to mobilize the nerves. (**A–C**) Brachial plexus stretch while sitting. (**D**) Brachial plexus stretch while leaning into a corner. (**E**) Brachial plexus stretch in supine position using wrist extension and external rotation at 90° of abduction.

I. History
   A. Onset. About three quarters of AC joint sprains are caused by a fall on the shoulder, with the arm at the side, as often occurs in football or after a fall from a horse.[171,239] The force drives the scapula downward, an action resisted by the coracoclavicular ligament. Other common injuries include a fall on the outstretched hand or elbow and repetitive overhead activities (swimmers, weightlifters, and body builders).[180] There is evidence that the AC joint as well as the sternoclavicular joint of the seat-belt shoulder may be injured with whiplash after road traffic accidents.[14,216]
   B. Site of pain. The lateral end of the clavicle is tender and severely painful at the exact site of the joint.[213]
   C. Pain and deformity are immediate and depend on the degree of ligamentous injury.

II. Physical Examination
   A. Inspection. The patient may present with a large lump over the AC joint. In a grade III lesion there is a noticeable step-off deformity. The deformity may occur later, if initial muscle spasms reduce the acromioclavicular separation.
   B. Active movements. The patient may complain of pain on moving the arm overhead or across the body into horizontal adduction; these movements compress the AC joint. Active shoulder adduction and depression may recreate instability and cause pain.
   C. Passive movements. Passive motions, especially at the extremes of motion, are quite painful. The shoulder–cross-body adduction maneuvers predictably exacerbate symptoms.
   D. Resisted motions are usually pain free.

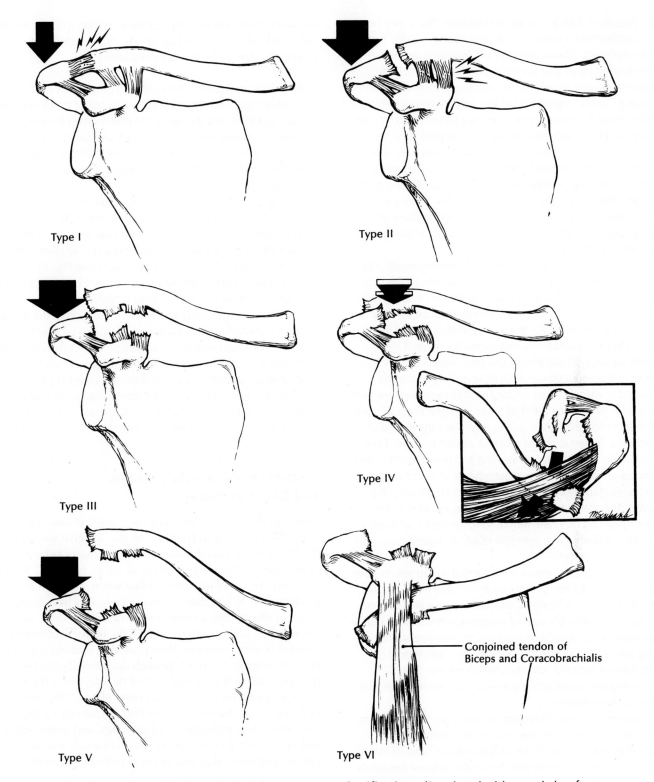

Type I

Type II

Type III

Type IV

Type V

Type VI

Conjoined tendon of
Biceps and Coracobrachialis

■ **FIG. 11-43.** Diagram of acromioclavicular joint separation classifications. (Reprinted with permission from Rockwood CA, Green DP: Fractures in Adults, 3rd ed. Philadelphia: Lippincott 1991:1193.)

E. Palpation. Pain at the site of the lesion. There may be crepitus when palpating the joint during mobility tests.

III. Management. Management of AC injuries is dependent on the type of injury that is inflicted on the patient. Initial treatment aims to reduce the symptoms. Ice and a sling support to take the weight of the arm are recommended. With grade I injuries, some relief may be provided by two strips of elastic adhesive taping over the joint from the sternum to the scapula. As inflammation subsides, exercise therapy is commenced to restore function, although a permanent step deformity is usual (in grade III), and joint degeneration may occur in later years. The deltoid and trapezius work should not be emphasized because this may apply disruptive forces to the AC joint capsule and ligament complex.[213]

Grades I and II sprains are treated nonoperatively. Friction massage is often used in Grade I lesions to the superior ligament (see Box 8-3). Cure is normally obtained after 10 to 15 sessions.[180] Range of motion exercises are started as soon as tolerated for the patient with a grade I injury and after the appropriate rest period for grade II injury. Early on patients are usually taught to mobilize their AC joint in full adduction and full flexion. They should be taught to carry out low-velocity oscillatory movement, with the joint held at the point of tension several times per day. Patients should be given advice to protect the joint during recovery, by reducing the strain of weight bearing. They should be asked to avoid reaching and lifting, and leaning on the affected arm. In the later phases of treatment dynamic stability of the proximal musculature is emphasized. The scapular stabilizers should be included in the strengthening program. Return to full activity is allowed when the goals of full pain-free ROM, strength power, and endurance are met.

Grade III sprains remain controversial. Good results have been reported after both surgical[250,251] and nonsurgical treatment.[57,259] If treated conservatively, grade III sprains may require 4 to 6 weeks of immobilization. Passive mobility exercises and resistive exercises are progressed, respecting the healing constraints. Initially exercises should be performed with the arm elevated no greater than 90°, avoiding horizontal active depression of the shoulder and horizontal adduction.

Grades IV, V, and VI require surgery (open reduction and internal fixation. Operative procedures are designed to attempt realignment of the clavicle with the scapula. After immobilization, the concerns are similar to those previously discussed.

AC JOINT DEGENERATION

Multiple authors have reported changes at the AC joint by age 40 in the average healthy adult.[54] Degenerative arthritis of the AC joint has been postulated to be age related or it may be secondary to trauma as in AC separation and intra-articular fractures. Subacromial impingement symptoms may coexist independently or secondary to AC joint osteophytes that reduce the size of the supraspinous outlet.[49]

I. Physical Examination. The condition presents as pain, which is usually dull and aching in nature, brought on by activities such as lifting and throwing. On examination there is point tenderness over the joint, with pain and crepitus to passive horizontal adduction.[177] If there is associated impingement of the rotator cuff, then impingement signs will also be positive.

II. Management. Initially, rest, nonsteroidal anti-inflammatory medications, and immobilization in a sling may be required in the very acute lesion. Movements that stress the joint (for example, push-ups or throwing) should be avoided. Later, joint mobilization provides good results (see Fig. 11-51). Injections of corticosteroid may give many months of relief. If symptoms fail to improve after prolonged conservative treatment, surgery may be indicated. Excision of the distal clavicle (Mumford procedure) usually yields excellent results for relief of pain and return to function.[236] Certain surgical fixations for acromioclavicular separation, such as those involving insertion of a screw from the clavicle to the coracoid, may permanently restrict normal clavicular axial rotation. As long as such a screw is still in place, full elevation of the arm should not be expected; it can occur only if the screw breaks.

Sternoclavicular Joint Sprains and Degeneration

Injury to this sternoclavicular (SC) joint is unusual. Normally the clavicle will fracture, or the AC give way, before the SC joint is seriously injured. Next to motor vehicle accidents, the most common source of injury to the SC joint is in sports (i.e., cycling, horse riding when sufficient force is produced).[181] When damage does occur, it is frequently the result of direct lateral compression of the shoulder, such as occurs when falling onto the side of the body.[177] Anterior dislocation is more common than posterior, and many dislocations are actually fractures through the physeal plate because the epiphysis at the medial end of the clavicle is the last to close, at approximately 23 to 25 years of age.[94] Because several important structures lie in close proximity to the joint (including the esophagus, trachea, lungs, and major arteries and veins) initial examination must obviously rule out lifethreatening injury that may occur in posterior dislocations.[177]

I. Physical Examination
   A. Inspection. Local swelling is sometimes present, with crepitus and pain on motion, especially horizontal adduction. Anterior dislocations leave a visible step deformity. In posterior dislocation, the medial end of the clavicle is palpable and is displaced posteriorly. The shoulder is frequently held in a protracted position.

B. Active and passive movements of the scapula and shoulder. There is pain on full active and passive elevation of the scapula and pain on active and passive movement of the arm because almost all arm movements have some influence on the SC joint. Pain is generally well localized, and may become progressively more limiting with time.

C. Active and passive or resisted movement of the neck that involves the SC muscles may also provoke some pain.

II. Management. Closed reduction is often possible for both anterior and posterior dislocation immediately after injury if pain is not too severe and before muscle spasm sets in.[177] Initial treatment consists of rest, nonsteroidal anti-inflammatory medications, and immobilization in a sling. Grade I sprains are immobilized for 5 to 10 days, with gradual return of use of the arm. Grade II (subluxation) may require reduction. Protection with a sling or a clavicle strap for a period of 4 to 6 weeks is recommended. Grade III (dislocations) are reduced. Posterior dislocations usually remain reduced, but anterior dislocations are apt to recur.

Even though the joint is frequently hypermobile, joint mobilization may be used to relieve pain (see Fig. 11-50).[158] Selective strengthening of the coracoclavicular ligament's dynamic synergists (i.e., the pectoralis minor and subclavius muscle) diminishes disruptive forces and further strain to the already frayed fiber of the SC ligamentous support.[213] In cases of ligamentous instability as well as disk degeneration, the rehabilitation should focus on strengthening the muscles attached to the clavicle in a range that does not further stress the joint.[217] Muscles such as the upper trapezius, pectoralis minor, and sternal fibers of the pectoralis major are strengthened to aid in controlling motions of the shoulder girdle complex.

Patients with a forward head posture, neurologically involved children with lack of disassociation of the shoulder girdle complex, and patients with degenerative arthritis of the SC joint secondary to trauma often present with hypomobility.[14,25,175] The seat-belt shoulder after whiplash leads to numerous degenerative restrictions of the anterior thorax, particularly the sternoclavicular and acromioclavicular joints and the ribs.[14] Clavicular fractures often involve injuries to the acromioclavicular, sternoclavicular, and coracoclavicular ligaments. Joint mobilization techniques should be started immediately after the immobilization period to restore normal arthrokinematics (see Figs. 11-50 through 11-52).

It is important to address the function of the SC joint on shoulder complex movement and to identify the cause of pain—ligamentous instability, disk degeneration, or ligamentous trauma.[217] The SC joint acts as the sole passive attachment of the shoulder complex to the axial skeleton.

Other Lesions

Other, more serious lesions commonly affect the shoulder, such as glenohumeral anterior dislocation. These are usually not seen by the physical therapist until they have been treated with prolonged immobilization, or perhaps surgery followed by immobilization. At this point, the therapist no longer deals with the original injury so much as with the effects of immobilization. As a result, the goals and techniques of management in such cases are often essentially the same as those for a patient with capsular tightness. There are, however, special considerations with which the therapist should be familiar, depending on the original problem. For example, surgery for recurrent anterior dislocation may be performed with the specific intent of limiting external rotation to help provide anterior stabilization.[40,56] Or, after an anterior dislocation, it may be desirable for the sake of preventing recurrence to allow the anterior capsule to heal in a tightened state. In both cases emphasis on regaining external rotation will be less than what it might be in other cases of capsular tightness. Although it is not within the scope of this book to discuss them at length, the therapist must be familiar with these other types of injuries, current surgical procedures, and such special considerations as those mentioned above.

PASSIVE TREATMENT TECHNIQUES

Joint Mobilization Techniques

(For simplicity, the operator will be referred to as the male, the patient as the female. P—patient; O—operator; M—movement.)

It is always difficult to determine which techniques are likely to be the most effective. Hundreds of techniques are described in the literature. Each technique is either an accessory motion or a particular capsular stretch, and can be applied with any grade of movement. These are also evaluative techniques when performed in the resting position. They should first be used to determine reactivity and the need for mobilization. To reduce the chances of being too aggressive, the operator should try to determine what stage of the healing process the involved joint is in: acute with extravasation, fibroplasia, or chronic with scar formation (see Chapter 1, Properties of Dense Connective Tissue).

Techniques performed with the arm at the side of the body or in prone position with the arm in flexion are primarily used to promote relaxation of the muscles controlling the joint, to relieve pain, and to prepare for more vigorous stretching techniques. In relatively acute cases of adhesive capsulitis, they may constitute the primary techniques used until resolution of the acute state allows more aggressive mobilization. In more chronic cases, they are typically used at the initiation of the mobilization session, between techniques, and at the end of the session to prevent and reduce reflex muscle cramping. As these techniques are performed, the arm may be gradually moved from the side of the body toward positions in which more vigorous techniques may be applied. For chronic conditions, these techniques should be used on a continuing basis in conjunction with the stretching techniques described. A very effective general capsular stretch (see Fig. 8-21) for the glenohumeral joint is described in Chapter 8, Soft Tissue Manipulations.

I. Glenohumeral Joint. General techniques for elevation and relaxation
    A. Distraction, in flexion (Fig. 11-44A)
        P—Prone, arm in 90° flexion over the edge of the table
        O—Sitting on a stool, facing the patient's arm. The hands contact the distal humerus.
        M—The hands apply distraction along the long axis of the arm, applying a caudal force to the glenohumeral joint. This technique may be interspersed with pendulum exercises. While maintaining traction, one may also apply lateral glide (Fig. 11-44B).
    B. Inferior glide, in flexion (Fig. 11-44C)
        P—Prone, arm in 90° flexion over the edge of the table
        O—Sitting on a stool. Legs contact the patient's arm and fixate it. The mobilizing hand is positioned with the web space over the cranial surface of the proximal humerus.
        M—The mobilizing hand glides the humerus in a distal direction, while the legs guide and control the position of the arm.
            These are useful techniques for relaxation of spasm, relieving pain, and facilitating flexion, along with inferior glide with the arm at the side (see below). These techniques should be used before and after treatment sessions and between other techniques.
    C. Inferior glide, arm at side (Fig. 11-44D)
        P—Supine, with arm resting at side of body
        O—Stabilizes the scapula with his foot in the patient's axilla and grasps her distal forearm above the wrist with both hands
        M—By applying gentle traction to the arm and carefully adjusting the angle of his foot, the glenohumeral joint can be distracted. The patient's scapula may also be stabilized using a strap around the axilla as both hands grip the humerus (Fig. 11-44E), or the operator can stabilize the scapula by putting one hand in the axilla against the coracoid process of the scapula and use the other hand to grip the humerus (Fig. 11-44F). The patient's forearm is tucked between the operator's mobilizing arm and trunk, and the operator fixes the patient's arm against his trunk. The mobilizing hand(s) glides the humerus caudally as the operator rotates his trunk away from the joint. Progressive long-axis extension moving toward abduction may be performed by the operator shifting his trunk into outward rotation. As the patient relaxes, the arm may be gradually moved toward abduction. This technique may be performed up to about 80° abduction. Note: This is an important technique for relaxing spasm and relieving pain, to be used before and after a treatment session and between other techniques. For greater ranges of elevation, see Techniques.

II. Glenohumeral Joint. Inferior glide techniques for elevation
    A. Inferior glide, resting position (Fig. 11-45A)
        P—Sitting with arms relaxed
        O—Patient's arm is supported in resting or neutral position by the operator's forearm and hand. The mobilizing hand is placed on the lateral surface of the upper humerus (just lateral to the acromion process).
        M—Mobilizing hand depresses the head of the humerus inferiorly and anteriorly. This technique may be used for assessment of inferior instability (multidirectional) or for loss of joint play, and as a technique to promote flexion and abduction. The limb may be moved out of the resting position and toward 90° of abduction if more aggressive techniques are indicated.
    B. Inferior glide, moving toward flexion (Fig. 11-45B)
        P—Supine, with the humerus flexed 60 to 100° and the elbow bent, with the wrist resting across the clavicular region
        O—Grasps the proximal humerus with both hands, the fingers interlaced. The patient's elbow region is contacted with the clavicular region of the operator's shoulder closest to the patient.
        M—The operator pulls caudally with his trunk to produce a movement of combined flexion of the humerus and inferior glide at the glenohumeral joint. The arm is gradually moved toward greater ranges of flexion, up to about 110°. For greater degrees of flexion, see Technique IID (below).
    C. Inferior glide, in abduction (Fig. 11-45C)
        P—Supine, elbow bent. The arm is close to the limits of abduction and external rotation, but comfortable.
        O—Approaches the arm superiorly. He supports the elbow with the left hand at the distal humerus. The patient's forearm is tucked and supported between the operator's arm and trunk. The right hand contacts the superior aspect of the proximal humerus with the heel of the hand, with the forearm supinated and the elbow bent.
        M—Inferior glide of the humeral head is produced by the right hand as the left hand applies a grade I traction simultaneously. As the patient relaxes, the arm can be guided into gradually increasing degrees of abduction with the stabilizing hand.
            This may be performed up to about 90°. The choice of position is guided by the ease with which a relaxed movement can be produced. This technique is used to increase abduction, allowing stretching into abduction while avoiding impingement of the greater tubercle on the acromial arch.
    D. Inferior glide, in more than 90° elevation (Fig. 11-45D)
        P—Supine, with arm elevated comfortably but close to the limits of full elevation in a somewhat horizontally abducted position, between flexion and abduction. The elbow is bent. Note: When moving into ranges past 90°, the patient's forearm may be supported on

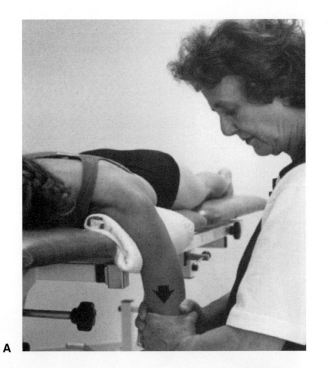

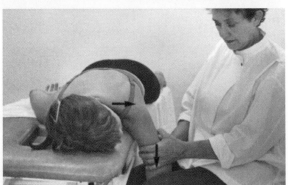

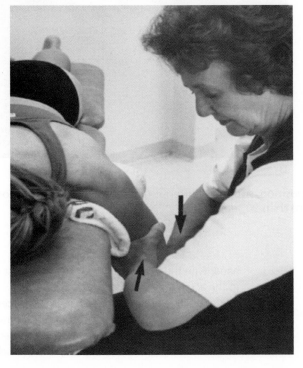

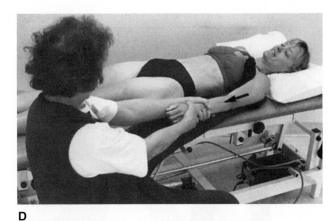

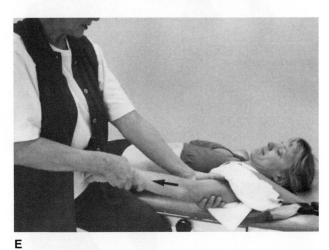

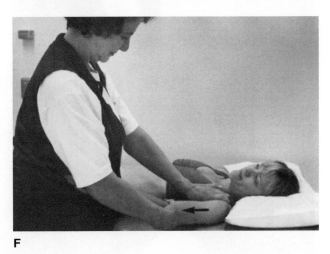

■ **FIG. 11-44.** General techniques for elevation and relaxation of the shoulder. **(A)** Distraction in flexion. **(B)** Distraction with lateral glide. **(C)** Distraction with inferior glide. **(D)** Inferior glide, arm at side. **(E)** Inferior glide, arm at side, alternative technique (with a halter). **(F)** Progressive long-axis extension moving toward abduction.

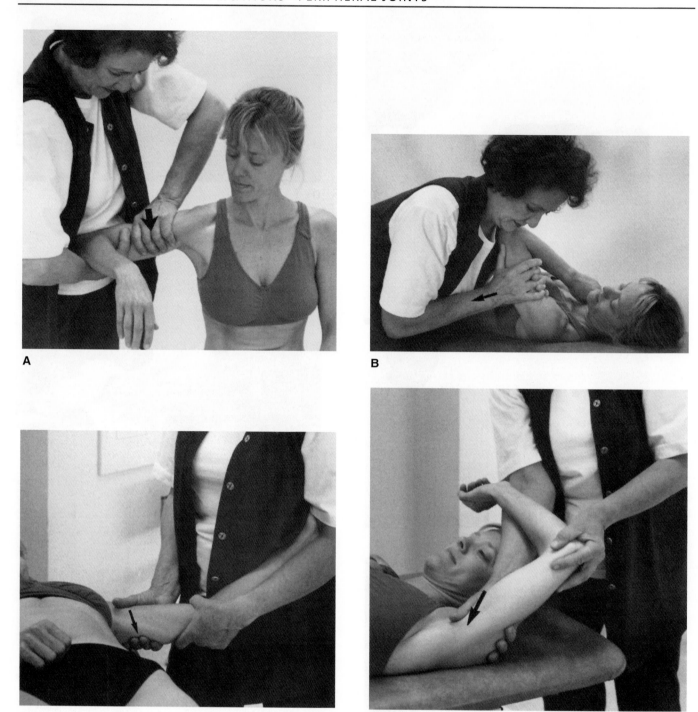

■ **FIG. 11-45.** Inferior glides. **(A)** Inferior glide in the resting position, sitting. **(B)** Inferior glide moving toward flexion. **(C)** Inferior glide in abduction, supine. **(D)** Inferior glide in more than 90° elevation.

her forehead or on a pillow above her head, or the operator may support it, as shown.

O—Approaches the arm superiorly. He supports the elbow with the left hand, supporting the patient's arm on his right arm. The operator contacts the superior aspect of the proximal humerus with the right

hand, with the thumb positioned ventrally just distal to the acromion.

M—Inferior glide of the humeral head is produced with the right hand. The arm can be guided into gradually increasing degrees of elevation. Note: The direction of movement is performed caudally and in a somewhat lateral direction, in keeping with the relationship of the joint surfaces in this position.

Movements in elevation beyond 90° are particularly useful as stretching techniques and may be used even when only a few degrees of elevation are restricted; however, they have no place in the treatment of a very painful shoulder.

III. Glenohumeral Joint. Internal rotation

A. Posterior glide, arm in various degrees of abduction (10 to 55°; Fig. 11-46A)

P—Supine, with the arm slightly abducted

O—Standing between the patient's arm and body, supporting the patient's elbow with his right hand. The hand, wrist, and forearm are supported by tucking them between his elbow and side. The left hand contacts the anterior aspect of the upper humerus with the heel of the left hand, with the forearm pronated and the elbow straight.

M—A posterior glide is produced by leaning forward slightly and flexing the knees, transmitting the force through the straight arm. This technique is used to increase joint play necessary for internal rotation and flexion.

B. Anterior glide, arm close to the limits of internal rotation (Fig. 11-46B)

P—Lying on uninvolved side with the arm behind the back so it rests comfortably, but close to the limits of internal rotation

O—Standing behind the patient with both thumb pads over the posterior humeral head. The fingers of the right hand grasp around anteriorly to stabilize at the anterior aspect of the acromion and clavicle. Elbows remain almost fully extended. The left knee may be brought up onto the plinth to support the patient's arm.

M—An anterior glide is produced by leaning forward with the upper trunk, transmitting the force through the thumbs. Internal rotation is gradually increased by progressively moving the patient's hand up the back. This technique results in a posterior capsular stretch, stretching into internal rotation while avoiding posterior impingement of the humeral head on the glenoid labrum.

C. Internal rotation technique, arm close to 90° abduction (Fig. 11-46C)

P—Supine, with the arm resting comfortably but as close to 90° abduction as possible, the elbow bent to 90°, and the forearm pronated

O—Supports the wrist with the left hand; supports under the elbow with the fingers of the right hand from the medial side. He positions the right upper arm in front of and just medial to the shoulder.

M—The right upper arm provides only enough counterpressure to the shoulder to prevent lifting of the shoulder girdle; the hand maintains the arm in abduction.

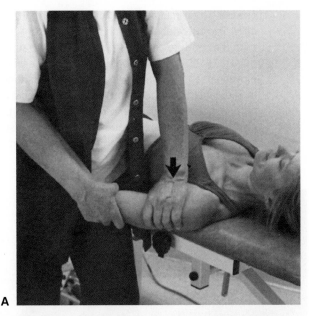

A

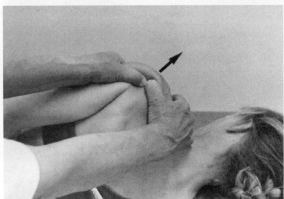

B

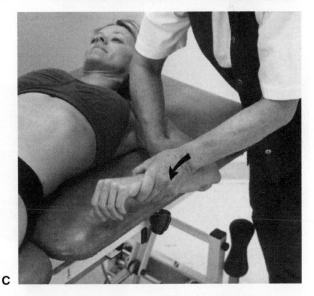

C

■ **FIG. 11-46.** Techniques for internal rotation of the shoulder joint. **(A)** Posterior glide, arm slightly abducted. **(B)** Anterior glide, arm close to the limits of internal rotation, at side or behind back. **(C)** Internal rotation, arm close to 90° abduction.

The left hand simultaneously rotates the arm internally. The operator's left thigh may be brought up onto the plinth to act as a stop to internal rotation (see Fig. 7-2). The stop should be close to the limit of movement so as to minimize anticipatory guarding by the patient. The stop is progressively moved as motion increases. This is an oscillatory movement.

Methods for internal rotation are useful for restoring necessary joint-play movements with the arm near the side or in various degrees of abduction (see Technique IIIA), or as a stretching technique in functional position (see Technique IIIB). Internal rotation is accompanied by scapular retraction and associated clavicular movements. Normal internal rotation at the glenohumeral joint, therefore, is not possible without adequate scapular mobility.[114]

IV. Glenohumeral Joint. External rotation
    A. Anterior glide, arm at side (Fig. 11-47A)

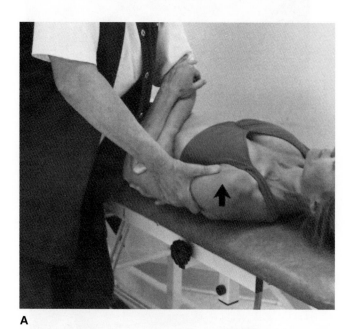

A

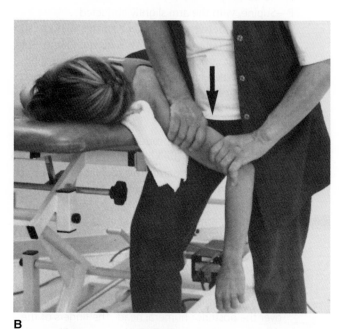

B

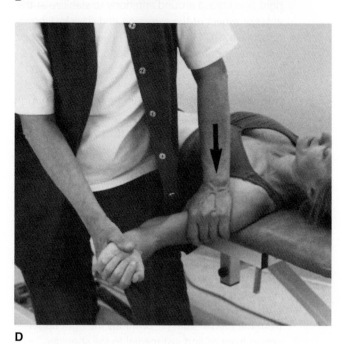

C

D

■ **FIG. 11-47.** Techniques for external rotation of the shoulder joint. **(A)** Anterior glide, arm at side (supine). **(B)** Anterior glide (prone). **(C)** Anterior glide near the limits of external rotation. **(D)** Posterior glide, arm close to 90° of abduction (capsular stretch).

P—Supine, arm at the side, elbow bent, forearm supported by operator's arm

O—Stabilizes with the right hand, grasping the distal humerus just proximal to the elbow. He grasps around the posterior aspect of the proximal humerus with the right hand.

M—An anterior glide is effected with the right hand after the slack in the shoulder girdle has been taken up. This is an oscillatory mobilization. This technique is used to increase the joint-play movement necessary for external rotation.

B. Anterior glide, prone (Fig. 11-47*B*)

P—Lies prone with the humerus positioned off the edge of the table; a pad supporting the coracoid process provides some stabilization of the scapula.

O—Standing, facing the medial side of the upper arm. The glenohumeral joint is positioned in the resting position (if conservative techniques are indicated) or approximating the restricted range (if more aggressive techniques are indicated, such as capsular stretch). He supports the patient's elbow against his body with the left hand, maintaining the arm in abduction and neutral rotation. The upper limb is lowered slightly into a position in the plane of the scapula (30 to 45° anterior to the coronal plane).[84,116,198] The mobilizing hand is placed over the posterior aspect of the proximal humerus close to the joint.

M—Grade I traction is maintained throughout with the left hand. An anterior glide is produced by leaning forward with the trunk, transmitting the force through the straight arm and flexion of the knees. This technique is used to increase joint play necessary for external rotation, extension, and horizontal abduction.

C. Anterior glide, near the limits of external rotation (Fig 11-47*C*)[136]

P—Prone, lying as above

O—Standing, facing the table. The patient's flexed elbow rests on the operator's distal thigh. The outside hand supports the distal forearm above the wrist. The mobilizing hand contacts the proximal dorsal aspect of the humerus.

M—The mobilizing hand glides the humerus in the anterior direction. The amplitude and velocity of this technique is graded according to the patient's symptoms.

D. Posterior glide, arm close to 90° abduction (Fig. 11-47*D*)

P—Supine, with the arm resting comfortably but as close to 90° abduction as possible; elbow bent to 90°

O—Supports the wrist with his right hand. He contacts the anterior aspect of the proximal humerus with the heel of the left hand. The thigh may be brought up onto the plinth to act as a stop (see Fig. 6-3).

M—Posterior glide is produced with the left hand, while the right hand simultaneously rotates the arm externally. The thigh provides a stop to external

rotation close to the limit of movement. This minimizes anticipatory guarding by the patient. The stop is progressively moved as motion increases. This is an oscillatory movement, produced synchronously with posterior glide.

This method results in an anterior capsular stretch, stretching into external rotation while avoiding anterior impingement of the humerus on the glenoid labrum.

V. Glenohumeral Joint. General capsular stretch and techniques for horizontal adduction

A. Posterior glide or shear (Fig. 11-48*A*)

P—Supine, with the arm flexed to 90°. The arm may also be placed in various degrees of horizontal adduction. A pad is placed under the scapula for stabilization.

O—One or both hands are placed over the patient's elbow.

M—Posterior glide is directed through the long axis of the humerus in a slightly lateral direction. This technique is used to increase horizontal adduction, extension, and flexion. Direction of movement may also be directed in a posterior cranial direction.

B. Lateral glide, arm at side (glenohumeral distraction; Fig. 11-48*B*)

P—Supine, arm at the side, with the elbow bent and the hand resting on her stomach or on the operator's forearm

O—The operator is at the patient's side facing the glenohumeral joint. Both hands grasp the humerus medially, as far proximally as possible.

M—A lateral glide is effected by moving the upper humerus laterally with both hands. The arm should be allowed to move laterally through the same excursion as the humeral head, avoiding a tilting maneuver, unless it is specifically intended to stretch the superior joint capsule. (Anterior, posterior, and inferior glides may also be carried out with this hand placement.)

This technique (performed at the side of the body) is used to promote relaxation, to relieve pain, to prepare for more vigorous stretching techniques, and to provide a general capsular stretch. As the latter, it may be useful in increasing movement toward the close-packed position by helping to prevent premature compression of the joint.

C. Lateral glide, in flexion (Fig. 11-48*C*)

P—Supine, with the arm flexed comfortably to 90° and the elbow bent so that the hand rests on the upper chest

O—Stabilizes the distal humerus with his left hand at the elbow. The right hand is placed against the medial surface of the upper end of the humerus. By bending forward, the arm is placed in a horizontal position in line with the movement.

M—The proximal humerus is moved laterally. This technique is used to restore joint play necessary for

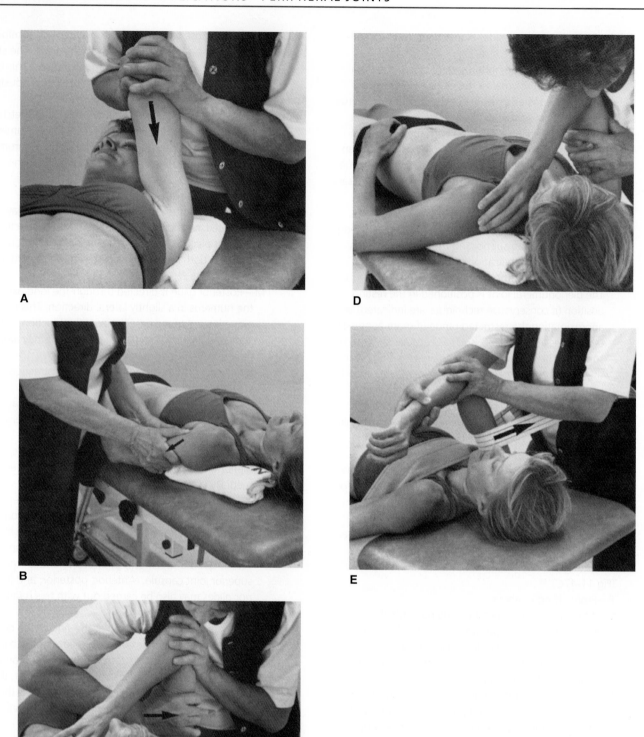

■ **FIG. 11-48.** General capsular stretch and techniques for horizontal adduction. **(A)** Posterior glide or shear. **(B)** Lateral glide, arm at side. **(C)** Lateral glide in flexion. **(D)** Lateral and backward glide in flexion. **(E)** Lateral glide in flexion with a belt.

horizontal adduction. It results in separation of the joint surfaces (lateral distraction).

D. Lateral and backward glide, in flexion (Fig. 11-48D)

P—Supine, with the arm flexed comfortably to 90° and the elbow bent so that the hand rests on the upper chest

O—Stabilizes the distal humerus and elbow by resting them against his trapezial ridge. He grasps the medial aspect of the proximal humerus with both hands, interlacing the fingers.

M—The proximal humerus is moved backward, toward the plinth, and outward simultaneously in a rocking forward and downward movement of the operator's trunk. The arm may be progressively moved toward increased horizontal adduction as the patient relaxes. This technique is used to increase joint play necessary for horizontal adduction by using lateral glide with a backward glide simultaneously. A belt placed around the patient's proximal humerus and around the operator's pelvis (or waist) may be used to apply lateral glide (traction) by backward leaning of the operator's trunk (Fig. 11-48E).[118]

VI. Glenohumeral Joint. Anteroposterior glide for the last few degrees of elevation

A. Anterior glide, in supine (Fig. 11-49A)

P—Supine, arm at end range of flexion or abduction

O—Standing, facing the patient's feet. Both hands grip the proximal humerus. The humerus is externally rotated to its limit. The patient's arm is cradled by the operator's arm and body to maintain the plane of scapula position.

M—The hands glide the humerus in a progressively anterior and posterior direction. During anterior glide, the force directs the head of the humerus against the inferior folds of the capsule.

B. Anterior glide, in sitting (Fig. 11-49B)

P—Sitting with the shoulder in maximum flexion or abduction and externally rotated

O—Standing next to the patient with the humerus against his chest and arm to maintain plane of scapula position. The stabilizing hand contacts the clavicle and scapular girdle proximal to the glenohumeral joint. The mobilizing hand grips the posterior proximal humerus.

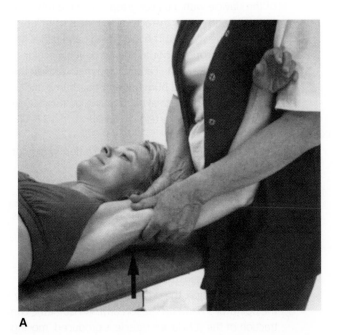

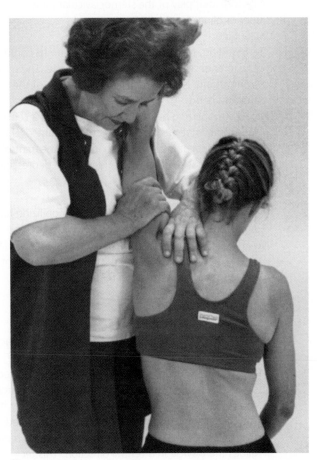

A   B

■ **FIGURE 11-49.** Anterior glides for the last few degrees of elevation (flexion, abduction) in supine (**A**) and sitting (**B**) positions.

M—The mobilizing force is directed anteriorly and slightly distally against the inferior folds of the capsule.

Scapulothoracic, acromioclavicular, and sternoclavicular mobilizations may also be performed in certain circumstances. However, these are rarely necessary in cases of glenohumeral capsular tightness, because these joints tend to become hypermobile by compensating for the restriction at the glenohumeral joint. They may be useful after immobilization of the entire shoulder complex or in other disorders, such as arthritis or injury in the different joints (i.e., fractures and dislocations) as well as neuromuscular dysfunction.

VII. Sternoclavicular Joint
  A. Distraction (Fig. 11-50*A*)[86]
     P—Supine
     O—Standing on the opposite side of the table. The index and middle fingers rest on the first costal cartilage and manubrium sterni to fixate the proximal aspect of the joint. The heel of the mobilizing hand contacts the lateral anterior concavity of the clavicle.
     M—Distraction force is applied in the lateral direction. This is considered a test and general technique to restore joint play of the sternoclavicular joint.
  B. Superior glide (Fig. 11-50*B*)
     P—Supine
     O—Standing, facing the patient. Both thumbs contact the inferior aspect of the proximal clavicle. The mobilizing thumb is positioned over the thumb of the guiding hand.
     M—The mobilizing hand glides the clavicle in a cephalad, somewhat medial direction in the plane of the joint. This technique is used to increase the joint play of the sternoclavicular joint and increase depression.
  C. Inferior glide (Fig. 11-50*C*)
     P—Supine
     O—Standing at the patient's head. The mobilizing hand is placed over the thumb of the guiding hand.
     M—The mobilizing hand glides the clavicle in a caudal, somewhat lateral direction in the plane of the joint. This technique is used to increase joint play and increase elevation.
  D. Posterior glide (Fig. 11-50*D*)
     P—Supine
     O—Standing, facing the patient. Both thumbs contact the proximal end of the clavicle.
     M—The thumbs glide in a posterior direction. This technique is used to increase retraction. Gliding anteriorly can be achieved by gripping around the clavicle with the fingers while the stabilizing hand is positioned over the sternum (Fig. 11-50*E*). The mobilizing hand glides the clavicle in a ventral direction. This technique is used to increase protraction.

VIII. Acromioclavicular Joint. All of the following techniques are considered general techniques to restore joint play of the acromioclavicular joint. The amplitude and velocity of the techniques vary according to the joint's irritability.
  A. Distraction (Fig. 11-51*A*)[86]
     P—Supine
     O—Standing on the opposite side of the table. The clavicle is grasped between the index finger and thumb to provide fixation. The mobilizing hand contacts the shoulder distal to the joint over the acromion.
     M—Distraction pressure is applied with the heel of the hand. This technique is considered a test and a general technique to restore joint play of the acromioclavicular joint.
  B. Anteroposterior glide (Fig. 11-51*B*)
     P—Sitting, the joint in the resting position
     O—Facing the ventral surface of the acromion. The thumbs are placed over the anterolateral surface of the clavicle. The medial hand provides stabilization over the dorsal aspect of the scapula.
     M—The thumbs glide the clavicle posteriorly.
  C. Posteroanterior glide
     P—Sitting (Fig. 11-51*C*) or sidelying (Fig. 11-51*D*), the joint in the resting position
     O—Standing, facing the dorsal surface of the acromioclavicular joint. The mobilizing hand is positioned with the thumb over the thumb of the gliding hand, which is positioned over the dorsolateral aspect of the clavicle.
     M—The clavicle is glided in a ventral, slightly lateral direction. Note: Anterior and posterior glide may also be performed in sidelying. The thumb and index finger of the stabilizing (cranial) hand contact the distal end of the clavicle with a pincer grasp, while the mobilizing (caudal) hand grasps the acromion process and lateral border of the scapula. The mobilizing hand glides the scapula anteroposterior at the acromioclavicular joint. Alternatively, the caudal hand may stabilize the scapula and proximal humerus and the thumb and index finger of the cranial hand may glide the clavicle anteriorly or posteriorly (Fig. 11-51*D*).

IX. Clavicle
  A. Inferior glide, active physiologic mobilization or isometric technique (Fig. 11-52)[175]
     P—Supine
     O—Standing, facing the patient. The medial hand grasps the posterior proximal aspect of the humerus and lifts the shoulder girdle into some protraction. The lateral hand holds the distal forearm above the wrist.
     M—The patient is instructed to lift the upper limb straight up against the unyielding resistance given by the operator's hand on the forearm. An isometric contraction of the subclavius muscle is produced, moving the clavicle inferiorly. This is a useful technique in patients with forward head postures. Superior sub-

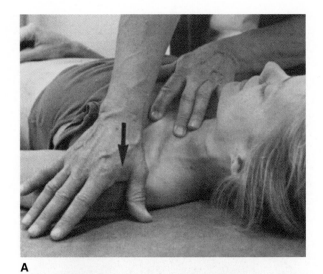

A

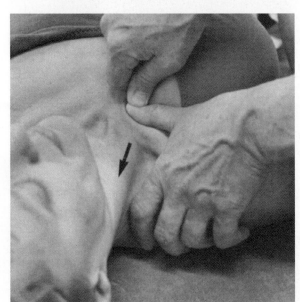

B

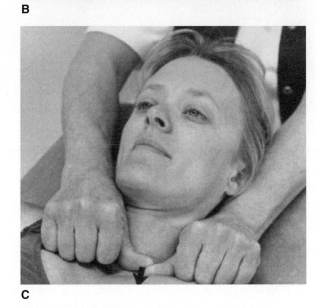

C

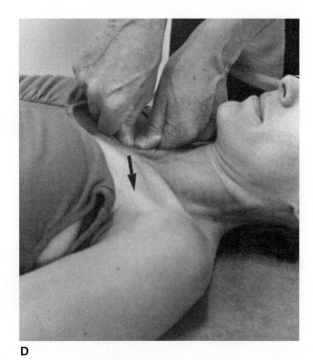

D

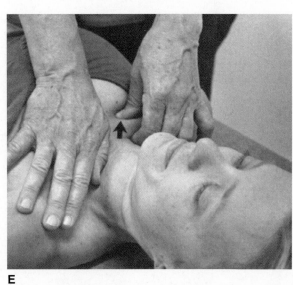

E

■ **FIG. 11-50.** Sternoclavicular joint: distraction (**A**), superior glide (**B**), inferior glide (**C**), posterior glide (**D**), and anterior glide (**E**).

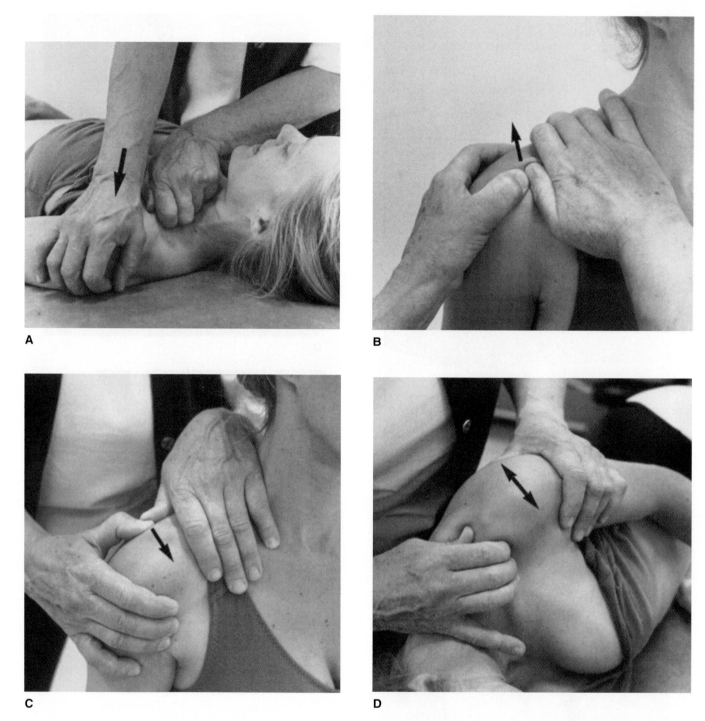

■ **FIG. 11-51.** Acromioclavicular joint: distraction (**A**), anteroposterior glide (**B**), posteroanterior glide (**C**), and anterior and posterior glide (**D**) in sidelying.

luxation of the clavicle may result from tightness of the sternocleidomastoid.[175] Soft tissue mobilizations and stretching of the sternocleidomastoid and other restricted soft tissues should be done concurrently.

X. Scapulothoracic Joint. Distraction techniques. (This is not a true joint, but the soft tissue is stretched to obtain normal shoulder girdle mobility.)

A. Distraction of the medial border of the scapula (Fig. 11-53A)
    P—Prone or sidelying
    O—Standing at the patient's side. The pads of the fingers of both hands contact the medial border of the scapula.
    M—Very slowly the scapula is distracted or lifted from the thorax, while simultaneously working the fingers

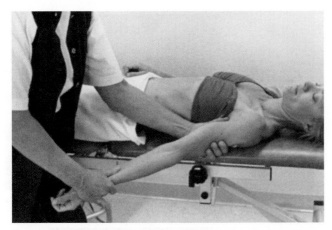

■ **FIG. 11-52.** Inferior glide of the clavicle using isometric technique.

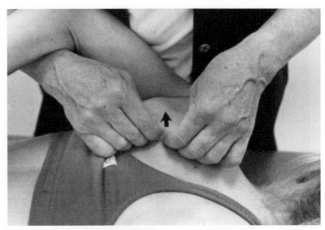

A

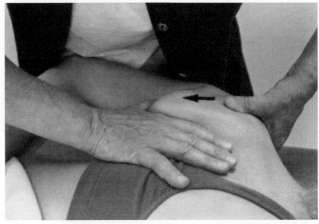

B

■ **FIG. 11-53.** Scapulothoracic joint distractions: medial border (**A**) and inferior border (**B**).

under the scapula. This is considered a general technique. The winging or distractive motion is an important movement for reaching behind the back. If there is little mobility, begin in prone position and progress to sidelying.

B. Distraction of the inferior border of the scapula (Fig. 11-53*B*)

P—Prone or sidelying

O—The mobilizing hand is placed over the acromion process while the web space of the guiding or stabilizing hand is positioned under the inferior border of the scapula.

M—The mobilizing hand moves the scapula medially and caudally over the guiding or stabilizing hand. The guiding hand assists in lifting the scapula away from the rib cage. Winging is an accessory motion that occurs when a person attempts to place the hand behind the back, accompanying shoulder internal rotation and scapular downward rotation.[131]

C. Scapulothoracic articulations, medial-lateral glide, superior-inferior glide, rotation, and diagonal patterns (Fig. 11-54)

P—Sidelying, the upper limb supported and draped over the operator's arm

O—Standing, facing the patient. The cranial hand is placed across the acromion process to guide and control the direction of motion. The caudal hand contacts the inferior angle of the scapula.

M—The scapula is moved in the desired direction by lifting from the inferior angle or by pushing on the acromion process (Fig. 11-54).

Self-Mobilization Techniques[204]

(For simplicity, all the techniques described in this section are applied to the patient's *right* extremity, except where indicated. In the self-mobilization techniques, the left hand usually is performing the mobilizations. E—equipment; P—patient; MH—mobilizing hand; M—movement.)

I. Inferior Glide. Long-axis extension (Fig. 11-55)

E—A high-back chair that is well padded with a blanket or towel on the back of the chair

P—Sitting, with the right arm over the back of the chair, the axilla firmly fixed over the back of the chair

MH—Grasps the arm just proximal to the humeral epicondyles so as to gain a purchase on them. An alternate handhold would be to grasp the forearm just above the styloid processes.

M—An inferior glide is produced by pulling directly downward toward the floor while using rhythmic oscillations (Fig. 11-55*A*). A variation of this technique is to use a weight in the hand (e.g., a bucket of sand) and to perform gentle, pivotlike motions at the end (Fig. 11-55*B*).

II. Inferior Glide. Shoulder adduction with distraction (Fig. 11-56)

E—A firm pillow or towel roll placed in the axilla

P—Standing, with the arm positioned across the chest

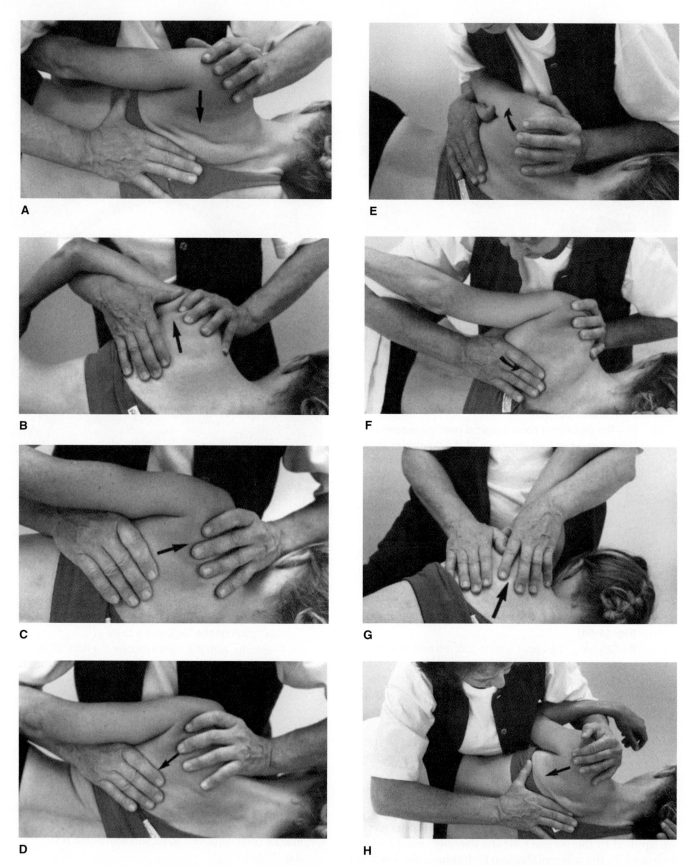

■ **FIG. 11-54.** Scapulothoracic joint. **(A)** Medial glide. **(B)** Lateral glide. **(C)** Superior glide. **(D)** Inferior glide. **(E)** Upward rotation. **(F)** Downward rotation. **(G)** Elevation and protraction. **(H)** Depression and retraction.

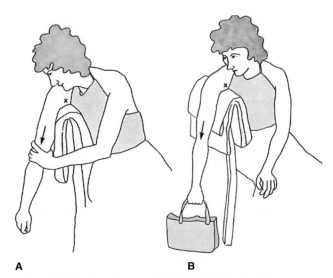

■ **FIG. 11-55.** Inferior glide (long-axis extension) of glenohumeral joint may be performed manually (**A**) or by using weights (**B**).

MH—Grasps the forearm just above the styloid processes. MH pulls the arm rhythmically across the chest (into adduction) and downward, resulting in a slight separation of the head of the humerus in the glenoid cavity (Fig. 11-56*A*). Note: Distraction dorsally may be carried out in a similar fashion if the patient has sufficient internal rotation to place the forearm behind the back. In this case, the elbow is flexed and the MH uses rhythmic oscillations behind the patient's back in a downward direction dorsally (Fig. 11-56*B*).

III. Inferior Glide. Glenohumeral abduction when the patient has less than 90° abduction (Fig. 11-57*A*)

P—Sitting sideways at a table, the right arm is positioned comfortably at the end of painless abduction

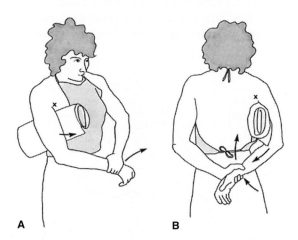

■ **FIG. 11-56.** Inferior glide of the glenohumeral joint. (**A**) Shoulder adduction with distraction ventrally. (**B**) Shoulder adduction with distraction dorsally.

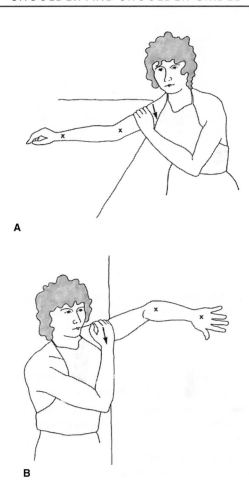

■ **FIG. 11-57.** Inferior glide of the glenohumeral joint. (**A**) Shoulder abduction for 90° or less. (**B**) Shoulder abduction for 90° or more.

with the muscles relaxed. The elbow is extended with the hand and the forearm fixed on the table.

MH—Contacts the anterior-superior aspect of the proximal humerus below the acromion

M—An inferior glide is produced by pushing directly downward toward the floor, with rhythmic oscillations

IV. Inferior Glide. Glenohumeral abduction when the patient has more than 90° abduction (Fig. 11-57*B*)

P—Standing with the right side facing a wall. The arm is positioned comfortably in abduction so that the forearm rests on the wall, with the elbow in 90° flexion.

MH—Contacts the anterior-superior aspect of the proximal end of the humerus below the acromion

M—An inferior glide is produced by pushing directly downward toward the floor with rhythmic oscillations. A stronger capsular stretch can be performed by bending the knees and using body weight to assist in the movement.

V. Inferior Glide. Glenohumeral flexion when the patient has less than 90° flexion (Fig. 11-58*A*)

P—Sitting facing a table. The right forearm is positioned comfortably at the end of painless flexion with the

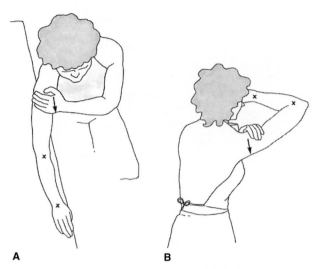

A   **B**

■ **FIG. 11-58.** Inferior glide of the glenohumeral joint.
(A) Shoulder flexion for 90° or less. **(B)** Shoulder flexion for
90° or more.

muscles relaxed. A pillow wedge is used under the
forearm to provide fixation of the hand and forearm.
MH—Contacts the anterior-superior aspect of the
proximal humerus below the acromion
M—An inferior glide is produced by pushing directly
downward toward the floor, with rhythmic oscillations
VI.   Inferior Glide. Glenohumeral flexion when the patient has
more than 90° flexion (Fig. 11-58*B*)
P—Standing facing a wall. The right forearm, with the
elbow bent to 90° flexion, is positioned at the end of
range on the wall for fixation.
MH—Contacts the anterosuperior aspect of the proximal end of the humerus below the acromion
M—An inferior glide is produced by pushing directly
downward toward the floor, with rhythmic oscillations. A stronger capsular stretch may be performed
by lowering the body weight.
VII.   Anterior Glide. Shoulder extension (Fig. 11-59)

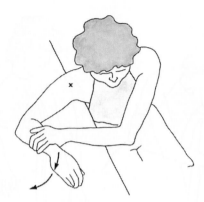

■ **FIG. 11-60.** Internal rotation of the glenohumeral
joint.

P—Sitting, with the back to a table. The right arm is
positioned comfortably at the limits of painless extension with the muscles relaxed. The elbow is extended
with the right hand fixed on the table. The trunk is
flexed.
MH—Contacts the posterosuperior aspect of the proximal humerus just below the acromion
M—An anterior glide is produced by moving the arm in
a ventral-caudal direction, with rhythmic oscillations.
VIII.   Shoulder Internal Rotation (Fig. 11-60)
P—Sitting sideways to a table. The right upper arm is
positioned so that its entire extent is braced against the
table. To do this, the patient bends the trunk to the
side toward the upper arm. The elbow is flexed to 90°.
MH—Grasps the dorsal aspect of the wrist with the
thumb, and with the fingers wrapped around the
ventral aspect
M—The arm is internally rotated as far as possible with
rhythmic oscillations performed at the end of the range.
IX.   Shoulder External Rotation (Fig. 11-61)
P—Sitting sideways to a table. The right upper arm is
positioned so that its entire extent is braced against the
table. To do this, the patient bends the trunk to the
side toward the upper arm. The elbow is flexed to 90°.

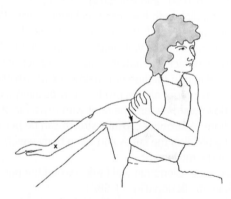

■ **FIG. 11-59.** Anterior glide (shoulder extension) of the
glenohumeral joint.

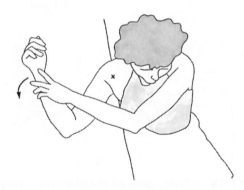

■ **FIG. 11-61.** External rotation of the glenohumeral
joint.

MH—Grasps the ventral aspect of the wrist

M—The forearm is externally rotated, and rhythmic oscillations are performed at the end of the range.

Note: Hold–relax techniques are particularly useful with rotation techniques of the shoulder.

Self Capsular Stretches

A more aggressive approach to stretching the joint capsule and surrounding musculature usually commences when the patient has attained flexibility of at least 90° abduction. The end feel is firm, and the end point is no longer painful. The patient may be instructed to hold at the end range for 10 seconds, with a 5-second rest between consecutive stretches (10 to 15 repetitions), or to apply a longer-duration, low-load stretch. Low-load, long-duration stretches are more efficient in elongating soft tissue than high-load, short-duration stretches.[144,247] Heat in conjunction with low-load, long-duration stretching can be used to facilitate shoulder flexibility.[142] Thus, the patient can be put in a comfortable elongation position with a slight load with heat for 40 seconds or longer.

I. Anterior Capsule Stretch (Fig. 11-62A)

    P—Supine with the involved shoulder over the edge of the table, the elbow flexed to 90°, and the shoulder in a comfortable position of abduction, depending on the portion of the capsule that is tight. A weight is placed in the hand (starting with 1 or 2 pounds or less), or tubing may be used (with tubing securely in the hand and the opposite end attached to the table or bed). Padding should be used under the upper limb to position the shoulder in the plane of the scapula.

    M—The patient allows the weight or tubing to pull the shoulder into maximum external rotation and some extension. As an exercise to stretch the anterior-inferior capsule, have the patient lie supine with the shoulder over the table edge in a position of about 135° abduction (Fig. 11-62B). Again, padding is used under the upper limb to maintain the plane of scapula position.

II. Inferior Capsule Stretch (Fig. 11-62C)

    P—Supine on the table with the shoulder at comfortable end range of flexion. Padding should be used under the upper limb to maintain the plane of scapula position.

    M—A weight or tubing is used to facilitate stretch into fuller flexion.

III. Posterior Capsule Stretch. The posterior capsule can be stretched by holding the involved arm in horizontal adduction and by placing the hand near the opposite shoulder (Fig. 11-62D). A gentle pull is applied with the opposite hand.

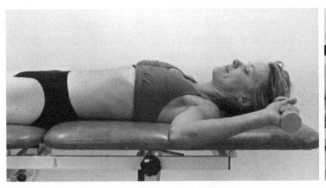

A

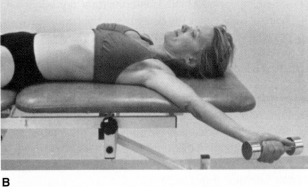

B

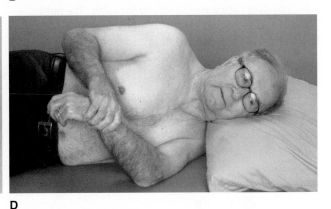

C

D

■ **FIG. 11-62.** Self capsular stretches. **(A)** Anterior capsular. **(B)** Anterior-inferior capsular. **(C)** Inferior capsular. **(D)** Posterior capsular stretch.

Self Range of Motion

Other exercises particularly useful in a home program for painful extremity joints have been advocated by Dontigny[61] and Grimsby.[87] They allow the patient to stretch his or her joints passively by moving the body in relation to the stabilized extremity. This type of movement affords an excellent stretch, minimizes incorrect movements by the patient, and allows a greater degree of pain-free movement. Grimsby[87] maintains that when passive exercise is used for the hip, shoulder, or ankle, the patient uses the concave surface of the joint to mobilize. In so doing, the patient avoids considerable pain and achieves a greater range of motion, because rolling and gliding occur in the same direction. If we compare these exercises to the traditional approach of movement of the extremity in relation to the body, it also appears that using a closed kinetic chain (through the stabilized extremity) provides greater joint stability and a more normal pattern of movement. Examples of these types of exercises are described for the shoulder.

I. Shoulder Flexion
   A. Sitting (Fig. 11-63)
      P—Sitting at the side of a table with the forearm resting on the table
      M—Patient flexes the trunk and head while sliding the arm forward along the edge of the table, so that the shoulder is moved passively into flexion
   B. Standing (Fig. 11-64)
      P—Standing, facing a high countertop (or a high window ledge or bookshelf). The patient rests the hand, palm down, on the edge of the counter with the elbow extended.
      M—The patient lowers the body weight to move the shoulder passively into flexion.
         Weight-bearing stretches may be done in the all-fours or crawling position. The upper limbs are gradually stretched forward as the body sinks into a prone position (sitting on the heels) to eventually achieve full forward flexion.
II. Shoulder Extension (Fig. 11-65)
      P—Standing with the right side to the table. The right hand is placed on the table, with the arm at the side and the elbow extended.

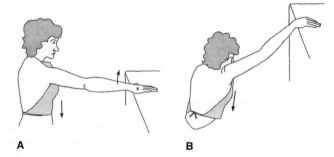

■ **FIG. 11-64.** Passive shoulder flexion (standing). **(A)** Starting position. **(B)** End position.

      M—Maintaining the right hand in a fixed position on the table, the patient walks forward to produce shoulder extension through the painless range of motion.
III. Shoulder Abduction
   A. Sitting (Fig. 11-66)
      P—Sitting at the side of a table and resting the forearm on the table, with the forearm supinated and the shoulder slightly abducted
      M—The patient sidebends the upper trunk to the left from the waist while sliding the arm across the table so that the shoulder is moved into abduction as the lower trunk moves away from the table.
   B. Standing (Fig. 11-67)
      P—Standing with the right side facing a high countertop (or a high window ledge or bookshelf). The patient rests the hand on the surface with the forearm slightly supinated, elbow extended, and shoulder abducted through partial range.
      M—The patient lowers the body weight, allowing the shoulder to move passively into abduction and external rotation.

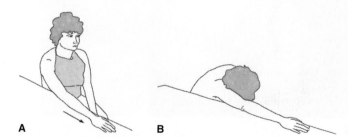

■ **FIG. 11-63.** Passive shoulder flexion (sitting). **(A)** Starting position. **(B)** End position.

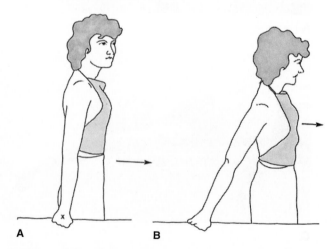

■ **FIG. 11-65.** Passive shoulder extension. **(A)** Starting position. **(B)** End position.

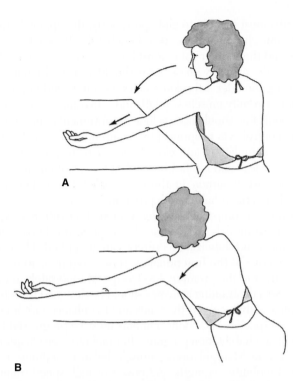

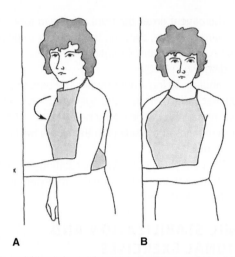

■ **FIG. 11-68.** Passive internal rotation of shoulder. **(A)** Starting position. **(B)** End position.

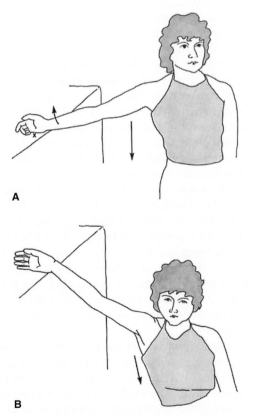

■ **FIG. 11-66.** Passive shoulder abduction (sitting). **(A)** Starting position. **(B)** End position.

IV. Shoulder Internal Rotation (Fig. 11-68)
   P—Standing with the left side toward a door frame. The patient places the back of the hand against the frame so that it will remain fixed with his elbow flexed 90°. The upper arm remains at the side with the elbow held close to the trunk.
   M—The patient walks forward, rotating toward the left forearm to produce passive internal rotation of the shoulder.
   Internal rotation may be done in a standing position, with the patient attempting to reach behind and up the back as far as possible. The opposite limb grasps the involved side at the wrist and attempts to stretch it further. A hand towel can be used behind the back in a similar fashion.
V. Shoulder External Rotation
   A. Sitting (Fig. 11-69)
   P—Sitting at the side of a table, with the forearm resting on the table, the shoulder abducted, and the elbow flexed

■ **FIG. 11-67.** Passive shoulder abduction (standing). **(A)** Starting position. **(B)** End position.

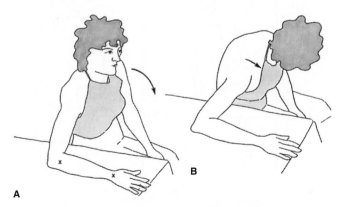

■ **FIG. 11-69.** Passive external rotation of shoulder (sitting). **(A)** Starting position. **(B)** End position.

M—The patient flexes the trunk and head forward toward the table, allowing the shoulder to be moved passively into external rotation.

B. Standing (Fig. 11-70)

P—Standing, facing a door frame. The patient places the palmar surface of the hand against the frame so that it will remain fixed. The elbow is flexed 90°. The upper arm remains at the side with the elbow held close to the trunk.

M—The patient walks backward, rotating the body away from the left arm to produce passive external rotation of the shoulder.

DYNAMIC STABILIZATION AND FUNCTIONAL EXERCISES

Combining functional (see Chapter 10, Functional Exercise) and stabilization exercises with manual therapy, and various other exercise models (i.e., plyometrics, concentric and eccentric isotonics, therapeutic exercises in functional kinetics, stretch-shortening exercises, closed kinetic chain exercises, proprioceptive neuromuscular facilitation exercises, and neuromuscular control exercises) will augment the rehabilitation of the patient with shoulder dysfunction.[1,4,5,27,31,42,44,59,66,82,83,89,90,95,114,129–133,137,163,182,199,212,229,240,241,244,253–255,257]

There has been increased attention to the development of balance and proprioception in the rehabilitation of patients after injury.[27,112,113,130,241] It is believed that injury results in altered somatosensory input that influences neuromuscular control. In addition to local treatment, evaluation and possible rehabilitation of the distant contributors to shoulder function should be done. Deficits in strength, neuromuscular control, strength balance, and flexibility in the legs, hips, and trunk should be sought. To complete humeral elevation beyond 120°

the ribs must be able to glide posteriorly, the upper thoracic spine must be able to extend and sidebend to the contralateral side, and the lumbar spine must be able to actively extend.[120] During the recovery phase of the shoulder, in addition to normalizing shoulder arthrokinematics, regaining and improving upper extremity muscle strength and active and passive range of motion, one should also include improvement of neuromuscular control (via proprioceptive neuromuscular facilitation, sensory stimulation, and closed chain activities) and normal back, cervical, and hip flexibility. Restrictions of hip and neck motions are common in throwing athletes and should be included in the rehabilitation program.[130]

Although comprehensive description of the different types of exercise models are beyond the scope of this book, a few functional and stabilization exercises are described. The overall objective of the functional exercise program is to return the patient to the preinjury level as quickly and safely as possible. Specific training activities should be designed to restore dynamic stability about the joints and to enhance motor control and specific ADL skills. Patients must be progressed forward in a rehabilitation program after mobility (see Chapter 8, Soft Tissue Manipulations), muscle balance, stability, controlled mobility, strength, and power or high-speed training formulas. Functional exercises are integrated, multiplanar movement patterns that require stabilization in all three planes (triplanar) versus isolated movement patterns.

I. Exercise procedures to reestablish neuromuscular control and promote stability in weight bearing. Compression into or through a joint stimulates the joint receptors and facilitates stability of the joint.[229]

A. Push-offs (Fig. 11-71). Push-offs allow the patient to perform a closed kinetic chain exercise (*A*). Progression to wall push-offs, challenged by a therapist, allows the patient to perform isometric, concentric, and eccentric contractions (*B*). These exercises will strengthen all shoulder girdle muscles with emphasis pectoralis major and minor and facilitate stability and controlled mobility of the shoulder girdle complex.

B. Shoulder abduction, in standing (Fig. 11-72). Abduction of the arms is performed by sliding the forearms and hands up the wall to 90° abduction followed by shoulder shrugs while continuing abduction. At the end of elevation, the hands are lifted off the wall by adducting the scapulae. The hands are returned to the wall and lowered back to the starting position with control. This technique is used to improve the performance of upper trapezius and control of humeral lateral rotation (after Sahrmann[212]).

C. Closed-chain exercises for scapular control with 90° of elevation (Fig. 11-73). Scapular elevation (*A*), scapular depression (*B*). Scapular and rotator cuff stability is initially developed by performing low-intensity isometric contraction, first in shortened range and then in more lengthened range and finally dynamically with an unstable surface (i.e., a ball).

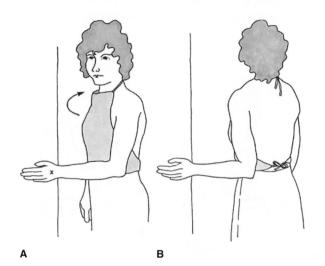

A **B**

■ **FIG. 11-70.** Passive external rotation of shoulder (standing). **(A)** Starting position. **(B)** End position.

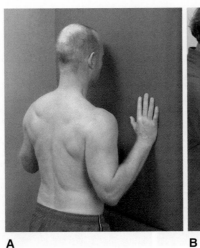 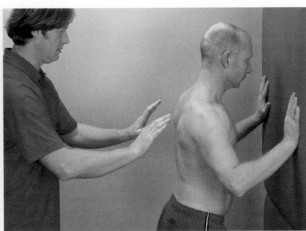

■ **FIG. 11-71.** **(A)** Push-offs allow the patient to perform a closed kinetic chain exercise. **(B)** Progression to a therapist-assisted wall push-off.

A   **B**

D. Exercise variations of modified plantigrade (Fig. 11-74) with arm supported on a stable surface while rocking forward and backward (*A;* four-point position), with the stronger arm up (*B;* three-point position), and lifting up against a band (*C;* Thera-Band or surgical tubing) while holding the band down with the weaker arm. These static–dynamic activities increase the dynamic stability of the weight-bearing segments. The arm that is supported in a closed kinetic chain is using shoulder force-couples to maintain neuromuscular control.

E. Seated push-up (Fig. 11-75) for scapular depression strength. Body weight is lifted upward off a stable sur-

face (*A*). A greater challenge for lower trapezius push-up strength and control can be achieved using stability (Swiss ball or therapeutic ball) balls (*B*).

F. Prone push-up (Fig. 11-76). Push-up with a plus: a normal push-up, followed by an extra "push" to the ceiling to allow full protraction (*A*). This exercise was shown by Mosely et al.[166] to have the highest electromyographic activity for the serratus anterior. Push-ups on a stability ball add more issues of stability and balance (*B*).

G. Scapular neuromuscular control drills in sidelying (Fig. 11-77). The shoulder is abducted to 90° and internally rotated, and the hand is placed on the plinth (*A*). Manual resistance is applied to the cardinal and diagonal scapular patterns of motion (*B*), that is, anterior elevation, posterior depression, posterior elevation, and anterior depression. A variety of manual therapy techniques, such as rhythmic stabilization, slows reversal holds, and timing for emphasis can be used to intensify dynamic control of the scapulothoracic joint.[1,256] Using the trunk with scapular motion, one can extend their action into such functional activities as rolling forward and backward. Scapular patterns can be done sitting and standing.

H. Quadruped stabilization (Fig. 11-78). Weight shifting can begin on a stable surface in a four-point position (*A*) or three-point position and progress to weight shifting on unstable surfaces such as a balance board (*B*) or ball (*C*). In the three-point position a free weight, Thera-Band, or an oscillating body blade (*D*) can be used while working on neuromuscular control on the weight-bearing shoulder. manual resistance produced by the therapist (*E*) can be applied to the non–weight-bearing arms as the patient focuses on controlling scapular movements.

I. Front bridge with four points of stable contact (Fig. 11-79) may be performed from the knees (*A*), from the toes

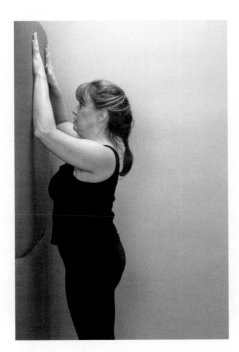

■ **FIG. 11-72.** Shoulder abduction in standing: upper trapezius exercise.

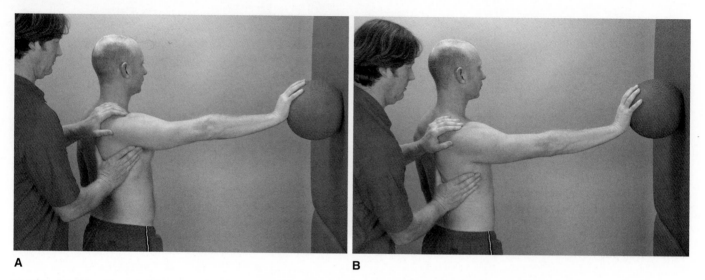

■ **FIG. 11-73.** Closed-chain exercise for scapular control. **(A)** Scapular elevation. **(B)** Scapular depression.

with a wide base of support (*B*), or from the toes with a narrow base of support. Performing these exercises correctly will develop the shoulder stabilizers as well as the trunk. Progression might include a front bridge with three points of contact (i.e., on the toes of one leg), and two points of contact with the thighs or feet on a stability ball. Repeated exercises are started for 5 to 10 seconds and work up to 10 repetitions. Repetitions may then be advanced for longer duration

(20 to 45 seconds) but with fewer repetitions (3 to 5 repetitions).[5]

II. Functional Exercise and PNF Strengthening Techniques. Methods of complex functional motions (triplanar) and diagonal patterns of motion are optimal preparations or training methods for both the athlete and nonathlete. The use of complex motions is based on the principles of stimulation of the neuromuscular apparatus with the additional help of entire body movement. Diagonal patterns can be initiated in

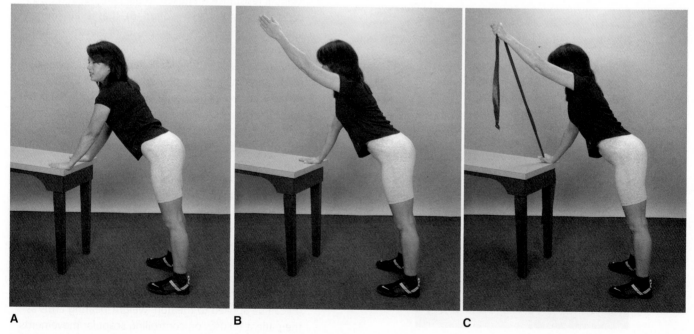

■ **FIG. 11-74.** Exercise variation of modified plantigrade, with the arms supported on a stable surface **(A)**, lifting up with one arm **(B)**, and lifting up against a therapeutic band **(C)**.

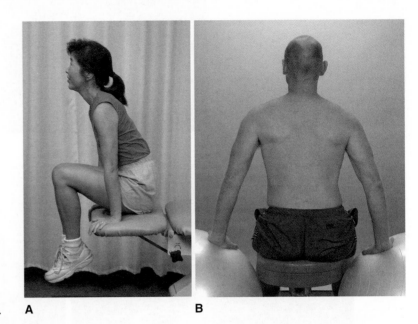

■ **FIG. 11-75.** Seated push-ups. Body weight lifted upward off a stable surface (**A**), and progression to an unstable surface (stability balls; **B**).

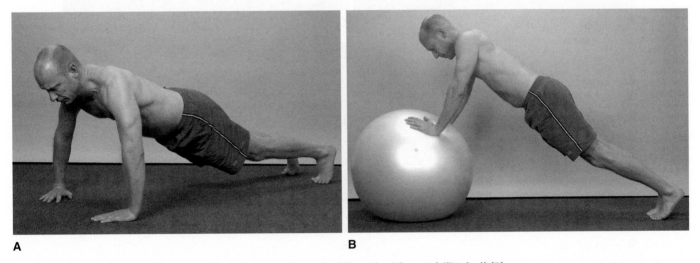

■ **FIG. 11-76.** Prone push-ups. Basic push-up with a plus (**A**) and with a stability ball (**B**).

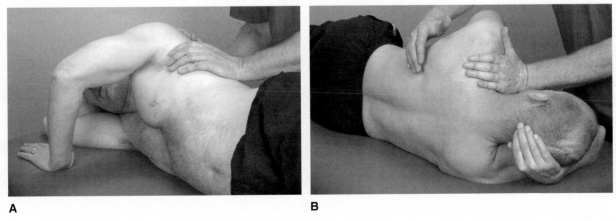

■ **FIG. 11-77.** Scapular neuromuscular control drill in sidelying. (**A**) The shoulder is abducted to 90° and the hand placed on the plinth. (**B**) Manual resistance is applied to cardinal and diagonal scapular patterns of motion.

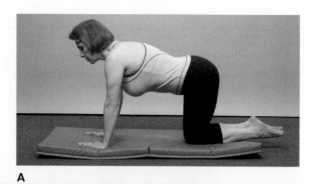

A

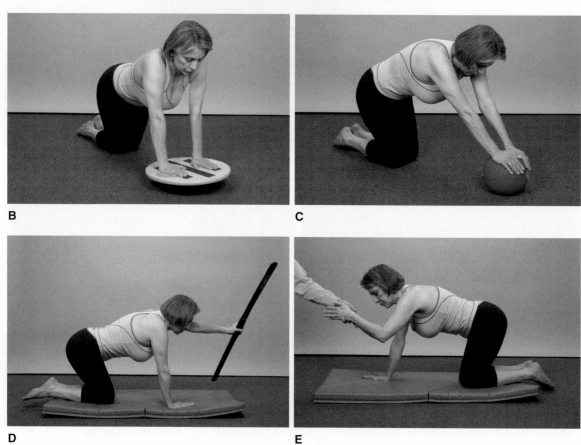

B

C

D

E

■ **FIG. 11-78.** Quadruped stabilization. Weight shifting in a four-point position on a stable surface (**A**), on a balance board (**B**), and on a ball (**C**). Three-point position using an oscillatory body blade (**D**) and with manual resistance (**E**).

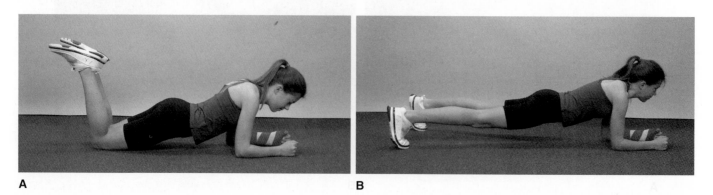

A

B

■ **FIG. 11-79.** Front bridge performed from the knees with four points of stable contact (**A**) and from the toes with a wide base of support (**B**).

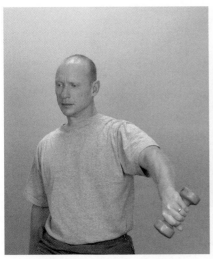
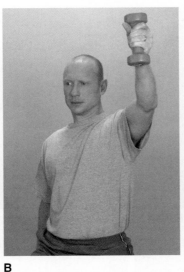
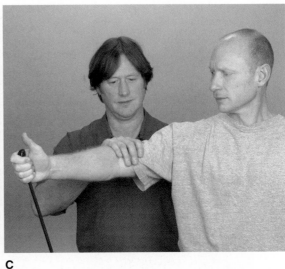

A   **B**   **C**

■ **FIG. 11-80.** Shoulder flexion in the plane of the scapula ("scaption") below 80° of flexion (**A**), from neutral to 120° (**B**), and with the application of resistance (**C**).

supine, sitting, and then standing with resistance applied manually, with free weights, or with elastic resistance. Use the actual patterns and type of contraction required in the desired outcome and progress to the desired speed first in a controlled manner, then with less control. Increase endurance and initiate stretch-shortening drills (plyometrics) in a safe, controlled pattern with light resistance; then progress speed and resistance as tolerated.

A. Shoulder flexion in the plane of the scapula with relative internal rotation and forearm pronation (Fig. 11-80), emphasizing supraspinatus activity and high activity levels of the deltoid below 80° (*A;* "empty can") and neutral to 120° (*B;* "scaption"). Rhythmic stabilization (*C*) can be performed as the patient holds a specific position in the plane of the scapula with or without the use of surgical tubing and force applied by the therapist. The alternating efforts of the patient mobilize the glenohumeral joint in all the involuntary motions (joint play).

B. Manually resisted scapular patterns (after Einhorn et al.[66]; Fig. 11-81) with Thera-Band or surgical tubing for scapula stabilization using other muscles to add stability (i.e., paraspinals and contralateral scapular muscles).

C. Combination exercises and the use of the stability ball and assistive devices to train strength, balance, and proprioception (Fig. 11-82). (*A*) Sitting on the ball while pulling a resistive band (Thera-Band or surgical tubing) in a diagonal pattern (one hand stabilizes while the other hand pulls into forward flexion, abduction, and external rotation of the shoulder). (*B*) Prone on the ball using a resistive band challenging the back extensors and trapezius (one arm moves into forward flexion and abduction while the other arm moves into extension

and adduction). (*C*) Supine on the ball (using dumbbells) and diagonal arm patterns (one arm is in extension while other arm moves in forward flexion, adduction, and external rotation). (*D*) Supine on the ball (using dumbbells) in chopping and lifting patterns (bilateral asymmetrical upper limb patterns), which are reinforced by upper trunk head and neck flexion patterns.

D. Diagonal upper quadrant pattern (Fig. 11-83). Trunk extension and rotation combined with D1 flexion pattern of the upper limb, starting position (*A*) and end position (*B*). Note the functional involvement of the lower quadrant: hip, knee, and ankle.

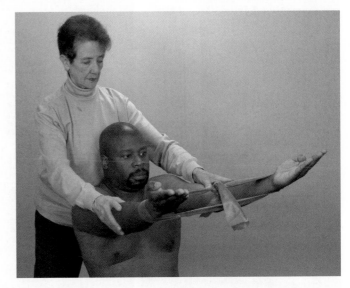

■ **FIG. 11-81.** Manually resisted diagonal scapular patterns with a therapeutic band or surgical tubing.

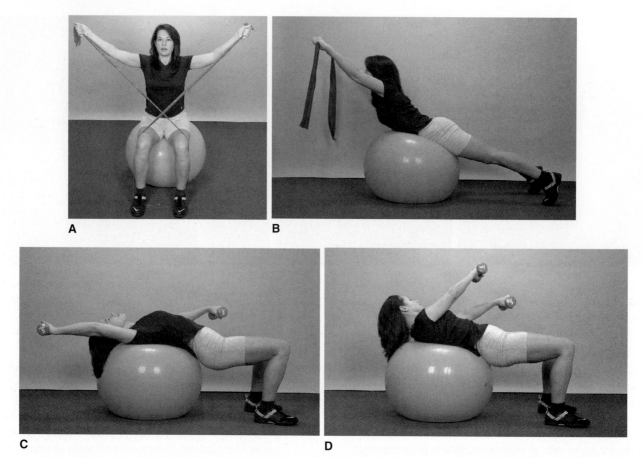

■ **FIG. 11-82.** Combination exercise on the stability ball. **(A)** Sitting on the ball while pulling a resistive band in diagonal arm patterns. **(B)** Prone on the ball using a resistive band challenging the back extensor and the trapezius. **(C)** Supine on the ball while carrying out diagonal arm patterns (with dumbbells). **(D)** Supine on the ball while using chopping and lifting patterns of the arms (with dumbbells).

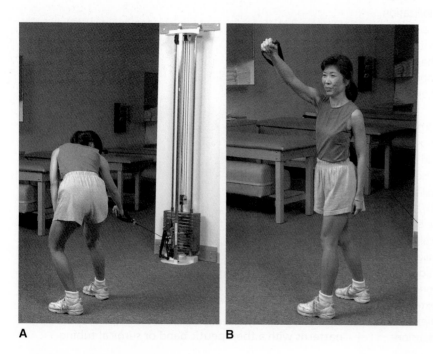

■ **FIG. 11-83.** Diagonal upper quadrant pattern. Trunk extension and rotation combined with D1 flexion pattern. **(A)** Starting position. **(B)** End position.

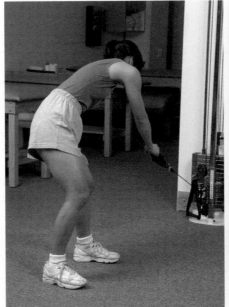
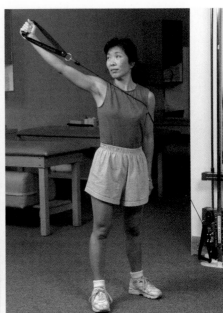

■ **FIG. 11-84.** Diagonal upper quadrant pattern. Trunk extension and rotation combined with D2 flexion pattern. (**A**) Starting position. (**B**) End position.

A

B

E. Diagonal upper quadrant pattern (Fig. 11-84). Trunk extension and rotation combined with D2 flexion pattern of the upper limb, starting position (*A*) and end position (*B*). Note the use of the head and cervical spine in these exercises.

F. Diagonal upper quadrant pattern (Fig. 11-85). Trunk flexion and rotation combined with the D2 extension pattern, starting position (*A*) and end position (*B*). This pattern emphasizes the posterior rotator cuff and posterior deltoid, which are often deficient with shoulder instability.

G. The lawnmower exercise (Fig. 11-86). Starting position (*A*) to simultaneously strengthen and facilitate scapular control and trunk extension, and end position (*B*) of the lawnmower exercise. Note the use of scapular retraction and elbow flexion as if tucking the elbow into the back pocket.

H. Combination exercise of squatting with lifting and chopping using a Plyoball or medicine ball (Fig. 11-87). Starting position (*A*) holding a medicine ball across to the

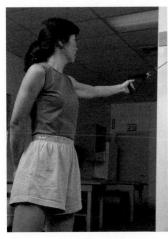
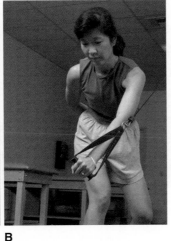

A

B

■ **FIG. 11-85.** Diagonal upper quadrant pattern. Trunk flexion and rotation combined with D2 arm extension pattern. (**A**) Starting position. (**B**) End position.

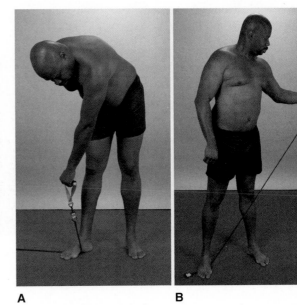

A

B

■ **FIG. 11-86.** The lawnmower exercise. (**A**) Starting position. (**B**) End position.

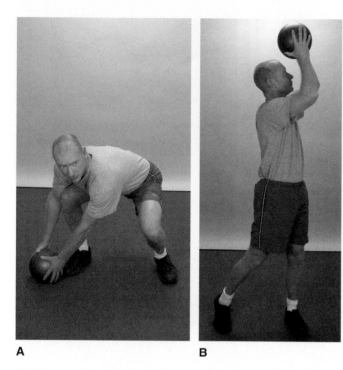

A   **B**

■ **FIG. 11-87.** Combination exercise of squatting, with lifting and chopping patterns (bilateral asymmetrical pattern: D1 R; D2 L) using a Plyoball or medicine ball.

right (bilateral asymmetrical pattern (D1 R; D2 L) and end position (*B*). The arms are lifted up and across to the left with hip and knee extension and trunk rotation and extension. The movement is followed with the head and neck. The exercise is repeated to the opposite side.

I. The Egyptian (Fig. 11-88; after Chasan[43]). (*A*) Bilateral reciprocal arm patterns with the elbows bent. Head, neck, and trunk follow the arm moving into external rotation. The reverse Egyptian (*B*), with the head, neck, and trunk following the arm moving into internal rotation. The lower quadrant (hip, knee, and foot) are also actively involved. These patterns facilitate cervical and upper trunk mobility and strengthen the rotator cuff.

J. Stretch-shortening drills (plyometrics; Fig. 11-89).[11,28,131,243,256–258] Catching a weighted Plyoball (*A*) with the body supported by the floor, using the ball to create overload into external rotation requiring the patient to stabilize the shoulder, (*B*) in free-standing position using PNF drills in a diagonal extension pattern, and (*C*) a diagonal flexion pattern. Various arm positions can be used with immediate toss back using the reciprocal pattern. Plyometrics should be initiated in a safe, controlled pattern with light resistance, then with increased speed and resistance as tolerated.

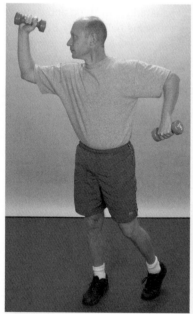
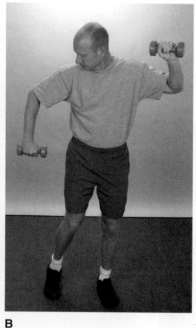

A   **B**

■ **FIG. 11-88.** The Egyptian. (**A**) Bilateral reciprocal arm patterns with head, neck, and trunk rotation following the arm moving into lateral rotation. (**B**) Reverse Egyptian with the head and neck following the arm moving into medial rotation.

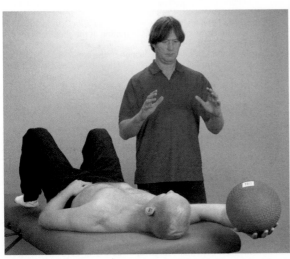
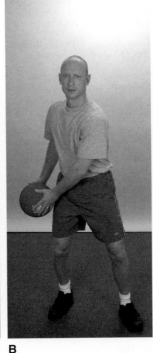
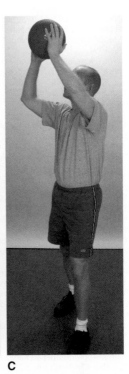

A   **B**   **C**

▪ **FIG. 11-89.** Stretch-shortening drills (plyometrics). Catching a ball with body weight supported by the plinth (**A**), and in freestanding position using proprioceptive neuromuscular facilitation (PNF) drills in a diagonal extension pattern (**B**) and in a diagonal flexion pattern (**C**).

Goals of plyometric drills are to improve the patient's proprioception skills and to enhance the neuromuscular control of the glenohumeral joint in positions that are dynamically challenging and place the patient in susceptible postures.

REFERENCES

1. Adler SA, Beckers D, Buck M: PNF in Practice: An Illustrated Guide. Berlin, Springer-Verlag, 1993
2. Adson AW, Coffey JR: Cervical rib: A method of anterior approach for relief of symptoms by division of the scalenus anticus. Ann Surg 85:839–857, 1927
3. Akeson WH, Woo SLY, Amiel D: The connective tissue response to immobility: Biomechanical changes in periarticular connective tissue of the immobilized rabbit knee. Clin Orthop 93:356–362, 1973
4. Albert M: Eccentric Muscle Training in Sports and Orthopaedics. New York, Churchill Livingstone, 1991
5. Alfiera RMG: Functional Training: Everyone's Guide to the New Fitness Revolution. New York, Hatherliegh Press, 2001
6. Allen EV: Peripheral Vascular Disease, 4th ed. Philadelphia, WB Saunders, 1970
7. Almekinders LC, Temple JD: Etiology, diagnosis, and treatment of tendinitis: An analysis of the literature. Med Sci Sports Exerc 30:1183–1190, 1998
8. Anderson MK, Hall SJ, Martin M: Sports Injury Management, 2nd ed. Philadelphia, Lippincott Williams & Wilkins, 2000
9. Andrews JR, Gillogly S: Physical examination of the shoulder in throwing athletes. In: Zarins B, Andrews JR, Carson WG, eds: Injuries to the Throwing Arm. Philadelphia, WB Saunders, 1985
10. Andrews JR, Wilk KE, eds: The Athlete's Shoulder. New York, Churchill Livingstone, 1994
11. Arrigo CA, Wilk KE: Shoulder exercises: A criteria-based approach to rehabilitation. In: Kelly MJ, Clark WA: Orthopedic Therapy of the Shoulder. Philadelphia, JB Lippincott, 1995:337–370
12. Bajelis D: The Biomechanical Assessment of the Myofascial System: A Practical Manual for Body Therapists. Mount Shasta, CA, Hellerwork, 1995
13. Barbis J: Therapist's management of thoracic outlet syndrome. In: Hunter JM, Schneider LH, Mackin EJ, Callahan AB, eds: Rehabilitation of the Hand: Surgery and Therapy, 3rd ed. St. Louis, Mosby. 1990:540–562
14. Barrel JP: The Thorax. Seattle, Eastland Press, 1991
15. Basmajian JV: Factors preventing downward dislocation of the abducted shoulder joint. J Bone Joint Surg Am 41:1182–1186, 1959
16. Basmajian JV: Weight bearing by ligaments and muscles. Can J Surg 4:166–170, 1961
17. Basmajian JV: Surgical anatomy and function of the arm-trunk mechanism. Surg Clin North Am 43:1471–1482, 1963
18. Basmajian JV: Muscles Alive: Their Functions Revealed by Electromyography, 4th ed. Baltimore, Williams & Wilkins, 1977
19. Bateman JE, Welsh RP: Surgery of the Shoulder. St. Louis, CV Mosby, 1984
20. Bechtol CO: Biomechanics of the shoulder. Clin Orthop 146:37–41, 1980
21. Beighton PH: Articular mobility in an African population. Ann Rheum Dis 32:413–418, 1973
22. Bell RH, Noble JB: Biceps disorders. In: Hawkins RJ, Misamore GW, eds: Shoulder Injuries in the Athlete. New York, Churchill Livingstone, 1996
23. Blackburn TA: Throwing injuries to the shoulder. In: Donatelli R, ed: Physical Therapy of the Shoulder, 2nd ed. New York, Churchill Livingstone, 1991:239–270
24. Blakely RL, Palmer ML: Analysis of rotation accompanying shoulder flexion. Phys Ther 64:1214–1216, 1984
25. Boehme R: Improving Upper Body Control: An Approach to Assessment and Treatment of Tonal Dysfunction. Tucson, AZ, Therapy Skill Builders, 1988
26. Booth RE, Marvel JP: Differential diagnosis of the shoulder pain. Orthop Clin North Am 6:353–379, 1975
27. Borsa PA, Lephart SM, Mininder SK, et al: Functional assessment and rehabilitation of shoulder proprioceptors for glenohumeral stability. Am J Sports Med 25:336–340, 1997
28. Bosco C, Koni P: Potential of the mechanical behavior of the human skeletal muscle through pre-stretching. Acta Physiol Scand 106:467–472, 1979
29. Bradley JP, Tibone JE: Electromyographic analysis of muscle action about the shoulder. Clin Sports Med 10:789–805, 1991
30. Brewster CE, Shields CL, Seto JL, et al: Rehabilitation of the upper extremity. In: Shields CL, ed: Manual of Sports Surgery. New York, Springer-Verlag, 1987:62–90
31. Brownstein B, Bronner S, eds: Evaluation, Treatment and Outcomes. Functional Movement in Orthopaedic and Sports Physical Therapy. New York, Churchill Livingstone, 1997
32. Brunnstrom S: Clinical Kinesiology. Philadelphia, FA Davis, 1962
33. Burdett-Smith P: Experience of scapula winging in an accident and emergency department. Br J Clin Pract 44:643–644, 1990

34. Burkhead WZ, Rockwood CA: Treatment of instability of the shoulder with an exercise program. J Bone Joint Surg Am 74:890–896, 1992
35. Butler DS: Mobilization of the Nervous System. Melbourne, Churchill Livingstone, 1991
36. Butler DS: The upper limb tension test revisited. In: Grant R: Physical Therapy of the Cervical Spine and Thoracic Spine, 2nd ed. New York, Churchill Livingstone, 1994:217–244
37. Cahill BR: Understanding shoulder pain. In: Stauffer ES, ed: Instructional Course Lectures. American Academy of Orthopaedic Surgeons. St. Louis, CV Mosby, 1985
38. Cahill BR, Palmer RE: Quadrilateral space syndrome. J Hand Surg 8:65–69, 1983
39. Calliet R: Neck and Arm Pain, 3rd ed. Philadelphia, FA Davis, 1991a
40. Calliet R: Shoulder Pain, 3rd ed. Philadelphia, FA Davis, 1991b
41. Calliet R: Soft Tissue Pain and Disability, 3rd ed. Philadelphia, FA Davis, 1996
42. Carriere B.: The Swiss Ball: Theory, Basic Exercise and Clinical Application. Berlin, Springer-Verlag, 1998
43. Chasan N: The Swing Reaction System. Seattle, Biomechanical Golf Exercise Video. 1996
44. Chasan N, Kane M: Functional training for the low back patient. Orth Phys Ther Clin North Am 8:451–477, 1999
45. Cipriani D: Open and closed chain rehabilitation for the shoulder complex. In: Andrews JR, Wilk LE, eds: The Athlete's Shoulder. New York, Churchill Livingstone, 1994:577–588
46. Codman EA: The Shoulder. Boston, Thomas Todd, 1934
47. Cole JH, Furness AL, Twoney LT: Muscles in Action, an Approach to Manual Muscle Testing. Edinburgh, Churchill Livingstone, 1988
48. Corrigan B, Maitland GD: Practical Orthopaedic Medicine. Boston, Butterworths, 1985
49. Cosgarea AJ, Sebastianelli WJ: The shoulder: Common pathologies. In: Canavan PK: Rehabilitation in Sports Medicine. Stamford, CT, Appleton and Lange, 1998:173–182
50. Cunningham J: Applying the Bad Ragaz method to the orthopaedic client. Orthop Phys Ther Clin North Am 3:251–260, 1994
51. Davies GJ, Gould JA, Larson RL: Functional examination of the shoulder girdle. Phys Sports Med 9:82–104, 1981
52. De Luca CJ, Forrest WJ: Force analysis of individual muscles acting simultaneously on the shoulder joint during isometric abduction. J Biomech 6:385–395, 1973
53. Dempster WT: Mechanisms of shoulder movement. Arch Phys Med Rehabil 46:49–67, 1965
54. DePalma AF: Surgery of the Shoulder, 2nd ed. Philadelphia, Lippincott, 1973
55. Deplane AF: Surgical anatomy of the rotator cuff and natural history of degenerative periarthritis. Surg Clin North Am 43:1507–1521, 1963a
56. Deplane AF: Surgical anatomy and function of the acromioclavicular and sternoclavicular joints. Surg Clin North Am 43:1541–1521, 1963b
57. Dias JJ, Steingold RF, Richardson RA et al: The conservative treatment of acromioclavicular dislocation. Review after five years. J Bone Joint Surg 69:719–722, 1987
58. Dickhoff-Hoffman S: Neuromuscular control exercises of shoulder instability. In: Andrews JR, Wilk KE, eds: The Athlete's Shoulder. New York, Churchill Livingstone, 1994:435–449
59. Dines DM, Levinson M: The conservative management of the unstable shoulder including rehabilitation. Clin Sports Med 14:797–814, 1995
60. Dominguez RH, Gajda R: Total Body Training. New York, Warner Books, 1982
61. Dontigny RL: Passive shoulder exercises. J Phys Ther 50:1707–1709, 1970
62. Dutton M: The cervicothoracic junction. In: Dutton M: Manual Therapy of the Spine: An Integrated Approach. New York, McGraw-Hill, 2002:379–407
63. Dvorak J, Dvorak V: Manual Medicine, Diagnostic. Stuttgard, Georg Thieme Verlag, 1990
64. Edgelow PI: Neurovascular consequences of cumulative trauma disorders affecting the thoracic outlet. A patient centered treatment approach. In: Donatelli RA, ed: Physical Therapy of the Shoulder, 3rd ed. New York, Churchill Livingstone, 1997:153–178
65. Ehgartner K: Has the duration of cast fixation after shoulder dislocations had an influence on the frequency of recurrent dislocations? Arch Orthop Unfallchir 89:187–190, 1977
66. Einhorn AR, Mandras M, Sawyer M, et al: Evaluation and treatment of the shoulder. In: Brownstein B, Bonner S, eds: Evaluation, Treatment and Outcomes, Functional Movement in Orthopaedic and Sports Physical Therapy. New York, Churchill Livingstone, 1995:89–139
67. Elvey RL: Painful restriction of shoulder movement: A clinical observation study. In: Proceedings: Disorders of the Knee, Ankle and Shoulder. Perth, Western Australian Institute of Technology, 1979
68. Elvey RL: Brachial plexus tension test and the pathoanatomical origin of arm pain. In: Idczack RM, ed: Aspects of Manipulative Therapy. Carlton, Australia, Lincoln Institute of Health Sciences, 1981
69. Elvey RL: The investigation of arm pain. In: Grieves GP, ed: Modern Manual Therapy of the Vertebral Column. New York, Churchill Livingstone, 1986a:530–535
70. Elvey RL: Treatment of arm pain associated with abnormal brachial plexus tension. Aust J Physiother 32:224–229, 1986b
71. Elvey RL, Hall T: Neural tissue evaluation and treatment. In: Donatelli R: Physical Therapy of the Shoulder. New York, Churchill Livingstone, 1997:131–152
72. Exelby L: Peripheral mobilisations with movement. Man Ther 1(3):118–126, 1996
73. Falconer MA, Weddell G: Costoclavicular compression of the subclavian artery and vein. Relation to scalenus anticus syndrome. Lancet 2:539–544, 1943
74. Falkel JE, Murphy TC: Common injuries of the shoulder in athletes. In: Malone TR, ed: Sports Injury Management: Shoulder Injuries. Baltimore, William & Wilkins, 1998:66–108
75. Fiddian NJ, King RJ: The winged scapula. Clin Orthop 185:228–236, 1984
76. Fish GH: Some observations of motion at the shoulder joint. Can Med Assoc J 50:213–216, 1944
77. Freedman L, Munro R: Abduction of the arm in the scapular plane: Scapular and glenohumeral movements. J Bone Joint Surg Am 48:1503–1510, 1966
78. Gamble JN: Strength and conditioning for the competitive athlete. In: Kulund DN: The Injured Athlete, 2nd ed. Philadelphia, JB Lippincott, 1988:111–150
79. Gerber C, Ganz R: Clinical assessment of instability of the shoulder, with special reference to the anterior and posterior drawer tests. J Bone Joint Surg Br 66:551–556, 1984
80. Gergoudis R, Barnes R: Thoracic outlet arterial compression prevalence in normal persons. Angiology 31:538–541, 1980.
81. Gozna ER, Harris WR: Traumatic winging of the scapula. J Bone Joint Surg Am 61:1230–1233, 1979
82. Gray G: Chain Reaction: Successful Strategies for Closed Chain Testing and Rehabilitation. Adrain MI, Wynn Marketing, 1989
83. Gray G: Lower Extremity Functional Profile. Adrian MI, Wynn Marketing, 1995
84. Greenfield B: Special considerations in shoulder exercises: Plane of the scapula. In: Andrews JR, Wilk KE, eds: The Athlete's Shoulder. New York, Churchill Livingstone, 1994:513–522
85. Gregg JR, Labosky D, Harty M, et al: Serratus anterior paralysis in the young athlete. J Bone Joint Surg Am 61:825–832, 1979
86. Grieve GP: Mobilisation of the Spine: A Primary Handbook of Clinical Method, 5th ed. Edinburgh, Churchill Livingstone, 1991
87. Grimsby O: Personal communication, 1977
88. Grimsby O: Fundamentals of Manual Therapy: A Course Workbook. Everett, WA, Sorlandets Institute, 1985
89. Gustavsen R: Fra Aktiv Avspenning. Oslo, Olaf Norlis Bokhandel, 1977
90. Gustavsen R, Streek R: Training Therapy: Prophylaxis and Rehabilitation, 2nd ed. Stuttgart, Georg Thieme Verlag, 1993
91. Halbach JW, Tank RT: The Shoulder. In: Gould JA, Davies GJ, eds: Orthopaedic and Sports Physical Therapy. St. Louis, CV Mosby, 1990:483–522
92. Hall CM: The shoulder girdle. In: Hall CM, Thein Brody L: Therapeutic Exercise, Moving Toward Function. Philadelphia, Lippincott Williams & Wilkins, 1998:575–626
93. Hall TM, Elvey RL: Evaluation and treatment of neural tissue pain disorders. In: Donatelli RA, Wooden MJ: Orthopedic Physical Therapy, 3rd ed. New York, Churchill Livingstone, 2001
94. Halpern BC: Shoulder injuries. In: Birrer RB, ed: Sports Medicine for the Primary Physician, 2nd ed. Boca Raton, CRC Press, 1994:411–433
95. Hanson C: Proprioceptive neuromuscular facilitation. In: Hall CM, Thein Brody L: Therapeutic Exercise, Moving Toward Function. Philadelphia, Lippincott, Williams & Wilkins, 1998:233–251
96. Hart DL, Carmichael SW: Biomechanics of the shoulder. J Orthop Sports Phys Ther 6:229–234, 1985
97. Hawkins RJ, Bokor DJ: Clinical evaluation of shoulder problems. In: Rockwood CA, Matsen FA III, eds: The Shoulder, vol 1. Philadelphia, WB Saunders, 1990:149–177.
98. Hawkins RJ, Hobeika PE: Impingement syndrome in the athletic shoulder. Clin Sports Med 2:391–405, 1983
99. Hawkins RJ, Kennedy JC: Impingement syndrome in athletes. Am J Sports Med 8:151–158, 1980
100. Heppenstall RB: Fractures of the proximal humerus. Orthop Clin North Am 9:467–475, 1975
101. Hirsh LF, Thanki A: The thoracic outlet syndrome: Meeting the diagnostic challenge. Postgrad Med 77:197–207, 1985
102. Hislop HJ, Montgomery J: Daniels and Worthingham's Muscle Testing, Techniques of Manual Examination, 6th ed. Philadelphia, WB Saunders, 1995
103. Holten O: Medisinsk Trenigsterapi Trykk Fugseth and Lorentzen. Medical Training Course. Salt Lake City, March 1–4, 1984
104. Host HH: Scapular taping in the treatment of anterior shoulder impingement. Phys Ther 75:803–811, 1995
105. Hovelius L: Recurrence after initial dislocation of the shoulder. J Bone Joint Surg Am 65:343–349, 1983
106. Howell JW: Evaluation and management of thoracic outlet syndrome. In: Donatelli R, ed: Physical Therapy of the Shoulder, 2nd ed. New York, Churchill Livingstone, 1991:151–190
107. Howell SM, Imobersteg M, Seger DH, Marone DJ: Clarification of the role of the supraspinatus muscle in shoulder function. J Bone Joint Surg Am 68:398–404, 1985
108. Inman VT, Saunders JB, Abbott LC: Observations of the function of the shoulder joint. J Bone Joint Surg Am 26:1–30, 1944

109. Jackson P: Thoracic outlet syndrome: Evaluation and treatment. Clin Manag 7:6–10, 1987
110. Janda V: Muscle Function Testing. London, Butterworth, 1983
111. Janda V: Muscles and motor control in cervicogenic disorders: Assessment and management. In: Grant R, ed: Physical Therapy of the Cervical and Thoracic Spine, 2nd ed. New York, Churchill Livingstone, 1994:195–216
112. Janda V, Vavrova M: Sensory motor stimulation: A video. Presented by Bullock-Saxton JE. Brisbane, Australia, Body Control System, 1990
113. Janda V, Vavrova M: Sensory motor stimulation. In: Liebenson C: Rehabilitation of the Spine. Philadelphia, Lippincott Williams & Wilkins, 1996:319–328
114. Jemmett R: Spinal Stabilization: The New Science of Back Pain. Minneapolis, OPTP, 2001
115. Jobe FW, Moynes DR: Delineation of diagnostic criteria and rehabilitation program for rotator cuff injuries. Am J Sports Med 10:336–339, 1982
116. Johnston TB: Movements of the shoulder joint—plea for use of "plane of the scapula" as the plane of reference for movements occurring at humeroscapular joint. Br J Surg 25:252–260, 1937
117. Jull GA, Janda V: Muscles and motor control in low back pain. In: Twomey LT, Taylor JR, eds: Physical Therapy of the Low Back. New York, Churchill Livingstone, 1987:253–278
118. Kaltenborn FM: Manual Mobilization of the Extremity Joints: Basic Examination and Treatment. Oslo, Olaf Norlis Bokhandel, 1989
119. Kaltenborn FM: The Spine: Basic Evaluation and Mobilization Techniques, 2nd ed. Oslo, Olaf Norlis Bokhandel, 1993
120. Kapandji IA: The Physiology of the Joints: Upper Limb, vol 1. New York, Churchill Livingstone, 1970
121. Karas SE: Thoracic outlet syndrome. Clin Sports Med 9:297–310, 1990
122. Kase K: Illustrated Kinesio-Taping, 2nd ed. Albuquerque, NM, Ken'kai Information, 1997
123. Kebaetse M, McClure P, Pratt N: Thoracic position effect on shoulder range of motion, strength, and three-dimensional scapular kinetic. Arch Phys Med Rehabil 80:945–950, 1999
124. Kelly MJ: Anatomic and biomechanical rationale for rehabilitation of the athlete's shoulder. J Sports Rehabil 4:122–154, 1995
125. Kendall FP, McCreary EK, Provance PG: Muscle Testing and Function, 4th ed. Baltimore, Williams & Wilkins, 1993
126. Kenneally M, Rubenach H, Elvey R: The upper limb tension test: The SLR test of the arm. In: Grant R, ed: Physical Therapy of the Cervical and Thoracic Spine. New York, Churchill Livingstone, 1988:167–194
127. Kent BE: Functional anatomy of the shoulder complex: A review. Phys Ther 51:867–888, 1971
128. Kessell L, Walson M: The painful arc syndrome. J Bone Joint Surg Br 59:166–172, 1977
129. Kibler WB: Role of the scapula in the overhead throwing motion. Contemp Orthop 22:525–532, 1991
130. Kibler WB: Rehabilitation of the shoulder. In: Kibler WB, Herring SA, Press JM: Functional Rehabilitation of Sports and Musculoskeletal Injuries. Gaithersburg, MD, Aspen Publications 1998:149:170
131. Kisner C, Colby LA: Therapeutic Exercise: Foundations and Techniques, 3rd ed. Philadelphia, FA Davis, 1996
132. Klein-Vogelbach S: Therapeutic Exercises in Functional Kinetics. Berlin, Springer-Verlag, 1986
133. Knott M, Voss DE: Proprioceptive Neuromuscular Facilitation, 2nd ed. New York, Harper & Row, 1968
134. Kondo M, Tazoe S, Yamda M: Changes of the tilting angle of the scapula following elevation of the arm. In: Bateman JE, Welsch PR, eds: Surgery of the Shoulder. St. Louis, CV Mosby, 1984:12–16
135. Leadbetter WB: Cell-matrix response in tendon injury. Clin Sports Med 11:533–578, 1992
136. Lee D: A Workbook of Manual Therapy Techniques for the Upper Extremities. Delta, BC, Canada, Delta Orthopaedic Physiotherapy Clinic, 1989
137. Lefever-Button S: Closed kinetic chain training. In: Hall CM, Thein Brody L: Therapeutic Exercise, Moving Toward Function. Philadelphia, Lippincott Williams & Wilkins, 1998: 252–273
138. Leffert RD: Neurological problems. In: Rockwood CA, Matsen FA: The Shoulder, vol 2, 2nd ed. Philadelphia, WB Saunders, 1998:965–988
139. Leffert RD, Gumley G: The relationship between dead arm syndrome and thoracic outlet syndrome. Clin Orthop Relat Res 23:20–31, 1987
140. Lehmann F, Warren CG, Scham SM: Therapeutic heat and cold. Clin Orthop 99:207–245, 1974
141. Lemos MJ: The evaluation and treatment of the injured acromioclavicular joint in athletes. Am J Sports Med 26: 137–144, 1998
142. Lentell G, Hetherington T, Eagan J, et al: The use of thermal agents to influence the effectiveness of a low-load prolonged stretch. Orthop Sports Phys Ther 5:200–207, 1992
143. Letournel E, Fardeau M, Lytle JO, et al: Scapulothoracic arthrodesis for patients who have fascioscapulohumeral muscular dystrophy. J Bone Joint Surg Am 72:78–84, 1990
144. Light LE, Nuzik S, Personius W, et al: Low-load prolonged stretch vs. high load in treating knee contractures. Phys Ther 64:330–338, 1984
145. Lippman RK: Frozen shoulder, peri-arthritis, bicipital tenosynovitis. Arch Surg 47:283–296, 1943
146. Lockhart RD: Movements of the normal shoulder joint. J Anat 64:288–302, 1936
147. Lord JW, Rosati LM: Neurovascular compression syndromes of the upper extremity. Clin Symp 23:3–23, 1971
148. Lucas DB: Biomechanics of the shoulder joint. Arch Surg 107:425–432, 1973
149. Ludington NA: Rupture of the long head of biceps flexor cubiti muscle. Ann Surg 27:358–363, 1923
150. Lutz FR, Geck JH: Thoracic outlet compression syndrome. Athl Train 21:302–310, 1986
151. MacConnaill MH, Basmajian JV: Muscles and Movements: A Basis for Human Kinesiology. Baltimore, Williams & Wilkins, 1969
152. Mackinnon SE, Dellon AL: Surgery of the Peripheral Nerve. New York, Thieme, 1988
153. MacNab I: Local steroids in orthopaedic conditions. Scott Med J 17:176–186, 1972
154. MacNab I: Rotator cuff tendinitis. Ann R Coll Surg Engl 53:271–287, 1973
155. Magee DJ: Orthopedic Physical Assessment, 3rd ed. Philadelphia, WB Saunders, 1997
156. Mahj JY, Otsuka NY: Scapular winging in young athletes. J Pediatr Orthop 12:245–247, 1992
157. Maitland GD: Vertebral Manipulations, 5th ed. Boston, Butterworths, 1986
158. Maitland GD: Peripheral Manipulations, 3rd ed. London, Butterworths, 1991
159. Matsen FA III, Harryman DT, Sidles JA: Mechanics of glenohumeral instability. Clin Sports Med 10:783–788, 1991
160. Matsen FA III, Lippitt SB, Sidles JA, et al: Practical Evaluation and Management of the Shoulder. Philadelphia, WB Saunders, 1994
161. Matsen FA III, Thomas SC, Rockwood CA, et al: Glenohumeral instability. In: Rockwood CA, Matsen FA, eds: The Shoulder, vol 2, 2nd ed. Philadelphia, WB Saunders, 1998:611–754
162. McNair JFS, Maitland GD: Manipulative therapy in the management of some thoracic syndromes: In: Grant R, ed: Physical Therapy of the Cervical and Thoracic Spine. New York, Churchill Livingstone, 1988:243–270
163. Meisser L: Proprioceptive neuromuscular facilitation: PNF complex motions. In: Kuprian W: Physical Therapy for Sports, 2nd ed. Philadelphia, WB Saunders, 1995:99–120
164. Moore KL: Clinically Oriented Anatomy. Baltimore, Williams & Wilkins, 1980
165. Morehouse L, Gross L: Maximum Performance. New York, Simon & Schuster, 1977
166. Mosely BJ, Jobe FW, Pink M, et al: EMG analysis of the scapular muscles during a baseball rehabilitation program. Am J Sports Med 20:128–134, 1992
167. Moseley HF: Disorders of the shoulder. Clin Symp 12:1–30, 1960
168. Moseley HF: The natural history and clinical syndromes produced by calcific deposits in the rotator cuff. Surg Clin North Am 43:1489–1492, 1963
169. Moseley HF: Shoulder Lesions, 3rd ed. Edinburgh, Churchill Livingstone, 1969
170. Mulligan BR, Manual Therapy 'Nags', 'Snags' 'MWMs' etc, 4th ed. Plant View Services, New Zealand, 1999
171. Neer C, Welsh P: The shoulder in sports. Orthop Clin North Am 8:183–191, 1977
172. Neer OS II. Anterior acromioplasty for chronic impingement syndrome in the shoulder. J Bone Joint Surg Am 54:41–50, 1972
173. Neer OS II: Impingement lesions. Clin Orthop 173:70–77, 1983
174. Neviaser JS: Adhesive capsulitis of the shoulder: a study of pathological findings in periarthritis of the shoulder. J Bone Joint Surg Am 27:211–222, 1945
175. Nicholson GG, Clendaniel RA: Manual techniques. In: Scully RM, Barnes MR, eds: Physical Therapy. Philadelphia, JB Lippincott, 1989:926–989
176. Nirschl R: Rehabilitation of the athlete's elbow. In: Morrey BR, ed: The Elbow and Its Disorders. Philadelphia, WB Saunders, 1985:524–525
177. Norris CM: Sports Injuries: Diagnosis and Management for Physiotherapists. Oxford, Butterworths-Heinemann, 1993
178. Norris TR: Diagnostic technique for shoulder instability. In: Sauffer ES, ed: Instructional Course Lectures. St. Louis, CV Mosby, 1985:239–257
179. Norwood LA, Terry GC: Shoulder posterior subluxation. Am J Sports Med 12:25–30, 1984
180. Ombregt L, Bisschop P, ter Veer HJ, et al: A System of Orthopaedic Medicine. London, WB Saunders, 1995
181. Omer GE: Osteotomy of the clavicle in surgical reduction of anterior sternoclavicular dislocation. J Trauma 7:584–590, 1967
182. O'Sullivan SB, Schmitz TJ: Physical Rehabilitation Laboratory Manual: Focus on Functional Training. Philadelphia, FA Davis, 1999
183. Paine RM: The role of the scapula in the shoulder. In: Andrews JR, Wilk KE: The Athlete's Shoulder. New York, Churchill Livingstone, 1994:495–512
184. Paine RM, Voight M: The role of the scapula. J Orthop Sports Phys Ther 18:386–391, 1993
185. Palmer L, Blakely R: Documentation of medial rotation accompanying shoulder flexion: A case report. Phys Ther 68:55–58, 1988
186. Palmer ML, Epler ME: Fundamentals of Musculoskeletal Assessment Techniques, 2nd ed. Philadelphia, Lippincott Williams & Wilkins, 1998
187. Palmittier RA, An KN, Scott SG, et al: Kinetic chain exercise in knee rehabilitation. Sports Med 11:402–413, 1991
188. Pappas AM, Zaacki RM, McCarthy CF: Rehabilitation of the pitching shoulder. Am J Sports Med 13(4):223–235, 1985
189. Peat M: Functional anatomy of the shoulder complex. Phys Ther 66:1855–1865, 1986
190. Perry J: Anatomy and biomechanics of the shoulder in throwing, swimming, gymnastics and tennis. Clin Sports Med 2:247–270, 1983
191. Perry J, Glousman RE: Biomechanics of throwing. In: Nicholas JA, Hershman EB, eds: The Upper Extremity in Sports Medicine. St. Louis, CV Mosby, 1990:727–751

192. Petty NJ, Moore AP: Neuromusculoskeletal Examination and Assessment: A Handbook for Therapist. Edinburgh, Churchill Livingstone, 1998

193. Phillips H, Grieve GP: The thoracic outlet syndrome. In: Grieve GP, ed: Modern Manual Therapy of the Vertebral Column. Edinburgh, Churchill Livingstone, 1986:359–369

194. Pink M, Jobe FW, Perry J, et al: The normal shoulder during the butterfly stroke: an EMG and cinematographic analysis of twelve muscles. Clin Orthop 288:48–59, 1993

195. Pink M, Jobe FW, Perry J, et al: The painful shoulder during the butterfly stroke: an EMG and cinematographic analysis of twelve muscles. Clin Orthop 288:60–72, 1993

196. Pink M, Perry J, Browne A et al: The normal shoulder during freestyle swimming. Am J Sports Med 19: 569–575, 1991

197. Pink M, Perry J, Browne A, et al: The normal shoulder during free style swimming: an EMG and cinematographic analysis of twelve muscles. Am J Sports Med 19:569–576, 1991

198. Poppen NK, Walker PS: Normal and abnormal motion of the shoulder. J Bone Joint Surg Am 58:195–201, 1976

199. Prentice WE: Proprioceptive neuromuscular facilitation techniques in rehabilitation. In: Prentice WE, Voight MI: Techniques in Musculoskeletal Rehabilitation. New York, McGraw-Hill, 2001:197–214

200. Protzman RR: Anterior instability of the shoulder. J Bone Joint Surg Am 62:908–918, 1980

201. Radin E: Relevant biomechanics in the treatment of musculoskeletal injuries and disorders. Clin Orthop 146:2–3, 1980

202. Riggins RS: The shoulder. In: D'Ambrosia RD, ed: Musculoskeletal Disorders, Regional Examination and Differential Diagnosis. Philadelphia, JB Lippincott, 1986

203. Rockwood CA: Subluxations and dislocations about the shoulder. In: Rockwood CA, Green DP, eds: Fractures in Adults. Philadelphia, JB Lippincott, 1984

204. Rohde J: Die Automobilisation der Extremitatengelenke (III). Z Physiother 27:121–134, 1975

205. Ross DB: The surgical anatomy of the scalene triangle. Contemp Surg 35:11–16, 1989

206. Ross DB, Owen JC: Thoracic outlet syndrome. Arch Surg 93:71–74, 1966

207. Rothman RH, Marvel JP, Heppenstall RB: Anatomical considerations in the glenohumeral joint. Orthop Clin North Am 6:341–352, 1975

208. Rothman RH, Parke BB: The vascular anatomy of the rotator cuff. Clin Orthop 41:176–186, 1965

209. Rowe CR: Dislocations of the shoulder. In: Rowe CR, ed: The Shoulder. Edinburgh, Churchill Livingstone, 1988:165–292

210. Rowe CR, Sakellarides HT: Factors related to recurrences of anterior dislocations of the shoulder. Clin Orthop 20:40–48, 1961

211. Sahrmann S: Diagnosis and treatment of muscle imbalances and associated regional pain syndromes. Level I and II Continuing Education Course, Seattle, Washington University School of Medicine, 1993

212. Sahrmann S: Diagnosis and Treatment of Movement Impairment. St. Louis, Mosby, 2002

213. Saidoff DC, Mc Donough AL: Critical Pathways in Therapeutic Intervention: Upper Extremity. St. Louis, Mosby, 1997

214. Sander J, Haug CE: Thoracic Outlet Syndrome. Philadelphia, JB Lippincott, 1991

215. Sarrafian SK: Gross and functional anatomy of the shoulder. Clin Orthop 173:11–18, 1983

216. Saunders L: Acromioclavicular joint sprain and its prevalence with whiplash injuries. Physiotherapy 87:587–592, 2001

217. Schneider R, Prentice WE: Rehabilitation of the shoulder. In: Prentice WE, Voight MI: Techniques in Musculoskeletal Rehabilitation. New York, McGraw-Hill, 2001:411–456

218. Schultz JS, Leonard JA Jr: Long thoracic neuropathy from athletic activity. Arch Phys Med Rehabil 73:87–90, 1992

219. Schumacher HR, Bomalski JS: Case Studies in Rheumatology for the House Officer. Baltimore, Williams & Wilkins, 1990

220. Sheldbourne DK, Nitz PA: Accelerated rehabilitation after anterior cruciate ligament reconstruction. Am J Sports Med 18:292–299, 1990

221. Shields CL: Manual of Sports Surgery. New York, Springer-Verlag, 1987

222. Silliman JF, Hawkins RJ: Current concepts and recent advances in the athlete's shoulder. Clin Sports Med 10:693–705, 1991

223. Skyhar MJ, Simmons TC: Rehabilitation of the shoulder. In: Nickel VL, Botte MJ, eds: Orthopaedic Rehabilitation, 2nd ed. New York, Churchill Livingstone, 1992:747–763

224. Slaughter D: Shoulder injuries. In: Sanders B: Sport Physical Therapy. Norwalk, CT, Appleton & Lange, 1990:343–367

225. Smith KF: The thoracic outlet syndrome, a protocol of treatment. J Orthop Sports Phys Ther 1:89–97, 1979

226. Spencer J, Turkel MA, Ithaca MC, et al: Stabilizing mechanism preventing anterior dislocation of the glenohumeral joint. J Bone Joint Surg Am 63:1208–1217, 1981

227. Steele R, Anthony J, Rice EL, et al: The winged scapula: Diagnosing the atypical case. Phys Sports Med 22:47–54, 1994

228. Stillman JF, Hawkins RJ: Current concepts and recent advances in the athlete's shoulder. Clin Sports Med 10:693–706, 1991

229. Sullivan PE, Markos PD, Minor MA: Clinical Decision Making in Therapeutic Exercise. Norwalk, CT, Appleton & Lange, 1994

230. Sutter JS: Conservative treatment of shoulder instability. In: Andrews JR, Wilk KE, eds: The Athlete's Shoulder. New York, Churchill Livingstone, 1994:589–604

231. Telford ED, Mottershead S: Pressure at the cervicobrachial junction: An operative and anatomical study. J Bone Joint Surg Am 30:2490, 1948

232. Todd TW: The decent of the shoulder after birth. Anatomischer Anzeiger Centralblatt fur die gesamte wissenschaftlichje. Anatomie 14:41, 1912

233. Totten P, Hunter J: Therapeutic techniques to enhance nerve gliding in thoracic outlet syndrome and carpal tunnel syndrome. Hand Clin 7:505–520, 1991

234. Travell JG, Simons DG: Myofascial Pain and Dysfunction: The Trigger Point Manual: Upper Half of the Body, vol I, 2nd ed. Baltimore, Williams & Wilkins, 1999

235. Turek SL: Orthopaedics: Principles and Their Applications, 3rd ed. Philadelphia, JB Lippincott, 1977

236. Turnbull JR: Acromioclavicular joint disorders. Med Sci Sports Exerc 30(Suppl):S26–S32, 1998

237. Uhl TM, Madaleno JA: Rehabilitation concepts and supportive devices for overuse injuries of the upper extremity. Clin Sports Med 20:621–639, 2001

238. Upton ARM, McComas AJ: The double crush in nerve entrapment syndromes. Lancet 2:359–362, 1973

239. Vandenbossche J, Raes R, Verdonck R: Acromioclaviculaire luxaties. Tijdschr Genneskd 4:393–398, 1990

240. Voight ML, Cook G: Clinical application of closed kinetic chain exercise. J Sport Rehabil 5:25–44, 1996

241. Voight ML, Cook G: Impaired neuromuscular control: Reactive neuromuscular training. In: Prentice W, Voight MI: Techniques in Musculoskeletal Rehabilitation. New York, McGraw-Hill, 2001:93–124

242. Voight ML, Dravitch P: Plyometrics. In: Albert MA, ed: Eccentric Muscle Training in Sports and Orthopaedics. New York, Churchill Livingstone, 1991:45–73

243. Voight ML, Tippet S: Plyometric Exercise in Rehabilitation. New York, McGraw-Hill, 2001:167–178

244. Voss DE, Ionta MK, Myers BJ: Proprioceptive Neuromuscular Facilitation Patterns and Techniques, 3rd ed. Philadelphia, Harper & Row, 1985

245. Walsh DA: Shoulder evaluation of the throwing athlete. Sports Med Update 4:24–27, 1989

246. Walsh MT: Therapist management of thoracic outlet syndrome. J Hand Ther 7:131–144, 1994

247. Warren CG, Lehmann JK, Koblanski JN: Elongation of rat-tail tendon: Effect of load and temperature. Arch Phys Med Rehabil 52:465–474, 1971

248. Warwick R, ed: Gray's Anatomy, 36th British ed. Philadelphia, WB Saunders, 1980

249. Watson-Jones RR: Fractures and Joint Injuries, vol II, 4th ed. Baltimore, Williams & Wilkins, 1960

250. Weaver JK, Dunn HK: Treatment of acromioclavicular injuries, especially complete acromioclavicular dislocation. J Bone Joint Surg Am 54:1187–1194, 1972

251. Weinstein DM, McCann PD, McIlveen SJ, et al: Surgical treatment of complete acromioclavicular dislocation. Am J Sports Med 23:324–331, 1995

252. Whiteneck SH, Hunter JM, Jaeger SH, et al: Thoracic outlet syndrome complex: Diagnoses and treatment. In: Hunter JM, Schneider LH, Mackin EJ, et al, eds. Rehabilitation of the Hand: Surgery and Therapy, 3rd ed. St. Louis, Mosby, 1990:530–539

253. Wilk KE: Current concepts in the rehabilitation of athletic shoulder injuries. In: Andrews JR, Wilk KE, eds: The Athlete's Shoulder. New York, Churchill Livingstone, 1994:335–354

254. Wilk KE, Arrigo C: Current concepts in rehabilitation of the athletic shoulder. J Orthop Sports Phys Ther 18:365–391, 1993

255. Wilk KE, Arrigo C: Closed and open kinetic chain exercises for the upper extremity. J Sports Rehabil 5:88–102, 1996

256. Wilk KE, Voight ML: Plyometrics for the shoulder complex. In: Andrews JR, Wilk KE, eds: The Athlete's Shoulder. New York, Churchill Livingstone, 1994:543–565

257. Wilk KE, Voight ML, Kerins MA, et al: Stretch-shortening drills for the upper extremities; theory and clinical application. J Orthop Sports Phys Ther 17:225–239, 1993

258. Wilt F: Plyometrics, what it is and how it works. Athl J 55:76–90, 1975

259. Wojtys EM, Nelson G: Conservative treatment of grade III acromioclavicular dislocations. Clin Orthop 268:112–119, 1991

260. Wolf WB: Shoulder tendinoses. Clin Sports Med 11:871–890, 1992

261. Woo SLY, Mathews SV, Akeson WH: Connective tissue response to immobility: Correlative study of biomechanical measurements of normal and immobilized rabbit knees. Arthritis Rheum 18:257–264, 1973

262. Wood VE, Twito R, Verska JM: Thoracic outlet syndrome. The result of first rib resection in 100 patients. Orthop Clin North Am 19:131–146, 1988

263. Wooden MJ: Isokinetic evaluation and treatment of the shoulder. In: Donatelli R, ed: Physical Therapy of the Shoulder. New York, Churchill Livingstone, 1987

264. Woolfenden JT: Aquatic physical therapy approaches for the extremities. Orthop Phys Ther Clin North Am 3:209–230, 1994
265. Wurnig C: Sonography of the biceps tendon. Z Orthop Ihre Grenzgeb 134:161–165, 1996
266. Wyke BD: The neurology of joints. Ann R Coll Surg Engl 41:25–50, 1967
267. Yackzan L, Adams C, Francis KT: The effects of ice massage on delayed muscle soreness. Am J Sports Med 12:159–165, 1984
268. Yergason RM: Supination sign. J Bone Joint Surg Am 13:160, 1931
269. Zuckerman JD, Matsen FA III: Biomechanics of the shoulder. In: Nordin M, Frankel VH, eds: Basic Biomechanics of the Musculoskeletal System, 2nd ed. Philadelphia, Lea & Febiger, 1989:209–247
270. Zuniga L: Management of thoracic dysfunction. In: Canavan PK: Rehabilitation in Sports Medicine: A Comprehensive Guide. Stamford CT, Appleton & Lange, 1997: 93–108

RECOMMENDED READINGS

Andrews JR, Wilk KE: The Athlete's Shoulder. New York, Churchill Livingstone, 1994
Conroy DE, Hayes KW: The effect of joint mobilization as a component of comprehensive treatment for primary shoulder impingement syndrome. J Orthop Sports Phys Ther 28:3–14, 1998
Dines DM, Levinson M: The conservative management of the unstable shoulder including rehabilitation. Clin Sports Med 14:797–815, 1995
Ghilarducci M: Rotator cuff repair and rehabilitation. In: Rehabilitation for the Postsurgical Orthopedic Patient. St. Louis, Mosby, 2001:46–70
Hau A, Hedman T, Chang JH, et al: Changes in abduction and rotation range of motion in response to simulated dorsal and ventral translation mobilization of the glenohumeral joint. Phys Ther 82:544–556, 2002
Jobe F, Schwab D, Brewster C: Anterior capsular reconstruction. In: Maxey L, Magnusson J: Rehabilitation for the Postsurgical Orthopedic Patient. St. Louis, Mosby, 2001:29–45
Jobe FW, Schwab D, Wilk KE, et al: Rehabilitation of the shoulder. In: Brozman SB, ed. Clinical Orthopedics Rehabilitation. St. Louis, Mosby, 1996
Johnson MP, McClure PW, Karduna AR: New method to assess scapular upward rotation in subjects with shoulder pathology. J Orthop Sports Phys Ther 31:81–89, 2001
Kibler WB: Rehabilitation of the shoulder. In: Kibler WB, Herring SA, Press J: Functional Rehabilitation of Sports and Musculoskeletal Injuries. Gaithersburg, MD, Aspen Publications, 1998, 149–170
Matsen FA, Lippitt SB, Sidles JA, et al: Practical Evaluation and Management of the Shoulder. Philadelphia, WB Saunders, 1994
McNab I, McCulloch J: Neck Ache and Shoulder Pain. Baltimore, Williams & Wilkins, 1994
Moynes DR: Prevention of injury to the shoulder through exercise and therapy. Clin Sports Med 2:413–422, 1983
Payne LZ, Deng X, Craig EV, et al: The combined dynamic and static contributions to subacromial impingement. Am J Sports Med 25:801–817, 1997
Rockwood CA, Matsen FA: The Shoulder. Philadelphia, WB Saunders, 1990
Sahrmann SA: Diagnosis and Treatment of Movement Impairment Syndromes. St. Louis, Mosby, 2002
Saunders L: Acromioclavicular joint sprain and its prevalence with whiplash injuries. Physiotherapy 87:587–591, 2001
Schneider R, Prentice W: Rehabilitation of the shoulder. In: Prentice WE, Voight MI: Techniques in Musculoskeletal Rehabilitation. New York, McGraw-Hill, 2001
Steinbeck J, Liljenqvist U, Jerosch J: The anatomy of the glenohumeral ligamentous complex and its contribution to anterior shoulder instability. J Shoulder Elbow Surg 7:122–126, 1998
Uhl TL, Madalleno JA: Rehabilitation concepts and supportive devises for overuse injuries of the upper extremity. Clin Sports Med 20:621–639, 2001
Wilk KE, Arrigo C: Current concepts in the rehabilitation of the athlete's shoulder. J South Orthop Assoc 3:216–231, 1994
Wuelker N, Korell M, Thren K: Dynamic glenohumeral joint instability. J Shoulder Elbow Surg 7:43–52, 1998

REVIEW OF FUNCTIONAL ANATOMY

Osteology

DISTAL HUMERUS

At the distal anterior end of the humerus there are two articular surfaces: the trochlea, which is pulley-shaped, somewhat like an hourglass or spool lying on its side, and the capitellum, which forms most of a sphere mediolaterally and half of a sphere anteroposteriorly. The lateral epicondyle extends laterally above the capitellum for attachment of the extensor muscles. The medial epicondyle is the site of attachment of the flexor–pronator group. The coronoid fossa lies immediately above the trochlea, and the radial fossa is immediately above the capitellum. These fossae receive the coronoid process and the anterior rim of the radial head, respectively, on full elbow flexion (Fig. 12-1).

If one looks laterally or medially, the distal humerus angulates anteriorly such that the longitudinal axis of the trochlea is directed anteriorly, 45° to the shaft of the humerus. As implied above, the hemisphere of the capitellum faces anteriorly, with the articular surface having an angular value of about 180° (Fig. 12-2).

Posteriorly (Fig. 12-3), the large, deep olecranon fossa accepts the olecranon process on full elbow extension. At times it communicates with the coronoid fossa. The trochlear articular surface, with its median groove, extends posteriorly. The medial half of the trochlea extends farther distally than does the lateral half. The groove usually runs obliquely, distally, and laterally; it dictates the path that the ulna must follow during flexion and extension of the forearm. The asymmetry of the trochlea causes the ulna to angulate laterally on the humerus when the elbow extends. This abduction of the forearm on full extension is referred to as the *carrying angle* of the elbow.

PROXIMAL RADIUS

The proximal end of the radius includes the head, neck, and bicipital tuberosity (Fig. 12-1). The radial head is concave on its superior surface for articulation with the convex capitellum. Viewed from above, the radial head is slightly oval, being longer anteroposteriorly, so that with pronation it is displaced slightly laterally (Fig. 12-4).

PROXIMAL ULNA

The proximal ulna consists of the olecranon and the coronoid process, between which is the trochlear notch. With the elbow extended, the trochlear notch faces anteriorly and superiorly, corresponding to the 45° angulation of the distal humerus (Fig. 12-2A). Lying inferiorly and medially to the trochlear notch is the radial notch, which faces laterally for articulation with the radial head (Fig. 12-1).

The angulation of the distal humerus and trochlear notch of the proximal ulna allows about 160° elbow flexion and 180° extension. The angulation is necessary to provide room for the anterior muscle groups of the arm and forearm, which approximate on elbow flexion (Fig. 12-5). Any bony malalignment

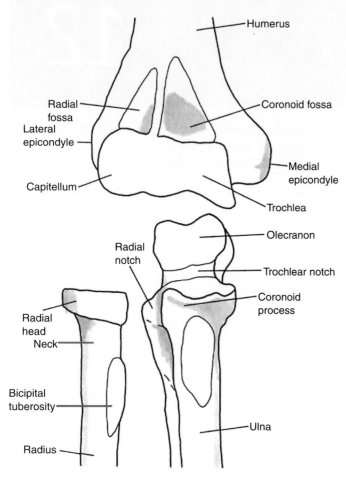

■ **FIG. 12-1.** Bones of the right elbow.

that interferes with these critical angles (e.g., after a supra-condylar fracture) will make normal movement impossible.

Joint Articulations

The elbow is a compound synovial joint composed of three joints: the humeroulnar, humeroradial, and superior radio-ulnar. These three joints make up the cubital articulations. The capsule and joint cavity are continuous for all three joints. MacConaill and Basmajian[97] have classified the cubital complex as a paracondylar joint in that one bone (the humerus) articulates with two others (the radius and ulna) by way of two facets. This enables one of the latter two bones to undergo movement independent of the other. The middle radioulnar joint should also be considered when examining the elbow.

HUMEROULNAR JOINT

The humeroulnar joint is a uniaxial hinge joint formed between the trochlear notch of the ulna and the trochlea of the humerus (Figs. 12-2A and 12-3). The ulnar trochlear notch, like the trochlea of the humerus with which it articulates, is a sellar surface. It is concave in the sagittal plane and convex in the frontal plane.[96] The trochlea covers the

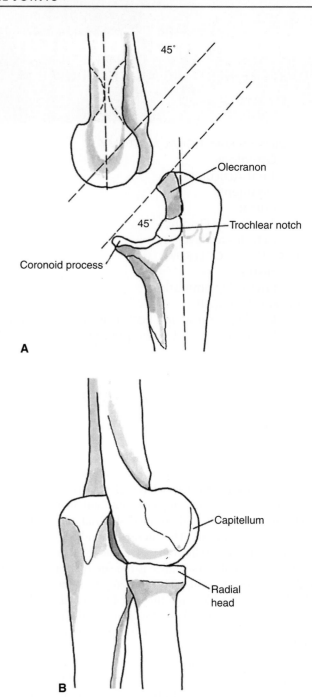

■ **FIG. 12-2.** Bones of the elbow, showing the relationship of the distal humerus and proximal ulna (**A**) and the proximal radius (lateral view; **B**).

anterior, inferior, and posterior aspects of the medial humeral condyle.[182] The trochlea of the humerus is asymmetrical. Its axis of motion points superolateral to inferomedial. This causes an angulation of the elbow, the carrying angle. When the arm is at the side, the carrying angle is 10 to 15° in men and 20 to 25° in women. The asymmetry of the trochlea allows for joint play needed for full range of motion. This incongruency produces the following accessory movements:

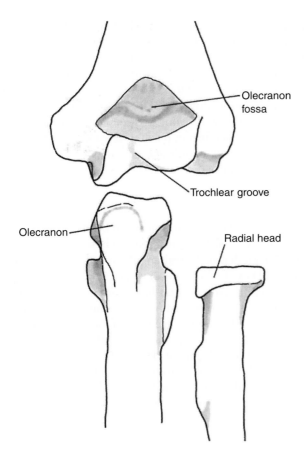

■ **FIG. 12-3.** Posterior view of bones of the elbow.

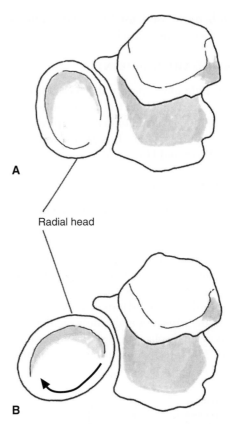

■ **FIG. 12-4.** Relationship of proximal radius and ulna in pronation (**A**) and supination (**B**), as viewed from above.

a slight screw action (the ulna is slightly supinated during flexion and pronated during extension) and abduction, adduction, and gliding of the radial head on both the humerus and ulna. On full extension, the medial part of the olecranon process is not in contact with the trochlea; on full flexion, the lateral part of the olecranon process is not in contact with the trochlea. This range allows the side-to-side joint-play movement necessary for supination and pronation. The ulna rotates internally 5° in early elbow flexion and externally 5° at end range of flexion.[25,187]

HUMERORADIAL JOINT

The humeroradial joint allows flexion and extension of the forearm and pronation and supination of the radius. In the humeroradial joint the convex-shaped capitellum articulates with the cup-shaped, concave proximal portion of the radial head (Fig. 12-2*B*). It is a triaxial ball-and-socket joint.

PROXIMAL RADIOULNAR JOINT

The articular surfaces of the superior radioulnar joint include the cylindrical rim of the radial head and an osseofibrous ring composed of the radial notch of the ulna and the annular ligament (Fig. 12-1). The spherical head of the radius allows the rotation needed for forearm pronation and supination. Move-

ment of the radius on the ulna reaches about 85° of both pronation and supination. Accessory movements include rotation and gliding of the radial head relative to the capitellum, lateral displacement of the radial axis during pronation owing to a larger anteroposterior head diameter (allowing room for

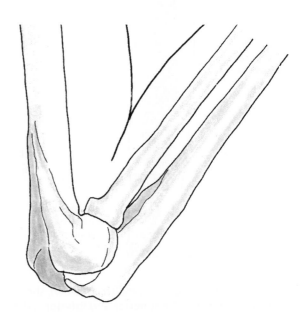

■ **FIG. 12-5.** Elbow in flexion.

the radial tuberosity), and distal-lateral tilt of the plane of the proximal surface of the radial head during pronation.[77,78]

INFERIOR RADIOULNAR JOINT

The inferior radioulnar joint is also a critical component in forearm rotation. It anchors the distal radius and ulna, and along with the superior radioulnar joint provides a pivot for radial movement (Fig. 12-6). This joint is discussed further in Chapter 13, Wrist and Hand Complex.

MIDDLE RADIOULNAR JOINT

The middle radioulnar syndesmosis includes the interosseous membrane and the oblique cord between the shafts of the radius and ulna (Fig. 12-6). Although this articulation is not really a joint, or part of the elbow joint complex, it is affected by injury or immobilization of the elbow; conversely, injury to this area can affect the mechanics of the elbow articulation. The oblique cord is a flat cord formed in the fascia overlying the deep head of the supinator and running to the radial tuberosity. It resists distal displacement of the radius during pulling movements. The interosseous membrane (a broad collage-

nous sheet) runs distally and medially from the radius and ulna. It provides stability for both the superior and inferior radioulnar joints. The interosseous membrane not only binds the joints together, but when under tension also provides for transmission of forces from the hand and distal end of the radius to the ulna.[119] The interosseous membrane stabilizes the elbow by resisting proximal displacement of the radius on the ulna during pushing movements. The fibers of the interosseous membrane are tight midway between supination and pronation.

Ligaments

The capsule of the elbow is reinforced by ulnar (medial) and radial (lateral) collateral ligaments. These ligaments serve to restrict medial or lateral angulation of the ulna on the humerus. They also help prevent dislocation of the ulna from the trochlea. Each collateral ligament consists of anterior, intermediate, and posterior fibers. The anterior fibers of both help reinforce the annular ligament of the radioulnar articulation (Fig. 12-7). The capsule is strengthened anteriorly by an anterior oblique ligament (Fig. 12-8).

The annular ligament runs from the anterior margin of the radial notch of the ulna around the radial head to the posterior

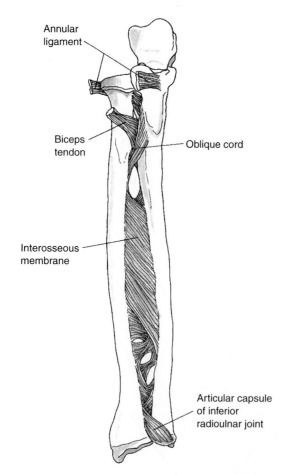

■ **FIG. 12-6.** Right radius and ulna (front view), showing structures that reinforce the superior and inferior radio-ulnar joints.

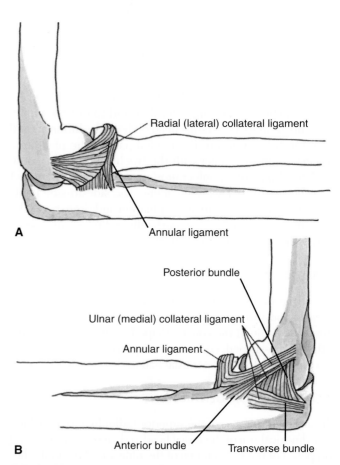

■ **FIG. 12-7.** Ligaments of the elbow viewed laterally (**A**) and medially (**B**).

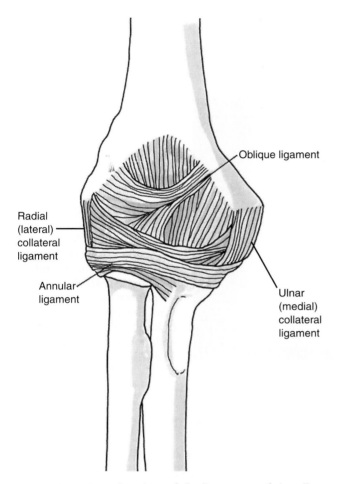

■ **FIG. 12-8.** Anterior view of the ligaments of the elbow.

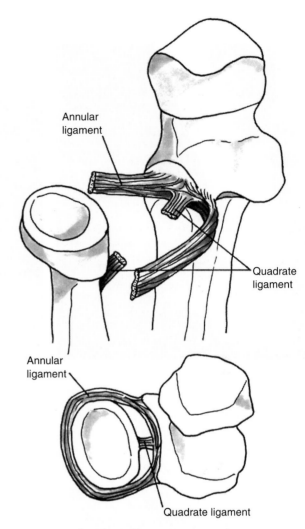

■ **FIG. 12-9.** Quadrate ligament.

margin of the radial notch. It is lined with articular cartilage so that with pronation and supination the radial head articulates with the capitellum of the humerus and the radial notch of the ulna, as well as with the annular ligament (Figs. 12-7 through 12-9). Some anatomists describe the existence of a quadrate ligament (ligament of Denucé) at the distal border of the annular ligament whose anterior fibers become taut on forearm supination and whose posterior fibers become taut on pronation (Fig. 12-9).[36,101,150]

The joint capsule of the elbow encloses the humeroulnar joint, the humeroradial joint, and the proximal radioulnar joint (Figs. 12-7 and 12-8). The anterior and posterior parts of the capsule are broad and thin. Forty-five degrees of flexion permits maximum volume of the joint, which is the position a patient assumes to accommodate diffuse swelling secondary to joint trauma or a supracondylar fracture.[69] Fat pads exist between the fibrous capsule and the synovial membrane over the fossae; thus, they are intracapsular but extrasynovial. The classic radiographic "fat pad sign" (used to detect effusion) is often associated with the presence of a fracture and is considered positive when a translucent area appears between the soft tissue and the bone in the area of the fat pad. In any condition leading to joint hemorrhage, effusion, or synovitis, the fat pad may be displaced so that it is visible (Fig. 12-10).

Bursae

The olecranon bursa overlies the olecranon posteriorly, lying between the superior olecranon and the skin (Fig. 12-11). It may become inflamed from trauma, prolonged pressure ("student's elbow"), or other inflammatory afflictions such as infection and gout.

Tendinous Origins

The flexor–pronator muscles of the wrist have their tendinous origins at a common aponeurosis that originates at the medial epicondyle of the humerus. The wrist extensor group has its common aponeurotic origin at the lateral epicondyle. From superior to inferior on the humerus, the brachioradialis inserts first, followed by the extensor carpi radialis longus, the extensor carpi radialis brevis, and the remaining extensor muscles (Fig. 12-12). The extensor carpi radialis brevis is the uppermost muscle to attach to the common extensor tendon. The extensor carpi radialis longus and the brachioradialis do not contribute to the common tendon but rather attach above the epicondyle.

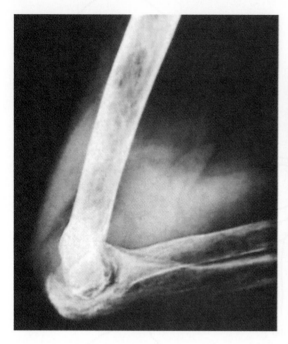
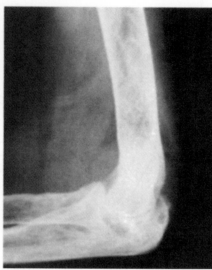

■ **FIG. 12-10.** Fat pad sign. Rheumatoid arthritis (elbow). Bilateral positive fat pad signs are seen; erosive changes of rheumatoid arthritis and osteoporosis are also noted. (Reprinted with permission from Greenfield GB: Radiology of Bone Diseases, 5th ed. Philadelphia, JB Lippincott, 1990:782.)

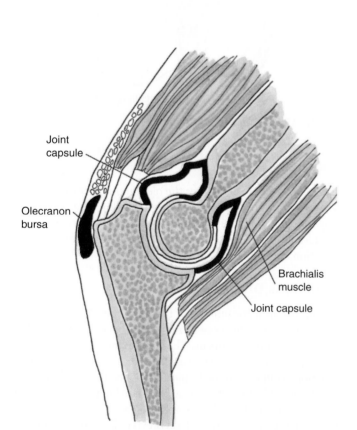

Joint capsule

Olecranon bursa

Brachialis muscle

Joint capsule

■ **FIG. 12-11.** Sagittal section through the elbow.

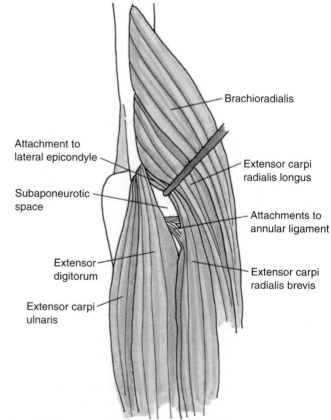

Brachioradialis

Attachment to lateral epicondyle

Subaponeurotic space

Extensor carpi radialis longus

Attachments to annular ligament

Extensor carpi radialis brevis

Extensor digitorum

Extensor carpi ulnaris

■ **FIG. 12-12.** Lateral view of the tendinous origin of the forearm muscles.

The extensor carpi radialis brevis is important clinically because its tendon is most frequently involved in cases of lateral tennis elbow. Although it originates in part from the common extensor tendon, the extensor brevis also has proximal attachments to the lateral collateral ligament of the elbow, and often to the annular ligament (Fig. 12-12).

Deep to the tendon of the extensor brevis, and just distal to its insertion at the lateral epicondyle, is a small space normally filled with loose, areolar connective tissue. This is termed the *subaponeurotic space*[56] and is bordered on the ulnar side by the extensor digitorum tendon and distally by the attachment of the brevis to the annular ligament (Fig. 12-12). Surgical findings commonly reveal granulation tissue in this space in cases of lateral tennis elbow. Histologic studies show hypervascularization and the ingrowth of numerous free nerve endings into this space with granulation.[32,56] The granulation probably represents the reactions of adjacent tissues to chronic irritation of the extensor brevis origin, resulting from tension stresses.[32,112]

On full forearm pronation, with the elbow extended, the orientation of the extensor carpi radialis brevis is such that proximally it is stretched over the prominence of the radial head (Fig. 12-4). This fulcrum effect from the radial head adds to the normal tensile forces transmitted to the origin of this muscle when stretched during combined wrist flexion, forearm pronation, and elbow extension.[112] This may in part explain the susceptibility of this tendon to chronic inflammation at or near its attachment.

Arteries and Nerves

BLOOD SUPPLY

Blood supply to the elbow joint is usually abundant. The medial portion of the elbow is supplied from superior and inferior ulnar collateral arteries and two ulnar recurrent arteries. The lateral portion is supplied by the radial and middle collateral branches of the profunda artery and the radial and interosseous recurrent arteries.[90,106]

INNERVATION

Joint branches are believed to be derived from all the major nerves crossing over this joint (i.e., radial, median, ulnar), including contributions from the musculoskeletal nerves. The variations and relative contributions have been documented by Gardner.[53] A detailed description of the nerves near the level of or close to the elbow joint can be found in other sources.[6,36,53,60,68,90,123,149,151] The reader will benefit from studying sagittal and anteroposterior diagrams that depict some of the anatomic relationships (Figs. 12-13 through 12-15).

Clinically, the examiner must be aware of potential injury or pinching of various nerves near the level of the elbow. For example, for the most part, resistant lateral tennis elbow may be caused by lateral epicondylitis and its associated fascial tears or calcification.[152] On occasion, persistent complaints may be related either to compression of the posterior interosseous

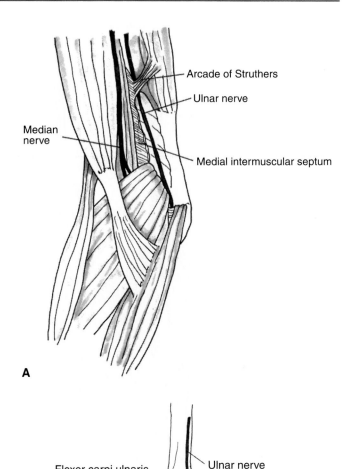

■ FIG. 12-13. Ulnar nerve. Anatomic distribution of the ulnar nerve crossing the intermuscular septum, passing under the arcade of Struthers (**A**) and the cubital tunnel at the elbow (**B**).

nerve or to a combination of persistent localized epicondylitis and nerve compression.[24,134,146]

Of the several entrapment syndromes near the level of the elbow, the ulnar tunnel syndrome is the most common.[35,66,84,148,151–153,171,173–175] The ulnar nerve at the elbow passes behind the medial epicondyle in a groove that is converted into an osseofibrous canal, the cubital tunnel, by the arcuate ligament, which runs from the medial epicondyle to the olecranon process (Fig. 12-13B).[35,175] The arcuate ligament is taut at 90° flexion and lax in extension. An entrapment neuropathy of the ulnar nerve is common especially after prolonged sitting, overuse of the elbow, or repeated microtrauma from occupations that involve leaning on the elbow.[35]

Next in frequency of occurrence is the posterior interosseous nerve syndrome, or radial tunnel syndrome.[24,42,57,64,95,108,111,123,145,147,152,153,160,171,172] The most common

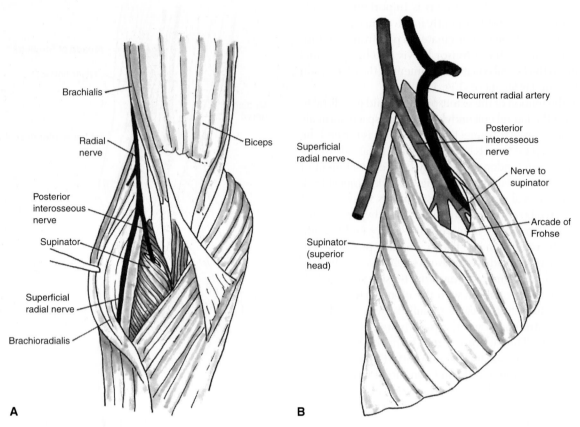

■ **FIG. 12-14.** **(A)** Radial nerve and its major forearm branches, the posterior interosseous nerve and the superficial radial nerve. **(B)** Enlarged view of the posterior interosseous nerve and its relationship to the supinator muscle and the arcade of Frohse.

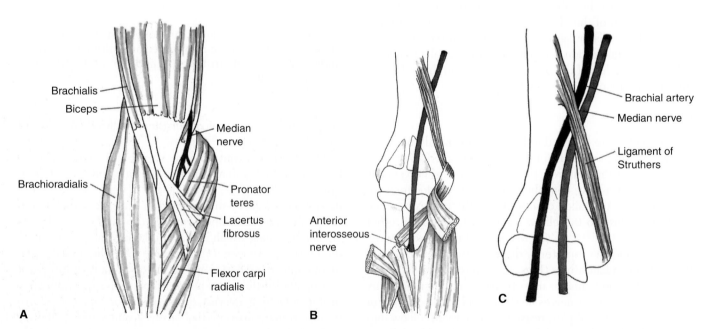

■ **FIG. 12-15.** Median nerve, proximal to the lacertus fibrosus **(A)**, the lacertus fibrosus released exposing the anterior interosseous nerve **(B)**, and the ligament of Struthers, an anomalous structure **(C)**.

compression site of the posterior interosseous nerve is as it passes under the fibrous origin of the extensor carpi radialis and then pierces the supinator muscles (in the region of the arcade of Frohse) to pass along the interosseous membrane, where it supplies the extensor muscles of the forearm, to reach the wrist (Fig. 12-14).[13,111,131,144,147]

The anterior interosseous nerve syndrome and the pronator syndrome, which involves the median nerve, are less common. The median nerve may be compressed just before the anterior interosseous branch on entering the forearm beneath the edge of the lacertus fibrosus of the biceps, resulting in the pronator syndrome (Fig. 12-15),[85,107,143] whereas the anterior interosseous nerve is occasionally pinched or entrapped as it passes between the two heads of the pronator teres.[48,89,98,136,145,149,152,179] Other types of entrapment neuropathies are much rarer. Median nerve entrapment is occasionally combined with that of the brachial artery, caused by a supracondylar spur or ligament of Struthers (Fig. 12-15C).[54,68,151,160] Ulnar nerve entrapment is caused by the arcade of Struthers, made up of fibers arising from the medial head of the triceps that interweave to the intermuscular septum (Fig. 12-13A).[76,151,152]

EVALUATION OF ELBOW

History

Routine questions to be asked when evaluating patients with common musculoskeletal disorders are discussed in Chapter 5, Assessment of Musculoskeletal Disorders and Concepts of Management. The following questions are of particular concern when evaluating patients with elbow disorders:

1. What activities (e.g., athletic or occupational) do you engage in that involve vigorous or repetitive use of the arm? (Except for the arthritides, most elbow conditions are traumatic or degenerative conditions, such as tennis elbow, that become active with certain activities.)
2. Are any other joints involved? (Except for the degenerative or traumatic lesions, rheumatoid arthritis is one of the few remaining causes of elbow pain of local origin.)

The elbow is largely derived from C6 and C7 and may, therefore, be the site of referred pain from other structures of the same segmental derivation; it may also refer pain to other structures in these segments.

Physical Examination

I. Observation
   A. Posture and attitude in which the arm is held. The normal carrying angle is approximately 5° in males and 10 to 15° in females.[69]
   B. Functional use of the arm during gait, dressing, and other activities. Clues for appropriate tests can be obtained from the subjective examination findings, particularly aggravating factors.
II. Inspection (include the entire extremity)
   A. Structure. Observe the extremities with the patient in a relaxed standing position.
      1. Shoulder height
      2. Elbow carrying angle (valgus–varus angle)
      3. Elbow flexion–extension angle
      4. Positions of medial and lateral epicondyles, radial head, and olecranon
   B. Soft tissue
      1. Muscle form. Examine the muscle bulk and muscle tone, comparing left and right sides. Observe for any evidence of atrophy and measure the girth of the arm or forearm.
      2. Swelling
         a. Marked posterior swelling is usually bursal swelling.
         b. Articular effusion is often visible anteriorly and posteriorly.
      3. General contours
   C. Skin
      1. Color changes
      2. Scars or blemishes
      3. Moisture
      4. Texture
III. Joint Tests
   A. Joint integrity tests
      1. Observe the relative position of the olecranon and the medial and lateral epicondyles. They should form a straight line with the elbow in extension and an isosceles triangle with the elbow in 90° flexion (Fig. 12-16).[69]
      2. Joint and ligamentous tests. To assess the integrity of the medial and lateral collateral ligaments, varus and valgus stress tests may be performed.
         a. Valgus stress (Fig. 12-17). To test the integrity of the ulnar collateral ligament (Fig. 12-7B), the examiner applies a valgus stress to the elbow with the arm slightly flexed (slightly out of the close-packed position), thus attenuating the anterior bundle (Fig. 12-17A). The test is repeated with the forearm flexed to 90°, to stress the transverse bundle, and fully flexed, to stress the posterior bundle.[92]
         b. Varus stress. To test the integrity of the radial collateral ligament (Fig. 12-7A), the examiner applies a varus stress to the elbow with the arm slightly flexed (slightly out of the close-packed position), thus stressing the anterior band of the radial collateral ligament (Fig. 12-17B). The test is repeated with the forearm flexed to 90°, to stress the medial band, and fully flexed, to stress the posterior band.[92] Excessive movement or reproduction of the client's symptoms is a positive test and is indicative of elbow joint instability.
      3. Anterior capsule test. Hyperextension test.[83] Elbow extension beyond 0° is considered hyperextension. A

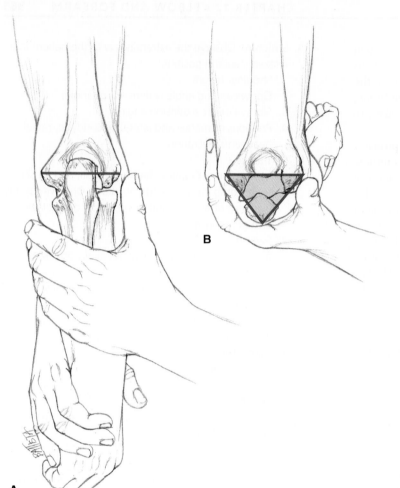

■ **FIG. 12-16.** Position of the medial and lateral epicondyle should form a straight line with the elbow in extension (**A**) and an isosceles triangle when the elbow is flexed (90°; **B**).

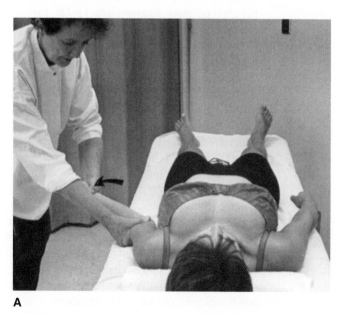

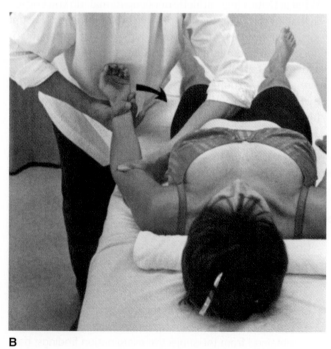

■ **FIG. 12-17.** Testing the collateral ligaments of the elbow. (**A**) Ulnar collateral ligament. (**B**) Radial collateral ligament.

positive finding of hyperextension may be attributed to a torn or stretched anterior capsule of the elbow. The examiner grasps the distal humerus at the medial and lateral condyle with one hand, while the other hand grasps the distal forearm and passively extends the elbow until no further motion is available.

B. Active and passive physiologic movement (sitting). For both active and passive physiologic movement, the examiner should note the following.
- the range of movement
- the quality of movement
- the resistance throughout the range of movement and at the end range of movement
- the behavior of pain through the range of movement and any provocation of muscle spasm

1. Active physiologic movements with passive overpressure.
2. Observe
   a. Elbow flexion–extension
   b. Forearm pronation–supination (with elbow at 90°)
   c. Wrist flexion–extension
3. Apply slight overpressure. Assess effect on pain; assess end feel; feel for crepitus.
4. Record significant findings relating to range of motion, pain, end feel, and crepitus.
5. Modification of active physiologic movements can be carried out for further information about active range of movement such as repeated movements, sustained movements, alteration of the speed of movement, adding compression and distraction, or combining two or more physiologic movements together, e.g., flexion with pronation or supination.

B. Passive movements (supine for optimal stabilization)
1. Tests
   a. Elbow flexion–extension with the shoulder flexed, extended, and in neutral position for constant-length phenomenon in case of muscular pain and tightness. This phenomenon results when the limitation of one joint depends on the position in which another joint is held.
   b. Elbow pronation–supination
   c. Wrist flexion with ulnar deviation (The elbow is held extended and the forearm pronated, stretching the common extensor tendon.)
   d. Wrist extension with the forearm supinated and the elbow extended (common flexor–pronator tendon stretched)
2. Record range of motion, pain, crepitus, and type of end feel. Characteristics of normal end feel are:
   a. Extension: bone-to-bone
   b. Flexion: soft-tissue approximation
   c. Pronation–supination: leathery or elastic
   When motion of the joint is restricted, a pathologic motion barrier impedes movement of the joint before the anatomic barrier is reached. Com-

mon pathologic barriers (abnormal end feel) encountered at the elbow are a springy block, suggesting a loose body,[38] and muscle guarding, suggesting an acute inflammation of the joint or extra-articular tissues. The comparison of the response of symptoms to the active and passive movements can help determine whether the structure at fault is noncontractile or contractile.[38]

C. Other joints. Other joints apart from the elbow and wrist need to be examined to prove or disprove their relevance to the patient's condition. The most likely joints suspected to be a source of the symptoms are the cervical spine, shoulder, and thoracic spine. These joints can be tested fully (see relevant chapters), or if these joints are not suspected to be a source of symptoms then the relevant clearing tests can be used (see Chapter 21, Cervicothoracic–Upper Limb Scan Examination).

D. Joint effusion. Measure the circumference of the joint using a tape measure and compare left with right.

E. Joint-play movements
1. Joint-play movements of the elbow are the same as the mobilization techniques (see Treatment Techniques below) except that they are always performed in the resting position. The clinician should note the following:
   - the range of movement
   - the quality of movement
   - the resistance through range and at the end of range of motion
   - the behavior of pain through the range and any provocation of muscle spasm
   Specific joint-play (accessory) motions to be tested include:
   a. Distraction of the humeroulnar joint (see Fig. 12-19A)
   b. Medial-lateral tilt of the humeroulnar joint (see Fig. 12-20)
   c. Superior (approximation) glide for humeroradial joint (see Fig. 12-22)
   d. Distal glide of radius on ulna for proximal radioulnar joint (see Fig. 12-23)
   e. Dorsal-ventral glide at the proximal radioulnar joint (see Fig. 12-24A)
   f. Dorsal-ventral glide of the distal radioulnar joint (see Fig. 13-37)
   g. Mobilization with movement (MWMs). Lateral glide of the humeroulnar joint (see Fig. 12-26). An increase in the range of movement and no pain or reduced pain on active flexion or extension of the elbow are positive examination findings indicating a mechanical joint problem.[109,126]
   For the patient with suspected tennis elbow, who is requested to make a fist (as lateral glide is performed), relief of pain is a positive finding, indicating a positional fault at the elbow, which is

contributing to the soft tissue lesion or a tracking fault.

2. Record significant findings related to degree of mobility and presence of pain and muscle guarding. For further information when examining the joint play movements, alter the:
   - direction of the applied force
   - point of application of the applied force
   - position of the joint. The elbow joint can be placed in a variety of resting positions, such as flexion, extension, supination, or pronation.

F. Other joint-play movements as applicable. Joints likely to be examined are the cervical spine, thoracic spine, shoulder, wrist, and hand.

IV. Muscle Tests. Muscle tests include muscle resistive isometric movements, muscle strength, functional strength testing or control, and muscle length.

A. Resisted isometric movements (supine)

1. Resisted wrist movements. The patient grips the examiner's hand and squeezes strongly. If elbow pain is reproduced, additional isometric contractions of the wrist are examined.
   a. Medial tennis elbow. The pain of medial tennis elbow may be reproduced by resisting wrist flexion.
   b. Lateral tennis elbow. Pain of lateral tennis elbow may be reproduced at the site of the common extensor tendon. Resistance to wrist extension and radial deviation is applied as the patient attempts to make a fist and pronate the forearm.

2. Resisted elbow movements. The four elbow movements of flexion, extension, supination, and pronation are tested using isometric contractions.

3. If referred pain from more proximal regions is suspected, include resisted isometric contraction tests of the shoulder and cervical spine movements.

4. Record whether the resisted isometric contraction is strong or weak and whether it is painful or painless.

B. Muscle strength. A routine examination of the elbow should include strength testing of the upper quadrant muscles beginning at the shoulder. This is particularly important because any weakness of the shoulder musculature will lead to altered throwing mechanics, potentially leading to increased stress in the soft tissue of the elbow. The examiner tests the elbow extensors, flexors, forearm supinators, forearm pronators, wrist flexors and extensors, and radial and ulnar deviations. For details of these tests, the reader is directed to Clarkson and Gilewish,[26] Cole et al.,[27] Hislop and Montgomery,[67] Kendall et al.,[81] and Palmer and Epler[124] to determine exactly which muscles are at fault. Grip strength (median nerve), thumb abduction strength (radioposterior interosseous nerve), and intrinsic muscle strength (ulnar nerve) should be tested to ensure that distal motor function is intact.

C. Motor control and functional strength testing. Some authors advocate functional strength testing of the elbow because the length of the forearm magnifies the load applied at the hand.[26,121] Examples of functional strength testing at the elbow include holding a light weight in the hand of the involved limb while bringing that hand to the mouth (testing extension and flexion, respectively), performing wall push-ups, seated push-ups, or activities demanding fast or powerful movements such as pitching.[9,137] Many activities such as pitching ball and self-maintenance activities including writing and dressing involve the pronators. The pronators are functionally linked to medial rotation of the shoulder, as pronation and medial rotation occur simultaneously in many activities.[93] Movement combinations required for specific tasks of the upper limb are helpful in analyzing motor control and movement compensations caused by weakness.

D. Muscle length. Muscle length of the elbow flexors (biceps brachii [long and short head]) are assessed with the shoulder joint in hyperextension and forearm pronation as the elbow is extended. The elbow extensors (triceps brachii and anconeus) are assessed with the shoulder completely flexed. If elbow flexion limitation exists without the shoulder completely flexed then the one-joint muscles or posterior capsular structures are limiting the motion.

1. Tennis elbow length testing is performed by stretching the extensor muscles of the wrist and hand, by extending the elbow, pronating the forearm, and then flexing the wrist and fingers. A positive sign (i.e., muscle shortening) is indicated if the patient's symptoms are reproduced or if range is limited compared with the other side.[126]

2. Tests for golfer's elbow or medial tennis elbow are performed by stretching the flexor muscles of the wrist and hand by extending the elbow, supinating the forearm, and then extending the wrist and hand. A positive test is indicated if the range of motions is limited compared with the other side or if the patient's symptoms are reproduced.[126]

V. Palpation

A. Skin
1. Temperature, especially over brachialis and joint
2. Moisture, especially over hand and forearm
3. Texture
4. Mobility of skin over subcutaneous tissues, especially after immobilization
5. Tenderness, primarily if neurologic involvement is suspected (e.g., ulnar nerve lesion)

B. Subcutaneous soft tissues
1. Consistency, tone, mobility
2. Swelling. Joint effusion is often palpable anteriorly by ballottement.
3. Tenderness
   a. Common tendon insertions

b. Tendon sheaths

c. Ligaments

d. Subcutaneous olecranon bursa

e. Relevant trigger points or points of fibromyalgia

C. Bones

1. Bony relationships, especially position of the radial head

2. Tenderness, tenoperiosteal junctions of common flexor and common extensor groups

3. Bony contours

VI. Neuromuscular Tests. The neurologic examination includes examination of the integrity of the nervous system, the mobility of the nervous system, and specific diagnostic tests.[58]

A. Integrity of the nervous system is tested if the examiner suspects that the symptoms are emanating from the spine or from a peripheral nerve.

1. Dermatomes or peripheral nerves (see Tables 5-7 and 5-8). Light touch and pain sensations of the upper limb are tested. In the limbs, neurologic tissue plays a significant role in function. Peripheral nerves may be traumatized about the elbow. Knowledge of the cutaneous distribution of nerve roots (dermatomes) and peripheral nerves (see Fig. 5-8) enables the examiner to distinguish the sensory loss caused by a root lesion or peripheral nerve.

2. Reflex testing. The following deep tendon reflexes are tested:

• C5–C6: biceps (see Fig. 11-24*A*)

• C7: triceps (see Fig. 11-24*B*)

B. Mobility of the nervous system. The upper limb tension test (ULTT) may be carried out to determine the degree that neural tissue is responsible for the production of the patient's symptoms. These tests are described in Chapter 11, Shoulder and Shoulder Girdle.

C. Other diagnostic tests for peripheral nerves.

1. Ulnar nerve (Fig. 12-13)

a. Sustained elbow flexion for 5 minutes producing paraesthesia in the distribution of the ulnar nerve is a positive test for cubital tunnel syndrome.[99]

b. Tinel's sign. The Tinel sign is a test designed to elicit tenderness over a neuroma within a nerve, to assess peripheral nerve entrapment, or to determine the distal point of sensory nerve regeneration. With the wrist stabilized, tapping the area of the nerve in the ulnar notch between the olecranon and the medial condyle with the index finger will send a tingling sensation down the forearm to the ulnar distribution of the nerve (hands and finger).[69]

2. Test for posterior interosseous nerve syndrome (PINS) or radial tunnel syndrome. This involves compression of the posterior interosseous nerve between the two supinator heads in the canal of Frohse (Fig. 12-14*B*).[99] Forearm extensor muscles are affected, weakening the strength of wrist and finger extension. A com-

plete history and thorough physical examination is the best way to diagnose PINS. This syndrome can mimic tennis elbow.

3. Median nerve (Fig. 12-15)

a. Pinch grip test. The pinch grip test of the thumb–index finger increases pressure in the anterior compartment, testing for entrapment of the anterior interosseous nerve branch of the median nerve as it passes through the interosseous membrane. The test is considered positive if the patient is unable to pinch tip-to-tip the index and thumb, which is caused by impairment of the flexor pollicis longus, the lateral half of the flexor digitorum profundus, and the pronator quadratus.[20]

b. Pronator syndrome tests.[20,51,74,75,138,151,159,186] These tests are for pronator teres syndrome (median nerve entrapment in the pronator teres muscle). One provocative test is strongly resisted pronation of the elbow as the patient extends from 90° flexion toward full extension to compress the median nerve at the interval between the superficial and deep heads of the pronator teres. Another maneuver uses resisted elbow flexion and forearm supination to stress the nerve as it passes under the lacertus fibrosus. The third maneuver calls for resisted flexion of the middle finger proximal interphalangeal joint while stabilizing the proximal metacarpal–phalangeal joint. This stresses the flexor digitorum superficialis arch and suggests entrapment at this location. Additional tests for pronator syndrome include weakening of grip strength and sensory loss in the distribution of the median nerve.

4. Tinel's sign. Tapping at the radial head and radial tunnel (radial nerve) and the carpal tunnel (median) may also reproduce the symptoms in entrapment syndromes of the peripheral nerves.

VII. Special Tests

A. Valgus extension overload test.[45,183] Valgus extension overload of the elbow is commonly seen in overhead-throwing athletes. This results in impingement of the posteromedial aspect of the olecranon tip on the soft tissue or bony architecture of the medial brim of the olecranon fossa. The valgus extension overload test is performed by repeatedly forcing the elbow into full extension with a valgus stress applied.

B. Thoracic outlet syndrome. These tests are described in Chapter 11, Shoulder and Shoulder Girdle.

C. Palpation of pulses. If there is any question about the integrity of the forearm circulation, the brachial pulse may be palpated in the cubital fossa medial to the biceps tendon, as well as the radial pulse lateral to the flexor carpi radialis tendon at the wrist. The brachial artery pulse can also palpated on the medial aspect of the humerus in the axilla if circulation is suspected of being compromised.

VIII. Other Tests. Results of roentgenograms, laboratory tests, and electromyograms should be reviewed if available.

COMMON LESIONS

Medial, Lateral, and Posterior Tendon Injuries

The most common contractile lesions occurring at the elbow involves the proximal attachments of the wrist extensors and flexors. Both are overuse syndromes involving strain and inflammation of a common tendon and share a common mechanism of disorder. The pull of many muscles on a small origin creates a high load per unit area.

The terms *golfer's elbow, medial epicondylitis*, and *medial tennis elbow* have been used by various authors in reference to tendinosis of the forearm flexors and pronators,[10,91,117,184] whereas strain of the extensor musculature leading to pathologic changes in tendons is often referred to as *tennis elbow, lateral tennis elbow*, and *lateral epicondiylitis*.[18,88,118]

Although the condition of lateral tendon injury is often referred to as lateral epicondylitis, researchers have failed to detect signs of an inflammatory process in chronic tennis elbow.[8] Elbow lateral tendon injury is a common disorder affecting the elbow. The tendon most commonly involved is the extensor carpi radialis brevis, at or near its insertion at the lateral epicondyle.[16,17,32,38,56,112] At times, other common extensor tendons are also involved concurrently or, rarely, by themselves. Much less frequently, the common flexor tendon is involved at the tenoperiosteal junction. Even more uncommon is tendinitis of the triceps at its attachment to the olecranon.

Tendinitis affecting the elbow is rarely of acute traumatic origin. Except in sports clinics, most patients presenting with tennis elbow, for example, do not relate the onset or aggravation of the problem to athletic endeavors such as tennis. Even when the chief complaint is the development of pain during some activity, the onset is usually gradual and pain is felt most after the activity. This is because tendon injuries are usually a "degenerative" disorder: it represents tissue response to fatigue stresses. The inflammatory response that characterizes the disorder is an attempt to speed the rate of tissue production to compensate for an increased rate of tissue microdamage (e.g., collagen fiber fracturing). The microdamage rate is increased because of greater internal strain to the tendon fibers over time. This might occur from some increase in use of the tendon—for example, with carpentry, pruning shrubs, needlework, or playing tennis. It may also occur with normal activity levels if the tendon's capacity to attenuate tensile loads is reduced. This typically occurs with aging, in which a loss of the mucopolysaccharide chondroitin sulfate makes the tendon less extensible; more of the energy of tensile loading must be absorbed as internal strain to collagen fibers rather than by deformation of the tissue.

Confusion about the pathology and treatment of tennis elbow has plagued the medical community since the 19th century. Surgical studies have clearly identified classic tennis elbow as tendon involvement (tendinitis), which Nirschl[114] and Nirschl and Pettrone[118] have divided into lateral, medial, and posterior areas and have classified on an anatomic basis.

LATERAL TENDON INJURIES (TENNIS ELBOW)

Tennis elbow is the most common problem of the elbow, accounting for 7% of all sports injuries; peak age at which it occurs is 40 to 50 years.[65]

Lateral tendinitis or tennis elbow involves primarily the extensor carpi radialis brevis and occasionally the extensor digitorum, extensor carpi radialis longus, and, more rarely, the extensor carpi ulnaris.[114,118] The susceptibility of the extensor carpi radialis brevis to excessive force overload, particularly with hyperpronation, is probably related to the added tensile load imposed on the tendon by the radial head when the tendon is stretched (e.g., wrist flexion, elbow extension, and forearm pronation). In this position the tendon is further stretched over the prominence of the radial head.[112] Because the development of tennis elbow may be caused by age-related tissue changes, most patients presenting with this problem are 35 years or older.[17,32,38]

Lateral tendon injuries are classically a persistent disorder that does not tend toward spontaneous resolution. If the patient with tennis elbow continues to perform activities that stress the tendon, the immature collagen produced in an attempt at repair continues to break down before it has the chance to mature adequately, and the chronic inflammatory process continues. If the part is completely immobilized, there may not be adequate stress to the new collagen to stimulate maturation, in which case the scar will again break down on resumption of activities. For treatment to be successful, this dilemma must be resolved.

The sequential progression of this overuse syndrome commonly follows the patterns or grades below[139]:

Grade 1. Generalized elbow soreness with activity, which is most often ignored.[113] A vicious cycle of irritation, inflammation, pain, weakness, and inadequate healing is initiated and gains full expression in subsequent grades of injury.

Grade 2. Working or playing through the soreness may increase pain, which becomes localized at the lateral condyle or radial head and persists after activity.[132] The lateral aspect of the joint below may become swollen and warm and tender to touch. Pain will interfere with work or athletic activity. As the condition persists, pain may radiate down the forearm to the wrist and may extend upward into the upper arm and shoulder.

Grade 3. Simple activities of daily living become more painful and difficult (i.e., shaking hands and turning a doorknob). Continued activity leads to secondary problems such as rotator cuff or low back pain as other joints attempt to compensate. If ignored, arthritic changes in the proximal radial or humeral ulnar joint may occur.[139]

MEDIAL TENDON INJURY (MEDIAL TENNIS ELBOW OR GOLFER'S ELBOW)

Medial tendon injuries or tendinitis (also known as golfer's elbow or medial epicondylitis) may occur in tennis (faulty forehand stroke), throwing (acceleration phase), swimming (faulty pull-through), golf ("hitting from the top"), and occupations such as carpentry that involve repetitive hammering or screwing.[22,116,129] The mechanism of injury is caused by medial tension overload of the elbow from repeated microtrauma to the flexor–pronator musculature at its insertion onto the medial epicondyle. It involves primarily the pronator teres and flexor carpi radialis and occasionally the palmaris longus, flexor carpi ulnaris, and flexor digitorum superficialis. Provocation occurs with resisted wrist flexion and forearm pronation, passive wrist extension, and supination. An additional factor is compression neurapraxia of the ulnar groove.[115] Typically it occurs in middle-aged patients, often those involved in sports or occupational activities that require a strong handgrip and an adduction movement of the elbow.

POSTERIOR TENDON INJURIES (POSTERIOR TENNIS ELBOW)

Tendinitis of the triceps at its attachment to the olecranon is rare. It typically follows sudden severe strain to the triceps tendon as the arm is fully extended and can result from throwing a javelin or from a twisted serve in competitive tennis players.[35,125] Pain is provoked on resisted elbow extension. The perception of snapping over the posteromedial aspect of the elbow may develop spontaneously during the second decade of life (snapping triceps tendon).[44,73,135] This may be the result of subluxation or dislocation of a portion of the triceps mechanism or subluxation or dislocation of the ulnar nerve.[130,154-156] Most or these patients will remain asymptomatic, but others may experience secondary irritation of the ulnar nerve, resulting in ulnar neuritis.

According to Nirschl,[112] the primary overload abuse in tendinitis is caused by intrinsic concentric muscular contraction. Curwin and Standish[37] maintain that decreased flexibility causes the muscles to be overstretched during eccentric contraction and overloading of the extensors. They argue that maximum strengthening of the muscles must necessarily include eccentric work because this is the nature of the force producing the injury and because eccentric exercise produces greater tensile force on the tendon.

Examination and Management

I. History
   A. Site of pain
      1. Lateral tennis elbow. Over the lateral humeral epicondyle, often referred into the C7 segment, down the posterior forearm into the dorsum of the hand, and perhaps into the ring and long fingers
      2. Medial tennis elbow. Over the medial epicondyle, rarely referred into the ulnar aspect of the forearm
      3. Posterior tennis elbow. Over the posterior compartment of the elbow
   B. Onset of pain. Usually gradual. May be related to wrist extension activities in lateral tennis elbow, such as grasping, hitting a backhand stroke in tennis, or pruning shrubs, or to wrist flexion and pronation activities in medial tennis elbow. The patient rarely recalls a sudden onset of pain during these activities, however. At times a direct blow to the epicondyle initiates the problem.
   C. Nature of pain. Varies from a dull ache or no pain at rest to sharp twinges or a straining sensation with activities, as mentioned above. Grasping activities because the wrist extensors must contract to stabilize the wrist during use of the finger flexors particularly aggravates lateral tennis elbow. Medial tennis elbow is worsened by repeated wrist flexion and gripping.

II. Physical Examination
   A. Active movements. Usually fairly painless. In more severe cases of lateral tennis elbow, there may be some pain with active wrist flexion with the elbow in extension from the stretch placed on the tendon. Active wrist extension does not usually produce enough tension to reproduce the pain. Similarly, there may be some pain with active wrist extension with the elbow extended in medial tennis elbow, but usually not on active wrist flexion.
   B. Passive movements
      1. One of the key tests that should reproduce the pain in lateral tennis elbow is full passive wrist flexion with ulnar deviation, forearm pronation, and elbow extension. Passive elbow movements alone are painless.
      2. Full wrist extension with supination and elbow extension reproduces the pain in medial tennis elbow.
   C. Resisted isometric movements. The other key test is resisted wrist extension (with the elbow extended), reproducing the pain in lateral tennis elbow; resisted wrist flexion reproduces pain in medial tennis elbow. At times, resisted pronation is painful in medial tennis elbow. Resisted elbow extension with the elbow in flexion and the forearm fully supinated is a key test for posterior tennis elbow.
   D. Joint-play movements. Should be full and painless
   E. Palpation
      1. Exquisite tenderness occurs usually over the epicondyles in medial and lateral tennis elbow. An area of tenderness may be palpated over the insertion of the triceps tendon into the olecranon in posterior tennis elbow.
      2. In lateral tennis elbow, the tenderness may often extend down into the muscle belly. Less often, the tenderness is felt superior to the epicondyle at the insertion of the extensor carpi radialis longus.
      3. Warmth may be noted over the respective epicondyle and olecranon.
   F. Inspection. Usually no significant findings
   G. Differential diagnoses. Other entities include De Quervain's tenovaginitis (see Chapter 13, Wrist and Hand Complex) and extensor carpi ulnaris tendinitis at the wrist, pronator

syndrome in the forearm, and radial nerve entrapment accompanying lateral epicondylitis at the elbow.[33,84] Associated problems can appear either independently or in combination with the various forms of tennis elbow tendinitis.[115] These may include ulnar nerve neurapraxia,[115] carpal tunnel syndrome,[112,118] intra-articular abnormalities, joint laxity,[72,110,182] and associated soft tissue or myofascial trigger point syndromes.[12,57,64,71,80,165,169] The multiplicity of conditions and treatments found in the literature is typified by the coverage of tennis elbow by Cyriax.[38]

Gunn[62,63] attributed the tennis elbow symptoms in one group of patients to reflex localization of pain from radiculopathy of the cervical spine. Maigne[100] has observed that about 60% of cases with clinical epicondylitis have minor intervertebral derangement at C5–C7 or C6–C7 levels on the side of the tennis elbow. About half of these cases are associated with some degree of periarthritis of the elbow and thus are considered mixed forms.

III. Management
  A. Goals
    1. To restore normal, painless use of the involved extremity
    2. To restore normal strength and extensibility of the musculotendinous unit
    3. To encourage proper maturation of scar tissue and collagen formation, and to allow extensibility and the ability of the tendon to attenuate tensile stresses
  B. Objectives
    1. Resolution of the chronic inflammatory process
    2. Maturation of the scar (healed area of the tendon). The new collagen must be sufficiently strong and extensible to withstand the tensile stresses imposed by activity. There must be an appropriate amount of tissue that is oriented to attenuate tensile stresses with a minimum of internal strain.
    3. Restoration of strength and extensibility to the muscle–tendon complex
  C. Techniques
    1. Acute cases. Tendon injuries of the elbow are by nature chronic disorders, but some patients may present with acute symptoms and signs associated with lateral or medial tennis elbow; pain is referred into the entire forearm and perhaps the hand, and occasionally up the back of the arm. There may be some pain at rest, and some degree of muscle spasm is elicited when the tendon is stressed passively or by resisted movements. In such cases, the immediate goal is to promote progression to a more chronic state, assisting in the resolution of the acute inflammation.
      a. Instruct the patient to apply ice to the site several times a day. The physical therapy modality of high-voltage galvanic stimulation has been helpful in relieving pain and inflammation.[115]
      b. Continued stress to the tendon must be prevented. If the patient presents with acute symptoms and signs as outlined above, this is best achieved by immobiliz-

ing the wrist, hand, and fingers (not the elbow) in a resting splint. In some cases a simple wrist cock-up splint will suffice because this obviates the need for the wrist extensors to contract when the finger flexors are used. Activities involving grasping, pinching, and fine finger movements must be restricted. This is often the most difficult component of the program to institute but at the same time the most important at this stage. The effectiveness of any other treatment measures will be compromised if the patient continues to engage in activities that stress the lesion site. For example, a carpenter must take some time off from work or temporarily change duties, a tennis player must abstain from playing for a while, and persons who enjoy knitting, sewing, or gardening must temporarily alter their activities.
      c. A few times a day, the patient should remove the splint and actively move the wrist into flexion, the forearm into pronation, and the elbow into extension, simultaneously, to minimize loss of extensibility of the muscle and tendon. This should be done gently, avoiding significant discomfort, and slowly to prevent high strain-rate loading of the tissue.

      If appropriate instructions are given and the patient faithfully follows the outlined program, progression to a more chronic status should occur during a period of a few (3 to 5) days.
    2. Chronic cases (lateral tennis elbow). If the pain is fairly localized over the lateral elbow region and there is little or no pain at rest, the disorder should be treated as chronic tendinitis.
      a. Advise the patient explicitly as to the appropriate level and type of activity that may be performed. Strong, repetitive, grasping activities, such as hammering, and activities that particularly stress the tendon, such as tennis, must be restricted until there is little pain on resisted isometric wrist extension and little or no pain when the tendon is passively stretched (wrist flexion, forearm pronation, and elbow extension). Such activities must be resumed gradually, with some protection of the part. Protection may be provided by counterforce bracing with an inelastic cuff worn firmly around the proximal forearm (the forearm extensors for lateral tennis elbow and the forearm flexors for medial tennis elbow). Ilfeld and Field[70] initially introduced the concept of elbow bracing for tennis elbow in 1966. Nirschl[112] later introduced a wider device, curved for better fit and support of the conical shape of the forearm.

      In theory, constraining full muscle expansion when muscles contract should diminish the potential force generated in the muscle. Cybex testing and biomechanical studies have demonstrated both angular velocity and the sequence of the electro-myographic recording of muscular activity, and have confirmed the clinical validity of this concept.[114,115] If such a device is used, the clinician should gradually wean the patient from it as strength, mobility, and painless function increase.

Also, as normal activities are resumed, certain adaptations may be implemented to minimize the stresses imposed on the wrist extensors. For example, the tennis player typically receives high strain-rate loading to the wrist extensor group when using a backhand stroke if the ball strikes the racquet above the center point of the strings. This produces a moment arm about which the force of the ball hitting the racquet can create a high pronator torque. If the wrist extensors are weak, the wrist might also be forced into flexion. The combined effects of the active and passive tension created in the wrist extensor group result in high loading of the extensor tendons. The passive component can be minimized by hitting the ball on center and by having adequate wrist extensor strength to keep the wrist from flexing. Increasing the diameter of the racquet handle can also reduce the passive pronator torque. Other considerations would include the tension of the strings on the racquet and the flexibility of the racquet shaft. High string tension and low racquet flexibility will result in reduced attenuation of forces by the racquet and, therefore, greater transmission of high strain-rate forces to the arm. Also, the larger the racquet head, the greater the potential moment arm about which pronatory forces can act. Thus, a tennis player might benefit from taking lessons to improve the likelihood of hitting the ball on center, reducing string tension, and using a relatively flexible racquet with a handle of maximum tolerable diameter and a head of standard size.

Each patient's activities should be similarly assessed for ways to reduce the loads imposed on the wrist extensor group.

b. Two rehabilitation approaches may be taken in treating lateral and medial tennis elbow. The first approach involves using all the normal measures to reduce inflammation and pain. Treatment may include rest and restriction of activities, using therapeutic modalities such as cryotherapy, electrotherapy, iontophoresis, and ultrasound, and using nonsteroidal anti-inflammatory drugs. The second approach would be to realize that the patient has a chronic inflammation, which is not going anywhere and is in effect stuck.[189] The goal of this approach is to "jump start" the inflammatory process, in effect, using techniques that are likely to increase the inflammatory response and allowing healing to progress as normal to the fibro-

plastic and remodeling phases.[189] To increase the inflammatory response, deep transverse friction massage may be used (see Box 8-1). The beneficial effects of friction massage in cases of tendinitis are not well understood but are probably related to the induced hyperemia and the mechanical influence it may have on tissue maturation (see Chapter 8, Soft Tissue Manipulations). The hyperemic effects are of greatest importance in cases of tendinitis that may be related to hypovascularity, for instance, at the shoulder. Hyperemia does not seem to be a significant factor in the origin of tennis elbow, however, and this may in part explain why friction massage is effective for a shorter period of time in cases of rotator cuff tendinitis than it is in cases of tennis elbow. The mechanical effects of the deep massage may promote orientation of immature collagen along the lines of stress. This would be an important factor in pathologic disorders, such as tennis elbow, in which some type of mechanical stimulus is necessary for adequate tissue maturation. Use of deep transverse massage may assist in tissue maturation without imposing a longitudinal stress to the healing tendon tissue and, therefore, without continued rupturing of fibers at the site of the lesion. Thus, the defect heals with a maximum degree of tissue extensibility and is less likely to be overstressed as use of the part is resumed. This seems to be a solution to the dilemma mentioned above. If the patient continues to use the part, he or she perpetuates the problem by producing continued damage at the lesion site; if the patient completely immobilizes the part, there is no stimulus for tissue maturation, and as soon as activity is resumed, the healed tissue begins to break down.

c. Strength and mobility must be restored. As symptoms and signs indicate improvement, the patient must resume activities gradually. Excessive internal strain to the tendon can be minimized during stressful activities by optimizing tissue extensibility. No vigorous activities should be allowed until it is determined whether the muscle–tendon complex has sufficient extensibility. To facilitate mobility, the clinician should gently and slowly stretch the tissue by holding the elbow extended, the forearm pronated, and the wrist ulnarly deviated, while flexing the wrist and fingers. The patient is instructed to perform this stretch at home, emphasizing that it must be performed slowly and gently. The patient should notice a stretching sensation but no pain. As vigorous activities such as tennis, carpentry, and gardening are resumed, the patient may be taught to administer friction massage for a few minutes before engaging in the activity.

Also, before a normal activity level is resumed, it is important to ensure that good forearm strength has been restored. In lateral tennis elbow, wrist extensor strengthening exercises are always necessary because the muscles invariably undergo atrophy from disuse and reflex inhibition. Good extensor strength is necessary to protect the tendon from high strain-rate passive loading, which may occur with many types of activities. A convenient method of wrist extensor strengthening is to have the patient tie a rope 3 feet long to the center of a 1-inch dowel and add a weight to the end of the rope; the patient grasps both ends of the dowel and rotates it toward him or her until the entire rope becomes wrapped around the dowel. This can be repeated as appropriate; the weight may be varied as necessary.

Forearm rehabilitative exercises to increase muscle power, flexibility, and endurance are important. Continued strengthening of uninjured areas and protective exercises for the injured area are necessary. Isometric, isotonic, isokinetic, and isoflex exercises are all used. Isoflex exercises consist of muscle strengthening, using both concentric and eccentric training with the resistance of an elasticized tension cord.[115] Maximum strengthening of the muscles must necessarily include eccentric exercise.[37] Plyometric exercises and functional training activities should progressively incorporate the stresses, strains, and forces that occur during normal activity, gradually increasing the frequency, intensity, and duration of exercise (see Dynamic Stabilization and Functional Exercises below).

Local anti-inflammatory therapy, such as infiltration with a corticosteroid, is commonly used in cases of tendinitis. Although symptomatic improvement is often dramatic; such treatment has only temporary value. It has no lasting beneficial effect on the pathologic process and does not influence etiologic factors. At best, it should be considered an adjunct to management in the acute state. Too often other important components of the treatment program are ignored when an apparent "cure" is heralded by dramatic symptomatic improvement.

In those individuals who have persistent pain that does not resolve after 1 year of conservative treatment, surgery should be considered.

Medial Tension Overload Syndromes

MEDIAL COLLATERAL LIGAMENT INJURIES (VALGUS OVERLOAD TRIAD)

The syndrome includes problems relating to the posterior medial joint capsule, the ulnar nerve, and medial collateral (ulnar) ligament of the elbow. The medial collateral ligament (MCL) has been clearly documented as a frequent site of serious injury in the overhead athlete.[2,7,11,29,40,41,120,161,162,167,185] It is mostly seen in repetitive activities of throwing (baseball, javelin), hitting, and racquet sports. These repetitive stress levels can affect all athletes, from youth to adults. Traumatic valgus thrust to the elbow either during a fall or after being hit while the arm is outstretched (associated with elbow dislocation) may be another mechanism of injury.[116,142] Valgus overload mechanism is common to many pathologic entities that have been described in the literature, including osteochondritis, medial epicondyle apophysitis, and Little League elbow (see below).[28,49,178]

Any of the structures on the medial aspect of the elbow may become injured. Repetitive stress applied to the medial elbow joint frequently results in ligament failure, tendinitis (wrist flexor), or osseous changes. The flexor–pronator muscles may tear, or a partial avulsion of one of these tendons or muscle insertion may occur with valgus overload injuries. Tension stress that the capsule and ligaments put on the ulna and humerus can lead to spur formation and possibly compression of the ulnar nerve.[82] These injuries can result in elbow flexion contracture or potentially increase instability of the elbow.

I. History. Typically there is a gradual onset of symptoms. The first symptoms appear to indicate a tendinitis, but other complaints of the syndrome then become apparent: medial elbow pain, "popping" sensation worsened by activities causing valgus stress, relieved by rest. Over time medial elbow pain may be accompanied by ulnar nerve irritability or posterior elbow pain caused by olecranon impingement.

II. Physical Examination
   A. Observation may reveal swelling in the form of effusion if acute tissue injury has occurred.
   B. Active and passive movements. Range of motion is frequently diminished. Clients may present with a loss of elbow extension and supination owing to flexor and pronator contractors.
   C. Joint-play movements reveal valgus laxity (see medial-lateral tilt of the humeroulnar joint; Fig. 12-20).
   D. Resisted movements. If the flexor–pronator tendon is involved, resisted forearm pronation will reproduce pain on this maneuver. Pain may also be reproduced on making a fist.
   E. Palpation
      1. Point tenderness over the ulnar collateral ligament
      2. Ulnar nerve hypersensitivity in the groove and possible subluxation
      3. The medial epicondyle insertion of the flexor–pronator tendon is often tender.
   F. Special tests
      1. Valgus stress. A positive elbow abduction stress test (valgus stress test at 20 to 30° of flexion) produces pain and medial opening (Fig. 12-17A) when compared with the opposite side. Stability of the elbow in this partially flexed position to valgus stress is depen-

dent on a competent MCL. This test can also be performed arthroscopically at 70 and 90° of flexion.[133]

2. Valgus extension overload tests.[162] This test is used to detect whether posterior (olecranon) impingement is present. The examiner stabilizes the humerus with one hand and, with the opposite hand, pronates the forearm and applies a valgus force while quickly extending the elbow. A positive test reproduces pain posteromedially around the olecranon.

G. Tissue overload of the upper limb may reveal shoulder muscle weakness (internal rotators) and decreased range of motion.

III. Management. Treatment options for the client with an MCL injury include conservative treatment, repair, and reconstruction.[133] Milder forms of the valgus overload syndrome can be treated with the medial tendon injury protocol (see above) emphasizing:

A. Pain reduction around the inflamed tissue. Initial treatment should included relative rest and judicious use of anti-inflammatory medication.

B. Proximal control of the scapula and rotator cuff muscles. Fatigue of the shoulder musculature is thought to affect arm angle during throwing, increasing the load to the medial elbow.[133]

C. Maintaining and regaining normal range of motion of the flexors and pronator.

D. Strengthening both concentrically and eccentrically the pronators and supinators. Grip exercises and a progressive strengthening program of the extensor and flexor using high-repetition, low-weight isotonic and isokinetic programs provide further strengthening. Strengthening of the flexors should be emphasized, particularly the flexor carpi ulnaris and flexor digitorum superficialis, which can help prevent medial injury by providing additional support of the medial elbow structures.[157] Exercises to increase both static and dynamic flexibility of the elbow without producing valgus stress should be incorporated.

E. The patient may then advance to functional patterns, plyometrics, and progressive throwing.[104,183]

Advanced cases will require surgical stabilization of the underlying MCL instability and posterior medial bony impingement.

LITTLE LEAGUER'S ELBOW

The young pitcher or tennis player is exposed to the risks already discussed above as well as the additional risk of epiphyseal injury. The clinical features of Little Leaguer's elbow include pain and tenderness with loss of full extension. Common characteristic changes are accelerated growth of the medial side or hypertrophy of the medial epicondyle as well as fragmentation of the medial epicondylar epiphysis. The term *Little Leaguer's elbow* is a wastebasket term that may encompass not only the accelerated growth of the medial side and fragmentation of the medial epicondylar epiphysis but

also the following: (1) delayed closure of the medial epicondylar apophyseal line, (2) osteochondritis of the capitellum, (3) osteochondritis of the radial head, (4) hypertrophy of the ulna, and (5) olecranon apophysitis with or without delayed closure of the olecranon apophysis.[19] The term should be abandoned in favor of a specific pathologic diagnosis.[43]

Medial Epicondylar Apophysitis. Medial epicondylar apophysitis is characterized by insidious onset of progressive medial elbow pain that occurs with throwing activities. A triad of symptoms is often present, including medial pain localized to the medial epicondyle, diminished throwing effectiveness, and delayed throwing distance or velocity.[19] The cause of injury includes repetitive valgus stress with tension forces on the medial epicondyle via the MCL and the flexor–pronator muscle mass. These valgus stresses result in repetitive microtrauma and ultimate stress fracture failure of the medial epicondylar apophysis.[39]

The mainstay treatment of medial epicondylar apophysitis is elimination of the repetitive valgus stress. This may mean eliminating throwing. Initially ice, combined with nonsteroidal anti-inflammatory drug therapy, can help alleviate symptoms. This is followed by a course of physical therapy for stretching and strengthening. A gradual return to throwing is initiated when the patient is completely symptom free. Nondisplaced stress fractures of the medial epicondyle respond well to conservative treatment.[61]

Osteochondrosis Dissecans of the Capitellum. Osteochondrosis of the capitellum (Panner's disease, osteochondrosis deformans, osteochondritis dissecans) may be directly related to trauma or to changes in the circulation; this is the so-called Panner's disease of aseptic or avascular necrosis. Panner's disease is the most common cause of lateral elbow pain in the young child and is typically seen in patients younger than 10. It represents a benign self-limited process characterized by fragmentation of the entire ossific center of the capitellum.[43] The cause is uncertain but is thought to mimic Perthes disease of the hip. Whatever the underlying cause, the ultimate outcome may be healing, nonhealing, or loose body formation.

The main presenting symptoms are usually pain, swelling, limitation of range of motion in a noncapsular pattern of restriction, and sometimes locking or clicking. Osteochondritis dissecans has been classified into three stages[106]:

1. Lesions in which there is no radiographic evidence of subchondral displacement or fracture.
2. Lesions in which there is evidence of subchondral detachment or articular cartilage fracture.
3. Lesions in which chondral or osteochondral fragments become detached and result in intra-articular loose body or bodies.

Treatment is dependent on the clinical and radiographic findings. Conservative treatment is indicated in stages 1 and 2 when the subchondral bone or articular cartilage has not become detached fragments. Patients with loose bodies and closed epiphyses do not fare well and may require surgical intervention.

Conservative treatment includes rest and avoidance of valgus stress. Occasionally a short period of immobilization with a splint may be required. Treatment is the same as outlined for throwing injuries. Usually, joint motion is restored or improved with manual therapy, strengthening, range of motion, and a stretching program. Flexibility exercises should be performed for the entire upper limb. Typically, a prolonged period of healing of up to 3 years can be expected, with excellent long-term clinical and radiographic results.[127] Once the patient is pain free and range of motion is normalized, plyometrics and high-speed drills can be added, as well as aggressive eccentric strengthening.

Internal Derangement

In patients with internal derangement (noncapsular limited range of motion, loose bodies in the joint with limitation of flexion or extension in isolation), the joint periodically locks, with full extension or flexion being limited. Range of motion returns gradually over several days. It then changes the hard end feel of extension into a rather soft one. The patient will exhibit a noncapsular pattern: the joint is limited in full extension (soft end feel) or full flexion (hard end feel). Frequent occurrences can set up a reactive osteoarthritis, even in adolescents.[31]

Three different clinical pictures can be considered depending on the age group in which they appear: adolescents, adults, or the elderly.[122]

In adolescence the condition does not occur before the age of 14 and usually results from osteochondritis dissecans, mostly on the humeral capitellum (see above),[5,103] or an intra-articular chip fracture.[94] Arthroscopic or surgical removal of the loose piece(s) is advised as the loose body has an osseous nucleus and still lies within its nutrient synovial fluid; it may grow and the condition may worsen with each attack.[14]

In a normal joint in adulthood the cause is usually traumatic, the injury having chipped off one or more pieces of cartilage. A very clear noncapsular pattern is found with limitation on either flexion or extension, depending on the position of the fragment. A loose body that limits extension can usually be reduced. Manipulation under strong traction shifts the loose piece of cartilage to a position at the back of the joint. It then no longer blocks movement, which becomes normal again.[122] The manipulation can be repeated each time that derangement occurs. Refer to Ombregt et al.[122] for a detailed description of the technique.

A loose body that limits flexion cannot be reduced by manipulation, but limitation of flexion, unless gross, is not of major concern. The alternatives are arthroscopic or surgical removal.

In an arthrotic joint in middle age or older, the symptoms are of repeated attacks of pain lasting for about a week.[122] Between attacks, the elbow presents with a capsular pattern and a hard end feel at the end of the achievable range. During the attacks, the limitation becomes of the noncapsular type with a soft end feel. The fragments are osseous and visible on radiograph. It is possible to have loose bodies in the joint without having attacks of internal derangement. Manipulative treatment can be considered during the attacks, although it is not strictly necessary, as the condition subsides spontaneously.

Subluxation of the Radial Head

Subluxation of the radial head (pulled elbow or nursemaid's elbow, acute limitation of extension and supination in children) is a common condition that occurs in young children before the age of 8 years, with a peak incidence between 2 and 3 years.[35] The history is a sudden traction injury that has been applied to the child's arm while held in an extended and pronated position above the child's head by an adult, who then lifts the child's arm suddenly upward. This may occur in many different situations, such as swinging the child by the arms, or when lifting the child up from the floor or lifting the child's arm as the adult goes up a step or down a curb. The imperfectly formed radial head in this age group may allow subluxation in association with damage and unfolding of the immature annular ligament.[129]

The child presents with a painful inability to use the arm, which may be accompanied by an audible or palpable click in the elbow. The child holds the elbow flexed at about 90° and in pronation. Because pain may be poorly localized, the diagnosis may be difficult; either the wrist or elbow, or the shoulder, may be considered as the site of the lesion. Once the diagnosis is clear, the pulled elbow is completely and rapidly cured by manipulation. With suitable encouragement normal shoulder and wrist movement may be demonstrated, but there may be a small loss of range of passive elbow extension and flexion. However, any attempt to produce passive supination is violently resisted.

Reduction is usually easily accomplished by elbow flexion and rotation of the forearm. One hand of the operator supports the elbow with the thumb over the head of the radius while the child's hand is held by the other hand. After gaining the child's confidence, the forearm is suddenly and firmly pulled into full supination. A palpable and sometimes audible click can usually be detected in the region of the radial head as the subluxation is reduced.[35] The main features of successful reduction are restoration of full range of motion, prompt resolution of pain, and demonstration of reduction by a normal radiograph. Sometimes spontaneous reduction occurs just by bringing the forearm into supination and flexion, as in examining for passive flexion of the elbow.[86]

The child usually does not require active treatment after the reduction, but the parents should be carefully instructed in the mechanism of the injury to prevent the possibility of a recurrence. Occasionally immobilization is advisable if reduction is delayed for more than 12 hours or reduction is unstable. Immobilization in an above-elbow posterior mold or cast with the forearm in full supination and the elbow in 90° of flexion is usually recommended.

Trauma

Trauma to the elbow may result in major impairment and disability, because it hinders functional use of the hand and fingers. Examination and treatment of fractures are beyond the scope of this text, but when fractures are suspected, such patients should be immediately referred to an orthopedic surgeon.

Sprains are examples of subluxation (dislocations) and injury to the ligaments and the joint capsules. They become clinically evident from a meaningful history and physical examination. Results of radiologic examination can eliminate the possibility of bony injury.

Joint stiffness after trauma, fracture, surgery, or sprained collateral ligaments at the elbow that involve the capsule itself are a major concern. A capsular pattern is the usual objective finding, although surgical repair may alter it. Diffuse swelling may be present. See Postimmobilization Capsular Tightness (below) for management of capsular tightness.

Postimmobilization Capsular Tightness

Patients with restricted movement at the elbow from capsular tightness are often referred to physical therapists. Because capsular restriction from degenerative joint disease at the elbow is rare, patients with capsular restriction seen by physical therapists are usually those whose elbows have been immobilized. Degenerative joint disease of the elbow when it occurs is almost always of the secondary type and frequently posttraumatic.[140] It can occur prematurely in certain athletes such as football linemen, gymnasts, and throwers.[3,11,59,180,181] The other frequent cause of capsular restriction at this joint is inflammatory arthritis (usually rheumatoid arthritis but occasionally traumatic arthritis).

The common injuries for which management may involve elbow immobilization include dislocations (usually posterior dislocation of the ulnar on the humerus) and fractures of the arm or forearm (humeral shaft fractures, supracondylar fractures, and Colles' fractures). Colles' fractures are the most common.

I. History. Determine the date of injury, dates of subsequent surgery (if any), duration of immobilization, and date of removal of supports or splints. Any suggestion of complications after the injury or immobilization, such as vascular dysfunction, should be noted. Determine whether there have been previous attempts at remobilization, and if so, what these entailed. Assess the patient's functional disability in terms of limitations on dressing or grooming and on occupational and recreational activities. These should be documented and used as a means by which to judge progress.

II. Physical Examination. The key sign is limitation of motion in a capsular pattern. However, note any complication that may have ensued.
   A. Reflex sympathetic dystrophy (see Chapter 13, Wrist and Hand Complex)
   1. Key signs include capsular restriction of all or most upper extremity joints to varying degrees; generalized edema of the forearm and hand; trophic changes in skin and nails (glossy smooth skin, hyperhidrosis, hypohidrosis, cyanosis, brittle or ridged nails); and dysesthesias, with pain hypersensitivity even to light touch. Roentgenograms often reveal marked osteopenia, especially of the bones of the hand and wrist.
   2. The exact cause of this disorder is unknown. It is especially prevalent in patients who have sustained a Colles'-type fracture. It is believed to be related to nerve trauma (such as trauma to the median nerve in Colles' fracture), the degree of edema, immobilization, and psychological factors. Preventive measures to be taken during immobilization should include frequent active exercise of the free joints (usually the shoulder and fingers) and regular periods of elevation of the involved extremity.

   Development of a true reflex sympathetic dystrophy, often referred to as a shoulder–hand syndrome, can be a significant complicating factor in the rehabilitation program after immobilization. The marked articular restrictions and pain hypersensitivity make efforts at remobilization especially difficult.
   B. Malalignment of bony fragments. This is occasionally seen after a supracondylar fracture at the elbow and invariably follows a Colles' fracture (see Chapter 13, Wrist and Hand Complex).

   Elbow malalignment is easily detected by observing the carrying angle of the arm and by assessing structural alignment. With a supracondylar fracture, the distal fragment tends to displace posteriorly and medially with an angulation medially. Rotational displacement, medial or lateral displacements, and posterior or anterior displacements are not significant in the young person, because these usually resolve with bone remodeling. Angular displacements, however, tend to persist. Typically, the malalignment after a supracondylar fracture presents as a decrease or reversal of the normal carrying angle. The medial epicondyle is positioned higher than the lateral epicondyle, and the olecranon becomes directed medially. Such malalignment usually does not result in a functional deficit but may be cosmetically unacceptable.
   C. Brachialis contusion. The displacement of bony parts that accompanies supracondylar elbow fractures and elbow dislocations may result in a contusion to the distal brachialis muscle belly, which overlies and is in close contact with the distal end of the humerus (Fig. 12-18). The consequence of such a contusion may be eventual metaplasia of the contused portion of this muscle into osseous tissue, a condition referred to as myositis ossificans.[1,55] Myositis ossificans usually results in permanent restriction of motion at the elbow; extension is restricted more than flexion.

   It is questionable whether mobilization of the part (active, passive, prolonged, or otherwise) actually affects the eventual outcome. Some believe that the condition is often the

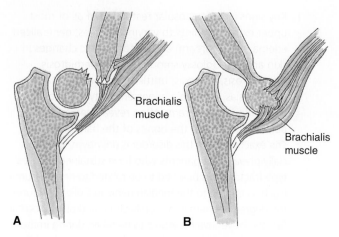

■ FIG. 12-18. Two common injuries of the elbow that result in displacement of bony parts: **(A)** supracondylar fracture; **(B)** posterior dislocation of ulna on humerus.

result of overzealous attempts to remobilize the part. This may be the case if the brachialis muscle is stretched. In cases of capsular restriction, however, in which the stretch is applied to the anterior capsule rather than the brachialis muscle, it is doubtful that any form of mobilization would predispose to development of myositis ossificans of the brachialis muscle. Myositis ossificans after injuries in which the brachialis muscle is traumatized probably develops as an inevitable event resulting from the original injury.

The clinician must be protected medicolegally in the event that myositis ossificans should occur. This can be done by recognizing the two common conditions (supracondylar fracture and posterior dislocation) that especially predispose to development of myositis ossificans, and by distinguishing between capsular and muscular restriction of motion at the elbow. Fortunately, fractures and dislocations at the elbow occur primarily in children; because of this, remobilization is not a major problem and passive mobilization is seldom required. However, if mobilization procedures are requested for a patient whose extremity has been immobilized after a supracondylar fracture or elbow dislocation, the clinician must take certain precautions.

First, the cause of the restriction is determined. Limitation of extension more than flexion with an elastic end feel suggests a muscular restriction. The constant-length phenomenon is used to determine whether it is the biceps or brachialis. Limitation of motion in a capsular pattern with a capsular end feel suggests a capsular restriction. Stretching a tight elbow flexor muscle in such a case must not be done vigorously, except in cases of persistent restriction of elbow extension, and then only with agreement of the referring physician and with the patient's understanding.

Second, whether the restriction appears capsular or muscular, the clinician must attempt to detect any signs of inflammation of the brachialis muscle. This is done by palpating for a hematoma or excessive tenderness over the distal brachialis muscle belly. Any suggestion of inflam-

mation or hematoma of the distal brachialis muscle belly should preclude vigorous mobilization, barring the stipulations indicated above. Regardless of the intensity of the mobilization program, the clinician would do well to record thermistor readings over the distal brachialis region before and after each treatment session. A rise in temperature that persists for a 24-hour period, for example, might indicate that the intensity of the program should be reduced, especially if a muscular restriction is at fault.

III. Management of Capsular Tightness. Wilk et al.[180] cite three predisposing factors for the onset of capsular elbow restrictions and flexion contractures of the elbow: (1) the congruency of the joint capsule, (2) a tight capsule, and (3) the scarring tendency of the anterior capsule. This only emphasizes the importance of early intervention.

A. Acute. Because most capsular elbow restrictions are those that follow immobilization after injury, they are rarely found in an acute stage, as the acute inflammatory process subsides during immobilization.

1. Provide relief of pain and muscle guarding using ice, superficial heat, and grades I and II joint-play movements.

2. Maintain existing range of motion and increase movement as pain and guarding abate.

   a. Use gentle joint-play movements, grades I and II. Restoration of joint motion is vital to the nutrition of articular cartilage and the prevention of adhesion formation.

   b. Soft tissue techniques (see Chapter 8, Soft Tissue Manipulations)

   c. Initiate a home exercise program of pain-free active, active-assistive, and passive elbow flexion, extension, pronation, and supination.

3. Strengthen progressively the muscles controlling the shoulder, elbow, forearm, and wrist as necessary. Use isometrics in the acute stage because joint movement might cause reflex inhibition of the muscles to be strengthened.

B. Chronic

1. Ultrasound to tight capsular tissues along with or followed by capsular stretching, with joint-play mobilization techniques. If the therapist is treating a stiff elbow after a radial head resection, special attention should be given to preventing the development of a valgus contracture at the elbow by use of the "varus tilt" (lateral tilt) mobilization technique (see Fig. 12-20*B*). The radius tends to migrate superiorly because the radial head no longer abuts the capitellum of the humerus. This may also result in problems at the distal radioulnar joint.

2. Joint distraction techniques to increase capsular extensibility are particularly advocated (Fig. 12-19).

3. Therapeutic techniques to enhance motion include stretching, proprioceptive neuromuscular facilitation stretching, muscle energy, and soft tissue manipulations.

4. Low-load, long-duration stretching has been proven to be extremely beneficial and superior to other tech-

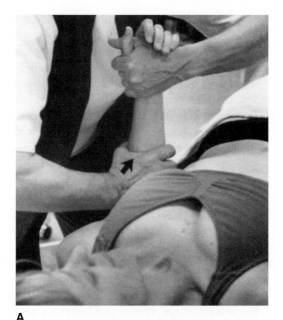

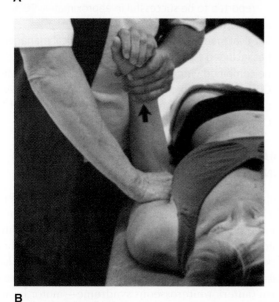

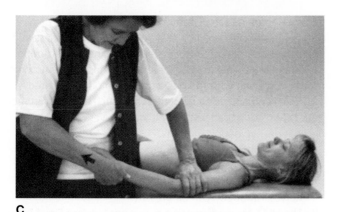

■ FIG. 12-19. Techniques for distraction of the humero-ulnar joint: **(A)** joint distraction in flexion (ulna moved inferiorly); **(B)**, joint distraction in flexion (ulna moved superiorly); **(C)** joint distraction, moving toward extension.

niques in restoring elbow motion.[4,15,87,141,176,177,181] Existing techniques such as dynamic splinting and skin traction rely on a time-dependent material property, creep, which applies a continuous load. Skin traction, therapeutic bands, and cuff weights can be successfully used at home (see Fig. 12-29). The three most important components of this technique are intensity (low to moderate), duration of the stretch (10 to 15 minutes), and frequency (five to six times daily).[4]

5. Progressions of home program to include stretching exercises, especially to improve elbow extension and forearm supination and pronation.

6. Progression of home strengthening program, including exercises to increase flexibility, endurance, and eccentric control. Total arm strength should be included in the program. Any elbow rehabilitation program is not complete without the inclusion of a shoulder girdle complex and hand rehabilitation program. This involves the development of proximal stability for distal mobility. Proximal stability of the upper limb depends on the strength and balance of the scapular stabilizers and rotator cuff musculature.

Nerve Entrapments

A variety of nerve injuries occur in and around the elbow (see Arteries and Nerves above). Of the several entrapment syndromes near the level of the elbow, ulnar nerve injury is the most common.

ULNAR NERVE ENTRAPMENT

Ulnar nerve entrapment (cubital tunnel syndrome, ulnar tunnel syndrome, ulnar neuritis) may occur from a number of causes, including (1) osseous degenerative changes, (2) compression caused by a thickened retinaculum or hypertrophied flexor carpi ulnaris muscle, (3) recurrent subluxations or dislocation, (4) direct trauma, and (5) traction caused by an increased laxity of the medial complex that causes a compressive force on the nerve resulting in a tension neuropathy.[34]

The term **cubital tunnel syndrome** is used to identify a specific anatomic site for entrapment of the ulnar nerve, the most common site of entrapment of the ulnar nerve at the elbow.[105,173–175] The ulnar nerve can be compromised by any swelling that occurs within the tunnel, with inflammatory changes that result in thickening of the fascial sheath, and because of constriction by the aponeurosis (tendinous insertion) of the flexor carpi ulnaris, located about 2 to 3 cm below the medial epicondyle (Fig. 12-13B).[79,189] Ulnar entrapment in the cubital tunnel is common after prolonged flexion of the elbow, such as in throwing athletes (most commonly), racquet sports enthusiasts, weightlifters, and manual laborers.[65,166] The nerve may be damaged by a single traumatic episode as it lies superficially in its groove, by repeated trauma from occupations that involve leaning on the elbow, by previous trauma that has resulted in a cubitus valgus deformity that gradually stretches the nerve, or by overuse of the elbow, resulting in entrapment as the nerve is tethered in its groove.[35] Ligamentous laxity, hyperflexed elbow posturing, recurrent subluxation or dislocation of the nerve out of the ulnar groove, tethering of the nerve at the arcade of Struthers (Fig. 12-13), muscle hypertrophy, tumors, ganglions, or restriction of the nerve by adhesions in the cubital tunnel may result in nerve compression.[65,166,170,171,173–175]

I. Physical Examination. Symptoms are mainly sensory, with pain or paresthesias in the sensory distribution of the nerve to the medial one and a half fingers.[35] Other symptoms include clumsiness of the hand as a result of weakness, hyperesthesia, or numbness, and complaints of muscle cramping. There may be a dull ache after activity or at rest. Pain may radiate up the forearm to the elbow and as far as the shoulder. Symptoms are aggravated by activity and relieved by rest.

   A. On examination, there may be weakness and wasting of the hypothenar eminence and of the adductor muscles of the thumb (clawing of the ring or little finger and grade III paresis).[23] The lack of the ability to adduct the little finger may be the first sign of ulnar compression. Grip and thumb–index finger pinch weakness become apparent. Sensation may be disturbed in the hand.

   B. Positive elbow flexion test. Three minutes of elbow hyperflexion and full wrist extension produces dysesthesias, pain, and numbness in the distribution of the ulnar nerve.[65]

   C. Positive Tinel's sign along the cubital tunnel.

   D. Sensory symptoms may be reproduced by pressure over the ulnar nerve behind the medial epicondyle, where tenderness or thickening of the nerve may be found. The ULTT for an ulnar nerve bias is positive (see Fig. 11-28).[21] Elbow hyperflexion usually elicits symptoms.

   E. Nerve conduction studies and appropriate electromyographic tests must confirm diagnosis because similar symptoms may arise from lesions in the neck, such as thoracic outlet syndrome or cervical nerve root entrapment from diskogenic disease.[23]

II. Management

   A. Conservative treatment. Conservative treatment should be tried initially, consisting of relief of symptoms with physical agents, extra rest to the elbow, and education of the patient to avoid aggravating activities or postures (especially repeated or excessive flexion).

     1. Soft elbow pads are helpful and should be worn continuously.

     2. Exercises to increase flexibility of the forearm muscles and functional activities are introduced slowly.[164]

     3. Appropriate neck and shoulder girdle postures are considered throughout the therapy program.

     4. Nerve gliding (see Fig. 8-62) may be started when symptoms are intermittent with elbow extension, forearm supination, and wrist extension.

     5. Soft tissue manipulations for release of the flexor muscles of the forearm and focal release proximally at the site of entrapment is clearly indicate.[158] There is often

an association of medial epicondylitis with cubital tunnel syndrome.[50] In such cases inflammation can lead to prominence of the pronator teres and flexor carpi radialis that compresses the ulnar nerve. Manual release of these muscles also may be indicated (see Chapter 8, Soft Tissue Manipulations).

     6. Training modification should include avoidance of hyperflexion and valgus stress. Dynamic stability drills should be initiated for the elbow stabilizers, specifically pronator teres and wrist flexor muscles. These muscles assist the ulnar collateral ligament in stabilizing the medial side of the elbow especially during the cocking and acceleration phase of throwing. Rhythmic stabilization drills can be performed to enhance dynamic stabilization.

     7. Once symptoms are resolved, a comprehensive rehabilitation program should be started with gradual return to athletic or work activities (see Rehabilitation Progression below). Nonsurgical treatment has been reported to be successful in approximately 90% of patients in the general population.[47]

   B. Surgical management. In the past surgical management has included translocation of the ulnar nerve, which may be combined with excision of the medial epicondyle. Currently division of the tendinous origin of the flexor carpi ulnaris from the humerus is the procedure of choice in most cases.[29,30]

MEDIAN NERVE ENTRAPMENT (PRONATOR SYNDROME)

Compression injuries involving the median nerve at the elbow are far less common. The median nerve can be compressed under the ligament of Struthers (Fig. 12-15C), within the pronator teres (Fig. 12-15A), and under the superficial head of the flexor digitorum superficialis. Other sites include the lacteus fibrosis (Fig. 12-15A) or bicipital aponeurosis and in the midforearm (anterior interosseous syndrome—motor branch).

I. Physical Examination. Symptoms consist of forearm pain that worsens with exertion (e.g., pronation), numbness and paresthesias in all or part of distal median nerve distribution, and fatigue or weakness of the forearm muscles. Symptoms seem to worsen with repetitive pronation or grip-related activities and extension of the forearm such as occurs in racquet sports or in patients whose job involves repetitive pronation–supination motions.

   A. On examination there may be weakness of thenar intrinsic, and variable weakness of median-innervated extrinsic muscles. Sensory deficit in all or part of distal median nerve distribution can be present.

   B. The ULTT for median nerve bias is positive (see Fig. 11-26) as well as Tinel's sign.

   C. Localized pressure at compression site causes discomfort.

   D. Specific tests on the basis of site.[128]

1. Pronator teres syndrome
   a. Pronator teres. Resisted forearm pronation and flexion with wrist and fingers flexed aggravates pain.
   b. Flexor digitorum superficialis arcade. Resisted flexion of the middle finger worsens symptoms.
   c. Lacertus fibrosis. Increased pain with elbow flexion and supination
2. Anterior interosseous syndrome
   a. Reduced thumb–index pinch strength
   b. Weakness of the flexor pollicis longus and flexor digitorum profundus

II. Treatment. Most compressive neuropathies are treated conservatively with good results.[20] Unlike the treatment of carpal tunnel syndrome, steroid injections have little to offer in the nonoperative treatment of proximal median nerve compression.[72]
   A. Initial treatment in the acute setting: relative rest, elevation, nonsteroidal anti-inflammatory drugs, and immobilization. Typically immobilization consists of a removable splint fashioned with the elbow in flexion, the forearm in slight pronation, and the wrist in slight flexion.[20] This allows the forearm musculature to relax in a favorable position relieving the suspected anatomic compression.
   B. Soft tissue manipulations, stretching to pronator and supinator muscles, and nerve gliding exercises (see Fig. 8-62) should be considered.
   C. Long-term treatment (see Rehabilitation Progression below)

RADIAL NERVE ENTRAPMENT

Entrapment of the radial nerve (radial nerve compression syndrome), specifically the posterior interosseous nerve, occurs with the radial tunnel and has been referred to as the **radial tunnel syndrome.** Five sites of entrapment in the radial tunnel have been recognized: (1) proximal fibrous band of the extensor carpi radialis, (2) extensor carpi radialis brevis margin (hypertrophy), (3) radial recurrent vessel arch, (4) arcade of Frohse, and (5) distal edge of supinator (Fig. 12-14B).[128] Radial nerve compression occurs in throwing and overhead activities.[189] Repetitive pronation and supination can also cause similar symptoms. It is important to examine the cervical spine and the radial nerve both proximal and distal to the elbow.[163] It has been postulated that a proximal compression can make the distal nerve more susceptible to injury. This is known as the double-crush theory.[168]

I. Physical Examination. Symptoms consist of lateral elbow pain, paresthesias, and weakness of finger extensors and supinator. The syndrome somewhat resembles tennis elbow. A decrease in grip strength or a subtle fall in performance may be the only presenting symptom. There is tenderness distal to the lateral epicondyle over the supinator muscle. There are sensory defects in the thumb, index, and long fingers.
   A. Positive resisted forearm supination with worsening of the symptoms
   B. Resisted middle finger extension with elbow fully extended aggravates the symptoms.

II. Treatment
   A. Initial treatment begins with avoidance of muscular activities that aggravate the symptoms. This includes action involving forceful repeated wrist and finger extension with supination. An extensor tenodesis splint or splinting with the wrist extended, the forearm supinated, and the elbow flexed may be effective.[46]
   B. Stretching to restore full intrinsic wrist extensors, and tendon excursion
   C. Radial nerve gliding techniques to encourage adequate gliding
   D. Soft tissue mobilization to improve extensibility
   E. Activity modification to prevent reoccurrence and progressive therapy (see Rehabilitation Progression below)

REHABILITATION PROGRESSION AFTER NERVE ENTRAPMENTS

After a course of conservative treatment (see initial treatments above), the rehabilitation program should consist of progressive therapy, which should concentrate on strengthening the involved muscles to maintain balance between agonist and antagonist muscles, stretching, and assessment of sports-specific or work-related functional activities. Soft tissue manipulations can prevent adhesions from developing, thus restricting the nerve. Mobility of the nerve is critical in reducing nerve entrapment. Functional activities can be incorporated, including exercises to establish neuromuscular control, proprioceptive neuromuscular facilitation (PNF) diagonal strengthening patterns (see Figs. 11-82 through 11-86), and closed-kinetic chain activities (see Figs. 11-71 through 11-76, 11-78, and 12-30 through 12-33).

Once an athlete regains full range of motions with protective strength, sports-specific drills and plyometrics are begun.

PASSIVE TREATMENT TECHNIQUES

(For simplicity, the operator is referred to as the male, the patient as the female. All the techniques described apply to the patient's *left* extremity except as indicated. P—patient; O—operator; M—movement; MH—mobilizing hand.)

Joint Mobilization Techniques

I. Humeroulnar Joint. Distraction
   A. Joint distraction, in flexion (ulna moved inferiorly; Fig. 12-19A)
      P—Supine with arm at side, elbow bent, forearm supinated
      O—Stabilizes the wrist with the left hand. He grasps the proximal forearm high up in the antecubital space with the right hand in a pronated position, using the web of the hand for contact.

M—The proximal ulna is moved inferiorly, affecting a joint distraction, with perhaps some inferior glide. As movement increases, the elbow can be progressively flexed.

This technique is used as a general capsular stretch, primarily to increase elbow flexion.

B. Joint distraction, in flexion (ulna moved superiorly; Fig. 12-19B)

P—Supine, with arm at side, forearm supinated, elbow flexed

O—Stabilizes the upper arm by holding the distal humerus at the elbow down against the plinth with the right hand. With the left hand, he grasps the back of the supinated wrist.

M—The proximal ulna is moved superiorly (toward the ceiling), producing joint distraction. Note: By holding the forearm against his body, the operator can combine distraction with increasing flexion (oscillatory movement) by a rocking motion of his body, while maintaining constant stabilization of the humerus.

This technique is also used to increase elbow flexion.

C. Joint distraction, moving toward extension (Fig. 12-19C)

P—Supine, with arm at side, elbow bent, forearm in neutral position

O—Stabilizes the distal humerus against the plinth with the left hand, forearm pronated. He grasps the distal ulna with his right hand, using primarily the thumb and index finger.

M—Ulnar distraction is effected as a distal pull and by a little outward rotation of the operator's entire body. The elbow may be gradually extended as movement increases.

This technique may be considered an inferior glide of the coronoid on the trochlea or, in a sense, a joint distraction. When used at the limit of extension it becomes an anterior capsular stretch.

II. Humeroulnar Joint. Medial-lateral tilt (Fig. 12-20)

P—Supine, with arm at side, forearm supinated, elbow close to the limit of extension

O—Supports the forearm with the caudal hand; grasps the humeral epicondyles, supporting the olecranon in the palm of the mobilizing hand

M—Keeping the patient's forearm stationary, the mobilizing hand moves medially or laterally, producing a medial (Fig. 12-20A) or lateral (Fig. 12-20B; valgus or varus) tilt of the patient's humeroulnar joint. The elbow is gradually extended as movement increases.

These techniques are used only when the elbow lacks a few degrees of extension. It is intended to increase a joint-play movement necessary for full elbow extension.

III. Humeroulnar Joint. Anterior glide (Fig. 12-21A)

P—Prone

O—Standing, facing the head of the table. With the medial hand, stabilize the distal (right) humerus. With the heel of the lateral hand, contact the posterior aspect of the olecranon process. The forearm is

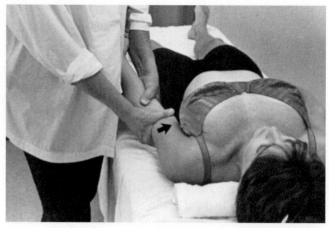

A

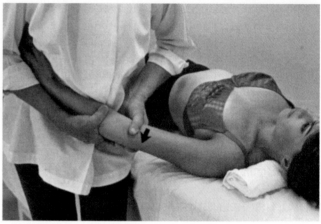

B

■ **FIG. 12-20.** Medial-lateral tilt of humeroulnar joint: **(A)** medial tilt (glide); **(B)** lateral tilt (glide).

supported on the operator's thigh at the limit of the physiologic range of motion.

M—From this position, glide the ulna anteriorly (toward the floor).

This technique is used to increase flexion. This technique may also be performed in supine position, with the head of the treatment table elevated, the upper arm supported on the table, and the forearm over the edge of the table and supported at the wrist (Fig. 12-21B).

IV. Humeroradial Joint. Approximation (Fig. 12-22)

P—Supine with the humerus on the table and elbow flexed to 90°

O—The stabilizing hand grips the distal humerus while the mobilizing hand grasps the patient's hand, thenar to thenar and thumb around thumb.

M—The shaft of the radius is moved downward indirectly through the wrist by the operator leaning his shoulder on the interlocking hands, causing the radius to approximate into the humerus. The forearm may be alternately pronated and supinated.

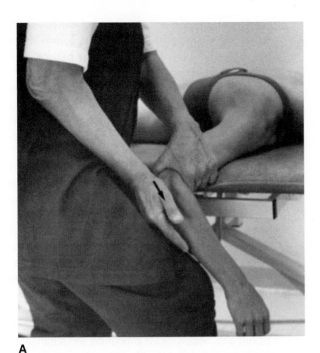

■ **FIG. 12-21.** Humeroulnar joint: **(A)** anterior glide in prone; **(B)** anterior glide in supine.

This technique may be used to reduce a distal positional fault of the radius and, when combined with pronation and supination, to increase pronation and supination, respectively.

V. Proximal Radioulnar Joint. Distal glide of radius on ulna (Fig. 12-23)

P—Supine, with arm resting at the side, elbow bent, and forearm in neutral position

O—Stabilizes the distal humerus against the plinth with his left hand, forearm pronated. He grasps the distal radius with his right hand, using primarily the thumb, index, and long fingers.

M—The radius is pulled distally with the right hand and by a little outward rotation of the operator's entire body. The elbow may be gradually extended as movement increases.

This technique may also be considered distraction at the radiohumeral joint and is intended to increase joint-play movement necessary for full elbow extension.

VI. Proximal Radioulnar Joint. Dorsal-ventral glide (Fig. 12-24A)

P—Supine, arm at side, elbow slightly flexed, forearm in slight supination. The patient's forearm is supported by placing her hand lightly on the operator's left forearm.

O—Supports the medial aspect of the distal humerus and proximal surface of the upper forearm with his left hand. The right hand holds the ventral surface of the proximal radius with the thumb and the dorsal surface with the crook of the flexed proximal interphalangeal joint of the index finger.

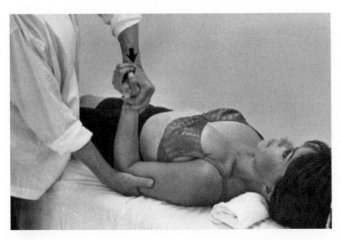

■ **FIG. 12-22.** Humeroradial joint: approximation.

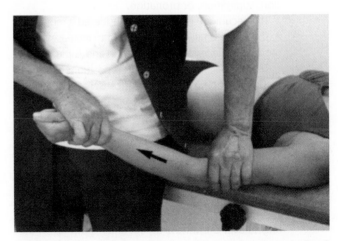

■ **FIG. 12-23.** Distal glide of radius on ulna for proximal radioulnar joint.

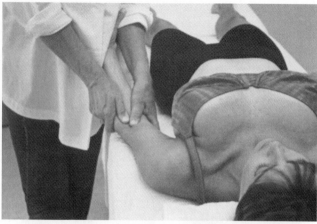

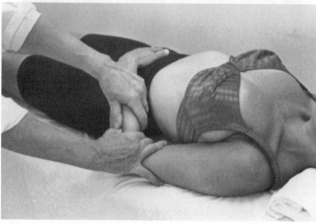

■ **FIG. 12-24.** Dorsal-ventral glide of proximal radio-ulnar joint: (**A**) dorsal glide in resting position; (**B**) ventral glide in restricted range.

M—The radial head may be moved dorsally or ventrally as separate motions. These movements can be performed in varying degrees of elbow flexion, extension, supination, or pronation.

This technique may also be considered a movement at the radiohumeral joint. It is used to increase joint movement necessary for pronation and supination.

The proximal radioulnar joint is positioned in the resting position (Fig. 12-24A) if conservative techniques are indicated, or approximating the restricted range if more aggressive range techniques are indicated (Fig. 12-24B).

VII. Proximal Radioulnar Joint. Technique to regain pronation (after Zohn and Mennell[188]; Fig. 12-25)

P—Supine, with arm in full supination and slightly abducted

O—With his left hand, he supports the wrist with his fingers over the ventral aspect and his thumb on the dorsal aspect. He places the thenar eminence of his right hand over the anterior aspect of the head of the radius and maintains the patient's upper arm on the plinth. The position of the head of the patient's radius is maintained with his thenar eminence.

M—The carrying angle of the patient's elbow is increased by the operator's hand at the wrist while maintaining full supination (Fig. 12-25A). Maintaining both supination and the carrying angle of the forearm, the operator flexes the patient's elbow until the head of the radius is felt to press firmly against his right thenar eminence (Fig. 12-25B). While maintaining the forearm in this position with firm pressure against the radial head, the forearm is moved into pronation (Fig. 12-25C). Note: This technique requires considerable practice to be effective. If supination, flexion, and pressure of the thenar eminence are not maintained throughout the technique, the proper movement will not be achieved. The angle of flexion should not be altered while the forearm is moved from supination to pronation.

This is a valuable technique in regaining joint-play movements necessary for pronation and supination. It is particularly helpful with dysfunction of the radial head. This dysfunction usually presents with a history of forceful pronation–supination of the elbow and forearm.[52]

VIII. Mobilizations With Movement (MWMs): Humeroulnar Joint. Lateral glide (after Mulligan[109]; Fig. 12-26)

P—Supine, with the arm in abduction and the forearm supinated

O—The right hand supports the upper arm while the left hand contacts the humeroulnar joint.

M—A lateral glide is applied to the ulna as the patient concurrently flexes the elbow (provided there is no pain) as the medial glide is sustained until the elbow returns to mid range. A seat belt can be used to apply the force if preferred.

For patients with suspected tennis elbow, the clinician applies a lateral glide to the ulna as the patient makes a fist.

For additional techniques using mobilizations with movement, see Mulligan.[109]

Self-Mobilization Techniques

I. Humeroulnar Joint
   A. Medial-lateral tilt (sidebending oscillations; Fig. 12-27)
      P—Standing in a doorway with the right forearm and hand fixed against the wall. The elbow is in slight flexion or close to the limit of extension.
      MH—Grasps the upper arm near the humeral epicondyles
      M—Keeping the forearm stationary, the MH moves the humerus medially or laterally, effecting a medial or lateral tilt of the humeroulnar joint.
   B. Distraction in flexion (Fig. 12-28)
      P—Sitting, with the shoulder abducted 90°. The upper arm is supported on a table. (A kitchen counter is usu-

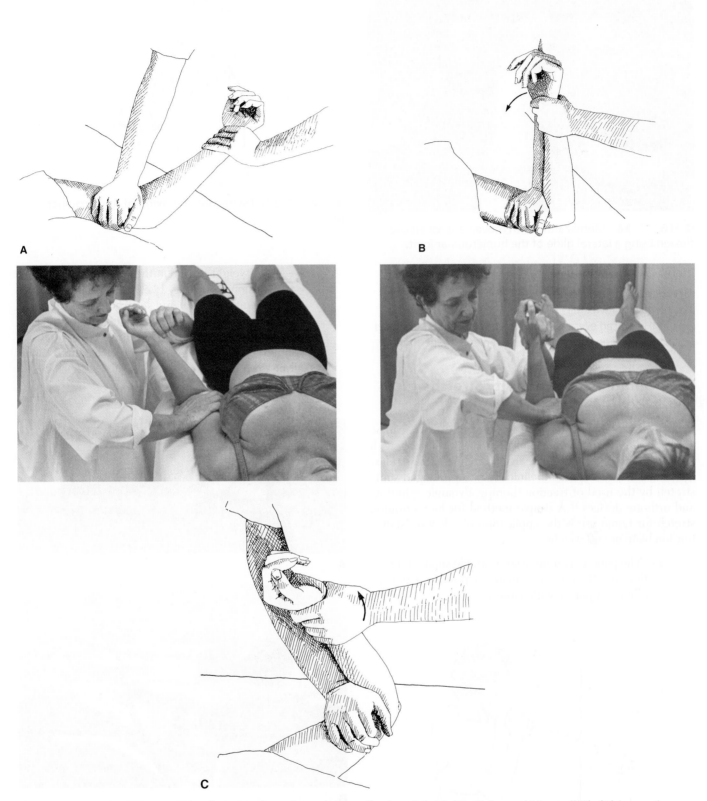

■ **FIG. 12-25.** Technique to regain pronation of proximal radioulnar joint (after Zohn and Mennell[188]): (**A**) increasing the carrying angle of the elbow; (**B**) moving the arm toward flexion; (**C**) pronation of arm near the end of motion.

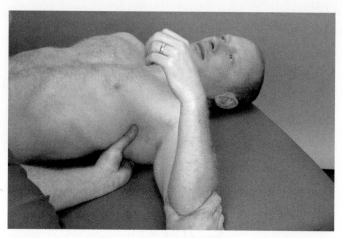

■ **FIG. 12-26.** Mobilization with movement for elbow flexion using a lateral glide of the humeroulnar joint.

ally a good height.) The elbow is flexed over a firm pillow or towel roll.

MH—Placed over the lower arm and dorsum of the hand

M—Slow, gentle, oscillating movements are performed downward in the direction of flexion.

Long-Duration, Low-Intensity Stretch (Fig. 12-29)

Prolonged stretching of the joint capsule of the elbow can be applied manually or by mechanical means, preferably with joint distraction. Static progressive stretching (stress relaxation) is easily incorporated clinically into prolonged static stretch by the used of traction therapy, dynamic splinting, and orthotic devices.[15] A simple method for long-duration stretch for home use is the application of a low-resistance tension band or cuff weight.

P—The patient assumes a comfortable supine position with the arm in an anatomic position with the elbow supported with a towel or pad.

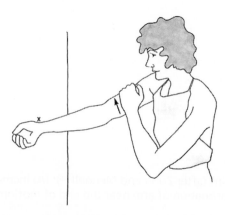

■ **FIG. 12-27.** Medial-lateral tilt (sidebending oscillations) of humeroulnar joint.

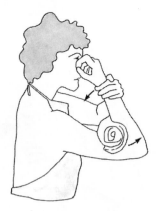

■ **FIG. 12-28.** Distraction in flexion of humeroulnar joint.

M—A cuff weight is used at the wrist (Fig. 12-29A) or a tension band (Fig. 12-29B) is applied around the patient's forearm and secured at one end of a table or attached to a weight that is almost resting on the floor as a safety precaution. The stretch should be a mild-intensity stretch sustained for a long duration (8 to 12 minutes).[176,181,189]

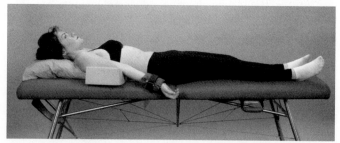

A

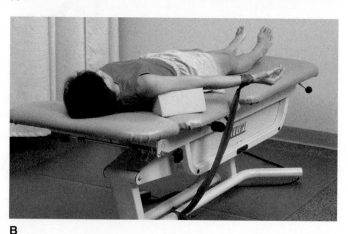

B

■ **FIG. 12-29.** Long-duration, low-intensity stretch to improve elbow extension with the use of a cuff weight (**A**) or low-resistance tension band (**B**). A mild-intensity stretch is sustained for several minutes (10 to 15 minutes).

DYNAMIC STABILIZATION AND FUNCTIONAL EXERCISES

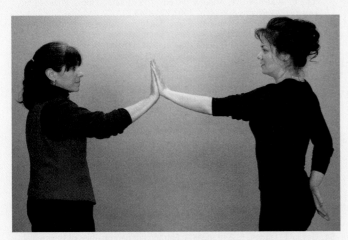

■ **FIG. 12-30.** Shadowing. The patient resists multiplanar movements initiated by the clinician.

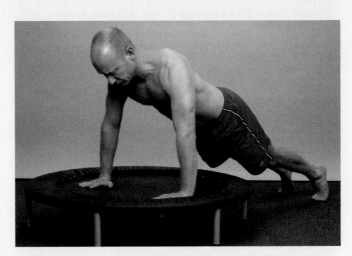

■ **FIG. 12-32.** Mini-trampoline push-ups for upper limb stability and strengthening. This exercise develops strength of the entire shoulder girdle as well as the muscles in the arm that cross the elbow and wrist.

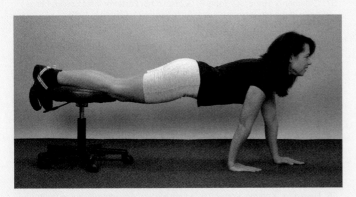

■ **FIG. 12-31.** Stool walking in all directions (forward, backward, or circular motions).

As with all areas of the body, rehabilitation of the elbow begins at the onset of symptoms or injury. With respect to tendon injuries, because there is a loss of tensile adaptation with age and the mechanism of injury involves tensile overloading of the tendons a logical strategy would emphasize eccentric work, as this in large part is the nature of the force producing the injury. Open kinetic chain strengthening exercises are described in numerous texts and will not be addressed here.

Proximal stability of the upper limb depends on the strength and balance of the scapular stabilizers and rotator cuff musculature. Weakness of these muscles may alter forces applied to the elbow during overhead motion and other activities. Scapular stabilization exercises should be introduced early into the rehabilitation program as long as symptoms are not invoked in the injured area and emphasized throughout the rehabilitation program (see Figs. 11-71, 11-73, and 11-75 through 11-81).

For the throwing athlete, Wilk et al.[180] emphasize the importance of biceps strengthening. During the follow-through phase of throwing motions, the biceps eccentrically contract to decelerate the elbow and prevent hyperextension. In addition to their role at the elbow, the biceps also act as humeral head depressor and therefore may help prevent impingement of the shoulder during active motion.[180]

Neuromuscular control may be gained by using PNF techniques. Submaximal PNF is indicated as long as care is taken to avoid valgus stress on the elbow. These exercises may be advanced to PNF with tubing, which allows the patient to incorporate the exercise into a home program (see Figs. 11-82 through 11-87).

Many upper limb closed-chain exercises and exercise procedures to promote stability in weight bearing and combined patterns of motion of the upper limb are described in Chapter 11, Shoulder and Shoulder Girdle (see Figs. 11-71 through 11-76, and 11-78). Additional examples of closed-chain activity for the upper limb include "shadowing" against the clinician's hand (Fig. 12-30),[130] stool walking (Fig. 12-31),[102] and mini-trampoline exercises (Fig. 12-32).

A graded program of stretch-shortening drills such as such as throwing and catching weighted balls (see Fig. 11-89) or practicing specific sports-related or occupational tasks that include pushing, pulling, lifting, or swinging may be appropriate in the late stage of rehabilitation.

REFERENCES

1. Ackerman LV: Extra-osseous localization non-neoplastic bone and cartilage formation (so-called myositis ossificans). J Bone Joint Surg Am 40:279–298, 1958
2. Adams JE: Injury to the throwing arm-a study of traumatic changes in the elbow joints of boy pitchers. Calif Med 102:127–132, 1965
3. Adams JE: Bone injury in very young athletes. Clin Orthop 58:129–140, 1968
4. Andrews J, Hurd WJ, Wilk KE: Reconstruction of the ulnar collateral ligament with ulnar nerve transition. In: Maxey L, Magnusson J, eds: Rehabilitation for the Postsurgical Orthopedic Patient. St. Louis, Mosby, 2001
5. Angelo RL: Arthroscopy. Advances in elbow arthroscopy. Orthopedics 16:1037–1046, 1993
6. Anson BJ, McVay CB: Surgical Anatomy, vol. 2, 5th ed. Philadelphia, WB Saunders, 1971
7. Azar FM, Andrews JR, Wilk KE, et al: Operative treatment of ulnar collateral ligament injuries of the elbow in athletes. Am J Sports Med 28:16–23, 2000
8. Baker CL, Nirschl RP: Lateral tendon injury: Open and arthroscopic treatment. In: Altchek DW, Andrews JR, eds: The Athlete's Elbow. Philadelphia, Lippincott Williams & Wilkins 2001:91–104
9. Basmajian JV, DeLuca CJ: Muscles Alive: Their Function Revealed by Electromyography, 5th ed. Baltimore, Williams & Wilkins, 1985
10. Bennett JB: Lateral and medial epicondylitis. Hand Clin 10:157–163, 1994
11. Bennett JB, Tullos HS: Ligamentous and articular injuries in the athlete. In: Morrey BF, ed: The Elbow and Its Disorders. Philadelphia, WB Saunders, 1985:502–522
12. Bernhang AM: The many causes of tennis elbow. NY State J Med 79:1363–1366, 1979
13. Blom S, Hele P, Parkman L: The supinator channel syndrome. Scand J Plast Reconstr Surg 5:71–73, 1971
14. Boe A, Molster A: Albueartroskopi. Tidsslr Nor Laegeforen 112:493–494, 1992
15. Bonutti PR, Windau JE, Ables BA, et al: Static progressive stretch to reestablish elbow range of motion. Clin Orthop 303:128–134, 1994
16. Bowden BW: Tennis elbow. J Am Osteopath Assoc 78:97–102, 1978
17. Boyd HB: Tennis elbow. J Bone Joint Surg Am 55:1183–1187, 1973
18. Boyer MI, Hasting H: Lateral tennis elbow: Is there any science out there? J Shoulder Elbow Surg 8:481–491, 1999
19. Bradley JP: Upper extremity: elbow injuries in children and adolescents. In: Stranitski CL, DeLee JC, eds: Orthopedic Sports Medicine: Principles and Practice, vol. 3: Pediatric and Adolescent Sports Medicine. Philadelphia, WB Saunders, 1994
20. Burke D, Meister K: Median nerve injuries about the elbow. In: Altchek DW, Andrews JR, eds: The Athlete's Elbow. Philadelphia, Lippincott Williams & Wilkins, 2001:131–138
21. Butler D: Mobilisation of the Nervous System. Melbourne, Australia, Churchill Livingstone, 1991
22. Cabrera JM, McCue FC: Nonosseous athletic injuries of the elbow, forearm and hand. Clin Sports Med 5:681–700, 1986
23. Cailliet R: Elbow pain. In: Cailliet R: Soft Tissue Pain and Disability. Philadelphia, FA Davis, 1988:209–222
24. Capener N: The vulnerability of the posterior interosseous nerve of the forearm. J Bone Joint Surg Br 48:770–783, 1966
25. Chiao E, Morrey B: Three-dimensional rotation of the elbow. J Biomech 11:57–73, 1978
26. Clarkson HM, Gilewish GB: Musculoskeletal Assessment, Joint Range of Motion and Manual Muscle Strength. Baltimore, Williams & Wilkins, 1989
27. Cole JH, Furness AL, Twoney LT: Muscles in Action, an Approach to Manual Muscle Testing. Edinburgh, Churchill Livingstone, 1988
28. Congeni J: Treating and prevention Little League elbow. Physician Sportsmed 22:54–64, 1994
29. Conway JE, Jobe FW, Gousman RE, et al: Medial instability of the elbow in throwing athletes. Treatment by repair or reconstruction of the ulnar collateral ligament. J Bone Joint Surg Am 4:67–83, 1992
30. Conway RR, Tanner ED: Elbow pain. In: Kaplan PE, Tanner ED, eds: Musculoskeletal Pain and Disability. Norwalk, CT, Appleton & Lange, 1989:133–142
31. Cookson JG: Musculoskeletal analysis: The elbow and hand. In: Scully RM, Barnes MR, eds: Physical Therapy. Philadelphia, JB Lippincott, 1989: 351–368
32. Coonard RW: Tennis elbow: Its course, natural history, conservative and surgical management. J Bone Joint Surg 55:1177–1182, 1973
33. Cooney WP III: Bursitis and tendinitis in the hand, wrist and elbow. Minn Med 8:491–494, 1983
34. Cordasco F, Parkes J: Overuse injuries of the elbow. In: Nicholas J, Hershman E, eds: The Upper Extremity in Sports Medicine. St. Louis, Mosby, 1995:335–346
35. Corrigan B, Maitland GD: Practical Orthopaedic Medicine. Boston, Butterworths, 1983
36. Cunningham DJ: Myology. In: Romanes GJ, ed: Textbook of Anatomy, 12th ed. New York, Oxford University Press, 1981
37. Curwin S, Standish WD: Tendinitis: Its Etiology and Treatment. Lexington, MA, The Collator Press, 1984:115–132
38. Cyriax J: Textbook of Orthopaedic Medicine, vol. 1: The Diagnosis of Soft Tissue Lesions, 8th ed. Baltimore, Williams & Wilkins, 1982:168–181
39. DaSilva MF, Williams JS, Fadale PD, et al: Pediatric throwing injuries about the elbow. Am J Orthop 27:90–96, 1998
40. David TS, Bast SC, Gambardella RA: Medial tendon injury. In: Altchek DW, Andrews JR, eds: The Athlete's Elbow. Philadelphia, Lippincott Williams & Wilkins. 2001:81–89
41. DeHaven KE, Evart CM: Throwing injuries of the elbow in athletes. Orthop Clin North Am 1:801–806, 1973
42. Dharapak C, Nimberg GA: Posterior interosseous nerve compression: Report of a case caused by traumatic aneurysm. Clin Orthop 101:225–228, 1974
43. Difelice GS, Meumier MJ, Paletta GA: Elbow injury in the adolescent athlete. In: Alatchek DW, Andrews JR, eds: The Athlete's Elbow. Philadelphia, Lippincott Williams & Wilkins, 2001:231–248
44. Dreyfuss U, Kessler I. Snapping elbow due to dislocation of the medial head of the triceps. A report of two cases. J Bone Joint Surg Br 60:56–57, 1978
45. Dugas JR, Andrews JR: Physical examination of the elbow. In: Altches DW, Andrews JR, eds: The Athlete's Elbow. Philadelphia, Lippincott Williams & Wilkins, 2001:49–58
46. Eaton CJ, Lister GD: Radial nerve compression. Hand Clin 8:345–357, 1992
47. Eisen A, Danon J: The mild cubital tunnel syndrome. Its natural history and indications for surgical intervention. Neurology 24:608–613, 1974
48. Farber JS, Bryan RS: The anterior interosseous nerve syndrome. J Bone Joint Surg Am 50:521–523, 1968
49. Field LD, Savoie FH: Common elbow injuries in sports. Sports Med 26:193–205, 1998
50. Gabel GT, Morrey BF: Operative treatment of medial epicondylitis: Influence of concomitant ulnar neuropathy at the elbow. J Bone Joint Surg Am 77:1065–1069, 1995
51. Gainor BJ: The pronator compression test revisited. A forgotten physical sign. Orthop Rev 19:888–892, 1990
52. Gale PA: Joint mobilization. In: Hammer WI, ed: Functional Soft Tissue Examination and Treatment by Manual Methods. Gaithersburg, MD, Aspen, 1991
53. Gardner E: The innervation of the elbow joint. Anat Rec 102:161–174, 1948
54. Gessini L, Jandolo B, Pietrangeli A: Entrapment neuropathies of the median nerve at and above the elbow. Surg Neurol 19:112–116, 1983
55. Gilmer WS, Anderson LD: Reaction of soft somatic tissue which may progress to bone formation: Circumscribed myositis ossificans. South Med J 52:1432–1448, 1959
56. Goldie I: Epicondylitis lateralis humeri. Acta Chir Scand Suppl 339:3–119, 1964
57. Goldman S, Honet JC, Sobel R, Goldstein AS: Posterior interosseous nerve palsy in the absence of trauma. Arch Neurol 21:435–441, 1969
58. Goodgold J, Eberstein A: Electrodiagnosis of Neuromuscular Diseases. Baltimore, Williams & Wilkins, 1972
59. Gore RM, Rogers LF, Bowerman J, et al: Osseous manifestations of elbow stress associated with sports pitchers. Am J Roentgenol 134:971–977, 1980
60. Grant JCB: Upper limb. In: Basmajian JV, ed: Grant's Methods of Anatomy, 10th ed. Baltimore, Williams & Wilkins, 1980
61. Gugenheim JJ Jr, Stanley RF, Woods GW, et al: Little League survey: the Houston study. Am J Sports Med 4:189–200, 1976
62. Gunn CC, Milbrandt WE: Tennis elbow and the cervical spine. Can Med Assoc J 114:803–809, 1976
63. Gunn CC, Milbrandt WE: Tennis elbow and acupuncture. Am J Acupunct 5:61–66, 1977
64. Hagert CG, Lunborg G, Hansen T: Entrapment of the posterior interosseous nerve. Scand J Plast Reconstr Surg 11:205–212, 1977
65. Halpren BC: Elbow and arm injuries. In: Birrer RB, ed: Sports Medicine for the Primary Physician, 2nd ed. Boca Raton, CRC Press, 1994:435–448
66. Hayashi Y, Kohimc, Kohno TH: A case of cubital syndrome caused by the snapping of the medial head of the triceps brachii muscle. J Hand Surg 9A:96–99, 1984
67. Hislop HJ, Montgomery J: Daniels and Worthingham's Muscle Testing, Techniques of Manual Examination, 6th ed. Philadelphia, WB Saunders, 1995
68. Hollinshead WH: Anatomy for Surgeons, vol. 3: The Back and Limbs, 3rd ed. New York, Harper & Row, 1982
69. Hoppenfeld S: Physical Examination of the Spine and Extremities. New York, Appleton-Century-Crofts, 1976
70. Ilfeld FW, Field SM: Treatment of tennis elbow. Use of special brace. JAMA 195:67–70, 1966
71. Indelicato PA, Jobe FW, Kerlan RK, et al: Correctable elbow lesions in professional baseball players: A review of 25 cases. Am J Sports Med 7:72–75, 1979
72. Jaeger SH, Sunger DI, Mandel S, et al: Nerve injury complications. Management of neurogenic pain syndromes. Hand Clin 2:217–234, 1986
73. Johnson DC, Answorth AA: Biceps and triceps tendon injuries. In: Altchek DW, Andrews J, eds: The Athlete's Elbow. Philadelphia, Lippincott Williams & Wilkins, 2001:105–120
74. Johnson RK, Spinner M, Shrewbury MM: Median nerve entrapment syndrome in the proximal forearm. J Hand Surg 4:48–51, 1989
75. Jones NF, Ming NL: Persistent median artery as a cause of pronator syndrome. J Hand Surg 13:728–732, 1988
76. Kane E, Daplan EB, Spinner M: Observation of the course of the ulnar nerve in the arm. Ann Chir 27:487–496, 1973
77. Kapandji IA: The inferior radioulnar joint and pronosupination. In: Tubiana R, ed: The Hand, vol. 1. Philadelphia, WB Saunders, 1981
78. Kapandji IA: The Physiology of the Joints, vol. 1, 2nd ed. London, E & S Livingstone, 1987

79. Katz RT, Marciniak CA: Electrodiagnosis in musculoskeletal medicine. In: Kaplan PE, Tanner ED, eds: Musculoskeletal Pain and Disability. Norwalk, CT, Appleton Lange, 1989:259–289

80. Kelly M: Pain in the forearm and hand due to muscular lesions. Med J Aust 2:185–188, 1947

81. Kendall FP, McCreary EK, Provance PG: Muscle Testing and Function, 4th ed. Baltimore, Williams & Wilkins, 1993

82. Kibler WB, Press JM; Rehabilitation of the elbow. In: Kibler WB, Herring SA, Press JM, eds: Functional Rehabilitation of Sports and Musculoskeletal Injuries. Gaithersburg, MD, Aspen Publication, 1998:171–187

83. Konin JG, Wiksten DL, Isear JA: Special Tests for Orthopedic Examination. Thorfare, NJ, Slack, 1997

84. Kopell HP, Thompsen WAL: Pronator syndrome. N Engl J Med 259:713–715, 1958

85. Kopell HP, Thompsen WAL: Peripheral Entrapment Neuropathies. Baltimore, Williams & Wilkins, 1963

86. Kosuwon W, Mahaisavariya S, Saengnipanthkul S, et al: Ultrasonography of the pulled elbow. J Bone Joint Surg Br 75:421–422, 1993

87. Kottke FJ, Pauley DL, Ptak RA: The rationale for prolonged stretching for correction of shortening of connective tissue. Arch Phys Med Rehabil 47:345–352, 1966

88. Kraushaar BS, Nirschl RP: Tendinosis of the elbow (tennis elbow). Clinical features and findings of histological, immunohistochemical, and electron microscopy studies. J Bone Joint Surg Am 81:259–278, 1999

89. Lake PA: Anterior interosseous nerve syndrome. J Neurosurg 41:306–309, 1974

90. Langman J, Woerdeman MW: Atlas of Medical Anatomy. Philadelphia, WB Saunders, 1976

91. Leach RE, Miller JK: Lateral and medial epicondylitis of the elbow. Clin Sports Med 6:259–272, 1987

92. Lee D: A Workbook of Manual Therapy Techniques for the Upper Extremity. Delta, BC, Canada, Delta Orthopaedic Physiotherapy Clinic, 1989

93. Lehmkuhl LD, Smith LK: Brunnstrom's Clinical Kinesiology, 4th ed. Philadelphia, FA Davis, 1983

94. Lindholm TS, Osterman K, Vankka E: Osteochondritis dissecans of the elbow, ankle and hip: A comparative survey. Clin Orthop 148:245–253, 1985

95. Lister GD, Belsole RB, Kleinert HE: The radial tunnel syndrome. J Hand Surg 4:52–60, 1979

96. London JT: Kinematics of the elbow. J Bone Joint Surg Am 63:529–535, 1981

97. MacConaill MA, Basmajian JJ: Muscles and Movement: A Basis for Human Kinesiology. Baltimore, Williams & Wilkins, 1969

98. Maeda K, Miura T, Komada T, et al: Anterior interosseous nerve paralysis—Report of 13 cases and review of Japanese literature. Hand 9:165–171, 1977

99. Magee DJ: Orthopedic Physical Assessment, 3rd ed. Philadelphia, WB Saunders, 1997

100. Maigne R: Tennis elbow (epicondylitis). In: Liberson WT, ed: Orthopedic Medicine, A New Approach to Vertebral Manipulations. Springfield, Charles C. Thomas, 1972:244–254

101. Martin BF: The annular ligament of the superior radioulnar joint. J Anat 92:473–482, 1958

102. Massie DL, Sager J, Spiker JC: Rehabilitation of the injured elbow. Orthop Clin North Am 3:385–401, 1994

103. McManama GB, Micheli LT, Berry MV, et al: The surgical treatment of osteochondritis of the capitellum. Am J Sports Med 13:11–21, 1985

104. Miller CD, Savoie FH III: Vagus extension injuries of the elbow in the throwing athlete. J Am Acad Orthop Surg 2:261–269, 1994

105. Miller RG: The cubital tunnel syndrome: precise localization and diagnosis. Ann Neurol 6:56–59, 1979

106. Morrey BF: The Elbow and Its Disorders. Philadelphia, WB Saunders, 1985

107. Morris HH, Defers BH: Pronator syndrome: Clinical and electrophysiological features in seven cases. J Neurol Neurosurg Psychiatry 39:461–464, 1976

108. Mulholland RC: Nontraumatic progressive paralysis of the posterior interosseous nerve. J Bone Joint Surg Br 48:781–785, 1966

109. Mulligan BR: Manual Therapy ("Nags", "Snags", "MWMS" etc.), 4th ed. New Zealand, Plant View Services, 1999

110. Newman JH, Goodfellow JW: Fibrillation of the head of the radius: One cause of tennis elbow. Br Medical J 10:328–330, 1975

111. Nielson HO: Posterior interosseous nerve paralysis caused by a fibrous band compression of the supinator muscle—A report of four cases. Acta Orthop Scand 47:304–307, 1976

112. Nirschl RD: Tennis elbow. Orthop Clin North Am 4:787–798, 1973

113. Nirschl RD: The etiology and treatment of tennis elbow. Am J Sports Med. 2:308–319, 1974

114. Nirschl RD: Medial tennis elbow: The surgical treatment. Annual Meeting of the American Academy of Orthopedic Surgeons. Atlanta, March 1, 1980

115. Nirschl RD: Muscle and tendon trauma: Tennis elbow. In: Morrey BF, ed: The Elbow and Its Disorders. Philadelphia, WB Saunders, 1985

116. Nirschl RD: Soft-tissue injuries about the elbow. Clin Sports Med 5:637–652, 1986

117. Nirschl RD: Elbow tendinosis/tennis elbow. Clin Sports Med 11:851–870, 1992

118. Nirschl RD, Pettrone F: Tennis elbow: The surgical treatment of lateral epicondylitis. J Bone Joint Surg Am 61: 832–839, 1979

119. Norkin CC, Levangie PK: Joint Structure and Function: A Comprehensive Analysis, 2nd ed. Philadelphia, FA Davis, 1992

120. Norwood LA, Shook JA, Andrews JR: Acute medial elbow ruptures. Am J Sports Med 9:16–19, 1981

121. O'Donoghue DF: Treatment of Injuries to Athlete, 2nd ed. Philadelphia, WB Saunders, 1970

122. Ombregt L, Bisschop P, ter Veer H, et al: Disorders of the inert structures. In: Ombregt L, Bisschop P, ter Veer H, et al., eds: System of Orthopaedic Medicine. London, WB Saunders, 1995:305–312

123. Omer G, Spinner M: Peripheral Nerve Problems. Philadelphia, WB Saunders, 1980

124. Palmer ML, Epler ME: Fundamentals of Musculoskeletal Assessment Techniques, 2nd ed. Philadelphia, Lippincott Williams & Wilkins,1998

125. Peterson L, Renstrom P: Sports Injuries: Their Prevention and Treatment. London, Martin Dutz Ltd, 1986

126. Petty NJ, Moore AP: Neuromusculoskeletal Examination and Assessment: A Handbook for Therapists. Edinburgh, Churchill Livingstone, 1998

127. Poehling GG: Osteochondritis dissecans of the elbow. In: Norris TR, ed: OKU Shoulder and Elbow. Rosemont, IL, American Academy of Orthopaedic Surgeons, 1997

128. Posner MA: Compressive neuropathies of the median and radial nerve at the elbow. Clin Sports Med 92:343–363, 1990

129. Reid DC, Kusher S: The elbow region. In: Donatelli RA, Wooden MJ, eds: Orthopaedic Therapy, 3rd ed. New York, Churchill Livingstone, 2001:182–204

130. Reis ND: Anomalous triceps tendon as a cause of snapping elbow and ulnar neuritis: a case report. J Hand Surg Am 5:361–362, 1980

131. Riordan DC: Radial nerve paralysis. Orthop Clin North Am 5:283–287, 1974

132. Rodman GP, Schumacher HR: Primer on Rheumatic Diseases, 8th ed. Atlanta, Arthritis Foundation, 1983

133. Rohrbough JT, Altchek DW, Cain EL, et al: Medial collateral ligament injury. In: Altchek DW, Andrews JR, eds: The Athlete's Elbow, Philadelphia, Lippincott Williams & Wilkins, 2001:153–173

134. Roles NC, Maudsley RH: Radial tunnel syndrome, resistant tennis elbow as a nerve entrapment. J Bone Joint Surg Br 54:499–508, 1972

135. Rolfsen L: Snapping triceps tendon with ulnar neuritis. Report on a case. Acta Orthop Scand 1:74–76, 1970

136. Rosk MR: Anterior interosseous nerve entrapment: Report of seven cases. Clin Orthop 142:176–181, 1979

137. Rosse C: The Musculoskeletal System in Health and Disease. New York, Harper & Rowe, 1980

138. Safran MR: Elbow injuries in athletes. Clin Orthop 310:257–277, 1995

139. Saidorff DC, McDonough AL: Bilateral epicondylar elbow pain. In: Saidorff DC, McDonough AL: Critical Pathways in Therapeutic Intervention: Upper Extremity. St. Louis, Mosby, 1997:66–79

140. Salter RB: Degenerative disorders of joint and related tissues. In: Salter RB: Textbook of Disorders and Injuries of the Musculoskeletal System, 3rd ed. Baltimore, Williams & Wilkins, 1999

141. Sapega AA, Quedenfeld TC, Moyer RA, et al: Biophysical factors in range of motion exercise. Arch Phys Med Rehabil 57:122–126, 1976

142. Schemmel SP, Andrew JR, Clancy WG: Acute ulnar collateral ligament injury in a baseball pitcher. Physician Sportsmed 16:133–138, 1988

143. Seyffarth H: Primary myoses in the m. pronator teres as a cause of lesions of the n. medianus (the pronator syndrome). Acta Psychiatr Scand Suppl 74:251–256, 1951

144. Sharrard WJW: Posterior interosseous neuritis. J Bone Joint Surg Br 48:777–780, 1966

145. Sharrard WJW: Anterior interosseous neuritis—Report of a case. J Bone Joint Surg Br 50:804–805, 1968

146. Somerville EW: Pain in the upper limb. Proceedings of the British Orthopaedic Association. J Bone Joint Surg Br 45:620–621, 1963

147. Spinner M: The arcade of Frohse and its relationship to posterior interosseous nerve paralysis. J Bone Joint Surg Br 50:809–812, 1968

148. Spinner M: The anterior interosseous nerve syndrome with special attention to its variations. J Bone Joint Surg Am 52:84–94, 1970

149. Spinner M: Injuries to the Major Branches of the Peripheral Nerves of the Forearm, 2nd ed. Philadelphia, WB Saunders, 1978

150. Spinner M, Kaplan EB: The quadrate ligament of the elbow: Its relationship to the stability of the proximal radio-ulnar joint. Acta Orthop Scand 41:632–647, 1970

151. Spinner M, Kaplan EB: The relationship of the ulnar nerve to the medial inter-muscular septum in the arm and its clinical significance. Hand 8:239–242, 1976

152. Spinner M, Linschied RL: Nerve entrapment syndromes. In: Morrey BF, ed: The Elbow and Its Disorders. Philadelphia, WB Saunders, 1985:691–712

153. Spinner M, Spencer PS: Nerve compression lesions of the upper extremity—A clinical and experimental review. Clin Orthop 104:46–67, 1974

154. Spinner RJ, Davids JR, Goldner RD: Dislocating medial triceps and ulnar neuropathy in three generations of one family. J Hand Surg Am 22:132–137, 1997

155. Spinner RJ, Goldner RD: Snapping of the medial head of the triceps and recurrent dislocation of the ulnar nerve. Anatomical and dynamic factors. J Bone Joint Surg Am 80:239–247, 1998

156. Spinner RJ, Goldner RD, Fada RA, et al: Snapping of the triceps tendon over the lateral epicondyle. J Hand Surg Am: 24:381–385, 1999
157. Stoyan M, Wilk KE: The functional anatomy of the elbow complex. J Orthop Sports Med Phys Ther 17:279–288, 1993
158. Sucher BM, Glassman JH: Upper extremity syndromes. Phys Med Rehabil Clin North Am 7:784–810, 1996
159. Szabo RM, Gelberman RH: Peripheral nerve compression. Etiology, critical pressure threshold, and clinical assessment. Orthopaedics 7:1416–1466, 1984
160. Tajima T: Functional anatomy of the elbow joint. In: Kashiwagi D, ed: Elbow Joint. Amsterdam, Elsevier, 1985
161. Timmerman LA, Andrews JR: Undersurface tear of the ulnar collateral ligament in baseball players. A newly recognized lesion. Am J Sports Med 22:33–36,1994
162. Timmerman LA, Schwartz ML, Andrews JR: Preoperative evaluation of the ulnar collateral ligament by magnetic resonance imaging and computed tomography arthrography. Evaluation in 25 baseball players with surgical confirmation. Am J Sports Med 22:26–32, 1994
163. Tolo ET, Weiland AJ: Posterior interosseous nerve compression. In: Altchek DW, Andrews JR, eds: The Athlete's Elbow. Philadelphia, Lippincott Williams & Wilkins, 2001:137–152
164. Tomberlin JP, Saunders HD: The elbow. In: Tomberlin JP, Saunders HD, eds: Evaluation, Treatment and Prevention of Musculoskeletal Disorders, vol. 2: Extremities. Chaska, MN, The Saunders Group Inc, 1994:249–274
165. Travel JG, Simons DG: Myofascial Dysfunction—The Trigger Point Manual. Baltimore, Williams & Wilkins, 1983
166. Tullos HS, Bryan WJ: Examination of the throwing elbow. In: Zarins JR, Andrews JR, eds: Injuries to the Throwing Athlete. Philadelphia, WB Saunders, 1985
167. Tullos HS, Erwin WD, Woods GW, et al: Unusual lesions of the pitching arm. Clin Orthop 88:169–182,1972
168. Upton AR, McComas AJ: The double crush in nerve entrapment syndromes. Lancet 2:359, 1973
169. Van Rossum J, Buruma OJS, Kamphuisen HAC, et al: Tennis elbow—A radial tunnel syndrome. J Bone Joint Surg Br 60:197–198, 1978
170. Vanderpool DW, Edinburg JC, Lamb DW, et al: Peripheral compression lesion of the ulnar nerve. J Bone Joint Surg 50:792–803, 1968
171. Wadsworth TG: The external compression syndrome of the ulnar nerve at the cubital tunnel. Clin Orthop 124:189–204, 1977
172. Wadsworth TG: The Elbow. New York, Churchill Livingstone, 1982
173. Wadsworth TG: Entrapment neuropathy in the upper limb. In: Birch R, Brook D, eds: Operative Surgery, The Hand. London, Butterworths, 1984:469–486
174. Wadsworth TG: The cubital tunnel syndrome. In: Kashiwagi D, ed: Elbow Joint. Amsterdam, Elsevier, 1985
175. Wadsworth TG, Williams JR: Cubital tunnel external compression syndrome. Br Med J 1:662–666, 1973
176. Warren CG, Lehmann JF, Koblanski JN: Elongation of rat tail tendon: effect on load and temperature. Arch Phys Med Rehabil 52:465–474, 1971
177. Warren CG, Lehmann JF, Koblanski JN: Heat and stretch procedures. An evaluation using rat tail tendon. Arch Phys Med Rehabil 57:122–126, 1976
178. Wells MJ, Bell GW: Concerns of Little League elbow. J Athl Train 30:249–256,1995
179. Wiens E, Lau SCK: The anterior interosseous nerve syndrome. Can J Surg 21:354–357, 1978
180. Wilk KE, Arrigo C, Andrews JR: Rehabilitation of the elbow in throwing athletes. J Orthop Sports Phys Ther 14:100–105, 1993
181. Wilk KE, Levinson M: Rehabilitation of the athletes elbow. In: Altchek DW, Andrews JR, eds: The Athlete's Elbow, Philadelphia, Lippincott Williams & Wilkins, 2001:249–273
182. Williams PL, Warwick R, eds: Gray's Anatomy, 36th ed. Philadelphia, WB Saunders, 1989
183. Wilson FD, Andrews JR, Blackburn TA, et al: Valgus extension overload in the pitching elbow. Am J Sports Med 11:83–88, 1982
184. Wittenberg RH, Schaal S, Muhr G: Surgical treatment of persistent elbow epicondylitis. Clin Orthop 278:73–80, 1992
185. Woods GW, Tullos HS, King JW: The throwing arm—Elbow joint injuries. J Sports Med 4(Suppl 1):43–47, 1973
186. Wright TW: Chronic Nerve Injuries and Neuropathies. Orthopaedic Surgery: The Essentials. New York, Thieme Medical Publishers, 1999:761–775
187. Youm Y, Dryer R, Thambyrajan K, et al: Biomechanical analyses of forearm pronation-supination and elbow flexion-extension. J Biomech 12:245–255, 1979
188. Zohn DA, Mennell JM: Musculoskeletal pain conditions. In: Musculoskeletal Pain: Diagnosis and Physical Treatment. Boston, Little, Brown, 1975
189. Zulia P, Prentice WE: Rehabilitation of the elbow. In: Prentice WE, Voight MI, eds: Techniques in Musculoskeletal Rehabilitation. New York, McGraw-Hill, 2001:457–482

RECOMMENDED READINGS

Altchek DW, Andrews JR, eds: The Athlete's Elbow. Philadelphia, Lippincott Williams & Wilkins, 2002
Andrews J, Hurd WJ, Wilks KE: Reconstruction of the ulnar collateral ligament with ulnar nerve transposition. In: Maxey L, Magnusson J, eds: Rehabilitation for the Surgical Orthopedic Patient. St. Louis, Mosby 2001: 82–100
Calandruccio, Akin K, Griffith K: Extensor brevis release and lateral epicondylectomy. In: Maxey L, Magnusson J, eds: Rehabilitation for the Surgical Orthopedic Patient. St. Louis, Mosby, 2001:71–81
Corrigan B, Maitland GD: Practical Orthopedic Medicine. Boston, Butterworths, 1983
Kisner C, Lynn AC: Therapeutic Exercises—Foundations and Techniques, 3rd ed. Philadelphia, FA Davis, 1996:332–351
London JT: Kinematics of the elbow. J Bone Joint Surg Am 63:529–535, 1981
Morrey BF, ed: The Elbow and Its Disorders, 2nd ed. Philadelphia, WB Saunders, 1993
Nirschl R: Rehabilitation of the athlete's elbow. In: Morrey BF, ed: The Elbow and Its Disorders. Philadelphia, WB Saunders, 1985:523–529
Nirschl RP, Sobel J: Conservative treatment of tennis elbow. Phys Sports Med 9:43–54, 1981
Thein Brody L: The elbow, forearm, wrist, and hand. In: Hall CM, Thein Brody L, eds: Therapeutic Exercise. Moving Toward Function. Philadelphia, Lippincott Williams & Wilkins, 1998

Wrist and Hand Complex

13

DARLENE HERTLING AND RANDOLPH M. KESSLER

FUNCTIONAL ANATOMY

Wrist Complex

OSTEOLOGY

Distal End of Radius. The radius flares distally, and this end is much larger than the distal end of the ulna. It extends farther laterally than medially. The distal lateral extension of the radius is the radial styloid process. The radial styloid normally extends about 1 cm farther distally than the ulnar styloid (Fig. 13-1).

The medial aspect of the distal radius is a concave surface anteroposteriorly. The medial concavity is the ulnar notch, which articulates with the head of the ulna, allowing pronation and supination to occur. The distal end of the radius is triangular in its transverse cross section. The distal articular surface of the radius is composed of two concave facets, one for articulation with the scaphoid and one for articulation with the lunate (Fig. 13-2). The distal articular surface of the radius faces slightly palmarly (average of 10°) and somewhat ulnarly (average of 20°; Fig. 13-3).

Distal End of Ulna. The distal end of the ulna flares only mildly compared with the distal end of the radius. The ulnar styloid process is a small conical projection from the dorsomedial aspect of the distal end of the ulna. The radial aspect of the ulnar head is convex anteroposteriorly. It is cartilage-covered for articulation with the ulnar notch of the radius during pronation and supination (Figs. 13-1 and 13-2).

The distal end of the ulna is somewhat circular on transverse cross section, except for the irregularity formed by the styloid process dorsomedially. The ulna's distal surface is covered with articular cartilage for articulation with the articular disk (not with the carpals). There is movement between the ulna and disk primarily on pronation and supination, during which the disk must sweep across the distal end of the ulna.

Carpals. The proximal row of carpals consists of the triquetrum, pisiform, lunate, and scaphoid bones. The scaphoid has a biconvex articular surface proximally for articulation with the lateral facet of the distal end of the radius. The lunate is also convex proximally and articulates with the medial facet of the distal radius and with the articular disk in positions of radial deviation. The triquetrum has a small convex articular surface proximally. This surface is in contact with the ulnar collateral ligament when the wrist is in neutral position and articulates with the articular disk primarily in positions of ulnar deviation. The flexor carpi ulnaris tendon inserts onto the pisiform bone, which lies palmarly over the triquetrum.

The distal end of the scaphoid consists of two distal articular surfaces. The radial surface of the distal scaphoid is convex for articulation with the concave surface formed by the

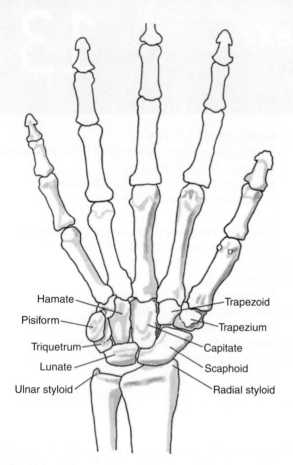

■ FIG. 13-1. Palmar aspect of the bones of the right wrist and hand.

combined proximal ends of the trapezoid and trapezium. The ulnar articulating surface of the distal scaphoid is concave and faces somewhat palmarly and ulnarly. It articulates with the proximal end of the capitate. The distal surface of the lunate is quite concave anteroposteriorly but less so mediolaterally. It grasps the convex proximal end of the capitate and also

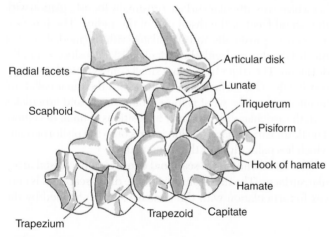

■ FIG. 13-2. Inferior aspect of the lower end of the radius and ulna and the carpal bones of the hand.

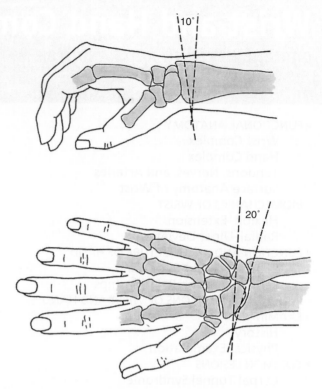

■ FIG. 13-3. Normal wrist alignment.

articulates, to a lesser extent, with the hamate. The distal surface of the triquetrum is concave for articulation with the hamate (Figs. 13-1 and 13-2).

There is some movement between the bones of the proximal row of carpals. For this reason each of the proximal carpals is lined with articular cartilage on its radial or ulnar surfaces, or both, to allow for such movement.

Ulnarly to radially, the distal carpals are the hamate, capitate, trapezoid, and trapezium (Fig. 13-1). The combined proximal surfaces of the hamate and capitate form a convex surface that articulates with the concave surface formed by the combined distal surfaces of the triquetrum, lunate, and scaphoid (Fig. 13-2). The combined proximal surfaces of the trapezoid and trapezium form a concave surface for articulation with the convex distal articular surface of the scaphoid. The distal end of the trapezium is a sellar surface that articulates with the corresponding sellar surface of the proximal aspect of the first metacarpal. The trapezoid articulates distally with the second metacarpal, the capitate with the third metacarpal, and the hamate with the fourth and fifth metacarpals (Fig. 13-1).

Because there is a small amount of movement between adjacent bones of the distal row, these are also lined with articular cartilage radially and ulnarly to allow for such intercarpal movement.

The carpals, taken together, form an arch in the transverse plane that is concave palmarly. This arch deepens with wrist flexion and flattens on wrist extension. The "hook" of the hamate, a large prominence on the palmar aspect of the hamate, and the pisiform bone, situated on the palmar aspect of the triquetrum, form the ulnar side of this arch. The trapezium, which tends to be oriented about 45° from the plane of the palm, and the radial aspect of the scaphoid, which curves palmarly, form the radial side of the arch. The flexor retinaculum, or transverse carpal ligament, traverses this arch (Fig. 13-4). The flexor ulnaris tendon inserts onto the pisiform. When this muscle contracts it pulls on the pisiform, causing tightening of the flexor retinaculum. This tightening deepens the transverse carpal arch.

LIGAMENTS, CAPSULES, SYNOVIA, AND DISK

The articular cavity of the distal radioulnar joint is usually distinct from the articular cavity of the radiocarpal joint, which is also separate from that of the midcarpal joint. The carpometacarpal joints often share a common joint cavity; in some cases this communicates with the midcarpal joint (Fig. 13-5).

The distal radioulnar joint is bordered proximally by the lax sacciform recess in the capsule, which loops proximally between the radius and ulna. Distally this joint is bordered by the triangular articular disk. This fibrocartilaginous disk attaches ulnarly to the ulnar styloid process and radially to the ulnar margin of the distal radial articular surface. It separates the distal radioulnar joint from the radiocarpal joint. Anteriorly and posteriorly the margins of the disk attach to the joint capsule. The superior aspect of the disk is a cartilage-lined concave surface for articulation with the distal end of the ulna. The disk moves with the radius on pronation and supination and must therefore sweep across the distal end of the ulna on these movements. During flexion and extension of the wrist, the disk remains stationary relative to the ulna. With this movement the lunate or triquetrum, or both, articulates with the distal surface of the disk, which is also concave

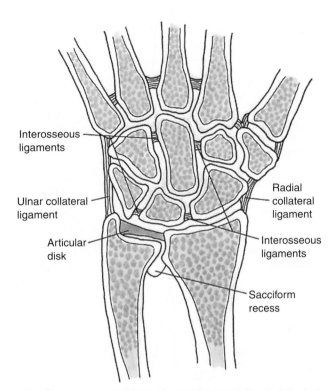

■ FIG. 13-5. Cross section through the articulations of the wrist, showing the synovial cavities.

and cartilage-covered. The disk, then, provides two articular surfaces for the ulna and carpals, separates the adjacent joint cavities, and binds together the distal ends of the ulna and radius (Fig. 13-5).

The radiocarpal joint is bordered proximally by the radius and the articular disk. Distally it is bordered by the three proximal carpals and their respective interosseous ligaments, which are flush with the continuous convex articular surface formed by the proximal carpals. Medially and laterally the joint is bordered by the strong ulnar and radial collateral ligaments. Both collateral ligaments attach proximally to the styloid processes. Distally, the ulnar ligament attaches to the triquetrum and pisiform; the radial ligament attaches to the scaphoid and trapezium. Palmarly and dorsally the capsule of this joint is reinforced by the palmar and the dorsal radiocarpal ligaments (Fig. 13-6). Palmarly, there is also an ulnocarpal ligament. These ligaments ensure that the carpals follow the radius during pronation and supination. Synovium lines the capsuloligamentous structures mentioned, as well as the interosseous ligaments between the triquetrum and lunate and between the scaphoid and lunate.

The articulations between the proximal and distal carpal bones are enclosed in a common joint cavity. Anatomically, the midcarpal joint is considered the compound joint between the two rows of carpals. However, functionally the distinction is not so simple. Proximally the midcarpal joint is bordered by the scaphoid, lunate, and triquetrum and their interosseous ligaments, which intervene between the proximal ends of these

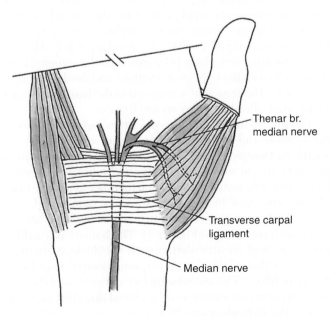

■ FIG. 13-4. Transverse carpal ligament and median nerve.

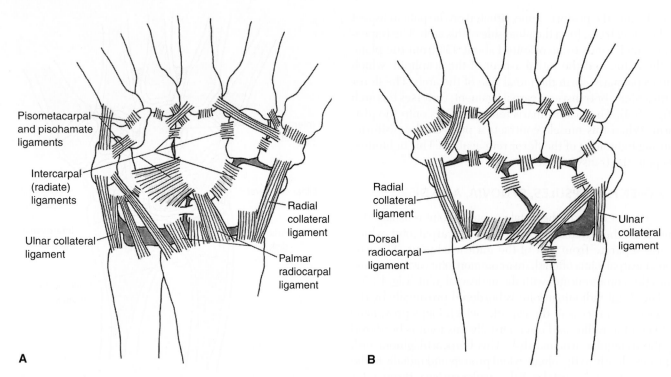

FIG. 13-6. Palmar aspect (**A**) and dorsal aspect (**B**) of the ligaments of the right wrist and metacarpus.

bones. In this way the intercarpal articulations between the proximal carpals are enclosed within the midcarpal joint cavity. Distally the midcarpal joint is bordered by the distal carpals and their interosseous ligaments, which intervene about midway, or further distally, between the distal carpals. Occasionally an interosseous ligament intervenes between the capitate and scaphoid, dividing the midcarpal joint into medial and lateral cavities. Because an interosseous ligament is often missing between the trapezoid and trapezium, the midcarpal joint often communicates with the common joint cavity of the carpometacarpal joints (Fig. 13-5). Medially and laterally, extensions of the ulnar and radial collateral ligaments connect the triquetrum to the hamate and the scaphoid to the trapezium. There are also dorsal and palmar intercarpal ligaments between the bones of the two rows. Palmarly these intercarpal ligaments are often referred to as the "radiate ligament" because they tend to radiate outward from the capitate (Fig. 13-6).

Palmar and dorsal intercarpal ligaments also connect the carpals within a row. The pisohamate ligament (from the pisiform to the hook of the hamate) and the pisometacarpal ligament (to the base of the fifth metacarpal) are believed to be continuations of the flexor carpi ulnaris tendon that attaches to the pisiform (Fig. 13-6). The joint between the pisiform and triquetrum is usually distinct from the other joints mentioned, having its own joint capsule and synovium-lined cavity.

Hand Complex

The hand consists of five digits, or four fingers and a thumb. There are 19 long bones distal to the carpals and 19 joints that

make up the hand complex. These are divided in five rays, with each ray making up a polyarticulated chain comprising the metacarpals and phalanges. The base of each metacarpal articulates with the distal row of carpals.

CARPOMETACARPAL JOINTS OF FINGERS

In the carpometacarpal joint area there are two stable joints that permit little or no motion: the carpometacarpal joints of the index and middle fingers. There are also two very mobile joints: the carpometacarpal joints of the thumb and the little finger.[151] Because thumb function differs significantly from that of the other digits, it will be examined separately. The second metacarpal articulates primarily with the trapezoid and secondarily with the trapezium, capitate, and third metacarpal (Fig. 13-1). The trapezoid is mortised in the base of the index metacarpal, affording a very secure fixation.

The middle or third metacarpal articulates primarily with the capitate and is also bound to the adjacent second and fourth metacarpal (Fig. 13-1). Therefore, all the carpals in the distal carpal row and the index and middle metacarpal bases are firmly joined and function together as a single osseoligamentous unit, the fixed stable portion of the hand.[107]

The little finger metacarpal articulates with the hamate and fourth metacarpal (Fig. 13-1). The hamate is a saddle-like joint, and its articulation with the little metacarpal resembles that of the thumb carpometacarpal joint but is not as mobile.[151] The articular surface of the base of the fifth metacarpal is convex in the volar-dorsal direction and concave in the radioulnar axis.[161]

The ring finger metacarpal base articulates with the hamate primarily in a joint similar to that of the little finger but with even less motion permitted. It also articulates with the capitate, as well as the middle and little finger metacarpals (Fig. 13-1).

Although the little finger carpometacarpal joint is considered a saddle joint with two degrees of freedom, the other finger carpometacarpal joints are plain synovial joints with one degree of freedom: flexion–extension.[82,133] Their proximal surface may be considered concave, the distal end convex.

The capsular pattern of restriction is limitation of motion equally in all directions. All are supported by strong transverse and weaker longitudinal ligaments volarly and dorsally (Fig. 13-6). This ligamentous structure controls the total range of motion (ROM) available at each carpometacarpal joint. The function of the carpometacarpal joints of the fingers is primarily to contribute to the hollowing of the palm to allow the hand and digits to conform optimally to the shape of the object being held.[133]

CARPOMETACARPAL JOINT OF THUMB

The carpometacarpal joint of the trapezium–thumb metacarpal joint is a very mobile articulation. Although described as a saddle-type joint, it is actually a reciprocally biconcave joint resembling two saddles whose concave surfaces are opposed to each other at right angles or 90° rotation (Fig. 13-7). All motions are possible, including circumduction.[26,151] The carpometacarpal articulation is specialized to produce automatic axial rotation of the first metacarpal during angular movements. Zancolli and associates[198] proposed the concept that the trapezium is formed by two different types of joints. One part, the saddle area, occupies the center of the articular surfaces and takes part in simple angular movements. The other part, located on the palmar side, is an ovoid area that represents a ball-and-socket joint for complex rotatory movements. The saddle part of the joint favors the circumduction motion to the motion of opposition. The trapezium is firmly bound to the trapezoid and indeed to the entire distal carpal row and has virtually no independent motion.

According to Zancolli and colleagues,[198,199] the greatest stability of the first metacarpal is achieved after complete pronation in the position of full opposition when ligamentous tension, muscular contraction, and joint congruence produce the maximal effect in achieving stabilization of pinch. Opposition with simultaneous pronation (or axial rotation) is sequentially abduction, flexion, and adduction of the first metacarpal. Axial rotation occurring in the carpometacarpal joint is made possible because of the laxity of the joint capsule and the joint configuration.[32,133,198,199] The tension in the ligaments combined with muscle activity of opposition and reposition form couples (paired parallel forces) that produce this axial rotation. The function of muscles crossing the joint is essential. According to Kauer,[85] the close structural relationship between the tendon of the abductor pollicis longus and the first carpometacarpal joint influences the restraining and directing function of the ligamentous system. The functional significance of the movement of opposition can be appreciated when one realizes that use of the thumb against a finger occurs in almost all forms of prehension.[133]

The strongest carpometacarpal joint ligament is the deep ulnar or anterior oblique carpometacarpal ligament that unites the tubercle of the trapezium and the volar beak of the metacarpal base (Fig. 13-8).[161] The abductor pollicis longus and the origin of the thenar muscles provide extrinsic support.

METACARPOPHALANGEAL JOINTS OF FINGERS

The distal metacarpophalangeal (MCP) joints of the fingers are made of an irregular spheroidal (convex) metacarpal head proximally and the concave base of the first phalanx distally (Fig. 13-9A). They are multiaxial condyloid joints and allow primarily flexion and extension, but also abduction, adduction, and some axial rotation. The most extensive movements are flexion and extension. The average flexion range is 90 to 95°, but hyperextension of 20 to 30° and even as much as 45° is common. The articular surface of the metacarpal head is rounded dorsally and is flat volarly (Fig. 13-9B). It has 180° of articular surface in the sagittal plane, with the predominant portion lying volarly. This is apposed to about 20° of

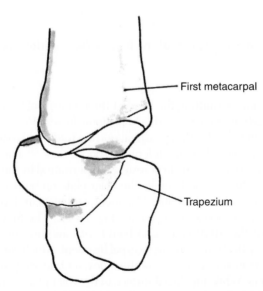

■ FIG. 13-7. Saddle-shaped carpometacarpal articulation of the thumb.

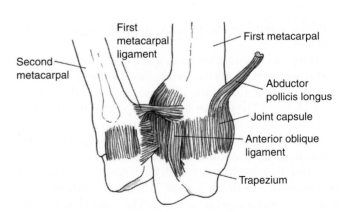

■ FIG. 13-8. Volar view of the right first carpometacarpal joint and the arrangement of the ligaments.

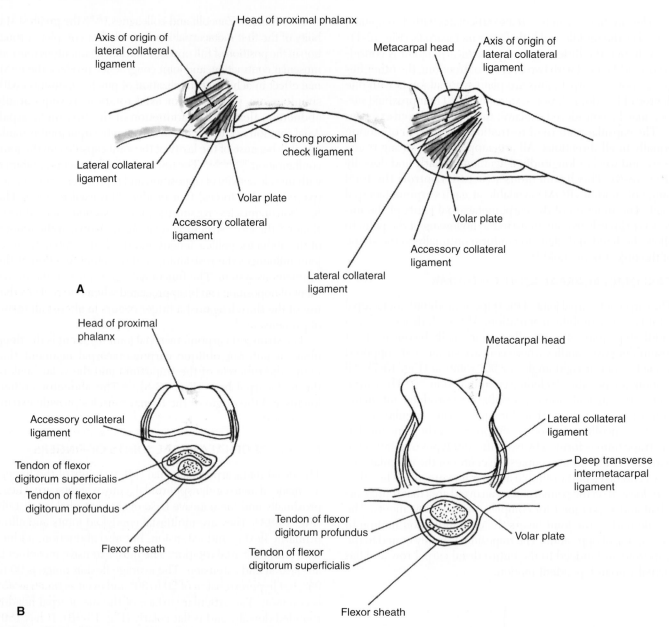

■ FIG. 13-9. **(A)** Sagittal view of the metacarpophalangeal and interphalangeal joints of the fingers. **(B)** Anterior view of metacarpal and proximal phalanx head.

articular surface on the phalanx, resulting in poorly mated surfaces.[133]

The joint is surrounded by a capsule that is lax in extension and in conjunction with the poorly mated surfaces allows some passive axial rotation of the proximal phalanx in this position (Fig. 13-10).[133] The primary ligament support of the MCP joint includes two lateral collateral ligaments, two accessory collateral ligaments, and the volar plate (Figs. 13-10 and 13-11). The volar plate or ligament is a thick, tough fibrocartilaginous structure that firmly inserts into the volar base of the proximal phalanx. Proximally it thins to become nearly membranous at its metacarpal attachment. The volar plate with the two accessory ligaments on the sides enlarges the cavity of the

MCP joint, permitting the head of the metacarpal to remain in the articular cavity as the MCP joint flexes (Fig. 13-10). During flexion, this thin proximal portion folds in like the billows of an accordion or a telephone-booth door.[151] The plate also helps to restrict the hyperextension permitted by the loose capsule. Distally and laterally the volar plate on both sides is attached to a lateral collateral ligament, and in its midposition laterally to an accessory ligament (Fig. 13-11). The four volar plates of the MCP joints also blend with and are interconnected by the transverse metacarpal ligament, which connects the adjacent lateral borders of the index, middle, ring, and little fingers. While the dorsal surface of the volar plate is in contact with the head of the metacarpal, the volar surface of this

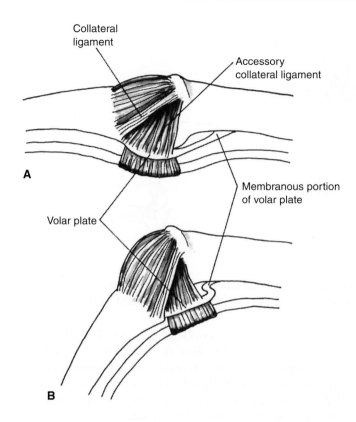

A

B

Collateral ligament

Accessory collateral ligament

Membranous portion of volar plate

Volar plate

■ **FIG. 13-10.** The metacarpophalangeal joint during extension (**A**) and flexion (**B**).

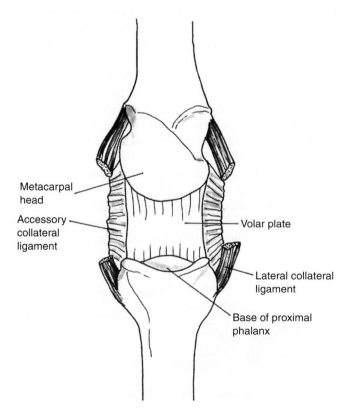

Metacarpal head

Accessory collateral ligament

Volar plate

Lateral collateral ligament

Base of proximal phalanx

■ **FIG. 13-11.** Metacarpophalangeal joint with collateral ligaments divided.

ligament is in contact with the flexor tendon. The volar plate and transverse metacarpal ligament form the dorsal wall of the vaginal ligament, which forms a tunnel and completely surrounds the flexor tendons (Fig. 13-9). The flexible attachment of the volar plate to the phalanx permits the plate to glide distally along the volar surface of the metacarpal head without restricting motion during flexion, and also prevents impingement by the joint of the long flexor tendons (Fig. 13-12).

The MCP joint is the most stable in maximal flexion because the lateral collateral ligaments are stretched tautly in this position and the accessory collateral ligaments offer additional stability by firmly holding the volar plate against the volar surface of the metacarpal head (Fig. 13-12). The capsule also becomes taut in this close-packed position (Fig. 13-10). In extension the capsule and lateral collateral ligaments are lax and the MCP joint is relatively mobile, permitting abduction and adduction as well as some axial rotation by the intrinsic muscles. Disparity of the articular surfaces and laxity of the ligaments at these joints allow for considerable passive range of movement in all positions of these joints except the close-packed position. Together with the transverse metacarpal arch, the passive movements at the MCP joints enhance the plasticity of the hand and facilitate its adaptability to the size and shape of the object being grasped.[148]

The asymmetry of the metacarpal heads, as well as the difference in length and direction of the collateral ligaments, explains why the ulnar inclination of the digits normally is greater than the radial inclination.[179] The normal ulnar inclination of the fingers occurs at the MCP joints and is most marked in the index finger. Inclination is less in the middle and little fingers and almost nonexistent in the ring finger. Normal ulnar inclination is related to several anatomic factors, which have been the subject of numerous studies in recent years.[55,63,66,159,199]

MCP JOINT OF THUMB

The MCP joint of the thumb is a semicondyloid-type articulation between the head of the first metacarpal and the base of its proximal phalanx. Two sesamoid bones are constantly present extracapsularly on its volar surface: a somewhat larger lateral sesamoid and a medial sesamoid (Fig. 13-13).[161] The joint has two degrees of freedom (flexion–extension, abduction–adduction) and limited axial rotation.[84] The capsule is inserted in the ridge separating the articulation of the proximal phalanx and the metacarpal. The capsule is reinforced on each side by the collateral ligaments, similar to those of the other MCP joints. Each collateral ligament is inserted into a tubercle on the base of the phalanx and into the corresponding sesamoid (Fig. 13-14). The two sesamoids are incorporated into the fibrocartilage of the volar plate.[154] The tunnel of the flexor pollicis longus is intimately connected to the volar plate, so the tunnel is an integral part of the apparatus, connecting the lateral ligaments and the volar plate with the sesamoids. The volar plate is attached firmly to the proximal phalanx but loosely to the metacarpal; it is the proximal attachment that has given way with irreducible dislocation.[26]

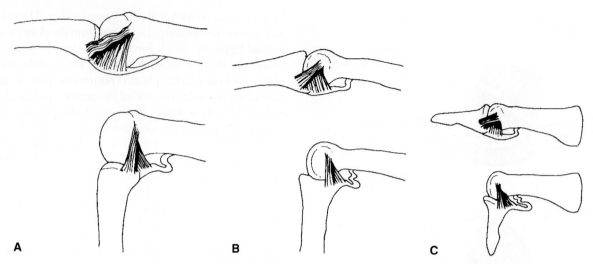

■ FIG. 13-12. Lateral view showing the volar plate and the two parts of the collateral ligament of the metacarpophalangeal (**A**), proximal interphalangeal (**B**), and distal interphalangeal joints with the joints extended and flexed (**C**).

There is considerable individual variation in joint ranges, depending on the anatomic configuration of the single broad condyle of the metacarpal.[17] Flexion ranges from 5 to 100°, with an average of about 75°.[151] If the head is round, 90 to 100° flexion is achieved. If it is flat (only 10 to 15% of cases), little flexion is possible. The main functional contribution of

the first MCP joint is to provide additional range to the thumb pad in opposition and to allow the thumb to grasp and contour to objects.[133] The literature contains little information on the function of the sesamoids. The most common belief is that they increase the leverage of certain muscles connected with the tendons running to these joints.[161]

INTERPHALANGEAL ARTICULATIONS OF FINGERS

The interphalangeal joints of the digits are each composed of the head of a phalanx and the base of the phalanx distal to it (Fig. 13-9). Each is a true synovial hinge joint that functions uniquely in flexion and extension with one degree of freedom. From a clinical standpoint, each phalanx has a head (caput) or a distal end with a convex surface and a body (corpus) and a base or proximal end with a concave surface.[80] The head of each phalanx, divided into two condyles separated by a cleft, fits the contiguous articular surface of the phalangeal base and articulates in a tongue-and-groove configuration (Fig. 13-9).[151] Their trochlea-shaped articulations are closely congruent through excursion of the joint.[179]

The proximal interphalangeal (PIP) joint has the greatest range of flexion and extension of any digital joint, with an average of 105°. The intrinsic ligamentous support of the PIP

Abductor pollicis brevis

Flexor pollicis brevis

Collateral ligament

Base of proximal phalanx

Sesamoids

Adductor pollicis

Collateral ligament

■ FIG. 13-13. Inner view of the metacarpophalangeal joint of the right thumb. The capsule and lateral ligaments are excised with the parts attached shown. The volar plate with the sesamoids is shown at the bottom of the joint.

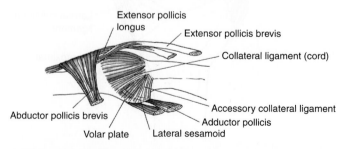

Extensor pollicis longus

Extensor pollicis brevis

Collateral ligament (cord)

Accessory collateral ligament

Adductor pollicis

Lateral sesamoid

Abductor pollicis brevis

Volar plate

■ FIG. 13-14. Metacarpophalangeal joint of the right thumb, radial aspect.

joint resembles that of the MCP joint and includes two lateral collateral ligaments, two accessory collateral ligaments, and a volar plate (Fig. 13-12*B*). The volar plate, which prevents hyperextension, has a thick distal insertion and two check ligaments proximally inserted on the middle phalanx (Fig. 13-15). Traumatic ruptures of the volar plate occur in the thicker distal insertion rather than the proximal insertion.[179] The fibrous flexor sheath is inserted on the volar plate on the base of the phalanx proximally and distally. This differs from the insertion at the MCP joint, where the flexor sheath inserts on the volar plate and base of the proximal phalanx but not on the metacarpal. This arrangement involving the collateral ligaments, volar plate, and flexor sheath is the key to interphalangeal stability.[26] Little hyperextension of this joint is possible, in contrast to the MCP joint.

The distal interphalangeal (DIP) joint resembles the PIP joint in function and ligamentous structure but has less stability and allows some hyperextension, giving a larger pulp contact (Fig. 13-12*C*). DIP flexion rarely exceeds 80°, but hyperextension is greater than at the PIP joint because the DIP joint's volar plate does not have the check ligaments proximally.[151]

The total range of flexion–extension available to the index finger is 100 to 110° at the PIP joint and 80° at the DIP joint.

The range at each joint increases ulnarly, with the proximal and distal joints achieving 135 and 90°, respectively, in the little finger.[133]

INTERPHALANGEAL JOINT OF THUMB

The interphalangeal joint of the thumb is structurally and functionally similar to the DIP joints of the fingers. It is a trochlear type of articulation, allowing mainly flexion and extension, with a slight degree of axial rotation toward pronation. Axial rotation, in fact, occurs at all three joints of the thumb: (1) trapeziometacarpal—automatic longitudinal rotation at a saddle joint; (2) MCP—active longitudinal rotation at a condylar joint through the action of the lateral thenar muscles; and (3) interphalangeal joint.[81,83]

At the end of the extension range, motion is restricted by the volar plate. There is considerable variation in the amount of extension permitted: many normal persons can hyperextend the joint.[26] Lack of extension of this joint, if greater than 15°, is functionally more disabling than lack of flexion.[179]

Tendons, Nerves, and Arteries

These structures are not discussed in detail here, but the reader will benefit from studying cross-sectional diagrams showing the anatomic relationships of these structures (Fig. 13-16). The relationships described below are most important clinically.

The transverse carpal ligament (flexor retinaculum) forms a roof over the palmar arch of the carpal bones (Figs. 13-4 and 13-16). Through the resulting tunnel pass the tendons of the flexor digitorum profundus and flexor digitorum superficialis. These tendons are all enclosed in a common synovial sheath. The flexor carpi radialis tendon and the flexor pollicis longus tendon also pass through the carpal tunnel, each enclosed in a separate sheath. Superficial to the common

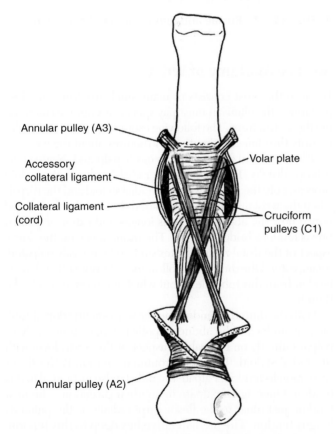

■ **FIG. 13-15.** Proximal interphalangeal joint and the arrangement of the components of the flexor sheath and volar plate.

Annular pulley (A3)

Accessory collateral ligament

Collateral ligament (cord)

Volar plate

Cruciform pulleys (C1)

Annular pulley (A2)

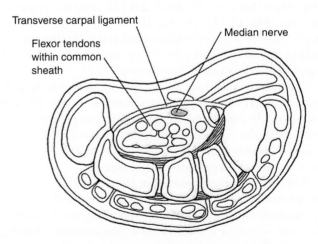

Transverse carpal ligament

Flexor tendons within common sheath

Median nerve

■ **FIG. 13-16.** Cross section of the wrist through the carpus, demonstrating the relationship of the median nerve to the flexor tendons and transverse carpal ligaments (flexor retinaculum).

flexor tendon sheath and deep to the flexor retinaculum passes the median nerve. At the distal end of the tunnel the nerve divides into several digital branches, one of which turns rather sharply around the distal border of the flexor retinaculum to innervate the thenar muscle (Fig. 13-4). Carpal tunnel syndrome is the result of compression of the median nerve within the tunnel or, occasionally, of just the thenar branch of the nerve as it turns around the distal border of the retinaculum. The palmaris longus tendon and the ulnar nerve and artery pass superficially to the flexor retinaculum. The nerve and artery travel beneath the flexor carpi ulnaris tendon, then radially to the pisiform bone before dividing to enter the hand.

The tendons of the extensor pollicis brevis and the abductor pollicis longus are enclosed in a common sheath as they pass across the lateral aspect of the distal radius. Inflammation of this sheath, or of the tendons within the sheath, is a fairly common disorder known as *De Quervain's disease,* or tenosynovitis. These tendons form the radial side of the anatomic snuffbox. The extensor pollicis longus tendon passes around Lister's tubercle on the dorsal aspect of the distal radius in a pulley-like fashion. It turns obliquely toward the thumb to form the ulnar side of the snuffbox. The radial artery travels laterally to the flexor carpi radialis tendon before turning deep beneath the abductor pollicis longus and extensor pollicis brevis tendons. It becomes superficial dorsally and can be palpated in the snuffbox (see Fig. 13-35).

At the level of the fingers, the long flexor tendons are attached to the volar aspect by three fibrous sheaths: the first lies just proximal to the metacarpal head, the second on the palmar surface of the proximal phalanx, and the third on the same surface of the second phalanx (Fig. 13-17). These form fibrous tunnels or digital pulleys along with the slightly concave osseous palmar surface of the phalanges. Between these three sheaths the tendons are held down by annular oblique and cruciate fibers that cover the MCP and PIP joints in a crosswise position (Fig. 13-15). The two digital pulleys are the most important elements of the flexor tendon sheaths; the cruciate pulleys play an accessory role.[96,158] Synovial sheaths allow gliding of the tendons within their tunnels.

The synovial sheaths of the flexor tendons start in the forearm proximal to the flexor retinaculum (Fig. 13-16). The skin creases on the flexor aspect of the fingers, except for the proximal crease, lie immediately proximal to the corresponding joints. At this level the skin is directly in contact with the synovial sheath, which can be readily infected.[82]

The long extensor muscles of the hand also run along fibroosseous tunnels, but because their course on the whole is convex these tunnels are less numerous. They are seen only at the wrist, where the tendons become concave outward during extension.[82]

A more detailed description of the anatomy of the hand and wrist complex can be found in other sources.[14,62,68,81,82,85,101,124,171,178]

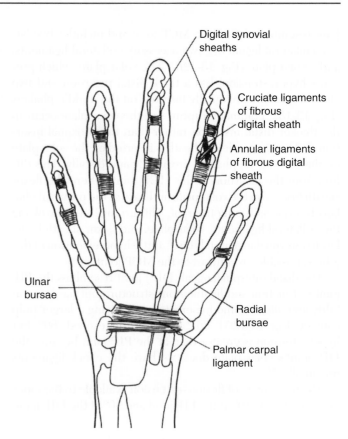

■ **FIG. 13-17.** Bursae and lumbrical sheaths of hand.

Surface Anatomy of Wrist

Because the wrist consists of many small structures in close proximity, the clinician must pay special attention to identifying these structures. The following exercise can help the reader identify the clinically significant structures about the wrist.

The distal end of the radius is easily palpated. Notice how it flares distally. Palpate along its radial border to the styloid process; note the gap between the radial styloid and the carpals when the wrist and thumb are relaxed. Extend the thumb and notice how the abductor pollicis longus and extensor pollicis brevis tendons bridge this gap. The prominence on the dorsal aspect of the distal radius, Lister's tubercle, is easily palpated. Again, extend the thumb and follow the extensor pollicis longus tendon from this tubercle, about which it curves, down to the thumb.

With the thumb extended and the wrist slightly dorsiflexed, once again locate the abductor pollicis longus tendon. Now palpate ulnarly on the palmar aspect of the wrist, level with the radial styloid. The next prominent tendon is the flexor carpi radialis tendon. Palpate the radial pulse just radial to this tendon. Once again palpate in an ulnar direction. The next tendon, just ulnar to the flexor carpi radialis, is the palmaris longus tendon. The median nerve lies deep to this tendon, beneath the flexor retinaculum.

The distal end of the ulna is also easily palpated. Feel the interval between it and the distal radius. Notice how much smaller the distal ulna is than the radius. The ulnar styloid process is quite prominent on the dorsoulnar aspect of the distal ulna. Palpate to the end of the ulnar styloid, and notice the gap between it and the carpals, which opens with radial deviation and closes with ulnar deviation. With the wrist in radial deviation, the ulnar collateral ligament can be felt bridging this gap.

From the ulnar styloid process dorsoulnarly, palpate distally to the next large prominence—the dorsal aspect of the triquetrum. From the dorsal aspect of the triquetrum, palpate around palmarly to the prominent pisiform, situated in the palmoulnar corner of the palm. Grasp the pisiform with two fingers and notice how it can be wriggled back and forth with the wrist in flexion, but not with the wrist in extension. This is because of the increased tension on the flexor carpi ulnaris tendon that attaches to the pisiform. Palpate the flexor carpi ulnaris tendon proximal to the pisiform. Feel the pulse from the ulnar artery just radial to this tendon. The ulnar nerve is situated just deep to and between the ulnar artery and the flexor carpi ulnaris tendon. Once again, locate the dorsal aspect of the triquetrum, the large prominence just distal to the prominent ulnar styloid. Slide your palpating finger distally over the dorsal aspect of the triquetrum. Feel the small interval or "joint line" between it and the hamate. With the index finger over the dorsal aspect of the hamate, bring the thumb around palmarly at the same level. With the thumb, palpate the prominent hook of the hamate deep in the hypothenar eminence; it is usually slightly tender to palpation. Between the hook of the hamate and the pisiform, beneath the pisohamate ligament, is the tunnel of Guyon. The ulnar nerve and artery pass through this tunnel.

Now imagine a line running dorsally from the base of the middle finger to Lister's tubercle. At the midpoint of this line, or just radial to it, the base of the third metacarpal can be felt as a prominence. The capitate lies just proximally to this prominence. With the wrist in neutral position, the dorsal concavity of the capitate can be palpated as a depression at the dorsum of the wrist. Just proximal to this depression is the lunate. If a palpating finger is placed over the lunate and capitate while passively flexing and extending the wrist, the distal end of the lunate can be felt to slide into the depression in the capitate on extension and out on flexion.

In the deepest portion of the anatomic snuffbox, the dorsoradial aspect of the scaphoid bone can be palpated. It is most easily felt with the wrist in ulnar deviation. Just distal to the scaphoid you can feel the trapezium. You should be able to identify the trapezium–first metacarpal articulation. The trapezoid is easily palpated as a prominence at the base of the second metacarpal.

BIOMECHANICS OF WRIST

The wrist is composed of three joints: the distal radioulnar joint, the radiocarpal joint, and the midcarpal joint. With this description it is understood that the radiocarpal joint includes the articulation between the disk and the carpals because the disk acts as an ulnar extension of the distal radial joint surface. From a functional standpoint, however, it is best to speak of an ulnomeniscotriquetral joint in addition to the three joints listed above. In this way the movements of the ulna and the carpals can be better considered in relation to the disk. (Refer to Appendix A for a description of the movements that occur at these joints and the arthrokinematic motions that accompany these movements.)

The movements among the many bones of the wrist are complex. The clinician must have a basic knowledge of the major interarticular movements to be successful in evaluating painful conditions affecting the wrist and in restoring movement when it is lost.

Flexion–Extension

The primary axis of movement for wrist flexion–extension passes through the capitate. The wrist close-packs in full dorsiflexion because it must assume a state of maximal intrinsic stability to allow one to transmit pressure from the hand to the forearm. In functional activities, such force transmission usually occurs with the wrist in dorsiflexion—for example, when pushing a heavy object or walking on all fours. As with any synovial joint, the close-packed position at the wrist is achieved by a "screw home" movement—a movement involving a conjunct rotation (see Chapter 3, Arthrology). The carpus, on dorsiflexion, moves in a supinatory rotation. This is easily observed by watching the wrist as it passes from neutral to full extension. The reason for this rotation is that the scaphoid moves in a manner different from that of other proximal carpal bones.[111] As the wrist moves from a position of flexion to neutral, the distal row of carpals remains relatively loose-packed with respect to the proximal row, and the proximal row remains loose-packed with respect to the radius. Disk movement occurs at both the radiocarpal joint and the midcarpal joint. At about the neutral position, or just slightly beyond, as the wrist continues into dorsiflexion, the distal row of carpals becomes close-packed with the scaphoid but not with the other proximal carpals (lunate and triquetrum). Because of this close-packing, the scaphoid moves with the distal row of carpals as the wrist moves into full dorsiflexion. During this final stage of dorsiflexion, then, movement must occur between the scaphoid and lunate as the distal row continues to dorsiflex against the lunate and triquetrum. Looking at it another way, the scaphoid moves more with respect to the radius than do the lunate and triquetrum. This asymmetry of movement results in a supinatory twisting of the carpus that twists capsules and ligaments to close-pack the remaining joints at full dorsiflexion (Fig. 13-18).

As in any joint, the bones forming the wrist are most susceptible to fracture or dislocation when in the close-packed position. Most frequently fractured are the scaphoid and the

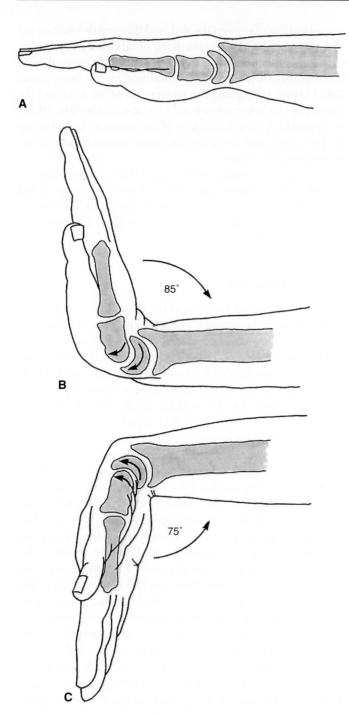

■ **FIG. 13-18.** Flexion–extension of the wrist showing neutral position (**A**), dorsiflexion with carpus moving palmarly and in supinatory rotation (**B**), and palmar flexion with carpus moving dorsally (**C**).

distal end of the radius. The most common dislocations are a palmar dislocation of the lunate relative to the radius and remaining carpals and a dorsal dislocation of the carpals with respect to the lunate and the radius. The common mechanism of injury for all the above injuries, as would be expected, is a fall on the dorsiflexed hand.

Radial–Ulnar Deviation

The axis of movement for radial–ulnar deviation also passes through the capitate. Ulnar deviation occurs over a much greater range of movement than radial deviation. This is because radial deviation is limited by contact of the scaphoid tubercle against the radial styloid process, whereas the triquetrum easily clears the ulnar styloid process, which is situated more dorsally and is less prominent than the radial styloid process. Both radial and ulnar deviation involve movements at the radiocarpal and midcarpal joints.[197] The associated arthrokinematic movements are not pure, but rather involve rotary movements between the proximal row and the radius, and between the distal row and the proximal row. As described by Kapandji,[83] the proximal row tends to move into pronation, flexion, and ulnar glide during radial deviation with respect to the radius and disk (Fig. 13-19). At the same time, the distal row moves into supination, extension, and ulnar glide with respect to the proximal row. The opposite movements occur during ulnar deviation (Fig. 13-20). This can be easily observed on a cadaver and seems to be related entirely to the shapes of the joint surfaces rather than the capsuloligamentous influences. Radial deviation involves close-packing of primarily the midcarpal joint.

FUNCTION AND ARCHITECTURE OF HAND

The hand is a complex machine: it may be used as a means of expression, a tactile organ, and a weapon. The study of the hand is inseparable from that of the wrist and forearm, which function as a single physiologic unit, with the wrist being the key joint. In pronation–supination the movement of the radius in relation to the ulna is in fact the movement of the hand around its longitudinal axis.[78,178] The entire upper limb is subservient to the hand.

Functional Arches of Hand

To grasp objects the hand must change its shape. Cupping of the hand occurs with finger flexion, and flattening of the hand occurs with extension. Cupping improves the mobility of the hand for functional use, and flattening is used for release of objects. Structurally the hand and wrist conform to three basic physiologic functional arches, which are concave palmarly. Usually three transverse arches (two carpal and one metacarpal arch) and one longitudinal arch are described (Fig. 13-21). To these the oblique arches of opposition between the thumb and each of the fingers may be added.[82,83] These arches allow coordinated synergistic digital flexion and thumb–little finger opposition. Usually the distal phalanges flex toward the scaphoid tubercle or obliquely; only the index ray flexes in a sagittal plane. Full thumb–little finger opposition usually achieves parallel pulp-to-pulp contact of the distal phalanges of these two digits.

The longitudinal arch (or arches, since each ray with its corresponding metacarpal and adjacent carpal forms its own

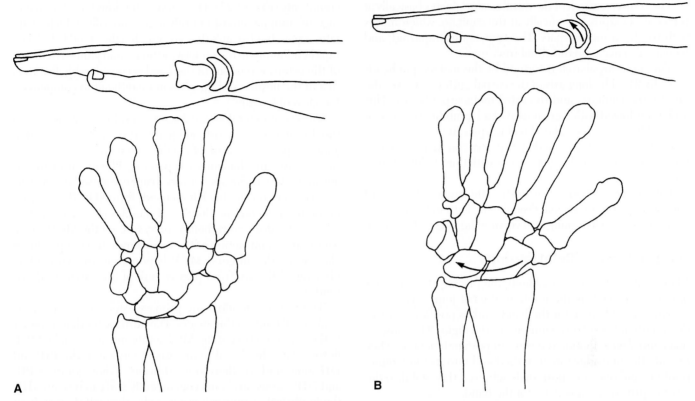

A   **B**

■ **FIG. 13-19.** Radial deviation of the wrist. **(A)** The wrist is shown in neutral position. **(B)** With radial deviation, the proximal row of carpals moves into dorsal and ulnar glide.

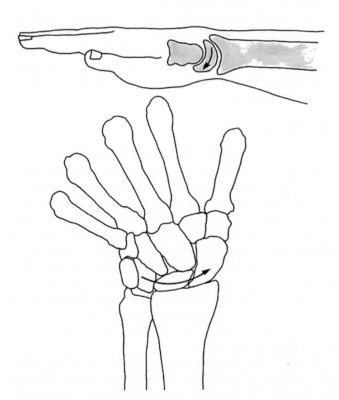

■ **FIG. 13-20.** Ulnar deviation of the wrist. The proximal row of carpals moves into palmar and radial glide.

arch) is centered about the MCP articulations, whose thick anterior glenoid capsules and volar plates prevent excessive hyperextension. The long finger ray and the capitate are the focal point.[151]

Two transverse carpal arches may be considered the proximal and distal carpal arch (Fig. 13-21). The proximal arch is more mobile than the distal carpal row because of its connections to the radius and the distal row. The scaphoid, lunate, and triquetrum, which make up this row, have their own distinct movements.

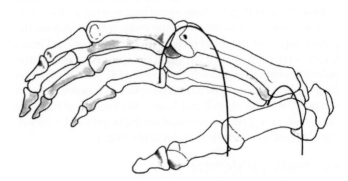

■ **FIG. 13-21.** Longitudinal and transverse arches of the hand, side view.

The transverse arch of the distal row originates basically at the central carpus, specifically at the capitate, which moves with the fixed metacarpals. The trapezium, trapezoid, and hamate also make up this distal row.

The metacarpal arch is formed by the metacarpal heads (Fig. 13-21). The long axis of the carpal gutter traverses the lunate, the capitate, and the third metacarpal bones. This arch is endowed with a great deal of adaptability because of the mobility of the peripheral metacarpals. It is relatively flat when the hand is at rest but demonstrates considerable curvature with strong clenching of a fist or with thumb–little finger opposition.

Pathologic conditions may destroy the arches of the hand and cause severe functional disability by flattening the transverse arches and flattening or reversing the longitudinal arch.

Length–Tension Relationships

Flatt[54] states, "In the normal limb, the placing of the hand is largely controlled by the multi-axial wrist joint." The wrist provides a stable base for the hand, and its position controls the length of the extrinsic muscles to the digits. The muscles that control wrist motion serve two important functions. They provide the fine adjustment of the hand into its functioning position, and once this position is achieved they stabilize the wrist to provide a stable base for the hand.

As the fingers flex, the wrist must be stabilized by the wrist extensor muscles to prevent the long finger flexor muscles from simultaneously flexing the wrist, and allow for optimal length–tension in the long finger muscles. As the wrist position changes, the effective functional length of the finger flexors change, and hypothetically the magnitude of force should also change. As grip becomes stronger, synchronous wrist extension lengthens the extrinsic flexor tendons across the wrist and maintains a favorable length of the musculotendinous unit for a strong contraction.

Hazelton and associates[66] investigated the peak force that could be exerted at the interphalangeal joints of the finger during different wrist positions. They found the greatest interphalangeal flexion force occurred with ulnar deviation of the wrist (neutral flexion–extension). The wrist position in which the least force is generated is volar flexion. For strong finger or thumb extension, the wrist flexor muscles stabilize or flex the wrist so the long finger extensors can function more efficiently.

When the wrist is extended, the pulp (soft cushion on the palmar aspect of the distal phalanges) of the thumb and index finger is passively in contact; when the wrist is in flexion, the pulp of the thumb reaches the level of the PIP joint of the index finger. The position of the wrist has important repercussions on the position of the thumb and finger. Movements of the wrist are usually in reverse of movements of the fingers and reinforce the action of the extrinsic muscles of the fingers.

EXTENSOR MECHANISM

The extensor mechanism, also called the dorsal finger mechanism or extensor apparatus, is a subject of great interest and complexity (Fig. 13-22). The extensor tendons have the advantage of running almost entirely extrasynovially, which facilitates repair, but because they are also thin they tend to become rapidly adherent to the underlying bones and joints. Excursion of the extensor tendons of the hand is considerably less than that of the flexors, and thus it is more difficult to compensate for a loss of length.[178]

The extensor tendons are discrete and obvious at the level of the dorsal forearm, wrist, and hand. At the level of the MCP joint it is proper to speak of the dorsal tendinous structures as the extensor mechanism or apparatus. The extensor mechanism is a broad, flat aponeurotic band composed of extrinsic extensor tendon and the lateral bands formed by the tendons of the interosseous and lumbrical muscles (Fig. 13-22). The extrinsic tendons exert their primary force at the MCP joints. An isolated contraction of the extensor digitorum produces clawing of the fingers (MCP hyperextension with interphalangeal flexion from passive pull of the extrinsic flexor tendons).

The intrinsic tendons are primary extensors of the interphalangeal joints of the fingers. The intrinsic tendons lie volar to the axis of motion of the MCP joints and are actually MCP flexors. They lie dorsal to the axis of motion of the PIP and DIP joints and are, therefore, extensors of those joints.[132] PIP and DIP extension occurs concurrently and can be caused by the lumbrical or interosseous muscles through their pull on the extensor hood (a flattened portion of the communis tendon just distal to the MCP joint; Fig. 13-22). There must be tension in the extensor digitorum.

The thumb has a similar anatomic situation, with one important exception. The thumb has an extrinsic extensor (extensor pollicis longus) that exerts its force on the distal phalanx. Forceful hyperextension of the interphalangeal joint is prevented and thumb extension is reduced with the loss of this tendon.[132]

PREHENSION

The major musculoskeletal function of the hand lies in its ability to grip objects. Prehension is seen in all forms of the animal world. According to Rabischong,[144] forms of prehension may be divided into four types: organs that pinch (i.e., pincers of the lobster), encircle, push, and adhere. Usually an animal can use only one of these forms of prehension; only in humans has it obtained perfection. This is largely because of opposition of the thumb, which brings it into contact with each finger.[81,83] Because this requires the hand to function as a unit, prehension can never be fully measured in terms of the movement of an individual joint. Many classifications of these movements were used until Napler[130] divided them into two categories: power grip and precision grip.

Power Grip. Power grip is a forceful act resulting in flexion at all fingers: the thumb, when used, acts as a stabilizer to the object held between the fingers and the palm (Fig. 13-23). This typically involves clamping an object with partially flexed fingers against the palm of the hand, with counterpressure

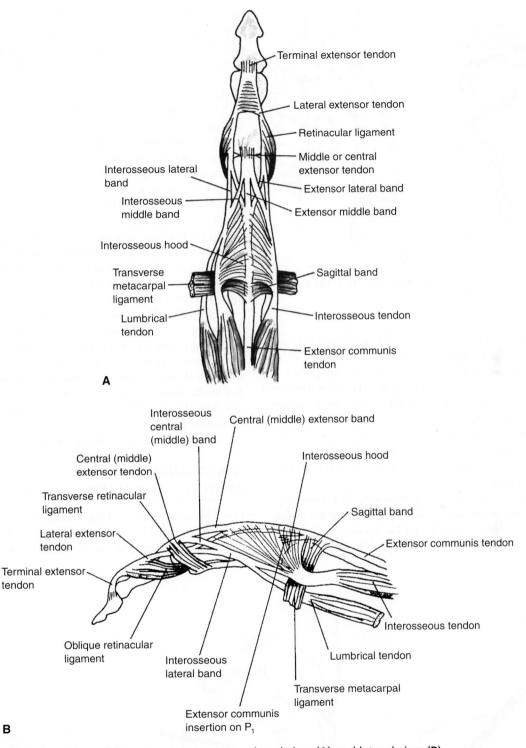

■ FIG. 13-22. Main insertions of the extensor apparatus: dorsal view (**A**) and lateral view (**B**).

from the adducted thumb. The fingers assume a position of sustained (isometric function) flexion that varies with the weight, size, and shape of the object. The ulnar two fingers flex across toward the thenar eminence. In the final posture the hypothenar and the thenar eminences are used as buttresses as the fingers flex around the object to be grasped.[33] With all power grips the hand is kept stable and the power movements are produced by either radial or ulnar deviation of the wrist, as in the action of hammering, by supination and pronation of the wrist, and by extension of the elbow. Varieties of power grip include cylindrical grip, spherical grip, hook grip, and lateral prehension.[108]

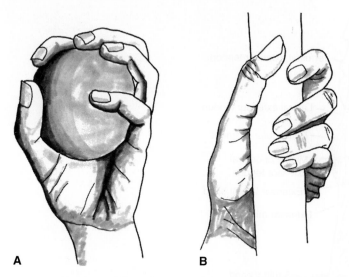

■ **FIG. 13-23.** Modes of power grip: spherical (**A**) and cylindrical (**B**) grip positions.

A crude form of this grip (cylindrical) is used while gripping a heavy object—for example, forcefully driving a nail with a hammer, using the thumb to provide stability and power. A more refined power grip is the ulnar grip, used when a lighter object lying across the palm is gripped mainly by the two ulnar fingers; the thumb is used for control.[33]

Power grip is the result of a sequence of (1) opening the hand, (2) positioning the fingers, (3) approaching the fingers to the object, and (4) maintaining a static phase, which actually constitutes the grip.[96]

Precision Grip. Precision grip shares the first three steps of the power grip sequence but does not have a static phase. The first three steps are followed by dynamic movement rather than a static phase; *precision handling* may be a bet- ter term. The muscles primarily function isotonically.[96] The object must be picked up and manipulated by the fingers and thumb (Fig. 13-24). The object is not in contact with the palm of the hand but is manipulated between the opposing thumb and against the fingers—mainly against the next two fingers or the index finger.

The sensory surface of the digits is used for maximum sensory input to influence delicate adjustments. Varieties of precision grip include (1) palmar pinch, in which the pad of the thumb is opposed to the pad of one or more fingers—this is used for picking up and holding an object; (2) lateral pinch or opposition, in which the palmar aspect of the thumb pad presses on the radial surface of the first phalanx of the index finger—for instance, holding a coin or a sheet of paper; and (3) tip prehension, in which the tip of the pad or even the edge of the thumbnail is opposed to the tip of the index finger (or middle finger)—it allows one to hold a thin object or pick up a very fine object such as a pin.[81,83] Tip prehension is the finest and most precise grip and is easily upset by any disease of the hand because it requires a whole range of movements and fine muscle control.

The functions of the digits can be related to the patterns of the nerve supply. Opening the hand depends on the radial nerve. Both the median and ulnar nerves innervate the muscles of the thumb required for opposition. Flexion and sensation of the radial digits, important in precision grip, are controlled chiefly by the median nerve, whereas flexion and sensation of the ulnar digits depend on the ulnar nerve.

FUNCTIONAL POSITIONS OF WRIST AND HAND

The functional position of the wrist and hand is that which is naturally assumed by the hand to grasp an object or the position from which optimal function is most likely to occur.[83,133]

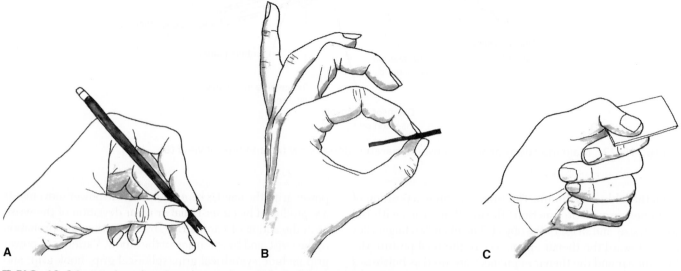

■ **FIG. 13-24.** Modes of prehension: palmar (**A**), tip (**B**), and lateral (**C**).

From this position it is possible to grasp an object with minimal effort. The functional position is one in which (1) the wrist is slightly extended (20°) and ulnarly deviated (10°); (2) the fingers are slightly flexed at all their joints, with the degree of flexion increasing somewhat from the index to the little finger; and (3) the thumb is in midrange opposition, with the MCP joint moderately flexed and the interphalangeal joints slightly flexed (Fig. 13-25).

This is not necessarily the position in which a hand should be immobilized. The preferred position for immobilization depends on the disability. However, this position is often the position of choice because other positions may result in serious functional sequelae. For example, if a finger is immobilized in extension it may become ankylosed.

The wrist and hand have a fixed and a mobile segment. The fixed segment consists of the distal row of carpal bones (hamate, capitate, trapezoid, and trapezium) and the second and third metacarpals. This is the stabilizing segment of the wrist and hand (Fig. 13-1), and there is less movement among these bones than among the bones of the mobile segments. The mobile segment is made up of the five phalanges and the first, fourth, and fifth metacarpals. This arrangement allows stability without rigidity.

EXAMINATION

The wrist structures are innervated primarily from C6 through C8. Lesions affecting structures of similar segmental derivation may refer pain to the wrist; conversely, lesions at or about the wrist may refer pain into the relevant segments. Because the wrist is located distally, and pain is more commonly referred in a proximal-to-distal direction than in a retrograde direction, pain from lesions at or about the wrist is fairly well localized. A more proximal origin, however, must always be suspected with symptoms experienced at the wrist or hand. Common lesions that often refer pain to this region include lower cervical pathologic processes (e.g., spondylosis, disk disease), tendinitis or capsulitis at the shoulder, thoracic outlet syndrome, and tennis elbow.[12] If subjective findings do not seem to implicate a local problem, a scan examination of the neck and entire extremity may be warranted before proceeding with an in-depth evaluation of the wrist (see Chapter 21, The Cervicothoracic–Upper Limb Scan Examination).

History

A structured line of questioning should be pursued, as set out in Chapter 5, Assessment of Musculoskeletal Disorders and Concepts of Management.

MUSCULOSKELETAL DISORDERS

Common lesions at or about the wrist vary in onset from insidious (carpal tunnel syndrome, De Quervain's tenosynovitis, rheumatoid arthritis) to those in which an incident of trauma is definitely recalled (Colles' fracture, scaphoid fracture, lunate dislocation, or capsuloligamentous sprains). Again, the clinician must be prepared to direct the line of questioning to elicit information concerning more proximal regions, especially if the onset is insidious. If a traumatic event is cited, the examiner should attempt to determine the exact mechanism of injury. Because rheumatoid arthritis is not uncommon at the wrist, questions might be asked about possible bilateral problems and problems with the MCP joints and the joints of the feet.

Physical Examination

The order and detail of the physical tests described below need to be appropriate to the patient being examined. Some tests will be irrelevant, others will only need to be carried out briefly, whereas others will need to be fully investigated. Throughout the physical examination the clinician must aim to find physical tests that reproduce the patient's symptoms.

I.   Observation
   A. General appearance and body build
   B. Functional activities. Observe the way the person shakes hands, noting the firmness of grasp and temperature and moisture of the hand. Note during dressing activities whether one hand tends to be favored. Observe for fumbling with fasteners or small objects—a problem typical of carpal tunnel syndrome or neurologic dysfunction of more proximal origin. Note whether the patient willingly puts pressure through the wrist, as when standing up from a chair.
   C. General posture and positioning of body parts. Note how the arm and hand are carried, and especially whether they swing naturally when walking. The person with a reflex sympathetic dystrophy, not an infrequent complication after healing of a Colles' fracture, invariably walks in with the elbow flexed and the forearm held across the upper abdomen.
   D. General posture of the hands. The hands should be observed in their resting position. The dominant hand

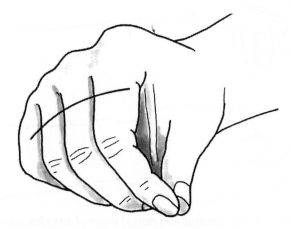

■ FIG. 13-25. Functional position of a hand.

is usually larger. The posture at rest will often demonstrate common deformities.

1. An abnormal hand posture may be characteristic and establish the diagnosis, as with a typical ulnar claw, or as with wrist drop and flexion of the wrist and MCP joints, pathognomonic of radial nerve palsy.[179]
2. Somewhat less typical is the dissociated radial palsy simulating an ulnar claw, in which extension of the thumb and index and middle fingers is preserved.[117]
3. Dissociated median nerve forearm palsy commonly results from compression of the anterior interosseous nerve supplying the flexor pollicis longus, the radial half of the flexor digitorum profundus, and the pronator quadratus. It also produces a characteristic deformity known as the anterior interosseous nerve syndrome.[88,176] During pinch the distal phalanges of the thumb and index finger cannot flex and stay in extension.
4. Clawing of the two ulnar digits, caused by paralysis of the interosseous muscle, is variable (ulnar nerve palsy). This deformity is often referred to as "bishop's hand" or "benediction hand" deformity.
5. Dupuytren's contracture is a contracture of the palmar aponeurosis, which pulls the fingers into flexion.
6. An avulsion fracture or a tear of the distal extensor tendon causes mallet finger, which results in flexion of the DIP joint, from the distal phalanx.
7. Swan-neck deformity presents as flexion of the MCP and DIP joints, and is caused by trauma with damage to the volar plate or by rheumatoid arthritis.
8. Boutonnière deformity—extension of the MCP and DIP joints and flexion of the PIP joint—is usually the result of a rupture of the central tendinous slip of the extensor hood. It is common after trauma or in rheumatoid arthritis.

II. Inspection
A. Bony structure and alignment. This is especially important after a fracture of the distal radius. The most common complication after Colles' fracture is healing of the fragments in a malaligned position, resulting in a "dinner fork" deformity (Figs. 13-26 and 13-27). In such a deformity the distal end of the radius is displaced and angulated dorsally, foreshortened, and often rotated into supination. Such a deformity must be considered when determining treatment goals, because normal ROM can never be obtained in such cases.
1. Note the structural alignment of the head, neck, shoulder girdle, arm, and forearm.
2. Note carefully the structural alignment and relationships of the distal end of the radius and ulna, the carpals, and the metacarpals (see section on the surface anatomy).
3. Note any structural deformities of the hands and fingers, such as boutonnière or swan-neck deformities, ulnar drift, claw hand, or ape hand.

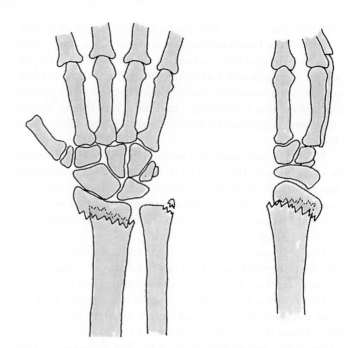

■ **FIG. 13-26.** Dorsal and lateral views of a Colles' fracture, showing extension fracture of the lower end of the radius.

B. Soft tissue
1. Muscle contours
a. Note especially any atrophy of the thenar muscles (this may accompany carpal tunnel syndrome), the hypothenar muscles (suggestive of an ulnar nerve lesion), and intrinsics.
b. Note any generalized atrophy of the arm or forearm (this invariably occurs with immobilization but may be masked by edema).
c. Note any localized atrophy about the shoulder girdle and the rest of the limb, which may

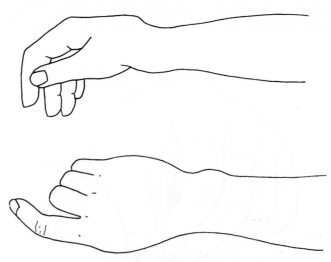

■ **FIG. 13-27.** Lateral and dorsal views of the characteristic dinner fork deformity resulting from a Colles' fracture.

suggest neuromuscular involvement of related segments.

2. Joint regions
   a. Inspect for effusion of any upper limb joints.
   b. Notice other periarticular swellings: Heberden's nodes about the DIP joints are characteristic of osteoarthrosis of those joints.
   c. Small pea-sized ganglia are commonly found on the dorsal or palmar aspect of the wrist and are usually of little significance.
   d. Large nodules about the wrist, extensor surface of the forearm, and elbow are characteristic of rheumatoid arthritis.
3. General soft tissue inspection
   a. Generalized edema of the distal extremity is invariably present after immobilization in all but younger patients.
   b. Localized edema over the dorsum of the hand suggests an infection involving any part of the hand.
   c. If swelling or edema is present, volumetric measurements and girth measurements should be taken to document a baseline.

C. Skin
   1. Color
      a. Redness with inflammation
      b. Often cyanotic in reflex sympathetic dystrophy
      c. Colorless with severe neurologic deficit
   2. Texture (see under Palpation)
   3. Moisture (see under Palpation)
   4. Scars, blemishes

D. Nails
   1. Splitting, ridging (typical in reflex sympathetic dystrophy)
   2. Clubbing (may suggest a cardiopulmonary disorder)
   3. Hollowing

III. Joint Tests. Joint tests include active and passive physiologic movements of the elbow, wrist, and hand joints and other relevant joints. Joint integrity and joint-play (accessory) movements complete the joint tests.

A. Joint integrity tests. Ligamentous instability is diagnosed by passive movement tests, as routine radiographs are normal.[172] The scapholunate and the lunotriquetral joints are commonly affected.[172]

   1. "Piano keys" test. The patient sits with both hands in pronation. The examiner stabilizes the patient's arm with one hand so that the examiner's finger can push down on the distal ulna. The other hand supports the patient's hand. The examiner pushed down on the distal ulna as one would push down on a piano key. A positive test is indicated by a difference in mobility and the production of pain or tenderness when compared with the opposite side. A positive test indicates instability of the distal radioulnar joint.[116,145]

   2. Watson (scaphoid shift) test: Watson's test assesses scaphulolunate ligament stability. The scaphoid is palpated anteriorly and posteriorly on its distal aspect as the wrist is moved from ulnar deviation to radial deviation. The test is positive if there is pain or a palpable displacement of the scaphoid posteriorly, which sometimes occurs with a "clunk."[172,173,189]

   3. Lunotriquetral ballottement test. The integrity of the lunotriquetral can be tested by immobilizing the lunate and moving the triquetrum and pisiform up and down on the lunate. The test is positive if it produces pain or excessive mobility.[103,173]

   4. Midcarpal joint test. The examiner applies an anteroposterior force to the scaphoid while distracting the flexing the wrist. Reproduction of the patient's pain indicates a positive test, suggesting instability between the radius, scaphoid, lunate, and capitate.

   5. Also ask the patient to place the hand flat on a table with the wrist dorsiflexed and the elbow extended and to lean forward so as to transmit body weight through the forearm and wrist. This maneuver is most likely to reproduce pain from a lesion of the palmar radiolunate or dorsal lunocapitate ligaments (see Ligamentous Sprains below).

   6. Murphy's sign. The subject is instructed to make a fist. If the subject's third metacarpal is level with the second and fourth metacarpal, a dislocated lunate is indicated.[92]

   7. Grind test. The grind test is used to test for abnormality of the thumb carpometacarpal joint. The examiner holds the patient's hand with one hand and grasps the patient's thumb below the metacarpophalangeal joint with the other hand. The examiner then applies an axial load to the thumb metacarpal (pushing proximally) and gently rotates it side to side. Positive findings include significant pain, crepitans, and lateral subluxation of the metacarpal.[156]

   All the joints of the wrist and hand can be checked for instability. Any of the joint-play movements (see Joint Mobilization Techniques below) can be used to assess stability. At the wrist, the ulnar collateral ligament can be checked by radially deviating the wrist in a neutral position. The radial collateral ligament is tested by ulnarly deviating the wrist in neutral. The integrity of the collateral ligaments of thumb and fingers can be assessed by applying ulnar and radial stresses. Overpressure can be applied to any of the carpals to test their stability. These tests are positive if there is excessive joint mobility.

B. Active and passive physiologic joint movements. For both active and passive physiologic joint movement, the examiner should note the following:
   • the range of movement
   • the quality of movement

- the resistance through range of movement and at the end range of movement
- the behavior of pain through the range and the end range of movement

    Both tendon excursion (active ROM) and joint motion (passive ROM) are evaluated by computing total active motion and total passive motion, as recommended by the Clinical Assessment Committee of the American Society for Surgery of the Hand. This method is used to measure and record finger and thumb motions.[4] If joint stiffness is present, closely examine the end feel of each joint before measuring passive ROM with a goniometer.

1. Active physiologic movements with overpressure. Establish the patient's symptoms at rest. Record ROM, pain, and crepitus. The following joints should be tested as indicated:
   - Superior and inferior radioulnar joint pronation and supination
   - Radiocarpal joints
     - flexion and extension
     - radial and ulnar deviation
   - Carpometacarpal joint of the thumb
     - flexion and extension
     - abduction and adduction
     - opposition
   - Distal intermetacarpal horizontal flexion and extension
   - Metacarpophalangeal joints
     - flexion and extension
     - abduction and adduction
   - Proximal and distal interphalangeal joints flexion and extension

    For further information about active range of movement, movements can be combined together, compression or distraction can be added, and various differentiation tests can be performed.

2. Passive physiologic joint movements. All the active movements described above can be examined passively. A comparison of the response of symptoms to the active and passive movements helps to determine whether the structure at fault is noncontractile (articular) or contractile (extra-articular).[34] If the lesion is noncontractile, then active and passive movements will be painful or restricted in the same direction. If the lesion is in a contractile tissue, active and passive movements are painful or restricted in opposite directions. Record ROM, pain, crepitus, and end feel.

    Capsular patterns for this joint are as follows:
   - distal radioulnar joint—full range with pain at the extremes of pronation and supination
   - wrist—equal limitation of flexion and extension
   - trapeziometacarpal joint—more limited abduction then extension, flexion free

   - thumb and finger joints—more limitation of flexion than extension

3. Other joints. The most likely joints suspected to be a source of the symptoms are the cervical spine, thoracic spine, and elbow complex. These joints can be tested fully or if these joints are not suspected to be a source of symptoms then relevant clearing tests can be performed. Fully test shoulder and elbow movements, after immobilization and when reflex sympathetic dystrophy is suspected.

C. Joint-play movements. Joint-play movements of the wrist and hand complex are the same as the mobilization techniques (see Treatment Techniques below) but are performed in the resting position. Record mobility and irritability (pain or muscle guarding).

1. Specific joint-play (accessory) motions to be tested include:
   a. Distal radioulnar joint: dorsal and ventral glide and distraction (see Figs. 13-37 and 13-38)
   b. Radiocarpal joint: dorsal and palmar glide, ulnar glide, and radial glide (see Figs. 13-40 and 13-41)
   c. Midcarpal joint: traction, dorsal and volar glide
   d. MCP joint: distraction, dorsal and palmar glide, radioulnar glide (or tilt), and rotation (see Figs. 13-49 to 13-52)
   e. Interphalangeal joint: distraction, dorsal–volar glide, side tilt, and rotation. The joint-play movements for the fingers are the same for the metacarpophalangeal; the hand position of the examiner simply moves further distally.

2. Special intercarpal movements should be performed if an intercarpal ligament sprain is suspected. Kaltenborn[80] has developed a systematic approach to examination of joint play of the individual carpal bones (Fig. 13-1).
   a. Stabilize the capitate and move the trapezium and trapezoid as a unit.
   b. Stabilize the capitate and move the scaphoid.
   c. Stabilize the capitate and move the lunate.
   d. Stabilize the capitate and move the hamate.
   e. Stabilize the scaphoid and move the trapezium and trapezoid as a unit.
   f. Stabilize the radius and move the scaphoid (see Fig. 13-43).
   g. Stabilize the radius and move the lunate.
   h. Stabilize the ulna with the articular disk and move the triquetrum.
   i. Stabilize the triquetrum and move the hamate.
   j. Stabilize the triquetrum and move the pisiform.

3. Mobilization with movement. Theses sustained mobilizations can also be carried out for additional information.[49,129,140]
   a. Forearm pronation and supination (Fig. 13-28). The patient actively supinates or pronates the forearm while the examiner applies a sustained anterior or posterior force to the distal end of the

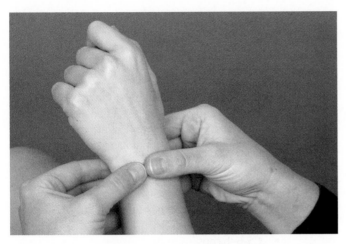

■ **FIG. 13-28.** Mobilization with movement for supination. A posteroanterior force is applied to the ulna as the patient actively supinates.

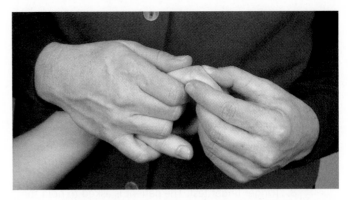

■ **FIG. 13-30.** Mobilization with movement for finger extension. The stabilizing hand supports the metacarpal as the mobilizing hand applies a medial glide just distal to the distal interphalangeal joint as the patient actively extends the joint.

ulnar at the wrist. An increase in range and no pain or reduced pain on active supination or pronation indicates a mechanical joint problem.
   b. Wrist flexion and extension (Fig. 13-29). The patient actively flexes or extends the wrist while the examiner applies a sustained lateral or medial glide to the carpal bones. An increase in range and no pain or reduced pain are positive examination findings.
   c. Interphalangeal flexion and extension (Fig. 13-30). The patient actively flexes or extends the fingers while the examiner applies a sustained medial or lateral glide just distal to the affected joint. An increase in range and no pain or reduced pain are positive examination findings.
   D. Joint effusion. Measure the circumference of the joint using a tape measure.

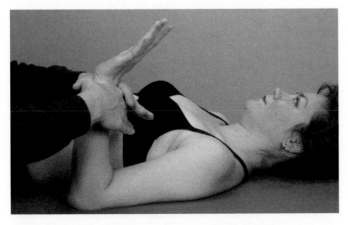

■ **FIG. 13-29.** Mobilization with movement for wrist flexion. A lateral glide is applied to the ulnar aspect of the wrist as the patient actively extends the wrist.

IV. Muscle Tests. Muscle tests include resistive isometric movements, muscle strength, functional strength testing or control, and muscle length.
   A. Resisted isometric movements. Record as strong or weak, painful or painless.
      1. Resist isometrically all wrist, forearm, finger, and thumb movements. The flexor and extensor tendons of the wrist and hand can be tested individually for tenosynovitis. To test for involvement of these structures, the muscle's action is isometrically resisted while palpating the tendon. The test is positive if it provokes pain or crepitus.[177]
      2. If referred pain from more proximal regions is suspected, include resisted elbow and shoulder movements.
   B. Muscle strength. Manual muscle tests should include the upper limb muscles beginning at the shoulder. For details of these tests the reader is directed to Clarkson and Gilewish,[30] Cole et al.,[31] Hislop and Montgomery,[67] Kendall et al.,[86] and Palmer and Epler[136] to determine exactly which muscles are at fault. Gross grip strength can be measured by a dynamometer. Force generated by the normal man is about 46 kg, that by the normal woman about 23 kg.[169,196] If the subject cannot grip the dynamometer, a sphygmomanometer may be used—the normal male grip usually exceeds 300 mm Hg, and the female grip is about 300 mm Hg.[182] A pinch meter is used to test pinch strength.
   C. Muscle length and musculotendinous tests
      1. Finkelstein's test. The classic test for the first extensor compartment tenosynovitis—de Quervain's disease—is called *Finkelstein's test*. The patient makes a fist with the thumb inside the fingers, and the examiner adds passive ulnar deviation of the wrist. Reproduction of the patient's pain is indicative of de Quervain's disease (tenosynovitis of the abductor

pollicis longus and extensor pollicis brevis tendons). The clinician should note that the test is not definitive for de Quervain's disease. This test also stretches the superficial radial nerve and may cause symptoms as a result of mechanical neural tension.[153]

2. Linburg's sign. The thumb is flexed into the hypothenar eminence and the index finger is extended. Limited range of index finger extension and pain is a positive test. This test is for tendinitis at the interconnection between the flexor pollicis longus and the flexor indices.[102,116]

3. Trigger finger test. The patient is asked to hold the digit extended. The examiner palpates over the anterior surface of the interphalangeal joints. The patient is asked to actively flex and extend the interphalangeal joint.[69,177] The test is positive if there is a palpable audible snapping or "triggering." Snapping is most often caused by a nodule in the flexor tendon that catches on a narrower annular sheath or pulley opposite the metacarpal head.

4. Tennis elbow syndrome (medial and lateral tendon injuries). It may be necessary to test for these. Tests are described in Chapter 12, Elbow and Forearm.

D. Other tests. The status of the motor system can be further described in terms of muscle tone. Coordination can be tested by performing activities such as tracing a diagram or buttoning a button. Standardized tests such as the Jebson Hand Function Test, the Minnesota Rate of Manipulation Test, the Purdue Pegboard Test, the Valpar Work Sample Series, and the O'Conner Dexterity Test are available for more detailed evaluation of manual dexterity and coordination.[8,51,75]

V. Neuromuscular Tests. The neurologic examination should be carried out as outlined in Chapter 5, Assessment of Musculoskeletal Disorders and Concepts of Management, if neurologic involvement is suspected. Indications for neurologic testing include complaints of paresthesia or anesthesia. The examiner should correlate the finding to patterns of cervical disk, nerve root, peripheral nerve entrapment, or other peripheral neurovascular problems that coincide with the patient's complaints and examination. Involvement of the cervical nerve roots and peripheral nerves may affect both muscle strength and sensation of the upper extremity. The level of the cervical nerve root or peripheral nerves may be determined by identifying key muscles or joint actions and sensory areas, which are representative.

A. Integrity of the nervous system

1. Dermatomes and peripheral nerves. A knowledge of the cutaneous distribution of peripheral nerves and cutaneous distribution of nerve roots (dermatomes) enables the examiner to distinguish the sensory loss attributable to a root lesion from that attributable to a peripheral nerve lesion. Light touch and pain sensation of the upper limb are tested, respectively. A knowledge of nerve roots (dermatomes) and periph-

eral nerves enables the examiner to distinguish the sensory loss attributable to a peripheral nerve lesion from that attributable to a root lesion (see Fig. 5-8 and Table 5-8).

2. Myotomes and peripheral nerves. A working knowledge of muscular distribution of the nerve roots (myotomes) and peripheral nerves enables the clinician to distinguish the motor loss attributable to a root lesion from that attributable to a peripheral nerve lesion (see Table 5-7). See Table 5-8 and Fig. 5-9 for myotomal testing for the cervical spine and upper thoracic nerve roots.

3. Reflex testing. Deep reflex testing should include upper limb reflexes (see Fig 11-24).
   • C5-6–biceps
   • C7–triceps

4. Other tests for sensation. The hand has many different types of sensation besides light touch that can be tested. Numerous tests have been described to evaluate the various sensory modalities of the hands. Two-point discrimination, vibratory threshold, temperature, and sudomotor activity may assist in lesion identification.[39,52,196]

   • Stereognosis is the ability to identify common objects by touch. To test stereognosis, an object is placed in the patient's hand, and the patient is not permitted to see the object. Patients with normal sensation should be able to name the object within 3 seconds of touching it.[79]

   • Semmes-Weinstein monofilament discrimination testing. The test assesses the threshold stimulus necessary for the perception of light touch to deep pressure. It is tested by using a pressure esthesiometer. This instrument consists of varying thicknesses of nylon monofilament, which are applied to the skin perpendicularly until the filament bends. The patient is not permitted to watch and is asked to identify when the filament bends. Normal values are 2.36 to 2.83 g/mm^2 pressure.[24]

   • Vibratory sense, which is closely allied with position sense, is tested using 30-cP or 256-cP tuning forks or vibrometers. Vibratory testing evaluates the threshold of stimulus needed to elicit vibration perception; this test is useful for monitoring nerve compression.[39,58] The examiner applies the vibratory instrument to one of the patient's fingertips and asks him or her to discern the differences between quality of vibration in the involved and noninvolved areas.

   • Two-point discrimination tests a patient's ability to feel one versus two blunt points placed simultaneously on the skin. This test assesses innervation density and is useful in charting nerve regeneration. A caliper or discrimination device marked in millimeter increments should be used; it should be applied to the palmar surface of the supported hand while the patient's vision is occluded.[39,109] The goal is to find the minimal distance the patient can distinguish between two stimuli. Patients with normal sensation should be able to distinguish between points 3 mm apart on the pulps of the fingers.[177]

- Moving two-point discrimination test is an indicator of functional recovery and clinically measures the quickly adapting fiber–receptor system.[39] A two-point stimulus starting at an 8-mm distance is moved from a proximal to a distal direction along the fingertip. The normal value is 2 mm; usually 7 to 10 trials are performed.[11,24,39]
- Applying warm or cold objects to the skin and asking the patient to discriminate between the two temperatures can test temperature sensation.
- Sudomotor (sweat) test. Sympathetic nerve function corresponds to sensory nerve function only initially after a lesion or in cases of complete loss of nerve function. Ninhydrin applied to the palm reacts with certain amino acids in sweat, if present, to produce a colored print; areas devoid of color can be assumed to be denervated.[79] The wrinkling test also correlates with sensory innervation. The digital pulp skin will wrinkle only if innervated, after being submerged in warm water for 5 minutes.[134]

B. Mobility of the nervous system

The upper limb tension test (ULTT) may be carried out to ascertain the degree to which neural tissue is responsible for the production of the patient's symptoms. These tests are described in Chapter 11, Shoulder and Shoulder Girdle. The suggested approach incorporates provocative maneuvers directed to the median, radial, and ulnar nerves.

C. Other diagnostic tests for peripheral nerves

1. Median nerve. Carpal tunnel syndrome is the most common compressive neuropathy affecting the median nerve.[181] The following tests may be considered:

a. Phalen's modified test (three-jaw-chuck test; Fig. 13-31). This test aids in the diagnosis of carpal tunnel syndrome. The patient performs a "three-jaw-chuck" pinch with both hands and maintains both wrists in extreme flexion by pressing the dorsum of the hands against one another. This position is held for 30 to 60 seconds. The production of pain or paresthesias into the first three or four fingers during the test suggests carpal tunnel syndrome.

b. Reverse Phalen's sign.[103] The patient makes a fist with the wrist in extension and the examiner applies pressure over the carpal tunnel for

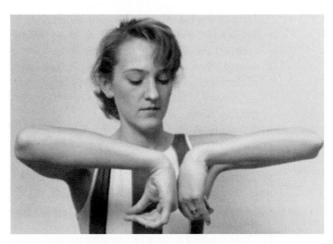

■ **FIG. 13-31.** Phalen's modified test.

1 minute. Paraesthesia in the distribution of the median nerve indicates a positive test.

c. Carpal compression test.[44] Using both thumbs, the examiner applies direct pressure on the carpal tunnel and the underlying median nerve for as long as 30 seconds. Durkan[44] found this test more accurate then the Tinel or Phalen test in diagnosing a carpal tunnel syndrome. The onset of median nerve symptoms usually occurs with 16 seconds of compression.

d. Tinel's sign. The examiner taps over the flexor retinaculum at the wrist. Paraesthesia felt distally in the hand in the distribution of the median nerve indicates a positive test. The most distal point of paraesthesia indicates the limit of nerve regeneration.[140] A positive test at the wrist may appear if the median nerve is disrupted at any point of its path. Therefore, a positive finding should warrant the examiner to assess the integrity at the neck, shoulder, and elbow to rule out other pathologic processes.

2. Ulnar nerve

a. Froment's sign. The patient is instructed to hold a piece of paper between the thumb and index finger. The examiner then tries to pull the paper out. Flexion of the patient's DIP joint of the thumb is indicative of adductor pollicis muscle paralysis as a result of ulnar nerve damage. Simultaneous hyperextension of the MCP joint of the thumb is indicative of ulnar compromise. This is known as *Jeanne's sign.*[156]

b. Wartenberg's sign. This is a finding that characterizes ulnar nerve-related motor weakness. The patient is asked to hold his or her fingers fully adducted with the MCP, PIP, and DIP joints fully extended. If the third palmar interosseus is weak (usually because of ulnar nerve dysfunction), the force of the extensor digiti minimi tendon is unopposed and the small finger tends to deviate (abduct) away from the ring finger.[156]

   c. Egawa's sign for ulnar nerve paralysis. Inability to abduct and adduct the flexed middle finger indicates paralysis of the interossei muscles because of ulnar nerve paralysis.[116]

3. Radial nerve. Wartenberg's syndrome involves entrapment of the radial sensory nerve where the nerve emerges between the tendons of the extensor carpi radialis longus and brachioradialis in the distal third of the forearm.[187]

   a. Tinel's sign may be positive along the course of the radial sensory nerve.

   b. There maybe a positive Finkelstein's test (see above).

   c. Mackinnon and Dellon[114] describe a provocative test in which the patient places the arm in front and hyperpronates the forearm with the wrist in ulnar deviation. With a positive test, the patient feels numbness and tingling over the dorsoradial aspect of the hand in 1 minute.

VI. Palpation. The elbow regions, cervical spine, thoracic spine, shoulder, and hand are palpated as appropriate.

  A. Skin
    1. Moisture
    2. Texture
    3. Temperature
    4. Mobility
    5. Tenderness. Dysesthesias, such as burning on light palpation, suggest nerve root or peripheral nerve disease (e.g., pressure).
    6. A common condition after immobilization (especially after Colles' fracture) is a reflex sympathetic dystrophy. The exact cause is unknown. Many believe it to be related to the development of edema during immobilization. Some believe it results from trauma to a nerve from the original injury (e.g., contusion of the median nerve from the displaced distal fragment in Colles' fracture). Others believe psychological factors also play an important role. In early phases of this disorder the skin may be dry, rough, and warm from decreased sympathetic activity. Later, increased sympathetic activity, with hyperhidrosis and vasoconstriction, seems to predominate. Skin palpation reveals several findings in this disorder:
      a. Hyperhidrosis
      b. Smooth, glossy skin
      c. Decreased temperature (cold, clammy hands)
      d. Hypersensitivity to normally nonnoxious sensory stimuli; even light touch may be painful.
      e. Loss of mobility of the skin in relation to subcutaneous tissues from interstitial fibrosis accompanying tissue edema

  B. Soft tissues
    1. Tenderness. Palpate tendons and ligaments, especially for local tenderness.

    2. Mobility, consistency. Soft tissues feel indurated and adherent in reflex sympathetic dystrophy from interstitial fibrosis, as well as atrophied fibrotic muscle.

    3. Edema and swelling (common with reflex sympathetic dystrophy)

    4. Pulse, radial and ulnar arteries. This may be performed in conjunction with various maneuvers of the arm (hyperabduction), shoulder girdle (depression, elevation, and retraction), and neck if thoracic outlet syndrome is suspected. The Allen test is usually performed to determine the patency of the radial, ulnar, and digital arteries: the patient pumps the blood out of the hand and then maintains a fist while the examiner occludes both arteries at the wrist; when the hand is opened it will appear white, and arterial filling on the respective side can be observed as pressure is released from one artery at a time.[44]

  C. Bones
    1. Tenderness. The radial styloid process is often the site of referred tenderness from more proximal lesions, usually within the C5 or C6 segment. It is usually also tender in de Quervain's tenosynovitis.
    2. Relationships. Palpate for structural alignment and positioning of the bony components of the wrist.

VII. Special Tests
  A. Bunnell Littner test. A test for intrinsic tightness was first described by Bunnell.[18] This test is performed by holding the patient's MCP joint in extension (stretching the intrinsics) and then passively flexing the PIP joint. The intrinsics are then relaxed by flexing the MCP joint. If the PIP joint can be passively flexed more with the MCP joint in flexion than when it is in extension, there is tightness of the intrinsics. Capsular or collateral ligament tightness of the PIP joint will limit proximal phalangeal motion, regardless of the position of the MCP joint. Loss of flexion at the DIP joint can also be caused by a joint contracture or a contracture of the oblique retinacular ligament.[69,97]

  B. Allen test (circulatory problems). This test determines the efficacy of blood flow in the radial and ulnar arteries. The patient makes a fist, then releases it several times. Next the patient makes a fist and holds it so that the venous blood is forced from the palm. The examiner locates the radial artery with his or her thumb and the ulnar artery with the index and middle fingers. Pressure is exerted on these arteries to occlude them, and the patient opens the hand. The examiner releases the pressure on one of the arteries and watches for immediate flushing. If this does not occur, or the response is slow, there is interference with the normal blood supply to the hand. The procedure is repeated for the other artery.

  C. Tests for thoracic outlet syndrome have been described in Chapter 11, Shoulder and Shoulder Girdle.

  D. Hand volume and circumferential measurements. Edema is a common problem in hand injuries. There are two popular methods of objectively measuring changes in hand sizes.[5,9,25] A volumeter is used and differences of 30 to 50 mL between one measurement and the next indicates significant hand swelling. The other method is circumferential measurements. Measurement are performed at designated sites and recorded. The sites may vary, depending on the areas of edema.

VIII. Functional assessment of the patient with a hand disability is done most effectively by using a variety of testing methods.[3,4,154] Functional assessment of the hand can include the following:

- ability to perform coordination movements may be tested by asking the patient to perform simple activities such as tying a shoelace, fastening a button, or tracing a diagram.
- ability to perform various power grips: fist, hook, and spherical and cylindrical grasp (Fig. 13-23)
- ability to perform prehension (or pinch) grips: tip pinch, and palmar and lateral prehension (Fig. 13-24).

COMMON LESIONS

Carpal Tunnel Syndrome

Carpal tunnel syndrome is very common. It is more common in women than men, and it rarely affects young people. So-called idiopathic or classic carpal tunnel follows certain patterns and is endemic in people with certain occupations such as keyboard operators, hairdressers, and dental hygienists.[28] The cause varies. Carpal tunnel syndrome occurs primarily as a thickening of the transverse carpal ligament.[28] In certain instances it is attributable to some known disorder involving increased pressure within the carpal tunnel. Such situations include a displaced fracture of the distal radius, a lunar or perilunar dislocation, and swelling of the common flexor tendon sheath. Excessive wrist flexion and extension will also increase pressure in the carpal tunnel. Conditions associated with carpal tunnel include tenosynovitis from overuse or from rheumatoid arthritis or internal pressures such as lipoma, diabetes, and pregnancy.[192] In most cases, the cause is not readily determined. Some believe it to be a vascular deficiency of the median nerve at the carpal tunnel, whereas others believe direct pressure to the nerve is the cause. Symptoms and signs accompanying this disorder are more suggestive of a pressure phenomenon.[34]

I. History

A. Onset of symptoms—usually insidious, unless they follow trauma resulting in fracture, dislocation, or swelling of the wrist

B. Nature of symptoms—The complaint is most often that of paresthesias (pins and needles) felt into the first three or four fingers. The patient is most troubled by being awakened at night, usually in the early morning, from paresthesias in the hand. The onset of paresthesias often occurs with activities involving prolonged use of the finger flexors, such as writing and sewing. Symptoms may

also increase with static positioning (e.g., driving or reading a newspaper).[71] Often the patient complains of clumsiness on activities requiring fine finger movements. At times a burning sensation is felt in the median nerve distribution of the hand as well. Subjective complaints of actual weakness are rare. The problem can be unilateral or bilateral.

C6 or C7 nerve root involvement and thoracic outlet syndrome often present as paresthesias in a similar distribution as that of carpal tunnel syndrome. In the case of nerve root involvement, however, the patient is rarely awakened by paresthesias, and use of the hand does not bring on symptoms. Differentiating carpal tunnel from thoracic outlet syndrome, based on subjective findings, is more difficult because these patients are usually awakened at night with paresthesias, and paresthesias may occur with certain activities involving use of the upper extremity. In thoracic outlet syndrome, paresthesias are more likely to involve the entire hand—although often the patient is not sure in just how many fingers paresthesias are felt—or perhaps just the more ulnar side of the hand from lower cord involvement only. The objective examination will help differentiate the two conditions in any case.

II. Physical Examination

A. Observation. There may be some clumsiness with activities requiring fine finger movements, such as handling buttons or other fasteners.

B. Inspection. Some thenar atrophy may be noticed, but usually only in chronic cases.

C. Joint tests. Joint tests include active and passive ROM of the elbow, forearm, wrist, and digits and other relevant joints including a cervical scan examination.

D. Muscle tests. Thenar weakness is the first objective sign of carpal tunnel syndrome. According to Chow,[28] it is the most valuable guide for evaluation of response to conservative therapy, and if thenar weakness is significant and persists, it indicates the need for surgery.

E. Neuromuscular tests

1. Careful sensory testing may reveal some deficit in the tips or dorsal ends of the first three or four fingers (usually the second or third). However, mild or early cases sufficient to cause significant symptoms may not present with a detectable sensory deficit. Moving two-point discrimination test has been found to be faster and more reliable than static two-point discrimination test and should read less than 4 mm (see above).[28]

2. Tinel's sign (reproduction of paresthesias by tapping the median nerve at the wrist) may be positive.

3. Modified Phalen's test (Fig. 13-31) and reverse Phalen's sign are positive. A positive test produces numbness, tingling, or pins-and-needles within 30 seconds. The more inflamed the nerve, the faster the onset.

4. Carpal compression test and the forearm compression test will produce numbness and tingling in the fingers somewhat faster than Phalen's tests.[28,44] A forearm

compression test is accomplished with the examiner's thumb compressing the median nerve at the pronator level.

5. Upper limb tension tests for the median, radial, and ulnar nerves.

6. Nerve conduction studies of the median nerve are very reliable but are often unnecessary for diagnosis.

F. Palpation—usually noncontributory. If the skin is tight and cannot be pinched by the examiner, diabetes should be suspected.[28]

III. Management. Nonsteroidal anti-inflammatory drugs are a standard part of conservative therapy, and help to reduce the edema and inflammation of the synovium in the tunnel. It has been well documented that changing activities, such as providing exercise, or interruption of activities, whether assembly line work or keyboarding, is extremely effective in relieving symptoms. Advise the patient regarding activities requiring grasping, pinching, or fine finger movements such as needlework or woodworking.

SPLINTING

These patients often do remarkably well simply by wearing a resting splint for the wrist at night. The reason why this helps is not entirely clear, except that it maintains the wrist in a neutral position, the position of least pressure within the carpal tunnel. (For this reason it seems more likely that this disorder is a pressure phenomenon rather than a release phenomenon.) The patient can be shown how to don the splint without impairing venous return from fastening straps or wraps too tightly. The splint may or may not include the fingers. It is usually unnecessary to wear the splint during the day. However, if night use does not provide relief of symptoms, a several-day trial of continuous use of the splint followed by gradual weaning should be instituted. Whether the splint is worn continuously or at night only, after 1 or 2 weeks of relief from symptoms, use of the splint can gradually be decreased and eventually discontinued.

MANUAL THERAPY

Nerve gliding exercises for mobilization of the median nerve described by Butler[19] (see Fig. 8-62), tendon gliding exercises (see Fig. 8-63), and soft tissue manipulation of carpal tunnel syndrome according to Sucher[165] and Sucher and Glassman[166] (see Fig. 8-64) also help to relieve symptoms. Quantitative rating of restriction directly over the canal can be used to monitor progress and assess the effectiveness of soft tissue manipulations. The most significant restrictions are (1) transverse extension, (2) thenar radial abduction and extension, and (3) thenar axial rotation.[165,166] The key to successful conservative treatment is early intervention addressing all structural components (i.e., muscles, joints, nerve, and skin).

Other considerations include joint mobilization, including distraction of the radiocarpal joint (see Fig. 13-39), dorsal-palmar glide of the radiocarpal joint (see Fig. 13-40), and

mobilization of the pisotriquetral joint (see Fig. 13-44). Progressive strengthening exercises in pain-free, symptom-free range of (1) elbow flexion–extension, (2) forearm pronation and supination, (3) wrist flexion and extension, and (4) grip should be included.

Only in persistent cases is surgery required to divide the flexor retinaculum and effectively relieve the pressure. Rehabilitation after release consists of wound care, if necessary; scar massage; and mobilization of the neurolyzed nerve.[114] Tendon gliding exercises (see Fig. 8-63) are used to improve ROM and isolation of tendons.

Other neurovascular syndromes, often associated with overuse syndromes of the wrist and hand, include:

- Ulnar neuropathy: Guyon canal syndrome.[146,157] Ulnar neuropathy affects individuals involved in cycling, martial arts, and other sports and activities requiring repetitive wrist motions similar to carpal tunnel syndrome. Clinically, patients present with paresthesias in the ulnar nerve distribution and variable amounts of weakness, depending on the motor involvement. Froment's sign and Wartenberg's sign can be present (see above). Grip strength testing is important because 40% of the grip strength is attributable to ulnar-innervated muscles.[146]
- Radial nerve compression at the wrist (Wartenberg syndrome) involves compression of the superficial branch of the radial nerve, also know as "handcuff neuropathy."[42,114,146,160] This may occur in sports requiring repetitive ulnar, pronation, and supination because of shear stress or may be attributable to direct compression from wristbands and taping.[42,160]

Ligamentous Sprains

The term "sprain" is often used when patients complain of pain and have a history of minor trauma. The diagnosis should be one of exclusion. Injuries that must be ruled out include fractures, traumatic instability patterns, and ligament tears.

WRIST SPRAIN

Ligamentous sprains of the wrist are common and often lead to chronic wrist pain unless treated appropriately. Ligaments most commonly involved are the lunate-capitate ligament, dorsally, and the radiocarpal ligament, palmarly. However, any of the ligaments about the wrist may conceivably be sprained.

I. History
A. Onset of pain. Ligamentous lesions are invariably of traumatic, not degenerative, onset. The patient usually recalls the traumatic event. Some impact such as striking the ground with a club or a fall on the outstretched hand may rupture one or more of several ligaments about the wrist, but often one of the ligaments attached to the lunate is sprained. This is because of the tendency toward a lunar or perilunar dislocation with such an injury. In fact, at this point in the examination, such a dislocation cannot

be ruled out. Because a fall on the outstretched hand tends to force the wrist into hyperextension, the palmar radiolunate and palmar lunocapitate ligaments tend to be sprained. However, if the lunate partially dislocates palmarly with spontaneous reduction, the dorsal radiolunate ligaments may also be sprained (Fig. 13-32).

Occasionally the fall is such that the person strikes the dorsum of the hand, forcing the wrist into extreme palmar flexion. This usually results in a sprain of one of the ligaments attached dorsally to the capitate. The ulnar collateral ligament is often sprained with a Colles' fracture.
  B. Site of pain. The pain is usually well localized to a small area that corresponds well to the site of the lesion.
  C. Nature of pain. The pain is felt with use of the wrist. Often a particular activity is cited as being most aggravating; the activity stresses the involved ligament. In the case of a dorsal radiocarpal sprain, often the activity that tends to reproduce the pain puts pressure down through the hand (as when doing push-ups).
II. Physical Examination
  A. Observation—usually noncontributory
  B. Inspection—usually noncontributory. Localized swelling after an injury to the wrist almost never accompanies a ligamentous injury only. Fracture or dislocation should be suspected.
  C. Joint test
    1. Active movements. Some pain may be noted on the extreme of a movement that stresses the ligament.

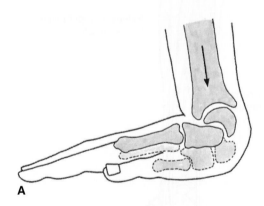

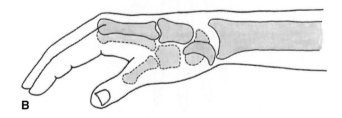

■ **FIG. 13-32.** Lunate dislocation. The injury occurs when the radius forces the lunate in a palmar direction (**A**), resulting in dislocation (**B**).

  2. Passive movements
    a. A ligamentous lesion may exist that is not stressed at the extreme of any passive anatomic movement.
    b. Often the only maneuver that reproduces the pain, other than some specific joint-play movement test, is having the patient lean forward, transmitting the body weight through the arm, forearm, extended wrist, and hand. This is most likely to reproduce pain from a lesion of the palmar radiolunate or dorsal lunocapitate ligaments.
    c. The dorsal radiocarpal ligament may be stressed on full passive pronation (applying the force through the hand and wrist to the forearm), and the palmar radiocarpal ligament may be stressed on full passive supination.
  3. Joint-play movements
    a. The specific intra-articular movement that stresses the involved ligament is likely to reproduce the pain, but again joint-play movement in itself may not be sufficient to reproduce the pain.
    b. The most important movements to perform are dorsal–palmar glide of the capitate on the lunate and the lunate on the radius.
    c. Some hypermobility of the lunate may be detected after partial dislocation and spontaneous reduction of the lunate with a fall on the dorsiflexed hand.
    d. Some hypermobility of the capitate may be detected after a fall on the palmarly flexed hand in which a lunocapitate or capitate–third metacarpal ligament may be ruptured.
  D. Muscle test—resisted movements. Strong and painless. Note: Resist pronation and supination at the distal forearm, not at the hand, to avoid stressing the radiocarpal ligaments.
  E. Neuromuscular tests—noncontributory
  F. Palpation. Localized tenderness usually corresponds well with the site of the lesion.
III. Management. The primary concern is ruling out more serious injury. Once other diagnoses are ruled out, treatment is focused on edema control, pain control, and maintaining (or increasing) active or passive ROM to the wrist and to the noninvolved joints.
  A. If necessary, splint immobilization may also be tried for pain relief. Taping the wrist may help provide support and help to decrease pain.
  B. Temporary restriction of activities that tend to stress the involved ligament. Activities that increase pain should be examined to determine whether modifications can be made to decrease pain.
  C. Friction massage to the site of the lesion to increase mobility of the collagen fibers without longitudinally stressing the ligament. As an adjunct, ultrasound may be used to assist in the resolution of chronic inflammatory exudates.
  D. After decrease in pain and edema, and return of ROM, strengthening should be performed to all wrist motions, and if necessary, to grip strength and the entire arm.

E. Joint mobilization for the wrist can help improve joint arthrokinematics and ROM.

ULNAR COLLATERAL LIGAMENT SPRAIN— FIRST MCP JOINT

An injury to the ulnar collateral ligament of the thumb at the MCP joint is sometimes called "skier's thumb" because of the high incidence of this injury in skiers. Situations in which this injury has been associated include skiers who fall on their ski pole, baseball players who slide head first into a base with their arms extended outward, soccer goalies catching a ball, and hockey players involved in a fight in which their thumb gets caught in a opponent's jersey.[41] It is also known as gamekeeper's thumb. The severity of this injury can range from a slight tear to an avulsion and dislocation of the MCP joint. Determination of instability is made clinically by weakness in pinch, swelling over the joint, and tenderness over the joint that is aggravated by excessive passive motion.[1] Surgical repair is recommended for complete rupture (grade III, unstable MCP joint). Treatment of incomplete tears (grade I or II) involves protected ROM and strengthening exercises of the thumb, with stability taking precedence over mobility.

I. Physical Examination. Request a radiographic examination to rule out the possibility of fracture.
   A. Test for ulnar collateral ligament: If radial deviation is greater than 35° (with the patient under local anesthesia) when the thumb is tested in 15° of MCP flexion, then complete rupture of the ligament is present.
   B. Partial ruptures produce local tenderness but not instability.
II. Management of Minor Sprains. Minor sprains without instability will heal if hyperabduction stress to the MCP joint of the thumb is avoided.
   A. Various strapping techniques include a "pancake" taping and a standard thumb spica, which help to prevent abduction.[41] A thumb spica splint is also useful in these injuries to shorten the ulnar collateral ligament and place it in an optimal position for healing.
   B. Therapeutic exercises after immobilization (surgical or nonsurgical) include pain-free thumb MCP flexion and extension and gradually adding pain-free rotation and opposition.[16] Grip and pinch strengthening exercises are initiated after 4 to 6 weeks. Exercises that simulate functional activities should be added as symptoms allow.
   C. Soft tissue techniques and joint mobilization should be encouraged as soon as possible to prevent contractures.

Tendinitis and Tenosynovitis of Wrist and Hand

Tendinitis can occur as a result of tension overload or shear stress. Clancy[29] noted that tension overload occurs in muscle, at the musculotendinous junction, in the tendon substance itself, or at its bony attachment to bone. Shear stress can occur where tendons pass in close proximity to fixed structure (e.g., de Quervain's syndrome [see below]).[146]

WRIST TENDINITIS OR TENOSYNOVITIS

Many of the wrist tendons can be involved, but the major involvement is from the extensor carpi radialis, extensor carpi ulnaris (Fig. 13-33), flexor carpi radialis (Fig. 13-34), the finger flexors, or the thumb extensors (Fig. 13-35).[87] Usually, some transitional elements, such as excessive amount of work, a change in throwing or hitting pattern, or traumatic injury, is the inciting incident.

I. History. The patient will report a history of repetitive use or trauma to the involved structure. Pain worsens with the provoking activity of the wrist and hand, which may affect the grip or repetitive hand motions.
II. Objective findings. Pain whenever the related muscle contracts or whenever there is movement of another joint that causes gliding of the tendon through the sheath.
   A. Warmth and point tenderness over the tendon itself, usually in association with the extensor retinaculum or flexor

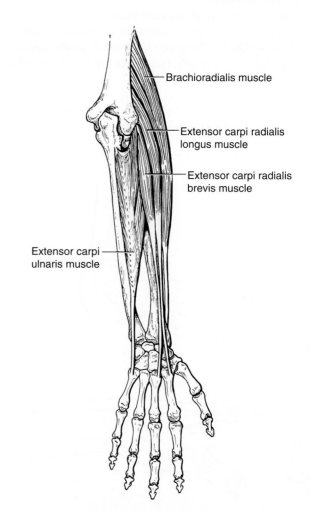

■ FIG. 13-33. Superficial muscles and tendons of the posterior compartment of the forearm. (Reprinted with permission from Pratt NE: Clinical Musculoskeletal Anatomy. Philadelphia, JB Lippincott, 1991:118.)

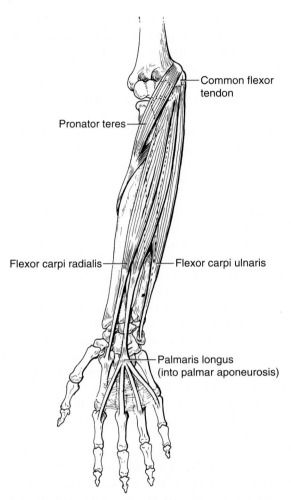

■ FIG. 13-34. Superficial muscles and tendons of the anterior compartment of the forearm. (Reprinted with permission from Pratt NE: Clinical Musculoskeletal Anatomy. Philadelphia, JB Lippincott, 1991:110.)

Labels (Fig. 13-34):
- Common flexor tendon
- Pronator teres
- Flexor carpi radialis
- Flexor carpi ulnaris
- Palmaris longus (into palmar aponeurosis)

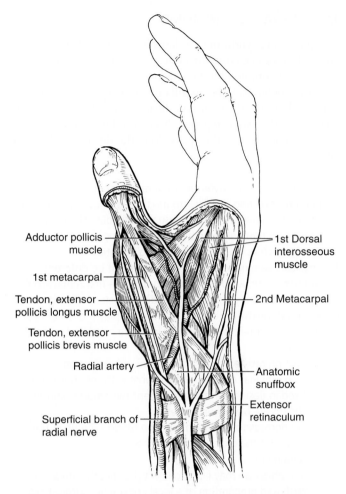

■ FIG. 13-35. Lateral view of the distal forearm, wrist, and hand. (Reprinted with permission from Pratt NE: Clinical Musculoskeletal Anatomy. Philadelphia, JB Lippincott, 1991:125.)

Labels (Fig. 13-35):
- Adductor pollicis muscle
- 1st metacarpal
- Tendon, extensor pollicis longus muscle
- Tendon, extensor pollicis brevis muscle
- Radial artery
- Superficial branch of radial nerve
- 1st Dorsal interosseous muscle
- 2nd Metacarpal
- Anatomic snuffbox
- Extensor retinaculum

retinaculum.[87] There maybe crepitus and soreness to direct pressure, with occasional snapping or locking of the tendon as it runs through the irritated area.
B. Resisted motion is strong and painful.
C. Passive stretch in the opposite direction may also hurt.
D. Frequently there is an imbalance in muscle length and strength or poor endurance in the stabilizing muscles. The fault may be more proximal in the elbow or shoulder, thus causing excessive load and substitute motion at the distal end of the chain.[89]

III. Management
A. Acute phase rehabilitation consists of relieving the stress in the involved muscles and maintaining a healthy environment for healing with nondestructive forces.
1. The wrist may be supported by taping, splinting, or casting in severe cases. Cryotherapy and oral anti-inflammatory agents are generally used.
2. If the tendon is in a sheath, apply cross-fiber massage while the tendon is in an elongated position (see Figs. 8-25 and 8-26).
3. Perform multi-angle muscle setting techniques in pain-free positions followed by pain-free ROM.
B. Subacute and chronic phases
1. Progress the intensity of exercises and stretching techniques. Increases in passive motion are best achieved through low-intensity, long-duration stretches. Strengthening should be started isometrically and progress throughout the entire ROM, concentrically and eccentrically as tolerated.
2. Assess the biomechanics of the functional activities provoking the symptoms and design a program to regain balance in length, strength, and endurance of muscles. Most cases of wrist tendinitis should respond to appropriate treatment within 14 to 21 days.[87]

DE QUERVAIN'S SYNDROME

De Quervain's syndrome is relatively common. Tenovaginitis of the first dorsal compartment, or de Quervain syndrome, is the most common tendinitis of the wrist in athletes.[146] It is generally believed to be an inflammation and swelling of the synovial lining of the common sheath of the abductor pollicis longus and the extensor pollicis brevis tendons (see Figs. 8-24, 13-14, 13-35), where they pass along the distal-radial aspect of the radius.

I. History. Pain is felt over the distal-radial aspect of the radius, perhaps radiating distally into the thumb or even proximally up the forearm. The onset is usually insidious. The patient notes pain primarily with activities involving thumb movements, such as wringing or grasping activities.

II. Physical Examination. This condition must be differentiated from osteoarthrosis of the trapezium–first metacarpal joint, also a fairly common disorder. In osteoarthrosis, A. and B. below are negative and joint-play movements at the trapezium–first metacarpal joint are restricted and painful.
   A. Pain on resisted thumb extension and abduction
   B. Pain on ulnar deviation of the wrist with the thumb held fixed in flexion. On this movement the tendons and the sheath are placed on a stretch.
   C. Tenderness to palpation over the tendon sheath in the region of the radial styloid process

III. Management
   A. The physician may elect to inject the sheath with a corticosteroid preparation or a local anesthetic. Surgical incision of the sheath is occasionally performed.
   B. If injection is not contemplated or if it is unsuccessful, a trial of ultrasound and friction massage (to the shared sheath) where the muscles pass over the wrist extensors; (see Fig. 8-24) for a 1- or 2-week period, on a basis of three to five times a week, is warranted. The goal of this program is to maintain and increase mobility of the tendons within the sheath and to help resolve the chronic inflammatory process. In more severe or persistent cases, temporary restriction of thumb movements with a small opponens splint should be considered to prevent continued irritation to the inflamed sheath process.

TRIGGER FINGER

Trigger finger, also known as digital tenovaginitis stenosans, is the result of thickening of the flexor tendon sheath. The function of the digital flexor tendon retinacular sheath (that is, the annular ligament) is to tightly restrain the tendon as it crosses the flexed MCP joint, serving as a simple pulley to prevent bowstringing from origin to insertion during contraction. Repetitive gliding of the tendon under the restraining sheath as from excessive repetitive handwork or unconscious fist clenching may exceed the lubricating capacity of synovial fluid and produce trigger finger.[149] The resulting friction generates localized inflammation at the point where the tendon enters the sheath, causing swelling of the tendon (tendinitis), which over time irritates the opening of the sheath causing inflammation and thickening (tenosynovitis).[36] Trigger finger progresses to the development of a fusiform swelling—a nodule in either the deep or superficial tendon or tendons at the metacarpal heads.[131]

Although tenovaginitis is usually secondary to degenerative changes in the A-1 pulley and flexor tendons, direct pressure on the distal palm and metacarpophalangeal flexion crease from a racquet, golf club, or bat can cause acute inflammation and produce trigger finger in the athlete.

Impairment associated with trigger finger includes pain and tenderness in the finger from the volar MCP to the PIP level and intermittent triggering or "snapping" of the finger. The digit often locks in flexion when the patient arises from sleep.[147] The triggering usually occurs with flexion, and it may require passive assist to fully extend the finger.

Early treatment consists in tapping or splinting the finger in extension at night along with nonsteroidal anti-inflammatory medication. Active interphalangeal flexion and tendon gliding exercises (see Fig. 8-63) on an hourly basis are recommended.[16] Ultrasound, soft tissue mobilization, and icing can be used to relieve symptoms of pain and swelling. When more chronic, a corticosteroid injection into the sheath is recommended, with cure rates from 36 to 84% reported in the literature.[119,143]

If conservative management is unsuccessful, surgical release by longitudinal incision of the thickened sheath is indicated. Postoperative therapy includes the same active exercise program and potential splinting as conservative management.

Extensor Tendon Injuries

A brief review of some common finger injuries is instructive because it emphasizes the functional importance of various structures of the extensor apparatus (Fig. 13-22).

MALLET FINGER

When the extensor tendon is evulsed from the distal phalanx, with or without a chip of bone, or when the lateral bands are ruptured or cut, flexion deformity results at the DIP joint (*baseball* or *mallet finger*). The torn ligament or the fracture may heal if the finger is immobilized with the DIP in extension.

Treatment (in the absence of a large fracture) is splinting the DIP joint in neutral to slight hyperextension for 6 to 8 weeks with no flexion of the DIP joint.[43,162] If the DIP joint is flexed even once during this period, the 6 weeks starts again at that time. ROM of noninvolved fingers and joints should be maintained.

Once the tendon is healed and splinting discontinued, active ROM to DIP joints is started. No attempts to passively flex the finger to regain ROM should be attempted for 4 weeks after splinting is discontinued.[155] Full ROM is usually gained by blocking exercises and regular functional use of the hand. Blocking DIP exercises encourage flexor digitorum profundus pull-through. Stabilizing the middle phalanx allows flexion force to concentrate at the DIP joint. Blocked DIP exercises are most often done with extensor tendon injuries, flexion tendon injuries, or finger fractures.

BOUTONNIERE DEFORMITY

If the central slip of the digital expansion is ruptured, minimal deformity results as long as the transverse fibers of the expansion remain in tact. If they are also torn, a deformity is produced at the PIP joint, which the English-speaking orthopaedic community calls the *boutonniere deformity* whereas the French call it the buttonhole.[148] In this case, all extensor force will be transmitted to the distal phalanx by intact lateral bands, producing hyperextension of the DIP joint. The PIP joint buckles into flexion and protrudes through the breech in the extensor hood. The two lateral bands will now run on the palmar aspect of the PIP joint and will exaggerate flexion. Treatment options include prolonged splinting or surgery for patients who present for evaluation with a chronic injury.

Treatment for acute injury is uninterrupted splinting of the PIP in full extension for 6 weeks.[156] After 6 weeks of immobilization, exercises as described by Burton and Melchior[19] are begun. The exercise involves two sequential maneuvers. The first is active assisted PIP joint extension. This will stretch the tight volar structures, will cause the lateral bands to ride dorsal to the PIP joint axis, and will put longitudinal tension on the lateral bands and oblique retinacular ligaments.[61] The second maneuver is maximal active forced flexion of the DIP joint while the PIP joint is held at 0° or as close to that position as the PIP will allow. This will gradually stretch the lateral bands and oblique retinacular ligaments to their physiologic length. Continue splinting 2 to 4 weeks when not exercising.[155] When full PIP joint extension can be maintained throughout the day, then night splinting only is appropriate. Length of treatment and splinting may be several weeks.

Flexor and Extensor Tendon Repair

One area of challenge to clinicians who see hand patients is that of postoperative management of flexor and extensor tendon repairs. The mechanism of injury and status of the patient influence the management and method of repair, which is beyond the scope of this chapter (see suggested reading list).

Dupuytren's Contracture

A contracture of the palmar aponeurosis with insidious onset and no history of injury are suggestive of Dupuytren's contracture.[113] Early in the course of this disease there is painless proliferation of fibroblasts, histologically manifesting as a low-grade inflammatory fibrosis that results in the transformation of noncontractile tissue into contractile tissue. A small node in the palm of the hand is the initial symptom. Further

contraction of the palmar fascia leads to flexion contracture of the fingers, especially the ring and little fingers, which are affected in 85%.[110]

The cause is still unknown, but it seems to occur more often in combination with alcoholism, disorders of the liver, diabetes, and epilepsy.[70,74,95,180] Microtrauma may play a role. This disorder may also appear as a late sequela to shoulder–hand syndrome after myocardial infarction.[149] It is common in men after the age of 30, whereas in women it does not occur younger than the age of 45. One or both hands may be affected, although the right hand is more frequently affected when the involvement is unilateral. In 5% of patients similar contractures occur in the feet.[131]

I. Physical Examination
    A. Observation. Pitting, fissuring, puckering, and dimpling over the palmar crease on the ulnar side of the hand with flexion contractures, typically involving the MCP and PIP joints of the ring or little finger.
    B. Palpation. Prominent nodules are felt at the ring and the little fingers, and the involved fingers cannot be passively straightened.
II. Management
    A. Conservative management in milder cases before surgical treatment. Ultrasound therapy and ionization have been said to lead to a certain amount of softening of nodules but have not been effective on cords.[99] Orally administered vitamin E, posterior extension splints, moist heat, and stretching to elongate the palmar fascia have all been advocated.[121]
    B. Postoperative therapy (after partial or complete fasciectomy). Prolonged postoperative therapy may be required for several months and is necessary to obtain optimal results.[149]
        • Edema control including elevation and muscular activity (i.e., bilateral overhead actively making a fist 10 times each hour). In cases of severe pitting edema, external compression using an intermittent compression unit is helpful to reduce edema. Soft tissue manipulation and string wrapping or the use of Coban wraps (Minnesota Mining and Manufacturing Co., 3M, St. Paul, MN) applied to the digits and hand also assist in reduction of edema.[112] An Isotoner glove (Aris Isotoner Glove, New York, NY) may also be helpful in controlling edema while allowing the patient to use the hand with minimal restrictions.[53,112]
        • Active exercise, tendon-gliding exercises (see Fig. 8-63), and finger blocking exercises. Progress to more difficult exercises (i.e., sustained grip–strengthening exercises), including functional exercises when indicated.
        • Gentle passive ROM of all joints
        • Splinting. Posterior extension splints or if flexion is a problem flexion splinting may be necessary.
        • Scar tissue massage with lanolin (see Box 8-5)
        • Desensitization programs if appropriate

- The importance of a carefully supervised early post-operative active-motion exercise and splinting program cannot be overemphasized.

Colles' Fracture

In most outpatient settings, patients who have sustained a Colles' fracture make up the largest proportion of those with wrist disorders. The term *Colles' fracture* is usually used to refer to fractures of the distal end of the radius, with or without an associated fracture at the distal ulna. This is one of the most common of all fractures. It affects primarily older people. Women are afflicted more often than men because of the prevalence of osteoporosis, especially in older women. These patients are often referred to therapists after the period of immobilization because of complications resulting in residual loss of function. The two most common complications after these injuries are malunion (*not* nonunion) of bony fragments, and development of a reflex sympathetic dystrophy. Pain and loss of movement are the major factors limiting function after immobilization of a Colles' fracture.

MECHANISM AND NATURE OF INJURY

Colles' fracture usually results from a fall on the outstretched hand in an older person. The patient lands with the wrist in dorsiflexion and the forearm in pronation. The lunate acts as a wedge to shear the distal 2 cm or so of the radius off in a dorsal direction. The momentum of the body weight causes the distal fragment to displace radially and rotate in a supinatory direction with respect to the proximal bone end (Fig. 13-26). Because this metaphyseal area of bone is typically osteoporotic, the compression force often results in comminution and impaction of the distal fragment. The major fracture line runs transversely across the distal radius, usually about 2 cm proximal to the radiocarpal joint. The momentum that results in radial displacement may also cause a sprain of the ulnar collateral ligament and an avulsion fracture of the ulnar styloid process.[39]

The characteristic dinner fork deformity results from the wrist and hand being displaced dorsally with respect to the forearm (Fig. 13-27). Often included in the deformity is radial displacement of the wrist and hand.

MANAGEMENT BY PHYSICIAN

Closed manipulative reduction is usually performed in an effort to bring the fragments back into anatomic alignment unless surgical intervention is indicated. Reduction is usually not so much of a problem as is maintenance of reduction. In unstable, comminuted fractures the distal fragment tends to slip back into its postinjury position of dorsal, radial, and supinatory displacement. In an attempt to maintain anatomic reduction, the wrist is usually splinted in a position of flexion and ulnar deviation, with pronation. The elbow is usually left free. Because the elbow is left free, splinting in a

position of excessive pronation may result in a force tending to pull the distal fragment into radial displacement and supination from tension on the brachioradialis with elbow extension. This would defeat the original purpose of positioning the part in pronation and ulnar deviation.

The plaster splint is left on for at least 4 weeks. Nonunion is rare as this fracture occurs in highly vascularized, metaphyseal bone.

COMPLICATIONS

Malunion. A Colles' fracture rarely heals without some residual malalignment. The radius invariably ends up foreshortened such that the radial styloid process no longer extends beyond the ulnar styloid process. The distal end of the radius also tends to be angulated and displaced dorsally; the distal radial articulation surface no longer faces 10 to 15° in a palmar direction. The malalignment described above will result in a permanent loss of full wrist flexion and ulnar deviation. In addition, there may be some residual malalignment of the distal fragment toward supination, resulting in a permanent loss of pronation. The distal fragment may also heal when displaced radially, but this would have little effect on motion.

Reflex Sympathetic Dystrophy. Reflex sympathetic dystrophy is not uncommon after Colles' fracture; in our experience it develops more often after Colles' fracture than after any other injury. Most patients sent to therapy after immobilization of a Colles' fracture have this condition to some degree; otherwise they probably would not require ongoing therapy.[22,40,126,127,163,164,194]

The pathophysiology is not well understood. It is generally agreed, however, that sympathetic dysfunction occurs as part of a vicious circle initiated reflexly by some alteration in afferent input from the periphery. Several proposals have been offered as to the precipitating factor, including direct trauma to a peripheral nerve, edema from prolonged immobilization, pain, and psychological predisposition. The characteristic features of the disorder are hyperalgesia, edema, and capsular tightness of the joints of the hand, wrist, and often the shoulder—it is often referred to as shoulder–hand syndrome, although the shoulder is not always involved. The elbow occasionally stiffens as well. In other than the early phases of this condition, there is usually increased sympathetic activity involving the distal part of the extremity, with vasoconstriction and hyperhidrosis. The vasoconstriction causes a cyanotic appearance and atrophy of the musculoskeletal tissues; the skin becomes glossy and thin, the nails brittle, and the bones osteoporotic. Early osteopenia, seen on roentgenography, is often marked. This early bone atrophy is believed to be a result of the hyperemia often present in the earlier stages; excessive blood flow to bone causes increased resorption.

Carpal Tunnel Syndrome. The median nerve may be traumatized at the time of injury. Prolonged pressure to the nerve may occur from malalignment of bony fragments, persistent edema involving the carpal tunnel, or both. (See the section on carpal tunnel syndrome above for a discussion of symptoms and signs.)

Late Rupture of Extensor Pollicis Longus Tendon. The extensor pollicis longus tendon normally takes quite a sharp turn around Lister's tubercle at the dorsum of the distal radius on its way to inserting at the thumb (Fig. 13-35). Malalignment of bony parts after Colles' fracture may cause excessive friction to this tendon, which may result in fraying of the tendon and eventual rupture. Pain on active and passive thumb flexion or opposition and pain on resisted thumb extension suggest such a problem before actual rupture. Painless weakness of thumb extension, at some time after the injury, is characteristic of rupture of the tendon.

I. History
   A. Determine the date of the initial injury, subsequent treatment, the length of time the part was immobilized, and the dates of splint removal. Ask whether exercise and elevation activities were performed while the part was immobilized. A patient whose wrist has been immobilized for 8 weeks with no instruction in shoulder exercises and elevation activities and who has not used the part since removal of the splint 2 weeks ago will present with more dysfunction and disability than the patient who has just come out of the splint after having had the wrist immobilized for 6 weeks, during which time ROM for the shoulder was performed, along with intermittent periods of elevation and active finger movements.
   B. Ask the standard questions relating to the patient's pain (see Chapter 5, Assessment of Musculoskeletal Disorders and Concepts of Management). Any acute inflammatory process, initiated at the time of injury, should have resolved during immobilization. Considering this, any residual pain would be expected to be related primarily to stiffness and would be associated with use of the part. Complaints of pain at rest, pain that awakens the patient at night, and inability to use the part because of pain suggest reflex sympathetic dystrophy in this case. Note any complaints of shoulder pain because of the possibility of stiffening of the shoulder from immobilization and perhaps shoulder–hand syndrome. Pain on use of the thumb may suggest involvement of the extensor pollicis longus tendon. Complaints of burning pain or paresthesias into the median nerve distribution of the hand should lead one to suspect carpal tunnel syndrome.
   C. Determine and document the patient's present functional status.
      1. What specific daily activities cannot be performed with the involved hand that could be performed before the injury?
      2. What activities can be performed but with difficulty or pain?
      3. Consider, especially, eating, grooming, dressing, household chores, occupational activities, and recreational activities.

II. Physical Examination
   A. Observation. Typically these patients walk into the room holding the hand and forearm out in front of them, across the chest or abdomen.
      1. Is the arm used when rising from a chair?
      2. Does the arm hang normally to the side and swing freely and normally when walking?
      3. Does the patient use the hand and arm during dressing activities, or does he or she guard it carefully?
      4. Observe the face for wincing during movement of the part.
   B. Inspection
      1. Posture. The patient should be evaluated for the presence of spinal scoliosis, thoracic kyphosis, forward head, and forward internally rotated shoulders. If these postural deviations develop after injury, pertinent therapeutic intervention can be added to the program.
      2. Skin and nails. Note especially trophic changes suggestive of a reflex sympathetic dystrophy: brittle, split nails; smooth, glossy skin; cyanotic appearance to skin in the distal part of the extremity.
      3. Subcutaneous soft tissue. Atrophy of the forearm muscles is invariably found but may be masked by edema, which is usually noticed most in the hand and forearm.
      4. Bony structure and alignment. Some degree of malalignment is likely to be present. In the classic dinner fork deformity, the wrist and hand are offset dorsally with respect to the forearm. There is usually some displacement radially also. The radial styloid process may no longer extend further distally than the ulnar styloid process, as it should, because of impaction of the distal fragment.
   C. Joint tests
      1. Active and passive ROM
         a. The interphalangeal and MCP joints of the hand are usually restricted in a capsular pattern—the MCP joints are especially restricted in flexion, the interphalangeal joints especially restricted in extension.
         b. Wrist and forearm movements are restricted in all planes. Flexion, ulnar deviation, and pronation are likely to be restricted from bony malalignment; check for bony end feel. Extension, radial deviation, and supination are likely to be limited because the hand is usually immobilized in a position opposite each of these movements (see above).
         c. All movements are likely to be painful at the extremes, especially in the presence of a reflex sympathetic dystrophy.
         d. Check shoulder ROM for possible capsular tightening.
      2. Joint-play movements. Considerable restriction of all joint-play movements of the wrist and hand is likely to be found.
   D. Muscle tests
      1. Resisted movements

a. Pain on resisted thumb extension may suggest involvement of the extensor pollicis longus tendon secondary to bony malalignment.

b. Otherwise, resisted movements should be strong and painless.

2. Muscle strength. A routine examination should include testing the strength of the upper limb muscles beginning at the shoulder. Prehensile (grip and pinch) strength should be determined: mean for age and sex norms or comparison with uninvolved side.

E. Neuromuscular tests. Here concern is primarily with the function of the median nerve. The special tests mentioned under carpal tunnel syndrome should be performed.

F. Palpation
1. Skin
a. The skin is likely to feel cool, moist, smooth, and tight, especially in the presence of a reflex sympathetic dystrophy.
b. Tenderness to light palpation of the skin is characteristic of a reflex sympathetic dystrophy.
2. Subcutaneous soft tissue. Pitting-type edema is very often present distally. The tissues may feel tight and bound down in the hand and forearm because of the fibrosis accompanying prolonged edema.
3. Bones. Careful bony palpation will reveal the extent of residual malalignment.

G. Other. A radiologist's report should be ordered so that the therapist can determine the degree of bony malalignment. This is helpful in setting treatment goals. Also, marked osteoporosis usually accompanies a reflex sympathetic dystrophy. As much as 40% of bone resorption may occur before osteopenia shows up on roentgenograms. If roentgenograms suggest considerable osteoporosis, techniques to regain ROM must not be performed using forces applied over a long lever arm.

MANAGEMENT

Functional use of the part is lost or restricted primarily because of pain and loss of motion. As in any joint in which motion is lost from capsular tightening, much of the pain may be caused by joint stiffness; the joint capsule is stretched excessively during use of the part. However, these patients often complain of pain out of proportion to the extent of the dysfunction. Such an abnormal pain state is characteristic of a reflex sympathetic dystrophy. In such situations the patient may complain of severe pain to light touch or another normally nonnoxious stimulation. This complaint may act as a considerable barrier to efforts to regain joint motion.

Pain Management. If such an abnormal pain state is apparent, special care must be taken not to reinforce the patient's pain behavior and not to allow such reinforcement by family members, so as to avoid development of an operant pain problem. On the other hand, the patient's very real pain problem cannot be ignored. The patient must be advised that although he or she is not imagining the pain, it does not serve

a useful function by signaling potential harm to tissues. Unless the problem is carefully explained to the patient, he or she cannot be expected to follow home instructions that may include exercises and other activities that may be painful. The patient will also doubt the therapist's professional judgment if certain techniques that cause considerable discomfort are used, unless the rationale of their use is carefully explained.

The therapist must also try to make the treatment sessions as painless as possible. This is one disorder in which some modality or procedure might be used solely for its effect to reduce pain, so as to allow the therapist to perform other treatment procedures, such as joint mobilization. A whirlpool bath during or just before mobilization procedures may act as a counterirritant, as well as increasing blood flow to the part. The part may be kept in the water for application of ultrasound in preparation for mobilization procedures.

Restoration of Joint Motion. These patients require an intensive mobilization program. All the joints of the extremity, with the possible exception of the elbow, are likely to be restricted in the case of reflex sympathetic dystrophy.[20] It is usually desirable to have the patient come in for treatment at least three times a week for joint mobilization. Treatment should include ultrasound to help increase the extensibility of capsular tissue, followed by specific joint mobilization techniques. Such techniques are especially indicated because they are performed with forces applied over very short lever arms.

A home program of active and active-assisted ROM exercises should be instituted. Take care to show the patient exercises that do not involve forces applied over long lever arms, especially when working on finger flexion and extension. These patients usually have some degree of tissue edema that contributes to the restriction in ROM. Frequent elevation of the part with activation of the muscle pump should be included in the home program. Encourage use of the part for dressing, grooming, and light activities.

Simple strengthening exercises for finger, wrist, and shoulder muscles should also be instituted. Strengthening the rotator cuff is especially important because of the important role these muscles play biomechanically. Exercises should be kept simple, and the number of exercises should be minimized. The patient who becomes confused or exhausted with a home program is likely to abandon the program completely. This is an important consideration: these patients need to perform ROM exercises for most of the upper extremity joints, in addition to strengthening exercises and elevation activities. Whenever possible, exercises should be designed that incorporate strengthening, ROM, and elevation so as to keep the program simple and concise.

If a marked or persistent reflex sympathetic dystrophy presents a major obstruction to rehabilitation, the patient may undergo a series of sympathetic blocks. In such a program the patient may be admitted to the hospital or to ambulatory surgery. The stellate ganglion is injected with an anesthetic in an attempt to reduce sympathetic activity to the part and to break up the cycle. Typically, a series of five injections is given on a daily basis. Such a program in no way precludes continuation of the normal physical therapy program. In fact, the ideal situation is for the patient to be seen in physical therapy each day after the block for mobilization procedures. Treating associated findings in the thoracic spine may also indirectly reduce sympathetic activity.[20] Obviously, close communication and cooperation among orthopaedics, anesthesiology, and physical therapy personnel is important here.

The active phase of a reflex sympathetic dystrophy after a Colles' fracture tends to resolve during several months. However, the patient may be left with some residual disability. Some residual loss of motion is not unlikely because of the often-extensive fibrosis of joint capsules as well as extra-articular structures. Goals, in these cases, should be set toward restoring *functional* motion, not necessarily *physiologic* motion. In older persons, the two are less likely to coincide. Of more significance, however, is the tendency for a chronic pain state to develop. Operant management at this point may be indicated over, or in addition to, continued physical treatment. The possibility of psychological consultation should be discussed with the physician.

Too often these patients continue to come in for treatment for a prolonged period without demonstrable improvement in function. Although vigorous treatment is indicated in the early phase after immobilization, once improvement plateaus for, say, a 2- or 3-week period, treatment should gradually be discontinued in favor of a progressive home program. However, improvement is rarely linear in such cases, and some fluctuation between spurts of improvement and periods of plateauing can be expected. Until satisfactory, functional use of the part is regained, intermittent follow-up visits should be arranged for reassessment and progression of the home program. As usual, improvement should be based primarily on objective findings and subjective reports of increased function, not on subjective reports of decreased pain.

Scaphoid Fracture and Lunate Dislocation

In an older person, a fall on the outstretched hand results in a Colles' fracture because the proximal carpals are jammed into the weak osteoporotic radius. However, in a younger person, in whom the radius is strong and healthy, the scaphoid may fracture on impact, or the radius may force the lunate palmarly, resulting in lunate dislocation in a palmar direction (Fig. 13-32).

LUNATE DISLOCATION

A lunate dislocation may be detected on a standard anteroposterior roentgenogram by the lunate appearing triangular rather than quadrangular and, in a lateral view, by its abnormal position. The therapist should always palpate for lunate positioning in patients referred to physical therapy after a fall on the outstretched hand. It may be reduced if seen early by placing the wrist in extension and putting pressure on the dorsal aspect of the lunate. Subluxations may be treated by a high-velocity, low-amplitude thrust technique.[80]

If repaired surgically, progression is very similar to the rehabilitation of distal radius fractures and other wrist injuries. Motions that need to be addressed for ROM and strengthening are flexion, extension, radial and ulnar deviation, supination, and pronation.

SCAPHOID FRACTURE

A scaphoid fracture is not always so obvious (Fig. 13-36). Often a fracture here does not show up on standard roentgenograms. A key clinical sign is localized bony tenderness in the anatomic snuffbox on palpation. When this is found in a patient referred after a fall on the outstretched hand, the therapist should suspect a scaphoid fracture and should consult the physician. The incidence of avascular necrosis of the proximal fragment of the scaphoid is high with this fracture because the blood supply to the scaphoid often enters only from the distal aspect of the bone. The fracture, then, cuts off the blood supply to the proximal fragment. Strict, prolonged immobilization of the wrist and thumb is necessary to minimize the possibility of avascular necrosis and nonunion.

Treatment of the nondisplaced scaphoid is casting. After casting, an additional 2 to 4 weeks of splinting may be used (i.e., thumb spica), with the removal of the splint for the exercise program.[155] Active ROM exercises of the wrist, thumb are initiated after immobilization. After approximately 2 weeks (sooner if cleared by the physician), passive ROM to the wrist and thumb is begun. Gentle strengthening with weights or putty may be started around the same time frame. Strength-

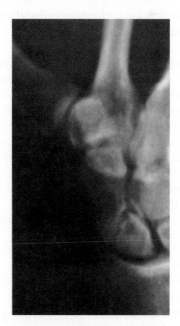

■ **FIG. 13-36.** Transverse fracture at the level of the proximal third of the scaphoid. (Reprinted with permission from D'Ambrosia RD, ed: Musculoskeletal Disorders: Regional Examination and Differential Diagnosis, 2nd ed. Philadelphia, JB Lippincott, 1986:440.)

ening is progressed accordingly and may include weight-bearing activities, general arm conditioning, and plyometrics.

Surgical repair rehabilitation is the same progression as nonsurgical.

Secondary Osteoarthritis of Thumb

The carpometacarpal joint of the thumb is particularly susceptible to osteoarthrosis. Women are more predisposed to this disorder than are men, and it can occur without evidence of osteoarthrosis in any other joint.[21,22] Typically it is bilateral, although it can be unilateral and may occur after prolonged overuse or trauma. It is a common finding after Bennett's fracture.[196]

The key structures in the trapeziometacarpal joint are the palmar or ulnar ligaments, which hold the beak of the thumb metacarpal down to the ridge on the trapezium, and the intermetacarpal ligaments, which hold the first to the second metacarpal (Fig. 13-8).[135] In normal flexion and extension these ligaments undergo very little stress. However, in opposition and power pinch the joint surfaces twist one on the other and are prevented from coming apart by these ligaments.[94] Unequal stresses over time, an incongruency resulting from injured joint surface, or ligamentous disruption can result in osteoarthrosis (as the initial stage) with the ultimate development of osteoarthritis.[58,104]

Initially, erosion of the joint surfaces causes pain. After a time, the joint commonly subluxates because of degenerative changes, causing a gradual proximal travel of the metacarpal base of the saddle of the trapezium, together with an adduction deformity.[26] A secondary hyperextension deformity of the MCP joint may develop with attempted abduction, resulting in weakness and loss of function.

I. History. The patient's first complaints are usually of pain aggravated by use. Advice is often sought long before destructive changes occur. Typical symptoms include:
   A. Pain on extremes of movement of the thumb or when gripping or holding tools for long periods. The pain is usually localized to the base of the thumb, just anterior and distal to the anatomic snuffbox (Fig. 13-35).
   B. Marked instability and weakness of the hand, with a tendency to drop things and difficulty guiding or manipulating tools
   C. Occasional subjective complaints of numbness of the thumb and stiffness
   D. Deep-seated grinding, which is particularly uncomfortable
   E. Occasional swelling
II. Physical Examination
   A. In later stages the patient may present with an adduction deformity and hyperextension of the MCP joint.
   B. Active ROM will often reveal crepitus and increased motion.
   C. Passive backward stretching of the thumb in abduction brings on the pain. The grind test is positive (see Joint Integrity Tests above).

D. Joint-play motions, particularly axial rotation, reproduce the pain. Later instability of the joint is evidenced by the prominence of the metacarpal base and hypermobility.[104]
   E. Resisted motions are painless. Pinch strength will progressively decrease.
   F. Tenderness is well localized over the joint on its anterior aspect. Osteophytes are sometimes palpable anteriorly.
III. Management
   A. In the early stages the physician may elect to use corticosteroid injections. In advanced cases intra-articular silicone is often effective, and for this reason arthroplasty and arthrodesis are required less often than formerly.[35] If arthritis clearly involves other trapezial joints, arthrodesis of the trapeziometacarpal joint will give only limited relief of symptoms, as will arthroplasty of that joint. Excision of the trapezium may be necessary, and good results have been reported from this procedure alone.[26,37,59] If the joint remains unstable, replacement of the excised trapezium by rolled tendon[123] or fascia[195] or with a Silastic prosthesis is increasingly practiced.[45,46,50,105,141,170]
   B. In the early stages, osteoarthrosis or traumatic arthritis responds well to friction massage.[35] Joint compression treatment can also provide relief.[128] At any point, fitting the patient with a splint can also provide relief. Patients often find it useful to continue to use the splint for many months or even years while undertaking heavy work. Mobilization techniques, when indicated, and isometric exercises are useful.

Patient education should include emphasis on avoiding positions of stress and activities that provoke the symptoms.

STIFF HAND

Stiffness and capsular restriction at the wrist and hand proper are common clinical problems seen by physical therapists. Whether caused by fracture immobilization, soft tissue contractures (Dupuytren's disease), burns, reflex sympathetic dystrophy, postoperative reconstructive hand surgery, complications of mastectomy, joint disease, peripheral nerve injury, or constriction by a cast or poorly applied dressing, the stiffness of the fingers and hand proper (metacarpals) that may result can be ruinous. Mobility is essential in normal function, and it can be disastrous when roentgenographic results of a fracture of the hand are normal but the patient is left with a stiff "frozen" hand.[196]

The major contributor to the stiff or frozen hand is edema. Postoperative or posttraumatic edema of the hand has been shown to be a normal physiologic response to injury. Edema is reversible; the degree and rapidity of reversibility determine its deleterious effect. If edema can be controlled early, subsequent scar formation is minimized in comparison with scar that forms if edema is prolonged and brawny. Persistence of edema may lead to joint stiffness and a reflex sympathetic dystrophy.

The measures against persistent posttraumatic or postsurgical edema merit particular attention. Edema is usually the result of an impairment of the microcirculation combined with the release of vasodilatating substances such as histamine and kinins, which also increase the vascular permeability.[125] Vascular dilation evoked by pain receptors also plays a role. Abnormal autonomic reflexes are believed to be a major contributor in the early and later stages of reflex sympathetic dystrophy, in which edema is the most constant physical finding (see Colles' Fracture above). As time passes, the swelling worsens rather than improves.[98] Later motion is further inhibited by joint stiffness and brawny edema. Boyes[13] and Bunnell[18] have described the sequence of events after edema as follows: When a hand remains swollen, from whatever cause, the movable parts are bathed in serofibrinous exudate. Fibrin is deposited between the various tissue layers and the folds of the joint capsules, between the tendons and their sheaths, throughout the ligamentous tissue itself, and between and within the muscles. While soaked in the exudate, all of these tissues swell with edema and become shorter and thicker. The fibrin seals them in this condition, and soon as the fibroblastic growth transforms all to connective tissue, ligaments become shorter and thicker. The folds of synovial membrane, the capsules of the joints, the plicae of tendon sheaths, and the tendons and their sheaths become plastered together with organized adhesions.

Typically in the hand proper, edema is localized to the dorsum of the hand, where the tissues are most easily distended. The swelling of the dorsal aspect causes MCP joint extension, which predisposes to stiffness, scar formation, and contractures. Then fibrosis ensues, and a vicious circle begins.

Finger joints may stiffen after injury even though the insult was distant. The tendency toward stiffness of the fingers is greatest in adults and the aged but varies among individuals. Some persons tend to form scar tissue in the periarticular tissues, whereas others form keloids in the skin.[178] Anatomic factors that can cause limitations of motion include joint or capsular restriction, scar contraction of the skin (burns), contracted muscle, or an adherent tendon and a bony block or exostosis. All tissues can contract or become adherent: subcutaneous tissue, fascia, nerves, vessels, and cartilaginous and bony structures.

Stiffness of the hand resulting from edema, scar formation, muscle contraction, or a combination of these problems renders the hand stiff by interfering with either joint mobility or power gliding of the musculotendinous unit. The effects of edema on tendon gliding result in fluid collection in the layered paratenon, causing increased work to effect tendon gliding and a decrease in longitudinal paratenon gliding. Consequently, edema forming even after a minor injury may restrict gliding even though the joints exhibit a near-normal ROM.[190] Full passive extension of the joints may be impossible because the swollen paratenon restricts gliding of the flexor tendons. The degree of joint impairment depends more on the anatomy of the joint, its supporting structures, and the position of the joint when the cicatrix was forming and maturing. Scar formation is particularly disabling in regard to tendon gliding because no matter what the position of the tendons, tendon gliding is impaired. Scar forms not only at the site of the lesion but also at many sites far removed. For example, a tendon lacerated in the fibroosseous tunnel may evoke scar formation in the paratenon of the flexor tendons proximal to the wrist.[190,191]

Involvement of muscle compounds functional loss. Muscles may become involved by internal or external cicatrix formation or by myostatic contracture. Muscle imbalance in nerve palsy can result in contractures combined with the effects of edema and cicatrix reaction to the initial injury.[190,191]

Examination

HISTORY

The patient presents with a primary complaint of loss of hand function because of stiffness after posttraumatic or postsurgical immobilization or lack of immobilization. Stiffness alone is usually not painful; the presence of pain poses a diagnostic problem. Nonunion of a fracture, neuroma, or degenerative arthritis must be considered. Once these causes have been eliminated, the distinction is made between pain that occurs during mobilization, which appears to be caused by traction at the gliding planes or irregularities of the articular surfaces, or pain presenting in the absence of mobilization. The latter may be related to sympathetic dystrophy.

INSPECTION

A stiff hand may restrict the normal swinging movement of the arm as the hand is held stiffly by the side. Some swelling may be present; it may be intra-articular or extra-articular. Synovitis of the MCP and PIP joints bulges into the looser tissues on the extensor surface of the hand. Its shape is determined by the synovial attachments around the joints, which tend to spread on either side of the tendon in a proximal direction. Synovitis produces a diffuse swelling and can be easily differentiated from traumatic swelling of the joint structures, which usually forms a localized swelling on one side of the joint.

Extra-articular swelling may be either localized or diffuse. Diffuse swelling of a digit produces a sausage-shaped deformity. Localized swelling may involve the soft tissues around a joint and tendon sheath. In the palm and fingers it usually involves the flexor tendon sheath and may then be associated with nodule formation and triggering of the thumb or finger.[26,33,104]

Localized swelling may be caused by ganglia or cystic swellings associated with Heberden's nodes.

KEY OBJECTIVE TESTS AND NEUROLOGIC TESTS

Assessment of ROM, strength, sensibility, and ability to perform activities of daily living completes the evaluation. Knowledge of the causes of joint stiffness is essential before evaluating the ROM of the chronically stiff hand. Testing for skin tightness is routinely done.[3,4,154] The capsular and extracapsular structures contributing to joint stiffness will be discussed according to the position of stiffness of the joint.

MCP JOINT

The initial response after trauma to a hand is an increase in tissue fluid (lymph, hemorrhage, or both). Fluid increases in the tissues of the joints. The fluid in the tissue of the capsule and collateral ligaments tends to produce an effective shortening of the structures. Fluid in the joint distends the capsule, and the joint assumes a position of maximum capacity. The anatomic positions are greatest in the MCP joints, and these joints are the key to the resultant negative hand: MCP extension, interphalangeal flexion, and wrist flexion.[188] Left in this attitude, certain periarticular changes occur and contractures develop.

Stiffness in Extension. Stiffness in extension can be caused by contraction of the dorsal skin, extensor apparatus, capsular restriction (dorsal aspect), contraction of the collateral ligaments, or lesions of the joint structures. The joint factors that contribute to stiffness of the joint include capsular restriction, pannus formation in the volar synovial pouch, and articular surface erosions with or without pannus invasion. Extracapsular factors that can contribute to stiffness of the MCP joint in extension include skin contractures, extensor tendon adhesions at the dorsum of the wrist, unopposed extension (loss of active MCP flexion), and forearm extensor muscle contractures.

Stiffness in Flexion. Capsular factors that can contribute to stiffness of the MCP joints in flexion include deformities of the MCP joints, contractures or binding of the proximal sinus of the volar plate, contraction of the collateral or accessory collateral ligaments, and erosion of the articular surfaces with or without fusion.[178,190] Extracapsular factors contributing to MCP joint stiffness in flexion include contractures of the palmar skin and fascia, adhesions or contractures of the flexor tendons, and intrinsic muscle contractures.

PIP JOINT

At the PIP joint, the flexor superficialis comes into contact with the distal portion of the volar plate and may become adherent to it. The same is true of the flexor profundus at the DIP joint. The fibrous sheath of the flexor tendon extends from the PIP joint to the MCP joint. It inserts on the volar plate and on the phalanges but not on the metacarpal. This explains the important role it may play in stiffness in flexion of the PIP joint but not in stiffness of the MCP joint.[178] Other problems limiting extension of the PIP joints include adherence of the retinacular ligament to the collateral ligaments, adherence of the collateral ligaments, a bony block or exostosis, scarring of the skin on the volar surface of the finger and contraction of the superficial fascia or forearm musculature, and contraction of the fibrous portion of the fibroosseous tunnel.

Abnormalities limiting flexion of the PIP joints include scar contracture of the dorsal skin of the finger, an adherent extensor tendon, capsular restriction, adherence of the collateral ligaments or retinacular ligament to the lateral capsular ligament or of the volar capsular ligament to the proximal phalanx, interosseous or lumbrical tendon adherence, intrinsic muscle contracture exostosis, a bony block, or articular surface erosion or pannus formation.[178]

Management

An understanding of the capsular and extracapsular factors responsible for normal joint stability and the factors responsible for the development of stiff joints is required in posttraumatic and postoperative mobilization of stiff joints. It is obviously better to prevent stiffness than to have to treat it. One of the most important aspects is to prevent edema; such action is taken as soon after the injury or elective surgery as possible. Active motion, elevation, manual lymph drainage,[175] anti-inflammatory medications, the use of a continuous passive-motion device,[150] intermittent compressive therapies, ice immersions, compressive wrapping or gloves, elastic tape for wrapping of individual fingers, and string wrapping may be considered.[23,27,72,139] Placing the hand in a protective position with a functional resting splint (secured with a figure-of-eight elastic wrap to help distribute pressure over a wide area) should be considered with severe edema.[120]

ACTIVE MOBILIZATION

The mainstay of the therapeutic program is active exercise. Early active mobilization should be started as soon as the lesions allow, but two extremes must be avoided: prolonged immobilization and excessive painful mobilization. The need for active use of the hand in mobilizing stiff joints cannot be overemphasized. Voluntary exercises, tendon gliding exercises (see Fig. 8-63), and the use of the hand by the patient throughout the day produce far better results than does forceful passive ROM applied for brief periods per day. Daily forcing of the finger joints causes reactive pain and swelling and is equivalent to spraining them daily, according to Bunnel.[13] Correct motions of the fingers and wrist are more important than strength of motion. Cocontraction of the agonist and antagonist should be prevented. Biofeedback often helps prevent unwanted muscle activity. Certain activities such as precision tasks can be done in elevation. Active exercises should include full ROM to the elbow and shoulder of the involved arm.

MODIFICATION OF SCAR TISSUE

The most accepted clinical method of accelerating the modification of scar tissue is the application of stress to the scar. Treatment by mobilization is based on concepts that were initially empiric but that have more recently been proved in laboratory studies.[15,115,138,193] Slight persistent tension can remodel the collagen within scar tissue. Active mobilization can be profitably combined with massage to increase suppleness and prevent contractures.[171] Direct application of stress to the scar tissue can be accomplished in several ways: (1) direct pressure by soft tissue manipulations (see Box 8-5) or bandages, (2) serial or dynamic splints, (3) joint mobilization techniques in the presence of capsuloligamentous tightening or adherence, and (4) passive ROM or stretching techniques.

SOFT TISSUE MANIPULATIONS AND MASSAGE

According to Wynn-Parry,[196] massage has no place in hand therapy to reduce muscle spasm, relieve pain, or improve circulation. Ice and active mobilization are the best means of reducing spasm. Pain is more efficiently and less expensively relieved by analgesia or other methods of modulation. Active exercises are infinitely better at increasing circulation than massage. Massage (soft tissue manipulations) is most effective in breaking down adhesions and fibrosis; mobilizing scar tissue; stretching restricted fasciae, skin, joint capsules, and ligaments; and helping to reduce edema. Soft tissue manipulation applies compressive and distractive forces directly to the scar and also helps to alter the fibrotic process and reduce any edema present. Deep friction massage is particularly useful for managing tenosynovitis (see Figs. 8-25 and 8-26) and for decreasing the adhesions that form at ligaments after a sprain (see Box 8-3).[35] Joint massage[137] and joint compression techniques[128] are valuable adjuncts in treating degenerative joints with stiffness or pain.

Connective tissue massage often can provide gentle stretch of the capsule without traumatizing the joint structures.[47,175] A common problem in the management of the hand is overstretching of the capsules in the small joints of the fingers. These joints must be stretched gently—forceful stretching causes reactive pain and swelling, with the joints becoming stiffer than ever. Various soft tissue mobilization techniques have been used effectively through the years to stretch abnormal fibrous tissue and to increase flexibility and ROM (see Chapter 8, Soft Tissue Manipulations).[6,77,106]

SPLINTING

Between physical therapy sessions, when retraction is marked, serial splints as advocated by Wynn-Parry[197] and dynamic or static splints can be used to provide a prolonged pull or traction on the scar tissue. In longstanding contractures, elongation by slow traction is necessary. Continuous mild traction provides a light prolonged stretch on the restraining tissues until, by cell multiplication, they actually grow longer, so that lengthening is permanent.[93,152]

Dynamic splints must be well adapted to the patient. If limitation in the ROM is strictly related to a soft tissue contracture around a particular joint, a splint must be designed to apply traction to that specific joint. Traction must be perpendicular (at a right angle to the treatment plane) to the involved phalanx.

When restrictions in active ROM are caused by a combination of joint contracture and muscle tightness, a two-stage splinting program is required.[120] Initially a splint is designed to increase the passive ROM of the involved joint. Later, when normal joint mechanics have been restored, the splinting program is directed at providing stretch to the involved intrinsic or extrinsic musculature.

JOINT MOBILIZATION

Free joint play within a useful or functional ROM is necessary to avoid joint trauma. If joint play is restricted, joint-mobilizing techniques should be used.[80] When pain is the dominant factor, grade I and II mobilization techniques are appropriate. If these techniques are successful and pain-free active motion increases, treatment is taken further into the range. Chronically, these stretching techniques can be vigorous as long as pain and irritation are avoided. Before initiating stretching techniques to muscle or inert tissue, there should be normal gliding of the joint surfaces to avoid joint damage. Both joint dynamics and muscle strength and flexibility must be balanced as the hand is restored to functional use.

PASSIVE RANGE OF MOTION AND STRETCHING TECHNIQUES

In vitro research has shown that prolonged low-intensity stretching at elevated tissue temperatures maximizes permanent lengthening of connective tissue and minimizes deterioration in tensile strength.[7,10,56,57,60,73,93,100,152,183,185,186] When using this principle of combining heat and stretch to a stiff hand, McEntee[120] suggests applying an elastic tape to the involved finger(s) in the direction in which increased motion is desired to maintain a prolonged stretch. Once the hand is stretched with the tape, it can be dipped in paraffin or placed under a hot pack for the desired time. Active exercises should follow immediately for the best results. As an adjunct to prolonged stretch, manual passive ROM or stretching techniques may be used.

The complexity of the joints and multijoint muscles of the fingers requires careful evaluation and management. Fingers should always be stretched individually, not grossly. When stretching the extrinsic muscles (which are multijoint muscles), elongation over all the joints, simultaneously, should be avoided. Stretching in this manner can result in joint compression and damage to the smaller or less stable joints. Gently distract the joints to avoid compressing the segments being mobilized. Use short levers whenever possible and apply the stretch force in a gentle, slow, sustained manner. Hold the patient in the stretched position for at least 15 to 30 seconds.

Muscles are more amenable to stretch after some form of warm-up exercise. The best and most specific warm-up exercise is contraction against resistance. Successive techniques of isometric contractions, relaxation, and stretching (contract–relax method), followed by stimulation of the antagonist, help relax the muscles so they are more easily stretched.[48,65,76,90,91,118,174,184,195]

Therapy is more effective if supplemented by frequent self-stretching. In general, the more frequent the stretching, the more moderate the intensity. The principle of moving the body in relationship to the stabilized extremity affords an excellent stretch and allows a greater degree of pain-free movement. For example, to stretch the long finger flexors, have the patient (in a standing position) rest the palm of the involved hand on a table. Using the other hand the patient extends the joints from distal to proximal in succession, or actively extends them, unassisted, when possible. When the joints are extended, the patient fixates or maintains this position with the other hand as he or she actively moves the trunk forward; this brings the arm (with the elbow extended) up over the hand, resulting in wrist extension.[58] Motion is taken to the point of discomfort and maintained. Motion is progressed as the length improves.

Reverse stretching techniques can also be used. For example, to stretch the extensor digitorum communis, the patient maximally flexes the elbow and then actively flexes the fingers to their maximum range, beginning with the most distal joint and progressing proximally until the wrist is simultaneously flexed. Once all the slack is taken up in the hand, the elbow is straightened. As a result, the stretch is primarily directed at the muscle belly rather than the tendons and joint structures of the hand.

RESISTIVE EXERCISE

Joint motion without adequate muscle support can cause additional trauma to the joints as functional activities are resumed. Initially isometric exercises are recommended to increase strength when there is a loss of joint play and when there is significant pain. Once joint play is restored, resistive isotonic exercises are recommended within the available range.[89] This does not imply that normal ROM needs to be present, but that joint play, within the available range, must be present. Graded resistive activity, progressing from manual resistive exercises using proprioceptive neuromuscular facilitation techniques to progressive resistive exercises using weights, the resistance of an elasticized tension cord (Isoflex exercises) or self-resistance, and activities such as woodworking can help increase the strength of the hand. Squeezing activities, such as squeezing a rubber ball or a bit of putty, should be forbidden: they prevent full range of flexion, which is one of the goals of treatment.

Full ROM is the primary target. Therapeutic and functional activities, as well as early return to work, are preferred to increase strength, endurance, and active motion of the chronically stiff hand. Acceptance of the hand by the patient, motivation, reeducation, and preparing the patient to return to a former job and activities are all responsibilities of the hand-care team.

Management of the postsurgical hand is beyond the scope of this book, but details of preoperative and postoperative care are readily available in the literature.[2,13,26,37,46,50,59,72,105,107,123,141,170]

PASSIVE TREATMENT TECHNIQUES

(For simplicity, the patient is referred to as female, the operator as male. P—patient; O—operator; M—movement)

Underwrap placed between the skin and the operator's mobilizing hand or the use of surgical gloves may allow the operator to obtain a firmer grip by reducing slippage against the patient's skin.

Joint Mobilization Techniques

WRIST AND HAND

I. Distal Radioulnar Joint. Dorsal-ventral glide (Fig. 13-37)

P—Supine, with the arm somewhat abducted and the elbow bent, so that the forearm may rest on the plinth in a neutral position with respect to pronation and supination

O—Stabilizes the distal radius against the plinth, grasping it between the heel of his hand and the pads of the second through fifth fingers. He grasps the distal ulna dorsally with the thumb pad and ventrally with the pads of the index and long fingers.

M—The distal ulna may be moved dorsally or ventrally relative to the distal radius. These motions should be performed separately. Note: Alternatively, the distal ulna may be stabilized and the distal radius moved by reversing the handholds. The movement may also be performed with the forearm vertical.

These techniques are used to increase joint-play motions necessary for pronation and supination.

II. Ulnomeniscotriquetral Joint. Dorsal glide (Fig. 13-38)

P—Supine or sitting, with the elbow resting on the plinth or table and the forearm vertical

O—Stabilizes the radial side of the wrist and hand with his left hand. The right hand contacts the dorsal aspect of the head of the ulna with the thumb, and the palmar aspect of the triquetrum and the pisiform with the radial aspect of the crook of the flexed PIP joint of his index finger.

M—A dorsal glide of the pisiform and triquetrum on the ulna is produced by a squeezing action between the thumb and the crook of the index finger.

This technique is used to increase joint-play movements necessary for pronation and supination.

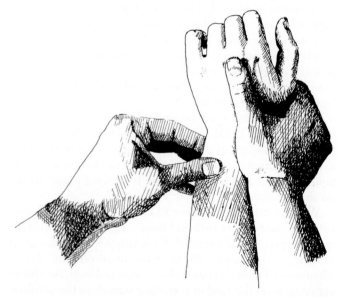

▪ **FIG. 13-37.** Dorsal-ventral glide of distal radioulnar joint.

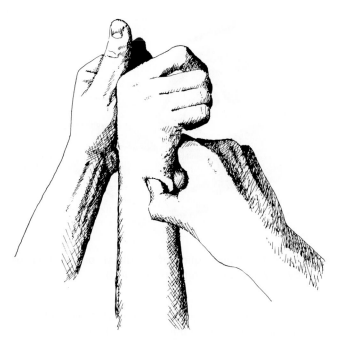

■ **FIG. 13-38.** Dorsal glide of ulnomeniscotriquetral joint (right hand).

III.   Radiocarpal Joint (and Ulnomeniscotriquetral Joint). Joint distraction (Fig. 13-39)

P—Sitting or supine, with the elbow bent and resting on the plinth, and the forearm in neutral pronation and supination

O—Stabilizes the distal humerus and elbow against the plinth with his right hand at the antecubital space. The left hand grasps around the proximal row of carpals, just distal to the styloid processes.

M—A distraction is produced with the left hand, paying particular attention to the radiocarpal joint.

This technique is used as a general mobilization procedure to increase joint play at the radiocarpal joint. Distraction tends to occur with palmar flexion of the wrist. By increasing the amount of joint distraction, movement toward the close-packed position, dorsiflexion, may be increased. This prevents premature compression of joint surfaces.

IV.   Radiocarpal Joint. Dorsal-palmar glide (Fig. 13-40)

P—Sitting with the arm somewhat abducted, the elbow bent, and the forearm resting on the plinth in pronation. The hand extends over the edge of the table or plinth.

O—Stabilizes the distal end of the forearm with his right hand, just proximal to the styloid processes. He grasps the proximal row of carpals with his left hand using the styloid processes and pisiform for landmarks.

M—The proximal row of carpals may be moved dorsally or palmarly, paying particular attention to the radiocarpal joint. Dorsal glide and palmar glide should be performed as separate techniques. Note: Dorsal glide may be performed more effectively with the arm in full supination and the hand extended over the edge of the plinth or table.

Palmar glide is used to increase joint-play movements necessary for dorsal flexion. Dorsal glide is used to increase joint-play movements necessary for palmar flexion.

V.   Radiocarpal Joint (and Ulnomeniscotriquetral Joint). Radial-ulnar glide (or tilt; Fig. 13-41)

P—Sitting, with the arm near the side, the elbow bent, and the forearm resting on the plinth in neutral pronation and supination. The radial aspect of the forearm faces superiorly.

O—Stabilizes the distal end of the forearm with the left hand, just proximal to the styloid processes. He grasps the proximal row of carpals with his right hand.

M—The proximal row of carpals may be glided radially or ulnarly on the distal ends of the radius and ulna (articular disk). Alternatively, a radial tilt or ulnar tilt may be produced.

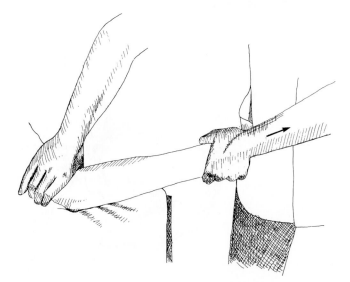

■ **FIG. 13-39.** Distraction of radiocarpal joint (and ulnomeniscotriquetral joint; right hand).

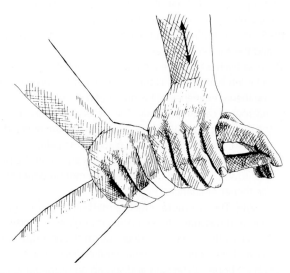

■ **FIG. 13-40.** Dorsal-palmar glide of radiocarpal joint.

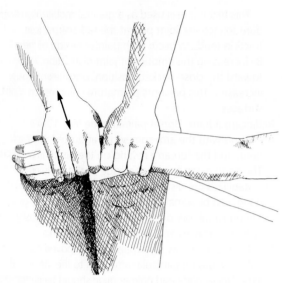

■ **FIG. 13-41.** Radial-ulnar glide (or tilt) of radiocarpal joint (and ulnomeniscotriquetral joint).

Radial glide and ulnar tilt are joint-play movements necessary for ulnar deviation. Ulnar glide and radial tilt are joint-play movements necessary for radial deviation.

VI. Midcarpal Joint. Joint distraction
    This technique is produced in exactly the same way as that for the radiocarpal joint, except that the left handhold moves distally to grasp the distal row of carpals. This technique is used for general mobilization to increase joint play at the midcarpal joint.

VII. Midcarpal Joint. Dorsal-palmar glide
    This technique is produced in exactly the same way as that for the radiocarpal joint, except that the left handhold moves distally to grasp the distal row of carpals. Palmar glide is used to increase the joint-play movements necessary for dorsal flexion. Dorsal glide is used to increase the joint-play movements necessary for palmar flexion.

VIII. Midcarpal Joint. Palmar glide of the distal row of carpals on the proximal row of carpals (Fig. 13-42)
    P—Sitting or supine, with the elbow resting on the plinth and the forearm vertical
    O—Approaches from the ulnar aspect. The thenar eminence of his left hand contacts the distal row of carpals dorsally. The thenar eminence of his right hand contacts the proximal row of carpals palmarly. The fingers are interlaced over the radial aspect of the wrist. The forearms are directed outward, perpendicular to the plane of the palm.
    M—A palmar glide of the distal row of carpals on the proximal row is produced by a squeezing motion between the thenar eminences.
      Note: This is a more effective method of palmar glide than that described for dorsal-palmar glide. The performance of this movement depends on the accurate placement of the operator's thenar eminences over the correct bones. Extension and spreading of the patient's fingers should occur when this movement is done cor-

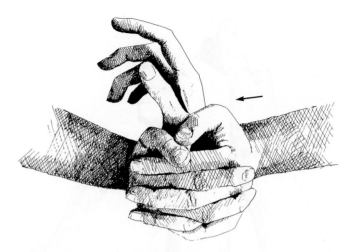

■ **FIG. 13-42.** Palmar glide of the distal row on the proximal row for midcarpal joint (right hand).

rectly.[18] This technique is used to increase joint-play motion necessary for dorsal flexion of the wrist.

IX. Intercarpal Joints
    Specific movements between adjacent bones of the wrist and carpal joints may be indicated. Mobility between the triquetrum and lunate, the lunate and radius, or the capitate and lunate, for example, can be tested and mobilized. In general, one joint partner is always fixated while the other is moved. The individual carpal bones can be mobilized by placing the thumb and index finger on the volar and dorsal sides of two adjacent carpal bones (e.g., the lunate and capitate), respectively. The thumbs may mobilize one carpal while the index fingers stabilize the other carpal bone, or vice versa. The reader is referred to detailed descriptions of these advanced techniques by Kaltenborn[80] and others.[122,168] Two examples will be described.
    A. Intercarpal joints. Palmar glide of the scaphoid on the radius (Fig. 13-43)

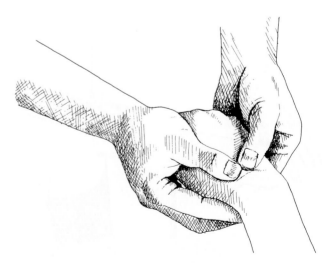

■ **FIG. 13-43.** Palmar glide of scaphoid on radius for intercarpal joints.

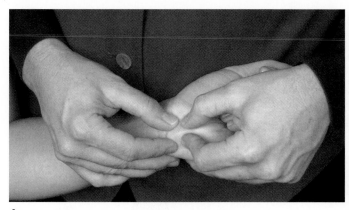

A

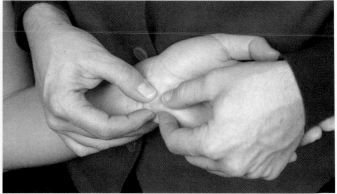

B

■ **FIG. 13-44.** Pisotriquetral joint. **(A)** Medial, lateral, cephalad and caudal glides, and **(B)** distraction.

P—Sitting or supine, with the forearm resting on the table, or with the arm held forward by the operator

O—Stands or sits facing the hand. Both hands hold the patient's thenar and hypothenar eminence. The index fingers are placed on the proximal palmar surface of the radius, stabilizing it in this position. The thumbs contact the scaphoid dorsally.

M—The scaphoid is moved palmarly relative to the distal end of the radius.

This technique is used to increase joint-play motion necessary for dorsal glide of the scaphoid on the radius.

B. Intercarpal joints. Pisotriquetral joint (Fig. 13-44).

P—Sitting

O—Stands supporting the patient's supinated hand and forearm against his body.

M—The pisiform is pinched between the index and thumb of the left hand and moved gently in a medial, lateral, and longitudinal cephalad and caudal direction while the opposite hand stabilizes the triquetrum (Fig. 13-44A). To perform distraction (Fig. 13-44B), the pisiform is gently pinched between the index and thumb and pulled away from the triquetrum.

X. Trapeziometacarpal Joint. Distraction (Fig. 13-45)

P—Sitting or supine with the ulnar aspect of the forearm resting on the table

O—The stabilizing hand grips the trapezium with the thumb on the dorsal surface and the index finger on the volar surface. The mobilizing hand grips the proximal metacarpal, with the thumb on the dorsal surface and the index finger on the volar surface.

M—A long-axis distraction is produced by the mobilizing hand moving the metacarpal distally.

Note: The metacarpal may be moved dorsally or ventrally relative to the trapezium using the same hand grips. These techniques are used to decrease pain and increase joint play of the trapeziometacarpal joint. Dorsal-volar glides are used to increase ROM into trapeziometacarpal abduction and adduction. The trapeziometacarpal joint is in the resting position if conservative techniques are indi-

cated or approximates the restricted range if more aggressive techniques are indicated.

XI. Trapeziometacarpal Joint. Dorsal-palmar glide

The handholds are exactly the same as for distraction of the trapeziometacarpal joint (Fig. 13-45). Dorsal-palmar glide is produced by gliding the metacarpal in a dorsal or palmar direction.

Dorsal glide is used to increase motion into trapeziometacarpal abduction. Palmar glide is used to increase motion into trapeziometacarpal adduction.

XII. Trapeziometacarpal Joint. Radial and ulnar glide (Fig. 13-46)

P—Sitting or supine with the ulnar aspect of the forearm resting on the table

O—The stabilizing hand grips the trapezium with the thumb on the radial surface and the index finger on the ulnar surface. The mobilizing hand grips the proximal metacarpal on the radial and ulnar surfaces.

M—Radial or ulnar glide or tilt may be produced with the thumb pad in one direction and the index finger in the other.

Radial glide (ulnar tilt) is necessary for trapeziometacarpal extension. Ulnar glide (radial tilt) is necessary for trapeziometacarpal flexion.

XIII. Carpometacarpal–Intermetacarpal Joints (II Through V). Distraction (Fig. 13-47)

P—Sitting with the forearm resting on the table, palm down

O—Stabilizes the respective carpal with one hand, grasping with the thumb on the dorsal aspect and the index finger

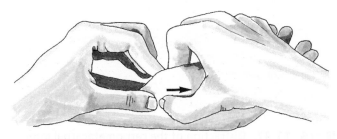

■ **FIG. 13-45.** Distraction of the trapeziometacarpal joint.

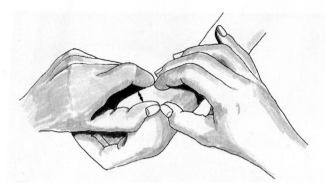

■ **FIG. 13-46.** Radial-ulnar glide of the trapezio-metacarpal joint.

on the volar aspect. The mobilizing hand grips the base of the metacarpal of the joint being mobilized, with the thumb on the dorsal surface and the index finger on the volar surface.

M—Long-axis distraction is applied to the metacarpal; the second metacarpal is moved distal on the trapezoid, the third metacarpal distal on the capitate, the fourth metacarpal distal on the hamate, and the fifth metacarpal on the hamate.

    Note: Volar glide may also be performed using the same stabilization and hand placement. Movement in these joints is minimal, especially in the second and third carpometacarpal joints. These techniques are used to increase joint play in the carpometacarpal joints and increase mobility of the arch of the hand.

XIV. Intermetacarpal Joints. Dorsal-palmar glide (Fig. 13-48; These joints between the metacarpal heads are not true synovial joints, but movement must occur here during grasp and release, as described in Appendix A.)

  P—Sitting or supine, with the elbow resting on the plinth, the forearm pronated

  O—Approaches from the dorsal aspect. The left hand stabilizes the head and neck of the third metacarpal. The thumb pad contacts dorsally, the pads of the index and long fingers palmarly. The left hand grasps the head and neck of the fourth metacarpal in similar fashion.

  M—The head of the fourth metacarpal can be moved palmarly or dorsally with respect to the third metacarpal. Similarly, the right hand can stabilize the third metacarpal, while the left hand moves the second

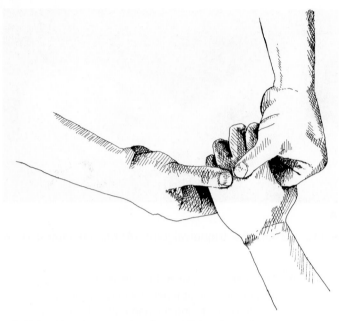

■ **FIG. 13-48.** Dorsal-palmar glide of intermetacarpal joints.

metacarpal. The third metacarpal is the "center of movement" as the hand flattens and arches during release and grasp. It is always stabilized, while the other metacarpals are moved relative to it.

    These techniques are used to increase joint-play movements necessary for the arching and flattening of the hand that occur with grasp and release.

FINGERS

Note: Traction grade 1 should be used with most gliding and mobilizing techniques of the fingers.

I. MCP or Interphalangeal Joints. Distraction (Fig. 13-49)

  P—Sitting or supine

  O—Supports the forearm and elbow by tucking them between his forearm and side. To treat the more radial

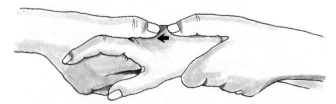

■ **FIG. 13-47.** Distraction of the carpometacarpal inter-metacarpal joints, II through V.

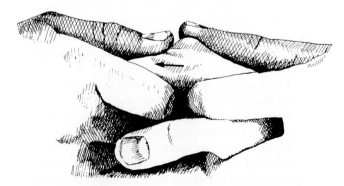

■ **FIG. 13-49.** Distraction of metacarpophalangeal or interphalangeal joints (right hand).

joints, the operator approaches from the ulnar side for the thumb, index, and long fingers, and from the radial side for the ring and small fingers. He grasps the head of the proximal bone dorsally with the thumb pad and palmarly with the crook of the index finger. He grasps the base of the distal bone in a similar manner.

M—Keeping the joint in slight flexion (avoiding the close-packed position), a long-axis distraction is produced with the operator's more distal hand.

These techniques are used for general joint mobilization to increase joint play. Distraction is necessary, especially during flexion at the MCP joints and extension at the interphalangeal joints, since these are movements toward the close-packed position. Premature compression of joint surfaces will result if sufficient joint play into distraction cannot occur.

II. MCP or Interphalangeal Joints. Dorsal-palmar glide (Fig. 13-50)
P—Supine or sitting
O—The handholds are essentially the same as those for distraction, except that during dorsal glide the palmar contact of the more distal hand is with the pad of the index finger.
M—The base of the distal bone may be moved palmarly or dorsally.
Palmar glide is necessary for flexion. Dorsal glide is a joint-play movement necessary for extension.

III. MCP or Interphalangeal Joints. Radioulnar glide (or tilt; Fig. 13-51)
P—Supine or sitting
O—The handholds are similar to those used for distraction, except that the thumbs are brought around to the aspect of the bones closest to the operator, and the crooks or pads of the index fingers are brought around to the aspect of the bone farthest from the operator. The contacts are then made on the radial and ulnar sides of the joint.
M—Radial or ulnar glide or tilt may be produced by the thumb pad in one direction, and by the index pad in the other. While one pad is producing the movement, the other moves to the more distal part of the bone.
Ulnar glide (radial tilt) is necessary for extension at the interphalangeal joints. Radial glide (ulnar tilt) is necessary

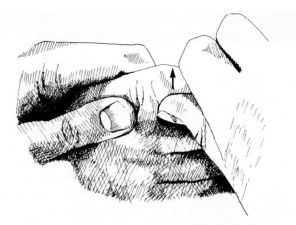

■ **FIG. 13-51.** Radial-ulnar glide of metacarpophalangeal or interphalangeal joints (right hand).

for flexion at the interphalangeal joints. The same is true, but to a lesser extent, at the MCP joints.

IV. MCP or Interphalangeal Joints. Rotation (pronation and supination; Fig. 13-52)
P—Supine or sitting
O—The proximal handhold is the same as that for distraction. The distal hand-holds are also similar to those used for long-axis distraction, except the operator may gain some leverage by holding the more distal segment of the digit, semiflexed, in his remaining fingers. This must be performed with caution.
M—A pronation or supination of the distal end of the bone is produced by the operator's more distal hand.
Supination is a joint-play movement (conjunct rotation) necessary for flexion, especially at the interphalangeal joints. Pronation occurs during extension. Note: The same techniques may be used at the carpometacarpal joint of the thumb. As for their specific uses in this case, consider the convex–concave rule and how it applies to this sellar joint.

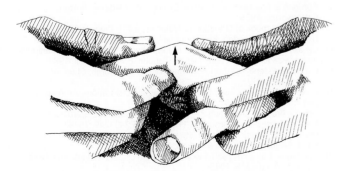

■ **FIGURE 13-50.** Dorsal-palmar glide of metacarpophalangeal or interphalangeal joints (right hand).

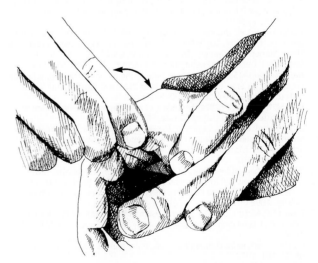

■ **FIG. 13-52.** Rotation (pronation and supination) of metacarpophalangeal or interphalangeal joints (right hand).

DYNAMIC STABILIZATION EXERCISES AND FUNCTIONAL EXERCISES

Open kinetic chain strengthening and endurance exercises are described in numerous texts and will not be addressed here.[64,89,142,167] These exercises include wrist and finger proprioceptive neuromuscular facilitation patterns, progressive resistive exercises with weights or tubing, putty and rubber band exercises, hand dexterity tasks, eccentric work, and graded programs of stretch-shortening drills such as throwing and catching ball. Overhead plyometrics encourage both endurance and strength of the entire upper extremity. Occupational tasks that include pushing and pulling may be appropriate in the late stage of rehabilitation.

Treatment of the wrist and hand also must restore normal joint stability. Most of the time, this can be done by improving ROM, allowing healing of the tissues and rehabilitation in cocontraction-stabilizing fashions. Surgical stabilization of the ligamentous or bony constraints may be necessary to achieve joint stability. Once stability has been established, work on the kinematic chain can help to optimize the efficiency of the physiologic and biomechanical patterns across the wrist and hand.

Closed-kinetic chain exercises might include:

- Floor push-ups (see Fig. 11-76), wall push-ups (see Figs 11-71), or mini-trampoline push-ups (see Fig. 12-32) to encourage wrist motion, general strengthening, and weight bearing
- Therapeutic ball or stool walking (see Fig.12-31; in all directions) with weight bearing through the wrists and arms to reestablish neuromuscular control, weight shifting, and balance
- Quadripod stabilization (see Fig. 11-78) with weight bearing through the wrists and arms to reestablish neuromuscular control, weight shifting, and balance

REFERENCES

1. Abrahamsson SO, Sollerman C, Lundborg G, et al: Diagnosis of displaced collateral ligament of the metacarpophalangeal joint of the thumb. J Hand Surg Am 15:457–460, 1990
2. American Academy of Orthopedic Surgeons: Symposium on Tendon Surgery in the Hand. Philadelphia, CV Mosby, 1975
3. American Society for Surgery of the Hand: The Hand: Examination and Diagnosis. Aurora, CO, American Society for Surgery of the Hand, 1978
4. American Society for Surgery of the Hand: The Hand: Examination and Diagnosis. New York, Churchill Livingstone, 1983
5. Aulicino P: Clinical examination of the hand. In: Hunter JM, Schneider LH, Mackin EJ, et al, eds: Rehabilitation of the Hand. Surgery and Therapy, 4th ed. St. Louis, CV Mosby, 1995:53–75
6. Bajelis D: Myofascial release, IV: Management of sports injuries. Presented at a course on physical therapy, management of the extremities, Seattle, July 1986
7. Barcroft H, Edholm OG: The effect of temperature on blood flow and deep temperature in the human forearm. J Physiol (Lond) 102:5–20, 1943
8. Baxter PL, Ballard MS: Evaluation of the hand by functional tests. In: Hunter JM, Schneider LH, Mackin EJ, et al, eds: Rehabilitation of the Hand. St. Louis, CV Mosby, 1984:91–101
9. Baxter-Petralia PL, Bruening LA, Blackmore SM, et al: Physical capacity evaluation. In: Hunter JM, Schneider LH, Mackin EJ, et al, eds: Rehabilitation of the Hand. Surgery and Therapy, 3rd ed. St. Louis, CV Mosby, 1990:93–108
10. Becker AH: Traction for knee-flexion contractures. Phys Ther 59:1114, 1979
11. Bell-Krotoski JA: Sensibility testing: state of the art. In: Hunter JM, Schneider LH, Mackin EJ, eds: Rehabilitation of the Hand. Surgery and Therapy, 3rd ed. St. Louis, CV Mosby, 1990: 575–584
12. Blair SJ, McCormick E, Bear-Lehman J, et al: Evaluation of impairment of the upper extremity. Clin Orthop 221:42–58, 1987
13. Boyes JH, ed: Bunnell's Surgery of the Hand. Philadelphia, JB Lippincott, 1970
14. Brand PW: Hand rehabilitation management by objectives. In: Hunter JM, Schneider LH, Mackin EJ, et al, eds: Rehabilitation of the Hand. St. Louis, CV Mosby, 1978
15. Brand PW: Clinical Mechanics of the Hand. St. Louis, CV Mosby, 1985
16. Brody LR: The elbow, forearm, and hand. In: Hall CM, Brody LR: Therapeutic Exercise: Moving Toward Function. Philadelphia, Lippincott Williams & Wilkins, 1998
17. Brown CP, McGrouther DA: The excursion of the tendon of the flexor pollicis longus and its relation to dynamic splintage. J Hand Surg Am 9:787–791, 1984
18. Bunnell S: Ischaemic contracture, local, in the hand. J Bone Joint Surg Am 35:88–101, 1953
19. Burton RI, Melchior JA: Extensor tendons—late construction. In: Green DP, Hofschkiss RV, Pederson WC, eds: Green's Operative Hand Surgery, vol. 2, 4th ed. New York, Churchill Livingstone, 1999:1988–2021
20. Butler RS: Mobilisation of the Nervous System. Melbourne, Churchill Livingstone, 1991
21. Cailliet R: Reflex sympathetic referred pain. In: Shoulder Pain, 2nd ed. Philadelphia, FA Davis, 1991:108–124
22. Cailliet R: Hand Pain and Impairment, 4th ed. Philadelphia, FA Davis, 1994
23. Cain HD, Liebgold HB: Compressive centripetal wrapping technique for reduction of edema. Arch Phys Med 48:420–423, 1967
24. Callahan AD: Sensibility testing, clinical method. In: Hunter JH, Schneider LH, Mackin EJ, eds: Rehabilitation of the Hand: Surgery and Therapy, 3rd ed. St. Louis, CV Mosby, 1990:594–610
25. Cambridge-Keeling CA: Range-of-motion measurements of the hand. In: Hunter JH, Schneider LH, Mackin EJ, et al, eds: Rehabilitation of the Hand. Surgery and Therapy, 4th ed. St. Louis, CV Mosby, 1995:93–107
26. Campbell-Reid DA, McGrouther DA: Surgery of the Thumb. Boston, Butterworths, 1986
27. Carter PR: Common Hand Injuries and Infections: A Practical Approach to Early Treatment. Philadelphia, WB Saunders, 1983
28. Chow JCY: Carpal tunnel syndrome. In: Watson HK, Weinzweg J, eds: The Wrist. Philadelphia, Lippincott Williams & Wilkins, 2001
29. Clancy WG: Tendon trauma and overuse injuries. In: Leadbetter W, Buckwalter J, Gordon S, eds: Sports-Induced Inflammation. Park Ridge, IL, American Academy of Orthopaedic Surgeons, 1990:609–618
30. Clarkson HM, Gilewish GB: Musculoskeletal Assessment, Joint Range of Motion and Manual Muscle Testing. Baltimore, Williams & Wilkins, 1989
31. Cole JH, Furness AL, Twoney LT: Muscle in Action, an Approach to Manual Muscle Testing. Edinburg, Churchill Livingstone, 1988
32. Cornacchia M: Considerazioni sulla meccanica articolare del pollice. Chir Organi Mov 33:137–153, 1949
33. Corrigan B, Maitland GD: Practical Orthopaedic Medicine. Boston, Butterworths, 1985
34. Cyriax J: Textbook of Orthopaedic Medicine, vol. 1: Diagnosis of Soft Tissue Lesions, 8th ed. London, Bailliere Tindall, 1982
35. Cyriax J: Textbook of Orthopaedic Medicine, vol. 2: Treatment by Manipulation, Massage and Injection, 11th ed. London, Bailliere Tindall, 1984
36. Dandy DJ: Essential Orthopaedics and Trauma. Edinburgh, Churchill Livingstone, 1989
37. De Palma F: The Management of Fractures and Dislocations: An Atlas, 2nd ed. Philadelphia, WB Saunders, 1970
38. Dell PC, Brushart TM, Smith RT: Treatment of trapeziometacarpal arthritis. Results of resection arthroplasty. J Hand Surg 5:243–249, 1978
39. Dellon AL: Evaluation of Sensibility and Re-Education of Sensation in the Hand. Baltimore, Williams & Wilkins, 1981
40. deTakas G: Nature of painful vasodilatation in causalgic states. Arch Neur Psychiat 50:318–326, 1943
41. Dickoff S: Elbow, wrist, and hand injuries. In: Sanders B, ed: Sports Physical Therapy. Norwalk, CT, Appleton & Lange, 1990:369–395
42. Dorfman LJ, Jayram AR: Handcuff neuropathy. JAMA 239:957, 1978

43. Doyle JR: Extensor tendons—acute injuries. In: Green DP, Hofschkiss RV, Pederson WC: Green's Operative Hand Surgery, vol. 2, 4th ed. New York, Churchill Livingstone, 1999:1950–1987

44. Durkin JA: A new diagnostic test for carpal tunnel syndrome. J Bone Joint Surg Am 73:535–538, 1991

45. Eaton RG: Joint Injuries of the Hand. Springfield, IL, Charles C. Thomas, 1971

46. Eaton RG: Replacement of the trapezium for arthritis of the basal articulation. A new technique with stabilization by tenodesis. J Bone Joint Surg Am 61:76–83, 1979

47. Ebner M: Connective Tissue Manipulation, Therapy and Therapeutic Application. Malabar, FL, Robert Knieger, 1985

48. Evjenth O, Hamberg J: Muscle Stretching in Manual Therapy: A Clinical Manual—The Extremities, vol. 1. Alfta, Sweden, Alfta Rehab Forleg, 1984

49. Exelby L: Peripheral mobilizations with movement. Man Ther 1:118–126, 1996

50. Ferlic DC, Busbee GA, Clayton ML: Degenerative arthritis of the carpometacarpal joint of the thumb. A clinical follow-up of 11 Niebauer prostheses. J Hand Surg 2:212–215, 1977

51. Fess EE, Harmon KS, Strockland JW, et al: Evaluation of the hand by objective measurement. In: Hunter JM, Schneider LH, Mackin EJ, et al, eds: Rehabilitation of the Hand. St. Louis, CV Mosby, 1978:70–96

52. Fess EE, Moran CA: Clinical Assessment Recommendations. Aurora, CO, American Society of Hand Therapists, 1981

53. Fietti VG Jr, Mackin EJ: Open-palm technique in Dupuytren's disease. In: Hunter JM, Schneider LH, Mackin EJ, et al, eds: Rehabilitation of the Hand. Surgery and Therapy, 4th ed. St. Louis, CV Mosby, 1995:981–994

54. Flatt AE: The Pathomechanics of Ulnar Drift. Final Report. Washington DC, Department of Health, Education, and Welfare, 1971

55. Flatt AE, Fischer GW: Stability during flexion and extension at the MCP joints. In: La Main Rheumatoide, Monographie du GEM. Paris, L'Expansion Scientifique Franáaise, 1967:51–61

56. Flax HJ, Miller RV, Horvath SM: Alterations in peripheral circulation and tissue temperature following local application of short-wave diathermy. Arch Phys Med Rehabil 3:630–637, 1949

57. Gersten JW, Wakin KG, Herrick JF, et al: The effect of microwave diathermy on the peripheral circulation and on tissue temperature in man. Arch Phys Med Rehabil 30:7–25, 1949

58. Gerstner DL, Omer GE: Peripheral entrapment neuropathies in the upper extremity: Part 1. Key differential findings, median nerve syndromes. J Musculoskeletal Med 5:14–29, 1988

59. Gervis WH: A review of excision of the trapezium for osteoarthritis of the trapeziometacarpal joint after 25 years. J Bone Joint Surg Br 55:56–57, 1973

60. Glazer RM: Rehabilitation. In: Happenstall RB, ed: Fracture Treatment and Healing. Philadelphia, WB Saunders, 1980

61. Gonzalez-King BZ, Syen DB, Burgess BL: Dysfunction, evaluation, and treatment of the wrist and hand. In: Donatelli RA, Wooden MJ, eds: Orthopaedic Physical Therapy, 3rd ed. New York, Churchill Livingstone, 2001:205–243

62. Grant JCB, Basmajian JV: Grant's Method of Anatomy, 9th ed. Baltimore, Williams & Wilkins, 1991

63. Hakstian RW, Tubiana R: Ulnar deviation of the fingers. The role of joint structure and function. J Bone Joint Surg Am 49:299–316, 1967

64. Hall CM, Brody LT: Therapeutic Exercise, Moving Toward Function. Philadelphia, Lippincott Williams, & Wilkins, 1998

65. Haugen P, Stern-Knudsen O: The effect of a small stretch on latency relaxation and the short-range elastic stiffness in isolated frog muscle fibres. Acta Physiol Scand 112:121–128, 1981

66. Hazelton FT, Smidt GL, Flatt AE: The influence of wrist position on the force produced by the finger flexors. J Biomech 8:301–306, 1975

67. Hislop HJ, Montgomery J: Daniels and Worthingham's Muscle Testing, Techniques of Manual Examination, 6th ed. Philadelphia, WB Saunders, 1995

68. Hollinshead WH: Anatomy for Surgeons, vol. 3: The Back and Limbs, 4th ed. New York, Harper Medical, 1985

69. Hoppenfeld S: Physical Examination of the Spine and Extremities. New York, Appleton-Century-Crofts, 1976

70. Hueston JR: Dupuytren's contracture. In: Flynn JE, ed; Hand Surgery, 3rd ed. Baltimore, Williams & Wilkins, 1982:797–822

71. Hunter JM, Davlin LB, Fedus LM: Major neuropathies of the upper extremity: The median nerve. In: Hunter JM, Schneider LH, Mackin EJ, et al, eds: Rehabilitation of the Hand. Surgery and Therapy, 4th ed. St. Louis, Mosby, 1995: 917–922

72. Hunter JM, Schneider LH, Mackin EJ, et al, eds: Rehabilitation of the Hand. Surgery and Therapy, 4th ed. St. Louis, CV Mosby, 1995

73. Jackman RV: Device to stretch the Achilles tendon. J Am Phys Ther Assoc 43:729–735, 1963

74. James JIP. The genetic pattern of Dupuytren's disease and idiopathic epilepsy. In: Hueston JT, Tubiana R, eds: Dupuytren's Disease, 2nd ed. Edinburgh, Churchill Livingstone, 1985:94–99

75. Jebson RH, Taylor N, Trieschman RB, et al: An objective and standardized test of hand function. Arch Phys Med Rehabil 5:311–319, 1969

76. Jenkins RB, Little RW: A constitutive equation for parallel-fibered elastic tissue. J Biomech 7:397–402, 1974

77. Johnson G: Functional orthopedics II: Advanced techniques of soft-tissue mobilization for evaluation and treatment of the extremities and trunk. Presented at a course at the Institute of Physical Arts, San Francisco, 1985

78. Johnson RK, Shrewsbury MM: The pronator quadratus in motions and in stabilization of the radius and ulna at the distal radioulnar joint. J Hand Surg 1:205–209, 1976

79. Jones LA: The assessment of hand function. A critical review of techniques. J Hand Surg Am 14:221–228, 1989

80. Kaltenborn FM: Mobilization of the Extremity Joints, 3rd ed. Oslo, Olaf Norlis Bokhandel, 1980

81. Kapandji IA: Biomechanics of the interphalangeal joint of the thumb. In: Tubiana R, ed: The Hand, vol. 1. Philadelphia, WB Saunders, 1981a

82. Kapandji IA: Biomechanics of the thumb. In: Tubiana R, ed: The Hand, vol. 1. Philadelphia, WB Saunders, 1981b

83. Kapandji IA: The Physiology of the Joints, vol. 1: Upper Limb, 5th ed. New York, Churchill Livingstone, 1982

84. Kaplan EB: The participation of the MCP joint of the thumb in the act of opposition. Bull Hosp Joint Dis 27:39–45, 1966

85. Kauer JMG: Functional anatomy of the carpometacarpal joint of the thumb. Clin Orthop 220:7–13, 1987

86. Kendall FP, McCreary EK, Provance PG: Muscle Testing and Function, 4th ed. Baltimore, Williams & Wilkins, 1993

87. Kibler WB: Rehabilitation of the wrist and hand. In: Kibler WB, Herring SA, Press JM, et al: Functional Rehabilitation of Sports and Musculoskeletal Injuries. Gaithersburg, MD, Aspen Publications, 1998:183–187

88. Kiloh LG, Nevin S: Isolated neuritis of the anterior interosseous nerve. Br Med J 1:850–851, 1952

89. Kisner C, Colby LA: Therapeutic Exercise: Foundations and Techniques, 3rd ed. Philadelphia, FA Davis, 1996

90. Knott M, Voss DE: Proprioceptive Neuromuscular Facilitation, Patterns and Techniques. New York, Hoeber & Harper, 1956

91. Knutsson E: Proprioceptive neuromuscular facilitation. Scand J Rehabil Med Suppl 7:106–112, 1980

92. Konin JG, Wiksten DL, Iseaar JA: Special Tests for Orthopedic Examination. Thorefare, NJ, Slack, 1997

93. Kottke FJ, Pauley DL, Ptak KA: The rationale for prolonged stretching for correction of shortening of connective tissue. Arch Phys Med Rehabil 47:345–352, 1966

94. Kuckynski K: The thumb and saddle. Hand 7:120–195, 1975

95. Lamb DW: Dupuytren's disease. In: Lamb DW, Kuczynski K, eds: The Practice of Hand Surgery. Oxford, Blackwell Scientific, 1981:470

96. Landsmeer JMF: The anatomy of the dorsal aponeurosis of the human finger and its functional significance. Anat Rec 104:431–453, 1949

97. Landsmeer JMF: Power grip and precision handling. Ann Rheum Dis 22:164–197, 1962

98. Lankford LL: Reflex sympathetic dystrophy. In: Green LL, ed: Operative Hand Surgery, vol. 1. New York, Churchill Livingstone, 1982

99. Leclercq C, Hurst L, Badalamente MA: Treatment. In: Tubiana R, Leclercq C, Hurst LC, et al, eds: Dupuytren's Disease. London, Martin Dunitz, 2000:121–138

100. Lehmann JF, DeLateur BJ, Silverman DRT: Selective heating effects of ultrasound in human beings. Arch Phys Med Rehabil 47:331–339, 1966

101. Lewis OJ, Hamshere RJ, Bucknill TM: The anatomy of the wrist joint. J Anat 106:539–552, 1970

102. Linburg RM, Comstock BE: Anomalous tendon slips from the flexor pollicis longus to the flexor digitorum profundus. J Hand Surg Am 4:79–83, 1989

103. Linscheid RL, Dobyns JH: Physical examination of the wrist. In: Post M, ed: Physical Examination of the Musculoskeletal System. Chicago, Year Book Medical Publishers, 1987:80

104. Lister GD: The Hand. Diagnosis and Indications, 2nd ed. New York, Churchill Livingstone, 1984

105. Lister GD, Kleinert HE, Kutz JE, et al: Arthritis of the trapezial articulations treated by prosthetic replacement. Hand 9:117–129, 1977

106. Little KE: Toward more effective manipulative management of chronic myofascial strain and stress syndromes. J Am Osteopath Assoc 68:675–685, 1969

107. Littler JW: Principles of reconstructive surgery of the hand. In: JM Converse, ed: Reconstructive Plastic Surgery. Philadelphia, JB Lippincott, 1977

108. Long C, Conrad DW, Hall EA: Intrinsic-extrinsic muscle control of the hand in power grip and precision handling. J Bone Joint Surg Am 52:853–867, 1970

109. Lovett WL, Mc Calla MA: Nerve injuries: Management and rehabilitation. Orthop Clin North Am 14:767–778, 1983

110. Lukes RJ, Collins RD: New approaches to the classification of lymphomata. Br J Cancer 31:1–28, 1975

111. MacConaill MA: Mechanical anatomy of the carpus and its bearing on surgical problems. J Anat 75:166–175, 1941

112. Mackin EJ, Byron PM: Postoperative management. In: McFarlan RM, McGrouther DA, Flint MH, eds: Dupuytren's Disease. Edinburgh, Churchill Livingstone, 1990:368–378

113. Mackin EJ, Skirven TM: Hand therapy. In: Tubiana R, Leclercq C, Hurst LC, et al, eds: Dupuytren's Disease. London, Marin Dunitz, 2000:250–263

114. Mackinnon SE, Dellon AL: Surgery of the Peripheral Nerve. New York, Thieme, 1988

115. Madden JW, de Vore G, Arem AJ: A rational postoperative management program for MCP joint implant arthroplasty. J Hand Surg 2:358–366, 1977

116. Magee DJ: Orthopedic Physical Assessment, 3rd ed. Philadelphia, WB Saunders, 1997

117. Marie P, Meige H, Patrikiou S: Paralysie radiale dissocice simulant une griffe cubitale. Rev Neurol 24:123–124, 1917
118. Markos P: Ipsilateral and contralateral effects of proprioceptive neuromuscular facilitation techniques on hip motion and electromyographic activity. Phys Ther 59:1366–1373, 1979
119. Marks M, Gunther SF: Efficacy of cortisone injection in treatment of trigger fingers and thumbs. J Hand Surg 14:722–727, 1989
120. McEntee PA: Therapist's management of the stiff hand. In: Hunter JM, Schneider LH, Mackin EJ, et al, eds: Rehabilitation of the Hand. St. Louis, CV Mosby, 1984
121. McFarlane RM, Albion U: Dupuytren's disease: In: Hunter JM, Schneider LH, Mackin EJ, et al, eds: Rehabilitation of the Hand: Surgery and Therapy, 3rd ed. St. Louis, CV Mosby, 1990:867–872
122. Mennell JMCM: Joint Pain. Boston, Little, Brown & Co, 1964
123. Menon J, Schoene H, Hohl J: Trapeziometacarpal arthritis. Results of tendon interpositional arthroplasty. J Hand Surg 6:442–446, 1981
124. Milford LW: Restraining Ligaments of the Digits of the Hand: Gross and Microscopic Anatomic Study. Philadelphia, WB Saunders, 1968
125. Mittelbach HR: The Injured Hand: A Clinical Handbook for General Surgeons. New York, Springer-Verlag, 1979
126. Moberg E: Objective methods for determining the functional value of sensibility in the hand. J Bone Joint Surg Br 40:454–476, 1958
127. Moberg E: Shoulder–hand–finger syndrome. Surg Clin North Am 40:367–373, 1960
128. Mulligan BR: Manual Therapy 'Nags,' 'Snags,' 'MWMs' etc, 3rd ed. New Zealand, Plant View Services. 1995
129. Mulligan BR: Manual Therapy 'Nags,' 'Snags,' 'MWMs' etc, 4th ed. New Zealand, Plant View Services. 1999
130. Napler JR: The prehensile movements of the human hand. J Bone Joint Surg Br 38:902–913, 1956
131. Netter FH: The CIBA Collection of Medical Illustrations, vol. 8: Musculoskeletal System, Part 2. Summit, NJ, CIBA-Geigy Corp, 1990
132. Newmeyer WL: Primary Care of Hand Injuries. Philadelphia, Lea & Febiger, 1979
133. Norkin C, Levangie DK: Joint Structure and Function: A Comprehensive Analysis, 2nd ed. Philadelphia, FA Davis, 1992
134. Omer GE: Acute management of peripheral nerve injuries. Hand Clin 2:193–206, 1986
135. Pagalidis T, Kuczynski K, Lamb DW: Ligamentous stability of the base of the thumb. Hand 13:29–35, 1981
136. Palmer ML, Epler ME: Fundamentals of Musculoskeletal Assessment Techniques, 2nd ed. Philadelphia, Lippincott Williams & Wilkins, 1998
137. Paris SV: The Spinal Lesion. Christ Church, New Zealand, Pegasus Press, 1965
138. Peacock EE: Some biomechanical and biophysical aspects of joint stiffness; role of collagen synthesis as opposed to altered molecular bonding. Ann Surg 164:1–12, 1966
139. Perry JF: Use of a surgical glove in treatment of edema in hand. J Am Phys Ther Assoc 54:498–499, 1974
140. Petty NJ, Moore AP: Neuromusculoskeletal Examination and Assessment. Edinburgh, Churchill Livingstone, 1998
141. Poppen N, Niebauer J: "Tie in" trapezium prosthesis: Long-term results. J Hand Surg 3:445–450, 1978
142. Prentice WE, Voight ML: Techniques in Musculoskeletal Rehabilitation. New York, McGraw-Hill, 2001
143. Quinnell R: Conservative management of trigger finger. Practitioner 224:187–190, 1980
144. Rabischong P: Les problèmes fondamentaux du rétablissement de la préhenisme. Ann Chir 25:927–933, 1971
145. Rettig AC: Wrist injuries. Avoid diagnostic pitfalls. Phys Sports Med 22:33–39, 1994
146. Rettig AC: Wrist and hand overuse syndromes. Clin Sports Med 20:591–636, 2001
147. Rodman GP, Schumacher HR: Primer on the Rheumatic Diseases, 8th ed. Atlanta, The Arthritis Foundation, 1983
148. Rosse C: The hand. In: Rosse C, Clawson DK, eds: The Musculoskeletal System in Health and Disease. Philadelphia, Harper & Row, 1980:227–251
149. Saidoff DC, McDonough AL: Hand and wrist. In: Saidoff DC, McDonough AL: Critical Pathways in Therapeutic Intervention: Upper Extremities. St. Louis, Mosby, 1997:7–14
150. Salter RB: Textbook of Disorders and Injuries of the Musculoskeletal System, 2nd ed. Baltimore, Williams & Wilkins, 1983
151. Sandzen SC: Atlas of Wrist and Hand Fractures. Littleton, MA, PSG Publishing Co, 1979
152. Sapega AA, Quedenfeld TC, Moyer RA, et al: Physiological factors in range-of-motion exercises. Physician Sportsmed 9:57–65, 1981
153. Saplys R, Mackinnon SE, Dellon AL: The relationship between nerve entrapment versus neuroma complications and the misdiagnosis of de Quervain's disease. Contemp Orthop 15:51–57, 1987
154. Schamber D: Simply Performed Tests of the Hand. New York, Vantage Press, 1984
155. Schneider AM: Rehabilitation of the wrist, hand and fingers. In: Prentice WE, Voight ML, eds: Techniques in Musculoskeletal Rehabilitation. New York, McGraw-Hill, 2001:483–507

156. Seiler JG: Extensor tendon injuries. In: Seiler JG: Essentials of Hand Surgery, American Society for Surgery of the Hand. Philadelphia, Lippincott Williams & Wilkins, 2002
157. Shea JD, McClain EF: Ulnar-nerve compression syndrome at and below the wrist. J Bone Joint Surg Am 51:1095–1103, 1969
158. Simmons BP, De La Caffiniere JF: Physiology of flexion of the fingers. In: Tubiana R, ed: The Hand, vol. 1. Philadelphia, WB Saunders, 1981
159. Smith EM, Juvinall R, Bender L, et al: Role of the finger flexors in rheumatoid deformities of the MCP joints. Arthritis Rheum 7:467–480, 1964
160. Smith MS: Handcuff neuropathy. Ann Emerg Med 10:668, 1981
161. Spinner M: Kaplan's Functional and Surgical Anatomy of the Hand. Philadelphia, JB Lippincott, 1984
162. Stark HH, Bayer JH, Wilson JN: Mallet finger. Bone Joint Surg 44:1061–1068, 1962
163. Steinbrocker O, Argyros TG: The shoulder–hand syndrome: Present status as a diagnostic and therapeutic entity. Med Clin North Am 42:1533–1553, 1958
164. Steinbrocker O, Spitzer N, Friedman NH: The shoulder–hand syndrome in reflex dystrophy of the upper extremity. Ann Intern Med 29:22–52, 1948
165. Sucher BM: Palpatory diagnosis and manipulative management of carpal tunnel syndrome. J Am Osteopath Assoc 94:647–663, 1994
166. Sucher BM, Glassman JH: Upper extremity syndromes. Man Med 7:787–810, 1996
167. Sullivan PE, Markos PD: Clinical Decision Making in Therapeutic Exercise. Norwalk, CT, Appleton & Lange, 1994
168. Svendsen B, Moe K, Merritt R: Joint Mobilization, Laboratory Manual. Loma Linda, CA, Loma Linda University, 1981
169. Swanson AB, Goran-Hagert C, Swanson G: Evaluation of impairment of hand function. In: Hunter JM, Schneider LH, Mackin EJ, et al, eds: Rehabilitation of the Hand. St. Louis, CV Mosby, 1978
170. Swanson AB, Swanson G, Watermeier JJ: Trapezium implant arthroplasty—long-term evaluation of 150 cases. J Hand Surg 6:128–141, 1981
171. Taleisnik J: The ligaments of the wrist. J Hand Surg 1:110–118, 1976
172. Taleisnik J: Carpal instability. J Bone Joint Surg Am 70:1262–1268, 1988
173. Taleisnik J: Soft tissue injuries of the wrist. In: Strickland JW, Rettig AC, eds: Hand Injuries in Athletes. Philadelphia, WB Saunders, 1992:104–128
174. Tanigava MC: Comparison of the hold–relax procedure and passive mobilization on increasing muscle length. Phys Ther 52:725–735, 1972
175. Tappan FM: Holistic, Classical Massage and Emerging Methods, 3rd ed. Norwalk, CT, Appleton-Lange, 1998
176. Tinel J: Le signe du "fourmillement" dans les lesions des nerf peripheriques. Presse Med 47:388–389, 1915
177. Tomberlin JP, Saunders HD: Evaluation, Treatment and Prevention of Musculoskeletal Disorders, vol. 2: Extremities, 3rd ed. Chaska, MN, The Saunders Group, 1994
178. Tubiana R: The Hand, vol. 1. Philadelphia, WB Saunders, 1981
179. Tubiana R: Examination of the Hand and Upper Limb. Philadelphia, WB Saunders, 1984
180. Tubiana R, Leclercq C, Hurst LC, et al: Dupuytren's Disease. Malden, MA, Blackwell Science, Inc, 2000
181. Vastamaki M: Extraarticular etiologies of wrist pain. In: Watson HK, Weinzweig J, eds: The Wrist. Philadelphia, Lippincott Williams and Wilkins, 2001:95–106
182. Wadsworth CT: Wrist and hand examination and interpretation. J Orthop Sports Phys Ther 5:108–120, 1983
183. Wakim KG, Krusen FH: Influence of physical agents and of certain drugs on intra-articular temperature. Arch Phys Med Rehabil 32:714–721, 1951
184. Wallin D, Ekblom B, Grahn R, et al: Improvement of muscle flexibility: A comparison between two techniques. Am J Sports Med 13:263–268, 1985
185. Warren CG, Lehmann JF, Koblanski JN: Elongation of rat tail tendon: Effect of load and temperature. Arch Phys Med Rehabil 52:465–474, 1971
186. Warren CB, Lehmann JF, Koblanski JN: Heat and stretch procedures: An evaluation using rat tail tendon. Arch Phys Med Rehabil 57:122–126, 1976
187. Wartenberg RL: Cherialgia paresthetica (Isolierte Neuritis des Ramus Superficialis Nerve Radialis). A Ges Neurol Psychiatr 141:145–155, 1932
188. Watson HK: Stiff joints. In: Green DP, ed: Operative Hand Surgery, vol. 1. New York, Churchill Livingstone, 1982
189. Watson HK, Ashmead D, Makhlouf MV: Examination of the scaphoid. J Hand Surg Am 13:657–660, 1988
190. Weeks PM, Wray R, Kux M: The results of nonoperative management of stiff joints in the hand. Plast Reconstr Surg 62:58–63, 1978
191. Weeks PM, Wray RC: Management of Acute Hand Injuries. St. Louis, CV Mosby, 1973
192. Weinstein SM, Herring SA: Nerve problems and compartment syndromes in the hand, wrist, and forearm. Clin Sports Med 11:161–188, 1992
193. Wilson J: Arthroplasty of the trapeziometacarpal joint. Plast Reconstr Surg 49:143–148, 1974
194. Woolf D: Shoulder–hand syndrome. Practitioner 213:176–183, 1974
195. Wright V, Johns R: Physical factors concerned with stiffness of normal and diseased joints. Bull Johns Hopkins Hosp 106:215–231, 1960

196. Wynn-Parry CB: Rehabilitation of the Hand. Toronto, Butterworths, 1973
197. Youm Y, McMurtry RY, Flatt AB, et al: Kinematics of the wrist. I. An experimental study of radioulnar deviation and flexion–extension. J Bone Joint Surg Am 60:432–434, 1978
198. Zancolli EA: Structural and Dynamic Bases of Hand Surgery. Philadelphia, JB Lippincott, 1979
199. Zancolli EA, Ziadenberg C, Zancolli E: Biomechanics of the trapeziometacarpal joint. Clin Orthop 220:14–26, 1987

RECOMMENDED READINGS

Burton RI, Melchior JA: Extensor tendon—late construction. In: Green DP, Hofschkiss RV, Pederson WC, eds: Green's Operative Hand Surgery, vol. 2, 4th ed. New York, Churchill Livingstone, 1999:1988
Culp RW, Taras JS: Primary care of flexor tendon injuries. In: Hunter JM, Schneider LH, Mackin EJ, et al, eds: Rehabilitation of the Hand. Surgery and Therapy, 4th ed. St. Louis, Mosby, 1995:417
Doyle JR: Extensor tendon—acute injuries. In: Green DP, Hofschkiss RV, Pederson WC, eds: Green's Operative Hand Surgery, vol. 2, 4th ed. New York, Churchill Livingstone, 1999:1950
Evans RB: An update on extensor tendon management. In: Hunter JM, Schneider LH, Mackin EJ, et al, eds: Rehabilitation of the Hand. Surgery and Therapy, 4th ed. St. Louis Mosby, 1995:565
Hunter JM, Taras JS, Mackin EJ, et al: Staged flexor tendon reconstruction using passive and active tendon implants. In: Hunter JM, Schneider LH, Mackin EJ, et al, eds: Rehabilitation of the Hand. Surgery and Therapy, 4th ed. St. Louis, Mosby, 1995:477

Jacobs JL: Hand and wrist. In: Richardson JK, Iglarsh ZA, eds: Clinical Orthopaedic Physical Therapy. Philadelphia, WB Saunders, 1994
Keinert HE, Kutz JE, Ashbell TS, et al: Primary repair of lacerated flexor tendons in no-mans's land. J Bone Joint Surg Am 49:577, 1967
Kobus RJ, Kirkpatrick WH: The superficialis finger: An alternative in flexor tendon surgery. In: Hunter JM, Schneider LH, Mackin EJ, et al, eds: Rehabilitation of the Hand. Surgery and Therapy, 4th ed. St. Louis, Mosby, 1995:515
Lister GD, Kleinert HE, Kutz JE, et al: Primary flexor tendon repair followed by immediate controlled mobilization. J Hand Surg 2:441, 1977
Rosenthal EA: The extensor tendons: Anatomy and management. In: Hunter JM, Schneider LH, Mackin EJ, et al, eds: Rehabilitation of the Hand. Surgery and Therapy, 4th ed. St. Louis, Mosby, 1995:519
Schneider LH, Berger-Fledscher S: Tenolysis: Dynamic approach to surgery and therapy. In: Hunter JM, Schneider LH, Mackin EJ, et al, eds: Rehabilitation of the Hand. Surgery and Therapy, 4th ed. St. Louis, Mosby, 1995:463
Schneider LH, Hunter JM: Flexor tendons—late reconstruction. In: Green DP, Hotchkiss RV, Pederson WC, eds: Operative Hand Surgery, vol. 2, 4th ed. New York, Churchill Livingstone, 1999:1969:1898
Seiler JG III: Essentials of Hand Surgery, American Society for Surgery of the Hand. Philadelphia, Lippincott Williams & Wilkins, 2002.
Stewart KM, van Strien G: Postoperative management of flexor tendon injuries. In: Hunter JM, Schneider LH, Mackin EJ, et al, eds: Rehabilitation of the Hand. Surgery and Therapy, 4th ed. St. Louis, Mosby, 1995:443
Strickland JW: Flexor tendons—acute injuries. In: Green DP, Hotschkiss RV, Pederson WC, eds: Green's Operative Hand Surgery, vol. 2, 4th ed. New York, Churchill Livingstone, 1999:1851

DARLENE HERTLING AND RANDOLPH M. KESSLER

14

REVIEW OF FUNCTIONAL ANATOMY

Osteology

The acetabulum is formed superiorly by the ilium, posteroinferiorly by the ischium, and anteroinferiorly by the pubis. The acetabulum faces laterally, anteriorly, and inferiorly (Fig. 14-1A). It is deepened by the fibrocartilaginous acetabular labrum, allowing it to enclose slightly more than half a sphere. The bony, fibrocartilaginous labrum and cartilaginous constituents of the acetabulum are interrupted inferiorly by the acetabular notch (Fig. 14-1B). This notch is traversed by the transverse ligament of the acetabulum (Fig. 14-1C).

The head of the femur constitutes about two thirds of a sphere. Slightly below and behind the center of the articular surface of the head is a roughened indentation termed the *fovea*, to which the ligament of the head of the femur attaches (Fig. 14-1B). The neck of the femur connects the head and shaft of the femur. In the frontal plane, the angle formed by the neck and shaft of the femur is about 125° in the adult but closer to 150° in the young child. This is often termed the *angle of inclination* (Fig. 14-2). In the transverse plane, the neck forms an angle of about 15° with the transverse axis of the femoral condyles, such that with the transverse axis of the condyles lying in the frontal plane, the neck of the femur is directed about 15° forward (Fig. 14-3). This is referred to as the *angle of torsion* or *angle of declination* of the hip.

In the anatomic position, both the acetabulum and the neck of the femur are directed anteriorly. Because of this, in the normal standing position, a large area of the articular surface of the head of the femur is exposed anteriorly, and the effective weight-bearing surface of the head is confined to a relatively small area on the posterosuperior aspect of the head.

An increase in degrees of the normal inclination angle is referred to as *coxa valgum;* a decrease in the angle is called *coxa varum* (Fig. 14-2). When an increased torsion angle is present, we speak of antetorsion; when the torsion angle is less than normal, it is called retrotorsion (Fig. 14-3B). The term *antetorsion* should not be confused with *anteversion.* Anteversion is not associated with alignment of any other part of the femur, but is a feature of the hip joint alone.[59,83] Anteversion is a positional change in which either the acetabulum or the head and neck of the femur are directed anteriorly relative to the frontal plane.[22] Antetorsion is a medial twist of the shaft of the bone, distal on proximal. When the transcondylar axis is aligned on the frontal plane, the femoral head and neck are directed anteriorly, indicating the existence of torsion in the femoral shaft. The result is a medially displaced patella. More distally, the feet are aligned either in a noncompensatory toe-in stance or in a compensatory toe-out stance.[22]

A patient with an anteverted hip will appear to lack external rotation, and a patient with a retroverted hip will appear to lack internal rotation. Also, the person with an anteverted hip will tend to walk with a toe-in gait; with retroversion, a toe-out gait is characteristic.

The greater trochanter is a prominence projecting laterally and superiorly from the junction of the neck and shaft of the femur. It serves as an area for attachment of many of the muscles controlling movement at the hip. Situated posteromedially to the junction of the neck and shaft is a smaller

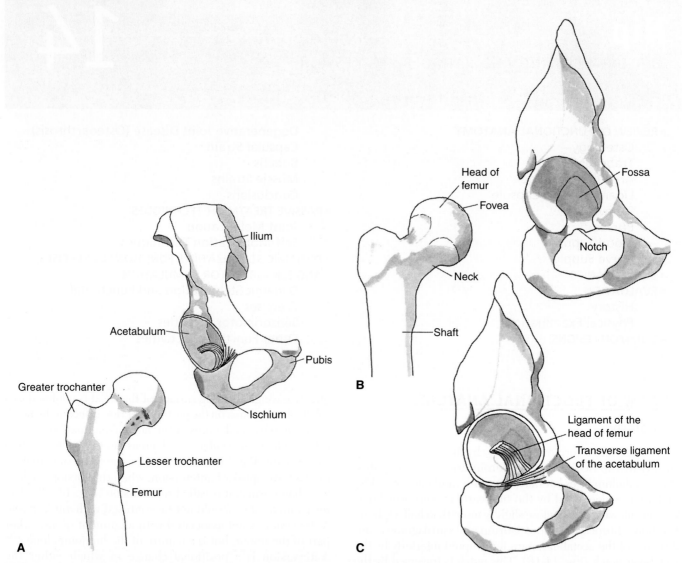

■ **FIG. 14-1.** Components of the right hip joint, showing the relationship of the acetabulum to the femur (**A**), the acetabular fossa to the proximal femur (**B**), and the ligaments of the acetabulum (**C**).

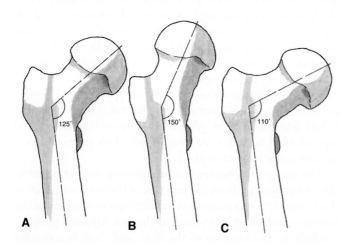

■ **FIG. 14-2.** Angle of inclination of the femur: (**A**) normal, (**B**) coxa valgum, and (**C**) coxa varum.

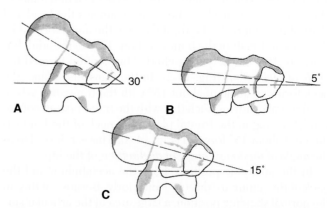

■ **FIG. 14-3.** Angle of torsion or declination of the femur in the transverse plane: (**A**) antetorsion, (**B**) retrotorsion, (**C**) normal angle.

prominence, the lesser trochanter; it also provides an area of insertion for muscles controlling the hip (Fig. 14-1A).

Trabeculae

The trabecular patterns of the upper femur reflect the normal stresses sustained by the hip; they correspond to the normal lines of force in this area (Fig. 14-4). The main system of trabeculae consists of two sets of trabeculae. The arcuate bundle resists a bending moment or a tendency for the weight of the body to shear the head and neck inferiorly with respect to the shaft of the femur; this bending moment is brought about by the lever arm created by the medially projecting neck of the femur. The vertical bundle resists vertical compressive forces through the head of the femur. The arcuate bundle runs from the lateral cortex of the shaft of the femur, just inferior to the greater trochanter, upward and medially to the middle and inferior cortical region of the head of the femur. The vertical bundle is contiguous with the medial cortex of the shaft of the femur, running straight upward to the superior cortex of the head.

Another trabecular system runs from the medial cortex at the base of the neck, upward laterally through the greater trochanter. These trabeculae resist the tensile forces from the muscles attaching to the trochanter.

The areas where the vertical bundle and the trochanteric bundle intersect the arcuate bundle are areas of particular strength. The intervening region is an area of relative weakness, made weaker by osteoporosis in older people. This region is often the site of femoral neck fractures.

Articular Cartilage

The area of the acetabulum covered by articular cartilage is horseshoe-shaped. The area not covered by articular cartilage corresponds to the total sweep of the ligament of the head of the femur when the hip is moved through a full range of movement in all planes. This nonarticular portion is the acetabular fossa and is lined by a fat pad (Fig. 14-1B). The entire head of the femur is covered by articular cartilage except for the small fovea where the ligament of the head attaches.

Ligaments and Capsule

The joint capsule of the hip joint is thick and strong and is reinforced by strong ligaments. Its fibers run longitudinally, parallel to the neck of the femur (Fig. 14-5). The capsule runs from the rim of the acetabulum and labrum to the intertrochanteric line anteriorly and to about 1 cm proximal to the intertrochanteric crest posteriorly. Much of the neck of the femur, then, is intracapsular. Some deep fibers of the joint capsule run circularly around the neck of the femur, forming the zona orbicularis.

The iliofemoral ligament is one of the strongest ligaments in the body. It is sometimes referred to as the Y ligament of Bigelow because it resembles an inverted Y. It attaches proximally to the lower portion of the anteroinferior iliac spine and to an area on the ilium just proximal to the superior and posterosuperior rim of the acetabulum. The ligament, as a whole, spirals around to overlie the anterior aspect of the joint, attaching to the intertrochanteric line. The more lateral fork of the Y attaches to the anterior aspect of the greater

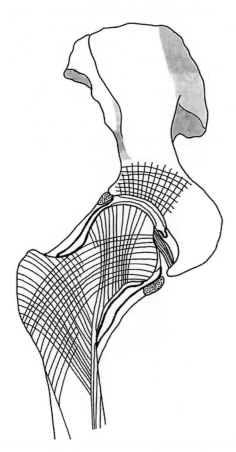

■ **FIG. 14-4.** Trabecular patterns of the upper femur.

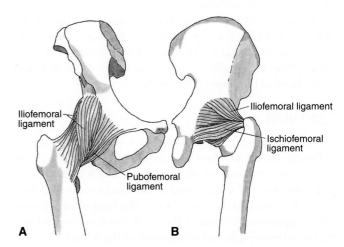

■ **FIG. 14-5.** Anterior (**A**) and posterior (**B**) views of the joint capsule of the hip joint.

trochanter, whereas the more medial fibers twist around to attach just anterior to the lesser trochanter (Fig. 14-5A).

This ligament primarily checks internal rotation and extension. It allows a person to stand with the joint in extension using a minimum of muscle action; by rolling the pelvis backward, a person can "hang" on the ligaments. The ligament prevents excessive movement in the direction toward the close-packed position of the hip joint. Looking at it another way, with movement toward the close-packed position, this ligament becomes taut and twisted on itself, causing an approximation of the joint surfaces and a "locking" of the joint. Some of the lateral fibers of the iliofemoral ligament probably pull tight on adduction.

The ischiofemoral ligament attaches proximally to an area of the ischium just posterior and posteroinferior to the rim of the acetabulum. Its fibers run upward and laterally to attach to the posterosuperior aspect of the neck of the femur, where the neck meets the greater trochanter (Fig. 14-5B). The ischiofemoral ligament also pulls tight on extension and internal rotation of the hip.

The pubofemoral ligament runs from the pubis, near the acetabulum, to the femur, just anterior to the lesser trochanter. It tightens primarily on abduction but also helps check internal rotation of the hip (Fig. 14-5A).

The ligament of the head of the femur (ligamentum teres) attaches to the roughened nonarticular area of the acetabulum inferiorly near the acetabular notch, to both sides of the notch, and to the transverse ligament that traverses the notch. It lies in the nonarticular acetabular fossa as it runs up and around the head of the femur to the fovea (Fig. 14-1C).

Although the ligament of the head of the femur pulls tight on adduction of the hip, its mechanical function is relatively unimportant. Of more significance is its role in providing some vascularization to the head of the femur and perhaps in assisting with lubrication of the joint. The ligament of the head of the femur is lined with synovium. It is believed that this ligament may act somewhat similarly to the meniscus at the knee by spreading a layer of synovial fluid over the articular surface of the head of the femur as it advances to contact the opposing surface of the acetabulum.

As mentioned, the transverse ligament crosses the acetabular notch to fill in the gap. It converts the notch into a foramen through which the acetabular artery (from the obturator artery) runs, eventually becoming the artery of the ligament of the head of the femur (Fig. 14-1C).

Synovium

The synovial membrane of the hip joint lines the fibrous layer of the capsule. It also lines the acetabular labrum and, inferiorly, continues inward at the acetabular notch to line the fat pad in the floor of the acetabular fossa and to cover the ligament of the head of the femur. From the femoral attachment of the capsule at the base of the neck, the synovium reflects backward proximally to line the neck of the femur.

The synovial "cavity" of the joint often communicates anteriorly with the iliopectineal bursa. It does so through a gap between the pubofemoral ligament and the medial portion of the iliofemoral ligament.

Bursae

The rather large iliopectineal bursa overlies the anterior aspect of the hip joint and the pubis and lies beneath the iliopsoas muscle as it crosses in front of the hip joint. This bursa often communicates with the hip joint anteriorly through a space between the pubofemoral and iliofemoral ligaments. This may be a factor in the characteristic anterior pain experienced by patients with hip joint disease (Fig. 14-6).

One or more trochanteric bursae overlie the greater trochanter, reducing friction between it and the gluteus maximus, which passes over the trochanter, and the other gluteals, which attach to the trochanter. This bursa is most extensive posterolaterally to the trochanter, where it underlies the gluteus maximus. It is important clinically because of the prevalence of trochanteric bursitis.

Blood Supply

The blood supply to the head of the femur is of particular importance because of its significance in common pathologic conditions at the hip, including fractures and osteochondrosis of the femoral head (Legg-Perthes disease). The head of the femur receives its vascularization from two sources, the artery of the ligament of the head of the femur and the arteries that ascend along the neck of the femur (Fig. 14-7). The importance of the artery of the ligament of the head of the femur is variable, but for the most part it supplies only a small area adjacent to the fovea. In as many as 20% of persons it fails to anastomose with the other arteries supplying the head of the femur.

The primary blood supply to the head of the femur, then, is derived from the arteries that ascend proximally along the neck of the femur to pierce the head of this bone just distal to

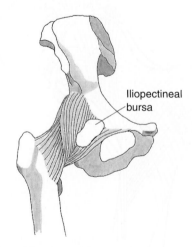

Iliopectineal bursa

■ **FIG. 14-6.** Anterior aspect of the hip joint showing the iliopectineal bursa.

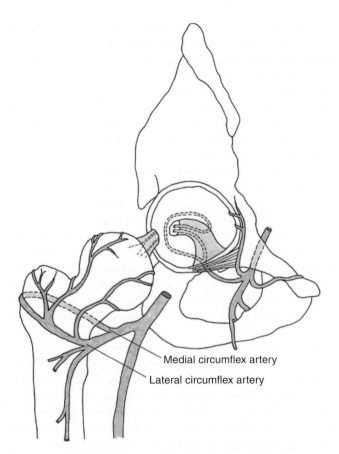

■ FIG. 14-7. Blood supply to the head of the femur.

Medial circumflex artery
Lateral circumflex artery

the margin of the articular cartilage. These are branches of the medial and lateral femoral circumflex arteries. The medial circumflex artery passes around posteriorly to give off branches that ascend along the posteroinferior and posterosuperior aspects of the neck of the femur. The lateral circumflex artery crosses anteriorly to give off an anterior ascending artery at about the level of the intertrochanteric line. The ascending arteries pierce the joint capsule near its distal attachment to the femur and run proximally along the neck of the femur intracapsularly. They run deep to the synovial lining of the neck. Because of their relationship to the neck, they are subject to interruption in the case of a femoral neck fracture. Also, because they are intracapsular, it is believed that increased intracapsular pressure caused by joint effusion may stop flow. This is believed to be a factor in osteochondrosis and in some cases of idiopathic avascular necrosis of the head of the femur. The circumflex vessels give off extracapsular branches to the trochanteric regions of the femur. This area also receives vascularization from the superior gluteal artery and a perforating branch of the profunda.

Nerve Supply

Innervation to the hip joint is supplied by branches from the obturator nerve, the superior gluteal nerve, and the nerve to the quadratus femoris and by branches from the femoral nerve, both muscular and articular. These nerves represent segments L2 through S1.

BIOMECHANICS

The hip joint, being a ball-and-socket joint, exhibits three degrees of freedom of motion. In this respect it is analogous to the glenohumeral joint. Unlike the shoulder, however, the hip is intrinsically a very stable joint. This is owing, in part, to the fact that the acetabulum forms a much deeper socket than the glenoid cavity; the head of the femur comes closer to forming a full sphere than does the head of the humerus. The acetabulum, with its labrum, can enclose more than half a sphere and can grasp passively the head of the femur to maintain joint integrity; it is difficult to pull the head from the acetabulum without removing or tearing the acetabular labrum.

Coaptation of joint surfaces is also maintained, in part, by atmospheric pressure. Because of the relatively large surface area of contact between joint surfaces, the atmospheric pressures holding the joint surfaces together may be as much as 25 kg. This is sufficient to maintain coaptation of the joint with all soft tissues about the joint removed and the limb hanging freely. Only when the vacuum created between the joint surfaces (by the close fit) is released (by, say, drilling a hole through the acetabulum) will the limb drop free.

Intrinsic stability at the joint is further enhanced by the strong ligamentous support at the hip. Because the major ligaments at the hip pull taut and are twisted on themselves with extension, the hip joint is particularly stable in the standing position. As mentioned, the twisting of the capsule that occurs with movement toward the close-packed position effects a type of "screw home" movement at the hip in which the joint surfaces become tightly approximated. As with any joint, the close-packed position at the hip (extension–abduction–internal rotation) is the position of maximal congruence of joint surfaces.

Because the acetabulum and the neck of the femur are both directed anteriorly, their respective mechanical axes are not coincidental. There are two positions of the hip in which these axes are brought into alignment. One position is attained by flexing the hip to about 90°, abducting slightly, and rotating slightly externally. The other position is one of extension, abduction, and internal rotation. The former position is the one that the hip would assume in a quadruped situation, and the latter is the close-packed position of the joint. As mentioned, in the upright position, a considerable portion of the articular cartilage of the head of the femur is exposed anteriorly. During normal use of the joint, as in walking, there is a relatively small contact area between the acetabulum and the femoral head. This may be a factor in the prevalence of degenerative hip disease in humans; stresses of weight bearing are borne by a small surface area of cartilage, and a relatively large area of cartilage may not undergo the intermittent compression necessary for adequate nutrition (see Chapter 3, Arthrology).

The smaller the torsion angle at the hip (the less it is anteverted), the greater the stability of the bone because the axes of the acetabulum and neck of the femur are closer to being in alignment. A smaller torsion angle also favors an increase in the effective contact area between joint surfaces for the same reason.

Because of its intrinsic stability, the normal hip joint rarely dislocates when compared with, say, the shoulder or elbow. The shoulder, elbow, or any other joint usually dislocates when a force is applied over the joint when it is in its close-packed position. This is not true at the hip, which will usually dislocate only when its capsule and major ligaments are lax and its joint surfaces and bony axes are out of congruence. Thus, the hip is most prone to dislocation when in a position of flexion (ligaments lax), abduction, and internal rotation (noncongruence). Dislocation usually occurs with a force driving the femur backward on the pelvis with the hip in this position—for example, striking the knee on the dashboard of a car in a head-on collision. With such an injury, the head of the femur is driven posteriorly through the relatively weak posterior capsule.

Because the hip is freely movable in all vertical planes, it is not subject to capsuloligamentous strain from horizontal forces applied to it in most positions, even though, owing to the length of the leg, these forces acting over a long lever arm are potentially quite large. However, because the hip is a weight-bearing joint, it is subject to vertical loading that must be borne by its bony and cartilaginous components.

In the case of a person bearing equal weight through both legs, the vertical force on each femoral head is equal to half the weight of the body minus the weight of the legs. When standing on one leg, however, the weight-bearing femoral head must support more than the weight of the body. This is because the center of gravity (at about S2) is located some distance medially to the supporting femoral head. This lever arm through which the force is acting causes a rotary moment about the supporting femoral head, with a tendency for the opposite side of the pelvis to drop. This rotary moment must be countered by the hip abductor muscles, primarily the gluteus medius, gluteus minimus, and tensor fasciae latae, on the weight-bearing side. The point of application of this counterforce provided by the abductor pull is at the greater trochanter, which is considerably closer to the fulcrum (femoral head) than is the center of gravity line that represents the force produced by the body weight. Because the distance from the femoral head to the trochanter is about half the distance from the femoral head to the center of gravity line, the abductors must pull with a force equal to two times the superincumbent body weight to prevent the pelvis from dropping to the non–weight-bearing side. The total force acting vertically at the femoral head is equal to the force produced by the pull of the abductors plus the force produced by the body weight, or up to *three times* the body weight.[52,70,74,113] In this case "body weight" is actually the total body weight minus the weight of the supporting leg.

During stance phase of the normal gait cycle, the vertical forces acting at the femoral head are substantial. If the abductors are not strong enough to counter the forces tending to rotate or tilt the pelvis downward to the opposite side, an abnormal gait pattern results. Either the pelvis will drop noticeably to the opposite side of the weakness, usually resulting in a short swing phase on that side, or the person will lurch toward the side of weakness during stance phase on the weak side. The effect of the lurch is to shift the center of gravity toward the fulcrum (femoral head), reducing the moment arm about which the forces from the body weight may act, thereby reducing the necessary counterpull by the abductors. In fact, a marked lurch may actually shift the center of gravity lateral to the fulcrum, allowing gravity to substitute for the hip abductors, thus preventing the pelvis from dropping to the opposite side. This lurching gait is often referred to as a "compensated gluteus medius gait." It is usually seen in patients with painful hip conditions, such as degenerative joint disease, in which there is some weakness of the abductors and in which it is desirable to reduce compressive forces acting at the joint for relief of pain. It is also seen in patients with abductor paralysis.

The "abductor lurch" may be prevented by providing an external means of preventing the pelvis from dropping toward the uninvolved side during stance phase on the involved side. This external force may be provided by using a cane on the uninvolved side. An upward force is transmitted from the ground through the cane to counter the weight of the body tending to rotate the pelvis downward on that side. The forces acting through the cane do so about a moment arm even longer than that about which the force of gravity on the body weight acts because the point of contact of the hand on the cane is farther from the supporting femoral head than is the center of gravity line. For this reason, a relatively small force applied through the cane is required to compensate for the abductors and relieve the vertical forces acting at the involved hip. The forces acting upward through the cane must be transmitted to the pelvis through contraction of the lateral trunk muscles, shoulder depressors, elbow extensors, and wrist flexors on the side of the cane.

Clearly, forces of muscle contraction contribute significantly to compressive loading at the hip. This is not only true in a weight-bearing situation. Studies in which strain gauges have been inserted into prosthetic hips suggest that supine straight-leg raising causes a compressive force to the hip that is greater than the body weight.[87] This is an important consideration in the early management of patients who have undergone an internal fixation for a hip fracture.[57]

EVALUATION

History

The hip joint is derived from segments L2 through S1. Clinically, however, pain of hip joint origin is primarily perceived as involving the L3 segment. Typically, the patient with hip joint disease complains first of pain in the midinguinal region. As the process progresses, or as the painful stimulus intensifies, pain is likely to be felt into the anterior thigh and knee. At this point pain may also be described in the greater trochanteric region and buttock as well. In some instances (and not uncommonly) pain is felt most in the knee, and the patient may actually believe the knee is at fault. In general, pain in the trochanteric region spreading into the lateral thigh is more suggestive of trochanteric bursitis. Pain in the buttock spreading into the lateral or posterior thigh is more suggestive of pain of lower spinal origin.

Because of its freedom of movement in all planes and its great stability, the hip is seldom afflicted by disorders of acute traumatic origin. The hip is a common site, however, of degenerative joint disease and, to a lesser extent, rheumatoid arthritis. The clinician should ask whether the patient suffered any childhood hip disorders such as congenital dysplasia, osteochondrosis (Legg-Perthes disease), or slipped capital epiphysis, as these may predispose to early hip degeneration. Bursitis, either trochanteric or iliopectineal, is also fairly common at the hip.

The clinician must also determine whether the patient has a history of back problems. Low back disorders may mimic hip disease and vice versa because of the segmental relationships. Also, hip disease often leads to back problems because of the biomechanical relationships. See Chapter 5, Assessment of Musculoskeletal Disorders and Concepts of Management, for a complete list of questions to be included in the history.

Physical Examination

The order and detail of the physical tests described below need to be appropriate to the patient being examined. Some tests will be irrelevant, others will only need to be carried out briefly, whereas others will need to be fully investigated. Throughout the physical examination the clinician must aim to find physical tests that reproduce the patient's symptoms.

I. Observation
    A. Gait. Analyze gait (including walking backward) on even and uneven ground, slopes, stairs, running, and so on. Note the stride length and weight-bearing ability. Inspect the feet, shoes, and any walking aids.
        1. A lurch to one side during stance phase suggests hip pain, abductor weakness, or both on the side to which the lurch occurs.
        2. Dropping of the pelvis on the opposite side of the stance leg suggests abductor weakness (uncompensated) on the side of the stance leg.
        3. Development of an excessive lordosis during stance phase may suggest hip flexion contracture on the side of the stance leg.
        4. A backward lurch of the trunk during stance phase may suggest hip extensor weakness on the side of the stance leg, or hip flexor weakness on the side of the swing leg.
        5. A persistent inclination of the pelvis to one side during all phases of the gait cycle, combined with a lack

of heel-strike on the side of inclination, suggests an adduction contracture on the side of the inclination.
    B. Functional activities. The emphasis is on assessing functional activities involving use of the hip. Functional activities (in addition to gait) should include the following:
        1. Activities of daily living. Loss of hip motion may result in considerable difficulty removing and donning shoes, socks, and slacks.
        2. Sitting. The patient may "sacral sit" to compensate for a lack of hip flexion.
        3. Forward bending. Bending forward to touch the toes and crossing the legs may be difficult.
        4. Balance. One-legged standing (with the eyes open and then closed). One should observe for dropping of the pelvis to the opposite side—Trendelenburg's sign and the patient's proprioceptive control in the joints being assessed. The *Trendelenburg test* is used to evaluate the functional force or torque capability of the hip abductor group. The use of stork standing has also been advocated for testing proprioception.[117]
        5. Balance and reach test (see Chapter 10, Functional Exercise)[40]
            a. Unilateral stance on involved extremity, reach in various directions with uninvolved extremity to assess both proprioception and strength in various muscles depending on direction of reach; compare distance reached to similar reaches in unilateral stance on uninvolved extremity.
            b. Unilateral stance on involved extremity, reach in various directions with one or both arms to assess proprioception and trunk and lower extremity strength; compare distance reached with similar reaches in unilateral stance on uninvolved extremity.
        6. Squatting and sitting on the heels
        7. Full rotation, and other movements of the trunk, while standing on one leg.
    C. Note general posture and body build. Note whether there is even weight bearing through the left and right leg. Passively correct any asymmetry to determine its relevance to the patient's problem. The assessment of posture should include both static (standing, sitting, and supine) and dynamic postural analysis (see Chapter 7, Myofascial Considerations and Evaluation in Somatic Dysfunction).
II. Inspection
    A. Skin. Usually noncontributory in common hip disorders. Observe for old surgical scars.
    B. Soft tissue
        1. Observe for muscle bulk and muscle tone of the patient, comparing left and right sides. Document thigh atrophy by girth measurements.
        2. Hip joint effusion is usually not visible owing to heavy soft-tissue covering.
    C. Bony structure and alignment. Measure and record deviations.

1. Use plumb bob to assess mediolateral and antero-posterior alignment in the standing position (including the spine).
2. Assess relative heights of the following structures:
   a. Navicular tubercles
   b. Medial malleoli
   c. Fibular heads
   d. Popliteal folds
   e. Gluteal folds
   f. Greater trochanters
   g. Anterosuperior iliac spines
   h. Posterosuperior iliac spines
   i. Iliac crests

Note: A vertical structural deviation arising from some abnormality at the hip joint or upper end of the femur is suggested if, from the floor upward, all of the above-mentioned landmarks are level up to the trochanters, but the anterosuperior iliac spines, posterosuperior iliac spines, and iliac crests are not. Note whether the relative levels of the anterosuperior and posterosuperior iliac spines on one side are the same as the levels on the opposite side. If not, the asymmetry may be caused by a sacroiliac torsion rather than some abnormality at the hip joint or upper femur. If the trochanters are level and the anterosuperior and posterosuperior iliac spines and iliac crest on one side are lower by the same amount than their counterparts on the opposite side, one may suspect one of several possibilities: coxa varum on the low side, coxa valgum on the high side, a shortened femoral neck on the low side or a lengthened neck on the high side (rare), or cartilaginous narrowing from hip joint degeneration on the low side. The two most common of these are coxa varum and hip joint degeneration. Coxa varum is usually associated with a decreased angle of declination (torsion angle); hip joint degeneration may be sufficient to cause clinically detectable vertical asymmetry and other signs of degenerative joint disease (see Common Lesions below).

The extent of coxa varum, hip joint narrowing, or other cause of asymmetry may be documented by assessing the position of the greater trochanter relative to a line drawn from the anterosuperior iliac spine to the ischial tuberosity (Nélaton's line). The "normal" trochanter should lie about on this line. This measurement is primarily useful in unilateral conditions in which it may be compared with the "normal" side. Documentation of total leg-length discrepancy should be made by measuring from the anterosuperior iliac spine to the medial malleolus of the same side.

III. Joint Tests. Joint tests include active and passive physiologic movements of the hip and other relevant joints. Joint-play (accessory) movements complete the joint tests.
   A. Active movements and passive physiologic joint movements. For both active and passive physiologic joint movement, the examiner should note the following:
      • the range of movement
      • the quality of movement
      • the resistance through the range of movement and at the end range of movement

   • the behavior of pain through the range and at the end range of movement
   B. Active physiologic movements with passive overpressure. Active hip movements commonly tested in standing are flexion and extension. The normal range of hip flexion (knee bent) is 120°, but there is a wide variation. Establish the patient's symptoms at rest. Record range of motion, pain, and crepitus. For the hip joint, the following should be tested:
      • flexion
      • extension
      • abduction
      • adduction
      • medial rotation
      • lateral rotation

      If the history has indicated that repetitive movements, sustained postures, or combined movements have caused symptoms, the examiner should ensure that these movements are tested. For further information compression or distraction can be added as well as repetitive movements. Numerous differentiation tests can be performed; the choice depends on the patient's signs and symptoms.[78] For example, when trunk rotation, with the patient standing on one leg (causing rotation in the lumbar spine and hip joint), reproduces the patient's buttock pain, differentiation between the hip joint and lumbar spine may be required.
   C. Passive physiologic joint movement. Passive physiologic joint movements should be compared with the uninvolved side. The type of end feel and the results of passive overpressure are noted. Although the movement must be gentle, the examiner should apply passive overpressure at end range to find out the type of end feel, whether there is any limitation of motion (hypomobility) or excessive range (hypermobility), and whether it is painful.
      1. Flexion–extension. Joint motions are best assessed with Mundale's pelvic femoral angle measurement using the standardized sidelying position.[90] Draw a transverse line for the pelvis, connecting the anterosuperior and posterosuperior iliac spines (line *AB* in Fig. 14-8*A*), with the hip in full flexion (with the knee flexed) or extension (with the knee straight). Construct a perpendicular line *CD* from this line to the most superior point of the greater trochanter; the angle between this line and the long axis of the femur, *DE*, is measured in full flexion and extension. By using the same landmarks the clinician can assess other hip positions, including weight-bearing flexion.

      Considering the ease of measurement, reliability, and reproducibility, the use of the prone extension test is recommended to measure hip extension in children with cerebral palsy and those with meningomyelocele. The Thomas test is recommended in the supine position as an alternative for nonspastic patients.[4,122]
      2. Abduction–adduction. When measuring, be sure to prevent internal-external hip rotation and lateral tilt-

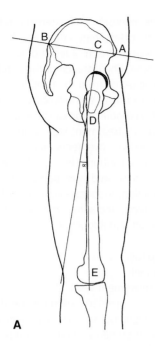

A

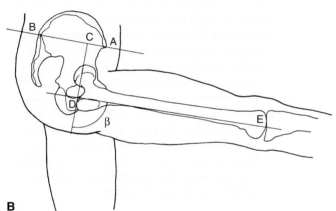

B

■ **FIG. 14-8.** Reference lines for the measurement of hip extension (**A**) and in the position of maximal hip flexion with the straight leg (**B**) as described by Mundale and coworkers.[90]

ing of the pelvis. The examiner must first fix the pelvis with one hand while the extended leg is then passively abducted with the other hand. When assessing abduction (supine), the leg to be tested should be close to the edge of the plinth so that when full abduction of the extended leg is reached, the knee can be passively flexed to assess one-joint adduction (mainly pectineus and the adductors) versus two-joint adduction (gracilis, biceps femoris, semimembranosus, and semitendinous).[54]

Adduction of the hip is normally limited by one leg coming into contact with the other. One leg should be held in slight flexion so as to cross over the other leg.

a. Capsular restriction will result in marked limitation of abduction and mild limitation of adduction.

b. Full motion with pain at the extremes of adduction, abduction, or both may be present with trochanteric bursitis.

3. Internal-external rotation. Passive hip rotation may be tested by three methods.

a. Assess while the patient lies supine with the hip and knees extended. The examiner rapidly rotates the leg inward and outward via the ankle. In the early stages of hip disease, before hip deformity develops, a characteristic type of end feel caused by loss of normal fluid type is perceived.[21] This test also becomes a useful mobilization technique.

b. Measure sitting with hips and knees flexed.

c. Measure prone with the knee flexed (this is a more "functional" measurement because the hip is extended as in walking).

d. Limited internal rotation and *excessive* external rotation suggest retrotorsion (decreased angle of torsion). Limited external rotation and *excessive* internal rotation suggest increased antetorsion (increased angle of torsion). If internal rotation is considerably limited and external rotation somewhat limited, capsular tightening is likely.

4. Combined hip flexion–adduction–rotation. This test uses the femur as a lever and stretches the posterolateral and inferior capsule and compresses the superior and medial portions of the capsule. With the patient supine, the examiner flexes the patient's knee and hip fully and then adducts the leg. As the knee is moved fully toward the patient's opposite shoulder, the examiner compresses the hip joint. The examiner should stabilize the pelvis and apply passive overpressure at the end of range. This test will also reveal tightness of the external rotators, particularly the piriformis.[54] If a tight piriformis is present, adduction and internal rotation range are decreased and painful. This test may produce pain in the buttock if a tight piriformis is impinging on the sciatic nerve or if an inflamed bursa is compressed beneath the stretched gluteus maximus. The distance of the knee from the chest is noted.

5. Scouring (quadrant test; Fig. 14-9) stresses the posterior and lateral hip capsule. It also reveals an abnormal end feel as the hip is rotated.[41,78,117] Normally the end feel is that of a smooth arc. In early joint changes, a clearly perceived bump in the arch is noted. A grating sensation or sound may be elicited in an osteoarthritic hip.

a. The subject lies supine with the hip flexed and adducted and the knee fully flexed. The examiner stands on the same side of the table, hands clasped over the patient's anterior knee.

b. The examiner passively flexes, adducts, medially rotates, and longitudinally compresses the femur to scour the inner aspect of the joint. The examiner then takes the femur into abduction and lateral

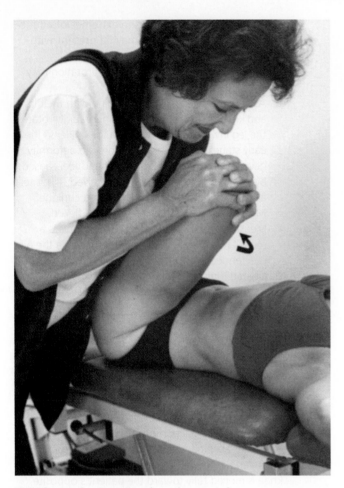

■ **FIG. 14-9.** Scouring (quadrant test).

rotation. The femur is rotated repetitively in the acetabulum between 90 and 140° of hip flexion.

    c. Compare the movement with that of the contralateral side to determine whether symptoms are reproduced or whether there is just routine discomfort. Both the quality of motion and the presence and location of pain are noted.

  6. Figure-of-four stretch test.[82] With the patient in a figure-of-four position (Fig. 14-10), the examiner can also evaluate the flexibility of the anterior hip structures and the medial rotators. This position tests the

available extension and external rotation at the hip, which are often limited because of shortening of the anterior structures as a result of underlying femoral antetorsion. The distance of the anterior superior iliac spine (ASIS) from the plinth is measured to provide the examiner with an objective measure of change. A modification of the test position can also be used as a treatment technique.

  7. On all passive movements, note the following:

    a. Range of motion. The capsular pattern of restriction is a marked limitation of internal rotation and abduction, moderate limitation of flexion and extension, and some limitation of external rotation and adduction.

    b. Pain

    c. Crepitus

    d. End feel

D. Joint-play movement tests

  1. The same movements used for specific joint mobilization techniques are used as examination maneuvers, except when evaluating joint play the femur should be in its resting position (30° of flexion and abduction; slight external rotation).

    a. Distraction (Fig. 14-11) With the patient lying supine, the joint is distracted by applying a distolateral force parallel to the neck of the femur. The operator's hands are placed around the subject's thigh.

    b. Inferior glide (Fig. 14-12). With the patient lying supine and the femur in its resting position, the examiner's hands are placed around the subject's thigh. An inferolateral force (inferior femoral glide) is applied along the longitudinal axis of the femur by the examiner leaning backward.

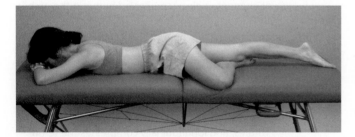

■ **FIG. 14-10.** Figure-of-four stretch test. This test is used to assess the flexibility of the anterior structures of the hip.

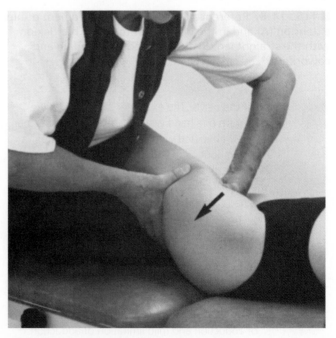

■ **FIG. 14-11.** Distraction of the hip joint.

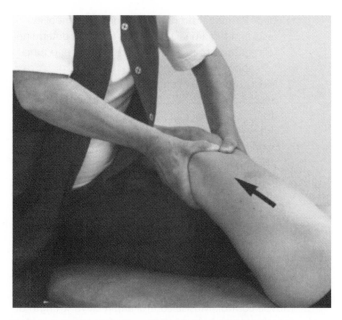

■ **FIG. 14-12.** Inferior glide of the hip joint.

c. Posterior glide (Fig. 14-13). With the hip maintained in its resting position, a posterior glide is performed with the examiner's hands by leaning forward with the trunk.

d. Anterior glide. With the subject in the same position as in Figure 14-13, the slack is taken up, and an anterior glide of the femur is performed with the examiner's hands by leaning backward with the trunk (see Fig. 14-29A).

2. The examiner should note:

a. Amplitude of movement: hypomobile, normal, hypermobile

b. The quality of movement, and the resistance through the range and at the end range of movement

c. The behavior of the pain through the range and any provocation of protective muscle spasm

3. Mobilization with movement (MWMs).[89] With the patient supine, the examiner stabilizes the pelvis and uses a belt to apply a lateral glide to the femur while the patient actively moves the hip into medial rotation or flexion (Fig. 14-14). An increase in the range of movement and no pain or reduced pain on active flexion or medial rotation of the hip joint in the lateral glide position are positive findings, indicating a mechanical joint problem.[104] When using this as a technique it will improve the range of rotation thus improving the patient's function with reducing the pain.[89]

4. Other joints as applicable. Joints likely to be examined are the lumbar spine, sacroiliac spine, knee, ankle, and foot.

IV. Muscle Tests. Muscle tests include resistive isometric, muscle strength, functional strength testing or control, and muscle length.

A. Resisted isometric movements

1. Resist maximal isometric contraction of muscles controlling all major hip movements, allowing no motion of the joint. Resisted knee flexion and extension should be done as well as the six isometric tests of the hip:

a. Flexion (supine) with the legs extended or with the hip and knee flexed to 90°. Resistance is applied above the knee. Painful weakness may indicate a psoas tendinitis; a painless weakness may be caused by rupture of the psoas or an L2 nerve root lesion.[21]

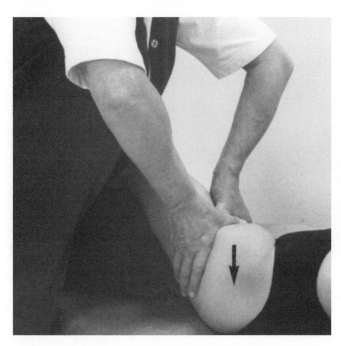

■ **FIG. 14-13.** Posterior glide of the hip joint.

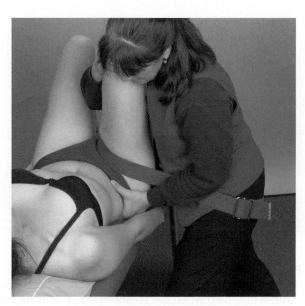

■ **FIG. 14-14.** Mobilization with movement for hip flexion.

b. Extension (supine) with an extended knee. Apply resistance at the heel. Pain in the upper thigh may be caused by a lesion of the origin of the hamstrings.

c. Adduction (supine) bilaterally. The knees are squeezed against the examiner's closed fist. Pain on resisted adduction suggests a lesion of the adductors (rider's sprain).[23]

d. Abduction (prone) with the opposite leg well stabilized. The hand around the patient's knee resists the patient's attempt to abduct the thigh. Resisted abduction can compress the gluteal bursa, as may passive abduction. A painful weakness may be caused by a gluteus medius tendinitis.[21]

e. Internal and external rotation (prone) with a flexed knee. Resistance is applied at the ankle. Pain, on resisted rotation, is considered an accessory sign in gluteal bursitis.[23]

2. Bursitis about the hip is very rare, but resisted hip flexion may reproduce pain in the presence of iliopectineal bursitis, and resisted hip abduction, or resisted hip extension and external rotation, may reproduce pain in trochanteric bursitis.

B. Muscle strength

1. Assess the hip flexors, extensor, adductors, abductors, medial and lateral rotators, and any other relevant muscle group. For details of these tests the reader is directed to Clarkson and Gilewish,[18] Cole et al.,[20] Hislop and Montgomery,[49] Kendall et al.,[63] and Palmar and Epler[101] to determine exactly which muscles are at fault. Positional strength testing can determine the length–tension properties of the relevant muscle. If a muscle tests weak in the short range but strong in a middle range, it is most likely an elongated muscle.[63] Positional strength combined with mobility tests and functional movement tests can determine relationships of muscle length, strength, and function about the hip joint.[46]

2. Most chronic joint conditions result in some weakness of the muscles controlling the joint because of disuse and reflex inhibition. At the hip some muscle groups are so powerful that mild or even moderate weakness may not be detected by manual muscle testing. Even if detected, manual testing does not permit documentation of the extent of weakness (or strength). For this reason, it is best to test each of the major muscle groups controlling the hip—abductors, adductors, flexors, and extensors—by determining the number of repetitions that can be performed against a constant load—for example, by determining the 10 repetition maximum. This allows for comparison with the "normal" side.

C. Muscle control. Muscle control and relative strength of muscles are considered to be more important than the overall strength of a muscle group according to many authors.[35,53,60,71,114,136] Relative strength and muscle control are assessed indirectly by observing posture, the quality of active motion, noting any changes in muscle recruitment patterns, and by palpating muscle activity in various positions. The following are examples:

1. Hip abduction assessment.[8,35,60,71,73] The patient lies on the contralateral side with the bottom knee flexed and the top leg fully extended. The examiner then observes and palpates the firing pattern, which will show gluteus medius to fire first, followed by the tensor fascia lata (TFL), in the normal firing pattern (Fig. 14-15A). A common substitution pattern is for the TFL to fire first rather than the gluteus medius.

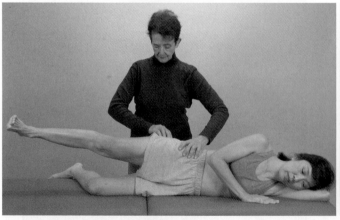 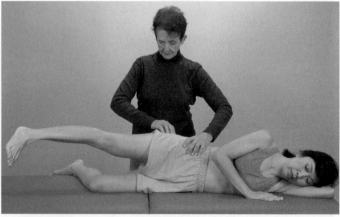

A   B

■ **FIG. 14-15.** Hip abduction assessment. **(A)** Firing patterns are monitored with hand placement over the gluteus medius and low back while visual observation of the low back and leg occur simultaneously. **(B)** Abnormal muscle contraction is observed when the tensor fascia latae contracts before the gluteus medius, introducing slight hip flexion and internal rotation.

When the gluteus medius is inhibited or weak, this test produces flexion and internal rotation of the hip that can be noted during active hip abduction movement (Fig. 14-15B). Other overactive muscles in the firing pattern that may be observed include the quadratus lumborum and piriformis.

2. Prone hip extension test.[8,35,60,71,73] The patient lies in a prone position and attempts to raise the leg into extension with the knee held in extension. Observe the activation sequence of (1) hamstrings and gluteus maximus, (2) contralateral lumbar paraspinals, and (3) ipsilateral paraspinals (Fig. 14-16). Use palpation to confirm. A positive test is noted if the paraspinal musculature contracts before the gluteus maximus, indicating overactivity of the lumbar paraspinal musculature with inhibition of the gluteus maximus. Also note overactivity of the hamstrings.

3. Sahrmann's[115] movement impairment tests of the hip during active hip flexion and extension are used to determine whether pain that seems to arise from musculotendinous injury is associated with impairment of accessory movements of the hip. An alteration of the path of the instant center of rotation (PICR) of the hip joint during hip flexion and often extension by monitoring of the greater trochanter is used to determine whether there is insufficient posterior glide.

  a. Hip flexion in supine. Monitoring the axis of rotation during hip flexion by palpation and following the path of the greater trochanter during active straight-leg raising can determine whether the greater trochanter is moving in a normal or an altered direction. During active flexion of the normal hip in supine, the greater trochanter main-

tains a relative constant position (Fig. 14-17A). When there is inadequate posterior glide of the femoral head during hip flexion, the greater trochanter moves in an anterior medial direction (Fig. 14-17B).

  b. Hip extension in prone. Palpating the greater trochanter during hip extension in the prone position indicates whether its movement is maintaining a relatively constant position (normal; Fig. 14-18A) or moving in an anterior or anterior medial direction (Fig. 14-18B).

    In the anterior glide syndrome with rotation, the anterior joint capsule and its associated soft tissue structures become stretched and the posterior structures become tight.

D. Muscle length

1. The Thomas test. The Thomas test detects a fixed hip flexion deformity in patients who have developed a compensatory lumbar lordosis that then masks the hip flexion.[126] It can also be used to assess the extensibility of the tensor fasciae latae and the adductors. With the patient lying at the end of a firm treatment table, one leg is flexed toward the chest and maintained in this position by the examiner or by the patient holding onto the knee, allowing the pelvis to tilt back and the lumbar spine to assume a flattened or neutral position. Monitor the low back position. If the knee is pulled too far forward and the back is allowed to assume a kyphotic position, the result is that the one-joint hip flexors, which may be normal length, will appear to be short. The flexed leg may be supported against the examiner's trunk (Fig. 14-19A). The leg to be tested must hang free of the table.

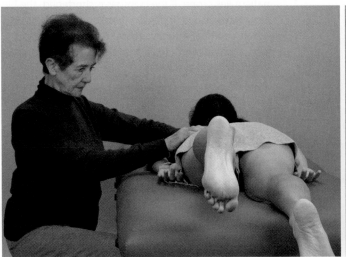
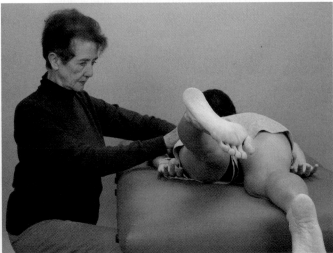

A   **B**

■ **FIG. 14-16.** Prone hip extension assessment. **(A)** Firing patterns are monitored by hand placement over the hamstrings and gluteus maximus while visual observation of the lumbar paraspinals simultaneously occurs. **(B)** Abnormal firing pattern. The gluteus maximus contracts after the lumbar paraspinals, rather than before.

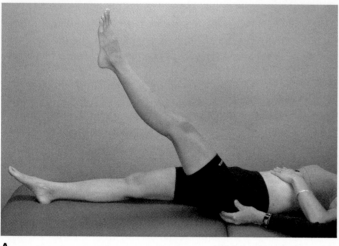
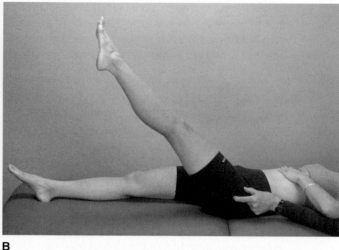

A   **B**

■ **FIG. 14-17.** Impairment of the movement pattern of the greater trochanter during hip flexion. **(A)** Correct movement of the greater trochanter during hip flexion. **(B)** Impaired movement pattern showing anterior medial displacement of the greater trochanter associated with hip rotation.

a. Initially observe the position of the leg to assess the length of the iliopsoas and the relative length of the rectus femoris. A tight iliopsoas muscle will restrict extension of the femur; a tight rectus will restrict knee flexion. A flexed hip position and a tendency toward simultaneous extension in the knee joint points to shortening of both the iliopsoas and the rectus femoris. End feel is noted, and passive overpressure is applied to hip extension and knee flexion.

b. If the anterior band of the tensor fasciae latae is tight, full femoral extension and knee flexion will occur; however, knee flexion will be possible only in conjunction with lateral tibial torsion.[69] If tibial rotation is passively blocked during the test, knee flexion will be restricted. Passive overpressure should also be applied to adduction. Hip adduction of less than 15 to 20°

indicates tightness of the tensor fascia latae and iliotibial band.[60] There will also be an associated increased deepening on the outside of the thigh over the iliotibial tract.

c. To isolate the two-joint hip adductors, the leg is abducted with the knee in extension (Fig. 14-19*B*), and the test is repeated with the knee flexed to 90°. A decreased range of abduction with the knee straight is a sign of shortness of the long adductors (two-joint adductors); a decreased range and compensatory flexion of the hip joint are signs of shortness of the one-joint thigh adductors.[54]

2. Ely's test for the iliopsoas and rectus femoris.[44] The patient lies prone. If the iliopsoas is shortened, the hip remains in flexion. If passive flexion of the knee provokes a compensatory increase of flexion in the hip joint and hyperlordosis of the lumbar spine, the rectus femoris muscle is tight.

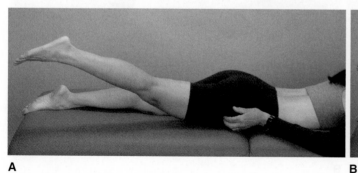
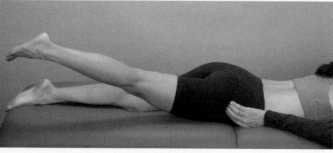

A   **B**

■ **FIG. 14-18.** Impairment of the movement pattern of the greater trochanter during hip extension. **(A)** Correct movement of the greater trochanter during hip extension. **(B)** Impaired movement pattern showing anterior displacement of the greater trochanter during hip extension.

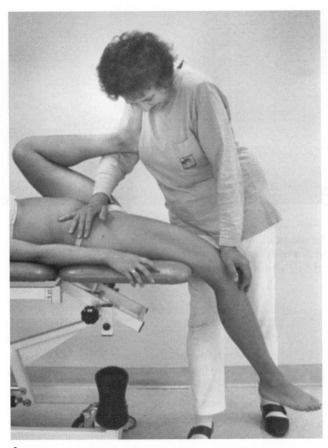

A

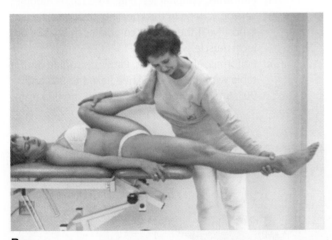

B

■ **FIG. 14-19.** Muscle length test: **(A)** iliopsoas, rectus femoris, tensor fascia latae, and **(B)** two-joint hip adductors.

3. Weight-bearing test with the patient assuming normal standing posture, using the pelvic femoral angle to assess the hip flexion angle in relationship to the floor (Fig. 14-8).[90]

4. Hamstrings (supine)
   a. 90°–90° straight-leg raise.[117] The patient flexes the hip to 90° and grasps behind the knee with both hands. The examiner then extends the knee through the available range. A measurement of 20° from full knee extension is within normal limits Fig. 15-27).

   b. Straight-leg raising test. The examiner flexes the hip so the knee is kept in extension. To avoid error, the lumbar spine should be monitored and kept flat on the plinth so there is no lordosis or kyphosis of the lumbar spine. When the hip flexors are shortened, the contralateral leg should be flexed at the hip and the knee joint passively flexed with the sole of the foot on the plinth so the lumbar spine is kept flat. The conventional straight-leg raise (SLR) is measured with a goniometer to determine the flexibility of the hamstrings and the status of the sciatic nerve.

   c. Straight-leg raising test (alternate method). Measurement of hamstring flexibility can be determined by using the same sidelying positioning and landmarks as in the measurement by Mundale and coworkers[90] (see above). Between lines *CD* and *DE,* an angle alpha exists in the resting position (Fig. 14-8*A*). In maximum flexion an angle beta is obtained between the reference lines (Fig. 14-8*B*). To obtain the result of isolated coxofemoral flexion, α must be subtracted from β. Once the angle alpha is determined, the subject is asked to perform maximal hip flexion without bending the knee. Supporting the leg on a powder board table eliminates abduction of the subject's leg. Instruct the subject not to perform movements of knee flexion, hip rotation, or movements of the ankle joint during hamstring measurement. Finally, the angle beta is determined (Fig. 14-8).[130]

5. Tensor fasciae latae (iliotibial band). A positive Ober test indicates a contracture of the iliotibial band.[96] It is performed in the sidelying position with the lower leg fully flexed to eliminate lumbar lordosis and stabilize the pelvis. The examiner then passively flexes the hip and knee to 90° of the leg to be tested (Fig. 14-20*A*). The hip is then abducted and extended to neutral (Fig. 14-20*B*). If the hip cannot extend to neutral consider the possibility of hip flexion contracture. Do not allow the pelvis to rotate externally during this maneuver. During positioning of the tested hip into full extension, stabilize the pelvis to maintain neutral femoral rotation. Once the upper leg is maximally abducted and extended, allow it to passively drop (adduct) by gravity toward the plinth while gently maintaining the knee flexion and femoral rotation (Fig. 14-20*C*). This position places the iliotibial band on stretch, and flexibility is assessed by observing how much adduction is possible. Generally the thigh should adduct to a position at least parallel to the

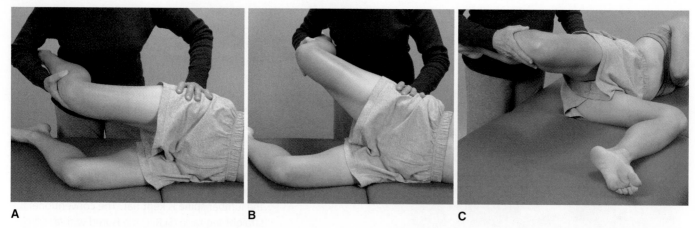

A   **B**   **C**

■ **FIG. 14-20.** Ober's test. **(A)** The supporting hip is maximally flexed to eliminate lumbar lordosis while the leg to be tested is flexed at the hip and knee. **(B)** Hip is abducted and extended maximally while stabilizing the pelvis to keep it perpendicular to the examination table. **(C)** Thigh is allowed to adduct while controlling femoral rotation in neutral.

examination table. If shortening is present, the leg will remain abducted. Palpation of the entire length of the iliotibial band allows the examiner to determine where excessive tightness exists. Palpation of the iliotibial band just lateral to the patella during maximal stretch usually reproduces pain in patients with excessive iliotibial band or lateral retinacular tightness.[105] The movement may reproduce pain associated with trochanteric bursitis.

6. Piriformis
   a. Piriformis: standard test position. To assess the extensibility of the piriformis the patient is positioned in sidelying with the test leg uppermost. The test leg is positioned in 60° of flexion with the knee in 90° of flexion. The examiner stabilizes the hip with one hand and applies downward pres-

sure at the knee (Fig. 14-21A). The quality and the end feel of motion are noted. This test is repeated on the opposite side. If the piriformis is tight, pain is elicited in the muscle. The production of pain in the buttock and along the course of the sciatic nerve represents a positive test, resulting from compression of the sciatic nerve by the piriformis muscle.[101,117] Tightness or pain in the hip and buttock areas is indicative of piriformis tightness.
   b. Piriformis: optional test (Fig. 14-21B). A modified version is done in the kneeling position. The test is positive if the patient complains of sciatica or local muscle symptoms.[129]
   c. Piriformis: alternate test. Patient is supine on the table with the hip and knee flexed to 90° and 90°. Internally rotate the femur to the first resis-

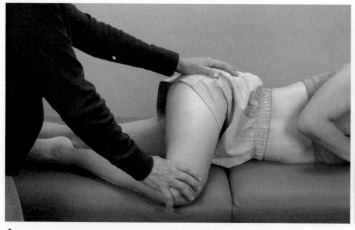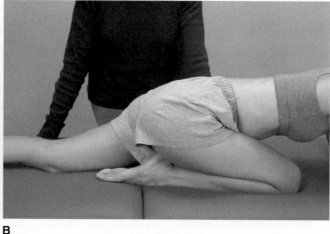

A   **B**

■ **FIG. 14-21.** Piriformis. **(A)** Standard test. Patient in sidelying position, the hip is positioned in about 60° of flexion and slight internal rotation. **(B)** Optional test. Patient in kneeling position.

tance barrier, while monitoring the pelvic movement (Fig. 14-22A). Normal is 45°.[16] In the supine position, tightness below 90° of hip flexion can be identified, with 60° of hip flexion and slight adduction while introducing internal rotation (Fig. 14-22B).[35] Flexion of the hip at greater than 90° with full external rotation and some adduction allows for detection of tightness of the piriformis greater than 90° (Fig. 14-22C).[35] The piriformis can be palpated for tightness by applying deep pressure at the point at which an imaginary line between the iliac crest and ischial tuberosity crosses a line between the posterosuperior iliac spine and the greater trochanter. The piriformis is often tight as it tries to substitute for an inhibited gluteus.

    7. Other individual muscles, prone to shortness, which may need to be checked, include the erector spinae, quadratus lumborum (see Fig. 23-32), tibialis posterior, gastrocnemius, and soleus.[60]

  E. Muscle bulk. The examiner may measure the circumference of the muscle bulk of the thigh with a tape measure if a difference between the left and right sides is suspected. Measurements are usually taken 5, 8, 15, and 23 cm above the base of the patella.[77]

V. Neuromuscular Tests. Neurologic examination involves examining the integrity and mobility of the nervous system.

  A. Integrity of the nervous system. The integrity of the nervous system is tested if the examiner suspects that the symptoms are emanating from the spine or peripheral nerves.

    1. Dermatomes and peripheral nerves. Light touch and pain sensation of the lower limb is tested (see Chapter 5, Assessment of Musculoskeletal Disorders and Concepts of Management). Knowledge of the cutaneous distribution of nerve roots (dermatomes) and peripheral nerves enables the enables the examiner to distinguish the sensory loss caused by a root lesion from that caused by a peripheral nerve lesion (see Tables 5-7 and 5-8 and Figs. 5-5 through 5-8).

    2. Myotomes and peripheral nerves. A working knowledge of the muscular distribution of nerve roots (myotomes) and peripheral nerves enables the examiner to distinguish the motor loss caused by a root lesion from that caused by a peripheral nerve lesion. Peripheral nerve distribution is shown in Figure 5-8. Myotome testing of the lumbar spine and sacral nerve root is performed (see Fig. 5-10).

    3. Reflex testing. The deep tendon reflexes are elicited by tapping the tendon a number of times to uncover the fading reflex response, which indicates developing root signs. The following reflexes are tested routinely:
- L3–L4—knee jerk (Fig. 14-23A)
- S1—ankle jerk (Fig. 14-23B)

  B. Mobility of the nervous system. Examination of the extensibility of the nervous system may be carried out to ascertain the degree to which neural tension is responsible for the production of the patient's symptom(s). Tests may include passive neck flexion, the slump test (see Chapter 22, Lumbar Spine), prone knee bend, and straight-leg raise (SLR).

    1. If the SLR is positive, the examiner can differentiate between a lesion in the lumbar spine and the buttock. The leg is taken to the end range of the SLR, and knee flexion is added. If there is further hip flexion available, this suggests pathologic involvement in the buttock such as bursitis, abscess, or tumor.[77]

    2. A modified SLR can also rule out piriformis involvement. The piriformis is placed on slack by externally

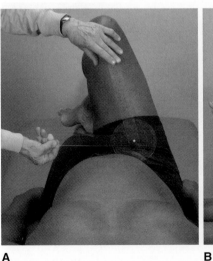
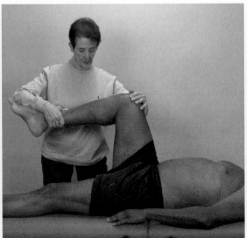
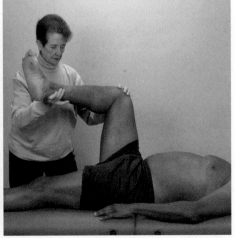

A   **B**   **C**

■ **FIG. 14-22.** Piriformis: alternative tests in supine. **(A)** For detection of tightness at 90° of hip flexion. **(B)** For detection of tightness at less than 90° of hip flexion. **(C)** For detection of tightness at greater than 90° of hip flexion.

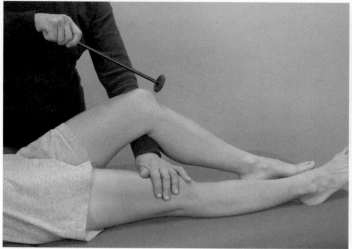

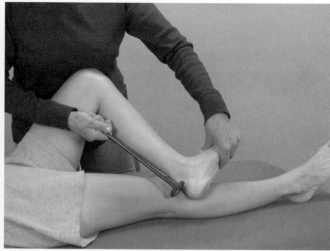

A

B

■ **FIG. 14-23.** Reflex testing. **(A)** Knee jerk (L3 and L4). **(B)** Ankle jerk (S1).

rotating the hip during SLR. The range obtained is compared with that obtained from SLR with the hip in internal rotation. If the piriformis is involved, more range will be obtained with the hip in external rotation, which places the piriformis on slack.

VI. Palpation. The examiner palpates the hip region and any other relevant area.

A. Skin. Palpate hip girdles and lower extremities (usually noncontributory in local lesions at or about the hip because of heavy soft tissue covering).

1. Temperature
2. Moisture
3. Tenderness
4. Texture
5. Mobility

B. Soft tissue

1. Mobility and consistency
2. Swelling (joint effusion usually cannot be palpated at the hip)
3. Tenderness

a. There may be localized tenderness anteriorly if the iliopectineal bursa is inflamed or distended. It may be distended with joint effusion as it often communicates with the joint.[134]

b. There may be localized tenderness laterally if the trochanteric bursa is inflamed.

c. There may be areas of referred tenderness (so-called trigger points) in the related segments (L2–S1) if a lesion is affecting any of the deep somatic tissues at or about the hip.

d. Baer's sacroiliac point is tender in the presence of sacroiliac lesion or iliacus flexor spasms. This point is located about 2 inches from the umbilicus on an imaginary line drawn from the anterosuperior iliac spine to the umbilicus.[85]

e. The sciatic nerve can be tender with muscle spasm of the piriformis muscle.

4. Test for relevant trigger points and tender points of fibromyalgia.

C. Bony structures (see under Inspection)

1. Tenderness of bone: the greater trochanter may be tender as a result of trochanteric bursitis and the ischial tuberosity as a result of ischiogluteal bursitis.

2. Increased or decreased prominence of bone

VII. Special Tests

A. Noble's compression test[93] is used to reveal an iliotibial band friction syndrome near the knee (Fig. 14-24). With the patient supine and the knee and hip flexed to 90°, thumb pressure is applied lateral to the femoral epi-

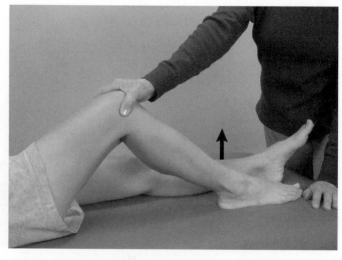

■ **FIG. 14-24.** Noble's compression test for iliotibial band friction syndrome. The patient extends the knee. The examiner is indicating where pain is felt.

condyle (or 1 to 2 cm proximal to it). While maintaining thumb pressure, the patient slowly extends the knee. Severe pain elicited at about 30° flexion indicates a positive test.

B. Joint-clearing tests. Take other joints in question to end range and stretch the capsule or other soft tissues to reproduce symptoms. If no symptoms are reproduced and range is within normal limits, the joint is cleared from involvement in the problem being assessed. These tests are important because pain may be referred to the hip from joints above and below the hip. For example, the lumbar spine may project pain via the sciatic or femoral nerve, and knee pain may be projected up to the hip via the obturator nerve. Tests such as squatting and valgus–varus stress tests may be used to clear the knee. Full active flexion, extension, and lateral flexion may be used to clear the lumbar spine.

C. Femoral torsion tests. Various clinical tests (Craig's test or Ryder's method) have been proposed to assess the degree of hip antetorsion.[22,129] For Craig's test, the patient lies prone with the knee flexed to 90°. The examiner palpates the posterior aspect of the greater trochanter of the femur. The hip is passively rotated (medially and laterally) until the greater trochanter is parallel to the examination table or in its most lateral position. The degree of antetorsion or retrotorsion can be measured on the angle of the lower leg to vertical (Fig. 14-25).

In weight bearing, the appearance of the patellae often suggests excessive femoral torsion when the patient stands with the knees in full extension and the feet pointing straight ahead. In excessive anteversion, the patellae face inward (squinting patellae). When the hips are externally rotated until the patellae are facing to the front, the feet and legs will be pointed outward.

D. Torque test. The torque test assesses the integrity of the capsular ligaments of the hip.[69] The patient's leg is extended over the edge of the examination table until the pelvis begins to move. The examiner applies a slow posterolateral stress to the femoral neck for 20 seconds while internally rotating the femur to the end range (Fig. 14-26).

E. Assessment of leg-length equality. Several anatomic (a decrease in the vertical dimensions of bony structure) and functional (a right–left asymmetry in joint position) methods have been proposed for assessing true and apparent leg-length discrepancies.[17,29,51,88,92,137] From a clinical standpoint, limb-length assessment should be done with the patient in a weight-bearing position with measurements determined by placing a calibrated block under the sole of the foot to level the pelvis. A gravity goniometer or level placed between the posterosuperior iliac spine can be used to assess when the pelvis is level. Discrepancy is determined by the height of the calibrated blocks needed for correction. Assessment should be accompanied by palpation and additional tests, if indicated, to determine the source of discrepancy (i.e., foot, ankle, knee, sacroiliac, and lumbar spine tests). With the exception of one tape-measure method, clinical tests for determining leg length have been shown to be inaccurate when compared with radiographic measurements.[5] Observer error of up to 10 mm has been found in clinical methods for assessing leg length.[17,88,92] When using the tape-measure method for determining leg length, an average of two tests may improve validity.[5]

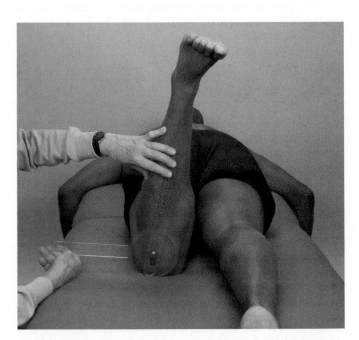

■ FIG. 14-25. Craig's test for femoral torsion. Align the greater trochanter in the midfrontal plane (parallel to the table). The degree of femoral torsion can be measured based on the angle of the lower leg to vertical.

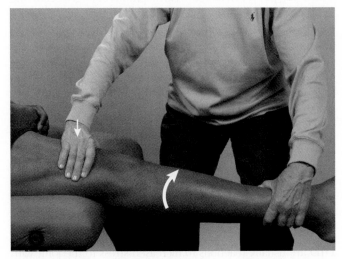

■ FIG. 14-26. Torque test of anterior stability of the hip joint.

1. Cartilaginous narrowing. Compare clinical with roentgenographic findings.
2. Coxa varum or coxa valgum. Malleoli, fibular heads, and trochanters are level. Posterosuperior and anterosuperior iliac spines and iliac crests are lower on the varus side and higher on the valgus side. Coxa varum is often associated with retroversion; coxa valgum is usually associated with increased anteversion. In coxa varum, the trochanter lies above Nélaton's line; in coxa valgum, it lies below. Compare clinical findings with roentgenograms.
3. Short femoral shaft. Malleoli, fibular heads, and popliteal folds are level. The greater trochanter and pelvic landmarks are lower on the short side.
4. Short tibia. The malleoli are level. The popliteal folds, fibular heads, and tibial tubercles are lower on the short side.
    Note: Dynamic evaluation should include a gait analysis and assessment of shoes.

COMMON LESIONS

Degenerative Joint Disease (Osteoarthrosis)

Degenerative joint disease (DJD) at the hip often progresses to a point at which it results in significant disability. This is true at the hip more so than at any other joint. Clinically, persons with DJD of the hip frequently present to outpatient healthcare services because of pain and disability. DJD is the most common disease process affecting the hip. Primary DJD is distinguished from secondary DJD by eliminating predisposing factors and is considered a result of aging alone; *secondary osteoarthritis* is the term used when the condition follows previous damage by disease or mechanical disorders.

The origin of DJD of the hip varies, and in many patients the cause is unclear. Age is an important factor, but the pathologic process of DJD is not a result of tissue changes with aging per se. In fact, the cartilaginous changes occurring with normal aging are seen first in the nonarticular areas of cartilage, whereas changes found in DJD are seen first in areas of cartilage that undergo most frequent contact—for example, during weight bearing.[3,11,30,80,81,87,111,132] DJD is a disease of older persons because it takes a long time to cause the fatigue of tissue, such as fibrillation of articular cartilage, characteristic of the disease.[52]

The asymptomatic changes occurring with normal aging of articular cartilage probably result from a nutritional deficiency; the areas of cartilage not undergoing frequent intermittent compression do not undergo the absorption and squeezing out of synovial fluid necessary for adequate nutrition. This is especially true in older persons because they tend to use their joints less frequently and through smaller ranges of movement.

The degenerative tissue changes that occur with primary DJD are usually reactions to increased stress to the joint with time.[30,36–39,80,87,91,110] The tissue changes may be of a compensatory hypertrophic nature, such as the bony proliferation that typically occurs at the joint margins and subchondral bone or capsular fibrosis. They may also be of an atrophic nature, such as the fatigue of cartilaginous collagen fibers or the degradation of cartilage ground substance (proteoglycan). Perhaps the most disputed issue with respect to pathogenesis is whether the first tissue changes occur in the subchondral bone or in the articular cartilage. It is generally accepted, however, that regardless of which tissue changes occur first, they take place first and foremost in the regions undergoing greatest stress with normal activities, and changes in subchondral bone will, with time, result in changes in articular cartilage, and vice versa.[111,121] Normal attenuation of the forces applied to a joint depends on the elastic properties of subchondral bone as well as those of articular cartilage. If stresses are not normally attenuated in one of these tissues, the other will undergo increased stresses.[108,109] Thus, with subchondral bony sclerosis, the overlying articular cartilage undergoes increased stress, as the subchondral bone becomes stiffer and less elastic. With fibrillation and softening of articular cartilage, increased stress is transmitted to the subchondral bone. Such abnormal stresses inevitably lead to progression of the process (see Chapter 3, Arthrology). It is interesting to note the difference in eventual reaction to increased stress between subchondral bone and articular cartilage: subchondral bone becomes denser (sclerotic), whereas articular cartilage breaks down. This difference reflects the differences in the vascularity and regenerative capacities of the two tissues.

If one accepts that in many, if not most, cases of DJD the pathogenesis is closely related to increased stress to joint tissues with time (or fatigue), then conditions that may predispose the joint to increased stresses must be considered as possible contributors to the causes of DJD. Perhaps the most important condition at the hip to consider in this regard is congenital hip dysplasia.[11,37,38,50,87] A deficient acetabular roof and increased femoral antetorsion angle are common sequelae of this condition. The resultant decrease in effective weight-bearing surface area at the joint predisposes the posterosuperolateral femoral head and superolateral acetabulum to early degenerative changes. Residual structural changes in joint components that may follow osteochondrosis or slipped femoral capital epiphysis—both of which affect younger persons—may have similar effects.

Leg-length disparity may be a factor in predisposing to unilateral DJD of the hip on the side of the longer leg.[37,39] In the standing position, the pelvic obliquity produced by the leg-length discrepancy would cause the long limb to assume a position of relative adduction with respect to the acetabulum. The increased adduction angulation on weight bearing results in an increased joint incongruence, causing greater stress to the lateral roof of the acetabulum. In addition, the center of gravity is shifted toward the short-leg side, increasing the moment arm about which the force of the superincumbent body weight acts at the supporting femoral head on the long-leg side (see Biomechanics). A greater pull by the abductors on the long side then is required to prevent the pelvis from dropping to the

short side during stance on the long side. This would increase the vertical compressive force acting at the femoral head during weight bearing on the long-leg side.

Another condition that may contribute to accelerated hip degeneration is capsular tightness.[11,75,103] Traditionally, capsular tightness has been regarded as more of a *result* than a *cause* of hip degeneration. Although this is true, the clinician must consider the role that capsular tightening may play in accelerating the progression of the disease and in some cases in actually initiating the degenerative process. The hip, unlike the shoulder, is a joint that is continually brought close to its close-packed position during normal functional activities, such as walking. With every step, at push-off, the hip is brought into a position of extension, internal rotation, and abduction, taking up most of the slack in the joint capsule by twisting the capsule on itself. The twisting of the capsule effects a compression of the joint surfaces. The compression force is normally in addition to, but acts after, the peak vertical compressive force of weight bearing. In other words, the peak compressive loading attributable to capsular twisting is normally not superimposed on that of weight bearing; rather, these forces are successively applied to the joint during the stance phase.[87,103] This is in accordance with the viscoelastic property of articular cartilage, which favors gradual loading over time as opposed to quick shock-loading with respect to its ability to attenuate compressive forces.[108–110] If for whatever reason the hip joint capsule loses extensibility, the slack will be taken up in the joint capsule sooner and the joint surfaces will become *prematurely* approximated during walking. This premature approximation causes the peak compressive loading from capsular twisting to become closer to being superimposed on the peak compressive loading of weight bearing. It causes a greater magnitude of compressive forces to be applied to the articular cartilage during a shorter period, approximating a situation of shock-loading. Certain studies suggest that shock-loading, even more than loss of normal lubrication, is one of the most important factors in fatigue of articular cartilage.[110]

Symptoms of pain on weight bearing in the presence of hip DJD are not related to compressive forces per se but result from strain to the capsuloligamentous structures as they pull prematurely tight with each step (recall that articular cartilage is aneural). Such capsular pain is enhanced by the low-grade capsular inflammation that tends to develop as the disease progresses.[11] Studies in which compressive forces have been calculated in degenerated hips before surgery and then determined after total hip arthroplasty suggest that such surgery does reduce the flexor moment acting at the hip from a tight capsule.[103] This may explain the often dramatic symptomatic improvement enjoyed by these patients soon after surgery.

A major goal of conservative management in the earlier stages of hip DJD should be prevention and reduction of capsular tightening of the joint. Such an approach, in addition to providing symptomatic improvement, may help slow the acceleration of the degenerative process; the effective weight-bearing surface area of cartilage is increased, and shock-loading is decreased.

Longstanding obesity may also contribute to accelerated degenerative changes at the hip. Because of the moment arm about which the force of gravity on the body weight acts at the femoral head during stance phase, an additional 3 pounds may act at the supporting femoral head for each added pound of body weight.

I. History
   A. Onset of symptoms. The patient is usually a middle-aged or older person who describes an insidious onset of groin or trochanteric pain. The pain is first noticed after use of the joint, such as long periods of walking, hiking, or running. The patient may relate some childhood hip problem or an old injury, but more often does not.
   B. Site of pain. The pain is typically felt first in the groin. As the problem progresses, the pain is more likely to be referred farther into the L2 or L3 segment, to the anterior thigh and knee. Later, other segments may become involved, with pain felt laterally and posteriorly. An occasional patient presents with a primary complaint of knee pain—this is because both the knee and the hip are largely derived embryologically from the same segment. Rarely is pain referred below the knee in a person with only hip joint disease.
   C. Nature of pain. The pain is noticed first at the end of the day, after considerable use of the joint; relief is obtained by rest. Later, as some low-grade inflammation develops, the patient notices some morning stiffness. At this point, pain and stiffness are noticed when getting up from sitting; the pain largely subsides after several steps (after "getting the joint loosened up"), then returns again after walking a certain distance. As the degeneration becomes more advanced, some constant aching may be noticed. The pain is increased by any amount of walking, and the patient is frequently awakened with pain at night.

      With progressive capsular tightness, the patient first notices some difficulty squatting—for instance, when picking up an object from the ground. Gradually, it becomes more difficult to put on stockings and tie shoes. The ability to climb stairs may be lost in the later stages, and the patient may be able to ambulate only with the assistance of canes or crutches. Some discomfort with sitting may develop as hip flexion becomes restricted.

II. Physical Examination
   A. Observation
      1. The patient may hesitate or have difficulty when rising from sitting and initiating ambulation.
      2. An abduction or antalgic gait, a swinging type of gait if the hip is stiff, a lurching of the trunk toward the affected side if there is any shortening of the limb, or a Trendelenburg gait if any weakness of the abductors is present may be noted.
      3. The patient may have some difficulty removing shoes, socks, and slacks.
      4. Note use of aids.

B. Inspection
1. Some localized (abductor or gluteal) or generalized atrophy may be noticed on the involved side. Document thigh girth, if appropriate.
2. If significant adduction and flexion contractures are present, the patient may tend to stand with the heel raised, the hip laterally rotated, and the pelvis elevated on the involved side.
3. If a flexion contracture and adduction contracture are present, and the patient stands with both feet flat and knees extended, the lumbar spine will be in some hyperlordosis, the pelvis will be shifted laterally toward the involved side (noticed in plumb-bob alignment), and the spine will be functionally scoliotic so as to bring the upper trunk back to the midline.
4. Assess levels of bony landmarks for leg-length equality. If this is unequal, attempt to determine the source of the discrepancy.

C. Joint tests. The capsular pattern of restriction of the hip is one in which the greatest loss is that of abduction, flexion, and internal rotation. These motions are always limited, although the order of restriction may vary. The one exception is the medial type of osteoarthritis in which the head of the femur is displaced into the deepened acetabular cavity, so that rotation, in both directions, and abduction tend to be most limited.[21]
1. Active movements
   a. Assess functional activities
      i. Squatting—usually unable to perform in moderate to advanced cases
      ii. One-legged stance. Pelvis will drop to the opposite side if the abductors are significantly weak (positive Trendelenburg sign).
      iii. Balance or reach test
      iv. Stair climbing—may be restricted in advanced cases
      v. Sit and bend forward—usually painful or restricted
   b. Note ability to perform, pain, and crepitus.
2. Passive movements
   a. Limited in a capsular pattern of restriction
      i. May be limited by pain and spasm—acute
      ii. May be limited by soft tissue restriction and discomfort—chronic
   b. Passive movement tests to determine status of joint surface scouring (quadrant test) (Fig. 14-9)
   c. Note pain, crepitus, range of motion, and end feel.
3. Resisted movements—strong and painless
4. Joint-play movements
   a. Hypomobility of all joint-play movements
   b. Note whether they are restricted by pain and spasm or by soft tissue restriction.
D. Muscle tests
1. Muscle strength. Mild to even moderate muscle weakness of the large muscle groups controlling the hip

must be tested by heavy, repetitive loading. Weakness, especially of the abductors, will be found in all but minor cases.
2. Muscle length. Consideration of age-related tightness resulting in positive results
   a. Thomas test (Fig. 14-19)
   b. Ober test (Fig. 14-20)
   c. Straight-leg raise test
   d. Gastrocnemius and soleus
E. Neuromuscular tests
1. If at this point a possible coexistent spinal lesion is suspected, motor, sensory, and reflex testing, in addition to other tests, may be warranted.
2. Assess the patient's balance (e.g., one-legged standing with eyes closed); this is often affected because of alteration in afferent input from the joint capsule receptors and controlling muscles.[25]
F. Palpation
1. Often noncontributory
2. Possibly some warmth anteriorly
3. Usually some tenderness anteriorly, over the trochanter and buttock; possibly some trigger points of referred tenderness elsewhere in the thigh
G. Other
1. Compare roentgenographic findings with clinical findings. However, early DJD can be detected clinically before roentgenograms show positive findings, and rather extensive changes may show on roentgenograms in the absence of significant symptoms. Migration of the femoral head upward in relation to the pelvis, which may be observed on radiographs owing to degeneration as seen in osteoarthritis, is referred to as the teardrop sign (Fig. 14-27).[44]
2. Because of the loss of hip extension characteristic of DJD and the compensatory hyperlordosis that develops when standing, these patients are predisposed to the development of back problems. A back evaluation may be warranted.

III. Management. Management depends on the stage of the disease as determined by the extent of the lesion and the degree of disability. In early disease, pain is noticed only with fatigue. There is only mild limitation of internal rotation, extension, and abduction associated with pain at the extremes of these movements. The patient walks with little or no limp. In advanced disease, there is constant aching, the patient is often awakened at night, and there is considerable morning stiffness. Motion is markedly limited in a capsular pattern. Ambulation is performed with a marked limp or with the use of canes or crutches.

These criteria reflect the two extremes; many patients fall somewhere between them. Information from roentgenograms is not included as a criterion because it cannot be reliably correlated to symptoms, signs, degree of disability, or prognosis.

The major difficulty facing the clinician is that rarely is a patient with *mild* DJD of the hip seen—and this is the patient

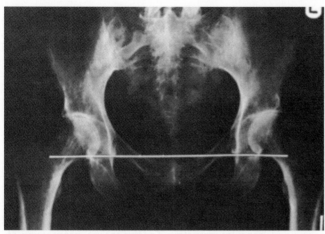

A

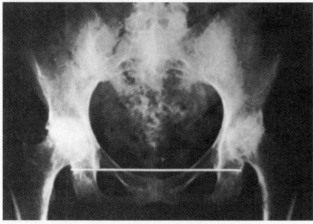

B

■ **FIG. 14-27.** Bilateral osteoarthritis of the hip. **(A)** A line has been drawn between the two teardrops and extended into the femoral neck. Note the left hip has migrated more superiorly than the right. **(B)** At a later date, both hips have moved upward as a result of loss of bone at the apex. The left hip is now higher than the right, confirming the original observation that the process of destruction in the left hip was ahead of that in the right. (Reprinted with permission from Bruebel-Lee DM: Disorders of the Hip. Philadelphia, JB Lippincott, 1983:61.)

to whom the clinician ultimately has the most to offer. The reason for this is twofold: (1) considerable progression of the disease may ensue before the patient experiences sufficient pain or disability to warrant seeking medical help, and (2) physicians often do not refer patients with symptoms and signs of early DJD to physical therapists because therapists in the past have not met their potential in managing these patients. Too often the patient is issued a cane and advised to return if the condition worsens, at which time surgical intervention may be indicated.

A. Early stages
 1. Goals

a. Restore normal joint mechanics
b. Prevent further progression of the disease—capsular tightness or other possible causes of increased stress to the joint
c. Functional strength—independent transfers to and from sitting
d. Decrease pain
e. Normal gait patterns with assistive device as needed
2. Therapeutic procedures
a. Restore normal capsular mobility with joint mobilization and active and active-assisted range of motion program. Ultrasound should be helpful in increasing capsular mobility when used during or before mobilization procedures.
b. Restore normal muscle strength with progressive-resistive exercise program. Emphasize abductor strengthening.
c. Restore extensibility of the soft tissues with soft tissue manipulations.
d. Range of motion exercises to be done indefinitely, instruction in appropriate levels, and other measures to minimize compressive stress to the hip
e. Attempt to determine whether there is an underlying biomechanical or constitutional factor that may predispose the joint to abnormal stresses.
   i. Obesity. For each additional pound of body weight, an additional 3 pounds is applied to each hip joint during the stance phase of normal walking. Although few physical therapists are qualified to institute a weight-loss program, the patient can be directed to the appropriate services, on agreement by the physician. A general conditioning program may be supervised by the therapist as an adjunct to a weight-loss program. The patient must be shown simple exercises to help maintain hip range of motion; these are to be done indefinitely on a regular basis.
   ii. Leg-length disparity. Inequality of leg length may be a factor in development of DJD on the long-leg side. Gradual, serial elevation of the heel and sole on the uninvolved (short) side, by one-fourth inch at a time, may be indicated, along with regular range of motion exercises.
   iii. Congenital hip dysplasia and epiphyseolysis (slipped capital epiphysis). Both of these conditions result in permanent structural abnormalities that often lead to increased stress to joint surfaces at the superolateral aspect of the hip joint. Some increased congruity of joint surfaces may be achieved by elevating the heel and sole of the shoe on the uninvolved side in unilateral cases. This places the involved hip in a relative position of abduction, as well as automatically shifting the center of gravity line closer to the involved hip so as to reduce the

moment arm about which it acts during stance phase on the involved side.

Because these patients are more or less permanently predisposed to accelerated degenerative changes, they should be encouraged to avoid activities that may be particularly stressful to the hip. Jogging and long-distance walking should be abandoned in favor of swimming and non–weight-bearing exercises. For patients whose regular activities involve considerable walking, alternative modes of travel and perhaps use of a cane should be encouraged.

These patients especially must maintain good strength and motion at their hips for maximal stabilization and maximal distribution of weight-bearing forces over joint surfaces.

B. Moderate to advanced stages. Unfortunately, the patient is often given the impression that he or she must simply wait until the disease progresses to a point at which surgery is indicated. Accordingly, the patient is often not referred to rehabilitative services, again because therapists have not demonstrated in the past that they have much to offer these patients. When these patients are referred to physical therapy, it is often simply for instruction in the use of a cane.

Our approach to these patients must be more comprehensive and vigorous. Surgery becomes inevitable unless appropriate measures are taken in the early or moderate stages of the disease. Even so, one may simply be delaying a potentially inevitable event. But one must also consider that these patients are usually middle-aged or older and that if progression of the disease can be retarded and a satisfactory level of function maintained, the patient may very well live out his or her life without undergoing major surgery.

1. Goals
   a. Restore function to optimal level
   b. Restore joint mechanics to optimal level
2. Therapeutic procedures
   a. Instruct the patient in the use of the appropriate walking aid to reduce compressive loading at the hip, to relieve pain on ambulation, and to increase ambulation endurance.
   b. A raised toilet seat may be desirable.
   c. Exercise and home program including cardiovascular conditioning, aquatic activity, closed kinetic chain exercises, progression of flexibility exercises, and neuromuscular balance and proprioceptive reeducation
   d. The patient may be made aware of special adaptations in shoe fasteners and devices to help put on and take off shoes and socks. An occupational therapist can be of assistance.
   e. The use of other adaptive aids and devices should be instituted if they may help the patient to per-form daily activities with less pain or difficulty. Integration of specific structural or biomechanical components that may relieve symptoms, including the choice of shoes or custom biomechanical orthoses to control excessive compensatory pronation, should be considered.
   f. Primary considerations in regard to improving joint mechanics include increasing capsular extensibility and increasing the strength of the muscles controlling the hip. The basic program is outlined above under management in the early stages. In moderate or advanced stages, however, the joint is likely to be more irritable in that motion tends to be limited more by pain and muscle spasm than by a pure capsular restriction. For this reason, progression of the mobilization program must often proceed more slowly. In addition, at some point in more advanced cases, motion in some planes may reach a point at which it is restricted by bony impingement because of the bony hypertrophic changes characteristic of the disease.

In most respects, the approach to management of these patients should closely resemble that of patients with a frozen shoulder. The primary differences are functional considerations and the concern for reducing compressive forces in patients with hip disease. However, there is no reason not to proceed with an intensive mobilization and strengthening program in cases of capsular hip restriction, as is done routinely with patients with capsular tightness at the shoulder. Remember that it is the tight capsule in cases of DJD at the hip that is a primary source of pain; it is a chief factor in intensifying and localizing compressive forces at the hip joint during walking.

Surgery should be considered in patients with severe pain or disability or who fail to respond to conservative treatment. Total hip replacement is the treatment of choice in older patients, whereas a femoral osteotomy may still have a role in surgical management.[21]

Capsular Strain

Hip joint disease is frequently seen without severe trauma or osteoarthrosis. With a capsular sprain, the injury may have occurred insidiously or with a minor twisting motion during weight bearing. Athletes frequently suffer from capsular sprains at the hip joint. Generally, the acute symptoms from these problems resolve, even without intervention; however, residual capsular tightness may predispose the patient to further hip problems including osteoarthrosis.[75] Hypomobility impairments, particularly in the direction of flexion and medial rotation, can be found in young, middle-aged, and elderly adult hip joints. Subtle losses in mobility may be caused by chronic lack of use as a result of altered movement patterns.[46] Subtle capsular pattern findings are common in young and middle-aged women with a history of hip-related conditions (e.g., groin pain, posterior buttock pain, hip bursitis, iliotibial band [ITB] fasciitis).[46] This may be the result of hypermobility causing intra-articular inflammation, which leads to capsular changes.

Hip joint hypomobility may also develop as a result of altered lumbopelvic movement patterns because of a combination of anthropometric, occupational, and environmental factors. It is hypothesized that ultimately as hip mobility decreases, lumbar mobility increases. This finding has been demonstrated in measuring lumbopelvic rhythm during forward bending,[28,72,84,98,127] The investigation of these studies found a significant relationship between a relative loss of hip flexion mobility and relative increased lumbar flexion mobility.

I. History
  A. Onset of symptoms The patient may present with or without a history of significant trauma. If there is a traumatic event, the injury usually involves a twisting motion usually in weight-bearing activities.[129] Often acute symptoms resolve quickly, and the patient does not seek medical care.
  B. Signs and symptoms. The patient may complain of problems in daily activities, especially after periods of inactivity such as prolonged sitting. Typical sites of pain are the anterior hip and groin, but some patients will complain of pain in the buttock. Ambulating, especially running, may be painful.[129] The patient may have decreased tolerance of weight-bearing activities, transfers, and functional activities. The presence of altered lumbopelvic movement patterns (because of hip joint hypomobility) may lead to microtrauma and macrotrauma of the lumbar spine.

II. Physical Examination
  A. Observation and inspection
    1. The gait pattern is antalgic on the involved side. Decreased stride length is present.
    2. There may be other contributing features such as leg length or pelvic asymmetry.
    3. Muscle guarding can be present with attempts to move into a painful range.
  B. Joint tests
    1. Findings show a capsular pattern of restriction of motion of the hip.
    2. Joint-play movements are restricted; they may be limited by pain and have a spongy end feel.[129]
    3. Overpressure is painful, especially in the direction of combined flexion and internal rotation.
    4. There may be altered lumbopelvic movement patterns with increased lumbar mobility.
    5. Another joint in the kinetic chain that may become stressed because of loss of mobility in the hip joint is the knee. During squatting movements, loss of motion at the hip may impose increased motion on the lumbar spine and the knee joint.[46]

  C. Muscle tests
    1. Weakness in the lateral hip rotators
    2. Loss of hip extension range of motion is another common finding; the pelvis may rest in a relative anterior tilt in relaxed standing. This posture may contribute to a relative increase in lumbar extension to achieve an upright position.
    3. With a chronically anterior tilted pelvis and associated loss of hip flexion range of motion there may be positional weakness in the external obliques, lower rectus abdominis, and transversus abdominus.[46]
    4. Muscle length tests may reveal loss of extensibility of the hip flexors (i.e., rectus femoris, TFL and ITB).
    5. Hamstrings have been also implicated as a potential source of hip stiffness.[128]
III. Management. Management of capsular strains and hip joint hypomobility is similar to treatment of early DJD (see above). The patient should be taught about controlled weight-bearing activities as soon as possible. Therapeutic procedures (from the findings) include:
  A. Physical agents can be used as needed to decrease pain and to increase the extensibility of the joint capsule.
  B. Manual therapy (as appropriate per differential diagnosis)
    1. Soft tissue techniques: myofascial release, friction massage, and soft tissue mobilization
    2. Passive range of motion and pain-free stretching as identified in evaluation
  C. Joint mobilization techniques for symptom relief include grade I and II joint distraction, with progression to higher grades to improve joint lubrication and prevent residual capsular tightness.[14,140]
    1. Other joint mobilization techniques: grades I and II oscillations for pain relief
    2. Progressive grades as tolerated to increase pain-free range of motion
  D. Exercise and home program (from findings)
    1. Acute phase
      a. Closed kinetic chain strengthening without exacerbation of pain (e.g., partial squats, weight shifting, gait drill)
      b. Open kinetic chain strengthening (e.g., use of pillow adductor squeezes and elastic bands in pain-free positions)
    2. Subacute phase
      a. Manual resistive activities
      b. Closed kinetic chain exercises
      c. Progression of flexibility exercises (e.g., hip flexors, hamstrings, TFL or ITB)
      d. Cardiovascular conditioning
      e. Neuromuscular, balance, and proprioceptive education (e.g., gait drill, balance board)
      f. Lumbar and pelvic stability exercises combined with retraining lumbopelvic rhythm (e.g., impairment associated with altered lumbopelvic movement patterns; see Chapters 22 and 23)

g. Positional strengthening of the appropriate abdominal muscle groups

E. Functional biomechanics. Integration of specific structural or biomechanical components that may relieve symptoms, including the choice of shoes or biomechanical orthoses to control excessive compensatory patterns, needs to be considered.

Bursitis

There are numerous bursae about the hip joint. All of these bursae are subject to various inflammatory processes, and the cause varies from infection to systematic diseases but most often is nonspecific.

TROCHANTERIC BURSITIS

Trochanteric bursitis is one of the few other common musculoskeletal disorders affecting the hip region for which patients are often referred to physical therapy.[116] It is a common misdiagnosis and differentiation of many other causes of lateral hip pain. The lateral hip is a common site for referred pain from the sacroiliac joint, deep external rotators of the hip, and lumbar spine.

I. History
   A. Onset—usually insidious. Occasionally an acute onset is described in association with a particular activity, such as getting out of a car, during which a "snap" is felt at the lateral or posterolateral hip region. Presumably such an incident involves a snapping of a portion of the iliotibial band over the trochanter, with mechanical irritation of the intervening bursa.
   B. Site of pain—primarily over the lateral hip region. It tends to radiate distally into the L5 segment; the patient describes pain over the lateral aspect of the thigh to the knee and occasionally into the lower leg. Some patients also experience pain referred into the lumbosacral region on the side of involvement. This pain pattern closely resembles that of an L5 spinal lesion, which is a more common disorder than trochanteric bursitis and which must be differentiated by means of careful examination.
   C. Nature of pain—aggravated most by ascending stairs (the strongly contracting gluteus maximus compresses the inflamed bursa) and by rolling onto the involved side at night. Indeed, the greatest complaint is often that of being awakened at night with pain. The pain is a deep, aching, scleratogenous pain rather than the sharp, lancinating, dermatomal pain characteristic of L5 nerve root irritation.
II. Physical Examination
   A. Observation—usually noncontributory. The lesion is not severe enough to cause a limp.
   B. Inspection—usually noncontributory. If the iliotibial band is tight, the patient may stand with the pelvis shifted laterally, away from the involved side on mediolateral plumb-bob assessment, with perhaps some increased valgus of the knee on the involved side.

C. Joint tests
   1. Active movements—no functional limitations
   2. Passive movements
      a. Full passive abduction may cause pain from squeezing of the bursa between the trochanter and the lateral aspect of the pelvis.
      b. Placement of the hip into full passive flexion combined with adduction and internal rotation compresses the inflamed bursa beneath the stretched gluteus maximus.
   3. Joint-play movements—mobility is normal and painless.
D. Muscle tests
   1. Resisted movements
      a. Resisted abduction will reproduce the pain by squeezing the bursa beneath the strongly contracting gluteals.
      b. Resisted extension and resisted external rotation may cause pain if the bursa underlying the gluteus maximus is involved.
   2. Muscle length—the Ober test may reveal iliotibial band tightness.
E. Neuromuscular examination—noncontributory
F. Palpation. A discrete point of tenderness is found over the site of the lesion, usually over the posterolateral aspect of the greater trochanter. Other areas of referred tenderness are often found elsewhere in the L5 segment, usually over the lateral aspect of the thigh. No increased temperature can be detected.
III. Management
   A. Goals
      1. Resolve the chronic inflammatory process.
      2. Prevent recurrence.
   B. Techniques
      1. Temporarily avoid continued irritation to the bursa.
         a. Arrange pillows so as to avoid rolling onto the painful side.
         b. Avoid climbing stairs and long walks.
         c. Ultrasound to the site of the lesion. Ultrasound is often dramatically effective over the course of three to six sessions. The increase in blood flow apparently assists in the resolution of the inflammatory process.
      2. A tight iliotibial band may be the cause or the result of the disorder.[116] Full mobility of the iliotibial band should be restored as the condition resolves. Ensure that good muscle strength of the gluteals is restored because they may weaken in longstanding cases.

ILIOPECTINEAL BURSITIS

Iliopectineal bursitis is less common than trochanteric bursitis. It presents in a similar manner, but resisted hip flexion and full passive hip extension reproduce the pain. The onset is insidious. The pain is felt most in the groin, with a tendency toward radiation into the L2 or L3 segment. Because this bursa often communicates with the joint, ascertain whether involvement of the bursa is a manifestation of hip joint effusion by checking for a capsular pattern of pain or restriction. Management should follow the same approach as for trochanteric bursitis.

ISCHIOGLUTEAL BURSITIS

The ischiogluteal bursa lies between the tuberosity of the ischium and the gluteus maximus. A sterile inflammation of the bursa often develops in persons whose occupation requires prolonged sitting. Ischiogluteal bursitis may be caused by direct trauma, such as falling or a direct hit when the hip is in a flexed position.[79] The name originally given to this bursitis was weaver's bottom.[24] The pain usually appears as soon as the ischium touches the chair and is relieved the minute the patient arises. The patient will report pain with walking, climbing stairs, and flexion of the hip and trunk.[117] The cause is similar to that of trochanteric bursitis. Clinical and physical findings are pain and tenderness over or just above the ischial tuberosity. Pain often radiates into the hamstring muscles.

After the initial phase of treatment with anti-inflammatory medications and ice, the patient may begin a pain-free stretching program of the lower limb. Sitting should be minimized; chair padding, prone lying over a wedge (to provide use of the hands), and other appropriate positioning to prevent aggravation of the bursa is most helpful.

Muscle Strains

The muscle of the hip can easily be strained in work and recreational activities. The causes of muscle strain are multifactorial: the muscle tendon unit can be susceptible to overload and injury owing to muscle imbalances, overstretching, violent muscle contraction against heavy resistance, poor flexibility, adverse neural tension, and leg-length discrepancies.[31,65,66] *Strains* may be defined as damage of some part of the contractile unit caused by overuse (chronic strain) or overstress (acute strain). Strains are graded as mild (first degree), moderate (second degree), and severe (third degree).[97] In severe strains, there is a loss of function of the muscle, tendon, or its attachment caused by a complete tear. The strain occurs at the weakest link of the muscle–tendon unit. Under stress, the muscle may tear, the musculotendinous junction may give way, or the tendon or its bony attachment may be damaged.

A typical client who has incurred a muscle strain has localized pain at the muscle belly, the point of insertion, or the origin of the muscle, and increased stiffness. Resisted isometric muscle contraction will reproduce the pain as will passive stretch (except in a complete tear). For a definitive diagnosis of the lesion, muscles must be isolated one at a time. The involved structures are tender to palpation and may reveal some apparent knotting or hardening in the muscle belly.

Management of muscle strain follows a common pattern.

I. Goals
   A. Pain-free range of motion of the hip, knees, ankle, and foot as compared with the uninvolved limb
   B. Pain-free normal gait pattern with assistive devices on all surfaces
   C. Return to previous functional status for activities of daily living, vocational, recreational, and sports activities as identified by the patient

II. Acute Phase. Initial treatment consists of rest, anti-inflammatory agents, and physical methods as indicated.
   A. Modalities. Initially ice and compression may be indicated. Up to 5 to 7 days after the injury, the muscle remains vulnerable to reinjury because of the loss in healing capabilities and the risk of intermuscular hemorrhage.[67] The clinician can also incorporate the use of modalities such as electrical stimulation, phonophoresis, and ionophoresis to control pain. Initially, electrical stimulation can be used in conjunction with ice, provided that the injured tissue can be effectively cooled with the electrical stimulation electrodes in place.[62]
   B. Manual therapy (as appropriate per differential diagnosis)
      1. Soft tissue techniques. To prevent random alignment of new collagen fibers, soft tissue manipulations follow. The consequences of inelastic scar tissue formation within the muscle belly must be minimized. Soft tissue manipulations, friction massage, and gentle stretching can be initiated early to reduce the risk of this occurrence.
      2. Pain-free stretching (self, proprioceptive neuromuscular facilitation [PNF] stretching) and passive range of motion. Although restoration of muscle length is important, it should not interfere with healing; therefore, the patient should feel a stretching sensation rather then pain when performing mobility exercises and stretching techniques. Carefully assessing the tissues involved and treating all contributing factors are critical to success of treatment and prevention measures.
      3. Joint mobilization as indicated
   C. Exercise and home program. Pain-free exercise early in the rehabilitation process also helps in the formation of scar tissue along the lines of force instead of randomly.[141]
      Within 24 to 48 hours if exercises are pain free, the client should start with submaximal isometrics exercises, progressing to isometrics with increasing load.[58]
      1. Open kinetic chain exercises. Short-arc active exercises with resistance followed by a pain-free isotonic exercise program
      2. Closed kinetic chain strengthening exercise without exacerbation of pain
         • Balance and reach
         • Weight shift
         • Squats
         • Lunges (anterior, posterior, lateral)
         • Gait drill
         • Step up and step down

III. Recovery phase
   A. Modalities and manual therapy techniques as indicated
   B. Exercises and home program
      • Cardiovascular conditioning
      • High-repetition strength training

- Endurance exercise (stationary bike, treadmill, stair-climbing)
- Progression of closed kinetic chain exercises
- Open kinetic chain exercises (free weights)

C. Neuromuscular, balance, and proprioceptive reeducation
- Gait skills
- Agility and plyometric exercise

Integration of specific or biomechanical components that may relieve symptoms, including the choice of shoes, or biomechanical orthoses to control excessive compensatory pronation should be performed.

With chronic strains, prevention is more important than cure. Gradually building up activities so that the muscle–tendon unit can withstand a heavier workload is a key component of rehabilitation. Closed kinetic chain exercises and eccentric and plyometric training in late-stage rehabilitation for the athlete should be considered.[32,94,131,133]

The most commonly strained muscles of the hip are the hamstrings, adductor longus, iliopsoas, and rectus femoris.[112,116]

HAMSTRING STRAIN

Perhaps the muscle strain most dreaded by the athlete is that of the hamstring muscle group.[68] Rehabilitation time is from 2 to 3 weeks for mild injuries, 2 to 6 months for severe conditions. The hamstrings may be injured either at their attachment to the ischial tuberosity or within their midbelly, or less commonly at the knee.[95] Garrett[33] found that the injuries were primarily proximal and lateral in the hamstring group. The biceps femoris is thought to be the most commonly injured muscle.[31]

The patient presents with pain in the posterior thigh region, usually proximal or middle third. With a hamstring injury, pain is apparent on straight-leg raising and resisted knee flexion. Resisted flexion and tibial rotation determine whether the biceps femoris or inner hamstrings are affected. In severe cases, ecchymosis, hemorrhage, and a muscle defect may be visible several days after the injury. Crutches may be necessary for ambulation. Concurrent complaints of a neurologic nature may be present if the neural tissues are involved. Neural tissue stretching has been shown to alter the sympathetic outflow to the lower limbs,[66] thus there may be a physiologic rationale for nerve stretching to treat and prevent grade I hamstring injuries.[65]

Potential causes of this injury include decreased flexibility, comparative bilateral strength deficits, and lack of coordination, poor posture, fatigue, and inappropriate quadriceps to hamstring strength ratios.[27] The optimum value of the hamstrings to that of the quadriceps muscles (HQ ratio) varies from 50 to 80%; the average is about 60%.[61] After knee injury, quadriceps wasting may result in the two muscle groups producing the same power, giving an HQ ratio of 100%.[10] A deficit greater than 10% between the two sets of hamstrings also has been cited as a predisposing factor in hamstring strain.[9]

Hamstring weakness has been described as a predisposing factor in hamstring strains.[9,13,138,139] Therefore, it is important to maximize strength to prevent reinjury. Because most hamstring injuries occur eccentrically, it is important to incorporate eccentric hamstring strengthening into the patient's program. Eccentric exercises are initially done at low, controlled speeds. According to Stanton and Purdam,[123] the use of eccentric exercises as part of a general leg-conditioning program may strengthen the elastic components within the hamstrings, making them better equipped to withstand loading at heel-strike. Schwane and Armstrong[118] showed that eccentric training by downhill running could prevent ultrastructural muscle injury in rats. A study by Jensen and DiFabio[57] indicated that training for eccentric strength can be an effective treatment for patellar tendinitis, and Jonhagen and associates[58] found that sprinters with a history of hamstring injury had tight hamstring muscles and were weaker in eccentric contractions at all velocities (30, 180, and 230° per second) compared with uninjured sprinters. Improper management can lead to recurrent tears and, in the case of the hamstrings, to a condition known as the hamstring syndrome (entrapment of the sciatic nerve).[68,107]

Other functional deficits of this injury include decreased flexibility of the iliopsoas and inhibition of the gluteus maximus.[35] Any anterior tilting of the pelvis resultant from gluteus maximus inhibition or sacroiliac dysfunction may also place the hamstrings at risk because of abnormal length. Cibulka et al.[15] showed that manipulation of patients with sacroiliac dysfunction increased the peak torque in injured hamstring muscles compared with injured patients who were not manipulated. Proper muscle balance must be restored to the iliopsoas owing to its inhibitory effects on the gluteus maximus. The gluteus maximus must also be reeducated to fire and unload the hamstring muscles.

In the early phases of treatment after hamstring injury, the guidelines for initial treatment (see above) should be followed. The use of transverse friction massage is important in the alignment of scar tissue along normal lines of force to prevent abnormal cross-linkage (see Box 8-5). Eventually, high-speed eccentric exercises should be incorporated in the final stages of rehabilitation.

QUADRICEPS STRAINS

The rectus femoris section of the quadriceps is the most commonly strained. Because of its combined action of hip flexion and knee extension it is at risk of tearing during sprinting, kicking, and jumping. Ruptures are not uncommon at the proximal or distal ends of the muscle. As with the more common hamstring strain, a "pop" or snapping is often reported. Treatment is the same as for other muscle strains (see above). See Chapter 15, Knee, for a discussion of quadriceps contusions.

ADDUCTOR STRAINS

Adductor strain often involves the muscles arising at the pubis, such as the adductor longus, adductor brevis, and gracilis. The most frequently injured of the hip adductors is the adductor longus.[2,34,48,86,120,125] Damage is usually to the musculotendinous junction about 5 cm from the pubis, or more rarely the teno-osseous junction giving pain directly over the pubic tubercle (adductor longus) or body of the pubis.[95] The condition tends to result in chronic injury, especially if adequate strengthening and stretching of the adductors are neglected. It may be associated with a periostitis, and it may take 6 months to 1 year to heal.[47]

The condition is more common in sports requiring a rapid change of direction and in which the adductors are used for propulsion. Pain is often experienced with sprinting, lunging, and twisting. Lesions are common in soccer players, ice hockey players, and other players of ball games, and may result from a sudden slip on a muddy field or slippery court, causing tearing or stretching of muscle or tendon fibers.[1,2,86,120] Alternatively, the lesions may start as an overuse phenomenon, which occurs in ballet dancers and in athletes (high-jumping).[19]

The adductor muscles are often neglected with respect to strengthening and flexibility. Functional tests reveal pain on resisted hip adduction and probable pain on passive abduction. Deficits include tightness of the ipsilateral adductors and contralateral tensor fascia latae.[35] The inhibited or weak muscles are the lower abdominals and the ipsilateral gluteus medius and minimus.[35] The ipsilateral piriformis substitutes as an abductor for the inhibited gluteus maximus and gluteus medius. This results in ipsilateral hip external rotation that may interfere with running and normal walking.

Treatment. See protocol above for muscle strains. The patient may need a thigh strap. Stretching plus active-resistance exercise is necessary; friction massage is essential.[47,99] Adductor stretching is begun in a non–weight-bearing position with the effects of gravity reduced, and progressed to more aggressive stretching techniques including standing and supine adductor stretching as the client tolerates (see Box 8-9). PNF stretching is incorporated. Muscle strengthening emphasizing eccentric training is introduced when the client tolerates isotonic exercises well. Resistive hip adductor exercises are initially introduced in the frontal plane and progressed to more functional patterns including hip rotation and diagonal patterns. Balance must also be restored between the ipsilateral lower abdominals and the adductors, along with the lateral pelvis and the thigh muscles.[35] Functional training is a crucial component of the rehabilitation program.

GROIN STRAIN

The anterior groin muscles (adductors, iliopsoas, sartorius, rectus femoris, and the intrinsic internal rotators) can be irritated by any activity that stretches and strains this area. Pain in the groin may result from a lesion of the lumbar spine, the hip joint, or uncommonly the sacroiliac joint. However, it frequently results from a tendinous or muscular lesion, when resisted movements provoke pain. If resisted flexion is painful the following conditions should be considered.

- Tendinitis of the rectus femoris
- Psoas tendinitis
- Tendinitis of the sartorius

Other possibilities include femoral anterior glide syndromes, an avulsion fracture of the anterosuperior iliac spine, and obturator hernia.

Tendinitis of the Upper Rectus Femoris. The rectus femoris (a two-joint muscle) is a weak hip flexor and a strong knee extender and can be overstressed in any sport or action requiring the normal action of hip flexion and knee extension. It is frequently injured by a mistimed kicking action. When dysfunctional, this muscle becomes facilitated, short, and tight. The other three components of the quadriceps group are one-joint muscles, and when dysfunctional become inhibited. A lesion involving the upper rectus femoris is located just below the inferior iliac spine (in the body of the tendon).[99] Alternatively, the tender point lies at the proximal part of the muscle belly.[76] Functional tests reveal definite pain on resisted knee extension, probable pain on passive flexion, extension, or rotation, and inability of the prone patient to flex the knee more than 120°, possibly indicating a tight quadriceps.[47]

Treatment. See protocol for hip strains above. Stretching must involve both knee flexion and hip extension and can be carried out in a sidelying position by the client himself or herself. Lunging actions are also helpful. The unaffected knee is flexed, forcing the affected knee into extension. Two-joint action of the muscle can be worked with resistance applied to the foot as the knee is extended and the hip is flexed.

Tendinitis of the Psoas. Strain of the psoas is usually caused by overactive contraction of the muscle, then the thigh is flexed and then forced into extension. The most frequent site of iliopsoas strain is the insertion at the lesser trochanter or the musculotendinous junction.[97] Patients present with pain in the anterior aspect of the thigh that tends to be made worse with activity. Functional tests reveal pain on resisted hip flexion, probable pain on passive hip extension, and aggravation on passive flexion and adduction.

Treatment. See protocol for hip strains above. Deep friction massage is a very effective treatment (see Box 8-2),[23,99] as is mobilization by oscillatory movements through an arc of the last 40° of hip extension.[21]

Femoral Anterior Glide Syndromes. On the basis of Sahrmann's[115] primary premise that compensatory joint motion in a specific direction is a cause of pain, syndromes of the hip are named for the direction of the movement most consistently associated with pain. A major source of groin pain, according to Sahrmann,[115] is femoral anterior glide syndrome. Femoral anterior glide syndrome may occur with or without medial or lateral rotation. The most common form of femoral medial glide syndrome is with hip medial rotation. Kinesiologic principles indicate that during flexion the femur should glide posteriorly, but in this syndrome posterior glide is insufficient. The anterior joint capsule and its associated soft tissue structures become stretched; the posterior structures become short and stiff.

Although the iliopsoas tendon may be a source of symptoms, the cause of the tendinous disease is pressure exerted by the femoral head against the anterior tissues of the joint capsule, which may occur when the postural alignment of the hip is hyperextended. This syndrome is common in activities that emphasize hip extension, such as dancing and long-distance runners. This impaired movement pattern can also contribute to iliopsoas tendinitis and iliopsoas bursitis.

Monitoring the greater trochanter during hip flexion (Fig. 14-17) and hip extension (Fig. 14-18) assesses movement impairment. Impairments of muscle length and strength as well as joint-play movements of the hip should be included in the evaluation. Functional deficits of the femoral anterior glide with medial rotation include weak or weak and painful iliopsoas, posterior gluteus medius, or intrinsic hip lateral rotators and weak gluteus maximus. Contributing factors may include short length of the tensor fascia lata and iliotibial band, short hamstring muscles (medial shorter than lateral), and apparent leg-length discrepancy.

Treatment. See suggested protocol for hip strains above. It is necessary that a balance of strength and flexibility be sought. Improvement of posterior glide of the femur is essential to correct impaired hip flexion motion and stretching of the posterior capsule (see Fig. 8-39).

Other overuse syndromes of the lower quadrant that have a significant impact on the hip, the lumbar–pelvic–hip complex, and the lower extremity kinetic chain include the ITB overuse syndrome, piriformis muscle syndrome, and the gluteus medius syndrome (see Chapter 8, Soft Tissue Manipulations).

ILIOTIBIAL BAND AND RELATED DIAGNOSES

A tight ITB with tight TFL or tight gluteus maximus are often associated with postural dysfunction of an anterior pelvic tilt posture, slouched posture, or flat back posture.[64] Associated lower limb compensations, commonly found in an anterior pelvic tilt posture, include medial rotation of the femur, genu valgum, lateral tibial rotation, pes planus, and hallux valgus. Because of the vast functional roles of the TFL and ITB, it is prone to overuse and sprain injuries. A few of the more common TFL- and ITB-related diagnoses are discussed in Chapter 8, Soft Tissue Manipulations, and include:

- Sprain of the iliotibial tract and ITB fascitis (see below)
- Greater trochanter bursitis and femoral anterior glide syndrome (see above)
- ITB friction syndrome and patellofemoral dysfunction (see Chapters 8 and 15)
- Low back and sacroiliac dysfunction (see Chapters 8, 22, 23)

Sprain of Iliotibial Tract. This may occur in athletes and dancers or may develop after a fall on the hip. Localized pain is felt in the trochanteric area. The signs are characteristic; pain on side flexion of the trunk toward the painless side, while the other movements are free.[99] When sprain of the iliotibial tract is suspected, an accessory test is performed: in a standing position, the patient crosses the painful leg behind the other and bends sideways toward the painless side, taking all the body weight on the affected limb.[99] Pain, sometimes severe pain, indicates a lesion of the iliotibial tract. Palpation reveals a painful spot, just behind or above the greater trochanter.

Iliotibial Band Fascitis. A condition, sometimes mistakenly diagnosed as sciatica, is the pain associated with inflammation of the fascial band from overuse of the TFL, commonly called ITB fascitis.[46] Pain may be limited to the area covered by the fascia along the lateral surface of the thigh or may extend upward over the buttock and involve the gluteal fascia or distally below the knee, with associated symptoms of paresthesia in the lateral calf. Peroneal nerve irritation can result from pressure from rigid bands of fascia in a short ITB or from the effect of traction from taut bands of fascia in an overstretched ITB. Peroneal nerve irritation can manifest as symptoms in the lateral calf.[63]

Treatment of numerous diagnoses associated with the TFL and ITB should be related to the presenting functional limitation, related impairments, and the stage of healing. A major focus of manual therapy includes soft tissue techniques (friction massage, soft tissue manipulations, stretching) and specific joint mobilization techniques as indicated by positive findings in the biomechanical examination. Improving the force-generating capabilities of the underused synergists is an important prerequisite to neuromuscular training. Progressive gluteus medius, gluteus maximus, quadriceps, and iliopsoas strengthening may be required to reduce the load on the TFL and ITB.[46] At times, one may actually need to strengthen the TFL and ITB if the condition is chronic.[115]

Conclusions

The lumbar spine, sacroiliac, and hip joint function as a mechanical unit and should not be assessed or treated in an isolated fashion. Rehabilitation programs for the client with hip, pelvic, and thigh pain must deal effectively with the relationship of the lumbar–pelvic–hip complex and the lower extremity kinetic chain. Many abnormalities presenting apparently simply as joint pain may be the expression of a comprehensive imbalance of the musculoskeletal system—articulations,[4,12,42,45] ligaments, muscles, fascial planes,[85] intermuscular septa, tendons, and aponeuroses, together with defective neuromuscular control.[53] A thorough understanding of muscle imbalances should serve as the basis of functional rehabilitation.[6,55,60,63,71,115] The iliopsoas is usually the first contracture to develop at the hip and can affect the lumbar spine, pelvis, and hip. The inhibitory effect of a tight postural muscle is evidenced when weakness of the gluteus maximus accompanies tightness of the iliopsoas. Many patients with a lateral pelvic tilt of 1 to 2 cm present with early degenerative changes of the hip on the longer side as well as low back and sacroiliac problems.[41,42,102]

PASSIVE TREATMENT TECHNIQUES

Joint Mobilization

Like the shoulder joint, techniques performed with the hip in a neutral position are used primarily to promote relaxation of the muscles controlling the joint, to relieve pain, and to prepare for more vigorous stretching techniques. The hip joint is, however, much more stable than the shoulder joint.

(For simplicity, the operator will be referred to as the male, the patient as the female. All the techniques described apply to the patient's *right* extremity, except where indicated. P—patient; O—operator; M—movement.)

I. Hip Joint. Elevation and relaxation
    A. Inferior glide, in neutral with a belt (Fig. 14-28A)
        P—Supine, with hip in resting position and knee extended. A stabilizing belt may be applied to the pelvis.
        O—Standing at the end of the treatment table. A belt describing a figure-of-eight is placed around the operator's waist and above the patient's ankle. The operator's hands are placed under the belt and around the distal end of the tibia and fibula.
        M—A distractive force is applied by leaning backward, thereby creating a pull through the belt to the operator's hands.
    B. Inferior glide, in abduction and external rotation (Fig. 14-28B)
        P—Supine. A belt may be used to keep the upper body from sliding inferiorly on the plinth. The leg is in slight abduction, external rotation, and flexion.
        O—Grasps the patient's ankle just proximal to the malleoli with the left hand, behind the back. He grasps the femur distally, just proximal to the condyles and from the medial aspect, with the right hand.
        M—The operator's arms remain fixed. An inferior glide is produced by leaning backward with the trunk. This may be done through various degrees of abduction.
            These techniques are used as general mobilization to increase joint play. Inferior glide is a joint-play movement necessary for hip flexion and abduction. It is also used for relaxation of muscle spasm and pain relief and may be used before and after a treatment session and between other techniques. These procedures should be used on a continuing basis and in conjunction with the stretching techniques described in Techniques I, C and D.
            Note: If there is a knee dysfunction, Techniques I, A and B should not be used; the evaluation position and handholds (Fig. 14-12) may be used as an alternate technique.
    C. Inferior glide, in flexion (Fig. 14-28C)
        P—Supine, with hip and knee each flexed to 90°. A belt may be used to stabilize the upper body.
        O—Supports the lower leg by letting it rest on his shoulder. He grasps the anterior aspect of the proximal femur as far proximally as possible, using both hands with the fingers interlaced.
        M—An inferior glide is imparted with the hands. This may be performed while simultaneously rocking the thigh into flexion.
            This technique is used to increase joint-play movement necessary for hip flexion. An alternative technique is to use a belt around the operator's trunk and the patient's thigh (Fig. 14-28D). Traction is applied by means of the operator's trunk.
    D. Inferior glide, in extension
        P—Supine. A belt may be used to keep the upper body from sliding inferiorly on the plinth. The leg is extended over the side of the plinth and positioned in various degrees of abduction and internal rotation.
        O—Same as for Technique I, B.
        M—The operator's arms remain fixed. An inferior glide is produced by leaning backward with the trunk. The leg may be progressively moved into various degrees of abduction and internal rotation combined with extension, working toward the close-packed position of the hip joint.
            This technique is particularly useful for capsular stretching.

II. Hip Joint. Anterior glide
    A. Anterior glide, in supine (Fig. 14-29A)
        P—Supine. A belt may be used to stabilize the pelvis.
        O—Grasps around posteriorly with both hands to the posterior aspect of the proximal femur, level with the greater trochanter. The fingers are interlaced or overlapping. He stabilizes the distal thigh and knee against the plinth with his trunk.
        M—The slack is taken up, and an anterior glide of the proximal femur is imparted with the hands.
            This technique is used to increase the joint-play movement necessary for external rotation.
    B. Anterior glide, in prone (Fig. 14-29B)
        P—Prone, with the knee bent to 90°. A 1-inch thickness of toweling may be placed under the anterior aspect of the pelvis, just proximal to the acetabulum, for extra stabilization.
        O—Supports the knee with the right hand by grasping around medially to the anterior aspect of the distal femur. He supports the lower leg by tucking it between his elbow and side. The left hand contacts the posterior aspect of the proximal femur with the heel of the hand. It is level with, and medial to, the greater trochanter.
        M—The left hand imparts an anterior glide to the proximal femur. The right hand may simultaneously glide the leg into internal rotation or abduction.
            Techniques II, B and C are considered more progressive than Technique II, A. They are used to increase joint play necessary for external rotation. They also

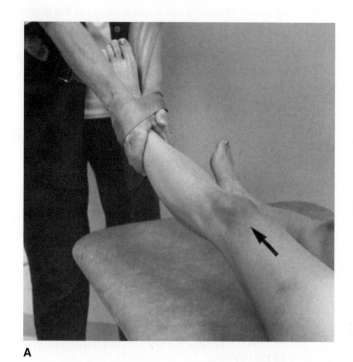

A

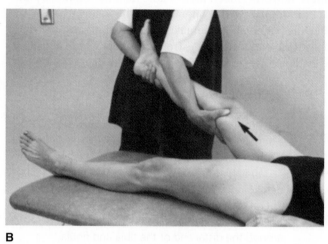

B

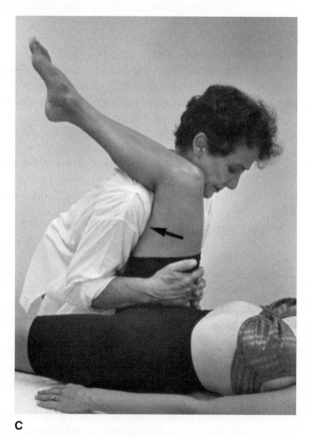

C

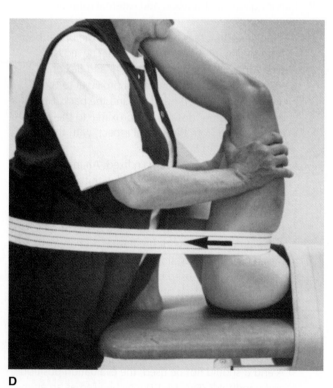

D

■ **FIG. 14-28.** Inferior glide of hip joint in neutral with a belt (**A**), in abduction and external rotation (**B**), in flexion (**C**), and in flexion with a belt (**D**).

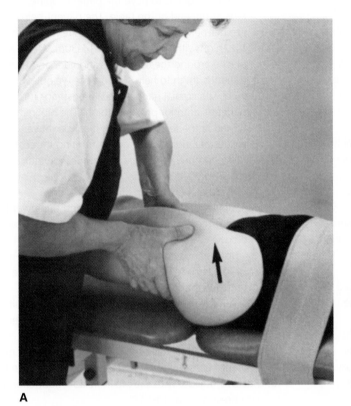

A

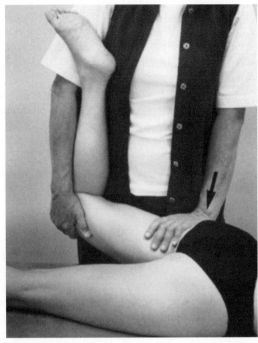

B

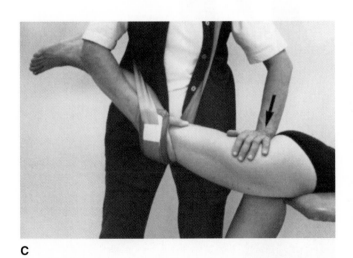

C

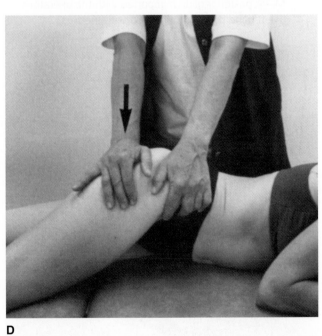

D

■ **FIG. 14-29.** Anterior glide of hip joint in supine (**A**), in prone (**B**), in prone with a belt (**C**), and in sidelying (**D**) positions.

provide a specific capsuloligamentous stretch by internally rotating the femoral head while simultaneously preventing its impingement on the acetabulum.

An alternative technique is to have the patient lie prone with the anterior pelvis at the edge of the table and the limb not being treated resting on the floor. In this position, a belt is placed around the operator's shoulder and the patient's thigh to help support the weight of the limb as force is applied in an anterior direction (Fig. 14-29C).

C. Anterior glide, in sidelying (Fig. 14-29D)

P—Lying on the left side, the bottom limb comfortably positioned and the right leg supported on the table near the limit of hip extension

O—Standing behind the patient. The pelvic girdle is supported with the cranial hand.

M—With the pelvis stabilized, posteroanterior pressure of the femur is applied into the capsule with the caudal hand.

III. Hip Joint. Posterior glide

P—Supine (Fig. 14-30A). An inch of padding is placed beneath the pelvis just proximal and medial to the acetabulum.

O—Supports the knee and distal thigh with the right hand by grasping around medially to the posterior aspect. He contacts the anterior aspect of the proximal femur with the heel of his left hand, with the forearm supinated.

M—A posterior glide is imparted with the operator's left hand by leaning forward with the trunk.

This technique is used to increase a joint-play movement necessary for internal rotation. An alternative technique is to have the patient supine, with the hips at the end of the table. The patient helps stabilize her pelvis by flexing the opposite hip and holding the thigh with the hands (Fig. 14-30B). A belt is placed around the operator's shoulder and under the patient's thigh to help support the weight of the limb. The cranial hand applies a posterior force to the patient's anterior proximal thigh. The hip joint is positioned in the resting position if conservative techniques are indicated or approximating the restricted range if more aggressive techniques are indicated.

IV. Hip Joint. Backward glide (Fig. 14-31A)

A. Backward glide, with hip in 90° of flexion

P—Supine, with the hip flexed 90° and the lower leg supported comfortably on the crook of the operator's elbow

O—Both hands contact the distal end of the femur. He places one hand over the other to provide reinforcement.

M—A backward (dorsal) glide is effected by leaning forward with the trunk, and is assisted by the operator's body weight.

This technique is used to increase joint-play movement necessary for horizontal adduction of the thigh.

B. Backward glide, with the hip in flexion–adduction with compression (Fig. 14-31B)

P—Supine, with the hip flexed and adducted and the knee fully flexed

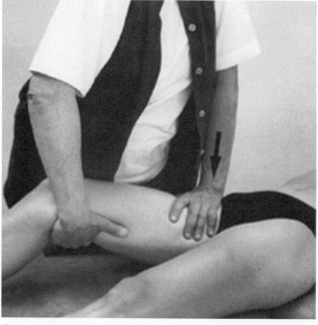

A

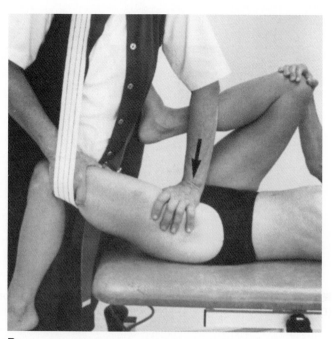

B

■ **FIG. 14-30.** Posterior glide of hip joint in supine (**A**) and in supine with a belt (**B**) positions.

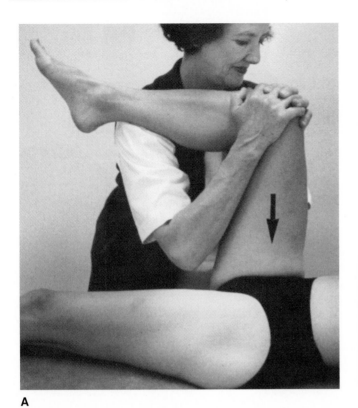

A

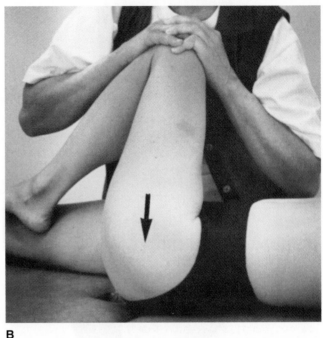

B

■ **FIG. 14-31.** Backward glide of the hip joint with hip in 90° of flexion (**A**), and with hip in flexion–adduction with compression (**B**).

O—Standing on the opposite side of the table, hands clasped over the anterior knee

M—The operator begins by allowing body weight to compress through the long axis of the femur in a backward and lateral direction. The hip is taken into adduction until resistance is felt. The hip is moved further into flexion while adduction and compression are maintained.

Scouring (the quadrant test; Fig. 14-9) may be used as a treatment technique. The operator attempts to identify the small arc of pain and stiffness. Once this arc is identified, the operator may rock back and forth over it, trying to smooth it out. This technique is useful in restoring osteokinematic function of the femur but should not be used when pain is the predominant factor.

V. Distraction Techniques

A. Distraction, in neutral (Fig. 14-32A)

P—Sidelying

O—Standing behind the patient. The fingers are interlocked so that the anterior aspect of the forearm is in contact with the patient's thigh.

M—The operator lifts (distracts) with his clasped hands while simultaneously depressing the patient's knee with his elbow. An alternative technique uses the patient's knee as a fulcrum against the operator's

lower abdomen (Fig. 14-32B).[43] With the elbows extended, the operator contacts the medial aspect of the upper thigh (a towel is placed on the medial aspect). By backward leaning of the trunk, distraction is performed in the line of the head of the femur.

B. Distraction (lateral glide), in flexion (Fig. 14-32C)

P—Supine, hip and knee flexed, leg positioned against the operator's trunk

O—Both hands grasp the upper adductor mass with clasped hands.

M—Mobilization force is applied by leaning at an angle that is lateral and distal (parallel with the neck of the femur). An alternative technique is to use a belt (Fig. 14-32D).

Distraction techniques are used to increase range of motion into hip adduction and internal rotation, to increase joint play, and to decrease pain in the hip joint.

VI. Medial Glide (Fig. 14-33A)

P—Sidelying with the lower leg bent, hip at end range abduction

O—The caudal hand cradles the lower leg or knee and supports the weight of the limb. The cranial hand contacts the lateral aspect of the hip at the greater trochanter.

M—Glide the femoral head inferiorly and medially.

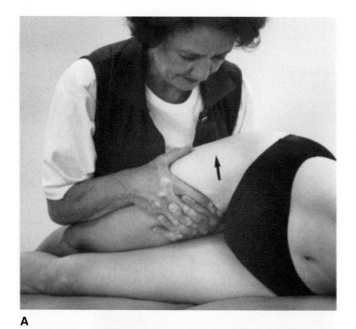

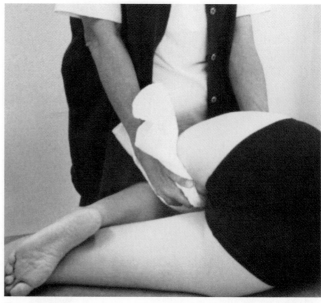

A

B

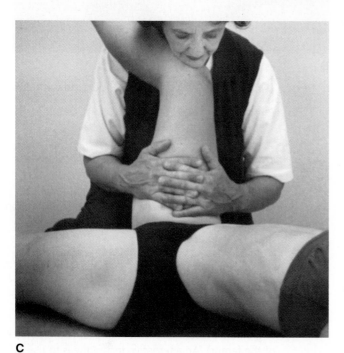

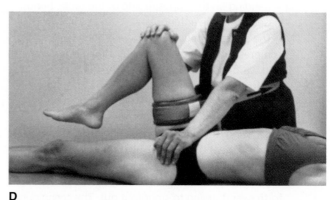

C

D

■ **FIG. 14-32.** Distraction of the femur in neutral (**A**), in neutral (alternative technique; **B**), in flexion (**C**), and in flexion with a belt (**D**).

This is primarily a medial capsular stretch to help restore abduction. A more vigorous capsular stretch may be achieved by abducting and rotating the limb near its end range (Fig. 14-33B).

VII. Rotation Techniques
   A. Lateral rotation (Fig. 14-34A)
      P—Prone, knee flexed to 90°

O—Rotates the lower leg until the buttock rises slightly from the table
M—While maintaining the position of the lower leg, the cranial hand applies downward pressure over the ipsilateral buttocks to the table.
   B. Medial rotation (Fig. 14-34B)
      P—Prone, knee flexed to 90°

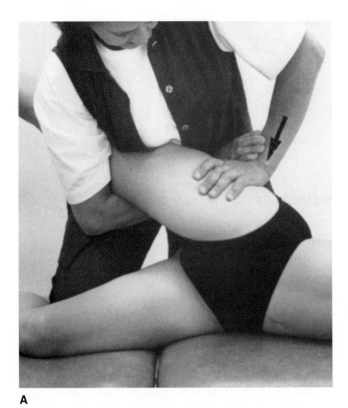

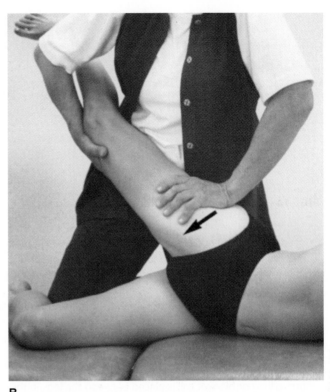

■ FIG. 14-33. Medial glide of the femur: **(A)** support above the knee, **(B)** support at the knee.

O—Rotates the lower leg until the contralateral buttock comes slightly off the table

M—While maintaining this position with the caudal hand, the cranial hand applies downward pressure toward the table over the contralateral buttock.

These techniques are used primarily to stretch the soft tissues of the hip joint, using a short lever system to help restore internal and external rotation.

Self-Mobilization Techniques

I. Inferior Glide or Long-Axis Extension (Fig. 14-35)
P—A comfortable, snug-fitting ankle strap and a stationary wall or table hook for attachment to the ankle strap are

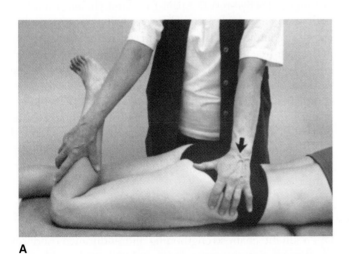

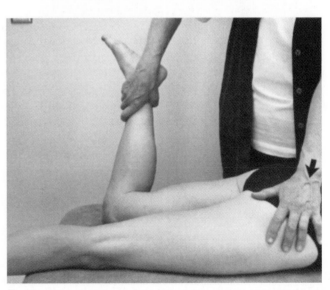

■ FIG. 14-34. Rotation techniques: **(A)** lateral, **(B)** medial rotations.

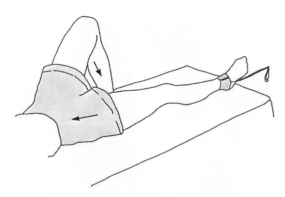

■ **FIG. 14-35.** Inferior glide or long-axis extension.

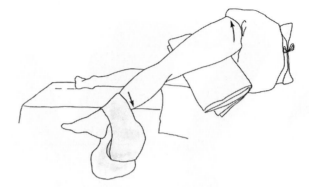

■ **FIG. 14-36.** Distraction in sidelying.

needed. The patient lies supine with the right leg extended and the ankle strap attached to the end of the table or wall hook. The left lower extremity is flexed, with the foot on the table or floor.

M—The left leg pushes downward and upward to push the body away from the fixed point, thus transmitting a traction force on the right lower extremity.

II. Distraction in Sidelying (Fig. 14-36)

P—Lying on the right side, close to one side of the table. A firm pillow or blanket roll is placed between the legs in the groin area. The left hip is extended at the hip with the

lower leg off the edge of the table. A sandbag or ankle cuff with a weight is applied to the left ankle.

M—The left leg is actively raised against the pull of the weight and held for a few seconds; the patient then relaxes, allowing the leg to fall into adduction, with the hip in slight extension, over the edge of the table. Slight oscillatory motion will occur naturally at the end of range.

This technique is a combination of distraction and a muscle-strengthening exercise. In this case, the gluteus medius, which is commonly weak in most hip conditions, is exercised.

DYNAMIC STABILIZATION, FUNCTIONAL EXERCISES, AND SENSORIMOTOR STIMULATION

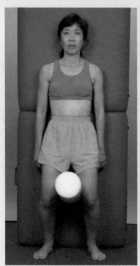
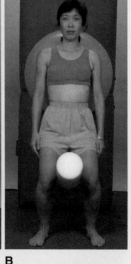

A   B

■ **FIG. 14-37.** Wall slides using an adductor pillow. **(A)** The patient bends the knees to a 45° angle, tightens the thighs, and squeezes the pillow. The patient holds for 10 seconds, then extends the knees and slides up the wall. **(B)** Same as **(A)** but with a therapeutic ball between the wall and the patient.

A primary goal in hip rehabilitation is the return of normal strength and stability of the musculature surrounding the hip and pelvic girdle. After the acute phase, the clinician should use modalities in combination with active range of motion and the beginning of active-resistive pain-free strengthening exercises, both open chain and closed chain, as well as concentric and eccentric contractions. Isometric and concentric strengthening in the pain-free range is started before eccentric work. Generally, the quadriceps and in particular the vasti are inhibited. The vasti are best stimulated in a closed-kinetic chain using glutei contraction to facilitate the quadriceps (Fig. 14-37).[35] Biomechanical deficits of tight hamstrings, gastrocsoleus, and rectus femoris should be dealt with. Additional stretches as indicated by the examination may include stretching exercises for the hip medial and lateral (Fig. 14-34), hip flexors, adductors, and piriformis (see Box 8-9).

Dynamic Stabilization and Functional Exercises

Open kinetic chain strengthening and endurance exercises are described in numerous texts and will not be addressed here.[46,64,100,106,115,124] Closed kinetic chain activities may involve isometric, isotonic, plyometric,[119,135] and even isokinetic techniques. Functional exercises and plyometric exercises are dis-

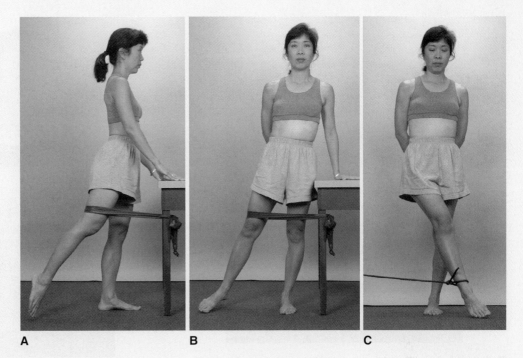

■ **FIG. 14-38.** Closed-chain kinetic exercise with elastic resistance. **(A)** Resisting hip extension requires stabilization of the anterior muscles of the standing leg. **(B)** Resisting abduction requires stabilization of the frontal plane muscles on the standing leg. **(C)** Resisting adduction requires stabilization for the frontal plane muscles on the standing leg.

A   B   C

cussed in Chapter 10, Functional Exercise. Additional closed kinetic chain exercises might include:

- Lumbopelvic stability exercises. Lumbopelvic stability training can be achieved by using a cross-country ski machine, a stationary bike, a fitter, or sliding board (see Fig. 10-6). All these activities are done in a closed-chain kinetic fashion. Controlled stabilization posture of the pelvis may be indicated early on when patients are unable to perform controlled anteroposterior tilt or diagonal patterns of the pelvis. Pelvis control activities can be used to establish kinesthetic awareness of this region (see Chapter 23, Sacroiliac Joint and Lumbar–Pelvis–Hip Complex).
- Closed-chain resistance exercise. Hip extension, (Fig. 14-38A), abduction (Fig. 14-38B), adduction (Fig. 14-38C), and flexion exercises may be included (open-chain movement). Stabilization is required in the weight-bearing leg.
- Gluteus medius training in weight bearing (Fig. 14-39)
- Hamstring eccentric training in kneeling (Fig. 14-40). With the patient in kneeling position on a treatment table, the clinician stabilizes the lower legs as the patient lowers the body to the prone position, eccentrically contracting the hamstrings while maintaining a neutral spine and staying erect. Hip flexion should be avoided.[26]
- Step-ups using repetitions. The patient can step up sideways (Fig. 14-41), forward, or backward.
- Lunges. A cane or rod can be used for balance initially. Progression might include assisted lateral lunges and resisted lateral lunges (Fig. 14-42), lunging in different planes, and lunging forward onto a step.
- Weight-bearing control and stability exercises using manual resistance, starting with rhythmic stabilization exer-

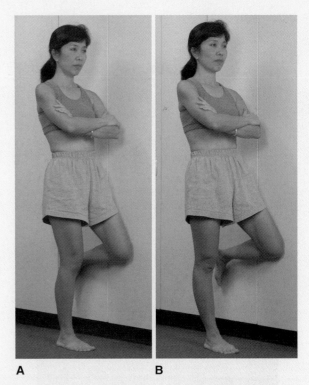

A   B

■ **FIG. 14-39.** Gluteus medius training. The patient stands with the non–weight-bearing knee touching the wall. **(A)** The femur of the standing leg is rotated laterally without moving the hip or foot by using the glutei muscles. **(B)** After lateral rotation of the femur, the next step is to introduce knee flexion to approximately 20 to 30°. Then the knee is extended using the gluteal muscles. A biofeedback device may be positioned on the gluteus medius.

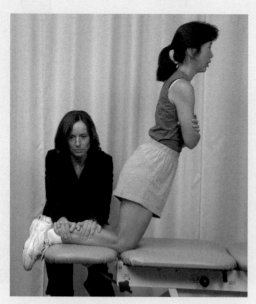

■ **FIG. 14-40.** Hamstring leans. Kneeling eccentric hamstring lowering exercises.[26]

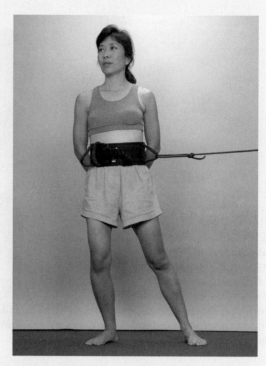

■ **FIG. 14-42.** Resisted lateral lunge.

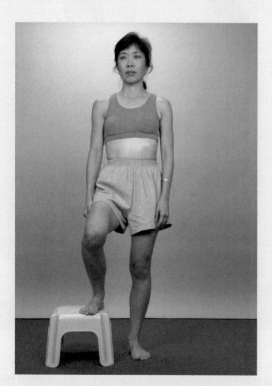

■ **FIG. 14-41.** Lateral step-ups (gluteus maximus, gluteus medius, tensor fasciae latae, quadriceps, and hamstrings).

cises to develop postural adjustments and progressing to resisted walking with manual resistance at the pelvis (Fig. 14-43A). Resisted progression might include sidestepping (Fig. 14-43B) and braiding (Fig. 14-43C).[124]

• Commercial hip machines, leg press, and Smith press squats

Sensorimotor Activities

Sensorimotor activities with increasing difficulty help to restore subcortical reflexes through balance and coordination activities, allowing the glutei muscles and other muscle groups of the lumbar–pelvic–hip complex to begin to fire more on a reflex basis.[35] The idea of neural plasticity is relevant to the orthopaedic patient, who in pain relies on a few stereotyped movement patterns and has lost the richness and relief of movement alternatives.[7] More desirable patterns either are not within the individual's experience or are no longer available voluntarily to the individual. Balance and coordination exercises include static and dynamic activities, on stable and unstable surfaces, on two or one leg, with and without visual input, and adding arm movements with or without weights. As the patient advances through this training the therapist can introduce forces with many different directions or planes of movement. Any of the PNF patterns are helpful (Fig. 14-44). Using a balance beam, fitter or slide board, small trampoline (Fig. 14-45A), wobble boards (Fig. 14-45B), Uniplane rocker board (Fig. 14-45C), foam padding or a DynaDisc (Fig. 14-45D), or training on balance shoes (wobble shoes;

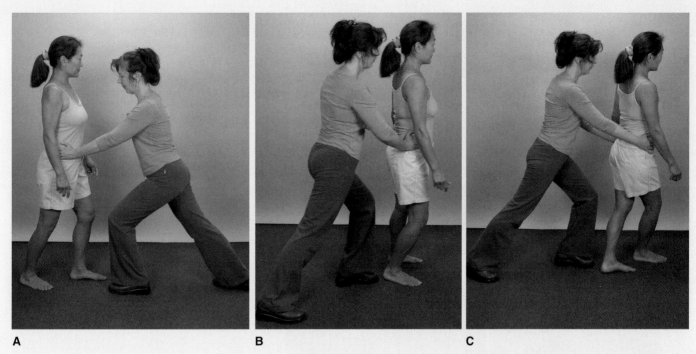

A   **B**   **C**

■ **FIG. 14-43. (A)** Walking forward, resisted progression. **(B)** Walking in sidesteps, resisted progression. **(C)** Braiding, resisted progression.

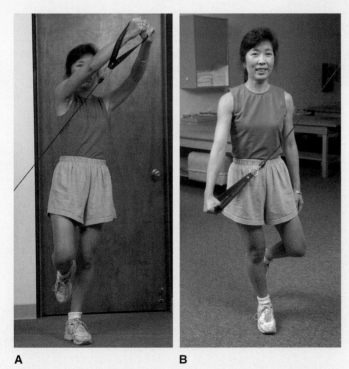

A   **B**

■ **FIG. 14-44.** Sensorimotor stimulation. **(A)** Using multiplanar proprioceptive neuromuscular facilitation (PNF) lift technique to provide rotation stress. **(B)** Using multiplanar PNF chop techniques to provide rotational stress.

Fig. 14-45*E*) are ideal for these activities. Training on balance shoes for 1 week was found to facilitate a significant increase in gluteal activity in normal subjects when measured with surface electromyography.[8] Patients demonstrate improvement in postural stabilization as they attempt progressively more difficult patterns on the balance shoes: walking, high marching, and heel–toe balance. When using balance shoes, several important aspects must be considered: (1) lateral and vertical shift of the pelvis should be avoided, (2) the client should try to control his or her posture, in particular the pelvis and shoulder girdles, (3) the feet should be parallel, (4) the steps should be short but quick, and (5) the small (short) foot must be maintained, if possible, during the activities.[56]

The term *small (short) foot* (Fig. 14-46) is used to describe the shortening and narrowing of the foot with the toes as relaxed as much as possible. The small foot improves the position of the body segments and the stability of the body in the upright position.[56] The small foot also helps to increase afferent input, mainly from the sole and helps to improve the required springing movement of the foot during walking.

Other Functional Activities

Activities including walking, running, starting, and stopping as well as sprinting can be considered as well as sport-specific activities. Agility training is a vital component in the athlete's rehabilitation to fully repair for the increased demands of

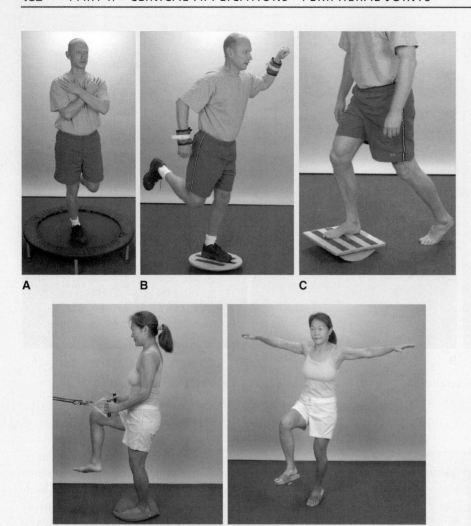

■ **FIG. 14-45.** Sensorimotor stimulation using unstable surfaces: **(A)** small trampoline, **(B)** wobble board, **(C)** Uniplane rocker, **(D)** foam padding or DynaDisc, and **(E)** balance shoes.

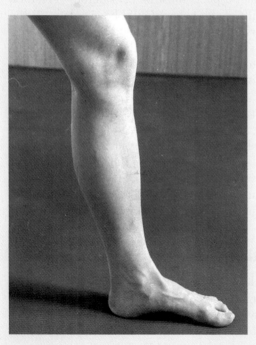

■ **FIG. 14-46.** The short foot. (Reprinted with permission from Liebenson C: Rehabilitation of the Spine: A Practical Manual. Philadelphia: Lippincott Williams & Wilkins, 1996:322.)

return to competitive sports. With advanced training, use an obstacle course requiring changing direction, variable surfaces, changing speed, and other adaptations based on return-to-function needs of the client. Goals in the final stages of rehabilitation are to maximize strength, flexibility, and muscular endurance, and to improve power and coordination.

When discussing the hip, we must always consider the interrelatedness of the lumbar–pelvic–hip complex in the client's rehabilitation program. Overuse injuries, especially, should be approached from a more global understanding of the influence of other biomechanical factors and muscle imbalances and their relationship to the entire lower limb kinetic chain.

REFERENCES

1. Adams RJ, Chandler FA: Osteitis pubis of traumatic etiology. Am J Bone Joint Surg 35:685–696, 1953
2. Akermark C, Johansson C: Tenotomy of the adductor longus tendon in the treatment of chronic groin pain in athletes. Am J Sports Med 20:640–643, 1992
3. Barnett CH: Effects of age on articular cartilage. Res Rev 4:187, 1963
4. Bartlett MD, Wolf LS, Shurtleff D: Hip flexion contractors: A comparison of measurement methods. Arch Phys Med Rehabil 66:620–625, 1985
5. Beattie P, Isaacson K, Riddle DL, et al: Validity of derived measurement of leg-length differences obtained by use of a tape measure. Phys Ther 70:150–157, 1990
6. Bookhout MR: Examination and treatment of muscle imbalances. In: Bourdillon JF, Day EA, Bookhout MR, eds: Spinal Manipulation. Oxford, Butterworth-Heinemann Ltd, 1992:313–333
7. Bronner S: Functional rehabilitation of the spine: The lumbopelvis as a key point of control. In: Brownstein B, Bronner S, eds: Evaluation, Treatment and Outcomes. Functional Movement in Orthopaedic and Sports Physical Therapy. New York, Churchill Livingstone, 1995:141–190
8. Bullock-Saxton JE, Janda V, Bullock MI: Reflex activation of gluteal muscles in walking. Spine 18:704–708, 1993
9. Burkett LN: Causative factors in hamstring strains. Med Sci Sports Exer 2:39–42, 1970
10. Burnie J, Brodie DA: Isokinetic measurement in preadolescent males. Int J Sports Med 7:205–209, 1986
11. Cameron HU, MacNab I: Observations on osteoarthritis of the hip joint. Clin Orthop 108:31–40, 1975
12. Chadwick P: The significance of spinal joint signs in the management of groin strain and patellofemoral pain by manual techniques. Physiotherapy 73:507–513, 1987
13. Christensen CS, Wiseman DC: Strength. The common variable in hamstring strain. Athl Train 7:36–40, 1972
14. Cibulka MT, DeLitto A: A comparison of two different methods to treat hip pain in runners. J Orthop Sports Phys Ther 17:172–176, 1993
15. Cibulka MT, Rose SJ, Delitto A, et al: Hamstring muscle strain treated by mobilizing the sacroiliac joint. Phys Ther 66:1220–1223, 1986
16. Clark MA: Muscle energy techniques in rehabilitation. In: Prentice WE, Voight ML, eds: Techniques in Musculoskeletal Rehabilitation. New York, McGraw-Hill, 2001:215–233
17. Clarke GR: Unequal leg length: An accurate method of detection and some clinical results. Rheumatol Phys Med 11:385–390, 1972
18. Clarkson HM, Gilewish GB: Musculoskeletal Assessment, Joint Range of Motion and Manual Muscle Testing. Baltimore, Williams & Wilkins, 1989
19. Cochrane GM: Osteitis pubis in athletes. Br J Sports Med 5:233–235, 1971
20. Cole JH, Furness AL, Twoney LT: Muscle in Action, an Approach to Manual Muscle Testing. Edinburg, Churchill Livingstone, 1988
21. Corrigan B, Maitland GD: Practical Orthopedics. Boston, Butterworths, 1985
22. Cusick BD: Progressive Casting and Splinting for Lower-Extremity Deformities in Children with Neuromuscular Dysfunction. Tucson, AZ, Therapy Skill Builders, 1990
23. Cyriax JH, Cyriax PJ: Illustrated Manual of Orthopedic Medicine. Boston, Butterworths, 1983
24. D'Ambrosia RD: The hip. In: D'Ambrosia RD, ed: Musculoskeletal Disorders: Regional Examination and Differential Diagnosis, 2nd ed. Philadelphia, JB Lippincott, 1986:447–490
25. Dee R: Mechanoreceptors of the hip joint capsule and their reflex contribution to posture. In: Callayhan JJ, Dennis DA, Paprosky WG et al: Symposium on Osteoarthritis. St. Louis, CV Mosby, 1976:52–65
26. DePalma B: Rehabilitation of the groin, hip and thigh. In: Prentice WE, Voight ML, eds: Techniques in Musculoskeletal Rehabilitation. New York, McGraw, 2001:509–540
27. Ellison AE, Boland AL, DeHaven KE, et al, eds: Athletic Training and Sports Medicine. Chicago, American Academy of Orthopaedic Surgery, 1986
28. Esola MA, McClure PW, Fitzgerald GK, et al: Analysis of lumbar spine and hip motion during forward bending in subjects with and without a history of significant low back pain. Spine 21:71–78, 1996
29. Fisk JW, Balgert ML: Clinical and radiological assessment of leg length. NZ Med J 81:477–480, 1975
30. Freeman MAR: The fatigue of cartilage in the pathogenesis of osteoarthritis. Acta Orthop Scand 46:323–328, 1975
31. Gallaspy JB: Hamstrings, quadriceps, and groin rehabilitation. In: Andrews G, Harralson G, eds: Physical Rehabilitation of the Injured Athlete, 2nd ed. Philadelphia, WB Saunders, 1998:405–424
32. Gamble JN: Strength and conditioning for the competitive athlete. In: Kulund DN, ed: The Injured Athlete, 2nd ed. Philadelphia, JB Lippincott, 1988:11–150
33. Garrett WE Jr: Basic science of musculotendinous injuries. In: Nicholas JA, Herschmann EB, eds: The Lower Extremity and Spine in Sports Medicine, vol. 1, 2nd ed. St Louis, Mosby-Yearbook, 1995:39–51
34. Garrett WE Jr, Mumma M, Lucareche CL: Ultrastructural differences in human skeletal muscle fiber types. Orthop Clin North Am 14:412–425, 1989
35. Geraci MC: Rehabilitation of the hip, pelvis and thigh. In: Kibler WB, Herring SA, Press JM, eds: Functional Rehabilitation of Sports and Musculoskeletal Injuries. Gaithersburg, MD, Aspen Publications, 1998:216–243
36. Gofton JP, Trueman GE: Studies in osteoarthritis of the hip: I. Classification. Can Med Assoc J 104:679–683, 1971a
37. Gofton JP, Trueman GE: Studies in osteoarthritis of the hip: II. Osteoarthritis of the hip and leg-length disparity. Can Med Assoc J 104:791–799, 1971b
38. Gofton JP, Trueman GE: Studies in osteoarthritis of the hip: III. Congenital subluxation and osteoarthritis of the hip disparity. Can Med Assoc J 104:911–915, 1971c
39. Gofton JP, Trueman GE: Studies in osteoarthritis of the hip: IV. Biomechanics and clinical considerations. Can Med Assoc J 104:1007–1011, 1971d
40. Gray G. Lower Extremity Functional Profile. Adrian, MI, Wynn Marketing, 1995
41. Grieve GP: Common Vertebral Joint Problems. Edinburgh, Churchill Livingstone, 1981
42. Grieve GP: The hip. Physiotherapy 69:196–204, 1983
43. Grieve GP: Mobilisation of the Spine: A Primary Handbook of Clinical Method, 5th ed. Edinburgh, Churchill Livingstone, 1991
44. Gruebel-Lee DM: Disorders of the Hip. Philadelphia, JB Lippincott, 1983
45. Gunn CC, Milbrandt WE: Bursitis around the hip. Am J Acupunct 5:53–60, 1977
46. Hall C: The hip. In: Hall CM, Brody LT, eds: Therapeutic Exercise, Moving Toward Function. Philadelphia, Lippincott Williams & Wilkins, 1998
47. Hammer WI: The hip and the thigh. In: Hammer WI: Functional Soft Tissue Examination and Treatment by Manual Methods. Gaitherburg, MD, Aspen Publishers, 1991:105–122
48. Hasselman CT, Best TM, Garrett WE Jr: When groin pain signals an adductor strain. Physician Sportsmed 23:53–60, 1995
49. Hislop HJ, Montgomery J, eds: Daniels and Worthingham's Muscle Testing, 6th ed. Philadelphia, WB Saunders, 1995
50. Hoagland FT: Osteoarthritis. Orthop Clin North Am 2:3–19, 1971
51. Hoppenfield S: Physical examination of the hip and pelvis. In: Hoppenfield S, ed: Physical Examination of the Spine and Extremities. New York, Appleton-Century-Crofts, 1976:143–170
52. Inman VT: Functional aspects of abductor muscles of the hip. J Bone Joint Surg Am 29:607–619, 1947
53. Janda V: Muscles, central nervous motor regulation and back problems. In: Korr I, ed: The Neurobiologic Mechanisms in Manipulative Therapy. London, Plenum Press, 1978
54. Janda V: Muscle Function Testing. Boston, Butterworths, 1983
55. Janda V: Evaluation of muscular imbalance. In: Lieberson C, ed: Rehabilitation of the Spine: A Practitioner's Manual. Baltimore, Williams & Wilkins, 1996:97–112
56. Janda V, Va Vrova M: Sensory motor stimulation. In: Lieberson C, ed: Rehabilitation of the Spine: A Practitioner's Manual. Baltimore, Williams & Wilkins, 1996:319–328

57. Jensen K, DiFabio RP: Evaluation of eccentric exercise in treatment of patellar tendinitis. Phys Ther 69:211–216, 1989
58. Jonhagen S, Nemeth G, Eriksson E: Hamstring injuries in sprinters: The role of concentric and eccentric hamstring muscle strength and flexibility. Am J Sports Med 10:75–78, 1994
59. Jordon RP, Cusack J, Rosseque B: Foot function and its relationship to posture in the pediatric patient with cerebral palsy and other neuromuscular disorders. Lecture notes and instructional materials from Neurodevelopmental Treatment Association meeting, New York, 1983
60. Jull GA, Janda V: Muscles and motor control in low back pain: assessment and management. In: Twomey LT, Taylor JR, eds: Physical Therapy of the Low Back. New York, Churchill Livingstone, 1987:253–278
61. Kannus P: Hamstring/quadriceps strength ratios in knees with medial collateral ligament insufficiency. J Sports Med Phys Fitness 29:194–198, 1989
62. Kelly RG: Management of hip and pelvic injuries. In: Canavan PK, ed: Rehabilitation in Sports Medicine, A Comprehensive Guide. Stamford, CT, Appleton & Lange, 1998:269–292
63. Kendall FP, McCreary EK, Provance PG: Muscle Testing and Function, 4th ed. Baltimore, Williams & Wilkins, 1993
64. Kisner C, Colby LA: Therapeutic Exercise: Foundations and Techniques, 3rd ed. Philadelphia, FA Davis Co, 1996
65. Kornberg C, Lew P: The effect of stretching neural structures in grade 1-hamstring injuries. J Orthop Sport Phys 10:481–487, 1989
66. Kornberg C, McCarthy T: The effect of neural stretching structures on sympathetic outflow to the lower limbs. J Orthop Sports Phys16:269–274, 1992
67. Krejci V, Koch P: Muscle and Tendon Injuries in Athletes. Chicago, Year Book Medical Publishers, 1979
68. Lambert SD: Athletic injuries to the hip. In: Echternach JL, ed: Clinics in Physical Therapy: Physical Therapy of the Hip. New York, Churchill Livingstone, 1990:143–164
69. Lee D: The Pelvic Girdle: An Approach to the Examination and Treatment of the Lumbopelvic region. Edinburgh, Churchill Livingstone, 1989
70. LeVeau B: Application of statics. In: Lissner HR, Williams M, eds: Biomechanics of Human Motion, 2nd ed. Philadelphia, WB Saunders, 1977:100–102
71. Lewit K: Manipulative Therapy in Rehabilitation of the Motor System. London, Butterworth, 1991
72. Li Y, McClure PW, Pratt N: The effect of hamstring stretching on standing posture and on lumbar and hip rotation in forward bending. Phys Ther 76: 836–849, 1996
73. Liebenson C: Active rehabilitation protocol. In: Liebenson C, ed: Rehabilitation of the Spine: A Practitioner's Manual. Philadelphia, Lippincott Williams & Wilkins, 1996:355–387
74. Lissner HR, Williams M: Biomechanics of Human Motion. Philadelphia, WB Saunders, 1962:44–45
75. Lloyd-Roberts GC: The role of capsular changes in osteoarthritis of the hip joint. J Bone Joint Surg Br 35:627–642, 1953
76. Lotke PA. Soft tissue afflictions. In: Steinberg ME, ed: The Hip and Its Disorders. Philadelphia, WB Saunders, 1991:669–682
77. Magee DJ: Orthopedic Physical Assessment, 3rd ed. Philadelphia, WB Saunders, 1997
78. Maitland GD: Peripheral Manipulations, 3rd ed. London, Butterworths, 1991
79. Malone T: Orthopedic and Sports Physical Therapy. St Louis, Mosby, 1996
80. Mankin HJ: Biochemical and metabolic aspects of osteoarthritis. Orthop Clin North Am 2:19–31, 1971
81. Mankin HJ: Biochemical changes in articular cartilage in osteoarthritis. In: Callayhan JJ, Dennis DA, Paprosky WG et al: Symposium on Osteoarthritis. St. Louis, CV Mosby, 1976:1–23
82. McConnell J, Fulkerson J: The knee: patellofemoral and soft tissue injuries. In: Zachazewski JE, Magee DJ, Quillen WS, eds: Athletic Injuries and Rehabilitation. Philadelphia, WB Saunders, 1996
83. McCrea JD: Pediatric Orthopedics of the Lower Extremity: An Instructional Handbook. Mount Kisco, NY, Futura, 1985
84. Mellon G: Correction of hip mobility with degree of back pain and lumbar spine mobility in chronic low back patients. Spine 13:668–670, 1988
85. Mennell JB: Physical Treatment, Movement, Manipulation, and Massage. Philadelphia, Blakiston Co, 1947
86. Merrifield HH, Cowan RF: Groin strain injuries in ice hockey. J Sports Med 1:41–42, 1973
87. Morris JM: Biomechanical aspects of the hip joint. Orthop Clin North Am 2:33–55, 1971
88. Morscher E, Figner B: Measurement of leg length. Prog Orthop Surg 1:21–27, 1977
89. Mulligan BR: Manual Therapy, 'Nags', 'Snags', 'MWMs' etc., 4th ed. New Zealand, Plant View Services, 1999
90. Mundale MO, Hislop HJ, Rabideau RJ, et al: Evaluation of extension of hip. Arch Phys Med Rehabil 37:75–80, 1956
91. Murray RO, Duncan C: Athletic activity in adolescence as an etiological factor in degenerative hip disease. J Bone Joint Surg Br 53:406–419, 1971
92. Nichols PJ: The short leg syndrome. Br Med J 1:1963, 1960
93. Noble HB, Hajek MR, Porter M: Diagnosis and treatment of iliotibial band tightness in runners. Phys Sports Med 10:67–74, 1982
94. Norris CM: Physical training and injury. In: Norris CM, ed: Sports Injuries: Diagnosis and Management for Physiotherapists. Oxford, Butterworth-Heinemann, 1993:89–116
95. Norris CM: The hip. In: Norris CM, ed: Sports Injuries: Diagnosis and Management for Physiotherapists. Oxford, Butterworth-Heinemann, 1993:160–168
96. Ober FB: The role of the iliotibial and fascia lata as a factor in causation of low-back disabilities and sciatica. J Bone Joint Surg Am 18:105–110, 1936
97. O'Donoghue DH: Treatment of Injuries to Athletes, 4th ed. Philadelphia, WB Saunders, 1984
98. Offerski CM, Macnab I. Hip-spine syndrome. Spine 8:316–321, 1983
99. Ombergt L, Bisschop P, ter Veer HJ, et al: The hip and buttock, disorders of the contractile structures. In: Ombergt L, Bisschop P, ter Veer HJ, et al: A System of Orthopaedic Medicine. London, WB Saunders, 1995:750–758
100. O'Sullivan SB, Schmitz TJ: Physical Rehabilitation Laboratory Manual: Focus on Functional Training. Philadelphia, FA Davis Company, 1999
101. Palmer ML, Epler ME: Fundamentals of musculoskeletal Assessment Techniques, 2nd ed. Philadelphia, Lippincott Williams & Wilkins, 1998
102. Patriquinn D: Differential diagnosis of lateral hip, inguinal and proximal anterior thigh pain. Proceedings of the 7th International Congress, Physical Medicine and Rehabilitation, Stockholm, 1980
103. Paul JP: Forces transmitted at the hip and knee of normal and disabled persons during a range of activities. Acta Orthop Belg Suppl 41:78–88, 1975
104. Petty NJ, Moore AP: Neuromusculoskeletal Examination and Assessment, A Handbook for Therapists. Edinburgh, Churchill Livingstone, 1998
105. Post R: History and physical examination. In: Fulkerson JP, ed: Disorders of the Patellofemoral Joint. Baltimore, Williams & Wilkins, 1995: 39–71
106. Prentice WF, Voight MI: Techniques in Musculoskeletal Rehabilitation. New York, McGraw-Hill, 2001
107. Puranen J, Orava S: The hamstring syndrome: A new diagnosis of gluteal sciatic pain. Am J Sports Med 16:517–521, 1988
108. Radin EL, Paul IL: Does cartilage compliance reduce skeletal impact loads? Arthritis Rheum 13:139–144, 1970
109. Radin El, Paul IL: Response of joints to impact loading. Arthritis Rheum 14:356–362, 1971
110. Radin El, Paul IL: The mechanics of joints as it relates to their degeneration. In: Callayhan JJ, Dennis DA, Paprosky WG et al: Symposium on Osteoarthritis. St. Louis, CV Mosby, 1976:34–44
111. Reiman I, Mankin HJ: Quantitative histological analysis of articular cartilage and subchondral bone from osteoarthritic and normal human hips. Acta Orthop Scand 48:63–73, 1977
112. Renstram P, Petyerson L: Groin injuries in athletes. Br J Sports Med 14:30–36, 1980
113. Rydell N: Forces acting on the femoral head prosthesis: A study on strain-gauge supplied prostheses in living persons. Acta Orthop Scand Suppl 88:1–132, 1966
114. Sahrmann SA: A program for identification and correction of muscular and mechanical imbalance: principles and methods. Clin Manage 3:23–28, 1987
115. Sahrmann SA: Diagnosis and Treatment of Movement Impairment Syndromes. St Louis, Mosby, 2002
116. Sammarco G: The hip in dancers. Med Probl Performing Artists 2:5–14, 1987
117. Saudek CE: The hip. In: Gould JA, Davies GJ, eds: Orthopedic and Sports Physical Therapy. St. Louis, CV Mosby, 1990:345–394
118. Schwane JA, Armstrong RB: Effect of training on skeletal muscle injury from downhill running in rats. J Appl Physiol 55:969–975, 1983
119. Seger JY, Westing SH, Hanson M, et al: A new dynamometer measuring concentric and eccentric muscle strength in accelerated, decelerated, or isokinetic movements. Eur J Appl Physiol 57:526–530, 1988
120. Smodlaka VN: Groin pain in soccer players. Physician Sportsmed 8:57–61, 1980
121. Sokoloff LS: The general pathology of osteoarthritis. In: Callayhan JJ, Dennis DA, Paprosky WG et al: Symposium on Osteoarthritis. St. Louis, CV Mosby, 1976:23–24
122. Stanton P, Purdam C: Hamstring injuries in sprinting: The role of eccentric exercise. J Orthop Sports Phys Ther 10:343–349, 1989
123. Staheli LT: Prone hip extension test: Method of measuring hip flexion deformity. Clin Orthop 123:12–15, 1977
124. Sullivan PE, Markos PD: Clinical Decision Making in Therapeutic Exercise. Norwalk, CT, Appleton & Lange, 1994
125. Symeonides PP: Isolated traumatic rupture of the adductor longus muscle of the thigh. Clin Orthop 88:64–66, 1972
126. Thomas HO: Diseases of Hip, Knee, and Ankle Joints, with Their Deformities (Treated by New and Efficient Method), 2nd ed. Liverpool, Dobb, 1876
127. Thurston AJ: Spinal and pelvic kinematics in osteoarthritis of the hip joint. Spine 10:467–471, 1985

128. Tinetti ME, Ginter SF: Identifying mobility dysfunctions in elderly patients: Standard neuromuscular examination or direct assessment. JAMA 259:1190–1193, 1988

129. Tomberlin JP, Saunders HD: Evaluation, Treatment and Prevention of Musculoskeletal Disorders, vol. 2, 3rd ed. Chaska, MN, The Saunders Group, 1994

130. Van Roy P, Borms J, Haentjens A: Goniometric study of the maintenance of hip flexibility resulting from hamstring stretches. Physiother Pract 3:52–59, 1987

131. Verhoshanski Y, Chornonson G: Jump exercises in sprint training. Track Field Q 9:1909–1912, 1976

132. Vignon E, Arlot M, Meunier P, et al: Quantitative histologic changes in osteoarthritic hip cartilage. Clin Orthop 103:269–278, 1974

133. Voight ML, Dravitch P: Plyometrics. In: Albert MA, ed: Eccentric Muscle Training in Sports and Orthopaedics. London, Churchill Livingstone, 1991:45–73

134. Warren R, Kaye JJ, Saluiati EA: Arthrographic demonstration of an enlarged iliopsoas bursa complicating osteoarthritis of the hip: A case report. J Bone Joint Surg Am 57:413–415, 1975

135. Westing SH, Thorstensson A: Iso-acceleration: A new concept in resistive exercise. Med Sci Sports Exer 23:631–635, 1991

136. White SG, Sahrmann SA: A movement system balance approach to musculoskeletal pain. In: Grant R, ed: Physical Therapy of the Cervical and Thoracic Spine. 2nd ed. Edinburg, Churchill Livingstone, 1994:339–358

137. Woerman AL, Binder-Macleod SA: Leg-length discrepancy assessment: Accuracy and precision in five clinical methods of evaluation. J Orthop Sports Phys Ther 5:230–236, 1983

138. Worrell TW: Factors associated with hamstring injuries: An approach to treatment and preventative measures. Sports Med 17:338–345, 1994

139. Worrell TW, Perrin DH: Hamstring muscle injury: The influence of strength, flexibility, warm up, and fatigue. J Orthop Sports Phys Ther 16:12–18, 1992

140. Yoder E: Physical therapy management of non-surgical hip problems in adults. In: JL Echternach, ed: Physical Therapy of the Hip. New York, Churchill Livingstone, 1990

141. Zarins B, Ciullo J: Acute muscle and tendon injuries in athletes. Clin Sport Med 2:167–172, 1983

Knee

DARLENE HERTLING AND RANDOLPH M. KESSLER

REVIEW OF FUNCTIONAL ANATOMY

Osseous Structures

The distal end of the femur consists of two large condyles, separated posteriorly by the very deep intercondylar notch and anteriorly by the patellar groove, in which the patella glides. The anterior condylar surface is called the *trochlear surface* of the femur.

Looking anteriorly (Fig. 15-1), the medial condyle extends farther distally than does the lateral condyle, so that when standing with the distal surfaces of the condyles level, the femur and tibia form a valgus angle of about 10°. Both condyles have epicondyles extending from their sides. Medially, the adductor tubercle lies just superior to the medial epicondyle. The articular cartilage extends farther superiorly on the anterior surface of the lateral condyle than it does on the same aspect of the medial condyle.

Looking inferiorly (Fig. 15-2), the articular surface of the distal femur forms a U about the deep intercondylar notch. The lateral condyle extends considerably farther anteriorly than does the medial condyle, helping to prevent lateral dislocation of the patella caused by the horizontal component of the direction of quadriceps pull. The medial condyle angles backward and medially. The lateral condyle lies in the sagittal plane.

Looking medially or laterally (Fig. 15-3), the condyles do not describe part of a circle; rather, their radius gradually decreases from anterior to posterior. The medial condyle is longer anteroposteriorly, with a more gradual change in radius from back to front. The small lateral condyle tends to flatten

sooner as one follows the curvature from back to front. The difference in the two condyles plays a part in the length rotation and locking mechanism of the knee, as discussed in the section on biomechanics.

The upper end of the tibia (Fig. 15-4) consists of two large condyles with joint surfaces superiorly for articulation with the femur. Both condyles are offset posteriorly to overhang the tibial shaft. They are also angulated 5 to 10° downward anteroposteriorly. The medial tibial condyle is larger; its superior surface is concave in all directions. The smaller lateral tibial condyle is actually convex anteroposteriorly. However, the lateral meniscus forms a concave articular surface for articulation with the convex lateral femoral condyle. Posterolaterally on the lateral tibial condyle is an articular facet for the head of the fibula, which faces somewhat downward. At the anteroinferior junction of the tibial condyles is the tibial tuberosity, an eminence onto which the patellar tendon inserts. Superiorly, between the condyles, is the roughened intercondylar area. The medial and lateral intercondylar tubercles, or eminences, lie centrally in the intercondylar area.

The patella (Fig. 15-5) is a triangular sesamoid bone, its apex lying inferiorly, embedded in the back of the quadriceps tendon. The posterior surface of the patella is cartilage-covered for articulation in the patellar groove of the femur, between the femoral condyles. The patellar articular surface consists of a lateral facet, a medial facet, and a small odd medial facet. The patella gives extra purchase to the quadriceps tendon in producing knee extension, especially toward the limits of extension.

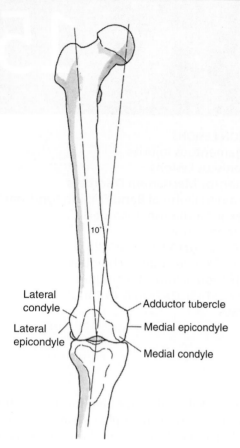

■ **FIG. 15-1.** Anterior view of the right femur.

Menisci

The medial meniscus is semicircular, being larger posteriorly than anteriorly. Its anterior horn inserts onto the intercondylar area of the tibia, in front of the attachment of the anterior cruciate ligament (ACL), and its posterior horn inserts in front

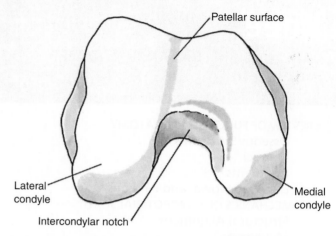

■ **FIG. 15-2.** Inferior aspect of the distal end of femur.

of the attachment of the posterior cruciate ligament (PCL). Peripherally, it is attached to the joint capsule, to the short capsular fibers of the medial collateral ligament (MCL), and to the outer margin of the superior aspect of the medial tibial condyle by the coronary ligament. The coronary ligament constitutes the inferior aspect of the joint capsule (Fig. 15-6).

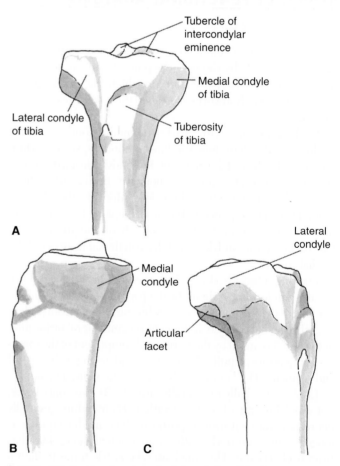

■ **FIG. 15-4.** Proximal end of the right tibia from anterior (**A**), medial (**B**), and lateral (**C**) aspects.

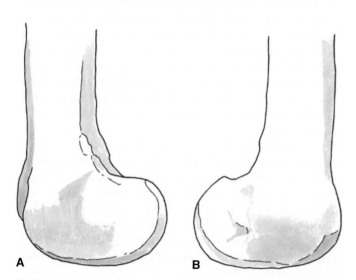

■ **FIG. 15-3.** Medial (**A**) and lateral (**B**) aspects of distal end of the right femur.

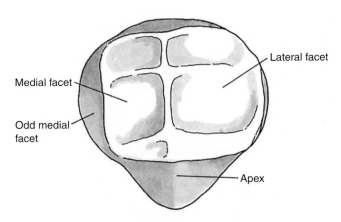

■ **FIG. 15-5.** Posterior aspect of the right patella.

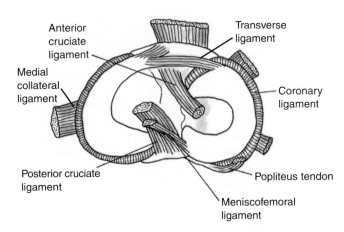

■ **FIG. 15-7.** Superior aspect of the right tibia, showing the ligaments.

The medial meniscus forms part of a larger circle, but the lateral meniscus forms almost all of a smaller circle. Its two horns attach close to each other, just in front of and just behind the intercondylar eminence. The periphery of the lateral meniscus attaches to the tibia, the capsule, and a coronary ligament, but not to the lateral collateral ligament (LCL). The lateral meniscus is more mobile than the medial meniscus as a result of its shape and less extensive peripheral attachments. A ligament usually runs from the posterior aspect of the lateral meniscus to the medial condyle of the femur. This meniscofemoral ligament runs behind the PCL, while another may run in front (Fig. 15-7). The popliteus tendon also attaches to the lateral meniscus; this attachment is said to assist in posterior movement of the meniscus during knee flexion.[195] Usually a transverse ligament connects the two menisci anteriorly.

In recent years the meniscus, formerly considered an unimportant appendage within the knee, has been recognized as one of the prime protectors of knee use and function.[193] The menisci serve several functions in the knee. They act as shock absorbers, spreading the stress over the joint surface and decreasing cartilage wear. They aid in the lubrication and nutrition of the joint, reduce friction during movement, and improve weight distribution by increasing the area of contact between the condyles. They are vascular in their cartilaginous inner two thirds and are partly vascular and fibrous in their outer

third.[14] Because most recent literature indicates that removal of the total meniscus can lead to early degeneration of the joint,[78,202,286,301] most surgeons today remove only the torn portion of the meniscus, not the entire structure.

Ligaments

The MCL is a long, flat band attached above to the medial epicondyle and below to the medial aspect of the shaft of the tibia, about 4 cm below the joint line (Fig. 15-8). Its fibers run somewhat anteriorly, from top to bottom. Older descriptions often refer to *deep, shorter fibers* and *posterior oblique fibers* of the MCL, but these are both considered part of the joint capsule (see below) in more recent literature.[145,356] The deep capsular fibers are attached to the medial meniscus.

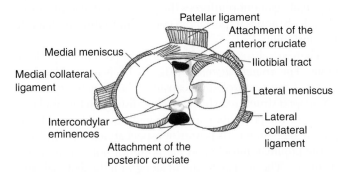

■ **FIG. 15-6.** Superior aspect of the right tibia, showing the menisci and tibial attachments of the cruciate ligaments.

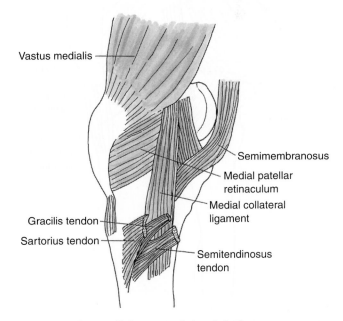

■ **FIG. 15-8.** Medial aspect of the right knee.

The MCL becomes tight on extension of the knee, abduction of the tibia on the femur, and outward rotation of the tibia on the femur. Some of the anterior fibers become tight on knee flexion. The MCL also helps prevent anterior displacement of the tibia on the femur.

The LCL is a shorter, round bundle of fibers running from the lateral epicondyle to the fibular head (Fig. 15-9). It does not attach to the lateral meniscus. The popliteus tendon runs underneath the ligament between it and the meniscus. The LCL is largely covered by the tendon of the biceps femoris. The LCL runs slightly posteriorly from top to bottom and is tight on extension of the knee, adduction of the tibia on the femur, and outward rotation of the tibia on the femur.

The ACL runs from the anterior intercondylar area of the tibia backward, upward, and laterally to the medial aspect of the lateral femoral condyle in the intercondylar notch (Fig. 15-7).[107] It acts primarily to check extension of the knee, forward movement of the tibia on the femur, and internal rotation of the tibia on the femur. Because the ACL pulls tight on internal tibial rotation and as the knee extends, some

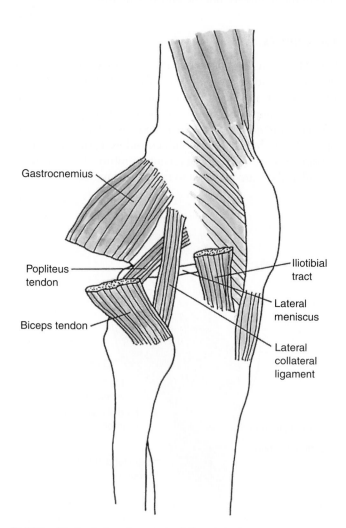

Gastrocnemius

Popliteus tendon

Biceps tendon

Iliotibial tract

Lateral meniscus

Lateral collateral ligament

■ **FIG. 15-9.** Lateral aspect of the right knee.

have proposed that this ligament guides the tibia into outward rotation during knee extension.[303]

The PCL runs from the extreme posterior intercondylar area of the tibia forward, medially, and upward to the lateral aspect of the medial femoral condyle in the intercondylar notch (Fig. 15-7). As it travels from the tibia to the femur, the ligament twists in a medial spiral. The posterolateral part of the PCL is taut in extension and the anteromedial portion is lax.[180,251,252] In flexion, all the fibers except the anteromedial portion are lax. It primarily checks backward movement of the tibia on the femur and helps check internal rotation of the tibia on the femur. It also tightens on full knee extension, although some fibers may be tight throughout the range of flexion–extension of the knee. It is aided by the popliteus muscle in checking forward sliding of the femur on the tibia when squatting.

The patellofemoral ligament is a thickening of the patellar retinaculum. It passes from the adductor tubercle of the femur to the medial aspect of the patella. Its femoral attachment often becomes irritated and tender in cases of patellofemoral tracking dysfunction.

A fibrous capsule surrounds the knee joint, attaching at the margins of the articular cartilage. The superior aspect of the capsule runs from the articular margin of the femur to the periphery of the menisci. The inferior fibers run a short distance from the menisci to the tibia. The inferior capsule is often called the *coronary ligament*.

The fibrous capsule receives extensive passive and dynamic reinforcement (Figs. 15-8 and 15-9). Passive reinforcement is provided by the above-mentioned ligaments and by what are referred to in older texts as the *deep layer* and *posterior oblique fibers* of the MCL. These are thickenings of the medial and posteromedial aspects of the joint capsule that provide added stabilization against valgus and external rotatory stresses. The posterior oblique fibers of the posterior capsular ligament are now referred to as the *posterior oblique ligament* (Fig. 15-10; also Fig. 15-8). The short capsular fibers deep to the MCL are attached to the medial meniscus. The posterior oblique popliteal ligament attaches to the posterior medial aspect of the meniscus and intersperses with the semimembranosus muscle (Fig. 15-10). Along with the MCL, the pes anserinus tendons, and the semimembranosus, the posterior oblique popliteal ligament reinforces the posteromedial joint capsule (Fig. 15-8) and is important in controlling anteromedial rotatory instability.[147]

There are also some thickenings of the posterior capsule laterally. The *arcuate ligament* (Fig. 15-10) is formed by thickening of the posterolateral capsule. The arcuate ligament is a Y-shaped structure, which attaches distally on the fibula and fans over the posterior capsule to joint the posterior oblique popliteal ligament. Its posterior aspect attaches to the fascia of the popliteal muscle and the posterior horn of the lateral meniscus. The arcuate ligament along with the iliotibial band, the popliteus, the biceps femoris, and the LCL reinforce the posterolateral joint capsule. Collectively, the posterior third of

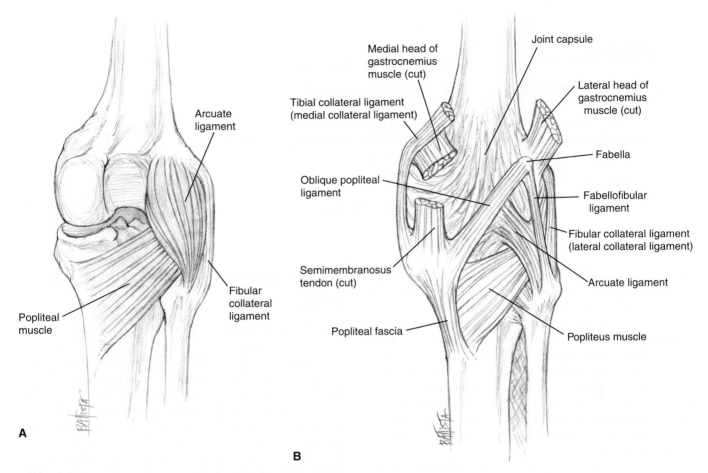

■ FIG. 15-10. Posterior aspect of the knee showing the arcuate ligament (**A**) and the posterior oblique popliteal ligament (**B**).

the lateral capsular ligament and the aponeurosis of the popliteus muscle are known as the *arcuate complex*.[361]

Dynamic capsular reinforcement is provided to all aspects of the joint capsule. Anterior reinforcement is provided by the patellar tendon inferiorly and the quadriceps tendon superiorly (see Fig. 7-19*B*). These constitute the anterior capsule because a fibrous capsule per se is absent anteriorly. Anteromedial and anterolateral reinforcements are provided by the medial and lateral patellar retinacula, which are superficial to and may blend with the fibrous capsule (see Fig. 7-19*B*). These help stabilize the patellofemoral joint during loaded knee extension.

The distal aspect of the iliotibial band provides anterolateral reinforcement. This stabilizes against excessive internal rotation of the tibia on the femur and thus works in conjunction with the cruciate ligaments.

The pes anserinus tendons (semitendinosus, gracilis, and sartorius) and the semimembranosus tendon give medial and posteromedial reinforcement (Fig. 15-8). These help prevent abnormal external rotation, abduction, and anterior displacement of the tibia on the femur. In doing so they dynamically reinforce the MCL, the posteromedial capsule, and to a certain extent the ACL.

Posterolateral support comes from the biceps femoris tendon. This helps check excessive internal rotation and anterior displacement of the tibia on the femur, providing reinforcement to the functions of the cruciate ligaments. It also may assist the LCL in preventing adduction of the tibia on the femur.

Finally, posterior reinforcement is provided by the insertions of the gastrocnemius muscles and from the popliteus muscle (Fig. 15-10). The popliteus helps check external rotation of the tibia on the femur and backward displacement of the tibia on the femur. Contraction of the popliteus muscle internally rotates the tibia on the femur to unlock the knee joint from the screw-home position at the beginning of knee flexion.[117] Contraction of the popliteus muscle also helps to pull the posterior horn of the lateral meniscus posteriorly during flexion of the knee.

Bursae, Synovia, and Fat Pads

The synovium of the knee joint, in addition to lining the fibrous capsule, forms several large recesses (Fig. 15-11). Anteroinferiorly, it extends inward to line the back of the infrapatellar fat

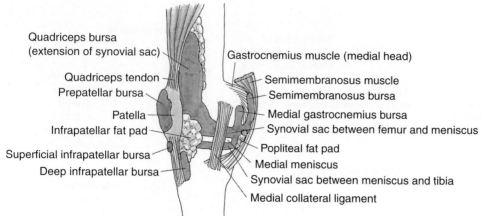

Quadriceps bursa
(extension of synovial sac)
Quadriceps tendon
Prepatellar bursa
Patella
Infrapatellar fat pad
Superficial infrapatellar bursa
Deep infrapatellar bursa

Gastrocnemius muscle (medial head)
Semimembranosus muscle
Semimembranosus bursa
Medial gastrocnemius bursa
Synovial sac between femur and meniscus
Popliteal fat pad
Medial meniscus
Synovial sac between meniscus and tibia
Medial collateral ligament

■ **FIG. 15-11.** Medial aspect of the knee, showing the synovia and bursae.

pad. The medial and lateral aspects of this lining unite centrally to form the ligamentum mucosa, which extends into the joint to attach to the intercondylar notch of the femur. Anterosuperiorly, the synovium runs from the superior aspect of the patella upward beneath the quadriceps tendon, then folds back on itself to form a pouch and inserts on the distal femur above the condyles. This suprapatellar pouch is part of the joint cavity and provides sufficient slack in the synovium to allow full knee flexion. Posteriorly, the synovium invaginates into the intercondylar notch to pass in front of the cruciate ligaments. In this way the cruciate ligaments are intracapsular but extrasynovial.

In addition to the suprapatellar pouch, which also serves as a bursa, there are three additional major bursae anteriorly. The prepatellar bursa lies over the patella, and may become inflamed with prolonged kneeling ("housemaid's knee"). A bursa also lies between the patellar tendon and the tibia (deep infrapatellar bursa) and between the patellar tendon and skin (superficial infrapatellar bursa).

Posteriorly, a main bursa lies between the semimembranosus tendon and the medial origin of the gastrocnemius muscle. This bursa often communicates with the joint and may become swollen with articular effusion ("Baker's cyst"). This bursa may also extend between the gastrocnemius and the capsule, or a separate bursa may be situated here.

Bursae may also exist beneath the tendons of the pes anserinus and the iliotibial band, just proximal to their insertions. These can become irritated with high levels of activity. There may also be other bursae about the knee joint, but these are of little clinical significance.

The large infrapatellar fat pad is situated deep to the patellar tendon and in front of the femoral condyles. When the knee is flexed, it fills the anterior aspect of the intercondylar notch. With the knee extended, it occupies the patellar groove and covers the trochlear surface of the femur. The back of the fat pad is lined with synovium. It is thought that as the fat pad sweeps across the condyles during knee flexion and extension, it helps to spread a lubricating layer of synovial fluid over the joint surface of the femur before contact with the tibia.

BIOMECHANICS OF FEMOROTIBIAL JOINT

Structural Alignment

Because the medial femoral condyle extends farther distally than does the lateral condyle, there is usually a slight valgus angulation of about 5 to 10° between the tibia and the femur. With the transcondylar axis of the femur in the frontal plane the patella faces straight forward. In this position, the neck of the femur is directed about 20° forward as a result of the normal internal torsion of the femoral shaft with respect to the femoral neck. Also in this position, the transmalleolar axis at the ankle is rotated outward about 25° as a result of the normal external torsion of the tibial shaft, and the long axis of the foot is directed 5 to 10° outward.

Movement

The knee is normally biaxial; it flexes and extends around an axis that is horizontally oriented in the frontal plane in the standing position, and it rotates about a vertical axis. Knee flexion–extension is polycentric, the axis of movement shifting backward along a curved centroid as the knee moves from extension into flexion.

FLEXION–EXTENSION

Osteokinematics. The total range of knee flexion–extension in the healthy knee is from about 5 to 10° of hyperextension to 140 to 150° of flexion. Flexion is limited by soft-tissue approximation of the calf and posterior thigh. Extension is terminated by locking of the joint in its close-packed position as the capsules and ligaments draw tight and become twisted. As the knee approaches full extension, it also assumes a valgus angulation because the medial femoral condyle extends farther distally than the lateral condyle.

Arthrokinematics. The femorotibial joint is markedly incongruent in positions of flexion, but becomes progressively more congruent as the knee extends. In the flexed position, the small convex radius of the posterior femoral condyles contacts a relatively large radius on the tibial condyles. In fact, the lateral tibial condyle is actually a convex surface. Because the radius of curvature of the femoral condyles progressively increases anteriorly, the joint becomes more congruent as the contacting area on the femur moves anteriorly during knee extension (Fig. 15-12).

The fibrocartilaginous menisci reduce joint surface incongruency. Their mobility and deformability allow them to conform to the shape of the contacting femoral joint surfaces. The anterior segments of the menisci are somewhat mobile, whereas the posterior horns are comparatively fixed. Thus, as the knee extends and the contacting radius of the femoral condyle increases, the anterior aspects of the menisci glide forward. Conversely, as the knee flexes, the anterior segments of the menisci recede to conform to the smaller radius of curvature of the contacting femoral condyles (Fig. 15-13). By reducing joint surface incongruency, the menisci help distribute the forces of compressive loading over a greater area, thus reducing compressive stresses to the joint surfaces of the knee.

As indicated by the instant centers of motion, flexion and extension of the knee occur with a combination of rolling and sliding at the joint surfaces. The closer the instant center is to the contacting joint surfaces, the greater the amount of rolling that occurs at a particular point in the range of movement. An instant center that lies some distance from the contacting surfaces indicates considerable sliding between the surfaces. Because the normal axes of movement for flexion and extension of the knee lie within the condylar region of the femur—not on the joint surfaces or a long distance away—it follows

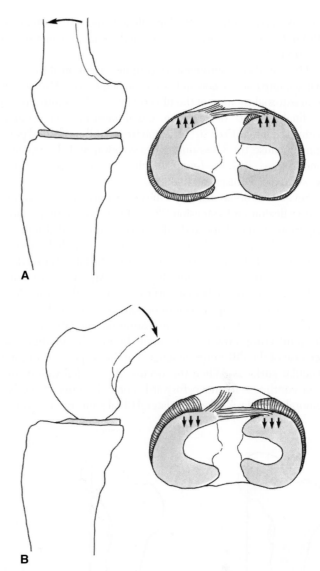

■ **FIG. 15-13.** During extension (**A**), the menisci glide forward, while during flexion (**B**), the menisci recede to conform to the radius of curvature of the connecting femoral condyles.

that both sliding and rolling accompany the movement. It can be seen from the loci of normal instant centers that the axis of movement shifts farther away from the joint surface as the knee extends, indicating that relatively more sliding is occurring as extension takes place (Fig. 15-12).[93,94,95] Considering that the tibia moves on the fixed femur, the direction of sliding and rolling of the tibial joint surface is anterior during extension and posterior during flexion.

TRANSVERSE ROTATION

Because the femorotibial joint surfaces are incongruent in all positions except full extension, and because the menisci are semimobile, the knee joint can undergo rotation in the transverse plane. This rotary movement can easily be produced

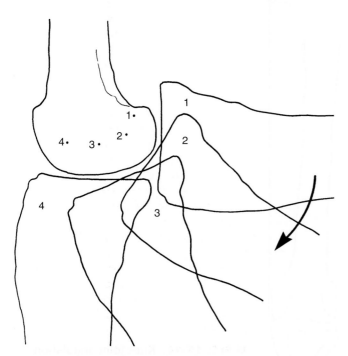

■ **FIG. 15-12.** Diagram showing loci of normal instant centers and congruency during flexion and extension of the knee.

actively or passively with the knee flexed, and is important for attenuation of rotary forces acting on the knee during normal function.

There is also an automatic, or conjunct, rotation at the knee that accompanies flexion and extension of the joint. This occurs as an external rotation of the tibia relative to the femur during the final 15 to 20° of extension, and an internal tibial rotation during the initial 15 or 20° of flexion from a fully extended position. Because the knee undergoes rotation and the menisci tend to move with the femur, much of the movement occurs between the menisci and the tibia.

Several factors contribute to the occurrence of knee rotation during flexion and extension.[17,303,347] First, and perhaps most important, is the shape and orientation of the medial femoral condyle. Looking at the femur end on, the medial condyle is curved and obliquely oriented, whereas the lateral condyle is situated in the sagittal plane (Fig. 15-2). Also of significance is the fact that the articular surface of the medial condyle is longer, in an anteroposterior direction, than that of the lateral condyle. As the tibia moves into extension, the lateral side of the joint completes its movement before the medial side because of the difference in lengths of the respective femoral articular surfaces. When this occurs, the medial side of the tibia continues to move forward along the curved medial femoral condyle, whereas the lateral tibial joint surface under-

goes a lateral spin. The net effect is an external rotary movement of the tibia on the femur. This movement reverses when the knee flexes from a fully extended position.

The cruciate ligaments are also thought to play a role in guiding rotary movement at the knee. The cruciate ligaments tighten as the knee extends and are twisted in a direction to rotate the tibia externally as they tighten.

Pathomechanics

STRUCTURAL ALTERATIONS

Frontal Plane. Although the knee joint normally assumes a valgus angulation, the line of application representing the weight-bearing force acting on the knee tends to bisect the joint. This is because the femoral head is offset medially from the shaft of the femur (Fig. 15-14). Excessive genu valgum causes the weight-bearing force to be shifted to the lateral side of the joint; genu varum results in a medial shift of the weight-bearing force line. Such alterations in force distribution may lead to accelerated wear on one side of the joint.[86] Common factors contributing to genu valgum are iliotibial band tightness, abnormal foot pronation, and femoral anteversion. Femoral retroversion tends to result in genu varum.

Transverse Plane. In increased femoral anteversion, the femoral condyles are rotated too far internally with respect to

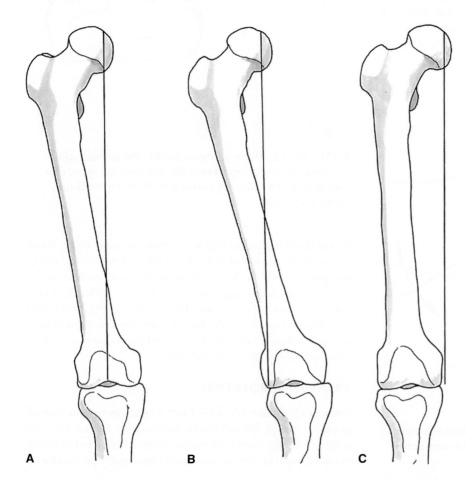

A   **B**   **C**

■ **FIG. 15-14.** Knee joint angulation showing normal valgus angulation (**A**), excessive valgus angulation (**B**), and varus angulation (**C**).

the femoral neck. Thus, with the hip joint in a neutral position, the condyles and patellae face inward, or, conversely, with the patellae and condyles facing forward, the hip joint assumes an externally rotated position. Because the tendency during gait is to maintain normal alignment of the hip joints, the person with increased femoral anteversion tends to walk with the knee rotated inward. This inward rotation may be transmitted to the foot as a toe-in stance or as abnormal foot pronation. At the knee, inward rotation results in a valgus angulation when the knee is semiflexed, as it is during most of the stance phase of gait. In a similar manner, abnormal retroversion of the hip causes a tendency for the patella to face outward during gait, for the knee to assume a varus position, and for the feet to either toe-out or supinate. In some persons with torsional deviations of the femur, compensatory structural rotation of the tibia develops. Thus, the child with femoral anteversion may also develop increased external tibial torsion to achieve normal foot placement. Similarly, internal tibial torsion may develop in association with femoral retroversion. Such torsional compensation at the tibia seems to enhance valgus–varus deviations.

INTRINSIC MOVEMENT ABNORMALITIES

Capsular Tightness. One of the most common causes of gross restriction of knee motion is capsular tightness. Fibrosis and subsequent loss of extensibility of the joint capsule frequently follow immobilization after trauma or surgery, and usually accompany the progression of chronic joint diseases such as degenerative joint disease (DJD) or rheumatoid arthritis. Capsular tightness at the knee results in a characteristic pattern of restriction in which knee extension is limited by 20 to 30°, and flexion is possible to only 80 or 100°. The functional disability resulting from capsular restriction varies with the patient's activity level, but ambulation is inevitably altered because nearly full knee extension is necessary for normal gait. According to Laubenthal and coworkers,[196] the mean total flexion–extension necessary for the stance phase of gait is 21°; for the swing phase of gait, 67°; for stair climbing, 83°; and for sitting and rising, 83°. Because capsular restriction at the knee typically allows only 50 to 80° of flexion–extension, some functional alteration is likely.

Of great significance during walking is the effect of reduced knee extension on the stresses imposed on the articular surfaces of the joint. Normally, during the stance phase of gait, peak weight-bearing forces are borne with the joint just short of full knee extension, a position in which the tibiofemoral contact area is greatest, and a position in which the joint capsule has not been drawn completely tight.[86,181] As stress equals force divided by unit area, the compressive stress of weight bearing is minimized by a relatively large tibiofemoral contact area. Furthermore, the joint is not "shock-loaded" by having the slack in the joint capsule suddenly taken up as the knee moves toward extension. If, however, knee extension is lacking because of capsular tightness, the joint cannot move to a position of maximal tibiofemoral contact, and as the knee extends, the joint capsule

suddenly pulls tight. Stress to the joint surfaces is increased in magnitude, and the joint is shock-loaded. The long-term effect is likely to be accelerated wear of joint surfaces.

Rotatory Dysfunction. A more subtle yet common movement disorder affecting the knee is loss of normal rotatory mechanics. The pathologic implications of rotatory dysfunction at the knee were proposed by Smillie[323] and confirmed by Frankel and colleagues.[94] The nature and the extent of rotation accompanying knee flexion and extension are governed by the shapes of the articular surfaces and are influenced by capsuloligamentous configurations. Alteration in normal rotatory mechanics may reflect articular surface abnormalities or capsuloligamentous disorders. Similarly, rotatory dysfunction produces abnormal stresses to the joint surfaces and the capsuloligamentous structures. Smillie[322,323] proposed that because normal rotatory movement is small and occurs at the very limits of knee extension, full knee extension is possible in the absence of normal rotation, but at the expense of increased deformation to articular tissues. Thus, knee extension occurring without normal external tibial rotation results in abnormal stresses to the medial joint surfaces, which are oriented to move into rotation, and in increased tensile stresses to the cruciate ligaments, which pull tight on extension and internal tibial rotation. Furthermore, the tibia must rotate externally as the knee approaches full extension to prevent the lateral side of the medial femoral condyle from contacting the medial edge of the ACL.

Several types of disorders may cause altered rotatory mechanics at the knee. Smillie[322,323] cites meniscal displacements, such as those associated with meniscus tears, as a frequent causative factor. Because knee rotation, when combined with flexion or extension, requires meniscofemoral as well as meniscotibial movement, alterations in the structural configuration of the menisci probably interfere with normal rotatory mechanics.

Another common cause of restricted external tibial rotation is reduced extensibility of the medial or posteromedial capsuloligamentous structures. This typically occurs after injury or surgery, in which the posteromedial capsule or MCL may heal in an adhered or shortened state. Laxity of these same structures will also lead to abnormal rotatory mechanics, because external tibial rotation may be excessive or premature.[178,320] This would especially be true if a secondary external rotation contracture developed.

In recognition of the pathomechanics and pathologic implications of rotatory dysfunction at the knee, Helfet[131] has described a simple means of detecting this problem clinically. The method involves comparing femorotibial rotatory alignment in a semiflexed and fully extended position. Using this test, in addition to instant center analysis, Frankel and associates[94] demonstrated a positive correlation between reduced femorotibial rotation and abnormal compression of the joint surfaces during terminal knee extension. In most of the patients evaluated, meniscal derangement was the underlying cause. Arthrotomy revealed abnormal wearing in localized areas of the medial articular surfaces in 22 of 30 knees. These findings confirm the nature of the kinematic abnormality associated with altered rotatory mechanics and also suggest that such disorders, over a long period, may predispose to progressive DJD.

Smillie[323] believes that kinematic disturbance resulting from rotatory dysfunction at the knee may also lead to fatigue disruption and fraying of the ACL. He supports this contention with surgical case studies of isolated ACL lesions associated with chronic meniscal derangements.

The significance of rotatory dysfunction at the femorotibial articulation is becoming better appreciated as our knowledge of detailed knee biomechanics improves. Because the disturbance is subtle, it is not readily recognized unless femorotibial rotatory function is carefully examined. This type of assessment should become a routine component of knee examination in the rehabilitation period after capsuloligamentous injury or internal derangement.

PATHOMECHANICS OF COMMON LOADING CONDITIONS

Trauma. Knee joint injuries are commonly of traumatic origin. This stems, in part, from the fact that the knee is freely movable in only the sagittal plane (flexion–extension). Thus, forces acting to move the knee in the frontal or transverse planes are largely attenuated by internal strain to the soft tissues about the joint. Furthermore, such forces may act over the relatively long lever arms provided by the femur and the tibia, thereby increasing the potential loading of the joint structures.

Valgus–External Rotation. Because of the exposure of the lateral side of the knee to external forces, compared with that of the protected medial aspect, traumatic valgus stresses are much more common than varus stresses. Usually such forces also involve components acting in the transverse and sagittal planes, thus causing rotatory and flexion–extension displacements. The knee is usually in some position of flexion when acted on by a force from the lateral aspect; thus, the direction of rotary movement is usually such that the tibia is rotated laterally with respect to the femur.

Valgus–external rotation injuries are most common in contact sports (especially football) and skiing. The degree of loading of the joint is accentuated by the fixation of the foot to the ground (e.g., by a cleated shoe) and by forces acting over a long lever arm (e.g., a ski). This does not allow rotary forces to be attenuated by movement of the foot with respect to the ground, and more of the energy is absorbed as internal strain to joint structures. Because valgus and external rotations are primarily checked by the posteromedial capsule and the capsular and superficial fibers of the MCL, these structures are most commonly damaged. The menisci, especially the medial meniscus, may be injured because of the rotary stress component. With marked separation of the medial side of the joint, the ACL may be torn as well. With progressive force in a valgus–external rotation direction, first the deep capsu-

lar fibers of the MCL are torn, then the long superficial fibers of the MCL and the posteromedial capsule, and finally the ACL. A torn medial meniscus would complete the so-called terrible triad of O'Donoghue.

Hyperextension. Because the knee is used in a position close to its physiologic limits of extension for most functional activities, hyperextension injuries are quite common. Again, those involved in violent contact sports and skiers are particularly vulnerable to such injuries. Forced hyperextension of the knee results in tearing first of the posterior capsule, followed by the ACL, then the PCL.[180]

Anteroposterior Displacement. Forces producing a pure translatory movement between the tibia and femur in an anteroposterior direction are less common than the aforementioned injuries. Of these, perhaps the "dashboard injury" is most common: the victim, in a suddenly decelerating auto, is thrust forward, striking the tibial tubercle of the bent knee on the dashboard. The tibia is forced posteriorly on the femur, stressing the PCL, often to the point of rupture.

Isolated ACL tears, resulting from forces in the opposite direction, are rare; in fact, there is controversy about the frequency of isolated ACL lesions. The mechanism of injury is more likely to be a force stressing the tibia into internal rotation on the femur.[180,355]

Rotation. Forced external rotation of the tibia on the femur tends to stress the collateral ligaments and the posteromedial capsule. As mentioned above, these forces usually occur in conjunction with valgus stresses and therefore typically affect the medial stabilizing structures.

The cruciate ligaments check internal rotation of the tibia on the femur. It is believed that forced internal rotation is the primary mechanism in isolated ACL injuries.[180,355]

Forced rotation may also injure the menisci. The medial meniscus, being less mobile by virtue of its attachment to the capsular fibers of the MCL, is much more frequently injured than the lateral meniscus. The menisci are particularly stressed when the knee is forced into rotation in an improper direction during flexion or extension. Thus, when the tibia, which is supposed to rotate internally during initial knee flexion, is forced externally as the knee goes into flexion, the menisci are caught between trying to move into flexion with the tibia and into rotation (in the wrong direction) with the femur. The result is often excessive deformation and tearing of a meniscus. If, as typically occurs, there is a valgus component to the rotary force, the medial meniscus is additionally stressed through its attachment to the MCL.

Rotary stresses sufficient to produce meniscal damage do not necessarily require external forces: often the victim simply twists suddenly on the weight-bearing leg. This usually occurs during athletics, but may also occur with less vigorous activities. Occupations or activities involving rotation of the fully flexed knee (e.g., wrestling, mining in cramped quarters) particularly predispose to meniscus tears because when the knee is fully flexed, the menisci reach their limit of posterior excursion. Rotation, which involves posterior movement of

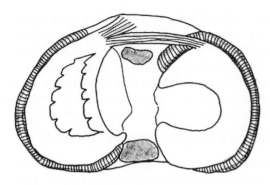

■ **FIG. 15-15.** Longitudinal tear of the medial meniscus.

one condyle and simultaneous anterior movement of the other, may further stress one meniscus posteriorly or cause the condyle to grind over the relatively fixed meniscus.

Most traumatic medial meniscus tears affect the posterior segment of the meniscus, with the tear running in a longitudinal direction.[323] Successive injury to the same meniscus may cause the tear to extend sufficiently anteriorly to allow the lateral segment of the torn structure to flip centrally into the intercondylar region—a "bucket-handle" tear (Fig. 15-15). This produces a mechanical block to full knee extension, and the knee is locked; full extension can occur only at the expense of further damage to the meniscus or excessive stretching of the ACL.

EVALUATION

Many common lesions affect the knee joint. Athletes as well as more sedentary persons may suffer traumatic injuries. Symptomatic degenerative disorders involving the knee are not uncommon in middle-aged or older persons, and "overuse" fatigue syndromes may affect virtually any age group. The approach to the evaluation of knee disorders must be flexible enough to accommodate such a broad spectrum of disorders. Presented here is an assessment scheme that includes most of the evaluative procedures needed to perform a thorough clinical examination of virtually any patient presenting with a common knee disorder. Practically speaking, the therapist will rarely use all the tests and procedures outlined here in any one examination. However, he or she should become proficient in all the tests, and must know the rationale for each to perform the most efficient knee examination.

History

The key to an efficient yet comprehensive examination of the knee is the patient interview. The information gained about the nature and extent of the physical problem is necessary so that the therapist can select the most appropriate objective evaluative procedures. Subjective data are also important in determining the degree of disability and in documenting a baseline.

Follow the format set out in Chapter 5, Assessment of Musculoskeletal Disorders and Concepts of Management, when conducting the subjective portion of the knee examination. Certain other questions depend on the nature of the disorder.

If the problem is of recent traumatic onset, ask:

1. What was the exact mechanism of injury? Did you feel a "pop"?
2. Did the knee swell? If so, how long after the injury did you notice the swelling? Where was it observed?
3. To what extent could you continue activities immediately after the injury? Could you walk? If the injury occurred during athletics, was a litter or some other form of passive or assisted transport required?

If the problem is of a chronic nature, ask:

1. Does the knee click, grind, grate, or pop? If so, was the onset of these symptoms associated with the onset of the present problem?
2. Has the knee ever locked, buckled, or given way? If so, under what specific circumstances? Is there some particular activity that tends to cause it?
3. Is going up or down stairs a problem?
4. Can you run? What is the effect of running backward, stopping quickly, or changing directions quickly?

Interpretative Considerations

SITE OF PAIN

The knee joint receives innervation from the L3 through S2 segments of the spinal column, and depending on the site of the pathologic process, pain from knee disorders may be referred into any of these segments. Most common knee problems affect the anteromedial or medial aspect of the joint, which is largely innervated by L3. Because the L3 segment usually does not extend much below the knee, it is rare for a patient with a common knee disorder to experience pain radiating farther distally than midleg. It is more common for pain originating at the knee to be referred proximally into the anterior or anteromedial thigh. The anterior aspect of the hip joint is also innervated primarily by L3, so referred pain of hip joint origin may be similar in site to that arising from the knee. In fact, it is not unusual, especially in children, for a patient with a hip joint problem to complain of "knee pain."

In the patient with nontraumatic onset of pain about the knee, lesions situated elsewhere in the L3 through S2 segments must be ruled out. The two common sources of referred pain to the knee are the lumbosacral region and the hip region.

Pain felt over the posterior aspect of the knee is often secondary to effusion causing distension of the posterior capsule. Because the S1 and S2 segments, which innervate the posterior knee region, extend well down into the foot, posterior knee pain may be referred some distance distally.

Pain of nontraumatic onset felt over a generalized region at the anteromedial aspect of the knee is most commonly from patellofemoral joint dysfunction. This is especially likely when the pain is aggravated most by descending stairs and prolonged sitting with bent knees.

Localized anteromedial pain felt at the joint line, usually of sudden onset, is often related to meniscus injuries. The pain arises from the anteromedial coronary ligament. A sprain of the coronary ligament may be the sole lesion, or it may be associated with a tear of the body of the meniscus.

Medial knee pain of traumatic onset after a valgus or rotary strain is usually of capsuloligamentous origin. A tear of the meniscus must also be ruled out.

ONSET OF PAIN

Sudden, Traumatic Onset. Sudden injuries caused by trauma are common, especially from sports activities involving contact or sudden changes in direction. A sudden twisting injury, in which the tibia is rotated externally on the femur without an external source of force, may tear either the capsular fibers of the MCL (grade I tear), the coronary ligament (peripheral attachment of the meniscus), or the body of the medial meniscus. When some external force is involved, such as in contact sports, and the knee is also forced into valgus position, the posteromedial capsule, MCL, or ACL may also be damaged.

Valgus–external rotation injuries are the most common traumatic knee disorders. In other types of injuries the mechanism should be determined, when possible, to estimate the nature of the stresses and to identify which structure may have been traumatized.

Gradual, Nontraumatic Onset. In middle-aged and older patients, symptomatic DJD must be ruled out. Pain from DJD is typically noticed first near the end of the day or after long periods of walking. Later, pain and stiffness are felt on rising in the morning, easing somewhat after getting up and about.

Possible precipitating factors, such as recent immobilization, alteration in activities, past injuries, and previous surgeries, should be considered. Patellofemoral joint dysfunction, a common knee problem, is frequently related to quadriceps insufficiency. This may include true quadriceps weakness, as from disuse, or some increase in loaded knee-extension activities in the presence of inadequately trained quadriceps muscles. Typical activities would be hiking, bicycling, or skiing.

Effusion. Articular effusion commonly follows traumatic injury to the knee joint. This may be the result of blood filling the joint or of overproduction of synovial fluid. The time frame of the onset of the effusion often provides important insight into its nature. Hemarthrosis tends to develop during a relatively short period after injury, from several minutes to a few hours; synovial effusion occurs during a longer period, perhaps 6 to 12 hours, before it is noticed. Synovial effusion causes a dull, aching pain from the distension of the joint capsule. Hemarthrosis may be associated with more severe discomfort caused by chemical stimulation of capsular nociceptors.

Clinically it is important to differentiate the nature of the effusion because in hemarthrosis an intra-articular fracture must be ruled out. Some relatively severe joint injuries, such as a complete rupture of the MCL, may not be followed by significant effusion because of leakage of fluid through the defect out from the confines of the joint capsule.

More subtle joint effusion may accompany chronic, nontraumatic knee disorders. The patient often describes posterior knee discomfort from posterior capsular distension.

NATURE OF PAIN AND OTHER SYMPTOMS

Pain of Traumatic Origin. Pain secondary to trauma is typically felt immediately at the time of injury. In ligamentous injuries the severity of the pain and resulting immediate disability do not necessarily reflect the severity of the injury. A minor or moderate sprain of the medial capsule or ligament is often more painful and more disabling at the time of injury than a complete MCL rupture.[263] This is because with a complete rupture, there are no longer intact fibers from which pain of mechanical origin can arise. Furthermore, later development of pain from joint effusion may not be significant because of leakage of fluid through the defect. Thus, after the initial pain from the ligament rupture, the patient may feel relatively little pain, especially if he or she is involved in a highly motivating activity such as an athletic competition.

Patellofemoral Joint Pain. Pain felt when sitting for long periods with the knee bent or when descending stairs is typical of patellofemoral joint problems.[23,113] Both these functions involve high and prolonged patellofemoral compressive loading. Pain is felt more on descending than on ascending stairs because greater passive tension is developed in the quadriceps mechanism during eccentric contraction than during concentric contraction. Sitting is a problem because of prolonged patellofemoral compression. Bone, being viscoelastic, undergoes "creep" or continued deformation with prolonged loading.[94] Bone is also weaker, or more likely to yield, with slowly applied loads. Thus, the likelihood of trabecular breakdown is greater with loading for a long time than with a similar load applied quickly.

Morning Pain. Pain that is present on wakening, subsides with initial use of the joint, and then increases again after some period of use is typical of DJD.

Buckling or Giving Way. A joint that buckles or gives way suggests structural or functional instability. The common structural disorder that causes giving way is loss of ligamentous integrity. In such circumstances the patient may cite a particular activity that is a problem, usually one that stresses the joint in a direction the involved ligament is supposed to check. Thus, persons with chronic MCL ruptures find it difficult to turn abruptly away from the involved leg because of the valgus–external rotation stress imposed on the leg.[263,320] Similarly, persons with loss of cruciate integrity may have problems descending inclines or squatting.

Functional buckling occurs as a result of reflex muscle inhibition, presumably from abnormal joint receptor activity. A common cause is internal derangement from a meniscus tear or loose body. In such cases, an abnormality in arthrokinematics resulting from the mechanical derangement may reflexively incite a sudden inhibition of the quadriceps muscles, causing the joint to give way. The patient usually cannot attribute the incidence of buckling to any consistent situation or activity, but claims that the joint gives way for no apparent reason.

Physical Examination

OBSERVATION

Record any functional deficits noted throughout the patient's visit. When possible, analyze and document the nature and extent of the deficit for future comparison. If the patient mentions a particular functional problem during the interview, ask him or her to attempt the particular activity or task to evaluate the problem more objectively. This is especially important for patients with relatively chronic problems who may not spontaneously demonstrate functional deficits during the evaluation.

Gait. Common gait abnormalities and their possible causes are discussed in Chapter 24, Lumbosacral–Lower Limb Scan Examination. The ability to hop, run, change directions quickly, stop abruptly, and climb stairs might be specifically evaluated.

Proprioception. The patient stands on each leg in turn with his or her eyes open and then closed. There will be greater difficulty balancing on the affected leg and differences between situations with eyes open and closed if proprioception is impaired.

Function. In a joint of low irritability, the patient may be asked to demonstrate the movements that produce the pain and the specific movement or action that produced the injury. Additional considerations include:

- With the patient squatting, note patellofemoral tracking—normally the patella should track freely and smoothly and describe a straight line over the second ray or midline of the foot. Also check to see whether both knees flex symmetrically.
- Balance reach tests, lunge distance, single-leg squat excursion, single-leg hope test (see Chapters 10 and 14).
- Other useful maneuvers include having the patient squat and bounce, and stand from a sitting position; observing him or her climb and descend steps; having the patient change direction quickly or stop abruptly during movement; observing the patient run forward or backward, hop, and so forth; and having the patient jump into a full squat.

INSPECTION

Examine and record specific alterations in bony structure or alignment, soft tissue configuration, and skin status.

I. Inspection of Bony Structure and Alignment. The section on assessment of structural alignment in Chapter 24, Lumbosacral–Lower Extremity Limb Examination, offers a complete discussion of this part of the examination. In many chronic knee problems, especially disorders of uncertain origin, a complete structural assessment of the lower extremities and lumbosacral region should be done. In traumatic disorders of recent onset, the examination is often confined to the knee area. The following assessments are particularly relevant to examination of the knee:

A. Standing examination
1. Frontal alignment. The patient is viewed from behind. Use a plumb line that bisects the heels. Vertical or horizontal asymmetries in the frontal plane are detected by determining the positions of the navicular tubercles, medial malleoli, fibular heads, popliteal and gluteal folds, greater trochanters, posterosuperior iliac spines, and iliac crests. Document vertical disparities (leg-length differences) or lateral shifts from a plumb line that bisects the heels. Note abnormal or asymmetric valgus–varus angulations. Differentiate tibial valgum or varum from genu valgum or varum; these are often confused. The knee is normally positioned in slight genu valgum because the medial condyle extends farther distally than the lateral condyle.
   a. Excessive genu valgum may be documented by measuring the distance between the malleoli, with the medial femoral condyles in contact.
   b. Excessive genu varum is noted by measuring the intercondylar distance at the knee, with the medial malleoli in contact.
   c. Vertical disparities are documented by measuring the distance from the lowest asymmetric landmark to the floor.
   d. Horizontal deviations from the plumb line can be documented by measuring distances from the plumb line.
2. Transverse rotary alignment. The patient is viewed from the front with the feet at a normal stance width and pointed outward 5 to 10° from the sagittal plane.
   a. The intermalleolar line is normally rotated outward 25 to 30° from the frontal plane.
   b. The tibial tubercles should be in line with the midline or lateral half of the patellae.
   c. With the feet in normal stance position, the patellae should face straight forward. A "squinting" patella may indicate medial femoral or lateral tibial torsion. The normal patellar posture for exerting deceleration forces in the functional position of 45° knee flexion places the patellar articular surface squarely against the anterior femur; a lower posture represents patella baja, a higher posture patella alta. Normally, the length of the patella and patellar tendon should be roughly equal. In patella alta, the patellar tendon is excessively long (Fig. 15-16A). When viewed from the side, a "camel" or double hump may be apparent, resulting from the uncovered infrapatellar fat pad.[150] Patella alta makes the patella less efficient in exerting normal forces, and lateral displacement occurs easily.[150,155]
   d. The quadriceps angle (Q angle or patellofemoral angle) is formed by a line drawn from the center of

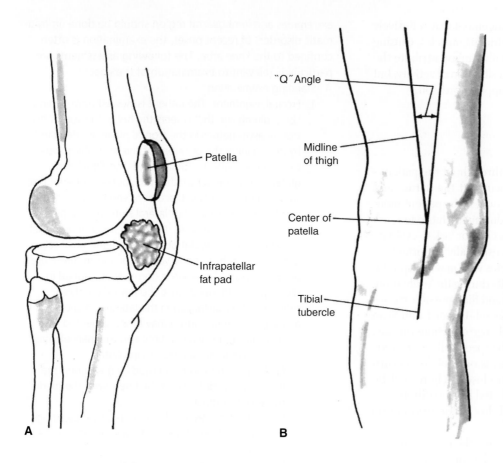

■ FIG. 15-16. Conditions predisposing the patient to recurrent subluxation of the patella. (**A**) The "camel" sign with a high-riding patella and uncovered fat pad. In a normal knee, the patella–patellar tendon ratio is approximately equal. (**B**) The quadriceps angle (Q angle) measures the divergence of the quadriceps from the sagittal plane. Normally, the Q angle should be 13 to 18° when the knee is straight and 0° in flexion.

the patella proximally toward the anterosuperior iliac spine, and a second line drawn from the center of the patella distally toward the tibial tubercle with the foot in the subtalar neutral position and the knee extended (weight bearing). Normally the Q angle is 13 to 18° (13° for males, 18° for females). An angle above 14° indicates a tendency toward less patellar stability (Fig. 15-16*B*). An angle above 18° is often associated with patellar tracking dysfunction, subluxating patella, increased femoral anteversion, or increased lateral tibial torsion. Hughston and coworkers[150] have advocated measuring the Q angle with the patient sitting and the quadriceps contracted; if the quadriceps is contracted and the knee fully extended, the normal Q angle is 8 to 10° (with 10° or more considered abnormal). If the patient is sitting and the quadriceps is relaxed (knee at 90°), the Q angle should be 0°.[150]

e. A line drawn between the left and right anterosuperior iliac spines should be parallel to the frontal plane.

3. Anteroposterior alignment. The patient is viewed from the side. A plumb line facilitates assessment and measurement of deviations. In a relaxed standing position it is normal for the knee to assume a position of slight recurvatum. With the plumb line about 1 cm anterior to the lateral malleolus, the lateral femoral condyle should be slightly posterior to the plumb line. Abnormal angulation in the sagittal plane can be documented by measuring from some anatomic landmark to the plumb line.

B. Sitting examination. The patient sits with the legs hanging freely over the edge of the plinth.

1. Femoropatellar alignment. Assess the position and size of the patellae.

a. A small, high-riding, outward-facing patella may predispose to a lateral patellar tracking disorder.

b. A laterally facing patella suggests that the medial femoral condyle is considerably longer than the lateral condyle. This is likely to be associated with a valgus angulation when the knee is straightened.

c. The inferior pole of the patella should be about level with the femorotibial joint line. A high-riding patella may be significant with respect to patellofemoral joint problems.[230]

2. Femorotibial alignment. Assess the position of the tibial tubercles with respect to the patellae in the sitting, knee-bent position. The tubercle usually lines up with the midline or lateral half of the patella. Most important here is symmetry.

a. A tubercle positioned too far medially may represent posteromedial capsular tightness, as may occur with healing of a sprain or rupture of one of the cruciate ligaments.

b. A tubercle situated too far laterally may suggest laxity (e.g., rupture) of the posteromedial capsule or MCL.

C. Supine examination

1. Legs straight

a. Valgus–varus angulations may be measured with a goniometer.

b. Leg-length disparities are documented by measuring from the anterosuperior iliac spines to the medial malleoli.

2. Knees bent 60°, feet flat on the plinth

a. Tibial lengths are compared by noting the heights of the tibial tubercles.

b. Leg-length disparities of more proximate origin are detected by observing the lengths of the femurs. This is done by siting a plane across the faces of the patellae.

c. Anteroposterior femorotibial displacements are detected by comparing the prominences of the tibial tubercles. This must be done before anteroposterior stability tests are performed. With a PCL rupture the tibia sags back and the tibial tubercle is less prominent. This is often associated with a false-positive anterior drawer test for ACL damage.

d. An excessively prominent tibial tubercle suggests previous osteochondrosis of the tibial apophysis (Osgood-Schlatter disease). This may lead to a high-riding patella.

II. Soft Tissue Inspection

A. Muscle contours

1. Have the patient maximally contract the quadriceps and calf muscle groups by fully extending the knees and plantar-flexing the ankle. Carefully assess the muscle contours for obvious atrophy or asymmetry. Often significant atrophy can be observed before it can be documented by girth measurements. When asymmetries can be measured, record baseline values so changes can be noted later.

2. Assess other muscle groups in a similar manner, including the hamstrings and the anterior and lateral compartments of the leg.

B. Swelling. If significant swelling exists, record baseline girth measurements when possible.

1. Generalized edema of the lower leg may accompany various metabolic or vascular disorders. If it occurs soon after a surgical procedure, it may indicate venous thrombosis, in which case a physician should be notified. Edema persisting some time after trauma or surgery may be associated with a reflex sympathetic dystrophy.

2. Localized swelling may be articular or extra-articular.

a. Articular effusion is manifest as swelling of the suprapatellar pouch and loss of definition of the peripatellar landmarks. Often the posterior capsule becomes distended, causing mild popliteal swelling. This swelling may be localized at the semimembranosus bursa, even in the case of articular effusion, because this bursa often communicates with the synovial cavity. If there is sufficient intracapsular swelling, the knee assumes a flexed or resting position (15 to 25°).

b. Extra-articular effusion is most often noted in the prepatellar bursa. This may swell after sudden or repeated trauma (e.g., housemaid's knee). Occasionally the distal belly of a hamstring muscle will herniate through the superficial fascia when contracted. This may appear as a pronounced popliteal "swelling," but disappears when the muscle is made to relax.

III. Skin Inspection

A. Color

1. Localized erythema may suggest an underlying inflammatory process.

2. Ecchymosis about the knee is most commonly associated with:

a. Contusion. The injury is usually over the lateral aspect.

b. Ligamentous damage, in which the ecchymosis is usually noted medially

c. Recent patellar dislocation, in which the ecchymosis is seen medially

3. Cyanosis over the lower leg after trauma or surgery may be associated with a reflex sympathetic dystrophy.

B. Scars. The cause should be determined. If surgical, the reason for the surgery should be discovered.

C. Texture. In the presence of dystrophic changes, the skin of the lower leg becomes smooth and glossy.

IV. Joint Tests. Joint tests include integrity tests, active and passive physiologic movements of the knee and other relevant joints. Joint-play (accessory movements) tests complete the joint tests.

A. Joint integrity tests (ligamentous instability tests). For all of the tests below, a positive test is indicated by excessive movement relative to the unaffected side. Because the knee, more than any other joint in the body, depends on ligaments to maintain its integrity, the status of the ligaments must be tested. In assessing joint laxity in the anterior, posterior, medial, or lateral direction, the four primary restraints by the MCL, LCL, ACL, and PCL are tested. The extent to which these four ligaments restrain their respective motions depends on the knee flexion angle. As the knee approaches extension, the participation of isolated ligaments lessens and the role of secondary restraints increases.[275]

When testing the ligaments of the knee, watch for one-plane instabilities as well as rotational instabilities. Evaluate anterior and posterior motions of the tibia in varying degrees of rotation. Always compare the measurements obtained with those from the normal knee.

It is important to grade the amount of laxity in a knee. In most clinical grading systems, grade I laxity represents up to 5 mm of motion; grade II, 6 to 10 mm; grade III,

11 to 15 mm; and grade IV, more than 15 mm.[275] However, instrumental measurements are challenging these concepts, and more accurate classification systems are being adopted.[41,228,229,248]

1. Straight instabilities

   a. Tests for anterior instability (one plane)

      i. Straight anterior drawer test (see Fig. 15-45B). The classic anterior drawer tests are done in the supine position with the knee flexed 90° and the examiner sitting on the patient's foot to stabilize the tibia as described by Slocum and Larson[320] and Furman and colleagues,[102] or with the patient supported in a semireclining sitting position (lower leg over the edge of the table) with the patient's foot stabilized between the examiner's legs to prevent rotation.[133] In either test, the hamstring muscles must be relaxed. The examiner's hands are placed around the proximal tibia (over the gastrocnemius heads and hamstrings) with the thumbs over the tibial plateau and the joint line. The tibia is then drawn forward on the femur. The test is positive when the anterior displacement exceeds 6 mm. If the test is positive with both tibial condyles displaced anteriorly, the usual mechanism is a tear of the posterolateral and posteromedial medial capsule and the medial and lateral capsular ligaments. This produces a combined anteromedial–anterolateral rotational instability. If the degree of subluxation is significant, the ACL is also ruptured.[252]

      ii. Flexion–rotation drawer test. This test is performed exactly like the straight anterior drawer test except the foot and leg are first externally rotated, allowing the examiner to assess rotatory instability as well. In each position, the examiner provides a gentle pull repeatedly in an anterior direction. The test is repeated with the foot in neutral. Each lower extremity is tested and the results are compared. A positive anterior drawer test with the foot in external rotation indicates anteromedial rotatory instability; with the foot in neutral position, a positive test indicates anterolateral rotatory instability; and with the foot in internal rotation, a positive test indicates a cruciate tear. A reliability of 62% has been reported for the flexion–rotation drawer test, rising to 89% with the anesthetized patient.[165]

      iii. Lachman test. The Lachman test, described by Tory and associates,[341] is considered the best indicator of ACL injury, especially the posterolateral band.[168,170,174,275] It is essentially an anterior drawer test with the knee near full extension (flexed 15 to 20°). The test can be performed with the patient in a semisitting position (with the back supported) and the ankle stabilized between the examiner's legs, or with the patient in supine. In the supine position one of the examiner's hands stabilizes the patient's femur laterally and gently applies an anterior translation force to the tibia from the medial side with the other hand (Fig. 15-17). The amount of anterior translation is compared with the uninjured knee, and the quality of end feel is assessed. The Lachman test is graded from 0 to 4+ (1+ = 5 mm; 2+ = 10 mm; 3+ = 15 mm; 4+ = 20 mm).[112] Fetto and Marshall[90] emphasize the importance of noting the type of end feel, for example, a 1+ Lachmann test with a soft end feel is diagnostic of an ACL tear. Positive results from the Lachman test may also reflect possible injury to the posterior oblique ligament and the arcuate–popliteus complex.

According to Henning and associates,[133] the Lachman test is positive in 92% of acute ACL tears and in 99% of chronic ACL tears. Positive results reflect anterior displacement, not reduction of a posteriorly displaced tibia.

The ACL has two functionally separate portions, so depending on the knee angle at the time of injury, only one portion may be damaged, thus resulting in a partial ligament tear.[251] If the posterolateral band is disrupted (more common), the anterior drawer test may be negative but the Lachman test is positive, as the posterolateral band becomes tighter as the knee approaches extension. Similarly, if only the anteromedial band is damaged, the Lachman test may be negative but the anterior drawer test positive.

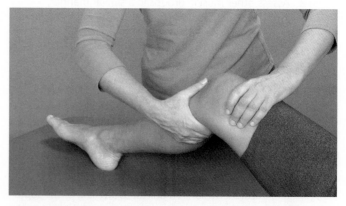

■ **FIG. 15-17.** Lachman's test. The patient's knee rests over the examiner's thigh and is stabilized by the proximal hand. The caudad hand applies an anterior translation force to the tibia.

b. Tests for posterior instability (one plane). PCL instability is best measured by performing the posterior drawer test at 70 and 90° flexion.[275] When this ligament is torn, carefully observe the profile of the knee from the lateral view during the drop-back test and palpate the joint line during the posterior drawer test.

i. Drop-back test (gravity drawer test) and Godfrey's chair test. Posterior tibial translation can be observed with the patient supine, the knee flexed 90° and the hip 45°, and the foot resting with the heel supported on the seat of a chair with the hip and knee in 70 to 80° flexion (Fig. 15-18A, B).[82,109] Observe the positions

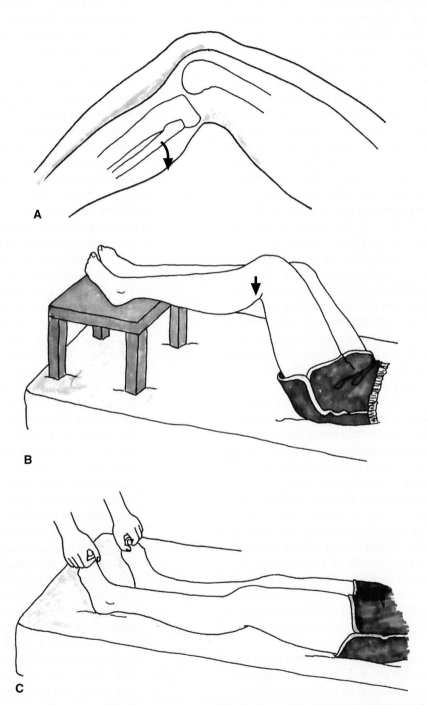

■ **FIG. 15-18.** The sag signs. **(A)** Posterior sag sign. Note profile of the two knees: the left (nearer) sags backward compared with the normal right knee. **(B)** The Godfrey chair test also is used to identify posterior sag of the tibia. **(C)** The external rotation recurvatum test: Apparent recurvatum and external tibial rotation demonstrate posterolateral rotatory instability.

of the patella and the tibial tubercle or recurvatum.[121] Compare one side with the other. Subtle degrees of hyperextension can be determined by holding the knee against the table and elevating the heel.[82] Measure the height of the heel over the table edge.

ii. Posterior drawer tests

    (a) Passive posterior drawer test. The patient is placed in the same position as for the anterior drawer test with the hip flexed 45° and the knee 90° (see Fig. 15-44B). The unaffected leg is examined first to determine the normal degree of laxity. The patient's foot is fixed in neutral rotation, and the examiner sits on the dorsum of the foot to stabilize it. The hands are used to push the tibia to and fro to reveal any backward movements of the tibia on the femur. This test is positive after disruption of the PCL with a tear of the posterior capsular ligament.

    (b) Active posterior drawer test. For the 90° active drawer test, the patient is in the same position as for the passive drawer test, with the examiner holding the foot against the table.[275] Have the patient contract the quadriceps and try to extend the knee by pushing the foot down toward the end of the table. With a torn PCL, the tibia will either remain in neutral or move slightly posteriorly. With a torn PCL, the tibia will move forward because of the unbalanced force vectors of the quadriceps and patellar tendon.[275]

c. Valgus stress test for medial instability (one plane). Medial instability is secondary to disruption of the ligaments of the medial tibiofemoral compartment and results in a valgus subluxation of the tibia on the femur. MCL laxity is best evaluated by the valgus stress test performed at 30 and 0° flexion.[275]

With the patient supine and the knee flexed 30°, apply a valgus stress at the knee (push the knee medially) while hugging the lower leg to steady it (see Fig. 15-50B). Repeat the test with the knee at 0°.

If the test is positive with the knee flexed to 30° but negative with the knee fully extended, the MCL has been damaged. If the test is positive with the knee at both 30° flexion and full extension, both the medial capsular and cruciate ligaments are damaged.

If a stress roentgenogram is obtained when the test is performed in full extension, a 5-mm opening indicates a grade I injury; up to 10 mm, grade II injury; and more than 10 mm, grade III injury.[133,177,244]

d. Varus stress test for lateral instability (one plane). Lateral instability is caused by disruption of the lateral compartment and results in a varus subluxation

of the tibia on the femur. The varus stress test is similar to the valgus stress test, but the hands are changed to apply varus stress (i.e., lateral push) to the knee (see Fig. 15-50A). The test is done in 30° flexion and in full extension.

If the test is positive with the knee flexed to 30° but negative with the knee fully extended, the LCL probably has been injured to some degree. If it is also positive in extension, this implies damage to the cruciate ligaments and lateral capsule.

Laxity is graded the same as for valgus stress test. When more than grade II laxity is present, there is a very high incidence of associated PCL and ACL laxity.

2. Rotatory instability. Various rotational instabilities may be present in an injured knee. There may be an isolated rotatory instability, or one associated with other forms of straight instabilities. A rotatory instability secondary to a ligamentous injury results in an excessive degree of rotation of the tibia on the femur. Typically the patient presents with a history of the knee suddenly giving way without any warning. The may occur while descending stairs or when a runner suddenly changes directions.

a. Anteromedial rotatory instability. Anteromedial instability, initially described by Slocum and Larson,[320] is an anterior subluxation of the medial tibial condyle that also moves into external rotation on the femur. Anteromedial rotatory instability is increased with a tear of the capsular ligament of the medial joint compartment or with loss of the ACL or the medial meniscus.[201] This instability is diagnosed clinically in the presence of a positive anterior drawer test performed while the tibia is held in external rotation.

b. Anterolateral rotatory instability. Anterolateral instability is caused by insufficiency of the ACL.[103,104,319] The degree of instability is increased if the LCL is also torn. Anterolateral rotatory results in anterior subluxation of the lateral tibial plateau, which also moves into internal rotation on the femur. Several tests are used to diagnose this condition. Tests demonstrating translation of the tibia include the presence of a 90° positive anterior drawer with the tibia held in neutral rotation[145,146] and the Lachman test with the knee in about 20° flexion.[252] Tests demonstrating anterolateral rotation laxity include a 90° flexion–rotation drawer test with the tibia rotated medially by 15° and various pivot-shift tests.[39,257] The pivot-shift or jerk test, a confirmatory test of the ACL, results in the tibia being subluxed anteriorly when the knee is straighter than 125°.[90,103,146,206,209] One or more of these maneuvers can be used (pivot-shift test of Galway and MacIntosh,[103,104] the Losee test,[206,207] the Slocum test, the crossover test, or Hughston's jerk test),[145,146,165] as well as the flexion–rotation drawer test designed to detect rotatory laxity.

i. Pivot-shift test (Fig. 15-19).[103,159] The patient is supine with the knee in full extension. The tibia of the affected knee is grasped at the proximal tibiofibular joint by the examiner's cranial hand. The caudad hand grasps the ankle and applies maximal internal rotation, subluxing the lateral tibial plateau (Fig. 15-19A). The knee is then slowly flexed as the proximal hand applies a valgus stress to the knee (Fig. 15-19B). If the test is positive, tension in the iliotibial band (ITB) will reduce the tibia, causing a sudden backward shift. The major disadvantage of the test is that the patient must be relaxed, which often is impossible because of pain. Donaldson and colleagues[79] tested more than 100 ACL-deficient knees and found that the pivot-shift test was positive in only 35% of the cases. When the same test was done under anesthesia, the test gave 98% positive results. This test is the reverse in the jerk test.

ii. Slocum test. One advantage of the Slocum test over the previously described tests is that it allows hamstrings and quadriceps relaxation.[244,319,320] The patient lies on the unaffected side with the leg flexed 90° at the hip and knee (Fig. 15-20). The pelvis on the involved side is rotated slightly backward so that the weight of the leg, with the knee extended, is supported by the inner aspect of the foot and heel. The weight of the extremity creates a valgus stress at the knee, and the relative positions of the pelvis and foot cause a slight internal rotation of the leg. The examiner grasps the distal thigh with the cranial hand and the proximal part of the leg with the caudal hand while pressing behind the head of the fibula (with the caudal hand) and the femoral condyle (with the cranial hand). The examiner applies an additional valgus stress by pressing down on the tibia and femur while simultaneously flexing the knee from full extension to about 30° of flexion. When the test is positive, the lateral tibial plateau is reduced with a palpable "clunk" or thud as the iliotibial tract passes behind the transverse axis of rotation.

iii. Crossover test.[15] With the patient standing, the examiner fixes the foot of the affected leg by standing on it. The patient crosses the unaffected leg over the fixed foot and rotates the upper torso away from the fixed foot until it faces 90° in the opposite direction. When this position is achieved, the patient contracts the quadriceps muscle. The test is positive when the patient describes the same symptoms as in the jerk test. This functional crossover test reproduces the pivot-shift and indicates anterolateral rotatory instability.[11,340]

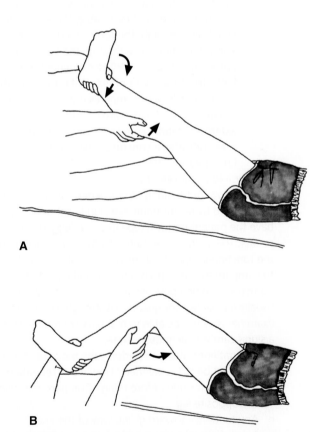

■ **FIG. 15-19.** The lateral pivot-shift. **(A)** With the knee in full extension, the examiner's cranial hand grasps the proximal tibia and applies a valgus force. The caudal hand grasps the ankle and maximally internally rotates the ankle. **(B)** The cranial hand then slowly flexes the knee. If the test is positive, a sudden posterior shift of the tibia on the femur will be noted.

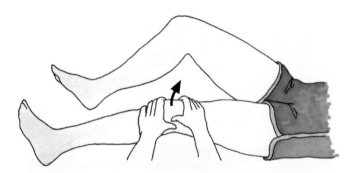

■ **FIG. 15-20.** Slocum's anterolateral rotary instability (ALRI) test. The patient lies on the uninvolved side, and the pelvis is rotated slightly posteriorly with the ankle and foot supported on the table. The weight of the extremity creates a valgus stress at the knee. When positive, as the extended knee is pushed into flexion and the iliotibial tract passes behind the transverse axis of rotation, the lateral tibial plateau is reduced with a palpable "clunk."

c. Posterolateral rotatory instability. This follows a tear of the arcuate ligament complex, including the PCL,[70,149] and results in posterior subluxation and internal rotation of the lateral tibial condyle. Several tests can be used to identify it.

   i. Reverse pivot-shift test, the primary test used to assess posterolateral rotatory instability.[158,244] The patient lies supine with the knees straight. The examiner places one hand around the patient's ankle and places the foot against the examiner's pelvis. Beginning at 80° flexion, with the leg externally rotated and a slight valgus force applied, the leg is slowly brought into extension (Fig. 15-21). If the test is positive, the lateral tibial plateau will suddenly move forward and internally rotate at about 20° flexion. This is the opposite of what happens in the true pivot-shift test, in which the tibia subluxates in extension and reduces in flexion.[31]

   ii. Posterolateral drawer test. Hughston and Norwood[149] described an alternate test for pos-

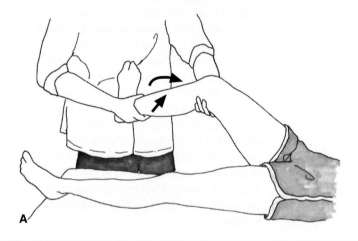

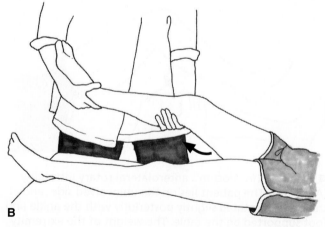

■ **FIG. 15-21.** Reverse pivot-shift test to detect posterolateral instability. Beginning at 80° flexion with the leg externally rotated and a slight valgus force applied (**A**), the leg is slowly brought into extension (**B**).

terolateral rotatory instability. The patient and examiner are in the same positions as for the previously described drawer tests, but the lower leg is slightly rotated externally. As the examiner pushes the tibia posteriorly, the lateral tibial condyle displaces posteriorly and the tibial tubercle displaces laterally.

   iii. External recurvatum test. This is used to identify tears of the arcuate complex and the anteromedial and intermediate fibers of the ACL.[149] The patient lies supine with the knees straight, and the examiner lifts the legs by the toes to produce hyperextension at the knee. The test is positive when the tibia rotates externally with posterolateral displacement of the tibial tuberosity (Fig. 15-18*C*).

   iv. The dial test or posterolateral rotation test. The dial test is done at 30 and 90° knee flexion. It has been found to provide a good assessment of the amount of posterolateral knee injury.[111,118,349] The test can be done either in prone or supine position. In the supine position with the knee flexed over the treatment table, the examiner stabilizes the thigh; the foot is then used to apply a rotation force through the foot and ankle (Fig. 15-22).[189,190] The examiner then looks for the amount of external rotation of the tibial tubercle, and compares it with the contralateral side. An increase of 100 to 150° external rotation, compared with the opposite side, indicates a concurrent posterolateral knee jury.[29,111,119]

B. Active physiologic movement

1. Unilateral weight-bearing flexion–extension. If not contraindicated by recent trauma or significant disability, have the patient perform repeated one-legged half-squats. This yields some useful information concerning the functional capacity of the part. It is also a good way to compare the strength of the involved knee to the normal side, when possible; manual muscle testing is usually a poor test for quadriceps strength because the examiner may not be able to manually overcome even a significantly weak muscle. Note:

   a. The patient's ability to perform the movement. Can the knee be fully extended? How many repetitions can be performed before tiring? Compare this with the opposite leg.

   b. Any tendency toward giving way of the knee

   c. Patellofemoral or femorotibial crepitus. Palpate at the medial and lateral patellar margins for the former and at the femorotibial joint line for the latter. It is normal for a knee to "pop" or "snap" during this movement. A grinding similar to "sand in the joint" is more likely to indicate articular surface degenerative changes.

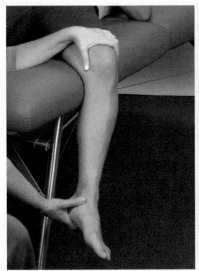
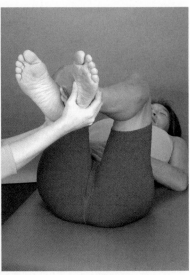

■ FIG. 15-22. Dial test or posterolateral rotational test in 30° of flexion (**A**) and in 90° of flexion (**B**).   **A**   **B**

d. Provocation of pain. If pain is experienced, determine the point in the range of movement at which it is felt.
2. Non–weight-bearing flexion–extension. If the patient cannot perform weight-bearing flexion–extension or cannot do it through a full range of movement, assess flexion and extension in a supine position. For extension, have the patient straighten the knee, then tell him or her to hold it extended and attempt to raise the leg against gravity (straight-leg raise). Then have the patient flex the knee as far as possible. Note:
    a. Range of motion. If the patient cannot fully flex or extend the knee, apply passive overpressure to determine whether the restriction is secondary to pain, weakness, or true tissue restriction. Compare the amount of passive extension to extension maintained against gravity. Document the degree of any extensor lag.
    b. Crepitus during movement. If joint crepitus is present determine whether it arises from the femorotibial or patellofemoral joint.
    c. The presence of pain and the point in the range at which it is felt
    d. If a capsular restriction exists, flexion is limited to 90 to 100° and extension is lacking by 20 to 30°.
    e. Loss of knee extension in the presence of full flexion is most often caused by an internal derangement such as a bucket-handle meniscus tear.
    f. Quadriceps lag. To complete the last 15° of knee extension, a 60% increase in force of the quadriceps muscles is required.[217] The loss of mechanical advantage, muscle atrophy, decreasing power of the muscle as it shortens, adhesion formation, effusion, or reflex inhibition may result in a quadriceps lag. This lag is usually associated with loss of accessory motion. Inability to extend the knee fully is

assessed by having the patient lie supine, with the heel supported on a small firm pillow or block so that the knee can sag into full extension. Have the patient lift the heel off the support (it should be possible to do this before the knee starts to lift). If a quadriceps lag is present, the knee lifts first.[53]
    g. Dynamic tibial rotatory function (Helfet test).[131] With the patient sitting, first assess the positions of the tibial tubercles, and then passively extend each knee repetitively for the final 25° of extension. Assess rotation of the tibia during extension by observing the tibial tubercle during the movement; normally the tubercle should rotate laterally through an angle of 10 to 15° during the final phase of extension. Compare the involved side with the opposite knee. Loss of dynamic tibial rotation may be secondary to one of several factors:
        i. The tibia may already be rotated at the starting position.
        ii. Tightness or adhesion of the medial capsuloligamentous structures, as may occur with immobilization during healing of a sprain
        iii. An internal derangement such as a meniscus displacement or a cartilaginous loose body
    h. Lateral and medial rotation of the tibia on the femur. With the patient seated and the knee flexed over the edge of the plinth, assess active axial rotation:
        i. Range of motion: Medial rotation should be about 30°, active lateral rotation about 40°.
        ii. Provocation of pain
        iii. End feel. The end normal feel of this movement is tissue stretch.
    i. Modifications to the examination of active physiologic movements. For further information about active range of movement the following can be carried out:

      i. The movements can be repeated.

      ii. The speed of movement can be altered.

      iii. Movements can be combined.

      iv. Movements can be sustained.

      v. Movements can be combined together, e.g., flexion–extension with rotation.

      vi. Compression or distraction can be added.

C. Passive physiologic joint movements. Comparison of the response of symptoms to active and passive movements can help to determine whether the structure at fault is noncontractile (articular) or contractile (extra-articular).[59]

1. Osteokinematic movements

    a. Flexion–extension. Passively flex and extend the knee and note:

      i. Range of motion. If movement is limited, determine whether the pattern of restriction is capsular or noncapsular.

      ii. Provocation of pain

      iii. End feel

      iv. Crepitus

    b. Combined movement. Combined movements or quadrants can be tested. Testing passive range of motion in combination may derive more information.

      i. Flexion–adduction movements are the most helpful in eliciting pain.[218]

      ii. Hyperextension.[49] With the patient lying supine, hold one hand over the patient's knee and use the other hand to lift the lower leg at the foot; repeat with the resting hand held over the tibial condyle. Normally up to 15° passive hyperextension is possible. Once the range of hyperextension has been determined, the test can be used in combination with abduction and adduction.

      iii. Compare both lower extremities; determine the range and pain response of performing combinations of flexion and extension.

    c. Passive lateral and medial rotation (axial rotation). To test axial rotation, the patient should be sitting. The knee is first flexed to 90°, then is nearly fully extended. The normal end feel of rotation of the tibia on the femur is tissue stretch. An increased range with the knee flexed may be associated with a rotatory instability of the knee. Loss of motion occurs in many intrinsic knee disorders.[49] With the patient supine, use a handhold at the foot, and then rotate the tibia internally and externally on the femur, with the knee close to full extension.

      i. Hypermobility of external rotation suggests an MCL or posteromedial capsule rupture.

      ii. Pain on external rotation may be present with a sprain of the coronary ligament or MCL. A valgus stress can be used to differentiate the two: it will stress the MCL but not the coronary ligament.

    d. Hip range of motion, including straight-leg raising and flexibility testing of adduction and abduction.

The Ober test is used to assess iliotibial band tightness (see Fig. 14-20). The assessment for flexibility should include hip rotation, spine extension, and examination of the hamstrings, hip flexors, iliotibial band, and rectus femoris. To assess for tight hamstrings, have the supine patient flex the hip to 90°. While maintaining this flexion, see how far the patient can extend the knee. A measurement of 20° from full knee extension is within normal limits.

According to Janda,[162] the first priority of treatment of motor imbalance is to lengthen the tight antagonist. Tight muscles not only increase the workload of the agonists, but also (according to Sherrington's law of reciprocal innervation) act in an inhibitory way on their antagonists.[313] This is an important factor in the quadriceps–hamstring relationship.[187,312,313]

2. Joint-play movements (stress tests). Assess the status of the capsuloligamentous structures by performing the following passive movements. Note the provocation of pain or muscle guarding and whether the movement is hypomobile or hypermobile. The latter can best be determined by comparing with a normal side, but experience is also helpful. Note and attempt to avoid eliciting protective muscle guarding when performing the joint-play tests; false-negative results may mask a serious injury that warrants immediate attention.

    a. Anterior glide of the tibia on the femur (see Fig. 15-45A)

    b. Posterior glide of the tibia on the femur (posterior drawer test; see Fig. 15-44A)

    c. Lateral-medial tilt (see Figs. 15-48 and 15-49)

    d. Internal and external rotation of the tibia on the femur (see Figs. 15-46B and 15-47B)

    e. Patellar mobility

      i. Medial-lateral (see Fig. 15-52A)

      ii. Superior-inferior (see Fig. 15-53A)

    f. Distraction of the femorotibial joint (see Fig. 15-43A); compare with the unaffected side.

    g. For further information when examining joint-play movements, alter the:

      i. Direction of applied force

      ii. Point of application of the applied force

      iii. Speed of applied force

3. Mobilizations with movement (MWMs).[246] Theses are sustained movements carried out with active movement. It is proposed that the mobilizations affect and correct a bony positional fault, which produces abnormal tracking of the articular surfaces during movement.[89,245,246] The examination tests can be used as treatment techniques, but details of these and other MWM techniques for the knee are outside the scope of this book.

    a. Proximal tibiofibular joint. This test is carried out if the patient has posterolateral knee pain. In weight bearing have the patient place his or her foot on a chair and then flex or extend the knee while the

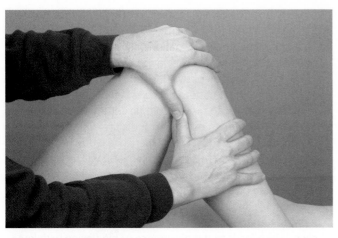

■ **FIG. 15-23.** Mobilization with movement for the proximal tibiofibular joint.

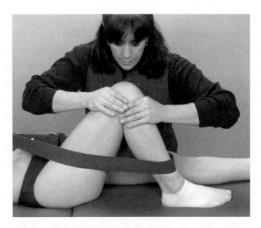

■ **FIG. 15-25.** Mobilization with movement for knee flexion. An anteroposterior glide to the tibia is applied as the patient actively flexes the knee.

examiner applies an anteroposterior or postero-anterior glide to the fibula head. This test can also be performed with the patient lying down (Fig. 15-23). Increased range of motion that is pain-free would indicate a mechanical joint problem.
  b. Femorotibial joint, medial or lateral glide. A medial glide is applied with medial joint pain and lateral glide with lateral joint pain. The patient lies prone and the examiner stabilizes the thigh and applies a glide to the tibia using a belt around the tibia (Fig. 15-24). A glide is then maintained as the patient actively flexes or extends the knee. Once again, increased range of motion indicates a mechanical joint problem.

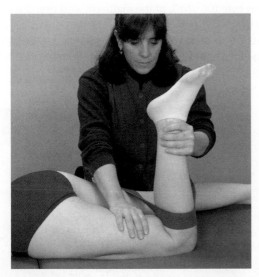

■ **FIG. 15-24.** Mobilization with movement for knee flexion. A belt around the lateral thigh allows the clinician to apply a medial glide while the patient actively flexes the knee.

  c. Femorotibial joint, posterior glide. Another MWM can be used for patients who have at least 80° knee flexion. In supine position with the knee flexed, foot flat on the plinth, a posterior glide of the tibia is applied by the examiner while the patient flexes the knee. A belt attached to the ankle of the patient allows the patient to apply some overpressure by cautiously pulling on the belt as active movement occurs (Fig. 15-25).
4. Other joints as applicable. Joint-play movements can then be tested for other joints suspected to be a source of symptoms. Joints likely to be examined are the hip joint, sacroiliac joint, lumbar spine, foot, and ankle.

MUSCLE TESTS

Muscle tests include examining muscle-resisted isometric contractions, muscle strength, control, length, and muscle bulk.

I. Resisted Isometric Movements. Lesions involving the muscles or tendons crossing the knee joint are not uncommon and are best detected by assessing the effect of maximal isometric contraction of the structure to be tested. Tendinitis most commonly affects the insertion of the iliotibial band, one of the pes anserinus tendons, or the insertion of the biceps femoris. The quadriceps are often contused in athletics, especially football.

   Provide manual resistance to the isometric contraction and determine whether the contraction is strong or weak and whether it is painless or painful. The most important movements to resist are knee flexion (for the biceps femoris and pes anserinus tendons), knee extension (for the iliotibial tendon and quadriceps muscles), external rotation of the tibia on the femur (for the biceps femoris tendon), and internal rotation of the tibia on the femur (for the pes anserinus tendon).

   If lesions involving other muscles or tendons are suspected, test the appropriate resisted movements. In relatively chronic tendinitis brought on by repetitive minor trauma (e.g., long-distance running), pain may not be elicited on resisted movement testing unless the patient has recently engaged in the provoking activity. To avoid false-negative findings, it may help to have the patient perform the relevant activity just before testing. Also, testing repeated contractions of the suspected structure may increase the likelihood of eliciting discomfort in chronic cases.

II. Muscle Strength. Manual muscle tests (MMT) should include the lower limb muscles beginning at the hip. The examiner tests the knee flexors and extensors and the ankle dorsiflexors and plantarflexors and any other relevant muscle groups. For details of these tests the reader is directed to Clarkson and Gilwish,[49] Cole et al.,[50] Hislop and Montgomery,[138] Janda,[163] Kendall et al.,[176] and Palmer and Epler[269] to determine exactly which muscles are at fault. To detect or quantify subtle losses in muscle strength—as may arise from disuse or segmental neurologic deficits—or strength increases resulting from training, repeated loading of the muscle to near-fatigue levels must be done. This is especially true for the large-muscle groups such as the quadriceps and calf muscles. Various exercise equipment may be used for this purpose. A convenient but expensive method is the use of an isokinetic apparatus, which gives a torque-curve readout. A simpler but useful method for the quadriceps and calf groups is to have the patient perform repeated half-squats and toe-raises, respectively, in a standing position. Most current reports support a quadriceps to hamstring strength ratio of 3:2.[275] Manual tests for smaller groups, used especially to detect myotomic weaknesses associated with nerve root lesions, are described in Chapter 24, Lumbosacral–Lower Limb Scan Examination.

Individual muscles prone to weakness in the lower quadrant include the gluteus maximus, medius, and minimus, vastus lateralis, medialis and intermedius, tibialis anterior, and peronei.

III. Muscle Control. Relative strength and muscle control is assessed indirectly by observing posture and the quality of active motion, noting changes in recruitment patterns, and palpating muscle activity in various positions. See Chapter 14, Hip, for the assessment of motor control of the hip abductors and hip extensors and motor impairment tests during active flexion and extension, which will have a significant influence on the knee and should be included in the evaluation of motor control.

An imbalance of the vastus medialis oblique (VMO) and vastus lateralis can occur in patients with extensor mechanism disorders and patellofemoral pain.[227,350] On quadriceps contraction, the patella may glide laterally because of weakness of the VMO and may contract after vastus lateralis.[236,350] In addition, the inferior pole of the patella may be displaced posteriorly as the quadriceps contracts, which may result in fat pad irritation.[236]

A method proposed by Beck and Wilderman[21] for assessing VMO dysfunction is as follows: The examiner places one rolled up fist under the supine patient's knee to flex the leg at the hip 11 to 20°. The patient is asked to extend the knee but not lift the knee from the examiner's fist (Fig. 15-26). Firing patterns are monitored by palpation over the hamstrings and quadriceps while visual observation of the hip, pelvis, and knee occurs simultaneously. One faulty abnormal firing pattern or substitution pattern occurs when the patient extends his or her hip first to prevent hip flexion by co-contracting the hamstrings, then extending the knee with the upper quadriceps. The examiner will experience a downward thrust of the knee against the fist, and palpation will reveal tension in the hamstrings. In severely inhibited cases the patient will demonstrate gluteal recruitment by lifting his or her pelvis off the table and arching the back. A second faulty recruitment pattern results from overuse of the proximal quadriceps, which leads to the occurrence of hip flexion with knee extension. The examiner will notice that the weight of the leg lightens on the hand and observe lateral patellar tracking. Sometimes an audible click or painful catch is experienced secondary to the lateral patellar tracking.

IV. Muscle Length. The examiner checks the length of individual muscles, in particular those muscles prone to become short, i.e., the iliopsoas, rectus femoris, tensor fascia latae, and hip adductors (see Figs. 14-19 and 14-20), piriformis (see Figs. 14-21 and 14-22), hamstrings (straight-leg raising and 90°/90° hamstring [Fig. 15-27]), quadratus lumborum (see Fig. 23-32), erector spinae, tibialis posterior, gastrocnemius, and soleus.[163] It has been demonstrated that muscle tightness alters neuromuscular control. Alterations in recruitment strategies and stabilization strength result. Such compensation and adaptations affect neuromuscular efficiency throughout the kinetic chain.[203,205,298]

V. Muscle Bulk. Although specific schemes may vary among practitioners, most take circumferential measurements with a tape measure at the knee joint line, at the suprapatellar region over the VMO, at the midthigh, and over the muscle belly of the gastrocnemius. The circumferential measurements are recorded on a relative scale that may be used to gauge the patient's progress through the rehabilitation

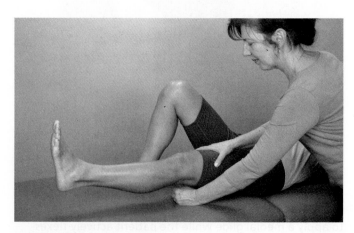

■ **FIG. 15-26.** Test for vastus medialis obliquus.

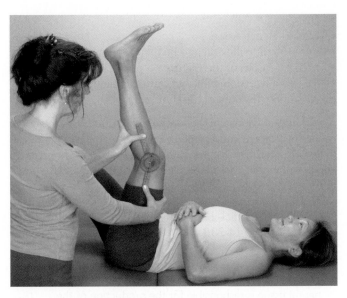

■ **FIG. 15-27.** 90°/90° hamstring assessment.

process; the joint line circumferential measurement should decrease as the problems of effusion and swelling are resolved, and the other measurements should increase as atrophied muscles are conditioned.

SPECIAL TESTS

I. Tests for Meniscal Injury. Clinical diagnosis of meniscal tears has been discussed by several authors, notably McMurray,[238] Apley,[12] Noble,[250] Barry et al.,[18] Anderson and Lipscomb,[10] and Ricklin et al.[291] Most of these meniscus signs are known by the names of their initiators. The maneuvers can help differentiate meniscus lesions from other knee joint lesions. Although a positive test can help diagnose a meniscus lesion, a negative test does not necessarily exclude the diagnosis of a torn meniscus. Most of these tests are similar, so any one can be used, although McMurray's is considered the best manipulative test.[10] Only some of the better-known meniscus signs are described below.

A. McMurray's test.[238] Nearly full range of knee flexion must be present to perform McMurray's test. The knee is fully flexed and the tibia fully rotated either internally or externally. The examiner places the thumb and index finger over the medial and lateral femorotibial joint lines and, while maintaining rotation of the tibia, extends the knee to 90°. This test does not pertain to extension beyond 90°. Provocation of a painful area of movement and a palpable click elicited during the movement may indicate a positive test, although there is some question as to the reliability.[247]

B. Apley's test.[12] The patient is prone with the knee bent to 90°. Joint distraction or compression can be maintained to help differentiate between ligamentous injuries and injuries to the menisci or coronary ligaments. Pain elicited

during external rotation with distraction suggests a collateral ligament injury. Pain on internal rotation with distraction may indicate a cruciate injury. Pain that is felt with rotation and compression, but not elicited when the joint is distracted, suggests a problem with a meniscus or a meniscal attachment (coronary ligament).[142]

C. Steinmann's sign.[291] If localized tenderness is present along the anterior joint line, Steinmann's sign may be useful. In the presence of a possible meniscus tear, pain appears to move anteriorly when the knee is extended and posteriorly when the knee is flexed. Rotating the tibia one way and then the other with the knee flexed 90° may localize pain to the joint line.

II. Plica Tests. A pathologic process affecting the synovial plica can mimic a meniscal injury and cause symptoms similar to those of other common internal derangements of the knee; this makes the differential diagnosis more difficult.[21,27,128] A symptomatic mediopatellar plica can often be palpated as a tender, bandlike structure paralleling the medial border of the patella (see Fig. 15-42). A palpable and sometimes audible snap is present during flexion and extension.

With the patient supine, check for the presence of a pathologic synovial plica by passively flexing and extending the knee from 30 to 90° flexion. Produce pressure on the patella medially with the heel of the hand while palpating the medial femoral condyle with the fingers of the same hand. Then flex the knee and medially rotate the tibia slightly with the opposite hand on the foot. A tender fold may often be palpated that recreates the patient's familiar, painful popping sensation.

III. Patellar Stability Tests
A. Patellar laxity, Fairbank's apprehension tests for patellar subluxation or dislocation. The patient's knee is positioned at 30° of flexion, and the examiner passively moves the patellar laterally.[83] A positive test is indicated by apprehension of the patient or excessive movement.

B. Passive medial-lateral glide. To determine the tightness of the medial and lateral restraints of the patellofemoral joint, perform passive glides (see Figs. 15-52A and 15-53). The tests can be performed in full extension and various degrees of flexion.

C. Passive patellar tilt test. To assess patellar laxity when the lateral patellar edge is elevated from the femoral condyle, passive patellar tilt is produced. A 0° or negative patellar tilt angle usually reflects excessive lateral retinacular tightness (Fig. 15-28A).[275]

D. Passive lateral glide test. To estimate lateral patellar excursion, the width of the patella is divided into fourths. Longitudinally, lateral overhang in excess of half the width of the patella usually indicates lax or torn medial patellofemoral restraints (Fig. 15-28B).[275] A Q angle exceeding 14° indicates a tendency toward patellar instability.

IV. McConnell Test for Chondromalacia Patellae. The patient isometrically contracts the quadriceps muscles for 10 seconds in various angles of knee flexion (0, 30, 60, 90, and 120°). If

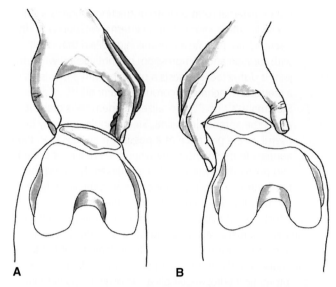

■ **FIG. 15-28.** Passive patellar tilt of +15° (**A**), and passive lateral glide test (**B**), demonstrating a patella being subluxated laterally to half its width.

pain is produced, the test is repeated with the examiner holding a medial glide to the patella, and if symptoms are eased this is indicative of chondromalacia patellae.[235,236]

V. Supine-to-Sit Test (see Fig. 23-30). This is where one leg appears longer in supine and shorter in long sitting or vice versa, suggesting innominate dysfunction (anterior or posterior rotation).[351]

VI. Leg Length (see Chapter 14, Hip). Check for sacroiliac dysfunction. Ipsilateral posterior rotation of the ilium on the sacrum or contralateral anterior rotation of the ilium will result in a decrease in leg length.[217]

VII. Vascular Tests. Palpate the pulses of the femoral, popliteal, and dorsalis pedis arteries if compromise is suspected. The state of the vascular system can also be determined by the response of symptoms to elevation of the lower limbs and to positions of dependency.[281]

Neuromuscular Testing. Neurologic tests involve examining the integrity and mobility of the nervous system.

I. Integrity of the Nervous System. The integrity of the nervous system is tested if the examiner suspects the symptoms are emanating from the spine or from a peripheral nerve.

Dermatomes and Peripheral Nerves. Light touch and pain sensation, respectively. A knowledge of the cutaneous distribution of nerve roots (dermatomes) and peripheral nerves enables the examiner to distinguish the sensory loss caused by a root lesion from that caused by a peripheral nerve lesion. The cutaneous and dermatome areas are shown in Figs. 5-5 and 5-8.

Myotomes and Peripheral Nerves. The following myotomes are tested and are shown in Figure 5-10.

- L2—hip flexion
- L3—knee extension
- L4—foot dorsiflexion and inversion
- L5—extension of the big toe
- S1—foot eversion, contract buttock, knee flexion
- S2—knee flexion and toe standing

A working knowledge of the muscular distribution of the nerve roots (myotomes) and peripheral nerves enables the clinician to distinguish the motor loss caused by nerve roots (myotomes) and peripheral nerve lesions. The peripheral nerves are shown in Figure 5-8.

Reflex Testing. Check the patellar (L3–L4; see Fig. 14-23*A*) and medial hamstring (L5), and Achilles reflex (S1–S2) (see Fig. 14-23*B*).

II. Mobility of Nervous System. The following neurodynamic tests may be carried out to ascertain the degree to which neural tissue is responsible for the production of the patient's symptoms.

- passive neck flexion (see Chapter 19, Cervical Spine)
- straight-leg raise (SLR)
- passive knee bend (PKB)
- slump test (see Chapter 22, Lumbar Spine)

PALPATION

Clinically, palpation is best done in conjunction with inspection and is organized similarly.

I. Bony Structures and Soft Tissue Attachments. Note any abnormalities in size, position, or integrity of bony structures. Determine the existence of tenderness, especially at tendon and ligament attachments, remembering that deep tenderness is often referred. With the patient sitting at the edge of the plinth, legs hanging freely, palpate the:

A. Patella. In terms of the position of the patella, the following should be noted:[281]

- The base of the patella normally lies equidistant (plus or minus 5 mm) to the lateral and medial femoral condyles when the knee is flexed 20°. If the patella lies closer to the lateral or medial epicondyle, it is considered to have a lateral or medial glide (see Fig. 15-37*A*).
- Lateral tilt is related to the distance of the medial and lateral borders of the patella to the femur. The patella is considered to have a lateral tilt when the distance is decreased on the lateral aspect and increased on the medial aspect such that the patella faces laterally. The opposite is true in medial tilt of the patella (see Fig. 15-37*B*).
- Anteroposterior tilt is the relative distance from the inferior and superior poles of the patella to the femur. Posterior tilt of the patella occurs if the inferior pole lies more posteriorly than the superior pole (see Fig. 15-37*D*)

- Patellar rotation is the relative position of the long axis of the patella to the femur, which should be parallel in the normal subject. The patella is considered to be laterally rotated if the inferior pole of the patella is placed laterally to the long axis of the femur (see Fig. 15-37C).
- The most common abnormality seen in patellofemoral pain is both a lateral tilt and a lateral rotation of the patella. This is thought to be the result of an imbalance of the lateral structures (tightness of the lateral retinaculum) of the patella and the medial structures (weakness of the vastus medialis oblique; see extensor mechanism disorders below).[236]

1. Note size, shape, and position. A small, high-riding patella may be a predisposing factor in patellofemoral joint problems. The proximal lateral pole of the patella may be enlarged in the presence of bipartite patella.[116,264] The inferior pole of the patellar tendon is a common location for "jumper's knee." With the knee in extension, the fat pad is normally extruded to either side of the taut patellar tendon. Hoffa[139] described tenderness on palpating the fat pad (fat pad syndrome).
2. Palpate the superior and inferior poles, where the quadriceps and patellar tendons attach, for tenderness.
3. Passively hold the knee extended, push the patella medially, and palpate the medial articular facets on the backside of the patella for tenderness.

B. Femoral condyles
1. Note the prominence of the anterior aspect of the lateral condyle.
2. Palpate the adductor tubercle, a major site of attachment for the medial retinaculum, as well as the site of insertion for the adductor magnus (Fig. 15-1).
3. Palpate the area over the medial femoral condyle for a snapping, tender medial patellar plica. Although a medial patella plica is present to some degree in nearly every knee, it is rarely symptomatic.
4. Palpate the medial and lateral joint lines. Cysts of the lateral cartilage are felt as hard lumps and are prominent at 45° flexion but disappear at both full extension and 90° flexion.

C. Proximal tibia
1. Palpate the area of insertion of the pes anserinus and MCL.
2. Palpate the tibial tubercle, where the patellar tendon inserts.
3. Palpate the lateral tibial tubercle, where the iliotibial band inserts.

D. Fibular head. The LCL inserts at its apex.

II. Soft Tissue Palpation
A. Muscles. Palpate the various muscle groups about the knee for:
1. Mobility. This is especially important after surgery or prolonged immobilization, which may lead to the development of adhesions between muscle planes or between muscles and other tissues.
2. Continuity. Severe trauma may cause palpable ruptures of muscles or tendons.
3. Consistency. Prolonged disuse and reflex sympathetic dystrophy predispose to stringy, fibrotic muscles. Contusions of the quadriceps often resolve with heterotopic bone formation, which may be palpable.

B. Ligaments
1. Anteromedial coronary ligament (anteromedial border of the medial meniscus; Fig. 15-7). This is palpated at the anteromedial joint line. It becomes more prominent here when the tibia is passively rotated internally with respect to the femur. This is a site of point tenderness after medial meniscus tears or isolated coronary ligament sprains.
2. MCL. The palpating finger follows the medial joint line from its anterior aspect a short distance posteriorly until it is felt to be obliterated by the anterior margin of the MCL (Fig. 15-8). The posterior margin of the ligament can be similarly palpated where it crosses the joint line. Estimate the course of the ligament and palpate along its extent. It cannot be distinguished as a discrete structure because of its flat configuration. Localized tenderness usually corresponds well with the site of MCL injuries.
3. LCL. This is best palpated with the patient's ankle crossed over the opposite knee. It is felt as a well-defined, round structure, crossing the lateral joint line between the femur and the fibular head (Fig. 15-9). This is one of the few sites at which a ligamentous rupture is palpable; however, at the LCL this is rare.

C. Tendons
1. Patellar tendon. This is easily palpated from the inferior pole of the patella to its insertion on the tibial tubercle.
2. Iliotibial band. From its insertion on the lateral tibial tubercle, the blunt, posterior edge of the iliotibial band can be felt well up into the lateral thigh region. Tenderness to palpation over the lateral femoral condyle in association with a tight iliotibial band suggests an iliotibial band friction syndrome (see Chapters 8 and 14).[250,288]
3. Popliteus tendon. Popliteus tendinitis is readily diagnosed by palpating the area of the fibular collateral ligament with the leg in the "figure-four" position (Fig. 15-9).[233]
4. Biceps femoris. This prominent tendon is easily felt at the posterolateral corner of the knee, inserting into the fibular head (Fig. 15-9).
5. Patellar retinaculum. Palpate this structure for mobility and tenderness. Palpate the lateral patellar retinaculum while attempting to displace the patella medially. A tight lateral retinaculum has been described as an important factor causing patellar pain.[91] Tension in the medial retinaculum can be tested between the medial edge of the medial border of the patella and the edge

of the medial condylar ridge. This area is often tender with patellofemoral joint dysfunction.

6. Medial retinaculum. The retinaculum is flat and cannot be distinguished as a distinct structure. It is palpated in a generalized area between the adductor tubercle and the medial border of the patella. It is often tender with patellofemoral joint dysfunction.

7. Pes anserinus tendons. The pes anserinus tendons join to give a flat tendinous insertion on the anteromedial aspect of the proximal tibia 5 to 7 cm below the joint line (Fig. 15-8).

   a. The semitendinosus tendon is easily felt as a prominent, cordlike structure at the posteromedial corner of the knee.

   b. The gracilis tendon is more difficult to distinguish, but can be felt as a "piano wire" between the semitendinosus tendon posteriorly and the sartorius tendon anteriorly.

   c. The sartorius tendon is a large, blunt structure crossing the posteromedial aspect of the knee, anterior to the semitendinosus and gracilis tendons.

8. Gastrocnemius heads. These are palpated deep in the popliteal fossa.

D. The popliteal space. The popliteal artery can usually be palpated at the midportion of the popliteal space. Comparing the popliteal artery pulse with the dorsal pedis and the posterior tibial pulses is helpful in assessing popliteal entrapment syndrome.[208] Swelling of the semimembranosus bursa (Baker's cyst) is best palpated with the knee fully extended.

E. Palpation for effusion. When a large volume of fluid accumulates within the confines of the synovial cavity, it is easily seen and palpated at the medial and lateral patellar margins, and distension of the posterior aspect of the joint is noted. Smaller quantities of fluid may be detected by:

1. Milking the fluid distally out of the suprapatellar pouch with one hand while palpating along the medial and lateral patellar margins with the other. Fluid will be felt to drain beneath the palpating fingers, and the patella may be felt to float up off the femoral condyles. Compare with the opposite knee.

2. After having milked the fluid distally, tap the patella posteriorly with the free hand. If fluid has caused the patella to float, a click will be felt as it is pushed down onto the femoral condyles. Palpate for distension of the semimembranosus bursa, which often communicates with the joint.

III. Skin Palpation. Palpate the skin about the knee area and the distal aspect of the leg lightly with the back of the hand, noting:

A. Temperature. Localized areas of increased temperature may signify underlying inflammation. In reflex sympathetic dystrophy or other vascular problems, the leg may feel abnormally cool.

B. Tenderness. Burning dysesthesias may be associated with neural disorders, such as nerve root impingement, or they may arise as referred tenderness from deep somatic pathologic processes.

C. Moisture. Hyperhidrosis is common with reflex sympathetic dystrophy. Abnormalities in skin moisture may also be associated with other vascular or metabolic disorders.

D. Mobility. Skin mobility is often impaired by adhesions after surgery or prolonged immobilization, and especially with development of a reflex sympathetic dystrophy.

Summary of Evaluation Procedures

The knee evaluation presented here is lengthy when considered in the context of a busy clinical practice. The experienced examiner rarely uses all these tests, but chooses the appropriate examination procedures on the basis of the patient interview and the general nature of the problem. To improve the efficiency of a knee examination, the clinician must organize the tests according to patient positioning. The standing tests are done first, then the sitting tests, the supine tests, and finally the prone tests. For each position, the relevant observations, inspection procedures, selective tissue tension tests, neuromuscular tests, and palpation procedures must be done before having the patient change position.

The following outline summarizes the knee evaluation according to patient positioning. It can be used as a checklist when performing the examination and as the basis for writing a knee evaluation form tailored to a particular clinical setting.

I. Standing
   A. Observation
      1. Gait
      2. Proprioception
      3. Special functions—running, stair climbing, abrupt stops, abrupt turns, hopping, squatting, balance reach tests, and so forth
   B. Inspection
      1. Standing structure and alignment
      2. Soft-tissue contours
      3. Swelling
      4. Skin
   C. Selective tissue tension tests—active weight-bearing flexion–extension
   D. Neuromuscular tests
      1. Repeated half-squats (L3; same as weight-bearing flexion–extension)
      2. Repeated toe-raises (S1–S2)
II. Sitting
   A. Inspection
      1. Patellar alignment and positioning
      2. Femorotibial rotatory alignment
      3. Muscle contours with maximal isometric contraction
      4. Skin
   B. Resisted isometric movements

1. Knee extension
2. Knee flexion
3. Internal tibial rotation
4. External tibial rotation

C. Neuromuscular tests—resisted hip flexion (L2, L3); patellar reflex (L3–L4)

D. Palpation
1. Bony structures and soft tissue attachments
2. Tendons
3. Ligaments

III. Supine
A. Inspection
1. Tibial lengths (knees bent)
2. Anteroposterior tibial alignment (knees bent)
3. Femoral lengths (knees bent)
4. Leg-length measurement (anterosuperior iliac spine to medial malleolus)
5. Valgus–varus angulation
6. Swelling or atrophy (girth measurements)
7. Skin

B. Selected tissue tension tests
1. Non–weight-bearing (active–passive) tests
   a. Flexion–extension—measured with goniometer
   b. Lateral and medial rotation
2. Joint-play movements
   a. Anterior–posterior glide
   b. Valgus–varus tilt
   c. Internal–external rotation
   d. Patellar mobility
   e. Distraction
3. Ankle range of motion
4. Passive hip flexion–extension, abduction–adduction, and straight-leg raise
5. Special tests for:
   a. Ligamentous instability
   b. Meniscal tears
   c. Patellofemoral joint involvement

C. Neuromuscular tests—resisted dorsiflexion (L5)

D. Palpation
1. Muscles
2. Effusion
3. Skin

IV. Prone
A. Inspection
1. Soft tissues
2. Skin

B. Selected tissue tension tests
1. Passive hip internal–external rotation
2. Resisted knee flexion

C. Neuromuscular tests—medial hamstring reflex (L5)

D. Palpation
1. Muscles
2. Skin

A knee examination is never done in isolation. The knee is only a single component of the closed kinetic chain, and pathologic processes may exist proximal or distal to the knee. Pelvic obliquity or leg-length inequality must be recognized, because these problems affect the knee. Abnormal foot function is not uncommon and causes various knee ailments, including patellar tendinitis and lateral knee pain.[235] Increased pronation of the foot or a rigid, supinated configuration contributes to knee problems.[34,210–213,226] Failure to recognize that a foot abnormality is causing a knee problem may delay treatment and recovery.

A patient with knee problems should be evaluated frequently with a motion examination both on and off a treadmill (using various speeds). A foot that looks as though it is one configuration often will actually function as the opposite when in motion.[212] Videotapes or films also help in diagnosing difficult problems.[34]

COMMON LESIONS

Ligamentous Injuries

HISTORY

The patient will invariably recall the traumatic event. The therapist should attempt to determine the exact mechanism of injury.

Onset. One of the most common mechanisms of injury occurs when a football player is tackled from the side with the foot planted and the knee slightly flexed. The victim is usually struck while trying to turn or cut away. The forces on the knee include a valgus stress, external rotation of the tibia on the femur, and usually an anterior movement of the tibia on the femur. With sufficient force, the medial capsule is torn first, followed by the MCL, then the ACL.[178] The medial meniscus is invariably torn as well, completing the "terrible triad of O'Donoghue."

A minor medial ligament sprain is a common lesion that usually results from an external rotation strain of the tibia on the femur. An external force may or may not be involved.

A force against the anterior thigh, which can drive the femur backward on the tibia, while the knee is close to full extension, tends to stress the ACL. This is especially true if the tibia is in a position—or forced into a position—of internal rotation with respect to the femur. In fact, forced internal rotation of the tibia on the femur in itself may tear the ACL. Internal rotary strains are thought by some to be the primary cause of isolated ACL lesions.[180,355]

A force driving the tibia backward on the femur will stress the PCL. This seems to be true regardless of whether or not the knee is flexed, because the PCL remains relatively taut in most positions of the knee. An example of such an injury is the previously described dashboard injury.

In the case of a force driving the knee into hyperextension, the posterior capsule tends to give way first, then the ACL, and finally the PCL.[180]

In cases of severe ligamentous injuries, sometimes the patient attempts to continue activities (e.g., return to the field in a football game) immediately after the injury. This is especially true in the case of a complete MCL rupture, as no fibers remain intact from which pain can arise. The pain often subsides after a few minutes if the patient is in a highly motivating situation. No effusion ensues because the capsule is usually torn, allowing the fluid to leak out of the joint cavity. In partial ligamentous injuries, the patient is less likely to continue activity because of persisting pain after the injury.

In severe injuries the patient may describe painful effusion occurring within a few minutes after the injury; this is highly suggestive of hemarthrosis, and an intra-articular fracture must be ruled out by the physician. Slower development of effusion (e.g., during several hours) suggests synovial effusion secondary to capsular irritation. This is common with mild and moderate ligamentous injuries.

Site of Pain. The patient usually will point to a localized area that corresponds well to the site of the tear as being the primary site of pain. The exception is an isolated ACL tear, which is relatively rare and may result in more generalized discomfort.

In the case of effusion, especially hemarthrosis, the entire knee area is likely to be painful; the patient is less able to localize the site of injury. Also, in severe injuries involving several structures, localization is less likely because of generalized pain.

The knee is largely innervated by the L3 segment, although it also receives contributions from L4 to S2. Referred pain into these segments is possible, although this does not seem to occur as frequently with acute ligamentous lesions as it does with chronic, degenerative problems.

Nature of Pain and Disability. In the absence of significant effusion, the pain is described as a continuous, deep, fairly localized pain, which is increased by any movement tending to further stress the ligament (partial tear). When considerable effusion exists, a more intense, aching, throbbing pain is described that is aggravated by weight bearing and virtually any movement. Hemarthrosis is, as a rule, more painful than synovial effusion.

If a moderately severe tear or complete rupture is left to heal, the pain will largely subside. The patient may walk quite comfortably but cannot perform some particular activity such as running, jumping, cutting, walking down stairs, or squatting without having the knee give way. If carefully assessed, the particular disabilities will correspond to activities that tend to move the knee into directions that the stretched or ruptured ligament is meant to check. Some examples include:

1. Inability to turn quickly—MCL or LCL
2. Inability to run forward—ACL
3. Inability to descend stairs easily, squat, or run backward—PCL or posterior capsule.

An MCL rupture will usually result in considerable disability, whereas isolated cruciate tears may cause little or no disability if quadriceps muscle function is good.[230]

PHYSICAL EXAMINATION

In the acute stage, once joint effusion, considerable pain, and significant muscle guarding have developed, it may prove very difficult to perform some of the evaluation procedures. In any case, the knee must be examined, sparing the patient as much discomfort as possible and ensuring that no harm is imposed by the tests. The value of immediate, on-the-spot examination before the onset of effusion cannot be overemphasized.

I. Acute Lesion with Effusion
   A. Observation. The patient may hobble into the office, perhaps on crutches. The knee is held slightly flexed with only toe-touch weight bearing, if any. The shoe, sock, and trousers are removed with difficulty.
   B. Inspection. Joint effusion is obvious, especially in the suprapatellar region. The patient stands with the leg held semiflexed, often unable to place the heel on the floor.
      1. The Helfet test cannot be done because the knee cannot be fully extended.
      2. Girth measurements at the suprapatellar region are increased from effusion.
      3. Some redness of the skin over the knee may be noticed. The skin may be somewhat shiny from being stretched.
   C. Selective tissue tension tests
      1. Active movement
         a. Weight-bearing flexion–extension is impossible.
         b. In the supine position, active movement is limited in a capsular pattern because of joint effusion, with pain especially at the extremes of both motions. Passive overpressure is met with a muscle-spasm end feel.
      2. Passive movements. Flexion–extension is limited in a capsular pattern (about 15° loss of extension and 60 to 90° loss of flexion) with no crepitus and a muscle-spasm end feel.
      3. Resisted movements
         a. Should be strong and painless, barring concurrent tendon injury
         b. Quantitative determination of muscle strength must be deferred because of the acute condition.
      4. Passive joint-play movements of the femorotibial joint may be hypermobile and painful. (Be aware of possible false-negative results from muscle guarding.)
         a. Anterior glide
         b. Posterior glide
         c. Medial-lateral glide
         d. Internal–external tibial rotation
         e. Patellar mobility cannot be validly assessed if significant effusion is present.
         f. Superior tibiofibular joint. Joint-play movement here may be painful in an LCL sprain.

D. Palpation
1. There is likely to be localized tenderness at the site of the tear. There may be referred tenderness in nearby areas as well.
2. Effusion is easily confirmed by the tap test or by emptying the suprapatellar pouch while palpating the lateral patellar margins. Posterior capsular distension may also be noted. Hemarthrosis may accompany (1) a cruciate tear, (2) a meniscus tear extending to the peripheral attachment, (3) a severe capsular tear, or (4) an intra-articular fracture.
3. The joint is warm and slightly moist.
E. Ligamentous stability and special tests (see Physical Examination, above)

II. Acute Lesion without Effusion. Some effusion follows most ligament injuries at the knee, but the absence of significant effusion does not necessarily mean that the injury is mild. On the contrary, complete medial capsular ruptures, usually with tearing of all or part of the MCL, may not be followed by much joint effusion because the fluid escapes the confines of the joint capsule through the defect.

There are two primary differences between a patient presenting with effusion and one presenting without. In the absence of effusion the patient presents with less of a gait disturbance—the knee is not maintained in as much flexion, and the patient may be able to walk without aids. Also, the available range of motion is greater. Generally, the patient who does not develop much joint swelling has less pain and disability. The clinician must carefully assess joint-play movements to determine whether the absence of effusion reflects a minor lesion or a very severe injury. Information acquired during the patient interview is also instructive.

If significant instability is present on one or more joint-play movements, a physician experienced in such injuries must be notified at once, because immediate surgery may be indicated.

III. Chronic Ligament Ruptures. Patients occasionally present with chronic ligament ruptures. The primary complaint is functional instability or giving way of the knee with particular activities. The patient may walk without a limp or obvious disability; the only significant findings may be (1) difficulty performing some specific function such as running, turning sharply, squatting, descending stairs, or running backward, (2) quadriceps muscle atrophy, especially if the joint was swollen or immobilized, (3) hypermobility on one or more joint-play movements or ligamentous stability tests, and (4) a positive Helfet test.

Laxity of one of the medial stabilizing structures—the medial capsule or MCL—is most likely to result in some disability. Often this is combined with ACL rupture. The result is instability of anterior glide and external rotation of the tibia on the femur. Functionally, the patient cannot turn away from the involved side without the leg giving way, a real problem for a young, active person. The medial meniscus may be torn at the time of injury or some time later from abnormal joint mechanics. The meniscus tear compounds the instability and the tendency for the knee to buckle.

MANAGEMENT

The approach to management of ligamentous injuries depends on several factors, including the patient's age and desired activity level and the nature of the pathologic process. It is important to determine the severity of the injury and whether the lesion is acute or chronic. Traditionally, ligamentous lesions have been graded as follows:

Grade I: Mild sprain, with no gross loss of integrity of the ligament fibers. On examination there is no joint-play hypermobility.
Grade II: Moderate tear, with partial loss of integrity of the ligament, manifested as mild joint-play instability
Grade III: Severe tear or complete rupture of the ligament resulting in moderate to marked joint-play hypermobility

This classification is useful for general communication purposes, but it cannot be used as an absolute guide to clinical management; it does not adequately represent the broad continuum of ligamentous injuries, nor does it take into account other individual factors such as the patient's age, activity level, motivational status, or the stage of the lesion.

The stage of the lesion—how acute or chronic it is—is also a somewhat arbitrary designation. For the sake of this discussion, we will base this classification on specific clinical criteria that may reflect the nature of the existing inflammatory process. In an *acute lesion*, the patient cannot bear weight without pain and a significant limp; there is significant loss of knee motion, with a painful, muscle-spasm end feel; and there is obvious swelling or effusion. In a *chronic lesion*, the patient can walk with minimal pain and without a significant limp; knee motion is relatively free, or, if restricted, is limited by stiffness (nonpainful end feel); and there is little or no swelling. A *subacute lesion* presents with some combination of acute or chronic criteria.

Grade I and II Sprains. After mild to moderate knee ligament injury, the patient should be able to return to a normal level of activity. In first-degree sprains, treatment is relatively unimportant and is designed mostly to prevent pain. In second-degree sprains, the critical factor in treatment is protection to allow healing. The rehabilitation program should be started early, with more progressive exercise techniques and functional activities added later. The general strengthening exercises usually do not need to be modified, although for medial lesions care must be taken to avoid valgus stress at the knee, and for lateral lesions varus stress should be avoided.

Friction massage at the site of the lesion, applied transversely to the direction of the ligament fibers with the knee in different degrees of flexion–extension, may help prevent the healing ligament from adhering to adjacent tissues and may help align newly produced collagen along the normal lines of stress (see Box 8-3).[60] Take care not to apply friction at the proximal attachment of the MCL, because occasionally a periosteal disruption results here in the development of a bony outcropping (Pellegrini-Stieda syndrome).[348] (Although this is undoubtedly an inevitable result of the original injury, the use of massage may be held suspect should some medicolegal question develop.)

MCL Tear (Grade III Sprain). MCL tears do not usually require surgical repair.[25,85,130,140,296,329] The normal course for these injuries is reexamination under anesthesia followed by arthroscopy of the knee.[240] It is necessary, however, to prove that an isolated MCL injury is present, with no involvement of the meniscal or cruciate structures. Patients with a combined MCL–ACL injury will most likely have an ACL reconstruction without MCL repair. The MCL has an excellent secondary support system. Weight-bearing forces tend to compress the medial side, thus aiding in stability, and the injury can be protected adequately with bracing. Three conditions must be met for healing to occur at the MCL: (1) the ligament fibers must remain in continuity or within a well-vascularized soft tissue bed; (2) there must be enough stress to stimulate and direct the healing process; and (3) there must be protection from harmful stresses.[360]

Whether surgical repair is used or not, the knee is usually immobilized in a hinge cast or brace cast to minimize atrophy and prevent valgus stress.[122] Rehabilitation after most MCL injuries can progress fairly rapidly (2 to 8 weeks). The treatment program is similar to that for second-degree sprains. Weight bearing with crutches is continued until full knee extension without an extension lag can be demonstrated and the patient can walk normally without gait deviations. Return to sports is not permitted until a normal gait pattern has been achieved. Functional proprioceptive neuromuscular facilitation (PNF) patterns stressing tibial rotation should be incorporated for strengthening with resistance as the patient becomes stronger. As strength improves, the patient should engage in functional activities to enhance dynamic stability of the knee. MCL sprains vary in severity and response to treatment. The physician and the patient's response to treatment will determine the timing of progression through the stages of treatment for a specific injury.

ACL Tear (Grade III Sprain). Ruptures of the ACL may occur as a result of a direct blow to the knee with the foot planted. Much more often, however, they are the result of a noncontact twisting injury associated with a hyperextension or varus or valgus stress to the knee. After the diagnosis of injury of the ACL, the patient is faced with various treatment options. The conservative approach is to allow the acute phase of the injury to pass and to then implement a vigorous rehabilitation program. If it becomes apparent that normal function cannot be recovered, and if the knee remains unstable, then reconstructive surgery to considered.

Nonoperative Rehabilitation. In the nonsurgical patient, after control of swelling and pain, treatment begins with iso-

metrics of the hamstrings and quadriceps to encourage co-contractions. Range of motion is limited and protected. Based on the studies of Daniels,[62] Daniels et al.,[63] Henning et al.,[132,133] and Paulos et al.,[278] the range is limited from 90° of flexion to 45° of extension. This is because the ACL undergoes a deceleration strain at about 30° with maximum strain at 0° extension. A protected exercise program is allowed in this range. Isometric internal and external rotation exercises, added once the patient has 90° flexion, decrease any abnormal tibial rotation.[320,321] Special emphasis is placed on hamstring exercises. During all phases of the exercise program, electrical stimulation with maximum contraction is desirable to maintain muscle integrity.[331]

Functional knee braces have been suggested for permanent use in sports activities involving cutting or rotational stresses.[20,81,329,334,339] There are two types, featuring hinge posts with or without shells to encompass the thigh. Gait studies have shown that under low loading conditions, most functional knee braces limit excessive anterior tibial translation. However, under conditions of high loading that more closely simulate high activity levels, there is little or no control of anterior tibial translation.

ACL repair or reconstruction, like nonsurgical rehabilitation, typically demands a protocol that minimizes any quadriceps muscle activity involving anterior translation of the tibia. This means using midrange quadriceps work, avoiding terminal knee extension, and emphasizing hamstring strengthening to provide active stabilization. The advanced phase of treatment features eccentric quadriceps exercise and the removal of the extension stop of the rehabilitative brace.[9,52,81,339]

Surgical Rehabilitation. The operative methods of stabilization are intra-articular or extra-articular. Extra-articular reconstruction involves taking a structure that lies outside of the joint capsule and moving it so that it can affect the mechanics of the knee in a manner that mimics normal ACL function.[157,222,223] The iliotibial band is the most commonly used structure. However, long-term results have been disappointing.[338] This procedure is effective in reducing the pivot-shift phenomena that is found in anterolateral rotational instability but cannot match the normal biomechanics of the ACL.[157,220–223] The rehabilitation after an extra-articular reconstruction is aggressive and permits an earlier return to functional activities but is not recommended for high-level patients.[285]

Intra-articular reconstruction involves placing a structure within the knee that will roughly follow the course of the ACL and will functionally replace the ACL. Bone–patellar tendon–bone grafts are the current state of the art, using human autografts or allografts.[75,76,87,96–98,101,157,261,262,295,359] Intra-articular ACL reconstruction using various tissues, including the patellar tendon, iliotibial band, and combinations of hamstring tendons (semitendinosus, semitendinosus–gracilis), has been extensively described in the literature.[3,4,7,33,46,54,92,96,115,123,137,156,167,249] Noyes and colleagues[258] reported that the patellar tendon graft had a strength of 168% of the ACL, whereas the semitendinosus had 70%, the gracilis 49%, and the quadriceps or patellar retinaculum only 21%. Currently, either the patellar tendon or semitendinosus autografts are the most widely used ACL substitutes to reconstruct the ACL-deficient knee.[282] In intra-articular procedures, the site must undergo revascularization followed by reorganization of collagen.[38,48,261] These procedures, therefore, usually necessitate a slower, longer rehabilitation process than extra-articular reconstruction.[37,38,260,277,330]

Allegoric tissue grafts from cadavers and amputation specimens pose an attractive option—they are readily available in various tissues (fasciae late, hamstring tendons) and because of lack of rigid size constraints may be used in quantities that provide greater mechanical strength than the corresponding autogenous tissue.[75,112,154,199,243,254,276,314–317] However, the enthusiasm surrounding the use of allograft replacement of the ACL has recently declined because of the small but tangible risk of infectious disease transmission.[282]

Much as been written regarding the rehabilitation of the patient who has undergone ACL reconstructive surgery. A body of literature has addressed the bone–patella tendon–bone complex (BPB) graft because this has been the gold standard. Many protocols have been presented to manage such patients.[65,74,97,98,129,219,222,223,255,256,276,279,282,290,294,297,302,305–311,337,359] With the use of securely fixed, high-strength, isometric grafts, the progressive rehabilitation protocol includes early protected motion, neuromuscular rehabilitation, and patellofemoral joint mobilization. Traditional rehabilitation after ACL reconstruction is lengthy: an athlete with such an injury will usually require a year before returning to full activity. Rehabilitation depends very much on the surgical procedure performed.[84,259,309,359] Traditionally, rehabilitation has been conservative, but in recent years the trend has been to become more aggressive in rehabilitation of the reconstructed ACL primarily as a result of the reports of Shelbourne and co-workers.[305–310] This has been referred to as an accelerated protocol. They have demonstrated that this program returns the patient to normal function early, results in fewer patellofemoral problems, and reduces the number of surgeries to obtain extension, all without compromising stability.[306] Rehabilitation proceeds through a controlled ambulation phase, light activity phase, and return to activity phase. The most frequent problems encountered after ACL surgery are quadriceps weakness, patellar irritability, flexion contractures, and joint stiffness.[359] Early restoration of full extension (1 to 4 weeks) is imperative to successful outcome, as is awareness of potential complications that may limit progress such as arthrofibrosis.[282] Joint mobilization is initiated in the form of early patellar mobilization and tibiofemoral mobilization to improve extension. The clinician instructs the patient in self-mobilization of the patella techniques as part of the home program.

The accelerated protocol emphasizes immediate motion, including full extension, immediate weight bearing within tolerance, and early closed-chain exercise for strengthening and neuromuscular control.

After reconstructive surgery, immobilization of the knee or restricted motion without muscle contraction leads to undesired outcomes for the ligamentous, articular, and muscular structures that surround the joint. It is clear that rehabilitation that incorporates early joint motion is beneficial for reduction of pain, minimizing capsular contractions and decreasing scar formation that can limit joint motion, and is beneficial for articular cartilage.[26] Aquatic therapy programs[342,359] and closed-chain kinetic exercises are often emphasized.[270] Aquatic therapy is often used to initiate a fast-paced walking or running program. A study by Tovin and associates[342] suggests that a rehabilitation program for patients with intra-articular ACL constructions performed in a pool is effective in reducing joint effusion and facilitating recovery of lower extremity function, as indicated by Lysholm scores.[216] The results also suggest that aquatic therapy is as effective as other exercise approaches for restoring knee range of motion and quadriceps femoris muscle strength, but not as effective in restoring hamstring muscle strength.

Rehabilitation with a closed kinetic chain program results in anteroposterior knee laxity values that are closer to normal, and earlier return to normal daily activities, compared with rehabilitation with an open kinetic chain program.[26] Closed-chain exercises appear to be more effective than open-chain exercises at increasing the joint compressive forces and, thus, minimizing the anteroposterior translation of the tibia.[107,270,352,353] Closed-chain knee extension has been advocated as a safe exercise for patients after ACL reconstruction, and research suggests that closed-chain exercises are safer than open-chain ones because there is less stress on the graft.[132,265,283] An open-chain action primarily emphasizes concentric work, but a closed-chain movement brings a more balanced action of concentric, eccentric, and isometric contraction. However, PNF strengthening patterns that stress tibial rotation are essentially the only way to concentrate on strengthening the rotation component of knee motion, which is essential to normal function of the knee. Because the PNF patterns are done in open kinetic chain, they should only involve active contraction through the functional movement pattern.[285]

Along with the early controlled weight bearing and closed-chain exercises, which act to stimulate muscle and joint mechanoreceptors, sensorimotor activities (e.g., balance board exercises, slide board training, mini-trampoline activities) to reestablish balance and neuromuscular control should also begin early in the rehabilitation process (see Figs. 14-44 through 14-46; also see Figs 15-63 through 15-65).[135] Training progression should begin with patients early in therapy with balance board activities with the patient in a bipedal stance and progress to single-leg stance in the more-advanced phase. Several authors advocate the use of balance board proprioceptive training well past the acute postsurgical rehabilitation phase, not only for restoration of function but for its prophylactic effect on ligament reinjury.[42,134,135,346]

An early goal of proprioceptive training is to achieve symmetric bipedal gait. Once achieved, a running gait retraining program improves symmetry of lower limb musculature contribution, which may prevent abnormal loading of the ligaments and soft tissue and increase strength and endurance during sports competitions.[136] Hewett et al.[136] suggest the use of gait training on a treadmill in front of a mirror to provide simultaneous visual and verbal trainer feedback to the patient. Incline treadmill running can increase range of motion across all joints, but especially at the hip. Backward incline training also should be used to increase range of motion and to increase quadriceps functional strength while simultaneously reducing patellofemoral stress (see Fig. 15-67).[47,324] For the athlete simultaneous gait retraining and a progressive plyometric program teaches the athlete to properly initiate, control, and decelerate ground reaction forces that will be encountered in running, jumping, cutting, and other activities. Functional exercises such as balance beam walking, vertical jumping, single-leg and double-leg hopping, shuttle runs, and rope skipping can be progressively incorporated into the training program. Return to sports depends on strength, skill acquisition, and response of the knee to activity.

PCL Tear (Grade III Sprain). Isolated tears of the posterior cruciate ligament are not common. It is more likely that the PCL is injured concurrently with the ACL, MCL, LCL, or menisci. The majority of PCL injuries result from a direct blow to the flexed knee. Hyperflexion and hyperextension injuries have also been shown to result in PCL ruptures. The PCL may also be injured when the tibia is forced posteriorly on the fixed femur or the femur is forced anteriorly on the fixed tibia.[220] Isolated PCL disruptions often have a good prognosis when treated nonoperatively.[55,61,66] Their prognosis after direct surgical repair is somewhat better than ACL repair because of a more generous blood supply; however, combined injuries to the PCL and posterolateral corner can be particularly troublesome (see Flexor Mechanism Disorders below). The knee with a torn ACL usually has symptoms of instability, but the knee with a torn PCL has symptoms of disability: medial compartment arthritis, patellofemoral arthritis, and swelling and pain related to activity. PCL rehabilitation closely follows ACL rehabilitation protocol, with a few exceptions:

- No isolated hamstring exercises are performed dung the first 6 to 8 weeks.
- Closed chain exercises are emphasized, allowing for hamstring strengthening but protecting against posterior tibial translation through the quadriceps–hamstring force–couple and compressive forces across the joint.

The recovery process proceeds essentially the same as the ACL rehabilitation program.

Acute PCL repair with augmentation appears to have a better success rate than does delayed reconstruction.[240,275] Early postoperative motion after PCL repair usually is not recommended. A period of 4 to 6 weeks of immobilization is advocated to allow the bone grafts to heal before initiating joint motion. The focus of rehabilitation for both surgical and nonsurgical patients is on quadriceps exercises. In conservative rehabilitation the hamstrings are omitted in the early exercise phase because they may accentuate posterior subluxation.

Eccentric quadriceps exercises are started as soon as the patient can tolerate them.

A common surgical procedure for PCL repair is repositioning of the origin of the medial gastrocnemius muscle.[179] This transfer acts dynamically during weight acceptance and the push-off phases of gait. In this case both quadriceps and gastrocnemius muscles are of primary importance with respect to exercise. Once the quadriceps have achieved 80% of the strength of the normal leg on Cybex or a similar testing device, hamstring exercises are added. The length of time to return to sports is about the same as for injury of the ACL.

In addition to hamstring training to prevent anterior subluxation for ACL injuries and quadriceps training to increase structural stiffness and knee strength for PCL injuries,[108,166,353] it is important to include dynamic joint control training.[56,153,352] Even if the hamstrings and quadriceps are strengthened, it is important that they function quickly and adequately during unexpected trauma by improving neuromuscular coordination. Training should consist of balance and proprioception activities, functional development of the feet to grasp the ground, stabilization of the stance position, and improvement of reactions to sudden additional forces applied by the clinician.[153]

LCL Tears (Grade III Sprain). The lateral aspect of the knee is well supported by secondary stabilizers and can be treated nonsurgically.[240,275] Isolated injury to the LCL is rare, and when it does occur, it is critical to rule out other ligamentous injuries. When the secondary restraints, lateral capsule, and cruciate ligaments are torn, functional instability is common and surgical correction is usually required. Rehabilitation after repair follows the guidelines for PCL rehabilitation and for posterolateral rotatory instability. Athletes or other persons placing unusual demands on the functional capacity of the knee must undergo a more rigorous retraining program. For these patients especially, exercises should approximate the type of loading normally imposed on the joint. Most athletic activities, as well as routine activities of daily living, involve relatively high loading conditions. Isokinetic exercise equipment with variable speed adjustments is a convenient means of providing high-speed resistance to various muscle groups, while monitoring the percent of maximal torque output. Such exercises result in strengthening and also optimize the training effect of the exercise program.

Running, jumping, and athletic activities are not permitted until strength is nearly normal, range of motion is full, and normal femorotibial rotation has returned. Such activities are gradually progressed from straight-ahead jogging to straight-ahead running, then running with gentle turns, and finally running with abrupt stops and turns. Clinical signs of healing, such as restoration of strength and range of motion with no pain on stress testing, in no way signify return of normal strength to the injured ligament.[253] Restoration of ligamentous strength requires a maturation process of collagen aggregation and realignment that may take several months to a year.[2,132]

Any advantages of returning to activities involving intermittent high loading of the knee must be weighed against the risk that the still-weakened structure may give way prematurely, possibly resulting in a more serious injury than the original one. In making judgments about appropriate activity levels, the desires of the coach and the highly motivated young athlete must often take second priority to knowledge of the rate and mechanisms of tissue healing.

Meniscus Lesions

Meniscus lesions affecting the knee are common, especially in athletes. Once it has been determined through examination that a meniscus lesion exists, it is important to classify the injury as a tear confined to the periphery or a tear involving the body of the meniscus. Often arthroscopy or arthrography will assist the physician in making this distinction. An anteromedial coronary ligament sprain accompanies most tears involving the body of the medial meniscus.

HISTORY

Onset. The menisci move with the tibia in flexion–extension and with the femur in rotation. If, during flexion, external tibial rotation is forced instead of the internal rotation that should normally occur, abnormal stresses are applied to the menisci, and a tear is possible. The same, of course, applies to the case of forced internal tibial rotation during knee extension. Similarly, flexion or extension in the absence of the normal rotary movement that should accompany it may result in a meniscus tear. The medial meniscus, being less mobile, is more susceptible to injury. Because tibial rotation is impossible in the fully extended knee, the history is one of twisting on a semiflexed knee. Again, athletes, especially those wearing cleated shoes and involved in contact sports, are particularly prone to meniscus injuries, occasionally in conjunction with ligament tears.

Meniscus tears may also occur with hyperflexion of the knee, especially during weight bearing. In this position, the femoral condyles have rolled back to articulate with the posterior aspects of the tibial articular surfaces. The menisci, then, must recede backward during flexion, but can recede only to a certain point before capsuloligamentous attachments restrict their further movement. If further flexion is forced once the menisci have reached their limit of backward movement, the menisci are susceptible to being ground between the femoral and tibial joint surfaces. This is especially true if rotation is forced in hyperflexion, because a rotary movement entails further backward movement of one condyle. Certain occupations, such as mining, in which one must move about in a squatting position, may predispose to development of meniscal tears from this mechanism. In athletics, the wrestler is classically prone to this type of injury.

Site of Pain. The person usually feels "something give" in the joint, often with an accompanying deep, sickening type of pain. If not masked by other injuries or extensive effusion, the patient often can point to the spot on the joint line corresponding to the site of the tear where the coronary ligament has been sprained.

Nature of Pain and Disability. The onset is usually sudden, with an immediate deep pain associated with giving way of the joint. If hemarthrosis occurs, pain is typically severe and generalized, arising within minutes of the injury. If a longitudinal tear of the medial meniscus extends anteriorly past the midpoint of the meniscus, the lateral portion may slip over the dome of the medial femoral condyle (Fig. 15-15). This grossly interferes with normal knee mechanics, with a resultant immediate locking of the joint so that the last 20 to 30° of extension are lost. An injury involving such immediate locking is usually preceded by one or more previous minor incidences of giving way followed by effusion; the developing longitudinal tear finally extends anteriorly far enough to cause such locking.

The person suffering a meniscus tear hesitates to resume activity immediately after the injury, unlike the person suffering a ligamentous sprain. Synovial effusion, causing a generalized pressure sensation, may arise within hours after the injury. Effusion nearly always accompanies a medial meniscus tear, but not always a lateral tear.

In an untreated meniscus tear, the acute stage may completely subside with restoration of motion. The person may resume normal activities with little or no pain. The complaint, however, is one of intermittent buckling of the joint for no apparent reason, even during simple walking. Occasional or persistent clicking of the joint may be reported. Chronic or intermittent effusion may also occur, probably from altered joint mechanics resulting in undue stress to the joint capsule.

PHYSICAL EXAMINATION

I. Acute Stage
  A. Observation
    1. The patient may hobble in on crutches with the knee held slightly flexed and touching down only the toe.
    2. Obvious effusion may be present.
    3. The patient may have difficulty removing the shoe, sock, and trousers.
  B. Inspection
    1. Effusion may be noted, especially in the suprapatellar region.
    2. The patient stands with the knee held semiflexed.
    3. The Helfet test may not be performed because of incomplete extension.
    4. The suprapatellar girth measurement may be increased from effusion.
    5. The skin may appear slightly red and shiny.
  C. Selective tissue tension tests
    1. Active movements
      a. Weight-bearing flexion–extension is impossible.
      b. Flexion–extension in supine reveals:
        i. A capsular pattern if effusion is present
        ii. Considerable loss of extension if the knee is locked, causing a distorted capsular pattern if

effusion is present, a noncapsular pattern if little or no effusion is present

   c. Passive overpressure reveals a muscle-guarding end feel at the extremes of flexion and extension.
   d. If the knee is locked, a springy rebound end feel will be noted moving into extension.
2. Passive movements
   a. Essentially the same as indicated above for active movement, with perhaps slightly greater range of movement
   b. McMurray's test may not be performed if considerable effusion restricts flexion, because it is applicable only from full flexion to 90°. If flexion is possible, a painful click may be elicited on combined external rotation and extension if a tear exists in the posterior portion of the medial meniscus, or on combined internal rotation and extension if a posterior lateral meniscus lesion exists.
3. Resisted isometric movements. These should be strong and painless unless a tendon or muscle has also been injured. Quantitative strength measurements cannot be made because of the acute condition.
4. Passive joint-play movements
   a. Rotation opposite the side of the lesion may be painful, especially during Apley's test with compression applied. Distraction with rotation should relieve the pain.
   b. Otherwise, these movements should be relatively normal unless a ligamentous injury also exists.
D. Palpation
   1. Tenderness is present at the joint line where a sprain of the peripheral attachment has occurred. This usually corresponds quite well with the side and site of the tear.
   2. Effusion, as mentioned, nearly always accompanies a medial meniscus tear, but not always a lateral tear. The tap test and emptying of the suprapatellar pouch will confirm the presence of minor effusion.
   3. The joint is warm, the skin somewhat moist.
II. Chronic Tear
   A. History. The patient describes intermittent giving way of the joint, often followed by some effusion, especially if the medial meniscus is at fault. There may be a history of locking with manipulative reduction by the patient, a friend, or physician, followed by immediate relief of pain and restoration of extension. The younger, active person is usually suffering from a longitudinal tear, beginning posteriorly and gradually extending anteriorly. The older person may have a degenerative horizontal tear, with sliding occurring between the upper and lower portions. The patient notes clicking when the femoral condyle passes over a centrally protruding piece of a meniscus.
   B. Objective signs
      1. Quadriceps atrophy, especially involving the vastus medialis

2. Full range of motion, but perhaps some difficulty or apprehension when performing weight-bearing flexion–extension
3. Possibly a positive Helfet test as a result of altered joint mechanics
4. Possibly a positive McMurray test if the posterior segment of the meniscus is torn
5. Pain on forced extension if the anterior segment of the meniscus is torn
6. Positive Apley test when the joint is compressed, but not when it is distracted
7. Tenderness to palpation at the joint line, usually corresponding to the site of the lesion
8. Perhaps some mild chronic effusion
9. Quantitative quadriceps weakness compared with the other leg
10. The clinical examination may be complemented by an arthrogram to give the examiner more information about the integrity of the menisci (Fig. 15-29).

III. Coronary Ligament Sprain
   A. History. The patient usually describes a twisting injury followed by some minor swelling and pain over the anteromedial knee region. Rarely is the victim significantly disabled immediately after the injury; he or she usually does not seek medical attention in the acute stage. Acute symptoms usually subside within a few days. If the meniscus maintains good mobility during healing, the patient should have no further problems. However, often the coronary ligament becomes adhered to the anteromedial margin of the medial tibial condyle as it heals, resulting in reduced mobility of this part of the meniscus. In such cases, the person develops a more chronic problem characterized by intermittent pain when the adhered tissue is stressed, usually with activities involving external rotation of the tibia on the femur. The persistent nature of the problem eventually prompts the person to seek medical assistance, even though the disorder is otherwise minor.

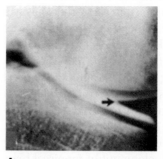
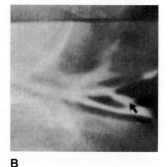

A　　　　　　　　　　　**B**

■ **FIG. 15-29.** Normal meniscus (**A**) appears as an uninterrupted dark wedge (*arrow*) on an arthrogram. An arthrogram of a torn meniscus (**B**) shows streaks of dye within the wedge. (Reprinted with permission from Kulund DH: The Injured Athlete, 2nd ed. Philadelphia, JB Lippincott, 1988:176.)

B. Objective findings
1. Consistent findings on physical examination:
a. Point tenderness over the anteromedial joint line
b. Pain on external rotation of the tibia on the femur, but no pain on valgus stress
2. Occasionally forced extension hurts as well. Rarely is effusion present by the time the person is seen clinically. There may be minimal quadriceps atrophy if the problem has been of long duration.

MANAGEMENT

Acute Tear of Body of a Meniscus. If an acute meniscus tear is suspected on examination, the referring physician should be consulted and notified of the positive findings. Usually after arthroscopic evaluation of the knee joint, if an isolated tear is encountered (i.e., one without concomitant ligament damage), a decision must be made as to whether repair or removal is the best treatment. Meniscal repair is a growing trend in orthopedics. Immobilization is necessary after meniscal repair. If the procedure is successful, recovery is expected in about 6 months. Most meniscal injuries still require removal of the torn portion of the meniscus; arthroscopy is the most effective way of doing this.[67,240]

If surgery is not planned, treatment in the acute stage is essentially the same as that discussed above for an acute, minor ligamentous sprain. Weight bearing must not be allowed on a locked knee and should be restricted on a knee that cannot fully extend because of effusion. Extension must not be forced in the locked knee, because if the displaced piece of meniscus does not slip back, extension may occur only at the expense of the ACL or articular cartilage.

Chronic Tear of Body of a Meniscus. Again, the physician should be notified if this is suspected. If arthroscopic surgery is not contemplated, the goal is restoration of optimal joint mechanics: mobilization, strengthening, and instruction in appropriate activity levels are necessary. A particular motion, especially extension, must not be encouraged if the restriction is secondary to an intra-articular block, as from a displaced piece of meniscus. Throughout meniscal rehabilitation, it is important to minimize compressive loading of the joint until adequate muscular protection and joint reorganization have been developed.

Meniscal Repair. Many options for meniscal repair exist for the orthopaedist. Options such as open repair or arthroscopically assisted inside-out technique have favorable long-term results.[234] Future directions include the potential use of growth factors and gene therapy to augment meniscus repair. There are many views on rehabilitation after meniscus repair. Traditionally, an individual with a meniscal tear has been treated with immobilization, no weight bearing, or both.[67-69] After repair, the repair should be protected until healing has occurred. The amount of protection required for meniscal repair can vary widely with surgical technique and the surgeon's experience. It is important for the clinician to obtain directions from the physician regarding the post-

operative treatment plan. Although long-term results are still unknown, the meniscus should be preserved whenever possible to avoid the late sequelae of meniscectomy.

Clinical, cadaveric, and biomechanical studies have all demonstrated significant shear and compression forces generated by open kinetic chain exercises that may potentially create deforming forces not only on reconstructed cruciate ligaments (see above) but also on healing meniscal injuries, repairs, or transplanted allografts.[119,132,175,214,215] For this reason closed kinetic exercises are emphasized. Early on in the rehabilitation program, manual resistance can be applied by the therapist to emphasize either a dynamic or static muscle contraction using PNF techniques. These exercises can be performed parallel to the floor, in half-kneeling, in supported plantigrade, or on a therapy ball (see Figs. 15-58 through 15-61) so that the actual compression loads placed on the knee are probably less than if performed in full weight-bearing positions.[43,335] Exercises are initially performed in the anatomic planes of motion and progressed to multiangled and diagonal patterns of motion. Exercises initially may be performed with double leg support and then single leg support (see Figs. 15-60 and 15-61). Once full weight-bearing restrictions have been lifted, the patient progresses to higher levels of full weight-bearing closed kinetic chain exercises. Therapeutic tubing can be used initially to provide some assistance. The patient can start with assisted squats and progress to assisted lunges. Progression to higher-level closed kinetic chain free-weight strengthening exercises depends on the patient's goals and abilities. Neuromuscular-proprioceptive training of patients after meniscal injuries is accomplished with a variety of balance boards and other sensorimotor activities (see Fig. 14-45). In patients who have a total meniscectomy or meniscal transplantation, a certain degree of activity modification is necessary. For the athlete who places higher functional demands on the knee, sports-specific agility training is necessary to ensure a safe return to athletic competition.

Coronary Ligament Tear. Cyriax[58] was the first to draw attention to sprains of the coronary ligaments, which is very common but mostly goes undiagnosed because the localization of the pain and nature of the onset resemble a meniscus lesion or sprain of the coronary ligament. The persistent intermittent knee pain is the result of adherence of the anteromedial coronary ligament to the underlying tibia (Fig. 15-7); the adhesion is broken with some sudden movement, then adherence recurs during healing. Scarring results in diminished movement of the meniscus during rotation, extension, and flexion.[124] The differential diagnosis from a meniscal lesion is extremely important and relies on history and clinical examination. In a chronic situation, the coronary findings will be painful on forced passive flexion or extension and on passive lateral knee rotation (lateral coronary problems are rare).[124]

The objective of treatment is to restore mobility gradually to this part of the meniscus. This is accomplished with ultrasound and transverse friction massage applied directly to the site of the lesion (see Box 8-3). Ten to fifteen minutes of massage, during three or four treatment sessions, are usually sufficient regardless of whether patients are seen the day after the sprain or many months later.[266] Attention should be paid to quadriceps weakness if present. The patient may be instructed in self-administered friction massage, to be applied before activity.

Extensor Mechanism Disorders

Of all the knee problems presenting to the physical therapist, the most common are disorders of the extensor mechanism.[322] The term *extensor mechanism* encompasses several anatomic structures: the patella and its articular surface as well as the trochlear surface of the femur, the patellar tendon and its attachment to both patella and tibial tuberosity, all of the associated supporting soft tissues (such as the retinaculum, peripatellar synovium, and the structures known as synovial plica), the various parts of the quadriceps musculature, and the quadriceps tendon attachment into the patella.

PATELLAR TRACKING DYSFUNCTION (CHONDROMALACIA PATELLAE)

Disorders of the patellofemoral joint constitute a large percentage of chronic knee problems of nontraumatic origin. Nonacute patellofemoral joint dysfunctions tend to be referred to as *chondromalacia patellae*, which literally means softening of the articular cartilage of the patella. Because articular cartilage is not a pain-sensitive structure, the term *chondromalacia* does not adequately describe the clinically significant features of the pathologic process, nor does it take into account etiologic considerations. In fact, surgical studies suggest that surface chondromalacia per se is a relatively normal characteristic of most adult patellae and probably has little relationship in cause or effect to symptomatic knee problems.[1,24,114,239,268,333]

Biomechanical Considerations. The patella is a triangular sesamoid bone receiving attachment from above by the quadriceps tendon, medially and laterally from the patellar retinacula, and inferiorly from the patellar tendon. The patella glides inferiorly with respect to the femoral condyles when the knee is flexed, and superiorly when the knee is extended.

Because the medial femoral condyle extends farther distally than does the lateral condyle, most knee joints assume a slight valgus angulation in the standing position (Figs. 15-1, 15-14*A*, and 15-30). The direction of pull of the quadriceps musculature tends to be in line with the femur, whereas the pull of the patellar tendon is in line with the long axis of the tibia. The angle formed between the line of pull of the quadriceps muscle and the patellar tendon is the Q angle.

The vector that represents the pull on the patellar tendon during loaded knee extension can be resolved into a longitudinal component and a lateral component (Fig. 15-30). The longitudinal component is in line with the direction of pull of the quadriceps and with the long axis of the femur. The lateral vectorial component causes a tendency for the patella to be pulled laterally with respect to the long axis of the femur during loaded knee extension.

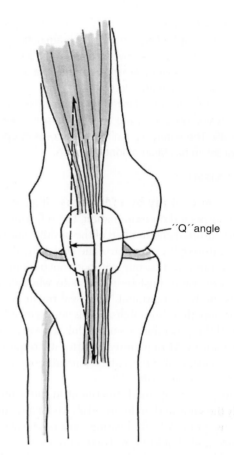

■ **FIG. 15-30.** Pull of the patellar tendon during loaded knee extension, showing the Q angle, and longitudinal and lateral vectoral components.

As the patella glides inferiorly and superiorly during knee flexion and extension, it should do so in line with the long axis of the femur. It is important then that excessive lateral patellar movement does not occur. Prevention of excessive lateral patellar movement during loaded knee extension depends on structural and dynamic mechanisms of patellar stabilization. Structural factors include:

1. Lateral femoral condyle, which, because it is prominent anteriorly, provides some abutment against lateral patellar movement (Fig. 15-2)
2. Deep patellar groove of the femur, in which the patella glides when the knee is in positions of flexion
3. Angle between the pull of the quadriceps and the pull of the patellar tendon. When the knee is in positions of flexion, there is an angle between the pull of the quadriceps and the pull of the patellar tendon, projected onto the sagittal plane (Fig. 15-31). The result of these pulls, represented vectorially, is a patellofemoral compressive force that holds the patella tightly against the patellar groove of the femur, disallowing extraneous movement.

The structural stabilizing mechanisms mentioned here are operational primarily in positions of some knee flexion. As the knee approaches full extension, the patella begins mov-

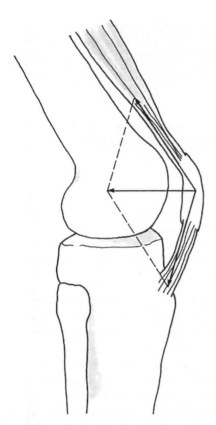

■ **FIG. 15-31.** Patellofemoral compression forces in the sagittal plane with the knee in a flexed position.

ing superiorly out of the deep part of the patellar groove of the femur. In this position the sagittally projected angulation between the quadriceps muscle and the patellar tendon decreases, thus reducing the patellofemoral compressive force that holds the patella firmly in the groove. As the knee moves into extension, especially when loaded, dynamic patellar stabilizing factors play an essential role.

The most important dynamic factor necessary to ensure normal patellofemoral joint function is contraction of the vastus medialis obliquus muscle. The distal fibers of the vastus medialis obliquus originate from the medial aspect of the distal femur and run almost horizontally to insert on the medial aspect of the patella. They attach to the patella by way of the medial retinaculum. The horizontal orientation of these fibers allows them to prevent excessive lateral movement of the patella during loaded knee extension (Fig. 15-32).

Etiology. Chronic patellar tracking dysfunction is a condition in which the patella tends to be pulled too far laterally each time the knee is extended under load. Causes, both structural and dynamic, might include:

1. An increase in the valgus angulation between the quadriceps muscle and the patellar tendon (increased Q angle; Fig. 15-30). Common causes are increased femoral anteversion, increased external tibial torsion, and increased foot pronation.

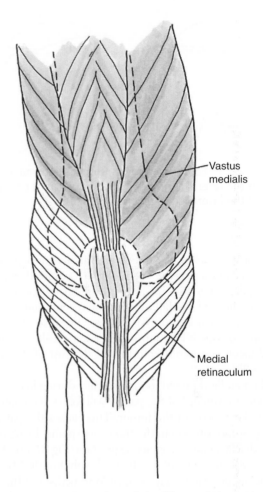

■ **FIG. 15-32.** Orientation of the fibers of the vastus medialis.

2. A lateral femoral condyle that is not sufficiently prominent anteriorly. This results in a loss of the abutment effect normally provided by the lateral condyle (Fig. 15-33).
3. A small, high-riding patella, often called *patella alta*. The more superiorly the patella moves on the femur during knee extension, the less time it spends in the deep portion of the patellar groove, where it is better stabilized.

Dynamically, the most important cause of reduced lateral patellar stabilization is vastus medialis obliquus insufficiency. This commonly occurs from disuse atrophy associated with immobilization or after knee injury. It may also occur when a person increases activities involving loaded knee extension and the vastus medialis is not adequately conditioned to meet the added loads imposed on the extensor mechanism.

Pathologic Process. To best understand the clinical manifestations of patellar tracking dysfunction, we must first discuss the pathologic implications of excessive lateral patellar movement. As the patella moves against the femoral condyles, the contact area on the back of the patella varies with the position of the knee. During normal knee function, both the medial and lateral facets of the patellar articular surface receive compressive stresses from contact with the femur. The small odd

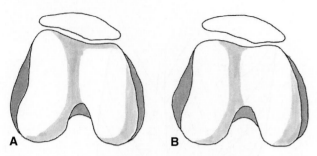

■ **FIG. 15-33.** Femoral condyles, showing normal prominence of the lateral condyle (**A**) and insufficient prominence of the lateral condyle anteriorly (**B**).

medial facet, however, makes contact only at extremes of knee flexion, a position that the knee seldom assumes during normal daily activities (Fig. 15-34).[114] Thus, during normal use of the knee, the odd medial facet is nonarticulating and does not receive much compressive stress. Because of this, the subchondral bone is less dense, softer, and weaker at the odd medial facet, compared with that of the rest of the patella (Fig. 15-35).[287,343–345]

If the patella is pulled too far laterally during loaded knee extension, movement of the patella will follow the contour of the patellar groove of the femur. This causes the patella to undergo some rotation in the transverse plane, bringing the odd medial facet into a contacting position (Fig. 15-36). Under such conditions the relatively weak subchondral bone of the odd medial facet may be unable to withstand the loads imposed on it. This results in an increased rate of trabecular microfracturing, which may incite a low-grade, painful inflammatory response. Trabecular breakdown may be further enhanced by shear stresses between the soft odd medial facet and the stiffer medial facet during compressive deformation.[345] For a particular load, the odd medial facet would deform more than the medial facet, resulting in shearing when the two are compressed simultaneously. This would cause the pathologic process to progress into the medial facet of the patella.

Excessive lateral patellar movement during repeated knee extension may also cause abnormal tensile stresses to the medial retinaculum of the knee. This could also be a source of low-grade inflammation and pain associated with patellar tracking dysfunction.

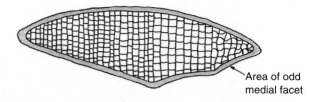

■ **FIG. 15-35.** Subchondral bone density of the patella. Density is reduced in the area of the odd medial facet.

Clinical Manifestations. The patient presenting with patellar tracking dysfunction usually demonstrates characteristic symptoms and signs consistent with the etiologic and pathologic factors mentioned. The consistent subjective complaints of a patient presenting with patellar tracking dysfunction include:

1. A gradual onset of pain. The patient often describes some recent increase in activities involving loaded knee extension or may report some knee injury or disuse preceding the onset of the problem.
2. Pain is felt primarily in a generalized area over the medial aspect of the knee and in the peripatellar regions.
3. The pain is aggravated by activities involving increased patellofemoral compressive stresses. These typically include descending stairs and sitting with the knee bent for long periods of time. Slowly applied loads, such as those involved with sitting with the knees bent, are likely to cause more discomfort than running or walking. This is because bone is stronger under fast strain rates for loads of equal magnitude.

The objective findings on physical examination of patients with patellar tracking dysfunction might include:

1. Rotatory limb malalignment—femoral antetorsion and lateral tibial torsion. Medial rotation of the femur is a common predisposing factor in patients with patellofemoral pain. The medial femoral torsion often causes a squinting of the patellae. Medial rotation of the femur is often associated with a tight iliotibial band and poor functioning of the posterior gluteus medius muscle. This gives rise to instability of the pelvis, causing an increase in

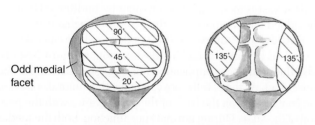

■ **FIG. 15-34.** Posterior aspect of the patella, showing contact areas of the facets during various degrees of flexion.

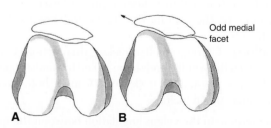

■ **FIG. 15-36.** (**A**) Position of patella during normal, loaded knee extension. (**B**) Abnormal lateral pull of the patella during loaded knee extension brings the odd medial facet into a contacting position.

dynamic Q angle, and increases the potential for patello-femoral pain.[237]

2. Abnormal position of the tibia relative to the femur (varus or valgus), and the presence or absence of torsion of the tibia. Common structural factors include lateral tibia torsion and marked tibia vara, especially when the varus is sharply localized to the tibia. If the lateral angulation of the tibia to the floor angle exceeds 10°, the extremity requires an excessive amount of subtalar joint pronation to produce a plantigrade foot. This can occur in both genu varum and tibia vara and may be a cause of peripatellar pain.[44]

3. Patellar malalignment. Quantifying the position of the patella is important because, as described above, exces-sive pressure on the odd facet may result if the patella's position is at fault. McConnell[235] described four abnormal patellar orientations: the glide component, tilt component, rotation component, and anteroposterior position (Fig. 15-37). By using the patellar poles as landmarks and comparing their positions with the planes of the femur, malalignment becomes apparent. These components can be assessed with the patient supine, knee extended, and quadriceps relaxed.

Patellar glide occurs when the patella moves from a neutral position. The distance from the center of the patella to the medial and lateral femoral condyles is assessed (Fig. 15-37A).[13] Typically the patient shows lateralization of the patella as a result of tightness of the

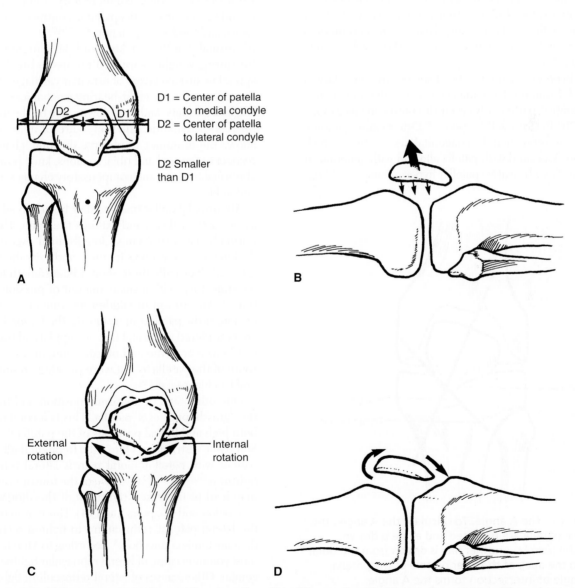

D1 = Center of patella to medial condyle
D2 = Center of patella to lateral condyle

D2 Smaller than D1

A

B

External rotation   Internal rotation

C

D

■ **FIG. 15-37.** Assessment of patella position. Patellar glide (**A**), patellar tilt (**B**), patellar rotation (**C**), and anteroposterior position (**D**). (Reprinted with permission from Arno A: A quantitative measurement of patella alignment. J Orthop Sports Phys Ther 12:237–242, 1990.)

lateral retinaculum. Patellar tilt evaluates the position of the medial and lateral facets of the patella. Patients with patellar tracking dysfunction frequently exhibit a more prominent medial facet (Fig. 15-37B). Patellar rotation occurs when the inferior pole deviates from the resting position. Rotations are described as internal (change to the medial side) or external (change to the lateral side; Fig. 15-37C). Anteroposterior position is assessed during quadriceps contraction. Normally the inferior pole should remain inferior and not tilt above the plane of the superior pole (Fig. 15-37D).

Arno[13] attempted to quantify the patellar position with a description of the A angle (Fig. 15-38). He argued that an A angle greater than 35° constituted malalignment when the Q angle remained constant. DiVeta and Vogelbach[77] showed A angle measurement to be reliable, with an average value of 12.3° for normal subjects and 23.2° for patients with patellar tracking dysfunction. This method relates patellar orientation to that of the tibial tubercle (Fig. 15-38).

4. Knee hyperextension may be observed with an enlarged fat pad. From this the clinician can infer that the quadriceps control, particularly eccentric control, in inner range (0 to 20° flexion) will be poor.[237] Other causes of knee hyperextension include congenital recurvatum, which may be associated with patella alta and with generalized joint laxity with relative patellar hypermobility.[278,354] Leg-length discrepancy may result in hyperextension on the shorter side during single-leg stance and at the push-off phase of gait, which may accelerate extensor mechanism difficulties.[30,352]

5. Increased foot pronation. Predisposing factors at the foot and ankle include increased foot pronation. To ascertain the weight-bearing status of the foot and detect any excessive pronation, determine the neutral position of the subtalar joint (see Chapter 16, Lower Leg, Ankle, and Foot). The normal weight-bearing foot should demonstrate a mild amount of pronation. If the patient is weight bearing or running with the foot out of neutral position and near full pronation, an obligatory medial tibial rotation occurs and is actually prolonged, resulting in an increased force that is absorbed by the soft tissues of the knee.[160,161] Entities that produce compensatory subtalar pronation include genu varum, triceps surae contractures, hindfoot varus, and forefoot supination.[35,155,160,161]

6. Abnormal patellar tracking and patellofemoral crepitus during weight bearing (if the tissue breakdown has spread to surface layers of articular cartilage). Observation of lower limb weight-bearing mechanics during gait, single-leg squats, and step-downs may be the most helpful test of dynamic function. Careful analysis of gait allows the examiner to observe dynamic changes with respect to femoral and tibial torsions, knee position, and abnormal tracking and compensatory changes in the foot and ankle.

   Abnormal patellar tracking may be observed in sitting as the patient flexes and extends the knee. The patella normally has 5 to 7 cm of longitudinal excursion with flexion and extension as it enters and exits the trochlear groove.[44] Normally there should be a smooth longitudinal trajectory, with a small amount of physiologic rotation.[194] Any abrupt or sudden movements at 10 to 30° flexion, as the patella enters or exits the femoral trochlea, are considered abnormal (i.e., abrupt lateral translations just before or at the end of extension, or a semicircular route of the patella as if it were pivoting around the lateral trochlear facet).[91]

   One other sign of abnormal position and tracking is the "grasshopper eye" patella. This is a combination of both high and lateral positions of the patella.[160]

7. Soft tissue restrictions. One of the frequent findings in the patient with patellofemoral pain is lateral retinaculum tightness.[91,99,100,182,267] Overuse of the tensor fasciae latae may lead to increased tightness of the iliotibial band (see below and Chapters 8 and 14). This may in turn cause the lateral patellar retinaculum to tighten secondary to their anatomic connection.[22] According to Merchant,[242] the most common cause of lateral retinacular tightness is congenital. Other causes of lateral retinaculum tightness are posttraumatic scarring, postsurgical fibrosis, and reflex sympathetic dystrophy.[242] Tightness of the lateral retinaculum is noted when the patella is assessed for passive

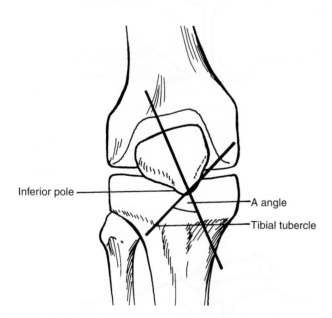

■ FIG. 15-38. The A angle. To calculate the A angle, the poles of the patella are palpated and a line is drawn bisecting the patella. Another line is drawn from the tibial tubercle to the apex of the inferior pole of the patella, and the angle of intersection forms the A angle. (Reprinted with permission from Arno A: A quantitative measurement of patella alignment. J Orthop Sports Phys Ther 12:237–242, 1990.)

medial excursion or glide of the patella, and when the retinaculum is palpated. Other soft tissue restrictions include:

- Tightness of the hamstrings places increased demand on the quadriceps during knee extension, which may increase patellofemoral joint reaction forces, whereas tight quadriceps increase compression of the patellofemoral joint.[22,144,251]
- Flexibility of the anterior hip structures. Available extension and lateral rotation of the hip are often limited because of chronic adaptive shortening of the anterior structures as a result of the underlying femoral antetorsion. Evaluate the patient in a figure-four position (Fig. 14-10) to assess available extension and lateral rotation.
- A tight gastrocnemius may make the patient walk with a slightly flexed knee, thereby putting more stress on the extensor mechanism about the knee.[144]

8. Visible vastus medialis obliquus atrophy when the patient is asked to contract the quadriceps strongly against resistance at 30° or in the presence of terminal extension lag. A useful method was proposed by Beck and Wildermuth[21] to assess a poorly functioning vastus medialis and to determine secondary substitutions (Fig. 15-26) and lack of muscle control (above) by using observation and palpation during active straight-leg raising. Substitutions that may occur include overuse of the proximal quadriceps and co-contraction by the hamstrings.

The strength of the hip abductors and lateral rotators warrants special attention, as weakness of these muscle groups has been associated with patellar tracking dysfunction.[22]

9. Discomfort when the patella is passively moved laterally (if the medial retinaculum is irritated) and tenderness to deep palpation of the backside of the medial patella and to palpation of the adductor tubercle, where the medial retinaculum attaches

10. Alterations in stability. Pelvic instability is often observed. Pelvic instability, depending on the tilt of the pelvis, may cause an increase in pelvic motion, and ultimately trunk rotation or lateral flexion. If the pelvis is anteriorly tilted, the patient exhibits an increase in pelvic rotation when walking because that individual has a lack of hip extension and external rotation. If the pelvis is posteriorly tilted, the patient presents with a Trendelenburg-like gait, including weakness of the gluteal muscles.[237] A patient with a short ITB demonstrates excessive medial rotation of the hip during stance phase of gait, allowing the pelvis on the opposite side to drop and giving a Trendelenburg appearance.[298]

11. Patellar discomfort elicited by provocation tests, which might include maintained inferior glide with an isometric contraction of the quadriceps, or resisted quadriceps contraction with the knee held at 30 to 45° flexion.

Management. The initial management for most patellar disorders is conservative. Sixty to 80% of knees treated respond favorably to nonoperative treatment.[182] The success of any conservative program relies on the compliance and cooperation of an informed patient. Treatment of patellar tracking dysfunction must take into account etiologic and pathologic factors. The most important early measure is to reduce activities involving high or prolonged patellofemoral compressive loads. This is necessary to prevent continued tissue trauma. The patient must understand the deleterious affects of such activities as descending stairs or bent-knee sitting, because these activities do not necessarily cause immediate pain.

Particular attention should be paid to strengthening the vastus medialis oblique (VMO). This may be necessary to correct insufficiency or as an attempt to compensate for structural causes of patellar tracking dysfunction. To strengthen the vastus medialis, it is often necessary to establish control of the muscle through techniques of neuromuscular facilitation (i.e., quick-stretch, cross-limb reversal, repeated contractions) and electrical stimulation.[292,328,336] For training to be effective, the patient must not experience pain while exercising, because this will have a strong inhibitory effect on muscle function.[326,332] The literature supports the concept of significant inhibition being present with pain and effusion.[219] Treatment to reduce pain and swelling result in enhanced strength measurements but no variation of the VMO or vastus lateralis (VL).

Traditionally, rehabilitation techniques for patients complaining of patellofemoral pain tended to strengthen the quadriceps group using open kinetic chain exercises. Straight-leg raising allows the least amount of patellofemoral contact force while maximally stressing the quadriceps muscle.[143,151] Vastus medialis activity is increased when performing straight-leg raising if the patient is instructed to "set" the quadriceps before lifting the leg.[197] Adding an adduction force while performing the exercise may facilitate the vastus medialis because muscle fibers have been found to originate from the tendon of the adductor magnus.[32,80,289] Doucette and Goble[80] describe this kind of vastus medialis exercise by performing straight-leg raising with the femur externally rotated. Selected hip adduction exercises have also been suggested as a means of increasing vastus medialis strength (squeezing a pillow between the knees positioned in about 20° of flexion).[32,34,127,289] Current literature suggests that although adduction of the hip shows overflow to the VMO, it is not sufficient to provide a strong training stimulus (greater than 70% of maximum voluntary contraction) to this structure.[219] Furthermore, the current literature does not support that isolated VMO exercises exist and that both the VMO and VL are highly active in terminal range of extension.[219]

The current treatment approach has a new direction and focus that includes strengthening of the quadriceps through closed kinetic chain exercises, regaining optimal patellar tracking, and regaining neuromuscular control.[358] Weight-bearing training is very important because the knee primarily functions in a closed kinetic chain. Training in weight bearing also places a major emphasis on eccentric control, thus facilitating muscle hypertrophy.[80,110,121] Closed kinetic chain exercises were discussed in Chapter 14, Hip. In the case of patellofemoral rehabilitation, mini squats and wall slides from 0 to 40° (see Fig. 14-37), lateral step-up (see Fig. 14-41), fitter or slide board exercises, a stationary bike, and leg presses from 0 to 60° are all examples of closed kinetic chain strengthening exercises.

Another goal in the current treatment approach is regaining optimal patellar positioning and tracking. This goal may be accomplished by stretching the tight lateral structures, correcting patellar orientation, and improving the timing and force of the VMO contraction.

Stretching. Assess the extensibility of the lateral retinaculum by noting the excursion of medial patellar movement with the knee close to full extension. If the lateral retinaculum appears tight, it should be stretched using the same technique as used to test its mobility. Medial-lateral tilt of the patellofemoral joint (see Fig. 15-52A) and strong medial glide techniques with the patient in sidelying (see Fig. 15-52B) have proved to be most effective at stretching the tight lateral structures around the knee.[235] According to McConnell,[235] this maneuver facilitates vastus medialis training because patellar movements are no longer restricted. The patient should be instructed in self-mobilization. Prior or simultaneous heating with ultrasound may enhance the effectiveness of stretching procedures.

Other consideration for successfully stretching the tight lateral structures involves a combination of soft tissue manipulations and active and passive stretching techniques. Longitudinal soft tissue stretching techniques of the retinaculum and insertion of the iliotibial band may be used applying traction with either passive or active motion of the knee (see Fig. 8-20) or in a closed kinetic chain while working on normal tracking of the patella. Manual stretch of the tensor fascia lata and ITB (see Figs. 8-69 through 8-72) and self-stretch can be used to manually stretch the entire band (see Box 8-9) when indicated. Mennell's selective stretching of various parts of the band and muscle belly may be used as well as other soft tissue mobilization techniques (see Figs. 8-14B, 8-70, and 8-71).[241]

Tight hamstrings have long been recognized as a cause of various extensor mechanism disorders.[21,152] Efficient lengthening can be accomplished by gentle, nonballistic techniques (i.e., reciprocal inhibition of antagonists: contract–relax, hold–relax), prolonged static stretch, and soft tissue mobilization techniques (see Fig. 7-32 and Box 8-9).[45,64,88,300,327,335]

Taping and Bracing. There is evidence that the application of patellar taping or a brace significantly reduces perceived pain and improves quadriceps output.[219] There is limited support that taping or bracing influence patellar alignment. Because a decrease in pain perception occurs, the application of taping or a brace can be an assistive measure enabling the inclusion of pain-free exercise.

On the basis of the works of McConnell[235] to enhance more normal tracking, the patella should be exercised during weight bearing, and it should be firmly taped in the direction of normal tracking during these exercises. The three components of the patella that must be assessed before taping are:

1. Glide. Most patients require mobilization of the patella; usually medial glide of the patella, which is most restricted (see Fig. 15-52B). Correction of the glide component involves placing the tape from the lateral border of the patella and firmly pulling it to just past the medial femoral condyle (Fig. 15-39).[235–237]

2. Tilt. Most patients present with a positive tilt sign (0° or less) because of tightness of the deep lateral retinacular fibers (Fig. 15-28A). Correction of this lateral tilt requires stretching and soft tissue mobilization (see Fig. 8-20). The patella should be firmly taped from the midline of the patella medially to lift the lateral border and provide a passive stretch to the lateral structures (Fig. 15-40).

3. Rotation (Fig. 15-37C). The longitudinal axis of the femur and the patella should be in line with one another. To correct any alterations in alignment, firm taping from either the superior or inferior poles can be used. To correct lateral rotation of the inferior pole, tape from the middle inferior pole upward (Fig. 15-41). For internal rotation of the inferior pole, tape from the middle superior pole downward.

Exercises and Home Program. Therapeutic exercise components of the rehabilitation program should include quadriceps reeducation using surface electromyography, pelvic, hip, and foot muscle reeducation, and activities of daily living or sports-specific retraining. The strategy for VMO rehabilitation is to restore strength gradually but painlessly. Once proficiency of muscle contraction is achieved, descending and ascending stairs and activities of daily living or sports-specific rehabilitation can continue. Isokinetic knee extension should not be used in the rehabilitation of patellofemoral joint injuries because of the stress they can place across the patellofemoral joint and the strain that these exercises produce in the patellar tendon and periretinacular tissues.[304]

McConnell[235] found the following exercises to be most useful:

1. With the patient in a walk-stance position (symptomatic leg forward) and the knee flexed to 30°, have him or her contract the vastus medialis and hold for a period of 10 seconds or so while the foot is supinated past subtalar neutral and then allowed to slowly return to partial pronation (slightly out of the resting position of pronation). This is repeated several times, then the knee is straightened and the exercise repeated. The object is to train the invertors of the foot, thus decreasing pronation.

2. The same exercise is repeated but with the knee flexed to about 70°. If the patient has difficulty achieving vastus medialis control with either of these exercises, a slightly turned-out position may facilitate control. Have the patient relax the vastus lateralis and hamstrings as much as possible with both these exercises. Pain-free progression may include half and three-quarter squats as greater control of the quadriceps is achieved.

3. Descending stairs is performed as an exercise to further facilitate eccentric and concentric quadriceps control. The

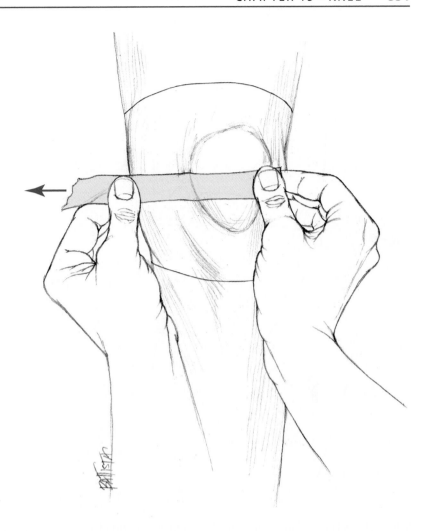

■ **FIG. 15-39.** Taping to correct positive patellar lateral glide component.

leg to be exercised remains on the top step while the patient steps down and then back up slowly, with the leg remaining on the step contracting eccentrically and concentrically. Emphasis is again placed on proper alignment and normal tracking. Progression can be made by altering the height of the step or providing resistance.

Neuromuscular Control. The rehabilitation program should include exercises to reestablish balance, neuromuscular control, and coordination activities in multiple planes. Neuromuscular control also involves improving the timing and force of VMO contraction. It is generally agreed that it is more important to emphasize the quality rather than the quantity of the contraction (concentrating more on motor skill acquisition) rather than on strengthening exercises. The use of dual-channel biofeedback capable of monitoring both VMO and VL electromyographic activity is recommended for the patient to gain control over both force of contraction and timing for the firing of the VMO.[285] The clinician should address concentric and eccentric control in a variety of functional tasks and position. Closed kinetic chain exercises can be performed using the biofeedback loop. Stepping, climbing, bicycling, and selective weightlifting can be performed, using the biofeed-

back sensor to assure the VMO is contracting during these activities.[304] Training on balance boards and unstable surfaces is useful for proprioceptive training (see sensorimotor activities in Chapter 14, Hip).

Functional Biomechanics. Integration of specific structural or biomechanical components that may relieve symptoms include the choice of shoes or custom biomechanical orthoses. If the condition is associated with abnormal foot pronation and does not respond to the treatment measures mentioned, consider stabilizing the foot to control pronation. This may be done with various orthotic devices, such as a contoured arch support, or shoe modifications, such as a medial heel wedge or lateral sole wedge. Shoe orthoses may be helpful in patients who have patellofemoral pain associated with pronated feet.[325]

Leg-length discrepancy and a hyperextended knee and abnormal gait can be corrected with a combination of a heel lift, gait training (using a program of resistive pelvic training and PNF techniques), and quadriceps control exercises.[184,185,260]

A few patients with patellar tracking dysfunction do not respond satisfactorily to a well-designed, appropriately instituted conservative treatment program. Common causes of failure include inadequate restriction of activities in the early

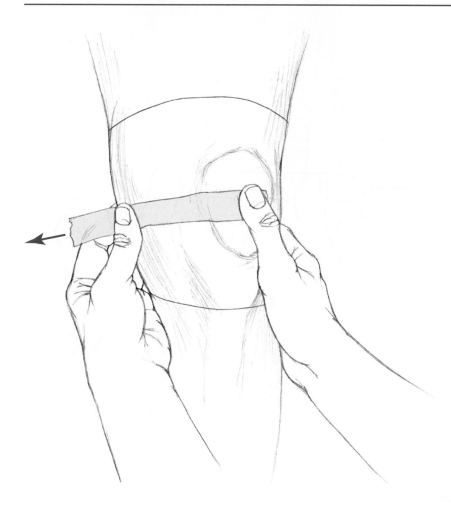

■ **FIG. 15-40.** Taping to correct positive lateral tilt.

stages of treatment and inadequate or inappropriate quadriceps strengthening.

QUADRICEPS CONTUSIONS (ANTERIOR THIGH)

A contusion to the lateral and, more importantly, the anterior
aspect of the thigh is often underestimated. It should be realized that this can be one of the most disabling injuries, and suspicion should be high after direct trauma in sports. A severe
blow to the thigh involves direct injury to the myofibrils and
blood vessels. Subsequently osteoblasts can replace fibroblasts
in myositis ossificans within the healing hematoma 1 week after
injury.[106] The patellofemoral joint can be directly involved,
especially if the contusion is in the distal third of the quadriceps. This is secondary to irritation when blood tracks down
the fascia planes to the knee.[106]

The clinical symptom complex involves a history of direct
blow to the anterior thigh, with resultant tenderness and
swelling. At the time of injury, the patient may develop pain,
loss of function to the quadriceps mechanism, and loss of knee
flexion range of motion. The thigh becomes progressively
stiffer while at the same time the quadriceps become more
and more unresponsive. If the injury is severe, swelling and
tightness of the thigh musculature are observed soon after-
ward. Worsening of symptoms is seen on active contraction of

the quadriceps or on passive stretching. How relaxed the
quadriceps was at the time of injury and how forceful the blow
will determine the grade of injury.

Physical Examination. Functional deficits may evolve
around preexisting tightness of the hamstring muscles, gastrocnemius and soleus muscles and in particular, the rectus
femoris.[106] The weak and inhibited muscles are generally the
vasti of the quadriceps.

I. Grade I Contusion. The patient may present a normal gait
    cycle, negative swelling, and only mild discomfort on pal-
    pation. Resisted knee extension may not cause discomfort,
    and active knee flexion in prone is usually within normal
    limits.[72]
II. Grade II Contusion. The patient may have a normal gait
    cycle. Attempting to continue activity will likely cause the
    injury to become progressively disabling.[72] If the gait cycle is
    abnormal, the patient may demonstrate ipsilateral anterior
    pelvic tilt in an attempt to slacken the fascia of the quadri-
    ceps and the rectus femoris.[106] The knee is generally held in
    an extended position, resulting in compensatory hip external
    rotation to use the hip adductors to pull the leg through dur-
    ing the swing phase of gait and premature plantar flexion of
    the ankle at heel strike. Swelling may be moderate to severe,

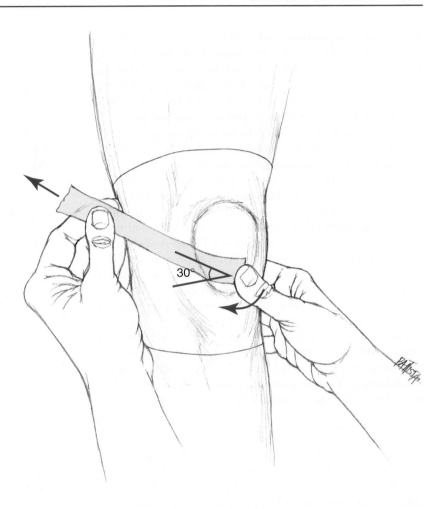

■ FIG. 15-41. Taping to correct positive lateral rotation.

with a noticeable defect and pain on palpation. Noticeable weakness of the quadriceps mechanism may be evident, and active range of motion of knee flexion limited (20 to 50% restriction of full range of motion).

III. Grade III Contusion. The patient may herniate the muscle through the fascia to cause a marked defect, severe bleeding, and disability.[106] The patient may not be able to ambulate without crutches. Severe swelling and a bulge of muscle tissue may be observed. Prone active knee flexion may be severely limited (50% or greater is noted), and resisted knee extension may not be tolerated.

Management. The sooner treatment is commenced the better the prognosis for the patient.[293] Immediately after the injury, it is usually not possible for either the client or the examiner to determine whether the injury will result in a major or minor hematoma. It is best to err on the conservative side and treat all contusions to the thigh as potentially serious. The following procedure is recommended:

- Acute phase (0 to 48 hours). During the first 24 to 48 hours, treatment consists of ice up to 20 minutes every hour, compression dressing, gentle active range of motion (in the pain-free range only), and electrical muscle stimulation modalities to decrease pain, bleeding, and swelling and to counteract atrophy. Evaluation should be instituted immediately. Soft tissue manipulations are contraindicated in the first 48 hours.

- Recovery phase (2 to 5 days to 3 to 4 weeks). In this phase, any functional deficits of tight hamstrings, gastrocnemius, soleus, and rectus femoris should be dealt with.[106] Crutches should be used until a normal gait can be accomplished free of pain. Soft tissue therapy such as manual lymphatic drainage, with the aim of promoting lymphatic drainage and reducing pain, may be introduced.[357] Modalities such as ultrasound and deep heating can be helpful in blood resorption but should be used with caution. Generally the quadriceps (particularly the vasti) are inhibited or weak. Within 3 to 5 days, active range of motion as well as PNF and reciprocal relaxation patterns are introduced. In the next several weeks (grade II and III contusions), crutches may be discontinued and increased resisted quadriceps exercises can be started. If should be noted that isometric and concentric strengthening in the pain-free range is started before eccentric exercises are permitted. As active range of motion increases and approaches 95 to 100° knee flexion, swimming, aquatic therapy, and cycling may be performed if the seat height is adjusted to the patient's available range.

Soft tissue manipulations and stretching of the hamstrings, gastrocnemius, soleus, and rectus femoris can also be started. The patient is then taught self-stretching and closed-chain kinetic exercises with an emphasis on quadriceps and glutei muscle strengthening (see Figs. 14-37, 14-40, and 14-42). Functional adaptations, such as ipsilateral anterior pelvic tilt and a resistance to flex the knee during the swing phase resulting in premature plantar flexion at heel strike, should be treated as well if these adaptations exist.[106]

It is important to rule out myositis ossificans. At 3 to 6 weeks, a plain radiographic examination can be done with concentration on the soft tissue. If this condition is present, activities are reduced along with the administration of nonsteroidal anti-inflammatory medications. Reassessment in 7 to 10 days is advised if myositis ossificans is present.[106] If the condition has not worsened, rehabilitation may restart. After 3 to 4 weeks, maintenance activities, including walking, slide board, plyometrics, and running with starting and stopping can be considered. Balance, proprioceptive, and sensorimotor retraining is critical and is almost always lost with this type of injury (see Figs 14-45 through 14-47). A patient with a grade III quadriceps contusion may require 3 weeks to 3 months for rehabilitation.[72] Compression and protective padding should be worn during all competition until the patient is symptom free.

PLICA SYNDROME

The medial synovial plica is found in 20 to 60% of knees[8] but does not necessarily cause symptoms (Fig. 15-42).[188] Occasionally this plica may become thickened and fibrotic, causing anteromedial knee pain and snapping or clicking, mimicking a patellofemoral or meniscal problem. These tissue changes are often initiated by trauma that results in synovitis; this is more common in athletes.[251] Joggers and swimmers (breast-strokers) commonly have symptoms.[274] Pain is usually intermittent and increases with activity and descending stairs.

Amatuzzi and associates[8] found conservative treatment to be effective in 60% of cases. Conservative treatment using extensor mechanism rehabilitative techniques and ice massage may reverse tissue changes. Treatment is directed at reducing compression over the anterior compartment of the knee by using stretching exercises (i.e., hamstrings, gastrocnemius, and quadriceps).

If conservative treatment fails, arthroscopic excision may be undertaken to relieve symptoms. It is often necessary to continue work on the extensor mechanism through exercise and perhaps external support. Several studies have found arthroscopic surgery to be efficacious in the treatment of pathologic plicae.[126,186,271–274]

PATELLAR TENDINITIS (JUMPER'S KNEE)

Repetitive jumping in sports such as volleyball and basketball can create chronic inflammatory changes of the patellar tendon either at the superior patellar pole (usually referred as quadriceps tendinitis), the tibial tubercle, or most commonly, at the distal pole of the patella (patellar tendinitis). It is there-

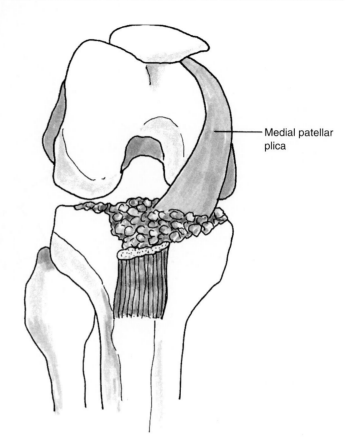

■ **FIG. 15-42.** Medial plica. (Adapted from Kulund DN: The Injured Athlete, 2nd ed. Philadelphia, JP Lippincott, 1988:468.)

fore an insertional tendinopathy resulting in derangement of the bone–tendon unit.[51] These changes are related primarily to overuse. Pain is the key complaint and is associated with swelling and joint tenderness. Pain may be described as burning pain with use or after prolonged sitting with the knee flexed.[125] Blazina et al.[28] describe four stages of jumper's knee. Stage 1 is pain only after activity. Stage 2 is pain at onset, disappearing during and reappearing after activity. Stage 3 is constant pain and inability to participate in sports. Stage 4 is complete rupture of the patellar tendon. Stage 3 may sometimes be irreversible and require surgery.[232]

Patellar tendinitis rarely, if ever, occurs in knees without predisposing physical findings found in tracking problems (i.e., patella alta, vastus medialis dysplasia).[354] Many factors known to aggravate extensor mechanism disorders can accentuate the symptoms of patellar tendinitis (changes in the hamstring to quadriceps ratio and inflexibility of hamstrings or triceps surae). Both intrinsic and extrinsic factors have been implicated as possible causes. Intrinsic factors include biomechanical alterations in the extensor mechanism, such as hypermobility, altered Q angle, and genu valgum or genu recurvatum.[251] Extrinsic factors include frequency and intensity of training, training surface (especially on hard surfaces), and training frequency.

Objective Findings

- Point tenderness occurs on the posterior aspect of the inferior pole of the patella, especially if the patella is pushed distally.
- Some swelling may be noticed around the patella in acute cases; quadriceps wasting is apparent in long-standing cases.
- Pain is reproduced on resisting active knee flexion with possible pain on passive knee flexion.
- Crepitus may be present on passive movement of the patellar tendon.

Management. Because patellar tendinitis involves a chronic inflammation, early management strategies may take one of two courses. One approach is the traditional approach designed to reduce inflammation, which includes rest, anti-inflammatory medication, cryotherapy, and ultrasound. Another approach would be to use deep friction massage (see Box 8-2) designed to exacerbate the acute inflammation, so that the healing process is no longer "stuck" in the inflammatory-response phase and can move on to the fibroblastic repair phase.[285] It has been recommended that deep transverse frictions be applied to the inferior pole of the patella for 5 to 7 minutes every other day for approximately 1 week.[285] Friction to the teno-osseous junctions attaching to the patella are only effective if the patella is tilted and the pressure from the clinician's finger is directed at a 45° angle rather than straight down. Ombergt et al.[266] recommend deep transverse friction massage over the tendinous fibers of the suprapatellar tendon for 20 minutes (10 to 20 sessions) to produce a good result (see Box 8-2). During deep friction massage treatment, all medications or modalities to reduce inflammation should be eliminated.[285]

Regardless of which of the two treatment approaches is used, once the problem begins to resolve a rehabilitation program should begin. Traditionally, extensor mechanism rehabilitation has been used with patellar tendinitis, but more recently work on the eccentric function of the quadriceps has been emphasized.[57,164,354] The basis of a knee program is to use activities that place maximal stress on the tendon to increase its tensile stress by performing variations of quick mini-squats.[57] Eccentric squats, called drop squats, are performed with the patient moving slowly from standing to a squat position and return.[285] To increase stress, the speed of the drop is increased until a mild level of pain is experienced. Biomechanical linkage with ankle mechanics has demonstrated that most patients present with weakness of the ankle dorsiflexors. Again, good results have been obtained with a program of eccentric work.[152,354]

Flexibility training is important: it increases the elasticity of the muscle–tendon unit and increases the tensile strength of the tendon. In chronic conditions in which scar tissue has formed at the teno-osseous junctions, limitation in flexion may be apparent. Flexibility exercises will increase range of motion, but more by stretching the quadriceps than the scar tissue. When this is the case, soft tissue manipulation may be required in an attempt to rupture the adherent scarring.[251] The patella should be mobilized using the techniques described in the joint mobilization section (see Figs. 15-52 and 15-53). As with any overuse syndrome, part of the management of this condition involves avoidance or modification of training. Strength must be developed symmetrically, and footwear should incorporate shock-absorbing materials.

OSGOOD-SCHLATTER DISEASE

Osgood-Schlatter disease used to be considered a form of osteochondritis associated with a partial avulsion of the patellar tendon at its insertion into the tibial tubercle before this apophysis unites. More recently the process has been viewed as one part of the spectrum of mechanical problems related to the extensor mechanism.[354] Almost all patients with this condition have some mechanical inefficiency of the extensor mechanism. In fact, it is now thought that this is not really a disease, but a form of tendinitis of the knee tendon. In young athletes, the tendon is attached to prebone, which is weaker than normal adult bone. With excessive stresses on the tendon from running and jumping, the structure becomes irritated and a tendinitis begins. This condition first appears in adolescents and usually resolves when the patient reaches the age of 18 or 19.

Objective findings include:

- A tender swelling over the tibial tubercle
- Pain reproduced on resisting quadriceps extension; squatting, running, and jumping may also reproduce the pain.
- Decreased flexibility. Most patients have significant restriction in the hamstrings, triceps surae, and quadriceps muscles.

Management. The mechanical inefficiencies of the extensor mechanism should be treated by appropriate rehabilitative exercises. Inflexibility should be addressed through stretching and ankle dorsiflexion strengthening if weakness is found. This condition usually resolves without any significant additional treatment. Complete immobilization is neither necessary nor practical. A simple patellar support, such as a Neoprene rubber knee sleeve, may help.

Strained Iliotibial Band Friction Syndrome

ITB syndrome is a common source of knee pain in competitive athletes, but may occur in workers and recreational athletes (see overuse syndromes of the lower quadrant, Chapter 8, Soft Tissue Manipulations).[71] The gluteus maximus and the tensor fascia lata, from which it arises, affect the mechanics of the ITB. The ITB is pulled anteriorly by the tensor fascia lata in flexion and posteriorly by the gluteus maximus in extension.[200] The iliotibial tract is pulled posteriorly by the biceps tendon, keeping it taut throughout knee flexion. Because of its angle of insertion, the ITB is a knee extensor from 0 to 30° and a knee flexor when the knee is flexed 30° or more.[231] The ITB crosses back and forth over the lateral femoral epicondyle with repetitive flexion and extension. The repetitive rubbing creates a friction syndrome and an inflammatory condition. The bursa beneath the ITB often becomes inflamed. Occasionally the popliteal tendon or the lateral ligament becomes inflamed.[293] A tight ITB, forefoot varus, tight hip adductors, leg-length discrepancy, or sudden increases in running distance or mileage can exacerbate this injury.

Signs and symptoms include:

- Lateral knee pain in activity, usually occurring at a fixed distance at a given pace; stinging during deceleration when the foot contacts the ground (foot strike). Pain may be localized to the lateral epicondyle or run diffusely along the iliotibial tract. Climbing stairs or running on inclines aggravates pain.
- Pain is usually elicited by full weight bearing with knee at 30° of flexion.
- There is tenderness over the lateral epicondyle (occasionally over the lateral joint line), at the origin of the popliteal tendon, or at Gerdy's tubercle. Because of its attachment to the ITB, the lateral retinaculum may also be tender.
- Frequently there is localized effusion and occasionally palpable crepitus over the femoral condyle on repeated flexion and extension of the knee.
- Most patients have a positive Ober's test (see Fig. 14-20) and Noble's compression test (see Fig. 14-24) the majority of the time.

MANAGEMENT

ITB syndrome management should address all contributing factors. Correction of training errors and any faulty biomechanics must be addressed in treatment. Symptomatic relief measures such as ice massage, ultrasound, and anti-inflammatory drugs can help control pain and inflammation and speed healing. During the subacute phase, treatment may include:

- Unloading the lateral structures of the knee (if the condition is severe) with taping
- Soft tissue manipulations to the gluteus medius, tensor fascia lata, and ITB as indicated
- Assisted stretching to all lower quadrant muscles as appropriate, using contract–relax and hold–relax techniques
- Home program of sustained static stretching of all lower limb muscle groups as indicated, as well as dynamic stretching of hamstrings and gluteals
- Strengthening using closed-chain kinetic exercises as indicated (e.g., squats, lunges, step-up and step-down, leg press)
- Agility drills, cardiovascular exercises, balance, and proprioceptive reeducation
- Abnormal foot mechanics should be addressed. Orthoses may decrease the lateral knee stresses by controlling the foot's position.

Flexor Mechanism Disorders

Flexor mechanism disorders encompass several anatomic structures. The popliteal area is surrounded superiorly and medially by the semimembranosus and semitendinosus muscle tendon, superiorly and laterally by the biceps femoris, and inferiorly by the two heads of the gastrocnemius muscle. Other anatomic structures that maybe involved in flexor mechanism disorders include a strained popliteal muscle, a sprained PCL (see above), or a lesion of the tibiofibular joint. Hamstring strains have been discussed in detail in Chapter 14, Hip.

HAMSTRING INSERTIONAL TENDINITIS

History of hamstring tendinitis will generally indicate that there has been a change in training (intensity, duration, or surface) with a gradual onset of symptoms.[279] When dealing with medial hamstring insertions differentiation must be made with a pes anserinus bursitis, which may refer pain to the distal medial hamstrings.[125] Tendinitis of the semimembranosus can also mimic a meniscal injury because of its proximity to the joint line. Long-distance runners are prone to tendinitis of the insertion of the semimembranosus on the posterior medial capsule of the knee.[36,152] The semimembranosus functions synergistically with the popliteus to prevent excessive lateral rotation of the tibia. Hyperpronating problems of the foot can stress the insertion of the semimembranosus. Medial rotation or antetorsion of the hip and femur may also stress the semimembranosus insertion.[152]

Biceps tendinitis usually occurs as an overuse lesion in athletes. Pain develops at the outer side of the knee, which may be confused with an irritated ITB. In palpating for involvement, the examiner should abduct the thigh with the patient prone to relax the ITB. Functional examination is entirely negative except that resisted flexion hurts at the outer side. Resisted lateral rotation is also painful. Tenderness is found at the biceps tendon, usually at the tenoperiosteal insertion at the head of the fibula.[266]

Key Objective Tests[125]

1. Pain on resisted knee flexion of medial and lateral sides
2. Possible pain on passive lateral or medial rotation of the tibia

Treatment. Along with the established methods of treatment of chronic hamstring strains (see Chapter 14, Hip), friction massage is a primary treatment for hamstring insertional tendinitis (see Box 8-2). Stretching, endurance strengthening of the hamstrings, and functional rehabilitation is necessary before returning to full activities. Hunter and Poole[152] also recommend resisted toe curls and posterior tibialis strengthening.

STRAINED POPLITEUS MUSCLE

Tendinitis of the popliteal follows overuse injuries, usually from long-distance running. Excessive quadriceps fatigue may predispose to popliteus involvement.[105] Hyperpronation of the foot may result in either popliteal or bicipital tendinitis at the knee secondary to overuse. The patient usually complains of pain on downhill running or walking but no pain on uphill running. Although the muscle is a flexor and medial rotator of the leg, its main function is to prevent a sliding forward of the lateral femoral condyle on the fixed tibia (an important active stabilizer) during the stance phase in walking or running, especially in running downstairs or descending stairs.[16,225,280] The prevention of forward sliding is also a function of the PCL (passive stabilizer), and a strained popliteus can closely simulate a ligamentous strain of the PCL.[266]

Key Objective Tests

- Resisted flexion and medial rotation hurt at the lateral or posterolateral aspect of the knee (patient is prone with the knee flexed 20°).[266] The patient rotates the tibia medially on the femur while the examiner resists against the distal medial foot with counterpressure against the lateral calcaneus.[19]
- Pain occurs on the lateral aspect of the knee on weight bearing with the knee flexed to 15 to 20°.[233] There may be pain on sitting cross-legged.[125]
- With the knee in the figure-four position, the LCL and popliteal tendon are stretched and can be palpated. When the popliteal tendon is inflamed, joint tenderness is noticed at its insertion on the lateral surface of the femoral condyle or the muscle belly.[148,233]

Foot and knee biomechanics and running gait should all be evaluated.

Treatment. Treatment consists of rest, ice for the first 72 hours, ultrasound, and flexibility and strengthening exercises. Lesions of the muscle belly and tendon respond to deep friction massage (see Box 8-4).[266] Proper training techniques and appropriate shoes should also be addressed. The patient should only run on level surfaces until the lesion is healed.

GASTROCNEMIUS INSERTIONAL TENDINOUS LESIONS (TENNIS LEG)

Tendinous lesions at the origin of the gastrocnemius are very uncommon. Ruptures or strains may occur at the origin near the popliteal space.[125] Tennis leg, a strain of the gastrocnemius normally involving the medial head at its musculotendinous insertion with the Achilles tendon, is far more common. Acute posterior knee pain is usually caused by a mild sprain of the posterior capsule, a PCL sprain, a strain to one of the gastrocnemius muscles, or rupture of the plantaris muscle.

Different types of treatment have been promoted for tennis leg. Most authorities advocate partial or plantarflexed position with 2 to 4 cm of heel lift,[59] although others claim that a neutral ankle total immobilization early on will prevent further tissue damage. Some authorities recommend that a 90° neutral position gives a better result by preventing contraction and tightening of the fascia to limit the spread of bruising.[105] Transverse friction and active contractions of the muscle are useful during the recovery phase (see Chapter 8, Soft Tissue Manipulations).[59,266] Massage involving calf-kneading and transverse frictions ensures adequate broadening of the mus-

cle. Stretching of the gastrocnemius and soleus muscles begins in sitting and progresses to standing. Strengthening exercises begin in open kinetic chain and progress to closed kinetic chain exercises. Gait reeducation is used to encourage equal stride length and adoption of a normal heel-toe rhythm avoiding lateral rotation of the leg.[251] When the calf is pain free, strength activities give way to power movements.

Occasionally the fabella, a sesamoid bone in the lateral head of the gastrocnemius (Fig. 15–10A), which articulates with the femoral condyle, may develop similar changes as the patella (chondromalacia fabellae).[53] Pain may be reproduced on full passive flexion or extension of the knee. Manual therapy intervention may include gentle transverse stretching of the lateral head of the gastrocnemius muscle and fabella mobilizations.[363] If symptoms are sufficiently severe the fabella should be removed.[53]

POSTEROLATERAL KNEE INJURIES AND LESIONS OF PROXIMAL TIBIOFIBULAR JOINT

Another possible cause of posterior knee pain on resisted flexion of the knee is a lesion of the proximal tibiofibular joint. Lesions of the superior tibiofibular joint include direct trauma, subluxation, and instability.[53] A sprain of the proximal tibiofibular joint can develop after a trauma to the ankle joint, or as the result of repetitive strains.[266] The findings on clinical examination are the same as in biceps tendinitis (see above). Because contraction of the biceps pulls the fibular backward on the tibia, resisted flexion and resisted lateral rotation hurt at the outer side of the knee. However, when biceps tendon is examined for tenderness none is found. Direct trauma may cause a hematoma formation and may result in calcification of the joint capsule.[53] Joint movements are then restricted and pain is reproduced, especially on ankle movements. Joint mobilization techniques include anterior and posterior glides (see Fig. 15-54).

Posterolateral knee injuries can be very debilitating. The majority of posterolateral knee injuries are caused by a blow to the anteromedial aspect of the knee, a contact or noncontact hyperextension injury, or a varus contact injury.[191] The fibular collateral ligament, popliteus tendon, and the popliteofibular ligament are the main static stabilizers against abnormal varus and posterolateral translational movements (Fig. 15-10).[192] The fibular collateral ligament is extra-articular, and if it is torn by itself there will not be an intra-articular effusion unless deeper structures are involved. The ligament can be easily palpated in the figure-four knee position. All of the stabilizers (see above) may be injured as well as the meniscotibial portion of the midthird lateral capsular ligament, coronary ligament of the posterior horn of the lateral meniscus, the popliteomeniscal fascicles, portion of the ITB, and the long and short head of the biceps femoris.[192]

A physical examination that includes the posterior lateral drawer test, reverse pivot-shift (Fig. 15-21), external recurvatum test (Fig. 15-18C), varus stress test at 30° (see Fig. 15-50), dial test at 30 and 90° (Fig. 15-22), and an assessment varus thrust gait are essential to properly diagnose a posterolateral knee injury.[192]

Treatment of the fibular collateral ligament alone is similar to that used for medial collateral ligament sprains. Treatment for patients with grade I to II posterolateral knee complex injuries are usually treated conservatively with a knee immobilizer in full extension for 3 to 4 weeks with no knee motion allowed.[192] The patient may do straight-leg raises and quadriceps sets in the knee immobilizer. After immobilization, weight-bearing, closed-chain quadriceps exercises (with the avoidance of active hamstring exercises for the first 6 to 10 weeks) are allowed. In general, patients who have grade III injuries have been found to do poorly with nonoperative treatment, resulting in an unstable knee with severe symptoms and posttraumatic osteoarthritis.[171] Kannus[171] emphasizes that in grade III sprains, the ACL is often injured as well, and the damage may be missed by clinical methods at the initial examination.

Osteoarthritis

Primary osteoarthritis has no known cause; secondary osteoarthrosis can be traced to abnormal joint mechanics. Whether posttraumatic (more common in men) or idiopathic (women), the salient clinical issues are the same: activity-related pain and swelling accompanied by radiographic changes.[105] Abnormal knee mechanics produce secondary changes in the articular cartilage, subchondral bone, and supportive structures of the knee. The knee is a common site of osteoarthritis of the femorotibial and patellofemoral joints, possibly because it is often subject to trauma.[173,224,318] Previous fractures of the joint surfaces, ligamentous instability, or tears of the meniscus may all be complicated by subsequent degenerative changes. Osteoarthritis may be a physiologic response to repetitive, longitudinal impulse-loading of the joint. Changes may involve either the medial or lateral tibiofemoral compartment, the patellofemoral joint, or any combination of these, or may be panarticular, involving all three areas.

Osteoarthritis usually begins in the medial or lateral tibiofemoral compartment, where it may be related to the articular cartilage damage that follows meniscal tears.[131] One of the compartments is usually involved if there is any knee deformity (e.g., the medial compartment is associated with a varus deformity, the lateral compartment with valgus deformity). As the disease progresses, the degenerative changes in either compartment tend to increase the degree of the existing deformity. If there is a leg-length disparity, the knee on the longer side is usually involved.[78] A flexed knee gait often results on the longer side, if the shorter side is not compensated for with a built-up shoe. This results in increased patellofemoral forces, leading to excessive wear and degenerative changes in the joint.

The most common alteration in alignment of the osteoarthritic knee is a varus deformity. This results in increased forces in the medial compartment, which creates a degenerative lesion of the medial meniscus and subsequent degenerative changes of the medial compartment, and eventually becomes panarticular. Varus deformity is often associated with internal femoral torsion. Because these persons tend to walk with their feet pointed straight ahead by externally rotating the tibia, torsional malalignment also produces patellofemoral arthritis and subsequent abnormal mechanics of the extensor mechanism.

Any condition resulting in a loss of rotation at the hip will eliminate the screw-home mechanism of the knee. This results in vastus medialis atrophy, lateral tibial rotation, increased ligamentous laxity of the knee, and eventual genu valgum deformity and degenerative changes in the knee.

In the tibiofemoral compartment, the meniscus is also usually involved in the degenerative process. As the joint space narrows, increased pressure is carried by the weight-bearing surface of the meniscus, which develops increased degenerative changes and, occasionally, a horizontal cleavage type of tear. The meniscus is slowly ground away, and the anterior part of the meniscus may actually disappear.[323]

HISTORY

The clinical features of primary and secondary osteoarthritis are the same. The major complaint is usually pain, which may be muscular, capsular, or perhaps venous in origin. The pain is usually medial and presents at both weight bearing and rest.[105] It often awakens the patient at night. The pain is frequently associated with an effusion, usually described by the patient as a sense of "tightness" or "fullness." Morning stiffness is also a common complaint. This is relieved after motion, but the knee becomes painful and stiff again once the weight-bearing tolerance of the joint is exceeded by prolonged standing or walking. A possible differentiation from rheumatoid arthritis is that in osteoarthritis the morning stiffness is milder and does not last long.[75] The muscles of the thigh, particularly the quadriceps, become painful as a fixed flexion contracture of the knee develops with resulting instability. An insecure knee results in episodes of giving way, secondary to muscle fatigue, and transient severe pain, secondary to minor trauma (which may be the result of impingement of degenerated menisci, the presence of loose bodies, or a misstep). Pain is aggravated by activity or weight bearing, but may also be aggravated at rest, particularly if the knee is held in one position for a prolonged time.

PHYSICAL EXAMINATION

Post[284] describes a particular gait that may occur with osteoarthritis of the knee depending on whether there is a collapse of the medial or lateral knee compartment owing to degeneration. Lateral knee degeneration would result in a varus knee, causing the knee to thrust medially during gait. Medial degeneration would result in a varus knee, causing the knee to thrust laterally during gait. Examination of the extensor mechanism may reveal quadriceps atrophy, parapatellar tenderness, retropatellar pain with compression, and retropatellar crepitation. If genu valgum is present, lateral subluxation of the patella is not unusual. In unicompartmental degenerative joint disease, joint compression with either a varus or valgus stress to the knee elicits pain. Marginal osteophytes along the femoral condyles may be palpable and are sites of capsular tenderness resulting from local irritation. The extremes of both flexion and extension are often limited. There is a loss of joint play.

MANAGEMENT

The general management of patients with osteoarthritis of the knee is similar to that previously outlined for osteoarthritis of the hip and includes anti-inflammatory drugs, rest, weight loss, aids, and physical therapy (see Chapter 14, Hip). Salicylates act as an enzyme inhibitor that prevents chondromalacia and, when given early and in adequate doses, prevents fibrillation. Ice for pain and spasm relief and heat applications are usually beneficial (hot moist packs or diathermy).[40] Patients also benefit from hydrotherapy. With bilateral involvement of the knees, weight loss allows muscle strengthening and reeducation of gait in the presence of pain relief, with resultant functional improvement.

Mobilization techniques aid in easing knee pain and stiffness. Small-amplitude stretching movements used at the limit of range are of most value.[53] One of the most common changes in the osteoarthritic knee is knee flexion contracture, so patients should be taught early how to avoid contracture. Stretching of the tight hamstrings may be as important as strengthening of the vastus medialis. Tight gastrocnemius muscles (common in women who wear shoes with heels higher than 1 inch) can also be detrimental.[172] Although it can be difficult to accomplish, stretching of the gastrocnemius often helps prevent ankle plantar-flexion or knee flexion contractures.

Exercises to strengthen the quadriceps group should be a daily ritual, beginning with setting exercises and increasing to full progressive resistive exercises as tolerated. Biofeedback can be of great value in strengthening the vastus medialis.[183] A training regimen should incorporate several types of exercise and might include isotonic exercises (with eccentrics) and isometric and isokinetic training.[5,6,198] Beneficial exercises include closed kinetic chain hamstring exercises (the patient stands and flexes one knee, then holds the contraction to the point of fatigue) and gastrocnemius and soleus exercises (the patient raises up on the toes bilaterally or unilaterally). Full weight-bearing strengthening exercises should be used judiciously in subacute and chronic phases and avoided in the acute phase. Unloading and weight bearing in water should be used as closed kinetic chain exercises in the more acute phases.[120,141,362]

The patient's daily activities must be evaluated and if necessary changed. In the morning, active flexion and extension exercises should be done before weight-bearing activities. Walking should be encouraged for daily activities but not forced. Deep knee bends, sitting in low chairs, and remaining in the same position for prolonged periods should be avoided. Faulty posture that strains the stance should be corrected. Biomechanical evaluation of the lumbar spine, sacroiliac joint, and lower limb is necessary, including angulation of the feet, which may benefit from orthoses. Heel wedges to unload the more sympathetic or collapsed side of the joint may be beneficial.[105] The combination of manual therapy and supervised exercise has been found to yield functional benefits for patients and may delay or prevent the need for surgical intervention.[73]

PASSIVE TREATMENT TECHNIQUES

Joint Mobilization Techniques

(For simplicity, the operator will be referred to as the male, the patient as the female. P—patient; O—operator; M—movement; MH—mobilizing hand.)

I. Femorotibial Joint. Distraction
    A. Distraction in prone (Fig. 15-43A)
       P—Prone with the thigh fixated with a belt
       O—Stands at the foot of the table and gently grasps the distal leg, proximal to the malleoli, with both hands. The present neutral (resting) position is found.
       M—Distraction is applied on the long axis of the tibia by the backward leaning of the operator's trunk.
       This technique is particularly well suited for treating pain but should not be used with forces beyond grade II traction.[299]
    B. Distraction in sitting (Fig. 15-43B)
       P—Sitting on the edge of the plinth, with several layers of toweling supporting the underside of the distal thigh
       O—Stands at the patient's side facing the patient's feet so as to direct his forearms in the line of force. Both hands grasp the tibia proximal to the malleoli to gain a purchase on them.
       M—A long-axis distraction is produced by leaning forward with the trunk. This may be performed through varying degrees of flexion and extension.
       This technique is used as a general mobilization to increase femorotibial joint play for pain control. Distraction at this joint tends to occur when moving into flexion (out of the close-packed position). As with any joint, if normal distraction does not occur, premature compression of joint surfaces will result when moving toward the close-packed position.
       If conservative techniques are indicated, the resting position of the tibiofemoral joint is used; if more aggressive techniques are indicated, a position approximating the restricted range is used. An alternative technique is to use an ankle strap with a stirrup attachment for placement of the operator's foot to apply distraction (Fig. 15-43C).[169,170] This allows the operator's hands to be free to palpate the joint space as the distraction is applied or to use soft tissue techniques (i.e., to a restricted lateral retinaculum). The operator may be either standing or sitting. Starting positions include neutral and internal and external rotation of the tibia, with various degrees of flexion or approaching extension of the knee.

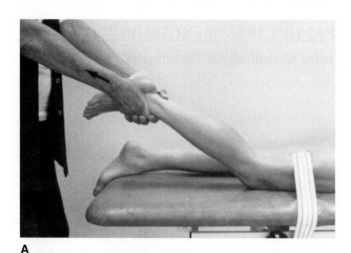

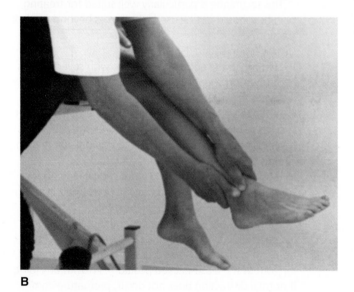

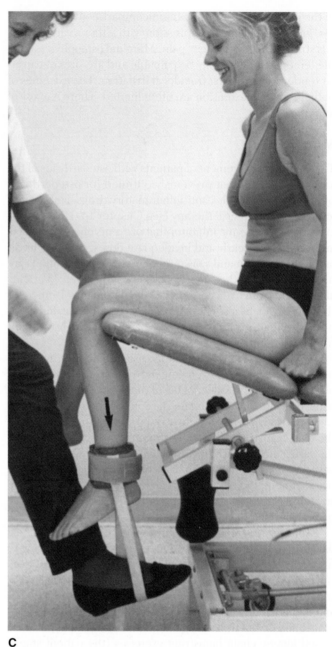

■ FIG. 15-43. Distraction of femorotibial joint in prone (**A**), in sitting (**B**), and in sitting with use of an ankle strap (**C**).

II. Femorotibial Joint. Posterior glide
    A. Posterior glide, resting position (Fig. 15-44*A*)
        P—Supine, leg beyond the end of the table
        O—Stands facing the medial aspect of the leg and
           places his caudal hand around the distal end of the
           leg above the ankle. The cranial hand is placed on the
           proximal aspect of the tibia, with the ulnar aspect of
           the hand just distal to the joint line of the knee. The
           present neutral (rest) position is found.
        M—With the elbow extended, the cranial hand applies
           a posterior glide by the operator leaning his body
           weight onto the tibia or by flexing his knees. Grade I

traction may be applied concurrently with the
caudal hand.
    This technique is used for assessment and pain con-
trol and to increase joint-play movement necessary for
flexion. The neutral position may change with the treatment, requiring repositioning.
    B. Posterior glide, of tibia on femur with knee flexed
       (Fig. 15-44*B*)
        P—Supine, with knee flexed 25 to 90°, foot flat on the
           plinth
        O—Stabilizes the anterior aspect of the distal femur by
           contacting it with his entire left hand. The forearm is

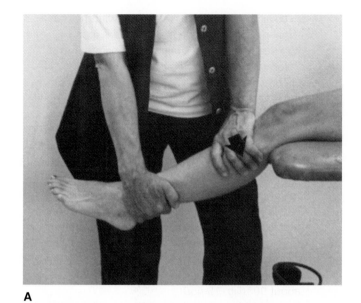

A

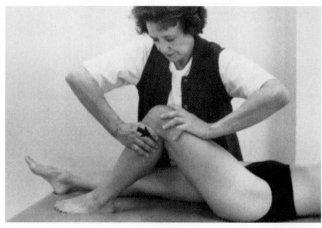

B

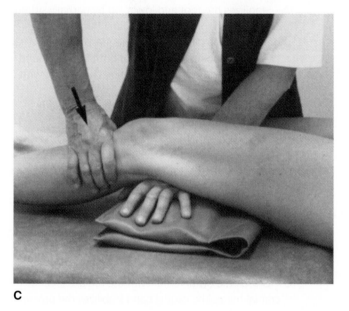

C

■ **FIG. 15-44.** Techniques for posterior glide of the femorotibial joint: tibia on femur near the resting position (**A**), with the knee flexed (drawer test; **B**), and with the knee approaching full extension (**C**).

directed horizontally. The operator contacts the proximal tibia with his caudal hand. The forearm is directed horizontally.

M—The caudal hand produces a posterior glide of the tibia while the cranial hand stabilizes the femur.

This technique is used to increase joint-play movement necessary for knee flexion. This position is also used for the drawer test (knee in about 90°) to evaluate the PCL.

C. Posterior glide, of tibia on femur with knee approaching full extension (Fig. 15-44C)

P—Supine, with knee slightly flexed from the limit of extension. A 1-inch thickness of toweling may be placed under the posterior aspect of the distal femur.

O—Supports the proximal tibia with the cranial hand placed over the distal femur. He uses the forearm to support and control the femur. The caudal hand is

placed on the proximal aspect of the tibia just distal to the joint space.

M—A posterior glide is produced with the caudal hand by moving the lower leg dorsally.

This technique is used to increase joint-play movement necessary for knee flexion. Because the knee is approaching full extension (close-packed position), it is considered more vigorous than Technique II, B.

III. Femorotibial Joint. Anterior glide

A. Anterior glide, of tibia on femur in prone, near the resting position (Fig. 15-45A)

P—Prone. A bolster may be placed under the distal femur for further stability and to prevent patellar compression.

O—Kneels on the table and supports the patient's leg across his thigh. The caudal hand grasps the proximal

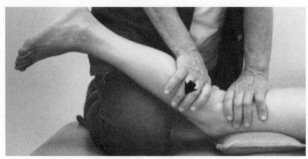

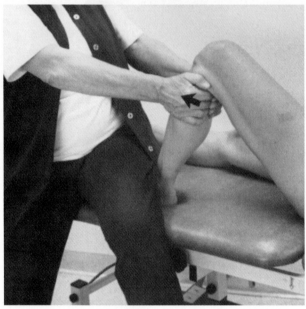

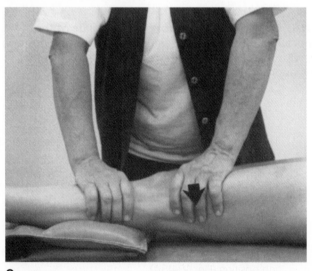

■ **FIG. 15-45.** Technique for anterior glide of the femorotibial joint: tibia on femur in prone near the resting position (**A**), in supine with the knee flexed (drawer test; **B**), and in extension (with posterior glide of the femur; **C**).

tibia. The distal thigh is stabilized with the cranial hand. The present neutral position is found.

M—Keeping the arm straight, the operator leans forward, gliding the tibia anteriorly.

This technique is used to increase joint-play movement necessary for knee extension. The tibiofemoral joint is positioned in the resting position if conservative techniques are indicated or approximating the restricted range of extension if a more aggressive technique is indicated. If grade I traction is also desired, the operator removes his thigh, stands facing the lateral aspect of the patient's leg, and places his cranial (mobilizing) hand over the proximal tibia. The caudal hand grasps the distal aspect of the patient's leg. The cranial hand then glides the tibia in an anterior direction as the caudal hand applies traction.

B. Anterior glide, of tibia on femur with the knee flexed about 90° (Fig. 15-45B)

P—Supine, knee flexed about 90°, foot flat on the plinth

O—Stabilizes the foot and lower leg by partially sitting on the plinth, placing the proximal thigh over the dorsum of the patient's foot. He grasps the proximal tibia by wrapping the fingers of both hands around posteriorly and contacting the tibial tuberosity with both thumbs anteriorly.

M—Anterior glide is produced by keeping the arms fixed and leaning backward with the trunk.

This technique is used to increase joint-play movement necessary for knee extension. This position is also used for the drawer test (knee in about 90°) to evaluate the ACL and as a technique to restore joint-play movement for knee extension. The operator leans backward and glides the tibia anteriorly.

C. Posterior glide of femur, anterior tibia glide (Fig. 15-45C)

P—Supine, knee approximating the restricted range of motion. The proximal aspect of the tibia is on a bolster.

O—Grasps the distal femur with the radial aspect of the cranial hand. The caudal hand stabilizes the proximal tibia on the bolster.

M—Keeping the arm straight, the operator leans down on the cranial hand, gliding the femur posteriorly.

This technique is used to increase joint-play movement for extension. This technique is particularly useful when the patient lacks the last few degrees of terminal knee extension.

IV. Femorotibial Joint. Internal rotation

A. Internal rotation, with the knee flexed about 90° (Fig. 15-46A)

P—Supine, knee flexed 90°, foot flat on the plinth

O—May stabilize the foot by sitting on the plinth, placing the proximal thigh over the dorsum of the patient's foot. The cranial hand grasps the proximal tibia laterally, with the fingers wrapped around posteriorly, the thumb contacting the lateral aspect of the tibial tuberosity so as to gain a purchase against

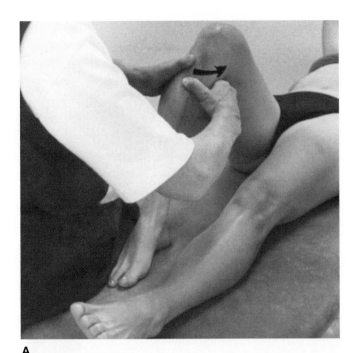
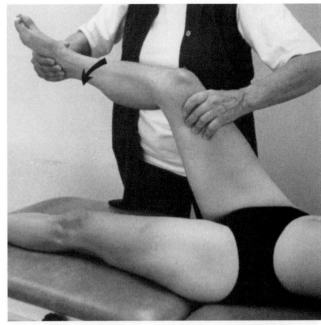

A   B

■ **FIG. 15-46.** Internal rotation of femorotibial joint with knee flexed to about 90° (**A**) and at varying degrees of flexion–extension (**B**).

it. The caudal hand grasps the tibia anteriorly and medially, just distal to the cranial hand, gaining a purchase on the tibial crest.

M—Both hands rotate the proximal tibia medially (internal rotation), gaining purchase on the tibial tuberosity and lateral tibial condyle with the cranial hand, and the tibial crest and medial tibial condyle with the caudal hand.

This technique is used to increase a joint-play movement necessary for knee flexion.

B. Internal rotation, at varying degrees of flexion and extension (Fig. 15-46B)

P—Supine

O—Controls the distal thigh with the cranial hand grasping from the lateral aspect, the thumb wrapping around posteriorly and the fingers anteriorly. The caudal hand grasps the heel of the foot. He must place the ankle in the close-packed position by fully dorsiflexing it so that the rotary force is transmitted to the tibia, not the ankle joint. His forearm is kept in close alignment with the patient's tibia.

M—The caudal hand rotates the foot medially, transmitting the movement to the tibia through the close-packed ankle. Starting with the knee slightly flexed, the movement can be applied at various degrees of flexion and extension. Do not, however, rotate and simultaneously flex or extend.

This technique is considered more vigorous than Technique IV, A. It increases joint-play movement necessary for flexion.

V. Femorotibial Joint. External rotation

A. External rotation, with the knee flexed to about 90° (Fig. 15-47A)

This is performed in the same manner as Technique IV, A. The handholds are reversed, however, so that the cranial thumb contacts the tibial tuberosity medially, while the caudal hand grasps the tibial crest and lateral aspect of the proximal tibia. This technique is used to increase joint-play movement necessary for knee extension.

B. External rotation, applied in various positions approaching full extension (Fig. 15-47B)

P—Supine

O—Supports the knee and distal end of the thigh with the cranial hand from the medial aspect, wrapping the fingers around anteriorly. The cranial hand primarily controls the position of the knee, keeping it from dropping into extension. He grasps the ankle and foot with the caudal hand, wrapping the fingers around the calcaneus. The ankle must be kept in the close-packed position so as to transmit the rotatory force to the tibia, not the ankle joint.

M—The caudal hand and forearm rotate the foot and ankle externally (lateral rotation), keeping the ankle in the close-packed position. The cranial hand controls the position of the knee. This may be performed at various positions approaching full extension. Do not rotate and simultaneously flex or extend the knee.

This technique is used to increase joint-play movement necessary for knee extension. It is considered more vigorous than Technique V, A.

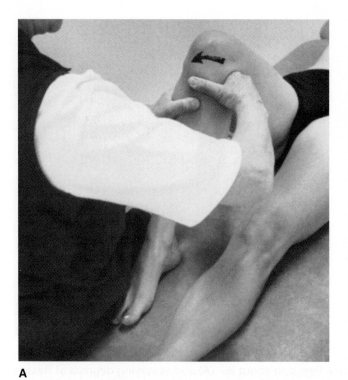

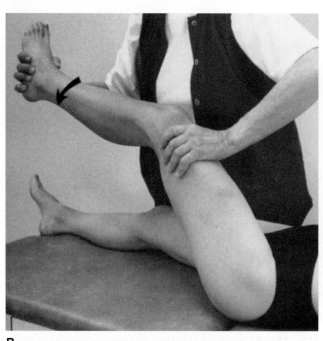

A

B

■ **FIG. 15-47.** External rotation of femorotibial joint with knee flexed to 90° (**A**) and at varying degrees of flexion–extension (**B**).

VI. Femorotibial Joint. Lateral (varus) tilt (Fig. 15-48)

P—Supine

O—Supports the lower leg by resting the leg on the proximal thigh. His knee is placed on the plinth. He supports the proximal tibia and knee with his caudal hand from the lateral side, wrapping the fingers around posteriorly and the thumb anteriorly. The cranial forearm is supinated and in line with the direction of force. The cranial hand contacts the medial aspect of the femoral and tibial condyles. The fingers wrap around posteriorly for additional support. The patient's knee is kept slightly flexed.

M—The cranial hand gently moves the knee into lateral tilt, taking care to avoid any flexion or extension of the knee. The operator's caudal hand supports the knee, but yields with the lateral movement.

This technique is used to increase joint play at the knee. As with any joint-play movement, it must not be moved past normal anatomic limits.

VII. Femorotibial Joint. Medial (valgus) tilt (Fig. 15-49)

This is performed in a similar manner to Technique VI. The handholds are reversed so that the caudal hand supports the proximal tibia and the knee. The cranial hand contacts the lateral condyle. The cranial forearm comes

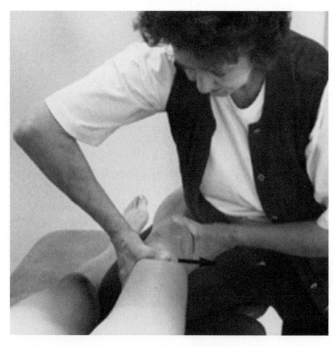

■ **FIG. 15-48.** Lateral (valgus) tilt of the femorotibial joint.

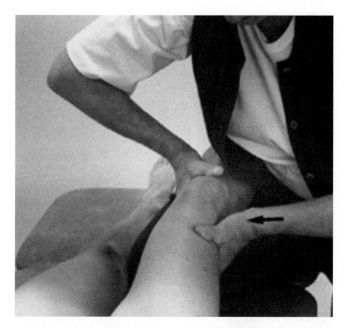

■ **FIG. 15-49.** Medial (varus) tilt of the femorotibial joint.

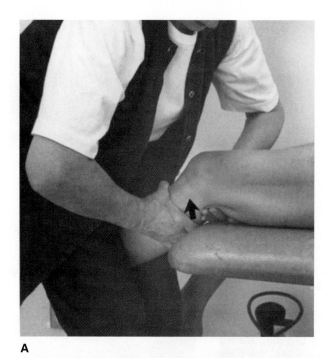

A

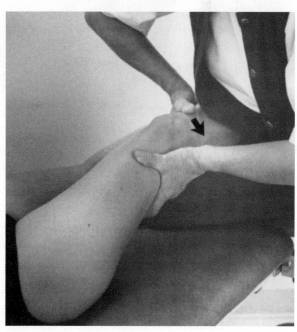

B

■ **FIG. 15-50.** Medial-lateral glide of the tibia: **(A)** medial glide, **(B)** lateral glide.

around and is in line with the mobilizing hand, which moves the knee in a medial direction, thus creating a medial gapping at the joint line.

VIII. Femorotibial Joint. Medial-lateral glide
   A. Medial (lateral) glide, in supine (Fig. 15-50A)
      P—Supine, leg extending over the edge of the table. The tibiofemoral joint is positioned in the resting position if conservative treatment is indicated or approximating the restricted range if more aggressive techniques are indicated.
      O—Stands at the foot of the table. The foot is held between his thighs or the lower leg is held between the arm and thorax. The cranial hand stabilizes the distal femur from the medial aspect. The caudal hand grips the proximal tibia and fibula from the lateral side.
      M—The mobilizing hand glides the proximal tibia and fibula in a medial direction.
      This technique is used to increase joint play at the knee. To perform lateral glide the handholds are reversed—the stabilizing hand grips the distal femur from the lateral aspect and the mobilizing hand grips the proximal tibia from the medial side (Fig. 15-50B). The mobilizing hand glides the tibia in a lateral direction while the trunk guides the motion.
   B. Medial (lateral) glide, in sidelying (Fig. 15-51A)[169,170]
      P—Sidelying on the uninvolved side, involved leg extending over the edge of the table. A bolster is placed under the medial aspect of the distal thigh.

      O—Stands facing the dorsal aspect of the leg. The caudal hand grasps the distal leg above the ankle. The cranial hand grips the proximal tibia and fibula from the lateral aspect. The knee is maintained in the resting position and the leg is held against the operator's trunk.

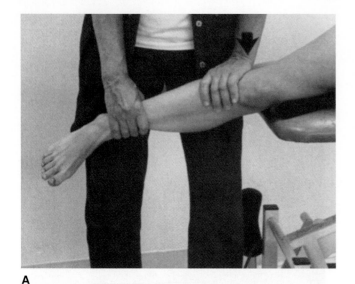

A

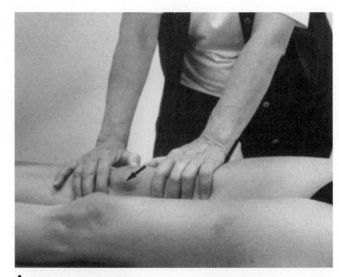

A

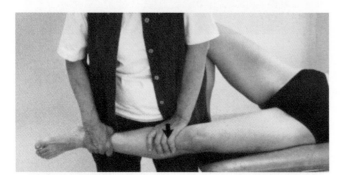

B

■ **FIG. 15-51.** Medial-lateral glide of femorotibial joint: **(A)** medial glide in sidelying, **(B)** lateral glide in sidelying.

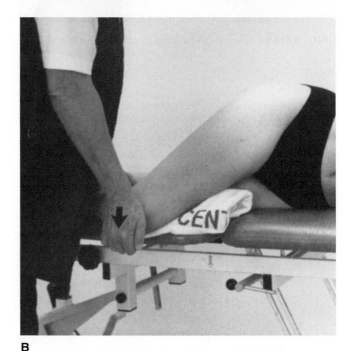

B

■ **FIG. 15-52.** Medial-lateral tilt **(A)** and medial glide **(B)** of the patellofemoral joint in sidelying.

M—The tibia is glided in the medial direction indirectly through the fibula while the trunk guides the motion (by flexing the knees).

Lateral glide is performed in the same manner as above, but the handholds are reversed and the patient lies on the involved side (Fig. 15-51*B*). These techniques are used to restore joint play for restricted flexion or extension.

IX. Patellofemoral Joint
A. Medial-lateral glide (tilt), in supine (Fig. 15-52*A*)
P—Supine, knee slightly flexed over a firm support of toweling
O—Contacts the lateral patellar border with the thumb pads or the heel of the hand. The remaining fingers rest over the anterior aspect of the patient's leg to help support the operator's hands. He keeps the elbows close to full extension.
M—A medial glide of the patella is produced with both hands. A lateral glide is produced by using the pads

of the index fingers. Both hands glide the patella in a lateral direction.

These techniques are used for general patellar mobilization in the presence of restricted patellar movement. Grades I and II should be applied to highly irritable joints in which pain is predominant. In less irritable joints, in which pain is a result of tight structures, grades III and IV should be considered.

B. Medial glide, in sidelying (Fig. 15-52*B*)

P—Lying on the unaffected side with the involved leg placed in hip and knee flexion. The affected patella is just over the edge of the table. A towel or bolster is placed under the knee.

O—Stands facing the leg. The stabilizing hand contacts the proximal tibia or distal femur. The mobilizing hand is positioned with the heel of the hand on the lateral border of the patella.

M—With the elbow extended, the mobilizing hand glides the patella in a medial direction. The force is produced by the operator's body weight.

In this position the lateral structures are under some degree of tension, allowing a more effective stretch to the lateral structures. Avoid compression.

X. Patellofemoral Joint. Superior-inferior glides

A. Inferior glide, in supine (Fig. 15-53A)

P—Supine, knee extended or in slight flexion with a towel under the knee

O—Stands next to the patient's thigh, facing her feet. The web space or heel of the near hand contacts the superior pole of the patella.

M—The mobilizing hand glides the patella in an inferior direction, parallel to the femur.

This technique is used to increase patellar mobility for knee flexion. Superior glide, to increase mobility for knee extension, is done in the reverse manner. The mobilizing hand is positioned with either the web space or the heel of the hand on the inferior pole of the patella. The patella is glided in the superior direction. Avoid compression of the patella into the femoral condyles. Grades I and II should be applied to highly irritable joints in which pain is predominant. In less irritable joints, in which pain is the result of tight structures, grades III and IV should be used.

B. Inferior glide, in knee flexion (Fig. 15-53B)

P—Supine, foot resting on the table, hip and knee in flexion

O—Stands next to the lower limb. The caudal hand stabilizes the leg by grasping the lower tibia. The heel of the mobilizing hand contacts the superior pole of the patella.

M—Glide the patella in a caudal direction, parallel to the femur.

This technique is considered more vigorous than Technique X, A. To selectively stretch the lateral or medial retinaculum, caudal glide may be directed in a more medial caudal or lateral caudal direction.

XI. Proximal Tibiofibular Joint. Anterior glide (Fig. 15-54A)

P—Assumes a half-kneeling position or stands at the side of the table, resting her leg on the table. The foot extends over the edge of the table.

O—Places the heel of the mobilizing hand over the posterior aspect of the fibular head. The other hand may be used to support or reinforce the mobilizing hand or stabilize the tibia. The thigh supports the patient's foot in plantar-flexion (10°).

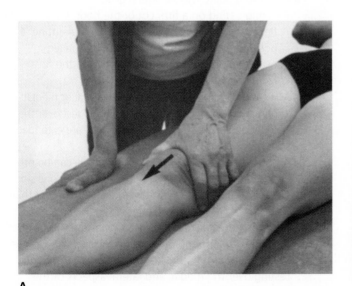

A

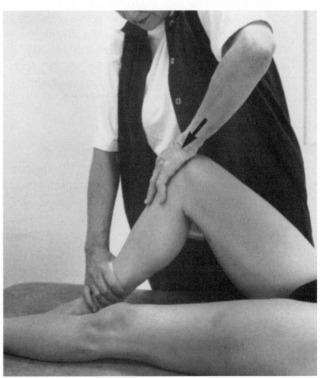

B

■ **FIG. 15-53.** Superior-inferior glide of patellofemoral joint with the knee in extension (**A**) and with the knee in flexion (**B**).

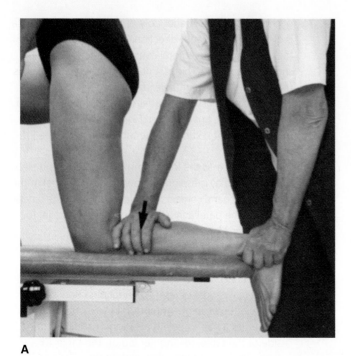

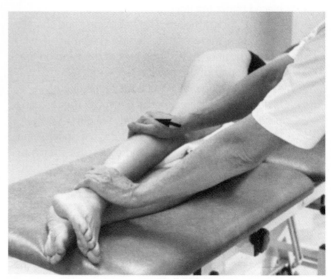

A   **B**

■ **FIG. 15-54.** Proximal tibiofibular joint: **(A)** anterior glide, **(B)** posterior glide.

M—An anterior lateral glide of the fibula is produced by leaning forward with the trunk. The operator must prevent pain or fibular nerve compression.

This technique is used to increase joint play in the proximal tibiofibular joint and to reduce a dorsal positional fault of the fibula. Lateral knee pain is often present when the proximal tibiofibular joint is affected.[299] Posterior mobilization may be performed in sidelying with the hip and knee slightly flexed (Fig. 15-54*B*). Both anterior and inferior glide may be performed in supine (see Chapter 16, Lower Leg, Ankle, and Foot).

Self-Mobilization Techniques

I. Femorotibial Joint. Forced (gentle) flexion (Fig. 15-55)
    P—Supine, hip flexed slightly above 90°. The knee is flexed over a firm pillow or towel roll, which acts as a fulcrum.

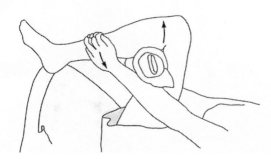

■ **FIG. 15-55.** Femorotibial joint: forced (gentle) flexion.

MH—Both hands contact the lower leg over the anterior aspect, with the fingers interlaced.
M—Gentle flexion, with oscillations, is performed.
    Note: Forced flexion may also be done in a sitting position. The right hip is completely flexed so that the thigh is supported on the chest. The knee is flexed over the right forearm, which now acts as a fulcrum and gives additional support. The left MH contacts the lower leg over the anterior aspect and carries out gentle flexion of the knee.

II. Patellofemoral Joint. Medial-lateral glide
    P—Long-sitting on a firm cot or the floor, knee slightly flexed over a firm pillow or towel roll. (A sitting position in a chair may be used, with the leg extended, the knee slightly flexed, and the foot fixed to the floor.)
    MH—Both thumb pads contact the lateral or medial patellar border. The remaining fingers rest over the anterior aspect of the leg. The elbows are extended as much as possible.
    M—A medial or lateral glide of the patella can be produced by leaning the trunk forward and to one side. The glide is effected by moving the trunk rather than any part of the hand.
    Note: Superior-inferior glide may also be performed by contact of the thumb pads on the superior or inferior borders of the patella, with the rest of the hand resting over the medial and lateral aspects of the knee.

DYNAMIC STABILIZATION AND FUNCTIONAL EXERCISES

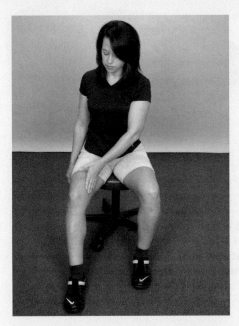

■ **FIG. 15-56.** Quadriceps and hamstring co-contraction exercise.

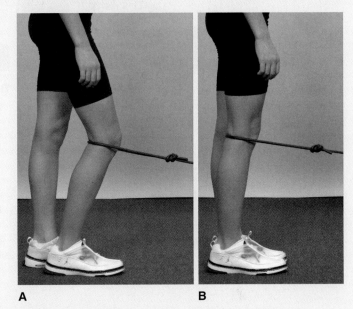

A   B

■ **FIG. 15-57.** Terminal knee extension using surgical tubing.

The concept of knee injury and its treatment is constantly evolving, and staying current is a challenge to those who treat the knee. Many changes in treatment have resulted from arthroscopic techniques.[193] Because the knee is just one part of the closed kinetic chain of the spine and lower limb, rehabilitation must always be directed toward the entire system as well as specific problems. Maintenance of optimal function as healing ensues is the cornerstone for rehabilitation. Unnecessary loss of strength and range of motion (ROM) must be minimized without imposing inappropriate stresses in the healing tissue. Throughout the entire program, appropriate warmup and aerobic activities are performed to maintain cardiovascular fitness. Current rehabilitation protocols are focusing more on functional training (see Chapter 10, Functional Exercise) including functional exercises, closed kinetic chain exercises, balance, and sensorimotor training and away from limited machines. Closed kinetic chain exercises and sensorimotor stimulation of the knee may include many of the exercises already described in Chapter 14, Hip (see Figs. 14-37, 14-38, 14-40, 14-41, 14-45, and 14-46).

Other exercises might include:

- Early phase quadriceps and hamstrings co-contraction exercise. Patient is seated with the involved knee flexed to a comfortable position. Patient palpates the vastus medialis oblique while applying pressure down through the heel (Fig. 15-56).
- Terminal knee extension using surgical tubing (Fig. 15-57)
- Gymnastic ball exercises for the hamstrings[204]

1. Bridge while rolling the ball in and out (Fig. 15-58)
2. 90°/90° bridge (Fig. 15-59)
3. One-leg bridge with roll (Fig. 15-60)
4. One-leg 90°/90° bridge (Fig. 15-61)
- Squatting movements using surgical tubing (Fig. 15-62). This exercise allows one to incorporate resistance with high-speed repetitions. Range of motion should be limited based on patellar crepitus and pain.
- Balance board squats (Fig. 15-63)
- One-leg half squat (Fig. 15-64). Changing the position of the bent leg allows the patient to work more for balance and stabilization.
- Step-ups: A simple exercise to isolate the quadriceps and gluteus maximus is to perform a step-up (on a slant board) with the ankle fixed in plantar flexion. This reduces the input from the gastrocnemius and soleus muscles while simultaneously reducing anterior shear of the femur on the tibia.[205] This step-up can be performed as front, back (Fig. 15-65), or lateral step-ups (see Fig. 14-41).

Lunges forward to strengthen quadriceps eccentrically (Fig. 15-66). Progression of lunges may include:

1. Lunges forward with hand weights or with resistance from behind.
2. Backward lunges
3. Sideways lunges (see Fig. 14-42)
4. Posterior lateral rotational lunges (see Fig. 10-4)
5. Anterior lunge off and onto a 4-inch step (see Fig. 10-5)

- Backward treadmill training (Fig. 15-67)[134]

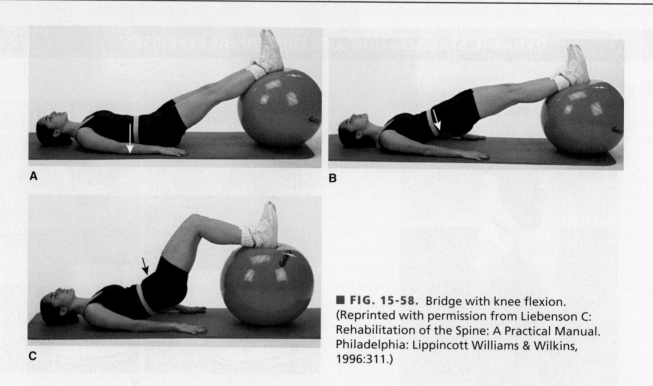

■ FIG. 15-58. Bridge with knee flexion. (Reprinted with permission from Liebenson C: Rehabilitation of the Spine: A Practical Manual. Philadelphia: Lippincott Williams & Wilkins, 1996:311.)

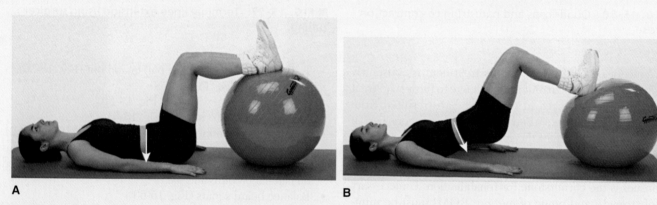

■ FIG. 15-59. 90°/90° bridge. (Reprinted with permission from Liebenson C: Rehabilitation of the Spine: A Practical Manual. Philadelphia: Lippincott Williams & Wilkins, 1996:312.)

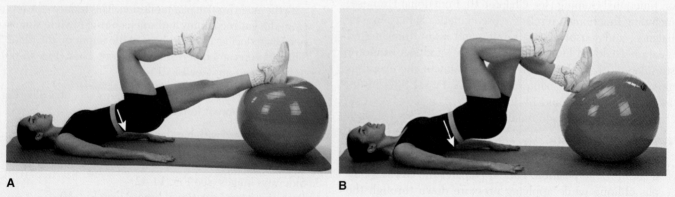

■ FIG. 15-60. One-leg bridge with roll. (Reprinted with permission from Liebenson C: Rehabilitation of the Spine: A Practical Manual. Philadelphia: Lippincott Williams & Wilkins, 1996:312.)

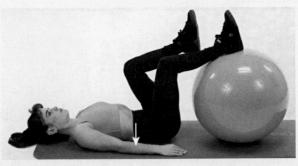 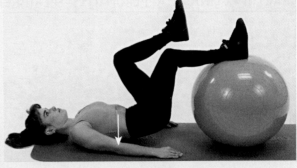

A   **B**

■ **FIG. 15-61.** 90°/90° one-leg bridge. (Reprinted with permission from Liebenson C: Rehabilitation of the Spine: A Practical Manual. Philadelphia: Lippincott Williams & Wilkins, 1996:312.)

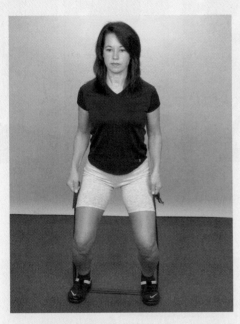 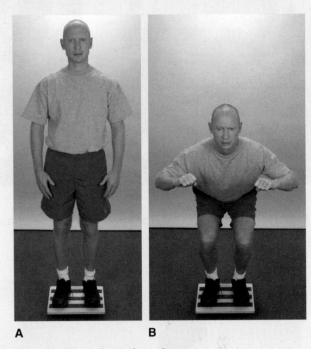

A   **B**

■ **FIG. 15-62.** Squatting movements using surgical tubing.   ■ **FIG. 15-63.** Balance board squat.

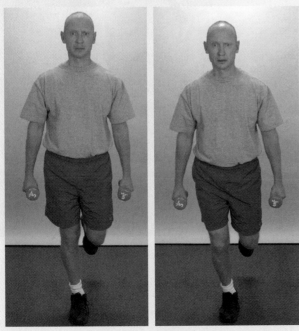

A   **B**   ■ **FIG. 15-64.** One-legged half squat.

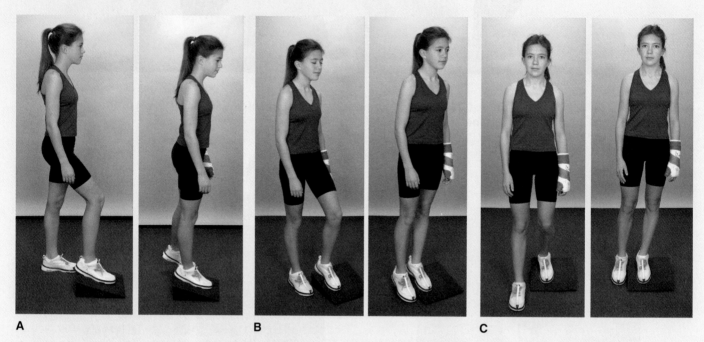

■ **FIG. 15-65.** Step-ups. **(A)** Front step-ups. **(B)** Side step-ups. **(C)** Back step-ups.

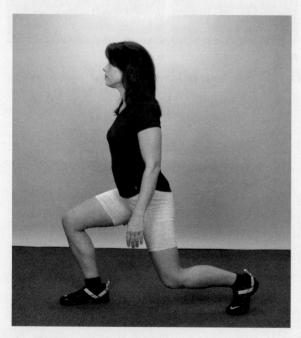

■ **FIG. 15-66.** Forward lunges.

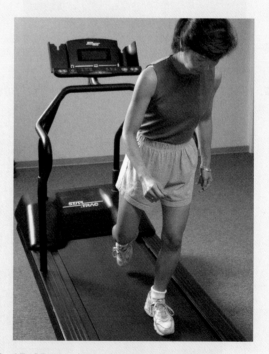

■ **FIG. 15-67.** Backward treadmill walking.

REFERENCES

1. Abernathy PJ, Townsend PR, Rose RM, et al: Is chondromalacia patellae a separate clinical entity? J Bone Joint Surg Br 60: 205–210, 1978

2. Adams A: Effect of exercise upon ligament strength. Res Q 37:163–167, 1966

3. Aglietti P, Buzzi R, Menchetti PM, et al: Arthroscopically assisted semitendinosus and gracilis tendon graft in reconstruction for acute anterior cruciate ligament injuries in athletes. Am J Sports Med 24:726–731, 1996

4. Aglietti P, Zaccherotti G, Buzzi R, et al: A comparison between patellar tendon and doubled semitendinosus/gracilis tendon for anterior cruciate ligament reconstruction. A minimum five-year-follow up. J Sports Trauma 19:57–68, 1997

5. Albert M: Eccentric Muscle Training in Sports and Orthopedics. London, Churchill Livingstone, 1991

6. Albert MS: Principles of exercise progression. In: Greenfield BH, ed: Rehabilitation of the Knee: A Problem-Solving Approach. Philadelphia, FA Davis, 1993:110–136

7. Alm A, Lijedalso SO, Stromberg B: Clinical and experimental experience in reconstruction of the anterior cruciate ligament. Orthop Clin North Am 7:181–186, 1976

8. Amatuzzi MM, Fazzi A, Varella MH: Pathologic synovial plica of the knee. Am J Sports Med 18:466–469, 1990

9. American Academy of Orthopaedic Surgeons: Knee Braces—Seminar Report. Rosemont, IL, The Academy, 1985

10. Anderson AF, Lipscomb AB: Clinical diagnosis of meniscal tears—Description of a new manipulative test. Am J Sports Med 14:291–293, 1986

11. Andrews JR, Mc Leod WD, Ward T, et al: The cutting mechanism. Am J Sports Med 5:111–121, 1977

12. Apley G: The diagnosis of meniscus injuries. J Bone Joint Surg Am 29:78–84, 1947

13. Arno S: The A angle: A quantitative measurement of patella alignment and realignment. J Orthop Sports Phys Ther 12:237–242, 1990

14. Arnoczky SP: The blood supply of the meniscus and its role in healing and repair. In: American Association of Orthopedic Surgeons: Symposium on Sports Medicine: The Knee. St. Louis, CV Mosby, 1985

15. Arnold JA, Coker TP, Heaton LM, et al: Natural history of anterior cruciate tears. Am J Sports Med 7:305–313, 1979

16. Barnett C, Richardson AT: The postural function of the popliteus muscle. Ann Phys Med 17:179, 1953

17. Barnett CH: Locking at the knee joint. J Anat 87:91–95, 1953

18. Barry OCD, McManus F, McCauley P: Clinical assessment of suspected meniscal tears. Ir J Med Sci 152:149–151, 1983

19. Basmajian JV, Deluca CJ. Muscles Alive, 5th ed. Baltimore, Williams & Wilkins, 1986

20. Beck C, Drez D, Young J, et al: Instrumental testing of functional knee braces. Am J Sports Med 14:253–256, 1986

21. Beck JL, Wildermuth BP: The female athlete's knee. Clin Sports Med 4:345–366, 1985

22. Beckman M, Craig R, Lehman RC: Rehabilitation of patellofemoral dysfunction in the athlete. Clin Sports Med 8:841–860, 1989

23. Bentley GL: Chondromalacia patellae. J Bone Joint Surg Am 52:221–232, 1970

24. Bentley GL: The surgical treatment of chondromalacia patellae. J Bone Joint Surg Br 60:74–81, 1978

25. Bergfeld J: Functional rehabilitation of isolated medial collateral ligament sprains. Am J Sports Med 7:207–209, 1979

26. Beynnon BD, Johnson RJ, Flemming BC: The science of anterior cruciate ligament reconstruction. Clin Orthop 402:9–20, 2002

27. Blackburn TA, Eiland WG, Brady WD: An introduction to the plica. J Orthop Sports Phys Ther 3:171–177, 1982

28. Blazina ME, Kerlan RK, Jobe FW, et al: Jumper's knee. Orthop Clin North Am 4:665–678, 1973

29. Bleday RM, Fanelli GC, Giannotti BF, et al: Instrumental measurements of the posterolateral corner. Arthroscopy 14:489–494, 1998

30. Blustein M, D'Amico JC: Limb-length discrepancy: Identification, clinical significance and management. Phys Ther 75:200–206, 1985

31. Bonnarens FO, Drez D: Clinical examination of the knee for anterior cruciate ligament laxity. In: Jackson DW, Drez D, eds: The Anterior Cruciate Deficient Knee: New Concepts in Ligament Repair. St. Louis, CV Mosby, 1987:72–89

32. Bose K, Kanagasuntherum R, Osman M: Vastus medialis oblique: An anatomical and physiological study. Orthopaedics 3:880–883, 1980

33. Brandsson S, Faxen E, Eriksson BI, et al: Reconstruction of the anterior cruciate ligament: Comparison of outside-in and all-inside techniques. Br J Sports Med 33:42–45, 1999

34. Brody D: Techniques in the evaluation and treatment of the injured runner. Orthop Clin North Am 13:541–558, 1982

35. Brownstein BA, Lamb RL, Magine RE: Quadriceps torque and integrated electromyography. J Orthop Sports Ther 6:309–314, 1985

36. Brubaker CE, Jame SL: Injuries to runners. J Sports Med 2:189–198, 1974

37. Cabaud HE, Feagin JA, Rodkey WG: Acute ACL injury and augmented repair. Am J Sports Med 8:395–401, 1980

38. Cabaud HE, Rodkey WG, Feagin JA: Experimental studies of acute ACL injury and repair. Am J Sports Med 7:18–22, 1979

39. Cabaud HE, Slocum DB: The diagnosis of chronic anterolateral rotary instability of the knee. Am J Sports Med 5:99–104, 1977

40. Cailliet R: Knee Pain and Disability, 2nd ed. Philadelphia, FA Davis, 1983

41. Cannon WD: Follow-up of ACL reconstructions and studies with the knee laxity tester. Presented at the ACL Study Group Meeting, Steamboat Springs, CO, 1984

42. Caraffa A, Cerulli G, Projetti M, et al: Prevention of anterior cruciate ligament injuries in soccer: A prospective controlled study of proprioceptive training. Knee Surg Sports Traumatol Arthrosc 4:19–21, 1996

43. Carriere B: The Swiss Ball: Theory, Basic Exercises and Clinical Applications. Berlin, Springer-Verlag, 1998

44. Carson WG: Diagnosis of extensor mechanical disorders. Clin Sports Med 4:231–246, 1985

45. Cavagna GA, Dusman B, Margaria R: Positive work done by a previously stretched muscle. J Appl Physiol 24:21–32, 1968

46. Cho KO: Reconstruction of the anterior cruciate ligament by semitendinosus tenodesis. J Bone Joint Surg Br 60:608–612, 1975

47. Cipriani D, Armstrong G, Gaul S: Backward walking at three levels of treadmill inclination: An electromyographic and kinematic analysis. J Orthop Sports Phys Ther 22:95–102, 1995

48. Clancy WG, Nelson DA, Reider B, et al: ACL reconstruction using one third of the patellar ligament augmented by extra-articular tendon transfers. J Bone Joint Surg Am 64:352–359, 1982

49. Clarkson HM, Gilewish GB: Musculoskeletal Assessment, Joint Range of Motion and Manual Muscle Testing. Baltimore, Williams & Wilkins, 1989

50. Cole JH, Furness AL, Twoney LT: Muscle in Action, an Approach to Manual Muscle Testing. Edinburg, Churchill Livingstone, 1988

51. Colosimo AJ, Bassett FH: Jumpers knee—Diagnosis and treatment. Orthop Rev 19:139–149, 1990

52. Colville MR, Lee CL, Ciullo V: The Lenox Hill brace: An evaluation of effectiveness in treating knee instability. Am J Sports Med 14:257–261, 1986

53. Corrigan B, Maitland GD: Practical Orthopaedic Medicine. London, Butterworths, 1985

54. Corry IS, Webb JM, Clingeleffer AJ, et al: Arthroscopic reconstruction of the anterior cruciate ligament: A comparison of patellar tendon autograft and four-strand hamstring tendon autograft. Am J Sports Med 27:444–454, 1999

55. Cross MJ, Powell JF: Long-term follow-up of PCL rupture: A study of 116 cases. Am J Sports Med 12:282–297, 1984

56. Curt WW, Markey KL, Mitchell WA: Agility training following ACL reconstruction. Clin Orthop 172:133–136, 1983

57. Curwin S, Stanish WD: Tendinitis: Its Etiology and Treatment. Lexington, MA, The Collamore Press, 1984

58. Cyriax J: Rheumatism and Soft-Tissue Injuries. London, Hamilton, 1947

59. Cyriax J: Textbook of Orthopaedic Medicine, vol. 1, Diagnosis of Soft Tissue Lesions, 8th ed. London, Bailliere Tindall, 1982

60. Cyriax J: Textbook of Orthopaedic Medicine, vol. 2: Treatment by Manipulation, Massage and Injections, 10th ed. London, Bailliere Tindall, 1984

61. Dandy DJ, Pusey RJ: The long-term results of unrepaired tears of the PCL. J Bone Joint Surg 64B: 92–94, 1984

62. Daniels DM: Instrumented measurement of anterior knee laxity. Presented at the ACL meeting, Steamboat Springs, CO, 1984

63. Daniels DM, Malcom LL, Losse G, et al: Instrumented measurement of anterior laxity of the knee. J Bone Joint Surg Am 67:720–726, 1985

64. Davis VB: Flexibility conditioning for running. In: D'Ambrosia R, Drez D, eds: Prevention and Treatment of Running Injuries, 2nd ed. Thorofare, NJ, Slack, 1989:12221–12232

65. DeCarlo MS, Shelborne KD, McCarroll JR, et al: Traditional versus accelerated rehabilitation following ACL reconstruction: one-year-follow up. J Orthop Sports Phys Ther 15: 309–316, 1992

66. Degenhardt TC: Chronic PCL instability: Nonoperative management. Orthop Trans 5:486–487, 1981

67. DeHaven KE: Rationale for meniscus repair or excision. Clin Sports Med 4:267–273, 1985

68. DeHaven KE, Black KP, Griffth HJ: Open meniscus repair: Technique and two to nine year results. Am J Sports Med 17:788–795, 1989

69. DeHaven KE, Bronstein RD: Arthroscopic medial meniscal repair in athletes. Clin Sports Med 16:69–86, 1997

70. DeLee JC, Riley MR, Rockwood CA: Acute straight lateral instability of the knee. Am J Sports Med 11:404–411, 1983

71. DePalma AF: Disease of the Knee. Philadelphia, JB Lippincott, 1954

72. DePalma B: Rehabilitation of the groin, hip and thigh. In: Prentice WE, Voight MI, eds: Techniques in Musculoskeletal Rehabilitation. New York, McGraw-Hill, 2001:509–540

73. Deyle GD, Henderson NE, Marekel RL, et al: Effectiveness of manual therapy and exercise in osteoarthritis of the knee. A randomized, controlled trial. Ann Intern Med 132:173–181, 2000

74. Dietrichson J, Souryal TO: Physical therapy after arthroscopic surgery, 'preoperative and post operative rehabilitation after anterior cruciate ligament tear.' Orthop Phys Ther Clin North Am 3:539–554, 1994

75. DiStefano V: Skeletal injuries of the knee. In: Nicholas JA Hershman EB, eds. The Lower Extremity and Spine in Sports Medicine. St. Louis, Mosby, 1986: 862–904

76. DiStefano V: ACL reconstruction: Autograft or allograft? Clin Sports Med 12:1–11, 1993

77. DiVeta JA, Vobelbach WD: The clinical efficacy of the A-angle measuring patellar alignment. J Orthop Sports Phys Ther 16:136–139, 1992

78. Dixon ASJ: Factors in the development and presentation of osteoarthritis of the knee. In: Roush PA, ed: Progress in Clinical Rheumatoid Arthritis. London, J & A Churchill, 1965:313–329

79. Donaldson WF, Warren RF, Wickiewicz T: A comparison of acute ACL examinations. Am J Sports Med 13:57–10, 1985

80. Doucette SA, Goble EM: The effect of exercise on patellar tracking in lateral patellar compression syndrome. Am J Sports Med 20:434–440, 1992

81. Drez D: Knee braces. In: Jackson DW, ed: The Anterior Cruciate Deficient Knee: New Concepts in Ligament Repair. St. Louis, CV Mosby, 1987

82. Drez D, Kinnard WH: Clinical examination. In: Shahriaree H, ed: O'Connor's Textbook of Arthroscopic Surgery. Philadelphia, JB Lippincott, 1984

83. Eifert-Mangine MA, Biblo JT: Conservative management of patellofemoral chondrosis. In: Mangine RE, ed: Physical Therapy of the Knee, 2nd ed. New York, Churchill Livingstone, 1995:113–142

84. Einhorn AR, Sawyer M, Tovin B: Rehabilitation of intra-articular reconstruction. In: Greenfield BH, ed: Rehabilitation of the Knee: A Problem-Solving Approach. Philadelphia, FA Davis, 1993:245–287

85. Ellsasser JC, Reynolds KC, Omohundro JR: The nonoperative treatment of collateral ligament injuries of the knee in professional football players. J Bone Joint Surg Am 56:1185–1190, 1974

86. Engin AE, Korde MS: Mechanics of normal and abnormal knee joint. J Biomechanics 7:325–334, 1974

87. Engle R, ed: Knee Ligament Rehabilitation. New York, Churchill Livingstone, 1991

88. Evjenth E, Hamberg J: Muscle Stretching in Manual Therapy: A Clinical Manual, vol. 1: The Extremities. Alfta, Sweden, Alfta Rehab Forhaj, 1984

89. Exelby L: Peripheral mobilisations with movement. Man Ther 1:118–126, 1996

90. Fetto JF, Marshall JL: The natural history and diagnosis of ACL insufficiency. Clin Orthop Relat Res 147:29–38, 1980

91. Ficat RP, Philippe T, Hangerford DS: Chondromalacia patellae. Clin Orthop 144:55–62, 1979

92. Fox JA, Nedeff DD, Bach BR, et al: Anterior cruciate ligament reconstruction with patellar autograft tendon. Clin Orthop 402:53–63, 2002

93. Frankel VH, Burstein AH: Orthopaedic Biomechanics. Philadelphia, Lea & Febiger, 1971

94. Frankel VH, Burstein AH, Brooks DB: Biomechanics of internal derangement of the knee. J Bone Joint Surg Am 53:945–962, 1971

95. Frankel VH, Nordin M: Basic Biomechanics of the Skeletal System, 2nd ed. Philadelphia, Lea & Febiger, 1980

96. Fu FH, Bennett CH, Ma CB, et al: Current trends in anterior cruciate ligament reconstruction. Part II: Operative procedures and clinical correlation. Am J Sports Med 28:124–130, 2000

97. Fu FH, Schulte KR: Anterior cruciate ligament surgery 1996 state of the art? Clin Orthop Rel Res 325:19–24, 1996

98. Fu FH, Woo S, Irrgang J, et al: Current concepts for rehabilitation following ACL reconstruction. J Orthop Sports Phys Ther 15:270–278, 1992

99. Fulkerson JP: Awareness of the retinaculum in evaluating patellofemoral pain. Am J Sports Med 10:147–149, 1982

100. Fulkerson JP: The etiology of patellofemoral pain in young active patients: A prospective study. Clin Orthop 179:129–133, 1983

101. Funk JF: Synthetic ligaments: Current status. Clin Orthop 219:107–111, 1987

102. Furman W, Marshall JL, Giris FG: The ACL: A functional analysis based on postmortem studies. J Bone Joint Surg Br 58:179–185, 1976

103. Galway HR, Beaupre A, MacIntosh D: Pivot-shift: A clinical sign of symptomatic anterior cruciate insufficiency. J Bone Joint Surg Br 54:763–764, 1972

104. Galway HR, MacIntosh DL: The lateral pivot-shift: A symptom and sign of ACL insufficiency. Clin Orthop 147:45–50, 1980

105. Garrick JG, Webb DR: Knee injuries. In: Garrick JG, Webb DR: Sports Injuries: Diagnosis and Management, 2nd ed. Philadelphia, WB Saunders, 1999:259–333

106. Geraci MC: Rehabilitation of the hip, pelvis, and thigh. In: Kibler WB, Herring SA, Press JM, eds: Functional Rehabilitation of Sports and Musculoskeletal Injuries. Gaithersburg, MD, Aspen Publishers, 1998:216–243

107. Girgis FG, Marshall JL, Morajem ARS: The cruciate ligaments of the knee joint: Anatomical, functional, and experimental analysis. Clin Orthop 106:216–231, 1975

108. Glove TP, Muller S, Barreck EK: Nonoperative treatment of the torn ACL. J Bone Joint Surg Am 65:184–192, 1983

109. Godfrey JD: Ligament injuries of the knee. In: Anstrom JP, ed: Current Practice in Orthopedic Surgery, vol. 5. St. Louis, CV Mosby, 1973

110. Goldberg A: Work-induced growth of skeletal muscle in normal and hypophysectomised rats. Am J Physiol 312:1193–1198, 1967

111. Gollehan DL, Torzilli PA, Warren RF: The role of the posterolateral and cruciate ligaments in the stability of the knee: A biomechanical study. J Bone Joint Surg Am 69:233–242, 1987.

112. Good L, Odensten M, Gillquist J: Sagittal knee stability after ACL reconstruction with a patellar tendon strip: A 2-year follow-up study. Am J Sports Med 22:518–523, 1994

113. Goodfellow J, Hungerford DS, Woods C: Patellofemoral joint mechanics and pathology, Part 2: Chondromalacia patellae. J Bone Joint Surg Br 58:291–299, 1976

114. Goodfellow J, Hungerford DS, Zindel M: Patellofemoral joint mechanics and pathology, Part 1: Functional anatomy of the patellofemoral joint. J Bone Joint Surg Br 58:287–290, 1976

115. Graham SM, Parker RD: Anterior cruciate ligament reconstruction using hamstring tendon grafts. Clin Orthop 402:64–75, 2002

116. Green WR Jr: Painful bipartite patellae. Clin Orthop 110:197–200, 1975

117. Greenfield BH: Functional anatomy of the knee. In: Greenfield BH: Rehabilitation of the Knee: A Problem Solving Approach. Philadelphia, FA Davis, 1992:3–42

118. Grood E, Noyes F, Butler D: Biomechanics of knee extension exercise. J Bone Joint Surg Am 66:725–734, 1984

119. Grood ES, Stowers SF, Noyes FR: Limits of movement in the human knee: Effects of sectioning the posterior cruciate ligament and posterolateral structures. J Bone Joint Surg Am 70:88–97, 1988

120. Gustavsen R, Streeck R: Training Therapy: Prophylaxis and Rehabilitation, 2nd ed. Stuttgart, Georg Thieme Verlag, 1993

121. Gutman E, Schiaffino S, Hazlikova V: Mechanism of compensatory hypertrophy in skeletal muscles of the rat. Exp Neurol 31:451–464, 1971

122. Haggmark TN, Eriksson E: Cylinder or mobile cast brace after knee ligament surgery. Am J Sports Med 7:48–56, 1979

123. Hammer DL, Brown JR CH, Steiner ME, et al: Hamstring tendon grafts for reconstruction of the anterior cruciate ligament: Biomechanical evaluation of the use of multiple strands and tensioning techniques. J Bone Joint Surg Am 81:549–557, 1999

124. Hammer W: Meniscotibial (coronary) ligament sprain: diagnosis and treatment. Chirop Sports Med 2:48–50, 1988

125. Hammer WI: The knee. In: Hammer W: Functional Soft Tissue Examination and Treatment by Manual Methods. Gaithersburg, MD, Aspen Publication, 1991:123–171

126. Hansen H, Boe S: The pathological plica in the knee—Results after arthroscopic resection. Arch Orthop Trauma Surg 108:282–284, 1989

127. Hanten WP, Schulthies SS: Exercise's effect on electromyographic activity of the vastus medialis oblique and vastus lateralis muscles. Phys Ther 70:561–565, 1990

128. Hardarkerwt WT, Whipple TL, Bassett FH: Diagnosis and treatment of the plica syndrome of the knee. J Bone Joint Surg Am 62:222–225, 1980

129. Hardin JA, Voight ML, Blackburn TA, et al: The effects of "decelerated" rehabilitation following anterior cruciate ligament reconstruction on a hyperelastic female adolescent: a case study. J Orthop Sports Phys Ther 26:29–34, 1997

130. Hastings DE: The nonoperative treatment of collateral ligament injuries of the knee joint. Clin Orthop 147:22–28, 1980

131. Helfet A: Disorders of the Knee. Philadelphia, JB Lippincott, 1974

132. Henning CE, Lynch MA, Glick K: An in vivo strain gauge study of elongation of the ACL. Am J Sports Med 13:22–26, 1985

133. Henning CE, Lynch MA, Glick K: Physical examination of the knee. In: Nicholas JA, Hershmann EB, eds: The Lower Extremity and Spine in Sports Medicine, vol. 1. St. Louis, CV Mosby, 1986:795–800

134. Hewett TE, Paterno MV, Myer GD: Strategies for enhancing proprioception and neuromuscular control of the knee. Clin Orthop 402:76–94, 2002

135. Hewett TE, Paterno MV, Noyes FR: Differences in single leg balance in an unstable platform between female and male normal, ACL-deficient and ACL reconstructed knees. The Twenty-fifth Annual Meeting of the American Orthopaedic Society for Sports Medicine. Traverse City, MI, 455, 1999

136. Hewett TE, Paterno MV, Noyes FR: Neuromuscular contribution to knee kinematics and kinetics: Normal versus pathological state. In: Lephart SM, Fu FH, eds:. Proprioception and Neuromuscular Control in Joint Stability. Champaigne, IL, Human Kinetics, 2000:77–88

137. Hiemstra LA, Webber S, MacDonald PB, et al: Knee strength deficits after hamstring tendon and patellar tendon anterior cruciate ligament reconstruction. Med Sci Sports Exerc 32:1472–1479, 2000

138. Hislop HJ, Montgomery J: Daniels and Worthingham's Muscle Testing. Techniques of Manual Examination, 6th ed. Philadelphia, WB Saunders, 1995

139. Hoffa A: The influence of the adipose tissue with regards to the pathology of the knee joint. JAMA 43:795–796, 1904

140. Holden DL, Eggert AW, Butler JE: The nonoperative treatment of grade I and II medial collateral ligament injuries to the knee. Am J Sports Med 11:340–344, 1983

141. Holten O: Medisinsk Treningsterapi Trykk Fugseth and Lorentzen. Medical Training Course, Salt Lake City, 1984

142. Hoppenfield S: Physical Examination of the Spine and Extremities. New York, Appleton-Century-Crofts, 1976

143. Huberti H, Hayes W: Patellofemoral contact pressures: The influence of the Q angle and tendofemoral contact. J Bone Joint Surg Am 66:715–724, 1984

144. Hughston JC: Extensor mechanism examination. In: Fox JM, Del Pizzo W, eds: The Patellofemoral Joint. New York, McGraw-Hill, 1993:63–74

145. Hughston JC, Andrews JR, Cross MJ, et al: Classification of knee ligament instability, Part I. J Bone Joint Surg Am 58:159–172, 1976a

146. Hughston JC, Andrews JR, Cross MJ, et al: Classification of knee ligament instability, Part II. J Bone Joint Surg Am 58:173–179, 1976b

147. Hughston JC, Eiler A: The role of the posterior oblique ligament in repairs of acute medial collateral ligament tears of the knee. J Bone Joint Surg Am 55:923–940, 1973

148. Hughston JC, Jackson KE: Chronic posterolateral rotatory instability of the knee. J Bone Joint Surg Am 67:351–359, 1985

149. Hughston JC, Norwood LA: The posterolateral drawer test for posterolateral rotatory instability of the knee. Clin Orthop 147:82–87, 1980

150. Hughston JC, Walsh WM, Puddu G: Patellar Subluxation and Dislocation. Philadelphia, WB Saunders, 1984

151. Hungerford DS, Barry M: Biomechanics of the patellofemoral joint. Clin Orthop 144:9–15, 1979

152. Hunter SC, Poole RM: The chronically inflamed tendon. Clin Sports Med 6:371–388, 1987

153. Ihara H, Nakayama A: Dynamic joint control training for knee ligament injuries. Am J Sports Med 14:309–315, 1986

154. Indelicato PA, Linton RC, Huegel M: The results of fresh-frozen patellar tendon allografts for chronic ACL deficiency of the knee. Am J Sports Med 20:118–121, 1992

155. Insall J, Falvo KA, Wise DW: Chondromalacia patellae, a prospective study. J Bone Joint Surg Am 58:1–8, 1976

156. Insall J, Joseph DM, Aglietti P, et al: Bone bock iliotibial-band transfer for ACL insufficiency. J Bone Joint Surg Am 63:560–569, 1981

157. Jackson D, Drez D: The Anterior Cruciate Deficient Knee. St. Louis, Mosby, 1987

158. Jakob RP: Observation on rotatory instability of the lateral compartment of the knee. Acta Orthop Scand 52(Suppl 191):1–32, 1981

159. Jakob RP, Staubli HU, Deland JT: Grading the pivot-shift. J Bone Joint Surg Br 69:294–299, 1987

160. James SL: Chondromalacia patella. In: Kennedy JC, ed: The Injured Adolescent Knee. Baltimore, Williams & Wilkins, 1979

161. James SL, Bates BT, Ostering LR: Injuries to runners. Am J Sports Med 6:40–50, 1978

162. Janda V: Treatment of Patients. International Federation of Orthopedic Manipulative Therapists, 4th Conference, Christchurch, New Zealand, 1980

163. Janda V: Muscle Function Testing. London, Butterworths, 1983

164. Jenkins D: Ligament Injuries and Their Treatment. Rockville, MD, Aspen, 1985

165. Jensen K: Manual laxity test for ACL injuries. J Orthop Sports Phys Ther 11:474–481, 1990

166. Jones AL: Rehabilitation for anterior instability of the knee—Preliminary report. J Orthop Sports Phys Ther 3:121–128, 1982

167. Jones KG: Reconstruction of the anterior cruciate ligament using the central one-third of the patella ligament, a follow up report. J Bone Joint Surg Am 52:1302–1308, 1970

168. Jonsson T, Alfhoff D, Peterson L, et al: Clinical diagnosis of ruptures of the ACL. Am J Sports Med 10:100–102, 1982

169. Kaltenborn FM: Mobilization of the Extremity Joints, vol. 1: Examination and Basic Treatment Techniques. Oslo, Olaf Norlis Bokhandel, 1980

170. Kaltenborn FM: Manual Mobilization of the Extremity Joints, vol. 2: Advanced Treatment Techniques. Oslo, Olaf Norlis Bokhandel, 1986

171. Kannus P: Nonoperative treatment of grade II and III sprains of the lateral ligament compartment of the knee. Am J Sports Med 25:596–602, 1989

172. Kaplan PE, Tanner ED: Musculoskeletal Pain and Disability. Norwalk, CT, Appleton &Lange, 1989

173. Karzel RP, Del Pizzo W: Patellofemoral arthritis—General considerations. In: Fox JM, Del Pizzo W, eds: The Patellofemoral Joint. New York, McGraw-Hill, 1993:243–248

174. Katz JW, Fingeroth RJ: The diagnostic accuracy of rupture of the ACL comparing the Lachman test, the anterior drawer sign, and the pivot-shift test in acute and chronic knee injuries. Am J Sports Med 14:88–91, 1986

175. Kaufman K, An KN, Lichy WJ, et al: Dynamic joint forces during knee isokinetic exercise. Am J Sports Med 19:305–316, 1991

176. Kendall FP, Mc Creary EK, Provance PG: Muscle Testing and Function, 4th ed. Baltimore, Williams & Wilkins, 1993

177. Kennedy JC: The Injured Adolescent Knee. Baltimore, Williams & Wilkins, 1979

178. Kennedy JC, Fowler PJ: Medial and anterior instability of the knee. J Bone Joint Surg Am 53:1257–1270, 1971

179. Kennedy JC, Galpin RD: The use of the medial head of the gastrocnemius muscle in the posterior cruciate-deficient knee: Indication, technique, results. Am J Sports Med 10:63–74, 1982

180. Kennedy JC, Weinberg HW, Wilson AS: The anatomy and function of the ACL, as determined by clinical and morphological studies. J Bone Joint Surg Am 56:223–234, 1974

181. Kettelkamp DB: Clinical implications of knee biomechanics. Arch Surg 107:406–410, 1973

182. Kettelkamp DB: Current concepts review—Management of patellar malalignment. J Bone Joint Surg Am 63:1344–1347, 1981

183. King AC, Ahles TA, Martin JE, et al: EMG biofeedback-controlled exercise in chronic arthritic knee pain. Arch Phys Med Rehabil 65:341–343, 1984

184. Kisner C, Colby LA: Therapeutic Exercise—Foundations and Techniques. Philadelphia, FA Davis, 1985

185. Knott M, Voss D: Proprioceptive Neuromuscular Facilitation, 2nd ed. New York, Harper & Row, 1969

186. Koshimo T, Okamoto R: Resection of painful shelf (plica synovialis mediopatellaris) under arthroscopy. Arthroscopy 1:136–141, 1985

187. Kottke FJ: Krusen's Handbook of Physical Medicine and Rehabilitation, 3rd ed. Philadelphia, WB Saunders, 1982

188. Kulund DK: The knee. In: Kulund DK: The Injured Athlete, 2nd ed. Philadelphia, JB Lippincott, 1988:435–512

189. LaPrade RF: The medial collateral ligament complex and the posterolateral aspect of the knee. In: Arednt EA, ed: Orthopaedic Knowledge Update, Sports Medicine 2. Rosemont, IL, American Academy of Sports Medicine, 1999:327–340

190. LaPrade RF, Hamilton CD, Engebretsen L: Treatment of acute and chronic combined anterior cruciate ligament and posterolateral knee ligament injuries. Sports Med Arthrosc Rev 5:91–99, 1997

191. LaPrade RF, Terry GC: Injuries to the posterolateral aspect of the knee: Association of injuries with clinical instability. Am J Sports Med 25:433–438, 1997

192. LaPrade RF, Wentorf F: Diagnosis and treatment of the posterolateral knee injuries. Clin Orthop 402:110–121, 2002

193. Larson RL: Overview and philosophy of knee injuries. Clin Sports Med 4:209–215, 1985

194. Larson RL, Cabaud HE, Slocum DB: The patella compression syndrome: Surgical treatment by lateral retinacular release. Clin Orthop 134:156–157, 1978

195. Last RJ: The popliteus muscle and lateral meniscus. J Bone Joint Surg Br 32:93–99, 1950

196. Laubenthal KN, Smidt GL, Kettelkamp DB: A quantitative analysis of knee motion for activities of daily living. Phys Ther 52:34–42, 1972

197. LeBrier K, O'Neill DB: Patellofemoral stress syndrome. Sports Med 16:449–459, 1993

198. Lechner DE: Rehabilitation of the knee with arthritis. In: Greenfield BH: Rehabilitation of the Knee: A Problem-Solving Approach. Philadelphia, FA Davis, 1993:206–241

199. Lephart SM, Kocher MS, Harner CD, et al: Quadriceps strength and functional capacity after ACL reconstruction: Patellar tendon autograft versus allograft. Am J Sports Med 21:738–743, 1993

200. Levandowski R: Knee injuries. In: Birrer RB, ed: Sports Medicine for the Primary Care Physician, 2nd ed. Boca Raton, FL, CRC Press, 1994:505–530

201. Levy IM, Torzilli PA, Warren RF: Effects of medial meniscectomy on anterior-posterior motion of the knee. J Bone Joint Surg Am 64:883–888, 1982

202. Lewis RJ: Degenerative arthritis. In: Nickel VL, ed: Orthopedic Rehabilitation. New York, Churchill Livingstone, 1982:515–524

203. Lewit K: Manipulative Therapy in Rehabilitation of the Locomotor System. 2nd ed. London, Butterworths, 1992

204. Liebenson CL: Active muscle relaxation techniques: Part II. Clinical application. J Manipulative Physiol Ther 13:2–6, 1990

205. Leibenson CL: Functional exercises. J Bodywork Movement Ther 6:108–113, 2002

206. Losee RE: Concepts of the pivot-shift. Clin Orthop 172:45–51, 1983

207. Losee RE, Johnson TR, Southwick WO: Anterior subluxation of the lateral tibia plateau. J Bone Joint Surg Am 60:1015–1030, 1978

208. Love JW, Whelan TJ: Popliteal artery entrapment syndrome. Am Med J Surg 109:620–624, 1965

209. Lucie RS, Wiedel JD, Messner DG: The acute pivot-shift: Clinical correlation. Am J Sports Med 12:189–191, 1984

210. Lutter L: Injuries in runners and joggers. Minn Med 63:45–51, 1980

211. Lutter L: Cavus foot in runners. Foot Ankle 1:225–228, 1981

212. Lutter L: Running athlete in office practice. Foot Ankle 3:52–59, 1982

213. Lutter L: The knee and running. Clin Sports Med 4:685–698, 1985

214. Lutz GE, Palmiter RA, An KN, et al: Comparison of tibiofemoral joint forces during open and closed kinetic chain exercise. J Bone Joint Surg Am 75:732–739,1993

215. Lutz G, Warren RF: Meniscal injuries. In: Griffin LY, ed: Rehabilitation of the Injured Knee, 2nd ed. St. Louis, Mosby, 1995:134–148

216. Lysholm J, Gillquist J: Evaluation of knee ligament surgery results with special emphasis on use of a scoring scale. Am J Sports Med 10:150–154, 1982

217. Magee DJ: Orthopedic Physical Assessment, 3rd ed. Philadelphia, WB Saunders, 1997

218. Maitland GD: Peripheral Manipulations, 3rd ed. London, Butterworth, 1991

219. Malone T, Davies G: Muscular control of the patella. Clin Sports Med 21:349–362, 2002

220. Mangine R: Physical Therapy of the Knee. New York, Churchill Livingstone, 1988

221. Mangine R, Heckman T: The knee. In: Sanders B, ed: Sports Physical Therapy, Norwalk, CT, Appleton & Lange, 1990:423–449

222. Mangine RE, Noyes FR: Rehabilitation of the allograft reconstruction. J Orthop Sports Phys Ther 15:294–302, 1992

223. Mangine RE, Noyes FR, DeMaio M: Minimal protection program: advanced weight bearing and range of motion after ACL reconstruction—weeks 1–5. Orthopedics 15:504–515, 1992

224. Mankin HJ: Articular cartilage, cartilage injury and osteoarthritis. In: Fox JM, Del Pizzo W, eds: The Patellofemoral Joint. New York, McGraw-Hill, 1993:49–62

225. Mann RA, Hagy JL: The popliteus muscle. J Bone J Surg Am 59:924–927, 1977

226. Mann R, Baxter D, Lutter L: Running symposium. Foot Ankle 1:190–224, 1981

227. Mariani PP, Caruso I: An electromyographic investigation of subluxation of the patella. J Bone Joint Surg Br 61:169–11, 1979

228. Markolf KL: Quantitative examination for anterior cruciate laxity. In: Jackson DW, Drez D, eds: The Anterior Cruciate-Deficient Knee: New Concepts in Ligament Repair. St. Louis, CV Mosby, 1987

229. Markolf K, Graff-Radford A, Amstutz H: In vivo knee stability: A quantitative assessment using an instrumented clinical testing apparatus. J Bone Joint Surg Am 60:664–674, 1978

230. Marks KE, Bentley G: Patella alta and chondromalacia. J Bone Joint Surg Br 60:71–73, 1978

231. Marshall JL: The biceps femoris tendon and its functional significance. J Bone Joint Surg Am 54:1444–1450, 1972

232. Martins M, Wouter P, Brussens A, et al: Patellar tendinitis: pathology and results of treatment. Acta Orthop Scand 53:445–450, 1982

233. Mayfield G: Popliteus tendon tenosynovitis. Am Sports Med 5:31–36, 1977

234. McCarty EC, Max RG, DeHaven KE: Meniscus repair. Considerations in treatment and update of clinical results. Clin Orthop 402:122–134, 2002

235. McConnell J: The management of chondromalacia patellae: A long-term solution. Aust J Physiol 2:215–223, 1986

236. McConnell J: Management of patellofemoral problems. Man Ther 1:407–414, 1996

237. McConnell J: The physical therapist's approach to patellofemoral disorders. Clin Sports Med 21:363–387, 2002

238. McMurray TP: The semilunar cartilage. Br J Surg 29:407–414, 1942

239. Meachim G, Emery IH: Quantitative aspects of patellofemoral cartilage fibrillation in Liverpool necropsies. Ann Rheum Dis 3:39–47, 1974

240. Mellion MB: Office Management of Sports Injuries and Athletic Problems. St. Louis, CV Mosby, 1988

241. Mennell JB: Physical Treatment by Movement, Manipulation and Massage, 5th ed. Philadelphia, Blakiston, 1947

242. Merchant AC: The lateral patellar compression syndrome. In: Fox JM, Del Pizzo W, eds: The Patellofemoral Joint. New York, McGraw-Hill, 1993:157–168

243. Meyer JF: Allograft reconstruction of the ACL. Clin Sports Med 10:487–498, 1991

244. Muller W: The Knee: Form, Function and Ligament Reconstruction. New York, Springer-Verlag, 1983

245. Mulligan BR: Mobilisation with movement (MWMs). J Man Manip Ther 1:154–156, 1993

246. Mulligan BR: Manual Therapy 'Nags,' 'Snags,' 'MWMs,' etc. 4th ed. New Zealand, Plant View Services, 1999

247. Nicholas JA: Injuries to the menisci of the knee. Orthop Clin North Am 4:647–664, 1973

248. Nicholas JA, Hershmann EB, eds: The Lower Extremity and Spine in Sports Medicine, vol. 1. St. Louis, CV Mosby, 1986

249. Nicholas JA, Minkoff J: Iliotibial band transfer through the intercondylar notch for combined anterior instability. Am J Sports Med 6:341–353, 1978

250. Noble CA: Iliotibial band friction syndrome in runners. Am J Sports Med 8:232–234, 1980

251. Norris CM: The knee. In: Norris CM: Sports Injuries: Diagnosis and Management for Physiotherapists. Oxford, Butterworth-Heinemann, 1993:169–192

252. Norwood LA, Cross MJ: The ACL: Functional anatomy of its bundles in rotatory instabilities. Am J Sports Med 7:23–26, 1979

253. Noyes FR: Functional properties of knee ligaments and alterations induced by immobilization—A correlative biomechanical and histological study in primates. Clin Orthop 123:210–242, 1977

254. Noyes FR, Barber SD, Mangine RE: Bone-patellar ligament-bone and fascia lata allografts for reconstruction of the ACL. J Bone Joint Surg Am 72:1125–1136, 1990

255. Noyes FR, Barber-Westin SD: Revision anterior cruciate ligament surgery: experience from Cincinnati. Clin Orthop Rel Res 325:116–129, 1996

256. Noyes FR, Barber-Westin SD: Revision anterior cruciate surgery with use of one-patellar tendon-bone autogenous grafts. J Bone Joint Surg Am 83:1131–1143, 2001

257. Noyes FR, Bassett RW, Grood ES, et al: Arthroscopy in acute traumatic hemarthrosis of the knee—Incidence of anterior cruciate tears and other injuries. J Bone Joint Surg Am 62:687–695, 1980

258. Noyes FR, Butler DL, Grood ES: Biomechanical analysis of human ligament grafts used in knee ligament repairs and reconstructions. J Bone Joint Surg Am 66:344–352, 1984

259. Noyes FR, Mangine RE, Barber S: Early knee motion after open and arthroscopic ACL reconstruction. Am J Sports Med 15:149–160, 1981

260. Noyes FR, Matthews DS, Mooar PA et al: The symptomatic anterior cruciate-deficient knee, Part II: The result of rehabilitation activity modification and counseling on functional disability. J Bone Joint Surg am 65:163–174, 1983

261. Noyes FR, Mooar PA, Matthews DS, et al: The symptomatic anterior cruciate-deficient knee, Part I: The long-term functional disability in athletically active individuals. J Bone Joint Surg Am 65:154–162, 1983

262. Noyes FR, Torvik PJ, Hyde WB, et al: Biomechanics of ligament failure: II. An analysis of immobilization, exercise, and reconditioning effects in primates. J Bone Joint Surg Am 56:1406–1418, 1974

263. O'Donoghue DH: Treatment of acute ligamentous injuries of the knee. Orthop Clin North Am 4:617–645, 1973

264. Ogden JA, McCarthy SM, Tokl P: The painful bipartite patella. J Pediatr Orthop 2:263–269, 1982

265. Ohkoshi Y, Yasada K: Biomechanical analysis of shear force exerted to ACL during half-squat exercise. Orthop Trans 13:310, 1989

266. Ombergt L, Bisschop P, ter Veer HJ, et al: A System of Orthopaedic Medicine. London, WB Saunders, 1995

267. O'Neill DB, Micheli LJ, Warner JP: Patellofemoral stress: A prospective analysis of exercise treatment in adolescents and adults. Am J Sports Med 20:151–156, 1992

268. Outerbridge REE: The etiology of chondromalacia patellae. J Bone Joint Surg Br 43:752–757, 1961

269. Palmer ML, Epler ME: Fundamentals of Musculoskeletal Assessment Techniques, 2nd ed. Philadelphia, Lippincott Williams & Wilkins, 1998

270. Palmittier RA, An KN, Scott SG, et al: Kinetic chain exercise in knee rehabilitation. Sports Med 11:402–413, 1991

271. Patel D: Arthroscopy of the plicae-synovial fold and their significance. Am J Sports Med 6:217–225, 1978

272. Patel D: Plica as a cause of anterior knee pain. Orthop Clin North Am 17:273–277, 1986

273. Patel D: Synovial lesions: Plicae. In: McGinty JB, ed: Operative Arthroscopy. New York, Raven Press, 1991:361–372

274. Patel D, Laurencin CT, Tsuchiya A, et al: Synovial folds—Plicae. In: Fox JM, Del Pizzo W, eds: The Patellofemoral Joint. New York, McGraw-Hill, 1993:193–198

275. Paulos LE: Knee and leg: Soft-tissue trauma. In: American Academy of Orthopedic Surgeons: Orthopedic Knowledge Update 2, 1987

276. Paulos LE, Cheri J, Rosenberg TD, et al: ACL reconstruction with autografts. Clin Sports Med 10:469–485, 1991

277. Paulos LE, Noyes FR, Grood E, et al: Knee rehabilitation after ACL reconstruction and repair. Am J Sports Med 9:140–149, 1981

278. Paulos L, Rusche K, Johnson C, et al: Patellar malalignment: A treatment rationale. Phys Ther 60:1627–1632, 1980

279. Peppard A: Knee rehabilitation. In: Canavan PK, ed: Rehabilitation in Sports Medicine. Stamford, CT, Appleton & Lange, 1998:301–323

280. Peterson L, Pitman MI, Gold J: The active pivot shift: the role of the popliteus muscle. Am J Sports Med 12:313–317, 1984

281. Petty NJ, Moore AP: Neuromusculoskeletal Examination and Assessment. Edinburgh, Churchill Livingstone, 1998

282. Podesta L, Magnusson J, Gillette T: Anterior cruciate ligament reconstruction. In: Maxey L, Magnusson J, eds: Rehabilitation for the Postsurgical Orthopedic Patient. St. Louis, Mosby, 2001:206–226

283. Pope MH, Stankewich CJ, Beynnon BD, et al: Effect of knee musculature on ACL strain in vivo. J Electromyog Kines 1:191–198, 1991

284. Post M: Physical Examination of the Musculoskeletal System. Chicago, Year Book Medical, 1987

285. Prentice WE, Davis M: Rehabilitation of the knee. In: Prentice WE, Voight ML, eds: Techniques in Musculoskeletal Rehabilitation, New York, McGraw Hill, 2001:541–582

286. Radin EL, de Lamotte F, Maquet P: Role of the menisci in the distribution of stress in the knee. Clin Orthop Relat Res 185:290–294, 1984

287. Raux P, Townsend PR, Miegel R, et al: Trabecular architecture of the human patella. J Biomech 8:1–7, 1975

288. Renne J: The iliotibial band friction syndrome. J Bone Joint Surg Am 57:1110–1115, 1975

289. Reynolds LR, Levin TA, Mederios JM, et al: EMG activity of the vastus medialis oblique and the vastus lateralis in their role in patellar alignment. Am J Phys Med Rehabil 62:61–70, 1983

290. Richards DB, Kibler WB: Rehabilitation of the knee injuries. In: Kibler WB, Herring SA, Press MD, eds: Functional Rehabilitation of Sports and Musculoskeletal Injuries. Gaithersburg, MD, Aspen Publishers, 1998:244–253

291. Ricklin P, Ruttmann A, Del Buno MS: Meniscus Lesions: Diagnosis, Differential Diagnosis, and Therapy, 2nd ed. Stuttgart, Thieme, 1983

292. Romero JA, Standford TL, Schroeder RV, et al: The effects of electrical stimulation of normal quadriceps on strength and girth. Med Sci Sports Exerc 14:194–197, 1982

293. Roy S, Irvin R: Thigh, knee and patella injuries. In: Steven R, Irvin R, eds: Sports Medicine: Prevention, Evaluation, Management, and Rehabilitation. Englewood Cliffs, NJ, Prentice Hall, 1983:293–368

294. Rubinstein RA, Shelborne KD, Van Meter CD, et al: Effect of knee stability if full hyperextension is restored immediately after autogenous bone-patellar anterior cruciate ligament reconstruction. Am J Sports Med 23:365–368, 1995

295. Saal J, ed: Physical Medicine and Rehabilitation: Rehabilitation of Sports Injuries. Philadelphia, Hanley & Belfus, 1987

296. Sandberg R, Balkfors B: Reconstruction of the anterior cruciate ligament: a 5 year follow-up of 89 patients. Acta Orthop Scand 59:288–293, 1988

297. Sandberg R, Balkfors B, Nilsson B, et al: Operative versus nonoperative treatment of recent injuries to the ligaments of the knee. J Bone Joint Surg Am 69:1120–1126, 1987

298. Sarhmann S: Diagnosis and Treatment of Movement Impairment Syndromes. St. Louis, Mosby, 2002

299. Schneider W, Dvorak J, Dvorak J, et al: Manual Medicine: Therapy. New York, Georg Thieme Verlag Stuttgart, 1988

300. Schultz P: Flexibility: The day of the static stretch. Phys Sports Med 7:109–117, 1979

301. Seedhom BB: Load-bearing function of the menisci. Physiotherapy 62:223–228, 1976

302. Seto JL, Clive E, Brewster MS, et al: Rehabilitation of the knee after anterior cruciate ligament reconstruction. J Orthop Sports Phys Ther 11:8–18, 1989

303. Shaw JA, Eng M, Murray DG: The longitudinal axis of the knee and the role of the cruciate ligaments in controlling transverse rotation. J Bone Joint Surg Am 56:1603–1609, 1974

304. Shea KP, Fulkerson JP: Patellofemoral joint injuries. In: Griffin LY, ed: Rehabilitation of the Injured Knee, 2nd ed. St. Louis, Mosby, 1995:121–133

305. Shelbourne KD, Gray T: Anterior cruciate ligament reconstruction with autogenous patellar tendon graft followed by accelerated rehabilitation. A two- to nine-year follow up. Am J Sports Med 25:786–795, 1997

306. Shelbourne KD, Klootwyk TE, DeCarlo MS: Update on accelerated rehabilitation after anterior cruciate ligament reconstruction. J Orthop Sports Phys Ther 15:303–308, 1992

307. Shelbourne KD, Klootwyk TE, Wilckens JH, et al: Ligament stability two to six years after anterior cruciate ligament reconstruction with autogenous patellar tendon graft and participation in accelerated rehabilitation program. Am J Sports Med 23:575–579, 1995

308. Shelbourne KD, Liotta FJ: Rehabilitation program for both knees when the contralateral autogenic patellar tendon graft is used for primary anterior cruciate ligament reconstruction; a case study. J Orthop Sports Phys Ther 29:144–153, 1999

309. Shelbourne KD, Nitz PA: Accelerated rehabilitation after ACL reconstruction. Am J Sports Med 18:292–299, 1990

310. Shelbourne KD, Nitz PA: Accelerated rehabilitation after ACL reconstruction. J Orthop Sports Phys Ther 15: 256–264, 1992

311. Shelbourne KD, Rubinstein RA, VanMeter CD, et al: Correlation of remaining patellar tendon width with quadriceps strength after autogenous bone patellar tendon-bone cruciate ligament reconstruction. Am J Sports Med 22:774–777, 1994

312. Shephard RJ: Physiology and Biochemistry of Exercise. New York, Praeger Press, 1982

313. Sherrington CS: The Integrative Actions of the Nervous System. New Haven, Yale University Press, 1906

314. Shino K, Horibe S, Nagano J, et al: Quantitative assessment of anterior stability of the knee following ACL reconstruction using allogeneic tendon. Trans Orthop Res Soc 12:130, 1987

315. Shino K, Inoue M, Horibe S, et al: Reconstruction of the ACL using allogeneic tendon—Long-term follow-up. Am J Sports Med 18:457–465, 1990

316. Shino K, Nakata K, Horibe S, et al: Quantitative evaluation after arthroscopic ACL reconstruction: Allograft versus autograft. Am J Sports Med 21:609–616, 1993

317. Shino K, Oakes BW, Inoue M, et al: Human ACL allograft-collagen fibril population studied as a function of age of the graft. Trans Orthop Res Soc 15:520, 1990

318. Shoji H: Chondromalacia patellae: Histological and biochemical aspects. NY State J Med 74:507–510, 1974

319. Slocum DB, James SL, Larson RL, et al: Clinical test for anterolateral rotary instability of the knee. Clin Orthop 118:63–69, 1976

320. Slocum DB, Larson RL: Rotary instability of the knee: Its pathogenesis and a clinical test to determine its presence. J Bone Joint Surg Am 50:211–225, 1968

321. Slocum DB, Larson RL, James SL: Late reconstruction procedures used to stabilize the knee. Orthop Clin North Am 4:679–689, 1973

322. Smillie IS: Injuries of the Knee Joint. New York, Churchill Livingstone, 1978

323. Smillie IS: Diseases of the Knee Joint, 2nd ed. Edinburgh, Churchill Livingstone, 1980

324. Snyder-Mackler L, Ladin Z, Schepsis AA, et al: Electrical stimulation of the thigh muscles after reconstruction of the anterior cruciate ligament: Effects of electrically elicited contraction the quadriceps femoris and hamstring muscles on gait and strength of the thigh muscles. J Bone Joint Surg Am 73:1025–1036, 1991

325. Sonzogni JJ: Physical assessment of the injured knee. Emerg Med 20:74–92, 1988

326. Spencer J, Hayes K, Alexander I: Knee joint effusion and quadriceps reflex inhibition in man. Arch Phys Med Rehabil 65:171–177, 1984

327. Stanish WD: Neurophysiology of stretching. In: D'Ambrosia R, Drez D, eds: Prevention and Treatment of Running Injuries. Thorofare, NJ, Slack, 1982:135–146

328. Steadman JR: Nonoperative methods for patellofemoral problems. Am J Sports Med 7:374–375, 1979a

329. Steadman JR: Rehabilitation of first- and second-degree sprains of the medial collateral ligament. Am J Sports Med 7:300–302, 1979b

330. Steadman JR: Rehabilitation of acute injuries of the ACL. Clin Orthop 172:129–132, 1983

331. Stillwell GK: Electrotherapy. In: Kottke FS, Stillwell GK, Lehmann JF, eds: Krusen's Handbook of Physical Medicine and Rehabilitation, 3rd ed. Philadelphia, WB Saunders, 1982

332. Stokes M, Young A: Investigation of quadriceps inhibition: Implications for clinical practice. Physiotherapy 70:425–428, 1984

333. Storigord J: Chondromalacia of the patella: Physical signs in relation to operative findings. Acta Orthop Scand 46:685–694, 1975

334. Stuller J: Bracing the unstable knee. Phys Sports Med 13:142–156, 1985

335. Sullivan PE, Markos PD: Clinical Decision Making in Therapeutic Exercise. Norwalk, CT, Appleton & Lange, 1994

336. Surburg RR: Proprioceptive neuromuscular facilitation. Phys Sports Med 9:115–127, 1981

337. Tegner Y: Strength training in the rehabilitation of cruciate ligament tears. Sports Med 9:129–136, 1990

338. Teitge RA, Indelicato PA, Kerlan RK: Iliotibial band transfer for anterolateral rotatory instability of the knee: summary of 54 cases. Am J Sports Med 8: 223–227, 1980

339. Teitz C, Larson R: Health Maintenance. In: American Academy of Orthopedic Surgeons: Orthopaedic Knowledge Update 2, 1987

340. Tibone J, Antich TJ, Fanton GS, et al: Functional analysis of ACL instability. Am J Sports Med 14:276–283, 1986

341. Tory JS, Conrad W, Kalen V: Clinical diagnosis of ACL instability in the athlete. Am J Sports Med 4:84–93, 1976

342. Tovin BJ, Wolf SL, Greenfield BH, et al: Comparison of the effects of exercise in water and on land on the rehabilitation of patients with intra-articular ACL reconstruction. Phys Ther 74:710–719, 1994

343. Townsend PR, Miegel RE, Rose RM, et al: Structure and function of the human patella: The role of cancellous bone. J Biomed Mater Res 7:605–611, 1976

344. Townsend PR, Raux P, Rose RM, et al: The distribution and anisotropy of the stiffness of cancellous bone in the human patella. J Biomech 8:363–367, 1975

345. Townsend PR, Rose RM, Radin EL, et al: The biomechanics of the human patella and its implications of chondromalacia. J Biomech 10:403–407, 1977

346. Tropp H, Askling C, Gillquist J: Prevention of ankle sprains. Am J Sports Med 13:259–262, 1985

347. Turner W, ed: Anatomical Memoirs of John Goodsir. Edinburgh, Adam & Black, 1968

348. Vaey FB: The painful knee. In: Germain BF, ed: Osteoarthritis and Musculoskeletal Pain Syndromes. Hyde Park, NY, Medical Examination Publishing, 1983

349. Veltri DM, Deng X-H, Torzilli PA, et al: The role of the cruciate and posterolateral ligaments in stability of the knee: A biomechanical study. Am J Sports Med 23:436–443, 1995

350. Voight ML, Wieder DL: Comparative reflex response times of vastus medialis obliquus and vastus lateralis in normal subjects and subjects with extensor mechanism dysfunction. Am J Sports Med 19:131–137, 1991

351. Wadsworth CT: Manual Examination and Treatment of the Spine and Extremities. Baltimore, Williams & Wilkins, 1988

352. Walker HL, Schreck RC: Relationship of hyperextended gait pattern to chondromalacia patellae. Physiotherapy 64:8–9, 1975

353. Walla DJ, Albright JP, McAuley E: Hamstring control and the unstable ACL-deficient knee. Am J Sports Med 13:34–49, 1985

354. Walsh WM: Office management of knee injuries. In: Mellion MB, ed: Office Management of Sport Injuries and Athletic Problems. Philadelphia, CV Mosby, 1988:213–230

355. Wang YJB, Rubim RM, Marshall JL: A mechanism of isolated ACL rupture—Case report. J Bone Joint Surg Am 57:411–413, 1975

356. Warren LF, Marshall JL: The supporting structures and layers on the medial side of the knee—An anatomic analysis. J Bone Joint Surg Am 61:56–62, 1979

357. Weiss JM: Treatment of leg edema and wounds in patients with severe musculoskeletal injuries. Phys Ther 78:1104–1113, 1999

358. Wilk KE: Challenging tradition in treatment of patellofemoral disorder. J Orthop Sports Phys Ther 28:275–276, 1998

359. Wilk KE, Andrews JR: Current concepts in the treatment of ACL disruption. J Orthop Sports Phys Ther 15:279–293, 1992

360. Wilk KE, Clancy W: Medial collateral ligament injuries: Diagnosis, treatment, and rehabilitation. In: Engle R, ed: Knee Ligament Rehabilitation. New York, Churchill Livingstone, 1991

361. Wooden MJ: Rehabilitation of lateral compartment injuries. In: Greenfield BH, ed: Rehabilitation of the Knee: A Problem-Solving Approach. Philadelphia, FA Davis Company, 1993:361–380

362. Woolfenden JT: Aquatic physical therapy approaches for the extremities. Orthop Phys Ther Clin North Am 3:209–230, 1994

363. Zipple JT, Hammer RL, Loubert PV: Treatment of fabella syndrome with manual therapy: A case report. J Orthop Sports Phys Ther 33:33–39, 2003

RECOMMENDED READINGS

Brotzman SB, Head P: The knee. In: Brotzman SB, ed: Clinical Orthopaedic Rehabilitation, St. Louis MO: Mosby, 1996

DeLeo A, Woodzell WW, Snyder-Mackler L: Resident's case problem: Diagnosis and treatment of posterolateral instability in a patient with lateral collateral ligament sprain. J Orthop Sports Phys Ther 33:185–191, 2003

James SL: Running injuries of the knee. AAOS Instructional Course Lectures 47:404–417, 1998

Macnicol MF: The Problem Knee. Oxford: Butterworth-Heinemann, 1995

Risberg MA, Mork M, Jenssen HK, et al: Design and implementation of a neuromuscular training program following anterior ligament reconstruction. J Orthop Sports Phys Ther 31:620–631, 2001

Tyler TF, McHugh MP: Neuromuscular rehabilitation of a female Olympic ice hockey player following anterior cruciate ligament reconstruction. J Orthop Sports Phys Ther 31:577–587, 2001

Williams GN, Chmielewski T, Rudolph KS, et al: Dynamic knee stability: Current theory and implications for clinicians and scientists. J Orthop Sports Phys Ther 31:546–566, 2001

Lower Leg, Ankle, and Foot

16

DARLENE HERTLING AND RANDOLPH M. KESSLER

FUNCTIONAL ANATOMY OF JOINTS

Osteology

FIBULA AND TIBIA

The two bones of the lower leg, the tibia and fibula, along with their articulations (superior and inferior joints) form a functional unit that is involved in movements of the ankle (Fig. 16-1). The tibia transmits most of the body weight to the foot. Proximally, an oval facet indents the tibia posterolaterally and provides an articular surface where the fibula joins the tibia as the superior tibiofibular joint. The fibula, the lateral bone of the leg, is more slender than the tibia for it is not called on to transmit body weight. With respect to the proximal end of the fibula, the medial part of the upper aspect of the head bears a circular articular surface for the lateral condyle of the tibia (see Fig. 15-4). Although the facets are fairly flat and vary in configuration among individuals, a slight concavity to the fibular face and a slight convexity to the tibial facet seems to predominate.[51] The surface of the fibular facet faces forward, upward, and medially. The shaft arches forward as it descends to the lateral malleolus.

The tibia or shinbone is, next to the femur, the longest and heaviest bone of the body.[62] The proximal end of the tibia (see Fig. 15-4) has been described earlier (see Chapter 15, Knee).

The tibia flares at its distal end (Fig. 16-1). As a result, the cross-section of the bone changes from triangular, in the region of the shaft, to quadrangular in the area of the distal metaphyseal portion of the bone. Medially there is a distal projection of the tibia, the medial malleolus; located laterally is the fibular notch, which is concave anteroposteriorly for articulation with the distal end of the fibula. Along the medial side of the posterior surface is a groove for the passage of the tibialis posterior tendon. The term *posterior malleolus* is often used to refer to the distal overhang of the posterior aspect of the tibia.

The lateral surface of the medial malleolus and the inferior surface of the tibia have a continuous cartilaginous covering for articulation with the talus. The articular surface of the inferior end of the tibia is concave anteroposteriorly. Mediolaterally, it is somewhat convex, having a crest centrally that corresponds to the central groove in the trochlear surface of the talus. This, then, is essentially a sellar joint surface. It is slightly wider anteriorly than posteriorly. The articular surface of the medial malleolus is comma shaped, with the tail of the comma extending posteriorly (Fig. 16-1).

The fibula, which is quite narrow in the region of its shaft, becomes bulbous at its distal end (Fig. 16-2A). This distal portion of the bone, the lateral malleolus, is triangular in cross-section. The lateral malleolus extends farther distally and is situated more posteriorly than the medial malleolus. The medial aspect of the lateral malleolus is covered by a triangular cartilaginous surface for articulation with the lateral side of the talus. Above this surface, the fibula contacts the tibia in the fibular notch of the tibia. The apex of this triangular surface points inferiorly. There is a fairly deep depression in the posteroinferior region of the lateral malleolus termed the *malleolar fossa* that can be easily palpated. The posterior talofibular ligament attaches in this fossa. There is a groove along the posterior

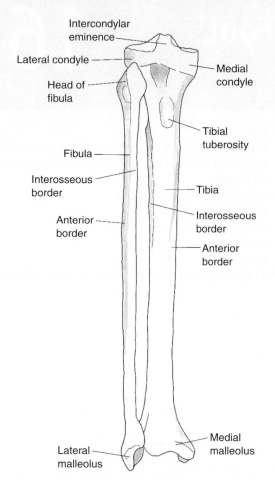

■ **FIG. 16-1.** Two bones of the lower leg: anterior view.

aspect of the lateral malleolus through which the peroneus brevis tendon passes.

TALUS

The talus constitutes the link between the leg and the tarsus (Fig. 16-3). It consists of a body, anterior to which is the head. The body and head of the talus are connected by a short neck.

The superior surface of the body of the talus is covered with articular cartilage for articulation with the inferior surface of the tibia. This articular surface is continuous with the articular surfaces of the medial and lateral aspects of the talus. The superior surface is somewhat wider anteriorly than posteriorly. It is convex anteroposteriorly and slightly concave mediolaterally, corresponding to the sellar surface of the inferior end of the tibia mentioned previously. In this sense, the superior talar articular surface is trochlear, or pulley-like, and is often referred to as the trochlea.

The lateral aspect of the body of the talus is largely covered by articular cartilage for articulation with the distal end of the fibula (Fig. 16-4). This articular surface is triangular, with the apex situated inferiorly. Just below this apex is a lateral bony projection to which the lateral talocalcaneal ligament attaches.

The articular surface of the medial aspect of the talus is considerably smaller than that of the lateral side, and it faces slightly upward (Fig. 16-5). It contacts the articular surface of the medial malleolus on the tibia. It is comma shaped, with the tail of the comma extending posteriorly. The roughened area below the medial articular surface serves as an attachment for the deltoid ligament. The medial and lateral talar articular surfaces tend to converge posteriorly, leading to the wedge shape of the trochlea. It should be emphasized, however, that the lateral articular surface of the talus is perpendicular to the axis of movement at the ankle joint, whereas the medial surface is not. This has important biomechanical implications, which are discussed in the following section.

If one views the profiles of the lateral and medial sides of the trochlea, the lateral profile is seen as a section of a circle, whereas the medial profile may be viewed as sections of several circles of different radii; the medial profile is of smaller radius anteriorly than posteriorly.[88] More precisely stated, the contour medially is of gradually increasing radius anteroposteriorly, forming a cardioid profile. The importance of this is described in the section on biomechanics.

Posteriorly, the body of the talus is largely covered by a continuation of the trochlear articular surface as it slopes backward (Fig. 16-6). At the inferior extent of the posterior aspect is the nonarticular posterior process. The posterior process consists of a lateral and a smaller medial tubercle, with an intervening groove through which passes the tendon of the flexor hallucis longus. The posterior talofibular ligament attaches to the lateral tubercle. The medial talocalcaneal ligament and a posterior portion of the deltoid ligament attach to the medial tubercle.

The neck and head of the talus are positioned anteriorly to the body. They are directed slightly medially and downward with respect to the body. The head is covered with articular cartilage anteriorly for articulation with the navicular and inferiorly for articulation with the spring ligament (plantar calcaneonavicular ligament).

The inferior surface of the talus has three cartilage-covered facets for articulation with the calcaneus (Fig. 16-7). The posterior facet, which is the largest of these, is concave inferiorly. The medial and anterior articular facets are continuous with each other and with the inferior articular surface of the head. Both the medial and the anterior facets are convex inferiorly and articulate with the superior aspect of the sustentaculum tali of the calcaneus. A deep groove, the sulcus tali, separates the posterior and medial facets on the inferior aspect of the talus. This groove runs obliquely from posteromedial to anterolateral. Where it is the deepest—posteromedially—it forms the *tarsal canal;* where it widens and opens out laterally it is referred to as the *sinus tarsi.* The interosseous talocalcaneal ligament and the cervical ligament occupy the sinus tarsi.

CALCANEUS

The calcaneus is situated beneath the talus in the standing position and provides a major contact point with the ground. It is the largest of the tarsal bones. The calcaneus articulates with the talus superiorly and with the cuboid anteriorly. Posteriorly

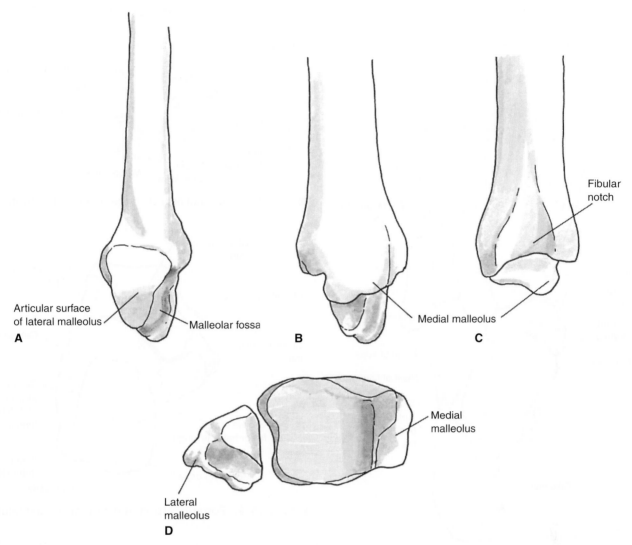

Articular surface
of lateral malleolus

Malleolar fossa

A

B

Medial malleolus

Fibular
notch

C

Medial
malleolus

Lateral
malleolus

D

■ **FIG. 16-2.** Distal right tibia and fibula, showing medial aspect of right fibula (**A**), tibia from the medial aspect (**B**), tibia from the lateral aspect (**C**), and the inferior end of the fibula and tibia (**D**).

it projects backward, providing considerable leverage for the plantar flexors of the ankle. The superior aspect of the calcaneus bears the posterior, medial, and anterior facets for articulation with the corresponding facets of the talus (Fig. 16-8). The posterior facet is convex, whereas the medial and anterior facets are concave. The medial and anterior facets are situated on the superior aspect of the sustentaculum tali, which is a bony projection of the calcaneus that overhangs medially. As with the corresponding facets on the talus, the medial and anterior facets of the calcaneus are usually continuous with each other. The medial and anterior facets are separated from the posterior facet by the *sulcus calcanei,* which forms the bottom of the sinus tarsi and tarsal canal, thus corresponding to the sulcus tali of the talus.

The posterior aspect of the large posterior projection of the calcaneus contains a smooth superior surface, which slopes upward and forward, and a rough inferior surface, which

slopes downward and forward. The upper surface is the site of attachment for the Achilles tendon (Fig. 16-6). The lower surface blends inferiorly with the tuber calcanei, which is the point of contact of the calcaneus with the ground in the standing position.

The tuber calcanei on the inferior aspect of the calcaneus consists of a medial tubercle and a lateral tubercle, of which the medial is the larger. Anterior to the tuber calcanei is a roughened surface for the attachment of the long and short plantar ligaments (Fig. 16-9). At the anterior extent of the inferior surface of the calcaneus is the anterior tubercle, which also serves as a point of attachment for the long plantar ligament. On the inferior aspect of the medially projecting sustentaculum tali is a groove through which runs the flexor hallucis longus tendon.

The lateral aspect of the calcaneus is nearly flat. There is a small prominence, the peroneal trochlea, that is located just

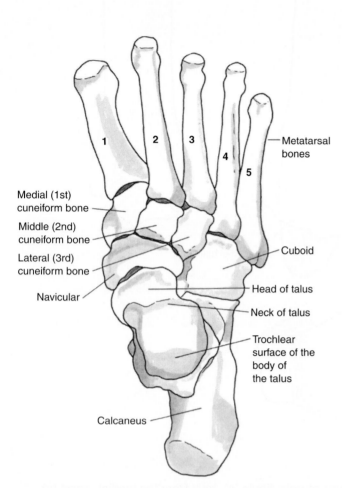

■ FIG. 16-3. Dorsal aspect of the bones of the right foot.

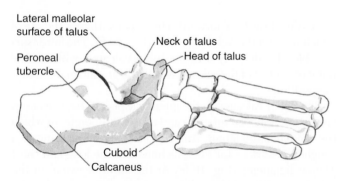

■ FIG. 16-4. Lateral aspect of the bones of the foot.

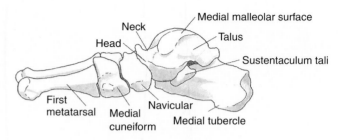

■ FIG. 16-5. Medial aspect of the bones of the foot.

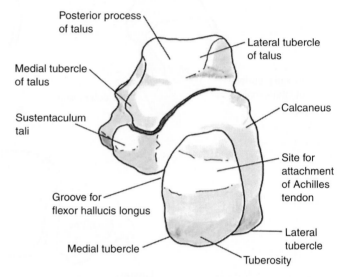

■ FIG. 16-6. Posterior aspect of the calcaneus and talus.

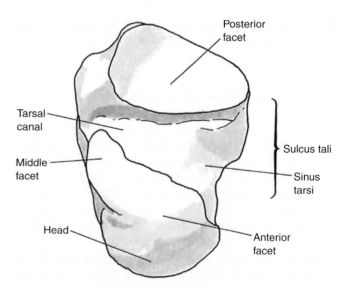

■ FIG. 16-7. Inferior surface of the talus.

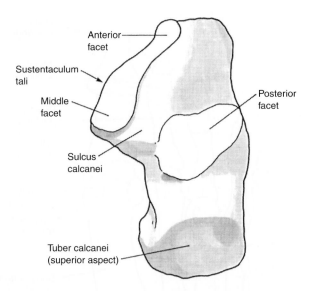

■ FIG. 16-8. Superior aspect of the calcaneus.

distal to the lateral malleolus (Fig. 16-4). The peroneus brevis tendon travels downward and forward, just superior to this trochlea, whereas the peroneus longus tendon passes inferior to it. The calcaneofibular ligament attaches just posterior and slightly superior to the peroneal trochlea, at which point there may be a rounded prominence.

From the anterosuperior extent of the medial aspect of the calcaneus, the sustentaculum tali projects in a medial direc-

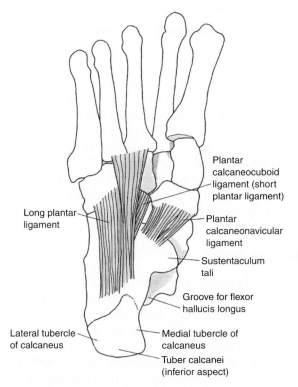

■ FIG. 16-9. Plantar surface of the foot.

tion (Fig. 16-8). The sustentaculum tali may be palpated just below the medial malleolus.

On the narrowed anterior aspect of the calcaneus is the cartilage-covered articular surface that contacts the cuboid bone. This is a sellar joint surface, being concave superoinferiorly and convex mediolaterally (Fig. 16-3).

The plantar surface of the calcaneus is protected and padded by a thick fat pad. The fat pad is encapsulated by a fibroelastic structure that attaches to the skin and the deepest layer to the calcaneus.[91,92] The foot pad may absorb up to 25% of the contact force at the heel.[164] The fat pad contains nerve endings that may cause pain if damaged or irritated.[92,92]

LESSER TARSUS

Distally, the three cuneiform bones (medial [first], intermediate [second], and lateral [third]) are interposed between the navicular proximally, the first three metatarsals distally, and the cuboid laterally (Fig. 16-3). The three cuneiforms and cuboid form an arcade or transverse arch that acts as a niche for the plantar musculotendinous and neurovascular structures (Fig. 16-10).[183] The middle cuneiform serves as the keystone. The cuneiforms, together with articulations of the metatarsal bones, form Lisfranc's joint.

The cuboid is intercalated between the calcaneus and the base of metatarsals 4 and 5 (Fig. 16-3). Medially, the cuboid has a fossa for the navicular and lateral cuneiform bones. On its plantar surface, there is a small groove for the peroneus longus tendon. Proximally, its articular surface with the calcaneus is saddle shaped, concave transversely and convex vertically.[183]

The navicular (scaphoid) articulates with the cuneiforms distally and with the talus proximally (Fig. 16-3). It establishes minimal articular contact with the cuboid and is firmly bound with ligaments to the os calcis. It is an integral part of the talotarsal joint. The midtarsal joint is formed by the articulations between the navicular and talus and between the cuboid and calcaneus. The proximal articular surface is biconcave, and

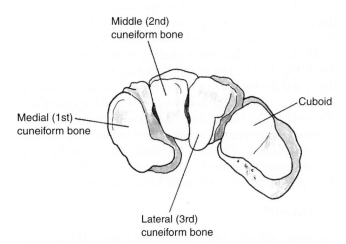

■ FIG. 16-10. Transverse arch formed by the cuneiforms (C1, C2, C3) and the cuboid.

in a few cases the surface is nearly flat.[131] It does not completely cover the navicular articular surface of the talus.[183] The distal articular surface to the three cuneiforms is faceted but is convex in its general contour.

METATARSALS

The metatarsals are the major stabilizers of the foot.[39] The five metatarsals articulate proximally with the three cuneiforms and the cuboid and form the tarsometatarsal or Lisfranc's joint (Fig. 16-3). Proximally, the bases of the metatarsals are arranged in an arcuate fashion, forming a transverse arch. The apex of this arch corresponds to the base of the second metatarsal. The metatarsals are also flexed, thus contributing to the formation of longitudinal arches.[183] The first metatarsal diverges slightly from the second metatarsal. The intermetatarsal angle formed by the long axis of these two metatarsals is 3 to 9° in the adult.[197] Any measurement in excess of 10° is indicative of varus deformity of the first ray.[104] Of all hallux valgus cases, 80% are caused by metatarsal primus varus, in which the intermetatarsal angle is increased to more than 15°.[46,169]

The first metatarsal is shorter than the second metatarsal. The metatarsal formula has been expressed in terms of the distal projections of the metatarsal heads relative to each other. Morton[148] introduced the formula of 1 = 2 > 3 > 4 > 5 and stated that "one of the requirements for ideal foot function is an equidistance of the heads of the first and second metatarsal bones from the heel." There are many variations, yet the metatarsal formula 2 > 3 > 1 > 4 > 5 is the one accepted by most anatomists.[98]

PHALANGES

The large toe has two phalanges: proximal and distal. The proximal base of the proximal phalanx bears an oval, concave articular surface with the glenoid cavity smaller than the corresponding articular surface of the metatarsal head (Fig. 16-11).[183] The articular surface of the head is trochlear and strongly convex in the dorsoplantar direction. The distal phalanx has an articular surface corresponding to the trochlear surface of the proximal phalangeal head. This surface is convex centrally and concave laterally.

The lesser toes have three phalanges: proximal, middle, and distal (Fig. 16-11). The proximal phalanx is the longest of the three, and the base has an oval (concave) articular surface for the metatarsal head. The head supports a trochlear type of articular surface. The base of the middle phalanx bears a transverse articular surface corresponding to the trochlear contour of the proximal phalangeal head.[183] The distal articular head presents a strong convexity in the dorsoplantar direction. The base of the distal phalanx corresponds to the head of the middle phalanx.

SESAMOIDS

The sesamoids are small, round bones so named because they resemble sesame seeds (Fig. 16-11). The sesamoids are embedded, partially or totally, in the substance of a corresponding ten-

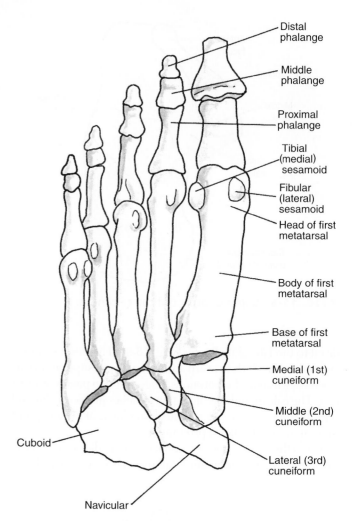

■ **FIG. 16-11.** Plantar aspect of the forefoot.

don juxtaposed to articulations and are anatomically a part of a gliding or pressure-absorbing mechanism. Structurally, some sesamoids always ossify, whereas others remain cartilaginous or fibrocartilaginous for life. The tibial (medial) and fibular (lateral) sesamoids of the flexor hallucis brevis are always present plantar to the first metatarsal head. Other locations where sesamoids may be found are in the plantar plates of the metatarsophalangeal and interphalangeal joints, the intrinsic tendons of the lesser toes, or in the tendons of the tibialis anterior, tibialis posterior, or peroneus longus.

ACCESSORY BONES

The accessory bones are developmental anomalies and appear in the foot between the ages of 10 and 20 years.[158,201] The most commonly occurring accessory bones are the os trigonum at the posterior plantar surface of the talus, the os tibiale externum (an accessory of the navicular bone), and the os intermetatarseum 1 through 2.[183] These accessory bones as well as the sesamoids become sources of irritation and may require excision.[201] Comprehensive accounts of the accessory bones of the foot can be found in the studies of Dwight,[48] Kohler and Simmer,[112] Marti,[136] O'Rahilly,[158] and Trolle.[208]

Ligaments and Capsules

SUPERIOR TIBIOFIBULAR JOINT

The superior tibiofibular joint is a plane synovial joint formed by the articulation of the head of the fibula with the postero-lateral aspect of the tibia (Fig. 16-12A). In about 10% of the population, the synovial membrane is continuous with the knee joint through the subpopliteal bursa.[70] Motion has been described as superior and inferior sliding of the fibula, antero-posterior glide, and fibular rotation.[7,100,216]

An interosseous membrane binds the tibia and fibula throughout their length and separates the muscles on the front from those on the back of the leg (Fig. 16-12A). The interosseous membrane forms a "Y" proximally to surround the upper tibiofibular joint, the anterior division being called the anterosuperior tibiofibular ligament and the posterior division being called the posterosuperior tibiofibular ligament

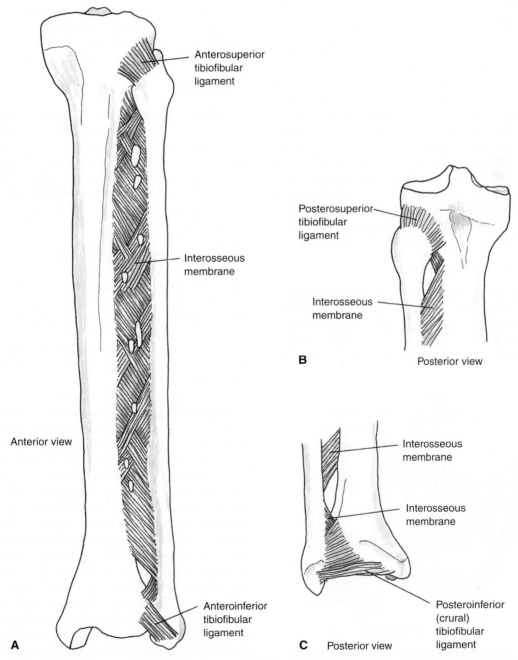

■ **FIG. 16-12.** Tibia and fibula, showing anterior aspect (**A**), ligaments of the proximal tibiofibular joint (**B**), and distal tibiofibular joints (**C**).

(Fig. 16-12*A, B*). A similar arrangement is formed below, where the interosseous membrane thickens and divides to surround the inferior tibiofibular syndesmosis (Fig. 16-12*A, C*). The two components are called the anteroinferior and posteroinferior tibiofibular ligaments.

The interosseous membrane serves as the floor of the anterior compartment of the leg (Fig. 16-13). This is a closed space; the boundaries are the anterior fascia of the leg in front, the interosseous membrane behind, the fibula laterally, and the tibia medially. This space as well as the lateral compartment permits little, if any, expansion of the structures contained within, whereas the posterior compartment is a loosely contained space with a relaxed and redundant fascia. The tight fascial investment of the muscles contained in the anterior and lateral compartments helps to prevent undue swelling of the muscles during exercise and thereby facilitates venous return.[62]

The ligaments of the inferior tibiofibular articulation are oriented to prevent widening of the mortise. They are also important in preventing posterior displacement of the fibula at the syndesmosis, which tends to occur when the leg is forcibly internally rotated on the tarsus. It should be realized that complete sectioning of the inferior tibiofibular ligaments alone allows only a minimal increase in the intermalleolar space.[1] This is because the two bones are indirectly held together by their mutual connections to the talus by way of the medial and lateral ligaments of the ankle. Significant diastasis, then, is usually accompanied by rupture of one or more of the talocrural ligaments, usually the deltoid ligament.

INFERIOR TIBIOFIBULAR JOINT

The inferior tibiofibular joint is a syndesmosis and lacks articular cartilage and synovium. The distal fibula is situated in the fibular notch of the lateral aspect of the distal tibia and is bound to it by several ligaments (Figs. 16-12*A, C*, 16-14, and 16-15). The anterior and posterior tibiofibular ligaments pass in front of and behind the syndesmosis. They are both directed downward and inward to check separation of the two bones. The inferior transverse ligament is a thickened band of fibers that is closely related to the posterior tibiofibular ligament (Fig. 16-12*C*). It passes from the posterior margin of the inferior tibial articular surface downward and laterally to the malleolar fossa of the fibula. This ligament is lined inferiorly with articular cartilage where it contacts the posterolateral talar articular surface during extreme plantar flexion. The interosseous ligament is a continuation of the interosseous membrane of the tibia and fibula (Fig. 16-12*C*). It extends between the adjacent surfaces of the bones at the syndesmosis.

The tibiofibular interosseous ligaments are considered the strongest and most important of the ligaments at the distal tibiofibular joint (Fig. 16-12*C*).[174] The tibia and fibula are separated at the syndesmosis by a fat pad.

ANKLE JOINT

Ankle Mortise or Talocrural Joint. The ankle joint is composed of the talocrural joint and distal tibiofibular joints. The talocrural joint also functions with the subtalar joint as part of the rear foot. The ankle joint is formed by the superior portion of the body of the talus fitting within the mortise, or cavity, formed by the combined distal ends of the tibia and fibula. The medial, superior, and lateral articular surfaces of the talus are continuous, as are those of the medial malleolus, the distal end of the tibia, and the lateral malleolus.

The fibrous capsule attaches at the margins of the articular surfaces of the talus below and to the tibia and fibula above, except anteriorly, where a portion of the dorsal aspect of the neck of the talus is enclosed within the joint cavity. The capsule extends somewhat superiorly between the distal ends of the tibia and fibula, to just below the syndesmosis. A synovial membrane lines the fibrous capsule throughout its entirety. The capsule is well supported by ligaments, especially medially and laterally.

The medial ligaments are collectively referred to as the *deltoid ligament* (Fig. 16-16). The anterior portion of the deltoid ligament consists of the tibionavicular ligament, superficially, and the deeper anterior tibiotalar fibers. The tibionavicular ligament blends with the plantar calcaneonavicular (spring) ligament inferiorly. The middle fibers of the deltoid ligament constitute the tibiocalcaneal ligament, with some tibiotalar fibers deep to it. The posterior tibiotalar ligament forms the posterior portion of the deltoid ligament. The deltoid ligament as a whole attaches proximally to the medial aspect of the medial malleolus and fans out to achieve the distal attachments described above. In this way, it is somewhat triangular, with the apex at its proximal attachment.

The lateral ligaments, unlike those of the medial side, are separate bands of fibers diverging from their proximal attachment at the distal end of the fibula (Fig. 16-14). The anterior talofibular ligament—the most frequently injured ligament about the ankle—passes medially, forward, and downward from the anterior aspect of the fibula to the lateral aspect of

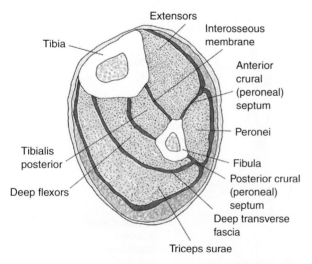

■ **FIG. 16-13.** Diagram of a horizontal section through the middle of the leg showing anterior compartment of the leg.

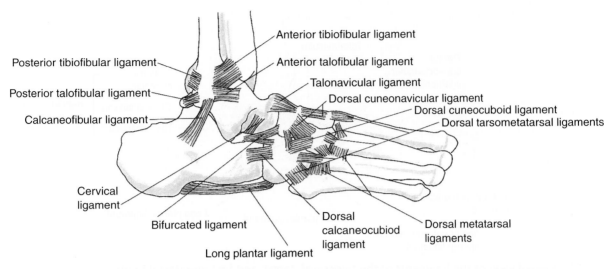

■ **FIG. 16-14.** Lateral view of the ligaments of the right talocrural, tarsal, and tarsometatarsal joints.

the neck of the talus. The calcaneofibular ligament runs from the tip of the lateral malleolus downward and backward to a small prominence on the upper lateral surface of the calcaneus. It is longer and narrower than the anterior and posterior talofibular ligaments. The posterior talofibular ligament passes from the malleolar fossa medially and slightly downward and backward to the lateral tubercle of the posterior aspect of the talus.

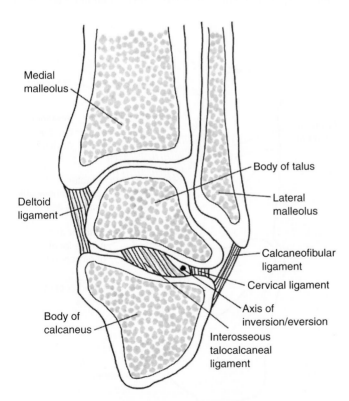

■ **FIG. 16-15.** Coronal section through the talocrural and subtalar joints.

It should be noted that the proximal attachments of both the medial and lateral ligaments of the ankle are near the axis of movement for dorsiflexion and plantar flexion. For this reason, these ligaments are not pulled tight to any significant extent during normal movement at the talocrural joint.[80] Also, the calcaneofibular ligament, which crosses both the talocrural and the talocalcaneal joints, runs parallel to, and inserts close to, the axis of movement at the subtalar joint. It, then, plays little or no role in restricting inversion at the subtalar joint. This is true in all positions of dorsiflexion and plantar flexion, as it maintains a parallel orientation to the subtalar axis throughout the range of movement.

The ligaments about the talocrural joint primarily function to restrict tilting and rotation of the talus within the mortise and to restrict forward or backward displacement of the leg on the tarsus. The main exception to this is the tibiocalcaneal portion of the deltoid ligament, which is so oriented as to help check eversion at the subtalar joint as well as an "eversion tilt" of the talus in the mortise.

In the neutral position, the anterior talofibular ligament can check posterior movement of the leg on the tarsus and external rotation of the leg on the tarsus because it is directed forward and medially. With the foot in plantar flexion, the anterior talofibular ligament becomes more vertically oriented and is in a position to check inversion of the talus in the mortise. This ligament is the most commonly injured of the ligaments of the ankle, the mechanism of injury usually being a combined plantar flexion–inversion strain.

The calcaneofibular ligament is directed downward and backward when the foot is in the neutral position. When the foot is dorsiflexed, the ligament becomes more vertically oriented and is in a better position to check inversion of the tarsus with respect to the leg.

The posterior talofibular ligament is oriented so as to check internal rotation of the leg on the tarsus and forward displacement of the leg on the tarsus.

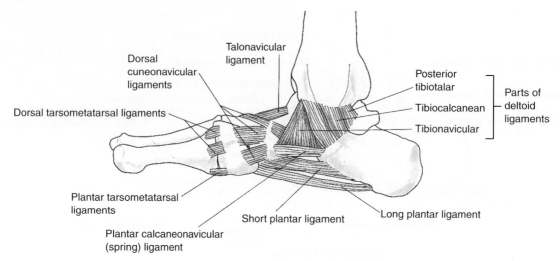

■ FIG. 16-16. Medial view of the ligaments of the talocrural, tarsal, and first metatarsal joints.

The deltoid ligament, considered as a whole, contributes to restriction of eversion, internal rotation, and external rotation, as well as forward and backward displacement of the tarsus. However, sectioning of the deltoid ligament alone apparently results primarily in instability of eversion of the tarsus on the tibia, the other motions being checked by other ligaments, as described previously.

Subtalar Joint. Functionally, the subtalar joint includes the articulation between the posterior facet of the talus and the opposing articular surface of the calcaneus, as well as the articulation between the anterior and medial facets of the two bones. These articulations move in conjunction with one another. Anatomically, the anterior and medial articulations are actually part of the talocalcaneonavicular joint; they are enclosed within a joint capsule separate from that of the posterior talocalcaneal articulation.

The joint capsules of the posterior portion of the talocalcaneal joint and the talocalcaneonavicular portion of the subtalar joint are separated by the ligament of the tarsal canal. This ligament runs from the underside of the talus, at the sulcus tali, downward and laterally to the dorsum of the calcaneus, at the sulcus calcanei. Because it is situated medially to the axis of motion of inversion–eversion at the subtalar joint, it checks eversion.[191] This ligament is often referred to as the *interosseous talocalcaneal ligament* (Fig. 16-15).

More laterally, in the sinus tarsi, is the cervical talocalcaneal ligament. It passes from the inferolateral aspect of the talar neck downward and laterally to the dorsum of the calcaneus. It occupies the anterior part of the sinus tarsi. Because the cervical ligament lies lateral to the subtalar joint axis, it restricts inversion of the calcaneus on the talus.[191]

Also, within the lateral aspect of the sinus tarsi, bands from the inferior aspect of the extensor retinaculum pass downward, as well as medially, to the calcaneus. These bands are considered part of the talocalcaneal ligament complex. They help check inversion at the subtalar joint.

MIDTARSAL JOINTS

Talocalcaneonavicular Joint. The talocalcaneonavicular joint includes the articulation between the anterior and medial facets of the talus and calcaneus (described previously as part of the subtalar joint), the articulations between the inferior aspect of the head of the talus and the subjacent spring ligament, and the articulation between the anterior aspect of the head of the talus and the posterior articular surface of the navicular (Fig. 16-17). The combined talonavicular and talo-spring

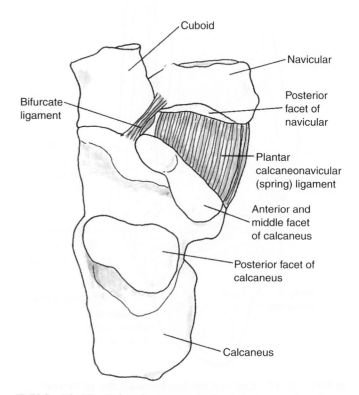

■ FIG. 16-17. Talocalcaneonavicular joint, superior view.

ligament portion of this joint is essentially a compound ball-and-socket joint; the head of the talus is the ball, whereas the superior surface of the spring ligament and the posterior surface of the navicular form the socket. It should be noted that the superior surface of the spring ligament is lined with articular cartilage. The talonavicular portion of this joint constitutes the medial half of the transverse tarsal joint.

The talocalcaneonavicular joint is enclosed by a joint capsule, the posterior aspect of which traverses the tarsal canal, forming the anterior wall of the canal. The capsule is reinforced by the spring ligament inferiorly, the calcaneonavicular portion of the bifurcate ligament laterally, and the tibionavicular portion of the deltoid ligament medially (Figs. 16-14 and 16-16).

The spring ligament passes from the anterior and medial margins of the sustentaculum tali forward to the inferior and inferomedial aspect of the navicular. As mentioned, its superior surface articulates with the underside of the head of the talus. This ligament maintains apposition of the medial aspects of the forefoot and hindfoot and in so doing helps to maintain the normal arched configuration of the foot. Laxity of the ligament allows a medial separation between the calcaneus and forefoot, with the forefoot assuming an abducted position with respect to the hindfoot. At the same time, the foot is allowed to "untwist," which effectively lowers the normal arch of the foot, and the talar head is allowed to move medially and inferiorly. Further discussion of the twisted configuration and arching of the foot is included in the section on biomechanics.

Calcaneocuboid Joint. The lateral portion of the transverse tarsal joint is the calcaneocuboid joint. The calcaneocuboid joint is a sellar joint in that the calcaneal joint surface is concave superoinferiorly and convex mediolaterally (Figs. 16-3 and 16-4); the adjoining cuboid surface is reciprocally shaped. This joint is enclosed in a joint capsule distinct from that of the talocalcaneonavicular joint and constitutes the lateral half of the transverse tarsal joint. The joint capsule is reinforced inferiorly by the strong plantar calcaneocuboid (short plantar) ligament and the long plantar ligament (Fig. 16-9). The short plantar ligament runs from the anterior tubercle of the plantar aspect of the calcaneus to the underside of the cuboid. The long plantar ligament runs from the posterior tubercles of the calcaneus forward to the bases of the fifth, fourth, third, and sometimes second metatarsals (Fig. 16-9). Both of these ligaments support the normal arched configuration of the foot by helping to maintain a twisted relationship between the hindfoot and forefoot. Dorsally, the joint capsule is reinforced by the calcaneocuboid band of the bifurcate ligament (Fig. 16-14).

ANTERIOR TARSAL AND TARSOMETATARSAL JOINTS

A common joint cavity connects the cuboid, navicular, three cuneiforms, and second and third metatarsal bones (Fig. 16-18). The first cuneiform and first metatarsal articulation has a separate cavity, as does the cuboid articulation with the fourth and fifth metatarsals.[216] Interosseous, dorsal, and plantar ligaments strengthen all of these small joints.

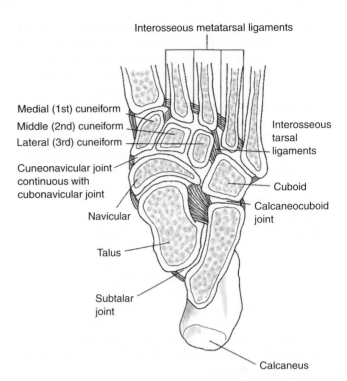

■ FIG. 16-18. Horizontal section through the foot joints from above.

Cubonavicular Joint. The cubonavicular joint is usually a fibrous joint, but not infrequently the syndesmosis is replaced by a synovial joint of an almost plane variety, with the capsule and cavity continuous with the cuneonavicular joint.[70] Ligaments include the plantar cubonavicular ligament, interosseus ligament, and dorsal cubonavicular ligament, which strongly unite the cuboid and the navicular (Fig. 16-19).

Cuneonavicular, Cuneocuboid, and Intercuneiform Joints. The cuneonavicular, cuneocuboid, and intercuneiform joints have a common articular and synovial capsule (Fig. 16-18). The navicular articulates with the three cuneiform bones and may be considered convex distally, being divided by low ridges into three facets that articulate with the first, second, and third cuneiforms to form the cuneonavicular joint.

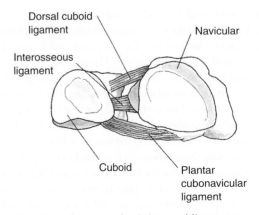

■ FIG. 16-19. Cubonavicular joint and ligaments.

Tarsometatarsal Joints. The tarsometatarsal (TMT) joints lie on a line, with the exception of the second cuneiform, which is located 2 to 3 mm proximal to the first and third cuneiform. This creates the cuneiform mortise, which enhances the stability of Lisfranc's joint (Fig. 16-18).[183]

The cuboid also shows three facets that articulate with the fifth metatarsal, the fourth metatarsal, and the lateral cuneiform (Fig. 16-3). The cuboid is in a slight proximal recess of at least 2 mm relative to the third cuneiform; this creates a shallow metatarsal mortise.[183] The ligaments connecting the cuboid and the cuneiforms of the metatarsal bases are the dorsal, plantar, and interosseous ligaments.

The first TMT joint (the articulations between the first metatarsal and medial cuneiform) has its own articular capsule (Fig. 16-18). The articular surface of the base of the first metatarsal presents a slight concavity transversely, the base of the second is concave with its articulation with the second cuneiform, the base of the third is flat, and the articular surface of the fourth is slightly convex with its articulation with the cuboid (Fig. 16-3).[183] The base of the fifth metatarsal is flat in a dorsoplantar direction and is projected laterally as the styloid apophysis or tubercle, which gives insertion to the peroneus brevis tendon.

The second TMT joint is the articulation of the base of the second metatarsal with a mortise formed by the middle cuneiform and the sides of the medial and lateral cuneiforms (Figs. 16-3 and 16-18). It is stronger and its motion more restricted than the other TMT joints. The third TMT joint shares its capsule with the second TMT joint, whereas the fourth and fifth TMT joints share a capsule with their articulation with the cuboid. There are small plane articulations between the bases of the metatarsals to permit motion of one metatarsal on the next. Slight gliding and rotation are possible at all of these joints. Although there is little movement between the individual tarsals and metatarsals, their collective movement can enhance either the foot's stability or flexibility. Dorsal and plantar ligaments join the bones (Figs. 16-14, 16-16, and 16-20). The plantar ligaments of the cuneocuboid and intercuneiform joints are strengthened by slips from the tendons of the tibialis posterior (Fig. 16-20).

METATARSOPHALANGEAL JOINTS

The first metatarsal head demonstrates a biconvex articular surface with its articular cap expanding inferiorly over the plantar condyles to the level of the anatomic neck and dorsally about one third of that distance.[214] The phalangeal base is correspondingly biconcave, and the capsular ligament inserts in close proximity with its articular outer edge. The compartment formed is reinforced by collateral ligaments (medial and lateral) and metatarsophalangeal ligaments (Fig. 16-21).[163] The dorsal capsule is reinforced by the extensor hood expansion.[214] The plantar plate (equivalent to the hand's volar plates) is the fibrocartilaginous plantar metatarsophalangeal ligament and is continuous with the plantar aponeurosis, so that toe dorsiflexion tenses the plantar aponeurosis and stabilizes the foot's longitudinal arch.[214,216] The articular surface of the head of the first

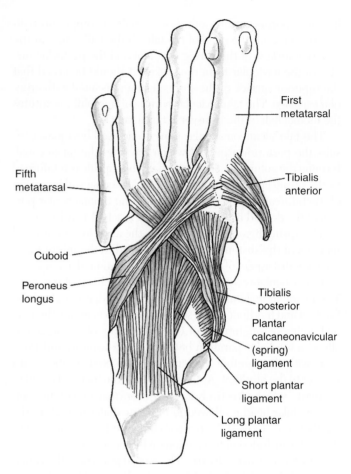

■ FIG. 16-20. Tendons and ligaments of the foot, plantar aspect. Note the widespread insertion of the tibialis anterior.

metatarsal presents with two fields in continuity: the superior phalangeal, which is convex, and the inferior sesamoidal, whose two sloped surfaces are grooved, and each corresponds to a sesamoid.[183] The heads of the lesser metatarsals are convex or condylar (Fig. 16-11).

INTERPHALANGEAL JOINTS

The articulations of the phalanges of the toes are essentially similar to those of the fingers (Fig. 16-11). On the plantar surface the capsule of each interphalangeal joint is thickened by a shallow concave plate, the plantar ligament; attached to its edges are the digital tendon sheaths as well as the lateral part of the fibrous capsule (Fig. 16-21).[83] The collateral ligaments of the interphalangeal joints extend from the lateral aspect of the head of the corresponding phalanx to the base of the distally located phalanx (Fig. 16-21). When sesamoid bones are present, they are an integral part of the plantar plate.[183]

PROXIMAL PHALANGEAL APPARATUS OF BIG TOE

The two sesamoids, embedded in the thick fibrous plantar plate and united to the proximal phalanx of the big toe, form

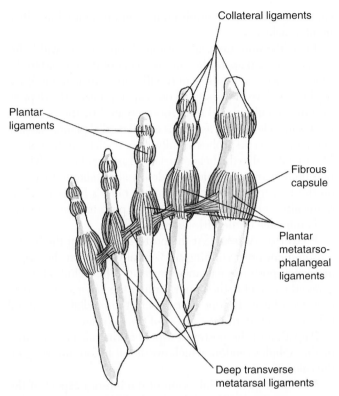

■ FIG. 16-21. Ligaments of the metatarsophalangeal and interphalangeal joints.

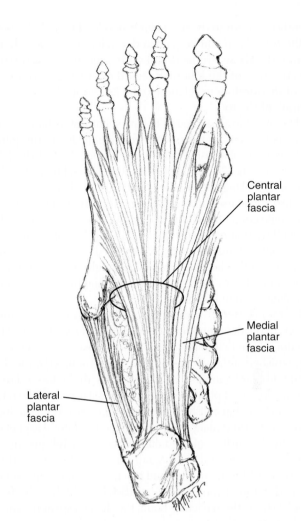

■ FIG. 16-22. Plantar fascia and its insertions.

an anatomic and functional unit called the *sesamophalangeal apparatus* (Fig. 16-11).[68] The sesamoids are foci of insertion: the flexor hallucis brevis inserts on the proximal segment of each sesamoid, the lateral head of the flexor hallucis brevis and abductor hallucis inserts on the medial sesamoid, and the lateral sesamoid gives insertion to the oblique and transverse components of the adductor hallucis muscle.[183] The deep transverse metatarsal ligament attaches longitudinally along the lateral sesamoid (Fig. 16-21). According to Sarrafian,[183] the sesamophalangeal apparatus moves backward or forward relative to the fixed metatarsal head; in hallux valgus the sesamoids follow the proximal phalanx and are displaced with the phalanx, not with the metatarsal head.

Plantar Fascia

Another structure playing an important role in maintaining the longitudinal arches in the foot is the plantar fascia (Fig. 16-22). This multilayered fibrous aponeurosis originates at the medial tuberosity of the calcaneus and passes anteriorly to split into five fibrous bands that attach to the digits in the following manner: each splits at the level of the corresponding metatarsophalangeal joint, to allow passage of the short and long plantarflexor tendons, and attaches at both sides of these joints and their ligaments. From the margins of the central part of the plantar fascia, vertical septa extend deeply to form three compartments of the sole of the foot: the medial compartment, lateral compartment, and central compartment.

The central portion of the fascia is usually the structure involved in subcalcaneal pain.[101] Hyperextension of the metatarsal joints during walking tenses the plantar fascia, raises the longitudinal arch of the foot, inverts the hindfoot, and laterally rotates the leg (see Fig. 16-29). This has been called the "windlass mechanism."[80]

Surface Anatomy

BONY PALPATION

Medial Aspect. The medial malleolus is easily palpated and observed as a large prominence medially. About 2 cm distal to the medial malleolus, the sustentaculum tali can be felt, especially if the foot is held in an everted position. The tibiocalcaneal portion of the deltoid ligament passes from the malleolus to the sustentaculum tali.

If the palpating finger is moved about 5 cm directly anterior to the sustentaculum, the *navicular tubercle* can be located as a prominence on the medial aspect of the arch of the foot. The tibionavicular portion of the deltoid ligament attaches just above the tubercle. Just superior and perhaps slightly posterior to the navicular tubercle, the medial aspect of the *talar head* can be palpated as a less prominent bony landmark. These two landmarks are important in assessing the structure of the foot with regard to the degree of twisting of the forefoot in relation to the hindfoot (the degree of arching of the foot).

The metatarsal can be felt to flare slightly at its base where it meets the first metatarsocuneiform joint. From the joint, one should probe distally along the medial shaft of the first metatarsal bone. The head of the first metatarsal bone and the metatarsophalangeal joint are palpable at the ball of the foot. The first metatarsophalangeal joint is the site of the common pathologic condition, *hallux abducto valgus*, characterized by lateral deviation of the great toe (see Fig. 16-33E). The first metatarsal shaft may be medially angulated (metatarsus primus varus) as well. The hallux abductus angle, intermetatarsal angle, and forefoot angles are increased, and the first metatarsophalangeal joint is subluxed.[220]

Dorsal Aspect. At the level of the malleoli, the anterior aspects of the distal ends of the tibia and fibula can be felt. The junction of the two bones, at the syndesmosis, can usually be distinguished, although it is considerably obscured by the distal tibiofibular ligament that overlies it. With the foot relaxed in some degree of plantar flexion, the dorsal aspect of the talar neck can be felt just distal to the end of the tibia. With the foot held inverted and plantarly flexed, the anterolateral aspect of the articular surface of the talus can be easily felt just distal and somewhat lateral to the syndesmosis. Between the dorsal aspect of the talar neck and the most prominent aspect of the dorsum of the foot farther distally, which is the first cuneiform, is the navicular bone, the dorsal aspect of which can be palpated.

The second and third cuneiform may be palpated distal to the navicular. One may palpate the cuboid by moving laterally from the third cuneiform or proximally from the styloid process at the base of the fifth metatarsal. By moving distally on the dorsum of the foot, the metatarsals and the phalangeal joints of each toe may be palpated.

Lateral Aspect. The lateral malleolus lies subcutaneously and so is easily palpated. The fairly flat lateral aspect of the calcaneus also has little soft tissue covering it and can be felt throughout its extent. About 3 cm distal to the tip of the malleolus, a small prominence can be felt on the calcaneus. This is the peroneal tubercle (Fig. 16-4). The peroneus brevis tendon passes superior to the tubercle, whereas the peroneus longus passes inferiorly. Occasionally a small prominence can be palpated just posterior to the peroneal tubercle; this is the point of insertion of the calcaneofibular ligament.

Just distal, and slightly anterior, to the malleolus, a rather marked depression can be felt if the foot is relaxed. This is the lateral opening of the sinus tarsi. Traversing the lateral aspect of the sinus tarsi are the inferior bands of the extensor retinaculum and the cervical talocalcaneal ligament. If the palpating finger is moved around dorsally and slightly superiorly from the sinus tarsi, the lateral aspect of the neck of the talus can be felt, where the often-injured anterior talofibular ligament attaches.

From the sinus tarsi, approximately one finger's width distally, one may palpate the lateral aspect of the cuboid to the styloid process at the base of the fifth metatarsal bone. Proximal to the flare of the styloid one can appreciate the depression of the cuboid and the groove created by the peroneus longus muscle tendon as it runs to the medial plantar surface of the foot. As one probes distally along the lateral shaft of the fifth metatarsal to the head, the lateral aspect of the fifth head may demonstrate a bunionette deformity similar to that seen on the first toe called a *tailor toe* or tailor's bunion.[128] The deformity is characterized by a painful prominence of the lateral eminence of the fifth metatarsal head.

Posterior Aspect. At the posterior aspect of the heel is a prominent crest running horizontally between the upper and lower posterior calcaneal surfaces. The Achilles tendon gains attachment to the upper surface; the lower surface, covered by a fat pad, slopes forward to the medial and lateral tubercles on the inferior aspect of the calcaneus.

Palpation of the posterior aspect of the talus is obscured by the Achilles tendon, which overlies it before inserting on the calcaneus.

Plantar Aspect. Palpation of the inferior aspect of the calcaneus is made difficult by the thick skin and fat pad that cover it. The weight-bearing medial tubercle can be vaguely distinguished posteriorly in most persons.

The calcaneus is palpated for point tenderness, which may be related to calcaneus periostitis (bone bruise), and also for a possible calcaneal spur (traction osteophytes), which may develop just anterior to the medial tubercle of the calcaneus where the long plantar ligament attaches. This is also called *heel-spur syndrome* and is more proximal than midfoot plantar fasciitis. Other bony structures that should be palpated include the sesamoid bones for possible sesamoiditis or displacement (which may occur in Morton's neuroma) and each metatarsal head. Metatarsalgia can develop if the transverse arch collapses, causing painful metatarsal heads and occasionally pinched digital nerves. The cause may be vascular, avascular, neurogenic, or mechanical, such as when the transverse arch collapses.[71] Generalized metatarsalgia often occurs secondary to a tight Achilles tendon, which restricts dorsiflexion.[115] One should palpate the shafts of the metatarsal bones and between the bones for evidence of pathology. Medially, on the plantar aspect of the first metatarsal, one may identify and palpate the two sesamoid bones just proximal to the head of the first metatarsal. This may be facilitated by dorsiflexing the big toe. In a similar fashion, the heads of the remaining four toes are palpated, and while doing so, it should be determined whether any are disproportionately prominent. If one is more prominent, it may bear an unaccustomed amount of weight, characterized by excessive callosities (keratoses) as a result of increased pressure. The various causes of plantar keratoses are numerous, and a significant differential diagnosis exists that needs to be taken into account when evaluating the patient.[128]

TENDONS AND VESSELS

Medial Aspect. The four ligaments that make up the deltoid (tibionavicular, tibiocalcaneal, and anterior and posterior tibiotalar) should be palpated for signs of disease (Fig. 16-16). Tenderness or pain elicited during palpation suggests an eversion ankle sprain.

The tendons of the tibialis posterior, flexor digitorum longus, and flexor hallucis longus muscles cross behind the medial malleolus (Fig. 16-23A). The tibialis posterior is the most anterior of these and is best visualized or palpated when plantar flexion and inversion are performed against some resistance. Posterior to the tibialis posterior tendon is the flexor digitorum longus tendon, which is less prominent. Palpation of the flexor digitorum is facilitated by providing some resistance to toe flexion. The flexor hallucis longus tendon is deeper and runs farther posteriorly; it is not usually palpable. Between the flexor digitorum and flexor hallucis longus tendons runs the posterior tibial artery. Its pulse is palpable behind the malleolus. The tibial nerve, which usually cannot be palpated, runs deep and posterior to the artery.

Just anterior to the medial malleolus is the long saphenous nerve; it can usually be visualized and palpated.

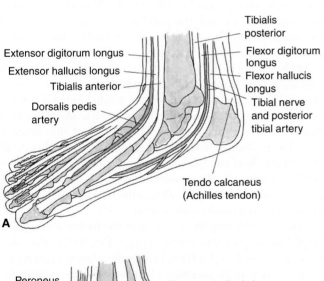

Tibialis posterior
Flexor digitorum longus
Flexor hallucis longus
Tibial nerve and posterior tibial artery
Extensor digitorum longus
Extensor hallucis longus
Tibialis anterior
Dorsalis pedis artery
Tendo calcaneus (Achilles tendon)
A

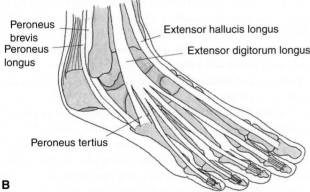

Peroneus brevis
Peroneus longus
Extensor hallucis longus
Extensor digitorum longus
Peroneus tertius
B

■ **FIG. 16-23.** Medial **(A)** and lateral **(B)** views of the tendons and vessels of the dorsum of foot.

Dorsal Aspect. Running along the medial side of the dorsum of the ankle is the tendon of the tibialis anterior, which is the most prominent tendon crossing the dorsal aspect of the foot. It is made especially prominent by resisting inversion and dorsiflexion of the foot. It attaches to the medial aspect of the base of the first metatarsal.

Just lateral to the tibialis anterior tendon, the extensor hallucis longus tendon can easily be seen and palpated as the subject extends the big toe.

Running laterally to the extensor hallucis longus tendon, passing distally from where it emerges at the ankle, is the dorsalis pedis artery. Its pulse can best be palpated over the dorsum of the foot, at about the level of the navicular and first cuneiform bones.

Farther laterally, the common tendon of the extensor digitorum longus is seen and felt when the subject extends the toes (Fig. 16-23B). Its four branches can be distinguished where they develop, just distal to the ankle.

If the subject everts and dorsiflexes the foot, the tendon of the peroneus tertius is usually observable just proximal to its insertion at the dorsum of the base of the fifth metatarsal.

Returning to the area of the medial and lateral malleoli, one may palpate the area of the inferior tibiofibular joint and follow the crest of the tibia superiorly while palpating the muscles of the lateral compartment (peroneals and posterior tibialis) and anterior compartment (tibialis anterior and long extensors) for swelling, tenderness, and signs of pathology (e.g., shin splints or stress fractures). About 75% of shin pain is caused by overuse of the posterior tibial muscle.[63] Patients with flexor compartment chronic syndrome or medial shin syndrome complain of pain over the posterior tibial and flexor tendons anywhere from the medial malleolus up to the medial tibial plateau.[107] There are usually palpable areas of maximum tenderness and nodules that represent fibrosis and scar tissue formation.

Lateral Aspect. The peroneus longus and peroneus brevis tendons cross behind the lateral malleolus, with the brevis running more anteriorly. The brevis passes superior to the peroneal tubercle on the lateral aspect of the calcaneus; the longus passes inferior to the tubercle. Some resistance should be applied to the plantar flexion and eversion of the foot when palpating these tendons.

Also one should palpate the peroneal retinaculum, which holds the peroneal tendons in place, for tenderness. The lateral ligaments (anterior tibiofibular, anterior talofibular, calcaneofibular, posterior talofibular, and posterior tibiofibular) are palpated for tenderness and swelling (Fig. 16-14). These ligaments will be point tender if they are sprained or partially torn. The most common sprain is of the anterior talofibular ligament. This injury occurs during plantar flexion and inversion. The bifurcate ligament (calcaneocuboid or calcaneonavicular portion) will be tender if sprained or partially torn from a plantar flexion injury (Fig. 16-14).[77]

The surrounding area of the calcaneus should be palpated for exostosis (e.g., pump bump) and swelling. Moving proximally, one may palpate the superficial (triceps surae) and posterior compartment muscles of the leg along their length. Ruptures or strains of the gastrocnemius usually occur to the medial muscle belly where the Achilles tendon joins the belly.[77] In addition to point tenderness, a gap can sometimes be felt in the muscle tissue.

Posterior Aspect and Posterior Compartment Muscles of Leg. The Achilles tendon is quite prominent and is easily seen and felt proximal to its insertion on the calcaneus. Deep to the tendon, between the tendon and the upper surface of the posterior calcaneus, is the retrocalcaneal bursa. There is also a calcaneal bursa between the Achilles tendon and the skin. These bursae cannot be distinguished on palpation.

Plantar Aspect. The intrinsic foot muscles and plantar aponeurosis (plantar fascia) should be palpated for tenderness, which may indicate midfoot plantar fasciitis, and for nodules in the fascia, which may indicate Dupuytren's contracture.[84,201] The plantar fascia (Fig. 16-22) should be palpated along its entire surface. Maintaining dorsiflexion of the toes will make the fascia more prominent and facilitate palpation. Nodules found on the skin, particularly on the ball of the foot (not usually on the weight-bearing area) are usually plantar warts.[128]

The plantar calcaneonavicular (spring) ligament is palpated for tenderness by applying pressure to the area immediately below the head of the talus, with the foot completely relaxed (Figs. 16-9 and 16-16). This ligament, which helps to support the longitudinal arch, can become strained and painful from overuse. Also one should probe the region of the long and short plantar ligaments, which also support the longitudinal arch of the foot, for point tenderness (Figs. 16-9 and 16-20). Foot pronation, sprain, or strain may result in acute pain.

BIOMECHANICS

The structural relationships and movements that occur at the ankle and hindfoot are complex. From a clinical standpoint, however, it is important that the clinician have at least a basic understanding of the biomechanics of this region. The joints of the foot and ankle constitute the first movable pivots in the weight-bearing extremity once the foot becomes fixed to the ground. Considered together, these joints must permit mobility in all planes to allow for minimal displacement of a person's center of gravity with respect to the base of support when walking over flat or uneven surfaces. In this sense, maintenance of balance and economy of energy consumption are, in part, dependent on proper functioning of the ankle–foot complex. Adequate mobility and proper structural alignment of these joints are also necessary for normal attenuation of forces transmitted from the ground to the weight-bearing extremity. Deviations in alignment and changes in mobility are likely to cause abnormal stresses to the joints of the foot and ankle as well as to the other weight-bearing joints. It follows that detection of biomechanical alterations in the ankle–foot region is often necessary for adequate interpretation of painful conditions affecting the foot and ankle, as well as conditions affecting the knee, hip, or lower spine in some cases.

Structural Alignment

In the normal standing position, the patella faces straight forward, the knee joint axis lies in the frontal plane, and the tibial tubercle is in line with the midline—or lateral half—of the patella. In this position, a line passing between the tips of the malleoli should make an angle of about 20 to 25° with the frontal plane.[7,79,88] This represents the normal amount of tibial torsion; the distal end of the tibia is rotated outward with respect to the proximal end. The lateral malleolus is positioned inferiorly with respect to the medial malleolus such that the intermalleolar line makes an angle of about 10° with the transverse plane.[88] The joint axis of the ankle mortise joint corresponds approximately to the intermalleolar line. With the patellae facing straight forward, the feet should be pointed outward about 5 to 10°.

If, when the feet are in normal standing alignment, the patellae face inward, increased femoral antetorsion, increased lateral tibial torsion, or both may be present. Clinically, the fault can be differentiated by assessing rotational range of motion of the hips and estimating the degree of tibial torsion by noting the rotational alignment of the malleoli with respect to the patellae and tibial tubercles. In the presence of increased hip antetorsion, the total range of hip motion will be normal but skewed such that medial rotation is excessive and lateral rotation is restricted proportionally. Similar considerations hold for a situation in which the patellae face outward when the feet are normally aligned; femoral retrotorsion, medial tibial torsion, or both are likely to exist.

With respect to the frontal plane, normal knee alignment may vary from slight genu valgum to some degree of genu varum. Because in most persons the medial femoral condyle extends farther distally than the lateral condyle, slight genu valgum tends to be more prevalent. At the hindfoot, the calcaneus should be positioned in vertical alignment with the tibia. A valgus or varus heel can usually be observed as a bowing of the Achilles tendon. A valgus positioning of the calcaneus on the talus is associated with pronation at the subtalar joint, whereas a varus hindfoot involves supination.

When considering the structure of the foot as a whole, it is helpful to compare it to a twisted plate (Fig. 16-24); the calcaneus, at one end, is positioned vertically when contacting the ground, whereas the metatarsal heads are positioned horizontally when making contact with a flat surface.[124] Thus, in the normal standing position on a flat, level surface, the metatarsal heads are twisted 90° with respect to the calcaneus.

To demonstrate this, a model can be constructed by taking a light rectangular piece of cardboard and twisting it so that one end lies flat on a table and the opposite end is perpendicular to the tabletop. Note the arching of the cardboard. This is analogous to the arching of the human foot. It should be realized that the term *arch* in this case applies to the configuration of the structure, which is dependent on the fact that it is twisted on itself. It does not refer to an arch in the true architectural sense, in which the arched configuration is dependent on the shapes of the component building blocks. In the

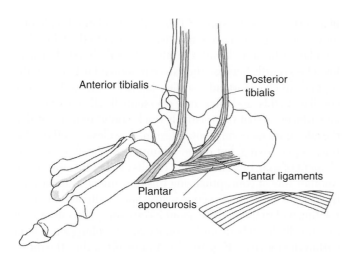

■ **FIG. 16-24.** "Twisted plate," which generates the medial arch.

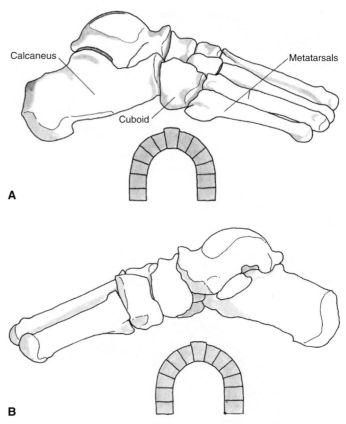

■ **FIG. 16-25.** **(A)** Lateral arch of the foot is a true arch. The calcaneus forms the ascending flank, the cuboid is the true keystone, and the fourth and fifth metatarsals are the descending flank. **(B)** Medial arch of the foot is not a true arch.

foot, both situations exist. On the medial side, there is little architectural arching and, therefore, little inherent stability of the medial arch. The medial arch is dependent almost entirely on the twisted configuration of the foot, which is maintained statically by the short and long plantar ligaments and dynamically by the anterior and posterior tibialis muscles. In contrast, the lateral side of the foot represents a true architectural arch (Fig. 16-25).[124] Here the cuboid, being wedged between the calcaneus and metatarsals, serves as the structural keystone. Only a small component of the lateral arch is a result of the twisted configuration of the foot.

Referring back to the cardboard model, notice that when the cardboard is allowed to untwist—by inclining the vertical end in one direction and keeping the other end flat on the table—the arch flattens. Inclining the vertical end in the opposite direction increases the twist and increases the arch. In the foot, inclination of the vertical component of the structure, the calcaneus, will result in similar untwisting or twisting; this results in a respective decrease or increase in the arching of the foot, if the metatarsal heads remain in contact with the ground (Fig. 16-26). The person who stands with the heel in a valgus position will have a relatively flat or untwisted foot, whereas a person whose heel is in a varus position when standing will appear to have a high arch because of increased twisting between hindfoot and forefoot. The former situation is often termed a *pronated foot* or *flatfoot*, and the latter is termed a *supinated foot* or *pes cavus*. In the situation of the heel remaining in a vertical position but the metatarsal heads are inclined, as on an uneven surface, the effect will also be to twist or untwist the foot, thereby raising or lowering the arch. For example, if the inclination is such that the first metatarsal head is on a higher level than the fifth, the forefoot supinates on the hindfoot, untwisting the foot and lowering the arch. Note that supination of the forefoot with the hindfoot fixed is the same as pronation of the hindfoot with the forefoot fixed; they both involve untwisting

of the tarsal skeleton from motion at the subtalar, transverse tarsal, and tarsometatarsal joints.

Reference is often made to a *transverse arch* of the foot, distinguishing it from the *longitudinal arch*. The cardboard model should help to make it clear that some transverse arching results from the twisted configuration of the foot. This is simply a transverse component of the arch discussed previously. This transverse component will increase and decrease along with twisting and untwisting of the foot. There is also a structural component to the transverse arching of the foot, resulting from the contours and relationships of the tarsals and metatarsals. It must be realized, however, that at the level of the metatarsal heads in the standing subject, no transverse arch exists, as each of the heads makes contact with the floor.

Arthrokinematics of Ankle–Foot Complex

ANKLE MORTISE JOINT

The superior articular surface of the talus is wider anteriorly than posteriorly, the difference in widths being as much as 6 mm.[7,88] The articular surfaces of the tibial and fibular malleoli maintain a close fit against the medial and lateral articular

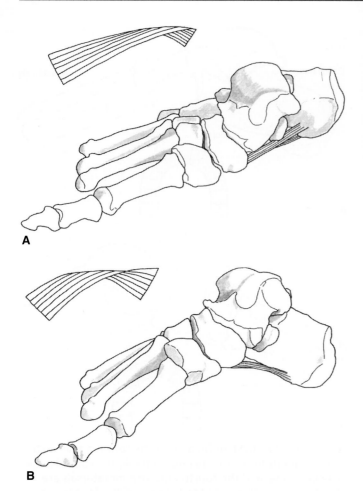

■ **FIG. 16-26.** Medial arch. When it is allowed to untwist, the arch flattens (**A**); when the medial arch is twisted, the arch increases (**B**).

surfaces of the talus in all positions of plantar flexion and dorsiflexion. As the foot moves from full plantar flexion into full dorsiflexion the talus rolls backward in the mortise. It would seem, then, that with ankle dorsiflexion the malleoli must separate to accommodate the greater anterior width of the talus. This separation could occur as a result of a lateral shift of the fibula, a lateral bending of the fibula, or both. However, it is found that the amount of separation that occurs between the malleoli during ankle dorsiflexion varies from none to only 2 mm, which is much less than would be expected, considering the amount of wedging of the superior articular surface of the talus. There appears to be a significant discrepancy between the difference in anterior and posterior widths of the trochlea of the talus and the amount of separation that occurs between the tibial and fibular malleoli with ankle dorsiflexion.

In understanding this apparent paradox, a closer look must be given to the structure of the trochlea and the type of movement the talus undergoes during ankle dorsiflexion. If both sides of the trochlea are examined it is evident that the lateral articular surface, which articulates with the fibular malleolus, is longer in its anteroposterior dimension than the medial artic-

ular surface. The reason for this is that the lateral malleolus moves over a greater excursion, with respect to the talus, during plantar flexion–dorsiflexion than does the medial malleolus. This is partly because the axis of motion is farther from the superior trochlear articular surface laterally than medially. The corollary to this (and this is true of essentially all joints with sellar surfaces) is that the relatively track-bound movement that the talus undergoes on plantar flexion–dorsiflexion at the ankle is not a pure swing, but rather an impure swing; it involves an element of spin, or rotation, that results in a helical movement. Another way of conceptualizing this movement is to consider the talus as a section of a cone whose apex is situated medially rotating within the mortise about its own long axis, rather than a truly cylindrical body undergoing a simple rolling movement within the mortise (Fig. 16-27). As a result of this, the intermalleolar lines projected onto the superior trochlear articular surface at various positions of plantar flexion and dorsiflexion are not parallel lines. Therefore, the degree of wedging of the trochlea does not reflect the relative intermalleolar distances in dorsiflexion and plantar flexion of the ankle. The true intermalleolar distances are represented by the length of these nonparallel lines projected onto the superior trochlear surface. The projected line with the foot in plantar flexion is only slightly shorter, if at all, than that for dorsiflexion, and the necessary separation of the malleoli during dorsiflexion is minimal.[88]

Up to this point, the ankle mortise joint axis has been considered as a fixed axis of motion. This has been done for the sake of simplicity and convenience using the approximate center of movement as the joint axis. But, as mentioned in Chapter 3, Arthrology, no joint moves about a stationary joint axis. As indicated by instant center analysis of knee joint motion, this is true of the ankle mortise joint as well.[181] The surface velocities determined from the instant centers of movement show that when moving from full plantar flexion to full dorsiflexion there is initially a momentary distraction of the tibiotalar joint surfaces, followed by a movement of combined rolling and sliding throughout most of the range, and terminating with an approximation of joint surfaces at the position of extreme dorsiflexion. These findings are consistent with the fact that the close-packed position of the ankle mortise joint is dorsiflexion; the tightening of the joint capsule that occurs

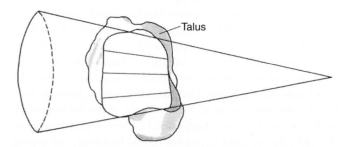

■ **FIG. 16-27.** Diagram to illustrate movement of the talus as a section of a cone, whose apex is situated medially, rotating within the mortise about its own long axis.

with movement of any joint into its close-packed position produces an approximation of the joint surfaces.

SUBTALAR JOINT

As discussed previously, this is a compound joint with two distinct articulations. From the outset, movement at this joint is somewhat difficult to conceptualize because the posterior articulation between the talus and calcaneus is concave superiorly and convex inferiorly, whereas the anteromedial articulation is convex on concave. Understanding talocalcaneal movement is perhaps facilitated by considering it analogous to movement at the proximal and distal radioulnar joints. The radioulnar joints, like the talocalcaneal joints, move in conjunction with one another and have only one degree of freedom of motion. The posterior calcaneal facet moving against the opposing concave talar surface can be compared with the radial head moving within the radial notch of the ulna. As this movement occurs, the anteromedial facet of the talus must move in relation to the concave anteromedial surface of the calcaneus, just as the head of the ulna must move within the ulnar notch of the radius at the distal joint of the forearm. In at least some persons, this type of movement at the subtalar joint is accompanied by a slight forward displacement of the talus during pronation and a backward displacement on supination, thus making the total movement a helical, or screwlike, motion.[124]

NEUTRAL POSITION OF A JOINT

To facilitate arthrometric studies and to correlate function of the joints, it is necessary to assign to joints certain reference points called the neutral positions of those joints. By definition these neutral positions are purely reference points. They are, however, significant in that they make it possible to measure and define positional and structural variances.

The neutral position of the first ray is that position in which the first metatarsal head lies in the same transverse plane as the central three metatarsal heads when they are at their most dorsiflexed position.[175] From this neutral position, the first metatarsal can move an equal distance above and below the transverse plane of the lesser metatarsal heads when the first ray is moved through its full range.

Root and coworkers[175] describe a neutral position of the subtalar joint as that position of the joint in which the foot is neither pronated nor supinated; another way to state this is the position from which the subtalar joint could be maximally pronated and supinated. From this position, full supination of the normal subtalar inverts the calcaneus twice as many degrees as full pronation everts it. Subtalar neutral is two thirds from inversion and one third from eversion of the calcaneus.

Clinically this is important because the subtalar neutral position provides a foundation for meaningful and valid measurements and observations with respect to the foot and entire leg. It is not only a basis for meaningful communication but also the foundation for the application of precise therapy, such as the fabrication of an effective biomechanical orthotic device.[72] There is also a direct clinical correlation between the subtalar joint and the midtarsal joint. When the subtalar joint is held in its neutral position, there is no longer the ability for the midtarsal joint to pronate. The midtarsal is unable to dorsiflex, evert, or abduct when the subtalar is in its neutral position. This position is termed the *normal locking position* of the midtarsal joint.

According to James,[93] the talar head in a pronated foot can be palpated as a medial bulge; in a supinated foot the talar head bulges laterally. In the neutral position the talar head can be palpated equally on the medial and lateral aspects of the ankle. The neutral position is usually present when the longitudinal axis of the lower limb and the vertical axis of the calcaneus are parallel. This method for establishing the subtalar neutral position is useful in both the open-chain and closed-chain positions.

A second method that is useful in the open-chain position involves visualizing and feeling the subtalar joint as it moves through its range of motion.[94] To begin, the examiner should place the ulnar surface of the thumb into the sulcus of the patient's fourth and fifth toes, moving the patient's foot from pronation to supination and back again. This movement is very similar in shape to that of a horse saddle, being very abrupt toward pronation and very flat and shallow toward supination (Fig. 16-28A). The bottom of this saddle is the neutral position of the subtalar joint. This can be confirmed visually by observing the lateral curves above and below the malleolus (Fig. 16-28B). If these curves are the same depth,

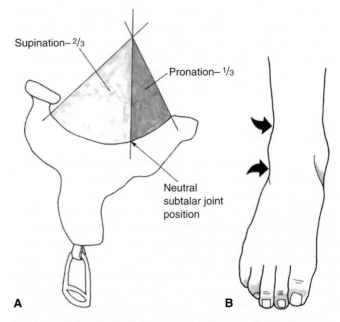

■ **FIG. 16-28.** Subtalar movement is very similar in shape to that of a horse saddle, being very abrupt toward pronation and flat and shallow toward supination. The bottom position is the neutral position of the subtalar joint (**A**), which can be visually confirmed by observing the lateral curves above and below the malleolus (**B**). These curves should be of the same depth.

this is the accurate neutral position. If the curve below the malleolus is deeper or shallower, then the foot is still in a pronated or supinated position and should be repositioned.

TALOCALCANEONAVICULAR JOINT

As the name implies, the talocalcaneonavicular (TCN) joint is a combination of the talonavicular joint and the subtalar (talo-calcaneal) joint, which are both anatomically and functionally related (Fig. 16-17).[157] The TCN synovial cavity is demarcated from the posterior subtalar cavity by the contents of the sinus and canalis tarsi. Ligamentous structures form an anatomic barrier between the posterior facet of the subtalar joint and its companion facets (the middle and anterior facets). This space houses the deep insertions of the inferior extensor retinaculum that cross anterior to the interosseous talocalcaneal ligament.

The plantar calcaneonavicular (spring) ligament spans the floor of this synovial cavity, enlarging the compartment and producing a functional anastomosis of sorts between the anterior portion of the sustentaculum tali and the navicular, known as the *acetabulum pedis*.[214] This unique space occupied by the talar head and neck is reinforced by the bifurcate ligaments laterally and the deltoid ligament medially.

The head of the talus and its large socket are enclosed by the same capsule that houses the anterior and middle facets of the subtalar joint. The capsule anatomically joins the subtalar joint and the talonavicular joints into the TCN joint.

The TCN joint, like its subtalar component, is a triplanar joint with one degree of freedom: supination and pronation.[157] Functionally, the subtalar joint and the talonavicular joint exist as components of the more complex TCN joint. The calcaneonavicular complex is a functional unit moving around the talus. The extracapsular ligaments of the sinus tarsi and tarsal canal are the major elements guiding the motion of the calcaneonavicular complex relative to the talus.

TRANSVERSE TARSAL JOINTS: TALONAVICULAR AND CALCANEOCUBOID

Although some movement may occur between the cuboid and navicular bones, movement of these two bones is considered here as a unit with respect to the calcaneus and the talus. The configuration of the talonavicular articulation is essentially that of a ball-and-socket joint. Because of this configuration, it potentially has three degrees of freedom of movement, allowing it to move in all planes. However, because the navicular is closely bound to the cuboid bone laterally, its freedom of movement is largely governed by the movement allowed at the calcaneocuboid joint.[52] The calcaneocuboid joint, having a sellar configuration, has two degrees of freedom, each of which occurs about a distinct axis of motion. The axis of motion of most concern here is the axis of pronation and supination. This axis is similar in location and orientation to the subtalar joint axis, the major difference being that it is not inclined as much vertically. It passes through the talar head, backward, downward, and laterally. Such an orientation allows a movement of

inversion–adduction–plantar flexion (supination) and eversion–abduction–dorsiflexion (pronation) of the forefoot. In the standing position, movement and positioning at the transverse tarsal joint occurs in conjunction with subtalar joint movement; when the subtalar joint pronates, the transverse tarsal joint supinates, and vice versa. Pronation of the forefoot causes close-packing and locking of the transverse tarsal joint complex, whereas supination results in loose-packing and a greater degree of freedom of movement.[124]

TARSOMETATARSAL JOINTS

The five metatarsals articulate with the three cuneiforms and the cuboid and form the tarsometatarsal (TMT) or Lisfranc's joint (Fig. 16-10). They are plane synovial joints. Proximally, the bases of the metatarsals are disposed in an arcuate fashion forming a transverse arch that is high medially and low laterally. The apex of this arch corresponds to the base of the second metatarsal. The metatarsals are also flexed, thus contributing to the formation of the longitudinal arch.

The tarsometatarsal joints allow flexion and extension of the metatarsal bones and a certain degree of supination and pronation of the marginal rays.[41] Sarrafian[183] describes the supination and pronation of the first and fifth rays as longitudinal axial rotations. The combination of the sagittal motions and the axial rotations of the first and fifth rays results in a supination and pronation twist of the forefoot, as defined by Hicks.[79] A pronation twist of the forefoot is the result of first ray flexion (plantar flexed) and fifth ray extension (dorsiflexed), whereas a supination twist is a result of first ray extension and fifth ray flexion.[79,183]

METATARSOPHALANGEAL AND INTERPHALANGEAL JOINTS

The five metatarsophalangeal (MTP) joints have two degrees of motion possible, either flexion–extension or abduction–adduction; the interphalangeal joints have one degree of motion, predominantly flexion and extension. In the weight-bearing foot, toe extension permits the body to pass over the foot while the toes dynamically balance the superimposed body weight as they press into the supporting surface through activity of the toe flexors.[157] The MTP joints serve primarily to allow the foot to hinge at the toes so that the heel may rise off the ground. This function is enhanced by the metatarsal break and the effect of MTP extension on the plantar aponeurosis (Fig. 16-29). The toes participate in weight bearing in giving hold against the ground and in stabilizing the longitudinal arch by tensing the plantar aponeurosis during the push-off phase of the walking cycle. Approximately 40% of the body weight is borne by the toes in the final stages of foot contact.[129]

Weight-bearing forces to the toes are attenuated by the tension in the toe flexor tendons and the tendon sheaths. The interosseous and lumbrical muscles dynamically stabilize the toes on the floor in the tiptoe position.[213] Failure of these muscles to function accounts for toe deformities such

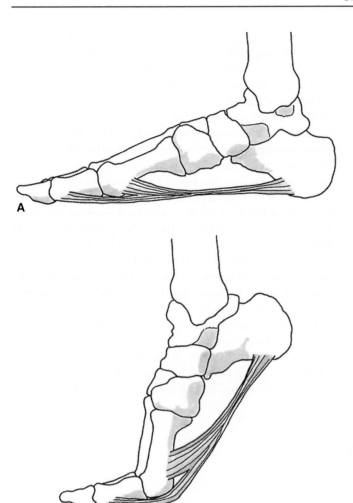

■ **FIG. 16-29.** **(A)** Foot is flat. **(B)** Toe-standing causes the aponeurosis to tighten. Tightening the plantar aponeurosis raises the arch and adds to the rigidity of the tarsal skeleton.

as claw toe. The long flexors of the toes act as plantar flexors of the ankle and invertors of the talocalcaneonavicular joint, whereas the long extensors of the toes act as dorsiflexors of the ankle and evertors of the talocalcaneonavicular joint.[183] Dorsiflexion of the toes, especially the first MTP joint, is important to the windlass mechanism (see ankle and foot during gait). Sixty to seventy degrees of dorsiflexion is necessary for tension to develop within the aponeurosis.[40,41]

Osteokinematics of Ankle–Foot Complex

TERMINOLOGY

At this point, some terms related to movement and positioning of various components of the ankle and foot must be clarified. Throughout this chapter the following definitions will hold:

Inversion–eversion—Movement about a horizontal axis lying in the sagittal plane. Functionally, pure inversion and eversion rarely occur at any of the joints of ankle or foot. More often they occur as a component of supination or pronation.

Abduction–adduction—Movement of the forefoot about a vertical axis or the movement of the forefoot that results from internal or external rotation of the hindfoot with respect to the leg.

Internal-external rotation—Movement between the leg and hindfoot occurring about a vertical axis. Pure rotations do not occur functionally but rather occur as components of pronation and supination.

Plantarflexion–dorsiflexion—Movement about a horizontal axis lying in the plane corresponding to the intermalleolar line. Functionally, these movements usually occur in conjunction with other movements.

Pronation–supination—Functional movements occurring around the obliquely situated subtalar or transverse tarsal joint axis. At both of these joints, pronation involves abduction, eversion, and some dorsiflexion; supination involves adduction, inversion, and plantar flexion of the distal segment on the proximal segment. This is because these joint axes are inclined backward, downward, and laterally. It must be appreciated that when the metatarsals are fixed to the ground, pronation of the hindfoot (subtalar joint) involves supination of the forefoot (transverse tarsal joint).

Pronated foot–supinated foot—Traditionally, a pronated foot (in the standing position) is one in which the arched configuration of the foot is reduced; the hindfoot is pronated and the forefoot is supinated. In a supinated foot (standing) the arch is high, the hindfoot is supinated, and the forefoot is pronated.

Valgus–varus—Terms used for alignment of parts. *Valgus* denotes inclination away from the midline of a segment with respect to its proximal neighbor, whereas *varus* is inclination toward the midline. At the hindfoot and forefoot, valgus refers to alignment in a pronated position and varus to alignment in a supinated position.

ORIENTATION OF JOINT AXES AND EFFECT ON MOVEMENT

In the normal standing position, the axis of movement for the knee joint is horizontal and in a frontal plane. With flexion and extension of the free-swinging tibia, movement will occur in a sagittal plane. The ankle mortise joint axis is directed backward mediolaterally about 25° from the frontal plane and downward from medial to lateral about 10 to 15° from horizontal. Movement of the free foot about this axis results in combined plantar flexion, adduction, and inversion or combined dorsiflexion, abduction, and eversion. Note that the above statements relate the movements at the respective joints to the orientations of the joint axes when the foot and leg are swinging freely. In this position, movements at one joint may occur independently of the other.

Clinicians must be more concerned, however, with what happens when the foot becomes fixed to the ground and movement occurs simultaneously at the joints of the lower limbs. This is the situation during weight-bearing activities or normal functional activities involving the leg. The obvious question in this regard would be, how is it possible to move both the tibia and femur in the sagittal plane, such as when performing a knee bend with the knee pointed forward, when movement is occurring at the ankle and knee about two non-parallel axes? The lifter of heavy weights largely avoids the problem by pointing the knees outward, thus using external rotation and abduction at the hip. This brings the knee and ankle axes closer to parallel alignment. The fact remains, however, that it is possible to perform a deep knee bend with the knee directed forward, and through a considerable range. Because the knee joint axis lies horizontally in the frontal plane, no problem would be expected there, as it is ideally oriented to allow rotation of the bones in the sagittal plane. It would seem, then, that by performing such a knee bend an internal rotatory movement must be applied to the ankle because the ankle joint axis is externally rotated with respect to the frontal plane. Surely

ankle mortise joints cannot be expected to withstand such stresses during daily activities. This apparent problem can be resolved by considering the orientation of the joint axis and associated movements at the subtalar joint.

The axis of motion for the subtalar joint is directed backward, downward, and laterally (Fig. 16-30).[25,88,132,134] The degree of inclination and mediolateral deviation of the axis varies greatly among persons. The average deviation from the midline of the foot is 16°, whereas the average deviation from the horizontal is 42°. Because the axis of motion for the subtalar joint deviates from the sagittal plane and from the horizontal plane, movement at this joint involves combined eversion, dorsiflexion, and abduction or combined inversion, plantar flexion, and adduction. Note that pure abduction and adduction of the foot are movements that would occur about a vertical axis and that inversion and eversion occur about a purely horizontal axis. Inasmuch as the subtalar axis is positioned about midway between horizontal and vertical, it follows that movement about this axis would include elements of adduction–abduction as well as eversion–inversion.

Consider again a situation of simultaneous knee and ankle flexion in the sagittal plane with the foot fixed (e.g., a deep knee bend). It was indicated that with such a movement an internal

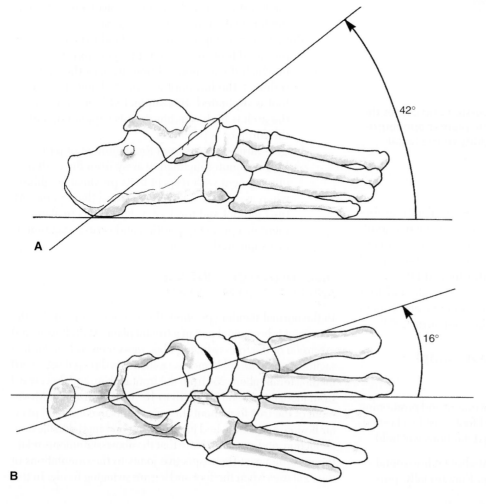

42°

16°

■ **FIG. 16-30.** Subtalar joint axis of movement. The subtalar joint axis is 42° from the transverse and 16° from the foot's midline, so the axis, as well as movement, is triplanar.

rotatory moment of the tibia on the talus would be applied to the ankle. Because the subtalar axis allows an element of movement about a vertical axis (rotation in the horizontal plane), this internal rotatory moment can be transmitted to the subtalar joint. Internal rotation of the tibia on the foot is, of course, equivalent to external rotation of the foot on the leg, which is referred to as abduction of the foot. Subtalar movement is essentially uniaxial, so that any movement occurring at the joint may occur only in conjunction with its component movements; that is, abduction can only occur in conjunction with eversion and dorsiflexion, the three together constituting pronation at the subtalar joint. Thus, with the foot fixed, simultaneous dorsiflexion of the ankle and flexion of the knee, keeping the leg in the sagittal plane, requires pronation at the subtalar joint. As a corollary to this, with such a movement, if pronation at the subtalar joint is restricted, an abnormal internal tibial rotatory stress will occur at the ankle mortise joint or an internal femoral rotatory stress will be placed on the knee, or both. The need for subtalar movement can be reduced by moving the leg out of the sagittal plane (by pointing the knee outward) and bringing the knee and ankle axes into closer alignment.

Similar considerations apply to the situation of a person rotating the leg over a fixed foot. Any rotation imparted to the tibia is transmitted to the subtalar joint (Fig. 16-31). For example, if one rotates the leg externally over a foot that is fixed to the ground, the subtalar joint undergoes a movement of supination. This is analogous to movement about a mitered hinge; movement of one component about a vertical axis is transmitted to the second component as movement about a horizontal axis. Supination causes the calcaneus to assume a varus position, which, because the metatarsals remain flat on the ground, increases the twist in the foot and raises the arch.[25] The opposite occurs with internal tibial rotation; pronation of

the hindfoot causes a relative supination of the forefoot; the foot untwists and the arch flattens. This can easily be observed if one attempts to rotate the leg with the foot fixed to the ground. With respect to the structural alignment, then, a person with excessive internal tibial torsion will tend to have a pronated hindfoot (calcaneus in valgus position) and a forefoot that is supinated with respect to the hindfoot. The resultant untwisting of the foot causes a flatfoot on standing. The person with excessive external tibial torsion will tend to have a varus heel and a high arch.

The degree of twisting and untwisting of the foot also varies with stance width.[124] When standing with the feet far apart, the heel tends to deviate into a valgus position with respect to the floor and the metatarsal heads remain flat; the metatarsals assume a position of supination with respect to the heel, thus untwisting the foot. The opposite occurs when standing with the legs crossed.

It should be noted that when standing with the hindfoot in pronation and the forefoot in supination, the medial metatarsals assume a position closer to dorsiflexion.[79] Because the joint axis of the first metatarsal is obliquely oriented (from anterolateral to posteromedial), dorsiflexion of the first metatarsal involves a component of abduction away from the midline of the foot. Therefore, in a pronated foot, the first metatarsal is usually positioned in varus. On the other hand, in a person with metatarsus primus varus, a condition in which the first metatarsal deviates into varus position, the foot will tend to assume a pronated position. This is because for the first metatarsal to be in a varus angle, it must also be in some dorsiflexion. This causes supination of the forefoot, which necessitates pronation of the hindfoot for the person to stand with the metatarsal head and calcaneus in contact with the ground.

ANKLE AND FOOT DURING GAIT

Clinicians must be concerned with the function of the joints of the ankle and foot during normal daily activities. The prime consideration here, of course, is walking. Again, because these are weight-bearing joints and because the foot becomes fixed to the ground during the stance phase, an understanding of the biomechanical interrelationships between these joints and the other joints of the lower extremity is necessary.

During the gait cycle, the leg progresses through space in a sagittal plane. To minimize energy expenditure, the center of gravity must undergo minimal vertical displacement. This is largely accomplished by angular movement of the lower extremity components in the sagittal plane, that is, flexion–extension at the hip, knee, and ankle complex. The hip has no trouble accommodating such movement as it is multiaxial, allowing some movement in all vertical planes. The knee, although essentially uniaxial, allows flexion and extension in the sagittal plane because its axis of movement is perpendicular to this plane and horizontally oriented. The ankle mortise joint, however, cannot allow a pure sagittal movement between the leg and foot because its axis of motion is not perpendicular to

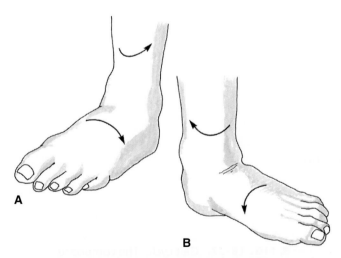

■ **FIG. 16-31.** **(A)** External rotation of the tibia over the fixed foot imparts a movement of supination to the foot, increasing the arch. **(B)** Internal tibial rotation flattens, or pronates, the fixed foot.

the sagittal plane; it is rotated outward about 25°. During the normal gait cycle, however, movement between the foot and leg in the sagittal plane does occur. This is only possible through participation of another joint, the subtalar joint. Movement of the tibia in a parasagittal plane over a fixed foot requires simultaneous movement at the subtalar and ankle mortise joints. This is consistent with the fact that no muscles attach to the talus. Those muscles that affect movement at the ankle mortise joint also cross the subtalar joint, moving it as well.

In considering the various movements occurring at each of the segments of the lower extremity during gait, it is con-venient to speak of three intervals of stance phase; these are (1) the interval from heel-strike to foot-flat, (2) midstance (foot-flat), and (3) the interval from the beginning of heel-rise to toe-off.

During the first interval, each of the segments of the lower extremity rotates internally with respect to its more proximal neighboring segment; the pelvis rotates internally in space, the femur rotates internally on the pelvis, and the tibia rotates internally on the femur (Fig. 16-32A).[117,119,184] It follows that the entire lower limb rotates during this phase and that distal segments rotate more, in space, than the more proximally situated

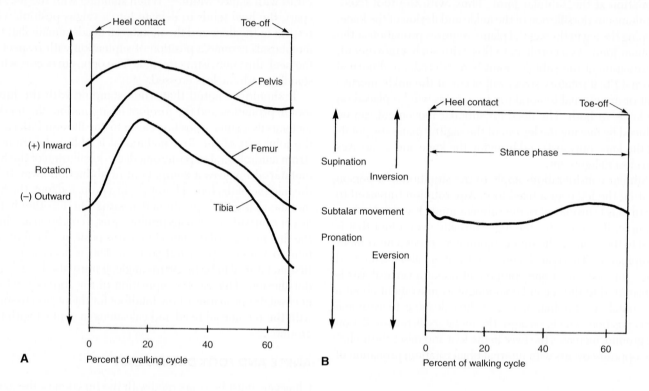

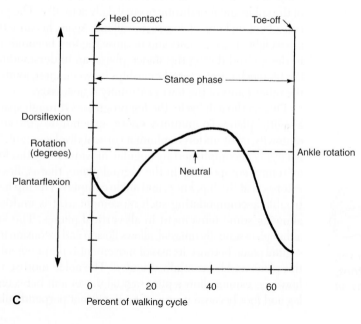

■ **FIG. 16-32.** Gait cycle. The composite curves show transverse rotations of the pelvis, femur, and tibia (stance phase; **A**), subtalar torsion (**B**), and ankle mortise rotation (sagittal plane; **C**).

segments. At the point of heel-strike, the foot becomes partially fixed to the ground, so that only minimal internal torsion between the heel and the ground takes place. Much of this internal rotation is absorbed at the subtalar joint as pronation (Fig. 16-32B).[199,222] Internal rotation of the leg with respect to the foot, occurring at the subtalar joint, makes the axis of the ankle mortise joint more perpendicular to the plane of progression. This allows the ankle mortise joint to provide for movement in the sagittal plane, which, of course, is the plantar flexion occurring at the ankle during this interval (Fig. 16-32C). Note that the foot tends to deviate slightly medially in this stage of stance phase. This is because the obliquity of the ankle axis, in the coronal plane, imposes a component of adduction of the foot during plantar flexion.

At heel-strike, a moment-arm equal to the distance between the point of heel contact and the ankle joint develops. The reactive force of the ground acting on the foot at heel-strike across this moment-arm will tend to swing the tibia forward in the sagittal plane. This results in some flexion at the knee, which is consistent with the fact that the tibia is rotating internally with respect to the femur. Knee flexion, from an extended position, involves a component of internal tibial rotation.

Note that at heel-strike, the hindfoot moves into pronation while the tibialis anterior muscle contracts to bring the forefoot into supination. This causes the foot to untwist, the transverse tarsal joint to unlock, and the joints to assume a loose-packed position. The foot at this point is in a position favorable for free mobility and is, therefore, at its greatest potential to adapt to variations in the contour of the ground.[52,222]

Once the foot becomes flat on the ground, movement at the ankle mortise joint changes abruptly from plantar flexion to dorsiflexion.[152,165] Through the early period of foot-flat, during which most of dorsiflexion occurs, the segments of the lower extremity continue to rotate internally. This rotation is transmitted to the joints of the ankle, as the foot is now fixed to the ground. Some internal rotation of the tibia automatically occurs at the ankle mortise joint during dorsiflexion with the foot fixed because the joint axis is inclined about 15° from horizontal, downward and laterally. However, most of the internal rotation takes place at the subtalar joint as a component of pronation.[25,222]

Throughout most of the period during which the foot is flat on the ground, the segments of the lower extremity rotate externally; the more distal segments rotate externally to a greater degree than their proximal neighbors.[121] Again, because the foot is fixed to the ground, the tibia rotates externally with respect to the foot. This occurs as supination at the subtalar joint. The change during foot-flat, from internal rotation to external rotation, takes place after most of ankle dorsiflexion is complete.

Because the forefoot is fixed to the ground, the inversion occurring at the subtalar joint imposes pronation at the transverse tarsal joint, causing a close-packing or locking of the tarsus. Consistent with this, the peroneus longus muscle contracts, maintaining a pronated twist of the metatarsals and bringing the foot as a whole toward its twisted configuration. The foot at this point is being converted into an intrinsically stable lever capable of providing for the thrust of pushing off.

During the final interval of stance phase, from heel-rise to toe-off, the segments of the lower limb continue to rotate externally. This external rotation of the tibia is again transmitted to the subtalar joint as supination of the hindfoot. With contraction of the calf muscle, the ankle begins plantar flexion, creating a thrust for push-off. This again creates a moment-arm acting on the knee, this time moving the tibia into extension with respect to the femur. Note that this is consistent with the external rotation of the tibia occurring during this phase because knee extension involves a component of external tibial rotation.

The extension of the metatarsophalangeal joints, occurring with heel-rise, causes a tightening of the plantar aponeurosis through a windlass effect because the distal attachment of the aponeurosis crosses the plantar aspect of the joints (Fig. 16-29).[80] This tightening of the aponeurosis further raises the arch and adds to the rigidity of the tarsal skeleton.

It should be emphasized that during this final phase of stance, the joint movements that occur automatically convert the foot into a stable lever system and require little, if any, muscle contraction to accomplish this.

In summary, then, the transverse rotations of the segments of the lower extremity that occur during stance phase of the gait cycle are transmitted to the ankle joints. This is because during the stance phase the foot is relatively fixed to the ground so that rotation between the foot and the ground is minimal. The ankle mortise axis is inclined slightly vertically (about 15° from the horizontal axis) whereas the subtalar joint axis is situated about midway between horizontal and vertical. Both joints are able to absorb rotatory movements transmitted to the ankle because of the vertical inclination of the joint axes. With the foot fixed to the ground, the tibia rotates slightly internally at the ankle mortise during dorsiflexion and externally during plantar flexion. Internal rotation of the talus with respect to the calcaneus occurs as pronation, whereas external rotation results in supination at the subtalar joint. Also, once the foot becomes flat on the ground, the metatarsal heads become fixed and the twisting and untwisting of the foot becomes dependent on the position of the hindfoot. At heel-strike, the tibia rotates internally, pronating the hindfoot, while the tibialis anterior contracts to supinate the forefoot; this results in an untwisted foot. During midstance, as the tibia rotates externally and the subtalar joint gradually supinates, the foot becomes twisted. This twisting is further increased by tightening of the plantar aponeurosis. The twisted configuration results in maximal joint stability with minimal participation of the intrinsic foot muscles. It is the twisted foot, then, that is best suited for weight bearing and propulsion. During midstance there is little activity of the intrinsic muscles in the normal foot because the twisted configuration confers a passive, or intrinsic, stability on the foot. However, in the flat-footed person, considerably more muscle action is required because the foot is relatively untwisted.[124] The flat-footed person must rely more on extrinsic stabilization by the muscles. An untwisted configuration is desirable in situations in which the foot must be mobile, such as in adapting to surface contours of the ground. Consistent with this is the fact that at heel-strike, the foot assumes an untwisted state in preparation for conformation to the contacting surface.

A relatively common condition that illustrates the biomechanical interdependency of the weight-bearing joints is femoral antetorsion. A person with femoral antetorsion must stand with the leg internally rotated to position the hip joint in normal (neutral) alignment. Conversely, if the leg is positioned in normal alignment with the patella facing straight forward, the hip joint assumes a position of relative external rotation. External rotation at the hip decreases the congruity of the joint surfaces. During stance phase, as the femur externally rotates on the pelvis, the hip of the person with femoral antetorsion will tend to go into too much external rotation. As the slack is taken up in the part of the joint capsule that pulls tight on external rotation, the joint receptors sense the excessive movement. To avoid excessive joint incongruity and to prevent abnormal stress to the joint capsule, the person with femoral antetorsion must *internally* rotate during stance phase. This internal rotation is transmitted primarily to the subtalar joint, which is best oriented to accommodate transverse rotations. Internal rotation at the subtalar joint causes pronation of the hindfoot; the foot untwists and the arch flattens. Thus, femoral antetorsion predisposes to pronation of the foot. Also, because of the internal rotatory movement transmitted through the knee, femoral antetorsion may be a causative factor in certain knee disorders. For example, internal rotation imposed on a semiflexed knee causes the knee to assume an increased valgus position. This may predispose to patellar tracking dysfunction (see Chapter 15, Knee). Because there is a tendency for the person with femoral antetorsion to walk with increased hip joint incongruity, the force of weight bearing is transmitted to a smaller area of contact at the articular surface of the hip. The result may be accelerated wear of the hip joint surfaces, perhaps leading to degenerative hip disease.

Femoral antetorsion provides a good example of how a structural abnormality in one region may lead to localized biomechanical disturbances as well as altered mechanics at joints some distance away. This, again, is especially true of the lower extremity and should emphasize that when evaluating many patients with foot disorders it may be appropriate, if not necessary, to examine the structure and function of the knee, hip, and lower back. Conversely, foot or ankle dysfunction may precipitate disturbances in more proximal joints.

EXAMINATION

The L4, L5, S1, and S2 segments contribute to the ankle and foot. Symptoms arising in the more proximal regions of these segments may refer to the ankle and foot, the most common of which might be paresthesias arising from lumbar nerve root irritation. Actual pain of more proximal origin is rarely felt in

the foot. Rather, foot and ankle pain usually arise from local pathologic processes. Pain arising from tissues of the foot or ankle may be referred a short distance proximally but almost never to the knee or above.

The common lesions affecting the ankle are of acute, traumatic onset, whereas those affecting the foot are more likely to be chronic disorders resulting from stress overload. Because of the biomechanical interdependency of the weight-bearing joints, attention must often be directed to the structure and function of more proximally situated joints during examination of patients with chronic or subtle foot disorders. Similarly, examination of the foot may well be in order in patients with disorders affecting more proximal regions.

History

A patient interview designed to elicit specific information related to the patient's pain, functional status, and other associated symptoms, as set out in Chapter 5, Assessment of Musculoskeletal Disorders and Concepts of Management, should be carried out. The following are general concepts that apply to information that may be elicited when a therapist interviews patients with common foot or ankle disorders.

If the disorder was of an acute, traumatic onset, an attempt can be made to determine the exact mechanism of injury. Plantar flexion–inversion strains are more likely to result in capsuloligamentous injury, whereas forces moving the foot into dorsiflexion and external rotation (abduction) are more likely to produce a fracture.

If the disorder is of a more chronic nature and of insidious onset, the therapist can attempt to determine whether a change in activity level or footwear may be associated with the onset of the problem. The effect of changing footwear should be ascertained. For example, a therapist might determine the effect of variations in heel height, including whether the problem is affected, for better or for worse, by going barefoot.

Chronic stress overload (fatigue) disorders may be classified as (1) those caused by high levels of activity in which the frequency or high rate of tissue stress is such that the body is unable to keep up with the increased rate of tissue microtrauma (the rate of tissue breakdown exceeds the rate of repair and the tissue gradually fatigues) and (2) those that occur with normal activity levels and are caused by some structural or biomechanical abnormality that subjects the affected tissue to mildly increased stresses for a long period. Such stresses may produce pain on an intermittent basis and, during a long time, may induce tissue hypertrophy. Because these are mild stresses acting for a long period, the body is able to respond by laying down an excessive amount of tissue in an attempt to strengthen itself against these abnormal stresses. Tissue hypertrophy such as corns and calluses may, in itself, lead to pain by allowing localized areas of stress concentration.

Patients incurring tissue damage from high stresses acting during a relatively short period are typically persons who have increased their activity level significantly. Often, but not always, the patient will blame a particular activity for contributing to the onset of the problem. Keep in mind that in such instances the patient may or may not be correct; the particular disorder may have been developing for some period, perhaps as a result of a biomechanical abnormality, and may simply be aggravated by a particular activity. By evaluating the mechanical effects of activities that reproduce the pain, the examiner can often find important clues as to the nature of a particular disorder.

Shoes tend to provide support for the twisted or arched configuration of the foot to varying degrees. A high heel causes the toes to dorsiflex when standing with the feet in contact with the ground. This raises the arch by tightening the plantar aponeurosis that crosses the plantar surface of the metatarsophalangeal joints (Fig. 16-29). Heels also reduce the passive tension on the Achilles tendon and gastrocnemius–soleus group and, by effectively reducing the toe lever-arm of the foot, reduce the active tension developed in the gastrocnemius–soleus muscle–tendon complex. Most shoes also provide some contoured base of support for the arch of the foot. This maximizes the contacting surface area of the foot and, therefore, distributes the stresses of weight bearing over most of the sole of the foot. Proper contouring of a shoe also minimizes the amount of tension that needs to be developed in the plantar aponeurosis, long and short plantar ligaments, tarsal joint capsules, and intrinsic muscles to maintain a normal twisted configuration to the foot. When a person walks barefoot, the effects of the heel and contoured support are lost. This usually creates no problem in a person with good bony alignment and ligamentous support. However, in a person with a tendency toward pronation (untwisting of the foot), the added tension to the plantar ligaments may lead to pain. Or, if the ligaments are already lax, increased intrinsic muscle activity will be necessary. If such muscular activity is prolonged, pain may also arise from muscular fatigue. These persons are often more comfortable wearing shoes than going barefoot. Even persons with normal foot structure may experience some foot pain with lower heel heights if they are accustomed to wearing a shoe with a heel. Lowering the heel reduces the support provided by the plantar aponeurosis, putting more tension on the plantar ligaments and joint capsules and calling for increased activity of the intrinsic muscles of the foot. This is why flat-soled shoes, especially, must have well-contoured arch supports.

Shoes also provide an interface for shear and compressive stresses. Foot pain arising from localized pressure concentration, from shear stresses between the skin and an exterior surface, or from shearing between skin and subcutaneous tissue may be alleviated by going barefoot. This is primarily true in cases in which such stresses occur over all but the soles of the feet. Pain from pressure concentration over the sole of the foot, as frequently occurs over the head of the second metatarsal, may be reduced by wearing shoes because the contouring of the shoe may serve to distribute the pressures of weight bearing over a broader area.

Complaints of cramping of the foot may accompany muscular fatigue usually associated with some biomechanical disturbance. Cramping may also accompany intermittent claudication from arterial insufficiency. Claudication should always be suspect when the patient relates a history of pain or cramping of the feet, and usually of the lower leg, after walking some distance, but the pain is relieved with rest. Cramping may accompany disk protrusions, presumably from altered conduction of fibers subserving motor control or muscle reflexes. This cramping is noticed more often at night.

Physical Examination

I. Observation
   A. General appearance and body build. Weight-bearing stresses will be increased in the presence of obesity.
   B. Functional activities. Clues for appropriate tests can be obtained from the subjective examination.
      1. Gait and activities of daily living. Dressing, grooming, gait, and transfer activities (see gait analysis discussion Chapter 24, Lumbosacral–Lower-Limb Scan Examination). With localized foot or ankle disorders, usually only the gait is affected. Observe the patient walking with and without shoes. An antalgic gait associated with foot or ankle lesions is typically one in which heel-strike or push-off, or both, is lacking. This results in a shortened stride on the affected side, which is accentuated at faster paces. Chronic disorders may produce no obvious gait disturbances. However, one should look carefully for more-subtle gait deviations, indicating a possible biomechanical abnormality of one or more of the weight-bearing joints that may be related to a foot problem. It is of primary importance to observe for abnormal rotatory movements of the weight-bearing segments. To assess rotations of the hindfoot into pronation and supination, look at the following:
      a. The patellae to judge rotary movements of the femur
      b. The position of the malleoli with respect to each other or the tibia
      c. The position of the calcanei
      d. The degree of toeing-in or toeing-out
      e. The degree of motion in ankle dorsiflexion and plantar flexion
      f. The angle and base of gait. Normally, this angle does not exceed 15° from the midline of the body.[175]
      g. Point of heel contact. The position of the calcaneus in either eversion or inversion during heel-strike[140]
      h. The approximate time of pronation. Normally, pronation will occur 15 to 20% into the contact phase of gait.[176,188]
      i. The approximate time of supination. Normally this will occur in the last half of stance.[176,188]
      j. For the foot, the critical periods to identify during gait include:[85]
         i. Contact (heel-strike or rear foot-strike to foot-flat)

ii. Midstance
iii. Lift-off (heel-rise to toe-off)

The patient's gait should be reviewed during both walking and running. Very frequently a foot that looks as though it is one configuration will actually function as the opposite in motion.[9] Videotape or film analysis with slow motion and the use of a treadmill, if available, are invaluable in diagnosing difficult problems.[123] The practical advantage of a treadmill is control of speed.

2. Proprioception and balance
   a. Ankle proprioception. Ankle proprioception should be checked in any patient with an ankle or foot injury. The literature suggests that proprioception is certainly a factor in recurrent ankle sprains.[54,56,57,69,103,171,209] While the patient stands on one foot, the examiner observes any difficulty the patient has maintaining balance. Proprioceptive tests can be made more difficult by having the patient stand on a foam pad or balance board. For more detailed information, assessment of reflex capabilities may be performed by measuring the latency of muscular activation to involuntary perturbation through electromyographic interpretation of firing pattern of those muscles crossing the respective joint.[215] One should also observe for evidence of a positive Trendelenburg sign.
   b. Balance reach tests (see Chapters 10 and 14)

Other useful maneuvers include having the patient squat and bounce, run forward or backward, hop, jump, and change directions quickly.

II. Inspection
A. Skin and nails
   1. If areas of abnormal callosities, redness, or actual skin breakdown are noted, suggesting excessive shear or compression forces, document the size of the involved area to serve as a baseline measurement. This can easily be done by tracing the perimeter of the involved area on a piece of acetate (such as old roentgenographic film).
   2. Excessive dryness or moisture may suggest abnormal vascularity or abnormal sympathetic activity to the part, or both.
   3. Note the site and size of hypertrophic skin changes, such as corns and calluses. These suggest mildly increased shear or compression forces acting during a longer period than those that might produce localized inflammation or actual breakdown. Keep in mind that a painful callus is one in which the underlying tissue is in the process of breaking down.
   4. Diffuse ecchymosis may be associated with common ankle sprains as well as more serious trauma.
   5. Inspect the toenails for splitting, overgrowth, inappropriate trimming, and inflammation of the nail beds.

B. Soft tissue
   1. Swelling (see under palpation)
   2. Wasting of isolated or generalized muscle groups
   3. General contours
C. Bony structure and alignment
   1. Note toe and metatarsal deformities such as claw toes, hammertoes, and varus–valgus deviations.[142]
      a. Claw toes are usually associated with a pes cavus deformity and may accompany certain neurologic disorders. The metatarsophalangeal joints are positioned in extension and the interphalangeal joints in flexion (Fig. 16-33A). Contracture of the long toe extensors causes extension of the toes, which increases the passive tension on the long toe flexors. The intrinsic muscles are overbalanced, both actively and passively, by these muscle groups.
      b. Hammertoes are a result of capsular contracture of the proximal interphalangeal joints (Fig. 16-33B). The involved joint or joints are fixed in some degree of flexion.

         Typically there is hyperextension of the metatarsophalangeal joint and distal interphalangeal joints and flexion of the proximal interphalangeal joint. It is usually only seen in one toe—the second toe, occasionally the third.
      c. Mallet toe is associated with a flexion deformity of the distal interphalangeal joint (Fig. 16-33C). The metatarsophalangeal joint and proximal interphalangeal joints usually are normal. There is usually a callus formation under the tip of the toe or a deformity of the nail.
      d. Tailor's bunions ("bunionette") are caused by irritation and pressure of the fifth metatarsal head. There may be an overlapping fifth toe or quinti varus deformity (often congenital) of the fifth toe (Fig. 16-33D).
      e. A hallux valgus is the most common deformity of the first MTP joint. Pathologically it is a lateral deviation of the proximal phalanx and medial deviation of the first metatarsal bone in relation to the center of the body (Fig. 16-33E). It may be associated with a pronated foot and is found most frequently in older women. The joint surfaces are no longer congruent and some may even go on to subluxation. Note the presence of any bursa over the MTP joint (bunion) and whether active inflammatory changes are present. The toe may be rotated with the toenail pointed inward.
      f. Assess the length of the metatarsals (Fig. 16-34). A line across the metatarsals should form a smooth parabola. The so-called Morton's, Grecian, or atavistic foot is a hereditary type, in which the second toe is longer than the first. With this condition, normal balance is disturbed and weight stress falls toward the inside arch (pronation).[82]

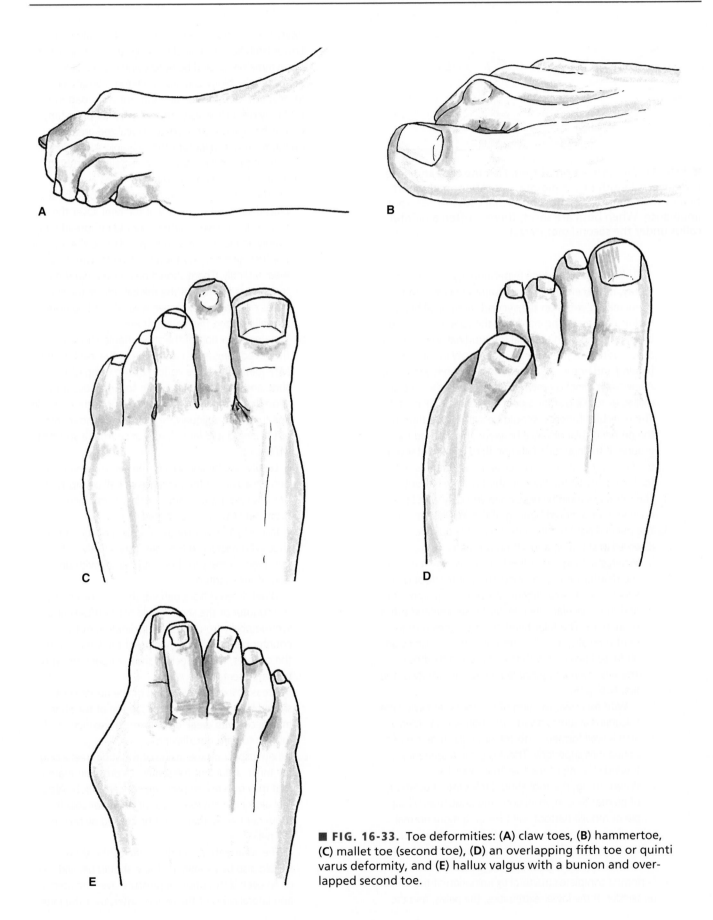

■ **FIG. 16-33.** Toe deformities: **(A)** claw toes, **(B)** hammertoe, **(C)** mallet toe (second toe), **(D)** an overlapping fifth toe or quinti varus deformity, and **(E)** hallux valgus with a bunion and over-lapped second toe.

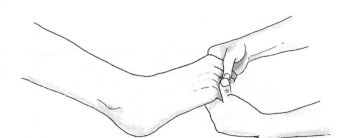

■ **FIG. 16-34.** Inspection of toes. Flex the toes and note the relative length of the metatarsals. Abnormally short first or fifth metatarsals are a potential cause of forefoot imbalance. When both are short, there is often a painful callus under the second metatarsal.

This tends to produce hypermobility of the first ray, displacement of the sesamoid bones, and increased stress on the second metatarsal head.

2. If indicated, assess pronation of the foot, manifested by a flattening of the medial longitudinal arch. The relative position of the navicular tuberosity in the weight-bearing and non–weight-bearing position is examined. A line (Feiss's line) is drawn from the tip of the medial malleolus to the plantar aspect of the first MTP joint.[162] The navicular tubercle should be within one third of the perpendicular distance between this line and the ground. If the navicular falls one third of the distance to the floor, the condition is referred to as first-degree flatfoot; if it rests on the floor, as third-degree flatfoot.

3. The calcanei should be positioned vertically with little or no inward or outward bowing of the Achilles tendon.

4. The general configuration of the foot should be assessed in standing and sitting positions.
   a. When standing, an untwisted foot is one in which the hindfoot is in pronation and the forefoot is in supination. The calcaneus will be in valgus position and the navicular tubercle will be sunken and often prominent. The talar head also becomes prominent medially, and the forefoot often assumes an abducted position with respect to the hindfoot. There is often an associated valgus deformity of the first MTP joint.

      With excessive twisting of the foot (pes cavus) the calcaneus assumes a varus position and the medial arch is well formed, with the navicular tubercle positioned well superiorly. There is often a tendency toward clawing of the toes in a cavus foot.
   b. When sitting, the foot should relax into a position of plantar flexion, inversion, and adduction. A supple or mobile flatfoot will take on a more normal configuration in sitting with the force of weight bearing relieved. A fixed or structural flatfoot will maintain its planus (untwisted) state.

5. Perform a complete structural examination of the remainder of the lower extremities, the pelvis, and the lower back, as discussed in Chapter 24, Lumbosacral–Lower Limb Scan Examination. Any structural deviations or asymmetries should be noted, and the possible effects on the biomechanics of the foot considered.

6. Inspect the shoes, inside and out, for wear patterns that may offer clues as to the presence of persistent biomechanical disturbances and localized areas of pressure. Also inspect for other possible sources of pain arising from the shoe, such as nails protruding through the insole and prominent seams.
   a. On the outer sole, the wear pattern should be displaced somewhat laterally at the heel. Over the front sole, the wear pattern should be spread fairly evenly across the area corresponding to the level of the first, second, and third MTP joints, with less wear laterally. There should be an even wear pattern across the rest of the medial side of the sole. Areas of localized excessive wear should be noted as well as abnormal wear patterns.
   b. The upper portion of the shoe should show a gently curved transverse crease line at the level of the MTP joints. Excessive curling of the vamp of the shoe and the front part of the sole may occur in a shoe that is too long, too narrow, or both. A crease line that runs obliquely, from forward and medial to backward and lateral, may arise from a stiff first MTP joint.

      Localized prominences of the vamp commonly occur medially in the presence of hallux valgus or dorsally with hammertoes or claw toes. Such prominences should be noted.

      Inspect for excessive overhanging of the upper shoe with respect to the sole. This is likely to be observed medially in shoes of patients with pronation of the hindfoot.

      When viewed from behind, the cup formed by the counter of the shoe should rise vertically and symmetrically from the sole. Inclination of the counter medially, with bulging of the lateral lip of the counter, will be seen in shoes of patients with pronated feet.

      Areas of excessive scuffing of the upper shoe should be noted. Scuffing of the toe of the shoe may occur with weak dorsiflexors or restriction of motion toward dorsiflexion.
   c. When inspecting the inside of the shoe, feel along the inner surface of the seams for prominent areas that may give rise to pressure concentration. Also feel along the entire surface of the inner sole for prominent areas that might be caused by protruding nails.

      The wear pattern on the inside of the shoe should also be examined. There should be evidence of an even distribution of pressure over the medial and lateral sides of the heel counter, over the inner sole at the heel, and over the inner sole at the metatarsal heads.

III. Joint Tests. Joint tests include integrity tests, active and passive physiologic movements of the foot and ankle, and joint-play (accessory) movements.

    A. Joint integrity tests

        1. Anterior drawer test. This test may be performed by using posterior glide accessory movement of the tibia on the talus as described in the joint mobilization section (see Fig. 16-50). An alternative anterior drawer test may be performed in prone (Fig. 16-35). While assuring stabilization of the distal tibia and fibula, the examiner applies an anterior force to the calcaneus and talus, to test the integrity of the medial and lateral ligaments. A positive sign is indicated by excessive anterior movement and a "sucking in" of the skin on both signs of the Achilles tendon.[75,113,125] This test should be performed bilaterally for comparison.

        2. Talar tilt.[105,113,125,144,166] These tests, valgus and varus tilt, (see Figs 16-53 and 16-54) may also be performed in prone or sidelying. The examiner first places the foot in the anatomic position (neutral plantar and dorsiflexion). The talus is then moved into abduction (valgus tilt) and adduction (varus tilt). Abduction stresses the deltoid ligament. Adduction tests the calcaneofibular ligament, and to some degree, the anterior talofibular by increasing the stress on the ligament by performing

this test in a more plantar flexed position.[113] These tests should be performed bilaterally for comparison.

    B. Active movements (functional movements)

        1. Barefoot walking

          a. Observe gait

          b. On toes. If unable to do so, determine whether it is because of pain, weakness, or restriction of motion. The heel should invert and the arch should rise.

          c. On heels. If unable to do so, determine whether it is because of pain, weakness, or restriction of motion.

        2. Standing with feet fixed

          a. Externally rotate the leg with respect to the foot. This should cause some varus deviation of the heels and raising of the arches. Compare one foot to the other.

          b. Internally rotate the legs on the feet. This should result in some valgus deviation of the heels and flattening of the arches. Compare one foot with the other.

        3. Standing, keeping knees extended

          a. Evert the feet by standing on medial borders of feet.

          b. Invert the feet by standing on lateral borders of feet.

        4. Assess active physiologic movements with passive overpressure. Sitting, with legs hanging freely. Compare range of motion of one foot to the other. Establish the patient's symptoms at rest and before the movement, and passively correct any movement deviation to determine the relevance to the patient's symptoms. Note the presence of crepitus, the end feel, and any capsular patterns of restriction (see Appendix).

          a. Dorsiflexion

          b. Plantar flexion

          c. Inversion

          d. Eversion

          e. Toe movements

            Numerous differentiation tests can be performed. Compression or distraction can be added. Movements can be sustained, or combined for further information.

    C. Passive physiologic movements

        1. Standing, before measurements are taken, determine the dynamic angle and base of walking using the patient's own line of progression as a reference.[141] A paper walkway (approximately 20 to 24 feet long) on which the patient's footprints can be recorded (after walking in a normal fashion) is most convenient.[11,141,189] Using the line of progression as a reference, select one left and one right footprint from the middle of the progression to use to construct a paper template of the footprints adjacent to each other. The dynamic foot angle and the distance between the middle of each heel are maintained (Fig. 16-36).

          Note: The paper walkway recording can be used for additional data collection such as stride length, velocity, and cadence in the gait analysis.

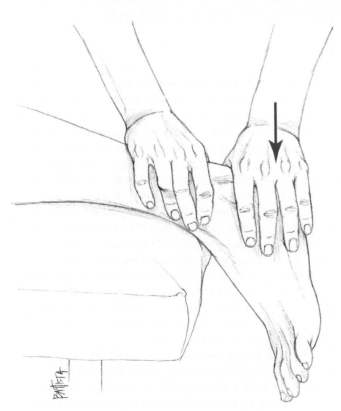

■ **FIG. 16-35.** Prone anterior drawer test.

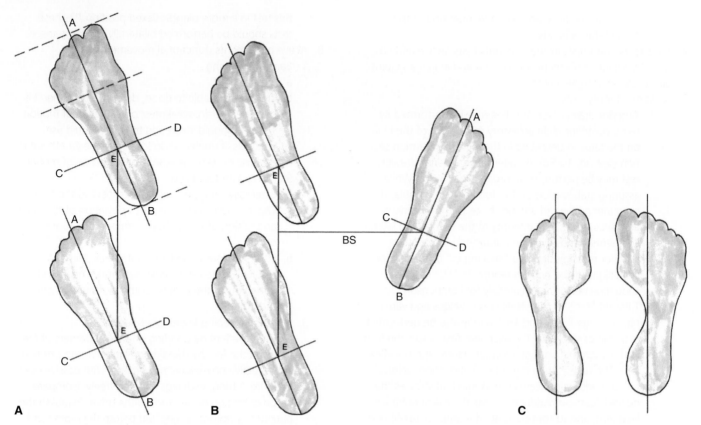

■ **FIG. 16-36.** **(A)** Computation of foot angle (AB, longitudinal line bisecting each foot; CD, horizontal line through posterior third of foot perpendicular to line AB; EE, connecting line of intersections of CD and AB of two ipsilateral feet [line of progression]; resulting angle is foot angle). **(B)** Computation of the base of support (BS, line drawn from intersection of CD and AB of contralateral foot perpendicular to line EE). **(C)** Computation of dynamic angle and base of walking template.

2. Measurement of subtalar joint in relaxed standing
   a. With a felt-tipped marking pen, bisect the middle one third of the posterior calcaneus.[175] Extend the bisection line plantarly to the base of the supporting surface and from the middle one third of the calcaneus superiorly approximately 1 inch; the point of bifurcation is located at the junction of the proximal and middle one third of the bisected calcaneus.
   b. Next, bisect the distal one third of the lower limb just proximal to the malleoli. Extension of this line superiorly should bisect the knee joint within the popliteal space. Calipers may be used to determine the center of the most proximal point of the lower one third of the leg and at the level of the malleoli. With a felt-tipped marking pen, these two points are then connected to form the bisector of the lower one third of the leg.
   c. Measure the neutral calcaneus stance (a relaxed foot with the subtalar joint allowed to pronate; Fig. 16-37).
      i. Have the patient stand in a normal angle and base of gait (see B, 1, above) and facing away

from the examiner.[175] Using a goniometer or protractor, place the straight arm along the supporting surface (transverse plane). The center point of the goniometer or protractor is placed at the apex point of the angle created by the calcaneal bisection and the supporting surface (frontal plane). Rearfoot valgus is then measured to the nearest degree.
      ii. The normal weight-bearing foot should demonstrate a mild amount of pronation but should still allow for additional pronation.[12] If the patient is bearing weight or walking with the foot out of neutral position and near full pronation, an obligatory internal tibial rotation occurs and is prolonged, resulting in an increased force that is absorbed by the soft tissues of the knee.[93,94]
3. Measurement of tibia varum
   a. Measure the tibia varum (tibiofibular varum), if indicated. If a lateral angulation of the tibia-to-floor angle is 10° or greater, the extremity requires an excessive amount of subtalar joint pronation to produce a plantigrade foot (Fig. 16-38).

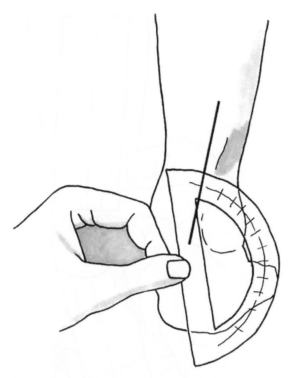

■ **FIG. 16-37.** Measurement of neutral calcaneal stance (a relaxed foot with subtalar joint allowed to pronate).

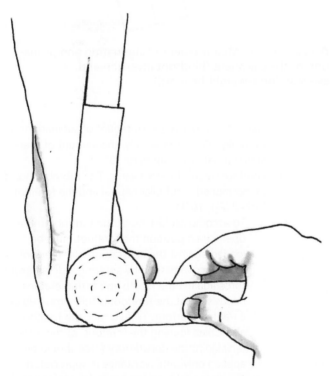

■ **FIG. 16-38.** Measurement of tibia varum in the resting calcaneal stance position.

i. Have the client stand in a normal angle and base of gait. With the feet in a resting calcaneal stance position, recheck the bisections of the calcaneus and lower leg. When the bisections are acceptable, measure the frontal plane relationship of the tibia to the transverse plane (or level ground). If a gravity goniometer is used, the angle between the bisection of the leg and vertical is read on the face of the goniometer. Tibia varum is present when the distal end of the bisecting line of the leg is closer to the midsagittal plane than the proximal end. Tibia valgum is present if the leg is angulated in the opposite direction.

Note: Tibia varum (tibiofibular varum) measurements can also be performed with the foot positioned in subtalar neutral by palpating for talar congruency as the patient rotates the trunk to the left and right, allowing the tibia to externally and internally rotate, thus supinating and pronating the subtalar joint. Once subtalar neutral is reached, the subject is then asked to maintain this position while measurements are recorded. According to McPoil and coworkers,[141] the best patient position for clinical measurement of tibiofibular varum is the neutral calcaneal stance position. It would appear that the measurement of true tibia varum cannot be done without obtaining roentgenograms of the lower extremities taken during weight bearing.[141]

4. Measurement of great toe extension
   a. Measurement of great toe extension can be made while the person is standing. The great toe is extended actively and assisted passively without dorsiflexing the first ray. Forty-five degrees has been found to be adequate for general ambulation.[130]
   b. Great toe extension test. Passive extension of the great toe at the MTP joint in the normal weight-bearing foot has two effects: elevation of the medial longitudinal arch (windlass effect) and lateral rotation of the tibia. The test is normal when both effects are seen (Fig. 16-39).[178]
5. Passive range of motion. The patient sits with legs hanging freely. Compare range of motion of one foot with the other. Note the presence of pain or crepitus. Note abnormalities or asymmetries in range of motion. Note the presence of pathologic end feels. Comparison of the response of symptoms with the active and passive movements can help to determine whether the structure at fault is noncontractile or contractile.[31]
   a. Hindfoot
      i. Plantar flexion
      ii. Inversion
      iii. Eversion

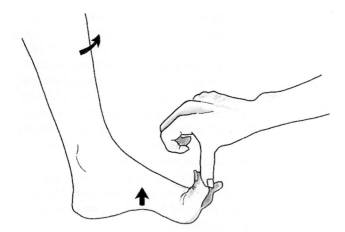

■ **FIG. 16-39.** Great toe extension test.

    b. Transverse tarsal
       i. Plantar flexion
       ii. Pronation (eversion)
      iii. Supination (inversion)
      iv. Abduction
       v. Adduction
6. Supine
  a. Hip flexion–extension
  b. Knee flexion–extension
  c. First ray: position and mobility
     i. Place the foot in a neutral subtalar position (Fig. 16-28). Load the forefoot (see 7, c, i, below). While maintaining the foot in neutral position, grasp the metatarsal heads (between the thumb and forefinger) with the loading hand. Grasp the first metatarsal head with the other hand.
     ii. Assess the position of the first metatarsal head in relationship to its neutral position and assess the end-range position of the first metatarsal head in relationship to the second metatarsal head.[176]
    iii. While maintaining the foot in neutral subtalar position, manually plantar flex and dorsiflex the first ray. Assess the motion of the first ray in relationship to its neutral position.
    iv. Limited range may result from a combination of biomechanical factors such as excessive pronation or a short tendon or from restriction of the joint proper.[58]
7. Prone, with the feet over the edge of the table
  a. Hip internal and external rotation with the knees flexed to 90°
  b. Supination and pronation of the calcaneus. The amount of supination and pronation that is available can be measured by lining up the longitudinal axis of the lower limb and vertical axis of the calcaneus (Fig. 16-40).[93,176] Passive movement of the

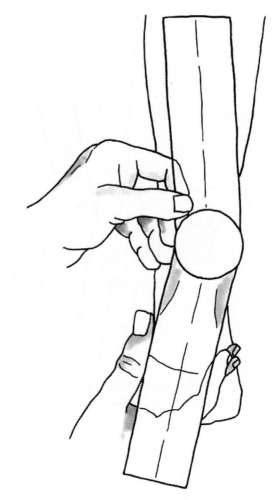

■ **FIG. 16-40.** Measurement of supination and pronation of the calcaneus (hindfoot inversion and eversion [non–weight bearing]).

calcaneus into inversion (amount of supination) is normally 20°.[176] Conversely, the amount of eversion (pronation) is normally 10°.[176]
  c. Forefoot valgus–forefoot varus. The subtalar should be positioned in subtalar neutral and the forefoot locked (Fig. 16-41).
    i. To accomplish locking of the forefoot in the open-chain position the forefoot must be loaded against the neutral subtalar rearfoot. This is accomplished by applying a dorsiflexory force against the fourth and fifth metatarsal heads so that the forefoot is fully pronated on a neutral rearfoot. To fully lock the forefoot, also called loading the forefoot, at the mid-tarsal joint the dorsiflexory force should be applied only until resistance is appreciated. The relationship of the neutral subtalar position and a fully pronated forefoot against the rearfoot results in the neutral position of the foot in the open-chain position. It is not neces-

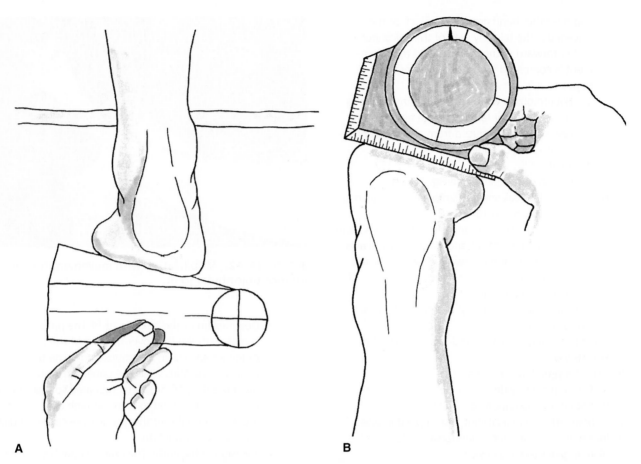

■ **FIG. 16-41.** Measurement of forefoot valgus or varus (non–weight bearing) with goniometer (**A**) or inclinometer (**B**).

sary to dorsiflex the foot to 90° or lift the leg from the supporting surface. Slightly adduct the forefoot to ensure complete midtarsal joint pronation.

ii. Place one arm of the goniometer along the posterior calcaneal bisection and the other arm along the plantar aspect of the heel (Fig. 16-41A). Align the latter arm with the plane of the forefoot (an imaginary line from the head of the fifth metatarsal to the head of the first) and read the degrees of forefoot deviation. An inclinometer may also be used with the knee in 90° of flexion (Fig. 16-41B). Deviation from a normal perpendicular relationship with a line bisecting the calcaneus represents a difference between alignment of forefoot to hindfoot.

iii. Forefoot valgus is commonly found in the varus foot. Forefoot varus may require increased pronation to adequately contact the surface while running or walking.[94,204]

iv. The calcaneal position, varus or valgus, can also be determined at this time.

d. Dorsiflexion

i. Position the patient prone with his or her foot over the edge of the table. Place a 4-inch roll underneath the distal anterior thigh to ensure full knee extension. Place the foot into subtalar neutral. While maintaining subtalar neutral, manually assist dorsiflexion of the foot on the leg while the patient actively dorsiflexes the foot to its end range.

ii. Repeat with the knee flexed to 90°.

iii. Dorsiflexion is measured to the nearest degree.
   Note: The subtalar joint must be maintained in a neutral position during these motions. Pressure applied to the first ray will help prevent pronation.[143]

D. Joint-play movements. Assess for hypermobility or hypomobility and presence or absence of pain.

1. Distal tibiofibular joint, anteroposterior glide (see Fig. 16-48)

2. Ankle mortise (talocrural) joint
   a. Distraction of talus (see Fig. 16-49)
   b. Anterior and posterior glide of talus. Anterior glide is an important test for integrity of the anterior talofibular ligament. The patient is supine. Place one hand over the dorsum of the distal tibia and

cup the other hand around the back of the calcaneus. The talus by way of the calcaneus is pulled forward in the mortise, and the movement is compared with the movement on the opposite side.

i. Hypermobility will be present in the case of a chronic anterior talofibular ligament rupture.

ii. Pain will be reproduced from a talofibular ligament sprain or adhesion.

3. Subtalar joint

a. Distraction of calcaneus (see Fig. 16-52)

b. Dorsal rock of calcaneus, plantar rock of calcaneus (see Figs. 16-55 and 16-56)

c. Varus–valgus tilts of calcaneus (see Figs. 16-53 and 16-54). The range of calcaneal inversion and eversion is assessed, and the two feet are compared. Capsular restriction will result in a greater loss of inversion than eversion.

4. Transverse tarsal joint, dorsal-plantar glides (see Fig. 16-57)

5. Naviculocuneiform joint, dorsal-plantar glides (see Fig. 16-58)

6. Cuneiform-metatarsal joints

a. Dorsal-plantar glides

b. Pronation–supination (see Fig. 16-59)

7. Cuboid–fifth metatarsal joint, dorsal-plantar glides

8. Intermetatarsal and tarsometatarsal joints, dorsal-plantar glides (see Fig. 16-61)

9. Metatarsophalangeal and interphalangeal joints

a. Dorsal-plantar glides (see Fig. 16-63)

b. Internal–external rotations

c. Medial–lateral tilts

d. Distraction (see Fig. 16-62)

E. Mobilization with movement (MWMs).[53,150,151] These examination tests can be used as treatment techniques, but details of the these and other techniques for the foot and ankle are outside the scope of this text. It is proposed that MWMs affect and correct bony positional faults, which produce abnormal tracking of the articular surfaces during movement.

1. Inferior tibiofibular joint. The examiner applies an anteroposterior glide to the fibula (Fig. 16-42) as the patient actively inverts the foot. Increases in range and no pain or reduced pain are positive findings indicating a mechanical joint problem.[150,151,166] When you glide the fibula, as a test or treatment, do so more or less along the line of the ligament. When used as a treatment technique it has been found to be most effective in repositioning the fibula after an inversion sprain.

2. Plantarflexion of the ankle joint. The knee is positioned in flexion with the heel resting on the table. The examiner with one hand applies an anteroposterior glide to the tibia and with the other hand rolls the talus anteriorly as the patient actively plantarflexes the ankle (Fig. 16-43).

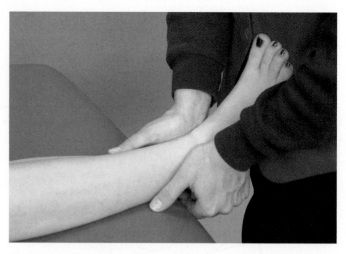

■ **FIG. 16-42.** Mobilization with movement for the inferior tibiofibular joint.

3. Dorsiflexion of the ankle joint.[166] The patient lies supine with the foot over the end of the table. The examiner applies an anteroposterior glide to the calcaneus and the talus while the patient actively dorsiflexes the ankle (Fig. 16-44). After repeated contractions the patient is then asked to relax, and the examiner moves the ankle into the further range of dorsiflexion gained during the contraction.

4. Inversion of the ankle. The examiner applies a sustained anteroposterior glide to the base of the first metatarsal and a posteroanterior glide on the base of the second metatarsal while the patient actively inverts the foot (Fig. 16-45). This test is carried out on patients with pain over the medial border of the foot on inversion owing to a positional fault of the first MTP joint.[166] Increases in range and no pain or reduced pain after the test are positive examination findings indicating a mechanical joint problem.

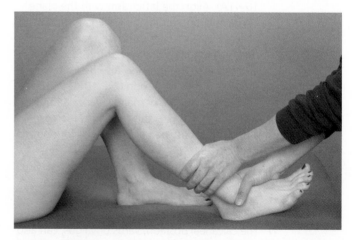

■ **FIG. 16-43.** Mobilization with movement for ankle plantar flexion.

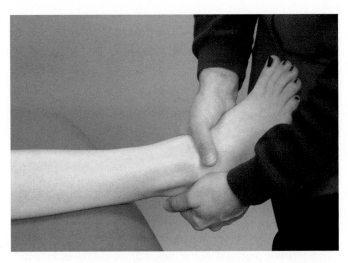

■ **FIG. 16-44.** Mobilization with movement for ankle dorsiflexion.

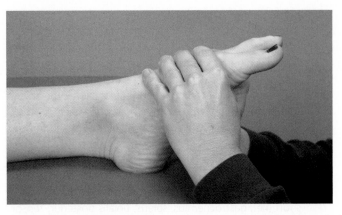

■ **FIG. 16-46.** Mobilization with movement for metatarsophalangeal joint.

5. MTP joints (anterior metatarsalgia). This test is carried out if the patient has pain under the transverse arch of the foot owing to a positional fault of the metatarsal head. The patient actively flexes the toes while the examiner applies a sustained anteroposterior glide to the head of the affected metatarsal (Fig. 16-46). Reduced pain and an increase in range are positive examination findings indicating a mechanical joint problem.

F. Other joints may need to be examined to prove or disprove their relevance to the patient's condition. The most likely joints suspected to be a source of the symptoms are the knee joint, hip joint, sacroiliac joint, and lumbar spine. Relevant clearing tests can be used.

IV. Muscle Tests. The muscle tests include resistive isometric muscle testing, muscle strength, functional muscle strength, muscle length, muscle bulk, and specific diagnostic tests (if indicated).

A. Resistive isometric muscle testing. Resisted isometrics are done in the supine or sitting position. Resisted isometric knee flexion should be included because of the triceps surae action on the knee. With the patient's foot placed in the anatomic position, the movements tested are as follows.

1. Dorsiflexion. Pain may be caused by a tendinitis. Painless weakness associated with a footdrop may be the result of a lesion of the lateral popliteal or the L5 nerve root. Painful resisted dorsiflexion and inversion occur in tendinitis of the anterior tibialis.

2. Plantar flexion. Test in weight bearing. Pain may be caused by a lesion of the Achilles tendon or a tear in the gastrocnemius. A painless weakness may be related to S1 nerve root pressure.

3. Inversion. A painful weakness of inversion is usually caused by tenosynovitis or tendinitis of the posterior tibialis muscle. Painless weakness may be related to a tendon rupture or L4 nerve root compression.

4. Extension of the great toe. A painful weakness occurs with tenosynovitis of the extensor hallucis longus muscle. Painless weakness may indicate an L5 nerve root compression.

5. Toe extension. A painful weakness may indicate a tenosynovitis of the extensor digitorum longus; painless weakness occurs in an L5 nerve root lesion.

B. Muscle strength. The examiner tests the muscle strength of the ankle, foot, and toes. For details of these tests the reader is directed to Clarkston and Gilewish,[23] Cole et al.,[26] Hislop and Montgomery,[81] Kendall et al.,[106] and Palmer and Epler[162] to determine exactly which muscles are at fault. Any other muscle groups influencing the foot and ankle should be included in the muscle tests as well as muscles prone to weakness, i.e., gluteus medius, gluteus maximus, and vastus medialis.[99]

C. Functional muscle strength. Some functional ability has already been tested by the general observation of the patient during active physiologic movements in weight

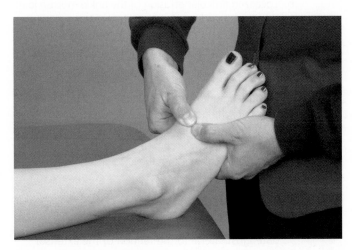

■ **FIG. 16-45.** Mobilization with movement for inversion of the ankle.

bearing during barefoot walking and activities in standing with the feet fixed. Additional tests may include repeated rising up on the toes and lifting the foot and toes in dorsiflexion while standing. These should be performed with the patient standing on one leg, using one hand to maintain balance. A typical criterion for normal function is the ability to perform 10 to 15 repetitions of each movement.[162] The functional strength of the toe flexors may be tested by having the client put a foot on a towel and scrunch it up or by having the patient pick up small objects with their toes.

D. Muscle length. The examiner checks the length of individual muscles, in particular those muscles prone to become short (i.e., gastrocnemius, soleus, tibialis posterior, tensor fascia lata, hamstrings, piriformis, and iliopsoas).[99] Limitation in dorsiflexion as a result of shortening of the gastrocnemius, plantaris, and soleus is not uncommon. The posterior joint capsular structures may also show tightness, along with the soleus muscle.[162]

E. Muscle bulk. Measure the circumference of the muscle bulk of the calf 15 cm below the apex of the patella or joint line. The examiner must also note, if possible, whether swelling or muscle bulk is being measured and remember that there is no correlation between muscle bulk and strength.

F. Diagnostic test. Thompson's test[207] for rupture of the tendocalcaneus should be performed in suspected Achilles tendon rupture. With the patient in prone, and the knee flexed to 90°, the examiner squeezes the calf of the leg being tested and observes the response. The absence of ankle plantarflexion indicates a positive test, suggesting rupture of the Achilles tendon.

V. Neuromuscular Testing. Neurologic tests involve the integrity and mobility of the nervous system.

A. Integrity of the nervous system. The integrity of the nervous system is tested if the examiner suspects the symptoms are coming from the spine or from a peripheral nerve. A knowledge of the cutaneous distribution of nerve roots (dermatomes) and peripheral nerves enables the examiner to distinguish the sensory loss as a result of a root lesion from that caused by a peripheral nerve lesion. The cutaneous and dermatome areas are shown in Tables 5-7 and 5-8 and Figures 5-5 and 5-8. Myotomes are tested for L2–L5, and S1 and S2 (see Fig. 5-10). A working knowledge of the muscular distribution of the nerve roots (myotomes) and peripheral nerves enables the clinician to distinguish the motor loss as a result of nerve root and peripheral nerve lesions. The peripheral nerves are shown in Figure 5-8.

B. Reflex testing. Check the patellar (L3–L4; see Fig. 14-23) and medial hamstring (L5), and ankle joint (S1) reflexes (see Fig. 14-23B)

C. Mobility of the nervous system. Neural tension tests may be carried out to ascertain the degree to which neural tissue is responsible for the patient's symptoms. The impor-

tant tests for the foot, ankle, and lower leg include the straight-leg raise (SLR), prone knee bend (PKB), and slump test (see Chapter 22, Lumbar Spine).

VI. Palpation

A. Skin

1. Moisture or dryness. Abnormal moisture, usually associated with pain and joint restriction, may accompany a reflex sympathetic dystrophy. Vascular disorders may also cause changes in the moisture or texture of the skin.

2. Texture

3. Mobility. Skin mobility may be restricted after prolonged immobilization, especially after a surgical procedure.

4. Temperature. Inflammatory lesions will often result in increased skin temperature over the site of the lesion. Fairly precise documentation of the degree of inflammation may be made by using a thermistor probe. This often offers a convenient guide as to the effect of treatment procedures on the state of the lesion as well as a guide to the state of the inflammatory process in general. For example, a baseline reading can be documented and measurements taken before and after each treatment session (these must be taken over precisely the same point and at the same time of day). A slight elevation of, say, 1°C can be expected after any treatment that imposes some mechanical stress, such as mobilization, massage, or exercise. However, it is important that the elevation does not persist for more than a few hours. If so, the treatment program may be too vigorous. If some decline in temperature is noted, it may be a sign that resolution is taking place. Thermistor readings, as with most tests, are significant when compared with a normal side.

B. Soft tissue

1. Swelling

a. Localized extra-articular swelling may accompany ankle sprains, usually involving the lateral aspect of the ankle below the lateral malleolus.

b. Localized articular effusion of the ankle mortise joint manifests as a loss of definition over the malleolar regions. Subtle joint effusion can be detected by applying firm pressure with the thumb and index fingers over the regions below the medial and lateral malleoli simultaneously. This will force the fluid into the anterior capsular region and cause a fullness over the dorsum of the ankle.

c. Generalized edema of the foot may follow major trauma, or it may accompany systemic, more generalized vascular or metabolic disorders.

2. Mobility

3. Consistency

4. Pulses

a. The pulse of the dorsalis pedis artery may be palpated just lateral to the tendon of the extensor hallucis longus over the dorsum of the foot.

b. The pulse of the posterior tibial artery is palpated behind the tendons of the flexor digitorum longus and flexor hallucis longus posterosuperior to the medial malleolus.
5. Other specific tendons, ligaments, and muscles should be palpated, as indicated by findings up to this point in the examination. A guide to palpation of these structures is included in the section on surface anatomy in this chapter.
C. Bony structures and tendon and ligament attachments
  1. Palpate joint margins to assess structural alignment and to note any hypertrophic changes.
  2. Palpate tendon and ligament attachments as indicated in the section on surface anatomy.

COMMON LESIONS AND THEIR MANAGEMENT

Probably the most common lower limb problem in amateur and professional athletics is that of overuse syndromes. The frequency of overuse injuries ensures that they will be a significant portion of the practice of the sports medicine clinic and the general orthopaedic clinic. Overuse injuries affect different anatomic sites and tissues and are usually secondary to training errors and accumulated microtrauma. In the lower leg group, specific syndromes include tibial stress syndrome, Achilles tendinitis, tibial stress fractures, compartment syndromes, and plantar fasciitis.

The common disorders affecting the foot are in the majority of cases the result of some biomechanical disturbance. As indicated in the preceding section, such biomechanical disorders may be of local origin, or the primary problem may involve one of the other weight-bearing segments. For this reason, evaluation of chronic, subtle foot disorders requires that structural and functional assessments of the other weight-bearing joints be made. Similarly, evaluation of patients with problems in these other regions may necessitate examination of the foot. In understanding the rationale of the evaluative and treatment procedures related to foot disorders, it is essential that the practitioner have a basic knowledge of the biomechanics of the foot and how they relate to the biomechanics of the other weight-bearing joints.

Because the numerous joints of the foot contribute to make it a very mobile structure as a whole, it has the ability to attenuate the energy of forces applied to it. For this reason, traumatic lesions affecting the foot are relatively rare. On the other hand, the common lesions affecting the ankle are usually of traumatic origin.[20] Whereas the individual joints making up the ankle are relatively track-bound or uniaxial, the ankle complex allows some movement in the sagittal, frontal, and transverse planes. However, transverse rotations are of limited range because they do not occur about a true vertical axis. Also, eversion is normally quite restricted because the fibular malleolus extends distally to create an abutment that limits this movement. Forces that move the ankle past its physiologic limits of motion will tend to cause damage, usually to the osseus or ligamentous components of the ankle complex, or to both. Excessive forces to the ankle producing such damage are often the result of forces from the ground acting over the lever-arm provided by the foot or forces of the center of gravity of the body acting over the lever-arm of the lower extremity with the foot fixed. Because of these lever-arms over which forces acting on the ankle may be applied and because certain ankle motions are normally limited, the ankle is often the site of acute traumatic injuries such as sprains and fractures.

Except in situations in which there is malalignment of bony constituents, such as after healing of a fracture, or in situations in which there is marked restriction of movement of one of the ankle joints, such as after arthrodesis of the subtalar joints, degenerative joint disease affecting the ankle is rare. Rheumatoid arthritis often affects the foot but less often the ankle.

Both the foot and ankle may be the site of fatigue disorders. Such disorders result from abnormally high stresses occurring for relatively short periods or from mildly abnormal stresses occurring for a long period. The former situation usually occurs in athletes or others who have undergone an abrupt increase in activity level. In such cases, the degree of microtrauma affecting certain tissues exceeds the rate at which the body is able to repair itself; the result is a fatigue-induced yielding of the involved tissue. Examples are stress fractures, blisters, and many of the tendinitis conditions affecting this region. Milder stresses occurring for longer periods tend to result in tissue hypertrophy that may contribute to certain painful disorders. Typical examples are heel spurs and various callus formations.

Overuse Syndromes of Leg and Foot

The pathophysiology of overuse injuries is a local inflammatory response to stress. The causes of overuse injuries are either intrinsic (malalignment syndromes, muscle imbalances) or extrinsic (training error).[73] A systematic musculoskeletal assessment is necessary to differentiate overuse injuries and to clarify the etiologic factors. Effective treatment is predicated on recognizing and correcting the underlying predisposing, precipitating, or perpetuating etiologic factors.

CHRONIC ANTERIOR LEG PAIN (SHIN SPLINTS)

The term *shin splints* is considered by many to be a catchall phrase applied to a number of different conditions limited to the legs and has generated much confusion.[179,190,193] Shin splints (idiopathic compartment syndrome) is used here to mean an etiologic subset of exercise-induced pain: mechanical inflammation caused by repetitive stress of the broad proximal portion of any of the musculotendinous units originating from the lower part of the leg or tibia during weight bearing.[97,107,190,217] This narrower definition is consistent with the American Medical Association's terminology.[2]

Depending on the affected muscles, shin splints can be anterolateral or posteromedial.[5,107,217] Anterolateral shin splints cause pain and tenderness lateral to the tibia over the anterior compartment and involve the pretibial muscles, including the anterior tibialis, extensor hallucis longus, and extensor digitorum longus. Anterolateral shin splints may occur secondary to heel contact on hard surfaces, or to wearing a shoe with a hard heel, or to biomechanical abnormalities such as forefoot varus.[73,107] A muscle imbalance between a weak pretibial muscle group and tight gastrocnemius–soleus muscles may result in overactivation of these muscles during heel-strike and swing phase.

Posteromedial shin splints cause symptoms along the posteromedial border of the middle to lower tibia over the posterior compartment, which is appreciated more during toe-off.[156] Research has shown a strong positive correlation between excessive pronation and posteromedial shin splints.[212]

In anterolateral and posteromedial shin splints, there is typically weakness of the affected muscles and pain reproduced by resisted active motion.[156] The condition may present as an acute myositis or strain of the posterior or anterior tibialis or peroneal muscles or as a chronic overuse condition termed *medial stress syndrome*.[120] This is the currently accepted term for shin splints.[196]

MEDIAL TIBIAL STRESS SYNDROME

Medial tibial stress syndrome (MTSS) or tibial periostitis presents as exercise-induced pain localized to the distal posteromedial border of the tibia. According to Walker,[217] the clinical distinction between posteromedial shin splints and MTSS is hazy, but the latter is usually more focal and more painful. The precise pathophysiology of MTSS is controversial, but it is most likely periosteal inflammation (periostitis) near the origin of the posterior tibialis or the medial soleus.[149] The soleus muscle syndrome has been identified as a cause of posteromedial shin splints through cadaver electromyography and open-biopsy analysis by Michael and Holder.[146] The differential diagnosis includes posterior tibial tendinitis (see below), anterior tibial tendonitis, exertional (chronic) compartment syndrome, and tibial stress microfractures.[177]

POSTERIOR TIBIAL TENDINITIS

Posterior tibial tendinitis is usually caused by overuse, which occurs frequently in a valgus deformity at the subtalar joint. Other etiologic factors include change in running terrain, poor flexibility, poor foot wear, and alignment abnormalities.[196] The tibialis posterior works in conjunction with the flexor hallucis longus and flexor digitorum as the dynamic stabilizer of the longitudinal arch together with the static restraints, spring ligament, and the deep plantar ligaments.[86] As a dynamic stabilizer, the posterior tibial muscle and tendon are especially important in foot-strike and stance. In these functions, they are continually being placed under tensile load and are commonly injured.[108]

With tibialis posterior irritation, the patient reports discomfort along the medial border of the tibia. There may be crepitus, swelling, or nodularity along the tendon. Palpation reveals tenderness along the middle and distal thirds of the tibia. Manual muscle testing of plantar flexion and inversion may elicit a report of pain or weakness. The evaluation should also include looking for possible hyperpronation.

The management program should focus on controlling inflammation, friction massage to the muscle or tendon (see Box 8-2), stretching and active range of motion to assist collagen production and remodeling, improving flexibility of the heel cord and the first MTP joint, joint mobilization as indicated to restore normal foot and ankle mobility, strength training of the calf muscles, and reducing excessive pronatory forces (possibly with different shoes or orthotics).[86,196] Loading should be done in eccentric fashion, with the heel in neutral. Progressive closed-chain activities work best.[109] Power and agility should be restored by short-duration, high-intensity exercises. Foot abnormalities and training errors should be addressed.

STRESS FRACTURE OF TIBIA

Stress fractures of the lower limbs account for 95% of all stress fractures in athletes.[159] About one half occur in the tibia or fibula. Stress fractures result from fatigue failure within the bone, although the surrounding muscle may actually fatigue first.[217] Increased or different activity results in an altered relationship of bone growth and repair (Wolff's law). The resulting stress fracture may run the spectrum from a microfracture with simple cortical hypertrophy to rupture of bony cortices with a fracture line.[133]

The factors that seem to be most clearly associated with the development of stress fractures are repetitiveness of activity and muscle forces acting across the bone. The muscle forces, or torque, across the bone may stress that bone if an imbalance between antagonistic muscles exists.[38]

Symptoms of stress fracture are usually gradual in onset during a 2- to 3-week period.[133] The patient complains of pain that initially occurs during activity and is relieved by rest. In the next stage the pain continues for hours, perhaps through the night, or it might become worse during the night, which is highly suggestive of bone pain.[183] Swelling may occur particularly after activity.

On clinical examination, localized tenderness with or without swelling is almost always present over the fracture. Common sites are the medial aspect of the tibia and 2 to 3 inches above the tip of the fibular malleolus above the joint line.[107] A positive percussion sign (transmission of pain to the fracture site area on percussion of the bone at a distance) and the tuning fork test may help to add weight to the presumptive diagnosis of stress fracture. The use of ultrasound over a stress fracture often causes rather acute pain 1 to 2 hours after the patient leaves a therapy session. This is believed to be secondary to increased hyperemia of the bone containing the stress fracture.[107]

A stress fracture may not be visible on ordinary x-ray films for 2 to 8 weeks after symptoms commence. Therefore, a technetium-99m diphosphonate bone scan is the gold standard in diagnosing stress fracture.[217] An increased uptake or hot spot on a positive bone scan can be seen within the first few days of the symptoms presenting, and false-positive scans are infrequent.[32,67,133,167] Stress fractures are managed with a period of prolonged rest to allow adequate healing of the fracture, with gradual return to activity. If activity is resumed too early, the fracture will recur or not heal. In some cases, operative fixation is indicated.[196]

CHRONIC EXERTIONAL COMPARTMENT SYNDROME

Exertional compartment syndromes of the leg are another common form of overuse injury. The anterior and deep posterior compartments are the most frequently involved. Chronic exertional compartment syndrome is caused by abnormally high intramuscular pressure during exercise in a closed fibro-osseous space, which causes ischemia of the muscles and nerves. Acute exertional compartment syndrome, which typically involves all four compartments, is extremely rare and needs to be emergently released with fasciotomies. Chronic exertional compartment syndrome, in stark contrast to acute exertional compartment syndrome, is not an emergency situation. An exertional compartment syndrome is usually associated with sports participation such as running and weight-lifting.[196]

The diagnosis of chronic compartment syndrome can be made with the history, physical examination, and pressure measurements before, during, and after exercise. Patients typically complain of a gradual onset of pain with exercise; the pain eventually reaches a level that precludes further exercise. Most agree that resting pressures greater than 15 mm Hg, pressures greater than 30 mm Hg during exercise, or a failure of pressures to decrease to less than 20 mm Hg 5 minutes after exercise are all very suggestive of exertional compartment syndrome.[177] Differential diagnosis includes MTSS, stress fractures, peripheral vascular disease (in older people), and popliteal artery entrapment.

Conservative rehabilitation differs little from rehabilitation of other overuse injuries. Emphasis is placed on soft tissue manipulations of the affected compartments, stretching inflexible muscles, eliminating training errors, and correcting biomechanical faults to reduce load on the muscles. Activity modification is key if the patient wishes to avoid surgery. It is generally suggested that the patient should exercise until pain is reached, then stop and rest approximately 10 minutes, then resume exercise.[120] If the pain is severe, the exercise should stop completely and ice should be applied with the leg elevated. Substitution activities such as cycling and swimming or deep-water running should be used to maintain aerobic conditioning when the patient is unable to train symptom-free.

ACHILLES TENDINITIS

Achilles tendinitis is the most common form of overuse tendinitis seen in athletes.[50,79,115] Because the Achilles tendon does not have a synovial sheath, this condition cannot be considered to be tenosynovitis. Inflammation, resulting from stress, often occurs in the loose connective tissue about the tendon known as the *paratenon.* Classification is based on whether this tissue, or the tendon itself, is involved.[182] The Achilles tendon possesses a zone of avascularity, which is the most common site of tendon microtrauma or rupture. Located 2 to 6 cm above the tendon insertion, this avascular zone also is an area in which the collagen fibers of the tendon rotate and are more prone to overuse and injury.[24]

Causes of Achilles tendinitis include overuse, excessive forced dorsiflexion (causing an eccentric contraction), an inflexible gastrocnemius–soleus complex, and hyperpronation.[24] Training errors, poor flexibility, and weakness of the Achilles tendon have also been implicated as predisposing factors in Achilles tendinitis.[73] Seen more often in men than women, Achilles tendinitis, with or without peritendinitis (involving the paratenon) is often associated with repetitive or high-impact sports such as running, basketball, or volleyball.[24] When overuse is a contributing factor, there will be a characteristic history of gradual onset of pain that may be accentuated by excessive pronation or supination.[201]

The pain may also be associated with underlying hyperostosis of the posterior surface of the calcaneus (Haglund's deformity or "pump bump") or inflammation of the infratendinous or supratendinous bursa.[115, 201] Bursitis alone may be present and should be included in the differential diagnosis for posterior heel and ankle pain. One should also consider in the differential diagnosis os trigonum problems.[201]

As with other overuse injuries, pain is aggravated by activity and relieved by rest. Evaluation of an inflamed Achilles tendon may reveal swelling, point tenderness, and discomfort with passive dorsiflexion or active plantar flexion. The patient presents with pain several centimeters proximal to the insertion of the tendon into the calcaneus, the area of poorest blood supply.[115] A presentation of considerable swelling and lumpiness of the Achilles tendon usually points to intratendinous damage. When there are superficial, isolated areas of pain and crepitation that are palpable, one may be sure of the diagnosis of paratenonitis. Dorsiflexion causes pain, and crepitus may be felt along the tendon at the most tender area.[115] If there is pain on excessive plantar flexion, especially with palpation at the lateral posterior aspect of the ankle, an os trigonum injury should be suspected.[201] A thorough examination should be conducted to identify any ankle, hindfoot, or forefoot abnormalities.

Treatment follows similar lines as that of other overuse injuries. The treatment should address any abnormal alignment in the foot or ankle while pursuing anti-inflammatory management. Short-term use of a heel lift may reduce tensile loading while allowing therapy.

Chronic paratenon lesions that do not respond to appropriate physical therapy, rest, and other adjunct measures will require a surgical tenolysis. Tendinosis or intratendinous lesions may require surgical exploration. Necrotic tissue is curetted and the tendon is repaired.[201] Rupture of the Achilles tendon requires immediate referral for consideration of a surgical repair. Rehabilitation concerns for the operative or nonoperative cases are the same—improvement in flexibility and normalization of muscle strength. Soft tissue techniques, including friction to the tendon (see Box 8-2), the surgical scar, and tendon repair, and myofascial techniques to the gastrocnemius and soleus muscle bellies are beneficial as well as joint mobilization (i.e., talocrural dorsiflexion, plantar flexion, and rearfoot and midfoot inversion–eversion). Concentric and eccentric loading in single and then multiple planes will encourage normal gastrocnemius and soleus function. Wobble board and slide board exercises are used to stimulate proprioception and neuromuscular control.

PLANTAR FASCIITIS (SUBCALCANEAL PAIN SYNDROME)

Plantar fasciitis is an inflammation of the plantar fascia and the perifascial structures. Chronic stress to the origin of this fascia on the calcaneus may cause calcium to deposit, forming a spur (plantar calcaneal spurs). Because plantar calcaneal spurs and plantar fasciitis involve basically the same symptoms, develop via similar mechanisms, and are treated in the same manner, these common disorders are often considered together. Frequently, heel spurs are not symptomatic. This has been shown to be the case with the discovery of calcaneal spurs on x-ray studies of nonsymptomatic heels. Roentgenograms may show big spurs without plantar fasciitis or no spurs in the patient with severe plantar fasciitis.

As is typical of any overuse injury, plantar fasciitis can be caused by an acute injury (strain) from excessive loading of the foot. More often the mechanical cause is related to chronic irritation from an excessive amount of pronation or prolonged duration of pronation, resulting in microtears at the plantar fascial origin (Fig. 16-22). A cavus or high-arched foot with its limited subtalar excursion is also at risk, because a tight plantar fascia is usually present in this type of foot. A cavus foot may develop plantar fasciitis owing to its intrinsic inability to dissipate force (lack of pronation) from heel-strike to mid stance, resulting in increased load in the plantar fascia.[116]

Plantar fasciitis occurs in patients of either sex, usually older than 40 years of age except in active sportsmen when the patient, usually male, may be in his twenties.[30] It is commonly found in people whose occupation involves prolonged standing or walking. Pain is made worse by activity, such as climbing stairs, walking, or running, may be present at night, and is often present when first getting out of bed in the morning. It tends to be relieved by rest.

Physical Examination. Physical examination should include the entire lower limb to check for hip, knee, and ankle alignment problems that may cause pes planus, pes cavus, or hyperpronation of the foot. Clinical examination usually localizes tenderness at the plantar fascial attachment of the calcaneus, just distal to this attachment, in the medial arch area and in the abductor hallucis muscle. Also, hyperextension of the MTP joints will increase the discomfort, as this tenses the plantar fascia by the windlass mechanism (Fig. 16-29). Pain to palpation of the posterior inferior origin of the abductor hallucis muscle has been theorized to be the result of overuse of the abductor hallucis muscle in its role to aid in producing forefoot supination to decrease loading on the plantar fascia.[22] Chronic partial ruptures have abundant scar tissue, which is palpable near the attachment of the plantar fascia to the plantar tubercle of the calcaneus or more distally, toward the mid aspect of the foot.[201] Range of motion of the great toe is usually limited in dorsiflexion, and ankle dorsiflexion is often less then 90°.[115] Swelling is rare, but occasionally a small granuloma is palpated on the medial fascial origin. With increased pain, the patient changes his or her gait pattern, keeping the foot in a rather supinated or inverted posture from foot-strike through to toe-off to minimize pain.[22]

This injury must be differentiated from tarsal tunnel syndrome and entrapment of the first lateral branch of the posterior tibialis nerve. Those with tarsal tunnel syndrome may also complain of burning pain with paresthesias of the heel. They usually have a positive Tinel sign and do not have pain to direct palpation of the plantar fascia. The cause in younger patients, particularly when the symptoms are bilateral and are unresponsive to the usual conservative treatments, may be seropositive and seronegative collagen vascular disorders (e.g., rheumatoid arthritis, spondylitis, and Reiter's syndrome).[16,65,66,187,211] The older patient with heel pain may have gout or osteomalacia.[161]

Management. When dealing with a mechanical cause, the treatment plan is directed at both a short-term goal (to control inflammation at the insertion of the fascia into the calcaneus in conjunction with relieving undue stress in the plantar fascia itself) and a long-term goal (correction of mechanical factors). Ice massage, rest, and anti-inflammatory medications should be used initially. Ultrasound and phonophoresis with 10% hydrocortisone have been used with limited success to control acute inflammation and pain.[89] A period of non–weight bearing is recommended until symptoms subside. Excessive pronation should be limited by use of low-dye strapping (see below), and if this is beneficial, an in-shoe orthotic device or over-the-counter arch support is recommended. The use of tension night splints has shown promising results. There is also an assortment of heel pads made specifically for heel pain.[210] In the case of a high-arched foot, a carefully selected in-shoe orthotic device with good shock absorbency should be considered.

Treatment of functional or structural leg-length discrepancy may also be indicated. Subcalcaneal pain syndrome is seen more frequently in the shorter leg.[192] A functional short leg may result from running in the same direction on the track on the same tilt of a road. Soft tissue techniques (see Box 8-10) that stretch the plantar fascia and progressive cross-friction massage at the origin of the fascia to break down the scar tissue can improve plantar fascia flexibility and joint mobilizations, which mobilize the hind foot, subtalar joint, and inferior navicular, and are usually the most effective treatment methods.[30,35] Local corticosteroid injections should be used judiciously. Strengthening exercises for the gastrocnemius and arch musculature should be incorporated into the rehabilitation program. Kibler and associates[109] report that lack of ankle dorsiflexion and weak plantar flexors manifests as a functional pronation. Eccentric loading seems to be the major factor as that allows increased velocity of pronation.[108] Closed kinetic chain activities and neuromuscular and proprioceptive control activities are effective for rehabilitation. Hip abduction exercises are very important to maintain proper leg posture. Surgery is rarely indicated.

TREATMENT OF OVERUSE INJURIES

The principles of treatment and rehabilitation of overuse injuries are the same as those related to the management of abnormal foot pronation and supination (see below). Rest of the affected muscle–tendon–bone unit is the mainstay of treatment in phase I. MTSS can progress to stress fracture, and stress fractures may progress to complete cortical break.[133] The duration of rest varies from 1 to 2 days for mild MTSS to several months for severe stress fractures.

In phase I, analogous to treatment of traumatic injuries (see management of ankle sprains below) compression, and elevation are used to reduce swelling and inflammation. Nonsteroidal anti-inflammatory drugs (NSAIDs) are believed to be beneficial in most types of overuse injury.[217] However, in stress fractures, they may have no advantage over simple analgesics.[137]

To prevent recurrence of overuse injury, it is imperative to review and correct faulty training methods and to evaluate for biomechanical factors. Of all running injuries, 60% result from training errors such as running on hard, uneven, or inclined surfaces, improper footwear, and overzealous training.[28]

Ankle Sprain

The most common lesion affecting the ankle is a sprain or tear of one of the ligaments.[20,59] Between 70 and 80% of the sprains involve the anterior talofibular ligament, calcaneal fibular ligament, or posterior talofibular ligament.[179,191,201,202,203] The next most frequently sprained ligaments at the ankle are the calcaneocuboid, the calcaneofibular and the bifurcate ligaments. Portions of the deltoid ligament may also be sprained, but more often a forceful eversion stress will result in an avulsion of the tibial malleolus rather than damage to the ligament.[21,37]

I. History
   A. Onset of pain. The patient will invariably recall the traumatic incident. The common mechanism of injury for an anterior talofibular ligament sprain is a plantar flexion–inversion stress.[64,74,111,155] Typical examples include an athlete who lands from a jump on the lateral border of the plantarly flexed foot, a person wearing high-heeled shoes or walking on uneven ground who catches a toe on the lateral side of the foot, or a person stepping off a curb or step who rolls over the lateral side of the plantarly flexed foot. If the forefoot is forced into supination or adduction, the calcaneocuboid ligament may be injured instead or as well. The calcaneofibular ligament restricts inversion with the foot in a more neutral or dorsiflexed position. It may be injured along with the talofibular ligament if, at the time of injury, the person retains good contact of the foot with the ground but continues to force the foot into inversion.

       When torn, the deltoid ligament is usually injured because the foot is forced into external rotation and eversion with respect to the leg. As mentioned, it is more common for a portion of the tibial malleolus to avulse with the deltoid ligament attachment. The anterior tibiofibular ligament may be torn with a similar mechanism, because as the talus rotates within the mortise, it tends to wedge the tibia and fibula apart, producing a diastasis.[1,21,37] For the talus to rotate enough to produce a diastasis and to tear the anterior tibiofibular ligament, the deltoid ligament is torn or the tibial malleolus is avulsed as well.[1]

   B. Site of pain. This usually corresponds well with the approximate location of the injury. Some pain may be referred distally into the foot or proximally into the lower leg.

   C. Nature of pain or disability. Similar to ligamentous lesions at the knee, the degree of pain and disability immediately after an injury to an ankle ligament does not necessarily correlate well with the severity of the lesion.[90] A person sustaining a mild or moderate sprain may describe more pain and be more reluctant to continue a particular activity than one who completely ruptures a ligament. This is because in the event of a rupture there is complete loss of continuity of the structure and there are no longer intact fibers to be stressed and from which pain can be elicited.

       Repeated episodes of anterior talofibular ligament sprains are not uncommon. Usually the initial injury results in somewhat more pain and disability than with subsequent occurrences. These patients typically describe intermittent giving way of the ankle, often during athletic activities, followed by pain and effusion lasting for a few days.[56,195]

II. Physical Examination
   A. Observation. A patient seen soon after injury may hobble into the office walking with a characteristic foot-flat, short-stance gait; both heel-strike and push-off are lacking. If the pain is more severe, the patient may walk in with the aid of crutches or hop on one leg.

   B. Inspection. Localized swelling over the region of the involved ligament is usually present within several hours after the injury. Because the anterior talofibular ligament and the deep fibers of the deltoid ligament blend with the ankle mortise joint capsule, there may be some associated articular effusion. Within a day or so after most ankle sprains, there is diffuse ecchymosis in the region of the injury, which may extravasate distally into the foot.

C. Selective tissue tension tests

1. Active movements. In the acute stage there is likely to be considerable difficulty in heel and toe walking and other weight-bearing activities involving ankle movements. The examiner must exercise judgment in requesting the patient to perform these movements to avoid undue discomfort or stress to the part.

2. Passive movements and joint-play movements (key objective tests)

a. If the ankle mortise joint capsule has been stressed with subsequent articular effusion, the ankle movements will be limited in a capsular pattern; plantar flexion will be slightly more restricted than dorsiflexion.

b. In the case of a mild or moderate ligamentous sprain, pain will be reproduced with movements that stress the involved ligament. There will usually be an associated muscle-spasm end feel. Painless hypermobility will be noted in the presence of chronic ruptures. Acute ruptures will also demonstrate hypermobility; however, a false-negative finding may be elicited because of protective muscle spasm. Take care to ensure maximal relaxation of the part when performing passive movements. The common ligaments injured and the passive movements used to test their integrity are as follows:

   i. Anterior talofibular ligament. Combined plantar flexion–inversion–adduction of the hindfoot and anterior glide of the talus on the tibia[20,122]

   ii. Calcaneocuboid ligament. Combined supination–adduction of the forefoot

   iii. Calcaneofibular ligament. Inversion of the hindfoot in a neutral position of plantar flexion–dorsiflexion

   iv. Deltoid ligament. Anterior fibers: combined plantar flexion–eversion–abduction of the hindfoot; middle fibers: eversion of the hindfoot

3. Joint instability tests, such as talar tilt and anterior drawer, are usually positive. There may be signs of internal derangement of the ankle joint if there are loose bodies, bone spurs, or interposed synovial tissue folds.[108]

4. Resisted movements. These should be strong and painless. Occasionally the peroneal tendons are strained in conjunction with an inversion ligamentous strain. In this case, isometric resistance to eversion will be strong and painful. Weakness of plantar flexion and eversion may be present.

D. Neuromuscular tests. Results are noncontributory.

E. Palpation

1. Tenderness will usually correspond to the site of the lesion in acute injuries. There is also likely to be diffuse tenderness in the presence of marked swelling from extravasation of blood into the tissues.

2. Joint effusion from synovitis or extra-articular swelling will be palpable in the acute stages.

3. Skin temperature will be elevated over the region of the involved structure in the acute stages.

III. Management

A. Acute sprains—immediate measures. At this early stage, there is little that needs to be done to, or for, the patient that he or she cannot do on his or her own. Ice, elevation, compression, mobility exercises, and strengthening can be carried out easily at home by most patients. This does, however, require very clear and precise instruction by the therapist. Do not spare words or time in making sure that the patient understands exactly what she or he should or should not be doing with the ankle. A follow-up visit after 2 or 3 days should be scheduled so that a reassessment can be made and the program appropriately progressed. At this point, there should be evidence of reduction of the acute inflammatory process; pain, temperature, and swelling should be decreased. It is important, in the subacute stage, to carefully reassess joint-play movements, because at this stage the therapist can determine more easily whether there has been some loss of integrity of the involved structure. Often in the acute stage, muscle spasm precludes accurate determination of the extent of the damage.

1. Reduction of stress to the ligament to allow healing without undue lengthening.

a. Ankle strapping will help reduce movement in response to mild (non–weight-bearing) stresses. Swelling should have stabilized by the time of application. A felt or foam rubber horseshoe pad should be used to fill in the submalleolar depressions to obtain even compressions of the area with tape or an elastic bandage.

b. Crutches should be used to relieve stress and pain during ambulation. A three-point, partial–weight-bearing crutch gait should be instituted; non–weight bearing is usually not necessary and should be avoided because of its nonfunctional nature.

2. Reduction of the acute inflammatory process to reduce pain and to prevent undue tissue damage from localized pressure and proteolytic cellular responses

a. Ice, to decrease blood flow and reduce capillary hydrostatic pressure, thus reducing extravasation of blood fluids

b. Compression. Increased external pressure to the area will minimize capillary leakage by effectively reducing the volume of the tissue spaces. This can be maintained by appropriate application of an elastic bandage with a horseshoe pad below the malleolus.

c. Elevation reduces capillary hydrostatic pressure to minimize fluid loss and assists venous and lymphatic return.

3. Prevention of residual disability

a. Motion of the part is instituted in planes that do not stress the healing ligament to minimize residual loss of movement and optimize circulation in the area.

   b. Isometric exercises to the muscles in the area should be started as early as pain allows, to maintain strength of the muscles of the lower leg and foot.

B. Acute sprains—subsequent measures

   1. Mild sprains. In the case of a simple sprain, in which there is no hypermobility on the associated passive movement tests, gradual return to normal activities should be allowed as the inflammatory process resolves. Weight bearing should be increased and the crutches discarded, usually by the fifth day. Range of motion, strength, and joint play should be restored to normal. Most patients may regain normal motion and strength with careful instruction in home exercises. Before discharging the patient from care, the therapist must ascertain that normal joint play has returned. If it has not, the restricted movements must be restored with passive joint mobilization techniques. Friction massage, initiated in the subacute stage, may promote healing of the ligament in a mobile state and prevent adherence to adjacent tissue.

     As the swelling subsides in the subacute stage, strapping should be substituted for the elastic bandage to provide support and to increase proprioceptive feedback as the patient resumes functional use of the part. Use of strapping should continue until good strength, range of motion, and joint play are restored. The athlete should continue to strap the ankle when participating in vigorous activities. Studies suggest that ankle strapping does play a role in preventing ankle sprains.[43] This is probably not because of actual mechanical support provided by the tape, as movement of the bones within the skin (to which the tape is adhered) is probably still sufficient to allow a ligament to be stretched. However, the added proprioceptive input provided by the tape may enhance protective reflexes (such as contraction of the peroneal muscles) in response to forces tending to stress the ankle ligaments.

     Return to vigorous activity must be gradual. Clinical evidence of healing does not indicate that a ligament has regained normal strength. In fact, maturation of the new collagen laid down during healing may take weeks or months. The necessary stimulus for maturation and restoration of normal ligamentous strength is stress to the ligament produced by functional use of the part. This induces formation of the appropriate collagen cross-links and realignment of the new collagen fibers along the normal lines of stress. However, the ligament must not be overstressed before normal strength is regained, as it is susceptible at this point to reinjury. The athlete should begin by jogging, then running, in straight lines. When normal muscle strength and joint motion have been regained, figure-of-eight patterns that impose some

lateral stress to the part may be initiated. Gradually, the patient should progress to sharp cutting drills. When these can be performed well and without pain, competitive activity may be resumed.

     Also during the later stages of rehabilitation, balance drills should be instituted to facilitate the restoration of normal protective reflexes.[55,57] Progression may proceed from challenging one-legged standing to one-legged standing on a rocking board to one-legged standing on a board supported on half a sphere (free to tilt in all planes).

   2. Moderate sprains and complete ruptures. The related literature reflects some controversy regarding the management of ruptured ligaments at the ankle. Most authorities would agree that injuries involving extensive damage, with rupture of both the anterior talofibular and calcaneofibular ligaments, should be repaired surgically to restore passive stability to the ankle.[4,195] Good results are favored by early surgery because the torn ends will tend to atrophy and retract with time, making apposition and suturing technically difficult or impossible. Similar considerations apply to rupture of the deltoid ligament.

     There is more divergence of opinion, however, with respect to management of isolated ruptures, in which some hypermobility of anterior glide of the talus in the mortise is demonstrable. Although some clinicians favor early surgical intervention to suture the torn ends and minimize residual and structural instability, others favor early return to function after some period of restricted activity and immobilization. There is evidence from studies by Freeman[55-57] that suturing of the ligament does result in a more stable joint, but in the end, the functional status of those undergoing surgery is really no better than those treated conservatively. In fact, those patients treated conservatively returned to normal function significantly sooner than those undergoing surgery, if they were not immobilized in plaster for a prolonged period of time. Of those treated conservatively, there was very little difference in residual mechanical stability between those who were immobilized in plaster for 6 weeks and those treated with strapping and early mobilization. The incidence of residual pain and swelling several months after injury was highest in the surgical group. The only way to guarantee increased mechanical stability after rupture of the anterior talofibular ligament is to reappose the torn ends with sutures. However, it seems that the residual disability resulting from prolonged immobilization in those treated with surgery outweighs whatever advantage this form of management may have in producing a more stable ankle. Further studies by Freeman[55-57] suggest that there is no correlation between mechanical instability, as determined by stress roentgenograms, and the incidence of residual disability resulting from chronic swelling and pain.

Conservative (nonsurgical) management of patients in whom there is evidence of actual loss of integrity of the ligament should follow the same approach as management for less serious injuries; the primary difference should be that those ankles with more extensive damage will need to be protected, by crutches and strapping, somewhat longer, perhaps as long as 2 weeks. However, early motion and strengthening at pain-free intensities should be initiated as resolution of the acute inflammatory process ensues. Also, in cases of more extensive damage, return to normal and, especially, to vigorous activity levels should be more gradual. Again, it must be emphasized that although new collagen is laid down within the first 1 or 2 weeks after injury, it takes months for this new tissue to mature to normal strength. During the period of maturation, the ligament is weaker than normal and, therefore, more susceptible to reinjury.

C. Chronic recurrent ankle sprains. After initial injury, especially to the anterior talofibular ligament, a certain number of patients will suffer recurrent giving way of the ankle, with subsequent pain and swelling. There are three possible causes of this to be considered and to which assessment should be directed.

1. Healing of the ligament with adherence to adjacent tissues. In this situation, the healed ligament does not allow the joint play necessary for normal functioning of the part.[37] With repetitive stress to the tightened structure, pain and swelling will result from a fatigue phenomenon. With forceful stress to the structure, the adhesion will rupture, producing another sprain. This type of problem will present as a painful, minor restriction on passive plantar flexion–inversion of the hindfoot and on anterior glide of the talus. Treatment consists of deep, transverse friction massage (see Fig. 8-27) to the ligament and specific joint mobilization in the directions of restriction. Normal mobility to the ligament is thus gradually restored.

2. Loss of protective reflex muscle stabilization. Normally, stress to some aspect of a joint capsule or to a joint ligament results in firing of specific receptors in the structure, through a reflex arc, to produce contraction of the muscles overlying the stressed structure. This booster mechanism of dynamic joint stabilization protects joint ligaments from injury under conditions of heavy loading. Thus, when the anterior talofibular ligament is stressed, the peroneus tertius is called on to reduce the load to the ligament. Damage to a ligament with subsequent immobilization may result in interference of this protective mechanism. Freeman[55] has shown good results in management of such cases by instituting a program of balance training. Emphasis should be placed on proprioceptive training and closed-chain strengthening. Mini-trampoline exercises are an excellent way to achieve both goals.[108] Jumping, crossover steps, and rotational jumps stimulate proprioception and require muscle contractions for stabilization. Closed-chain exercises have the distinct advantage of allowing concomitant training of the proprioceptive system. Poor proprioception is a major cause of repeat strains and functional instability.[209]

3. Gross mechanical instability of the joint. If both the anterior talofibular ligament and the calcaneofibular ligament are ruptured, or if there has been extensive capsular disruption with an anterior talofibular ligament rupture, the resultant mechanical instability of the joint may not allow certain functional weight-bearing activities to be performed without giving way. Such patients will present with obvious hypermobility on joint-play movement tests. If an aggressive muscle strengthening and balance training program is not sufficient to compensate for the instability, surgical reconstruction may be contemplated.

Thus, the therapist should direct assessment of the chronically unstable ankle toward determining whether there is some residual increase or decrease in joint play, whether good muscle strength has been regained, and whether the person is able to balance well during one-legged standing under various unstable conditions. It is important to realize that giving way of the joint is not necessarily the result of structural instability and that some degree of structural instability can be compensated for by muscle strengthening or balance training.

Foot Injuries

CUBOID DYSFUNCTION

Cuboid dysfunction also may be referred to as subluxation or the cuboid syndrome. The cause is uncertain but may be related to dysfunction of the calcaneocuboid joint or abnormal pull of the peroneus longus tendon through a groove on the inferior aspect of the cuboid dorsally, causing the medial aspect of the cuboid to sublux plantarward.[154] Newell and Woodie[154] found that 80% of cuboid subluxations occur in pronated feet. The patient presents with fairly acute, severe pain and sometimes swelling localized to the calcaneocuboid joint. He or she is unable to run, cut (do a lateral shift), jump, or dance without a marked increase in pain. There is localized tenderness to palpation in the plantar aspect of the foot and laterally over the joint.[179] Roentgenograms are negative.

Treatment by manipulation of the cuboid, using one of a number of methods, usually brings immediate relief (see Fig. 16-60).[35,61,115,126,134,135,144] Release of the long dorsiflexors and peroneals with deep massage should be performed before manipulation.[134] This should be followed by placement of a felt pad beneath the cuboid on the plantar surface of the foot, along with a low-dye strapping procedure to give the arch added support for 1 or 2 weeks.[115] Box 16-1 provides guidelines for preparing the foot for low-dye strapping. In long-standing cases resistant to other forms of therapy, surgical

BOX 16-1   MODIFIED LOW-DYE STRAPPING[221]

Rationale for Use
- To stabilize the head of the first metatarsal by plantar flexion
- To decrease pain
- To determine need for orthotic
- Materials
- Moleskin strapping
- Tape adherent (e.g., Tuf–skin)
- Tape—1 or 1½ inch
- Procedure
- Preparation
  1. Shave, clean, and thoroughly dry the forefoot.
  2. Apply tape adherent to dorsal, plantar, and medial aspects of foot.
  3. Place small piece of adhesive moleskin below the first and fifth metatarsal heads to reduce abrasion on these areas.
  4. Cut a 2-inch-wide adhesive moleskin strip to size of foot, measuring from the first to fifth metatarsal head. Cut a 3- × ½-inch angled piece from both sides of midportion of the moleskin (A).
- Tape application
  1. An anchor strip of 1-inch adhesive tape is applied loosely on the dorsal and plantar aspects of the foot just proximal to the metatarsal heads (B).
  2. Peel away the backing of the moleskin strip. Place one end on the head of the fifth metatarsal and secure it along the lateral aspect of the foot. Continue around the posterior aspect of the calcaneus (C).
  3. Ensure that the foot is in subtalar neutral position (Fig. 16-28). Stabilize the lateral four rays by placing your hand on the lateral aspect of the foot with your thumb on the plantar aspect of the foot. Plantar flex the first ray before securing the rest of the moleskin to the head of the first metatarsal (D).

  Note: If tape is used in place of the adhesive moleskin, second and third strips are placed around the foot, partially overlapping each other.

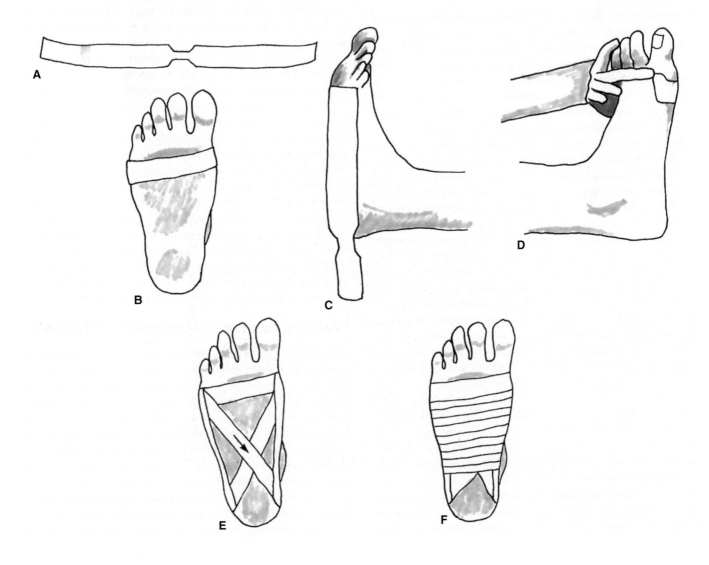

Box 16-1. continued

4. With 1-inch adhesive tape, strap the longitudinal arch with the "scissor" method or figure-of-eight. Half a figure-of-eight is performed by starting at the base of the great toe, angling across the longitudinal arch around the heel, and returning to the base of the little toe as the starting position (*E*). The steps are repeated once or twice.
5. A closing anchor is placed on the dorsum of the foot over the original anchor. Additional anchor strips may be placed on the plantar aspect of the foot with horizontal strips applied from one side of the moleskin to the other, along the entire length of the foot. These horizontal strips are placed by

pulling gently medially, from the heel to the ball of the foot (*F*).

Care must be taken to account for expansion of the foot on weight bearing. When the strapping is correctly applied, the great toe will be plantar flexed at the MTP joint and the medial longitudinal arch will be heightened and well maintained. A felt pad or a post under the medial aspect of the forefoot can be incorporated in the taping if a large deformity is present. The patient should be advised to keep the strapping dry. When weight bearing, shoes should be worn to help prolong the life of the strapping. The foot and limb posture should be reevaluated in stance and gait.

exploration of the cuboid and peroneus longus tendon has been undertaken.[179]

METATARSALGIA

Metatarsalgia is a syndrome describing pain over the metatarsal heads or in the MTP joints. The cause may be vascular, avascular, neurogenic, or mechanical.[71] It is most commonly caused by abnormal foot biomechanics and repetitive forces that cause stress to the metatarsal arch.[196] It is more common in the pes cavus foot, but many abnormal foot alignments of the hindfoot or forefoot contribute to metatarsalgia. Scranton[185] classifies metatarsalgia according to whether a weight-bearing imbalance exists between the metatarsals (primary) or whether the forefoot pain is caused by other factors, such as stress fractures or rheumatoid arthritis (secondary). Both primary and secondary metatarsalgia have characteristic associated keratosis. A third classification of forefoot pain is that without reactive keratosis such as neuromas, gout, and plantar fasciitis.[89]

Many theories have been developed to attempt to explain the origin of primary or generalized metatarsalgia. One theory suggests that a short first metatarsal will cause the second to have to bear a disproportionate amount of weight as the body propels over the foot and thereby result in ultimate dysfunction and the development of a painful callus.[89] A subluxing second or third MTP joint, or failure of the transverse metatarsal arch to be maintained by the transverse metatarsal ligaments and the transverse head of the adductor hallucis muscle, may also be the cause of metatarsalgia.

According to Kraeger,[115] generalized metatarsalgia often occurs secondary to a tight Achilles tendon, which restricts dorsiflexion. The loss of full dorsiflexion loads the weight onto the forefoot, thus applying pressure to the MTP joints. Any tendency toward excessive pronation will lead to hypermobile functioning of the first and fifth ray and thereby cause a relative depression of the transverse metatarsal arch. Metatarsalgia is common in middle-aged persons with a pronation tendency.[17] Other extrinsic factors such as excessive weight

gain and wearing high-heeled shoes have been suggested as causes for or aggravating circumstances of the condition.

The patient presents with an antalgic gait including diminished push-off. In some cases the patient may prevent any weight shift across the metatarsal heads by weight bearing exclusively on the lateral border of the foot.[89] Pain may occur at night, but the patient typically reports pain only on weight bearing. Palpation reveals point tenderness over the plantar surface of the metatarsal heads, usually the second and third. Compression to the involved metatarsal head will elicit pain.

Treatment of the different causes of metatarsalgia is similar, although it must be individualized to the exact problem. Treatment should include correction of any abnormal biomechanics, cord stretching, and exercises to strengthen the intrinsic toe flexors. Mobilization is suggested to reduce secondary fibrositis from spasm and joint dysfunction.[35] Metatarsophalangeal decompression (traction) and manipulation of the metatarsals (metatarsal whip) are recommended treatments. Metatarsal pads just proximal to the second or third metatarsal head or an external metatarsal pad should be considered. Another option is to place a pad beneath the first metatarsal to allow it to bear more weight.[115] Orthotics, shoe modification, or a reduction in heel height should be considered.

Problems Related to Abnormal Foot Pronation

Pronation of the hindfoot with respect to the forefoot is a relatively common disorder that may or may not give rise to foot pain. Also, because of the biomechanical interplay between the foot and other weight-bearing segments, the pronated foot may result in dysfunction in other regions of the lower limb, especially the knee. Similarly, a pronated foot may be caused by some local structural abnormality of the tarsal skeleton, or it may be caused by some structural deviation in segments either distal or proximal to the hindfoot.

Pain resulting from a pronated foot is usually of the fatigue type from prolonged increased stress on the affected tissues. In some patients, pain may arise with normal activity levels, whereas others may get along well until they engage in some activity, such as jogging, that involves increased stress levels or frequency. Pain of local origin usually has its source in one of the plantar structures responsible for maintaining the twisted configuration of the foot—the plantar aponeurosis, the short plantar ligament, or the long plantar ligament (see plantar fasciitis above). Pain may also arise from fatigue of the intrinsic muscles of the foot, in which activity may be increased in an attempt to prevent undue stress to the plantar aponeurosis and ligaments. Another source of local pain occurring in association with a pronated foot is pressure from the shoes against the talar head or the navicular, which becomes prominent medially when the foot untwists.

A pronated foot may be the cause of, or be associated with, pain in the forefoot, leg, or knee.[19] Pain from pressure over the first one or two metatarsal heads may result from increased weight bearing over the medial side of the forefoot. This occurs if the talar head and navicular drop downward and inward, shifting the center of gravity line medially. Because hallux valgus often accompanies pronation of the hindfoot, either as a cause or as a result, pressure over a prominent first MTP joint may also occur with increased pronation of the foot. Leg pain may result from increased tension on the anterior or posterior tibialis muscles, which are dynamic supporters of the arch of the foot (see above). The knee tends to assume a valgus position when the foot pronates. Such an angulation tends to increase the lateral pull on the patella during loaded quadriceps contraction. This may predispose to pain from patellar tracking dysfunction at the knee (see Chapter 15, Knee).

As mentioned, pronation of the hindfoot may occur from some local structural disorder or from structural deviations elsewhere. The common local causes are capsuloligamentous laxity and bony abnormalities. Capsuloligamentous laxity may be a hereditary condition, or it may accompany some specific disease state, such as rheumatoid arthritis. The common *bony* anomaly resulting in flatfoot is tarsal coalition, in which the talus and calcaneus are fixed to one another in a pronated orientation through fibrous or osseous union.[49] The common malalignment problems affecting other regions that predispose to abnormal pronation of the hindfoot are femoral antetorsion, internal tibial torsion, a shortened Achilles tendon, and adduction of the first metatarsal. The excessive internal rotation imposed by antetorsion of the femur or internal tibial torsion during stance phase is at least partially absorbed by the subtalar joint, bringing the hindfoot into pronation. In the presence of a short Achilles tendon, the midtarsal joint attempts to compensate for lack of dorsiflexion at the ankle; to do so, the foot must untwist to unlock the midtarsal joints. Because of the oblique orientation of the first cuneiform–first metatarsal joint, adduction of the first metatarsal also involves a component of dorsiflexion. This effectively supinates the forefoot, which necessitates a compensatory pronation of the hindfoot to get the foot flat on the ground. Each of these possible causes must be considered when examining the patient with a pronated foot.

Finally, it must be remembered that abnormal foot pronation during gait is not always associated with a pronated foot seen on structural examination with the patient standing. The typical example is a person with increased tibial varum. The foot usually appears normal or even supinated during relaxed standing. However, when running or walking there is a tendency to heel-strike on the lateral border of the heel, causing the foot to undergo increased hindfoot pronation to press the heel flat on the ground. Even though the foot appears not to be pronated, it will be subject to increased pronatory stresses. Similar considerations apply to the patient with either femoral retrotorsion or external tibial torsion, in which the cause of pronation is not localized to the foot itself.

I. History
    A. Onset of pain is usually insidious because the pathologic tissue conditions associated with biomechanical abnormalities such as a pronated foot are typically fatigue phenomena. Often the onset can be related to some increased activity level, such as long-distance running. Another common predisposing factor is a period of disuse, such as immobilization of the foot in a cast. In such cases, the muscles of the foot weaken, and when activity is resumed, they no longer contribute their share to stabilizing the arch of the foot. This results in increased stress to the capsuloligamentous structures. Occasionally, a change in footwear, for example, to a lower heel height, can be related to the onset. Lowering the heel height increases the tension on the Achilles tendon, which may in turn result in increased pronation of the hindfoot in the same way as described for a shortened Achilles tendon. A lowered heel also results in reduced dorsiflexion of the toes during the stance, decreasing the windlass effect on the plantar aponeurosis and reducing the twisted configuration of the foot.
    B. Site of pain. Foot pain associated with abnormal pronation usually is felt over the plantar aspect of the foot. Pain from calcaneal periostitis and heel spurs is fairly well localized over the bottom of the heel, often more medially; it may be referred anteriorly into the sole of the foot. Pain from fatigue stress to the plantar ligament or aponeurosis is felt over the sole of the foot, usually more medially. Keep in mind that the bony and soft tissue pathologic processes referred to previously may occur concurrently.

    Forefoot pain arising secondary to a pronated foot condition may be felt in the region of the medial metatarsal heads, if caused by abnormal weight distribution, or it may be felt over the medial aspect of the first MTP joint, if caused by pressure over the joint resulting from a hallux valgus deformity.

    Knee pain related to a pronated foot is typically from patellofemoral joint problems (see section on patellar tracking dysfunction in Chapter 15, Knee).
    C. Nature of pain. Pain is from increased stress to the plantar ligaments, fascia, capsules, or calcaneal periosteum under

conditions in which increased untwisting of the foot takes place. This typically occurs in a person whose foot undergoes an abnormal degree of pronation during stance phase or whose foot remains in a pronated position during prolonged standing. The muscles controlling the twist, or arch, of the foot will protect these structures for a certain length of time. However, once the muscles fatigue, more stress is transmitted to the ligaments and fascia, which are responsible for the passive stabilization of the arched configuration of the foot. In some cases, this may occur with normal activity levels, such as after walking some distance or after standing for a long time. In others, increased activity, such as long-distance running, provides the added stress to bring on the pain. Once a low-grade inflammation develops, the pain is brought on with less stress and may be relatively continuous during weight bearing. In these more severe cases, pain is typically pronounced on initial weight bearing, subsiding somewhat as the muscles contract more to protect the painful structures, then increasing again as the muscles fatigue.

II. Physical Examination
  A. Observation and inspection of structural alignment. Evidence of excessive pronation of the foot and associated biomechanical abnormalities may be noted when the patient walks or stands.
    1. Flattening of the medial arch. The region of the navicular and the talar head may appear to be prominent medially and depressed inferiorly.
    2. Abduction of the forefoot on the rearfoot
    3. Adduction of the first metatarsal, perhaps with a valgus deformity of the first MTP joint
    4. Valgus position of the heel maintained throughout stance phase
    5. Medial tibial torsion. The feet may be pointed inward while the patellae face straight forward.
    6. Femoral antetorsion. The patellae face inward when the feet are in normal alignment. This must be differentiated from lateral tibial torsion, which may present similarly. Lateral tibial torsion is evidenced by an increased external rotation of the intermalleolar line with respect to the frontal plane (in excess of about 25°). Femoral antetorsion is suggested when the total range of motion at the hip is about normal, but the range of internal rotation is increased and the range of external rotation is proportionally decreased.
    7. Genu valgum. This often exists in conjunction with femoral anteversion.
  B. Inspection (supine)
    1. Structural alignment
      a. Forefoot varus. This is the most common intrinsic deformity resulting from abnormal pronation.[39,176,206] Root and coworkers[175] describe it as a frontal plane deformity that is compensated at the subtalar joint by eversion or a valgus position of the calcaneus in weight bearing.

      b. Dorsiflexed and hypermobile first ray producing hallux valgus, which is subluxation of the MTP joint of the big toe in the sagittal and transverse plane[175]
    2. Skin. Inspect for signs of pressure over the navicular tubercle, first MTP joint, and medial metatarsal head. As a result of first ray insufficiency, callus or keratosis may develop under the head of the second metatarsal.[87]
    3. Soft tissue. Inspect for muscle atrophy that may relate to loss of dynamic support of the arch of the foot.
    4. Inspection of shoes (see physical examination section)
  C. Selective tissue tension tests
    1. Active movements. If inspection of structural alignment reveals a pronated position of the hindfoot, the patient is observed while raising up on the toes and externally rotating the leg over the fixed foot. Both of these movements should decrease the pronation and cause an increased twisting and arching of the foot. If not, a rigid flatfoot, caused by some fixed structural abnormality such as tarsal coalition, probably exists.
    2. Passive movements. Unless a rigid flatfoot exists (a relatively rare condition), a pronated foot is usually a hypermobile foot. Hypermobility, especially of the midtarsal joints, may be noted.
      a. If a tight heel cord or restricted ankle mortise joint capsule is a contributing cause, dorsiflexion of the hindfoot will be restricted. One must lock the foot by supinating the calcaneus and pronating the forefoot when testing ankle dorsiflexion to avoid misinterpreting movement of the forefoot as being movement at the ankle. There should be about 10 to 20° of dorsiflexion. If dorsiflexion and plantar flexion are both restricted, the joint capsule is probably at fault. If dorsiflexion is restricted with the knee straight, but not with the knee bent, the gastrocnemius is tight. If dorsiflexion is restricted regardless of the position of the knee, the soleus is probably at fault.
      b. If antetorsion of the hip is a contributing factor, hip range of motion will be relatively normal but skewed toward internal rotation with restriction of external rotation.
      c. Joint play. Movements of the tarsal joints are likely to be hypermobile. Excessive arthrokinematic movements typically occur among four bones: calcaneus, talus, navicular, and cuboid.[39]
      d. Pain from low-grade inflammation of the plantar fascia or ligaments, or from calcaneal periostitis, may be reproduced by passively everting the heel, supinating the foot, and dorsiflexing the toes.
    3. Resisted movements. Results are usually noncontributory.
  D. Neuromuscular tests. Determine whether weakness, either neurogenic or atrophic, of any of the muscles controlling movement and stability of the foot exists.
  E. Palpation. Localized tender areas may exist that relate to areas of low-grade inflammation occurring in response to

abnormal tissue stresses. As usual, the finding of localized tenderness to palpation, in itself, must not be taken to be diagnostic of any specific disorder because of the common phenomenon of referred tenderness associated with lesions of deep somatic tissue.

Typical areas of tenderness associated with abnormal foot pronation might include the calcaneal attachment of the plantar fascia and long plantar ligament, especially at the medial tubercle; the plantar fascia, usually over the medial aspect of the sole of the foot; the navicular tubercle; the spring ligament, between the sustentaculum tali and the navicular tubercle; the medial one or two metatarsal heads; and the medial aspect of the first MTP joint.

Areas of skin or subcutaneous tissue hypertrophy may be distinguished on palpation as localized indurated regions. Such calluses, associated with pronation, might be found over the medial one or two metatarsal heads or over the medial aspect of the first MTP joint.

III. Management. Symptoms arising in association with abnormal foot pronation are the result of increased stress to some pain-sensitive tissue. Proper management, then, must involve selective reduction of abnormal stresses. The approach used must be in accordance with findings on evaluation, including information relating to the patient's activity level. In developing a program of management, it must be kept in mind that the tissue disorder resulting in the painful condition may be caused by normal stresses occurring at too great a frequency, abnormally high stresses occurring at normal frequencies, or some combination thereof.[173] Either situation may result in tissue fatigue in which the rate of tissue breakdown exceeds the rate at which the tissue is able to repair itself. However, the approach to management will differ, depending on which condition prevails. In general, management of conditions associated with pronation of the foot involves measures to reduce either the frequency or the magnitude of stresses, or both.

In the case of the pronated foot, forces are typically increased by structural malalignments that cause changes in the direction in which forces occur and in the degree of movement of skeletal parts during functional activities. The most common postural malalignment causing abnormal foot pronation is probably increased femoral antetorsion, which is usually accompanied by increased genu valgum (knock knees). As mentioned earlier, the other common structural deviations predisposing to increased pronation of the foot are adduction of the first metatarsal and increased medial tibial torsion. Each of these conditions results in untwisting of the tarsal skeleton during ambulation, such that a greater tensile stress is imposed on the plantar ligaments, fascia, and joint capsules. Under such conditions, the foot loses the typical passive stability normally produced by becoming twisted during stance phase. To compensate, the intrinsic muscles of the foot must contract more to prepare the foot for push-off. Pain may arise from increased stress to the plantar capsuloligamentous structures, from fatigue of the abnormally contracting muscles, or both.

Persons with longstanding pronation from a congenital structural malalignment or from a malalignment acquired early in life are likely to have a permanent hypermobility of the joints of the foot. The ligaments and joint capsules will have been elongated from the chronic increased stresses applied to them throughout development. By the time they are adults, these persons are not likely to have pain arising from the already lengthened ligaments and fascia during normal activity levels. They are, however, likely to have feet that tire easily from increased activity of the intrinsics and other muscles supporting the arch during gait. They are also more predisposed to developing problems elsewhere, such as metatarsalgia, hallux valgus, and patellofemoral joint dysfunction.

Persons with more subtle structural deviations resulting in an increased tendency toward pronation are likely to have problems only with increased activity levels, such as long-distance running, that increase the magnitude and frequency of pronatory stresses. The mobility of the joints of the foot in these persons allowed by the capsules and ligaments is likely to be fairly normal. It is especially important in patients experiencing pain suggestive of increased pronation, but who have relatively normal structural alignment, to consider nonstructural causes. The most common of these would include a tight heel cord and inappropriate footwear. It is these patients, having subtle structural deviations or nonstructural causes of increased pronation, who are likely to experience pain and develop pathologic lesions associated with increased strain to specific tissues. The most common tissues involved are the supporting plantar structures of the foot, including the periosteum of the plantar aspect of the calcaneus, and the Achilles tendon.

A. Techniques

1. Instruction in appropriate activity levels. As in any common musculoskeletal disorder, appropriate instruction in exactly what the patient should and should not do, and to what degree, is an essential component of the treatment program too often overlooked. With respect to problems related to increased foot pronation, this is especially important in the person experiencing problems primarily with increased activity levels. Treatment of the long-distance runner experiencing pain from plantar fasciitis, Achilles tendinitis, or other pronation-related disorders simply involves advising the patient to not run so much. But this is not adequate management of the problem because, as with any disorder, the therapist must be concerned primarily with restoring optimal function. From the patient's standpoint, optimal function may be running long distances!

The role of the therapist should be first to decide whether the patient's functional expectations are realistic. The patient with considerably increased femoral antetorsion, knock knees, and hypermobile flat feet probably should not be engaging in activities such as long-distance running that involve high-frequency, weight-bearing stresses. However, this condition should not prevent the person from engaging in other vigorous conditioning exercise, such as swimming and bicycling.

If there are no gross structural malalignments predisposing to pronation-type problems, the therapist must then determine what can be done to reduce the stresses to the involved tissues, to allow them to heal, and to prevent further pathologic processes and pain. As far as healing is concerned, the most important step to be taken is to reduce the stresses that caused the problem. The most reliable method of doing this is to reduce the activity level. The long-distance runner experiencing chronic, persistent pain must be advised to markedly reduce or stop running for a period of 1 to 2 weeks to allow the tissue to heal. Complete immobilization, however, is seldom, if ever, indicated for fatigue disorders such as these. During this period of relative rest the therapist should determine what can be done to reduce stresses when the activity is resumed. Other procedures to help restore the involved tissue to its normal state may also be instituted.

2. Muscle strengthening and conditioning. Strengthening and endurance exercises for the intrinsic muscles of the foot as well as for the extrinsic muscles, such as the anterior and posterior tibialis that help maintain a twisted configuration of the foot, are important in the management of virtually all foot problems resulting from abnormal pronation. Improving the function of these muscles will allow the person with the hypermobile flat foot to stand or walk for longer periods of time before muscle fatigue sets in. It will also help relieve strain on the plantar fascia and ligaments in patients suffering from strain of these structures by increasing the dynamic support of the arch, thus allowing the muscles to take a greater portion of the load.

3. Proprioceptive balance training (see section on dynamic stabilization and functional exercises)
   a. Because the pedal intrinsic muscles appear to function similarly to the plantar fascia in stabilization of the foot, pedal intrinsic strengthening exercises should be prescribed.[134] Foot doming is a particularly beneficial exercise.[42,134]
   b. Dorsiflexors are often found to be weak. Before strengthening, according to Janda,[95] it is better to stretch the tight structures (gastrocnemius–soleus). Both eccentric and concentric exercises should be included.
   c. The tibialis posterior, flexor digitorum longus, and flexor hallucis longus exert a supinatory force at the subtalar joint. These muscles help control pronation by working eccentrically. Marshall[134] prefers to strengthen the supinators eccentrically by using the BAPS balance board (Camp International, Inc., Jackson, MI). One can begin closed-chain strengthening by adding weights to the BAPS or wobble board. The patient can progress as tolerated from a

seated position, to partial weight bearing, and finally, to a single-leg stance on the injured limb. Once the patient can perform a single-leg stance on the injured limb without pain, he or she can begin a progression of balancing activities specifically designed to improve proprioception.

4. Strapping. Strong muscles are of little use unless they contract with sufficient force and at the appropriate time to perform the desired function. Abnormal foot pronation can be controlled to varying degrees by contraction of the muscles that cause an increased twisted configuration of the foot. Most important among these are the anterior and posterior tibialis muscles and the peroneus longus. Theoretically, muscle function can be enhanced by providing additional input along the afferent limb of the reflex arcs that normally invoke muscle contraction during functional activities. One method of doing so is to strap the part in a manner that will cause increased tension to the straps, and therefore the skin, when movement occurs in the undesired direction. The added afferent input from the tension and pressure produced by the straps serves to enhance activity of muscles that normally check the undesired movement. This is apparently the means by which ankle strapping helps to stabilize the ankle against inversion sprains.[59] Although empirically there seems to be evidence for the efficacy of such procedures, electromyographic studies have yet to be performed to substantiate the proposed mechanism.

For an excellent review of the literature, the reader is referred to the work of Metcalf and Denegar.[145] The low-dye strapping technique that was designed by Ralph Dye in an attempt to provide functional mechanical support of the joints of the feet is recommended by Newell and Nutler[153] and by others (see Box 16-1)[3,6,45,82,114,186,219,221] to restrict abnormal foot pronation. The ability of low-dye strapping to modify forces on the medial arch during weight bearing has been clearly demonstrated by Scranton and colleagues.[186] It is meant to bring the ground up to the foot to eliminate the need for the foot to pronate to reach it.[219] It may be used to protect the passive stabilizing structures of the foot, such as the plantar fascia and associated structures, during the rehabilitation phase after injuries and to assess the effect of more permanent stabilizing measures, such as a biomechanical functional foot orthosis or shoe modification.

A number of variations have been developed (modified low-dye, cross-X technique, Herzog taping) and used in rehabilitating posterior tibial syndrome, posterior tibial tendinitis, peripatellar compression pain, Achilles tendon problems, and jumper's knee.[94,153,218,219] James and associates[94] demonstrated effectiveness of this type of treatment for overuse injuries when combined with rehabilitation exercises. These procedures pull the medial aspect of the foot toward the supportive surface and secure it in this position with tape (see Box 16-1 for one variation of this technique).

5. Ultrasound and friction massage. These may be important treatment measures in cases of plantar fasciitis, Achilles tendinitis, and tibialis periostitis. The resultant increased blood flow may assist in the healing process. Transverse frictions will promote the development of a mobile structure and help prevent adhesions as healing ensues.

6. Achilles tendon stretching. This is especially important when evaluation reveals a tight heel cord as a possible contributing cause of the patient's problem, and in cases of Achilles tendinitis.

McCluskey and coworkers[138] were one of the first groups to report the beneficial effects of calf muscle stretching to reduce ankle injuries. Ten degrees of dorsiflexion with the knee extended and the subtalar in neutral is the amount considered necessary for normal walking.[176] James[93] suggests at least 15° talocrural joint dorsiflexion is required for running. One must take care to ensure that the stretching force is applied to the hindfoot, as using the forefoot as a lever to stretch the heel cord will result in dorsiflexion of the transverse tarsal joint in addition to dorsiflexion at the ankle mortise (talocrural) joint. This may result in hypermobility of the transverse tarsal joint, which may add further to a tendency toward pronation of the foot.

When stretching of the calf muscle is attempted, it is important that the subtalar joint is maintained in a neutral position. To ensure that this position is maintained, the patient should either stretch out in a biomechanical orthotic device or place a lift under the medial aspect of the bare foot during stretch.

In the more acute stages of Achilles tendinitis, the therapist must not be overly vigorous in restoring mobility to the heel cord, as the condition could be aggravated. However, because most cases of Achilles tendinitis are fatigue disorders, an acute stage never exists. Some gentle stretching may be initiated carefully from the outset; the slow, short-termed stress produced by such stretching procedures in no way approximates the high-frequency, high strain-rate stresses that produce this type of disorder. In fact, early stretching, performed judiciously, will help prevent the fibers from healing in a shortened state.

Increasing the load and speed of contraction with an emphasis on eccentric training has been found to be particularly helpful.[194] This can be carried out with the rear foot over the edge of a step to allow for greater range of dorsiflexion–plantar flexion and eccentric control. To ensure normal weight-bearing alignment, a tennis ball can be placed between the patient's medial malleoli; the patient is instructed not to lose contact with the ball throughout the exercise, as this may invoke excessive supination or pronation.[147]

7. Shoe inserts and modifications. When abnormal foot pronation is caused by some structural malalignment, whether marked or subtle, only surgery can remedy the true cause of the disorder. However, nonsurgical management is effective in the majority of cases. To optimize function, while at the same time preventing stresses sufficient to cause painful pathologic processes, the excessive untwisting of the foot must be reduced. This can be accomplished by altering the orientation of the segments of the foot as they contact the ground during stance phase or by producing direct support to the arched configuration of the foot, or both.

If the joint capsules and ligaments of the foot are not elongated, as in the hypermobile flat foot accompanying gross malalignment, the twist in the foot during stance phase can be increased by increasing the pronatory orientation of the forefoot or by increasing the supinatory orientation of the hindfoot. This can be done by providing a lateral wedge for the forefoot or a medial wedge for the heel. A trial, temporary insert can be made by cutting such a wedge from a piece of felt, 1/8- to 3/16-inch thick, to fit inside the shoe. However, if it is to be used on a permanent basis, the wedge should be incorporated into the sole or heel of the shoe by one experienced in shoe modifications or should be incorporated into an orthosis.

If the tarsal joints of the foot are lax, then the twisted configuration cannot be restored by indirect means such as wedging because these rely on taking up the slack in the joint capsules to effect a twisting of the tarsal skeleton. In the case of a hypermobile, pronated foot, some direct support must be provided to prevent the head of the talus and navicular from dropping downward and medially in a pronatory fashion. For the severely pronated foot, an arch support may be used in conjunction with wedging of the sole or heel. Such wedging may be built into the orthosis or into the shoe. Regardless of the type of shoe modification or insert used, for the support to be effective the calcaneus must be stabilized by a firm shoe counter or a calcaneal cup built into an orthosis.[139] If the calcaneus is not held firmly, it will tend to compensate for attempts to increase the twist of the foot by rolling farther over into a valgus position (pronation). Thus, many orthoses now in use have a heel cup incorporated into the orthosis itself, obviating the need for an extra-firm shoe counter. Such an orthosis can be used, for example, in athletic shoes, which often do not have very stiff counters.

When chondromalacia of the knee occurs as a result of abnormal pronation of the foot, the use of arch supports or shoe modification may be a necessary component of the treatment program.

The progression of a hallux valgus deformity may also be retarded by use of orthoses or shoe modifications, if the adduction of the first metatarsal is a result of abnormal foot pronation.

In cases of metatarsalgia, if reducing the degree of pronation with appropriate orthotic devices or shoe modification does not adequately relieve the pressure over the metatarsal heads, a metatarsal insert may be used. This simply reduces the stress to the metatarsal heads by increasing the weight-bearing surface area behind the heads. Metatarsal pads are available with an adhesive backing, or a metatarsal support may be incorporated into an arch-supporting orthosis. To place the pad properly in the shoe, tape it to the patient's foot in place just behind the metatarsal heads with the widest dimension of the pad forward. Outline the bottom of the pad with lipstick or some substance that will leave a mark on the insole of the shoe when the patient steps down. The patient then puts on the shoes and walks about to make sure they are reasonably comfortable, realizing, of course, that they will at first feel somewhat peculiar. The shoes are then removed and the pad adhered to the insole of the shoe in the appropriate place as indicated by the marks left on the insole by the lipstick.

Several devices designed to modify forces in the foot have been reported to be helpful for the patient with plantar heel pain. Heel pads have been used to reduce the shock of weight bearing and to shift vertical forces forward and away from the heel.[6,8,60] Some authors have suggested the use of a heel cup to prevent calcaneal eversion and thus reduce tension on the plantar fascia.[18,47,102,186]

Problems Related to Abnormal Foot Supination

Abnormal supination of the entire foot occurs when the subtalar joint functions in a supinated position.[176] There are three basic classifications for abnormal supination: pes equinovarus, pes cavus, and pes cavovarus.[127,200,204] A pes equinovarus foot demonstrates a fixed plantar-flexed forefoot and an inverted forefoot; the rear foot in weight bearing is in neutral.[39] A pes cavovarus foot demonstrates a fixed medial column or first ray. In the weight-bearing position the calcaneus is in varus or inverted.

Root and coworkers[176] define forefoot valgus as eversion of the forefoot on the rear foot with the subtalar joint in neutral. The compensation for a forefoot valgus is inversion of the calcaneus in the weight-bearing position.[170,204] Forefoot valgus and a fixed plantar-flexed first ray are the most common intrinsic deformities resulting in abnormal supination of the subtalar joint.

Functionally abnormal supination is a failure of the foot to pronate, resulting in a foot unable to compensate normally. There is prolonged supination during the stance phase and a delayed pronation during the gait cycle. Stress fractures, metatarsalgia, plantar fasciitis, and Achilles tendinitis are common in this type of foot.

In general, treatment consists of stretching, mobilization, exercises, and orthoses.[206] The flexible cavus foot responds well to conventional biomechanical orthotic foot control. The rigid cavus foot requires a special orthosis or a shoe with shock-absorbing materials such as Spenco Insoles (SpencoMedical Corp., Waco, TX) or Sorbothane Inserts (Spectrum Sports, Twinsburg, OH) to lessen the strain on the lower extremities.

Orthoses

Ultimately, the patient exhibiting a true intrinsic biomechanical fault should be fitted with a custom-made functional biomechanical orthosis to correctly balance the foot during weight-bearing activities.[27] Orthotic devices are most often used to correct excessive pronation and thus may be effective in the management of related MTSS, chondromalacia, and, occasionally, trochanteric bursitis.

The orthosis made from a positive mold of the foot in its neutral position is designed for restoration of normal alignment of the subtalar and midtarsal joint by controlling excessive pronation and supination and reducing the abnormal forces through the kinetic chain. In basic terms, it is directed toward preventing the foot from compensating and allowing normal motion to take place in its proper sequence.

When the orthosis is in place, the foot should function near its neutral position. It is important to evaluate muscle imbalances extrinsic and intrinsic to the foot, in addition to evaluating forefoot and rear foot deformities. Softer flexible types of orthoses can be fabricated in the clinic as a temporary measure or may be made of flexible materials molded to a positive cast of the patient's foot. Most clinics are not equipped for fabrication of the rigid orthosis, which must be custom-made (from a positive model). There are a number of podiatry laboratories specializing in these types of orthotic appliances. Many excellent texts and articles have described orthotic fabrication and shoe modifications.[9,12,18,27,29,33,34,43,45,54,78,80,116,118,134,141,172,198,218]

Shoe styles and features are constantly being changed by the manufacturers so that it is almost impossible for the clinician to keep abreast of current shoe models, particularly the athletic shoe. The basic functions of any quality shoes are to enhance shock absorption and foot control and to provide good traction and protection. Lasting or curve of the sole of the shoe should generally conform to the patient's own foot shape. In general, most patients will do well with a relatively straight last. Many manufacturers now provide information on shoes that have been selectively designed to limit common foot abnormalities such as overpronation or oversupination of the subtalar joint.

Inasmuch as foot problems and related disorders are common and alteration of footwear is often an important component of management of these problems, it is important that the therapist develop a close working relationship with an orthotist, podiatrist, or other professional possessing these skills.

JOINT MOBILIZATION TECHNIQUES

Note: For the sake of simplicity, the operator will be referred to as the male, and the patient as the female. All of the techniques described apply to the patient's left extremity except where indicated. (P—patient; O—operator; M—movement.)

Tibiofibular Joint

I. Proximal Tibiofibular Joint. Anteroposterior glide (Fig. 16-47)
    P—Supine, with knee flexed about 90°, the foot flat on the plinth
    O—Stabilizes the knee with the right hand contacting the medial aspect of the knee area. He grasps the head and neck of the proximal fibula with the left hand, the thumb contacting anteriorly, the index and long finger pads contacting posteriorly. He takes care to avoid direct pressure to the common peroneal nerve.
    M—The left hand may move the proximal fibula posteriorly or anteriorly. This should be performed through a movement of flexion and extension at the shoulder, rather than through finger or wrist movements.

    This technique is used to increase joint play at the tibiofemoral joint. The fibular head must move forward on knee flexion and backward on knee extension. Dysfunction at the proximal tibiofibular joint commonly causes symptoms distally in the leg or ankle rather then proximally.
II. Leg, Involving the Entire Tibia and Fibula with the Crural Interosseous Membrane
    P—Sidelying with the leg supported on the table with the hip and knee in some flexion
    O—Stands facing the patient's leg

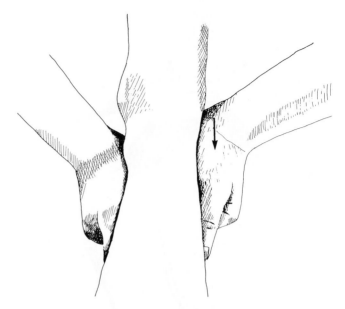

■ **FIG. 16-48.** Distal tibiofibular joint: anteroposterior glide.

    M—Apply ventral or dorsal gliding along the shaft of the fibula in the areas of restricted gliding
    The crural interosseous membrane (which has a little elasticity) may become restricted anywhere along the shaft of the fibula, particularly after tibiofibular fractures.
III. Distal Tibiofibular Joint. Anteroposterior glide (Fig. 16-48)
    P—Supine
    O—Cradles the ankle in his right hand, fixing it to the plinth, so that the fingers wrap around the heel posteriorly. The medial malleolus rests over the palmar aspect of his dorsiflexed wrist. The left hand contacts the lateral malleolus anteriorly with the heel of the hand.
    M—While the operator's right hand prevents downward movement of the medial malleolus, the left hand glides the lateral malleolus posteriorly in relation to the medial malleolus. The handholds may be reversed to move the medial malleolus posteriorly on the lateral malleolus.

    These techniques are used to increase joint play at the distal tibiofibular joint. This joint must spread slightly during ankle dorsiflexion, because the talus is wider anteriorly than posteriorly. Although spreading cannot be performed passively by the operator, increasing anteroposterior movement is likely to increase other joint-play movements such as spreading.

Ankle

I. Talocrural Joint. Distraction (Fig. 16-49)
    P—Supine, with the knee flexed about 90°, the hip flexed and somewhat abducted
    O—Half-sits on the edge of the plinth, with his back to the patient. He wraps the patient's leg around his right side to support the knee on his iliac crest, tucking the lower

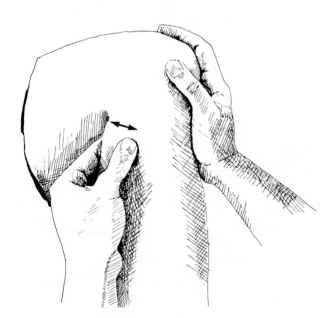

■ **FIG. 16-47.** Proximal tibiofibular joint: anteroposterior glide.

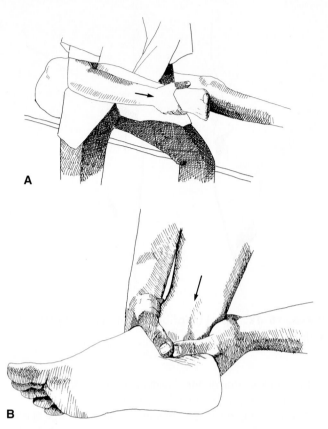

■ **FIG. 16-49.** Talocrural joint. Distraction: **(A)** position of the operator; **(B)** view of the operator's grip at the ankle.

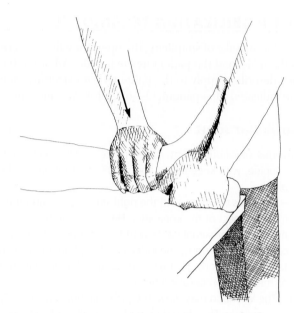

■ **FIG. 16-50.** Talocrural joint (left foot): posterior glide of tibia on talus.

leg between his elbow and side (Fig. 16-49*A*). The operator grasps the ankle with both hands so that the thumbs wrap around medially and the fingers laterally. The web of his right hand contacts the neck of the talus dorsally; the web of his left hand contacts the calcaneus posteriorly. The forearms are kept in line with the direction of force (Fig. 16-49*B*).

M—A distraction is imparted with both hands. The ankle may be slightly everted to help lock the subtalar joint.

  This technique is used to increase joint play at the ankle mortise joint. Distraction must occur here during plantar flexion, and is necessary for full movement toward the close-packed position, which is dorsiflexion.

II. Talocrural Joint. Posterior glide of tibia on talus (or anterior glide of talus on tibia; Fig. 16-50)

P—Supine

O—Stabilizes the talus and foot by grasping around medially to the posterior aspect of the calcaneus with the left hand. He contacts the distal tibia by placing his right hand over the anterior distal aspect of the tibia, just proximal to the malleoli.

M—The tibia is glided posteriorly on the talus with the right hand.

  Note: An anterior glide of the talus on the tibia may be performed by stabilizing the tibia with the one hand

and moving the talus anteriorly in the prone position (Fig. 16-35).

  Both of these techniques are used to increase joint-play movements necessary for plantar flexion at the ankle mortise joint.

III. Talocrural Joint. Posterior glide of the talus on the tibia (Fig. 16-51)

P—Supine, with the calcaneus hanging over the end of the plinth

O—Stabilizes the distal tibia against the plinth by grasping it with the left hand, wrapping the fingers around posteriorly. The left forearm rests over the dorsum of the

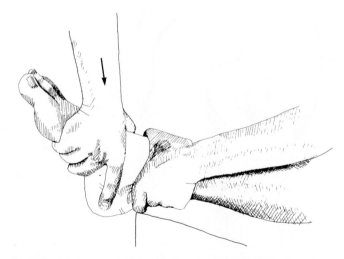

■ **FIG. 16-51.** Talocrural joint: posterior glide of talus on tibia.

patient's lower leg to prevent it from rising up from the plinth during the movement. He contacts the neck of the talus dorsally with the web of the right hand, bringing the thumb around laterally and the index finger medially. The remaining three fingers of the right hand wrap around the sole of the foot for support and control of the degree of plantar flexion.

M—The right hand moves the talus posteriorly on the tibia.

 This technique is used to increase joint-play movement necessary for ankle dorsiflexion.

IV. Subtalar Joint. Distraction

 This is performed in the same manner as distraction at the talocrural (refer to technique I), except that the dorsal handhold moves distally to contact the navicular. In this way the calcaneus is distracted from the talus by the navicular and cuboid. Alternatively, subtalar distraction may be performed in the prone position (Fig. 16-52). A sandbag is placed under the patient's talus. While one hand stabilizes the talus, the other hand glides the calcaneus distally (parallel to the sole of the foot).

V. Subtalar Joint. Valgus tilt (eversion; Fig. 16-53)

 P—Supine, with the knee flexed about 90°, the hip flexed and somewhat abducted

 O—Assumes the same position as for distraction (Fig. 16-49A) and grasps the ankle so that the thumb pads contact the medial aspect of the calcaneus and the remaining finger pads contact laterally, just proximal to the calcaneus and level with the sinus tarsi

 M—A valgus tilt of the calcaneus is produced by ulnar deviation of the wrists, transmitting the force through the thumb pads. The finger pads act as a fulcrum about which the movement occurs. This technique is used to increase eversion at the subtalar joint.

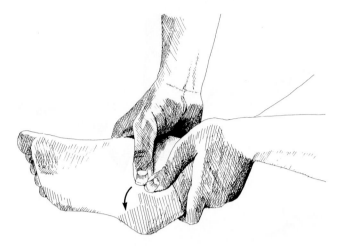

■ **FIG. 16-53.** Subtalar joint: valgus tilt (eversion).

VI. Subtalar Joint. Varus tilt (inversion; Fig. 16-54)

 This is carried out in the same manner as valgus tilt (refer to technique V). The operator's thumb pads move just proximal to the calcaneus; the finger pads move distally to contact the calcaneus laterally. The finger pads move the calcaneus into inversion about a fulcrum created by the thumb pads.

 This technique is used to increase inversion at the subtalar joint.

VII. Subtalar Joint. Dorsal rock of the calcaneus on the talus (Fig. 16-55)

 P—Supine, with the knee flexed about 90°, the hip flexed and somewhat abducted

 O—Assumes the same position as for distraction (Fig. 16-49A) and stabilizes the talus dorsally with the web of the right hand, wrapping the thumb around medially and the fingers laterally. He contacts the upper border of the calcaneus posteriorly with the web of his left hand in a similar fashion.

 M—While the right hand stabilizes the talus, the left hand rocks the calcaneus forward and dorsally.

 Note: According to Mennell,[144] a small amount of movement must occur at the subtalar joint at the

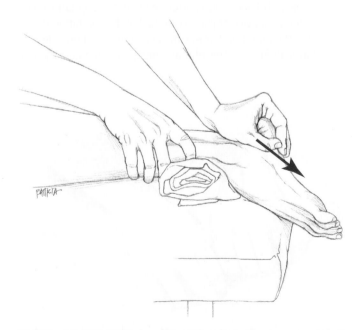

■ **FIG. 16-52.** Subtalar distraction in prone.

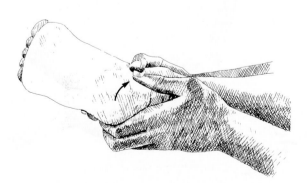

■ **FIG. 16-54.** Subtalar joint: varus tilt (inversion).

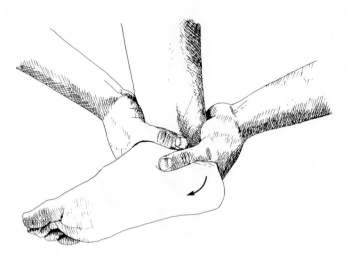

■ **FIG. 16-55.** Dorsal rock of the calcaneus on the talus.

extremes of plantar flexion and dorsiflexion. This technique, and the one that follows, have been developed to restore that movement.

VIII. Subtalar Joint. Plantar rock of the calcaneus on the talus (Fig. 16-56)

This is carried out in the same manner as dorsal rock (refer to technique VII), except the handholds are changed so that the right hand moves down to contact the navicular. The navicular tubercle is used as a landmark. The left hand moves just proximal to the posterior aspect of the calcaneus. The right hand rocks the calcaneus backward and plantarly via the navicular and cuboid. The web of the left hand acts as a fulcrum about which movement occurs.

IX. Dorsal Rock to Tibia (Fig. 16-43)

P—Supine with the knee flexed and the heel placed on the table (the ankle in the resting position). The calcaneus and indirectly the talus are fixated on the table.

O—Stands facing the patient with the hand wrapped around the lower leg (just proximal to the ankle joint)

M—Move the patient's tibia dorsally (by operator leaning forward and backward) in a repetitive fashion.

This is an effective way of restoring motion to the subtalar for plantar flexion as well as dorsiflexion (indirectly) by possibly breaking up adhesions that have formed in the talocrural joint.

Foot

I. Transverse Tarsal Joints (Talonavicular and Calcaneocuboid Joints). Dorsal-plantar glide (Fig. 16-57)

P—Supine, with the knee bent about 60°, the heel resting on the plinth

O—The left hand fixes the calcaneus and talus to the plinth by grasping dorsally at the level of the talar neck, the thumb wrapping around laterally and the rest of the fingers medially. The right hand grasps the navicular, using the navicular tubercle as a landmark. The web and the thumb contact dorsally, and the hand and fingers wrap around the foot medially and plantarly.

M—As the left hand stabilizes and prevents movement at the ankle, the right hand may move the navicular dorsally or plantarly on the talus.

The cuboid is moved in a similar manner, with one hand fixating the calcaneus and talus while the other hand moves the cuboid dorsally or plantarly on the calcaneus. These techniques are used to increase joint play at the forefoot.

II. Naviculocuneiform Joint. Dorsal-plantar glide (Fig. 16-58)

This is performed in the same manner as dorsal-plantar glide at the talonavicular joint (refer to technique I), with the handholds moved distally. The left hand stabilizes the navicular while the right hand moves the cuneiforms.

This technique is used to increase joint play at the forefoot.

III. Cuneiform–Metatarsal Joints. Dorsal-plantar glide

This technique is also performed in the same manner as for the talonavicular joint, with the handholds shifted distally. The right hand grasps the cuneiforms and provides stabilization while the left hand moves the metatarsal joints.

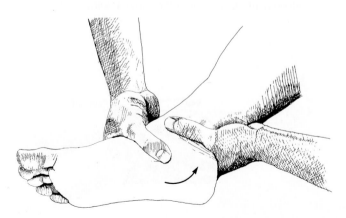

■ **FIG. 16-56.** Plantar rock of the calcaneus on the talus.

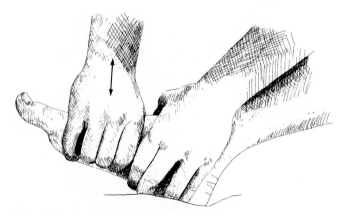

■ **FIG. 16-57.** Transverse tarsal joints: dorsal-plantar glide.

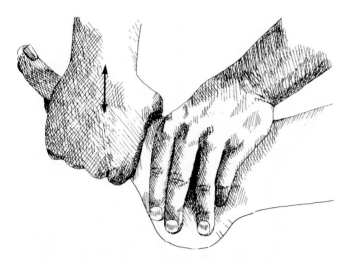

■ **FIG. 16-58.** Naviculocuneiform joint: dorsal-plantar glide.

This technique, like techniques I and II for the talonavicular and naviculocuneiform joints, is used to increase joint play of the forefoot.

IV. Cuneiform–Metatarsal and Cuboid–Metatarsal Joints. Rotation (pronation and supination; Fig. 16-59)

P—Supine, with the knee bent about 70°, the heel resting on the plinth

O—Stabilizes the cuneiforms and cuboid with the left hand, the thumb wrapping around the foot dorsally, the fingers plantarly. For pronation, the operator's right hand grasps the proximal metatarsal shafts from the lateral aspect, with the thumb contacting dorsally and the fingers plantarly. His forearm is supinated (Fig. 16-59A). For supination, the operator's right hand grasps the proximal metatarsal shafts from the medial aspect, with the thumb contacting dorsally and the fingers plantarly. His forearm is pronated (Fig. 16-59B).

M—The right hand rotates the metatarsals, as a unit, into pronation or supination.

These techniques are used to restore pronation and supination to the forefoot.

V. Cuboid–Metatarsal Joint. Dorsal-plantar glide

This technique is performed as dorsal-plantar glide at the calcaneocuboid joint (refer to technique I), with the handholds moved distally. The proximal hand stabilizes the cuboid while the distal hand moves the fourth and fifth metatarsal joints. This technique, like technique III for the cuneiform–metatarsal joints, is used to increase joint play of the forefoot.

VI. Manipulation of Cuboid and Navicular Joints. Whip and squeeze techniques (Fig. 16-60)

P—Prone with the thigh and leg beyond the table and flexed at 30° or, even better, standing and leaning forward on the table (Fig. 16-60A)

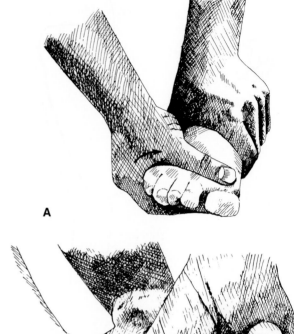

A

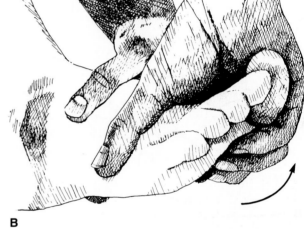

B

■ **FIG. 16-59.** Rotation of cuneiform–metatarsal and cuboid–metatarsal joints: (**A**) pronation and (**B**) supination.

O—Standing at the foot end of the table, the operator holds the foot, pressing on the cuboid with both thumbs superimposed (Fig. 16-60B)

M—The arms of the operator are extended so that the pressure on the cuboid causes knee flexion and dorsiflexion. Finally when the foot is relaxed, a thrusting movement similar to cracking a whip, is performed (tractional plantar-flexion thrust) laterally at a 45° angle.

This action usually allows the subluxed cuboid (inferolateral) to move dorsally back into place. Treatment is identical to that of the cuboid for manipulation of an inferior navicular when present in the pronated foot. Dorsal glide of the cuboid or navicular joints can be effectively applied in the prone position. Marshall and Hamilton[135] believe that a technique called the "cuboid squeeze" is far more effective than the cuboid whip. To perform the squeeze technique, the clinician gradually stretches the foot and ankle into maximum plantar flexion. When

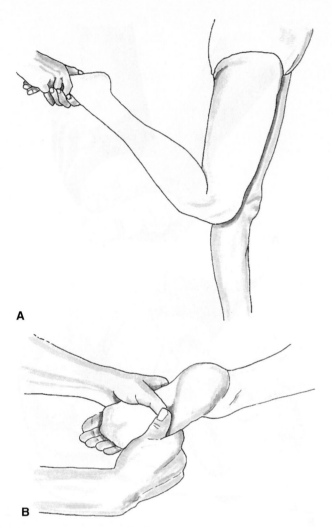

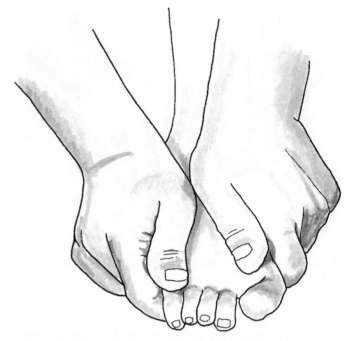

■ **FIG. 16-61.** Intermetatarsal and tarsometatarsal joints: dorsal-plantar glide.

■ **FIG. 16-60.** Manipulation of the cuboid and navicular joints: **(A)** whip and **(B)** squeeze techniques.

tion, the mobilizing hand glides the metatarsal in a dorsal or plantar direction.

Movements can be performed between the second and first, the third and fourth, and the fourth and fifth metatarsal bones. The purpose is to restore or increase joint play in the intermetatarsal articulations in the presence of hypomobility and to decrease pain in the forefoot. Movements will simultaneously take place in the tarsometatarsal joints and between the MTP joints.

Toes

Note: The use of a surgical glove, athletic underwrap used in adhesive taping, or a tongue blade taped to the toe may assist the operator in obtaining a stronger grip by reducing slippage and in directing a more precise mobilization of the toes.

the operator feels the soft tissues relax, the cuboid is reduced with a final squeeze of the thumbs.

These techniques should be followed with a low-dye strapping procedure to give added arch support for 1 to 2 weeks.[217] The management of chronic subluxations should include instruction in self-mobilization techniques.

VII. Intermetatarsal and Tarsometatarsal Joints. Dorsal-medial glide (Fig. 16-61)

P—Supine, with the foot in a neutral position

O—Facing the dorsal surface of the foot, the stabilizing hand grips the midshaft of one metatarsal with the thumb on the dorsal aspect and the index finger on the plantar aspect.

M—The mobilizing hand grips the midshaft of the adjacent metatarsal in the same manner as the stabilizing hand. While the stabilizing hand holds one metatarsal in posi-

I. MTP Joints. Distraction (Fig. 16-62)

P—Supine

O—Facing the dorsal aspect of the foot; the stabilizing hand holds the midfoot securely, while the thumb and forefinger of the mobilizing hand grasp the first phalanx at the MTP joint. The MTP joint is positioned in the resting position if conservative techniques are indicated or near the restricted end range if more aggressive techniques are indicated.

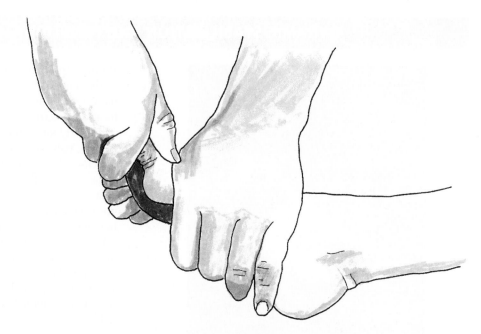

■ **FIG. 16-62.** Metatarsophalangeal joints: distraction.

M—The mobilizing hand moves the base of the proximal phalanx distally.

This is a useful technique in increasing joint play in the MTP joint and overall range of motion. A hallux valgus deformity is usually caused by improperly fitting shoes or has a genetic origin. Because of this, the treatment of choice is mechanical, such as orthotics or surgery. However, along with this, mobilization should be used to help increase the abduction of the first MTP joint.[35] Mobilization of the MTP joint—with oscillatory movements in dorsal-plantar glide, medial-lateral glide, abduction, adduction, rotation, and compression—may provide pain relief.

II. MTP Joints. Dorsal-plantar glide (Fig 16-63)

P—Prone or supine with the forefoot supported on the table or with a sandbag or wedge, toes extended over the edge of the table

O—Standing beside the patient and facing the foot; the stabilizing hand grips the head of the metatarsal between the thumb and index finger.

M—The mobilizing hand grips the proximal phalanx (dorsal and plantar aspect) between the thumb and index fingers. The MTP joint is positioned in the resting position or approximating the restricted range if more aggressive techniques are indicated. The mobilizing hand glides the proximal phalanx in a dorsal direction (Fig. 16-63*A,* patient prone) or plantar direction (Fig. 16-63*B,* patient supine) while using grade I traction.

The purpose of these techniques is to increase joint play in the MTP joints; plantar glide for restricted flexion and dorsal glide for restricted extension.

As to the remaining joints of the foot, the interphalangeal joints may be mobilized in the same manner as that described for the corresponding joints of the hand. Self-mobilization should be considered in chronic conditions.

The patient can be taught self-mobilization of arthrokinematic motions.

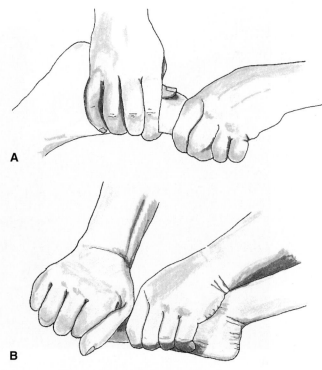

A

B

■ **FIG. 16-63.** Metatarsophalangeal joints: **(A)** dorsal and **(B)** plantar glide.

DYNAMIC STABILIZATION AND FUNCTIONAL EXERCISES

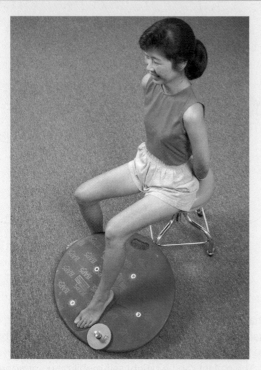

■ **FIG. 16-64.** Use of a balance board in a seated position allows early proprioceptive training.

Proprioception has been shown to be impaired after an injury to the ankle.[36,48] It is theorized that joint nerve receptors are damaged and must be retrained before one may safely return to activity. Exercises to improve proprioception might begin with short foot exercises (see Fig. 14-46) allowing focused training on balance and muscle coordination, which helps to increase afferent input, mainly from the sole.[15] Once the patient has achieved sufficient skill, exercises on rocker boards and later on a wobble board are added starting in sitting (Fig. 16-64), progressing to balancing on one foot and multidirectional board balancing (see Fig. 14-45), and eventually progressing to tubing-resisted hip motions while bearing weight on the involved ankle (standing on the injured leg forces this ankle to respond to the resistance applied to the other leg; see Fig. 14-38). This strengthen the involved leg and stimulates proprioception Additional exercises might include playing catch while balancing on the affected limb (Fig. 16-65), using multiplanar proprioceptive neuromuscular facilitation techniques to provided for rotational stress (see Fig. 14-44) and single-leg squats (see Fig. 15-64). Other activities such as balance beams, Pilates equipment, foam rolls, foam cushions, Swiss balls, and mini-trampolines provide proprioceptive and balance challenges.

Balance shoes (see Fig. 14-45E) are exceptionally useful, and increase demands on the entire postural mechanism and automatically, without conscious effort, help to correct pos-

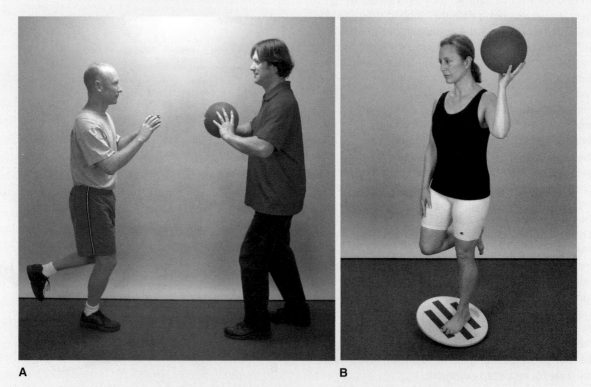

A   B

■ **FIG. 16-65.** Various activities with opposite and upper limbs can be performed to improve proprioception in the affected limb. **(A)** Single-leg stance on the affected limb while playing catch. **(B)** Playing catch while balancing on a wobble board.

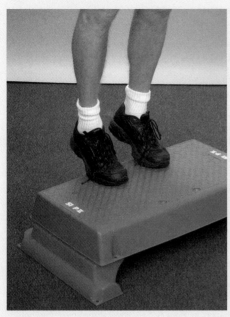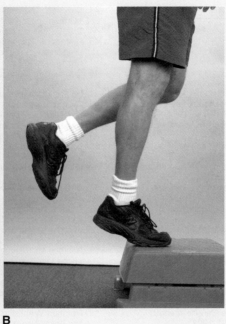

A   **B**

■ **FIG. 16-66.** Strengthening the gastrocnemius–soleus–Achilles complex through concentric (**A**) and eccentric contraction. (**B**) Performing the exercise with a single-leg stance provides greater resistance.

ture. When worn during the day, better coordination and increased speed of muscle contraction can be noticed within 1 week of training, attributed to improved activation of the gluteal muscles.[15,96] Subjects with grade II+ or ankle sprains demonstrated significant decreases in vibration perception and delayed recruitment of gluteus maximus during hip extension.[13,14] Gait should be trained in place first with some support to avoid instability and falls. Progressively more difficult gait patterns in the balance shoes can be added.

Open-chain strengthening exercises are described in numerous texts and will not be addressed here.[76,110,160,168,180,205] Closed kinetic chain exercises include strengthening of the gastrocnemius–soleus–Achilles complex through concentric and eccentric contractions (Fig. 16-66) and isolated soleus strengthening (Fig. 16-67). There are great demands on the

soleus as it decelerates the forward progressing tibia between initial contact and midstance running. After range of motion is within normal limits and strength has returned to normal, sport-specific and functional training can be implemented. Exercise options include plyometric, box drills, slide board, and lateral shuffles. The mini-trampoline allows early weight-bearing activities, enabling the patient to perform light jogging, jumping motions, and plyometric drills (Fig. 16-68).

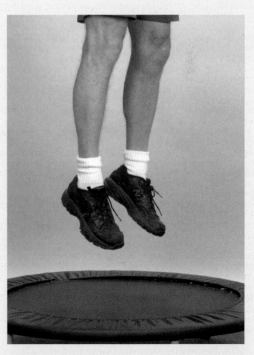

■ **FIG. 16-68.** Mini-trampoline to initiate light jogging and jumping activities to which other functional plyometric activities may be added.

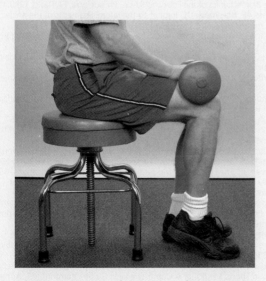

■ **FIG. 16-67.** Isolation of the soleus for strengthening.

REFERENCES

1. Alldredge RH: Diastases of the distal tibiofibular joint and associated lesions. JAMA 115:2136–2140, 1940
2. American Medical Association, Subcommittee on Classification of Sports Injuries: Standard Nomenclature of Athletic Injuries. Chicago, American Medical Association, 1966:122–126
3. Anderson JL, George F, Krakauer LJ, et al: Year Book of Sports Medicine. Chicago, Year Book Medical Publishers Inc, 1982
4. Anderson KJ, LeCocq JF: Operative treatment of injuries to the fibular collateral ligament of the ankle. J Bone Joint Surg Am 36:825–832, 1954
5. Andrews JR: Overuse syndromes of the lower extremity. Clin Sports Med 2:139–148, 1983
6. Appenzeller O, Atkinson R: Sports Medicine: Fitness Training, Injuries, 2nd ed. Baltimore, Urban & Schwarzenberg, 1983:413–414
7. Barnett CH, Napier JR: The axis of rotation at the ankle joint in man: Its influence upon the form of the mobility of the fibula. J Anat 86:1–9, 1952
8. Bateman JE: The adult heel. In: Jahss MH, ed: Disorders of the Foot, vol. 1. Philadelphia, WB Saunders, 1982
9. Bates B: Running biomechanics. Presented at American Orthopedic Foot Society Meeting, New Orleans, 1982
10. Bates BT, Osternig LR, James MS, et al: Foot orthotic devices to modify selected aspects of lower extremity mechanics. Am J Sports Med 7:338–342, 1979
11. Boeing DD: Evaluation of a clinical method of gait analysis. Phys Ther 57:795–798, 1977
12. Brody DM: Running injuries. Clin Symp 32:2–36, 1980
13. Bullock-Saxton JE: Local sensation changes and altered hip muscle function following severe ankle sprains. Phys Ther 74:17–31, 1994
14. Bullock-Saxton JE, Bullock MI: Changes in hip and knee muscle strength associated with ankle injury. N Z J Physiother 21:10–14, 1993
15. Bullock-Saxton JE, Janda V, Bullock MI: Reflex activation of gluteal muscles in walking. Spine 18:704–708, 1993
16. Bywater EG: Heel lesions of rheumatoid arthritis. Ann Rheum Dis 13:42–51, 1953
17. Cailliet R: Foot and Ankle Pain, 3rd ed. Philadelphia, FA Davis, 1997
18. Campbell JW, Inman VT: Treatment of plantar fasciitis and calcaneal spurs with the UC-BL shoe insert. Clin Orthop 103:57–62, 1974
19. Carson WG: Diagnosis of extensor mechanism disorders. Clin Sports Med 4:231–246, 1985
20. Cedell CA: Supination-outward rotation injuries of the ankle. Acta Orthop Scand Suppl 110:1–148, 1967
21. Cedell CA: Ankle lesions. Acta Orthop Scand 46:425–445, 1976
22. Clancy WG: Tendinitis and plantar fasciitis in runners. In: D'Ambrosia R, Drez D, eds: Prevention and Treatment of Running Injuries. Thorofare, NJ, Slack, 1982:77–87
23. Clarkston HM, Gilewish GB: Musculoskeletal Assessment, Joint Range of Motion and Manual Muscle Testing. Baltimore, Williams & Wilkins, 1989
24. Clement DB, Taunton JE, Smart GW: Achilles tendinitis and peritendinitis: Etiology and treatment. Am J Sports Med 12:179–184, 1984
25. Close JR, Inman VT, Poor PM, et al: The function of the subtalar joint. Clin Orthop 50:159–179, 1967
26. Cole JH, Furness AL, Twomey LT: Muscle in Action, an Approach to Manual Muscle Testing. Edinburgh, Churchill Livingstone, 1988
27. Colson JW, Berglund G: An effective orthotic design for controlling the unstable subtalar joint. Orthot Prosthet 33:39–49, 1979
28. Cook SD, Brinker MR, Poche M: Running shoes: Their relationship to running injuries. Sports Med 10:1–8, 1990
29. Cook SD, Kester MA, et al: Biomechanics of running shoe performance. Clin Sports Med 4:619–626, 1985
30. Corrigan B, Maitland GD: Practical Orthopaedic Medicine. London, Butterworth, 1985:212–213
31. Cyriax J: Textbook of Orthopaedic Medicine—Diagnosis of Soft Tissue Lesions, 8th ed. London, Bailliere Tindall, 1982
32. Daffner RH: Stress fractures: Current concepts. Skeletal Radiol 2:221–229, 1978
33. D'Ambrosia RD: Orthotic devices in running injuries. Clin Sports Med 4:611–618, 1985
34. D'Ambrosia RD, Drez D: Orthotics. In: D'Ambrosia RD, Drez D, eds: Prevention and Treatment of Running Injuries. Thorofare, NJ, Slack, 1982
35. Davis DG: Manipulation of the lower extremity. In: Subotnick SI, ed: Sports Medicine of the Lower Extremity. New York, Churchill Livingstone, 1989:397–417
36. Day RW, Wildermuth BP: Proprioceptive training in the rehabilitation of lower extremity injuries. Adv Sports Med Fitness 1:241–258, 1988
37. De Souza Dias DL, Foerster TP: Traumatic lesions of the ankle joint: The supination external rotation mechanism. Clin Orthop 100:219–224, 1974
38. Devas M: Stress Fractures. London, Churchill Livingstone, 1975:224–227
39. Donatelli R: Normal biomechanics of the foot and ankle. J Orthop Sports Phys Ther 7:91–95, 1985
40. Donatelli R: Abnormal biomechanics of the foot and ankle. J Orthop Phys Sports Ther 9:11–16, 1987
41. Donatelli R: Normal anatomy and biomechanics. In: Donatelli R, Wolf SL, eds: The Biomechanics of the Foot and Ankle. Philadelphia, FA Davis, 1990
42. Dowd I: In honor of the foot. Contact Q (Fall):33–39, 1986
43. Doxey GE: The semi-flexible foot orthotic, fabrication and guidelines for use. J Orthop Sports Phys Ther 5:26–29, 1983
44. Drez D: Running footwear. Am J Sports Med 8:140–141, 1980
45. Duggar GE: Plantar fasciitis and heel spurs. In: McGlawry ED, ed: Reconstructive Surgery of the Foot and Leg. New York, Intercontinental Medical Book Co, 1974:67–73
46. Durman DC: Metatarsus primus varus and hallux valgus. Arch Surg 74:128–135, 1957
47. DuVries HL: Surgery of the Foot, 4th ed. St Louis, CV Mosby Co, 1959:287–291
48. Dwight T: Variations of the Bones of the Hands and Feet: A Clinical Atlas. Philadelphia, JB Lippincott, 1907:14–23
49. Dwyer FC: Causes, significance and treatment of stiffness in the subtaloid joint. Proc R Soc Med 69:97–102, 1976
50. Eggnold JF: Orthotics in the prevention of runner's overuse injuries. Phys Sports Med 9:125–128, 1981
51. Eichenblat M, Nathan H: The proximal tibiofibular joint. Int Orthop 7:31–39, 1983
52. Eltman H: The transverse tarsal joint and its control. Clin Orthop 16:41–46, 1960
53. Exelby L: Peripheral mobilisations with movement. Man Ther 1:118–126, 1996
54. Forkin DM, Koczur C, Battle R et al: Evaluation of kinesthetic deficit indicative of balance control in gymnasts with unilateral chronic ankle sprains. J Orthop Sports Phys Ther 23:245–250, 1996
55. Freeman M: Treatment of ruptures of the lateral ligament of the ankle. J Bone Joint Surg Br 47:661–668, 1965a
56. Freeman M: Instability of the foot after injuries to the lateral ligament of the ankle. J Bone Joint Surg Br 47:669–677, 1965b
57. Freeman M: The etiology and prevention of instability of the foot. J Bone Joint Surg Br 47:678–685, 1965c
58. Fromherz WA: Examination. In: Hunt GC, ed: Physical Therapy of the Foot and Ankle. New York, Churchill Livingstone, 1988:59–90
59. Fulp MJ: Ankle joint injuries. J Am Podiatry Assoc 65:889–911, 1975
60. Furey JG: Plantar fasciitis: The painful heel syndrome. J Bone Joint Surg Am 57:672–673, 1975
61. Garbalosa JC: Physical therapy. In: Donatelli R, Wolf SL, eds: The Biomechanics of the Foot and Ankle. Philadelphia, FA Davis, 1990:217–247
62. Gardner E, Gray DJ, O'Rahilly R: Anatomy: A Regional Study of Human Structure, 4th ed. Philadelphia, WB Saunders, 1978
63. Garrick JG, Requa RK: Role of external support in the prevention of ankle sprains. Med Sci Sports 5:200–203, 1973
64. Gerbert J: Ligament injuries of the ankle joint. J Am Podiatr Assoc 65:802–815, 1975
65. Gerster JC: Plantar fasciitis and Achilles tendinitis among 150 cases of seronegative spondarthritis. Rheum Rehabil 9:218–222, 1980
66. Gerster JC, Vischer TL, Bennani A: The painful heel. Ann Rheum Dis 36:343–348, 1977
67. Geslien GE, Thrall JH, Espinosa JL: Early detection of stress fractures using 99m Tc-polyphosphate. Radiology 121:683–687, 1976
68. Gillette: Des os sesamoides chez l'homme. J Anat Physiol 8:506–538, 1872
69. Glenncross D, Thorton E: Position sense following joint injury. J Sports Med Phys Fitness 21:23–27, 1981
70. Gorman D: The Body Moveable. Guelph, Ontario, Ampersand Press, 1981
71. Gould JS: Metatarsalgia. Orthop Clin North Am 20:553–562, 1989
72. Gray GW: When the Foot Hits the Ground Everything Changes. Toledo, OH, The American Physical Rehabilitation Network, 1984
73. Greenfield B: Evaluation of overuse syndromes. In: Donatelli R, Wolf SL, eds: The Biomechanics of the Foot and Ankle. Philadelphia, FA Davis, 1990:153–177
74. Gross AE, MacIntosh DL: Injuries to the lateral ligaments of the ankle: A clinical study. Can J Surg 16:115–117, 1973
75. Gungor T: A test for ankle instability: Brief report. J Bone Joint Surg Br 53:333–337, 1988
76. Hall CM, Brody LT: Therapeutic Exercise: Moving to Function. Philadelphia, Lippincott Williams & Wilkins, 1998
77. Hartley A: Knee assessment. In: Hartley A, ed: Practical Joint Assessment. St Louis, Mosby Year Book, 1990
78. Henderson WH, Campbell JW: UC-BL shoe inserts: Casting and fabrication. Bull Prosthet Res 10:215–235, 1969
79. Hicks JH: The mechanics of the foot: I. The joints. J Anat 87:345–357, 1953
80. Hicks JH: The mechanics of the foot: II. The plantar aponeurosis and the arch. J Anat 88:25–30, 1954
81. Hislop HJ, Montgomery J: Daniels and Worthingham's Muscle Testing, Techniques of Manual Examination, 6th ed. Philadelphia, WB Saunders, 1995
82. Hlavac HF: The Foot Book. Mountain View, CA, World Publications, 1977
83. Hollinshead WH: Leg and foot. In: Hollinshead WH, ed: Textbook of Anatomy, 3rd ed. Hagerstown, MD, Harper & Row, 1974:423–490
84. Hoppenfeld S: Physical examination of the foot and ankle. In: Hoppenfeld S, ed: Physical Examination of the Spine and Extremities. New York, Appleton-Century-Crofts, 1976:197–236
85. Hunt GC: Examination of lower extremity dysfunction. In: Gould JA, Davies GJ, eds: Orthopaedic and Sports Physical Therapy. St Louis, CV Mosby, 1985:408–436
86. Hurwitz S, Ernst GP, Yi S: The foot and ankle. In: Canavan PK, ed: Rehabilitation in Sports Medicine: A Comprehensive Guide. Stamford, CT, Appleton & Lange, 1998:325–382

87. Hutton WC, Dhanedran M: The mechanics of normal and hallux valgus feet: A quantitative study. Clin Orthop 157:7–13, 1981

88. Inman VT: The Joints of the Ankle. Baltimore, Williams & Wilkins, 1976

89. Jablonowski GJ: Foot and ankle dysfunction. In: Kaplan PE, Tanner ED, eds: Musculoskeletal Pain and Disability. Norwalk, CT, Appleton & Lange, 1989:203–242

90. Jackson DW: Ankle sprains in young athletes: Relation of severity and disability. Clin Orthop 101:201–219, 1974

91. Jahss MH, Kummer F, Michelson JD: Investigations into the fat pads of the sole of the foot: Heel pressure studies. Foot Ankle 13:227–232, 1992

92. Jahss MH, Michelson JD: Investigations into the fats of the sole of the foot: Anatomy and histology. Foot Ankle 13:223–242, 1992

93. James SI: Chondromalacia of the patella in the adolescent. In: Kennedy JC, ed: The Injured Adolescent Knee. Baltimore, Williams & Wilkins, 1979:214–228

94. James SI, Bates BT, Ostery LR: Injuries to runners. Am J Sports Med 6:40–50, 1978

95. Janda V: Muscle Function Testing. Boston, Butterworth, 1983

96. Janda V, Va Vrova M: Sensory Motor Stimulation. In: Liebenson C, ed: Rehabilitation of the Spine: A Practitioner's Manual. Philadelphia, Lippincott Williams & Wilkins, 1996:319–328

97. Jones DC, James SL: Overuse injuries of the lower extremity. Clin Sports Med 6:273–290, 1987

98. Jones FW: Structure and Function as Seen in the Foot, 2nd ed. London, Bailiere, Tindall & Cox, 1949

99. Jull GA, Janda V: Muscles and motor control in low back pain: Assessment and Management. In: Twoney LT, Taylor JR, eds: Physical Therapy of the Low Back. New York, Churchill Livingstone, 1987: 253–278

100. Kapandji IA: The Physiology of Joints: The Lower Limb, vol. 2. Edinburgh, Churchill Livingstone, 1970

101. Karr SD: Subcalcaneal heel pain. Orthop Clin North Am 25:161–175, 1994

102. Katoh Y, Chao EY, Morrey BF, et al: Objective technique for evaluating painful heel syndrome and its treatment. Foot Ankle 3:227–237, 1983

103. Kay DB: The sprained ankle: Current therapy. Foot Ankle 6:22–28, 1985

104. Kelikian H: Hallux Valgus: Allied Deformities of the Forefoot and Metatarsalgia. Philadelphia, WB Saunders, 1965:102–112

105. Kelikian H, Kelikian AS: Disorders of the Ankle. Philadelphia, WB Saunders Co, 1985

106. Kendall FP, McCreary EK, Provance PG: Muscle Testing and Function, 4th ed. Baltimore, Williams & Wilkins, 1993

107. Key J, Jarvis G, Johnson D, et al: Leg injuries. In: Subotnick SI, ed: Sports Medicine of the Lower Extremity. New York, Churchill Livingstone, 1989:187–296

108. Kibler WB: Rehabilitation of the ankle and foot. In: Kibler WB, Herring SA, Press JM, eds: Functional Rehabilitation of Sports and Musculoskeletal Injuries. Gaithersburg, MD, Aspen Publishers, 1998:273–283

109. Kibler WB, Goldberg C, Chandler TJ: Functional biomechanical deficits in running athletes with plantar fasciitis. Am J Sports Med 19:66–71, 1991

110. Kisner C, Colby LA: Therapeutic Exercise: Foundations and Techniques. 3rd ed. Philadelphia, F.A. Davis, 1996

111. Kleiger B: Mechanisms of ankle injury. Orthop Clin North Am 5:153–176, 1974

112. Kohler A, Simmer EA: Borderlands of the Normal and Early Pathologic in Skeletal Roentgenology, 3rd ed. New York, Grune & Stratton, 1968

113. Konin JG, Wiksten DL, Isear JA: Special Tests for Orthopedic Examination. Thorofare, NJ, Slack, 1997

114. Kosmahl EM, Kosmahl HE: Painful plantar heel, plantar fasciitis, and calcaneal spur: Etiology and treatment. J Orthop Sports Phys Ther 9:17–24, 1987

115. Kraeger DR: Foot injuries. In: Lillegard WA, Rucker KS, eds: Handbook of Sports Medicine: A Symptom-Oriented Approach. Boston, Andover Medical Publishers, 1993:159–171

116. Kwong PK, Kay D, Voner RT, et al: Plantar fasciitis: Mechanics and pathomechanics of treatment. Clin Sports Med 7:119–126, 1988

117. Lamoreux L: Kinematic measurements in the study of human walking. Bull Prosthet Res 10:3–84, 1971

118. Langer S: Posting: Theory and practice. Langer Lab Bio Mech New Lett 1:3, Deer Park, New York, Professional Protective Technology, Inc., the Langer Group, 1973

119. Leonard MH: Injuries of the lateral ligaments of the ankle: A clinical and experimental study. J Bone Joint Surg Am 31:373–377, 1949

120. Levandowski R, Difort JP: Leg injuries. In: Birrer RB, ed: Sports Medicine for the Primary Physician, 2nd ed. Boca Raton, FL, CRC Press, 1994:531–541

121. Level AS, Inman VT, Blosser JA: Transverse rotation of the segments of the lower extremity in locomotion. J Bone Joint Surg Am 30:859–872, 1948

122. Lindstrand A: New aspects in the diagnosis of lateral ankle sprains. Orthop Clin North Am 7:247–249, 1976

123. Lutter LD: The knee and running. Clin Sports Med 4:685–698, 1985

124. MacConnaill MA, Basmajian JV: Muscles and Movements: A Basis for Human Kinesiology. Baltimore, Williams & Wilkins, 1969:74–84

125. Magee DJ: Lower leg, ankle, and foot. In: Magee DJ: Orthopedic Physical Assessment, 3rd ed. Philadelphia, WB Saunders, 1997:599–672

126. Maigne R: Manipulations and mobilization of the limbs. In: Rogoff JB, ed: Manipulation, Traction and Massage, 2nd ed. Baltimore, Williams & Wilkins, 1980:121–139

127. Mann RA: Biomechanics of running. In: Mack RP, ed: Symposium on the Foot and Leg in Running Sports. St Louis, CV Mosby, 1982:1–29

128. Mann RA, Coughlin MJ: Keratotic disorders of the plantar skin. In: Mann RA, Coughlin MJ: Surgery of the Foot and Ankle, vol. 1, 6th ed. St Louis, CV Mosby, 1993

129. Mann RA, Hagy JL: The function of the toes in walking, jogging and running. Clin Orthop 142:24–29, 1979

130. Mann RA, Hagy JL: Running, jogging and walking: A comparative electromyographic and biomechanical study. In: Bateman JE, Trott AW, eds: The Foot and Ankle. New York, Brian C Decker, 1980

131. Manner-Smith T: A study of the cuboid and os peroneum in the primate foot. J Anat Physiol 42:399–414, 1908

132. Manter JT: Movements of the subtalar and transverse tarsal joints. Anat Rec 80:397–410, 1941

133. Markey KL: Stress fractures. Clin Sports Med 6:405–425, 1987

134. Marshall P: The rehabilitation of overuse foot injuries in athletes and dancers. Clin Sports Med 7:175–191, 1988

135. Marshall P, Hamilton WG: Cuboid subluxation in ballet dancers. Am J Sports Med 20:169–175, 1992

136. Marti T: Die Skeletvarietaten des Fusses ihre Klinische und Unfallmedizinische Bedentug. Berne, Hans Uber, 1947:27–111

137. McBryde A: Stress fractures in runners. In: D'Ambrosia RD, Drez D, eds: Prevention and Treatment of Running Injuries, 2nd ed. Thorofare, NJ, Slack, 1989:43–82

138. McCluskey GM, Blackburn TA, Lewis T: Treatment of ankle sprains. Am J Sports Med 4:158–161, 1976

139. McKenzie DC, Clements DB, Taunton JE: Running shoes, orthotics and injuries. Sports Med 2:334–347, 1985

140. McPoil TG, Brocato RS: The foot and ankle: Biomechanical evaluation and treatment. In: Gould JA, Davies GL, eds: Orthopaedic and Sports Physical Therapy. St Louis, CV Mosby, 1985:313–341

141. McPoil TG, Schuit D, Knecht HG: A comparison of three positions used to evaluate tibial varum. J Am Podiatr Med Assoc 78:22–28, 1988

142. McRae R: Clinical Orthopedics. New York, Churchill Livingstone, 1983

143. Melillo TV: Gastrocnemius equinus: Its diagnosis and treatment. Arch Podiatr Med Foot Surg 2:159–205, 1975

144. Mennell JM: Joint Pain. Boston, Little, Brown and Co, 1964

145. Metcalf GR, Denegar CR: A critical review of ankle taping. Athl Train 187:121, 1983

146. Michael RH, Holder LE: The soleus syndrome: A cause of medial tibial stress (shin splints). Am J Sports Med 13:87–98, 1985

147. Molnar ME: Rehabilitation of the injured ankle. Clin Sports Med 7:193–204, 1988

148. Morton DJ: The Human Foot: Its Evolution, Physiology and Functional Disorders. New York, Columbia University Press, 1935

149. Mubarak SJ, Gould RN, Lee YF, et al: The medial tibial stress syndrome. Am J Sports Med 10:201–205, 1982

150. Mulligan BR: Mobilsations with movement (MWMs) J Man Manip Ther 1:154–156, 1993

151. Mulligan BR: Manual Therapy 'Nags,' 'Snags,' 'MWMs' etc., 3rd ed. New Zealand, Plant View Services, 1999

152. Murray MP, Draught AP, Kory RC: Walking patterns in normal men. J Bone Joint Surg Am 46:335–360, 1964

153. Newell SG, Nutler S: Conservative treatment of plantar fascial strain. Phys Sports Med 5:68–73, 1977

154. Newell SG, Woodie A: Cuboid syndrome. Phys Sports Med 9:71–76, 1981

155. Nicholas JA: Ankle injuries in athletes. Orthop Clin North Am 5:153–176, 1974

156. Nicholas JA, Hershmann EB, eds: The Lower Extremity and Spine in Sports Medicine. St Louis, CV Mosby, 1986:601–655

157. Norkin CC, Levangie PK: The ankle–foot complex. In: Norkin CC, Levangie PK, eds: Joint Structure and Function, 2nd ed. Philadelphia, FA Davis, 1992:379–418

158. O'Rahilly R: Developmental deviations in the carpus and tarsus. Clin Orthop 10:9–18, 1957

159. Orava PJ, Puranene J, Ala-Ketola L: Stress fractures caused by physical exercise. Acta Orthop Scand 49:19–27, 1970

160. O'Sullivan SB, Schmitz TJ: Physical Rehabilitation Laboratory Manual: Focus on Functional Training. Philadelphia, FA Davis, 1999

161. Paice EW, Hoffbrand BI: Nutritional osteomalacia presenting with plantar fasciitis. J Bone Joint Surg Br 69:38–40, 1987

162. Palmer ML, Epler M, eds: Clinical Assessment in Physical Therapy, 2nd ed. Philadelphia, Lippincott Williams & Wilkins, 1998

163. Patton GW, Tursi FJ, Zelichowski JE: The dorsal fold of the first metatarsal phalangeal joint. J Am Podiatr Med Assoc 26:210–212, 1987

164. Paul IL, Munro MB, Abernathy PJ et al: Musculoskeletal shock absorption: Relative contribution of bone and soft tissues at various frequencies. J Biomech 11:237–239, 1978

165. Peiyer E, Wright DW, Mason L: Human locomotion. Bull Prosthet Res 10–12:48–105, 1969

166. Petty NJ, Moore AP: Neuromusculoskeletal Examination and Assessment: A Handbook for Therapist. Edinburgh, Churchill Livingstone, 1998

167. Prather JL, Nusynowitz ML, Snowdy HA, et al: Scintigraphic findings in stress fractures. J Bone Joint Surg Am 59:869–974, 1977

168. Prentice WE, Voight ML, eds: Techniques in Musculoskeletal Rehabilitation. New York, McGraw, Medical Publishing Division, 2001
169. Price GFW: Metatarsus primus varus—including various clinicoradiologic features of the female foot. Clin Orthop Relat Res 145:217–223, 1979
170. Ramig D, Shadle J, Watkins A, et al: The foot and sports medicine: Biomechanical foot faults as related to chondromalacia patellae. J Orthop Sports Phys Ther 2:48–50, 1980
171. Rebman LW: Ankle injuries: Clinical observations. J Orthop Sports Phys Ther 8:153–156, 1986
172. Reed JK: Orthotic devices, shoes and modifications. In: Hunt GC, ed: Physical Therapy of the Foot and Ankle. New York, Churchill Livingstone, 1988
173. Reid DC: Sports Injury Assessment and Rehabilitation. New York, Churchill Livingstone, 1992
174. Rocce D: The leg, ankle and foot. In: Rocce D, ed: The Musculoskeletal System in Health and Disease. Hagerstown, MD, Harper & Row, 1980
175. Root ML, Orien WP, Weed JH: Biomechanical Examination of the Foot, vol. 1. Los Angles, Clinical Biomechanics Corp, 1971
176. Root ML, Orien WP, Weed JN: Clinical Biomechanics, Normal and Abnormal Function of the Foot, vol. 2. Los Angeles, Clinical Biomechanic Corp, 1977
177. Rorabeck CH, Fowler PJ, Nott L: The results of fasciotomy in the management of chronic exertional compartment syndrome. Am J Sports Med 16:224–227, 1988
178. Rose GK, Welton EA, Marshall T: The diagnosis of flat foot in the child. J Bone Joint Surg Br 67:71–78, 1985
179. Roy SM, Irvin R: Injuries to the running athlete—Particularly the long-distance runner. In: Roy SM, Irvin R, eds: Sports Medicine: Prevention, Evaluation, Management, and Rehabilitation Englewood Cliffs, NJ, Prentice-Hall, 1983:433–435
180. Sahrmann SA: Diagnosis and Treatment of Movement Impairment Syndromes. St Louis, Mosby, 2002
181. Sammarco GJ, Burstein AH, Frankel VH: Biomechanics of the ankle: A kinematic study. Orthop Clin North Am 4:75–95, 1973
182. Santilli G: Achilles tendinopathies and paratendinopathies. J Sports Med 19:245–259, 1979
183. Sarrafian SK: Anatomy of the Foot and Ankle, 2nd ed. Philadelphia, JB Lippincott, 1993
184. Saunders JB, Dec M, Inman VT, et al: The major determinants in normal and pathological gait. J Bone Joint Surg Am 35:543–558, 1953
185. Scranton PE: Metatarsalgia diagnosis and treatment. J Bone Joint Surg Am 62:723–732, 1980
186. Scranton PE, Pedegana LR, Whitsel JP: Gait analysis: Alterations in support phase using supportive devices. Am J Sports Med 10:6–11, 1982
187. Sewell JR, Black CM, Statham J: Quantitative scintigraphy in diagnosis and management of plantar fasciitis (calcaneal periostitis): Concise communication. J Nucl Med 21:633–636, 1980
188. Sgarlato TE: A Compendium of Podiatric Biomechanics. San Francisco, College of Podiatric Medicine Press, 1971
189. Shore M: Footprint analysis in gait documentation: An instructional sheet format. Phys Ther 60:1163–1167, 1980
190. Slocum DB: The shin splint syndrome: Medical aspects and differential diagnosis. Am J Surg 114:875–881, 1967
191. Smith JW: The ligamentous structures in the canalis and sinus tarsi. J Anat 92:616–620, 1958
192. Smith S, Hall C, Brody LT: The ankle and foot. In: Hall CM, Brody LT, eds: Therapeutic Exercise: Moving toward Function. Philadelphia, Lippincott Williams & Wilkins, 1998: 470–498
193. Southmayd W, Marshall H: The lower leg. In: Southmayd W, Marshall H, eds: Sports Health: The Complete Book of Athletic Injuries. New York, Quick Fox, 1981:300–309
194. Standish WD, Curwin S, Rubinovich M: Tendinitis: The analysis and treatment for running. Clin Sports Med 4:593–609, 1985
195. Staples OS: Ruptures of the fibular collateral ligaments of the ankle: Result study of immediate surgical treatment. J Bone Joint Surg Am 57:101–107, 1975
196. Stonnington MJ: Lower leg, ankle, and foot. In: Buschbacher RM, Braddom RL, eds: Practical Guide to Musculoskeletal Disorders: Diagnosis and Rehabilitation. 2nd ed. Boston, Butterworth Heineman, 2002:229–254
197. Straus WL Jr: Growth of the human foot and its evolutionary significance. Contrib Embryol 19:101–116, 1927
198. Subotnick SI: Orthotic foot control and the overuse syndrome. Phys Sports Med 3:75–79, 1975a
199. Subotnick SI: Biomechanics of the subtalar and midtarsal joints. J Am Podiatr Med Assoc 65:756–764, 1975b
200. Subotnick SI: The cavus foot. Phys Sports Med 8:53–55, 1980
201. Subotnick SI: Foot injuries. In: Subotnick SI, ed: Sports Medicine of the Lower Extremities. New York, Churchill Livingstone, 1989a:237–239

202. Subotnick SI: Ankle injuries. In: Subotnick SI, ed: Sports Medicine of the Lower Extremities. New York, Churchill Livingstone, 1989b:277–278
203. Subotnick SI, Jones RE: Normal anatomy. In: Subotnick SI, ed: Sports Medicine of the Lower Extremities. New York, Churchill Livingstone, 1989:74–112
204. Subotnick SI, Newell SG: Podiatric sports medicine. In: Fielding MD, ed: Podiatric Medicine and Surgery. Mount Kisko, NY, Futura, 1975
205. Sullivan PE, Markos PD: Clinical Decision Making in Therapeutic Exercise. Norwalk, CT, Appleton & Lange, 1994
206. Tax H: Flexible flatfoot in children. J Am Podiatry Assoc 67:616–619, 1977
207. Thompson T, Doherty J: Spontaneous rupture of the tendon of Achilles. A new clinical diagnostic test. Ant Res 158:126, 1967
208. Trolle D: Accessory Bones of the Human Foot: A Radiological, Histo-embryological, Comparative Anatomical and Genetic Study. Copenhagen, Munksgaard, 1948
209. Troop H, Askling C, Gillquist J: Prevention of ankle sprains. Am J Sports Med 13:259–262, 1985
210. Van Pelt WL: Accommodating, strapping, and bracing. In: Subotnick SI, ed: Sports Medicine of the Lower Extremity. New York, Churchill Livingstone, 1989
211. Vidigal E, Jacoby RK, Dixon AJ: The foot in chronic rheumatoid arthritis. Ann Rheum Dis 34:292–297, 1975
212. Viitasale JT, Kust M: Some biomechanical aspects of the foot and ankle in athletes with and without shin splints. Am J Sports Med 11:125–130, 1983
213. Viladot A: The metatarsals. In: Jahss MH, ed: Disorders of the Foot, vol. 1. Philadelphia, WB Saunders, 1982:659–710
214. Vogler HW, Bauer GR: Contrast studies of the foot and ankle. In: Weissman SD: Radiology of the Foot, 2nd ed. Baltimore, Williams & Wilkins, 1989:439–495
215. Voight ML, Nashner LM, Blackburn TA: Neuromuscular function changes with ACL functional brace use: A measure of reflex latencies and lower quarter EMG responses. Abstract: Conference Proceedings, San Francisco, American Orthopedic Society for Sports Medicine, 1998
216. Wadsworth CT: Manual Examination and Treatment of the Spine and Extremities. Baltimore, Williams & Wilkins, 1988
217. Walker WC: Lower leg pain. In: Lillegard WA, Rucker KS, eds: Handbook of Sports Medicine: A Symptom-Oriented Approach. Boston, Andover Medical Publishers, 1993:150–158
218. Wallace L: Lower quarter pain: Mechanical evaluation and treatment (Continuing education course). Bellingham, WA, 1984
219. Wallace L: Foot pronation and knee pain. In: Hunt GC, ed: Physical Therapy of the Foot and Ankle. New York, Churchill Livingstone, 1988:101–122
220. Weissman SD: Podiatric pathology. In: Weissman SD, ed: Radiology of the Foot. Baltimore, Williams & Wilkins, 1989:106–109
221. Whitesel J, Newell SG: Modified low-dye strapping. Phys Sports Med 8:129–131, 1980
222. Wright DG, Desai SM, Henderson WH: Action of the subtalar and ankle complex during stance phase of walking. J Bone Joint Surg Am 46:361–382, 1964

RECOMMENDED READING

Dananberg HJ, Shearstone J, Guiliano M: Manipulation method for the treatment of ankle equinus. J Am Podiatr Med Assoc 90:385–389, 2000
Digiovanni BF, Gould JS: Achilles tendonitis and posterior heel disorders. Foot Ankle Clin 2:441–428, 1997
Ferkel R, Donatelli R, Hall W: Lateral ligament repair. In: Maxy L, Magnusson J, eds: Rehabilitation for the Postsurgical Orthopedic Patient. St. Louis, Mosby, 2001a:288–301
Ferkel R, Donatelli R, Hall W: Open reduction and internal fixation of the ankle. In: Maxy L, Magnusson J, eds: Rehabilitation for the Postsurgical Orthopedic Patient. St. Louis, Mosby, 2001b:302–313
Frey C: Ankle sprains. In: Sim FH, ed: Instructional Course Lectures. 50:515–520, Rosemont, II, 2001
Gottsacker PA: Physical therapy following fractures and surgery. In: Hunt GC, McPoil TG, eds: Physical Therapy of the Foot and Ankle, 2nd ed. New York, Churchill Livingstone, 1995
Mandelbaum B, Gruber J, Zachazewski J: Achilles tendon repair and rehabilitation. In: Maxy L, Magnusson J, eds: Rehabilitation for the Postsurgical Orthopedic Patient. St. Louis, Mosby, 2001:323–349
Porter DA, Clanton TO: Primary care of foot and ankle injuries in the athlete. Clin Sports Med 16:435–466, 1997
Ranawat CS, Positano RG: Disorders of the Heel, Rearfoot, and Ankle. New York, Churchill Livingstone, 1999

Temporomandibular Joint and Stomatognathic System

17

DARLENE HERTLING

Disease and dysfunction of the temporomandibular joints and the adjacent structures affect a large number of persons. More than 20% of the average population at one time or another has symptoms relating to the temporomandibular joint (TMJ).[172] Practitioners of dentistry and medicine have long been aware that the TMJs are among the few joints in the body that, like the vertebral joints, function as a unit in a sliding–gliding action because of the mandible, which links the two condyles together. However, the many intricacies of the TMJ are just beginning to be appreciated.

The term **stomatognathic system** is used to refer to the TMJs, the masticatory systems, its component structures, and all the tissues related to it. The designation includes a number of systematically related organs and tissues that function as a whole. The components of this system include the following:

- Bones of the skull, mandible, maxilla, hyoid, clavicle, and sternum
- Temporomandibular and dentoalveolar joints
- Muscles and soft tissues of the head and neck and the muscles of the cheeks, lips, and tongue
- Vascular, lymphatic, and nerve supply systems
- Teeth

The stomatognathic system functions almost continuously, not only in mastication and swallowing but also in respiration and speech. It also directs the intricate postural relationships of the head, neck, tongue, and hyoid bone as well as movements of the mandible. One must remember that the entire system governs the movements of the mandible. Impaired physiologic function results in break down not only of an individual tissue, but also of the interdependent structures and eventual function of the other parts, thus setting up a chain reaction.

The relationship of the head and neck must be considered. Postural maintenance must consider the shoulder girdle, clavicle, sternum, and scapulae as the fixed base of operation. The head may be said virtually to teeter on the atlanto-occipital joint. Because the center of gravity of the head lies in front of the occipital condyles, it follows that a balanced force must be applied to hold the head erect. The large posterior muscles of the neck provide that force. Normal balance of the head and neck unit requires normal balance of the anterior and posterior muscles, mandible and cranial relationship, and occlusion of the teeth. If one element is off balance, the normal relationship is broken, leading to eventual dysfunction. To restore balance, the entire system must be evaluated and treated.

A faulty relationship of the mandible and maxilla may result in faulty posture of the cranium on the first and second cervical vertebrae, or an imbalance between these vertebrae may result in symptoms referable to the mouth, ear, face, or even the thoracic cavity. Furthermore, faulty curvature of the cervical spine, along with the strains it produces, often is responsible for pain and dysfunction of the head, TMJs, shoulders, upper extremities, and chest.[14]

Management of the stomatognathic system is not limited to the discipline of any one particular field but encompasses in part nearly every specialty within dentistry and medicine. Treatment involves a team approach that may include physical, myofunctional, and speech therapists; the general dentist; oral-maxillofacial surgeon; orthodontist; otolaryngologist; psychologist; neurologist; allergist; and others.

FUNCTIONAL ANATOMY

Osteology

The mandible, the largest and strongest bone of the face, articulates with the two temporal bones and accommodates the lower teeth. It is composed of a horizontal portion, the body, and two perpendicular portions, the rami, which unite with ends of the body nearly at right angles (Fig. 17-1).

The external surface of the body is marked by a midline, the mental protuberance, bilateral mental foramina (for passage of the mental artery and nerve), and the oblique line. Muscle attachments include the platysma, depressor anguli oris, depressor labii inferioris, mentalis, and buccinator. The internal surface is concave from side to side. The superior or alveolar border, wider posteriorly than anteriorly, consists of the dentoalveolar cavities for reception of the teeth. Extending upward and backward on either side of the internal surface is the mylohyoid line, to which the mylohyoid muscle attaches (Fig. 17-1). Other muscle attachments include the digastric and medial pterygoid muscles.

The ramus, which is quadrilateral in shape, has two processes, the coronoid process and the condylar process. The coronoid process serves as an insertion for the temporalis and masseter muscles. The triangular eminence varies in shape and size; its anterior border is convex, and its posterior border is concave. The condylar process consists of two portions, the neck and the condyle. The condyle, which is convex in shape, articulates with the meniscus of the TMJ. The mandibular condyle is 15 to 20 mm long and 8 to 10 mm thick and resembles a little cylinder laid on its side. Its long axis is directed medially and slightly backward. An imaginary line drawn

through the axis to the middle line would meet a line from the opposite condyle near the anterior margin of the foramen magnum (Fig. 17-2). (This relationship is an important consideration in the application of mobilization techniques.) The lateral pterygoid inserts into a depression on the anterior portion of the neck of the condyle.

Joint Proper

The TMJ is located between the temporal fossa (glenoid fossa) on the inferior surface of the temporal bone and the condylar process of the mandibular bone (Figs. 17-3 and 17-4). Just posterior to the joint is the external auditory meatus. The temporal portion consists of the temporal fossa, which is concave, and an anteriorly placed articular eminence, which is convex.

The temporal fossa is bounded in front by the articular eminence (tubercle) and posteriorly by the post-glenoid process (spine) (Figs. 17-3 and 17-4). The post-glenoid process separates the articular surface of the temporal fossa from the anterior margin of the tympanic part of the temporal bone (Fig. 17-3). The temporal fossa (squamous part of the temporal bone) is composed of thin compact bone. The articular surface, which is smooth, oval, and deeply concave, articulates with the articular disk or meniscus of the TMJ. The average person after his mid-twenties has no more fibrocartilage in the posterior portion of the mandibular fossa (Moffett BC: Personal communication, 1979.).

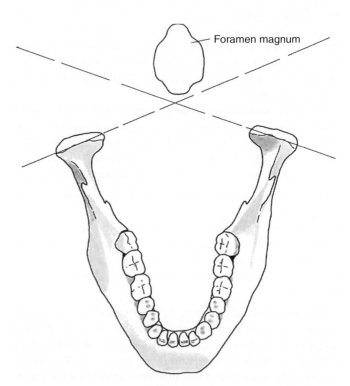

■ **FIG. 17-2.** Extensions of the long axis of the condyles meet near the anterior margin of the foramen magnum.

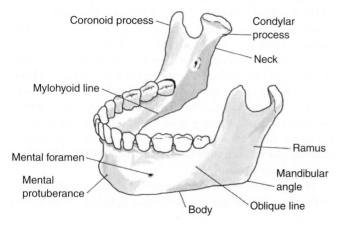

■ **FIG. 17-1.** Lateral and frontal aspects of the mandible.

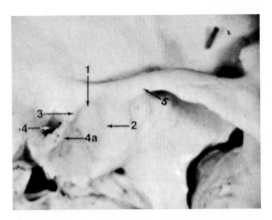

■ FIG. 17-3. Temporal bone, articular area. Temporal fossa (*1*), articular eminence (*2*), postglenoid process (*3*), external auditory meatus (*4*), tympanic bone (*4a*), and zygomatic arch (*5*). (Reprinted with permission from Alderman MM: Disorders of the temporomandibular joint and related structures. In: Lynch MA, ed: Burket's Oral Medicine: Diagnosis and Treatment, 7th ed. Philadelphia, JB Lippincott, 1994.)

From a functional point of view, the concave fossa serves as a receptacle for the condyles when the jaws are approximated and as a functional component in lateral movements of the jaw. During opening, closing, protrusion, and retrusion, the convex surface of the condylar head must move across the convex surface of the articular eminence. The existence of the interarticular disk (meniscus) compensates functionally for the incongruity of the two opposing convex bony surfaces. In addition, the disk divides the joint into two portions, sometimes referred to as the upper and lower joints. The disk is concavoconvex on its superior surface to accommodate the form

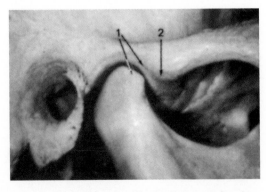

■ FIG. 17-4. Temporomandibular joint, right view of bony relations. Note the mandibular condyle and the incongruity of the articular surfaces (*1*) and the lateral view of articular eminence of temporal bone (*2*). (Reprinted with permission from Alderman MM: Disorders of the temporomandibular joint and related structures. In: Lynch MA, ed: Burket's Oral Medicine: Diagnosis and Treatment, 7th ed. Philadelphia, JB Lippincott, 1994.)

of the mandibular fossa and the articular tubercle. The inferior surface is concave over the condyle. In function both the condylar head and articular eminence of the temporal bone are not in contact with each other but with the opposing surfaces of the disk. The upper cavity is the larger of the two. The outer edges of the disk are connected to the capsule. Synovial membranes line the two cavities above and below the disk (Fig. 17-5). The superior portion of the joint acts as a gliding joint that allows forward, backward, and lateral movements of the joint. During horizontal lateral jaw movements, the ipsilateral condyle rotates with a slight lateral shift (Bennett movement), with a corresponding forward translation and rotation of the other condylar head. On opening of the mouth, the disk rotates and translates forward under the articular eminence. The lower joint, consisting of the mandible caudally and the disk cranially, is primarily responsible for rotation while the upper joint is primarily responsible for translation.

The disk follows the condyle closely in normal function, being pulled forward as the lateral pterygoid contracts to open the mouth and back by the elasticity of its posterior attachment. Arthrography has shown that the disk also changes shape during function while it moves bodily.[109]

Rees has described the disk or meniscus as having three parts: (1) a thick anterior band (pes meniscus), (2) a thicker posterior band (pars posterior), and (3) a thin intermediate zone (pars gracilis) between the two bands (Fig. 17-6).[199] It is the intermediate band that is both avascular and aneural, with its fibrous tissue being most dense. The intermediate band is positioned between the pressure-bearing articulating surfaces of the temporal bone and the mandibular condyle. The anterior and posterior bands have both vascular and neural elements present.

The disk envelops the condyle much as a cap envelops the head of a jockey, with the anterior and posterior bands converging medially and laterally to be inserted rigidly onto the medial and lateral poles.[151] The two terms **meniscus** and **disk** usually given to this structure do not describe it adequately. It is not the shape of a meniscus (a crescent-shaped body) or a disk (suggesting a flat structure interposed between the bony surfaces).[128] The articular disk or meniscus has the following attachments:[128,151,180,198]

- Anterior attachment (Fig. 17-6). Anteriorly, the disk is attached to the capsule. Fibers from the upper head of the lateral pterygoid muscle attach through the capsule into the medial part of the anterior edge of the disk.
- Medial and lateral attachments (Fig. 17-7). Medially and laterally, the disk inserts into the corresponding poles of the mandibular condyle, via the medial and lateral collateral ligaments.
- Posterior attachments (Figs. 17-6 and 17-7).[151,198] The posterior-superior disk attaches to the superior stratum, which then attaches to the postglenoid spine. The posterior-inferior disk attaches to the inferior stratum, which then attaches to the neck of the mandibular condyle. The disk

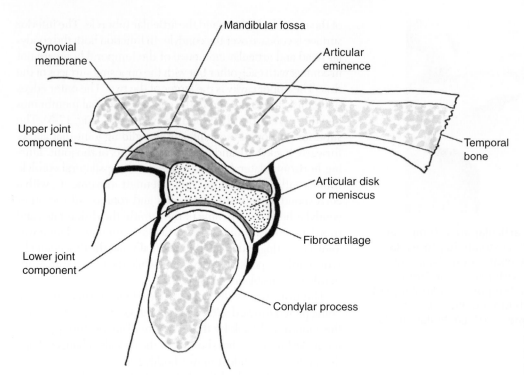

■ **FIG. 17-5.** Articular structures of the temporomandibular joint in the closed position.

also attaches to the posterior capsule. The superior and inferior (lower) strata or laminae enclose an area termed the **bilaminar zone.**[199] This bilaminar zone consists of loose neurovascular connective tissue referred to as the retrodiskal pad.[101] Since the retrodiskal pad consists of both vascularized and innervated tissue within the capsule it may be a source of nonarthritic intracapsular inflammation and arthralgia.

An excellent comprehensive study by Rees provides a more detailed analysis of the function and structure of the TMJ.[199]

Ligamentous Structures

The ligamentous structures around the TMJ include the following:

- Articular capsule (capsular ligament)
- Lateral ligament (temporomandibular ligament)
- Sphenomandibular ligament (internal lateral ligament)
- Stylomandibular ligament

The capsular ligament is attached to the circumference of the mandibular fossa and the articular tubercle superiorly and

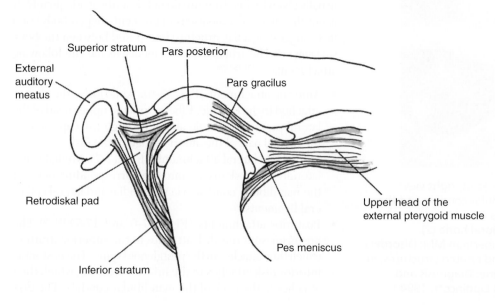

■ **FIG. 17-6.** Parasagittal section of the temporomandibular joint. The lower lamina of the bilaminar zone is inserted into the condylar neck, and the upper lamina is inserted into the squamotympanic fissure.

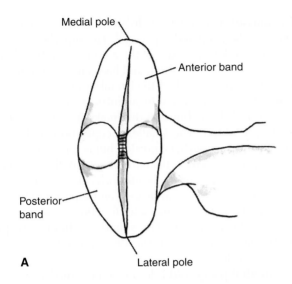

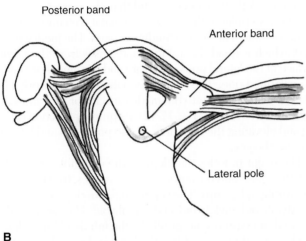

■ FIG. 17-7. Schematic drawing showing the normal disk (right side) seen from above (**A**) and from the side (**B**). The posterior and anterior bands are converging, to be inserted at the medial and lateral poles.

to the neck of the mandibular condyle inferiorly (Fig. 17-8). It is a sleeve of thin, loose, fibrous connective tissue. The capsule is especially lax anteriorly in the superior cavity but very taut in the inferior cavity between the head and disk. Therefore, when the condyle moves forward, the disk follows.

The temporomandibular ligament, a thickening of the joint capsule, is attached superiorly to the lateral surface of the zygomatic arch and articular eminence; inferiorly it attaches to the lateral surface and the posterior border of the neck of the mandible (Fig. 17-8). The ligament prevents extensive forward, backward, and lateral movements and is the main suspensory ligament of the mandible during moderate opening movements.

The sphenomandibular ligament, an accessory ligament, originates from the spine of the sphenoid and attaches to the lingula of the mandible at the mandibular foramen (Fig. 17-9). This ligament serves as a suspensory ligament of the

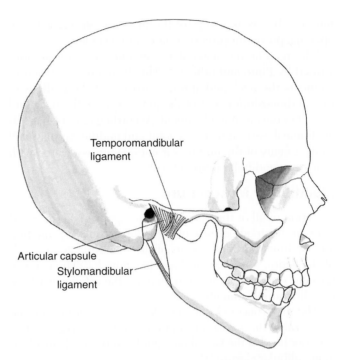

■ FIG. 17-8. Temporomandibular ligament and capsule.

mandible during wide opening. After moderate opening, the temporomandibular ligament relaxes and the sphenomandibular ligament becomes taut. The medial pterygoid is associated with the medial surface of the sphenomandibular ligament.

The stylomandibular ligament is also considered an accessory ligament (Fig. 17-9). It runs from the styloid process of the temporal bone to the posterior portion of the ramus of the mandible and separates the masseter and medial pterygoid

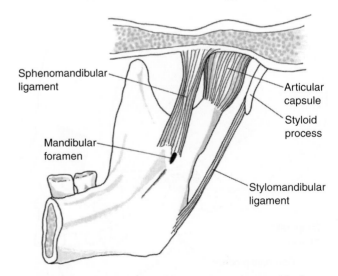

■ FIG. 17-9. Sphenomandibular and stylomandibular ligaments as viewed from the medial aspect of the mandible.

muscles. It acts as a stop for the mandible during extreme opening, preventing excessive anterior movement.

The mandibular-malleolar ligament has been demonstrated by Pinto and others.[191] This ligamentous structure connects the neck and anterior process of the malleus to the medioposterior part of the joint capsule, the disk, and the sphenomandibular ligament. According to Ermshar this anatomical association of the joint and middle ear may well explain many of the middle ear complaints associated with temporomandibular dysfunction.[67]

Mandibular Musculature

Function of all of the muscles of the upper quadrant need to be understood because of their impact on TMJ function and dysfunction. Movements of the mandible are a result of the action of the cervical and jaw muscles. The cervical muscles stabilize the head to increase the efficiency of the mandibular movements.

The three major closing muscles of the mandible are the temporalis, the masseter, and the medial pterygoid. The superior head of the lateral pterygoid is also actively involved in mandibular closure.[150,163]

The **temporalis** muscle, which is fan shaped, arises from the temporal fossa and deep surface of the temporal fascia. The anterior fibers of the muscle are vertical, the middle is oblique, and the posterior is nearly horizontal. The fibers converge as they descend, becoming tendinous, and insert into the medial and anterior aspects of the coronoid process of the ramus (Fig. 17-10). The temporalis muscle functions primarily as an elevator of the mandible, moving the jaw vertically and diagonally upward. The posterior fibers also retract the mandible and maintain the condyles posteriorly.

The **masseter** is a thick quadrilateral muscle composed of two bellies, the deep and superficial. The superficial portion arises from the lower border of the zygomatic arch and maxillary process; it extends down and back and inserts into the angle and the inferior half of the lateral surface of the ramus. The muscle itself is formed by an intricate arrangement of tendinous and fleshy bundles that make it extremely powerful (Fig. 17-11A). The smaller, deeper portion is fused anteriorly to the superficial portion but is separated from it posteriorly. It arises from the entire length of the zygomatic arch and passes anteriorly and inferiorly, inserting in the lateral surface of the coronoid process and superior half of the ramus (Fig. 17-11B). The masseter functions primarily as an elevator of the mandible. The superficial fibers also protrude the jaw a little, with the deep portion acting as a retractor as well.

The **medial pterygoid** is located on the medial aspect of the ramus. Although less powerful than the masseter, its construction is similar to the masseter in that it is characterized by an alternation of fleshy and tendinous parts. The medial pterygoid, which is quadrilateral in shape, arises from the medial surface of the lateral pterygoid plate and pyramidal process of the palatine bone. The fibers pass laterally, posteriorly, and inferiorly and insert onto the medial surface of the ramus and angle of the mandible (Fig. 17-12). Its primary function is closing and elevating the mandible. It also protrudes and laterally deviates the jaw.

The major muscles that depress the mandible are the lateral pterygoids and the anterior strap muscles, the suprahyoid and infrahyoid groups. The suprahyoid muscles are the digastric, stylohyoid, mylohyoid, and geniohyoid. They are all either opposed or assisted synergically by the infrahyoid muscles.

The lateral pterygoid is a thick conical muscle and consists of two bellies (Fig. 17-12). The superior head arises from the infratemporal crest of the greater wing of the sphenoid bone. The inferior head arises from the lateral surface of the pterygoid plate. The two heads form a tendinous insertion in front of the TMJ. The lower fibers run horizontally and insert on the neck of the condyle, with some fibers attaching to the medial portion of the condyle as well. Fibers from the superior head are attached to the articular disk and capsule as well as to the condylar head.[163,194] The attachment of the lateral pterygoid to the condyle and disk is significant in stabilizing the TMJ during bilateral protrusion, retrusion, and closing of the mandible. Lateral movement of the mandible is achieved by the action of the lateral and medial pterygoid on one side and the contralateral temporalis muscle. The lateral pterygoid, especially its inferior head, is also the primary muscle used in opening the mouth and in protruding the mandible. The superior head is believed to play an important role in stabilizing the condylar head and disk against the articular eminence during closing movement of the mandible.[163] This muscle is particularly important in cases of TMJ dysfunction and is the muscle most frequently involved.

The **digastric** muscle consists of an anterior and posterior belly connected by a strong round tendon. The anterior belly arises from the lower border of the mandible close to the sym-

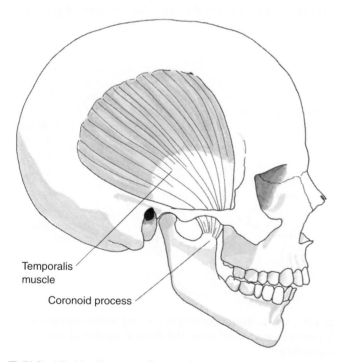

Temporalis
muscle

Coronoid process

■ **FIG. 17-10.** Temporalis muscle.

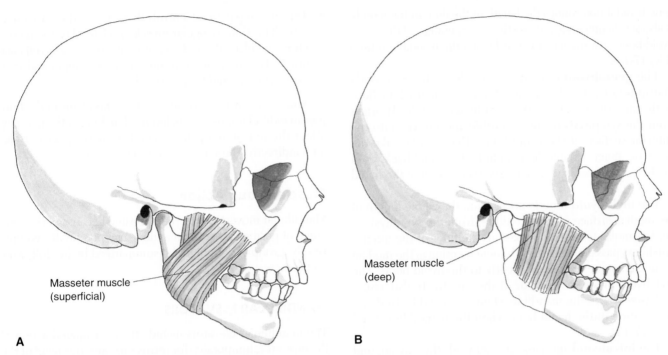

■ **FIG. 17-11.** Superficial (**A**) and deep (**B**) layers of masseter muscle.

physis. The posterior belly, which is considerably longer than the anterior one, arises from the mastoid process of the temporal bone. Both bellies descend toward the hyoid bone and are united by the intermediate tendon, which is connected to the hyoid bone by a loop of fibrous tissue (Fig. 17-13). The function of the digastric is to pull the mandible back and down. The digastric, assisted by the suprahyoids, plays a dom-

inant role in forced opening of the mandible when the hyoid bone is fixed by the infrahyoid muscle group. It also aids in retraction of the jaw and elevation of the hyoid bone.

The **stylohyoid** muscle arises from the styloid process of the temporal bone and inserts on the hyoid bone. Along with the

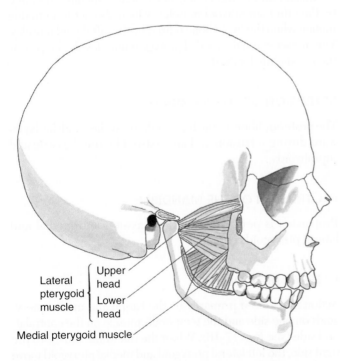

■ **FIGURE 17-12.** Medial and lateral pterygoid muscles.

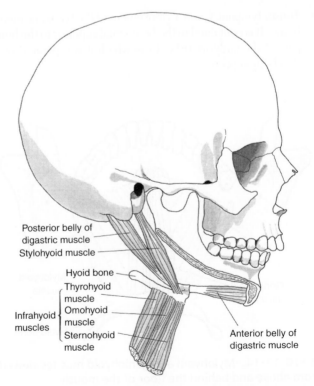

■ **FIG. 17-13.** Digastric, stylohyoid, and infrahyoid muscles.

geniohyoid it determines the length of the floor of the mouth. It also acts in initiating and assisting jaw opening and draws the hyoid bone upward and backward when the mandible is fixed (Fig. 17-13).

The **geniohyoid** is a narrow muscle, wider posteriorly than anteriorly, that lies adjacent to the midline of the floor of the mouth and above the mylohyoid muscle. It arises from the symphysis of the mandible and inserts onto the anterior surface of the hyoid bone (Fig. 17-14). Like the digastric, it acts to pull the mandible down and back when the hyoid bone is fixed and assists in elevation of the hyoid bone.

The **mylohyoid** muscle arises from the whole length of the medial surface of the mandible, from the symphysis to the last molar teeth, and makes up the floor of the mouth. The fibers pass downward, with some meeting in the median raphe and some attaching directly to the hyoid bone. The mylohyoid elevates the floor of the mouth. It also assists in depression of the mandible when the hyoid is fixed and in elevation of the hyoid bone when the mandible is fixed (Fig. 17-14).

The **infrahyoid** muscles (sternohyoid, thyrohyoid, and omohyoid) act together to steady the hyoid bone or depress it, thus allowing the suprahyoids to act on the mandible (Fig. 17-13). Of the extrinsic muscles of mastication, only the digastric and geniohyoid muscles exert a direct pull on the mandible, pulling it in a posterior and inferior direction, thereby retruding and depressing the mandible.[24]

Other muscles that have a close neurophysiologic relationship to the TMJ and that are innervated by the fifth cranial nerve include:

- Tensor tympani. Controls movement of the tympanic membrane. It is contained in the bony canal superior to the bony part of the auditory tube, from which it is separated by a thin bony septum.

- Tensor veli palatini. Controls diameter of the eustachian tube. This thin triangular muscle lies lateral to the medial pterygoid plate, the auditory tube, and the levator veli palatini. Its lateral surface is in contact with the upper and anterior part of the medial pterygoid.

Abnormal muscle contraction or spasms of any of the temporomandibular muscles, including clenching of the jaw, may affect the tensor veli palatini and tensor tympani muscles and, indirectly, the stapedius muscle of the ear.[39,125]

Muscle Group Action

Mandibular movements are complicated because of the wide range of positions that the mandible can potentially assume. Briefly, group action might be summarized by the following sections.

MANDIBULAR ELEVATORS

The mandibular elevators include the coordinated action of the masseter, temporalis (for retrusion), superior head of the lateral pterygoid (for stabilization), and medial pterygoid (for protrusion).

MANDIBULAR OPENING

The inferior head of the lateral pterygoid and the anterior head of the digastric are considered the primary muscles used in opening the mandible. The inferior head of the lateral pterygoid acts synergistically with the suprahyoid muscle group in the translation of the condylar head downward, inferiorly, and contralaterally during opening movements. Opening is assisted by the other suprahyoid muscles, which also act in initiating motion when the hyoid bone is fixed by the infrahyoid muscles. The masseter and the medial pterygoid muscles also help draw the jaw slightly forward.

RETRUSION OF THE MANDIBLE

The posterior fibers of the temporalis draw the condyles backward during retrusion and are assisted by the digastric and suprahyoids.

PROTRUSION OF THE MANDIBLE

Protrusion is performed by the masseter and medial and lateral pterygoids.

LATERAL MOVEMENTS

Action is achieved primarily by the lateral and medial pterygoids on one side and the temporalis muscle on the contralateral side (see Fig. 17-16). When the mandible moves to the right side, the left lateral pterygoid and medial pterygoid move

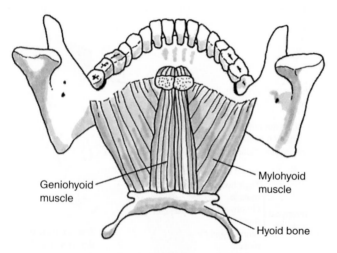

■ **FIG. 17-14.** Mylohyoid and geniohyoid muscles viewed from above and behind the floor of the mouth.

Geniohyoid muscle

Mylohyoid muscle

Hyoid bone

the chin across the midline toward the right side. The digastric, geniohyoid, and mylohyoid also are actively involved.

Dynamics of the Mandible and Temporomandibular Joints

POSITIONS OF THE MANDIBLE

Before evaluating the dynamics of the various mandibular movements, certain physiologic positions of the jaw should be defined. These are the rest position, occlusal positions, hinge position, and centric position. The terminology of some of these positions is confusing and controversial. No basic terminology has been universally adopted, and each investigator has had to establish his or her own.

The **rest position** of the mandible is considered the position the jaw assumes when there is minimal muscle-action potential. It usually implies that the head is also in its normal rest position when the person is in an upright posture. The mandibular rest position is considered to be an equilibrium between the tonus of the gravity, or jaw-opening muscles, and that of the antigravity, or jaw-closing muscles. The residual tension of the muscles at rest is termed **resting tonus.** In this position there is no occlusal contact between the maxillary and mandibular teeth. The space between the upper and lower teeth is called the **free-way space** or **interocclusal clearance.** It normally measures from 2 to 5 mm between incisors.

The rest position of the tongue, often referred to as the **postural position,** is up against the palate of the mouth.[74] The most anterosuperior tip of the tongue lies in the area against the palate just posterior to the backside of the upper central incisors. The rest position of the tongue by way of neuroreflexors (jaw–tongue reflex) provides a foundation for the resting muscle tone of the elevator muscles of the mandible and for the resting activity of the tongue.[5]

The importance of the rest position lies in the fact that it permits the tissues of the stomatognathic system to rest and thus repair themselves. If the vertical dimension is abnormally decreased (eliminating the interocclusal space), the teeth will be in constant contact. This eliminates the rest position and creates constant muscular tension and stress on the supporting structures and teeth. Factors that influence muscle tonus and the rest position are function, sleep, pathologic conditions, and the normal aging process.

Occlusal positions are functional positions in which contact between some or all of the teeth occur. One occlusal position, termed **median occlusal position** by Sicher and DuBrul, is highly significant.[226] This is the position in which the jaw is closed so that all upper and lower teeth meet, resulting in full occlusion with a balanced intercuspation of the upper and lower dental arches. From the median occlusal position, the mandible can move forward into protrusive occlusal positions, laterally, and backward to a limited extent in all normal jaws. Absent or abnormally positioned teeth can displace the mandible from the normal median occlusal position, disturbing the complete balance between the teeth, TMJs, and the musculature.

The **hinge position** is the position of the mandible from which a pure hinge opening and closing of the jaw can be made.[226] In the hinge position, the condyles are in the most retruded position that the muscles of the jaw can accomplish; the length of the temporomandibular ligaments determines it. The position is considered a retruded position or "strained relationship," which the mandible can assume actively or passively. Determination of this position is useful for some clinical procedures.

Centric position, or centric-relation occlusion, denotes a concept of normal mandibular posture. Centric position implies the most retruded, unstrained position of the mandible from which lateral movements are possible and the components of the oral apparatus are in balance. Normal centric position is slightly forward of the most posterior position that the mandibular musculature can actually achieve. Ideally, median occlusal position should coincide with centric position.

MOVEMENT PATTERNS

Mandibular movements are complicated because of the wide range of positions that the mandible can assume. Involved and integrated in mandibular movements are the shape of the fossae, the degree of tension of the associated ligaments, the menisci, the neuromuscular system, and the guiding incline of the teeth.

Kinematically, the mandible may be considered a free body that can rotate in any angular direction. It has, therefore, three degrees of freedom; each of these degrees of freedom of motion is associated with a separate axis of rotation.[253] The two basic movements required for functional motion are rotation and translation. The mandible is capable of affecting these movements in three planes: sagittal, horizontal, and frontal. The joint has three functional motions: opening and closing, protrusion and retrusion, and lateral motions. A considerable degree of rotation is also possible.

When the mouth is opened, the condyles first rotate around a horizontal axis. This motion is then combined with gliding of the condyles forward and downward with the lower surface of the disk at the same time as the disk slides forward and downward on the temporal bone. This movement results from the attachment of the disk to the medial and lateral poles of the head of the mandible and from the contraction of the lateral pterygoid, which carries the condyle with the disk onto the articular eminence. The forward sliding of the disk ceases when the fibroelastic tissue attached to the temporal bone posteriorly has been stretched to the limits. Thereafter, there is some further hinging and gliding forward of the condyle until it articulates with the most anterior part of the disk and the mouth is fully opened. The condyles essentially rotate on an axis in the horizontal plane and translate against the posterior slope of the articular eminence in the sagittal plane.

Opening movements of the mandible are caused by the synergistic action of the lateral pterygoid muscles and the depressors of the mandible. Although the lateral pterygoid pulls the condylar head and disk forward, the digastric and geniohyoid muscles pull the mandible downward and backward, affecting rotation. This blending of muscle action makes possible the rotatory and translatory movements of jaw opening. This motion affects all the other muscles anchored to the mandible. The elevators of the mandible must lengthen to ensure smoothness of performance, and the muscles of the cranium and hyoid bone must act as holders to establish a fixed position (Fig. 17-15).

In mandibular closure, the movements are reversed. In the first phase of the movement, the condyles glide backward and then hinge on the disks, which are held forward by the lateral pterygoids. The backward glide of the mandible results from interaction between the retracting portions of the masseter and temporalis muscles and the retracting portions of the depressors. During the second phase, the inferior head of the lateral pterygoids relaxes while the upper head allows the disks to glide backward and upward on the temporal bone along with the condyles.[150] The second phase begins with the contraction of the masseter, the medial pterygoid, and temporalis muscles; it ends with intercuspation of the teeth. The onset of superior head or lateral pterygoid function is usually concurrent with that of the elevator musculature.[163]

In protrusion, the teeth are retained throughout in the occlusal position, so far as possible, and the lower teeth are drawn forward over the upper teeth by both lateral pterygoids. In contrast to opening movements, the condyles and disks move downward and forward along the articular eminences without rotation of the condyles around a transverse axis. To prevent the mandible from falling, the elevating muscles exhibit some degree of contraction. They must make the necessary adjust-

ment with the balancing depressor–retractors as they lengthen to allow the mandible to slide forward just free of the interlocking dentition.

In retraction, the mandible is drawn backward by the deep portion of the masseter muscles and by the posterior fibers of the temporalis muscles to the rest position. At the same time, the geniohyoid, the digastric muscles, and the elevators synergistically balance each other to maintain the mandible in the horizontal position.

In lateral movements of the mandible, asymmetrical muscular patterns develop on both sides. In this movement, one condyle and disk slide downward and forward in the sagittal plane and medially in the horizontal plane along the articular eminence. At the same time, the other condyle rotates laterally on a sagittal plane around a shifting vertical axis and translates medially in the horizontal plane while remaining in the fossa. The condylar translation in the horizontal plane is known as the Bennett movement.[226,257,260] If one views the mandible from above, it will be seen that the medial pole of the condyle juts far medially from the plane of the jaw, while the coronoid process leans laterally. The lateral pterygoid muscle, inserted on the medial pole of the condyle, pulls inward and forward in the horizontal plane, while the horizontal fibers of the temporalis muscle, inserted on the coronoid process, pull outward and backward (Fig. 17-16). These muscles, operating as a force couple, contribute to the torque of rotating the condyle that is necessary to effect chewing on this side. This condyle is known as the working-side condyle. Therefore, in lateral deviation to the left, the lateral pterygoid on the right, together with the right and left anterior bellies of the digastric and geniohyoid, contract. This causes the right condyle to move downward, forward, and medially, while the actions of the left temporalis and the lateral pterygoid rotate the left condyle in the fossa and displace the mandible to the left. This is described as **left lateral excursion with a Bennett shift to the left.** The left condyle is called the **working-side condyle** and the right condyle is

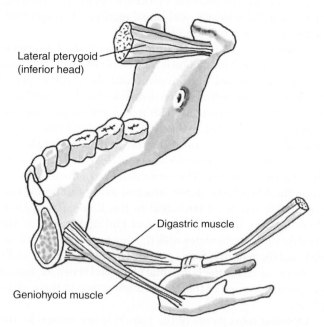

Lateral pterygoid
(inferior head)

Digastric muscle

Geniohyoid muscle

■ **FIG. 17-15.** Mandibular muscles involved in opening.

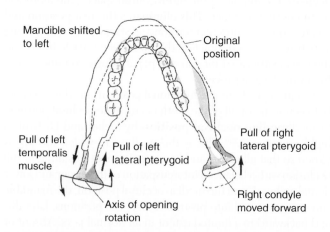

Mandible shifted
to left

Original
position

Pull of left
temporalis
muscle

Pull of left
lateral pterygoid

Pull of right
lateral pterygoid

Axis of opening
rotation

Right condyle
moved forward

■ **FIG. 17-16.** Mandibular muscles involved in lateral movement of the mandible to the left. The suprahyoid muscles are not shown.

the nonworking condyle or balancing condyle. Basic types of working condylar motions include the following[258]:

- Rotation with no lateral shift (Fig. 17-17A)
- Rotation with movement backward, upward, and/or laterally (Fig. 17-17B)
- Rotation with movement downward, forward, and laterally (Fig. 17-17C)
- Rotation with a lateral shift (Fig. 17-17D)
- Rotation with movement downward, backward, and laterally (Fig. 17-17E)

It is apparent that the right lateral pterygoid has also entered into the force-couple system. In the closing stroke, the force couple changes in direction and components. Thus, in the rotatory movements of grinding or chewing, these alternating movements swing the mandible from side to side.

Although masticatory movements are highly complex, they become automatic in each person as a result of the integration of the proprioceptive mechanism and muscular action. All the muscles of mastication are involved in the act of chewing because it involves all four movements of the mandible—elevation, depression, protrusion, and retrusion.

Nerve Supply

Three nerves that are part of the mandibular division of the fifth cranial nerve supply the innervation of the TMJ. The posterior deep temporal and masseteric nerves supply the medial and anterior regions of the joint. The auriculotemporal nerve supplies the posterior and lateral regions of the joint. The auriculotemporal nerve is the major nerve innervating the posterior lateral capsule, the retrodiskal pad, the temporomandibular ligaments, and the capsular blood vessels. The auriculotemporal nerve also sends a few branches to the tympanic membrane, the external auditory meatus, the superior one half of the auricle on its lateral aspect, and the skin of the temples and scalp.[56,99] The central part of the disk is not innervated.[198]

All four types of joint mechanoreceptors have been identified with respect to the joint structures of the TMJ. For a

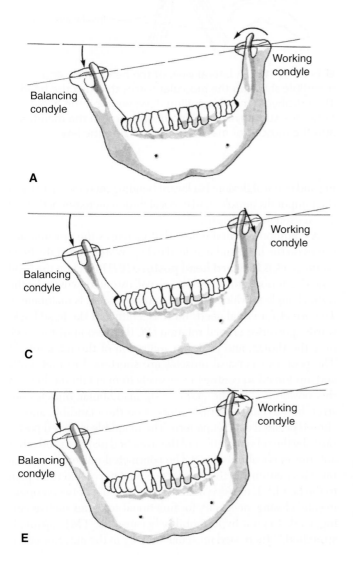

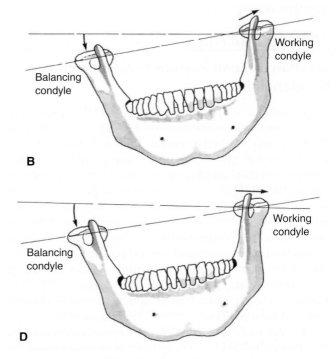

■ **FIG. 17-17.** The basic types of working condylar motions are (**A**) rotation with no lateral shift; (**B**) rotation with movement backward, upward, and/or laterally; (**C**) rotation with movement downward, forward, and laterally; (**D**) rotation with a lateral shift; and (**E**) rotation with movement downward, backward, and laterally. (Adapted from Weinberg LA: An evaluation of basic articulators and their concepts: I. Basic concepts. J Prosthet Dent 13:622–644, 1963.)

detailed understanding of their morphologic and functional characteristics see Chapter 3, Arthrology, and articles by Clark and Wyke,[46] Klineberg,[136] and Wyke.[268] The general characteristics of mechanoreceptor types I, II, and III are postural and kinesthetic perception, reflexive influence on motor neuron pool activity, and inhibition of nociceptor-mechanoreceptor activity. The major contribution to position sense of the mandible is believed to come from these joint receptors, although the presence of spindles in the muscles of mastication and pain impulses from the periodontal membrane also contribute to afferent information. This mechanoreceptor system is polysynaptic and heavily influences the reflex coordination of masticatory activity (both inhibitory and facilitory).

There is also an abundant supply of type IV, nonadapting, high-threshold pain receptors, which are nonactive under normal conditions. Abnormal activity of these receptors results when related tissue is subject to marked deformation or other noxious mechanical or chemical stimulation (e.g., intracapsular pressure changes, capsular tightness, and strained positions of the mandibular condyles).[131] As a result there will be altered perception of mandibular movement and positioning as well as altered muscle activity of those muscles innervated by the fifth cranial nerve.

APPLIED ANATOMY

Relation of Head Posture to Rest Position of the Mandible

Functionally the TMJ, the cervical spine, and the articulations between the teeth are intimately related (Fig. 17-18). Muscles attach the mandible to the cranium, the hyoid bone, and clavicle. The cervical spine is, in essence, interposed between the proximal and distal attachments so some of the muscles controlling the TMJ. Studies demonstrate high prevalence of cervical spine disorders associated with temporomandibular disorders.[182,186,207,238,265] The neuromuscular influence of the cervical and masticatory region actively participates in the function of mandibular movement and cervical positioning.[106,190,245,268] Many factors influence the masticatory muscles and affect the rest position and path of mandibular closure.[140,166,170,195,197] A change in head position caused by cervical muscles changes the mandibular position.[47,54,94,170,201] This change affects occlusion and the masticatory muscles, and the masticatory muscles then affects the TMJ.[82,206] The muscles of mastication and the suprahyoid and infrahyoid muscles affect the balance between the flexors and extensors of the head and neck.[203] Dysfunction in either the muscles of mastication or the cervical muscles can easily disturb this normal balance.

Cervical posture change affects the mandibular path of closure,[195] the mandibular rest position,[47] masticatory muscle activity,[106,161,195] and, subsequently, the occlusal contact pattern. Neurologically the cervical apophyseal joints and increased gravitational forces on the head can directly alter muscular activity about the jaw. Electromyographic studies have indicated increased masticatory levels with cervical backward bend-

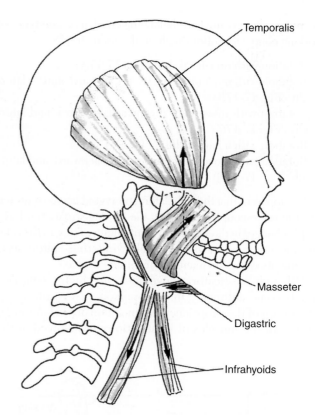

■ **FIG. 17-18.** A lateral view of the head, neck, and mandible showing the muscular forces that flex the head. The infrahyoid muscles pulling downward on the hyoid bone, the suprahyoids pulling downward on the mandible, and the muscles of mastication stabilizing the jaw.

ing and cervical flexion: backward bending increases activity of the temporalis muscles and cervical flexion increases activity of the masseter and digastric.[28,30]

A common postural defect that increases the gravitational forces on the head and may lead to hyperextension of the head on the neck is **forward head posture** (FHP). When the head is held anteriorly, the line of vision will extend downward if the normal angle at which the head and neck meet is maintained. To correct for visual needs there is a tilting of the head backwards (posterior cranial rotation [PCR]), flexion of the neck over the thorax, and posterior migration of the mandible.[206] The posterior cervical muscles are shortened isometrically and are forced to contract excessively to maintain the head in this position while the anterior submandibular muscles are stretched to cause retrusive forces on the mandible and an altered occlusal contact pattern. The mandible is forced posteriorly by the rebound effect of the stretched platysma and other anterior cervical muscles.[83] The contracted posterior cervical muscles may entrap the greater occipital nerve and refer pain to the head.[37] Excessive mandibular shuttling between opening and closing, necessary for functional activities such as eating, leads to joint hypermobility because the TMJ capsule is stretched.[82] Increased muscular activity in the anterior cervical (longus colli) and hyoid muscles will in turn cause tightness in the throat and difficulty swallowing.[206]

Among important environmental factors contributing to FHP are the many occupations and activities of daily living that require that the upper extremities and the head be positioned more anterior to the trunk than is either normal or comfortable (improper home, work, or driving postures).[55,62,155,156] Another contributing factor is mouth breathing. Various investigations have shown that postural relationships change to meet respiratory needs.[55] Breathing through the mouth facilitates FHP, lowered mandibular position, and a low and forward tongue position.[111,196]

Acute trauma (such as hyperextension injuries, in which reflex guarding of the longus colli, sternocleidomastoid, and scalenes occurs) is usually associated with a decrease in the cervical spine curvature approaching total flattening of the cervical lordosis—a straight form of FHP without PCR (Fig. 17-19B).[154,160] Any forward deviation of the head out of the long axis of the body should be considered pathologic, as this reduces the potential mobility of the cervical spine. Total flattening out of the physiologic cervical lordosis and any kyphosis of the lower cervical spine (cervical or neck kyphosis) must also be considered pathologic.[134] Kyphosis of the neck affects, roughly, the C5–T3 segments. It is seen in connection with a pronounced thoracic flat back, particularly in the midthoracic spine. Motions of all segments affected by the kyphosis of the neck are considerably restricted.

In the presence of a FHP with no significant PCR the suprahyoids shorten and the infrahyoids lengthen, consequently decreasing or eliminating the free-way space.[141,218] The hyoid bone is repositioned superiorly and the degree of elevation is proportional to the decrease in the cervical lordosis or increase in FHP.[141,202,205] An opposite action occurs at the mandibular condyles as they are forced to elevate and translate forward at the same time the mentum is depressed and retruded.[76,234] These repositioning effects are maximized when the FHP is associated with a significant degree of PCR.[156]

As the mandibular condyles assume a retro position in the joint, the superior head of the lateral pterygoid becomes stretched.[55] By reflex action, this stretch may lead to premature contraction, causing the disk to become anteriorly displaced.[32,95] With changes in the mandibular position and the length–tension relationship of the hyoid, the occlusal contact pattern and the arthrokinematics of the TMJ also change.[31,84,170,196] Mouth breathing may compound the situation with the tongue assuming a lowered position and causing abnormal swallowing patterns.[9] The position of the scapula, to which the omohyoid muscle is attached, will also influence the length–tension relationship of the hyoid muscles.[202,203] Shoulder girdle posture relates to the position of the head and neck in the same way that the sacral base rules the position of the lumbar spine.[203]

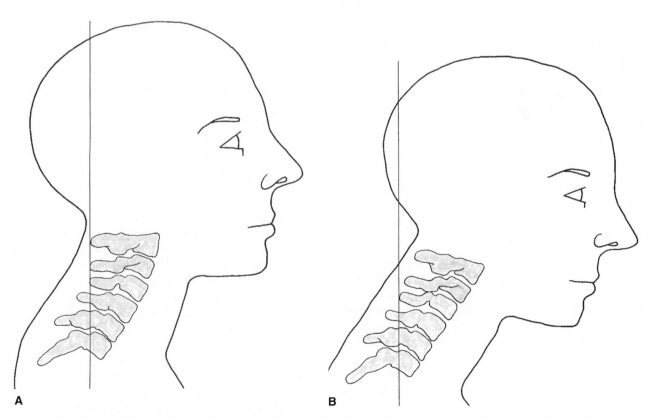

■ **FIG. 17-19.** Types of forward head. **(A)** Increased cervical lordosis with posterior cranial rotation. **(B)** Total flattening of cervical lordosis without posterior cranial rotation.

The effects of abnormal FHP may lead to an excessive amount of tension in the masticatory musculature, teeth, and supporting structures.[5] Abnormal position may lead to eventual osteoarthrosis and remodeling of the TMJ.[87,170]

One of the common neuroanatomical sequelae involving FHP is suboccipital impingement or entrapment. The neuroanatomical studies by Bogduk et al.[23–25] have clarified the numerous possibilities for muscular, osseous, and facial entrapments of C1, C2, and C3.

Subluxation and Premature Translation of the Jaw

The TMJ can subluxate itself through its own muscular dynamics. Subluxation occurs when the condyle translates onto the articular tubercle and then back to the articular eminence. Predisposing factors that allow the subluxation to occur more easily in some persons than others is a decrease in the slope of the articular eminence or a flattened articular eminence (Figs. 17-4 and 17-5) and stretching of the ligamentous attachments of the meniscus into the condylar pole.[127,128,269] Signs of subluxation include excessive mandibular opening (greater than 40 mm), movement of the lateral poles too far anteriorly (too much translation), and joint noise at the beginning of closing. If unilateral subluxation occurs, there will be a quick deviation from midline to the contralateral side at the end of opening.

In premature translation during jaw opening, translation occurs within the first 11 mm of opening. Such a movement is contrary to normal arthrokinematic movements of the jaw, in which translation begins only after the first 11 mm of opening.

Both translation occurring too soon and subluxations are conditions that are believed to involve muscle imbalances. There may be no actual TMJ dysfunction present with these two conditions, and they may occur separately or together in some patients. Their long-range effect on the TMJ, however, can lead to TMJ dysfunction. If either or both of these conditions are observed, it is important to control them to minimize the stress placed on the intracapsular tissues and prevent the perpetuation of TMJ dysfunction that is present and may be a hindering factor to treatment.

Dislocation of the Jaw

Dislocation may result from actual trauma to the chin during opening of the mouth, or it may occur without actual trauma, such as with a sudden muscular spasm during a yawn. This dislocation is always anterior and may be unilateral or bilateral, resulting in displacement of one or both condyles forward into the infratemporal fossa anterior to the articular eminences.[224] In bilateral dislocations, the chin is displaced forward so that the patient shows some degree of prognathism with an open bite. In unilateral dislocation the mandible is displaced toward the noninjured side.

Reduction is accomplished unilaterally by depressing the mandible with the thumb placed on the last molar teeth and at the same time elevating the chin. The downward pressure overcomes the spasm of the elevating muscles, and elevating the chin repositions the condyles backward behind the articular eminences. Reduction is usually followed by several days of rest.[220]

Habitual dislocation, subluxations, or self-reducing dislocations are not especially rare. According to Dufourmentel and Axhausen, there are two kinds of habitual subluxation that patients themselves may learn to adjust either by a special jaw movement or with the hand. These are luxation in the upper cavity (meniscotemporal) and luxation in the lower cavity (meniscocondylar).[7,61]

Derangement of the Disk

Trauma, overclosure of the mouth with backward displacement of the condyle, or malocclusion may cause derangement of the disk. Trauma to the disk can vary from an inflammatory condition to a complete or partial tearing of the disk from its capsular attachment. If the disk remains attached to the anterior capsule and the external pterygoid, an anterior dislocation of the disk occurs. It may be manifested by displacement of the mandible toward the affected side and possible blockage of mandibular opening and closing.[224] If the disk remains attached to the posterior capsule, a painful blockage in closing the mandible results.[224]

The most widely accepted view is that clicking is the result of derangement of the disk. However, many investigators have reported various other theories of its etiology in addition to derangement of the disk. Among these are incoordinate contraction of the two bodies of the lateral pterygoid, so that the disk snaps over the condyle rather than following the movement smoothly and coordinately when the mouth is open; deterioration of the disk and cartilaginous surfaces; and stretching of the joint ligaments by frequent subluxation.[225]

Clicking may occur as one or more clicks in one joint, or clicking may occur in both joints; it may or may not be associated with pain. Various types of clicking noises have been observed during sagittal opening, including an opening click, an intermediate click during the opening phase, and a full opening click. Each of these clicks appears to be associated with various pathologic occlusions.

An opening click is believed to be caused by an anterior displacement of the disk, with the condyle displaced posteriorly and superiorly. As the mandible opens, the condyle must pass over the posterior surface of the disk.[225]

Clicking during various parts of the opening of the mandible is believed to result from incoordinate movements of the upper and lower heads of the external pterygoid, so that the condyle cannot remain in its normal relationship with the disk.[225] More likely causes are possible anteroposterior displacement of the disk and ruptures or rents of the disk.[263]

A final click occurring in the full opening phase may be caused by the condyle passing over the anterior portion of the disk, by the disk being pulled forward of the condyle, or by both the disk or condyle passing over the articular eminence.[225]

In addition to clicks produced during mandibular opening, eccentric movements may produce clicks. Again, these may be largely owing to structural changes in disks or incoordinate functioning of the parts of the joint.[225]

Crepitus has been associated with perforation of the disk. Moffett and coworkers demonstrated that perforation of the disk is usually followed by osteoarthritic change on the condylar surface, which is, in turn, followed by similar bony alterations on the opposing surface of the fossa.[169] The most common disk–condyle derangements that present clinically are anterior disk derangements in which there are anterior disk dislocations that reduce and those that do not reduce.[71]

The classic signs of the type of anterior disk dislocation that reduces are (1) a distinguished, sometimes loud click or pop during mandibular opening, signifying that the disk has relocated itself with respect to the condyle, and (2) a more subtle click usually occurring during mandibular closing, signifying that the disk has displaced itself anterior to the mandibular condyle. The sign of an anterior disk dislocation that does not reduce is the absence of joint noises with a series of reproducible restrictions during mandibular movements. These restrictions are owing to the disk blocking translatory glide.

TEMPOROMANDIBULAR EVALUATION

History

The general format of the initial evaluation should follow the same lines of questioning as set out in Chapter 5. Information on when the problem started and how it occurred as well as previous management and the results obtained is helpful. If injury or surgical procedure caused the problem, the clinician will need to know what the attending personnel and physicians did. A most important aspect of taking the history is the attempt to clarify any emotional factors in the patient's background that may provoke habitual protrusion or muscular tension.

The history may be handwritten from answers to verbal questions. A more complete history may be obtained, however, by using a personal history form, which is completed by the patient. After reviewing the form, all pertinent facts may be reviewed in detail with the patient. The work of Day,[57] Shore,[225] and Morgan and Rosen[173] provides excellent detailed outlines and the rationale for obtaining such information as a means of compiling a complete history relating specifically to TMJ disorders. Such forms have been designed to include most of the information that will be found useful in treating TMJ disorders and related orofacial problems. Certainly no specific set of questions is adequate, and more detailed questioning will usually be necessary. It is also unlikely that the clinician will obtain all relevant information at the initial evaluation. A few pertinent questions that apply particularly to TMJ disorders include the following:

1. Does the joint grate, click, pop, snap, or lock?
2. Do you have difficulty opening and closing your mouth?
3. Do you have frequent headaches? What area of the head? How long do they last?
4. Have you ever had a severe blow to the head or a whiplash injury?
5. Are your jaws clenched or your teeth sore when you awaken from sleep?
6. Do you have frequent headaches?

Perhaps one of the most common complaints of head pain is what is generally termed **tension-type headache.**[183] Many studies reveal that headache is a common symptom associated with temporomandibular disorders.[15,36,77,78,89,96,123,142,200,216,254] Many different types of headaches originate from a variety of causes. Headaches may be the result of structural cervical disease, may be associated with vascular pain syndrome, or may occur as a separate entity (see Chapter 19, Cervical Spine).[14,57]

Physical Examination

The order and detail of the physical examination described below need to be appropriate to the patient being examined. Some tests will be irrelevant, others will only need to be carried out briefly, and others will need to be investigated fully.

I.   Observation
     Record significant findings. The physical examination, in a sense, occurs simultaneously when the clinician takes the history. The appearance, general posture, and characteristics of bodily movements are often revealing. Physically the typical patient with TMJ pain–dysfunction, with an emotional overlay, has a posture of elevated shoulders, forward head, stiff neck and back, and shallow, restricted breathing.[115] The patient is observed for facial expression and habits of the jaw (e.g., clenching or grinding the teeth, biting the fingers, or twitching the jaw muscles).
     The most common abnormality in the cervical spine with direct impact on the TMJ, cranial facial area, and temporomandibular area is the FHP. Any increase in the sternocleidomastoid angulation or distance from the thoracic apex to midcervical region manifested by forward inclination of the head and neck constitutes a FHP (Fig. 17-20). Optimal

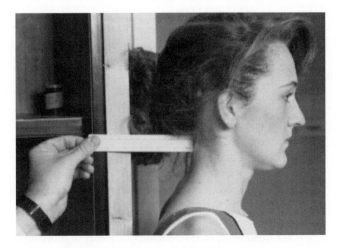

■ **FIG. 17-20.** Measurement of head posture.

posture is 4 to 8 cm from the apex of the thoracic kyphosis to the deepest point in the cervical spine.[203] Angulation of the sternocleidomastoid is considered to be minimal at 60°, moderate at 60 to 75°, and maximal at 75 to 90°.[155] Internal rotation of the glenohumeral joint and protraction of the shoulder girdle may also be observed. The scapulae may be protracted, retracted, elevated, or winged.

II. Inspection of the Head, Face, and Neck
   Record significant findings.
   A. Skin. Examine the face for blemishes, moles, pigmentations, scars, and texture.
   B. Soft tissue. Note any swelling. Swelling of the joint must be moderate or significant before it is apparent on inspection. If swelling is detectable, it appears as a rounded bulge just anterior to the external meatus. The face should be further examined for atrophies and hypertrophies. Asking the patient to clench his or her jaws together may help to disclose asymmetry.
   C. Bony structure and alignment. The profile of the face in both the frontal and sagittal planes will reveal the relative development of the skull, face, and mandible. The size of the mandible should be compared with that of the skull and abnormal positions or asymmetry of the jaw noted. Asymmetry may be indicative of a growth or developmental problem or unusual muscular activity.
   D. Functional mechanics. Take particular note of the occlusal and rest positions of the jaw. Note the following:
      1. Respiration, alteration in nasal diaphragmatic breathing
      2. Swallowing pattern
      3. Tongue rest position
      4. Lip closure position
      5. Mandibular and condylar rest position
      6. Presence of tongue thrust
         Part the patient's lips (or use a lip separator) to reveal the alignment of the incisors as well as any evidence of abnormal resting position of the tongue or a deviant swallow (see section on dynamics of the mandible and TMJ).
         The examiner should briefly inspect the upper spine, shoulder girdles, and arms for obvious muscle atrophy or deformities.

III. Joint Tests
   Joint tests include active and passive physiologic movements, joint-play (accessory) movements, and other relevant joints. If instability of the upper cervical spine is suspected, stress tests should be carried out; these are described in Chapter 19, Cervical Spine, on the examination of the upper cervical spine.
   A. Active physiologic joint movements. Observe the general patterns of active physiologic movements (depression, elevation, lateral deviation, protraction, and retraction) for freedom of movement, range, quality of movement, deviations, crepitus, or clicking on opening and/or closing

the mouth. Ascertain if any pain accompanies active movements and in what part of the range it occurs and where. Pain may be felt in the area of the joint and about the ear, but often it is felt diffusely through the face, teeth, jaws, and mouth. Masticatory pain is typically not well localized. (During the palpation portion of the examination, actual sites of tenderness can be established.)

Abnormal movements such as "jumps" or "facet slips" should be noted. In particular the patient is asked to open the mouth to a limited extent (approximately 1 cm) while the examiner observes whether the mandible is making an initial rotation or translatory movement. Forward movement will be revealed by a reduction in incisal overjet and by excessive prominence of the condylar heads.

The restriction of movement, deviations to one side, and asynchronous patterns of movement are recorded; the maximum opening the patient can achieve without pain is measured. Lateral movements to the left and right, using the bite position as the control as well as protrusion–retrusion, again using normal bite as control, should be recorded when restricted. Lateral motions may be lost earlier and to a greater degree than vertical motions.

A T bar is often used for recording active motion and abnormal tracking of the mandible during opening.

1. Mandibular opening and closing. The client should be able to put at least two of his or her knuckles between the upper and lower incisors for normal jaw opening. Measurement of maximal voluntary mandibular opening can be obtained by measuring between the maxillary and mandibular incisal edges with a ruler scaled in millimeters (Fig. 17-21). Measurements may be recorded on the vertical plane of the T bar. Normal mandibular opening has been reported to be between 35 and 50 mm[1,2,104] when using this method, and from 48 to 52 mm when measured from acquired occlusion (including vertical overlap).[70,71,119] To complete 40 mm of functional range, 25 mm is rotational and 15 mm occurs with anterior and inferior translational glide.[111,174,204]

The vertical path of the mandible during opening and closing should be recorded for deviations or deflections. A deviation is defined as a lateral movement of the mandible that returns to midline prior to maximal opening, whereas a deflection is a lateral movement without return to midline.[264] If deflection occurs to the right on opening with limited motion, the right TMJ is said to be hypomobile. If the mandible abnormally tracks (deviates) out of midline (i.e., in an S-type curve) the problem is probably caused by muscle imbalance.

2. Lateral characteristics (range of motion [ROM] and deviations or deflections). Lateral movements are normally 8 to 10 mm when the midline of the maxillary and mandibular incisors is viewed in the normal

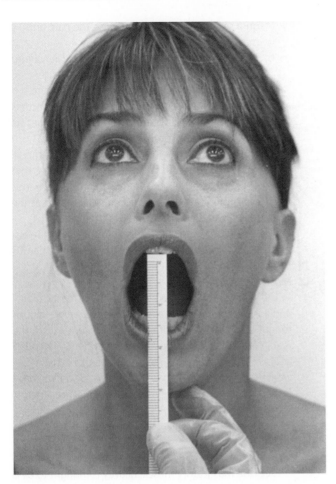

■ **FIG. 17-21.** Measurement of maximum intercisal distance.

adult.[264] Movement of 50% or less is indicative of an intracapsular restriction in the TMJ contralateral to the side of lateral movement.[264] Measurements may be recorded on the horizontal plane of the T bar.

3. Protrusion characteristics (ROM and deviations or deflections). Protrusion is defined as the distance through which the lower teeth can move horizontally past the maxillary teeth. It may be measured by the distance between the upper and lower central incisor teeth. The normal adult should have 5 mm of movement from the position of centric occlusion in which the front teeth are opposed.[248] Loss of movement in one TMJ will result in an ipsilateral deviation of the mandible ascertained by palpation and observation. Pain at the end of range or limitation can be owing to joint dysfunction (e.g., synovitis or a capsular sprain) or a displaced disk.[14,111]

4. Retrusion characteristics. Retrusion is measured the same way as protrusion. Full retrusion, or centric relation, places the TMJs in a close-packed position with the condyles resting on the center of the disk in the uppermost and most posterior position in the

fossa. Normally there is 3 to 4 mm of movement from the position of rest to the position of centric relation.[95] The muscles or their nerve supply can cause pain, weakness, or limitation of range. Intracapsular injury causes pain at the end of active retrusion.[14]

It should be noted whether pain is provoked when the jaws are in firm occlusion and when the patient is asked to bite against a tongue blade on one side. Such tests help distinguish muscle spasms from diskitis and retrodiskitis (see resisted movements below).[14]

B. Passive physiologic joint movements (with passive overpressure). With passive movements, in addition to seeing how easily the jaw can be moved and making a comparison with active ROM, note the resistance through the range and the type of end feel as well as the presence of pain and spasms. To determine the nature of the end feel, have the patient open the mouth and then apply additional pressure with the thumbs and index fingers on the edge of the upper and lower teeth, noting the type of end feel present. Passive movements should routinely include depression, elevation, protraction, retraction, and lateral movements.

One of the most common intracapsular dysfunctions of the TMJ is internal derangement of the articular disk. This is characterized by a posterior-superior displacement of the condyle and anterior displacement of the disk. The most common signs of internal derangements are (1) reciprocal clicking, (2) disk displacement without reduction (locking), or (3) subluxation indicating condyle/disk incoordination.[240]

Two specific pathologic conditions of the TMJ should be recognized: (1) hypermobility with excessive translational glide, clicking, and subluxation; and (2) locking of the joint that is characterized by hypomobility. Locking can be of two major types and present with different types of end feel.[26]

1. The first type of locking is caused by shortening of the periarticular connective tissues as a defensive mechanism. With passive stretch there is gummy end feel and a considerable increase in ROM after stretching.

2. Closed-lock caused by anterior displacement of the disk is characterized by a hard end-feel with limited motion. Passive stretch will produce little or no increase in ROM.

C. Joint-play movements. Because movements are small and difficult to feel, one can obtain more information by applying repeated gentle oscillations. The movements are classified as normal, hypomobile, or hypermobile. Many of the joint mobilizations for the TMJ are extensions of the mobility testing. For more details of carrying out the tests, see the joint mobilization section (see Figs. 17-33 to 17-37). The most common accessory movements tested are:

1. Caudal traction produced by distraction of the joint by pressure over the lower mandible (see Fig. 17-33).

2. Ventral glide (protrusion) produced by placing the index and third finger over the angle of the ramus (see Fig. 17-34).

3. Medial-lateral glide, produced by the fingers and hypothenar eminence around the patient's mandible (see Fig. 17-35).

4. Medial-lateral glide, produced by placing the thumb in the patient's mouth and over the medial surface of the mandible head (see Fig. 17-36).

5. Medial glide applied directly to the condyle by thumb pressure (see Fig. 17-37*A*).[153,249]

6. Anterior glide applied directly to the condyle by thumb pressure (see Fig. 17-37*B*).[153,249]

   Note stability, mobility, pain, guarding, spasm, and behavior.

D. Other Joints as Applicable

   Joints likely to be examined (if suspected to be a source of the symptoms) are the shoulder girdle as well as cervical and thoracic spine.

IV. Muscle Tests

   Muscle tests include examining muscle strength, control, length and resistive movements (static), and functional manipulation.

A. Resisted movement. Determine the presence of pain by applying resistance to mandibular opening, protrusion, and lateral deviations. For the assessment of the pterygoids musculature in addition to assessing resistive movement (static) a second method for evaluating symptoms, called **functional manipulation,** has been developed.[12,13,27,182,239] During functional manipulation each muscle is contracted and then also stretched.

1. Resisted mandible depression. Resistance is applied to the underside of the mandible while the client attempts to keep the mouth open (1 to 2 cm). The lateral pterygoids and hyoids can present with pain or weakness caused by injury to the muscle or nerve supply. Imbalance problems may cause TMJ problems or result from TMJ dysfunction.

2. Resisted mandible lateral excursion. With good stabilization of the head, the examiner should ask the patient to open her jaw slightly and then resist lateral excursion to each side. A weak lateral pterygoid may not be obvious on resisted depression but becomes evident with resisted lateral excursion when compared bilaterally.

3. Resisted protrusion. This motion tests the lateral and medial pterygoids, not the suprahyoids. Adding stretch (functional manipulation) following resisted motion confirms that the muscle is the true source of pain.[27,181,182]

   a. The lateral pterygoid (inferior fibers) should be checked. Have the patient protrude the mandible against resistance provided by the examiner; this activity increases pain if the muscle is the source of pain. When the teeth are clenched (stretched), pain increases if this is the source of pain; biting

on a separator does not increase the pain and may even decrease it.

   b. The lateral pterygoid (superior fibers). Clenching increases the pain. Stretching of the muscle occurs at maximum intercuspation; therefore, stretching and contraction of this muscle occurs during clenching. Opening of the mouth does not increase the pain and may even be painless.

   c. The medial pterygoid. Clenching increases the pain both with and without a separator. The muscle is stretched when the mouth is opened wide; therefore, opening the mouth wide increases the pain if the medial pterygoid is the source.

      Pain arising in the pterygoid muscles may also be provoked by resisted deviation to the painful side.

B. Muscle Strength

   The examiner should test the muscles of mastication, and if indicated the muscles of the cervical spine, mouth, tongue and palate. For details of these general tests, the reader is directed to Hislop and Montgomery,[117] Kendall et al.,[132] and Palmer and Epler.[85] Mandibular muscle weakness is considered to be rare in TMJ disorders, particularly the muscles that close the mouth, since strength is generally maintained by mastication. According to Janda,[121] the suprahyoid and mylohyoid muscles have a tendency to weaken.

C. Muscle Control

   Excessive masticatory muscle activity is thought to be a factor in TMJ conditions. An abnormal protrusive position may be associated with tongue thrust (deviant swallowing) or habitual protrusion. The evaluation described by Kraus to determine the presence of an acquired adult tongue thrust is helpful.[140] The patient is asked to swallow water several times, pausing between each swallow while the therapist palpates the hyoid bone and the suboccipital muscles (Fig. 17-22). Quick up and down movement of

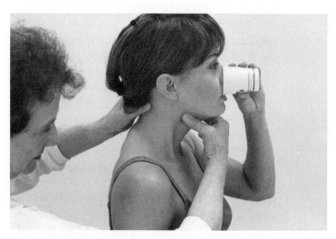

■ **FIG. 17-22.** Examination of altered swallowing sequence.

the hyoid should normally be felt with minimal contraction of the suboccipital muscles. With an acquired anterior adult tongue thrust, a slow up and down movement of the hyoid bone is felt along with significant suboccipital muscle contraction. Excessive forward movement of the entire head and neck and lip may be noted.

Another method of looking at muscle control is to observe for abnormal tracking during opening and closing of the mandible (see active physiologic motions above).

Testing the muscles of the shoulder girdle and cervical spine may be relevant for some patients and is described in Chapters 11, Shoulder and Shoulder Girdle, and 19, Cervical Spine.

V. Palpation
    The cervical spine, TMJ, and face are palpated.
    A. Skin. Palpate for warmth, tenderness, temperature, localized increased skin moisture, and mobility.
    B. Mobility and feel of superficial tissues (e.g., ganglion, nodules, thickening of deep suboccipital muscles, and the presence of edema or effusion).
    C. Muscles. Palpate for consistency, mobility, continuity, tenderness, pain, and signs of spasm. Palpation of the muscles of mastication should routinely include the origin, insertion, and muscle bellies of the masseter, temporalis, internal pterygoid, and the insertion of the external pterygoid (Fig. 17-23).[220]

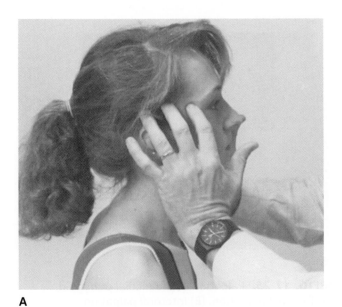

A

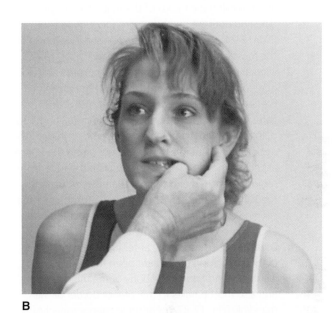

B

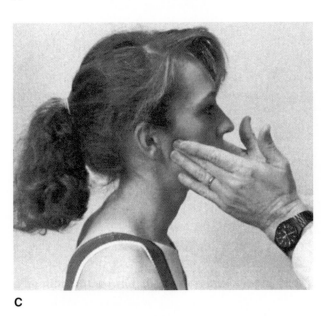

C

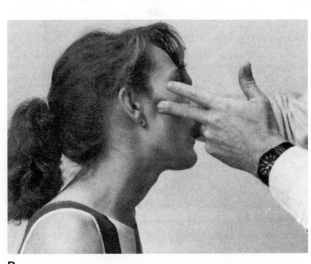

D

■ **FIG. 17-23.** Palpation of the muscles of mastication. **(A)** Belly of the temporalis muscle, **(B)** the masseter (inside the mouth), **(C)** the masseter (superficial fibers), and **(D)** the inferior lateral pterygoid.

When indicated, all the muscles of the maxillary facial region should be palpated including the facial muscles, sublingual, suprahyoids and the cervical muscles, especially the sternocleidomastoid and longus colli (Fig. 17-28). Various structural or functional cervical diseases may result in spasms of the masticatory muscles. A comprehensive thesis on the musculature and differential diagnosis of orofacial pain is described by Bell.[14] Always compare bilaterally. With respect to the TMJ itself, musculature and insertions that should be included are the following:

1. Insertion of the temporalis. Palpation of the insertion on the coronoid process is best achieved intraorally by placing the finger lateral to the first mandibular molar and following the ramus of the mandible in a posterior direction until the tip of the coronoid can be felt (Fig. 17-24). Tenderness is often caused by overuse of the muscles of mastication or bruxism.

2. Medial pterygoid. Palpate externally on the anterior edge of the ramus and intraorally to the lower medial surfaces of the ramus (Fig. 17-25).

3. Lateral pterygoid. Intraorally, use the index finger to palpate this muscle behind the last molar toward the neck of the mandible. Slide a finger along the buccal aspect of the maxillary dentition until the tuberosity region is reached and then palpate superiorly and medially in the region of the hamular process of the pterygoid process (Fig. 17-26). Wide opening will elicit point tenderness of the muscle.[33]

4. Digastric. Palpation of the anterior digastric is accomplished by having the patient open the jaw against resistance and finding the body of the muscle medial and also most parallel to the inferior border of the mandible (Fig. 17-27A). For the posterior aspect of the digastric, palpate near the angle of the ramus while

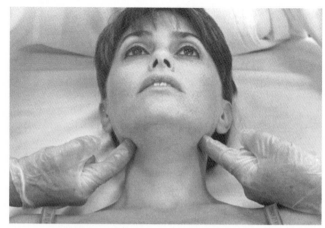

A

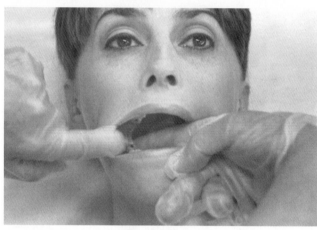

B

■ **FIG. 17-25.** Palpation of the medial pterygoid. **(A)** External palpation. **(B)** Interoral palpation.

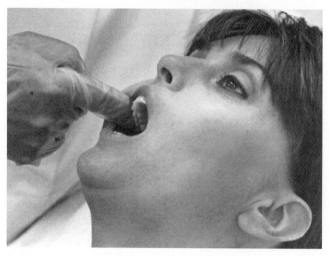

■ **FIG. 17-24.** Palpation of the insertion of the temporalis.

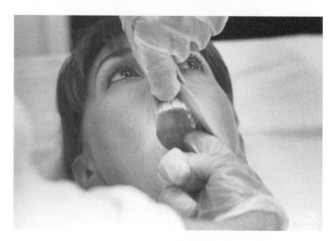

■ **FIG. 17-26.** Palpation of the lateral pterygoid (interorally).

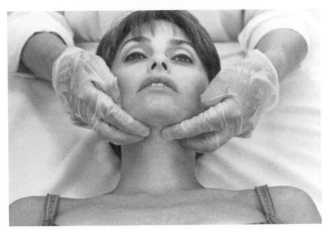

A

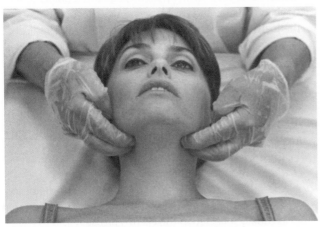

B

■ **FIG. 17-27.** Palpation of the **(A)** anterior digastric and **(B)** posterior digastric.

instructing the patient to swallow (Fig. 17-27B). The muscle felt to be contracting is the digastric. The hyoid bone can also be checked for mobility by manipulating it while asking the patient to swallow (Fig. 17-22). If there is greater tension of the digastric on one side, there may be lateral deviation of the hyoid and thyroid cartilage as well as increased resistance to shifting of midline structures away from the deviating side.

    5. Mylohyoid. This muscle, which forms the floor of the mouth, can be palpated easily intraorally and extraorally.

D. Palpate ligaments, tendon, tendon sheath, and nerve. Test for relevant trigger points and tender points of fibromyalgia. Determine if pain is provoked or reduced on palpation.

E. Temporomandibular joint. First, palpate the condylar heads laterally with the mouth closed; then palpate the distal aspect with the jaw apart for tenderness. Determine if any such tenderness is definitely accentuated when the mandible is moved contralaterally. This maneu-

ver brings the condyle more firmly under the palpating finger. The posterior aspect can be palpated through the external auditory meatus with the palpating finger. Pain and tenderness on palpation suggests a capsulitis, particularly if tenderness is found posteriorly. Abnormal capsular thickening, warmth, and swelling should also be noted. Moderate degrees of swelling in the joint prevent the fingertip from entering the depressed area overlying the joint. Swelling of a marked degree may be palpable as a rounded, often fluctuant mass overlying the joint.

    The range and dynamics of condylar motion can also be ascertained by means of palpation. From a position behind the patient, the examiner's forefingers are placed on the lateral aspects of the condylar heads as the patient actively opens his mouth. Inability to feel protrusion of the condylar head suggests a lack of forward movement.

    The examiner can determine the presence and the amount of rotation by placing the fingertips in the ear. Palpation should be done bilaterally so that a comparison of both joints can be made and any asymmetrical movements ascertained. Palpable snapping, clicking, or jumps should also be noted.

    During jaw opening, translation and rotation should occur simultaneously and at a similar ratio to one another throughout ROM.[164] The relative contribution of these two motions should be analyzed. Distraction techniques are somewhat more effective in restoring rotation while ventral glide is more helpful in restoring translation when it appears to be deficient.

F. Bony Palpation

    1. Palpate the posterior structures of the neck (spinous processes, facet joints) and the bones of the skull and temporal bone (including the mastoid process) for tenderness, deformity, and symmetry. Palpate along the entire length of the mandible, maxilla, and zygomatic bone for bony asymmetry, growth irregularities, and suspected fracture sites.

    2. Anteriorly, palpate the hyoid bone and note its relations to C2–C3. In FHP with shortening of the suprahyoids it is often elevated and may be displaced somewhat posteriorly. Ask the patient to swallow. Normally, the hyoid bone should move and cause no pain. With the neck in a neutral position, the thyroid cartilage can be easily moved back and forth with the index finger and thumb (Fig. 17-28). Motion may be limited with loss of normal crepitations following traumatic injury to the cervical spine and under circumstances of overuse (e.g., musicians who play wind instruments).[153] Palpate the thyroid cartilage for tenderness and the longus colli muscle for swelling, knots and taut bands. Avoid pressure on the vertebral artery.

G. Auscultation. Palpation of the temporomandibular movements often reveals the presence of clicking or crepitus. However, such sounds can be more accurately evaluated with the bell of a stethoscope placed over the

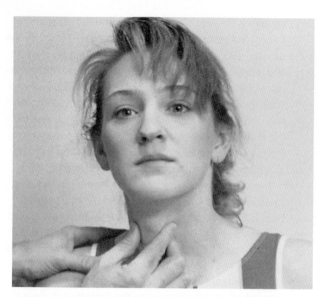

■ **FIG. 17-28.** Palpation of the thyroid cartilage and longus colli muscle. Slowly and slightly slide the fingers medial under the trachea toward the anterior bodies of the cervical vertebrae to gain access to the longus colli muscle.

condylar head as the patient actively opens his mouth. Note the type of sound associated with the movements and particular phase of movement in which it occurs. All movements—opening, closing, lateral deviation, protrusion, and retrusion—should be assessed.

The placement of a tongue depressor between the molar teeth, onto which the patient bites, occasionally eliminates the click, possibly because its presence frees the disk from the condyle before opening fully.[33]

VI. Selective Loading of the Temporomandibular Joint Can Aid in Determining Intracapsular Pathologic Conditions

Tests may include the following:

A. Dynamic loading of one joint. Have the patient bite forcefully on a cotton roll or tongue blade on one side. This procedure loads the contralateral TMJ and may elicit pain.

B. Posterior loading (compression) of both TMJs. Grasp the mandible with both hands. The thumbs are placed on the most distal molars or alveolar ridge with the fingers beneath the mandible. The mandible is then tipped down and back to compress the joints. The mandible may also be moved forward or backward to localize tenderness in the posterior or inferior parts of the joint.

C. Distraction (unloading) or caudal traction. Using the same handhold as above, distraction of both joints is performed at the same time or caudal traction of each joint is performed separately (Fig. 17-33).

Frequently the incisors are not aligned, with the mandible being deviated to one side. To assess the relevance of this deformity to the patient's symptoms, the examiner passively attempts to correct the deformity.[249] If the deviation is a protective deformity, then this test will increase the pain.

VII. Dental and Oral Examination

Make a general survey of the oral cavity, because both facial pain and TMJ disorders may have their origin in dental or oral lesions.[162] The examination of the teeth and their supporting structures, other oral structures, and mucosa is important.

By having the patient open his or her mouth maximally, the examiner is able to observe the oropharynx, tonsillar areas, and surfaces of the palate and tongue. Any alteration in the color and texture of the lingual tissues is noted.

Cavities, restored teeth, and missing teeth should be noted. Wear of biting edges and chewing surfaces that appears excessive for the patient's age often points to tensional oral habits such as bruxism. Also, the occlusion of the teeth, premature contact, overclosure of the vertical dimension, and the degree of overjet are noted.[49] Detailed occlusal analysis should always be deferred until muscle relaxation has been achieved.

Faulty occlusion may be the most common cause of TMJ dysfunction and pain. Malocclusion patterns are categorized according to the relationship of the first molars (upper and lower) to each other.

1. Class I. Mesiodistal first molar relationship is normal but there are tooth irregularities elsewhere.
2. Class II, division 1. The lower first molar is posterior to the upper first molar, causing mandibular retrusion that is usually reflected in the client's profile.
3. Class II, division 2. The lower first molar is posterior to the upper first molar but greater than in division 1, causing a large overbite.
4. Class III. The lower first molar is anterior to upper first molar, causing an underbite with mandibular protrusion.

A bimaxillary protrusion exists when the occlusion is normal but the entire dentition is forward with respect to the facial profile. When a vertical space exists between the upper and lower anterior teeth in centric occlusion, the condition is called an open bite.

Malocclusion can lead to temporomandibular disk problems, joint deterioration, and muscle imbalances. Individuals with class II malocclusion are more prone to muscle and joint dysfunction than clients with class I or class III.[111] Both the bimaxillary protrusion and anterior open bite encourage soft tissue disorders of the tongue and lips.

Other types of malocclusion causing temporomandibular symptoms include the loss of posterior teeth without replacement, loss of the vertical dimension of the jaw (**vertical dimension** is the distance from the bottom of the nose to the tip of the chin), and an off-center bite. Decreased vertical dimension will lead to excessive TMJ compression and shortening of the muscles of mastication, whereas an off-center bite (which can originate from or cause overwork to the muscles on one side of the jaw) typically results in compression on the shortened side and extension on the opposite side.

VIII. Neurologic Tests

Neurologic examination should be carried out as outlined in Chapter 5, Assessment of Musculoskeletal Disorders and Concepts of Management, if neurologic involvement is suspected. Neurologic examination involves examining the integrity of the nervous system and the mobility of the nervous system. Generally, if symptoms are localized to the upper cervical spine and head, neurologic examination can be limited to C1–C4 nerve roots. Masticatory and orofacial functioning and the neurologic system that integrates it are complex. Involvement of the muscles innervated by the fifth to 12th cranial nerves and at least the upper three cervical spinal nerves may be reflected in masticatory malfunctioning or pain. Not only the chief masticatory and secondary muscles but also the muscles of the lips, cheeks, tongue, floor of the mouth, neck, palate, and pharynx may be involved. Sensory and motor function testing may be indicated. The characteristic muscular imbalance is increased activity in the masticatory muscles, which are tight, whereas the muscles that govern the opening of the mouth (mainly the digastric and the deep neck flexors) are relatively weak.[148]

A. Integrity of the Nervous System

1. Dermatomes/peripheral nerves. Sensory testing of the cutaneous nerve supply of the face, scalp, and neck should be included if a neural deficit or neural problem is suspected (Fig. 17-29). A knowledge of the cutaneous distribution of nerve roots, dermatomes of the head and neck (see Fig. 5-4), and peripheral nerves enables the examiner to distinguish the sensory loss owing to root lesions from that owing to peripheral nerve lesions.

2. Myotomes/peripheral nerves. The following myotomes are tested and are shown in Figure 5-9:

   a. C1–C2. Upper cervical flexion.
   b. C2–5th cranial. Upper cervical extension.
   c. C3–5th cranial. Cervical lateral flexion.
   d. C4. Shoulder girdle elevation.

      The facial nerve (7th cranial) supplies the muscles of fascial expression, and the mandibular nerve the muscles of mastication.

3. Upper limb reflexes (see Fig. 11-24) and the jaw reflex should be tested for possible damage to the fifth cranial nerve. To test the jaw reflex, the examiner's thumb is placed on the patient's chin with his or her mouth slightly open. Tapping is done with the finger or reflex hammer (Fig. 17-30).

B. Mobility of the Nervous System[35]

The following neurodynamic tests may be performed to ascertain the degree to which neural tissue is responsible for the production of the patient's symptoms (see Chapters 11, Shoulder and Shoulder Girdle; 19, Cervical Spine; and 20, Thoracic Spine).

1. Passive neck flexion
2. Straight leg raise
3. Prone knee bend

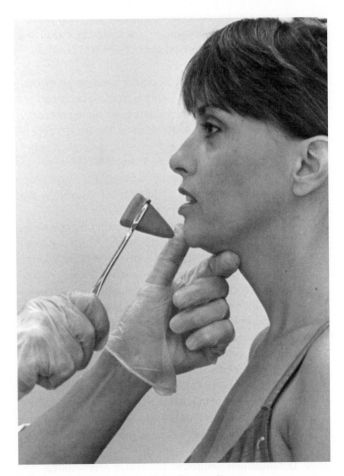

■ **FIG. 17-30.** Testing of the jaw reflex.

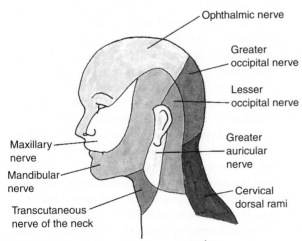

Ophthalmic nerve

Greater occipital nerve

Lesser occipital nerve

Greater auricular nerve

Cervical dorsal rami

Maxillary nerve

Mandibular nerve

Transcutaneous nerve of the neck

■ **FIG. 17-29.** Cutaneous nerve supply.

4. Slump test
5. Upper limb tension tests
C. Chvostek test for facial nerve palsy.[139] To carry out this test the examiner taps over the masseter muscle and parotid gland. Twitching of the fascial muscles, especially the masseter, is indicative of positive findings for facial nerve pathology.

IX. Other Tests
A. Vascular Tests
1. Vertebral artery test.[220] This is described in detail in Chapter 19, Cervical Spine, in examination of the cervical spine.
2. The examiner palpates the pulses of the carotid, facial, and temporal arteries if compromised circulation is suspected.
B. A cervical–upper extremity scan examination is frequently indicated in the evaluation of TMJ disorders (see Chapter 21, Cervicothoracic–Upper Limb Scan Examination). The upper cervical spinal nerves are more likely sources of pain that refers or spreads to the masticatory region than are the lower cervical nerves. The upper cervical joints (occipito-atlantal, atlanto-axial) and suboccipital muscles that are supplied by C1 to C3 nerves have been shown to refer pain into the frontal, retro-orbital, temporal, and occipital areas of the head.[50,72,82,147] Passive movements (physiologic) and passive joint-play movements of the upper cervical spine should be included (see Chapter 19, Cervical Spine).[153,249] Rule out thoracic outlet Syndrome.
C. Adjuncts, such as roentgenography and electromyography, may be indicated. Only electromyography can reveal how a muscle acts at any point during mandibular movements and postures; some researchers believe that electromyography is more reliable diagnostically than roentgenograms of the TMJs.[18,153,172]
D. Analgesic blocking of tender muscles of the joint proper may be needed to confirm the source of pain as well as to help identify secondary pain effects.[14]
E. Examination of the ear, nose, and throat may be necessary to exclude a variety of diagnosable and treatable conditions that may be confused with TMJ pathology. In addition to the history and clinical examination, further procedures are often necessary to evaluate tinnitus, hearing loss, and vertigo to establish or rule out an otologic or neurologic cause for these symptoms.

X. Interpretation of Findings
Bourbon[26] and others have found the use of the three types of syndromes of the spine, described by McKenzie, helpful in identifying the source of pain and a plan of care to reduce or eliminate pain and the effects of the pathologic mechanism in mechanical dysfunction of the TMJ. They are described below as they relate to TMJ pathology.
A. Derangement syndrome. The TMJ in which normal articular alignments are disrupted is prone to internal derangements. These are defined as some type of mechanical restriction that alters the TMJ function. Disk displacement with reduction (clicking) may manifest itself by the disk displacing in any of several directions. The most common direction of displacement is antero-medial.[240] Locking occurs when the disk becomes lodged anterior to the condyle.
B. Postural syndrome. A postural syndrome presenting as prolonged FHP is a classic example of a condition causing increasing stress to the joint and causing pain. Restoration of normal posture may help to normalize the joint. However, adaptive changes often lead to a dysfunction syndrome.
C. Dysfunction syndromes typically present with abnormal ranges of motion as the result of changes in the surrounding tissue. There are two major categories: hypermobility and hypomobility. Osteoarthritis, skeletal limitations, and reduced vertical dimensions secondary to poor posture are often followed by capsular restriction and muscle tightness leading to limited ROM.

COMMON LESIONS

Temporomandibular Joint Dysfunction Syndrome

A common TMJ disorder found clinically is TMJ dysfunction syndrome, also referred to as mandibular pain–dysfunction syndrome, arthrosis temporomandibularis,[225] TMJ arthrosis, and myofascial pain syndrome.

Temporomandibular joint dysfunction syndrome cannot be considered a disease of aging or senility, because it commonly occurs in patients between the ages of 20 and 40 years.[220] It is most frequently found among women. The early incoordination phase associated with clicking, subluxation, and recurrent dislocation is most commonly found among women in the third to fourth decade of life and in men during the third decade. The later limitation phase occurs most frequently in women in the fourth to fifth decade of life.[221]

Signs and symptoms of the early incoordination phase are usually unilateral but may be bilateral. They may include muscular tenderness, limited motion, and a dull aching pain in the periarticular area often radiating to the ear, face, head, neck, and shoulders and aggravated by function. Usually, the syndrome first manifests itself in the form of functional incoordination of the mandibular muscles with symptoms of clicking in the TMJ, which is otherwise asymptomatic, and subluxation or recurrent dislocation. Additionally, clinical examination often reveals hypermobility of the joints or a tendency to protrude the mandible or both during the initial opening movement.[235] These symptoms are followed in many cases by spasms of the masticatory muscles characterized by pain on movement of the joint, especially during mastication. Gradually, the pain becomes worse and is accompanied by decreased mobility. Pain and mobility tend to be worse in the morning. In unilateral conditions, the mandible deviates to the symptomatic side, resulting in compensation of the contralateral joint by hypermobility, subluxation, and irregular mandibular opening and closing movements. Mandibular "catching" or "locking" in certain positions may also occur on opening. Often pain may accompany movement of the hypermobile joint and may require treatment as well.

The TMJ dysfunction syndrome is usually reversible, but its perpetuation may and often does result in organic changes. When spontaneous recovery does not occur and when spasm is not relieved by treatment, such spasm may set up a sustaining cycle. If dysfunction is of a long duration, contracture of the masticatory muscles with limited painless mandibular movement may occur. This is referred to as the **limitation phase.** At this stage, pathologic changes are noted and are mainly degenerative. They are located in the fibrous covering of the articular eminence, in the condylar head, and in the fibrous articular disk. There is, however, little evidence to support the view that there is a relationship between degenerative changes within the joint and symptoms of TMJ dysfunction.[220] Significant changes are often seen without symptoms, and frequently significant symptoms are seen without radiographic evidence of changes in structure. When arthrosis of the TMJ shows extreme changes in the structure of the joint or joints, the disease is sometimes referred to as **arthrosis temporomandibularis deformans.**[225]

It is generally accepted that TMJ dysfunction–pain syndrome is a neuromuscular or joint dysfunction and that the etiology of pain is multicausal. The five major causes of pain may be neurologic, vascular, the joint itself, muscular, or hysterical conversion.[262] Pain that originates from the joints themselves can be caused by infection, disk derangement, condylar displacement, microtrauma, and traumatic injury.[259] Many patients, particularly those with painful limited mandibular movements, complain of sudden onset of symptoms on awaking, after rapid or extensive mandibular opening (e.g., yawning or after a long dental appointment), or when changes are made in occlusion (e.g., through restoration, grinding, or the use of a dental appliance).

Many authors point out that many conditions called TMJ disorders are not, in the strict sense of the word, disorders of the joint at all but simply dysfunction of the masticatory muscles.[177] The presence of painful areas within the muscles and signs of mandibular dysfunction were Schwartz's most constant finding.[220] Such painful areas and accompanying dysfunction have been given various names such as **myalgia, myositis, fibrositis,** and **myofascial pain syndromes.** The precipitating factor is believed to be motion that stretches the muscle, setting off a self-sustaining cycle of pain, spasm, and pain. The muscles that are commonly involved are the masseters, medial and lateral pterygoids, temporalis, suprahyoids, infrahyoids, sternocleidomastoids, scaleni, and rhomboids. The muscles most frequently involved are the lateral pterygoids.

Myofascial pain syndrome (MPS) has been defined as a regional pain syndrome accompanied by trigger point(s).[19,39,80,81,228,247] Diagrams have been published depicting the areas of trigger points and the zones of referred pain on palpation of these points.[38,80,81,228,246,247] Friction and coworkers[79,80,81] quantified the areas of pain with their trigger points among patients seen in a TMJ and craniofacial clinic. A large majority of the patients understandably had pain in the jaw (63%) and the TMJ area (56%).

Rheumatologists and clinicians have attempted to categorize myofascial pain into distinct syndromes, with specific criteria applying to each one. For categorization purposes, the syndromes are generally classified into two distinct categories, each with specific criteria: MPS and primary fibromyalgia (fibromyalgia syndrome [FMS]) (Table 17-1).[39,267,270–272] FMS is considered a form of nonarticular rheumatism characterized by widespread musculoskeletal aching and stiffness, as well as tenderness on palpation at characteristic sites, called tender points.[231,267,271] It occurs predominantly among females; only 5 to 20% of patients are males.[92,267,270–272]

The most common and characteristic symptoms of fibromyalgia are generalized pain, stiffness, fatigue, poor sleep, edema, and paresthesia. Associated symptoms include chronic headache, primary dysmenorrhea, and irritable bowel

TABLE 17-1 SOME DIFFERENCES BETWEEN MYOFASCIAL PAIN SYNDROME (MPS) AND FIBROMYALGIA SYNDROME (FMS)

SIGNS AND SYMPTOMS	MPS	FMS
Features	Regional pain	Diffuse, global pain
Physical signs		
• Tender-point palpation	Referred	Local
• Tender-point anatomy	Muscle belly	Muscle–tendon junction
• Stiffness	Regional	Widespread
Sleep patterns	Alpha; disruption of delta sleep in some cases	Alpha; disruption of delta sleep in most cases
Fatigue	Usually absent	Debilitating
Prognosis	Moderately poor; better than FMS	Poor, seldom cured

syndrome.[270,271] The most common sites of pain or stiffness are the neck, scapular girdle and shoulder region, arm, hand, low back, pelvic girdle, hips, and knees.[271] Other frequent sites include the anterior chest[189,271] and TMJ.[21,22,65,158,176,251,256] Although the cause of FMS is likely different than masticatory muscle pain disorders, these two conditions coexist in many chronic patients.[45,53,93,113,114,192,270–272] The most significant finding related to FMS is the presence of multiple tender points.[231,232,267,272]

Myofascial manipulations, flexibility, and low-grade strength training, cardiovascular training, transcutaneous nerve stimulation, biofeedback, cryotherapy, acupressure, stress management, and patient education all apply to the management of FMS and MPS. Myofascial manipulations become more regional than global in the management of MPS with specific emphasis on trigger point areas. It is possible to stimulate trigger points in a number of ways. These include deep pressure (acupressure), ultrasound, massage with an ice cube, dry needling with a hypodermic or acupuncture needle, laser therapy, and strain–counterstrain.[29,126,145] Another method, developed by Travell, is to spray the area from the trigger point to the reference zone with a vapocoolant spray while at the same time stretching the muscle to its fullest length. This is best followed by the application of moist heat and a home stretching exercise program. Since postural and muscle imbalances are more common in MPS, strengthening and elongation are emphasized.[39]

Emotional tension may also play a predominant role. With stress, the tension of the skeletal muscles increases, often with clenching of the teeth or bruxism resulting in local disharmony of the masticatory apparatus. When hypertonicity occurs in the masticatory muscles for a long period of time, pain-dysfunction syndrome, occlusal wear, and tooth mobility may be evident. Once the pattern is established, it appears to be self-perpetuating. Other habit manifestations seen in these patients that cause pathologic occlusal contact are numerous and include unilateral mastication, abnormal swallowing, and "tooth doodling" during the waking hours.[88,235] What the patient does to his or her occlusion in reaction to stress seems to be more important than any existing malocclusion. Certainly malocclusion, by mechanically increasing the amount of force or altering its direction, can make the chance of injury more likely. More important than the type of malocclusion, however, may be the amount and kind of muscular activity and the reaction of the person to such activity. In some persons, change in proprioception, no matter how slight, seems to be more important than a long-standing malocclusion, no matter how irregular.

Diagnostic procedures to establish the presence of TMJ dysfunction and a definitive diagnosis include the following:

- An accurate history
- Determination of the patient's emotional state and daily habits
- Examination of mandibular movements

- Measurement of mandibular opening, lateral deviation, and protrusion
- Palpation of the TMJ and muscles of mastication
- Dental and oral examination
- Occlusal analysis
- Roentgenograms
- Electromyography
- Physical examination of related structures (cervical spine)
- Neurologic testing

The primary methods of therapy revolve around the correction of occlusal disharmonies and tension habits as well as physical therapy to eliminate spasm and increase ROM through therapeutic exercise and mobilization techniques.

Hypermobility

Hypermobility of the TMJ is defined as a laxity of the articular ligaments. It may be localized or be part of a generalized hypermobility syndrome.[240] Localized hypermobility of the TMJ is believed to be the most common mechanical disorder.[174] It is characterized by early or excessive anterior translation, or both. Unfortunately, this permits hypertranslation of the condyle, which can lead to dysfunction. This excessive anterior glide results in the laxity of the surrounding capsule and ligaments. It is interesting to note that the TMJ has no capsule on the medial half of the anterior aspect.[111] The breakdown of these structures enables disk derangement in one or both TMJs. Ultimately, pain, functional loss, and possibly arthritic changes set in.

Generalized hypermobility, a disorder of increased mobility of multiple joints, has been suggested to be a predisposing factor in the development of degenerative TMJ disorders.[4,10,11,59,100,110,146,165,193,233,236,242] The results of a study by Dijkstra and colleagues,[58] however, did not support the hypothesis that generalized hypermobility predisposes to TMJ osteoarthrosis and internal derangement. Future research is necessary in order to determine whether local hypermobility of the TMJ may be a predisposing factor.

Parafunctional habits that appear to contribute to localized hypermobility of the TMJ include gum chewing, nail biting, mouth breathing, nocturnal bruxism, prolonged bottle feeding, and pacifier use.[119,209] Hypermobility can also occur when trauma subluxations and dislocations stretch the joint.

Presenting signs and symptoms clinically demonstrated by patients with TMJ hypermobility include the following[111,174]:

1. The ability to insert three or four knuckles between the incisors
2. Excessive joint mobility often characterized by large anterior translation at the beginning of opening when rotation should be occurring
3. Lateral deviation of the mandible during depression or elevation
4. Clicking, popping, or cracking with mandibular depression or elevation
5. Closed or open locking

6. Pain in one or both TMJs and the surrounding masticatory muscles
7. Tinnitus

Structures that are overstretched in hypermobile joints should be identified and stabilized. A program of muscle retraining in the control of joint rotation and translation and mandibular stabilization should be implemented. Avoiding excessive anterior translation and reestablishing normal head, neck, and shoulder girdle posture have been found to be particularly beneficial, as have splint therapy and stress management.[174]

Existing programs stress exercises that help normalize the position of the jaw, regain normal tracking, and restore the proper sequence of movement. According to Rocabado and Iglarsh,[209] hypermobile joints are best treated by avoiding excessive anterior translational glides of the condyle, controlling rotation, stabilizing the joint and reestablishing normal head, neck, and shoulder girdle posture.

Degenerative Joint Disease—Osteoarthritis

Although osteoarthritis may occur at any age, it is considered primarily a disease of middle or old age. It affects an estimated 80 to 90% of the population older than 60 years of age.[103,172]

The etiology is generally believed to be the result of normal wear and tear associated with aging and function, as well as the result of repeated minor trauma. The damage is speculated to consist primarily of degeneration of the chondroitin–collagen-protein complex.[102] Roentgenographic examination may reveal narrowing of the TMJ space with condensation of bone in the region of the articular cortex, spur formation, and marginal lipping at the articular margins of the condylar head.[102] In some cases there is considerable thickening of the synovial membrane owing to chronic synovitis. There may be perforation of the disk without bony changes. Erosion of the condylar head, articular eminence, and fossa may be noted.

Symptoms do not seem to be related to the extent of articular damage. Osteoarthritis may be asymptomatic even in the presence of extensive articular damage, while on the other hand, articular findings may be completely absent in patients with acute symptoms. The onset is generally insidious with mild symptoms. Pain, which is usually a dull aching in or around the joint, is usually not constant. Typically, painful stiffness of the jaw muscles is noted in the morning or following periods of rest. With use, the symptoms may disappear and then reappear with fatigue at the end of the day. Pain may be precipitated on opening or during mastication. Crepitation, crackling, or clicking may occur in one or both joints. Subluxation and locking of one or both joints during certain movements are common complaints. The patient may also complain of symptoms of the ear, impaired hearing, frequent headaches, and dizziness. At the onset, symptoms are usually short lived, but as degeneration progresses they occur more frequently and last longer. Crepitation and limited motion are the most constant findings.

Diagnostic procedures to establish the presence of osteoarthritis can be difficult but again depend on an accurate history, the determination of the patient's emotional state, physical examination, and roentgenograms. Physical examination may or may not reveal discrete painful areas in the musculature; minimal emotional tension may be noted. Loss of movement is greatest in the upper joint compartment. There is limitation in a capsular pattern of restriction. In unilateral conditions, contralateral excursions and opening are most restricted; protrusion and retrusion are both restricted. There is an ipsilateral deviation of the mandible at the extreme range of opening. Accessory movements are limited and reproduce temporomandibular pain.

The primary method of therapy is directed at symptoms and may involve correcting the occlusion of the teeth or prosthesis, drug therapy, and physical therapy. During the painful phase, the application of hot packs may help to reduce muscle spasm and pain. Active range-of-motion exercises (often in conjunction with ultrasound), passive ROM exercises, mobilization techniques (preceded by deep friction massage to the capsule),[51] and stretching may be used during the chronic phase. Graded exercises involving a few simple movements performed frequently during the day are often prescribed as a home treatment. Advanced bony changes within the joint may necessitate arthroplasty with joint debridement.

Rheumatoid Arthritis

There is little agreement regarding the incidence of patients with rheumatoid arthritis who also develop the disease in the TMJs; estimates vary from 20 to 51%.[102] Women are affected more often than men.

There are three groups of symptoms: transitory, acute, and chronic. Transitory symptoms include limitation of motion and referred pain. Acute symptoms consist of transitory symptoms plus joint pain, swelling, and warmth lasting 6 to 10 weeks. Chronic symptoms are characterized by severe pain and limitation of motion. The joint and muscle symptoms are most severe in the morning and diminish with the day's activity. Inflammatory changes are noted in the synovial membrane and periarticular structures by atrophy and rarefaction of bone. A serious sequela of ankylosis may restrict or even eliminate movement. If conservative management does not relieve symptoms, surgical intervention may be indicated.

The primary method of therapy is directed at symptoms and may involve drug therapy, if indicated by specific signs and symptoms, and physical therapy. In the acute phase, immobilization is contraindicated but rest in the form of a soft or liquid diet is advocated. After inflammation has subsided, treatment is directed at reducing muscle spasm and restoring mandibular movements by corrective exercises.

Surgical procedures such as condylectomies and condylotomies frequently used in the past are now believed to be obsolete for the most part but are occasionally performed.[214] After surgery, corrective exercises and exercises of mandibular excursions, using mouth props to ensure that ROM is not compromised, should be performed several times a day.[152]

Trauma and Disorders of Limitation

One of the most frequent causes of TMJ dysfunction is a direct or indirect blow to the area, including resultant fracture in the region of the condyle. When there is no fracture, injuries may result in edema and possible soft-tissue damage, such as tearing of the capsular ligaments or disk and simple dislocations and subluxations. Other causes of limitation include postoperative trismus following tooth extraction and whiplash injuries.

Early and late presentation following motor vehicle trauma is frequently theorized to include temporomandibular disorders.[30,68,85,107,116,138,144,211,215,261] Whiplash can be explained as a deceleration effect on the mandible and thus on the TMJ either through direct injury or through neurologic involvement. When the head is snapped back abruptly, the mouth flies open, evoking a stretch reflex of the masseter. The capsule, ligaments, and inter-articular disk act as a restraining ligament; tearing or stretching of these tissues may result. Immediately following, the jaw snaps shut; this may strain the attachment of the disk if malocclusion is present. Cervical traction, commonly used in the management of the cervical spine, may also produce TMJ dysfunction, or the primary TMJ dysfunction may be aggravated.

Treatment and management of such injuries will depend on the structures involved, the extent of displacement, the effect on function, and the degree of pain. During the acute phase, soft and liquid diets, head bandages or intermaxillary immobilization, and splints may be used to rest the joint. Surgical procedures, open and closed reduction, and manipulations may be necessary.

Physical therapy may consist of heat and other methods to reduce pain and muscle spasm, early mobility exercises after surgery or after immobilization to ensure ROM is not compromised, and muscle re-education and corrective exercises. Stretching and mobilization techniques may be necessary to treat contracture of the musculature or capsules. When mechanical cervical traction is considered necessary in the treatment of neck and whiplash injuries, the TMJ should be protected with bite plates or soft splints and the proper use of traction.

Other Conditions

Other conditions that may cause TMJ dysfunction include a variety of neurologic and muscular disorders, bone disease, tumors, infections, psychogenic disorders, growth and developmental disorders, diseases causing disturbance of the occlusion of the teeth or supporting structures, faulty habits of the jaw, and orofacial imbalance.

TREATMENT TECHNIQUES

Temporomandibular joint dysfunction, arthritic conditions, ankylosing diseases, traumatic injuries, and postsurgical enti-

ties may be a few of the causes that bring a patient to the physical therapist.

When degenerative disease, bony or fibrous ankylosis, fractures, occlusal disharmony, and other conditions necessitate surgery, follow-up physical therapy may become necessary to maintain or regain motion, as well as regain normal mandibular osteokinematics. In the majority of postsurgical cases, muscle tonus remains good, except after long-term ankylosis or degenerative joint disease. In these cases there is greater possibility that the muscles have atrophied, making rehabilitation more difficult and necessitating a more extensive program of therapeutic exercises to increase the physiologic elasticity and strength of the muscles.

After condylectomy the attachment of the lateral pterygoid to the condyle has been severed, so that the jaw will increasingly deviate ipsilaterally. Postoperative rehabilitation for the lost function should encourage the similarly functioning muscles of the masseter, temporalis, and suprahyoid muscles on the healthy side to perform with increased strength. At least partial use of the lateral pterygoid muscle should be stressed so that it is able to contribute to contralateral mandibular excursion and to prevent posterior drifting of the ramus in its tonic state.

Signs and symptoms of the TMJ syndrome vary but generally include a cluster of symptoms:

- Pain and tenderness of the masticatory muscles
- Limited or altered mandibular function (i.e., hypermobility or a tendency to protrude the mandible in the initial opening phase)
- Crepitation or clicking
- Deviation of the mandible on opening
- Disturbed chewing patterns
- Locking of the jaw
- Vague, remote subjective complaints

The means of treatment of TMJ syndrome is basically like that for other MPSs—anesthetics, exercise, and physical and pharmacologic agents. There are, however, additional considerations. There are two traditional concepts of the etiology of TMJ dysfunction. Some clinicians stress malocclusion as the causal factor. They advocate treatment involving mainly mechanical methods, such as equilibration of the occlusion.[51,105] Others emphasize that psychologic factors, especially response to stress, and harmful habits of the jaw may influence both the onset and course of symptoms. They advocate patient education, the elimination of habitual protrusion or other harmful habits, and muscular relaxation.

The effective management of TMJ disorders requires first of all a diagnosis based on a complete history, thorough physical examination, and when indicated, adjuncts such as a detailed study of the patient's occlusion, roentgenography, and electromyography.

Soft Tissue Techniques

Soft tissue manipulations may include deep friction massage to the capsule of the joint,[51] gentle kneading or stroking techniques interorally to inhibit pain (to the insertion of the temporalis and medial and lateral pterygoid musculature) (Figs. 17-23A,17-24 through 17-27), deep pressure joint massage,[44,159,217,243] connective tissue massage,[244] strain–counterstrain,[126] craniosacral therapy,[252] myofascial release, muscle energy or postisometric relation techniques,[148,149,168] and stretching techniques (see Chapter 8, Soft Tissue Manipulations, and Box 8-6).

Soft tissue manipulations have been found to be particularly helpful to release a tight masseter, the temporalis masseter complex and supra- and infrahyoid musculature.[62] Suprahyoid and infrahyoid release techniques are indicated for patients with lack of craniocervical extensibility and restriction of the infrahyoid muscles. These techniques assist in proper placement of the tongue in patients with abnormal tongue position or swallowing habits and are useful in patients with FHP either after traumatic injury or overuse through maladaptation.[62,252] Gentle tractions are held for a number of seconds to a minute or longer until a giving way is sensed (Fig. 17-31). Infrahyoid release may be used to decrease spasms in the overstretched infrahyoid muscles, often seen in patients with cervical whiplash (see Box 8-7).

A useful postisometric relaxation technique for increased tension of the digastric on one side (the main antagonist of the masticatory muscles) is to have the patient assume a supine position.[148] In this position, the clinician resists the opening of the mouth with one hand while the thumb of the other hand exerts minimal pressure on the hyoid on the side of increased tension (Fig. 17-32A). The patient is instructed to open the mouth gently and breathe in, to hold the breath, and then to breathe out and relax. During relaxation, resistance in the digastric will automatically give way under the clinician's thumb. This technique is also a useful self-treatment (Fig. 17-32B).

Treatment of Limitation Disorders

STRETCHING TECHNIQUES

To increase limited mandibular movements, a variety of exercises involving the muscles of mastication may be employed.

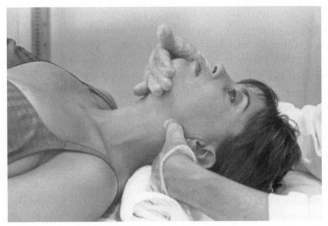

A

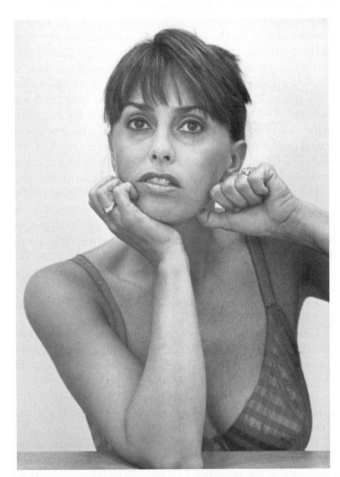

B

■ **FIG. 17-32.** Digastric. **(A)** Postisometric relaxation technique. **(B)** Self-treatment. One hand is placed under the chin, while the other hand contacts the lateral aspect of the hyoid bone (tense side) with the thumb. Following the resistance phase, the thumb gently moves the hyoid medially.

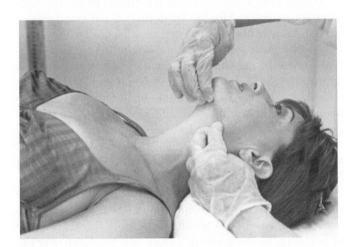

■ **FIG. 17-31.** Suprahyoid release technique.

They are used, on one hand, to help break up the muscle spasm, and on the other, to maintain and increase limited jaw movement to full physiologic function.

Active Stretch. The patient actively opens the mouth as wide as possible several times following a series of warm-up exercises.[221] By having the patient repeat a gentle, rhythmic, hingelike movement a number of times before active stretch, muscle spasm can be physiologically diminished or eliminated. With the patient in a comfortable, relaxed, reclining position or in a recliner chair, have the patient place the tongue in contact with the hard palate as posteriorly as possible, while keeping the mandible in a retruded position. In this position with the tongue on the hard palate, the patient's articular movements are mainly rotatory and early protrusion is avoided. It is helpful to have the patient palpate the condyles so that he or she can feel the movement. If glide occurs too early, with little or no rotatory motion, there is an early protrusion problem. Instruct the patient to open the mouth slowly and rhythmically within this limited range 10 times or so in succession. The patient then performs active stretch by opening the mouth as wide as possible within the pain-free limit, as slowly as possible two or three times. The opening position should be held for 5 seconds, followed by relaxation in the rest position for 5 seconds. In the case of unilateral limitation, the tip of the tongue is positioned on the palatal surface behind the canine teeth on the contralateral side. The application of a vapocoolant spray or ultrasound may be an effective adjunct during active stretch.

During normal mandibular opening, translation begins beyond 11 mm.[140] Improving translation is therefore accomplished by having the patient place a finger (six or so tongue blades, or a wooden pencil) horizontally between the teeth, which will open the mandible approximately 11 mm. The patient can then actively practice protrusive, retrusive, and lateral excursions of the mandible but avoid any jamming effects that might occur if translation is done within the first 11 mm of opening.

Lateral excursion exercises are frequently used during postoperative physical therapy. During the repair phase, lateral deviations should be limited to 5 mm on the side opposite the surgery to prevent overstretching of the repair site.[17,118,208,209]

Yawning is recommended as a home program exercise. It is an active stretching movement that is accomplished by strong reflex inhibition of the mandibular elevators.

These active exercises should be repeated often during the day for brief periods. These procedures must be applied cautiously in the presence of roentgenographic evidence of TMJ arthropathy and if done soon after disk plication or graft.

A variety of neuromuscular facilitation exercises may be used when ROM is limited by shortening, contracture, or spasm.[136,220,263] One of the most frequently used methods is hold–relax to make stretching of the masticatory muscles more effective. This technique implies a contraction of the antagonist against maximal resistance, followed by relaxation, and then active or assistive stretch of the agonist. For example, to increase mandibular opening, the patient is asked to close his mouth tightly as resistance is applied gently and slowly to the mandible. This is followed by a relaxation and then by active or passive motion. Isometric contraction of the mouth elevator muscles facilitates their relaxation. The resultant stimulation of the jaw-opening muscles permits increased active or passive stretch. The clinician might use the following commands:

1. "Just hold your jaw closed and don't let me move it." (Apply resistance gently and slowly to the mandible.)
2. "Let go." (Maintain gentle support of the mandible and wait for relaxation to occur.)
3. "Open your mouth." (Have the patient move the mandible actively with or without resistance.)

Unresisted reversing movements may also be used as a follow-up procedure by either active or assistive stretch.

A variety of similar techniques such as maximal resistance superimposed on an isotonic or isometric contraction, slow-reversal–hold, and contract–relax may be used.[136,220,263] Such exercises may also be used for increasing range of protrusion, retrusion, and lateral deviation. The clinician provides resistance, or the patient may be asked to do so with his or her own hand.[220] By using resistance, the patient effects an increased relaxation of the antagonist muscles. This sets up a reflex mechanism called **reciprocal inhibition.**

Passive Stretch. Prolonged static stretch is often advantageous and may be accomplished by using a series of tongue blades built up, one on top of the other, between the anterior incisors for bilateral limitation or between the upper and lower teeth (far back on the involved side) in the case of unilateral limitation.[153] This places the capsule and tight elevator muscles on moderate stretch. The tongue blades are not meant to be used as a forced stretch but rather to take up the slack and maintain the mandible in a relaxed open position. The use of cold (ice or vapocoolant spray) or ultrasound may be administered during the passive stretch. As the jaw begins to relax, additional tongue blades may be added. Prolonged stretch is usually applied for 15 to 20 minutes. Following TMJ surgery, no more than 1 or 2 minutes of stretching is recommended.

Tongue blades can also be used for home treatment, both as a static stretch and for briefer periods of active and passive stretch. Tongue blades, however, must be used with caution since too vigorous application may cause injury. Shore recommended the use of a tapered cork.[225] The cork, which is approximately 15 mm at its narrow end and 30 mm at its widest end, is gradually inserted (small end first) into the patient's mouth until the jaws are separated. Once the jaw begins to relax, the cork can be placed farther into the mouth, thus progressively opening the jaw wider and wider. Shore[225] recommends using this technique as a home treatment for 30-second periods every 2 hours.

Assistive Stretch (Direct Method). With the patient sitting, the clinician stands behind and places both thumbs over the patient's lower teeth and his index fingers over the upper teeth. Sterile gauze or a cloth may be placed over the lower teeth. The patient is instructed to support the mandible with one hand under the chin. The mandible is then opened with gentle but maximal effort. If a less vigorous stretch is indicated, the clinician uses one hand, with the index finger and thumb in the same position, and supports the patient's mandible with the opposite hand.[220]

The patient may be taught to use this method as a form of self-treatment, using the thumb and index finger in a reverse position and supporting the mandible with one or both hands.[220]

All these exercises should emphasize movement without pain or undue force. Stretching should be done slowly and can be done actively (with or without resistance to the mandible) or passively.

Reflex relaxation of the elevator muscles followed by active stretch, as used for the opening movement, as well as passive and assistive stretch may also be applied to lateral, protrusive, and retrusive movements. With instruction, the patient can carry out many of these exercises alone.

JOINT MOBILIZATION TECHNIQUES

Joint mobilization techniques in the treatment of TMJ disorders are aimed at restoring normal joint mechanics in order to allow full, pain-free osteokinematics of the mandible to occur. The techniques described are based on courses presented by Rocabado and the works of Kaltenborn.[130,202]

Temporomandibular Joint Mobilization

1. Caudal Traction (Fig. 17-33)
    Note: *P*, patient; *O*, operator; *M*, movement.
    P—Lies supine on a semireclining table or in dental chair that supports the head and trunk.

O—Stands at patient's side and faces left side of patient's head. Right hand and forearm are placed around patient's head, fixating head against the table. (A stabilizing belt across the forehead may be used instead.) Left hand holds, with thumb in the mouth over the left inferior molars and with the fingers outside around the patient's jaw.

M—Ask patient to swallow. While maintaining the forearm in a straight line (hand and forearm act as a unit), apply traction caudally. Reverse for the opposite side.

Note: Caudal traction may be combined with ventral and dorsal glide (protraction and retraction). The mandible is first distracted caudally, and while traction is maintained the mandible is glided ventrally, then dorsally, followed by a gradual release of caudal traction.

2. Protrusion—Ventral glide (Fig. 17-34)
    P—Lies supine on a semireclining table or in dental chair that supports the head and trunk.

O—Stands at patient's side and faces left side of patient's head. Right hand and forearm are placed around the patient's head, fixating against the operator's body. Left hand holds onto the angle of the ramus with index and third finger. The rest of the hand contacts the patient's jaw.

M—Ask patient to swallow. While maintaining the forearm in a straight line, glide the mandible ventrally into protrusion. Reverse for the opposite side.

Note: An alternative handhold would be to place the thumb in the mouth on the right inferior molars and the fingers outside around the right side of patient's jaw. This same handhold can be used for retrusion (dorsal glide).

Gliding movements ventrally may be combined with a little rotation. The right mandible is first glided forward, as described, and then rotated to the left by rotation of operator's body.

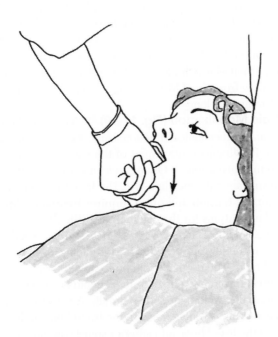

■ **FIG. 17-33.** Caudal traction.

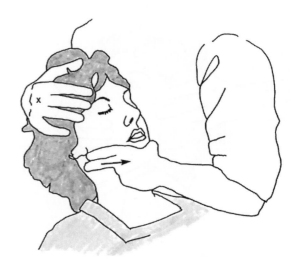

■ **FIG. 17-34.** Protrusion.

3A. Medial-Lateral Glide (Fig. 17-35)—Rotation of the left joint and forward glide of the right joint.

  P—Lies supine on a semireclining table or dental chair that supports the head and trunk.

  O—Stands behind patient. Right hand holds around the patient's head, fixating head against table. Left hand is positioned so that the hypothenar eminence is placed just caudal to the left TMJ with the fingers wrapped around the patient's jaw.

  M—Ask patient to swallow. The hypothenar eminence acts as a pivot point as the mandible is glided forward and medially to the left. Reverse for opposite side.

3B. Alternative Technique (Fig. 17-36)

  P—Lies supine on a semireclining table or in dental chair that supports the head and neck.

  O—Stands at patient's side and faces left side of patient's head. Right hand is placed around patient's head, fixating head against table. Left hand holds with thumb in mouth on medial aspect of body of mandible near the right inferior molars, with the fingers (outside) wrapped around the jaw.

  M—Ask patient to swallow. With the thumb acting as a pivot point, move the wrist ulnarly so that the right condyle moves outward, forward, and laterally as the mandible is moved medially to the left. Reverse for opposite side.

Many of the semireclining techniques described above may be carried out in a sitting position. The patient's head may be stabilized against the operator's body and supported with the free hand. However, the semireclining or supine position is preferred, since the head and mandible are in a better position for fixation. Furthermore, if a stabilizing belt is used, the operator's other hand is free to assist the mobilizing hand or to palpate the joint to determine if correct

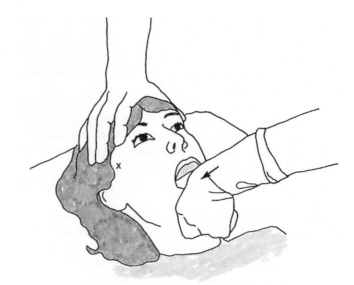

■ **FIG. 17-36.** Medial-lateral glide (alternative technique).

motion is obtained. Mobilization techniques using pressures against the head of the mandible, which has been developed by Maitland, is particularly useful (Fig. 17-37).[153,248] One of the greatest difficulties encountered when mobilizing the jaw is the patient's inability to relax the jaw completely. By mobilizing the condyle directly rather than through the mandible (which involves large movements), the patient is often able to relax more readily and treatment is often more successful. Also, overstretching of the upper joint compartment is avoided. Medial glide is particularly useful in restoring rotation (lower joint compartment).

Self-distraction (caudally directed traction to the TMJ via the mandible) can be performed easily by the patient.[62] Both palms of the hands are placed onto the side of the face with the forearms supported on the patient's chest or with the elbows resting on a table. Distraction occurs as the skin and fascia are taken to their elastic limits and the underlying structures are eased away from the TM joint (Fig. 17-38). This is held for a least 1 minute or longer.

Hyoid Mobilization (Fig. 17-39).[230] The hyoid bone is a significant biomechanical functional unit of the stomatognathic system. It influences movement of the mandible, swallowing and sound formation.[205] Owing to its anatomic relationship to the suprahyoids and digastric, the hyoid is often subject to abnormal tension and often requires treatment. Specific clinical indications for the can include difficulty swallowing, laryngitis, and hoarness.[229,230] Assessment is first carried out to determine the side of restriction by side gliding the hyoid to the left and right. The normal hyoid bone should move equally in both directions freely. The examiner should be able to palpate crepitus as the hyoid bone slides laterally. An absence of crepitus may indicate swelling beneath the hyoid bone in the tissue between the hyoid bone and anterior spinal column (i.e., muscle spasms of the longus colli or infrahyoid muscles).[205]

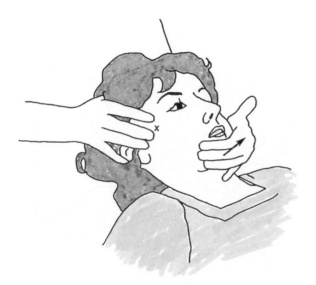

■ **FIG. 17-35.** Medial-lateral glide.

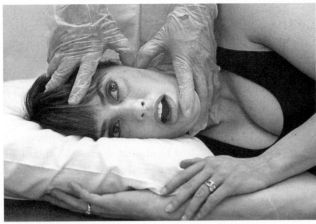
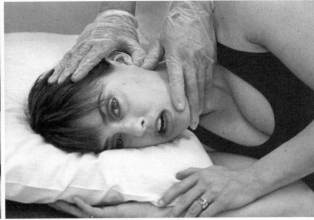

A   **B**

■ **FIG. 17-37.** Mobilization techniques may be applied directly to the condyle with the patient in sidelying. **(A)** Medial glide. Gentle oscillatory medial glides are performed over the lateral pole of the condyle with the thumbs. **(B)** Anterior glide. Gentle oscillatory mobilizations are performed over the posterior aspect of the condyle. (Reprinted with permission from Hall C, Brody L: Therapeutic Exercise: Moving Toward Function, 2nd ed. Baltimore, Lippincott Williams & Wilkins, 1998.)

P—Lies supine with the head well supported.

O—Sits at the head of the table. Light thumb contact is placed the side of the restriction.

M—The patient is asked to open the mouth slightly (being sure to obtain pure condylar rotation). As the patient gently tries to open the mouth, the operator applies resistance. The patient holds for 7 to 10 seconds and then relaxes the mandible. After waiting for relaxation the hyoid bone will move away from the thumb. The operator then takes up the slack to meet the new barrier. This procedure is repeated two to three times.

Suprahyoid release technique (Fig. 17-31) may be used to release the suprahyoid musculature. For home training the patient should carry out neuromuscular re-education for excessive translation (see Fig. 17-42), postisometric relaxation technique for the digastric (Fig. 17-32), isometric coordinating exercise (see Fig. 17-43) and digastric facilitation techniques (e.g., rhythmic stabilization) for the mandibular depressors.

TREATMENT OF TMJ DYSFUNCTION SYNDROMES, DISK DERANGEMENT, OR CONDYLAR DISPLACEMENT

Signs and symptoms of early TMJ dysfunction include primarily muscular hyperactivity and pain, disturbed chewing habits, clicking, "catching" or "locking" of the jaw (recurrent subluxations), and limited motion or hypermobility of the joints. Palliative therapy is directed at reducing muscle spasm (the pain–spasm–pain cycle) and relieving intrajoint symptoms

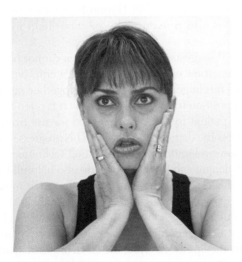

■ **FIG. 17-38.** Self-distraction. (Reprinted with permission from Hall C, Brody L: Therapeutic Exercise: Moving Toward Function, 2nd ed. Baltimore, Lippincott Williams & Wilkins, 1998.)

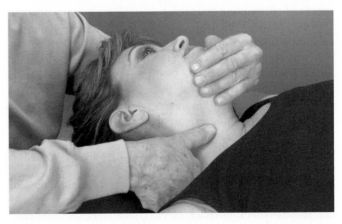

■ **FIG. 17-39.** Hyoid mobilization.

caused by trauma, inflammation, condylar displacement, or disk derangement.[262] Treatment may include drug therapy, injections, application of thermotherapy,[178] coolant therapy,[34,120,219,228,247] disengagement of the occlusion by prostheses or voluntarily disengagement, and alterations in dietary and oral habits.

Causative therapy procedures may include manipulations and joint mobilization techniques to restore normal joint mechanics; correction of condylar displacements with the use of occlusal repositioning splints or occlusal equilibration; and correction of disk derangement by mandibular manipulations or repositioning appliances.[143,153,187,225,262] Occasionally, surgical correction may be necessary.

Adjunctive therapy may include the use of ultrasound,[129] electrogalvanic electrical stimulation,[122,179,222] transcutaneous electrical nerve stimulation (TENS),[175] acupuncture,[64,124,255] cold laser,[18,20,108,184,213,255] patient education, relaxation techniques, psychotherapy, biofeedback, and exercises. According to Somers,[235] treatment directed toward patient education, the elimination of poor oral habits, and the acquisition of muscle relaxation is often all that is required to relieve the patient's symptoms.

Patient Education. A most important step is to educate patients regarding the functioning of their joints, the reason for their symptoms, and the means of removing those symptoms. Advice should include reassurance, which is often simply gained by understanding the anatomy of the joint and the physiologic mechanisms at work.

Use of a skull, the patient's roentgenograms, or simple diagrams will help the clinician explain the structure and function of the TMJs and the rationale for the various procedures that must be undertaken. Instructions should emphasize diet and careful use of the jaw.[159] The harmful effects of wide opening, yawning, biting off large mouthfuls of hard food, habitual protrusion, diurnal clenching, or nocturnal bruxism should be explained. Because an emotional overlay is often present, counseling on how emotional conflicts are translated into muscle tension and pain is usually an important consideration. Point out that methods to achieve muscle relaxation and abolish well-established patterns of inappropriate muscular activity and methods to acquire new ones are important means of eliminating symptoms.

Relaxation Training. In addition to patient education, relaxation training for jaw and facial muscles is often considered, although it may be difficult to achieve. Muscle tension is one of the most important contributing causes of muscular derangements of the TMJ, regardless of whether the derangement occurred through trauma. A report by Heiberg and colleagues[115] indicates that of a group of patients with a diagnosis of TMJ syndrome, almost all exhibited tense muscles in the neck and back as well, indicating that muscular tension is not confined to the masticatory muscles alone. Increased muscular tension, especially in the erector trunci, was present in 95% of these patients.[115] Typically they presented with a tightly closed jaw, stiffened neck and back, elevated shoulders, and a forward head. Faulty respiration patterns were also a common finding.[112]

Relaxation of the whole body or body regions is frequently indicated in the treatment of these overly tense patients. More often than not, general relaxation techniques will have to precede training for local relaxation (see Chapter 9, Relaxation and Related Techniques). Relaxation exercises such as those modified from Jacobson, autogenic training, and reflex relaxation exercises may all be used.

The clinician can show the patient the presence of unnecessary muscular contraction at the end of the initial physical examination or during the first treatment session. Most patients are unable to relax the jaw muscles so that the mandible can be moved freely by the therapist. They are unable to let the head loll back when the shoulders are supported, since the neck muscles remain rigid. They cannot permit their elevated arm to fall limply to the treatment table when requested by the examiner.

Perhaps one of the hardest of all relaxation procedures to achieve is elimination of overcontraction of the jaw muscles. An example of a local technique using a modification of Jacobson's approach (progressive relaxation) follows:

- Clench the jaw firmly and concentrate on feeling the sense of tightness in the temples as well as the jaw itself.
- Switch off and let the jaw fall open.
- Push the jaw open against the pressure of an assistant's hand.
- Relax completely.
- Move the jaw sideways to the left as far as possible with or without resistance and experience the sensation this gives to the jaw and temples before relaxing.
- Repeat the same exercise to the right.
- Complete the sequence by clenching the jaw firmly again, and let the jaw drop open loosely.

Another form of progressive relaxation uses a reverse approach. Instead of asking the patient to contract the muscle and then relax, the muscles are passively stretched and then relaxed.[41–43] Other training methods include self-hypnosis, meditation, and yoga.[91,157,233] Hypnosis provided by a trained therapist has also proven to be of some help in reducing pain.[60,227,237]

Somers[235] suggests that total relaxation cannot be assumed until the assistant can take the patient's chin between the thumb and forefinger and tap the tooth together rapidly without any opposition from the jaw muscles. It is often most helpful for the patient to adapt this method for use from time to time to assess the degree of tension and his progress in attempting to achieve relaxation. Autosuggestion techniques to guard against clenching and tooth contact are also helpful. He or she may be told to repeat the following after each meal, "Lips together, teeth apart." He or she should also be instructed to make frequent checks during the day for jaw clenching and to attempt to maintain the rest position of the mandible in which only the lips touch while the teeth are held apart. These methods of treatment are often considered the first line of defense against clenching and nocturnal bruxism.[225]

The use of biofeedback methods to guide the patient in controlling muscle activity and promoting relaxation is frequently used.[66,75,97,105,167,188,212,223,249,250] Feedback from electromyography of the frontal, temporal, and masseter muscles has been particularly useful.[48,66]

Posture Awareness and Balancing the Upper Quadrant. In addition to relaxation training and patient education, the clinician must spend time instructing the patient in good body mechanics, postural control, and correct body positioning for maximum relaxation of the cervical spine and masticatory muscles. Cervical traction, exercises, and mobilization may also be indicated when associated cervical symptoms or pathologic processes coexist. Occlusal splints may be indicated to create relaxation of the elevator muscles and to disorient an acquired noxious occlusal sensory input. Splints may also be used to disorient the sensory input in patients who clench, by changing the quality of afferent touch information.[143,225] Occlusal analysis and equilibration, if indicated, are usually best deferred until relaxation has been achieved.

Many clinical manifestations of pain in the upper quarter have their source not in an isolated joint disorder, but in chronic upper quarter dysfunction spanning several body segments. It is estimated that 70% of patients presenting with craniomandibular dysfunction (temporomandibular disorders) will also present with craniocervical dysfunction.[203] Based on clinical studies and experience of numerous practitioners, there are several findings that are common to a population of patients presenting with TMJ dysfunction. Some of the findings include the following:

- Abnormal forward or lateral head postures
- Compensatory abnormal shoulder girdle postures (protracted shoulders)
- Changes in the position of the mandible (condylar retrusion and diminished interocclusal distance)[63]
- Mouth and upper chest breathing
- Abnormal resting position of the tongue
- Deviant swallow

Postural or orthostatic evaluation and treatment of these patients is extremely important, because an altered biomechanical relationship will always produce accommodations and even subsequent adaptations if the accommodations are maintained.[171,206]

A system of upper quarter re-education methods has been developed by Rocabado[206] and Kraus[140] that addresses these common imbalances. Methods of treatment encompass correcting abnormal head posture and craniocervical dysfunction, instructions in the normal sequence of swallowing and the proper resting position of the tongue and mandible, and techniques to enhance proper use of the diaphragm (nasodiaphragmatic breathing) and thoracic spine mobility.[63,140,202,206]

Swallow Sequence. The presence of a residual pediatric tongue thrust or an acquired adult anterior tongue thrust secondary to FHP can affect the response to all treatment of the TMJ.[62,209] Treatment should include instruction in the normal resting position of the tongue and proper swallowing. Maintenance of the correct head-on-neck posture is essential. The

evaluation method (Fig. 17-22) of "water-sipping" can be used as an exercise in retraining aberrant swallowing patterns. As water is sipped during the initial phase of swallowing, the tip of the tongue should return to its resting position without putting pressure on the teeth. The main force of swallowing should be against the palate and is maintained by the middle third of the tongue.[62] The patient should sense a wavelike motion that starts at the tip of the tongue and ends with the middle third of the tongue against, and putting pressure on, the posterior part of the palate.[54,140,202]

A useful exercise to learn to alleviate symptoms of FHP and cervical syndromes in the region of the anterior neck (larynx and pharynx) and to facilitate normal swallowing is talking with a cork in the mouth (Fig. 17-40).[134] The musculature of the TMJ is designed not only to provide power (for chewing) but intricate control, as in speech.[13]

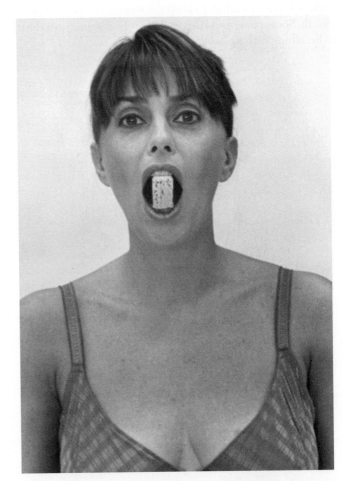

■ **FIG. 17-40.** Articulating with a cork exercise. The height of the cork depends on how far the patient can open the mouth (he or she should only open it halfway). The patient reads aloud or simply improvises for about 2 minutes; then, with the cork out of the mouth, the patient repeats what was just said and feels how easy it is now to articulate.

DIAPHRAGMATIC BREATHING

Proper diaphragmatic breathing is also important. Patients with allergies, asthma, or nasal obstructions often breathe through their mouths with increased activity of the accessory muscles of respiration (scalenes and sternocleidomastoids), which leads to FHP with PCR.[241] The patient should be instructed in nasodiaphragmatic breathing, which is best-learned supine, followed by sitting, and finally standing.[8,40,133]

Attempts to alter breathing patterns are often difficult. However, altering the head and neck posture can facilitate a more normal breathing pattern. An exercise proposed by Fielding[73] may help. A soft ball or equivalent is placed behind the patient's back at the level of the scapula as he or she sits in a straight chair (Fig. 17-41). The mechanism for this is not clear, but the patient is observed to reduce cervical lordosis, close the mouth, lower the elevation of the shoulders, and breathe at a slower deeper rate. A more normal breathing pattern can also be accomplished by suggesting that while sitting relaxed, the patient make a conscious effort to keep the tongue on the roof of the mouth. Some patients do this well, thereby resulting in a return to breathing with a closed mouth.[73]

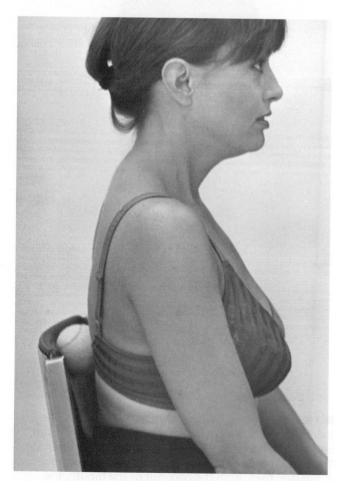

■ **FIG. 17-41.** Posterior contraction using a ball to facilitate a more normal breathing pattern.

Exercise Therapy. The use of retraining exercises to overcome spasm and incoordination of the mandibular musculature, to promote harmonious coordinated mechanisms, to reduce momentary luxation of the disk, and to increase muscle strength have long been advocated; however, they are now considered controversial.[16,52,187,220,221]

Cyriax[51] believed that strengthening the muscles of mastication could usually relieve clicking of the jaw caused by momentary luxation of the intra-articular disk. Opening, protrusion, and lateral resistive movements are performed. It is usually not necessary, he believed, to develop the jaw-closing muscles, because most patients usually maintain normal strength of these muscles by chewing.[51]

Schwartz[220,221] and Bertoft[16] recommend a training program of exercises against resistance to promote reflex relaxation of the antagonistic muscles. This stimulates the maximum number of motor units within the lateral pterygoids during opening and lateral mandibular movements.

Paris advises that major derangements should be treated in the same manner as subluxations by mobilization techniques. Minor derangements, however, are best treated by isometrics to the lateral pterygoids (i.e., protrusion and lateral movements).[187] Regardless of the type of exercises used, they should always be carried out without clicking and pain.

Such strengthening-resistive exercises, according to Weinberg, are not indicated in the TMJ pain–dysfunction syndrome because the neuromuscular mechanism involved is associated with overfunction rather than underfunction.[259,260] Such exercises do not seem to have a rational basis as an effective therapy. Strengthening and re-education exercises may be indicated when true muscle weakness is found (as in the limitation phase) or when habits such as deviant swallowing or habitual protrusion reverses normal muscle function and contributes to the TMJ pain–dysfunction syndrome.[235,262]

Treatment of Orofacial Imbalances

Muscles of the entire stomatognathic system and the orofacial complex play a major role in proper balance and function of the TMJ. It should be kept in mind that the orofacial muscles are under stress 24 hours a day. Swallowing takes place 2,000 times a day as a reflexive act. Forces during eating, drinking, speech, and the rest position of the tongue must be taken into consideration. If there is an imbalance of forces, there will be a tremendous amount of pressure against the TMJ that can cause malfunction of the joint apparatus.

Protrusion of the mandible resulting in an abnormal palatal swallow may be caused by ankylotic tongue, shortened frenulum, or abnormal use of facial muscles, particularly the mentalis.[86,98] Abnormal use or position of the tongue at rest, muscle imbalance of the masseter, decreased strength of the orbicularis oris, neuromuscular problems, posttraumatic and surgical conditions (e.g., unilateral condylectomies), pain conditions of the head, face, or cervical spine, and other pathologic processes can result in malfunction of the TMJ.

In many of these conditions, real or apparent reduction in muscle strength of one or more muscles may be disclosed during examination. This may point to lack of use (e.g., in unilateral function), atrophy of muscle fibers, muscular fibrositis, and other pathologic conditions localized in or near the muscle and its tendon, causing pain on contraction. Although strengthening–resistive exercises are usually not indicated in muscles that are already refusing to relax, they do need to be considered in the proper balance and function of the TMJ complex when weakness exists, from whatever cause.

FACILITORY EXERCISES

There is a wide variety of well-known facilitory and strengthening-resistive exercises that are at the clinician's disposal.[69,86,137,210,220,221] Exercises employing postural reflexes, brushing, vibration, synergistic muscle action of the facial and cervical muscles, and activities of daily living may be used as facilitory techniques. Stimuli—consisting of stretch, maximal resistance, pressures, stroking, or tapping—may be given manually. Popping or clucking of the tongue on the hard palate may be used to strengthen the muscle of the tongue and encourage greater ROM of the jaw. Gargling after each brushing helps facilitate mandibular depressors. Resistive tongue exercises may be used to facilitate the three major jaw muscles. Resisted neck motion may facilitate tongue motions as well as mandibular motions. In general, facial and mandibular motions that require depression or downward motions are facilitated by neck flexion; conversely, facial and mandibular motions that require elevation and upward motions are facilitated by neck extension. Neck rotation reinforces motion on the side of the face or the mandible toward which the head is turned.

NEUROMUSCULAR COORDINATION OF THE TEMPOROMANDIBULAR JOINT

Early protrusion of the mandible during opening that is owing to an imbalance of the synergistic action of the suprahyoids and lateral pterygoids is often revealed during examination. A translatory rather than a rotatory movement is occurring; its abolition should be a major step in management. An excellent, initial exercise requires the patient to place his or her tongue as posteriorly as possible in contact with the hard palate to effect retrusion (Fig. 17-42). By assuming this position, protrusion of the lower jaw is eliminated, since the patient's articular movements are mainly rotatory and limited by the constraints of the internal pterygoids. By limiting the movement to the interocclusal clearance, any subsequent translatory movement is eliminated. Instruct the patient to open his or her mouth slowly and rhythmically within the pain limits several times in succession. This simple exercise should be practiced frequently during the day.

The next step is to instruct the patient to repeat this exercise with the addition of one critical modification, voluntary resistance. The patient should grasp the chin firmly or position a closed fist under the mandible to resist the motion of pressing the jaw down and back.

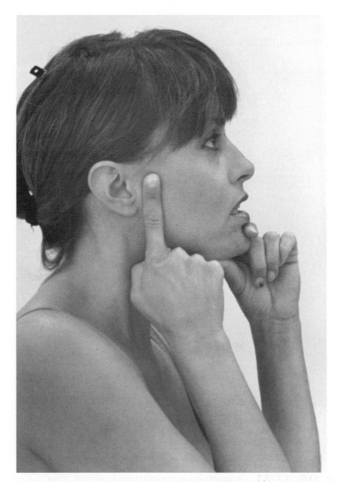

■ **FIG. 17-42.** Neuromuscular re-education for excessive translation. The index finger of one hand palpates the lateral aspect of the condyle of the temporomandibular joint, while the other hand contacts the chin. With the tongue on the hard palate, the patient practices mandibular opening with only condylar motions occurring.

Both these exercises rely on synergistic action of the suprahyoids and lower bodies of the lateral pterygoids. In normal opening, all of these muscle pairs contract strongly. However, when the lateral pterygoids contract more strongly than the suprahyoids, the mandible will protrude. These exercises are believed to help train the suprahyoids to contract more forcefully than the lateral pterygoids.

Another useful exercise for the development of the suprahyoids, described by Shore, consists of teaching the patient to perform isometric contraction of these muscles in front of a mirror (Fig. 17-43).[225] The patient is taught to contract these muscles with the mouth closed and the teeth in light contact. The patient then makes a conscious effort to retrude the jaw and depresses the floor of the mouth without actually moving it. Once acute spasms have subsided, the patient repeats the exercise with the mouth slightly open. Each day he or she can gradually increase the extent of mouth opening until coordinated mandibular muscular action is achieved.

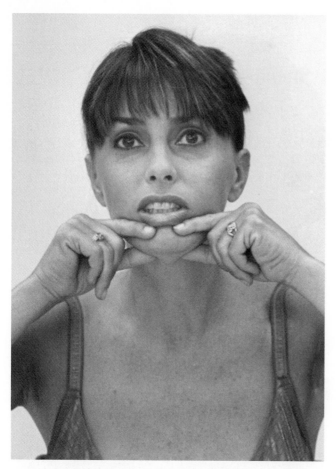

■ **FIG. 17-43.** Isometric coordinating exercise. The patient places the tip of the tongue against the hard palate and attempts to retrude and depress the floor of the mouth without moving it (additional isometrics can be performed moving the mandible in all directions).

After the patient has mastered rotation during limited opening without forward condylar movement, the range of opening is gradually increased. While the patient is looking in a mirror, he or she is asked to place the index finger over each condylar head, or the palms over the sides of the face, to monitor and correct any abnormal protrusion of the condylar head during opening and closing. The patient should also note any irregular movements such as one condylar head preceding movement of the other. Keeping the hands in place, the patient is instructed to carry out slow rhythmic full opening and closing within the pain-free range, avoiding any clicking, abnormal protrusion, or lateral deviation of the jaw. If abnormal deviation or protrusion does occur, she is taught to guide the motion with her thumb or forefinger positioned on her chin so that the mandible moves smoothly in a coordinated hingelike fashion without protrusion. Initially, this exercise should be performed with the clinician, who assists by guiding the motion of the mandible as the patient actively opens and closes the mouth.

An interesting variation of this exercise (for patients who can assume the position) is learning to move the TMJs freely and with precision with the head in the inverted position (Fig. 17-44).[134] Opening of the mouth in this position must be performed against gravity, providing eccentric isotonic work of the masseter muscle in opening and making its concentric work in closing superfluous.

Functional kinetic exercises developed by Klein-Vogelbach[134,135] have been found to be particularly helpful for the patient to learn to move the TMJs freely and with precision in all directions. In normal TMJ activity, it is the mandible that moves while the head remains relatively stationary. It is often helpful to reverse these roles. To functionally circumvent and break up faulty habit patterns and facilitate motion, the levers are reversed; the head (i.e., proximal lever) initiates the movement. The clinician or patient provides the fixation of the mandible while the head moves on the mandible. Exercises include opening and closing the mouth, lateral deviations, and protrusion and retrusion (Fig. 17-45). These unfamiliar movements are performed at low intensity and slowly. These exercises are followed with normal mandibular motions. Similar exercises have been developed based on the Feldenkrais method of sensory awareness.[266]

In the absence of obvious malocclusion and organic disease, simple exercises have been found to alleviate the annoying problem of TMJ clicking. Gerschmann[90] found that simple exercises such as lower jaw thrust exercises, in a forward, backward or anteroposterior direction with teeth disengaged, and the "chewing the pencil" exercise could alleviate this problem in about 2 weeks. The latter exercise consists of using a soft cylindrical rod (1.5 to 2 cm) placed horizontally at the

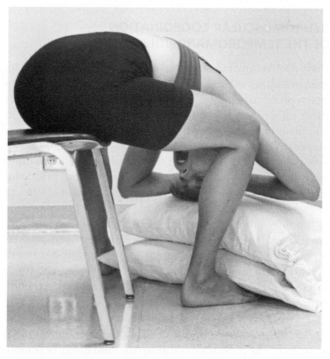

■ **FIG. 17-44.** Opening-the-mouth exercise with the long axis of the body inverted.

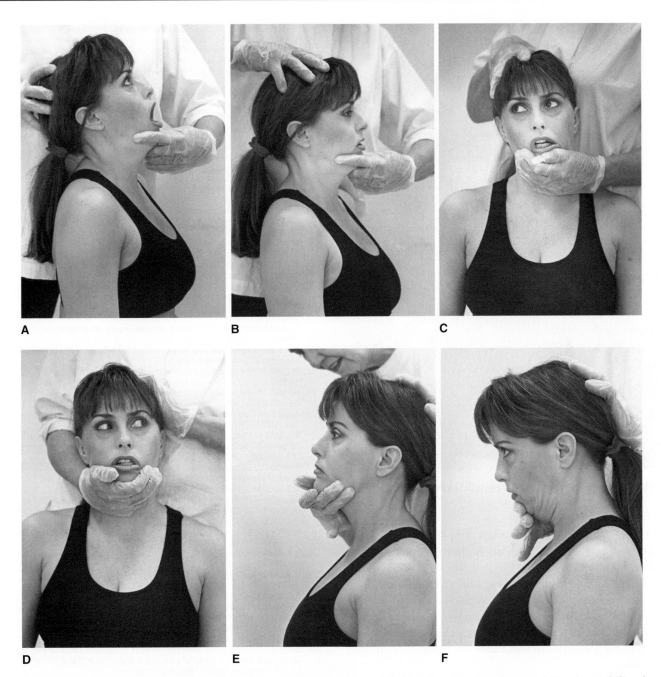

■ **FIG. 17-45.** Functional kinetic exercises using the proximal lever. (**A**) Opening. The head extends on the stabilized mandible. (**B**) Closing. The patient flexes the head as the mouth closes. (**C**) Lateral movements to the right. With the mandible stabilized, the maxilla (upper teeth) slides laterally. (**D**) Lateral movements to the left. The movement is one of the atlanto-occipital and atlanto-axial joints of the cervical spine and lateral translation of the TMJ. (**E**) Protrusion. The maxilla (upper teeth) slides dorsally in relationship to the stabilized mandible (lower teeth). (**F**). Retrusion. The maxilla (upper teeth) moves ventrally in relationship to the stabilized mandible. The movement is one of dorsal or central glide of the cervical spine and dorsal or ventral translation of the TMJs. (Reprinted with permission from Hall C, Brody L: Therapeutic Exercise: Moving Toward Function, 2nd ed. Baltimore, Lippincott Williams & Wilkins, 1998.)

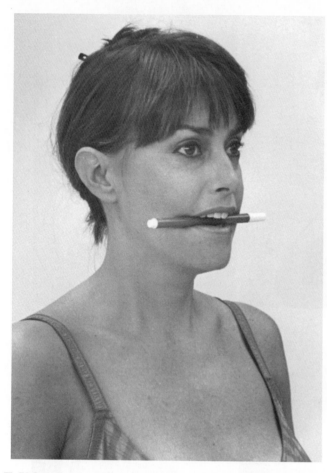

■ **FIG. 17-46.** "Chewing the pencil" exercise.

back of the mouth so that the molars grasp the object with the mandible thrust forward. The patient then rhythmically bites on the object with a grinding like movement (Fig. 17-46). Au and Klineberg[6] in a study in young adults found that clicking was a reversible condition that could be treated successfully with noninvasive isometric exercises (jaw opening as a hinge movement and lateral deviations), which helps to confirm that there is a neuromuscular cause for many TMJ clicking problems.

REFERENCES

1. Agerberg G: Maximal mandibular movements in young men and women. Sven Tandlak Tidskr 67:81–100, 1974
2. Agerberg G, Osterberg T: Maximal mandibular movements and symptoms of mandibular dysfunction in 70-year-old men and women. Sven Tandlak Tidskr 67:147–163, 1974
3. Alderman MM: Disorders of the temporomandibular joint and related structures. In: Lynch MA, ed: Burket's Oral Medicine: Diagnosis and Treatment, 8th ed. Philadelphia, JB Lippincott, 1994:485–519
4. Annandale T: Displacement of the inter-articular cartilage of the lower jaw, and its treatment by operation. Lancet 1:411, 1987
5. Atwood DA: A critique of research of the rest position of the mandible. J Prosthet Dent 16:848–854, 1966
6. Au AR, Klineberg IJ: Isokinetic exercise management of temporomandibular joint clicking in young adults. J Prosthet Dent 70:33–38, 1993
7. Axhausen G: Pathology and therapy of the temporomandibular joint. Fortschrite der Zahnaerz 6:101–215, 1932
8. Barlow W: Learning the principle. In Barlow W: The Alexander Technique. New York, Warner Communications, 1973:185–199
9. Barrett R, Hanson M: Oral Myofascial Disorders. St. Louis, CV Mosby, 1978
10. Bates R, Stewart CM, Atkinson WB: The relationship between internal derangements of the temporomandibular joint and systemic joint laxity. J Am Dent Assoc 109:446–447, 1984
11. Beighton P, Graham R, Bird HA: Hypermobility of Joints. Berlin, Springer Verlag, 1989
12. Bell WE: Orofacial Pains—Differential Diagnosis. Dallas, Denedco of Dallas, 1973
13. Bell WE: Temporomandibular Disorders: Classification, Diagnosis, Management, 3rd ed. Chicago, Yearbook, 1990
14. Bell WE: Orofacial Pains: Classification, Diagnosis, Management, 4th ed. Chicago, Yearbook, 1989
15. Berry DC: Mandibular dysfunction pain and chronic minor illness. Br Dent J 127:170–175, 1969
16. Bertoft G: The effect of physical training on temporomandibular joint clicking. Odontologisk Revy 23:297–304, 1972
17. Bertolucci LE: Postoperative physical therapy in temporomandibular joint arthroplasty. J Craniomand Pract 10:211–220, 1992
18. Bertolucci LE, Grey T: Clinical comparative study of microcurrent electrical stimulation to mid-laser and placebo treatment in degenerative joint disease of the temporomandibular joint. Cranio 13:116–120, 1995
19. Bessette RW, Mohl ND, DiCosimo CJ: Comparison of results of electromyographic and radiographic examination in patients with myofascial pain-dysfunction syndrome. J Am Dent Assoc 89:1358–1364, 1974
20. Bezuur NJ, Habets LL, Hansson TL: The effect of therapeutic laser treatment in patients with craniomandibular disorders. J Craniomandib Disord 2:83–86, 1988
21. Blasberg B, Chalmers A: Temporomandibular pain and dysfunction syndrome associated with generalized musculoskeletal pain. A retrospective study. J Rheumatol Suppl 19:87–90, 1989
22. Block SR: Fibromyalgia and rheumatisms. Common sense and sensibility. Rheum Dis Clin North Am 19:61–78, 1993
23. Bogduk N: The clinical anatomy of the cervical dorsal rami. Spine 7:319–330, 1982
24. Bogduk N: The cervical zygapophyseal joints as a source of neck pain. Spine 13:610–617, 1988
25. Bogduk N, Corrigan B, Kelly P, et al: Cervical headache. Med J Aust 143:2–207, 1985
26. Bourbon B: Musculoskeletal analysis: The temporomandibular joint and cervical spine. In: Scully RM, Barnes MR, eds: Physical Therapy. Philadelphia, JB Lippincott, 1989:415–420
27. Bourbon B: Craniomandibular examination and treatment. In: Sgarlat Myer, R, ed: Saunders Manual of Physical Therapy Practice. Philadelphia, WB Saunders, 1995:669–725
28. Boyd CH: The effect of head position on electromyographic evaluations of representative mandibular positioning of muscle groups. J Craniomandib Pract 5:51–53, 1987
29. Bradley JA: Acupuncture, acupressure, and trigger point therapy. In: Peat M, ed: Current Physical Therapy. Toronto, BC Decker, 1988:228–234
30. Bratzlavsky M, HanderEecken H: Postural reflexes in cranial muscles in man. Acta Neurol Belg 77:5–11, 1977
31. Brenman HS, Amsterdam M: Postural effects on occlusion. Dent Progr 4:43–47, 1963
32. Bronstein SL, Tomasetti BL, Ryan DE: Etiology of internal derangement of the temporomandibular joint: Correlation of arthrography with surgical findings. J Oral Surg 39:572–584, 1981
33. Brooke RI, Lapointe HJ: Temporomandibular joint disorders following whiplash. Spine: State of Art Review 7:443–454, 1993
34. Burgess JA, Sommers EE, Truelove EL, et al: Short-term effect of two therapeutic methods on myofascial pain and dysfunction of the masticatory system. J Prosthet Dent 60:606–610, 1988
35. Butler DS: Mobilisation of the Nervous System. Melbourne, Churchill Livingstone, 1991
36. Cacchiotti DA, Plesh O, Bianchi P, et al: Signs and symptoms in samples with and without temporomandibular disorders. J Craniomandib Disord 5:167–172, 1991
37. Cailliet R: Neck and Arm Pain, 3rd ed. Philadelphia, FA Davis, 1991
38. Campbell CD, Loft GH, Davis H, et al: TMJ symptoms and referred pain patterns. J Prosthet Dent 47(4): 430–433, 1982
39. Cantu RI, Grodin AJ: Myofascial Manipulation: Theory and Clinical Application. Gaithersburg, Aspen, 1992
40. Caplin D: Breathing Correctly to Ease Back Pain. Gainesville, Triad, 1987
41. Carlson CR, Ventrella MA, Sturgis ET: Relaxation training through muscle stretching procedures: A pilot study. J Behav Ther Exp Psychiatry 18:121–126, 1987
42. Carlson CR, Collins FL Jr, Nitz AJ, et al: Muscle stretching as an alternative relaxation training procedure. J Behav Ther Exp Psychiatry 21:29–38, 1990
43. Carlson CR, Okeson JP, Falace DA, et al: Stretch-based relaxation and reduction of EMG activity among masticatory muscle pain. J Craniomandib Disord 5:205–212, 1991
44. Chin LC, Jiang YH, Shen WW, et al: Kinesic press–finger compress method for TMJ treatment. J Craniomandib Pract 5:261–267, 1987

45. Cimino R, Michelotti A, Stradi R, et al: Comparison of clinical and psychologic features of fibromyalgia and masticatory myofascial pain. J Orofac Pain 12:35–41, 1998
46. Clark R, Wyke B: Contributions of temporomandibular articular mechanoreceptors to the control of mandibular posture: An experimental study. J Dent 2:121–129, 1974
47. Cohen S: A cephalometric study of rest position in edentulous persons: Influence of variations in head position. J Prosthet Dent 7(4):467–472, 1957
48. Crider AB, Glaros AG: A meta-analysis EMB biofeedback treatment of temporomandibular disorders. J Orofac Pain 13:29–37, 1999
49. Curnutte DC: The role of occlusion in diagnosis and treatment. In: Morgan DH, Hall WP, Vamvas SV, eds: Disease of the Temporomandibular Apparatus: A Multidisciplinary Approach. St. Louis, CV Mosby, 1977:117–131
50. Cyriax J: Rheumatic headache. Br Med J 2:1367–1368, 1938
51. Cyriax J: Textbook of Orthopedic Medicine: Diagnosis of Soft Tissue Lesions, vol. 1, 8th ed. London, Bailliere Tindall, 1982
52. Dachi SF: Diagnosis and management of temporomandibular dysfunction syndrome. J Prosthet Dent 2:53–61, 1968
53. Dao TT, Reynolds WJ, Tenenbaum HC: Comorbidity between myofascial pain of masticatory muscles and fibromyalgia. J Orofac Pain 11:232–241, 1997
54. Darling DW, Kraus S, Glasheen-Wray MB: Relationship of head posture and the rest position of the mandible. J Prosthet Dent 52:111–115, 1984
55. Darnell M: A proposed chronology for events for forward head posture. J Craniomandib Pract 1:50–54, 1983
56. Davis D: Gray's Anatomy Descriptive and Applied, 34th ed. London, Longmans Green, 1967
57. Day LD: History taking. In: Morgan DH, Hall WP, Vamvas SV, eds: Disease of the Temporomandibular Apparatus: A Multidisciplinary Approach, 2nd ed. St. Louis, CV Mosby, 1982:73–81
58. Dijkstra PU, Lambert GM, de Bont LGM, et al: Temporomandibular joint osteoarthrosis and generalized joint hypermobility. J Craniomandib Pract 10:221–227, 1992
59. Dolwick F, Katzberg RW, Helms CA: Internal derangement of the temporomandibular joint: Facts or fiction. J Prosthet Dent 49:315–418, 1983
60. Dubin LL: The use of hypnosis for temporomandibular joint (TMJ). Psychiatr Med 10:99–103, 1992
61. Dufourmentel L: Chirugie de l'articulation Temporo-maxillaire. Paris, Masson, 1920
62. Dunn J: Physical therapy. In: Kaplan AS, Assael LA, eds: Temporomandibular Disorders: Diagnosis and Treatment. Philadelphia, WB Saunders, 1991:455–500
63. Ellis JJ, Makofsky HW: Balancing the upper quarter through awareness of RTTPB. Clin Manage 7:20–23, 1987
64. Elsharkawy TM, Ali NM: Evaluation of acupuncture and occlusal splint therapy in the treatment of temporomandibular joint disorders. Egypt Dent J 41:1227–1232, 1995
65. Eriksson PO, Lindman R, Stal P, et al: Symptoms and signs of mandibular dysfunction in primary fibromyalgia syndrome (PSF) patients. Swed Dent J 12:141–149, 1988
66. Erlandson PM Jr, Poppen R: Electromyographic biofeedback and rest position training of masticatory muscles in myofascial pain-dysfunction patients, J Prosthet Dent 62:335–338, 1989
67. Ermshar CB: Anatomy and neuroanatomy. In: Morgan DH, Hall WP, Vamvas SV, eds: Disease of the Temporomandibular Apparatus: A Multidisciplinary Approach, 2nd ed. St. Louis, CV Mosby, 1982:8–25
68. Eversole JR, Machado J: Temporomandibular joint internal derangement and associated neuromuscular disorders. J Am Dent Assoc 110:69–70, 1985
69. Farber SD: Sensorimotor Evaluation and Treatment Procedures, 2nd ed. Bloomington, Indiana University Press, 1974
70. Farrar WB: Characteristics of the condylar path in internal derangements of the TMJ: J Prosthet Dent 39:219–323, 1978
71. Farrar W, McCarty W Jr: Outline of Temporomandibular Joint Diagnosis and Treatment, 6th ed. Montgomery, AL, Normandy Study Group, 1980
72. Feinstein B, Lanton NJK, Jameson RM, et al: Experiments on pain referred from deep somatic tissues. J Bone Joint Surg Am 36:981–997, 1954
73. Fielding M: Physical therapy in chronic airway limitation. In: Peat M, ed: Current Physical Therapy. Toronto, BC Decker, 1988:12–14
74. Fish F: The functional anatomy of the rest position of the mandible. Dent Pract 11:178, 1961
75. Flor H, Birbaumer N: Comparison of the efficacy of electromyographic biofeedback, cognitive behavioral therapy, and conservative medical interventions in the treatment of chronic musculoskeletal pain. J Consult Clin Psychol 61:653–658, 1993
76. Forsberg CM, Hellsing E, Linder-Aronson S, et al: EMG activity in the neck and masticatory muscles in relation to extension and flexion of the head. Eur J Orthod 7:177, 1985
77. Forssell H, Kangasniemi P: Correlation for frequency and intensity of headache to mandibular dysfunction in headache patients. Proc Finn Dent Soc 80:223–226, 1984
78. Forssell H, Kirveskari P, Kangasniemi P: Response to occlusal treatment in headaches patients previously treated by mock occlusal adjustment. Acta Odontol Scand 45:77–80, 1987
79. Friction J, Hathaway K, Bromaghim C: Interdisciplinary management of patients with TMJ and craniofacial pain: Characteristics and outcome. J Craniomandib Dis 1:115–122, 1987
80. Friction J, Kroening R, Haley D: Myofascial pain syndrome of the head and neck: A review of clinical characteristics of 164 patients. Oral Surg 60:615–623, 1985
81. Friction J, Kroening RJ, Hathaway KM: TMJ and Craniofacial Pain: Diagnosis and Management. St. Louis, Ishiyaku EuroAmerica, 1988
82. Friedman MH, Weisberg J: Temporomandibular Joint Disorders: Diagnosis and Treatment. Chicago, Quintessence, 1985
83. Friedman MH, Weisberg J, Agus B: Diagnosis and treatment of inflammation of the temporomandibular joint. Semin Arthritis Rheum 12:44–51, 1982
84. Funakoshi M, Fujita N, Takehana S: Relations between occlusal interference and jaw muscle activities in response to changes in head posture. J Dent Res 55:684–690, 1976
85. Garcia R Jr, Arrington JA: The relationship between cervical whiplash and temporomandibular joint injuries: A MRI study. Cranio 14:232–240, 1996
86. Garliner D: Myofunctional Therapy. Philadelphia, WB Saunders, 1976
87. Gattozzi JG, Nicol BR, Somes GW, et al: Variations in mandibular rest position with and without dentures in place. J Prosthet Dent 36:159–163, 1978
88. Gelb H: The craniomandibular syndrome. In: Garliner D, ed: Myofunctional Therapy. Philadelphia, WB Saunders, 1976:403–432
89. Gelb H, Tarte J: A two-year clinical dental evaluation of 200 cases of chronic headache: The craniocervical mandibular syndrome. Am J Dent Assoc 91:1230, 1975
90. Gerschmann JA: Temporomandibular dysfunction. Aust Fam Phys 17:274, 1988
91. Gershmann J, Burrows G, Reade P: Hypnotherapy in the treatment of oro-facial pain. Aust Dent J 23:492–496, 1978
92. Goldenberg DL: Fibromyalgia chronic fatigue syndrome, and myofascial pain syndrome. Curr Opin Rheumatol 5:199–208, 1993
93. Goldenberg DL, Felson DT, Dinerman H: A randomized, control trail of amitriptyline and naproxen in the treatment of patients with fibromyalgia. Arthritis Rheum 31:1535–1542, 1986
94. Goldstein DF, Kraus SL, Williams WB, et al: Influence of cervical posture on mandibular movement. J Prosthet Dent 52:421–426, 1984
95. Graber TM: Over-bite: The dentists' challenge. J Am Dent Assoc 79:1135–1139, 1969
96. Graff-Radford SB: Oromandibular disorders and headache: A critical appraisal. Neurol Clin 8:929–945, 1990
97. Grazzi L, Bussone G: Effect of biofeedback treatment on sympathetic function in common migraine and tension-type headache. Cephalalgia 13:197–200, 1993
98. Greene BJ: Myofunctional Therapy. In: Morgan DH, Hall WB, Vamvas SJ, eds: Disease of the Temporomandibular Apparatus: A Multidisciplinary Approach, 2nd ed. St. Louis, CV Mosby, 1982:512–525
99. Greenfield B, Wyke B: Reflex innervation of the temporomandibular joint. Nature 211:940–941, 1966
100. Greenwood LF: Is temporomandibular joint dysfunction associated with generalized hypermobility? J Prosthet Dent 58:701–703, 1987
101. Griffen C: A neuro-myo-arterial glomus in the temporomandibular meniscus. Med J Austr 48:113–116, 1961
102. Grokoest A: Osteoarthritis. In: Schwartz L, ed: Disorders of the Temporomandibular Joint. Philadelphia, WB Saunders, 1959:399–406
103. Grokoest A, Chayes CM: Rheumatic disease. In: Schwartz L, Chayes CM, eds: Facial Pain and Mandibular Dysfunction. Philadelphia, WB Saunders, 1968: 388–398
104. Gross A, Gale EN: A prevalence study of the clinical signs associated with mandibular dysfunction. J Am Dent Assoc 107:932–936, 1983
105. Grossan M: Biofeedback. In: Morgan DH, Hall WP, Vamvas SJ, eds: Disease of the Temporomandibular Apparatus: A Multidisciplinary Approach, 2nd ed. St. Louis, CV Mosby, 1982:327–334
106. Halbert R: Electromyographic study of head position. J Can Dent Assoc 23:11–23, 1958
107. Hand TP: Injury to the temporomandibular joint. In: Swerdlow B, ed: Whiplash and Related Headaches. Boca Raton, CRC Press, 1999:693–704
108. Hanson TL: Infrared laser in the treatment of craniomandibular arthrogenous pain. J Prosthet Dent 61:614–617, 1989
109. Hargreaves A: Dysfunction of the temporomandibular joints. Physiotherapy 72:209–212, 1986
110. Harinstein D, Buckingham RB, Braun T, et al: Systemic joint laxity (the hyper-mobile joint syndrome) is associated with temporomandibular joint dysfunction. Arthritis Rheum 31:1259–1264, 1988
111. Hartley A: Temporomandibular assessment. In: Hartley A, ed: Practical Joint Assessment: A Sports Medicine Manual. St. Louis, Mosby Year Book, 1990:33–43
112. Harvold EP: Primate experiments on oral respiration. Am J Orthod 79:359–372, 1981
113. Hedenberg Magnusson B, Ernberg M, et al: Symptoms and signs of temporomandibular disorders in patients with fibromyalgia and local myalgia of the temporomandibular system: A comparative study. Acta Odontol Scand 55:344–349, 1997

114. Hedenberg Magnusson B, Ernberg M, et al: Presence orofacial pain and temporomandibular disorder in fibromyalgia: A study in questionnaire. Swed Dent 23:185–192, 1999
115. Heiberg AN, Heloe B, Krogstad BS: The myofascial pain dysfunction: Dental symptoms and psychological and muscular function: An overview. Psychother Psychosom 30:81–97, 1978
116. Heir GM: Mandibular whiplash. In: Malanga GA, Nadler S, eds: Whiplash. Philadelphia, Hanley & Belfus, 2002:133–149
117. Hislop HJ, Montgomery J: Daniels and Worthingham's Muscle Testing: Techniques of Manual Examination, 6th ed. Philadelphia, WB Saunders, 1995
118. Iglarsh Z, Snyder–Mackler L: Temporomandibular joint and cervical spine. In: Richardson JK, Iglarsh ZA, eds: Clinical Orthopaedic Physical Therapy. Philadelphia, WB Saunders, 1994:1–72
119. Isberg-Holm A, Ivarsson R: The movement pattern of the mandibular condyle in individuals with and without clicking: A clinical cineradiologic study. Dentomaxillofac Radiol 9:55–65, 1980
120. Jaeger B: Overview of the head and neck region. In: Simons DG, ed: Travell & Simons' Myofascial Pain and Dysfunction: The Trigger Point Manual, vol. 1: Upper Half of the Body. Baltimore, Williams & Wilkins, 1999:237–277
121. Janda V: Muscles and motor control in cervicogenic disorders: Assessment and management. In: Grant R, ed: Physical Therapy of the Cervical and Thoracic Spine, 2nd ed. Edinburgh, Churchill Livingstone, 1994:195–216
122. Jankelson B, Swain CW: Physiological aspects of masticatory muscle stimulation: The Myo-Monitor, Quint Int 3:57–62, 1972
123. Jensen R, Rasmussen BK, Pedersen B, et al: Prevalence of oromandibular dysfunction in a general population. J Orofac Pain 7:175–182, 1993
124. Johansson A, Wenneberg B, Wagersten C, et al: Acupuncture in treatment of facial muscular pain. Acta Odontol Scand 49:153–158, 1991
125. Jonck LM: Ear symptoms in temporomandibular joint disturbance. S Afr Med J 54:782–786, 1978
126. Jones LH: Strain and Counterstrain. Colorado Springs, American Academy of Osteopathy, 1981
127. Juniper RD: Temporomandibular joint dysfunction: A theory based upon electromyographic studies of the lateral pterygoid. Br J Oral Maxillofac Surg 22:1–8, 1984
128. Juniper RD: The pathogenesis and investigation of TMJ dysfunction. Br J Oral Maxillofac Surg 25:105–112, 1987
129. Kahn J: Iontophoreses and ultrasound for postsurgical temporomandibular trismus and paresthesia, Phys Ther 60:307–308, 1980
130. Kaltenborn F: Manual Therapy for the Extremity Joints. Oslo, Olaf Norlis Bokhandel, 1974
131. Kawamura Y, Majina T, Kato I: Physiologic role of deep mechanoreceptors in temporomandibular joint capsule. J Osaka Univ Dent School 7:63–76, 1967
132. Kendall FP, McCreary WK, Provance PG: Muscle Testing and Function. 4th ed. Baltimore, Williams & Wilkins, 1993
133. Kisner C, Colby LA: Chest therapy. In: Kisner C, Colby LA, eds: Therapeutic Exercise: Foundation and Techniques. Philadelphia, FA Davis, 1990:577–616
134. Klein-Volgelbach S: Functional Kinetics: Observing, Analyzing, and Teaching Human Movement. Berlin, Springer-Verlag, 1990
135. Klein-Vogelback S: Therapeutic Exercises in Functional Kinetics: Analysis and Instructions of Individually Adaptive Exercises. Berlin, Springer-Verlag, 1991
136. Klineberg I: Structure and function of temporomandibular joint innervation. Ann R Coll Surg 49:268–288, 1971
137. Knott M, Voss DE: Proprioceptive Neuromuscular Facilitation. New York, Harper & Row, 1962
138. Kolbinson DA, Epstein JB, Senthilselvan A, et al: A comparison of the TMD patient with or without prior motor vehicle accident involvement: Initial signs, symptoms and diagnostic characteristics. J Orofac Pain 11:206–214, 1997
139. Konin JG, Wilsten DL, Isear JA: Special Test for Orthopedic Examination. Thorofare, Slack, 1997
140. Kraus SL, ed: TMJ Disorders: Management of Craniomandibular Complex, 2nd ed. New York, Churchill Livingstone, 1994
141. Kraus SL: Cervical spine influences on the craniomandibular region. In: Kraus SL, ed: TMJ Disorders: Management of the Craniomandibular Complex. New York, Churchill Livingstone, 1988:368–404
142. Kreisberg MK: Headache as a symptoms of craniomandibular disorders. II. Management. Cranio 4:219–228, 1986
143. Krogh-Poulsen WG: Management of the occlusion of the teeth. In: Schwartz L, Chayes CM, eds: Facial Pain and Mandibular Dysfunction. Philadelphia, WB Saunders, 1968
144. Kronn E: The incidence of TMJ dysfunction in patients who have suffered a cervical whiplash injury following a traffic accident. J Orofac Pain 7:209–213, 1993
145. Kusunose RS: Strain and counterstrain. In: Basmajian JV, Nyberg R, eds: Rational Manual Therapies. Baltimore, Williams & Wilkins, 1993:329–333
146. Laskin DM: Surgery of the temporomandibular joint. In: Solberg WK, Clark GT, eds: Temporomandibular Joint Problems. Biologic Diagnosis and Treatment. Chicago, Quintessence, 1980:111–128
147. Lazorthes G, Gaubert J: L'innervation des articulations interapophysaires vertebrales. Comptes Rendus de l'Association des Anatomistes, 1956: 488–494
148. Lewit K: Manipulative Therapy in Rehabilitation of the Locomotor System, 2nd ed. Oxford, Butterworth-Heinemann, 1991
149. Lewit K, Simons DG: Myofascial pain: Relief by post isometric relaxation. Arch Phys Med Rehabil 64:452–456, 1984
150. Luschei ES, Goodwin GM: Patterns of mandibular movement and muscle activity during mastication in the monkey. J Neurophysiol 35(5): 954–966, 1974
151. Mahan P: Temporomandibular problems: Biologic diagnosis and treatment. In: Solberg WK, Clark GT, eds: Temporomandibular Joint Problems. Chicago, Quintessence, 1980
152. Mahan PE, Kreutziger KL: Diagnosis and management of temporomandibular joint pain. In: Alling C, Mahan P, eds: Facial Pain, 2nd ed. Lea & Febiger, 1991:201–212
153. Maitland GDP: Peripheral Manipulations, 3rd ed. Boston, Butterworth, 1991
154. Mannheimer JS, Attanasio R, Cinotti WR, et al: Cervical strain and mandibular whiplash: Effects upon the craniomandibular apparatus. Clin Prev Dent 11:29–32, 1989
155. Mannheimer JS, Dunn J: Cervical spine. In: Kaplan AS, Assael LA, eds: Temporomandibular Disorders. Philadelphia, WB Saunders, 1991:50–94
156. Mannheimer JS, Rosenthal RM: Acute and chronic postural abnormalities as related to craniofacial pain and temporomandibular disorders. Dent Clin North Am 35:185–208, 1991
157. Manns A, Zuazola RV, Sirhan RM et al: Relationship between the tonic elevator mandibular activity and the vertical dimension during the states of vigilance and hypnosis. Cranio 8:163–170, 1990
158. Marylon F: Fibrositis (fibromyalgia syndrome) and the dental clinician. Cranial 9:63–70, 1991
159. Masunaga S, Ohashi W: Zen Shiatsu: How to Harmonize Yin and Yang for Better Health. New York, Japan Pub, 1977
160. McCall J: Electromyography of muscles of posture: Posterior vertebral muscles in man. J Physiol (London) 157:33, 1961
161. McLean LF, Brenman HS, Friedman MGF: Effects of changing body position on dental occlusion. J Dent Res 52:1041–1050, 1973
162. McNamara DC: Examination, diagnosis and treatment of occlusion pain-dysfunction. Aust Dent J 23:50–55, 1978
163. McNamara JA: The independent function of the two heads of the lateral pterygoid muscle. Am J Anat 138:197–205, 1973
164. Merlini L, Palla S: The relationship between condylar rotation and anterior translation in healthy and clicking temporomandibular joints. Schweiz Monatsschr Zahnmed 98:119, 1988
165. Merrill RG: Arthroscopic lysis, lavage, manipulation and chemical sclerotherapy of the TMJ for hypermobility and recurrent dislocation. In: Clark GT, Sanders B, Bertolami CN, eds: Advances in Diagnostic and Surgical Arthroscopy of the Temporomandibular Joint. Philadelphia, WB Saunders, 1992
166. Mintz VW: The orthopedic influence. In: Morgan DH, Hall WP, Vamvas SJ, eds: Disease of the Temporomandibular Apparatus: A Multidisciplinary Approach. St. Louis, CV Mosby, 1977:232–235
167. Mishra KD, Gatchel RJ, Gardea MA: The relative efficacy of three cognitive-behavioral treatment approaches to temporomandibular disorders. J Behav Med 23:293–309, 2000
168. Mitchell FL Jr, Moran PS, Pruzzo NA: An Evaluation and Treatment Manual of Osteopathic and Muscle Energy Procedures. Valley Park, MO, Mitchell, Moran and Pruzzo, 1979
169. Moffett BC, Johnson LC, McCabe JB, et al: Articular remodeling in the adult human temporomandibular joint. Am J Anat 115:10–130, 1964
170. Mohl ND: Head posture and its role in occlusion. NY State Dent J 42:17–23, 1976
171. Mohl ND: The role of head posture in mandibular function. In: Solberg W, Clark G, eds: Abnormal Jaw Mechanics: Diagnosis and Treatment. Chicago, Quintessence, 1984:97–116
172. Morgan DH, Hall WP, Vamvas SJ, eds: Disease of the Temporomandibular Apparatus: A Multidisciplinary Approach, 2nd ed. St. Louis, CV Mosby, 1982:166–120
173. Morgan DH, Rosen LM: Interpretation of radiograph. In: Morgan DH, Hall WP, Vamvas SJ, eds: Disease of the Temporomandibular Apparatus: A Multidisciplinary Approach, 2nd ed. St. Louis, CV Mosby, 1982:166–210
174. Morrone L, Makofsky H: TMJ home exercise program. Clin Manage 11:20–26, 1991
175. Moystad A, Krogstad BS, Larheim TA: Transcutaneous nerve stimulation in a group of patients with rheumatic disease involving the temporomandibular joint. J Prosthet Dent 64:596–600, 1990
176. Muller W: The fibrositis syndrome: Diagnosis, differential diagnosis and pathogenesis. Scand J Rheumatol Suppl 65:40–53, 1987
177. Munro RR: Electromyography of the masseter and anterior temporalis muscle in the open-close-clench cycle in the temporomandibular joint dysfunction. Monogr Oral Sci 4:117–125, 1975
178. Nelson SJ, Ash MM Jr: An evaluation of moist heating pads for the treatment of TMJ/muscle pain dysfunction. Cranio 6:355–359, 1988
179. Murphy GJ: Electrical physical therapy treating TMJ patients. J Craniomandib Pract 1:67–73, 1983
180. Norkin CC, Levangie PK: The temporomandibular joint. In: Norkin CC, Levangie PK, eds. Joint Structure and Function: A Comprehensive Analysis, 2nd ed. Philadelphia, FA Davis 1992:193–206
181. Okeson J: Orofacial Pain; Guidelines for Assessment, Diagnosis, and Management. Chicago, Quintessence Brooks, 1996

182. Okeson JP: Management of Temporomandibular Disorders and Occlusion. St. Louis, Mosby, 2003

183. Oleson J: Classification and diagnostic criteria for headache disorders, cranial neuralgias and facial pain. Cephalalgia 8:11–06, 1988

184. Palano D, Martelli M: A clinical statistical investigation of laser effect in the treatment of pain and dysfunction of the temporomandibular joint (TMJ). Med Laser Rep 2:21–23, 1985

185. Palmer ML, Epler ME: Fundamentals of Musculoskeletal Assessment Techniques, 2nd ed. Baltimore, Lippincott Williams & Wilkins, 1998

186. Pandamsee M: Incidence of cervical disorders in a TMD population. J Dent Res IADR, Abstract No. 680, 1994

187. Paris SV: The Spinal Lesion. Christchurch, New Zealand, Pegasus Press, 1965

188. Peck C, Kraft G: Electromyographic biofeedback for pain related to muscle tension: A study of tension headache, back, and jaw pain. Arch Surg 112:889–895, 1977

189. Pellegrino MJ: Atypical chest pain as an initial presentation of primary fibromyalgia. Arch Phys Med Rehabil 71:526–528, 1990

190. Perry C: Neuromuscular control of mandibular movements. J Prosthet Dent 30:714–720, 1973

191. Pinto OF: A new structure related to the temporomandibular joint and the middle ear. J Prosthet Dent 12(1):95–103, 1962

192. Plesh O, Wolfe F, Lane N: The relationship between fibromyalgia and temporomandibular disorders: Prevalence and symptoms severity. J Rheumatol 23:1948–1952, 1996

193. Plunkett GAJ, West, VC: Systemic joint laxity and mandibular range of movement. J Craniomandib Pract 6:320–326, 1988

194. Porter MR: The attachment of the lateral pterygoid muscle of the meniscus. J Prosthet Dent 24:555–562, 1970

195. Prieskel HW: Some observations on the postural position of the mandible. J Prosthet Dent 15:625–633, 1965

196. Profitt WR: Equalization theory revisited: Factors influencing position of the teeth. Am J Orthod 48:175–186, 1978

197. Ramfjord SP: Dysfunctional temporomandibular joint and muscle pain. J Prosthet Dent 11:353–374, 1961

198. Rayne J: Functional anatomy of the temporomandibular joint. Br J Oral Maxillofac Surg 25:92–99, 1987

199. Rees LA: The structure and function of the temporomandibular joint. Br Dent J 96:125–133, 1954

200. Reik L Jr, Hale M: The temporomandibular joint pain-dysfunction syndrome: a frequent cause of headache. Headache 21:151–156, 1981

201. Robinson MJ: The influence of head position on TMJ dysfunction. J Prosthet Dent 16:169–172, 1966

202. Rocabado M: Management of the temporomandibular joint. Presented at a course on physical therapy in dentistry. Vail, Colorado, January, 1978

203. Rocabado M: Advanced Upper Quarter Manual. Tacoma, Rocabado Institute, 1981

204. Rocabado M: Arthrokinematics of the temporomandibular joint. Dent Clin North Am 27(3):573–594, 1983

205. Rocabado M: Biomechanical relationship of the cranial, cervical and hyoid region. J Craniomandib Pract 1:61–66, 1983

206. Rocabado M: Diagnosis and treatment of abnormal craniomandibular mechanics. In: Solberg W, Clark G, eds: Abnormal Jaw Mechanics: Diagnosis and Treatment. Chicago, Quintessence, 1984

207. Rocabado M: Radiographic study of the craniocervical relation in patients under orthodontic treatment and the incidence of related symptoms. J Craniomandib Prac 5:36–48, 1987

208. Rocabado M: Physical therapy for the post-surgical TMJ patient. J Craniomandib Pract 3:75–82, 1989

209. Rocabado M, Iglarsh ZA: Musculoskeletal Approach to Maxillo-facial Pain. Philadelphia, JB Lippincott, 1991

210. Rood M: Neurophysiological reactions as a basis for physical therapy. Phys Ther 34:444–449, 1954

211. Roydhouse RH: Whiplash and temporomandibular dysfunction. Lancet 1:1394–1395, 1973

212. Santoro F, Maiorana C, Campiotti A: Neuromuscular relaxation and CCMDP: Biofeedback and TENS. Dent Cadmos 57:88–89, 1989

213. Satlerthwaite JR: Ice massage. Pain Manag Nurs 2:116, 1989

214. Scherman P: Surgery of the temporomandibular articulation. In: Gelb H, ed: Clinical Management of Head, Neck and TMJ Pain and Dysfunction: A Multidisciplinary Approach to Diagnosis and Treatment, 2nd ed. Philadelphia, WB Saunders, 1985;368–395

215. Schneider K, Zerneke RF, Clark G: Modeling of jaw-head-neck dynamics during whiplash. J Dent Res 68:1360–1365, 1989

216. Schokker RP, Hansson TL, Ansink BJ: Craniomandibular disorders in patients with different types of headaches. J Craniomandib Disord 4:47–51, 1990

217. Schultz W: Shiatsu: Japanese Finger Pressure Therapy. New York, Bell, 1976

218. Schwartz AM: Positions of the head and malrelationships of the jaws. Int J Ortho Oral Surg Radiol 14:56–88, 1928

219. Schwartz L: Ethyl chloride treatment of limited painful mandibular movement. J Oral Rehabil 48:497–507, 1954

220. Schwartz L, ed: Disorders of the Temporomandibular Joint. Philadelphia, WB Saunders, 1959

221. Schwartz L, Chayes CM, eds: Facial Pain and Mandibular Dysfunction. Philadelphia, WB Saunders, 1968

222. Sheehy K, Middeditch A, Wickham S: Vertebral artery testing in the cervical spine. Manip Physiother 22:15–18, 1990

223. Shaw RM, Dettmar DM: Monitoring behavioral stress control using a craniomandibular index. Aust Dent J 35:147–151, 1990

224. Shira RB, Alling CC: Traumatic injuries involving the temporomandibular joint articulation. In: Schwartz L, Chayes CM, eds: Facial Pain and Muscular Dysfunction. Philadelphia, WB Saunders, 1968

225. Shore MA: Temporomandibular Joint Dysfunction and Occlusal Equilibration. Philadelphia, JB Lippincott, 1976

226. Sicher H, DuBrul EL: Oral Anatomy, 8th ed. St. Louis, CV Mosby, 1988

227. Simon EP, Lewis DM: Medical hypnosis for temporomandibular disorders: treatment efficacy and medical utilization outcome. Oral Surg Oral Med Oral Pathol Oral Radiol Endod 90:5463, 2000

228. Simons DG: Muscular pain syndromes. In: Friction JR, Awad EA, eds: Advances in Pain Research and Therapy, vol. 1. New York, Raven Press, 1990:1–41

229. Simons DG, Travell JG, Simons L: The digastric muscle and other anterior neck muscles. In: Travell & Simons' Myofascial Pain and Dysfunction, 2nd ed. Baltimore, Williams & Wilkins, 1999:397–415

230. Skagg CD: Diagnosis and treatment of temporomandibular disorders. In: Murphy DR, ed: Conservative Management of Cervical Spine Syndromes. New York, McGraw-Hill, 2000:579–592

231. Smythe HA: Non-articular rheumatism and fibrositis. In: McCarty DJ, ed: Arthritis and Allied Conditions: A Textbook of Rheumatology. Philadelphia, Lea & Febiger, 1972:874–884

232. Smythe HA: Non-articular rheumatism and psychogenic musculoskeletal syndromes. In: McCarty DJ, ed: Arthritis and Allied Conditions: A Textbook of Rheumatology. 2nd ed. Philadelphia, Lea & Febiger, 1979:881–891

233. Solberg WK: Temporomandibular disorders: Clinical significance of TMJ changes. Br Dent J 160:231–236, 1986

234. Solow B, Kreiberg S: Soft tissue stretching: A possible control factor in craniofacial morphogenesis. Scand J Dent Res 85:505–507, 1977

235. Somers N: An approach to the management of temporomandibular joint dysfunction. Aust Dent J 23(1):37–41, 1978

236. Speck JE, Zarb GA: Temporomandibular dysfunction: A suggested classification and treatment. J Can Dent Assoc 6:305–310, 1976

237. Stam HJ, McGrath PA, Brooke RI, et al: Hypnotizability and treatment of chronic facial pain. Int J Clin Exp Hypn 33:182–191, 1986

238. Steenks MH, Wifer A, Bosman F: Orthopedic diagnostic tests for temporomandibular and cervical spine disorders. J Back Musculokel Rehabil 6:135–155, 1996

239. Svensson P, Aredt-Nielsen L, Nielsen H, et al: Effect of chronic and experimental jaw muscle pain on pain-pressure thresholds and stimulus response curves. J Orofac Pain 9:347–356, 1995

240. Talley RL, Murphy GJ, Smith SD, et al: Standards for the history, examination, diagnosis and treatment of temporomandibular disorders (TMJ): A position paper. J Craniomandib Pract 8:60–77, 1990

241. Tallgren A, Solow B: Hyoid bone position, facial morphology and head posture in adults. Eur J Orthod 9:1–8, 1987

242. Tanaka TT: A rational approach to the differential diagnosis of arthritic disorders. J Prosthet Dent 56:727–731, 1986

243. Tappan FM: Finger pressure to acupuncture points. In: Tappan FM, ed: Healing Massage Techniques: Holistic, Classic and Emerging Methods, 2nd ed. Norwalk, Appleton & Lange, 1988:133–166

244. Tappan FM: The bindegewebmassage system. In: Tappan FM, ed: Healing Massage Techniques: Holistic, Classic, and Emerging Methods, 2nd ed. Norwalk, Appleton & Lange, 1988:219–260

245. Thompson JR, Brodie AG: Factors in the position of the mandible. J Am Dent Assoc 29:925–941, 1942

246. Travell JG, Rinzler SH: The myofascial genesis of pain. Postgrad Med 11:425–434, 1952

247. Travell JG, Simons DG: Myofascial Pain and Dysfunction: The Trigger Point Manual. Baltimore, Williams & Wilkins, 1999

248. Trott PH: Examination of the temporomandibular joint. In: Grieves GP, ed: Modern Manual Therapy of the Vertebral Column. New York, Churchill Livingstone, 1986;521–529

249. Trott PH: Passive movements and allied techniques in the management of dental patients. In: Grieves GP, ed: Modern Manual Therapy of the Vertebral Column. New York, Churchill Livingstone, 1986:691–699

250. Trott PH, Goss AN: Physiotherapy in diagnosis and treatment of the myofascial dysfunction syndrome. Int J Oral Surg 7(4): 360–365, 1978

251. Truta MP, Santucci ET: Head and neck fibromyalgia and temporomandibular arthralgia. Otolaryngol Clin North Am 22:1159–1171, 1989

252. Upledger JE, Vredevoogd JD: Craniosacral Therapy. Chicago, Eastland Press, 1983

253. Viener AE: Oral surgery. In: Garliner D, ed: Myofunctional Therapy. Philadelphia, WB Saunders, 1976

254. Wanman A, Agerberg G: Recurrent headaches and craniomandibular disorders in adolescents: A longitudinal study. J Craniomandib Disord 1:229–236, 1987

255. Wang K: A report of 22 cases of temporomandibular joint dysfunction syndrome treated with acupuncture and laser radiation. J Tradit Chin Med 12:116–118, 1992

256. Waylonnis GW, Heck W: Fibromyalgia syndrome: New associations. Am J Phys Med Rehabil 71:343–348, 1992

257. Weinberg LA: An evaluation of basic articulators and their concepts: I. Basic concepts. J Prosthet Dent 13:622–644, 1963

258. Weinberg LA: The etiology, diagnosis, and treatment of TMJ dysfunction-pain syndrome: I. Etiology. J Prosthet Dent 42(6):654–664, 1979

259. Weinberg LA: The etiology, diagnosis and treatment of TMJ dysfunction-pain syndrome: II. Differential diagnosis. J Prosthet Dent 43(2):50–70, 1980

260. Weinberg LA: The etiology and treatment of TMJ dysfunction-pain syndrome: III. Treatment. J Prosthet Dent 43(2):186–196, 1980

261. Weinberg LA, Lapointe H: Cervical extension-flexion injury (whiplash) and internal derangement of the temporomandibular joint. J Oral Maxillofac Surg 45:653–656, 1987

262. Wetzler G: Physical therapy. In: Morgan DH, Hall WP Vamvas SV, eds: Disease of the Temporomandibular Apparatus: A Multidisciplinary Approach. St. Louis, CV Mosby, 1977:344–360

263. Whinery JG: Examination of patients with facial pain. In: Alling C, Mahan P, eds: Facial Pain. Philadelphia, Lea & Febiger, 1977:155–164

264. Widmer CG: Evaluation of temporomandibular disorders. In: Kraus SL, ed: TMJ Disorders: Management of the Craniomandibular Complex. Edinburgh, Churchill Livingstone, 1988:79–111

265. Wijer A, Leeuw R, Steenks MH, et al: Temporomandibular and cervical spine disorders. J Back Musculokel Rehabil 21:1638–1646, 1996

266. Wildman F: The TMJ Tape for the Jaw, Head and Neck Pain. The Intelligent Body Tape Series. Berkeley, Institute of Movement Studies, 1993

267. Wolfe F, Smythe HA, Yunus MB, et al: The American College of Rheumatology 1990 criteria for classification of fibromyalgia: Report of the Multicenter Criteria Committee. Arthritis Rheum 33:160–172, 1990

268. Wyke BD: Neuromuscular mechanisms influencing mandibular posture: A neurologist's review of current concepts. J Dent 2:111–120, 1972

269. Yale S, Allison B, Hauptfuehrer J: An epidemiological assessment of mandibular condyle morphology. Oral Surg 21:169–177, 1966

270. Yunus MB: Fibromyalgia syndrome and myofascial pain syndrome: Clinical features, laboratory tests, diagnosis, and pathophysiologic mechanisms. In: Rachlin ES, ed: Myofascial Pain and Fibromyalgia. St. Louis, CV Mosby, 1994:3–29

271. Yunus MB, Masi AT: Fibromyalgia, restless legs syndrome, periodic limb movement disorder and psychogenic pain. In: McCarty DJ Jr, Koopman WJ, eds: Arthritis and Allied Conditions: A Textbook of Rheumatology. Philadelphia, Lea & Febiger 1992:1383–1405

272. Yunus MB, Masi AT, Calbro JJ, et al: Primary fibromyalgia (fibrositis): Clinical study of 50 patients with matched normal controls. Semin Arthritis Rheum 11:151–171, 1981

RECOMMENDED READING

Dutton M: The temporomandibular joint. In: Dutton M, ed: Manual Therapy of the Spine: An Integrated Approach. Pittsburgh, McGraw, 2002:537–571

Okeson JP: Management of Temporomandibular Disorders and Occlusion. St. Louis, Mosby, 2003

Mannheimer JS, Rosenthal RM: Acute and chronic postural abnormalities as related to craniofacial pain and temporomandibular disorders. Dent Clin North Am 35:185–207, 1991

Rocabado M, Iglarsh: Musculoskeletal Approach to Maxillofacial Pain. Philadelphia, JB Lippincott, 1991

Sessle BJ, Bryant PS, Dionne RA, eds: Temporomandibular Disorders and Related Pain Conditions: Progress in Pain Research and Management, vol. 4. Seattle, IASP Press, 1995

Clinical Applications—Spine

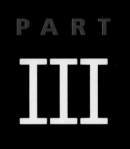

PART III

III

Clinical Applications—Spine

Spine: General Structure and Biomechanical Considerations

DARLENE HERTLING

GENERAL STRUCTURE

The spine is divided into five regions: cervical, thoracic (or dorsal), lumbar, sacral, and coccygeal (the "tail" or coccyx). The spine usually has 33 segments—7 cervical, 12 thoracic, 5 lumbar, 5 sacral, and 4 coccygeal (Fig. 18-1). The sacral vertebrae are fused together and serve as an attachment to the pelvic girdle. The "presacral" vertebrae, with which we are most concerned clinically, most often total 24.

Occasionally there are supernumerary thoracic or lumbar vertebrae, or perhaps an unfused sacral vertebra, rather than an actual additional segment. It is questionable whether these variations hold much clinical significance, although a spine in which a lumbar vertebra is sacralized is believed to gain stability at the expense of mobility, and a spine in which a sacral vertebra is not fused tends to be mobile but less stable.[6,31,59] Unilateral sacralization or lumbarization, in which only one side of the vertebra is involved, is often thought to be of more significance, presumably leading to asymmetry in mobility and stability. However, this may not always be the case, because osseous fusion on one side is often accompanied by fibrous fusion (not evident on roentgenograms) on the opposite side. Another not uncommon finding is fusion of two upper cervical vertebrae, which again may have little clinical significance.[28,57,62]

The spine is a flexible, multicurved column. When viewed in the sagittal plane, the cervical and lumbar regions are in lordosis (lordotic curve); the thoracic, sacral, and coccygeal regions are in kyphosis (kyphotic curve) (Fig. 18-1C). These normal anatomic curves give the spinal column increased flexibility and augmented shock-absorbing capacity while maintaining adequate stiffness and stability at the intervertebral joints.[3,177] In humans, the thoracic spine is partially splinted by the rib cage. The thoracic curve is structural and is secondary to less vertical height at the anterior thoracic vertebral border, as opposed to the posterior border. This is also true of the sacral curve. Although the sacrum is rigid, slight motions occur in vivo in the sacroiliac joint, which decrease with age (Fig. 18-1).[38,56,135,138,220] The coccyx, which is not well developed in humans, has no functional role (Fig. 18-1A, C).

In contrast, the cervical spine and lumbar spine are quite flexible yet still are able to support heavy loads. The demanding functional role they play is felt to be a major reason why these regions of the spine are the most likely to become symptomatic. Curvature of the cervical and lumbar regions is largely owing to the wedge-shaped intervertebral disks.[225] These disks are entirely responsible for the existence of a normal cervical lordosis, because the cervical vertebral bodies are actually shorter in height anteriorly than posteriorly (Fig. 18-1C). They are largely responsible for the lumbar lordosis in the upper lumbar spine, but less so in the lower lumbar spine, where the vertebral bodies are wedge-shaped so as to form the lordosis. Thus, in both the cervical and lumbar regions the disks are of greater height anteriorly than posteriorly. In the thoracic spine the kyphosis is almost entirely caused by the shape of the vertebral bodies—the disks being of equal height anteriorly and posteriorly.

The spine has at least four biomechanical functions: 1) housing and protection, 2) support, 3) mobility, and 4) control.[177,225] Its most important function is to protect the delicate spinal cord from potentially damaging forces or motions. From a support standpoint, it transfers the weight and bending movements of the head and trunk to the pelvis. Facilitated by the ribs, it functions as a framework for attachment of the internal organs.

The human neck has been described as a cylindrical conduit that supports the head and renders it mobile.[121] It provides avenues of passage for essential connections in the respiratory, gastrointestinal, nervous, and vascular systems and serves as a locus for vital ductless glands and for the organs

671

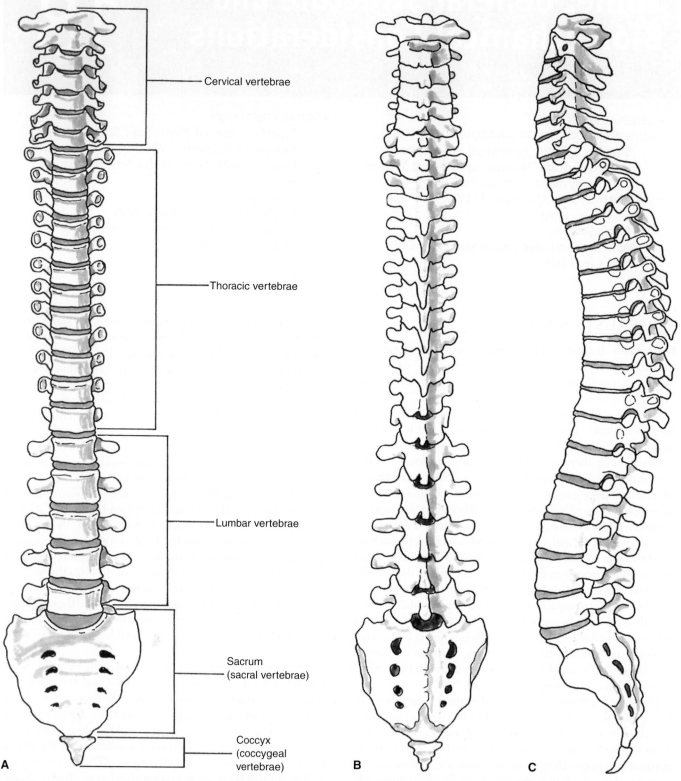

Cervical vertebrae

Thoracic vertebrae

Lumbar vertebrae

Sacrum
(sacral vertebrae)

Coccyx
(coccygeal
vertebrae)

A   B   C

■ FIG. 18-1. The vertebral column, including the sacrum and coccyx, as seen on (A) anterior, (B) posterior, and (C) left sagittal views.

of phonation, vocalization, and ventilation. As such, it is a compact aggregate of numerous critical structures related to the cervical spine, which serves as the major architectural member. The cervical spine is a highly mobile structure that functions principally to position the head in space, permitting effective adaptation of the organism to the environment. Motions of the neck are therefore inseparably linked with motions of the head, and this linkage is a critical concept in both normal and pathologic states.[121]

Mobility allows for physiologic motion to occur between the parts of the spine. Thus, instead of a single rigid column, the spine is a flexible stack of rigid blocks with flexible soft tissue in between. The basic functional unit of the spine is the **spinal motion segment,** which may be defined as comprising the adjacent halves of two vertebrae, the interposed disk and articular facet joints, as well as the supporting structures (i.e., ligaments, blood vessels, nerves, and muscles).[57,172,177,196] It should be noted that in the cervical spine there are no disks between the atlas and the occiput and the atlas and the axis. The disks permit intervertebral movement, while the posterior articulations control the amplitude and direction of the movement. This concept leads to a more functional than anatomical approach to pathology.

REVIEW OF FUNCTIONAL ANATOMY OF THE SPINE

Although a detailed description of the anatomy of the spine is beyond the scope of this chapter, the reader is referred to several other, comprehensive sources.[59,65,105,149,191,192,225,226] Briefly, the following constituents of the spinal segment and how they respond to motion and load are reviewed:

1. Support system. Vertebral bodies, posterior elements, articular facet (apophyseal) joints, intervertebral disks, and vertebral foramen
2. Control system. Both contractile (muscles) and noncontractile (ligaments, fascia, capsules, and vertebral innervations)

Support System: Individual Structures

VERTEBRAE

The special anatomic features of the vertebrae are probably best described in relation to their biomechanical functions. Probably Messerer[137] conducted the earliest biomechanical study of the human spine with respect to strength measurements of the vertebrae more than 100 years ago.

Each vertebra consists of two major parts—the anterior vertebral body, which is the major weight-bearing structure of the vertebra, and the posterior vertebral arch (Fig. 18-2). The vertebral arch is composed of the pedicle, which joins the arch to the body and to which the superior articular process is attached. This superior process articulates with the inferior articular process by means of the articular facet (apophyseal) joint and the transverse and spinous processes.

The basic design of the vertebrae in the various regions of the spine is the same. The size and mass of the vertebral bodies increase all the way from the first cervical to the last lumbar vertebra (Fig. 18-1A); this is a mechanical adaptation to the progressively increasing loads to which the vertebrae are subjected.[225] There are individual differences in the various regions of the spine. Unique to the typical cervical vertebrae (C2–C7) are lateral prominences called **uncinate processes;** the transverse processes contain **foramina** (foramina transversarii) through which the vertebral artery passes (Fig. 18-3B, C).

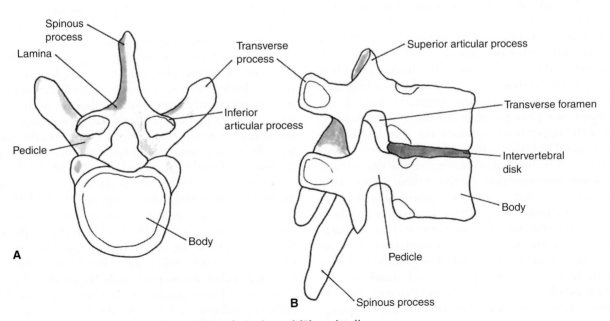

■ **FIG. 18-2.** Parts of a vertebra viewed **(A)** inferiorly and **(B)** sagittally.

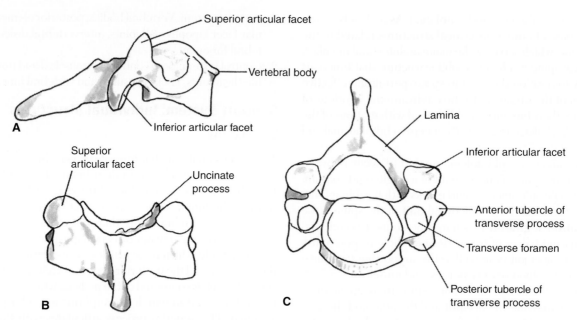

■ **FIG. 18-3.** Typical lower cervical vertebra. **(A)** Sagittal, **(B)** posterior, and **(C)** inferior views.

The thoracic vertebrae have articular facets for the ribs (Fig. 18-4A, C) and the lumbar spine has **mammary processes** (roughened raised areas on each articular pillar that serve for muscle attachment for the multifidi) (Fig. 18-5A, C). Of course the sacral spine, being fused, is unique.

ANTERIOR PORTION OF THE MOTION SEGMENT

Although the articular facets carry some compressive load, it is the vertebral bodies that are primarily designed to sustain these loads. A compressive load is transmitted from the superior end-plate of a vertebra to the inferior end-plate by way of two paths, the **cortical shell** and the **cancellous core.** The body consists of spongy bone covered with a thin, dense bony cortex, whereas the neural arch and its processes are thinner and have proportionally more cortical bone. The cortical bone of the upper and lower surfaces of the bodies (vertebral plateaus) reflects the structure of the overlying cartilaginous end-plate, with a somewhat concave center and a more dense, ringed epiphyseal plate peripherally. As the superimposed weight of the upper body increases, the vertebral bodies become larger. The bodies in the lumbar spine have a greater height and cross-sectional area than those in the thoracic and cervical spine; their increased size allows them to sustain the greater loads to which this part of the spine is subjected.[65]

The vertebral bodies are about six times stiffer and three times thicker than the disks. Thus the vertebral bodies deform about half as much as the disks under compression. Because the vertebrae are filled with blood, it is possible that they behave like hydraulically strengthened shock absorbers.[107,108]

Vertical and oblique trabecular systems that correspond to the stresses placed on the bodies are found within the spongy bone (Fig. 18-6).[70,105] Vertically directed trabeculae mainly support the body and the compressive forces and help to sustain the body weight (Fig. 18-6A). The other trabecular systems help to resist shearing forces. At both the lower and upper surfaces of the body there are oblique trabeculae, which aid in compressive load-bearing function and also serve to resist the bending and tensile forces that occur at the pedicles and spinous processes (Fig. 18-6B, C). In osteoporosis there is a greater loss of horizontal trabeculae in comparison to the vertical trabeculae of cancellous bone; the effect on the strength of the vertebrae is considerable. In pathologic processes of the spine, the type of failure may be related to whether the spine was loaded in flexion or extension, with flexion tending to cause anterior collapse where the trabeculae are weakest.[177] This also explains the wedge-shaped compression fracture of the vertebrae that occurs.[105]

Krenz and Troup[119] found that the pressure was higher in the center of the end-plate than in the periphery during compressive loading. This is a common site for failure in which the nucleus apparently ruptures the end-plate. Again, this may be a significant problem for those who have diminished bone strength, as in osteoporosis. Central fractures of the end-plate typically occur in nondegenerated disks, whereas peripheral fractures are found to be related to degenerated disks.[174,175,190]

Regionally, the lumbar vertebral bodies alter in shape from the first lumbar vertebra (more squared) to the fifth lumbar vertebra (more rectangular), giving the articular end-plate a broader surface area (Fig. 18-5C). The bodies of the middle thoracic vertebrae are almost heart-shaped because of the pressure of the descending aorta (Fig. 18-4C). The thoracic vertebral bodies are proportionally higher than the lumbar vertebrae and more squared in the transverse plane. Unique to the cervical spine (C2–C7) are lateral uncinate processes on the superior surface of each vertebral body, which articulate

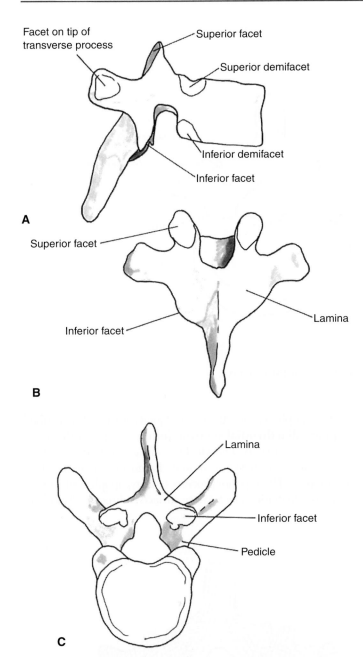

■ **FIG. 18-4.** Typical thoracic vertebra. (**A**) Lateral, (**B**) posterior, and (**C**) inferior views.

with the beveled edge of the inferior surface of the proximal vertebral body (Fig. 18-3*B*). At this junction there is usually a synovial joint called the **joint of Luschka.**[83,227]

The atypical cervical vertebrae (C1 and C2) are characterized by the absence of a vertebral body at C1 (the **atlas**) and by the embryologic fusion of the C1 body with C2 (the **axis**), forming a prominent pillar on the surface of C2 known as the **odontoid process** or **dens** (Fig. 18-7*B–D*).[227]

Each vertebral body has its primary nutrient foramen located in the center of the posterior aspect, and in situ it is covered by the posterior longitudinal ligament (Fig. 18-8*A, B*).[191,192]

In general the upper and lower surfaces of the vertebral bodies are slightly concave.

POSTERIOR ELEMENTS AND FACET JOINTS

The vertebral arch is more complex than the body, because it has many projections, including four articulating facet (apophyseal) joints and three processes (Fig. 18-2). The processes, two transverse and one spinous, provide for the attachment of ligaments and muscles. The arch is divided into a short anterior portion and a long posterior portion by the articulating projections and transverse processes. The anterior half of the arch consists of the pedicles, which attach the arch anteriorly to the upper posterior wall of the vertebral body (Fig. 18-2). The laminae join to form the peak of the arch and continue to form the spinous process. At the site where the lamina takes origin from the pedicle, the lamina is narrowed; this area is referred to as the **pars interarticularis or isthmus** (Fig. 18-5*B*). Whereas pedicles rarely fracture, the pars is a frequent site of a distinctive fracture, apparently secondary to fatigue of bone rather than a sudden or acute fracture; this defect is commonly found in athletes.[3] Because the pars interarticularis is actually part of the neural arch forming a part of the posterolateral boundary of the arch, these lesions are often referred to as **neural arch defects.**[76] These defects are known as either **spondylolysis,** which consists of a single fracture of the pars, or as **spondylolisthesis,** which consists of a bilateral fracture often accompanied by some degree of forward slippage of the vertebral body (see Chapter 22, Lumbar Spine).

The trabecular systems of the vertebral arch extend into the vertebral body (Fig. 18-6). The area where the transverse process and articular facets arise is reinforced by many crossing trabeculae. The alignment of the trabeculae in the vertebral body and posterior element indicates that the facet articulations must function to some extent as a fulcrum between the anterior vertebral body and the laminae and spinous processes, although the compression forces applied to the posterior elements in direct axial compression are significantly relieved by the compression strength of the body and disk system and by the potential for tensile elongation of the ligaments and muscles posteriorly.[105]

The articular facet joints are extensions of the laminae and are covered with hyaline cartilage on their articulating surfaces (Fig. 18-9*A, B*). The articular facets are particularly important in resisting torsion and shear, but they also play a role in compression. They may carry large compressive loads (25 to 33%), depending on the body posture, and they also provide (in equal proportion to the disk) 45% of the torsional strength of a motion segment.[59,95,112,127]

The amount of load bearing by the articular facet joints is related to whether the motion segment is loaded in flexion or extension. Differences in interdiskal loading between erect sitting and standing can be explained in part by load bearing of the articular facet joints while in extension or lordosis. Theoretically, the disk would be protected from both torsional

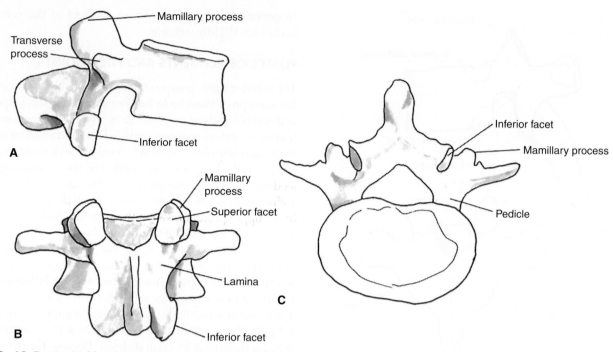

■ **FIG. 18-5.** Typical lumbar vertebra. **(A)** Lateral, **(B)** posterior, and **(C)** inferior views.

and compressive loads when the motion segment is in extension. However, excessive loading of the spine in extension may cause failure of this secondary load-bearing mechanism; that is, loads transmitted through the articular facet joints may produce high strains in the pars interarticularis, leading to spondylolysis.

The apophyseal or articular facet joints are usually described as **plane diarthrodial synovial joints** (except for the joints between the first two cervical vertebrae), although there is a "meniscus" (fatty synovial mass) in most of the joints (Fig. 18-9A, B).[113] The superior processes (prezygapophyseal) always bear an articulating facet whose surface is directed dorsally to

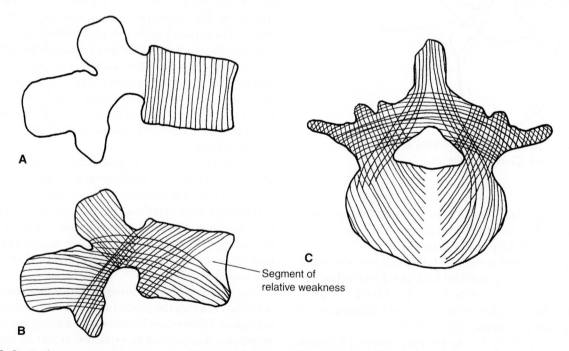

■ **FIG. 18-6.** Trabecular arrangement of vertebrae. **(A)** Vertical trabeculae, **(B)** inferior and superior oblique patterns (note segment of relative weakness), and **(C)** oblique patterns viewed from above.

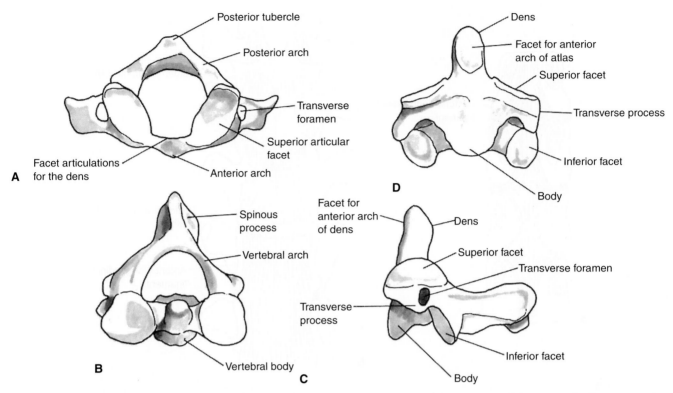

■ **FIG. 18-7.** First and second cervical vertebrae. **(A)** The atlas (C1), as viewed from above; **(B)** the axis (C2), as viewed from above; **(C)** anterior view of axis; and **(D)** sagittal view of axis.

some degree (Figs. 18-3A, B; 18-4A, B; and 18-5A, B); the inferior articulating processes (postzygapophyseal) direct their articulating surfaces ventrally (Figs. 18-3A, 18-4A, and 18-5A).[191,192] The joint consists of a cartilaginous articular surface, a fluid-filled capsule, and numerous ligaments surrounding and reinforcing the capsule. In degeneration the synovium is redundant, and the capsule frequently is redundant or torn and may contribute to malfunction as trapped menisci do in other joints.[113,172]

Generally motion between two vertebrae is extremely limited and consists of a small amount of gliding or sliding. The net effect of small amounts of gliding in a series of vertebrae produces a considerably large range of motion for the spinal column as a whole. The motions available to the column may be likened to that of a joint with three planes of motion: flexion–extension, lateral flexion (sidebending), and rotation.[163] In addition, a small amount of vertical compression and distraction is possible. The type and amount of motion that are available differ from region to region and depend on the orientation of the facets and the fluidity, elasticity, and thickness of the intervertebral joint. Although the degree of movement at the spinal segment is largely determined by the disks, the patterns of movement of the spine depend on the shape and orientation of the articular facet joint surfaces. If the superior and inferior articular facets of the three adjacent vertebrae lie in the sagittal plane, the motions of flexion and extension are facilitated. Conversely, if the articular facets are placed

in the frontal plane, the predominant motion is that of lateral flexion or sidebending.

Regionally (except for C1 and C2, whose articular facets are oriented in the transverse plane), the articular facets of the intervertebral joints of the cervical spine are oriented at 45° to the transverse plane and parallel to the frontal plane (Fig. 18-3A). This alignment of the intervertebral joints allows flexion, extension, sidebending, and rotation. The angle increases at descending levels, approaching vertical at C7 in the frontal plane. The superior articular facet surface is convex, and the inferior facet surface is concave. The articular facet joint surfaces tend to separate during forward bending and approximate during backward bending (Fig. 18-9C, D). Sidebending and rotation occur together to the same side. This is because the articular facet joint surfaces are positioned approximately halfway between the frontal and transverse planes. As one articular facet joint slides forward and upward, its mate slides backward and downward, translating to a sidebending component in the frontal plane and a rotatory component in the frontal plane and in the transverse plane. In this way, sidebending and rotation from C2–C3 to about T1 involve essentially an identical movement between articular facet joint surfaces. The only difference between sidebending and rotation of the cervical spine results from differences in movement at the upper cervical spine. The unique joint configuration found in the alanto-axial complex is discussed in Chapter 19, Cervical Spine. According to Kapandji,[105] combined movement of flexion and

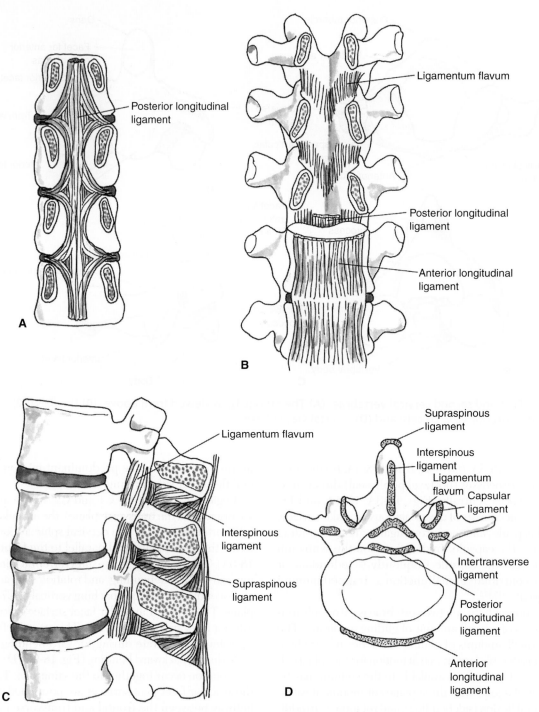

■ **FIG. 18-8.** The ligaments of the vertebral column include **(A)** the posterior longitudinal ligament (posterior view), **(B)** the ligamentum flavum and anterior longitudinal ligament (anterior view), **(C)** the supraspinous ligaments (sagittal view), and **(D)** the intertransverse ligaments (superior view).

extension for these segments is approximately 100° to 110°. When combined with movement of the atlanto-axial complex, the total range of motion is 130°.

In the erect spine, sidebending and rotation in the thoracic and lumbar regions tend to occur to opposite sides. The reasons may be more complex than at the cervical spine, but

again seem to be largely the result of the orientation of the articular facet planes (Figs. 18-4A and 18-5A). In the thoracic spine, all 12 thoracic vertebrae support ribs and show facets for the articulation of these structures. Unlike the spinous processes in the lumbar and cervical areas, where the tip of the spinous process is found directly posterior to the body of

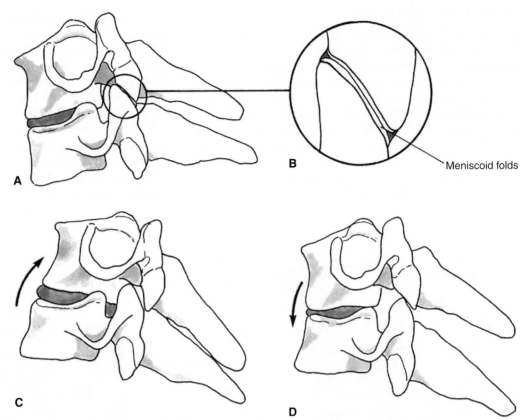

■ **FIG. 18-9.** Sagittal section of an articular facet joint (**A**), with an enlarged view (**B**) showing the meniscoid folds. The articular surfaces tend to approximate during extension (**C**) and separate during flexion (**D**).

Meniscoid folds

the vertebra, the tip of the spinous process lies posteriorly and inferiorly to the body (Fig. 18-4*A, B*). The spinous processes are long and triangular in section. Those of the upper and lower four thoracic vertebrae are more blade like and are directed downward at an angle of 60° so that their spines completely overlap the next lower segment (Fig. 18-1*C*).[191,192] This elongation limits the amount of extension possible at each segment. The thoracic pedicles are longer than in the cervical and lumbar areas, giving the vertebral canal an oval appearance and diminishing the possibility of stenosis of the canal (Fig. 18-4*C*). The transverse processes are characterized by having a concave facet that receives the tuberculum of the rib and being angled backward; this encourages rotatory movements by the attached muscles.

The articular facets of the thoracic vertebrae are oriented 60° to the transverse plane and 20° to the frontal plane (Fig. 18-4*A, B*),[65,114,131] which allows sidebending, rotation, and some flexion and extension. Because of the articular facet alignment and stabilization of the vertebral bodies laterally, rotation is the most accessible movement. Gregersen and Lucas[78] concluded from a study on rotation of the trunk that approximately 74° of rotation occurred between the first and twelfth thoracic vertebrae (the average cumulative rotation from the sacrum to the first thoracic vertebrae was 102°). The superior articular facets form a stout, shelflike projection. The ovoid surfaces of the superior articular facets are slightly convex, whereas the inferior articular facets are slightly concave (similar to the articular facet joint surfaces in the cervical spine), which is opposite to the articular facets in the lumbar spine.[72]

The majority of thoracic vertebrae adhere to the basic structural design of all vertebrae, except for some minor variations. The C7–T3 segments are a transitional zone between the cervical lordosis and thoracic kyphosis, with all ranges being diminished, although flexion and extension are freer than in the lower thoracic spine. The first thoracic vertebra is considered the transitional vertebra. The second thoracic vertebra (which can be distinguished by an enlarged pedicle) is thought to be developed to carry that portion of the weight borne by the articular facets into a more forward position. Thus, at levels below the second thoracic vertebra, the weight is carried principally by the vertebral bodies and disks.[172] The physiologic movement combinations are the same as for the typical cervical regions (i.e., sidebending accompanied by rotation).[81] At the T3–T10 segments, both sidebending and rotation are limited by the bony thorax. Amplitudes of movement, especially in the sagittal range, increase progressively as the restriction offered by the ribs begins to decrease. The T11–L1 segments are a transitional zone between the thoracic kyphosis and lumbar lordosis. While the articular facet joints remain vertically oriented, they begin to change from the frontal to the sagittal plane. The last thoracic vertebra (T12), acting as a bridge between the thoracic and lumbar regions, has its inferior articular facets in the sagittal plane to match those of L1.[105]

RIB CAGE ARTICULATIONS

According to Maigne, involvement of the rib cage in pathologic processes is often neglected; yet costal sprain is very frequent and is expressed by thoracic or upper lumbar pain.[131] It follows either a contusion, an unusual effort, or a faulty movement (generally in rotation). The ribs are thus mechanically significant articulations of the thoracic spine. The 12 pairs of thin arc-shaped bones form a protective cavity for the heart, lungs, and great vessels.[41] They also provide attachment for muscles necessary for respiration, posture, and arm function. The rib cage has several important biomechanical functions related to the spine. It acts as a protective barrier for any traumatic impact directed from the sides or anterior aspect, and it stiffens and strengthens the thoracic spine. The moment of inertia provided by the rib cage is its most important biomechanical aspect, according to White and Panjabi.[225] The increased moment of inertia stiffens the spine when it is subjected to any kind of rotatory forces, such as bending movements and torques.

The transverse dimensions of the thoracic spine are increased manifold by the inclusion of the sternum and ribs. Cartilaginous junctions fix the ribs to the sternum. Characterized as **true ribs,** the first seven are attached to the sternum by individual cartilages (Fig. 18-10A). The eighth, ninth,

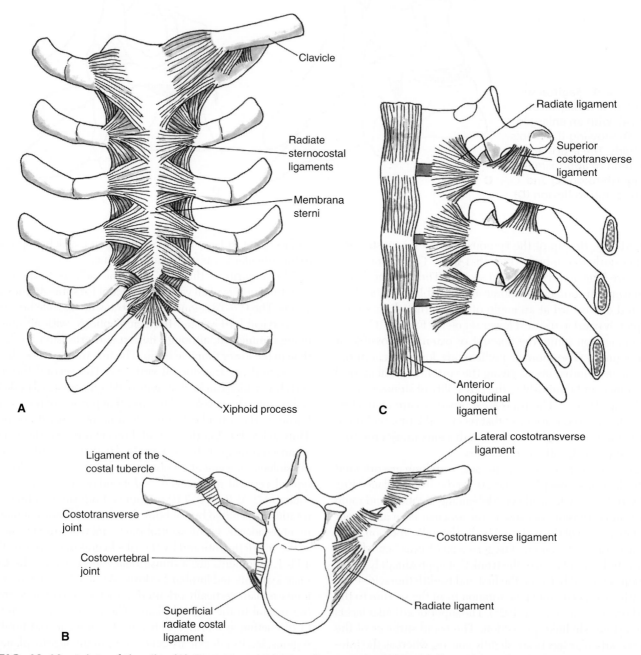

■ **FIG. 18-10.** Joints of the ribs. **(A)** Costosternal joints and connections. **(B and C)** Costovertebral joints on superior and sagittal views.

and tenth ribs have a common junction with the sternum and are called **false ribs.**

The ends of the true ribs join this costal cartilage by means of the costochondral joint. The first rib is joined firmly to the manubrium by a cartilaginous joint, while the second rib articulates with demifacets on both the manubrium and the body of the sternum by way of synovial joints (Fig. 18-10A). The cartilages of the third to seventh ribs have small synovial joints which attach to the body of the sternum.[225] Later in life these joints become ankylosed or obliterated.[80]

The ribs and vertebrae are united at two locations. The radiate ligament anchors each rib head to two adjacent vertebral bodies and the disk between them (Fig. 18-10B, C).[176] This occurs at the superior and inferior costal demifacets located at the junction of the vertebral body and posterior arch, and forms the costovertebral joint (a synovial joint) (Fig. 18-10B). Costotransverse ligaments join the rib tubercle and corresponding vertebral transverse process (Fig. 18-10B,C). To accommodate this articulation, each long transverse process is capped by a costal facet. The costotransverse joint is also a synovial joint surrounded by a capsule, but it is primarily strengthened by three costotransverse ligaments.[105]

Each rib is a curved lever which has its fulcrum immediately lateral to the costotransverse joint, and each has its own range and direction of movement differing slightly from the others. Although it is fair to surmise that each rib has its own pattern of movement, certain generalizations can be made. The first ribs form a firm horseshoe-shaped arch, which moves upward and forward as a unit (Fig. 18-11A, B). This movement occurs at the heads of these ribs and is a simple elevation of the manubrium upward and forward.[130] The false ribs combine the elevation of their anterior ends with a caliper-like opening (Fig. 18-11C).[130] Following direct trauma or secondary to some attempts at trunk rotation, the false ribs induce pain somewhat analogous to that of lumbago. The pain is typically located in the lumbar fossa, radiating toward the groin, and is acutely intensified by certain movements.[131]

The final two (eleventh and twelfth) ribs are free floating (termed **floating ribs**) and simply end in the trunk musculature of the abdominal wall. Their loose attachment at their heads and lack of union with the transverse processes leaves them subject to push and pull in any direction, hinging on the head.[130] The twelfth rib is the shortest and may be so short that it fails to project beyond the lateral border of the back muscles that cover it.[93]

With respect to spinal motion, both sidebending and rotation of the thoracic spine are limited by the rib cage. When a thoracic vertebra rotates, the motion is accompanied by distortion of the associated rib pair. The ribs on the side to which the body rotates become convex posteriorly, while the ribs on the contralateral side become flattened posteriorly.[163] The amount of rotation that is possible depends on the ability of the ribs to undergo distortion and the amount of motion available in the costovertebral, costotransverse, and costochondral joints.

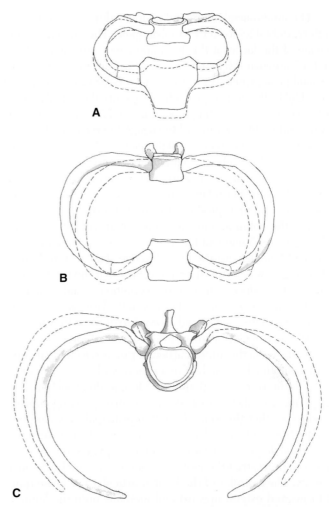

∎ **FIG. 18-11.** Movements of the ribs. **(A)** The first rib and manubrium with upward and forward movement. **(B)** The typical vertebrosternal ribs with bucket-handle movement. **(C)** The caliper-like movements of the lower ribs.

Because the rib cage actually encloses the thoracic spine, any external stabilizing force must be indirectly applied through the ribs. Because of their size and configuration, the ribs are more plastic than the vertebral bodies.[188] Therefore, they readily yield to applied forces, and their shape will be altered before any corrective effect is noted on a rigid spine.[41]

LUMBAR ARTICULATIONS

The average plane of inclination of the lumbar articular facets is almost 90° to the transverse plane and 45° to the frontal plane (Fig. 18-5A, B). The articular facets face in almost a lateromedial direction and are therefore aligned in the sagittal plane, whereas the articular facets of the fifth lumbar vertebra face obliquely forward and laterally toward the frontal plane.[191,192,225] This alignment allows flexion, extension, and sidebending, but almost no rotation. Sidebending is limited to a range of approximately 5° between each successive vertebra, whereas rotation is limited to approximately 3°.[3]

The lumbosacral intervertebral joints differ from the other intervertebral joints in the lumbar spine. The orientation and shape of the facets at this level allow more rotation.[128] Most L4–L5 articular facet joints are angled 43° from the coronal or frontal plane, whereas most L5–S1 articular facets are angled 52°. Unlike the more superior lumbar joints, the articular facets of the inferior articulating process of the L5 vertebra face forward and slightly downward to engage the reciprocally corresponding articular processes of the sacrum. The most essential function of the lumbosacral articulations involves their role as buttresses against the forward and downward displacement of the L5 vertebra relative to the sacrum.[191,192] Because the sacrovertebral angle produces the most abrupt change of direction in the column, and the center of gravity which passes through the L5 segment falls anterior to the sacrum, there is a marked tendency for the thick, "wedge-shaped" fifth lumbar disk to give way to the shearing vector that the lumbosacral angularity produces. The resulting condition, spondylolisthesis, most frequently reveals a deficiency in the laminae that fails to anchor L5 to the sacrum and allows it to displace forward.

All the articular pillars of the lumbar vertebrae have convex surfaces on the inferior articular process, forming in most cases one third or one half of a sphere with a greater curvature in the transverse than in the longitudinal section. The superior articular process carries a corresponding concave surface so that the joints have two principal movements—translation (slide) and distraction (gapping). Unlike the intervertebral disks, which allow motion in all planes, the articular facet joints restrict the motion segment, assisted by the ligaments. The capsules of the lumbar articular facets are quite fibrous and extend upward and medially onto the laminae above, which enables them to restrict forward bending.[49,172]

According to White and Panjabi,[225] "mechanical load-sharing" between the facets and disks is rather complex. Other authors have made quantitative estimates of the biomechanics, including Nachemson,[153] who found that 18% of the compressive load is borne by the articular facet; King et al.,[112] who reported that 0 to 33% of the axial load was borne by the facet, depending on the position or posture of the joint; and Farfan,[59] who attributed 45% of torsional stiffness to the articular facets and capsules. The articular facet joints make a major contribution to the rotational stiffness of the lumbar spine; this is important because in vitro testing of loaded motion segments in rotation alone and rotation with either flexion or sidebending can produce the types of disk lesions seen clinically. The importance of asymmetrical articular facet orientation for pathologic processes of the intervertebral disk has been well documented by Farfan and Sullivan,[61] who established a highly significant correlation between asymmetry of the articular facet joints and the level of disk involvement, and between the side of the more oblique articular facet orientation and side of sciatica. Most articular facet planes have a difference in angle of less than 10°, but "gross" asymmetry is seen in approximately 25% of an essentially random population by conventional roentgenography.[61] This may be associated with asymmetrical vertebral bodies or with unilateral laminar hypertrophy and is clearly associated with early disk degeneration at the level of the asymmetry. When such asymmetry is present, it is the side with the most oblique articular facet that acquires early posterolateral annular damage.

INTERVERTEBRAL DISKS

The spine, which is composed of alternating rigid and elastic elements, possesses a considerable degree of flexibility that is primarily attributable to the intervertebral disks. The amount of flexibility depends on the material characteristics, the size and shape of the disk, and the amount of restraint offered by the invertebral ligaments. Normally the disks may be considered to act as universal joints, permitting motion in four directions between vertebral bodies: (1) translational motion in the long axis of the spine, occurring because of compressibility of the disk; (2) rotary motion about a vertical axis; (3) anteroposterior bending; and (4) lateral bending.[149]

VERTEBRAL BODY RELATIONSHIP

Each successive vertebral body is linked by an intervertebral disk, which acts as a symphysis between the vertebrae. There are no disks between the occiput and atlas nor between the atlas and axis. The disk "spaces" in the young adult contribute to as much as 20 to 33% of total vertebral column height. The ratio between the height of the disk and the corresponding vertebral bodies, in part, determines the amount of motion that may occur in a particular region. Flexibility has been shown to vary directly with the square of the vertical height of the disk and indirectly with the square of the horizontal diameter of the body.[151] Because of the proportionally greater height in the lumbar region, the range of intervertebral motion is greater in the lumbar region; however, because of the greater horizontal diameter, the flexibility is less than in the thoracic region.[149] Motion is greatest in the cervical spine. The unique composition of the intervertebral disks allows for a more even distribution of weight transmitted to the adjacent vertebral bodies during movement.

It is often mentioned that the disks act as shock absorbers during vertical compressive loading. While this may be true to some extent, shock absorption on vertical loading is largely related to the fact that the spine is a curved, "spring-loaded," flexible column, rather than a rigid, rodlike structure.

The cervical disks are largely responsible for the existence of a normal cervical lordosis in the upper spine; the lumbar disks are somewhat less responsible for the normal lumbar lordosis, which is mostly caused by the wedged-shaped vertebral bodies. In the thoracic spine the normal kyphosis is almost entirely caused by the shape of the vertebral bodies.

DISK STRUCTURE

The disk is composed of several structures, including the nucleus pulposus, which is the central fluid-filled portion of the disk, and the annulus fibrosus, the series of elastic fibers that

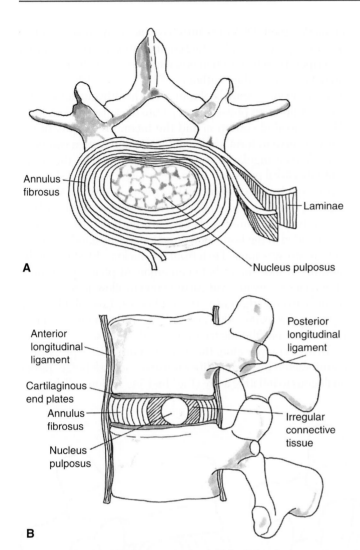

■ **FIG. 18-12.** The intervertebral disk. **(A)** Inferior and **(B)** sagittal views.

surround the nucleus (Fig. 18-12). The disk is bounded above and below by cartilaginous end-plates, to which the annular fibers are firmly anchored. These end-plates are then attached to the body surface of the vertebral bodies. The inner fluid nucleus (a remnant of the embryonic notochordal tissue) is surrounded by a zone of irregular connective tissue bands that are also rich in fluid and are, in turn, surrounded by the lamellae of the annulus fibrosus.[172] The overall shape of the nucleus mimics that of the body, and takes up about 25% of the disk area.[59] The fluid mass of the nucleus pulposus is composed of a colloidal gel rich in water-binding glucosaminoglycans with a few collagen fibers randomly embedded within. It is centrally located in the disk, except in the lower lumbar segments where it is located more posteriorly.

NUCLEUS PULPOSUS AND FLUID EXCHANGE

Both the relative size of the nucleus pulposus and its capacity to take on water and swell are greatest in the cervical and lumbar spine. It is well suited for its essential function to resist and redistribute compressive forces within the spine. Because of its high water content and plastic nature, its functions follow closely the laws of hydrodynamics. Typically, the nucleus pulposus occupies an eccentric position within the confines of the annulus, usually close to the posterior margin of the disk (Fig. 18-12B). Being avascular, the nucleus depends on nutrition from its exchange of fluid across the cartilaginous end-plate with the vascularized vertebral body. The tendency of imbibition of fluid by the nucleus is greatest when weight-bearing is reduced through the disk (as in sleeping). As a result, a young person tends to be taller (¼ to ¾ inch) in the morning than at the end of the day. During the day the disk fluid is expressed from the disk to complete the nutrient cycle. In addition to being expressed, the disk fluid can be relocated by the assumption of specific postures.[116] Examples of this include the loss of normal lordosis after assuming a flexed position when gardening, or a lateral shift associated with low back injury.[172] The mucopolysaccharide gel changes in its biochemical characteristics with damage and age. These biochemical changes decrease the water-binding capability of the nucleus. Hendry demonstrated that a disk will give up water more readily if it is degenerated because of damage or age.[86] Normally, the nucleus contains between 70 and 88% water, which makes it nearly incompressible; thus, it acts as a distributor of force at the vertebral level. As the disk becomes drier and its elasticity decreases, it loses its ability to store energy and to distribute stresses and is therefore less capable of resisting loads.

ANNULUS FIBROSUS

The annulus fibrosus consists of fibroid cartilage with bundles of collagen fibers arranged in a criss-cross pattern, which allows them to withstand high bending and torsional loads (Fig. 18-12A). These fibers run obliquely between vertebral bodies such that the fibers in one layer run in the opposite direction to the fibers in adjacent layers. The outer layer of fibers blends with the posterior longitudinal ligament posteriorly and with the anterior longitudinal ligament anteriorly. These outer fibers attach superiorly and inferiorly to the margins of the vertebral bodies by Sharpey's fibers. The fibers of the outermost ring of the annulus extend beyond the confines of the disk and blend with the vertebral periosteum and longitudinal ligaments. The inner fibers attach superiorly and inferiorly to the cartilaginous end-plates. The cartilaginous end-plate is composed of hyaline cartilage that separates the outer two components of the disk from the vertebral body (Fig. 18-12B). In addition to absorbing forces, the annulus contains the nucleus pulposus, which acts as the fulcrum of movement for the three planes of motion available at each vertebral level.[105] One of the major functions of the annulus is to withstand tension, whether the tensile forces are from the horizontal extension of the compressed nucleus, from torsional stress of the column, or from the separation of the vertebral bodies on the convex side of spinal flexion.[191,192] The entire unit is then ensheathed by the periosteum, which extends over the vertebrae (and, in effect, the intervertebral disks), displaying a thickening both anteriorly (anterior longitudinal ligament) and posteriorly (posterior longitudinal ligament).[200] According to Paris,[172] the area of the disk covered by this sheath has been found to be both innervated and vascularized and possesses, in effect, a neurovascular capsule. Innervation from the sinuvertebral nerve has been substantiated by findings of Cloward and others.[37] It is proposed that the diseased disk, in which parts of the annulus have been torn and repaired, contains a richer innervation from the ingrowth of nerve tissue with granulation.[37] This may be of some importance clinically in patients with spinal pain. Surgically removed disk tissue has been reported to contain some complex as well as free nerve endings.

DISK PRESSURES

The young healthy disk maintains a positive pressure within the nucleus pulposus at rest, which increases as loads are applied to the spine. This pressure approximates 1.5 times the mean applied pressure over the entire area of the end-plate.[161] These pressures have importance therapeutically when activity and exercise programs for patients with disk problems are being designed. Disk pressures have been extensively studied in various postures and seating configurations. A more detailed description can be found in other sources and will not be covered here (see other authors[5,7–15,79–81,84,85,144,148,150,153,155–159,161]) The "preloaded" spinal column in the healthy nucleus maintains a continuous pressure to separate the adjacent vertebrae. This preloaded condition and the incompressibility of the nucleus serve to form a self-righting system: with a compressive force or angular movement in any direction, the resultant intradiskal pressure changes are such that the disk favors movement back to the "neutral" position. However, this self-righting system also depends on the tensile strength and the elasticity of the annulus. Tensile strength or stiffness must be provided in the horizontal direction to withstand the intermittent stresses applied to it from the nucleus. Elasticity of the annulus or movement between adjacent planes of annular fibers is necessary in a vertical direction to allow angular movement between adjacent vertebral bodies. Loss of a balance between this extensibility and stability of the annular fibers is probably a contributing factor in disk disorders.

In axial compression, the increased intradiskal pressure is counteracted by annular fiber tension and disk bulge, rather analogous to inflating a tire (Fig. 18-13A).[177] Some disk-space

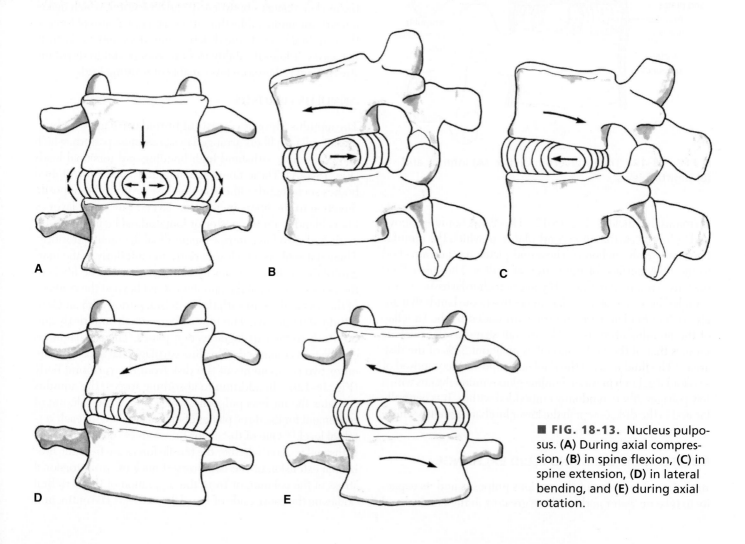

■ **FIG. 18-13.** Nucleus pulposus. **(A)** During axial compression, **(B)** in spine flexion, **(C)** in spine extension, **(D)** in lateral bending, and **(E)** during axial rotation.

narrowing also occurs. Because of the incompressibility of the fluid-like nucleus, forces acting on the nucleus will act to move it, change its shape, or both. In flexion, extension, and lateral bending, the same process occurs. Because the annular fibers are somewhat elastic and because the annulus allows vertical and tangential movements between vertebral bodies, the nucleus in the healthy disk may either change in shape or move within the limits allowed by the annulus.[198] Its volume, however, must remain the same. Displacement of the nucleus within the disk has been disputed.[80,114] Because the nucleus is roughly spherical, some have considered it as a ball that allows one vertebra to rotate over its neighbor. The nucleus is said to move backward during flexion and forward during extension. However, others have not confirmed this observation, and Krag and associates found little motion of the nucleus.[114,115]

In the consideration of an angular movement forward (flexion) of one vertebral body on another in a weight-bearing situation, the forward shift of weight will result in an increased compressive force on the anterior aspect of the disk. This causes the anterior annular fibers to bulge backward and causes the nucleus to shift backward, transferring the vertical compressive force to a horizontally directed force backward against the posterior annulus (Fig. 18-13*B*). Because the healthy nucleus is fluid-like, an even distribution of pressure results across the inner annular layers. The posterior annular fibers, which are normally bulged somewhat backward in the neutral position, tend to straighten because of the increase in distance between the posterior vertebral bodies. However, because of the pressure against the posterior annulus by the nucleus, there is also a tendency to maintain this posterior bulge and thus bring the vertebrae back to a neutral relationship (the self-righting mechanism discussed earlier). Looking at it from another perspective, the straightening of the annular fibers tends to increase the counterpressure against the posteriorly bulging nucleus, which effects a counterforce against the original vertical compressive force. In this way equilibrium must be reached between the transformation of the vertical loading to a horizontal pressure against the annulus and the tendency for the annulus to reconvert this pressure, in a self-righting manner, to counter the compressive loading. In extension and lateral bending, the same process occurs (Fig. 18-13*C, D*). Of clinical significance is the fact that changes in this equilibrium favor pathologic changes in the related tissues, while, conversely, pathologic tissue changes result in a change in the equilibrium; the resultant cycle of events should be obvious. For example, a weakening of the annular fibers results in less tendency to resist the horizontal forces exerted by the nucleus, which will result in further weakening of the annulus. Osteoporosis of the vertebral bodies results in a decreased ability to withstand reactive vertical forces with erosion of disk material into the vertebral bodies; the so-called vacuum phenomenon.

In axial rotation, a compressive force causes an increase in intradiskal pressure and tends to narrow the joint space (Fig. 18-13*E*). When rotation occurs, the annular fibers (which are oriented in the direction of rotary movement) become taut, while the fibers oriented in the opposite direction tend to slacken. Mathematical models based on the geometry of the disk demonstrate that torsion produces stress concentrated on the region of the posterior lateral annulus, which is a common site of disk herniation.[117,207] Torsional loading of spinal segments in vitro produces fissures in the annulus in the same posterolateral location and is thought to be one of the common early causes of acute low back pain.[178] During daily activities the disk is loaded in a complex manner, usually by a combination of compression, bending, and torsion.[133] Flexion, extension, and lateral flexion of the spine produce mainly tensile and compressive stresses in the disk, whereas rotation produces shear stress. The tensile stress in the posterior part of the annulus fibrosus in the lumbar spine has been estimated to be four to five times the applied axial load.[69,153] The thoracic annuli fibrosi are subjected to less tensile stress than the lumbar annuli fibrosi because of their geometric difference. The ratio of disk diameter to height is higher in the thoracic disk than the lumbar disk.[120]

The entire intervertebral disk in the adult is avascular. Up to the time of skeletal maturity, blood vessels do enter the disk from the vertebral bodies through the cartilaginous end-plates. These vessels are gradually obliterated, leaving scars in the end-plate where they penetrated.

INTERVERTEBRAL FORAMINA

The **intervertebral foramen** is the aperture that gives exit to the segmental spinal nerves and entrance to the vessel and nerve branches that supply the bone and soft tissues of the vertebral canal. This aperture or canal is superiorly and inferiorly bounded by the respective pedicles of the adjacent vertebrae (Fig. 18-2). Its ventral and dorsal relations involve the two major intervertebral articulations. Ventrally it is bounded by the dorsum of the intervertebral disk, covered by the posterior longitudinal ligament, and dorsally by the capsule of the articular facet and ligamentum flavum (Fig. 18-8). Spur formation within the foramen can decrease the available space and create compression forces on the spinal nerves exiting through the foramen or on the structures that reenter the foramen, such as the sinuvertebral nerve, which innervates the posterior longitudinal ligament (see below, Vertebral Innervation).

Nerve-root entrapment may also result from closure or narrowing of the vertebral foramen, through any of the following mechanisms: (1) approximation of the pedicles resulting from narrowing of the intervertebral disk, (2) hypertrophic degenerative arthritic changes of the articular facet joints, and (3) thickening of the ligamentum flavum. The existence of additional ligamentous elements in relation to the intervertebral foramen (e.g., the transforaminal ligaments, found frequently in the lumbar region) could be critical.[31,191,192] The transforaminal ligaments are strong, unyielding cords of collagenous tissue that pass anteriorly from various parts of the neural arch to the body of the same or adjacent vertebra.

Control System: Noncontractile Soft Tissues

LIGAMENTS

The ligaments are vital for the structural stability of the spinal system. Their principle role is to prevent excessive motion. The ligaments are also the principal tensile load-bearing elements and, along with the apophyseal capsules, provide the central nervous system with information in regard to posture and movement.[234] Unlike muscles; ligaments are passive structures so that their tension depends on their length. Ligaments are viscoelastic in nature, with their deformation and type of failure being dependent on the rate of loading. Like all materials, ligaments fatigue and can fail with repetitive loading.[177,221] They readily resist tensile forces but buckle when subject to compression.

The ligaments that connect the anterior elements of the spine are the broad **anterior longitudinal ligament,** which extends from the basiocciput to the sacrum, and the **posterior longitudinal ligament,** which also extends from the basiocciput to the sacrum on the anterior aspect of the neural canal, behind the vertebral bodies. These ligaments are interlinked at each level by the disk, which adds support to the disk and vertebral body network (Fig. 18-8). The annulus fibrosus of the intervertebral disk may be considered a part of the ligamentous structure. These ligaments deform with separation of the vertebrae and bulging of the disk.[225] Richly supported by nerve fibers, they respond to painful stimuli. The remaining ligaments of the spine support and link the posterior elements.

ANTERIOR LONGITUDINAL LIGAMENT

The anterior longitudinal ligament is one ligamentous structure placed anterior to the center of rotation of the intervertebral joint. It thus acts to prevent hyperextension, along with the capsular ligament of the articular facet joint (Fig. 18-8). It begins as a rather narrow band from the basiocciput and broadens as it descends from C3 to the sacrum. It consists of long fibers along its length and short, arched fibers coursing between individual vertebrae and inserting into the anterior aspect of the intervertebral disk (Fig. 18-10C).[105] Considered perhaps the strongest ligament in the body (with a tensile strength of nearly 3,000 pounds per square inch), the anterior longitudinal ligament, along with the muscles about the spine, keeps a preload beam condition in the spine that helps to strengthen the spine during lifting.[58] In the lumbar spine it also resists the weight of the spine in its tendency to slip into the pelvic cavity.[172] Because of its breadth and tensile strength, this ligament provides strong support and reinforcement to the anterior disk during lifting, and Harrington and others have used the strength of the anterior ligament combined with Harrington rods to apply traction to fracture dislocations of the low back.[225]

POSTERIOR LONGITUDINAL LIGAMENT

The posterior longitudinal ligament extends from the basiocciput to the sacrum on the anterior aspect of the neural canal behind the vertebral bodies (Fig. 18-8A, B, D). It is densely attached to the posterior annulus fibrosus at each level, with both vertical and transverse fibers that spread across the posterior annulus; however, as the posterior longitudinal ligament passes the vertebral bodies, it narrows and is not attached to them except at their margins.[191,192] This allows entrant arteries, veins, and lymphatics to pass in and out of the posterior portion of the vertebral bodies. In flexion the posterior longitudinal ligament becomes taut and serves as a valve on these vessels, which do not have a valve mechanism of their own. It, like the anterior longitudinal ligament, is thickest in the thoracic (dorsal) spine. It is often reduced to a cord-shaped filament in the lumbar spine. The lateral expansions over the disks are thin, whereas the central portions are much thicker. This is presumably why most posterior protrusions of the disk soon move laterally to become posterolateral protrusions. Although the posterior longitudinal ligament is not as massive as the anterior longitudinal ligament in terms of cross-sectional area, the tensile strength per unit area seems to be the same for both structures.[210] Functionally, the ligament limits forward bending and gives support to the disks except in the lumbar region. Of interest is that in the midline the ligament does have a small amount of elastic tissue.[172] In the cervical spine the ligament is a broad band on the entire posterior aspect of the bodies, but because it is attached only in the region of the disk, with disk degeneration it produces folds that can press into the spinal canal on backward bending; this movement is therefore to be avoided in such conditions.

SEGMENTAL LIGAMENTS

The segmental ligaments of the spine include the **ligamentum flavum,** the **interspinous** and **intertransverse ligaments,** and the **anterior and posterior capsular ligaments of the articular facet joints.** The biomechanical significance of these structures depends on their strength, stiffness, and distance from the axis of rotation of the joints they span.[225]

Ligamentum Flavum. The ligamentum flavum extends from the anteroinferior border of the laminae above to the posterior border of the laminae below (Fig. 18-8B–D). It connects the laminae from C2 to S1. The medial edges fuse with the contralateral ligament in midline and completely close the vertebral canal (a slight septum is provided for the passage of arteries and veins). At its lateral border, the ligamentum flavum blends with the capsules of the articular facets, particularly in the lumbar region (Fig. 18-8B, C).[92] Histologically, the ligamentum flavum has the highest percentage of elastic fibers of any tissue in the body.[30,160] It checks the movement of the articular facet joints by exerting a constant pull on the capsule and thus assists in preventing the synovial lining and intra-articular menisci from being painfully nipped between the articular joint surfaces.[172] It owes much of this function to its yellow elastic fibers (hence, *flavum,* meaning yellow).

During forward bending the ligamentum flavum permits considerable range and assists in return to neutral or the resting position of the spinal segments without the development of folds. It thus serves to protect the spinal canal from encroachment by soft tissues on flexion and extension. Nachemson and Evans[160] found that in neutral the ligamentum flavum is prestrained by approximately 15% and that full physiologic flexion can stretch it an additional 30 to 35%, whereas it retains a 5% stretch in full physiologic extension. This elasticity is lost to some extent in normal aging, but if the instant axis of rotation for flexion is in the region of the posterior annulus, the flexion–extension torque resistance in the ligamentum flavum is significant. There is appreciable strain of the ligamentum flavum on sidebending or lateral flexion.[170] The ligamentum flavum also provides some preloading of the disk (leading to disk nucleus pressures greater than atmospheric), even when there is no external load on the spine, which may reduce slack in the motion segment. In patients with severe spine degeneration, the ligamentum flavum may be thickened and less elastic and may produce narrowing of the spinal canal in extension. This narrowing occurs because of the buckling of the ligament. Thus, at the time of surgery for spinal stenosis, its excision may be necessary.

Intertransverse and Interspinous Ligaments. The intertransverse ligaments are well developed in the thoracic spine and are intimately connected with the deep muscles of the back.[225] They pass between the transverse processes and are characterized as rounded cords. These ligaments are barely mentioned in many texts on functional anatomy, particularly with respect to the lumbar spine, as being significant. Functionally, they tend to limit sidebending and rotation.

The interspinous ligaments, which connect the spinous processes, are important for the stability of the spinal column. They are reinforced, especially at the level of the thoracic and lumbar spine, by the supraspinous ligaments (Fig. 18-8C, D). Their attachments extend from the root to the apex of each spinous process, proceeding in an upward and backward direction, *not* an upward and forward direction, as often illustrated.[172] This upward and backward orientation permits increased range of motion during flexion while still resisting excessive range. Panjabi and associates found high strain in both the interspinous and supraspinous ligaments with flexion while these were relatively unstrained in rotation.[170] The interspinous ligaments are narrow and elongated in the thoracic region, only slightly developed in the cervical spine, and thicker in the lumbar spine.[225] In 90% of cadavers of persons older than 40 years of age, Rissanen[187] noted that the interspinous ligament between L4 and L5 had degenerated or was completely ruptured.

The supraspinous ligament is a strong fibrous cord that connects the apices of the spines from the C7 to L4, and occasionally to L5 (Fig. 18-8C, D).[172] At this level it is replaced by the interlocking fibers of the somewhat stronger erector spinae tendons of insertion. The supraspinous ligament is thicker and broader in the lumbar region than the thoracic, and it is intimately blended in both areas with the neighboring fascia. Between the spine of C7 and the external occipital protuberance, it is much expanded and called the **ligamentum nuchae** (see Fig. 19-4).[227] In the cervical region the spinous processes

are buried deeply between the heavy muscles on the back of the neck so that the supraspinous ligament is represented by a thin septum between the musculature of the two sides. In quadrupeds with heavy heads, the ligamentum nuchae is a strong, thick band of elastic tissue which aids the muscles in holding up the head.[93] In humans, however, the supraspinous and interspinous ligaments and the ligamentum nuchae are largely collagenous tissue, relatively inelastic and of little strength; in the cervical and lumbar regions, where they should be most important in limiting segmental flexion, the interspinous ligaments are frequently defective or lacking in one or several interspaces.[93] Because the supraspinous ligament is the most superficial of the spinal ligaments and farthest from the axis of flexion, it has a greater potential for sprains.[105]

FASCIAL ANATOMY

As in the limbs, the principle muscle masses, the viscera, and the main nerves and vessel of the neck and trunk are contained with fascial coverings. Of major significance in understanding musculoskeletal function and dysfunction is the fact that the fascia comprises one connected network from the fascia attached to the inner aspect of the skull to the fascia in the soles of the feet there exists just one fascial structure. Apart from its immense role of support, structural organization and motion of the body, fascia is involved in numerous complex chemical activities. Although not technically a ligament, the thoracolumbar fascia (lumbodorsal) fascia had a tensile strength of nearly 2,000 pounds per square inch and serves as on the most important noncontractile structures in the lumbar spine.[59] For a review of the fascial system of the spine see Chapter 7, Myofascial Considerations and Evaluation in Somatic Dysfunction.

CAPSULES

The joint capsule of the spinal articular facet joint is composed of two layers, an outer layer known as the **stratum fibrosum** and an inner layer called the **stratum synovium.** The outer layer is attached to the periosteum of the component bone by Sharpey's fibers and is reinforced by musculotendinous and ligamentous structures that cross the joint. The outer layer is poorly vascularized but richly innervated. The nerve endings that are located in and around the joint capsule are sensitive to the rate and direction of motion, tension and to compression and vibration.[82]

In contrast to the outer layer, the inner layer of the capsule is highly vascularized but poorly innervated.[87] The stratum synovium is insensitive to pain but undergoes vasodilatation and vasoconstriction in response to heat and cold. It produces the hyaluronic acid component of the synovial fluid and serves as an entry point for nutrients and an exit point for waste material.[87] The capsules of the articular facet joints possess two noteworthy recesses, one superior and one inferior, through which the synovium may distend during effusion or backward bending.[53,132] The superior recess is the weaker, and effusion here may protrude sufficiently to press on the mixed spinal nerve as it enters the intervertebral foramen.[53]

Capsules encompass all the articular facet joints in the spine including the articulation of the head with the atlas.[148] The capsules include separate thickenings, which have different functional roles. The capsules and their ligaments guide and restrict the motion segments. Because they are far from the disks and therefore act on long moment arms, these ligaments have an important functional role in resisting spinal flexion.[177] In full flexion of the lumbar spine, the capsules support 40% of the body weight.[72] These fibers are generally oriented in a direction perpendicular to the plane of the articular facet joints. They are broader and more taut in the cervical region than the rest of the spine.[170] The capsules of the lumbar spine, which are often illustrated as being short and bunchy, in fact have a considerable medial extent and are quite fibrous, possessing an upward and medial direction that ideally suits them to restricting forward bending.[172] The capsular ligaments, along with the anterior longitudinal ligament, also act to prevent hyperextension of the spine.[59]

Capsules are an important consideration with respect to the loose- and close-packed positions of the articular facet joints of the spine.[47,72] The concept of loose-packed and close-packed positions is useful in understanding when a joint may be less stable and more vulnerable. Loose-packed positions are those positions in a joint's range of motion in which the ligaments and capsules are slack; the area of contact with the articular surfaces is generally low, and the joints are more vulnerable and less able to resist an external force. Close-packed positions, on the other hand, are those in which there is maximum contact between articular surfaces and maximum tautness of the ligaments.[2] The close-packed position of the articular facet joints from C3 to L5 is extension, whereas the close-packed position for the atlas and axis is full flexion.[72] The close-packed position is often lost following a pathologic process, trauma, or prolonged periods of poor posture. Inability to assume a full close-packed position results in the potential for increased dysfunction, and as a result a more unstable, loose-packed position is maintained.

VERTEBRAL INNERVATION

Because of the high frequency of patients presenting clinically with complaints of spinal pain or pain appearing to be of spinal origin, it is necessary for the clinician to have a thorough knowledge of spinal innervation. More specifically, the clinician must be aware of what structures appear to lack innervation totally. This information must be combined with an understanding of common pathologic processes and their clinical manifestations. In this way a more reliable understanding may be acquired as to the nature and extent of various disorders and perhaps a better understanding of the often bizarre symptoms and signs that result.

Information relating to spinal innervation and pain-sensitive spinal tissues has come from two types of investigations:

(1) actual experiments with human subjects in which attempts are made to isolate noxious stimuli to a particular tissue, and (2) laboratory tissue studies in which sensory endings are identified and attempts are made to trace the afferent pathways from these endings to central connections. For obvious reasons, those studies belonging to the first category of investigation are relatively few and results have at times been inconsistent or highly criticized. There have been numerous studies of the second type, however, and the results (for the most part) seem to be consistent. One must realize, however, that there is a limit as to how much can be inferred from tissue studies with respect to clinical significance. This is especially true when considering pain-sensitive tissue, because there is no direct correlation between the type of ending found within a particular tissue and the capacity for the tissue, when stimulated, to send signals to higher centers, which result in the perception of pain.

Presented here is a summary of what seem to be reasonably well-accepted findings relating to spinal neurology. Spinal structures receive innervation largely from two sources, the sinuvertebral (recurrent meningeal) nerves and the medial branches of the posterior primary divisions of the segmental spinal nerves (Fig. 18-14A, B). Endings found in the dura mater and blood vessels are primarily of the free nerve plexus type (see Chapter 3, Arthrology). Endings found in the posterior longitudinal ligament and periosteum include free nerve endings and plexuses as well as encapsulated and nonencapsulated nerve endings. It is assumed that the larger encapsulated nerve endings act primarily as mechanoreceptors. It is important to realize that each sinuvertebral nerve tends to innervate the tissues at its own level as well as send ascending and descending branches to levels above and below (Fig. 18-14A). It follows that stimulation of endings supplied by a particular sinuvertebral nerve may result in the perception of pain or in reflex changes in muscle tone at levels of the spine other than the level at which the lesion lies. Also, because it is well documented that stimulation of deep somatic tissues often results in segmentally referred pain, one may assume that pain may be referred into a segment not corresponding to the vertebral segment (level) at which the lesion lies.

The posterior division of the spinal nerve divides into lateral, intermediate, and medial branches (Fig. 18-15). The lateral branch innervates the skin and deep muscles of the back segmentally, while the medial branch innervates the articular facet joint capsules, the posterior aspect of the ligamentum flavum, the interspinous ligaments, the supraspinous ligaments, and the blood vessels supplying the vertebrae. The medial branches of the posterior division also send ascending and descending branches to (usually) one level above and one level below, with the same clinical implications as discussed for the overlapping sinuvertebral nerves. Receptors found in the facet joint capsules, sending signals along the medial branch of the posterior division, include all four of the receptors discussed in the section on joint neurology (see Chapter 3, Arthrology).

Afferent fibers from both the sinuvertebral nerve and the medial branch of the posterior primary division approach the

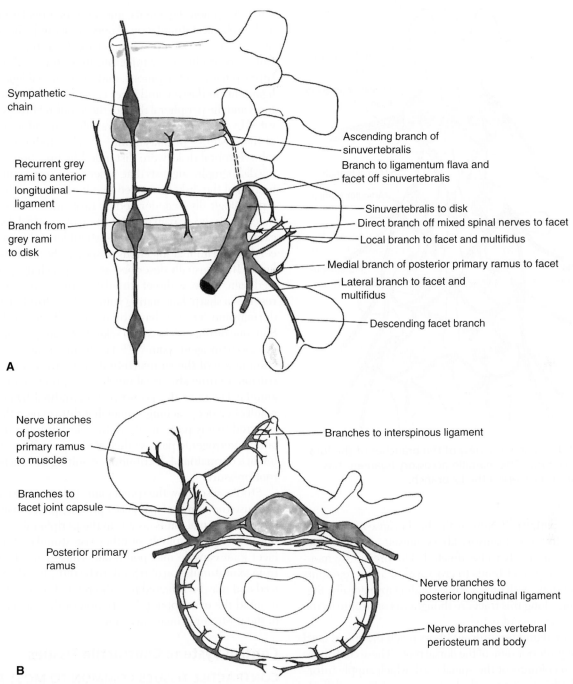

Sympathetic chain

Recurrent grey rami to anterior longitudinal ligament

Branch from grey rami to disk

Ascending branch of sinuvertebralis

Branch to ligamentum flava and facet off sinuvertebralis

Sinuvertebralis to disk

Direct branch off mixed spinal nerves to facet

Local branch to facet and multifidus

Medial branch of posterior primary ramus to facet

Lateral branch to facet and multifidus

Descending facet branch

A

Nerve branches of posterior primary ramus to muscles

Branches to facet joint capsule

Posterior primary ramus

Branches to interspinous ligament

Nerve branches to posterior longitudinal ligament

Nerve branches vertebral periosteum and body

B

■ **FIG. 18-14.** **(A)** Innervation of the posterior joints. (Adapted from Paris SV: Anatomy as related to function and pain. Orthop Clin North Am 14:476–486, 1983.) **(B)** Innervation of the spinal structures.

spinal cord through the dorsal roots. In the dorsal roots the small unmyelinated fibers, thought to be largely responsible for transmission of noxious stimuli, aggregate toward the anterior aspect of the dorsal root. These enter the spinal cord and send branches to Lissauer's tract, where they may ascend or descend for a few segments before sending fibers to the substantia gelatinosa at the tip of the dorsal horn. Other fibers may pass directly to the base of the dorsal horn of the gray matter. From

here they may ascend along the spinoreticulothalamic tract or through internuncial neurons and synapse with alpha motor neurons of segmentally related muscles (Fig. 18-14A). In this way, noxious stimulation of sensitive spinal tissues may result in reflex muscle spasm (or perhaps inhibition) of segmentally related muscles. Thus, muscle spasms—which are often a part of this clinical syndrome—may result from this proposed pathway or by yet an undetermined sensory or

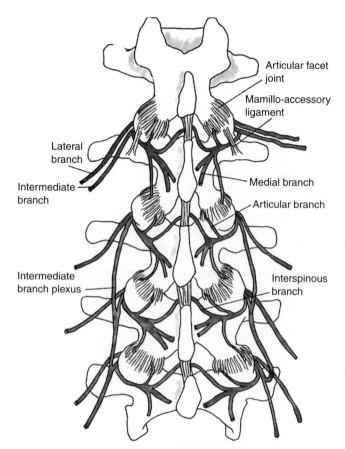

■ **FIG. 18-15.** Posterior view of the branches of the lumbar posterior rami. The mamillo-accessory ligament has been left in situ covering the L2 branch.

motor-reflex pathway.[68] Note again that because of the overlapping distribution of sensory fibers, muscles of more than one segment are likely to be affected. The previously mentioned ascending tract tends to cross within a few segments before ascending, with only a few ascending ipsilaterally. Signals traveling along this tract are thought to contribute to the conscious awareness of pain.

The larger-diameter afferent fibers reach the spinal cord through the posterior rami of the dorsal roots. These contribute to the dorsal columns of the spinal cord, which supply information to higher centers, including proprioceptive and "fast-pain" input. Other large fibers synapse at the tip of the dorsal horn of the gray matter, the substantia gelatinosa, to contribute to modulation of afferent input to higher centers. Recall, however, that ultimate perception of pain is, in part, determined by the relative balance of large-fiber and small-fiber input to the substantia gelatinosa, and that an imbalance in favor of small-fiber input tends to facilitate pain perception.

Selective stimulation of spinal structures has been carried out in a number of investigations. These studies include distention of normal and pathologic disks, needling of various aspects of intervertebral disks, injection of hypertonic saline

into interspinous ligaments, injections of articular facet joints, and mechanical stimulation of nerve roots and other structures during surgery carried out under local anesthesia. Back pain can be reproduced by injecting hypertonic saline into the supraspinatus, interspinous, and longitudinal ligaments; the ligamentum flavum; and facet capsules.[88,125,134] These structures and the peripheral third of the annulus fibrosus are innervated by nociceptive nerve fibers, which are afferent branches of the posterior primary rami.[22,235] The studies in which the intervertebral disks were distended by injection of dye during diskography suggests that, indeed, pain can result from distention of the disk. It is noted that in most cases distention of a pathologically degenerated or protruded disk resulted in much more severe pain than injection of a normal disk. In most cases pain was referred into the shoulder or hip girdles with cervical and lumbar injections, respectively, and often into the limbs. It was usually described as a deep, aching, poorly localized pain, whereas direct stimulation of a nerve root tends to result in a sharp, lancinating pain well localized to the related dermatome. On the basis of such findings, Rothman and Simeone distinguish between scleratogenous pain of spinal origin and neurogenic pain.[191,192] The former usually results from stimulation of the sinuvertebral nerve from a nuclear protrusion, putting abnormal mechanical pressure on the outer annular layers or the posterior longitudinal ligament. This results in a deep, aching, somewhat diffuse pain that may be referred to any part, or all, of the relevant sclerotomes. The latter, neurogenic pain, is that of sharp, well-localized pain felt in a dermatomal distribution, resulting from actual nerve-root pressure.

Studies also show the spinal joints to be sensitive to pain.[234] Because the fibrous capsule is a primary pain-sensitive structure of the spinal joints, as it is in the peripheral joints, conditions that stretch, pinch, or otherwise stimulate the articular facet joint capsule may potentially cause pain. Pain elicited from joint stimulation also tends to be diffuse and poorly localized and may be referred into the related segments, keeping in mind the overlapping distribution of the medial branches of the posterior primary divisions.

Control System: Contractile Tissues

CONTRACTILE TISSUES COMMON TO MOST AREAS OF THE SPINE

The spinal column is the vertical supporting structure of the body and the only rigid link between the upper and lower parts of the body. However, this structure is in itself unstable and so is supported by the major trunk muscles, which act as guidewires to prevent excessive movement in a direction of imbalance. Gregersen and Lucas[78] showed how an excised spine, with the ligaments intact but without muscles, buckles under even very small compressive forces, whereas a muscled spine can, with abdominal support, carry the weight of the trunk, head, and upper extremities in addition to hundreds of added pounds. These muscles also contract to produce motion of the trunk against the forces of gravity and may play a role in protecting the spine during trauma, if there is time for voluntary control, and possibly in the postinjury phase.[225] From a preventive and therapeutic standpoint, the muscles are very important structures of the spine. Under voluntary control they position the spine and stabilize it during awkward postures and provide the power necessary for lifting and carrying. Chaffin and Park[34] have demonstrated that workers with inadequate lifting strength who perform relatively stressful lifting tasks have higher low-back injury rates than workers with equally stressful lifting tasks but better strength. Apparently when lifting near the strength limit of these muscles, excessive strain may be transmitted to the other soft tissues, such as ligaments and disks.

The proper functioning of the mobile segment demands perfect synergy of the different muscles. A movement that is not anticipated or is poorly estimated can bring about a harmful distribution of forces on the intervertebral joints. Certain elements of the joints may be submitted to traction or compression forces beyond their capacity for resistance. The motor elements of the mobile segment comprise short and long paraspinal muscles. The former exert their action directly, whereas the latter act indirectly by affecting distal segments. These muscles are innervated by the posterior branches of the spinal nerves, which thus play a very important part in invertebral mechanical pathologic processes.

The posterior muscles are organized in three planes, with the shortest muscles being the deepest. Although they have different sources, the multifidi, semispinalis, and rotatores are often called the transversospinalis muscles (Fig. 18-16). The intermediate layer of the posterior musculature is massive and courses from transverse process to spinous processes two to four segments above (multifidi) or multisegmentally (Fig. 18-16). According to their regions, they are the multifidus (lumbosacral), semispinalis thoracis, semispinalis cervicis, and semispinalis capitis (cervical). The deep and intermediate layers are of most interest to the motion segment; in particular, the complex multifidus in the lumbosacral region. The multifidus is bipennate in both origin and insertion and is functionally significant with respect to its posterior insertion to the capsule of the articular facet joint.[172]

Overlying the multifidi are the longer and more lateral muscles that arise from the sacrum and adjacent connections to insert on the ribs and transverse process of the lower thoracic

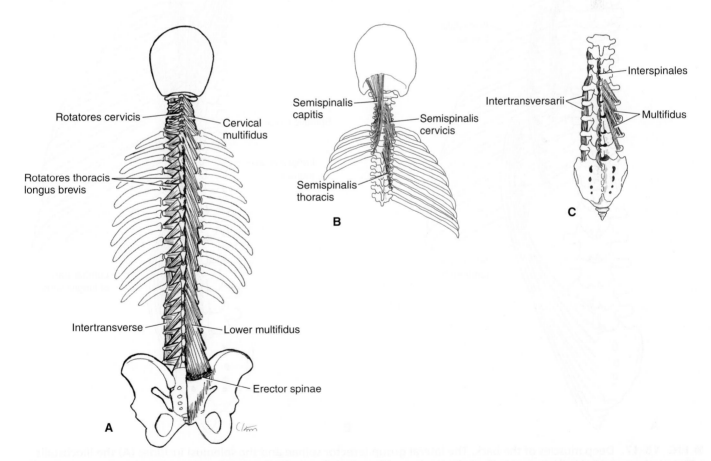

■ **FIG. 18-16.** **(A)** Deep muscles of the back. The medial group (the transversospinalis, interspinalis, and intertransversarii) includes **(B)** the semispinalis (head, neck, and thoracic sections) and **(C)** the intertransversarii, interspinales, and multifidus (lower thoracic and lumbar sections). (These muscles are only partially illustrated so that their relation to the bony structures of the spine can be seen.)

vertebrae (Fig. 18-17). These superficial and posterior muscles are collectively called the **erector spinae.**

The rotator muscles, although present at other levels, are most prominent in the thoracic region.[84] Theses muscles bring about rotation of the vertebrae in the direction opposite the side of the muscle and have a sensory role in monitoring rotation. Morris and colleagues found the longissimus thoracis and rotatores spinae to be continuously active during standing.[150] Wilke et al. determined the lumbar multifidus to be the back muscle most responsible for lumbar segmental stiffness, thus contributing to stability.[229] Many studies have demonstrated a tonic level of activation of the multifidus, which provides antigravity support of the spine with almost continuous activity.[4,19] Via electromyographic studies of the back muscles,

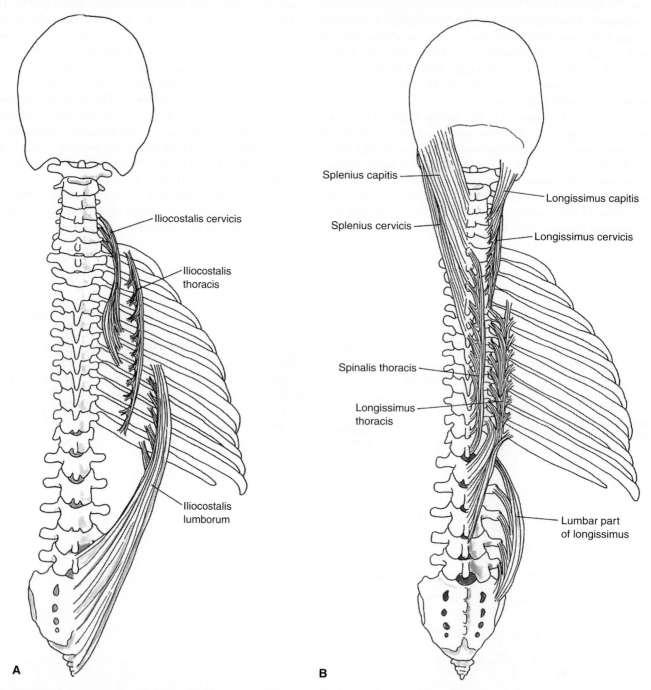

■ FIG. 18-17. Deep muscles of the back. The lateral group (erector spinae and the splenius) includes (**A**) the iliocostalis (cervical, thoracic, and lumbar sections) and (**B**) the longissimus (head and neck sections), splenius (head and neck sections), and spinalis thoracis. (These muscles are only partially illustrated in each section so that their relation to the bony structures of the spine and ribs can be seen.)

the multifidus showed silence infrequently compared other muscles.[212] This signified its stabilizing role.

The trapezius and latissimus dorsi are common to most areas of the spine (see Fig. 7-7A). Combined, the origin of the trapezius and latissimus dorsi span the entire spine from the occiput to sacrum. The trapezius spans from the occiput to T12, and the latissimus overlaps the six segments from T6 to the sacrum. The trapezius then inserts on the stable portion of the shoulder girdle complex (the scapula), whereas latissimus dorsi inserts onto the mobile humerus. Together they act to position the shoulder and retract it during lifting, spreading the load of the upper limb across the entire span rather then concentrating the force in the upper thoracic region.[72] The latissimus dorsi also produces extension of the lumbar spine, along with the serratus posterior. In addition, it acts in concert with the transverse abdominus, internal oblique, and gluteus maximus muscles as a dynamic stabilizer of the low back, by way of the attachments to the thoracolumbar fasciae or aponeuroses (see Figs. 7-8 through 7-12 and 18-18). The trapezius also serves as one of the suspensor motors of the shoulder girdle, along with the rhomboids and the levator scapulae (see Figs. 7-7A and 19-7). These muscles, taking origin from the cervical and thoracic spine, suspend and mobilize the scapula and thereby link thoracic and cervical spine motions with the upper limb motions.[121]

MUSCLES OF THE CERVICAL SPINE

The musculature of the cervical spine is complex, and anatomy texts should be consulted for descriptions of origins and

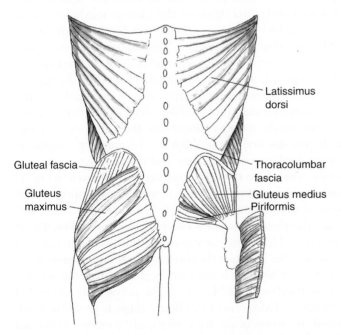

Latissimus dorsi

Gluteal fascia

Gluteus maximus

Thoracolumbar fascia

Gluteus medius
Piriformis

■ **FIG. 18-18.** Muscles of the posterior back and gluteal region.

insertions.[227] In the cervical area, special attention must be paid to balance of the length and strength of the posterior, anterior, and lateral musculature that control the movements of the head on the neck and the neck-on-thoracis spine.[105] The muscles best equipped to provide dynamic stability are the small intrinsic muscles.[36,167,168,231] The most important muscles are the multifidi (Figs. 18-8A and 19-8), suboccipitals (see Fig. 19-8), including the rectus capitis anterior, and the deep cervical flexors (see Figs. 7-22 and 19-10). The enhanced ability of small muscle to provide intersegmental stability is owing to the fact that they are positioned closer to the centers of rotation and provide less deformation to the neural arch.[168] In individuals with forward head posture, the deep anterior musculature lengthens and becomes functionally weak, but the posterior group tends to shorten.

The stabilizing effect of the intrinsic muscles is especially important in the upper cervical spine where, when only the larger muscles are used, focal areas of instability develop during normal motion.[231] The craniovertebral muscle (rectus capitis posterior major and minor, superior and inferior oblique and rectus capitus anterior) (see Fig. 19-8) enable fine movements of this region that are required for hearing, balance, and sight. They are richly supplied with mechanoreceptors, which are integrated to the muscles' strong propioceptive function and implicated in the production of dizziness in patients with dysfunction in this region.[111] The large muscles of the cervical spine are active intermittently, primarily playing a role of torque production, while the deeper muscles show more continuous activity, consisted with a tonic supporting role.[40]

The muscles that serve the function of ventilation, mastication, vocalization, and phonation are collectively known as the **suprahyoids** and **infrahyoids** (see Figs. 17-13 through 17-15, 17-18, and 19-9). These muscle groups are discussed in Chapter 17, Temporomandibular Joint and Stomatognathic System. Dysfunction of these muscle groups can have profound effects on cervical posture and should be assessed in patients with chronic neck dysfunction.

MUSCLES OF THE THORACOLUMBAR SPINE

Posterior Thoracolumbar Myology. The thoracolumbar fascia (TLF) and its powerful muscular attachments play an important role in stabilization of the thoracolumbar and pelvic region. Numerous muscular attachments into the TLF have been described including the attachments of the transversus abdominus and some fibers of the internal obliques and attachments of the gluteus maximus, latissimus dorsi, erector spinae, and biceps femoris into the posterior layer (see Chapter 7, Myofascial Considerations and Evaluation in Somatic Dysfunction, Figs. 7-8 through 7-12).

The lateral muscles of the trunk originate from the hypaxial portion of the lateral mesoderm, the quadratus lumborum, and psoas. The quadratus is the more posterior and is complex, filling the space between the iliac crest and the twelfth rib, while also attaching to the transverse processes of the lumbar vertebrae (see Figs. 7-16B and 23-8). It is a primary lateral bender of the lumbar vertebrae, assisted by the psoas muscle. It is also described as a "hip hiker" that is active in gait, during the swing phase, to hold the pelvis in a neutral position.[96] If painfully restricted, it can limit chest or rib cage expansion and can contribute to a leg-length discrepancy.

Anterior Thoracolumbar Myology. The human abdominal wall is developed from the body wall portion of the hyaxial mass of the lateral embryonic mesoderm. The two-paired rectus muscles run alongside the midline from the sternum and costal cartilage to the pubis and, although they flex the spine powerfully, they do not increase interabdominal pressure. The transverse abdominus is the deepest of the lateral abdominal muscles, and runs from the lumbar vertebrae forward around the abdominal wall to merge with the contralateral transverse abdominus (see Fig. 7-13). In the lower abdomen the lower fibers of the transverse abdominus and those of the internal oblique muscle form a conjoint tendon. The transverse abdominus has a major role in developing intra-abdominal pressure and is an important tie between the muscle–fascia column formed anteriorly by the rectus abdominus and posteriorly by the sacrospinalis muscles and the thoracolumbar fascia.[84]

The stabilizing roll of the transversus abdominis is well documented. Creswell and colleagues[43,44] found continuous activation of the transversus abdominus throughout trunk flexion and extension. In another study, they looked at the response of the trunk muscles to perturbation. The transversus abdominis is the first muscle in the trunk to be activated and it remains active through dorsal and ventral trunk loading.[43,44] During limb movement, the transversus abdominis also is the first trunk muscles to be active, irrespective of limb movement direction or the direction of forces acting on the spine.[91]

The internal oblique muscle is the intermediate layer and has its fibers from the iliac crest to the lower ribs and the lateral margin of the rectus sheath oriented to flex the trunk and turn the upper body to the contracting side (see Fig. 7-13). The external oblique muscle is the most superficial abdominal muscle layer, and its fibers also run from the lower ribs to the rectus, the pubis, and the iliac crest. However, these fibers flex and rotate the trunk away from the side that is contracting.

Associated Pelvic and Hip Myology. Four key muscle groups work in synergy to provide trunk stability: the transversus abdominus, the lumbar multifidus (Fig. 18-16), the pelvic floor (see Fig. 7-18), and the thoracoabdominal diaphragm (see Fig. 7-17).[185] Pelvic floor muscle strength is thus an integral part of spinal stability, as part of the central cylinder that requires support from all sides.[185] Hodges and Richardson,[91] Richardson et al.,[185] and Sapsford et al.[193] investigated the interaction among the muscles of the pelvic floor

and abdominal muscles. They found that activation of the transversus abdominis increased significantly when subjects performed pelvic floor contractions. Other researcher have noted that contraction of the abdominal muscles (in particular, the transversus abdominus) is associated with contraction of the pelvic floor muscles and aids in retraining the pelvic floor muscles to manage urinary stress incontinence.[193]

At the other end of the trunk cylinder, the thoracoabdominal diaphragm (see Chapter 7, Myofascial Considerations and Evaluation in Somatic Dysfunction, Fig. 7-17) plays a role in trunk stability.[89] Richardson et al.[185] found that when subjects performed shoulder flexion, both portions of the diaphragm contract at the same time as the transversus abdominus during inspiratory and expiratory phases of respiration. This suggests a connection with spinal control.

The psoas is considered, by some, primarily a limb muscle, but as Michele[139] has stated, it is also a potential extensor of the spine and a flexor of the lumbar spine on the pelvis depending on the relative positions of the spine, pelvis, and femur. The **psoas major** arises from the anterolateral aspect of the lumbar vertebral bodies and transverse processes, and then crosses the hip before inserting with the iliacus on the lesser trochanter (see Fig. 7-16). The **psoas minor** (not always present) lies ventral to the psoas major and courses from the vertebrae of the thoracolumbar junction to insert on the superior pubis ramus, which allows it to work with the abdominal muscles in upward tilting of the pelvis.

The extensive fascial attachment of the gluteus maximus muscle (see Figs. 7-2 and 18-18), both at its origin and insertion, is well known. The crescent-shaped origin has widespread bony aponeurotic and ligamentous attachments. Approximately two thirds of the gluteus maximus muscle ends in a thick tendinous lamina, which inserts into the iliotibial band of the fascia lata. This offers strong control of the lower extremity during stressful activity. A comparison of the magnitude of action potentials elicited in the gluteus maximus muscle during a variety of exercises and activities demonstrates that the greatest electrical activity occurs during muscle-setting contractions; these include exercises of hyperextension of the thigh accompanied by resistance, external rotation or abduction, and vigorous hyperextension of the trunk from the erect position.[63] The muscle seems to lack a major postural function in symmetrical upright positions at rest. Rotation of the trunk in a standing position activates the gluteus maximus contralateral to the direction of rotation, which is the corresponding function as an outward rotator of the leg when the trunk is flexed. Anteflexion of the trunk in the hip joint is attended by gluteus maximus activity, whose function probably is to fix the pelvis in its anteverted attitude.[106] Extension of the flexed thigh is performed primarily by action of the hamstrings, while extension beyond the relaxed standing position is associated with strong contraction of the gluteus maximus. Electromyographic studies recorded during lifting activities indicate that hamstrings are activated earlier and to a greater extent during straight-knee lifts than during flexed-knee lifts. In contrast, the gluteus maximus and adductor magnus are more activated initially in the flexed-knee lift than the straight-leg lift.[63,155,173]

There is a fair concurrence of opinion about muscular activity in human posture based on electromyographic studies by many investigators.[59,93,154,225] Briefly, the activity of the lumbar spine muscles is low in relaxed standing and alternates with low levels of activity during body sway. There seems to be somewhat more constant activity in the paralumbar portion of the psoas major, both in standing and sitting, which provides additional preload to the spine and helps to maintain normal lumbar lordosis. Roentgenographic studies have shown that the line of gravity in most adults is 1 cm ventral to the center of L4, and that gravity would tend to straighten the lumbar spine without psoas activity. There is a small increase in activity of the lumbar spine muscles in sitting compared with standing. In the unsupported sitting posture, the muscle activity in the lumbar region was found to be about the same as that in the standing posture. In the thoracic region, Andersson and colleagues[7,9] found higher activity of the back muscles compared with that found in the standing posture. These low levels of muscle activity imply that posture is maintained partly by active muscle contraction and partly by ligamentous and noncontractile support.

The lack of significant activity in the pelvic portion of the psoas major means that truncal equilibrium over the pelvis is fairly stable and is maintained by the strong ligaments anterior to this joint, as is also the case at the knee and sacroiliac joints. The line of force clearly falls behind the hip and in front of the knee, and there is no activity in the glutei at rest.

During flexion from standing to sitting the glutei and erectors are active until full flexion is reached, at which time they are again quiet. They are active while initiating extension and again at full extension. As the erector spinae muscles grade the rate of flexion, the abdominal muscles grade the rate of extension. During rotation, the longer erector muscles on the ipsilateral side, the short rotators and multifidi on the contralateral side, and the glutei on both sides are active, as is the tensor fascia lata on the ipsilateral side. Although the internal oblique muscles could assist with this motion, there is little abdominal activity in active rotation without resistance. Return to neutral is accomplished without significant muscular activity, evidently recovering some of the deforming force stored in the soft tissue. Sidebending is accomplished with ipsilateral activity of the back muscles, unless the person is very tall and limber or is supporting external weight, in which case the contralateral muscles become active as soon as the equilibrium position is overcome by ipsilateral contraction.

A number of studies have scrutinized muscular function in control of the spine.[5,7–15,29,64,71,97–103,150,151,164–166,170,173,181,202,218,232,233] Several studies have also reported results in patients with back disorders.[20,39,42,64,71,73,94,118,136,177,182,199,202,203,233]

Most would concede the importance of muscular function during both posture and functional activities. Whether or not injury to these muscles is a common cause of spinal pain is still controversial. Factors that protect the thoracolumbar spine in lifting include the following:

- Stabilization of the vertebral column through the action of the thoracolumbar fascia (see Chapter 7, Myofascial Considerations and Evaluation in Somatic Dysfunction).
- The lever action of the thoracolumbar fascia, erector spinae muscles, and supraspinous ligaments. These structures pass some distance posteriorly to the spinous processes (and far posterior to the anterior column of the spine). However, they are firmly attached to them; thus, passive stretch of these structures can reduce the tendency toward flexion and forward shear of the lumbar vertebrae that would otherwise occur during lifting because of the orientation of the spinal elements. A shear resistance is created by the curve of the back, which imparts a posteriorly directed vector to the pull of the erector spinae muscles and the posterior ligaments of the lumbar vertebrae. Although this mechanical feature is lost in the upper lumbar spine with flexion, it is preserved in the lower lumbar spine.[1,59]
- According to Adams and Hutton,[1] the flexion position may strengthen the spine and obviate the need for a great amount of relief from increased abdominal pressure. It is thought that the posture adopted by experienced weightlifters (i.e., flexed lower lumbar spine, extended thoracic spine, and weight as close to the body as possible to reduce the bending moment) is the most efficient one biomechanically. The authors do not feel their studies negate the importance of abdominal pressure in increasing the margin of safety; rather, they state that the role of abdominal pressure is better defined as increasing the margin of safety, not making the lift possible in the first place, as others have implied.[1]
- The lumbosacral rhythm, in which the spine does not perform its segmental motions in the most disadvantageous position of full trunk flexion, but waits until after the hip extensors have brought the trunk to approximately 45° and reduced the lever arm
- Action of the external and internal oblique muscles when asymmetrical loads are encountered. Although the line of action of these muscles is anterior to the axis of rotation for flexion, these muscles are critical in preventing buckling and overrotation with asymmetrical loading.

SACROILIAC JOINT AND BONY PELVIS

The base of support for spinal movement is the pelvis, to which many of the back muscles attach and through which the muscles of the thigh exert their influence on posture. The pelvis supports the abdomen and links the vertebral column to the lower limbs. It is a closed osteoarticular ring composed of three bony parts and three joints. The three bony parts are the two iliac bones and the sacrum, a solid piece of bone resulting from

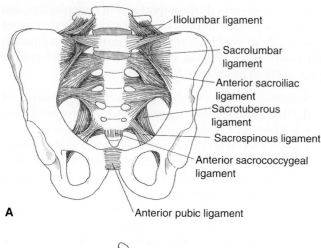

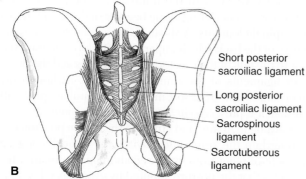

■ **FIGURE 18-19.** Pelvic joints and ligaments. **(A)** Anterior aspect. **(B)** Posterior aspect.

fusion of the five sacral vertebrae. The three joints consist of the two sacroiliac joints and the pubic symphysis, which links the iliac bones anteriorly (Fig. 18-19).[105]

Sacroiliac Joints

The major forces through the sacroiliac joints (SIJs) are borne by ligaments that tend to bind the sacrum into the ilia and lock together the unusually shaped articular surfaces (narrow, curving in an earlike shape in their plane, and deeply modified by depressions and elevations). The pelvis is usually described as a ring or arch with the innominate bones as lateral pillars and the sacrum as the keystone. This analogy only holds if it is appreciated that the sacroiliac ligaments hold the arch together; in usual engineering practice it is the superimposed and lateral masses that hold an arch together and there is usually no tension member. The pelvis is an extremely stable system of joints maintained by some of the strongest ligaments in the body.

Movement of the SIJs has been described by many authors, with considerable effort being expended to try to measure precisely these movements by roentgenographic and physical means (e.g., pins placed in bones).[35,38,56] It is quite clear from this latter type of study that some motion does occur, but it is of small amplitude, while at least one roentgenographic study indicated the potential for "significant" deflection of bones of

the pelvis during various static manipulations.[66,228] Even if the motions of the joint are of small amplitude, the joint is located and constructed to serve as a shock absorber and thus there is little reason that it should fuse. In fact, careful anatomical studies indicate that although the joint undergoes severe degenerative changes, fusion is relatively unusual, except in ankylosing spondylitis.[27] With respect to degenerative changes it is interesting that the iliac articular surface is fibrocartilaginous throughout life, whereas the sacral surface is hyaline cartilage. In general, the sacral cartilage is also about three times thicker in early adult life than the iliac cartilage. Resnick and associates[183] found that early degenerative changes occurred on the iliac surface rather than on both surfaces of the joint simultaneously.

Mitchell, in describing normal motion in the SIJs and in gait, suggests that the ilium rotates in a posterior direction at heel-strike and gradually moves from a posterior to an anterior direction as the person proceeds through the stance phase (see Fig. 23-4).[141] Elaborate descriptions of the possible axes and degree of motion have been postulated. These include a transverse axis through the pubic symphysis with rotation of the pubis to allow ilial motion in walking; a superior transverse axis, in the appropriate line of the second sacral segment, where some gross flexion occurs; a middle transverse axis, where additional gross flexion occurs; an inferior transverse axis, held to be the site of reciprocal motions of the joint during ambulation; and a set of oblique axes from the upper portion of one side of the sacrum to the lower portion of the contralateral joint.[141,222] Work by Weisl and others are not in total agreement about the amount and planes of motion.[38,143,219,228]

Kapandji describes the movements of nutation and counternutation (flexion and extension) of the sacrum within the ilia as being about a transverse axis posterior to the joint at the sacral tuberosity where the sacroiliac ligaments insert.[105] During nutation (flexion), movement of the sacral promontory is anterior and inferior, while the apex of the sacrum moves posteriorly (see Fig. 23-3A). The iliac bones approximate and the ischial tuberosities move apart (see Fig. 23-6). Conversely, during counternutation (extension), the sacral promontory moves superiorly and posteriorly and the apex of the sacrum moves anteriorly (see Fig. 23-3B). The iliac bones move apart while the ischial tuberosities approximate each other (see Fig. 23-7). These movements occur normally during the gait cycle and during activities such as forward and backward bending.

Understanding the position of the sacrum and ilia during gait and various body positions will help give the clinician an appreciation of the sacroiliac joint pain that may occur with locomotion. Despite differences of opinion regarding the movement center, most researchers agree that nutation and counternutation of the sacrum correspond to movements of the spine.[66,220] Therefore, in forward bending there is initially a backward bending (counternutation) of the sacrum, and as the spine completely flexes there is a resultant forward bending (nutation) of the sacrum. Whereas the position of the sacrum is determined by a force that reaches it from above, the ilium is controlled by movement of the femur. In standing, the base of the sacrum moves anteriorly. At heel-strike, the ipsilateral ilium is in a posteriorly rotated position. During the initial stance phase, sacral torsion occurs to that side. At midstance, increased tension of the iliopsoas encourages the ilium to move toward anterior rotation.[141]

Movement of the stable pelvic structure is made possible by the pelvic joints, consisting of the paired L5–S1 articular facet joints, the two SIJs, and the pubic symphysis. The two synovial SIJs are L-shaped when viewed from the side (see Fig. 23-2). The shorter and disposed cephalic limb of the sacral articulation is borne by the first sacral segment, while the longer and horizontally directed caudal limb is borne by the second and third sacral segments. Weisl has extensively studied these joints and has shown that a central depression can often be found at the junction of the two segments.[219,220] It has been noted that the cephalic limb of the sacral articular surface is more angled or wedged and is essentially vertical until it flares again inferiorly, as if to prevent it from sliding upward against the ilia.[203] The horizontal section of the sacrum has been described by Solonen[203] as wedged dorsally in the upper portion of the joint and ventrally in the lower portion, whereas the ilial surface is convex superiorly and concave inferiorly. The articular capsule is attached close to the margin of the articular surfaces of the sacrum and ilium.

The ligaments of the sacrum are a network of fibrous bands that fuse and intermingle to give added strength to the wedge of the pelvis. There are three main intrinsic and three main extrinsic ligaments. The three main **intrinsic ligaments** are the anterior sacroiliac, short posterior sacroiliac, and long posterior sacroiliac ligaments (Fig. 18-19A, B).

The **anterior sacroiliac ligaments** represent a thickening of the anterior and inferior parts of the fibrous capsule. They are particularly well developed at the level of the articular line but are thin elsewhere.[227] They stretch and tear easily on slight pubic separation and allow the SIJs to gap during pregnancy.[194]

The **short posterior sacroiliac ligaments** pass from the first and second transverse tubercle on the dorsum of the sacrum to the posterior ilium. They prevent anterior (flexion) motion of the sacrum (Fig. 18-19B).

The **long posterior sacroiliac ligaments** attach from the third transverse tubercle of the dorsum of the sacrum and the posterosuperior iliac spine, where they merge with the superior part of the sacrotuberous ligament and counteract the motion of downward slipping of the sacrum into the pelvis (Fig. 18-19B).

The three main **extrinsic ligaments** are the sacrospinous, sacrotuberous, and iliolumbar ligaments (Fig. 18-19A, B). The **sacrospinous ligaments,** which attach to the ischial spine and cross over to the anterior sacrum, and the sacrotuberous ligaments, which attach at the ischial tuberosity and traverse to the inferior sacrum, strongly stabilize the pelvis and anterior motion of the sacrum.

The **iliolumbar ligament** attaches from the iliac crest to the transverse processes of L4 and L5. It resists posterior

rotation of the ilium and forward gliding of L5 on the sacrum (Fig. 18-19A). According to Kapandji,[105] the function of the superior band of the iliolumbar ligament is to check forward flexion of the vertebrae while the inferior or second band checks extension of the vertebral bodies. Both bands of the iliolumbar ligament are also thought to be involved in lateral flexion (sidebending) and rotation of the lumbar spine.[179,180] According to Mitchell,[141] sacral movement is a result of forces carried to it through the pull of ligaments or gravitational forces, or both.

The reader is referred to Chapter 23, Sacroiliac Joint and Lumbar–Pelvic–Hip Complex, regarding myokinematics of the SIJ as well as articular and myofascial stability of the pelvis.

Pubic Symphysis

The pubic symphysis is an amphiarthrodial joint in the anterior aspect of the pelvis that forms a fibrocartilaginous union between the two pubic bones. A thin layer of hyaline cartilage covers the osseous surfaces and the joint is formed by a fibrocartilaginous disk that joins the bones. The four ligaments associated with the joint are the **anterior pubic ligament** (Fig. 18-19A), **superior pubic ligament,** the **inferior arcuate ligament** (see Fig. 23-1), and the posterior ligament.[122] The thick inferior pubic ligament or arcuate ligament forms an arch that spans both inferior rami and stabilizes the joint from rotatory, tensile, and shear forces.[75] Kapandji[105] describes the muscle expansions as forming an anterior ligament consisting of the internal obliquus abdominus, rectus abdominus, transversus abdominus, and the adductor longus.

The pubic symphysis permits tissue deformation and small translatory movements as a result of muscle, ground reaction, and trunk forces.[180] Many forces act on this joint, especially those exerted by the muscles of the lower limb when the foot is fixed to the ground. The pubic symphysis can be affected by excess motion in the SIJs and can be a source of symptoms.

Articular and Myofascial Stability of the Pelvis and SIJs

The strong ligamentous support system (see above) that allows for proper SIJ function is nevertheless felt to be inadequate to prevent dislocation of the joints under postural load unless supplemented by other forces. This has lead to the concept of a "self-bracing" or "self-locking" mechanism based on the fact that in combination with load transfer through the fascia, muscle forces that cross the SIJs can produce joint compression. Snijders et al.[205] and Vleeming et al.[216,217] coined the terms "form closure" and "force closure" to describe the passive and active forces that help to stabilize the pelvis and SIJs.

SIJ FORM CLOSURE

Form closure refers to a state of stability within the pelvic mechanism, with the degree of stability dependent on its anatomy, with no need for extra forces to maintain the stable state of the system.[206] The following anatomic structures assist with form closure:

- The triangular shape of the sacrum makes it fit between the ilia like a keystone in a Roman arch. The incongruent surfaces provide resistance against horizontal and vertical translation. Both the coarseness of the cartilage and the complimentary grooves and ridges noted with advancing age increase the friction coefficient and thus contribute to form closure.[203]
- The shape of the closely fitting articular surfaces. The interlocking of the variably oriented sacral and iliac articular surfaces helps to counter vertical and anterior-posterior translation.
- The integrity of the ligaments. The ligaments that influence the SIJ include the anterior and posterior SI ligaments and the pelvic floor ligaments.

The integrity of form closure is clinically evaluated by shear tests (see Chapter 23, Sacroiliac Joint and Lumbar–Pelvic–Hip complex).

SIJ FORCE CLOSURE

SIJ force closure is derived from two sources, the first of which is any active force that results in nutation of the sacrum (see Figs. 23-3A and 23-6). Nutation comes about by anterior rotation of the sacral base (e.g., multifidi, contraction of the extensor spinae or sacrospinalis) or posterior rotation of the ilia (e.g., contraction of the rectus abdominus or hamstrings).[195] Nutation results in a tightening of the sacrospinous and sacrotuberous ligaments (Fig. 18-19). This tightening appears to facilitate the force closure mechanism, thereby increasing the compression of the SIJ articular surfaces, which in turn increases the stability of the joint for load transfer.[215] Conversely, counternutation (see Fig. 23-3B) decreases tension in these ligaments and results in decreased stability. Second, kinetic analysis of the pelvic girdle highlights two muscle groups that resist translational forces and help to provide stability, the inner unit and the outer unit.

Inner Unit.   The inner unit consists of the following:

- Thoracic diaphragm
- Transverse abdominus
- Pelvic floor muscles
- Multifidus

The simultaneous contraction of some of the muscles that constitute this inner core may be able to set up a force couple capable of affecting the stability of the SIJ and lumbosacral junction. Hodges and Richardson[90,91] have shown that the transversus abdominis is an anticipatory muscle for stabilization of the low back and pelvis. Although it does not cross the SIJ, it has an impact on compression of the pelvis[186] through (in part) its direct pull on the middle and deep lamina of the posterior layer of the thoracolumbar fascia.[213]

The multifidus also plays a crucial role in stabilization of the pelvic girdle. It is contained between the lamina of the vertebrae, dorsal aspect of the sacrum, and the deep layer of the thoracolumbar fascia. When it contracts, it increases the tension of the thoracolumbar fascia and therefore compresses the posterior pelvis.[186]

Muscles of the pelvic floor also play a critical role in stabilization of the pelvic girdle. For example, simultaneous contraction of multifidi and the ilio and ischiococcygeus muscles of the plevic floor (which insert into the coccyx) (see Fig. 7-18C) may be able to set up a force couple capable of affecting the stability of the SIJ and lumbosacral junction.[195] Contraction of the multifidi causes sacral nutation; contraction of the ilio/ischiococcygeus causes counternutation. The balance of forces could move the sacrum into a stable or unstable position respectively.

According to Richardson and associates,[185] the thoracic diaphragm and muscle of the pelvic floor are activated in synergy with the transverse abdominus and lumbar multifidi during the action of drawing in the abdominal wall. Co-activation of the transversus abdominus and muscles of the pelvic and thoracic diaphragm is likely to act to maintain intrabdominal pressure at a critical level, thus allowing co-contraction to affect spinal support.

Outer Layer.   The outer unit consists of four systems (slings).[206,213,214]

- Posterior oblique system or sling contains connections between the latissimus dorsi, by way of the thoracolumbar fascia, to the contralateral gluteal maximus, which contributes to force closure of the sacroiliac joint posteriorly by approximating the posterior aspect of the innominates. This system also contributes to load transfer through the pelvic region with rotational activities[147] and during gait.[74,77]
- Anterior oblique system. The anterior oblique sling contains connections between the external oblique, the anterior abdominal fascia and the contralateral internal oblique and the adductors of the thigh. The oblique abdominals, acting as phasic muscles, initiate movement[184] and are involved in all movements of the trunk and upper and lower limb, except when the legs are crossed.[204] The lower horizontal fibers may augment transversus abdominis in its role of supporting the SIJ.[185]
- Deep longitudinal system. The longitudinal sling connects the peroneii, the biceps femoris, sacrotuberous ligament, deep lamina of the thoracolumbar fascia, and the erector spinae.[124] This system counteracts any anterior shear (sacral nutation) and facilitates the compression through the SIJs. The biceps femoris muscle will, on contraction, compress the SIJ and control the degree of nutation via its connection to the sacrotuberous ligaments.[230] This system also increases tension in the thoracolumbar fascia and thereby enhances the ability of the fascia to contribute to any SIJ force closure mechanisms acting across it.
- Lateral system. The lateral sling contains the primary stabilizers for the hip mainly the gluteus medius, gluteus minimus, tensor fascia lata, and the contralateral adductors of the hip. These muscles are more involved with

proper function of the pelvic girdle in standing and walking rather than with SIJ force closure. These muscles are reflexively inhibited with instability of the hip and may account for the feeling of hip "giving away," or "slipping clutch syndrome."[50–52,213]

This myofascial system is essentially an integrated system, which represents forces and is composed of several muscles that may participate in more than one of the systems or slings. These slings may overlap and interconnect depending on the activity. It is important that the length and strength of each of these structures are assessed, because weakness, insufficient length, or recruitment of these systems can reduce the force closure mechanism and lead to compensatory movement strategies.[204]

Not unlike the shoulder girdle, the pelvic girdle serves as the fixed base of support of operation of the lumbar and thoracic spine. Static and dynamic disorders that alter this fixed base of support, such as differences in leg length (real or apparent) or malpositions of the pelvic bones, may often elicit symptoms over time and result in degenerative changes of the lumbar spine, hip, and SIJs. The SIJ is a common site for referred pain and tenderness derived from segmental diskogenic backache.

SPINAL KINEMATICS

Motion in the spine is produced by the coordinated action of nerves and muscles. **Agonistic** muscles initiate and carry out motion, whereas **antagonistic** muscles often control and modify it. Although the disk–vertebral height ratio largely determines the degree of movement at spinal segments, the types of movement that may occur depend on the orientation of the articular facets of the intervertebral joints at each level. The motion between two vertebrae is small and does not occur independently. Obviously, the degree and combination of the individual types of motion vary considerably in the different vertebral regions.

Skeletal structures that influence motion of the spine are the rib cage, which limits thoracic motion, and the pelvis, whose tilting increases trunk motion.

Fryette's Laws of Physiologic Spinal Motions[67,142]

Theories related to spinal joint movement have developed gradually, beginning with Hippocrates or earlier and are still developing. Particularly useful guidelines in the evaluation and treatment concepts are the theories developed by Fryette.[67] In the early 1990s, he described coupling of the various spinal motions with one another. Fryette introduced the term **neutral** (articular facets not engaged) and **nonneutral** (articular facet joints not engaged). Although referred to as "laws," these statements are better viewed as concepts because they have undergone review and modification over time.

FRYETTE'S FIRST LAW

When any part of the thoracic or lumbar vertebral segments is in the neutral (or easy normal) position without locking of the

articular facets, rotation and sidebending are in the opposite directions (type 1 motion). The cervical spine is not included in this law, as the articular facet joints of this region are always engaged. Neutral sidebending produces rotation to the other side; in other words, the vertebral body will turn toward the convexity that is being formed, with maximum rotation occurring near the apex of the curve. Dysfunctions that occurs in the neutral range are termed type I dysfunction.

FRYETTE'S SECOND LAW

If the vertebral segments are in full flexion or extension with the articular facets locked or engaged (nonneutral), rotation and sidebending are to the same side, individual vertebral joints acting one at a time (type II motion).

Dysfunctions occurring in the flexion or extension range are described as **type II dysfunction.** Type I dysfunction in both flexion and extension occur in the thoracic spine and cervical spine in the C2 to T3 areas of the spine.[26] Despite the absence of experimental evidence, it is found clinically that type II dysfunctions of the lumbar spine do occur in extension, although not commonly except at the lumbosacral joint.[26]

FRYETTE'S THIRD LAW

This law tells us that if motion in one plane is introduced to the spine, motion in the other two planes is thereby restricted.

It is quite difficult to demonstrate the validity of the first two "laws" but they continue to be cited throughout many books when discussing spinal coupling and serve as a model for analysis of vertebral dysfunction. Lee[123] has proposed that at the T3 to T10 levels, the coupling depends on which of the two coupled motions initiates the movement (rotation or side-flexion). Lee and others propose that if side-flexion initiates the motion (latexion), then the side-flexion produce a contralateral rotation. However, if rotation initiates the motion (rotexion), then ipsilateral side-flexion is produced. See the Appendix for additional information regarding motion patterns of the thoracic spine.

Ranges of Segmental Motion

In three-dimensional space, the spine has six planes of freedom. A vertebra may rotate about or translate along a transverse, a sagittal, or a longitudinal axis or move in various combinations of these motions.[75,111]

Although the range of motion in an individual segment of the spine has been found to vary in different studies using autopsy material or roentgenographic in vivo measurements, there is agreement on the relative amount of motion at different levels of the spine. The phenomenon of **coupling,** in which two or more individual motions occur at the same time, has been well documented experimentally.[17,60,78,126,190,197,208,211] Frequently three motions will simultaneously take place during normal physiologic spinal movement or function. The coupling effect occurs in the thoracic spine[169,223,224] but is more common in the cervical[129] and lumbar spine.[114,171]

Pure movement in any of the three principle planes very seldom occurs, because orientation of facet joint surfaces does not exactly coincide with the plane of motion and therefore modifies it to a greater or lesser extent.[80] For example, when the lumbar motion segment is rotated axially, it simultaneously bends in the sagittal plane and rotates axially.[225] Spinal movement is complex, and the intricacies of changing relationships observed on cineradiographical and other studies are sometimes difficult to explain.[80]

The occipito-atlanto-axial joints are the most complex joints of the axial skeleton, both anatomically and kinematically. Although there have been some thorough investigations of this region, there is considerable controversy about some of the basic biomechanical characteristics. In Chapter 19, Cervical Spine, the best available information is analyzed with some discussion of representative values of range of segmental motion.

Representative values of other parts of the spine are presented here to allow a comparison of motion at various levels of the lower cervical (C2–C7), thoracic, and lumbar spine.[225] A representative value for flexion–extension is 8° at C2–C3, 13° at C3–C4, and 17° at C5–C6. A representative value for flexion–extension is 4° at T1–T4, 6° at T5–T10, and 12° at T11–T12. The range of flexion–extension progressively increases in the lumbar motion segments, reaching a maximum of 20° at the lumbosacral level (Fig. 18-20).

Lateral flexion shows the greatest range in the C3–C4 and C4–C5 segments, which reach 11°. The greatest range in the thoracic spine is in the lower segments, where 8° to 9° is possible. In the lumbar spine, 6° of lateral flexion is common, except for the lumbosacral segments, where only 3° of lateral flexion occurs (Fig. 18-20).[225]

Axial rotation is greatest in the midcervical spine, where 10° to 12° of motion is found. In the thoracic spine, axial rotation is greatest in the upper segments, where 9° is possible. The range of motion progressively decreases caudally, reaching 2° in the lower segments of the lumbar spine, but it again increases in the lumbosacral segment to 5° (Fig. 18-20).[225]

Segmental motion cannot be measured clinically and motion of the spine is a combined action of several segments. The degree of movement in the spinal segment has clinical meaning in relation to its immediate neighbor and in general terms of the patient's body type.

Regional movement characteristics should also be appreciated. In general it can be said that in all sagittal starting positions of the cervical spine and in the flexed thoracic (below T3) and lumbar spines, sidebending is unavoidably accompanied by rotation to the same side; in the neutral or extended thoracic (below T3) and lumbar spines, sidebending is accompanied by rotation to the opposite side.[80]

In the upper thoracic spine there appears to be less consistency. According to White, the direction of coupled axial rotation is probably dominated by the middle sections of the thoracic spine, but sometimes the reverse is true.[225]

Functional Motions of the Thoracolumbar Spine

Normal values of functional range of motion of the spine do not exist because there are great variations among individuals. In fact, the range of motion in each of the three planes shows a Gaussian distribution, according to Frankel.[65] The range of motion also differs between the sexes and is strongly age dependent, decreasing by approximately 50% in old age.[144]

FLEXION–EXTENSION

Flexion is the most pronounced movement of the vertebral column as a whole. It requires an anterior compression of the intervertebral disks and a gliding separation of the articular facets, in which the inferior set of an individual vertebra tends to move upward and forward over the opposing superior set of the adjacent inferior vertebra. Mainly the posterior ligaments and epaxial muscles check the movement. With respect to the thoracolumbar spine, the first 50 to 60° of spinal flexion occurs in the lumbar spine, mainly in the lower motion segments.[60] Forward tilting of the pelvis allows further flexion. There is an interconnection of movement between the spine and pelvis, particularly in total forward bending. Normally there is a synchronous movement in a rhythmical ratio of the lumbar spine to that of pelvic rotation about the hips. As forward bending progresses, the lumbar curve reverses itself from concave to flat to convex. The sacrum is also moving within the ilia during forward bending. Initially, the sacrum flexes. As the pelvis rotates anteriorly over the hips, the sacrum begins to counterextend within the ilia. The thoracic spine contributes little to flexion of the total spine because of the orientation of the facets, the almost-vertical orientation of the spinous processes, and the restriction of the rib cage. The abdominal muscles and

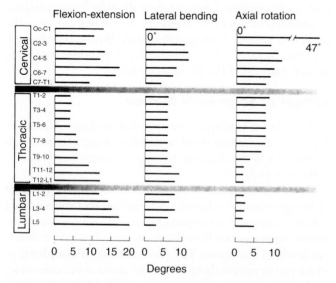

■ **FIG. 18-20.** Average ranges of segmental movement of spinal joints. (Reprinted with permission from White AA III, Panjabi MM: The basic kinematics of the human spine: A review of past and current knowledge. Spine 3:16, 1978.)

the vertebral portion of the psoas initiate flexion. The weight of the upper body then produces further flexion, which is controlled by the gradually increasing activity of the erector muscles as the movement force increases.

Extension tends to be a more limited motion, producing posterior compression of the disk with the inferior articular process gliding posteriorly and downward over the superior set below. It is checked by the anterior longitudinal ligament and all the ventral muscles that directly or indirectly flex the spine. The laminae and spinous processes may also limit extension.[181,182] A reverse sequence of flexion is observed as the trunk returns from full flexion to the upright position. The lumbar spine becomes concave and the pelvis derotates and shifts forward as the spine extends. In some studies the concentric work performed by the muscles involved in raising the trunk has been shown to be greater than the eccentric work performed by the muscles during flexion.[66,104] When the trunk is extended from the upright position, the back muscles are active during the initial phase of motion. Activity decreases during further extension, and the abdominal muscles become active to control and modify motion.[65]

This arc of movement in forward and backward bending should normally be smooth and rhythmical, with a balance between lumbar reversal and pelvic rotation.[31]

LATERAL FLEXION

Lateral flexion is accompanied by some degree of rotation. It involves a rocking of the vertebral bodies on their disks, with a sliding separation of the articular facets on the convex side and overriding of the articular facets related to the concavity.[191,192] Lateral flexion is limited by the intertransverse ligaments and the extension of the ribs. During lateral flexion, rotation may predominate in the thoracic or lumbar spine. In the lumbar spine the wedge-shaped spaces of the intervertebral joints show variation during motion. The spinotransversal and transversospinal systems of the erector spinae are active in lateral flexion of the spine. The motion is initiated by ipsilateral contraction of these muscles and modified by the contralateral side.[65]

Rotation

Rotation is consistently combined with lateral flexion. The entire vertebral column rotates approximately 90° to either side of the sagittal plane, but most of this transversion is accomplished in the cervical and thoracic spines. With respect to the thoracic spine, the combined motion is most marked in the upper segments. The vertebral body rotates toward the concavity of the lateral curve of the spine.[223] A combined pattern of rotation and lateral flexion also exists in the lumbar spine.[140] In this region the vertebral body rotates toward the convexity of the curve. Lumbar rotation is extremely limited at the lumbosacral level because of the orientation of the facets. Pelvic motion is essential to increase the range of trunk rotation. During rotation, back and abdominal muscles are active on both sides of the spine as both ipsilateral and contralateral muscles cooperate.[65]

Measurements obtained during walking indicate that the pelvis and lumbar spine rotate as a functional unit.[78] In the lower thoracic spine, rotation diminishes gradually up to T7. This vertebra represents the area of transition from vertebral rotation in the direction of the pelvis to rotation in the opposite direction—that of the shoulder girdle.

COMMON PATTERNS OF SPINAL PAIN

Anatomic and Pathologic Considerations

FACET (APOPHYSEAL) JOINTS

The facets have been clearly shown to be a source of referred pain. Like the synovial joints elsewhere in the body, the apophyseal joints can be a source of pain caused by trauma and various forms of arthritis, including degenerative arthritis. Inflammation of these joints produces dull to severe pain, depending on the extent of the inflammation. Inflammation can also lead to associated muscle spasm, which in itself is capable of causing pain.[33]

The cervical facet joint syndrome can cause both local and referred pain and is often indistinguishable from cervical disk disease.[16] Upper cervical facet joint irritation may be responsible for symptoms of upper neck pain, with referral to the occipital region and ipsilateral frontal area. Associated symptoms are occipital and vascular headaches.[201] Lower cervical facet joint irritation is characterized by referred pain to the shoulder and scapular girdle.[24] Often, cervical facet and disk disorders occur together. Facet joint irritation most commonly arises from facet joint thickening and hypertrophy initiated by trauma, spondylosis, excessive load-bearing stress, or disk degeneration.[23]

Two or three adjacent nerves originating from the dorsal nerves, which originate from the dorsal primary rami, innervate each lumbar apophyseal joint.[22,23,109,145,146] The joint capsules are also innervated by free nerve endings. Immunohistochemical studies of degenerated facets in low-back-pain patients have revealed erosion channels extending through the subchondral bone and calcified cartilage into the articular cartilage containing substance P nerve fibers.[21] This confirms that a component of low back pain resides in the facets.[33] Pain from these joints can be referred to any part of the lower limb as far distal as the calf and ankle, but most commonly to the gluteal region, groin, and proximal thigh.[110]

INTERVERTEBRAL DISK

Until recently, the intervertebral disk was generally believed to be a non–pain-sensitive structure. It has been found that the superficial layer (outer third) of the annulus fibrosis has significant innervation from the sinuvertebral nerves and stimulation of these nerves may result in pain.[25] Their function has not been clarified, but they appear to have a proprioceptive and nociceptive function. Thus, internal disk disruption may cause intrinsic disk pain.

However, the disk more commonly causes pain by its effect on pain-sensitive structures such as the anterior dura mater and posterior longitudinal ligament or by a posterior lateral prolapse against a nerve root. When a prolapsed disk exerts pressure on the posterior longitudinal ligament and the dura, the consequence is spondylogenic referred pain, which is usually experienced locally but can be referred over a wider area. The pain is usually dull, deep, and poorly localized. In the lumbar spinal region, the pain is typically experienced in the low back, buttocks, and sacroiliac. Less commonly it may be referred to both legs and to the calf but is not referred to the ankle or foot.

The concept of dural pain was introduced by Cyriax[46] and further expanded on in his many-edition *Textbook of Orthopaedic Medicine*[48] (see Fig. 20-2). On the basis of its innervation by the sinuvertebral nerve, dura mater has also been suggested as a source of primary pain by Edgar and Nundy,[55] Murphy,[152] Bogduk,[22] and Cuatico and coworkers.[45] Some elements of this concept may be usefully criticized, but there are many aspects of the interpretation of dural pain that are relevant and useful in assessment and treatment.[32]

According to Cyriax[48] and Cailliet,[31] if the disk exerts pressure on the dural sleeve of the nerve root only, the radicular pain is experienced along the course of the nerve root. Pain can be experienced in any part of the dermatome of the affected nerve root (see Fig. 5-5). Nevertheless, actual pain in the hand or foot owing to nerve root compression is unusual.[54] Rather, the radicular pain is proximal and only numbness is felt distally. With further mechanical pressure on the nerve dura there may be no pain and the following may occur[110]:

1. Motor weakness
2. Diminished or absent reflexes
3. Anesthesia or paresthesia in the distal end of the dermatome

TYPES OF SPINAL PAIN

The two basic types of mechanical spinal pain may be classified simply as radicular pain and nonradicular (or spondylogenic) pain.

Radicular pain is that caused by disorders of the spinal nerves and their root. Radicular pain is common in the cervical and lumbar spine but very rare in the thoracic spine.[110] Although the roots as they exit from the spinal canal can be compressed by numerous factors, by far the most common source of such irritation is either an acute disk herniation or a degenerative disk that in turn has caused focal osteoarthritic changes with foraminal stenosis.[18,209] The terms soft and hard disk disorders are commonly used. The soft disk (herniation) disorders tend to occur in patients younger than 50 years of age, and the hard disk/osteoarthritis tends to occur in the older population. The onset is often acute. Pain may be sharp, stabbing, or lancinating, and accompanied by anesthesia and numbness. It is often superimposed on the dull ache of referred pain.

Nonradicular (spondylogenic) pain is produced by stimuli within deep skeletal structures such as muscle attachments, ligaments, fascia, periosteum, joints, dura mater, and the intervertebral disk. Nonradicular pain tends to be a deep, dull, aching type of pain, vaguely localized, referring over a great distance, and relatively prolonged in duration. It is relieved by rest. There are no neurologic signs, dermatome reference, or localizing features. Such pain is usually insidious in onset.

Spinal pain is a complex phenomenon and it is not always possible to determine its source reliably. The possible causes are numerous and frequently originate from sources outside the spine. Nevertheless, diagnosis is possible in the majority of cases but depends on an orderly evaluation, including a careful history, a thorough physical examination, and routine laboratory and x-ray studies. At times, diagnostic tests such as nerve and joint blockade and computed tomographic scanning may be necessary to help establish the origin of the problem.

REFERENCES

1. Adams M, Hutton WC: Prolapsed intervertebral disc: A hyperflexion injury. Spine 7:184–191, 1982
2. Akeson WH, Amiel D, Woo SL: Immobility effect on synovial joints: The pathomechanics of joint contracture. Biorheology 17:95–110, 1980
3. Alexander MJL: Biomechanical aspects of the lumbar spine injuries in athletes: A review. Can J Appl Sci 10:1–20, 1985
4. Allen CEL: Muscle action potentials used in the study of dynamic anatomy. Br J Phys Med 11:66–73, 1948
5. Andersson GBJ: Interdiscal pressure, intraabdominal pressure and myoelectric back muscle activity related to posture and loading. Clin Orthop 129:156–164, 1977
6. Andersson GBJ: Epidemiology of low back pain. In: Bueger AA, Greenman PE, eds: Empirical Approach to the Validation of Spinal Manipulation. Springfield, Charles C. Thomas, 1985
7. Andersson GBJ, Jonsson B, Örtengren R: Myoelectric activity in individual lumbar erector spinae muscles in sitting. I: A study with surface and wire electrodes. Scand J Rehabil Med Suppl 3:91–108, 1974
8. Andersson GBJ, Örtengren R: Lumbar disc pressure and myoelectric back muscle activity during sitting. II: Studies on an office chair. Scand J Rehabil Med 6(3):115–121, 1974
9. Andersson GBJ, Örtengren R: Myoelectric back muscle activity during sitting. Scand J Rehabil Med Suppl 3:73–101, 1974
10. Andersson GBJ, Örtengren R: Lumbar disc pressure and myoelectric back muscle activity during sitting. III: Studies on a wheelchair. Scand J Rehabil Med 6:128–133, 1974
11. Andersson GBJ, Örtengren R, Herberts P: Quantitative electromyographic studies of back muscle activity related to posture and loading. Orthop Clin North Am 8:85–96, 1977
12. Andersson GBJ, Örtengren R, Nachemson A: Intradiskal pressure and myoelectric back muscle activity related to posture and loading. Clin Orthop 129:156–164, 1977
13. Andersson GBJ, Örtengren R, Nachemson A: Quantitative studies of the load on the back in different working postures. Scand J Rehabil Med 6:173–178, 1978
14. Andersson GBJ, Örtengren R, Nachemson A, et al: Lumbar disc pressure and myoelectric back muscle activity during sitting: Parts I–III. Studies on an experimental chair. Scand J Rehabil Med 6:104–127, 1974
15. Andersson GBJ, Örtengren R, Nachemson A, et al: Lumbar disc pressure and myoelectric back muscle activity during sitting: II. Studies on a car driver's seat. Scand J Rehabil Med 6(3):128–133, 1974.
16. Aprill C, Dwyer A, Bogduk N: Cervical zygapophyseal joint pain patterns: II. A clinical evaluation. Spine 15(6):458–461, 1990
17. Arkin AM: The mechanism of rotation in combination with lateral deviation in the normal spine. J Bone Joint Surg Am 32:180–188, 1950
18. Aryanpur J, Ducker TB: Differential diagnosis and management of cervical spine pain. In: Tollison CD, ed: Handbook of Chronic Pain Management. Baltimore, Williams & Wilkins, 1989:320–325
19. Asmussen E, Klausen K: Form and function of the erect human spine. Clin Orthop Rel Res 25:55–63, 1962
20. Basmajian JV: Electromyography of iliopsoas. Anat Rec 132:127–132, 1958
21. Beaman D, Glover R, Graziano G, et al: Substance P innervation of lumbar facet joints. International Society for the Study of the Lumbar Spine, Chicago, Illinois, May 20–24, 1991 [Abstract].
22. Bogduk N: The innervation of the lumbar spine. Spine 8:286–293, 1983
23. Bogduk N: Lumbar dorsal ramus syndromes. In: Grieve G, ed: Modern Manual Therapy of the Vertebral Column. Edinburgh, Churchill Livingstone, 1986:396–404

24. Bogduk N, Marsland A: The cervical zygoapophyseal joints as a source of neck pain. Spine 13:610–617, 1988
25. Bogduk N, Twomey LT: Clinical Anatomy of the Lumbar Spine. Melbourne, Churchill Livingstone, 1987:139–147
26. Boudillon JF, Day EA, Brookhout MR: Spinal Manipulation, 5th ed. Oxford, Butterworth-Heinemann, 1993
27. Bowen V, Cassidy JD: Macroscopic and microscopic anatomy of the sacroiliac joint from embryonic life until the eighth decade. Spine 6:620–628, 1980
28. Brain WR, Northfield D, Wilkinson M: The neurological manifestations of cervical spondylosis. Brain 75:187–225, 1952
29. Brasseur K, Melvin J: Myoelectric activity in deep muscles of the back: A review. Arch Phys Med Rehabil 59:546, 1978
30. Buckwalter JA, Cooper RR, Maynard JA: Elastic fiber in human intervertebral discs. J Bone Joint Surg Am 58:73–76, 1976
31. Cailliet R: Low Back Pain Syndrome, 4th ed. Philadelphia, FA Davis, 1988
32. Cailliet R: Tissue sites of low back pain. In: Cailliet R, ed: Low Back Pain Syndrome, 4th ed. Philadelphia, FA Davis, 1988:63–75
33. Cailliet R: Pain: Mechanisms and Management. Philadelphia, FA Davis, 1993
34. Chaffin JB, Park KS: A longitudinal study of low back pain as associated with occupational lifting factors. J Am Ind Hyg Assoc 34:513–525, 1973
35. Chamberlain WE: The symphysis pubis in the roentgen examination of the sacroiliac joint. J Bone Joint Surg Am 24:621–623, 1930
36. Cholewicki J, Mc Gill SM: Mechanical stability of the in vivo lumbar: Implications for injury and low back pain. Clin Biomech 11:1–5, 1996
37. Cloward RB: Cervical diskography. Ann Surg 150:1052–1064, 1959
38. Colachis S, Worden R, Bechtol C, et al: Movement of the sacroiliac joint in the adult male: A preliminary report. Arch Phys Med Rehabil 44:490–498, 1963
39. Collins G, Cohen M, Naliboff B, et al: Comparative analysis of paraspinal and frontalis EMG, heart rate and skin conductance in chronic low back pain patients and normals to various postures and stress. Scand J Rehabil Med 14:39–46, 1982
40. Conley MS, Meyer RA, Bloomerg JJ, et al: Noninvasive analysis of human neck muscle function. Spine 20:2505–2512, 1995
41. Cotch MT: Biomechanics of the thoracic spine. In: American Academy of Orthopedic Surgeons: Atlas of Orthotics: Biomechanical Principles and Applications. St. Louis, CV Mosby, 1975
42. Cram J, Steeger J: EMG scanning in the diagnosis of chronic pain. Biofeedback Self Regul 8:229–241, 1983
43. Creswell AG, Grundstrom A, Thorstensson A: Observation on interabdominal pressure and patterns of abdominal intramuscular activity in man. Acta Physiol Scand 144:409–418, 1992
44. Creswell AG, Oddsson L, Thorstensson A: The influence of sudden perturbations on trunk muscle activity and intra-abdominal pressure while standing. Exp Brain Res 98:336–341, 1994
45. Cuatico W, Parker JC, Pappert E, et al: An anatomical and clinical investigation of spinal meningeal nerves. Acta Neurochir 90:139–143, 1988
46. Cyriax J: Perineuritis. Br Med J 1:570–580, 1942
47. Cyriax J: Textbook of Orthopedic Medicine, 8th ed, vol. I. London, Bailliere Tindall, 1982
48. Cyriax J: Textbook of Orthopaedic Medicine, 11th ed, vol. 2. Treatment by Manipulation, Massage and Injection. London, Bailliere Tindall, 1984
49. Cyron BM, Hutton WC: The tensile strength of the capsular ligament of the apophyseal joints. Anatomy 132:145–150, 1981
50. Dorman TA. Failure of self-bracing at the sacroiliac join: The slipping clutch syndrome. J Orthop Med 16:49–51, 1994
51. Dorman TA: Failure of self-bracing at the sacroiliac joints: the slipping clutch syndrome. In: Vleeming V, Dorman T, Snijders CJ, eds: Second Interdisciplinary World Congress on Back Pain. San Diego, California, 1995:653–656
52. Dorman TA, Brierly S, Fray J, et al: Muscles and pelvic clutch: Hip abductor inhibition in anterior rotation of the ilium. In: Vleeming A, Mooney V, Tischler H, et al., eds: Proceeding of the Third Interdisciplinary World Congress on Low Back and Pelvic Pain. Vienna, 1998:140–148
53. Dory MA: Arthrography of the lumbar facet joints. Radiology 140:23–27, 1981
54. Dubuisson D: Pathophysiology of pain. In: Warfield CA, ed: Principles and Practice of Pain Management. New York, McGraw-Hill, 1993:13–25
55. Edgar MA, Nundy S: Innervation of the spinal dura mater. J Neurol Neurosurg Psychiatry 29:530–534, 1966
56. Egund N, Olsson TH, Schmid H, et al: Movements of the sacroiliac joints demonstrated with roentgen stereophotogrammetry. Acta Radiol 19:833–846, 1978
57. Ehni G: Cervical Arthrosis: Disease of the Cervical Motion Segments. Chicago, Year Book, 1984
58. Epstein BS: The Spine. Philadelphia: Lea & Febiger, 1962
59. Farfan HF: Mechanical Disorders of the Low Back. Philadelphia, Lea & Febiger, 1973
60. Farfan HF: Muscular mechanism of the lumbar spine and the position of power and efficiency. Orthop Clin North Am 6:135–144, 1975
61. Farfan HF, Sullivan JD: The relation of the facet orientation to intervertebral disc failure. Can J Surg 10:179, 1967
62. Fielding JW: Normal and selected abnormal motion of the cervical spine from the second cervical vertebra to the seventh cervical vertebra based on cineoentgenography. J Bone Joint Surg Am 46:1779–1781, 1964
63. Fischer FJ, Houtz SJ: Evaluation of the function of the gluteus maximus muscle: An electromyographic study. Ann Phys Med 47:182–191, 1968
64. Floyd WF, Silver PHS: Function of the erector spinae in flexion of the trunk. Lancet 1:133–134, 1951
65. Frankel V, Nordin M: Basic Biomechanics of the Skeletal System. Philadelphia, Lea & Febiger, 1980
66. Frigerio N, Stow R, Howe J: Movement of sacroiliac joint. Clin Orthop 100:370–371, 1974
67. Fryette HH: The Principles of Osteopathic Technique. Carmel, Academy of Osteopathy, 1954
68. Frymoyer JW: Back pain and sciatica. N Engl J Med 318:291–300, 1988
69. Galante JO: Tensile properties of the human lumbar annulus fibrosis. Acta Orthop Scand Suppl 100:9–96, 1967
70. Gallois J, Japoit T: Architecture interieuredes vertebre du point de vue statique et physiologique. Rev Chir Orthop (Paris) 63:689, 1925. (Cited in Steindler A, ed: Kinesiology of the Human Body. Springfield, Charles C. Thomas, 1958)
71. Golding JSR: Electromyography of the erector spinae in low back pain. Postgrad Med J 28:401–440, 1952
72. Gould JA: The spine. In: Gould JA, Davies GJ, eds: Orthopedics and Sports Physical Therapy, 2nd ed. St. Louis, CV Mosby, 1985:518–549
73. Grabel J: Electromyographic study of low back muscle tension in subjects with and without chronic low back pain. United States International University Dissertation Abstracts International (1973) 34:292–293, 1974 [Doctoral thesis].
74. Gracovetsky SA: Linking the spinal engine with the legs: A theory of human gait. In: Vleeming A, Mooney V, Dorman T, et al., eds: Movement, Stability and Low Back Pain. New York, Churchill Livingstone, 1997:243–251
75. Gracovetsky S, Farfan H, Helleur C: The abdominal mechanism. Spine 10:317–324, 1985
76. Grant JCB: Grant's Atlas of Anatomy. Baltimore, Williams & Wilkins, 1972
77. Greenman PE: Clinical aspects of sacroiliac joint in walking. In: Vleeming V, Dorman T, Snijders CJ, et al., eds: Movement, Stability & Low Back Pain: The Essential Role of the Pelvis. New York, Churchill Livingstone, 1997:235–242
78. Gregersen GG, Lucas DB: An in vivo study of the axial rotation of the human thoracolumbar spine. J Bone Joint Surg Am 49:247–262, 1967
79. Grew ND: Intra-abdominal pressure response to load applied to the torso in normal subjects. Spine 5:149–155, 1980
80. Grieve GP: Common Vertebral Joint Problems, 2nd ed. New York, Churchill Livingstone, 1988
81. Grieve GP: Diagnosis. Physiother Pract 4:73–77, 1988
82. Guyton AC: Basic Human Physiology: Normal Function and Mechanisms of Disease, 2nd ed. Philadelphia, WB Saunders, 1977
83. Hall MC: The Locomotor System: Functional Anatomy. Springfield, Charles C. Thomas, 1965
84. Hamilton WJ, ed: Textbook of Human Anatomy, 2nd ed. St. Louis, CV Mosby, 1976
85. Hemborg B, Moritz V: Intra-abdominal pressure and trunk muscle activity during lifting: II. Chronic low-back patients. Scand J Rehabil Med 17:5–13, 1985
86. Hendry NG: The hydration of the nucleus pulposus and its relation to intervertebral disc derangement. J Bone Joint Surg Br 40:132–144, 1958
87. Hettinga DL: I. Normal joint structures and their reaction to injury. J Orthop Sports Phys Ther 1:10, 1979
88. Hirsch C, Ingelmark BE. Miller M: The anatomical basis for low back pain: Studies on the presence of sensory nerve endings in ligamentous, capsular and intervertebral disc structures in the human lumbar spine. Acta Orthop Scand 33:1–17, 1963
89. Hodges PW, Butler JE, McKenzie D, et al: Contraction of the human diaphragm during postural adjustments. J Physiol 505:239–548, 1997
90. Hodges PW, Richardson CA: Inefficient muscular stabilization of the lumbar spine associated with low back pain: A motor control evaluation of transversus abdominis. Spine 21:2640–2650, 1996
91. Hodges PW, Richardson CA: Contraction of transversus abdominis associated with movement of lower limb. Phys Ther 77:132–143, 1997
92. Hollinshead WH: Anatomy for Surgeons, 2nd ed. New York, Harper and Row, 1969
93. Hollinshead WH, Jenkins DB: Functional Anatomy of the Limbs and Back. Philadelphia, WB Saunders, 1981
94. Hoyt W, Hunt H, De Pauw M, et al: Electromyographic assessment of chronic low back pain syndrome. J Am Osteopath Assoc 80:728–730, 1981
95. Hutton WC, Stott JRR, Cyron BM: Is spondylosis a fatigue fracture? Spine 2:202–209, 1977
96. Inman VT, Ralston HJ, Todd F: Human Walking. Baltimore, Williams and Wilkins, 1981
97. Iwasaki T, Ito H, Yamada M, et al: Electromyographic study of the lifting weights. J Jpn Phys Ther Assoc 4:52–61, 1978
98. Jonsson B: The Lumbar Part of the Erector Spinae Muscle: A Technique for Electromyographic Studies of the Function of its Individual Muscles. Gîteborg, Sweden, University of Gîteborg, 1970
99. Jonsson B: Topography of the lumbar part of the erector spinae muscle: An analysis of the morphologic conditions present for insertion of EMG electrodes into individual muscles of the lumbar part of the erector spinae muscle. Z Anat Entwickl Gesch 130:177–191, 1970
100. Jonsson B: The function of individual muscles in the lumbar part of the spinae muscle. Electromyogr Clin Neurophysiol 10:5–21, 1970

101. Jonsson B: Electromyography of the lumbar part of the erector spinae muscle. Medicine and Sport, vol. 6. In: Komi PV, eds: Biomechanics II. Basel, Karger, 1971:185–188

102. Jonsson B: Electromyography of the erector spinae muscle. Medicine and Sport, vol. 8. Biomechanics III. Basel, Karger, 1973:295–300

103. Jonsson B, Synnerstad B: Electromyographic studies of muscle function in standing: A methodological study. Acta Morphol Neerl Scand 6:361–370, 1966

104. Joseph J: Man's Posture: Electromyographic Studies. Springfield, Charles C. Thomas, 1960

105. Kapandji IA: The Physiology of the Joints, vol. 3: The Trunk and Vertebral Column. Edinburgh, Churchill Livingstone, 1974

106. Karlsson E, Jonsson B: Function of the gluteus maximus muscle: An electromyographic study. Acta Morphol Neerl Scand 6:161–169, 1965

107. Kazarian L: Dynamic response characteristic of the human vertebral column. An experimental study of human autopsy specimens. Acta Orthop Scand (Suppl) 146:1–186, 1972

108. Kazarian L: Creep characteristics of the human spinal column. Orthop Clin North Am 6:3–18, 1975

109. Keller TS, Holm SH, Hansson TH, et al: The dependence of intervertebral disc mechanical properties on physiological conditions. Spine 15:751–761, 1990

110. Kenna C, Murtagh J: Patterns of spinal pain. In: Kenna C, Murtagh J, eds: Back Pain & Spinal Manipulation. Sydney, Butterworths, 1989:1–10

111. Kennedy CN: The cervical spine. In: Hall CM, Brody LT, eds: Therapeutic Exercise: Moving Toward Function. Philadelphia, Lippincott Williams & Wilkins, 1998:525–548

112. King AI, Prasad P, Ewing CL: Mechanism of spinal injury due to caudocephalad acceleration. Orthop Clin North Am 6:19–31, 1975

113. Kraft, GL, Levinthal DH: Facet synovial impingement. Surg Gynecol Obstet 93:439–443, 1951

114. Krag MH, Wilder DG, Pope MH: Internal strain and nuclear movements of the intervertebral disc. Proceeding of International Society for Study of the Lumbar Spine, Cambridge, England, April 15, 1983

115. Krag MH: Three dimensional flexibility measurements of preload human vertebral motion segments. New Haven, Yale University School of Medicine, 1975 [PhD dissertation].

116. Krammer J: Treatment of the Lumbar Syndrome in Intervertebral Disk Disease. Chicago, Year Book, 1981

117. Kraus H: Stress analysis. In: Farfan HF, ed: Mechanical Disorders of the Low Back. Philadelphia, Lea & Febiger, 1973:112–133

118. Kravitz E, Moore M, Glaros A: Paralumbar muscle activity in chronic low back pain. Arch Phys Med Rehabil 62:172–176, 1981

119. Krenz J, Troup JDG: The structure of the pars interarticularis of the lower lumbar vertebrae and its relation to the etiology of spondylosis with a report of healing fracture in the neural arch of a fourth lumbar vertebra. J Bone Joint Surg Br 55:735–741, 1973

120. Kuluk RF, Belytshko TB, Schultz AB, et al: Non-linear behavior of the human intervertebral disc under axial load. J Biomech 9:377–386, 1976

121. La Rocca H: Biomechanics of the cervical spine. In: American Academy of Orthopedic Surgeons: Atlas of Orthotics: Biomechanical Principles and Application. St. Louis, CV Mosby, 1975

122. Lee D: Anatomy. In: Lee D, ed: The Pelvic Girdle. Edinburgh, Churchill Livingstone, 1989:17–38

123. Lee D: Manual Therapy for the Thorax: A Biomechanical Approach. Delta, BC, Canada, DOPC, 1994

124. Lee D: Pelvic Girdle, 2nd ed. Edinburgh, Churchill Livingstone, 1999

125. Lewis T, Kellgren JH: Observation relating to referred pain, visceromotor reflexes and other associated phenomena. Clin Sci 4:47–71, 1939

126. Loebl WY: Regional rotation of the spine. Rheum Rehabil 12:223, 1973

127. Lorenz M, Patwardhan A, Vanderby R: Load-bearing characteristics of lumbar facets in normal and surgically altered spinal segments. Spine 8:122–130, 1983

128. Lumsden RM, Morris JM: An in vivo study of axial rotation and immobilization at the lumbosacral joint. J Bone Joint Surg Am 50:1591–1602, 1968

129. Lysell E: Motion in the cervical spine. Acta Orthop Scand (Suppl) 123:1–61, 1969

130. MacConaill MA, Basmajian JV: Muscles and Movements. Baltimore, Williams & Wilkins, 1969

131. Maigne R: Orthopaedic Medicine. Springfield, Charles C. Thomas, 1976

132. Maldague B, Mathurin P, Malghem J: Facet joint arthrography in lumbar spondylosis. Radiology 140:29–36, 1981

133. Manning DP, Shannon HS: Slipping accidents causing low-back pain in a gearbox factory. Spine 6:70–72, 1981

134. McCall IW, Park WM, O'Brien JP: Induced pain referral from posterior lumbar elements in normal subjects. Spine 4:441–446, 1979

135. McGregor M, Cassidy JD: Post-operative sacroiliac syndrome. J Manip Physiol Ther 6:1–11, 1983

136. McNeill T, Warwick D, Andersson G, et al: Trunk and strengths in attempted flexion, extension and lateral bending in healthy subjects and patients with low-back disorders. Spine 5:527–538, 1980

137. Messerer O: Uber Elastizitat und Festigkeit der Menschlichen Knochen. Stuttgart, JG Cottasche Buchhandlung, 1880

138. Meyer GH: Der Mechanismus der symphysis sacroiliaca. Arch Anatom Physiol Leipzig 1:1–16, 1978

139. Michele AA: Iliopsoas. Springfield, Charles C. Thomas, 1962

140. Miles M, Sullivan WE: Lateral bending at the lumbar and lumbar sacral joints. Anat Rec 139:387–398, 1961

141. Mitchell FL: Structural Pelvic Function. Academy of Applied Osteopathy, vol. 2. Chicago, Year Book, 1965

142. Mitchell FL: An Evaluation and Treatment Manual of Osteopathic Muscle Energy Procedures. Valley Park, MO, Mitchell, Moran and Pruzzzo, 1979

143. Mitchell FL JR: Elements of Muscle Energy Technique. In: Basmajian JV, Nyberg R, eds: Rational Manual Therapies. Baltimore, Williams & Wilkins, 1993: 285–323

144. Moll JMH, Wright V: Normal range of spinal mobility: An objective clinical study. Ann Rheum Dis 3:381–386, 1971

145. Mooney V: The syndromes of low back disease. Orthop Clin North Am 14:505–515, 1983

146. Mooney V: Facet joint syndrome. In: Jayson MIV, ed: The Lumbar Spine and Back Pain, 3rd ed. Edinburgh, Churchill Livingstone, 1987:370–382

147. Mooney V, Prozos R, Vleeming A, et al: Coupled motion of the contralateral latissimus dorsi and gluteus maximus: Its role in sacroiliac stabilization. In: Vleeming A, Mooney V, Dorman T, et al., eds: Movement, Stability & Low Back Pain: The Essential Role of the Pelvis. New York, Churchill Livingstone, 1997:115–122

148. Mooney V, Robertson J: The facet syndrome. Clin Orthop 115:149–156, 1976

149. Morris JM: Biomechanics of the spine. Arch Surg 107:418–423, 1973

150. Morris JM, Benner G, Lucas DB: An electromyographic study of intrinsic muscles of the back in man. J Anat 96:509–520, 1962

151. Morris JM, Lucus DB, Bresler B: Role of the trunk in stability of the spine. J Bone Joint Surg Am 43:327–351, 1961

152. Murphy RW: Nerve roots and spinal nerves in degenerative disc disease. Clin Orthop 129:46–60, 1977

153. Nachemson AL: Lumbar interdiscal pressure. Acta Orthop Scand Supp 43:9–104, 1960

154. Nachemson A: The load on lumbar disc in different positions of the body. Clin Orthop 45:107–122, 1966

155. Nachemson A: Electromyographic studies on the vertebral portion of the psoas muscle with special reference to its stabilizing function of the lumbar spine. Acta Orthop Scand 37:177–190, 1966

156. Nachemson AL: The lumbar spine: An orthopaedic challenge. Spine 1:59–71, 1976

157. Nachemson A: Disc pressure measurements. Spine 6:93–97, 1981

158. Nachemson A: Low back pain including biomechanics of the intervertebral joint complex. In: Straub LR, Wilson PD, eds: Clinical Trends in Orthopaedics. New York, Theime-Stratton, 1982

159. Nachemson A, Elfstrom G: Intravital dynamics pressure measurements in lumbar discs. A study of common movements, maneuvers and exercises. Scand J Rehabil Med 2(Suppl 1):1–40, 1970

160. Nachemson AL, Evans J: Some mechanical properties of the third lumbar inter-laminar ligament (ligamentum flavum). J Biomech 1:211–219, 1968

161. Nachemson AL, Morris JM: In vivo measurements of intradiscal pressure. Discometry, a method for the determination of pressure in the lower discs. J Bone Joint Surg Am 46(5):1077–1092, 1964

162. Nemeth G, Ekholm J, Arborelius UP: Hip load moments and muscular activity during lifting. Scand J Rehabil Med 16:103–111, 1984

163. Norkin CC, Levengie DK: Joint Structure and Function: A Comprehensive Analysis, 2nd ed. Philadelphia, FA Davis, 1992

164. Okada M: Electromyographic assessment of the muscular load in forward bending postures. J Faculty Sci Univ Tokyo 3:311–336, 1970

165. Okada M: An electromyographic examination of the relative muscular load in different human postures. J Hum Ergol 1:75–93, 1972

166. Örtengren R, Andersson GBJ: Electromyographic studies of trunk muscles with special reference to the functional anatomy of the lumbar spine. Spine 2:44–52, 1977

167. Panjabi MM: The stabilizing system of the spine: Part I. Function, dysfunction, adaptation and enhancement. J Spinal Disord 5: 383–389, 1992.

168. Panjabi MM, Abumi K, Durenceau J, et al: Spinal stability and intersegmental muscle forces: A biomechanical model. Spine 14:194–200, 1989.

169. Panjabi MM, Brand RA, White AA: Mechanical properties of the human thoracic spine as shown by three-dimensional load-displacement curves. J Bone Joint Surg Am 8:642–652, 1976

170. Panjabi MM, Goel VK, Takata K: Physiologic strains in the lumbar ligaments: An in vitro biomechanical study. Spine 7:192–203, 1983

171. Panjabi MM, Krag MH, White AA, et al: Effect of preload on load displacement curves of the lumbar spine. Orthop Clin North Am 88:181–192, 1977

172. Paris SV: Anatomy as related to function and pain. Orthop Clin North Am 14:475–487, 1983

173. Pauly JE: An electromyographic study of certain movements and exercises: I. Some deep muscles of the back. Anat Rec 155:223–234, 1966

174. Perry O: Fracture of the vertebral end-plate in the lumbar spine. Acta Orthop Scand 25:34–39, 1957

175. Perry O: Resistance and compression of the lumbar vertebrae. In: Ranninger K, ed: Encyclopedia of Medical Radiology. New York, Springer-Verlag, 1974

176. Platzer W: Color Atlas and Textbook of Human Anatomy: Locomotion System, vol. 1. Chicago, Year Book, 1978

177. Pope MH, Lehmann TR, Frymoyer JW: Structure and function of the lumbar spine. In: Pope MH, Frymoyer JW, Andersson G, eds: Occupational Low Back Pain. New York, Praeger, 1984

178. Pope MH, Rosen JD, Wider DG, et al: The relation between biomechanical and psychological factors in patients with low back pain. Spine 5:173–178, 1983
179. Porterfield JA, DeRosa C: Articulations of the lumbopelvic region. In: Porterfield JA, DeRosa C: Mechanical Low Back Pain: Perspectives in Functional Anatomy. Philadelphia, WB Saunders, 1991:83–122
180. Porterfield JA: The sacroiliac joint. In: Gould JA, Davies GJ, eds: Orthopedics and Sports Physical Therapy. St. Louis, CV Mosby, 1985:550–580
181. Portnoy H, Morin F: Electromyographic study of postural muscles in various positions and movements. Am J Physiol 186:122–126, 1956
182. Poulsen E, Jorgensen K: Back muscle strength, lifting and stooped working postures. Appl Ergon 2:133–137, 1971
183. Resnick D, Niwayama G, Goergen TG: Degenerative disease of the sacroiliac joint. Invest Radiol 10:608–621, 1975
184. Richardson C, Jull GA: Muscle control—pain control. What exercise would you prescribe? Man Ther 1:2–10, 1995
185. Richardson C, Jull G, Hodges P, et al: Therapeutic Exercise for Segmental Stabilization in Low Back Pain: Scientific Basis and Clinical Approach. Edinburgh, Churchill Livingstone, 1999
186. Richardson CA, Snijders CJ, Hides JA, et al: The relationship between the transversely oriented abdominal muscles, sacroiliac joint mechanics and low back pain. Spine 27:399–405, 2002
187. Rissanen PM: Comparisons of pathological changes in the intervertebral discs and interspinous ligaments of the lower part of the lumbar spine. Acta Orthop Scand 34:54–65, 1964
188. Roberts S, Chen PH: Global characteristics of typical human ribs. J Biomech 5:191–201, 1972
189. Rolander SD: Motion of the lumbar spine with special reference to the stabilizing effect of posterior fusion. Acta Orthop Scand (Suppl) 90:1–144, 1966
190. Rolander SD, Blair WE: Deformation and fracture of the lumbar vertebral end-plate. Orthop Clinic North Am 6:75–81, 1975
191. Rothman RH, Simeone FA: The Spine, 2nd ed, vol 1. Philadelphia, WB Saunders, 1982
192. Rothman RH, Simeone FA: The Spine, 2nd ed, vol 2. Philadelphia, WB Saunders, 1982
193. Sapsford R, Bullock-Saxton J, Markwell S: Women's Health: A Textbook for Physiotherapist. London, WB Saunders, 1998
194. Sashin D: A critical analysis of the anatomy and pathological changes of the sacro-iliac joints. J Bone Joint Surg Am 12:891–910, 1930
195. Schamberger W: The Malalignment Syndrome: Implications for Medicine and Sport. Edinburgh, Churchill Livingstone, 2002
196. Schmorl G: Die pathologische anatomie der wirbelsaule. Vern Dtsch Orthop Ges 21:3, 1927
197. Schultz A, Andersson G, Örtengren R, et al: Loads on the lumbar spine. J Bone Joint Surg Am 64:713–720, 1982
198. Shah JS, Hampson WGJ, Jayson MIV: The distribution of surface strain in the cadaveric lumbar spine. J Bone Joint Surg Br 60:246–251, 1978
199. Sherman RA: Relationships between strength of low back muscle contraction and reported intensity of low back pain. Am J Phys Med 64:190–200, 1985
200. Shore LR: On osteoarthritis in the dorsal intervertebral joint. Br J Surg 22:833–849, 1935
201. Sluijter ME, Koetsvedl-Baart CC: Interruption of pain pathways in the treatment of the cervical syndrome. Anesthesia 35:302–307, 1984
202. Soderberg GL, Barr JO: Muscular function in chronic low-back dysfunction. Spine 8:79–85, 1983
203. Solonen KA: The sacro-iliac joint in the light of anatomical, roentgenological and clinical studies. Acta Orthop Scand Suppl 26:9–127, 1957
204. Snijders CJ, Slagter AHE, van Strik R et al: Why leg-crossing? The influence of common postures on abdominal muscle activity. Spine 20:1989–1993, 1995
205. Snijders CJ, Vleeming A, Stoeckart R: Transfer of lumbosacral load to iliac bones and legs. 2: Loading the sacroiliac joints when lifting in a stooped position. Clin Biomech 8:295–301, 1993
206. Snijders CJ, Vleeming A, Stoeckart R, et al: Biomechanics of the interface between the spine and pelvis in different postures. In: Vleeming A, Mooney V, Dorman T, et al., eds: Movement, Stability and Low Back Pain. Edinburgh, Churchill Livingstone, 1997:103–113
207. Spilker RL: Mechanical behavior of a simple model of an intervertebral disk under compressive loading. J Biomech 13:895–901, 1980
208. Stoddard A: Manual of Osteopathic Technique. London, Hutchinson, 1962
209. Tauber J: An unorthodox look at backaches. J Occup Med 12:128–130, 1970
210. Tkaczuk H: Tensile properties of human lumbar longitudinal ligament. Acta Orthop Scand Suppl 115:9–69, 1968
211. Troup JDG, Hood CA, Chapman AE: Measurements of the sagittal mobility of lumbar spine and hips. Ann Phys Med 9:308–321, 1976
212. Valencia EP, Munro RR: An electromyographical study of the lumbar multifidus in man. Electromyogr Clin Neurophysiol 25:205–221, 1985
213. Vleeming A, Pool-Goudzwaad AJ, Stoeckart R, et al: The posterior layer of the thoracolumbar fascia: its function in load transfer form spine to legs. Spine 20:753–758, 1995
214. Vleeming A, Snijder CJ, Stoeckart R, et al: A new light low back pain. Proceedings of the 2nd Interdisciplinary World Congress on Low Back Pain, Sydney, Australia, 1995
215. Vleeming A, Snijders CJ, Stoeckart R, et al: The role of the sacroiliac joint in coupling between spine, pelvis, legs and arms. In: Vleeming A, Mooney V, Dorman T, et al., eds: Movement, Stability, and Low Back Pain. New York, Churchill Livingstone, 1997:53–71
216. Vleeming A, Stoeckart R, Volkers ACW, et al: Relation between form and function in the sacroiliac joint 1: Clinical anatomical aspects. Spine 15:130–132, 1990
217. Vleeming A, Volkers ACW, Snijders CJ, et al: Relation between form and function in the sacroiliac joint. 2: Biomechanical aspects. Spine 15:133–136, 1990
218. Watanabe K: A study on the posture: The function of the human erector spinae. Jpn J Phys Educ 21:69–76, 1976
219. Weisl H: The articular surfaces of the sacro-iliac joint and their relation to the movement of the sacrum. Acta Anat 22:1–14, 1954
220. Weisl H: The movements of the sacro-iliac joint. Acta Anat 23:80–91, 1955
221. Weisman G, Pope MH, Johnson RJ: Cyclic loading in knee ligament injuries. Am J Sport Med 8:24–30, 1980
222. Weismantel A: Evaluation and treatment of sacroiliac joint problems. Bull Orthop Sect APTA 3:5–9, 1982.
223. White AA: Analysis of the mechanics of the thoracic spine in man. Acta Orthop Scand (Suppl)127:8–105, 1969
224. White AA, Hirch C: The significance of the vertebral posterior elements in the mechanics of the thoracic spine. Clin Orthop 81:2–20, 1971
225. White AA, Panjabi MM: Clinical Biomechanics of the Spine, 2nd ed. Philadelphia, JB Lippincott, 1990
226. White AA, Southwick WO, Panjabi MM, et al: Practical biomechanics of the spine for orthopaedic surgeons. Instr Course Lect 23:62–78, 1974
227. Williams P, Warwick R: Gray's Anatomy, 36th ed (Br). Philadelphia, JB Lippincott, 1980
228. Wilder DG, Frymoyer JW, Pope MH, et al: The functional topography of the sacroiliac joint. Spine 5:575–579, 1980
229. Wilke JH, Wolf D, Claes LE, et al: Stability increase of the lumbar spine with different muscle groups. A biomechanical in vitro study. Spine 20:192–198, 1995
230. Wingerden JP van, Vleeming A, Snijders CJ, et al: A functional-anatomical approach to the spine-pelvis mechanism: Interaction between the biceps femoris muscle and the sacrotuberous ligament. Eur Spine J 2:140–144, 1993
231. Winters JM, Peles JD: Neck muscle activity and 3-D head kinematics during quasi-static and dynamic tracking movements. In: Winters JM, Woo SLY, eds: Multiple Muscle Systems: Biomechanic and Movement Organization. New York, Springer-Verlag, 1990:461–480
232. Wolf SL, Basmajian JV: Assessment of paraspinal electromyographic activity in normal subjects and in chronic back pain patient using muscle biofeedback device. In: Asmussen E, Gorgensen J, eds: International Series in Biomechanics. Baltimore, University Paris Press, 1977:319–323
233. Wolf SL, Basmajian JV, Russe CTC, et al: Normative data on low back mobility and activity levels. Am J Phys Med 58:217–229, 1979
234. Wyke BD: The neurology of joints. Ann R Coll Surg Engl 41:25–50, 1967.
235. Wyke B: Receptor systems in lumbosacral tissues in relation to the production of low back pain. In: White AA, Gordon SL, eds: American Academy of Orthopaedic Surgeons Symposium on Idiopathic Low Back Pain. St. Louis, CV Mosby, 1982

Cervical Spine

DARLENE HERTLING AND MITCHELL BLAKNEY

REVIEW OF FUNCTIONAL ANATOMY

Osseous Structures

The seven vertebrae of the cervical spine are divided into two groups according to structure and function. The vertebrae of the **lower cervical spine** (C2–C7) are similar in structure to the vertebrae of the thoracic and lumbar spine with clearly defined vertebral bodies and spinous processes (Fig. 19-1).[136] The transverse processes are abbreviated to allow better mobility, and there is a foramen to allow passage of the vertebral artery (Fig. 19-1A). From C3–T1 there is a total of 10 saddle-shaped, diarthrodial articulations between the uncinate process (Fig. 19-1B) and the adjacent body know as uncovertebral joint, or joints of Luschka, which also facilitate mobility of the lower cervical spine.[106,136] The articular facet joints of the lower cervical spine are in the sagittal plane and incline forward at approximately 45° (Fig. 19-1C). This forward inclination allows the articular facet joints to bear weight and guides the motion of the segment.

The bony structure of the **upper cervical spine** (occiput–C1–C2) is specialized to allow a great deal of mobility and to protect the medulla oblongata (Fig. 19-2A, B). The inferior articular facet of C2 has the same form and function as the articular facets of the lower cervical spine. The joint surfaces of the superior articular facet of C2 are aligned in the horizontal plane to allow approximately 90° rotation. The dens portion of C2 is a vertical pin of bone that acts as a pivot around which the atlas rotates (Fig. 19-2C, D).[136] The atlas is a wide, thin ring of bone with a well-developed transverse process but no spinous process. There is no intervertebral disk between the C1 and C2 because the atlas, with concave joint surfaces above and below, serves the function of the disk. The anterior portion of the transverse ligament of the atlas forms a socket for the dens (Fig. 19-3).

The atlanto-occipital joint is the one true convex-on-concave joint in the spine. The superior articular facet surfaces of the atlas are oval, concave, and toed-in slightly (Fig. 19-2A). The convex condyles of the occiput are slightly larger than the joint surfaces of the atlas, making maximal congruence possible on only one side at a time, when the occiput is laterally bent on the atlas. The anterior placement of the center of rotation of the atlas causes a lateral movement to the opposite side whenever the atlas is rotated (Fig. 19-3). This can be palpated as the transverse process becoming more prominent on the side opposite rotation. When viewed from the side, the superior articular facet joint of C2 is rounded as the atlas rotates. It rolls down the shoulder of the side of rotation and climbs up the shoulder of the side opposite rotation. This can be palpated as the transverse process of the atlas becoming higher and farther forward on the side opposite rotation and lower and more posterior on the side of rotation.[136]

The atlanto-occipital, atlantoaxial, and, arguably, the Luschka joint surfaces are lined with articular cartilage. They have synovial membranes and, like other synovial joints, have rich proprioceptive and nociceptive innervation.[276]

Joints and Ligaments

The **anterior** and **posterior longitudinal** ligaments and the **ligamentum flavum** are present in the cervical spine from

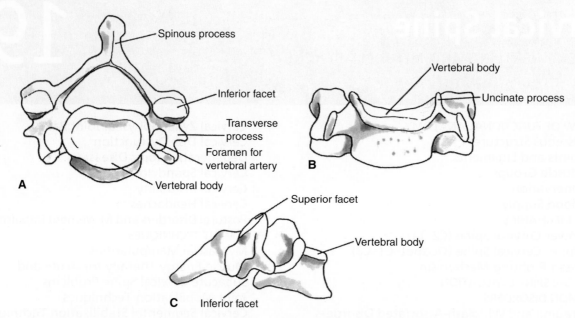

FIG. 19-1. A typical lower cervical vertebra. **(A)** Inferior, **(B)** anterior, and **(C)** sagittal views.

C2 through C7 and perform the same functions as in the thoracic and lumbar spine (see Fig. 18-8).

The **interspinous** and **supraspinous** ligaments blend with the nuchal ligament of the cervical spine (Fig. 19-4). The **nuchal** ligament has its origins on the spinous processes of the cervical spine and its insertion on the occiput. Its function in quadruped animals is to support the head. Its function in humans is to prevent overflexion of the neck. The nuchal ligament tightens at the extreme of neck flexion. It also becomes tight, flattening out the cervical lordosis, with approximately 15° of nodding of the upper cervical spine.[226]

The **posterior longitudinal** ligament ends at C2. The tectorial membrane, which is thin and diaphanous through the rest of the spine, thickens into the **tectorial** ligament

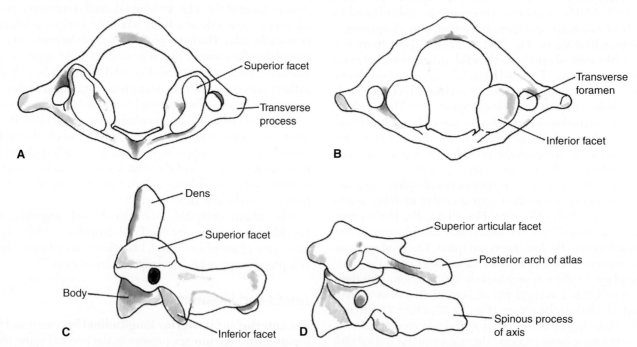

FIG. 19-2. The upper cervical spine. **(A)** Superior view of atlas, **(B)** inferior view of axis, **(C)** lateral view of axis, and **(D)** lateral view of atlantoaxial articulation.

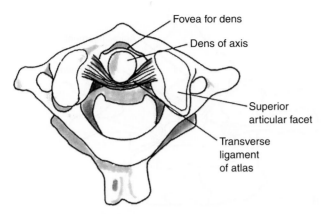

■ **FIG. 19-3.** The atlantoaxial joint from a superior view, showing the dens and the transverse ligament of the atlas.

arising from C2, bypasses the atlas, and inserts on the occiput (Fig. 19-5). The tectorial ligament becomes tight with flexion of the head.

Deep to the tectorial ligament is the **cruciform** ligament, which has both vertical and transverse portions (Fig. 19-5). The vertical portion of the cruciform ligament has its origin on C2 and has the same insertion and function as the

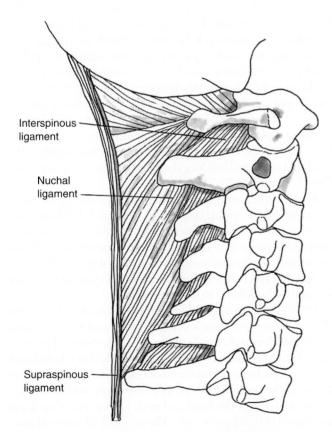

■ **FIG. 19-4.** A lateral view of the cervical spine, showing the interspinous, supraspinous, and nuchal ligaments.

tectorial ligament. It also bypasses C1. The horizontal portion of the cruciform ligament has its origin and insertion on the interior surface of the anterior ring of the atlas. It encircles the dens to reinforce the transverse ligament of the atlas (Fig. 19-3).

The **transverse** ligament of the atlas has its origin and insertion on the interior surface of the anterior ring of the atlas (Fig. 19-3). It encloses the dens and is lined with a synovial membrane and articular cartilage to provide lubrication as the atlas rotates around the dens. If the transverse ligament of the atlas and the horizontal portion of the cruciform ligament are weakened by systemic inflammatory disease or injured in an accident, there is danger of damage to the medulla oblongata by dislocation of the dens. If this is suspected, traction or mobilization of the cervical spine should be considered gravely dangerous.

The **alar** ligament is a winglike structure that has its origin on the lateral borders of the dens and its insertion on the occiput (Fig. 19-5B). It is a major portion of the stabilization system of the upper cervical spine. The configuration of the atlanto-occipital joints could allow considerable lateral flexion, which would damage the medulla oblongata. This lateral flexion is checked by the alar ligament. If the alar ligament is congenitally absent or damaged or if the dens is fractured or congenitally absent, mobilization or traction to the cervical spine should be considered gravely hazardous.

The **apical** ligament has its origin on the tip of the dens and inserts on the occiput (Fig. 19-5B). It becomes taut when traction is applied to the head. The joint capsule of the atlanto-occipital joint is reinforced with ligaments. The lateral placement of the atlanto-occipital joint capsules and ligaments severely limits rotation of the occiput on the atlas.

CLINICAL CONSIDERATIONS

To distract by traction the atlanto-occipital or atlanto-axial joint, the head must be in a neutral or slightly extended position to slacken the nuchal and posterior longitudinal ligaments.

The upper cervical spine can be thought of as an upper joint which flexes and extends and has some sidebending but no rotation, and as an inferior joint that allows approximately 90° rotation, no sidebending, and limited flexion–extension. Therefore, if the lower cervical spine is locked in full flexion or sidebending, movements of the atlanto-occipital joint are tested by lateral flexion, and movements of the atlanto-axial joint are tested by rotation.[136]

The ligaments of the upper cervical spine may be damaged in high-velocity accidents, weakened by rheumatoid arthritis or other types of systemic inflammatory diseases, or may be congenitally absent or malformed. Before any kind of mechanical treatment is begun, the integrity of the upper cervical ligament should be tested.[93]

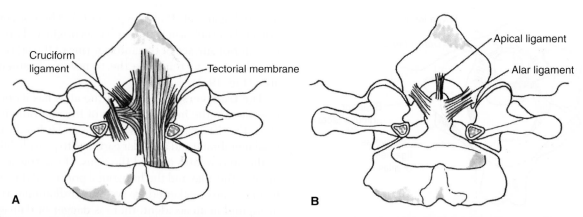

■ **FIG. 19-5.** A posterior view of the ligaments of the upper cervical spine: the more superficial tectorial and cruciform ligament (**A**) and the deeper alar and apical ligament (**B**). (Note: the cruciform ligament is not shown so that the deeper ligaments can be seen.)

The Sharp-Purser test has been described as a safe and effective method to evaluate alar ligament stability and correlates strongly (r = 0.88) with radiographic findings.[244,245] This test should be performed with extreme caution. To perform this test the patient should be sitting in a relaxed position with the cervical spine in a semiflexed position (Fig. 19-6). The examiner places the web space or thumb of one hand around the spinous process of the axis for fixation and then presses with the palm of the other hand on the patient's forehead dorsally. While the examiner presses dorsally with the palm, an excessive sliding motion of the head posteriorly in relation to the axis can be appreciated, which indicates atlanto-axial instability.[3,263] Symptoms exhibited when the head is in the forward-flexed position should be alleviated with posterior movement of the head.

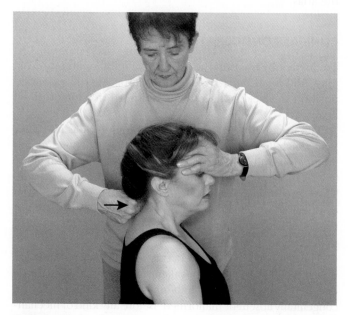

■ **FIG. 19-6.** The Sharp Purser test for subluxation of the atlas on the axis.

Muscle Groups

The muscles of the cervical spine can be considered in four functional groups: superficial posterior, deep posterior, superficial anterior, and deep anterior. Normal function of the cervical spine depends on proper flexibility and balance of these muscle groups.

The trapezius muscle is the largest, strongest, and most prominent of the posterior neck muscles (Fig. 19-7). It is very well developed in quadruped animals and serves to hold the head up against gravity. It inserts into the nuchal ligament and occipital ridge and extends the head and neck. In its function of maintaining the head in an erect position against the pull of gravity, the trapezius muscle works most efficiently when the head and neck are in their optimal position; that is, with the deepest part of the cervical lordosis no more than 4 to 6 cm from the apex of the thoracic kyphosis. The levator scapulae, splenius capitis, and splenius cervicis are other large superficial muscle groups that assist in extending the head and neck and holding the head up against gravity (see Figs. 7-7A and 19-7).

The multifidi and suboccipital muscles make up the deep posterior muscle group (Fig. 19-8). The multifidi have their origins on the transverse processes and insertions on the spinous process of the vertebra one to two segments above. When contracted together they extend the cervical spine; when contracted unilaterally they rotate the cervical spine to the opposite side and sidebend to the same side.

The sternocleidomastoid muscle is the largest and strongest of the anterior neck muscles (Fig. 19-9). From its dual origins on the sternum and clavicle, it inserts on the mastoid process, posterior to the center of gravity of the head. When both heads of the sternocleidomastoid are contracted together, they are flexors of the neck but extensors of the head. When only one side is contracted, the head and neck are laterally flexed and are rotated to the opposite side. The sternocleidomastoid muscles are very strong. When injured or in spasm, they hold the neck and head in the forward-head, chin-out posture.

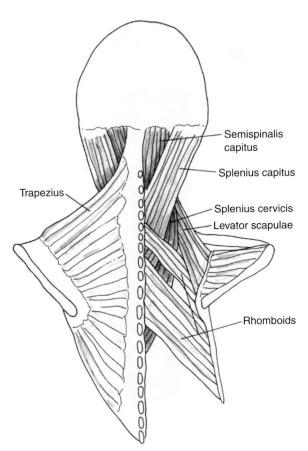

■ **FIG. 19-7.** The superficial muscles of the head, neck, and shoulders. This posterior view shows the trapezius, levator scapulae, splenius capitis, splenius cervicis, and rhomboid muscles.

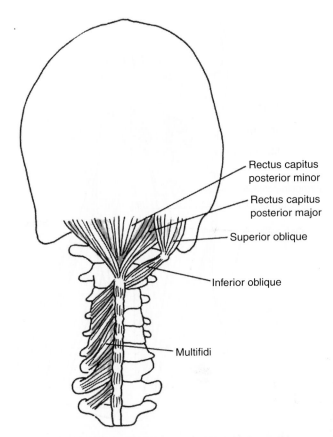

■ **FIG.19-8.** A posterior view of the deep posterior neck muscles, showing the multifidi and suboccipital muscles.

The other major neck flexors are the scalenus muscles, which have their origins on the first and second ribs and their insertions on the lateral tubercles of C2 to C7 (see Figs. 7-22 and 19-9). The scalenus anticus and scalenus medius are the anterior and posterior walls of the thoracic outlet. The first rib forms the bottom of the box, and the clavicle forms the top.[119] If the scalenus muscles are hypertrophied or in spasm, they may impinge on the lower roots of the brachial plexus or the subclavian artery as it passes through the thoracic outlet. Flexion of the head is accomplished by stabilization of the mandible by the muscles of mastication and a downward pull on the mandible by the strap (suprahyoid and infrahyoid) muscles (see Fig. 17-18).[136]

The deep anterior neck muscles are the longus colli and longus capitis (see Figs. 7-22 and 19-10). They are small muscles with origins and insertions on the bodies of the cervical vertebrae. In spite of their size, they are very strong and have very good leverage. Their function is to prevent anterior collapse of the cervical lordosis to resist the compressive force of the long cervical muscles. When these muscles are injured or in spasm, they exert a constant force that gradually flattens out the curve in the cervical spine.[136]

Innervation

Sensory and sympathetic innervation of the head and neck is a complex overlapping of cervical plexus and cranial nerves, making evaluation of pain complaints difficult. Sensory and sympathetic innervation of the face come from the facial and trigeminal nerves, both of which have sensory ganglia in the medulla oblongata and have anastomoses with sensory nerves of the cervical plexus (Fig. 19-11). The posterior portion of the head and upper cervical spine is primarily innervated by the greater and lesser occipital nerves, which arise from the cervical plexus but also have twigs from the trigeminal nerve. The joint and ligamentous structures and the segmental spinal muscles of the cervical spine are innervated by the recurrent fibers of the segmental spinal nerves. The brachial plexus arises from the roots of the fifth through eighth cervical nerves and provides the sensory and motor innervation to the scapula and upper extremity.[117]

CLINICAL CONSIDERATIONS

Mechanical irritation of deep somatic structures in the cervical spine may refer pain to the face, head, upper extremity, or interscapular area.[72]

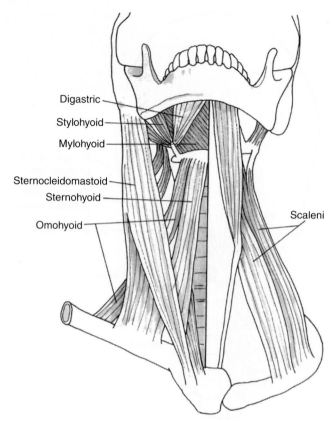

Digastric
Stylohyoid
Mylohyoid
Sternocleidomastoid
Sternohyoid
Omohyoid
Scaleni

■ **FIG. 19-9.** A frontal view of the superficial anterior neck muscles, showing the sternocleidomastoid, scaleni, suprahyoid, and infrahyoid muscles.

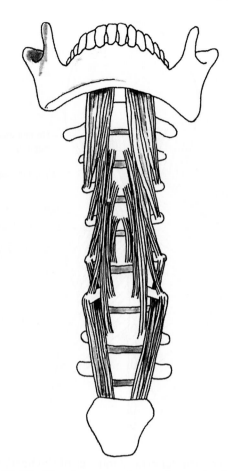

■ **FIG. 19-10.** The deep anterior neck muscles include the longus colli.

Neuritis and neuralgia of the cranial nerves, particularly V, VII, IX, and XI and also the greater and lesser occipital nerves, are common and may be mistaken for musculoskeletal pain.[10]

Peripheral entrapment of the brachial plexus is possible at the thoracic outlet, the shoulder, the elbow, and the carpal tunnel. This can produce symptoms that may be mistaken for shoulder tendinitis, elbow tendinitis, nerve root pain, or musculoskeletal pain of the neck or shoulder.

The nerve roots may be irritated by pressure from the bulging nucleus pulposus or by stenosis of the intervertebral foramen.

Blood Supply

The blood vessels in the cervical region of particular interest to physical therapists are the subclavian arteries, which pass between the scalenus anticus and scalenus medius and may be compressed (see Chapter 11, The Shoulder and Shoulder Girdle), and the vertebral arteries. The vertebral arteries pass upward through the lateral foramen of the cervical vertebrae. There is a redundant portion that allows full rotation of the atlas in both directions (Fig. 19-12). The vertebral arteries enter the cranium at the foramen magnum and come together to form the basilar artery.[148] The normal blood supply for the brain is through the carotid arteries if the circle of Willis is complete. If the circle of Willis is incomplete or if there is interruption of the blood supply through the carotid arteries, the vertebral arteries may form a major portion of the blood supply for the brain, particularly the brain stem and cerebellum. The vertebral arteries are at least partially occluded by extension and rotation of the cervical spine; maximum occlusion occurs with the combination of extension and rotation. Brief occlusion of the vertebral artery is not a problem in a patient who has normal carotid arteries and a normal circle of Willis; however, if there is interruption of the normal blood supply to the brain, occlusion of the vertebral artery may cause a reduction of blood flow to the brain stem and cerebellum, the symptoms of which are dizziness, nystagmus, slurring of speech, and loss of consciousness.[176]

There are many well-documented cases of coma and death secondary to vasospasm or thrombosis of the vertebral arteries caused by manipulation of the upper cervical spine.[51,148,184] The most common history of this type of catastrophe involves an attempt to rotate the atlas and usually involves an exceptionally forceful maneuver. In many cases the patient felt violently ill, dizzy, briefly lost consciousness after manipulation, was manipulated again, and died several hours later. Because death may occur several hours after manipulation, it is possi-

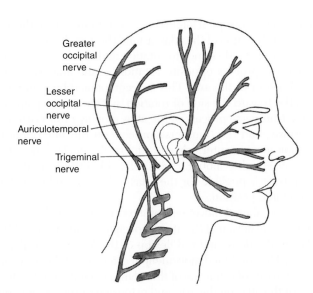

■ **FIG. 19-11.** Lateral view of the neck, head and face showing the cervical plexus, trigeminal, and occipital nerves.

ble that the number of catastrophic responses to upper cervical manipulation is actually underreported.

Blood vessels in the cervical spine have no nociceptive innervation per se, but when overdilated, intense headaches (migraines) are perceived. Migraine headaches may be accompanied by blurring of vision from pressure of the distended cranial blood vessel on the optic nerves. They may also be accompanied by nausea and muscle spasm in the neck. The migraine headache may be distinguished from the musculoskeletal headache in that the pain is generally throbbing

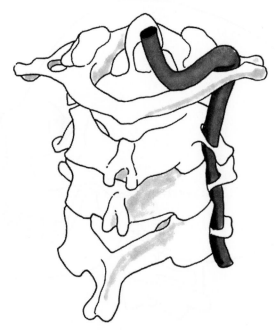

■ **FIG. 19-12.** A posterior view of the upper cervical spine, showing the vertebral artery emerging from C2 with a redundant loop that allows mobility of the atlas.

rather than constant, and the pattern of the headache is generally irregular and not related to trauma or activity.[10]

CLINICAL CONSIDERATIONS

Before using traction or mobilization techniques on the upper cervical spine, the vertebral arteries should be tested carefully one at a time by placing the neck in full rotation, extension, and lateral flexion to each side and holding for approximately 1 minute. The clinician should observe the patient for nystagmus, slurring of speech, blurring of vision, dizziness, or unconsciousness. Dizziness as a result of vertebral artery testing is fairly common and should be a warning sign to the practitioner to proceed very cautiously. Nystagmus, slurring of speech or loss of consciousness should be considered contraindications to traction and mobilization of the neck, and the practitioner should take care when treating the patient to make sure that the neck is not positioned in extension or the extremes of rotation.[211]

If a patient has a history of throbbing headaches or headaches accompanied by blurring of vision and nausea, or if the history of headaches is irregular and not related to activity, the possibility of migraine headaches should be investigated before investing in a long course of physical therapy treatment.

JOINT MECHANICS

Lower Cervical Spine (C2–T1)

The articular facet joints of the lower cervical spine are planar; at the single-joint level the only motions possible are superior and inferior glide. In inferior glide or extension the joint surfaces are maximally congruent, and the articular facets and joint capsules are maximally taut. Extension is the close-packed position and the position of maximal stability of the cervical spine. In full flexion the ligaments of the joint capsule are also taut, but the surfaces of the joint are barely engaged, making flexion the position of instability.[226]

CLINICAL CONSIDERATIONS

When the cervical spine is positioned in slight lordosis, there is good passive stability from the facet joints and supporting ligaments. When the cervical lordosis is lost or the cervical curve is reversed, passive stability is lost, and the segmental muscles must go into constant contraction to stabilize the spine. When there is slight lordosis in the cervical spine, the articular facet joints are able to bear approximately one third each of the compressive forces on the spine. When the cervical lordosis is lost, the entire compressive force is borne by the disk, causing excessive pressure and flattening.

Motion of a lower cervical segment involves movement of the vertebral bodies, which use the disk as a pivot, as well as movement of the joints of Luschka and the articular facet joints. Flexion of a cervical segment is superior glide of both articular facet joints. Extension of the cervical spine is inferior glide of both articular facet joints. Rotation and sidebending of the lower cervical spine are the same movements: there is inferior glide of the articular facet joint on the side to which the spine is rotated or sidebent, and superior glide of the articular facet on the side opposite rotation. Because of the 45° slope of the facet joints, the lateral tubercle on the same side moves downward and backward while that on the opposite side moves upward and forward. With either rotation or lateral flexion, there is always slight extension of the segment as well.[136]

Upper Cervical Spine (Occiput–C1–C2)

When the ring of the atlas lifts up posteriorly, there is approximately 20° of flexion–extension of the atlanto-occipital joint and approximately 15° of flexion of the atlanto-axial joint. When the atlanto-occipital joint is in extension, the ring of the atlas gets closer to the occiput and may compress the neurovascular structures in the suboccipital area. When the atlanto-occipital joint is flexed by nodding the head, the space between the atlas and occiput is maximally opened (Fig. 19-13). This can be seen clearly on mobility roentgenograms. Sidebending of the atlanto-occipital joint is always accompanied by a small conjunct rotation to the opposite side, which allows the condyle of the occiput on the side of lateral flexion to become congruent with the superior joint surface of the axis below. Lateral flexion is checked by the alar ligament, which because of its insertion on the dens, causes rotation of the axis toward the side of lateral flexion. This can be palpated as the spinous process of the axis swinging to the side opposite lateral flexion. Palpating for motion of the spinous process of the axis with sidebending

of the atlanto-occipital joint is one test for integrity of the alar ligament. Rotation of the atlas around the axis always involves a swing to the side opposite rotation and an elevation of the transverse process opposite rotation as the atlas slides up the shoulder of the axis. This is accompanied by a tilting of the atlas toward the side of rotation, which may be palpated as the transverse process of the atlas moving posteriorly and inferiorly, and the transverse process on the side opposite rotation moving anteriorly and superiorly. Because the atlas has considerable mobility with relatively little ligamentous stability, it is possible for the atlas to be jammed or locked in a rotated position.

The combined movement of flexion of the head and neck involves full flexion of the atlanto-occipital joint, flexion of the atlas on the dens, and full flexion of the lower cervical segments. The combined movement of extension of the head and neck consists of extension of the atlanto-occipital joint, extension of the atlas on the axis, and extension of the lower cervical segments. As mentioned above, in the lower cervical spine there is no difference between rotation and sidebending. In the upper cervical spine, rotation of the head and neck is rotation of the atlantoaxial joint to the same side and sidebending of the atlanto-occipital joint to the opposite side. Sidebending actually involves lateral flexion of only the atlanto-occipital joint, but rotation of the atlanto-axial joint to the opposite side. Both rotation and sidebending involve slight flexion of the atlanto-occipital joint to compensate for extension of the lower cervical spine (Fig. 19-14).[136]

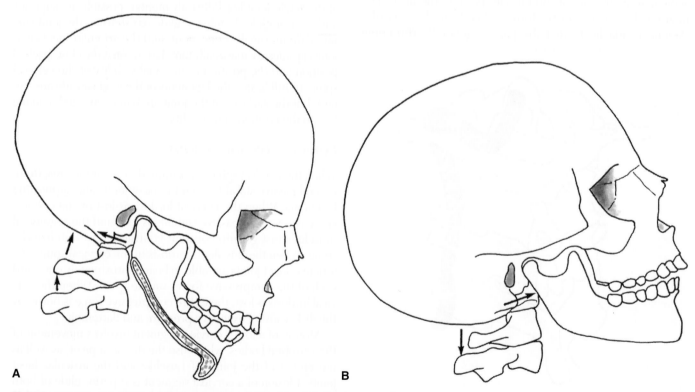

A   B

■ **FIG. 19-13.** Mobility of the upper cervical spine. **(A)** Flexion and **(B)** extension. (Note: In flexion, the space between the occiput and C1 increases, and it decreases with extension.)

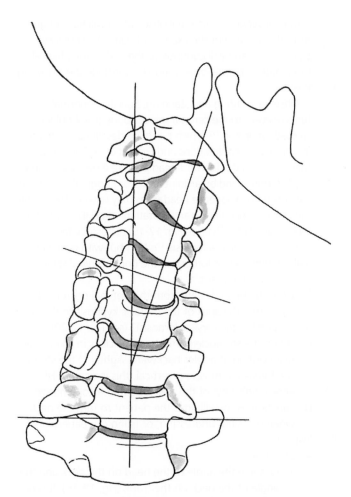

■ **FIG. 19-14.** An oblique view of the cervical spine showing full rotation: external rotation and lateral flexion of the lower cervical segments, rotation of the atlanto-axial joint, and flexion of the atlanto-occipital joint.

As an example, in left rotation of the head and neck, each segment of the lower cervical spine is in the combined movement of left lateral flexion and rotation, and each segment is slightly extended. The atlanto-axial joint is in full left rotation. The atlanto-occipital joint is in sidebending to the right and is slightly flexed. In left lateral flexion of the neck and cervical spine, each segment of the lower cervical spine is as in left rotation, with lateral flexion, rotation, and slight extension. The atlanto-axial joint is fully rotated to the right. The atlanto-occipital joint is in sidebending to the left and in slight flexion.

The only difference between left lateral flexion of the head and neck and left rotation of the head and neck is what happens in the upper cervical spine.

Head-Righting Mechanism

The posture and righting mechanism seen in infants and lower animals are present in adult human beings as well. There is a strong tendency for the eyes to face forward and level in the horizontal plane. This means that any lateral or rotational deviation from normal posture must be compensated for in the upper cervical spine. This also means that if there is a rotational or sidebending fault in the upper cervical spine, it will impart scoliosis to the rest of the spine. For example, in an atlanto-occipital joint locked in left lateral flexion, the cervical spine will move into right sidebending to bring the eyes level, thus producing an S-shaped scoliosis in the rest of the spine. Another example would be a left leg-length discrepancy that imparts a long C-shaped scoliosis; this is compensated for by left lateral flexion at the atlanto-occipital joint to bring the eyes level (Fig. 19-15).[226]

CERVICAL SPINE EVALUATION

The cervical and thoracic sections of the vertebral column are closely related functionally and anatomically and, in most instances, should be examined as a single unit (see Chapter 20, Thoracic Spine).

History
    In most situations an early priority is to establish the patient's functional limitations and/or disability (dysfunction), allowing the patient to report his or her problems,

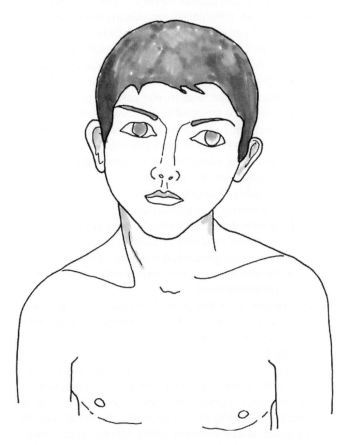

■ **FIG. 19-15.** Clinical appearance of a boy with a rotated atlas.

including the patient's understanding of and feeling about those problems and the effect they have had on the patient's life. In addition to the general musculoskeletal history (see Chapter 5, Assessment of Musculoskeletal Disorders and Concepts of Management), the following factors should be considered:

A. Routine screening questions. A number of postures or activities can provide useful information about potential source of symptoms within the cervicothoracic region. Therefore, screening to cover these should be included routinely if the patient does not address theses activities or postures spontaneously. For the cervical region, these might include the following:

   1. Activities involving sustained flexion, such as reading or driving.
   2. Activities involving cervical extension, such as hair washing in the hairdresser's wash basin or computer work.
   3. Effect of carrying loads or carrying a bag over the shoulder.
   4. Activities involving rotation, such as turning the body when driving the in reverse.
   5. Sleeping postures. Cervical symptoms are often increased when a firm or very firm pillow is used, as a result of loss of cervical lordosis or abnormal pressure placed against the neck or lack of support.[95]

B. Headaches. Is the patient experiencing headache? Several disorders can cause headache. Headaches from cervical spine problems usually present with specific referral patterns. Problems at the first cervical level cause headaches in a characteristic pattern at the top of the head. The second cervical level tends to refer ipsilateral pain retroorbitally in the temporal region. Lower cervical problems will frequently refer to the base of the occiput.[257] Characteristics of cervicogenic head pain include[128]:

   1. Moderate, nonthrobbing, nonlancinating pain, usually starting in the neck.
   2. Episodes of varying duration.
   3. Fluctuating, continuous pain.

C. Determine if neuritis or neuralgia causes pain.[10]

   1. Unrelated to activity or trauma.
   2. Superficial, stimulating in quality, or electric.
   3. Follows the pattern of innervation of a cranial or peripheral nerve.

D. Evaluate upper limb pain. If the patient is complaining of upper limb pain, is it in the pattern of a nerve root or peripheral entrapment?

Physical Examination

Although core examination procedures are undertaken with most patients, within the limitations of appropriate examination, the physical examination should be individualized, thus providing an assessment specific for each patient. Some tests will be irrelevant, others will need to be carried out briefly, whereas others will need to be investigated fully. The physical examination typically begins with informal and formal observation. Informal observation will have begun from the movement the examiner begins the subjective examination and will continue to the end of the physical examination. Formal observation may include the following.

I. Posture

   Observe in sitting and standing. Specific abnormal postures relevant to the cervical spine include the shoulder crossed syndrome,[122] which has been described in Chapter 7 (Myofascial Considerations and Evaluation in Somatic Dysfunction), and the forward head posture (FHP) (see Chapter 17, Temporomandibular Joint and Stomatognathic System). Patients who experience headaches may have a FHP.[269] Both the FHP with posterior cranial rotation and FHD without posterior cranial rotation (see Fig. 17-19) are associated with loss or reversal of cervical lordosis,[170,171,267] but with posterior cranial rotation there is lordosis in the upper cervical spine.

   A. General alignment.
   B. Does the head deviate from the optimal posture (4 to 8 cm from the apex of the thoracic kyphosis to the deepest point in the cervical lordosis)? (see Fig. 17-20)[226]
   C. When the sternocleidomastoid muscle is in its normal rest position, it angles backward slightly. If the sternocleidomastoid muscle is vertical, this indicates FHP and/or tightness of the sternocleidomastoid muscle.
   D. Function. How willing is the patient to turn the neck when dressing, undressing, or filling out paperwork?

II. Inspection

   A. Structure
      1. Observe the angle of the head on the neck and the angle of the neck on the trunk (Fig. 19-16). It is not uncommon for patient suffering from chronic cervical spine syndromes to exhibit a head tilt or slight rotation of the head in normal stance. This may be related to alteration of the head-righting mechanism (see above) or dysfunction of postural reflexes.[16,85,86]
      2. Are clavicles angled or horizontal?
      3. Do the scapulae lie flat against the thoracic wall or are they winged?

   B. Soft tissue signs. Observe muscle bulk and muscle tone comparing left and right sides of the patient. Some muscles are thought to shorten under stress (e.g., suboccipital muscles, levator scapulae, sternocleidomastoid, scalenes) whereas other muscles weaken (e.g., deep neck flexors, suprahyoids) producing muscle imbalance (see Table 5-6).[122,129] Note the following:
      1. Muscle spasm or parafunctional activity of the muscles of mastication, the facial muscles, or muscles of the cervical spine.
      2. Segmental guarding or hypertrophy of muscle.
      3. Atrophy of the muscles of the neck, upper extremity, or scapula.

   C. Skin. Neck, shoulder girdle, and upper extremity regions.
      1. Color.
      2. Moisture.

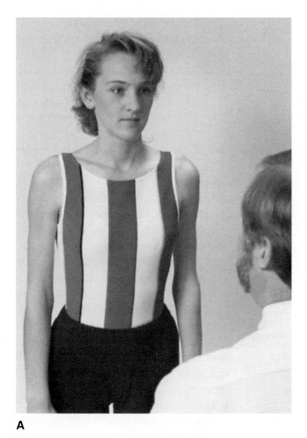
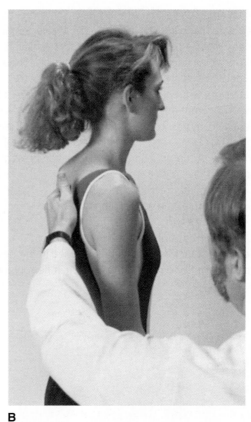

A   B

■ **FIG. 19-16.** Observation view of the head, neck, and shoulder girdle.

3. Redness or swelling.
4. Scars or blemishes.

III. Vertebral Artery and Craniovertebral Stability Tests

It is recommended that vertebral artery test[17] and craniovertebral stability tests be performed first on all patients with a cervical diagnosis, especially in the presence of trauma, subjective reports of cardinal signs or symptoms, or when testing or treatment will include manual therapy techniques which approach end ranges of balance.[238] Craniovertebral instability manifests itself with the presence of cardinal signs, which suggest either vertebral or basilar insufficiency or spinal cord compression.

A. Loss of balance or "drop attacks."
B. Nystagmus.
C. Bilateral or quadrilateral limb paresthesia.
D. Other noncardinal signs and symptoms that may be associated with craniovertebral instability include:
   1. Empty end feel.
   2. Significant muscle spasms.
   3. Severe headaches.
   4. Nausea or vomiting.
   5. Inconsistent swallowing.
   6. Lump in the throat.
E. Vertebral artery tests.

It is recommended that the vertebral artery be progressively stressed.[238] The patient keeps their eyes open during the entire test. Each position is held until the patient complains of arterial occlusion symptoms or for 30 seconds, whichever comes first. In sitting or lying:

1. Rotate the head as far as possible to one side, hold and repeat to the other side.
2. Maintaining lower cervical flexion, rotate and extend the upper cervical spine (this takes the stress off of the lower part of the vertebral artery while testing the upper portion). Repeat on the other side.
3. Maintaining upper cervical flexion, test the lower portion of the artery by rotating and extending the lower cervical spine.
4. Maintaining extension of the entire cervical spine, rotate the head to one side, hold and repeat to the opposite side.
5. If the above positions do not reproduce symptoms, the vertebral artery is maximally stressed by the addition of traction to the fully extended head and rotated cervical spine.
6. Note: Remember that in the presence of considerable loss of cervical range of motion (ROM), the ver-

tebral artery cannot be stressed fully. Therefore, as gains are made in the available ROM, the vertebral artery must be retested until full range is achieved.

F. Craniovertebral stability and joint integrity tests. These tests check the ability of the bony and ligamentous structures of the craniovertebral joints to prevent excessive accessory motions.

1. General compression. General compression of the spine (Fig. 19-17) provides an indication of vertical irritability. A reproduction of pain with compression suggests[58]:
   a. An end plate fracture.
   b. A fracture of the vertebral body.
   c. A disk problem.
   d. Acute arthritis of the zygapophysial joint.
2. General distraction. Distraction is applied in the neutral position first (Fig. 19-18) and then in flexion and extension.[57]

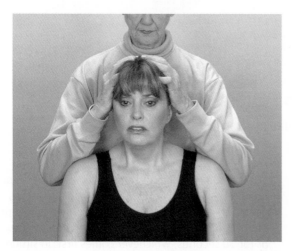

■ **FIG. 19-17.** General compression of the cervical structures.

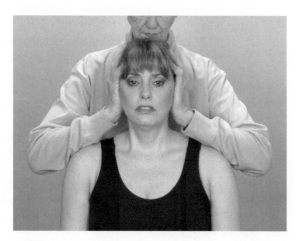

■ **FIG. 19-18.** General distraction of the cervical structures.

a. Distraction in extension produces a distraction of the zygapophysial joint surfaces and a compression of the disk.
b. Distraction in flexion increases the compression of the zygapophyseal joint and distracts the disk.
c. Reproduction of pain with distraction suggests:
   1. A tear of a spinal ligament, particularly implicating the tectorial membrane.[217]
   2. A tear or inflammation of the annulus fibrosis.
   3. An irritated dura.

IV. Joint Tests

Joint tests include joint integrity as well as active and passive physiologic movements of the cervical spine and other relevant joints. Joint play (accessory) movements complete the joint tests.

A. Joint integrity. Joint integrity tests for CO–C2 and C1–2 includes the Sharp-Purser test (Fig. 19-6) and the following tests for patients who have suffered trauma to the spine, such as an acceleration injury (or whiplash), or for patients in whom cervical spine instability is suspected. The Sharp-Purser test (see above) and the tests described below are considered positive if the patient experiences one or more of the cardinal signs described above.

1. Posterior stability (posterior-anterior shear) of the atlanto-occipital joint.[217] With the patient supine, the sides of the patient's cranium are gently compressed as the examiner applies an anterior force bilaterally to the atlas and axis on the occiput (Fig. 19-19). This has the effect of moving C1-2 anteriorly on the occiput.
2. Anterior stability (anterior-posterior shear) of the atlanto-occipital joint.[217] With the patient supine, the examiner applies a posterior force bilaterally to the anterolateral aspect of the transverse process of the atlas and axis on the occiput (Fig. 19-20). This has the effect of moving the occiput anteriorly on C1–C2.

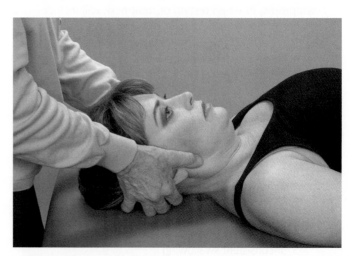

■ **FIG. 19-19.** Posterior stability test of the atlanto-occipital joint.

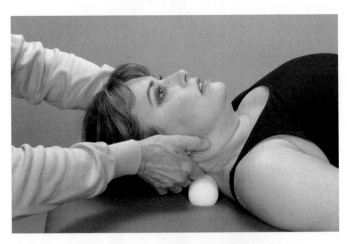

■ **FIG. 19-20.** Anterior stability test of the atlanto-occipital joint.

3. Transverse shear of the atlanto-occipital joint.[217] With the patient supine, stabilize the mastoid. C1 is moved in a transverse direction, using the soft part of the metacarpophalangeal joint of the index finger (Fig. 19-21). If instability can be demonstrated in every direction, the problem is true segmental instability. However, if the instability is just unilateral or bilateral, the more probable cause is a capsular tear.

4. Alar ligament stress tests. Two stress tests apply a lateral flexion and a rotation stress on the alar ligament. The alar ligaments limit contralateral flexion and rotation of the occiput on the cervical spine.

   a. Lateral flexion stress test for the alar ligaments.[218] With the patient supine, the examiner fixes C2 along the neural arch and attempts to flex the craniovertebral joint laterally. No movement of the head is possible if the contralateral alar ligament is intact. The test is repeated with upper cervical spine in neutral, flexion, and extension.

   b. Rotational stress test for the alar ligament.[217] This test is carried out if the lateral flexion stress test is positive, to determine whether the instability is owing to laxity of the alar ligament or instability at the C0–C1 joint. In sitting, fix C2 gripping the lamina and then rotate the head. More than 20 to 30° of rotation indicates damage to the contralateral alar ligament (Fig. 19-22). When the excessive rotational motion is in the same direction as the excessive lateral rotation (from the test above), this suggests damage to the alar ligament; when the excessive motions are in opposite direction, this suggests arthrotic instability. The same test can be performed using passive side-flexion of the patient's head.

B. Active physiologic joint movement. Test in sitting. An assessment of gross ROM of cervical flexion (Fig. 19-23A), extension (Fig. 19-23B), rotation (Fig. 19-23C), and lateral flexion (Fig. 19-23D) is performed, and the examiner makes note on any motion that reproduces or enhances the symptoms and the location of the symptoms. If lateral flexion is severely limited, suspect capsular tightness of the lower cervical spine. The weight of the head should provide sufficient overpressure for all motions except rotation (Fig. 19-23C). Three screening tests can be used to highlight the level of rotation. All of the tests use rotation of the neck in various amounts of flexion.

   1. Rotation with the neck in full flexion test the C1–C2 level (Fig. 19-23E).

   2. Rotation with the neck in a chin tuck position tests the C2–C3 level.[125]

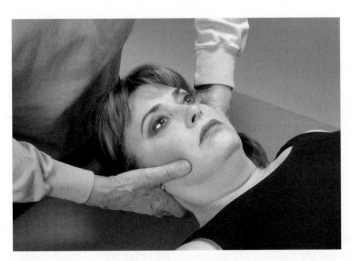

■ **FIG. 19-21.** Transverse shear test (lateral stability test) for the occipito-atlantal joint.

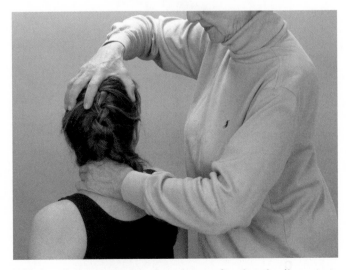

■ **FIG. 19-22.** Rotational stress test for the alar ligament.

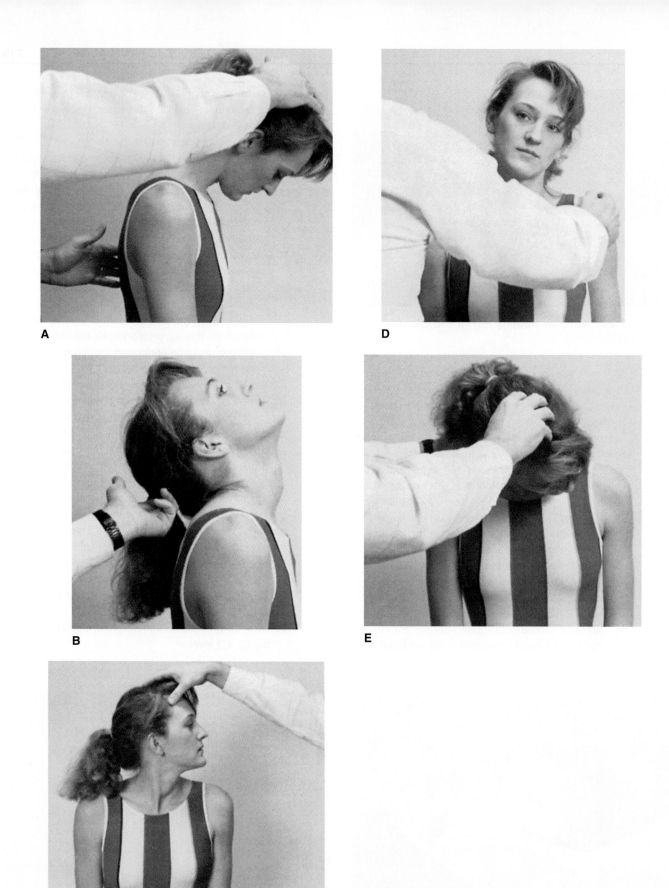

■ **FIG. 19-23.** Active movements of the cervical spine. **(A)** Flexion, **(B)** extension, **(C)** rotation, **(D)** sidebending, and **(E)** atlantoaxial rotation.

3. Rotation with the neck in full extension tests the levels below C3.[58] The more extension, the lower the level of involvement.

4. For further information about active range of movement, the following can be performed:

   a. Movements can be repeated; if there is no change in area of symptoms then the condition is categorized as a dysfunction syndrome.[177]

   b. The speed of movement can be altered; if peripheralization and centralization occur when the condition is characterized as one of several derangement syndromes.[177]

   c. Movements can be combined together.[63–65] Those described by Edwards are:

      i.   Flexion then rotation.
      ii. Extension then rotation.
      iii. Flexion then lateral rotation.
      iv. Extension then lateral flexion.

   d. Movement can be sustained. Sustained upper cervical extension or movement combinations with ipsilateral flexion or rotation often reproduce headaches.[159] Medial scapular pain or arm pain may be reproduced with sustained ipsilateral rotation, extension, or the combination of low cervical extension with ipsilateral rotation and lateral flexion.

C. Passive physiologic joint movement. Repeat tests for active cervical physiologic movements passively in supine, noting the ROM, end feel, muscle spasm, and any provocation of pain. Quadrant tests and upper cervical spine passive physiologic movements are carried out in sitting.

1. Upper cervical spine flexion. One hand cups around the anterior aspect of the mandible while the other hand grips under the occiput. Both hands guide the head forward on the upper cervical spine.

2. Lateral flexion. The hands grasp around the head at the level of the ears and apply a force to tilt the head laterally on the upper cervical spine.

3. Upper cervical extension One hand holds underneath the chin while the other hand and forearm lie over the head. The upper head and neck are displaced forwards on the upper cervical spine (Fig. 19-24*A*).

4. Upper cervical quadrant. The head position is the same as for upper cervical extension. The head is then moved into rotation and lateral flexion to one side (Fig. 19-24*B*).

D. Passive physiologic intervertebral movements (PPIVMs) which examine the movement at each segment level can be a useful adjunct to joint play movements to identify segmental hypomobility and hypermobility. PPIVMs can be performed in sitting or supine. The examiner palpates between adjacent spinous processes or articular pillars to feel the range of intervertebral movement during: cervical flexion and extension, lateral flexion, and rotation. Figure 19-25 demonstrates atlanto-occipital joint distraction and lateral flexion. Other tests include:

1. Rotation PPIVMs at the atlantoaxial joint (Fig. 19-26).

2. Lateral flexion PPIVMs of the lower cervical spine by placing the web space of the thumb over the joint and gently gliding each segment laterally (Fig. 19-27).

3. Rotation PPIVMs of the lower cervical spine.

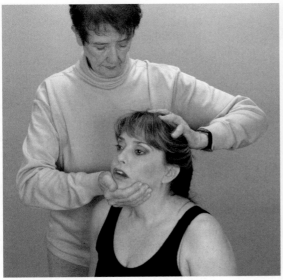
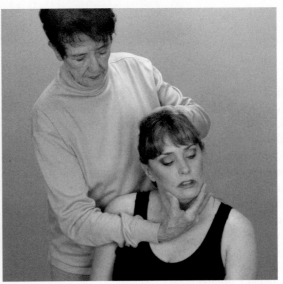

A   **B**

■ **FIG. 19-24.** Passive upper cervical spine movements. (**A**) Extension. (**B**) Upper cervical quadrant.

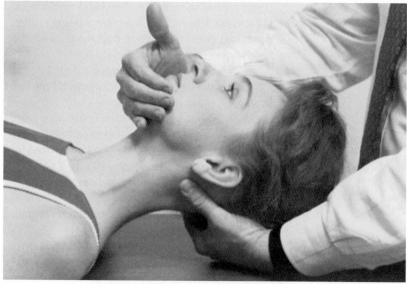

A

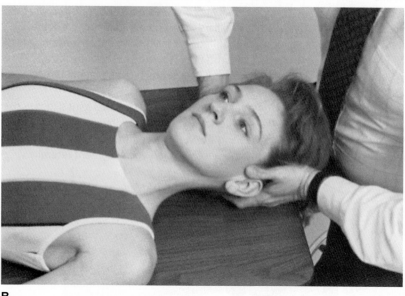

B

■ **FIG. 19-25.** PPIVMs of the atlanto-occipital joint. **(A)** Distraction and **(B)** lateral flexion.

E. Segmental mobility (accessory movements, joint play, or passive accessory intervertebral movements [PAIVMs]).[99,169,193,268] They consist of central postero-anterior (PA) pressures over the spinous processes and poster arch of C1, unilateral PAs over the facet joints, transverse pressures against the spinous processes or articular pillars and unilateral anteroposterior pressures to the articular pillars. To elicit an exact pain response from the patient, vary the pressure in different directions. The examiner should examine accessory movements in stages, observing the following points. Confirm any apparent vertebral rotational malpositions of the right and left facet.

1. Examine for bony alignment (position) on the sides of the spinous processes and laminae. One may note on palpation of the articular pillars on the involved segment that one articular pillar is more prominent posteriorly.

2. Gain a brief overall appraisal of the cervical segments by performing grades I–II central posteroanterior (PA) oscillations. Stand at the patient's head or to one side. Place the opposed straight thumbs over the posterior arch of C1 and direct upward and forward oscillations towards the patient's eyes. Then apply thumb pressure on the spinous process of C2, and methodically move down the midline on the spinous processes (see Fig. 19-50). Use each increasing oscillation to detect stiffness, pain, or muscle spasm.

3. Further examination of accessory motions may be undertaken using unilateral PA oscillations, which

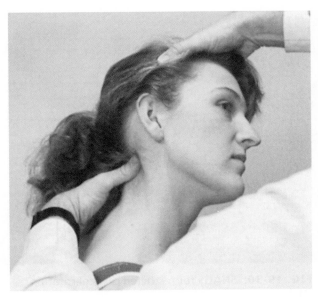

■ **FIG. 19-26.** Rotation PPIVMs at the atlantoaxial joint rotation.

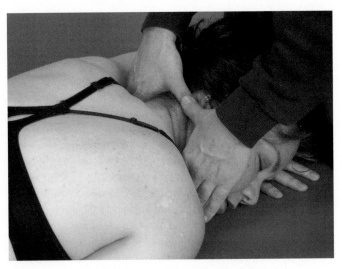

■ **FIG. 19-28.** Transverse pressures (rotational oscillations) for the atlanto-occipital joint.

contact each level of the right and left articular pillar. Press with opposed thumbs against the articular pillars about two to three centimeters from the midline. (see Fig. 19-51*B*) This will reproduce pain in the underlying apophyseal joints if they are abnormal. At the C1 level, unilateral PA oscillations are applied laterally over the posterior arch of C1 (see Fig. 19-51*A*).

4. Other accessory motions may be assessed are transverse (right to left, or left to right) pressures on the spinous processes of C2, the lower cervical segments (see Fig. 19-53), and the upper thoracic segments. For the atlanto-occipital joint, the head should be positioned in rotation and thumb pressure applied to the transverse process of C1 (Fig. 19-28). Unilateral anteroposterior (AP) oscillations should be assessed, especially in patients whose symptoms are anterior

in origin or in those with any upper limb related conditions. A double thumb contact can be used on the anterior aspect of the transverse process. Care in handling must be exercised because of the normal sensitivity in this area. Again, signs of restriction and pain provocation are sought.

5. One can also alter the position of the joint. In lying the cervical spine can be placed in a variety of resting positions. Commonly the spine is positioned flexion (see Fig. 19-50), extension (see Fig. 19-52), lateral flexion, flexion and rotation, flexion and lateral flexion, extension and rotation, and extension and lateral flexion. These positions are thought to increase and decrease the compressive and stretch effect at the intervertebral joints.[63–65]

Note: These palpatory/accessory motions are not only diagnostic but are also used for joint mobilization therapy.

6. Other joints as applicable. Other joints suspected to be a source of pain should also be tested. Joints likely to be examined are the temporomandibular joint, shoulder girdle, thoracic spine and ribs, glenohumeral joint, elbow joint, wrist, and hand.

F. Natural apophyseal glides (NAGS), sustained natural apophyseal glides (SNAGS), and mobilization with movement (MWM).[69,135,186,218] During examination with these accessory movements, it is the relief of symptoms, which implicates the joint as the source of pain. The examination tests can be used as a treatment technique, but details of these techniques are outside the scope of this book. For further details on these techniques refer to Mulligan.[186]

1. SNAGS. The painful cervical spine movements are examined in sitting. Pressure is applied to each transverse or spinous process by the examiner as the

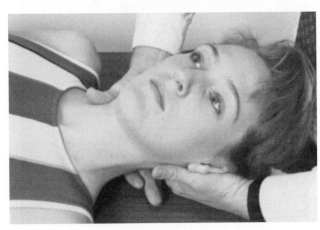

■ **FIG. 19-27.** Lateral flexion PPIVMs of the lower cervical spine.

patient moves slowly toward the pain.[186] Figure 19-29 demonstrates a posteroanterior pressure (SNAGS) applied to the cervical spine as the patient moves into flexion. Figure 19-30 demonstrates SNAGS for restricted cervical rotation at C1/C2. A posteroanterior pressure is applied to the articular pillow of C1 as the patient moves slowly into rotation. Figure 19-31 Demonstrates extension SNAG to the lower cervical spine. Thumb pressure is applied to the spinous process in question in the direction of the facet plane as the patient slowly extends.

2. Headache SNAGS. Figure 19-32A demonstrates a posteroanterior pressure applied to C2 using the heel of the hand. The other hand supports the head. Pressure is sustained for at least 10 seconds while the patient remains still. The test is considered positive if the headache is relieved and would indicate a mechanical joint problem. Reverse headache SNAGS uses one hand to palpate the transverse processes of C2 and the other hand supports and moves the head anteriorly on the stabilized C2 (Fig. 19-32B).

3. Upper cervical traction in slight extension is another test and often a treatment of choice for many headaches that would indicate a mechanical problem. The examiner maintains the patient's cervical lordosis by placing a forearm under cervical spine with the patient in supine (Fig. 19-33). Pronation of the forearm and a gentle pull on the chin produces cervical traction. The position is held for a least 10 seconds. Relief of symptoms indicates a positive test.

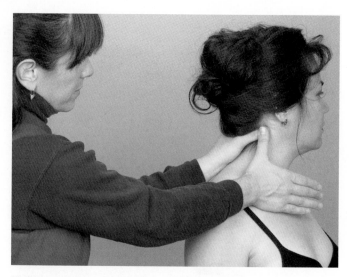

■ **FIG. 19-30.** SNAGS for restricted cervical rotation at C1/2.

4. NAGS. Theses can be applied to the apophyseal joints between C2 and T3. Static or oscillatory force is applied to the articular pillar in the direction of the facet joint plane of each symptomatic vertebrae. Figure 19-34 demonstrates a unilateral NAG applied to articular pillar as the patient laterally flexes to the opposite side.

V. Muscle Tests

Muscle tests include resistive isometric contractions, muscle strength, control, and length.

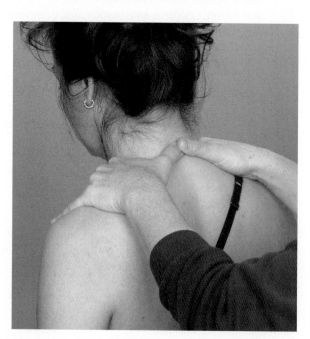

■ **FIG. 19-29.** Flexion SNAGS. Posterior-to-anterior pressure is applied to the spinous process as the patient flexes.

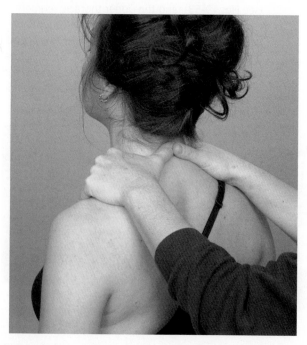

■ **FIG. 19-31.** Extension SNAGS to the lower cervical spine.

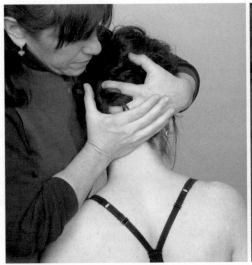 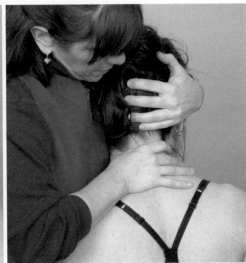

■ FIG. 19-32. (A) Headache SNAG. Posterior-to-anterior pressure is applied to C2. **(B)** Reverse headache SNAG applied to C2.

A   **B**

A. Isometrically resisted contractions. These tests are usually carried out in sitting. Isometrically resisted movements at mid range are performed in each direction to stress the contractile units of the neck for lesions of the cervical muscles.

   1. Cervical lateral flexion and rotation. One hand is placed on each side of the patient's head (without covering the auditory meatus). The forearms and elbows rest over the patient's trapezial ridges to help stabilize against trunk movements. From this position the examiner resists cervical rotation and lateral flexion to the left and right, without allowing movement of the head.

   2. Cervical extension. To resist cervical extension, the examiner places one hand over the back of the patient's head, such that the wrist lies over the patient's cervical spine and the forearm rests against the thoracic spine. The other hand reaches across the front of the patient to grasp the opposite shoulder. Extension of the patient's and neck is resisted without allowing movement.

   3. Cervical flexion. Flexion is resisted by approaching the patient from behind, resting the elbows against the back of the patient's shoulders, and placing both hands over the patient's forehead.

   4. Others. Test rotator cuff muscles, noting pain and/or weakness (see Chapter 11, Shoulder and Shoulder Girdle).

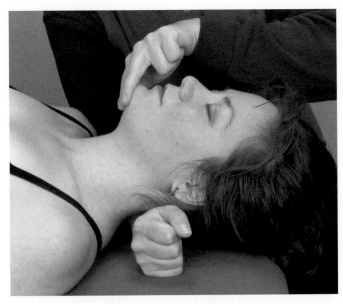

■ FIG. 19-33. Upper cervical traction.

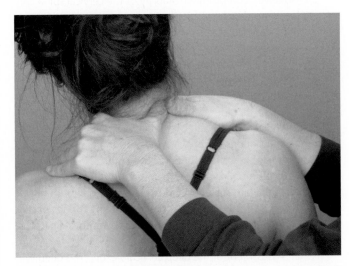

■ FIG. 19-34. Unilateral NAG. Thumb pressure is applied to the articular pillar (in line with the facet) as the patient laterally flexes to the opposite side.

B. Muscle strength. When indicated, the examiner should test the cervical extensors, flexors, rotators, capital extensors, capital flexors, combined neck extensors (capital plus cervical), combined flexors (capital plus cervical), and combined flexors to isolate a single sterno-cleidomastoid. For details of these tests, the reader is directed to Hislop and Montgomery.[115] All muscles that act on the head are inserted on the skull. Those that are anterior or in the coronal midline are termed capital extensors or flexors. Their center of motion is in the atlanto-occipital or atlanto axial joints.[73,216]

C. Muscle control and stability. As Panjabi et al.[209] have written, there are three subsets that interact to provide the spine with the necessary stability to avoid injury. These are (1) the active system (muscles), (2) the passive system (ligaments, joint capsules, bones, facet joints, discs, passive properties of muscles) and (3) the control system (mechanoreceptors in the locomotor system that direct force, direction and velocity of motion, neural control centers). The active and neural control systems function to prevent movement that exceeds the normal neutral zones when internal and external perturbations are introduced to the spine (dynamic stabilizers), while the passive system functions to prevent excessive motion at end range (passive stability). Both these dynamic and static processes provide stability in the cervical spine. Dynamic instability is defined by Panjabi as "a significant decrease in the capacity of the stabilizing system of the spine to maintain the intervertebral neutral zones within the physiologic limits so that there is no neurologic dysfunction, no major deformity, and no incapacity pain."[206,207] The size of the intervertebral neutral zone has been demonstrated to be a better indicator of spinal instability than gross ROM.[134,185,208,209,274] Unfortunately, there is no current method to measure the neutral zone. However, compromised stability of the cervical spine can be inferred by assessing those muscles that are the most important stabilizers of the cervical spine. Motion palpation may help assess the state of multifidus muscles.

1. To determine the dynamic stability of the cervical spine, the hypermobile segment(s) is (are) palpated during active motion of the neck or upper limbs (e.g., shoulder flexion) (Fig. 19-35). Special attention is given to the amount or inappropriate directions of translations, planes of laxity, and the type of end feel while the spine is under active control.[140] Slight hypermobilities (Class 4), although often asymptomatic, are still at risk for overstretching injuries during activities that place the joint at end ranges of movement and can progress to a symptomatic (Class 5) hypermotility.[135]

2. Assessment of the deep cervical flexors. The deep cervical flexors, when acting as stabilizers, must have both a short reaction time (brought about by the type II fibers) and a long endurance capacity (brought

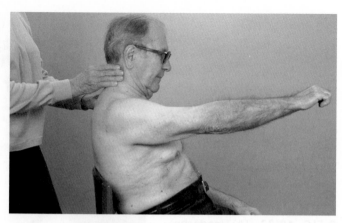

■ **FIG. 19-35.** Assessment of cervical spine segmental stability during arm motion.

about by type I fibers). Tests procedures may be used to determine both function as well as the balance between the deep cervical flexors and the sternocleidomastoid. Studies of patients with cervicogenic headache symptoms have found both decreased maximal isometric strength and isometric endurance of the short upper cervical flexor muscles (capital flexors) with those of normal subjects.[269] Treleavan et al.[259] found similar findings in patients with post-concussion headache. Silverman et al.[247] found true weakness (as opposed to inhibition, which they did no tests for) in the deep cervical flexors in patients with chronic pain as compared to controls. Several methods of testing the deep several flexors have been proposed.

a. These muscles are first tested by palpating and observing the pattern of movement, which occurs when the patient flexes his head from a supine position.[272] The patient lies supine with the cervical spine in a neutral position. The examiner places one hand under the occiput and the other hand beneath the cervical spine. Subsequently the patient is asked to perform upper cervical flexion ("chin-tuck") without lifting the head off of the table. On correct performance the examiner should feel a slight increase of pressure on the cervical hand while the pressure on the 'occiput hand' should remain unchanged. If the capital flexors are weak and the sternocleidomastoid is relatively strong, the latter muscle will increase the extension of the cervical spine and there will be a decrease of pressure on the "occiput" hand. This will only happen if the capital flexors are not active enough to pre-fix the head in flexion.[115] If the capital flexors are weak, the head can be raised off the table, but it will be in a position of capital extension with the chin leading.

b. Alternatively, with the patient in supine, the examiner may passively preposition the head in the neutral position with the chin slightly tucked.[189] The examiner tells the patient that he or she is going to let go of the head and that the patient should continue to hold it in the exact position. The clinician then lets go of the head suddenly and observes how well the position is maintained for 10 seconds. The normal pattern is maintained without excessive shaking. Any of the following responses is abnormal; they are listed from most to least common.[189]

 i. The chin pokes out.
 ii. The head shakes excessively
 iii. The entire cervical spine flexes
 iv. The head drops into extension.

These findings are indicative of hypertonicity of the sternocleidomastoids or inhibition of the deep cervical flexors or both. The presence of shaking suggests that transformation of type I to type II fibers has taken place in the deep cervical flexors.

c. A pressure biofeedback unit (PBU, Chattanooga, Australia) can be used to measure the function of the deep neck flexors more objectively (Fig. 19-36).[128] The patient is positioned in supine with the cervical spine in neutral. The PBU is positioned suboccipitally behind the neck to monitor the subtle flattening of the cervical spine (which occurs with the action of the longus colli). The PBU is inflated to baseline of 20 mm Hg, and the patient is then asked to slowly perform craniocervical flexion and to progressively increase the pressure to 22 to 30 mm Hg. (normal target level). Once the target level is reached the patient is asked to hold the position for a least 5 seconds.

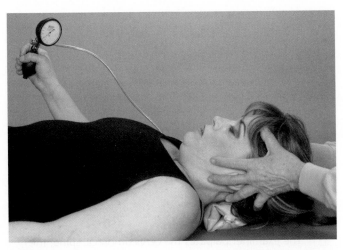

▪ **FIG. 19-36.** Craniocervical flexion test using a pressure biofeedback unit to measure function of the deep neck flexors.

D. Muscle length. The examiner tests the length of individual muscles, in particular those muscles prone to become short[122]; the deep occipital muscles, scalenes, upper trapezius, sternocleidomastoid, and levator scapulae. Testing for length of these muscles is described in Chapter 7, Myofascial Considerations and Evaluation in Somatic Dysfunction (see Figs. 7-34 through 7-37).

VI. Neurologic Tests

Neurologic examination involves examining the integrity and mobility of the nervous system and special diagnostic tests.

A. Integrity of the nervous system
 1. Dermatomes/peripheral nerves. A knowledge of the cutaneous distribution of peripheral nerves and cutaneous distribution of the nerve roots (dermatomes) enables the examiner to distinguish the sensory loss owing to root lesion from that owing to a peripheral nerve lesion (see Fig. 5-8 and Table 5-8).
 2. Myotomes/peripheral nerves. A working knowledge of muscular distribution of the nerve roots (myotomes) and peripheral nerves enables the examiner to distinguish the motor loss caused by a root lesion from that caused by a peripheral nerve lesion (see Table 5-7). (See Table 5-8 and Fig. 5-9 for myotomal testing for the cervical spine and upper thoracic nerve roots.) The facial nerve (seventh cranial) supplies the muscle of facial expression, while the mandibular nerve (fifth cranial) supplies the muscles of mastication.
 3. Reflex testing. The following deep tendon reflexes are tested (see Fig. 11-24):
   a. C5–C6—biceps.
   b. C7—triceps.
 4. Sensory testing. Test sensation, particularly around the hand (Fig. 19-37) (see Chapter 5, Assessment of Musculoskeletal Disorders and Concepts of Management)

B. Mobility of the nervous system. The following neurodynamic tests may be performed in order to ascertain the degree to which neural tissue is responsible for the production of symptom(s).[34,66,169]
 1. Passive neck flexion. In the supine position, the head is flexed passively. The normal response would be pain free full ROM. Sensitizing tests include the straight leg raise (SLR) or one of the upper limb tension tests (ULTTs). When symptoms are related to cervical extension, investigation of passive neck extension is included.
 2. ULTTs. These are described in Chapter 11, Shoulder and Shoulder Girdle.
 3. SLR. Although an integral part of the lumbar spine, the SLR should also be considered a routine neurodynamic test for the cervical spine.
 4. Slump test. The slump test is described in Chapters 20, Thoracic Spine, and 22, Lumbar Spine. The most commonly useful variation of the test for the cervical

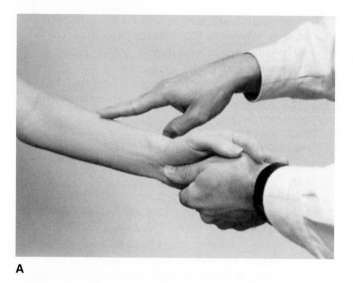

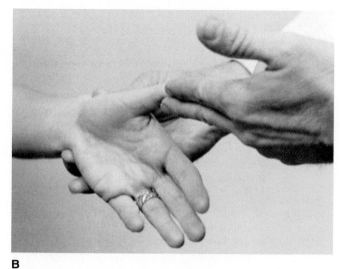

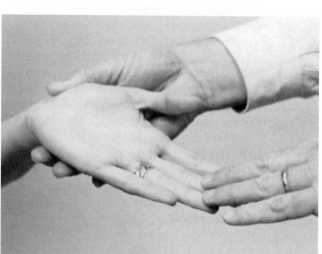

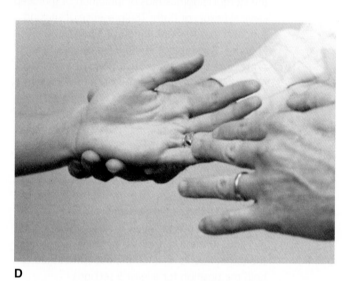

■ **FIG. 19-37.** Sensory testing of the dermatomes of the hand. (**A**) C5, (**B**) C6, (**C**) C7, and (**D**) C8 sensory areas.

and thoracic spine involves performing it in long sitting (see Fig. 20-34). The desensitizing tests may include cervical extension or one of the ULTTs.

C. Foraminal compression (Spurling test).[253] A progression of three stages, each of which is increasingly provocative is recommended with this test.[25] If symptoms are produced one does not proceed to the next stage. In the first two stages, the examiner carefully compresses straight down on the head in neutral (Fig. 19-17) and extension. If no symptoms were provoked in the first two stages, Spurling's test is performed. Spurling's test involved an axial compression loading, which is manually applied at the end of all four quadrants to fully open or close in the intervertebral foramina and stress the disk. It is only used if the patient does not report any arm symptoms before the examination; otherwise compression is applied only in neutral. Neck flexion,

combined with side-flexion away from the pain tests the integrity of the disk (Fig. 19-38A). Neck extension, combined with lateral flexion to the painful side, tests for foraminal encroachment. A test result is classified as positive if pain radiates into the arm toward which the head is flexed during compression: This indicates pressure on the nerve root (cervical radiculitis). The dermatome distribution of the pain and altered sensation can give some indication as to which nerve root is involved. Apply traction to the neck and watch for improvement of referred pain or neurologic symptoms (Fig. 19-38B).

VII. Palpation

The examiner palpates the cervicothoracic spine, the temporomandibular joint and musculature of the jaw (see Figs. 17-23 through 17-28), thoracic spine and any other relevant areas. The following structures should be care-

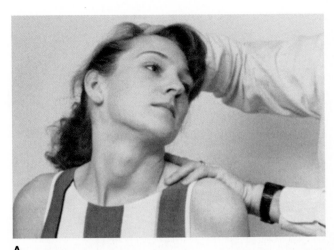

A

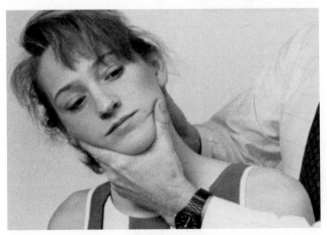

B

■ **FIG. 19-38.** Foraminal compression (Spurling's) test. **(A)** Compression test. **(B)** Distraction test.

fully palpated for guarding, spasm, and particularly to see if deep palpation reproduces pain referred to another area.

A. Trapezius—Palpate inferior, middle, and superior portions (Fig. 19-39A).
B. Levator scapula—Palpate particularly close to the origin
C. Multifidi—Should be palpated segmentally from C2–C7, particularly noting segmental guarding at the C4, C5, or C6 segments (Fig. 19-39B).
D. Lesser occipital nerve (Fig. 19-39C)
E. Greater occipital nerve and suboccipital musculature (Fig. 19-39D)
F. The sternocleidomastoid muscle (Fig. 19-39E)
G. The thyroid cartilage and longus colli muscle (Fig. 19-39F)
H. The suprasternal notch and sternoclavicular joint (Fig. 19-39G)
I. The acromioclavicular joint (Fig. 19-39H)
J. Simultaneous palpation of the sternocleidomastoid muscle (Fig. 19-40)

VIII. Special Tests
   Special tests that may need to be considered include:
   A. Carpal tunnel test (see Chapter 13, Wrist and Hand Complex).
   B. Tests for thoracic outlet syndrome. There are several tests for this syndrome, which are described in Chapter 11, Shoulder and Shoulder Girdle.
   C. Tests for thoracic pain of cervical origin.[161–163,166] See thoracic pain of cervical origin in Chapter 20, Thoracic Spine. Signs of cervical spine involvement include the presence of a painful unilateral point, precise and constant in the T5 or T6 region. Pressure with the thumb over the anterolateral portion of the cervical spine, maintained for a few seconds at the responsible cervical level, triggers the patient's thoracic pain.
   D. Pinch-roll maneuver of Maigne for headaches of cervical origin.[164–166] Maigne has found that occipitomandibular headaches of cervical origin typically present with a painful pinch roll maneuver of the eyebrow (see Fig. 7-42A) and the angle of the mandible (see Fig. 7-42B) on the same side of the headache compared with the opposite side. The anterior branches of C2–C3 supply the cutaneous area of the angle of the mandible. In these cases there is also unilateral articular sensitivity at the level of C2–C-3 or C3–C4.
   E. Tests to identify cervicogenic vertigo.[26,36,58,80,149] The following screen is a useful tool to determine the cause of the patient's dizziness. It should not take the place of a full neurologic exam.
      1. The patient attempts to follow the examiner's finger, using the eyes only. If dizziness is reproduced, it is the result of ocular incoordination.
      2. Ask the patient to close his or her eyes and shake the head from side to side as far and quickly as possible. Some patients will have minimal side to side movement because of pain. If vertigo is present, it may originate either from the vestibular nuclei or from the muscles and joints in the cervical spine.
      3. Rotating stool test. Instruct the patient to use his or her feet to rotate the entire body on the stool from side to side (Fig. 19-41). The patient is asked to keep the head still. The examiner stands behind the patient and cups the head to restrict its motion while applying slight traction to the head via the mastoid processes. The patient is instructed to close his or her eyes, while continuing to rotate the body from side to side. If the patient now experiences vertigo, it originates from the tissues of the cervical spine.[82]
      4. Rotation in standing. In a similar manner have the patient stand and rotate the body from side to side as the examiner stands behind the patient and stabilizes his or her head. This activates all the spinal, pelvic, and lower limb musculature. The working diagnosis of cervicogenic vertigo that was developed is founded

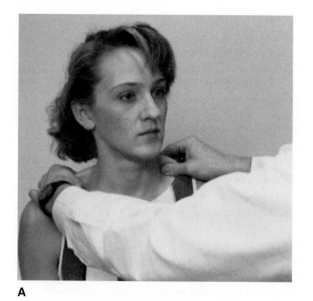

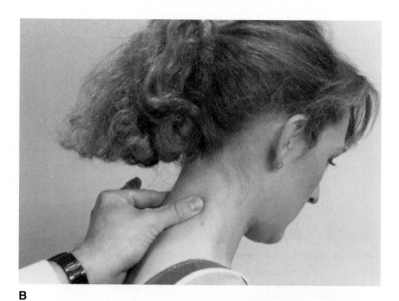

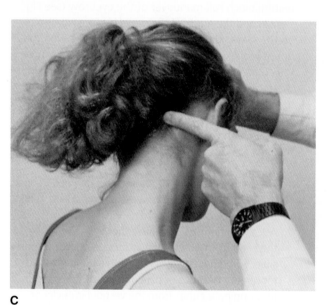

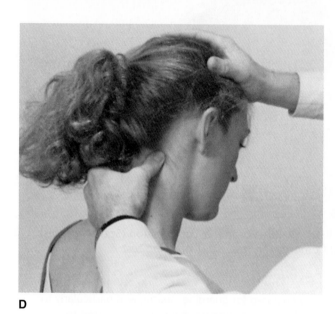

■ **FIG. 19-39.** Palpation of **(A)** the trapezius, **(B)** multifidi muscles (segmentally), **(C)** the lesser occipital nerve, **(D)** the greater occipital nerve and the suboccipital musculature

upon the report of a feeling of unsteadiness when standing or walking,[26] that can be induced by neck-body rotation with the head held stationary.

IX. Functional Tests

    A. Swallowing. Swallowing can contribute to instability of the cervical spine and persistent forward head. Examine the rest position of the tongue and the swallowing pattern (see Fig. 17-22).

    B. Breathing. Observe the patient's breathing pattern. Normal breathing is carried out primarily by the diaphragm. The shoulders and clavicle remain relaxed. With faulty breathing, the accessory breathing apparatus is utilized as the primary mechanism of breathing.

Contraction of the scalenes and sternocleidomastoids are used excessively on inhalation, with little or no movement of the abdomen and lower ribs. Although faulty breathing can place increased strain on the cervical spine owing to excessive activity in the accessory breathing muscles, the faulty pattern itself can arise as a result of joint or muscle dysfunction in the cervical spine.[189]

    C. Sit to stand. The movement pattern is very closely related to the cervical flexion pattern.[189] Observe the patient as he or she stands up from sitting. The normal pattern would be for the patient to lead with the posterosuperior aspect of the head. If the sternocleidomas-

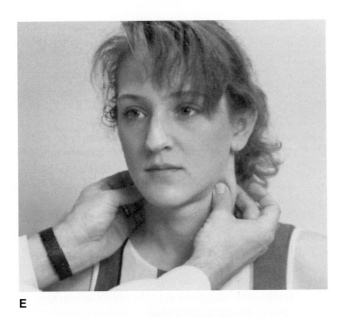

E

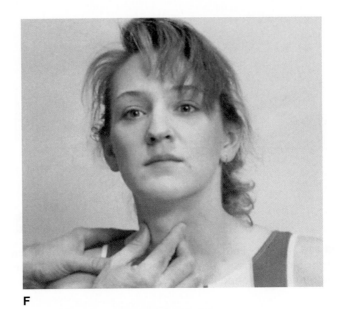

F

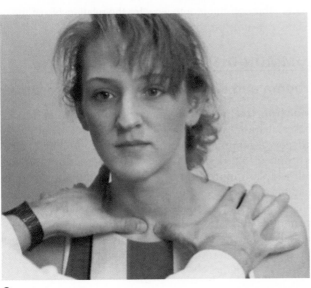

G

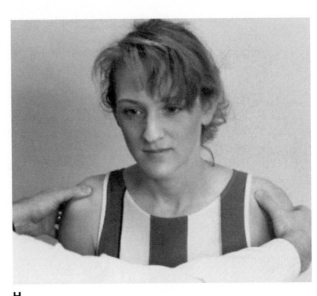

H

■ **FIG. 19-39.** (*continued*) **(E)** the sternocleidomastoid muscle, **(F)** the thyroid cartilage and longus colli muscle, **(G)** the suprasternal notch and sternoclavicular joint, and **(H)** the acromioclavicular joint.

toids or suboccipitals, or both, are dominant the patient will lead with the chin.

D. Postural foot reaction (Vele's test) The purpose of this test is to assess the automatic reaction of the intrinsic foot muscles to postural stress. This reaction is essential to maintaining stability of the locomotor system as a whole, and its has particular implications for the cervical spine.[123,189] For the nervous system to stabilize the head in space, it must be aware of the position of the head in space.[181–183,194] This requires not only the vestibular system, but also knowledge of the head position in relation to the trunk, which, in turn, is dependent on the knowledge of the position of the trunk to the ground.

To determine the position of the trunk relative to the ground, normal afferentation from the foot is essential. If there is dysfunction of the foot, this afferentation is compromised. Normal stability of the cervical spine is also dependent on a stable trunk in relation to the ground. The absence of normal stability reaction in the foot may be reflective of a disordered postural stability system as a whole.[201]

1. To assess postural foot reaction, the patient is standing and looking straight ahead. The examiner asks the patient to lean his or her body weight forward so the body weight shifts to the forefoot. An immediate reaction of the intrinsic muscles should occur

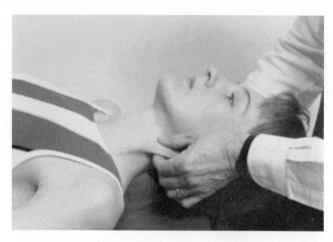

■ FIG. 19-40. Palpation of the sternocleidomastoid from its origin to its base. (Both sternocleidomastoids should be palpated simultaneously).

such that the toes flex at the distal interphalangeal joints.

   2. Abnormal findings. Anything that deviates from the normal is considered a faulty pattern. The common faults are:

     a. No reaction, with falling forward of the body.

     b. Flexion of the proximal interphalangeal joints with extension of the distal interphalangeal joints, creating a hammer toe position.

  E. Other functional test that may be considered is Revel's test, developed by Revel et al.[222] to evaluate the kinesthetic sensibility of the cervical spine and the stepping test to access the functional integrity of the tonic neck reflexes, as well as locomotor system afferent processing.[84,89,90]

X. Roentgenographic Analysis

A. Cervical curve. Normal or abnormal curvature.
   1. There should be a slight lordotic curve in the cervical spine.
   2. Note a straight or kyphotic spine suggesting spasms of the longus colli or overdevelopment of the anterior neck musculature.
   3. Ankylosis or instability on mobility films
B. Lipping or spurring of the vertebral bodies or uncinate processes indicating abnormal weight-bearing or degeneration of the disk.[100] Also note disk height (Fig. 19-42).
C. Intervertebral foramina. Look for opening on an oblique film. Note any narrowing or encroachment.
D. A 9- to 12-mm space between the ring of the atlas and the occiput. There should be a minimum of 9 to 12 mm of space visible on the x-ray film between the occipital bone and the posterior arch of the atlas. Less than 9 mm of space indicates extension of the upper cervical spine and possible compression of the neurovascular structures in the suboccipital area.
E. Through-the-mouth view for the relationship of the odontoid process to the adjacent bones.

COMMON DISORDERS

Trauma and Whiplash-Associated Disorders

Aside from fractures, discussion of which is beyond the scope of this chapter, a common clinical presentation of patients with cervical trauma is the whiplash syndrome. This term was introduced to describe the total involvement of the patient with whiplash injury and its effect.[116,158] The most common incident is the acceleration-deceleration injury after a motor vehicle accident. It usually results from the collision of two automobiles but also can result from contact sports such as football or high-velocity sports such as skiing. Whiplash associated injuries can result from all types of motor vehicle acci-

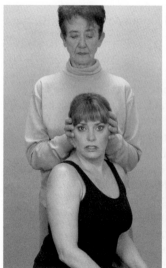 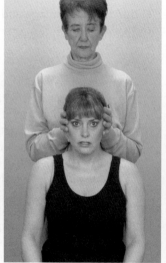 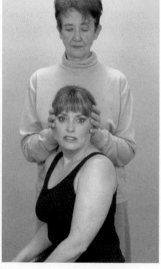

A   B   C

■ FIG. 19-41. A–C. Rolling stool test for cervicogenic vertigo. Patient rotates the body as the examiner holds the head steady.

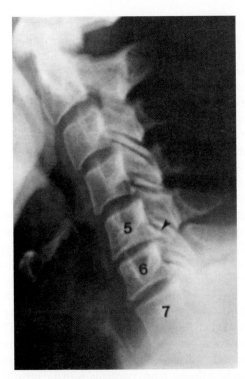

■ FIG. 19-42. Roentgenogram depicting posterior osteophytes in a patient with degenerative disk disease at the C5–C6 level. (Reprinted with permission from D'Ambrosia RD: Musculoskeletal Disorders: Regional Examination and Differential Diagnosis, 2nd ed. Philadelphia, JB Lippincott, 1986:256.)

dents, but the typical mechanism involves rear-end collision with neck hyperextension.[52,53,157,200] Rear-end collisions are responsible for about 85% of all whiplash injuries typically in the occupants of the vehicle that was struck.[52,214,215,244] At the moment of impact, the trunk of the body, which is supported by the car seat, moves rapidly forward. The moment of inertia of the head creates a relative backward acceleration of the head and neck.[244] Macnab[158] has reported that the rear-end collision hyperextension mechanism is significantly more likely to result in chronic soft tissue symptoms than flexion and lateral flexion injuries. Injuries include disruptions of the anterior longitudinal ligament, disk, or articular facet capsule, muscular strains (sternocleidomastoid, longus colli, scalene), retropharyngeal hematoma, intraesophageal hemorrhage, and cervical sympathetic chain reaction.[18]

The extent of damage seen in hyperflexion (head-on collisions) injuries is similar. Injuries include tears of the posterior cervical musculature, sprains of the ligamentum nuchae and posterior longitudinal ligament, articular facet joint disruption, and posterior intervertebral disk injury with nerve root hemorrhage.[6,22] Flexion at the atlantoaxial joint will stress the alar ligament complex as the atlas and head attempt to rotate anteriorly over the axis.[6]

Lateral flexion of the cervical spine between C2 and C7 is strictly coupled to rotation of the cervical disks. If an external

forces laterally flex the neck, the structures at risk of injury will be determined by the extent to which coupling occurs. If the force simply reproduces physiologic movements, the articular facet joint capsules on both sides and intervertebral disks will be most at risk from axial torque.[6] If there is little coupling, lateral flexion will compress the ipsilateral articular facet joint and distract the contralateral joint.

As with low back injuries, there is a natural history to acceleration injuries; 80% of patients reporting symptoms following a motor vehicle accident will be better within 3 to 4 weeks.[91,116,200] If this is so, are there any factors that would allow one to predict from the physical examination who the 20% will be who will not improve spontaneously? These questions have been partially answered by experimental animal research and longitudinal studies of patients injured in automobile accidents. In a study of 525 patients injured in automobile accidents, the **direction of the initial impact** was found to be an important predictor of prognosis. In this group, the 100 patients who were in cars involved in head-on collisions had no prolonged symptoms. The 200 patients for whom initial impact was from the side had lingering symptoms for a short period but no symptoms lasting more than a few months. Of the 250 patients in cars that were hit from the rear, 50% were still having symptoms 1 year after the accident.[157] The possibility of insurance compensation did not seem to be a factor in prognosis. Presumably, when the initial impact is from the front, the chin hits the chest before the cervical spine reaches its anatomical limit of motion. When the initial impact is from the side, the head hits the shoulder before the anatomical limit of ROM is reached. When the impact is from behind, however, unless the back of the car seat is high enough, there is no anatomical stop to prevent hyperextension. Other predictors of a poor prognosis are **roentgenographic evidence of degenerative joint disease** and **neurologic signs** soon after the accident.[200]

Other associated disorders following whiplash injury may include temporomandibular disorders,[11,28,47,48,87,103,109,147,228,242,270] whiplash induced headaches (posttraumatic headache),[4,5,47,74,137,174,205,214,229] spinal cord injuries,[75] traumatic brain injury and postconcussion syndrome. It is estimated that a velocity of only 20 mph can cause concussion for inertial loading (no head impact) for most healthy adults.[199]

Other common complaints following neck injury are reports of blurry vision, tinnitus, dizziness, or vertigo, either initially or in chronic stages.[160] Ryon and Cope[229] coined the term "cervical vertigo" in 1955 for this syndrome. It would appear that this form of dizziness results from disturbed sensory input from the mechanoreceptors of the neck. Sandstrom[236] found vertigo and postural nystagmus in about 20% of patients with cervicobrachial pain and cervical spondylosis. Dizziness and vertigo are reported by up to 80 to 90% of patients with chronic whiplash syndrome,[113,204] and in one study, 48% of consecutive patients and neck rotationally induced cervicogenic vertigo.[82] The physical examination of such patients usually reveals some neck muscle spasm and limited neck mobility. Cervicogenic dizziness is demonstrated best by rotational movements of the body, with the head stationary (Fig. 19-41).[57]

Fibromyalgia syndrome (FMS)[20,31,37,47,199,269,278] is a common posttraumatic diagnostic syndrome as well as thoracic outlet syndrome (cervicobrachial syndrome).[75,167,199,234,235] Several authors feel that FMS or myofascial pain is one of the most common causes of long term persistent pain following whiplash injuries.[76,146]

Although seat belts saves many lives they also leads to numerous osteoarticular restrictions of the anterior thorax, particularly the sternoclavicular and acromioclavicular articulations and ribs.[7] Seat belts and shoulder harness use have decreased the number of fatalities and serious facial and chest trauma but have significantly increased the number of minor and sometimes disabling cervical, thoracic, and lumbar injuries, as well as numerous types of abdominal and vascular injuries.[47,150,187] The primary reason that neck injuries are increased by restraint systems is because the shoulder harness abruptly restrains the decelerating trunk of the occupant while the head's inertia carries it forward unrestrained. This results in an exaggerated bending moment at the cervicothoracic region and is why, today the flexion injury is often as injurious or more so than the extension injury.[47]

CLINICAL CONSIDERATIONS: REAR-END COLLISIONS

Patients with injuries from initial impact from the rear should be followed more closely and should be considered to be at higher risk for having prolonged symptoms. Patients who have roentgenographic evidence of degenerative joint disease or neurologic signs soon after the accident must also be considered at higher risk and followed more closely. Acceleration injuries should be considered legitimate trauma with potential anatomic damage sufficient to cause the symptoms about which most patients complain. Muscle injury to the anterior neck must not be overlooked, particularly the sternocleidomastoid and deep anterior neck musculature.

Acceleration injury should be considered in three phases: acute, subacute, and chronic. The injury should be classified according to the findings from examination, rather than the length of time since the accident.

Acute Phase. The acute phase begins at the moment of the accident and may last as long as 2 to 3 weeks. The most severe injury is from a rear impact. As the head hyperextends on the trunk, the sternocleidomastoid muscle becomes tight and it is pulled or torn. With higher velocity impacts, the longus colli may be pulled or torn, the anterior longitudinal ligament may be pulled or torn, and the annulus of the disk may tear away from the vertebral body. The articular facet joints are hyperextended and their capsules may be strained or torn. There is generally little pain and fairly free ROM immediately after the accident, with painful stiffness gradually developing over 24 to 48 hours. There is a possibility of fracture, traction injury to the nerve roots, contusion to the spinal cord, head injury, or tearing of the supporting ligaments of the upper cervical spine. These conditions cannot be ruled out definitively without a roentgenographic evaluation. Consultation with a physician before mechanical treatment is wise.

Evaluation. The examination of the acute and recently traumatized neck is necessarily different from the routine examination because of the potential for the examination itself to be harmful. When possible, the patient should be examined for central and peripheral neurologic deficit, neurovascular compromise, and serious skeletal injury or craniovertebral ligamentous instability. The examination must be discontinued at the first signs of serious pathology.[179]

The patient will generally feel very little pain or stiffness immediately after the accident. As the large muscles swell and develop spasm, the patient will note onset of muscle soreness, stiffness, and swelling. The examiner may observe spasm of the sternocleidomastoid muscle, and the head will often be pulled into the forward-head posture. The skin may be red, and the muscles will be warm, rubbery, and tender to touch. Active ROM will be quite limited with muscle spasm end feel. Passive ROM will be greater than active. Joint play will be very difficult to assess because of muscle spasm. The sternocleidomastoid muscle will generally be warm, swollen, and in spasm. There may be palpable tears, particularly in the proximal third. There may be clearly delineated segmental spasm of the multifidi at the C4–C5 or C5–C6 level.

Treatment. The goal of treatment in the acute phase is to allow the cervical musculature to rest without becoming stiff and to progress to the subacute phase as rapidly as possible. Very little treatment is needed in the acute phase. Consider soft tissue techniques (e.g., soft tissue mobilization and strain/counterstrain) and joint mobilization (grades I–II) including specific traction with the intent of pain relief. The patient should be instructed in the use of heat or ice and supported postures at home and in the use of a soft cervical collar. The patient should also be instructed in active rotation of the cervical and thoracic spine, and upper limbs within limits of pain to maintain joint ROM. Mealy and colleagues[180] found that early active mobilization technique improved pain reduction and increased mobility compared with a control group receiving 2 weeks of rest with a soft cervical collar and gradual mobilization there after. The patient should be given an explanation of the mechanics of the acceleration injury, including the information that most cases are completely healed in 4 to 5 weeks. The patient should be encouraged to be as active as possible and should be rechecked at approximately 1-week intervals. Borchgrevink and associates[19] found that patients encouraged to continue with daily activities had a better outcome than patients prescribed sick leave and immobilization. The exercises are not intended to increase ROM. Consequently, they are gentle repetition within the pain-free range. Once a relatively pain-free passive ROM can be achieved, it is important to have the patient activate the cervical musculature to maintain motion. Active assisted range of motion (AAROM) can be accomplished with the patient in the supine position with the clinician supporting the head and assisting the patient to move through all planes of motion. Usually the easiest and most comfortable active exercise (AROM) the patient can perform independently is cervical rotation in supine with the head supported. A very effective and comfortable method to perform AROM is with the use of the Occipital Float (OPTP, Winnetonka, MN) (Fig. 19-43). Gradually AROM exercises can be performed on a foam wedge allowing non–weight-bearing motion, combing rotation and side flexion with flexion–extension. (Fig. 19-44). When the patient can perform a relatively pain-free ROM in all directions, weight-bearing movements can be added.

Subacute Phase. In the subacute phase, which usually lasts 2 to 10 weeks, the larger muscles have healed and are no longer swollen or tender. General muscle guarding will be reduced, and a more detailed evaluation of the cervical spine will be possible.

Evaluation. The patient will report that the muscle pain originally experienced has gone away but has been replaced by deep aching pain that may be referred to the head, the interscapular area, or the upper limbs. The large cervical muscles will no longer feel warm, rubbery, and swollen. There will be focal areas of intense tenderness in the sternocleidomastoid, suboccipital, multifidi, and deep anterior neck muscles. These areas of tenderness may refer pain to the head, shoulder, or upper limb when palpated. Active ROM will have increased considerably. The end feel will be capsular muscle guarding. If the articular facet joints have been injured, there will be capsular restriction of the neck with limitation of joint play when tested. The patient should be given a complete neurologic screening, which in most cases will be negative. The major muscle groups of the neck should be carefully palpated noting tenderness, guarding, spasm, or anatomical shortening. The longus colli should be carefully palpated. As the patient progresses through the subacute phase, the longus colli should become progressively less tender. Roentgenograms may show flattening of the cervical spine from spasm of the longus colli.

Treatment. The treatment goal in the subacute phase is to restore flexibility to the cervical muscle groups and articular facet joints, if they are involved. Mechanical treatment is most effective in the subacute phase because muscle guarding has subsided, and stretching and mobilization will be fairly comfortable, but adhesions between muscle and joint fibers will not have solidified into scars. Clinicians have many effective techniques for dealing with tight, painful muscles. The following principles will make treatment of the muscles of the cervical spine more effective:

1. The sternocleidomastoid muscles will be overshortened and very strong. Any strengthening program that increases the strength of the sternocleidomastoid musculature will contribute to muscle imbalance. In order to stretch the sternocleidomastoid, the head and neck must be put into an extreme of rotation and lateral flexion, which can be uncomfortable and can also be damaging to joints and smaller muscles. The sternocleidomastoid muscle can be easily treated by massage and soft tissue manipulations (see Figs. 8-44 and 8-45).

2. The most effective treatment for the longus colli and multifidi is to restore normal resting length (slight lordosis).[226] Retraining of motor control of the deep cervical flexor muscles (longus colli and longus capitis) can be facilitated with the use of a pressure biofeedback unit (Fig. 19-36).

3. Lordosis is a dynamic position and cannot be restored passively. Strengthening of the multifidi is the best way to restore cervical lordosis and to stabilize the midcervical spine. Multifidi strengthening through isometric exercise should be started as early as possible (see Figs. 19-61 through 19-63).

   The large posterior neck musculature should be strengthened but not stretched. These muscles need to be strong to counteract the anterior pull of the sternocleidomastoid muscle. Many of the muscles of the cervical spine are accessory muscles of respiration. They can be aerobically strengthened by any activity that increases heart rate above the target level. Aerobic training of muscle is very helpful in reducing lactic acid to carbon dioxide. Blood flow to muscle can be increased by a factor of one or two by massage, but by a factor of six with aerobic exercise.[13]

4. Sensorimotor training and cervical stabilization (see below) should be emphasized with the purpose of improving the

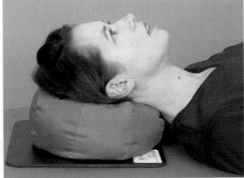 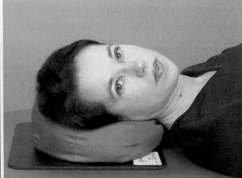

■ **FIG. 19-43.** Active range of motion exercises on an Occipital float. Allows early non weight-bearing rotation.   **A**   **B**

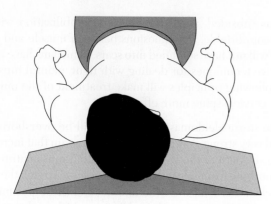

■ **FIG. 19-44.** Active range of motion exercises on a foam wedge. Allows non-weight bearing combined motions of the cervical spine. (Reprinted with permission from Hall C, Brody L: Therapeutic Exercise: Moving Toward Function, 1st ed. Baltimore, Lippincott Williams & Wilkins, 1998:535.)

efficiency and effectiveness of the common movement patterns in which the cervical spine and upper limbs engage on a regular basis. The ultimate goal is to bypass cortical involvement by creating a new automatic motor program by which the patient carries out movement correctly without having to think of them.[123]

In addition to muscle therapy, attention must also be directed toward the articular facet joints. The cervical articular facet joints are approximately the same size as the distal interphalangeal joint of the little finger. The capsule and ligaments are delicate, and the mechanical forces that the articular facet joints undergo in an acceleration injury are severe. Because the articular facet joints are so deep, swelling, warmth, and redness are not always apparent; however, the articular facet joints do go through the same stages that any acutely injured joint does. Mobilization or stretching that causes an increase in swelling will be harmful to the joint, because the presence of edema contributes to scarring. It is possible that overstretching or mobilization of swollen joints may lead to ankylosis or degenerative joint disease. Based on the information that we have about peripheral joint injuries, immobilization of injured joints also contributes to scarring.

The following guidelines are useful in treating the articular facet joints during the subacute phase:

1. During the acute phase, the patient should be instructed in active rotation within limits of pain to be done every hour (Figs. 19-43 and 19-44).
2. Joint mobilization in the subacute phase should not be painful to the patient or cause lingering discomfort after treatment.
3. Hypermobile areas should be identified and mobilization avoided.
4. Gross passive stretching of the head and neck should be avoided because of the possibility of overstretching hyper-

mobile segments. ROM should be restored by segmental joint mobilization (see Figs. 19-49 through 19-55) and gentle AROM exercises.

Chronic Phase. The chronic phase of an acceleration injury begins when the acute healing process is over. The large muscle groups will have completely healed, but they may be shortened and fibrotic. The longus colli may remains in chronic spasm and be acutely tender to palpation. The longus colli exerts a force that gradually flattens the cervical spine and may lead eventually to cervical instability. The multifidi at the C5 or C6 segment will be in constant contraction and may feel rubbery and inflamed as a result of overwork, in an attempt to stabilize the lower cervical spine.

Evaluation. The patient will complain of symptoms, which are consistent with irritation of the deep somatic structures. The pain will be deep, aching, vague, and often referred to the head, shoulders, interscapular area, or upper limb. It is very common to have a headache in the suboccipital area, which begins in the morning and gets gradually worse with the day's activity. The patient will have hypertrophy of the sternocleidomastoid muscles and may have parafunctional hyperactivity of the anterior neck muscles and muscles of mastication.

The patient often will have a forward-head posture with protraction of the scapula and superior angulation of the clavicles. Active range of motion of the neck may be limited by as much as 50%. Active and passive ranges of motion will be approximately the same. When tested segmentally, the upper and midcervical spine will be limited in a capsular pattern of restriction with segmental hypermobility of the C4, C5, or C6 segments. Neurologic testing will generally be negative, but there is the possibility of nerve-root irritation or thoracic outlet syndrome from shortening and hypertrophy of the scalenus muscles. On palpation there will generally be segmental guarding of the multifidus muscle at the C5 or C6 segment. There may be tenderness and spasm of the suboccipital muscles from overcontracting in a shortened position from the FHP. There may be tenderness of the greater or lesser occipital nerve from mechanical compression. The muscles of mastication should be carefully palpated if tenderness is present. A temporomandibular joint evaluation should be performed (see Chapter 17, Temporomandibular Joint and Stomatognathic System). The sternocleidomastoid muscle will be hypertrophied and may have palpable fibrous nodes. The longus colli will be acutely tender, particularly at the C4 through C7 segments.

Roentgenograms may begin to show flattening or kyphosis of the cervical spine. If retropharyngeal swelling is present, it may be seen along the anterior border of the cervical spine on the lateral roentgenogram. The intervertebral foramina will be open. There may be less than 8 mm of space noted on the lateral film between the occiput and atlas, indicating chronic extension of the upper cervical spine secondary to forward-head posture. If mobility films are taken, they may show hypermobility of C4, C5, or C6.

Treatment. The treatment approach in the chronic phase must be gradual. Rapid increases in ROM should not be expected because of fibrosis of joints. Muscles will respond well to gentle repetitive stretching, but attempts to overstretch will result in increased swelling and scarring. The emphasis of treatment must be to gradually restore cervical lordosis by mobilization into extension and specific segmental strengthening of the multifidus at the hypermobile segments. Normal muscle balance should also be restored by stretching the large anterior neck musculature, retraining motor control of the deep cervical flexors, and strengthening of the deep the posterior neck musculature.

Treatment of the acceleration injury in the chronic phase must be undertaken carefully and gradually, with a view not only to short-term symptoms but also to long-range outcome. A few precautions should be noted:

- Stretching of the posterior neck musculature, particularly by pulling the head into flexion, may give temporary reduction of muscular symptoms, but in the long run will contribute to cervical instability.
- The "chin-tuck" exercise (Fig. 19-45) may be helpful in stretching the suboccipital muscles, but it also completely flattens the curve in the cervical spine. When instructing a patient in this exercise, always give the precaution that it should be continued for no longer than 6 weeks.

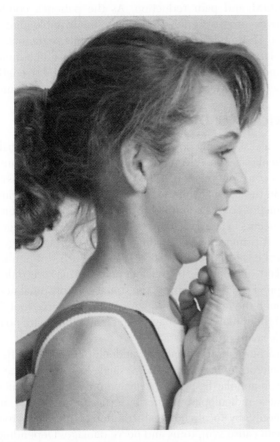

■ **FIG. 19-45.** The chin-tuck exercise.

- Strengthening exercises for the deep posterior cervical muscles should be light, as the multifidi are very small muscles. Reeducation of neuromuscular control of the deep neck flexors can be facilitated with the use of a pressure biofeedback unit (Fig. 19-36) and rhythmic stabilization (RS) techniques (see Fig. 19-64). Care should be taken in the exercise instruction to avoid strengthening of the sternocleidomastoid muscles and superficial neck flexors.
- Vigorous rotatory mobilization or passive stretching may overstretch segments that are already hypermobile, contributing to cervical instability.
- The patient should be encouraged to remain as active as possible and 20 minutes of aerobic activity should be a component of every treatment program.

Acute Locking of the Cervical Spine

Classically, acute locking of the cervical spine follows an unguarded movement of the neck, with instant pain over the articular pillar and an antalgic posture of lateral flexion to the opposite side and slight flexion, which the patient is unable to correct. Acute locking can occur at any intervertebral level but is most common at C2–C3.[98] Locking is more common in children and young adults. The literature to date reveals that authors are at variance when considering the underlying pathology, and the structure at fault, when spinal locking occurs. Some authors[46,50,98,104,178,261] suggest that either disk or apophyseal joint disorders may cause locking, while others[23,35,237,240] mainly implicate apophyseal joint disorders. Corrigan and Maitland[45] and Maitland[168] suggest that the problem within the intervertebral joint complex is owing to faulty mechanics.

The pathomechanical disorder of the disk is ascribed to the ruptures or tears of the annulus that enables the nucleus pulposus to ooze or extrude eccentrically[50,95,255] into theses breaches in the annulus, producing mechanical blocking to the movements on the side of the lesion. If the disk bulges anteriorly, it presses on the anterior longitudinal ligament and may cause spasm of the longus colli. The patient may have difficulty swallowing or have the sensation of a sore throat. If the disk bulges posteriorly, it may press on the posterior longitudinal ligament, the spinal cord, or the nerve root.

Postulated mechanical derangement of the apophyseal joint[178,237,261] include trapped or nipped synovial fringes, capsular tissue, villi or meniscoids,[23,95,144,145] trapped loose bodies, and mechanical sticking[256] of roughened and irregular arthrotic articular surfaces.

EVALUATION

Sudden onset of acute neck pain usually noticed early in the morning or else come on during a sudden unguarded movement during the day. The pain begins with clearly delineated, sharp neck pain and progresses during the day to generalized muscle spasm and inability to rotate the neck in one direction. The patient may be in acute distress. Both active and passive movements are found to be painfully limited. The usual pattern is restricted lateral flexion and rotation toward the painful side and loss of extension. An occasional variation of pain may be experienced at the end range of rotation and rotation to the opposite side.[45] ROM will be limited by pain and muscle spasm, with passive ROM usually considerably greater than active. The passive intervertebral movements and accessory movements are always found to be limited by pain and muscle spasms. Traction often makes the condition immediately more comfortable.

TREATMENT

These conditions generally resolve in a few days but if left untreated, there is an excellent treatment method described by Cyriax[50] that will provide greatly increased comfort and ROM for the first few days. This consists of placing the neck in as much extension as possible under fairly strong manual traction. ROM under traction is begun first to the pain-free side. When full ROM of the pain-free side is achieved, ROM under traction to the painful side is begun.[50] It is often wise to precede the mobilization or traction with ice or heat and soft tissue techniques to relieve the muscle guarding and spasm. Relaxation techniques directed towards the muscles in spasms should be performed and assessed.

Another excellent form of treatment is to apply muscle energy therapy. The cervical spine is the ideal area in which to apply muscle energy especially for acute or subacute problems involving muscle spasm (see Figs. 19-47 and 19-48).[193] It is very effective for problems that have a high level of irritability.

The patient should be instructed to avoid flexion of the neck. A soft collar will be helpful for the first few days. The patient should be reassured and encouraged to be as active as possible. When the acute symptoms subside, treatment for cervical instability should begin (see segmental stabilization section).

Cervical Zygapophyseal Joint Pain

Cervical zygapophyseal (articular facet) joints can be responsible for a significant portion of chronic neck pain, particularly in the upper cervical spine, where they can cause local neck pain and pain referred to the head.[261] Joints between C3–C7 can refer pain to the supraspinous process and into the arm.[2,60] If the patient has atlanto-occipital, atlanto-axial, C2–C6 zygapophyseal involvement, or a T4 syndrome,[34] the patient may experience headaches.[15,16,55] The atlanto-axial joint involvement may also cause ear pain.[55]

EVALUATION

Cervical zygapophyseal joint pain is typically unilateral and described as a dull ache. Limited range of cervical motion owing to soft tissue dysfunction and restrictions either diffusely or segmentally will be noticed by the patient or can be confirmed easily on examination.[42] Palpation just lateral to the midline often indicates regional soft tissue changes in response to the injured or involved zygapophyseal joint.[130] The spondylogenic reflex[55,59] may be responsible for the appearance of secondary zones of irritation with tender points or trigger points. Korr originally described this "facilitated segment" concept.[54,142,143] The affected tissues may be related to the dysfunctional articular facet, segmentally and sclerotomally.[55,59]

Occasionally the pain can be referred into the cranioverbral or interscapular regions and may mimic cervical disk disease or shoulder pain.[60] Osteoarthrotic changes (joint space narrowing, sclerosis and osteophytosis) may or may not be evident on plain radiography.[47] Rees[221] found these changes to be common features in his tomographic studies of 2,000 patients with cervical headaches. Patient history, mechanism of injury, pattern of painful and pain-free motion, and response to treatment are helpful in sorting out the source of pain (i.e., whether the source of pain is the cervical articular facet or the disk).

TREATMENT (SEGMENTAL ARTICULAR RESTRICTIONS)

Segmental articular restrictions generally respond well to manual therapy mobilization techniques unless there is excessive degeneration of the bony structures. Early on, grades I–II are used to relieve pain to the involved segments and grades III–V to hypomobile segments above and below. Specific traction may be performed at the involved segment(s). Other treatments may include soft tissue mobilization, strain-counterstrain and muscle energy or postisometric muscle relaxation therapy for ROM and pain reduction. As the patient's condition improves, progress graded traction to the irritable joints and graded II–V mobilization to the hypomobile segments. Self-articulations (mobilization) exercises are a useful adjunct to treatment (see Fig. 19-60) as well as self-resisted strengthening, active ROM exercises and cardiovascular conditioning.

Cervical Disk Dysfunction

Cervical disk dysfunction may cause symptoms similar to those of articular facet involvement and/or neurologic signs cause by root or cord compression. Although disk herniation is less common in the cervical spine than in the lumbar spine, various dysfunctions of the cervical disk do occur. Disk herniation typically occurs in a disk that has had some pre-existing degeneration. It primarily involves the 30- to 55-year age range and cervical levels of C5–C6, C6–C7, and C4–C5.[30] When radial annular tears coalesce; the nucleus pulposus may protrude into the spinal canal to compress the spinal cord or spinal nerves. Although the herniated disk may cause local nerve root damage of the spinal cord, it may also just cause pain with no neurologic symptoms.

Disk herniation can happen suddenly or insidiously. Repetitive microtrauma or an excessive single load occurrence may cause an annular fissure or herniated pulposus.[231] Herniation can cause radiculopathy either by local compression or, more commonly, by focal chemical irritation to the nerve root.[231] This can cause symptoms and nerve damage. Depending on the size and location of the lesions and the significance of any inflammation[231,232] or compression of local nervous or vascular tissue,[230] the patient may develop axial pain, referral zone pain,[49,51] radicular pain, radiculopathy, or even myelopathy if the spinal cord is compressed.

Chronic radiculopathy may develop because of progressive narrowing of the intervertebral foramen over time. Abnormal posture or trauma aggravates the symptoms and cause exacerbations.

The pain is usually unilateral and may be felt anywhere in the cervical or scapular area.[8,24,38] The pain usually starts in the cervical area and then diminishes and quickly extends in to the scapula, shoulder, upper arm, and then possibly the forearm and hand.[39] Patients with a herniated nucleus without radiculopathy will complain of increased pain with cervical extension or flexion and will usually experience relief with traction.[40,41,51,257]

EVALUATION

Radiculopathy will include radicular pain, paresthesia, and weakness in the appropriate myotome, as well as associated changes in reflexes. These findings may be subtle at times. In the acute stages, disk dysfunction can manifest with painful limitation of active ROM in all planes, pain on cough or sneeze, and painful cervical muscle contraction due to compression loading. The symptoms may be worsened by the Valsalva maneuver, with positional foraminal compression maneuvers (Fig. 19-38) and with cervical extension and rotation. The pain maybe relieved with cervical distraction (Fig. 19-18).

Diagnosis of cervical myelopathy owing to stenosis is made by the clinical picture (lower motor signs at the level of the cervical spine, upper motor neuron signs below this level), electromyography, and measurements of the diameter of the spinal canal through imaging studies.[30]

TREATMENT

In radiculopathy, early treatment involves resting the neck, which is achieved through education about proper resting positions to unload the compressive forces on the cervical spine. Aggravating activities such as straining, bending or lifting should be avoided. Stool softeners decreases the straining associated with bowel movements. A soft collar can help restrain the patient from aggravating movement and may give some support to the neck. Therapeutic modalities may be useful to help alleviate the inflammatory response and decrease muscle spasms. Diaphragmatic breathing exercises encourages an optimal breathing pattern and unloads the cervical spine. Soft tissue mobilization and joint mobilization (grade I or II) may be used with the intent of pain relief. Pain may also be relieved with specific traction at the involved segment performed in the position of comfort. Manual traction techniques seems to be better tolerated than is mechanical traction and help to decompress the disk and increase intervertebral space.[40–42,118,257,263] Self-positional traction may be used as a home technique (Fig. 19-59) Muscle energy cervical traction

(Fig. 19-57) and active joint mobilization techniques can also be used to mobilize and alter muscle activity at the involved segment (Figs. 19-48 and 19-54 through 19-55).

After a few days or weeks, gentle range-of-motion (avoiding excessive extension or extension/rotation) can be instituted. Joint mobilization may be progressed to grades III-V to appropriate cervical and upper thoracic segments. More vigorous exercises, including strengthening, stretching, cardiovascular conditioning and functional activities, are instituted over a period of 2-8, week as tolerated.[30] Stability testing at the affected segment may detect increased motion because of the disk's inability to control transitional forces in the spine. This impairment must be addressed with a progression of stabilization exercises (see Figs. 19-61 through 19-63). With a chronic cervical nerve root condition, it often necessary to assess neuromeningeal extensibility and to use ULTT as a form of treatment. For example, if there is no change in the ULTT following treatment to the intervertebral joint, one may choose to begin exercises to increase the mobility of this structure.

Mild, nonprogressive cases of cervical myelopathy can be treated similarly to radiculopathy. Gentle flexion exercises may help to open up the spinal canal. Most patients with conservatively treated cervical myelopathy see an improvement of their symptoms.[30] More significant cases benefit from early surgical decompression.[239]

It is important to point out the radiculopathy is pathology of the nerve root. Although commonly caused by disk herniation, the term is not synonymous with "herniated disk"; it can occur in the face of no disk pathology whatsoever.

Degenerative Joint Disease/Cervical Spondylosis

Degenerative joint disease is a chronic and commonly progressive degeneration of the cervical articular facet joints and/or the intervertebral disk (Fig. 19-42). The cause is unknown but may be accelerated by trauma, overuse, or genetic predisposition.[30] It is associated with heavy lifting, smoking, diving (from a board), and possibly with driving and operating vibratory equipment.[138] It preferentially affects the C5–C7 vertebrae and affects the intervertebral disk and the facet joints.[30] Degenerative joint disease must be considered a normal aging process. From in vitro studies[248] it has been noted that horizontal fissuring of the disk from the uncovertebral region begins in the first decade of life and is quite extensive by 20 to 30 years of age. In many cases, this degenerative process remains asymptomatic, but in others, symptoms develop spontaneously or after postures involving sustained extension or flexion.[261]

Lateral canal stenosis, which is frequently referred to as cervical spondylosis, is the second most common cause of cervical radiculopathy[277] and may cause symptoms of neck pain, shoulder pain, radiating pain in the arm, numbness in the extremity, or muscle weakness. These symptoms occur as a result of the degenerative process, which in part involves the development of hypertrophic spurs along the margins of the disk, the joints of Luschka, and along the articular facet joints.[190] This spur formation is often associated with hypertrophy of the ligamentum flavum. If the spurring continues, it eventually compresses the contents of the spinal canal. If it encroaches on the spinal canal, it is called central (or spinal) stenosis as opposed to narrowing of the intervertebral foramina as in lateral stenosis. Central stenosis can lead to cervical myelopathy, a condition of ischemic compression of the spinal canal. Lateral stenosis can result in radiculopathy.

In most people, degenerative joint disease is a painless process and occurs without consequence.[14,77] One of the paradoxes of degenerative joint disease is that the patient may have lateral stenosis for many years without symptoms and then suddenly begin to have neurologic signs and symptoms. After treatment with traction or passage of time, these signs or symptoms may resolve. Clearly the bony changes have not improved, so what accounts for the sudden appearance and disappearance of symptoms?

Pain from compression of nerve roots is complex. In an experimental study, ligatures were placed around nerve roots at the time of surgery so that pressure could be applied after the surgical incision had healed. When pressure was applied to the healthy nerve roots, there were no symptoms of pain or paresthesia. When pressure was applied to injured nerve roots, there was a gradual onset of anesthesia, diminished reflex, and eventually motor weakness. If, however, the nerve root was ischemic, very light pressure by the ligature produced immediate pain and paresthesia in the arm.[275,276] A model of nerve-root irritation then might be that some unusual activity, probably involving extension or sidebending of the neck causes the nerve root to swell. With impingement of the blood supply to the nerve root, it becomes extremely sensitive. When pressure is removed by traction or proper positioning, swelling of the nerve root diminishes, and the symptoms disappear. This would also seem to explain some of the complexities of peripheral entrapments. If the nerve root has slight compression and is ischemic, the nerve would be considerably more sensitive to pressure at the shoulder, wrist, or carpal tunnel.

EVALUATION

The diagnosis of degenerative spine disease is straight forward, because almost everyone older than 50 years of age has some evidence of it. It can be demonstrated on plain x-ray, computed tomography (CT), or magnetic resonance imaging (MRI).[30] The clinical picture varies considerably. Hypomobility of the lower cervical spine is common in all cases. This may progress to the stage at which loss of mobility interferes with daily activities; loss of extension and rotation make it difficulty to turn the head while driving. The patient will generally have a forward-head posture. Often stiffness of the cervicothoracic region causes the development of a kyphotic (dowager's hump) deformity. The pronounced kyphosis of the upper thoracic spine may cause the midcervical spine to increase its ROM. There will be capsular restriction of the lower cervical spine (limited active rotation and lateral flexion as well as extension) with possible ankylosis. The mobility of the upper cervical spine is generally quite good.

The stiff lower cervical joints may be a source of pain, which is often described as a burning pain across the base of the neck, or the mobile midcervical joints may become symptomatic, the typical complaint being central, deep midcervical pain.[261] Pain maybe experienced in the midcervical region.[38] Pain is worse in the morning and is improved with moderate activity. The area over the cervical facet joints may be tender to palpation. Compression testing worsens symptoms, whereas distraction may relieve them (Figs. 19-17 and 19-18). In most patients these symptoms and signs stabilize and lessen in time, as the spine becomes stiffer (but more stable).[30]

There may be diminished reflex, motor weakness, anesthesia, or muscle atrophy owing to osteophyte irritation and compression of the nerve roots.

TREATMENT

Conservative treatment is almost always successful in uncomplicated osteoarthritis of the neck. ROM exercises, nonsteroidal anti-inflammatory drugs (NSAIDs), and modalities such as heat and cold and cervical pillows are the mainstays of treatment. Many patients will respond well to cervical traction. In the case of nerve root pain positional traction is useful. The head is positioned in flexion and sidebending away from the painful side (Fig. 19-59) with reduction of symptoms being the best indicator of proper position. Mobilization of the hypomobile segments may reduce some of the mechanical forces on the involved segments of the lower cervical spine and the hypomobile segments of the kyphotic posture of the upper thoracic spine when present. Self-mobilization exercises are a useful adjunct to this treatment (Fig. 19-60). Segmental stabilization techniques are helpful for the hypermobile segments often found in the midcervical spine.

With a long-standing forward head posture, there is often an associated poking chin with posterior cranial rotation with adaptive shortening of the suboccipital muscles and weakness of the short flexor muscles group (see Fig. 17-19). One of the more common soft tissue manipulations used in myofascial release is the bilateral suboccipital release technique (Fig. 19-46), which releases some of the long and particularly the

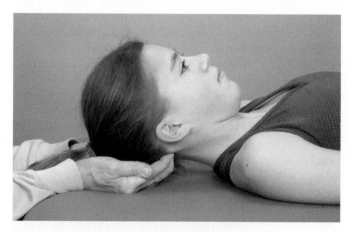

■ **FIG. 19-46.** Bilateral suboccipital release.

short muscles of the posterior cervical spine. Other soft tissue manipulations may be used for any myofascial restrictions. Specific training of the deep flexors may be necessary and consists of teaching the patient how to position his/her head and neck in a neutral position in supine, using towels under the occiput. Active or active assisted head-on-neck flexion (nodding) and extension can be practiced in this neutral position. The patient should be shown how to palpate for unwanted activity. This may be facilitated with the use of a pressure biofeedback unit to measure function of the deep neck flexors (Fig. 19-36). The patient should also be given instruction in activities of daily living to avoid long periods of extension. These may include thoracic extension exercises to improve back bending at the C5 through C7 segments, switching from bifocal glasses (which require extension of the neck to read) to reading glasses, and general avoidance of working above the head.

Cervical Instability

Stability is necessary for proper function of the kinematics of the spine. Many authors have identified common component of spinal stability.[13,110,188,209,210,265] Panjabi[207] conceptualized the components into three functionally integrated subsystems (passive, active, and neural control). Passive stability (passive subsystem) of the cervical spine comes from the tripod configuration of the two posterior facet joints and the anterior disk, capsules and spinal ligaments. When the cervical spine is in its normal rest position of slight lordosis, the cervical facet joints are engaged and bear approximately one third of the vertical compressive force. Very little muscle contraction is needed to maintain stability in this position. Passive stability may be lost as a result of an injury (see Trauma and Whiplash-Associated Disorder in this chapter) or may develop after years of poor posture or activities that involve flexion of the neck. If cervical lordosis is lost, the cervical facet joints disengage and are no longer capable of stabilizing rotational forces. The vertical compressive forces are shifted forward onto the disk, which gradually begins to lose height. Over time the annulus of the disk stretches out and weakens, and the vertebral bodies may show lipping and traction spurs as an attempt to compensate for increased vertical compressive forces (see degenerative joint disease in this chapter).

The active subsystem, which consists of spinal muscles and tendons, generates the forces required to stabilize the spine in response to changing loads. It is primarily responsible for controlling the motion occurring within the neutral zone (i.e., position of minimal passive resistance) and contributes to maintaining the size of the neutral zone.[202,206,207] Because of the large neutral zone in the cervical spine, much of the stability in this region is imparted by the dynamic control of the active muscular system. The spinal muscles along with the passive subsystem act as transducers and provides the neural control subsystem with information about vertebral position, motion and the forces generate by each muscle.[202] In the case of loss of integrity of the inert stabilizing structure,

training of neuromuscular control may result in a functionally stable spine.[140] With the loss of passive stability, the multifidus muscle must be in constant contraction to prevent overrotation or overflexion. The segmental muscle will progress from constant guarding to spasm and inflammation. The annulus of the disk is weakened, and there may be acute episodes of bulging of nuclear material, either anteriorly or posteriorly.

Strengthening exercises enhance the function of the active subsystem.[206,207] In the lumbar spine region, the multifidus and transversus abdominus play roles in spinal stabilization.[78,120, 131,224,225] The multifidus provides stability by segmental attachments to the lumbar spine, and the transversus abdominus provides anterior stability by increasing intra-abdominal pressure when contracted. It is hypothesized that an analogy can be made between the lumbar and cervical multifidus and the transversus abdominus and the longus colli and longus capitis muscle. Several authors have identified the particular role of these deep neck flexors, in the function of segmental and postural control.[43,173]

Patients with cervical instability have decreased cervical lordosis. Imaging studies may show facet subluxation, ligamentous damage, osteophytes, disk degeneration, and vertebral displacement.[83,206,207,219,246] They may have aberrant motions occurring in the mid-ranges of active cervical movements, chronic headaches (occipital and frontal or retro-orbital), neck pain, and shoulder or interscapular pain.[70,110,202,212] Patients may have asymptomatic periods and acute episodes of locking of the cervical spine that happen suddenly for no apparent reason.

EVALUATION

The patient may have a history of acceleration injury or an occupation that involves flexion of the neck such as office or laboratory work. Active and passive ranges of motion will be limited. The typical findings of a hypermobile C4 or C5 segment (when tested segmentally), is that the upper cervical spine and the segment(s) below C5 are restricted. The patient may have a forward-head posture but observation alone should not be relied on to determine cervical lordosis or compression of the upper cervical spine. There will generally be hypertrophy of the superficial anterior neck and anterior chest musculature and protraction of the scapula with elevation of the clavicles. The multifidi will be in segmental guarding or spasms and may feel rubbery or acutely inflamed. The sternocleidomastoid muscles are hypertrophied and may have localized areas of fibrosis that are acutely tender. The deep anterior neck musculature, particularly the longus colli will be in spasm and may be acutely inflamed. The assessment of motor control and stability should be carried out as described in the evaluation section of this chapter. The patient should be given a careful neurologic examination. Generally, results of neurologic tests will be negative. There may be nerve irritation from peripheral entrapment or a bulging disk but rarely from bony compression. Assessment of cervical spine segmental mobility by palpation (Fig. 19-35) and the craniocervical flexion test using a pressure biofeedback (Fig. 19-36) will reveal inferior performance. Unwanted contribution from the superficial neck flexors can be monitored clinically by palpation or measured with surface EMG.[128]

TREATMENT

The only effective conservative treatment for cervical instability is to restore the normal lordosis to the cervical spine. Posture correction exercises are an integral component of unloading the hypermobile segments in the cervical spine. This should be accomplished by mobilizing any restrictions of the upper and midcervical spine to restore ROM, segmental strengthening of the multifidi to hold the lordosis, followed by restoration of the muscular balance of the cervical spine. Strengthening of the longus colli muscle and longus capitis is imperative. Early on, the stabilization program is to isolate the short neck flexor using head nod exercises with progression for strengthening the longus colli with cocontraction of cervical extensor. Exercises can be progressed by integrating arm and leg motions while ensuring cervical stabilization (sees sensorimotor and cervical stabilization program below). As with chronic acceleration injuries, care must be taken when working with the neck to avoid strengthening the sternocleidomastoid musculature and to avoid stretching segments that are already hypermobile. The resting posture of the shoulder girdle also plays a role in imparting translational forces to the cervical spine and exercises should be developed to correct the impairments found on assessment of the shoulder girdle. Throughout this program, motion at the hypermobile segments must be controlled, particularly for excessive translation. Because of the large neutral zone of the cervical spine, much of the stability in this region is imparted by dynamic control of the active muscular system. Specialized muscle training and ergonomic instruction are important whether or not the hypermobility is symptomatic.

Cervical Headaches

Treatment of cervical headaches by manual and therapeutic methods has recently received a lot of attention in the literature.[9,71,92,121,124,126–128,132,172,195,197,198,220,243,264,271,273] Cervical headache (cervicogenic) is difficult to define and classify because of its distribution and character of symptoms, which are similar to those of other forms of headache. Cervical headache refers to headache arising from dysfunction or inflammation of the musculoskeletal structures of the upper cervical spine (i.e., the atlanto-occipital joints, atlanto-axial joints, C2–C3 zygapophyseal joints and disk, and the capsules, ligaments and muscle crossing these joint).[61,126] The pathogenetic mechanism of cervicogenic headaches is not well understood.[252] It is thought that the most common causes of cervicogenic headache are degenerative joint disease or trauma (e.g., whiplash injury) that is either sudden or gradual (repetitive occupational or postural strain).[16,251,260] Headache is the second most frequently reported symptom in the acute acceleration/deceleration injury.[47] It is almost invariably present with moderate to severe trauma to the cervical spine. Surprisingly, it is more common with low-velocity crashes than with more severe impacts.[174]

Clinicians may encounter other forms of headache (i.e., tension [muscle contraction], migraine, cluster, and temporomandibular headaches). The common factor among all of these forms of headache is that of a common relay for nociceptive transmission, the trigeminocervical nucleus. Bogduk[17] has described the trigeminocervical nucleus as a continuous column of gray matter extending through the brain stem to the upper three segments of the spinal cord. The trigeminocervical nucleus receives all the nociceptive afferents from the head and upper cervical spine.[17]

Other causes for cervical headache is involvement of the greater occipital nerve that supplies the posterior aspect of the skull as far forward as the vertex and extrasegmental headache. Entrapment of the greater occipital nerve (GON) can occur when the muscles that cross this joint compress it sufficiently or alter joint mechanics.[227] The GON commonly passes through the semispinalis muscle and in many cases the upper trapezius.[21] The symptoms of compromise of the GON are pain in the occipital, retroorbital, temporal, and parietal areas.

Extrasegmental headache (dural headache) results from compression of the dura at any cervical level.[203] The cranial and cervical dura are innervated, therefore, the dura can be considered a source of cervical headache.[15,17] The pain often radiates from the midneck up to the temples, the forehead and behind one or both eyes. According to Ombregt et al.[203] if, from this distribution, there is also downward reference of pain to the scapular area, the dural origin is clear. Signs and symptoms implicating the dura mater as a source of cervical headache tend to occur after traumatic injury to the nervous system (i.e., whiplash or an iatrogenic complication myelography, epidural block or lumbar puncture).[34]

EVALUATION

Typically patient with cervicogenic headache reports a dull aching pain of moderate intensity that begins in the neck and "spreading" forward. It is usually a unilateral headache or a headache that dominates on one side.[250] When severe, it may also be felt on the contralateral side, but to a lesser extent and may radiate behind one eye or both eyes. It never dominates on the contralateral side.[250] There are signs pertaining to the neck, such as reduced ROM in the neck, mechanical precipitating mechanisms, and ipsilateral shoulder/arm sensation or pain. Aggravating factors include certain neck movements, sustained postures (upper cervical extension), and abnormal postures. Cervicogenic headache sufferers have been shown to demonstrate weakness and loss of endurance of the upper cervical muscles and often exhibit a FHP.[268]

C0–1, C1–C2, and C2–C3 segments and the temporomandibular joint include the main musculoskeletal structures that may refer pain to the head and are the focal point of the physical examination.[17,126] Examination procedures include active, passive, and resistive movements and palpation to provoke symptoms or identify dysfunction that may cause a mechanical disturbance, resulting in tissue irritability. Assessment should include a postural assessment, manual examination of the cervical and thoracic joints, selected muscles lengths and activation and endurance capacity of the neck flexors and lower trapezius muscle. FHP is the most commonly described abnormality in cervicogenic headache patients[94,105,259,268] It is also necessary to screen the shoulders for ROM and to include an examination of jaw movements to identify any dysfunction of the temporomandibular joints or masticatory muscles.

The upper cervical joints are examined with passive physiologic and accessory movements for the amount and quality of movement and the reproduction of symptoms (see examination section earlier). The myofascia is important to examine as a direct source of pain with respect to traumatic injuries or myofascial trigger points. Common triggers associated with headaches are located in the upper trapezius, sternocleidomastoid, masseter, temporalis and other muscles of the face and neck.[249] Refer to Simons et al.[249] for details for each muscle. The myofascial system is also examined as an indirect contributor to headache symptoms by assessing length and strength. Imbalances of muscle length and strength may create mechanical stress on the other pain sensitive tissues. Strength and endurance of the upper cervical flexor muscles have been found to be less in headache groups[269] and are often associated with tightness or hypertonicity of the upper cervical extensors (i.e., sternocleidomastoid, suboccipitals, and upper trapezius). The pectorals are often tight with relative weakness of the middle and lower trapezius creating an imbalance of the shoulder girdle.[122]

Headaches resulting from dural irritation may continue despite manual treatment to address muscle and joint dysfunction. For headaches suspected to be of nervous system origin, all tension tests must be performed including straight leg raising, slump test and passive knee bend.[34] If the patient does not present with a headache, some of the tests may reproduce one.

Headache in this context is often related to sensory meningeal branches of vagus nerve, which are distributed in the dura mater covering the ipsilateral cerebellar cavity, with some fibers going to the lateral and occipital sinuses.[7] Other symptoms involving the vagus nerve may include difficulty swallowing, digestive problems such as heartburn, reflux and nausea, ringing in the ears, or heart palpations.[7,64] When organic cause cannot be found, it may because the soft tissues surrounding the vagus nerve have become restricted.

TREATMENT

The success of manual therapy treatment in the management of headache relies on accurate diagnosis of a cervical musculoskeletal origin to the headache. There is growing evidence to support the use of passive mobilization and manipulations in the treatment of cervical dysfunction associated with headache (see Figs. 19-28, 19-32–19-33, 19-49, 19-51A, 19-56A, and 19-57).[61,102,177,186,243,262] Treatment interventions should also target impairment of posture (see forward head posture below) and mobility. Mobility exercises may be performed as gener-

alized ROM exercises or designed to address the segmental mobility restrictions. Specific muscle stretches and soft tissue manipulation, particularly for the upper cervical extensors (Fig. 19-46), can address the myofascial restrictions and trigger points that may be contributing to the headache (see Box 8-7). Re-education of neuromuscular control of the deep neck flexors (using a pressure biofeedback unit) without dominant activity in the superficial neck flexors should be included. The goal of the exercise program is to reverse the impairments in the deep and supporting muscle system to enhance joint support and control.[126–128] Sensorimotor and kinesthetic training to retrain position sense and balance exercises may be necessary (see below).

Movements to mobilize the nervous system and interfacing structures (e.g., scalenes and the erector spine) should be considered in treatment for headaches suspected to have irritability of the dura.[34] Sensitizing maneuvers such as the slump test (see Fig. 20-34) can be used to maximally tense the dura from above and below. When involvement of the vagus nerve is suspected, elongation of the soft tissues in the front of the body may prove benificial.[7,27] This may include prone lying thoracolumbar extension (see Fig. 20-28) and tongue stretching.[27] In the comfortable supine position, the patient is instructed to stick out the tongue over the lower lip, as far as possible while at the same time gazing up and back as far as possible.

McKenzie's protocol in treatment of the cervical headache syndrome is similar for patients with derangement in that postural correction is performed along with sustained or repetitive movements in the preferred loading strategy indicated by the objective testing procedures (see Chapters 20, Thoracic Spine, and 22, Lumbar Spine).[107,177]

Another component of headache treatment is the identification of headache triggers. The autonomic regulatory systems of chronic suffers appears to be unstable.[195,271] Common headache triggers are caffeine, red wine and particular food products (e.g., cheeses with tyramine as a vasoactive substance). Other important triggers of headache are emotional stress and changes in sleeping patterns.[195]

Postural Disorders and Movement Impairments

Common postural syndromes of the cervical spine may be caused by facilitation of a spinal segment, neurologic or neurodevelopmental deficit, or direct biomechanical impairment affecting tissues remote from the impaired area.[58] Any or all of theses can lead to imbalances in the forces acting on the joint capsule, ligaments, muscle fascia, and nerve. The proximal or shoulder girdle crossed syndrome, muscle imbalance syndromes,[122,129] and FHP have been described earlier (see Chapters 7, Myofascial Considerations and Evaluation in Somatic Dysfunction; 8, Soft Tissue Manipulations; and 17, Temporomandibular Joint and Stomatognathic System) Although posture is affected by the whole of the axial skeleton, the cervical spine plays an important role in the control of posture. Any attempt to alter cervical spine posture must include an evaluation of the shoulder girdle, pelvis and thoracic spine (see Chapter 20, Thoracic Spine). Many of the involved muscles are multi-joint muscles, spanning all three regions. Changes in the length and strength of muscles of the shoulder girdle have a profound effect on the cervical spine and the shoulder complex.

TREATMENT

Treatment of the FHP should address muscle imbalances, loss of neuromeningeal extensibility, articular hypomobility, proprioception and sensorimotor deficits. Scapular control with retraining of the serratus anterior and lower trapezius should be incorporated into postural control and functional activities. Postural re-education with correction through pelvic position to upright neutral position adds in control of scapular position. In the forward head posture, the intrinsic neck flexors are elongated and usually test weak. During neck flexion, the activity of the extrinsic neck flexors (sternocleidomastoid and the scaleni) is dominant, and the intrinsic neck flexors do not exert counterbalancing control of the motion. To correct this imbalance, start with gentle active motions with lots of feed back (see cervical segmental stabilization techniques below).

Muscle imbalances as they relate to musculoskeletal pain syndromes of the cervical and thoracic spine have been described by Kendall et al.,[139] Jull and Janda,[129] McDonnell and Sahrmann,[175] and Sahrmann[233] (see Chapters 7, Myofascial Considerations and Evaluation in Somatic Dysfunction, and 8, Soft Tissue Manipulations). Two common cervical impairment syndromes described by McDonnell and Sahrmann,[175] in which cervical lordosis or the forward posture is common is the cervical extension and cervical rotation impairment syndromes. In both impairment syndromes the levator scapulae is usually dominant during neck extension. In individuals with elevated shoulder, the upper trapezius and levator scapulae are short, whereas in patients with depressed or downwardly rotated shoulders the upper trapezius is long. In these individuals, passive elevation of the shoulder by support under the forearm can help to alleviate the symptoms and is used as a confirming test for this syndrome. Exercises to improve the performance of the upper trapezius (see Fig. 11-72) and serratus anterior (see Fig. 11-76) are indicated.[233] Treatment should also include maintaining passive elevation of the shoulders for prolonged periods of time and practicing cervical rotation with the shoulders elevated. The primary purpose of this program is to decrease shoulder girdle muscle tension that restricts rotation and contributes to pain.

Local effects of FHP include[213]:

- Malalignment of the temporomandibular joint
- Hyperextension of the subcranial region causing compression and reduction of vertebral flow to the brain and brainstem.
- Hypermobility of the midcervical region cause by slackening the ligamentum nuchae
- Hypomobility of the upper thoracic region caused by locking it in forward bending

The posterior suboccipital muscle group can be lengthened and released by using the head nod exercise (Fig. 19-45), bilateral suboccipital release (Fig. 19-46), augmented postisometric relaxation (see Fig. 8-43), and specific stretching techniques to increase rotation and lateral flexion of the occiput on atlas and atlas on the axis (see Box 8-7).[56,67,249]

TREATMENT TECHNIQUES

Numerous manual therapy techniques are available to the clinician. These techniques can be used for hypomobility, hypermobility, instabilities, and soft tissue dysfunction.

For the sake of simplicity, the operator will be referred to as the male, and the patient as the female; (P = patient; O = operator; M = movement).

Myofascial Manipulations

Myofascial restrictions lend themselves well to soft tissue manipulations, stretching, strain–counterstrain, muscle energy, and postisometric relaxation techniques (see Chapters 7, Myofascial Considerations and Evaluation in Somatic Dysfunction, and 8, Soft Tissue Manipulations). According to Janda,[122] muscles that tend to become hypertonic are the temporalis, sternocleidomastoid, upper trapezius, rhomboids, masseter, suboccipital, levator scapulae, scalenes, and pectoralis minor and major. Myofascial restrictions most commonly occur between the neck and shoulder girdle, producing a raised shoulder posture, or between the neck and the upper thoracic spine, producing FHP. Treatment should include myofascial stretching techniques (see Figs. 8-43 through 8-45, 8-47 through 8-49, 8-52, 8-53, 8-58, and Boxes 8-6 through 8-8), posture re-education, and inhibitive distraction.

1. Bilateral suboccipital release and subcranial inhibitive distraction (Fig. 19-46).[56,196,212]

   P—Supine.

   O—Seated, the operator rests the back of the hands on the table and places the ends of the fingers of both hands on the inferior nuchal line of the patient's occiput. The fingers should be flexed at the IP joints to be oriented perpendicular to the posterior arch of C1. The palms of the hands are initially supporting under the occiput.

   M—The operator's shoulders are very slowly abducted so as to remove the palmar support from the occiput creating more pressure on the finger tips so that finally the occiput is entirely supported by the fingers. When the tissues are completely relaxed, long-axis distraction is applied. As the tension in the neck changes, the fingers take up the slack. The patient is encouraged to close her eyes and relaxation suggestion is used. Optimum time is usually 2 to 5 minutes.

   Comment: This procedure is effective in relaxing and releasing some of the long and particularly the short muscles of the posterior cervical muscles. These tissues are often responsible for nerve entrapment, encountered with FHP and with posterior cranial rotation (see Fig. 17-19A). This techniques is particularly valuable when treating patients with cervical headaches, craniofacial and craniovertebral pain.[56,196] Releasing of the soft tissue as well as decompressing of the atlanto-occipital joints frequently relieves difficult symptoms to treat such as tinnitus, dizziness, and blurred vision. It is often used as a preparatory treatment for other mobilization procedures.

Muscle Energy Techniques for Acute and Subacute Cervical Spine Problems[192,193]

The cervical spine is the ideal area, in which to apply muscle energy therapy or neuromuscular techniques especially for acute and subacute problems involving muscle spasm and for problems that have a high level of irritability (i.e., acute locking of the cervical spine [torticollis] or whiplash injury).[193,254] The objective of therapy is to relax the muscle at the affected level, increase its length and movement, and thus increase the range of movement of the joint. The contraction of the muscle should be synergized or reinforced by two simple functions: inspiration[151,152] and ocular movements (upward and towards the direction of activity of the contracting muscle). Alternatively the relaxation of the muscle is facilitated by looking downwards in the direction of which relaxation is desired. Two methods will be described: the standard contralateral method and ipsilateral method for muscles on the painful side exclusively.

1. Standard contralateral method (Fig. 19-47)[193]
   P—Sitting.
   O—Positions the neck at the pathologic motion barrier by passively flexing and rotating the head away from the painful side to the point of comfortable movement.

M—Place one hand on the side of the head opposite the painful side and push toward the direction of pain at the same time requesting the patient to resist this movement by pushing his or head gently into the operator's hand (Fig. 19-47A) The patient should be producing strong isometric contraction of the neck in rotation away from the painful side. During the contraction phase, the patient is instructed to inhale for 5 to 7 seconds (holding her breath) while looking upward in the direction of the contracting muscle.

After the contraction the patient is requested to relax (let go). As the muscle relaxes, the operator stretches the neck gently toward the painful side (namely rotation) while requesting the patient to slowly exhale and gaze downward in the direction of stretching (Fig. 19-47B) The procedure is repeated from the new starting position of the improved motion barrier. The sequence is repeated several times.

2. Ipsilateral methods.[193] In this method, after the neck is positioned to the painful limit the clinician achieves contraction of the muscles on that side by pushing the patient's head away from the painful side as the patient resists the movement. This causes the patient to contract the muscles directly responsible for the painful contraction (rotation or lateral flexion). In more chronic painful necks, a specific techniques directed at the painful segmental level can be performed as follows:
   P—Sitting.
   O—Stands behind the patient and grasps the lower two vertebrae at the painful level. The upper hand curves around the patient's head with the fingers resting on the caudal hand (fixating hand) (Fig. 19-48).
   M—The patient is instructed to rotate against the upper hand while inhaling and looking up in the direction of the

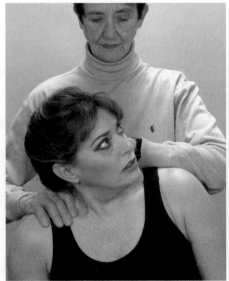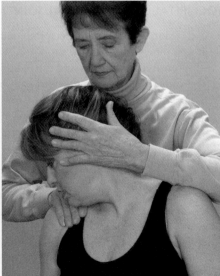

■ **FIG. 19-47.** Muscle energy therapy (standard contralateral method): **(A)** the contraction phase and **(B)** stretching phase.

A   B

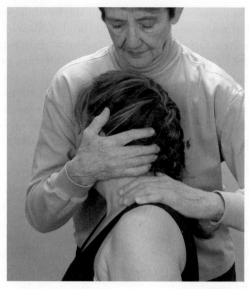

■ FIG. 19-48. Muscle energy therapy (a specific ipsilateral method) showing the contraction phase towards the painful left side against the resisting hand.

contraction for five to seven seconds against only mild pressure. As the patient exhales, the operator stretches the neck by rotating the head in the opposite direction to the contraction while the lower hand remains fixed.

Other combined movements may be used such as active proprioceptive neuromuscular facilitation (PNF) head and neck diagonal patterns For example, starting with left rotation and extension the patient actively moves into right rotation in and flexion. This can be used as a self-mobilization technique.

Joint Mobilization Techniques

CRANIOVERTEBRAL REGION (OCCIPITAL ATLANTO-AXIAL JOINT)

1. Extension at the atlanto-occipital joint (see Fig. 19-25A)
   P—Supine with the head supported midway between full extension and flexion and the head in a straight line.
   O—Stands at the patient's head and supports the patient's occiput dorsally. The other hand grasps the patient's chin with the forearm along the patient's face.
   M—The atlas is relatively flexed with bottom hand. The occipital condyles are moved by repetitive mandibular oscillations into extension.
   Comment: Note that Figure 19-25 is for evaluation of distraction of the atlanto-occipital joint. These same hand positions are used for extension mobilizations at the atlanto-occipital joint and manual traction of the upper cervical spine (occiput to C2–C3). To apply manual traction, the operator leans backward, thus moving the head in a cranial direction by a gentle longitudinal pull on the occiput and then followed by a controlled relaxation back to the starting

position. Most of the force exerted by the operator should be directed to the occiput not the mandible.

2. Flexion at the atlanto-occipital joint (Fig. 19-49).
   P—Supine with the occiput resting on a block.
   O—Stands at the patient's head. The operator stabilizes the atlas by a finger and thumb grip with the other hand placed on the patient's frontal bone.
   M—The operator flexes the cranium on the atlas by repetitive caudal oscillations on the patient's frontal bone.
   Comment: This technique can be used as an active mobilization by instructing the patient to hold her head still while the operator minimally releases the support of the cranium. This isometric contraction recruits the deep and superficial cervical flexors muscles. Full support is reapplied and the patient instructed to relax. The new flexion barrier is localized and the mobilization repeated two or three times.

3. Lateral flexion occipito-atlantal joint (Fig. 19-25B).
   P—Supine.
   O—The finger of both hands grasp behind the patient's occiput. The thumb on the side to which movement will occur rests along the body of the patient's mandible. The opposite hand rests across the patient's parietotemporal region.
   M—The head is tilted about an axis passing approximately through the patient's nose.

4. Transverse vertebral movement (rotational oscillations) of C1–C2. (Fig. 19-28)[169,193]
   P—Lies prone with the head turned approximately 30°.
   O—Stands at the head of the patient with both thumb pads placed against the articular pillar of C2. The long axis of the operator's thumbs is posteroanterior directed but tilted slightly toward the head.
   M—The oscillatory movement is transmitted through the thumbs. It is important to maintain a constant rhythm. Although the mobilization is created by a posteroanterior pressure against C2, it is in fact increasing the rotation between C1 and C2.

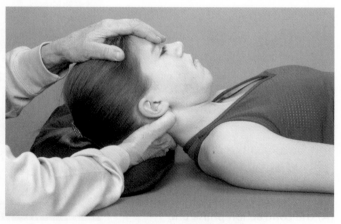

■ FIG. 19-49. Flexion at the occipito-atlantal joint.

Comment: This same position (or with the patient in sidelying) can be used to apply transverse vertebral movement of the atlas. Both of these techniques are very effective in the management cervical headaches. They are usually performed on the side of the restriction or pain. Other effective mobilizations and special tests found to be useful in restoring a loss of cervical C1–C2 rotation (often associated with headache of upper cervical origin) include "headache snags" (Fig. 19-32) and "reverse headache snags" (Fig. 19-33).[186] Other techniques include rotation mobilization of the atlanto-axial joint (see below) and upper cervical manual traction (see Figs. 19-56A and 19-57)

5. Rotation atlanto-axial joint (Fig. 19-26).
   P—Sitting, supported by a chair.
   O—Stand at the patient's side. With an open pinch grip of the dorsal hand, contact the posterior arch of axis. The other hand contacts the cranium.
   M—Fix the atlas and rotate the atlanto-axial joint.

Comment: See posteroanterior oscillation, lateral gliding/sidebending, and segmental traction below for additional techniques of the upper cervical spine.

MIDCERVICAL REGION

1. Posteroanterior vertebral central vertebral oscillations (PAs). Segmental flexion of the atlanto-axial joint and C2–C7 segments (Fig. 19-50).
   P—Prone, the head is positioned toward flexion.
   O—Stands next to the table, facing the P's head. The tips of both thumbs (with the nails back to back) are placed on the tip of the spinous process.
   M—Holding the thumbs in opposition, direct graded oscillations forward along the articular facet joint plane. Pressure is transmitted through the T's thumbs by movement of the trunk and arms. The depth and amplitude of the mobilization can be increase according to the response.
   Note: Posteroanterior central vertebral oscillations are of most benefit to those patients whose symptoms are situated either in the midline or distributed evenly to each side of the head, neck or upper trunk.[169]

2. Posteroanterior vertebral unilateral oscillations (PAs). Segmental flexion of the atlanto-axial joint and C2–C7 segments (Fig. 19-51).
   P—Lies prone, with two pillows under the chest and a small pillow under the forehead
   O—Stands next to the table, with thumb reinforced by a middle finger on the lamina of the joint to be mobilized.
   M—For the atlanto-axial and atlanto-occipital joints, oscillatory motion from grades I to IV should be applied in a direction perpendicular to the table (Fig. 19-51A). (The atlanto-axial, atlanto-occipital and facet joints are all oriented in the horizontal plane.) For C2 to C7 segmental flexion, the oscillation should be applied downward and forward at a 45° angle. (The lower cervical facet joints are aligned at 45° off the sagittal plane.) (Fig. 19-51B).

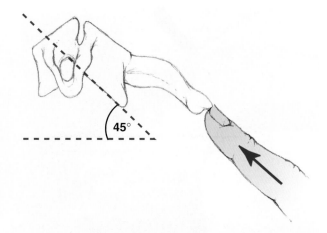

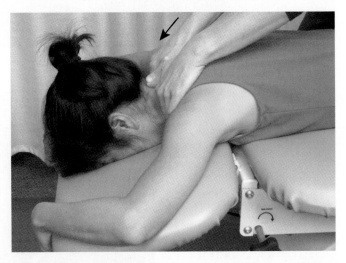

■ **FIG. 19-50.** Posteroanterior central oscillations (PAs) (segmental flexion of the C2–C7 segments).

3. Segmental extension of the C2–C7 segments (Fig. 19-52).
   P—Lie prone. The head is pre-positioned by extending it down to the level to be mobilized.
   O—Stands at the head of the table. The thumbs contact the facet joint or the spinous process as described for segmental flexion.
   M—Movement toward extension is performed by mobilizing backward about 45° from perpendicular, parallel to the plane of the cervical facet joint surfaces.

1. Transverse pressure (rotational oscillation). Rotational oscillations in prone C2–T3 (Fig. 19-53).
   P—Lies prone, with two pillows under the chest; forehead supported with a towel or the P's hands to establish the resting position of the cervical spine if conservative techniques are indicated or approximating the restricted range if more aggressive techniques are indicated.
   O—Stands beside table or at the patient's head facing the patient head, with thumb on the lateral side of the spinous process of the segment to be mobilized

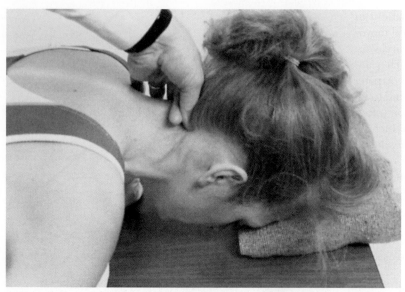

A

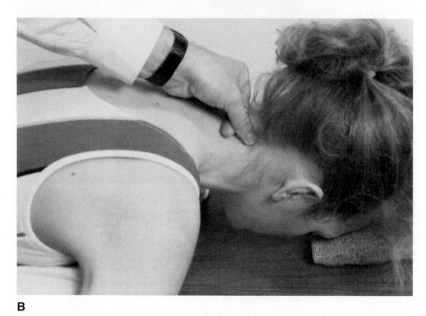

B

■ **FIG. 19-51.** Posteroanterior vertebral oscillations (PAs) (segmental flexion) of **(A)** the atlantoaxial, and **(B)** the C2–C7 segments.

M—The operator applies graded oscillating movements, from grades I–IV, in a direction to induce rotation of the segment.

Comments: Rotational mobilizations can employ both hands using one thumb to stabilize the caudal vertebra in position while the mobilizing hand glides the more cranial vertebra in a medial direction thus rotating and sidebending the vertebra being mobilized on the vertebra below it. (See Figs. 19-26 and 19-28 for rotational mobilizations of the atlanto-occipital joint.)

2. Rotational mobilization in sitting C2–T2 (Fig. 19-54).

P—Sitting, spine supported against a chair or the operators leg.

O—Standing at the patient's side with his arm supporting the patient's head with one hand. The stabilizing hand grips the more caudal vertebrae dorsally with the web space and laterally with the fingers The motion barrier is established by flexing down to the barrier (interbarrier zone), sideflexing and ipsilaterally rotating the joint complex to the physiologic limit.

M—As the stabilizing hand holds the caudal vertebra in position, passive mobilization is affected by the small finger of the mobilizing hand pulling in a rotational manner at the articular pillar of the superior vertebra while applying slight traction while the mobilizing hand rotates.

Comment: Pure rotation as a treatment technique is detrimental to the joint since this motion is unphysiologic. Active mobilization or muscle energy may be used by instructing the patient to hold the head still while the oper-

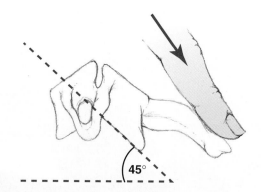

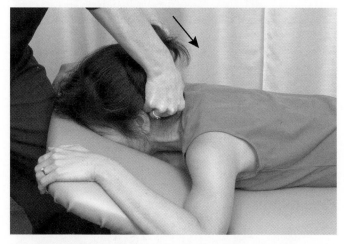

■ **FIG. 19-52.** Posteroanterior vertebral oscillations (segmental extension) of the C2–C7 segments.

ator applies gentle resistance to the cranium. The isometric contraction can be either toward or away from the desired direction and is held for 6 to 10 seconds followed by relaxation. The new barrier is localized and the mobilization repeated (three to six times). This technique can also be done with the patient supine.

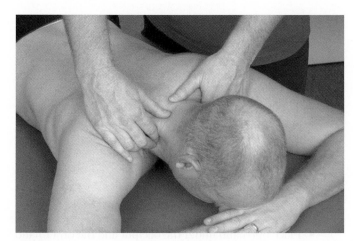

■ **FIG. 19-53.** Transverse pressures (rotational oscillations) in prone of the C2–T3 segments.

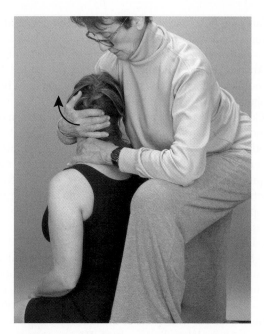

■ **FIG. 19-54.** Transverse pressures (rotational oscillations) in sitting of the C2–T3 segments.

3. Lateral flexion mobilizations C2–T3. Lateral flexion in sitting (Fig. 19-55).
   P—Sitting with the cervical spine in the resting position.
   O—Standing on the patient's side with the operator's arm supporting the patient's head. The stabilizing hand grips the more caudal vertebra with the web space and laterally with the fingers. The operator locks the more cranial vertebra by forward bending the neck or lateral flexing and/or rotating the neck to the same side as the direction of the mobilization to the extent that the motion segment above the one being mobilized is fully forward bent,

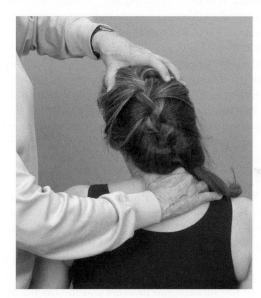

■ **FIG. 19-55.** Lateral flexion mobilizations C2–T3.

laterally flexed, and/or rotated, but the segment being manipulated has not yet moved.

M—The mobilizing hand laterally flexes the patient's head. An oscillatory movement produces the lateral flexion mobilization while the stabilizing hand acts as a fulcrum against the articular pillar.

Comment: Mobilization in lateral flexion is often underrated, but it can be a very effective technique. It can be used effectively when rotation is painful, combined with other movements, and be used as a specific or general technique. Muscle energy technique using an isometric contraction either away from the pathologic barrier or toward the pathologic barrier can be used.

4. Lateral flexion in supine C2–T3 (Fig. 19-27).

P—Lies supine

O—Sits at the head of the table, with the patient's head cupped in one hand and the web space of the other hand cupping below the facet joint of the segment to be moved.

M—The operator takes up the slack by sidebending the neck over the web space of the hand and applies oscillations into sidebending grades I–IV.

Comment: Cervical lateral glide mobilizations also uses the same basic position as cervical lateral flexion (in supine) as described above. The main difference between this technique and that in lateral flexion technique, the patient's head is carried to the side with the movement. This is accomplished by a shift of the operator's hips in the direction of the movement. In the lateral flexion technique, the head and neck actually tilt as sidebending occurs around the fulcrum created by the operator's index finger. When cervical dysfunction can be regarded as a cause of a neurogenic disorder or as a contributing factor that impedes natural recovery, cervical lateral glide mobilization has been found to have a positive immediate effect in patients with subacute peripheral neurogenic cervicobrachial pain.[44,266]

Manual Traction Techniques. Manual traction is infinitely more adaptable than mechanical traction, and changes in the direction, force, and patient position can be made instantaneously as the operator senses relaxation or resistance.[96,97,196,256] Cervical traction can be applied manually to the supine patient via a belt (modified car seat belt) or strap,[12,97,135] bath towel,[237,279] or cervical halter.[256] In most cases involving sprains and strains, simple manual traction used to produce a rhythmic longitudinal movement is very successful in reducing joint compression forces, and decreasing pain, muscle spasms, stiffness, and inflammation.

1. Supine cervical traction.

P—Variation of supine traction can be semi-specific for the three general areas of the cervical spine: upper, mid, and lower. As traction is applied for lower parts of the spine the neck should be flexed proportionally.

• The upper cervical spine (occiput to C2–C3). The head should be in slight extension to allow slackening of the suboccipital muscles and the nuchal ligament (Fig. 19-56A).

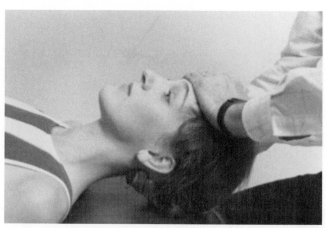

A

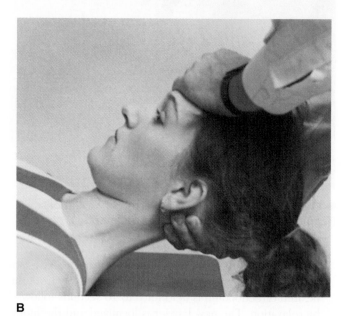

B

■ FIG. 19-56. Variations of manual traction (in supine) of **(A)** the upper cervical spine (occiput to C2–C3), and **(B)** the lower cervical spine (C5–C6 and C7–T1)

• The mid-cervical spine (C3–C4 and C4–C5). The head should be lifted off the table at an angle of 30° (not illustrated).

• The lower cervical spine (C5–C6 and C7–T1). The angle of the neck should be approximately 45° (Fig. 19-56B) The upper cervical spine is flexed, drawing the nuchal ligament tight and transferring the force to the lower cervical spine.

O—Stands at the head of the treatment table, supporting the weight of the patient's head in the O's hands. Suggestions include:

• Place one hand under the occiput and the other hand over the frontal region.

• Place the fingers of both hands under the occiput

M—Traction is achieved by using body weight, and not the arms. The operator applies force by fixing his arms isometrically as he leans backward in a controlled manner while gradually applying a gentle pull (3 to 5 lb) in a cephalic direction. The force is usually applied intermittently, with a smooth and gradual building up and releasing of the traction forces.

Comment: When traction is applied to the upper cervical spine, strong traction is not necessary. PIR (postisometric relaxation) is often the method of choice.[151] The operator simply cradles the head with both hands under the occiput and tells the patient to look up while breathing; when the operator see the scaleni and sternocleidomastoid automatically contract and feels resistance against the traction, the operator instructs the patient to hold her breath, and then to look down while breathing out and relaxing.

- Traction may be sustained (holding for several minutes) or intermittent (graded oscillations), depending on patient response. Although more difficult to "grade" than specific mobilization techniques, it is worth striving to do so.
- If a particular problem segment can be identified, then it should be positioned near its neutral range of flexion–extension. A palpating finger placed between the spinous processes of the dysfunction segment, while applying traction can be helpful to determine the angle of flexion when the separation occurs.
- Traction can also be localized by placing the web space of the hand at the desired level and laterally flexing the neck over the web space of the hand. A variety of head and neck positions can be used (e.g., head positioned in flexion and some neck rotation or flexed and laterally flexed to one side).
- Cyriax[49] often incorporated passive ROM with the cervical traction. This technique is used to distract the cervical vertebrae for brief periods to allow ROM or stretching to occur with less discomfort and through a greater ROM than is possible with ROM or stretching by itself.
- Satisfactory knowledge of cervical kinesiology and biomechanics and skill in joint mobilization is required when applying manual traction.

Sitting Traction. As with manual traction in supine, sitting traction can be performed in a variety of ways. It can be semi-specific to the upper and lower cervical spine or specific to selected level. Muscle energy and PIR methods can also be used.[151,193]

1. Manual cervical traction to the upper cervical spine (Fig. 19-57).
   P—Sitting on a low chair with the head in a neutral position.
   O—Stands behind the patient in the fall out position with all his weight on the forward leg and only toe touching the floor with the hind leg. The thenar eminence or

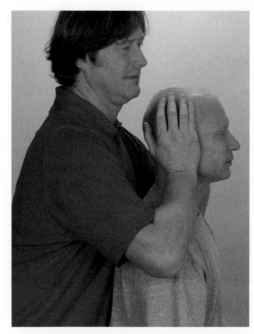

■ **FIG. 19-57.** Manual cervical traction to the upper cervical spine in sitting.

capitate is placed under the mastoid processes of the patient's skull with hand contact on the side of the P's face. The operator's forearms are placed on top of the patient's shoulders.
   M—The patient's body is drawn in close contact with the operator's body. Traction is applied upward with the head in neutral by rocking onto the hind foot. Traction is employed not by moving the elbows or hands but by the operator leaning backward.
   Comment: Muscle energy with coordination of breathing and eye movement is a very useful adjunct.[193] In the same positioning as above, the patient is asked to breathe in and look upward simultaneously (without extending the neck) as the operator holds the neck in a fixed position. The patient then exhales while looking down as the operator applies a gentle but firm upward stretch. This technique can be applied a number of times with traction being applied during the expiration phase.
2. Manual cervical traction to the mid–upper cervical spine (Fig. 19-58).
   P—Sits at end of table or chair.
   O—Stands in front of patient in the fall out position. The operator grasps the dorsal aspect of the patient's head with the ulnar sides of the hands under the mastoid processes. The patient's cervical spine is positioned in its resting position, which may involve some sidebending and rotation.
   M—Traction is applied by small backward movements of the operator's trunk. It is important to make only small excursions of movement.

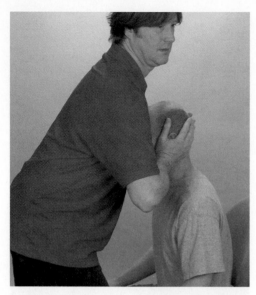

■ **FIG. 19-58.** Manual cervical traction to the mid cervical spine in sitting.

Positional Traction (Fig. 19-59)

1. This is a method of opening the intervertebral foramen by carefully positioning the head and neck.[212]

   P—Lies supine.

   O—Palpates the interspinous ligament at the segment to be distracted. The patient's head is elevated and supported by small blocks or pillows until the interspinous ligament at the desired segment becomes taut, indicating the segment has flexed. The operator then places a hand on the lateral portion of the desired segment and, taking care to keep the head flexed at the same level, laterally flexes the neck over the finger. The patient can rest indefinitely in this position.

   Comment: The primary value of positional traction is the traction force is isolated to a specific facet. This may be beneficial when selective stretching is necessary, as when the

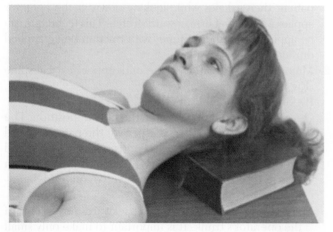

■ **FIG. 19-59.** Positional traction of the cervical spine.

segment above or on the contralateral side is hypermobile and should not be stretched. Manual or mechanical traction can be added to positional traction but the position itself is beneficial and can be used as a home treatment.

SELF-MOBILIZATION TECHNIQUES

Self-cervical traction,[62,133,186] self-articulations, auto-assisted exercises and self-stretching for joint dysfunction (see Box 8-7) have been advocated by numerous authors.[32,33,67,68,101,152,242] The patient is taught to localize the involved segment with her hand(s) using the ulnar border(s) to fix the lower vertebra of the segment to be treated or by using segmental locking techniques. To mobilize the atlanto-axial joint using ligamentous locking, the patient flexes the head fully to take up all the slack in the posterior longitudinal ligament and then actively rotates the head to the left and right (Fig. 19-60A). Muscle energy techniques can be used to facilitate further range. Localized occipito-atlantal joint (OA) flexion can be performed by having the patient rotate her head so as to lock atlas; she pulls the chin in to take up all the slack and while breathing out and looking down she moves into OA flexion (Fig. 19-60B). To mobilize into OA extension, she lifts her chin to take up the slack, looks up, and breathes in while moving into extension. When using the hands for segmental self-articulation both hands can be used to localize the segment (Fig. 19-60C–E, H) as the patient actively moves the head in the desired direction, or one hand can be used to localize the segment while the opposite hand passively moves the head in the desired direction (Fig. 19-60F, G). Unilateral extension techniques can be used for the OA (Fig. 19-60H) or midcervical extension (Fig. 19-60I). Self-headache SNAGS has been found to be invaluable in restoring loss of C1–C2 motion associated with headache.[186]

A very valuable technique for mobilizing the cervicothoracic junction is the combination of arm rotations in opposite directions while employing active cervical rotation (see Fig. 11-88). This technique can be carried out with the elbows flexed as illustrated in Figure 11-88 or with outstretched arms with the fingers spread while the arms rotate in an opposite direction; one arm supination into pronation as the other move in the opposite directions. The head rotates to the side that is pronating.

Cervical Segmental Stabilization Techniques

The management of a hypermobility is directed to limiting or minimizing joint movement in the excessively hypermobile direction through specialized muscle training, by increasing movement in the kinetically related joints, and taping or other supportive applications. It is common for the small one-and two joint spinal muscles (i.e., rotatores, multifidi) to be weak or atrophied at a hypermobile segment. This also includes the deep and short cervical flexors (see cervical instability above).

1. Training and strengthening of the multifidi muscle. Isometric strengthening of the multifidi muscle. This may be

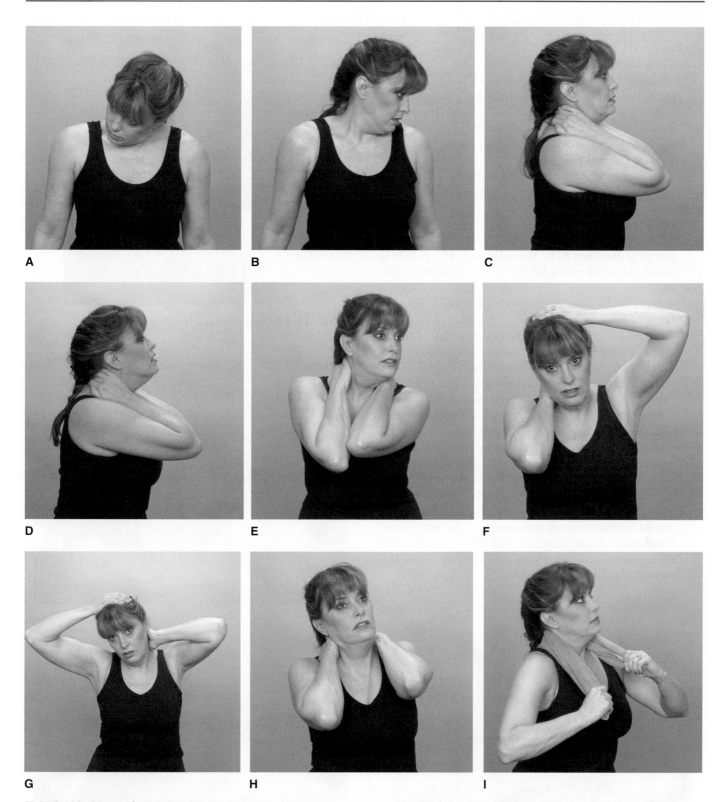

■ **FIG. 19-60.** Self-mobilization techniques. (**A**) Atlanto-axial rotation. (**B**) Occpito-atlantal flexion. (**C**) Backward cervical shift. (**D**) Forward cervical shift. (**E**) Segmental rotation (C2–C7). (**F**) Lateral flexion of the upper cervical spine. (**G**) Lateral flexion of the mid- and lower cervical spine. (**H**) Unilateral extension of the OA joint. (**I**) Unilateral extension of the mid-cervical spine.

performed by the clinician or taught as a home program (Fig. 19-61).

P—In a sitting position.

O—Stands behind and to one side. A hand is cupped behind the neck, forming a slight backward curve. Light pressure is applied to the back of the head. The patient is asked to hold. (Note: The pressure should be applied with one finger only to avoid the possibility of overworking the multifidus muscle.)

2. Specific segmental strengthening of the multifidi muscle. This may be done as a manual technique or taught as a home program (Fig. 19-62).[226]

P—In a sitting position.

O—Stands behind and to one side. One or two fingers are placed at the level to be strengthened. The patient is asked to extend and sidebend the neck over the fingers. The patient is asked to hold while the force is applied in the direction of flexion and sidebending to the opposite side. As progress is made, this exercise may be modified by having the operator give the command to "push" and allowing 10° or so of motion.

3. Antigravity strengthening of the multifidi (Fig. 19-63)

P—Lies prone, with head off the table. The top of the patient's head should be resting in the therapist's hand.

O—Sits at the head of the table with the patient's head resting in one hand, which is supported by the knee. The operator lifts the patient's head until a slight backward curve can be palpated. The operator gives the command to "hold" and allows the multifidi muscles to take some of the weight. As progress is made, the operator should allow the patient to accept more weight as long as the patient is strong enough to maintain a curve in the neck. (Precaution: If the patient's multifidus muscle is not strong enough to support the weight of the head, this exercise should not be done.)

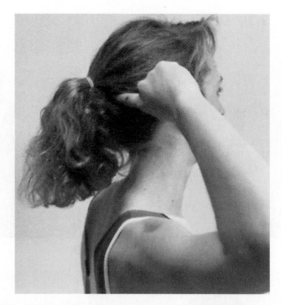

■ **FIG. 19-62.** Segmental strengthening of the multifidi.

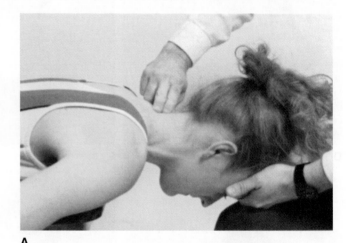

A

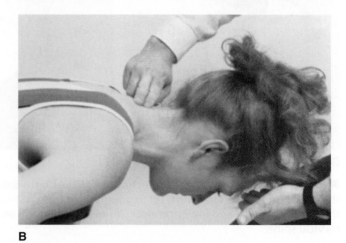

B

■ **FIG. 19-63.** Antigravity strengthening of the multifidi.

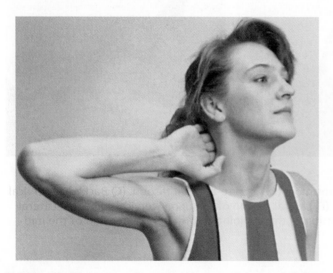

■ **FIG. 19-61.** Isometric strengthening of the multifidi.

TRAINING AND STRENGTHENING SHORT AND DEEP NECK FLEXORS

The primary exercise to recruit these muscles is the head nod exercise of craniovertebral flexion, continuing down into the midcervical flexion (see Fig. 19-45). It is important to control the tendency to excessively translate anteriorly during this exercise and not to substitute with the sternocleidomastoid. Assistance using a pressure biofeedback unit (Fig. 19-36) is often necessary until the correct patterns are learned. If the patient cannot tuck the chin and curl the neck to lift the head off the mat, begin the patient on a large wedge or slant board to reduce the effects of gravity. Progress by decreasing the angle of the board or wedge. In full supine, the muscles must work against gravity, making the exercise more difficult. At first, the head nod is performed with no lifting of the head off the pillow and progressed into 50% of the available craniovertebral forward bending motion. A small towel roll should be placed under the hollow of the midcervical spine to support the normal lordosis and to act as a fulcrum for active head nodding.[140] Head nodding into a flexion quadrant can be used in cases of asymmetric weakness. ROM can be gradually increased depending on the muscle strength and the ability to continue the head nod without excessive anterior translation.

Further progression includes training tonic endurance, cocontraction exercises of the neck flexors and low-resistance isometric rotation.[128] If the patient can not provide adequate resistance during manual resistance to the deep cervical flex-

ors and an alternate RS technique is often helpful. With this technique, a tongue depressor is placed in the patient's mouth and the patient instructed to gently bite down on it while pressing her tongue against it (Fig. 19-64).[191] The operator performs RS by gently pulling the tongue depressor out while the patient prevents chin poke.

The short neck flexors can also be trained in prone lying over a therapeutic ball or in four-point kneeling, in standing while superimposing arm motions, in supine (with no support of the head), and in prone lying (see cervicothoracic stabilization techniques below).

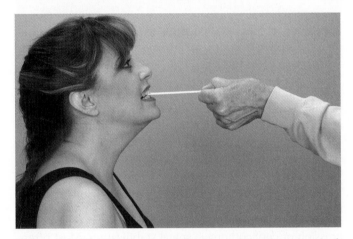

■ **FIG. 19-64.** Rhythmic stabilization of the deep cervical flexors using a tongue blade.

DYNAMIC CERVICOTHORACIC STABILIZATION TECHNIQUES AND SENSORIMOTOR TRAINING[123,191]

The purpose cervical stabilization techniques and sensorimotor training is threefold.[191] The first purpose is to improve the effectiveness and efficiency of the common movement patterns in which the cervicothoracic spine and upper limbs engage on a daily basis. The second purpose is to improve the efficiency of the reflexes that govern eye–head–neck–upper limb coordination. The third purpose is to improve certain key muscles involved in the stability of the cervical spine (see cervical segmental stabilization techniques above) and other strengthening and endurance exercises described in numerous texts.

The stabilization system of the cervical spine operates as an integrated system that encompasses the entire body. So when training this system, it is best to isolate certain parts of the system whose function may be impaired, followed by integrating these parts with the whole. Sensorimotor training as has been demonstrated in previous chapters, is a method of stimulating the central nervous system through the bombardment of afferent impulses to change the program for a certain

movement pattern from abnormal to normal. Sensorimotor training is designed to specifically correct altered programs, which may include compromised stability mechanisms but include other faulty movement patterns as well.[123,191]

DYNAMIC CERVICOTHORACIC STABILIZATION TECHNIQUES[140,141,191,258]

Cervicothoracic stabilization training focuses on balance of the neutral spine, restoration of segmental mobility, dynamic muscular control, and dynamic stabilization training. The components of training must therefore encompass mobility as well as stability. The early stabilization training is to isolate the short neck flexors and multifidi described earlier. The ability to cocontract the deep neck flexors and the scapular stabilizers (i.e., middle and lower trapezius and serratus anterior) is also a goal. Other important components that need to be addressed with regards to the stability of the cervical spine are the lumbar stabilizers (i.e., transverse abdominus, internal oblique,

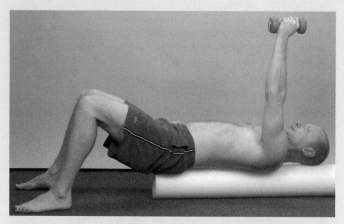

■ **FIG. 19-65.** Maintaining axial extension (cocontraction) on a half roll with overhead arm motion.

and multifidus) and pelvic stabilizers (i.e., gluteus maximus and medius) (see Chapters 20, Thoracic Spine; 23, Sacroiliac Joint and Lumbar–Pelvic–Hip Complex; and 24, Lumbosacral–Lower Limb Scan Examination). After the patient is able to maintain cocontraction of the anterior and posterior muscle of the cervicothoracic spine, exercises can be progressed by integrating arm movements while ensuring cervical stabilization by palpating the affected segments for translation. Advancing the exercise pattern, trunk positions, and resistance provides a progression of cervicothoracic spinal stabilization. Most often, because the most stable position is supine, it is used as the starting position with or without arm motions (Fig. 19-65). The same exercises as well as others can be progressed by having the patient do them in sitting and moving from sitting to a supine bridge position (Fig. 19-66). This later exercise is considered an advance exercise for strengthening the cervical and upper thoracic flexors and extensor as stabilizers.[141] Progression can be added by adding arm motions or arm motions with

weights. A variety of resistive and strengthening training exercises can be performed in standing, such as neck ball isotonic (Fig. 19-67) and isometric exercises (Fig. 19-68). RS can be applied in various trunk positions and quadruped for facilitation of specific stabilization responses, such as the deep cervical flexors and lower cervical/upper thoracic extensors and scapular stabilizers (Fig. 19-69). Therapy balls or foam rolls can be used at all levels of the program first by maintaining controlled cervical spine motions while performing simple rocking motions and advancing increased demands by adding arm motions with and without weights (Fig. 19-70).

To train and strengthen the muscles of the shoulder girdle that affect posture (particularly the forward head posture) emphasis is placed on the shoulder on the serratus anterior, scapular retractors and lateral rotators. See Chapter 11, Shoulder and Shoulder Girdle, for description of shoulder girdle exercises (see Figs. 11-71, 11-73, 11-76 through 11-78, and 11-81) and Chapter 12, Elbow and Forearm (see Figs. 12-31 and 12-32). The Brugger exercise[29] is an excellent shoulder girdle exercise to train the patient to facilitate the middle and lower trapezius and infraspinatus and inhibit the upper trapezius, levator scapulae, pectoralis minor and major (Fig. 19-71).[29] It is an exceptional exercise for improving spinal posture when done on a regular basis, particularly when sitting for long periods.[152–155,191]

SENSORIMOTOR TRAINING[123,191]

With sensorimotor training, an attempt is made to facilitate the autonomic, reflexogenic reactions that the locomotor system creates in response to unexpected stimuli from the periphery. The indications for the need for sensorimotor training is detection of a faulty movement pattern in which it has been determined that the central nervous system program for that pattern has been altered. In sensorimotor stimulation, an attempt is made to facilitate the proprioceptive system and those circuits

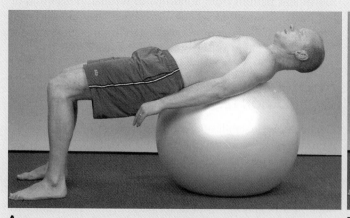

A

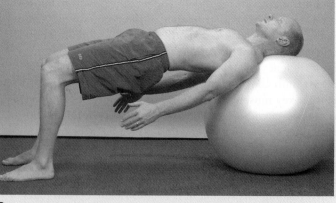

B

■ **FIG. 19-66.** Strengthening exercisers for the cervical and upper thoracic flexors and extensor as stabilizers. The patient begins by sitting on the ball, and **(A)** then walks forward while rolling the ball up the back to the mid-thoracic region. The patient continues walking forward until the ball **(B)** is under the head. The patient alternates control between the flexors and extensors.

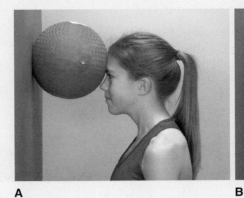
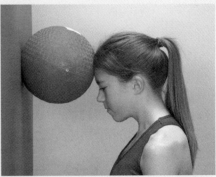

■ **FIG. 19-67.** Cervical ball isotonic exercises. **(A)** Starting position. **(B)** Capital flexion. Isotonic exercises can also be performed in axial extension (no capital extension).

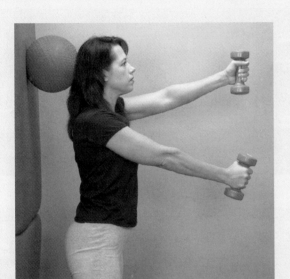

■ **FIG. 19-68.** Cervical ball isometric. Strengthening of the cervical and upper thoracic extensor muscles by maintaining control of the ball while varying the resistance and exercise pattern of the arms (e.g., unilateral arm movements, bilateral arm movements and reciprocal patterns).

that play a role in regulation of equilibrium and posture. From the point of view of afferent, receptors in the sole of the foot, from the neck muscles[1] and in the sacroiliac area have the main proprioceptive influence.[114] The foot is a very important source of sensory input to the central nervous system and appropriate afferentation from the foot is necessary for the proper elicitation of postural reflexes. The "small foot" exercise (see Fig. 14-46) described by Janda[123] is used throughout sensorimotor training. Repatterning activities include balance training as a way to increase or normalize joint and muscle afferent input, and trigger better-coordinated efferent responses. Balance activities attempt to challenge reorganization of the neuromuscular system to provide new behaviors that may be more efficient and preferable. Balance and coordination exercises include static and dynamic activities, on stable and unstable surfaces, on two or one leg, with and without visual input, and adding arm movements with or without weights and perturbations after the ability to maintain a quiet stance has been established. Using rocker boards (see Fig. 14-45C), wobble boards (see Fig. 14-45B) or training on balance shoes (see Fig. 14-45E) are ideal for these activities. Applying perturbations to the upper thoracic spine (Fig. 19-72) while the patient maintains

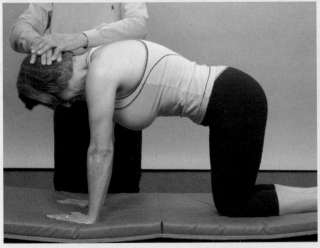
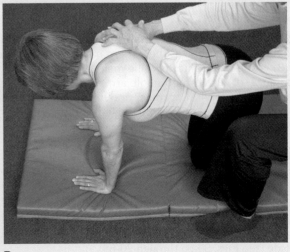

■ **FIG. 19-69.** Rhythmic stabilization for the **(A)** deep cervical flexors, and **(B)** serratus anterior in quadruped.

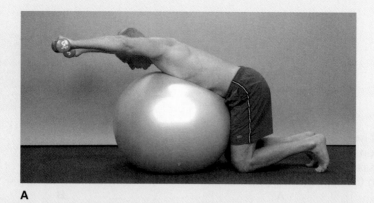

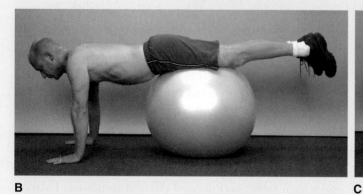

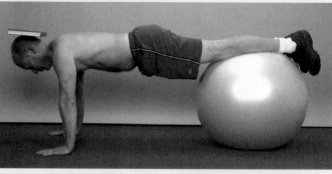

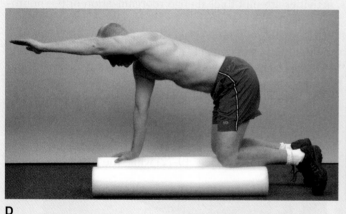

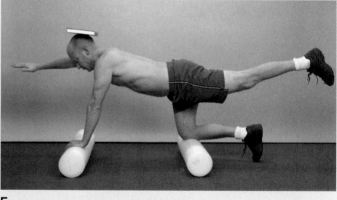

■ **FIG. 19-70.** Cervicothoracic stabilization training using therapeutic balls and rolls. **(A)** Developing cervicothoracic stabilization over a gym ball as the patient maintains the head and neck in neutral while arm motions provide varying resistance. **(B)** Prone ball walkouts while maintaining the cervical and abdominal brace position. **(C)** Prone static hold with book balance. **(D)** Quadriped single arm raise on foam rolls placed parallel. **(E)** Quadriped book balance as the patient maintains proper cervical, scapular and lumbar stability on foam rolls placed perpendicular (single arm raise, single leg raise or cross crawl [opposite arm and leg] can be added as illustrated).

balance on a wobble board can facilitate the deep cervical flexors.[191] Internal perturbations can be introduced via movements such as having the patient move the arms over head while maintaining a neutral head posture. Both internal and external perturbations can be stimulated in sequence by throwing an object such as a ball back and forth (see Fig. 16-65) or using a body blade (see Figs. 20-65 through 20-68).

Eye–head and neck coordination often must be trained in patients who have experienced cervical trauma.[79,81,156,222,223]

This involves all the mechanisms involved in coordination, which includes the visual, vestibular and somatosensory systems, which are essential to normal cervical function.[191] It has been demonstrated that these processes can become disturbed in cervical injury[6,88,111,112] and tension headaches.[36] Disruption to these reflexes can be corrected through sensorimotor training.[81,108,223] (See the works of Janda[122,123] and Murphy[191] for details of this training which is beyond the scope of this text.)

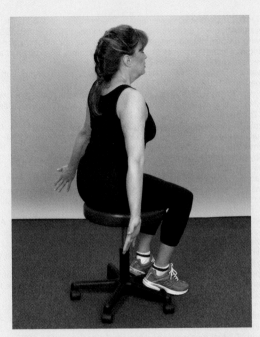

■ **FIG. 19-71.** The Brugger relief position. The patient sits on the edge of a chair with a neutral lumbar spine (the legs are abducted and in external rotation). The patient breathes in and then exhales slowly while at the same time he or she externally rotates the arms while spreading the fingers as wide as possible.

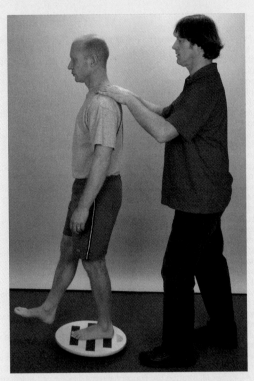

■ **FIG. 19-72.** Applying perturbations to facilitate stabilization responses in the deep cervical flexors.

There has been increased attention to the development of balance and proprioception in the rehabilitation and reconditioning of patients following cervical injury. It is believed that injury results in altered somatosensory input that influences neuromuscular control. If static and dynamic balance and neuromuscular control are not reestablished following injury, then the patient will be susceptible to recurrent injury. The inclusion of sensorimotor training and cervical stabilization can be instrumental in fully rehabilitating patients with cervical spine dysfunction.

REFERENCES

1. Abrahams VC: The physiology of neck muscles: Their role in head movement and maintenance of posture. Can J Physiol Pharmacol 55:332–338, 1977
2. Aprill C, Dwyer A, Bogduk N: Cervical zygapophyseal joint pain patterns. II: A clinical evaluation. Spine 15:458–561, 1990
3. Aspinall W: Clinical testing for the craniovertebral hypermobility syndrome. J Orthop Sports Physiother 12:47–54, 1990
4. Balla J: The late whiplash syndrome. Aust NZ Surf 50:610–614, 1980
5. Balla J, Karnaghan J: Whiplash headaches. Clin Exp Neurol 23:179–182, 1987
6. Barnsley L, Lord SM, Bogduk N: The pathophysiology of whiplash. In: Malanga GA, Nadler SF, eds: Whiplash. Philadelphia, Hanley & Belfus, 2002:41–77
7. Barral JP: The Thorax. Seattle, WA, Eastland Press, 1991
8. Bateman JE: The Shoulder and the Neck, 2nd ed. Philadelphia, WB Saunders, 1978
9. Beaton K, Jull G: Effectiveness of manipulative physiotherapy in the management of cervicogenic headaches: A single case study. Physiotherapy 80:417–423, 1994
10. Bell W: Temporomandibular Disorders. Classification, Diagnosis, Management. Chicago, Year Book, 1986
11. Bizzi E, Polit A: Characteristics of the motor program underlying visually evoked movements. In: Talbott RE, Humphrey DR, eds: Posture and Movement. New York, Raven Press, 1979:169–176
12. Blackburn J, Prip K: Mobilization Techniques, 2nd ed. Edinburgh, Churchill Livingstone, 1988
13. Blakney M: The cervical spine. In: Hertling D, Kessler RM, eds: Management of Common Musculoskeletal Disorder: Physical Therapy Principles and Methods, 2nd ed. Philadelphia, JB Lippincott, 1990:496–531
14. Boden SD, McCowin PR, Davis DO, et al: Abnormal magnetic resonance imaging scans of the spine in asymptomatic subjects. J Bone Joint Surg Am 72:1178–1184, 1990
15. Bogduk N: Cervical causes of headache. Cephalgia 9(Suppl 10):172–173, 1989
16. Bogduk N: Anatomy of headache. In: Dalton M, ed: Proceedings of Headache and Face Pain Symposium, Manipulative Physiotherapist Association of Australia, Brisbane, 1989
17. Bogduk N: Cervical causes of headache and dizziness. In: Boyling JD, Palastanga N, eds: Grieve's Modern Manual Therapy, 2nd ed. New York, Churchill Livingstone, 1994:317–322
18. Boon AJ, Smith J: Whiplash- associated disorders: Prognosis after injury. In: Malanga GA, Nadler SF, eds: Whiplash. Philadelphia, Hanley & Belfus, 2002
19. Borchgrevink GE, Kassa A, McDonagh D, et al: Acute treatment of whiplash neck sprain injuries. Spine 23:25–31, 1998
20. Borenstein D: Prevalence and treatment outcome of primary and secondary fibromyalgia in patients with spinal pain. Spine 20:796–800, 1995
21. Bovim G, Bonamico L, Fredriksen TA, et al: Topographic variations in the peripheral course of the greater occipital nerve. Autopsy study with clinical correlation. Spine 16:475–478, 1991
22. Bower KD: The patho-physiology and symptomatology of the whiplash syndrome. In: Grieve GP, ed: Modern Manual Therapy of the Vertebral Column. Churchill Livingstone, Edinburgh, 1986:342–349
23. Bourdillion JF: Spinal Manipulation, 5th ed. London, Butterworth-Heinemann, 1992
24. Brain WR, Northfield D, Wikinson M: The neurological manifestation of cervical spondylosis. Brain 75:187, 1952
25. Bradley JP, Tibone JE, Watkins RG: History, physical examination, and diagnostic tests for the neck and upper extremity problems. In: Watkins RG, ed: The Spine in Sports. St. Louis, Mosby-Year Book, 1996

26. Brandt T: Traumatic otolith vertigo. In: Vertigo: Its Multisensory Syndromes. London, Springer-Verlag, 1991:227–281

27. Brill PW: The Core Program, Fifteen Minutes a Day That Can Change Your Life. New York, Bantam Books, 2001

28. Brooke RI, Lapointe HJ: Temporomandibular joint disorders following whiplash. Spine: State of the Art Review 7:443–454, 1993

29. Brugger A. Die frunktionskrankheiten des bewegungsapparates. Funktionskrankheiten des Bewegungsapparates 1:69–129, 1986

30. Buschbacher RM: Head and neck. In: Buschbacher RM, Braddom RL, eds: Practical Guide to Musculoskeletal Disorders: Diagnosis and Rehabilitation. Boston, Butterworth-Heinemann, 2002:65–85

31. Buskila D, Neumann L, Vaisberg G: Increased rates of fibromyalgia following cervical spine trauma. A controlled study of 161 cases of traumatic injury. Arthritis Rheum 40:446–452, 1997

32. Buswell JS: A manual of home exercises for the spinal column. Auckland, Pelorus, 1977

33. Buswell JS: Exercises in the treatment of vertebral dysfunction. In: Grieve GP, ed: Modern Manual Therapy of the Vertebral Column. Edinburg, Churchill Livingstone, 1986:834–838

34. Butler DS. Mobilisation of the Nervous System. Melbourne, Churchill Livingstone, 1991

35. Caillet R: Neck and Arm Pain, 3rd ed. Philadelphia, FA Davis, 1991

36. Carlsson J, Rosenthal U: Oculomotor disturbances in patients with tension headaches. Acta Otolaryngol (Stockh) 106:354–360, 1988

37. Chester JB: Whiplash, postural control, and the inner ear. Spine 16:716–720, 1991

38. Cloward RB: Cervical discography: A contribution to the etiology and mechanism of neck, shoulder, and arm pain. Ann Surg 150:1052–1064, 1959

39. Cloward RB: The clinical significance of the sinuvertebral nerve. J Neurol Neurosurg Psychiatr 23:321–326, 1960

40. Colachis S, Strohm B: Cervical traction: Relationship of tractive force with constant angle of pull. Arch Phys Med Rehabil 46:815–819, 1965

41. Colachis S, Strohm B: A study of tractive forces and angle of pull on vertebral interspaces in the cervical spine. Arch Phys Med Rehabil 46:820–830, 1965

42. Cole AJ, Farrell JP, Stratton SA: Functional rehabilitation of cervical spine athletic injuries. In: Kibler WB, Herring SA, Press JM, eds: Functional Rehabilitation of Sports and Musculoskeletal Injuries. Gaithersburg, Aspen, 1998:127–148

43. Conley MS, Meyer RA, Bloomberg JJ, et al: Noninvasive analysis of human neck muscle function. Spine 20:2505–2512, 1995

44. Coppieters MW, Stappaets KH, Wouters LE, et al: The immediate effects of a cervical lateral glide treatment technique in patients with neurogenic cervicobrachial pain. J Orthop Sports Phys Ther 33:369–378, 2003

45. Corrigan B, Maitland GD: Practical Orthopaedic Medicine. London, Butterworth 1983

46. Crisp EJ: Disc Lesions. Edinburg, E & S Livingstone, 1960:106–110

47. Croft AC: Soft tissue injury: Long and short-term effects. In: Foreman SM, Croft AC: Whiplash Injuries: The Cervical Acceleration/Deceleration Syndrome, 3rd ed. Philadelphia, Lippincott Williams & Wilkins, 2002:335–428.

48. Curl D: Whiplash and temporomandibular joint injury: Principles of detection and management. In: Foreman SM, Croft AC, eds: Whiplash Injuries: The Cervical Acceleration/Deceleration Syndrome, 3rd ed. Philadelphia, Lippincott Williams & Wilkins, 2002:452–498

49. Cyriax J: Illustrated Manual of Orthopaedic Medicine. Boston, Butterworth, 1983

50. Cyriax J: Textbook of Orthopedic Medicine, 11th ed., vol. 2: Treatment by Manipulation, Massage, and Injection. London, Balliere Tindall, 1984

51. Davidson KC, Welford EC, Dixon GD: Traumatic vertebral artery pseudoaneurysm following chiropractic manipulation. Radiology 115:651–652, 1975

52. Dean G, McGalliard J, Rutherford W: Incidence and duration of neck pain among patients injured in car accidents. Br Med J 292:94–95, 1986

53. Dean GT, Maglliard JN, Kerr M, et al: Neck sprain–A major cause of disability following car accidents. Injury 18:10–12, 1987

54. Denslow JS, Korr IM, Krems AD: Quantitative studies of chronic facilitation in human motoneuron pools. Am J Physiol 150:229, 1947

55. Dreyfus P, Calodnex A: Cervical facet pain. Pain Digest 3:197–201, 1993

56. Dunn J: Physical therapy. In: Kaplan AS, Assel LA, eds: Temporomandibular Disorders. Philadelphia, WB Saunders, 1991:445–500

57. Dutton M: Whiplash-associated disorders. In: Dutton M, ed: Manual Therapy of the Spine: An Integrated Approach. New York, McGraw-Hill, 2002:524–536

58. Dutton M: Manual Therapy of the Spine: An Integrated Approach. New York, McGraw-Hill, 2002

59. Dvorak J, Dvorak V: Differential diagnosis and definition of the radicular and spondylogenic (nonradicular) pain syndromes. In: Manual Medicine—Diagnostics, 2nd ed. New York, Thieme, 1990:63–64

60. Dwyer A, Aprill C, Bogduk N: Cervical zygapophyseal joint pain patterns I: A study in normal volunteers. Spine 15–453–457, 1990

61. Edeling J: Manual Therapy for Chronic Headache. London, Butterworth-Heinemann, 1988

62. Edgelow PI, Neurovascular consequence of cumulative trauma disorders affecting the thoracic outlet: A patient centered treatment approach. In: Donatelli RA, ed: Physical Therapy of the Shoulder, 3rd ed. New York, Churchill Livingstone, 1997

63. Edwards BC: Combined movements in the cervical spine (C2–7): Their value in examination and technique choice. Aust J Physio 26:165–169, 1980

64. Edwards BC: Combined movements in the cervical spine (their use in establishing movement patterns). In: Glasgow EF, Twomey LT, Skull ER et al., eds: Aspects of Manipulative Therapy. Melbourne, 1985:128

65. Edwards BC: Manual of Combined Movements, 2nd ed. Oxford, Butterworth Heinemann, 1999

66. Elvey RL: Brachial plexus tension tests and the pathoanatomical origin of arm pain. In: Glasgow EF, Twomey LT, Scull ER, et al., eds: Aspects of Manipulative Therapy, 2nd ed. Melbourne, Churchill Livingstone, 1985

67. Evjenth O, Hamberg J: Muscle Stretching in Manual Therapy, vol. 2. The Spinal Column and the TM Joint. Sweden, Alfta Rehab Forlag, 1984

68. Evjenth O, Hamberg J: Autostretching. Sweden, Alfta Rehab Forlag 1997

69. Exelby L: Peripheral mobilisations with movement. Man Ther 1:118–126, 1996

70. Farfan HF, Gracovetsky S: The nature of instability. Spine 9:714–719, 1984

71. Farina S, Granella F, Malferrari G, et al: Headache and cervical spine disorders: Classification and treatment with transcutaneous electrical stimulation. Headache 26:431–433, 1986

72. Feinstein B: Referred pain from paravertebral structures. In: Buerger AA, Tobis JF, eds: Approaches to Validation of Manipulation Therapy. Springfield, Charles C. Thomas, 1977

73. Fielding JW: Sineroentgenography of the normal cervical spine. J Bone Joint Surg Am 39:1280–1288, 1957

74. Fishbone DA: A group of craniocervical acceleration/deceleration trauma patients who developed chronic post-traumatic headache. Eur Spine J 11:606, 2002

75. Foreman SM: Nervous system trauma. In: Foreman SM, Croft AC, eds: Whiplash Injuries: The Cervical Acceleration/Deceleration Syndrome, 3rd ed. Philadelphia, Lippincott, Williams & Wilkins, 2002:429–451

76. Friction JR: Myofascial pain and whiplash. Spine 7:403–422, 1993

77. Friedenberg ZB, Miller WT: Degenerative disc disease of the cervical spine: A comparative study of asymptomatic and symptomatic patients. J Bone Joint Surg Am 45:1171–1178, 1963

78. Fritz JM, Erhard RE, Hagen BF: Segmental instability of the lumbar spine. Phys Ther 78:889–896, 1998

79. Fritz-Ritson D: Neural mechanisms involved in the control of the eye-head-neck coordinated movement: A review of the literature with emphasis on future directions for the chiropractic profession. J Manip Physiol Ther 7:252–260, 1984

80. Fritz-Ritson D: Assessment of cervicogenic vertigo. J Manip Physiol Ther 14:193–198, 1991

81. Fritz-Ritson D: Phasic exercise for cervical rehabilitation after "whiplash" trauma. J Manip Physiol Ther 18:21–24, 1995

82. Fritz-Ritson D: Cervicogenic vertigo and disequilibrium. In: Murphy DR, ed: Conservative Management of Cervical Spine Syndromes. New York, McGraw-Hill, 2000:221–235

83. Frymoyer JW, Selby DK: Segmental instability: rationale for treatment. Spine 10:280–286, 1985

84. Fukuda T: Statokinetic Reflexes in Equilibrium and Movement. Tokyo, University of Tokuyo Press, 1984

85. Fukushima H, Hinoki M: Role of cervical and lumbar proprioceptors during stepping: An electromyographic study of muscular activities of the lower limbs. Acta Otolaryngol Suppl 419:91–105, 1985

86. Fukushima K, Fukushima J: Involvement of the interstitial nucleus of Cajal in midbrain reticular formation in the position-related, tonic component of vertical eye movement and head posture. In: Berthoz A, Graf W, Vidall PP, eds: The Head-Neck Sensory Motor System. New York, Oxford University Press, 1992:330–344

87. Garcia R JR, Arrington JA: The relationship between cervical whiplash and temporomandibular joint injuries: a MRI study. Cranio 14:233, 1996

88. Gimse R, Tjell C, Bjorgen I, et al: Disturbed eye movements after whiplash due to injuries to posture control system. J Clin Exp Neuropsychol 18:178–186, 1996

89. Gordon, CR, Fletcher WA, Jones GM, et al: Adaptive plasticity in the control of locomotor trajectory. Exp Brain Res 102:540–545, 1995

90. Gordon CR, Fletcher WA, Jones GM, et al: Is the stepping test a specific indicator of vestibular function? Neurology 45:2035–2037, 1995

91. Gotten N: Survey of one hundred cases of whiplash injury after settlement of litigation. JAMA 162(9):865–867, 1956

92. Graff-Radford SB, Reeves JL, Jaeger B: Management of chronic head and neck pain: Effectiveness of altering factors perpetuating myofascial pain. Headache 27:186–190, 1987

93. Grant R: Premanipulative testing of the cervical spine–Reappraisal and update. In: Grant R, ed: Physical Therapy of the Cervical and Thoracic Spine, 3rd ed. New York, Churchill Livingstone 2002:138–158

94. Griegel-Morris P, Larson K, Mueller-Klaus K, et al: Incidence of common postural abnormalities in the cervical, shoulder, thoracic regions and their association with pain in two age groups of healthy subjects. Phys Ther 72:425–431, 1992

95. Grieve GP: Common patterns of clinical presentation. In: Grieve GP, ed: Common Vertebral Joint Problems. Edinburgh, Churchill Livingstone, 1981:205–302

96. Grieve GP: Neck traction. Physiotherapy 6:260–265, 1982
97. Grieve GP: Belt traction. In: Grieve GP, ed: Modern Manual Therapy of the Vertebral Column. Edinburgh, Churchill Livingstone, 1986:716–718
98. Grieve GP: Common Vertebral Joint Problems, 2nd ed. Edinburgh, Churchill Livingstone, 1988
99. Grieve GP: Mobilization of the Spine: A Primary Handbook of Clinical Method, 5th ed. Edinburg, Churchill Livingstone, 1991
100. Greenfield GB: The joints. In: Greenfield GB, ed: Radiology of Bone Disease, 4th ed. Philadelphia, JB Lippincott, 1986:748–910
101. Gustavsen R: From active relaxation to training. Olso, Olaf Norlis Bokhandel, 1977
102. Hammill JM, Cook TM, Rosencrance JC: Effectiveness of a physical therapy regimen in the treatment of tension type headache. Headache 36:149–153, 1996
103. Hand TP: Injury to the temporomandibular joint. In: Swerdlow B, ed: Whiplash and Related Headaches. Boca Raton, CRC, 1999:693–704
104. Harris RI, Mcrab I: Structural changes in the intervertebral disk. J Bone Joint Surg Br 36:304–322, 1954
105. Haughie LJ, Fiegert IM, Roach KE: Relationship of forward head posture and cervical backward bending to neck pain. J Manip Physiol Ther 3:91–97, 1995
106. Hayashi K, Yabuki T: Origin of the uncus and of Luschka's joint in the cervical spine. J Bone Joint Surg Am 67:778–791, 1985
107. Heffner S: McKenzie protocol in cervical spine rehabilitation. In: Murphy DR, ed: Conservative Management of Cervical Spine Syndrome. New York, McGraw-Hill: 2000:641–661
108. Heikkila H, Astrom PC: Cervicocephalic kinesthetic sensibility in patients with whiplash injury. Scand J Rehabil 28:133–138, 1996
109. Heir GM: Mandibular whiplash. In: Malanga GA, Nadler SF, eds: Whiplash. Philadelphia, Hanley & Belfus, 2002:133–149
110. Herkowitz HN, Rothman RH: Subacute instability of the cervical spine. Spine 9:348–357, 1984
111. Hildingsson C, Wenngren B, Bring G, et al: Oculomotor problems after cervical spine injury. Acta Orthop Scand 60:513–516, 1989
112. Hildingsson C, Wenngren B, Bring G, et al: Eye mobility dysfunction after soft tissue injury of the cervical spine. A controlled prospective study of 38 patients. Acta Orthop Scand 64:129–132, 1993
113. Hinoki M, Hine S, Tada Y: Vertigo due to whiplash injury. In: Bustamante Gurria A, ed: Oto-Rhino-Laryngology. Proceeding of the Ninth International Congress. Amsterdam, Excerpta Medica, 1970:416–424
114. Hinoki M, Ushio N: Lumbosacral proprioceptive reflexes in body equilibrium. Acta Otolaryngol 330(Suppl):197, 1975
115. Hislop HJ, Montgomery J: Daniels and Worthingham's Muscle Testing: Techniques of Manual Examination, 6th ed. Philadelphia, WB Saunders, 1995
116. Hohl M: Soft tissue injuries of the neck in automobile accidents. J Bone Joint Surg Am 56:1675–1682, 1974
117. Hollinshead WH: Functional Anatomy of the Limbs and Back, 5th ed. Philadelphia, WB Saunders, 1981
118. Hooker DN: Spinal traction. In: Prentice Therapeutic Modalities for Allied Health Professionals. New York, McGraw-Hill, 1998:359–389
119. Hoppenfeld S: Physical Examination of the Spine and Extremities. New York, Appleton-Century-Crofts, 1976
120. Hides JA, Stokes MJ, Saide M, et al: Evidence of lumbar multifidus muscle wasting ipsilateral to symptoms in patients with acute/subacute low back pain. Spine 19:165–172, 1994
121. Jaeger B: Are cervicogenic headaches due to myofascial pain and cervical dysfunction. Cephalgia 9:157–164, 1989
122. Janda V: Muscles and motor control in cervicogenic disorders: assessment and management. In: Grant R, ed: Physical Therapy for the Cervical and Thoracic Spine, 2nd ed. New York, Churchill Livingstone, 1994:195–216
123. Janda V, Va Vrova M: Sensory Motor Stimulation. In: Liebenson C, ed: Rehabilitation of the Spine. Philadelphia, Lippincott Williams & Wilkins, 1996:319–328
124. Jensen OK, Nielsen FF, Vosmar L: An open study comparing manual therapy with the use of cold packs in the treatment of post-traumatic headache. Cephalgia 10:241–250, 1990
125. Jirout J: The rotational components in the dynamics of the C2-C3 spinal segment. Neuroradiology 17:177–181, 1979
126. Jull GA: Cervical headache: a review. In: Boyling JD, Palastanba N, eds: Grieve's Modern Manual Therapy, New York, Churchill Livingstone, 1994:333–347
127. Jull GA: Management of cervical headaches. Man Ther 2:182–190, 1997
128. Jull GA: Management of cervicogenic headaches. In: Grant R, ed: Physical Therapy of the Cervical and Thoracic Spine, 3rd ed. 2002:239–266
129. Jull GA, Janda V: Muscles and motor control in low back pain. In: Twomey LT, Taylor JR, eds: Physical Therapy of Low Back, New York, Churchill Livingstone, 1987:253–278
130. Jull GA, Bogduk N, Marsland A: The accuracy of manual diagnosis for cervical zygapophyseal joint pain. Med J Aust 148:233–236, 1988
131. Jull GA, Richardson CA: Rehabilitation of active stabilization of the lumbar spine. In: Twomey LT, Taylor JR, eds: Physical Therapy of the Low Back, 2nd ed. Edinburgh, Churchill Livingstone, 1994:251–283
132. Jull G, Trott P, Potter H, et al: A randomized controlled trial of exercise and manipulative therapy for cervicogenic headaches. Spine 27:1835–1843, 2002

133. Kabat H: Low Back and Leg Pain from Herniated Cervical Disc. St. Louis, Warren H. Green, 1980
134. Kaigle AM, Holm SH, Hansson TH: Experimental instability of the lumbar spine. Spine 20:421–430, 1995
135. Kaltenborn FM: The Spine: Basic Evaluation and Treatment, 2nd ed. Olaf Noris Bokhandel, Oslo, 1989
136. Kapandji IA: Physiology of the Joints, vol. 3: The Trunk and Vertebral Column. New York, Churchill Livingstone, 1974
137. Kash H, Stengaard-Pedersen K, Arendt-Neilsen L et al: Headache, neck pain and neck mobility after acute whiplash injury: a prospective study. Spine 26:1246–1251, 2001
138. Kelsey JL, Githens PB, Walter SD, et al: An epidemiological study of acute prolapsed cervical intervertebral disc. J Bone Joint Surg Am 66:907–914, 1984
139. Kendall FP, McCreary EK, Provance PG: Muscle Testing and Function. Baltimore, Williams & Wilkins, 1993
140. Kennedy CN: The cervical spine. In: Hall C, Brody LT, eds: Therapeutic Exercise: Moving Towards Function. Philadelphia, Lippincott, Williams & Wilkins, 1998:525–548
141. Kisner C, Colby LA: Therapeutic Exercise: Foundations and Techniques, 3rd ed. Philadelphia, FA Davis, 1996
142. Korr IM: The facilitated segment. In: Kent B, ed: Proceedings of the International Federation of Orthopaedic Manipulative Therapists. International Federation of Orthopaedic Manipulative Therapists, Hayward, CA, 1977
143. Korr IM, Thomas PE, Wright HM: Symposium on the functional implications of segmental facilitation. JAOA 54:265, 1955
144. Kos J, Wolf J: Intervertebral menisci and their possible role in intervertebral blockage. Bull Ortho Sec Am Phys Ther Assoc, Winter 1976
145. Kraft G, Levinthal S: Face synovial impingement. Surg Gynecol Obstet 93;439–443, 1951
146. Kraus H: Management of myofascial pain. In: Tollison CD, Saterthwaite JR, eds: Painful Cervical Trauma: Diagnosis and Rehabilitation Treatment of Neuromusculoskeletal Injuries. Baltimore, Williams & Wilkins, 1992
147. Kronn E: The incidence of TMJ dysfunction in patients who have suffered a cervical whiplash injury following a traffic accident. J Orofac Pain 7:209–213, 1993
148. Krueger BR, Okazak H: Vertebrobasilar distribution infraction following chiropractic cervical manipulation. Mayo Clin Proc 55:322–332, 1980
149. Kuilman J: The importance of the cervical syndrome in otorhinolaryngology. Pract Oto-Rhino-Larnyngol 21:227-281, 1959
150. Le Bourdais F: Cost of seat-belt–related whiplash injuries rising. CMAJ 160:1425, 1999
151. Lewit K: Manipulative Therapy in Rehabilitation of the Locomotor System, 2nd ed. Oxford, Butterworth-Heinmann, 1991
152. Lewit K, Kolar P: Chain reactions related to the cervical spine. In: Murphy DR, ed: Conservative Management of Cervical Spine Syndromes. New York, McGraw Hill, 2000:515–530
153. Liebenson CS: The Brugger relief position. J Bodywork Mov Ther 3:147–149. 1999
154. Liebenson CS: Self–treatment of the slump posture. J Bodywork Mov Ther 4:99–100, 2001
155. Leibenson CS: Micro-breaks. J Bodywork Mov Ther 6:154–155, 2002
156. Loudon JK, Ruhl M, Field E: Ability to reproduce head position after whiplash injury. Spine 22:865–868, 1997
157. Macnab I: Acceleration injuries of the cervical spine. J Bone Joint Surg Am 46:1797–1799, 1964
158. Macnab I: The whiplash syndrome. Orthop Clin North Am 2:389–403, 1971
159. Magarey ME: Examination of the cervical and thoracic spine. In: Grant R, ed: Physical Therapy of the Cervical and Thoracic Spine. New York, Churchill Livingstone, 2002:105–137
160. Magnusson T: Extracervical symptoms after whiplash trauma. Cephalagia 14:223–227, 1994
161. Maigne R: Sur l'origine cervicale de certaines dorsalgies rebelles et benignes. Ann Med Phys 1:1–18, 1964
162. Maigne R: Semeiologie clinique des derangements intervertebraus mineurs. Ann Med Phys 15:275–292, 1972
163. Maigne R: Fondamentos fisiopatologicos de la manipulacion vertebral. Rehabilitacion 4: 427–442, 1976
164. Maigne R: Un signe evocateur et inattendu des cephalees cervicales "la douleur au pince-roule du sourcil." Ann Med Phys 19:416–434, 1976
165. Maigne R: Orthopaedic Medicine, 3rd ed. Springfield, Charles C. Thomas, 1979
166. Maigne R: Manipulation of the spine. In: Rogoff JB, ed: Manipulation, Traction and Massage, 2nd ed. Baltimore, Williams & Wilkins, 1980:59–120
167. Mailis A, Papagapiou M, Vanderlinden RG, et al: Thoracic outlet syndrome after motor vehicle accidents in a Canadian pain clinic population. Clin J Pain 11:316–324, 1995
168. Maitland GD: Acute locking of the cervical spine. Aust J Physio 15:103–109, 1978
169. Maitland GD: Vertebral Manipulations, 6th ed. London, Butterworth, 2001.
170. Mannheimer JS. Prevention and restoration of abnormal upper quarter posture. In: Gelb H, Gelb M, eds: Postural Considerations in the Diagnosis and Treatment of Cranio-Cervical-Mandibular and Related Chronic Pain Disorders. St. Louis, Ishiyaku Euro America, 1991:93–161

171. Mannheimer JS, Rossenthal RM: Acute and chronic postural abnormalities as related to craniofacial pain and temporomandibular disorders. Dent Clin North Am 35:185–208, 1991

172. Martelletti P, La Tour D, Giacovazzo M: Spectrum of pathophysiological disorders in cervocogenic headache and its therapeutic indications. J Neuromusc Syst 3:182, 1995

173. Mayoux-Benhamou MA, Revel M, Vallee C, et al: Longus colli had a postural function on cervical curvature. Surg Radiol Ant 16:367–371, 1994

174. McCrory P: Whiplash-related headaches. In: Malanga GA, Nadler SF, eds: Whiplash. Philadelphia, Hanley & Belfus, 2002:125–131

175. McDonnell MK, Sahrmann S: Movement impairment syndromes of the thoracic and cervical spine. In: Grant R, ed: Physical Therapy of the Cervical and Thoracic Spine. New York, Churchill Livingstone, 2001: 335–354

176. McKenzie JS, Williams JF: The dynamic behavior of the head and cervical spine during whiplash. J Biomech 4:477–490, 1971

177. McKenzie RA: The Cervical and Thoracic Spine: Mechanical Diagnosis and Therapy. Spinal Publications, New Zealand, 1990

178. McNair JFS: Acute locking of the cervical spine. In: Grieve GP, ed: Modern Manual Therapy of the Vertebral Column, Edinburgh, Churchill Livingstone, 1986:350–358

179. Meadows J: Manual therapy: Biomechanical assessment and treatment: A rationale and complete approach to the acute and subacute post-MVA cervical patient. Supplement to Swodeam Consulting Video Series. Calgary AB, Swodeam Consulting 1995

180. Mealy K, Brennan H, Fenelon GC: Early mobilization of acute whiplash injuries. BMJ 292:656–657, 1986

181. Mergner T, Siebold C, Schweigart G, et al: Human perception of horizontal trunk and head rotation in space during vestibular and neck stimulation. Exp Brain Res 85:389–404, 1991

182. Mergner T, Hlavacka F, Schweigart G: Interaction of vestibular and propioceptive inputs. J Vestib Res 3:41–57, 1993

183. Mergner T, Huber W, Beckert W: Vestibular-neck interaction and transformation of sensory coordinates. J Vestib Res 7:347–367, 1997

184. Miller RG, Burton R: Stroke following chiropractic manipulation of the spine. JAMA, 229:189–190, 1974.

185. Mimura M, Panjabi MM, Oxland TR, et al: Disc degeneration affects the multidirectional flexibility of the lumbar spine. Spine 19:1371–1380, 1994

186. Mulligan BR: Manual Therapy 'Nags', 'Snags', 'MWMs' etc. Plant View Services, New Zealand, 1995

187. Mulhall KJ, Moloney M, Burke TE, et al: Chronic neck pain following road traffic accidents in an Irish setting and it's relationship to seat belt use and low back pain. Ir Med J 96:53–54, 2003

188. Munro D: The factors that govern the stability of the spine. Paraplegia 45:219–228, 1965

189. Murphy DR: Evaluation of posture and movement patterns related to the cervical spine. In: Murphy DR, ed: Conservative Management of Cervical Spine Syndromes. New York, McGraw-Hill, 2000:307–327

190. Murphy DR, Gruder MI, Murphy LB: Cervical radiculopathy and pseudoradicular pain syndromes. In Murphy DR: Conservative Management of Cervical Syndromes. New York, McGraw-Hill, 2000:189–219

191. Murphy JE: Sensorimotor training and cervical stabilization. In: Murphy JE, ed: Management of Cervical Spine Syndromes. New York, McGraw-Hill, 2000:607–640

192. Murtagh JE, Kenna CJ: Muscle energy therapy. Aus Fam Phys 16:756–765, 1987

193. Murtagh JE, Kenna CJ: Back Pain & Spinal Manipulations: A Practical Guide, 2nd ed. Oxford, Butterworth Heinemann, 1997

194. Nashner LM, McCollum G: The organization of human postural movements: A formal basis and experimental synthesis. Behav Brain Sci 8:135–172, 1985

195. Nelson D, Murphy DR, Flower J, et al: Headache. In: Murphy DR, ed: Conservative Management of Cervical Spine Syndromes. New York, McGraw-Hall, 2000:169–187

196. Nicholson GG, Clendaniel RA: Manual techniques. In: Scully RM, Barnes MR, eds: Physical Therapy. Philadelphia, JB Lippincott, 1989:926–985

197. Nicholson GG, Gaston J: Cervical headache. J Orthop Sports Phys Ther 31:185–193, 2001

198. Nilsson N, Christensen HW, Hartvigsen J: The effect of spinal manipulation in the treatment of cervicogenic headache. J Manip Physiol Ther 20:326–330, 1997

199. Nordhoff LS Jr: Cervical trauma following vehicle collisions. In: Murphy DR, ed: Cervical Spine Syndromes. New York, McGraw-Hill, 2000:129–151

200. Norris SH, Watt I: The prognosis of neck injuries resulting from rear-end vehicle collisions. J Bone Joint Surg Br 65:608–611, 1983

201. O'Connel A: Effect of sensory deprivation on postural reflexes. Electomography 197:519–527, 1971

202. Olson KA: Diagnosis and treatment of cervical spine clinical instability. J Orthop Sports Phys Ther 31:194–206, 2001

203. Ombergt L, Bisschop P, ter Veer HJ, et al: A System of Orthopaedic Medicine. London, WB Saunders, 1995

204. Oosterveld WJ, Kortschot HW, Kingma GG, et al: Electronystagmographic findings following cervical whiplash injuries. Acta Otolaryngol (Stockh) 111:201–205, 1991

205. Packard RC: Epidemiology and pathogenesis of post-traumatic headache. J Head Trauma Rehabil 14:9–21, 1999

206. Panjabi MM: The stabilizing system of the spine: Part I. Function, dysfunction, adaptation, and enhancement. J Spinal Disord 5:383–389, 1992

207. Panjabi MM: The stabilizing system of the spine: Part II. Neutral zone and instability hypothesis. J Spinal Disord 5:390–397, 1992

208. Panjabi M, Abumi K, Durenceau J, et al: Spinal stability and intersegmental muscle force: A biomechanical model. Spine 14:194–200, 1989

209. Panjabi MM, Lyons C, Vasavada A, et al: On the understanding of clinical instability. Spine 19:2641–2650, 1994

210. Panjabi MM, White AA, Johnson RM: Cervical spine mechanics as a function of transection of components. J Biomech 8:327–336, 1975

211. Paris S: Introduction to spinal evaluation and manipulation. Continuing education course, Institute of Graduate Health Sciences, Los Angeles, May 19, 1978

212. Paris S: Cervical spine. In: Payton OD, ed: Manual of Physical Therapy. New York, Churchill Livingstone, 1989:399–408.

213. Paris SV: Cervical symptoms of forward head posture. Topics Geriatr Rehabil 5:11–19, 1990

214. Pearce J: Post-traumatic syndrome and whiplash injuries. In: Kennard C, ed: Recent Advances in Clinical Neurology. New York, Churchill Livingstone, 1995:133–150

215. Pearce JM: Headaches in the whiplash syndrome. Spinal Cord 39:228–233, 2001

216. Perry J, Nickel VL: Total cervical-spine fusion for neck paralysis. J Bone Joint Surg Am 41:37–60, 1959

217. Pettman E: Stress test of the craniovertebral joins. In: Boyling JD, Palastanga N, eds: Grieve's Modern Manual Therapy, 2nd ed. Edinburgh, Churchill Livingstone, 1994:529

218. Petty NJ, Moore AP: Neuromusculoskeletal Examination and Assessment: A Handbook for Therapists. Edinburg, Churchill Livingstone, 1998

219. Pope MH, Frymoyer JW, Krag MH: Diagnosing instability. Clin Orthop 279:6–67, 1992

220. Radanov BP, Di Stefano, Augustiny KF: Symptomatic approach to post-traumatic headache and its possible implication for treatment. Eur Spine J 10:403–407, 2001

221. Rees S: Relaxation therapy in migraine and chronic tension headaches. Med J Aust 2:70, 1975

222. Revel M, Andre-Deshays C, Minguet M: Cervicocephalic kinesthetic sensibility in patients with cervical pain. Arch Phys Med Rehabil 72:288–291, 1991

223. Revel M, Minguet M, Gregory P, et al: Changes in cervicocephalic kinesthetic sensibility in patients with neck pain: A random controlled trial. Arch Phy Med Rehabil 75:895–899, 1994

224. Richardson CA, Jull GA: Muscle control-pain, control. What exercises would you prescribe: Man Ther 1:2–10, 1995

225. Richardson CA, Jull G, Hodges P, Hides J: Therapeutic Exercise for Spinal Segmental Stabilization in Low Back Pain: Scientific and Clinical Approach. Edinburg, Churchill Livingstone, 1999

226. Rocabado M: Advanced upper quarter. Continuing education course, Rocabado Institute, San Francisco, December 10, 1984

227. Rosenholtz C, Nelson D, Hambrick T, et al: Migraine headache. J Bodywork Mov Ther 7:30–45, 2003

228. Royhouse RH: Whiplash and temporomandibular dysfunction. Lancet 1:1394–1395, 1973

229. Ryan GMS, Cope S: Cervical vertigo. Lancet 2:1355–1361, 1955

230. Rydevik B, Brown M, Lundborg G: Pathoanatomy and pathophysiology of nerve root compression. Spine 9:7–15, 1984

231. Saal JS, Franson RC, Dobrow R, et al: High level of inflammatory phospholipase A2 in lumbar disk herniations. Spine 15:676–678, 1990

232. Saal JS, Saal J, Herzog R: The natural history of lumbar intervertebral disk extrusion treated nonoperatively. Spine 15:683–686, 1990

233. Sahrmann SA: Diagnosis and Treatment of Movement Impairment Syndromes. St. Louis, Mosby 2000

234. Sanders RJ, Pearce WH: The treatment of thoracic outlet syndrome: A comparison of different operations. J Vas Surg 10:626–634, 1989

235. Sanders RJ, Jackson CGR, Banchero N, et al: Scalene muscle abnormalities in traumatic thoracic outlet syndrome. Am J Surg 159:231–236, 1990

236. Sandstrom J: Cervical syndrome with vestibular symptoms. Acta Orolaryngo (Stockh) 54:207–226, 1962

237. Saunder DH, Saunders R: Treatment of the spine by diagnosis. In: Saunders SH, Saunders R: Evaluation, Treatment and Prevention of Musculoskeletal Disorders. vol. 1: Spine, 3rd ed. Claska, MN, Saunders Group, 1995:99–143

238. Schank C, Reed K, eds: Therapeutic Associates, Inc. Rehabilitation Guidelines. Beaverton, OR, Therapeutic Associates, 1995

239. Scherping SC, Boden SD, Borenstein DG, et al: Neck Pain, 3rd ed. New York, Lexis Publishing, 2000

240. Schmorl G, Junghanns H: The Human Spine in Health and Disease, 2nd ed. New York, Grune and Stratton, 1971

241. Schneider K, Zeneke RF, Clark G: Modeling of jaw-head-neck dynamics during whiplash. J Dent Res 68:1360–1365, 1989

242. Schneider W, Dvorak J, Dvorak V, et al: Manual Therapy. New York, Georg Thieme Verlag Stuttgart, 1988

243. Schoensee SK, Jensen G, Nicholson G, et al: The effect of mobilization on cervical headaches. J Orthop Sports Phys Ther 21:184–196, 1995

244. Severy DM, Mathewson JH, Bechtol CO: Controlled automobile rear-end collisions: An investigation of related engineering and medical phenomena. Can Serv Med J 11:727–759, 1955

245. Sharp J, Purser DW: Spontaneous atlanto-axial dislocation in ankylosing spondylitis and rheumatoid arthritis. Ann Rheum Dis 20:47–72, 1961
246. Shippel AH, Robinson GK: Radiological and magnetic resonance imaging of cervical spine instability: A case report. J Manip Physiol Ther 10:317–322, 1987
247. Silverman J, Rodriquez AA, Agre JC: Quantitative cervical flexor strength in healthy subjects and in subjects with mechanical neck pain. Arch Phys Rehabil 72:679–681, 1991
248. Simeone FA, Rothman RH: Cervical disk disease. In: Rothman RH, Simeone FA, eds: The Spine, vol. 1. Philadelphia, WB Saunders, 1975:387–434
249. Simons DG, Travell JG, Simons LS: Travell & Simon's Myofascial Pain and Dysfunction: The Trigger Point Manual, vol. 1. Upper Half of the Body. Baltimore, Williams & Wilkins, 1999
250. Sjaastad O, Fredriksen TA: Cervicogenic headache: Criteria, classification and epidemiology. Clin Exp Rheumatol (2 Suppl 19):S3–6. 2000
251. Sjaastad O, Fredriksen TA, Pfaffenrath V: Cervicogenic headache: Diagnostic criteria. Headache 38:442–445, 1998
252. Sjaastad O, Fredriksen TA, Stolt-Nielsen A, et al: Cervicogenic headache: A clinical review with a special emphasis on therapy. Funct Neurol 12:305–317, 1997
253. Spurling RG, Scoville WB: Lateral rupture of the cervical intervertebral disc. Surg Gynecol Obsetet 78:350–358, 1944
254. Stiles E: Manipulation: A tool for your practice. Patient Care 18:699–707, 1984
255. Stoddard A: The intervertebral disk. In: Stoddard A, ed: Manual of Osteopathic Technique, London, Hutchinson, 1959:230–259
256. Stoddard A: Manual of Osteopathic Practice, 2nd ed. London, Hutchinson, 1983:83–85
257. Stratton S, Bryan JM: Dysfunction, evaluation and treatment of the cervical spine and thoracic outlet. In: Donatelli RA, Wooden MJ, eds: Orthopaedic Physical Therapy, 3rd ed. New York, Church Livingstone, 2001:73–107
258. Sweeny T: Neck school: cervicothoracic stabilization training. Occupational Medicine: State of the Art Review 7:43–54, 1992
259. Treleavan J, Jull G, Atkinson L: Cervical musculoskeletal dysfunction in post-concussion headache. Cephalalgia 14:273–279, 1994
260. Trevor-Jones R: Osteoarthritis of the paravertebral joints of the second and third cervical vertebrae as a cause of occipital headache. S Afr Med 38–392–396, 1964
261. Trott PH: Management of selected cervical syndromes. In: Grant R, ed: Physical Therapy of the Cervical and Thoracic Spine. New York, Churchill Livingstone, 2002:272–294
262. Turk Z, Ratkolb O: Mobilization of the cervical spine in chronic headache. Man Med 3:15–17, 1987
263. Valtonen E, Kiun E: Cervical traction as a therapeutic tool: A clinical analysis based on 212 patients. Scand J Rehabil Med 2:29, 1970
264. Vernon H: Spinal manipulation and headaches of cervical origin: A review of literature and presentation of cases. J Manip Physiol Ther 12:455–468, 1989
265. Vicenzino G, Neal R, Collins D, et al: The displacement, velocity and frequency profile of the frontal plane motion produced by the cervical lateral glide treatment technique. Clin Biomech 14:515–521, 1999
266. Visscher CM, deBoer W, Naeije M: The relationship between posture and curvature of the cervical spine. J Manip Physiol Ther 23:388–391, 1998
267. Wadsworth CT: Manual Examination and Treatment of the Spine and Extremities. Baltimore, Williams & Wilkins, 1988
268. Watson DH, Trott P: Cervical headaches: An investigation of natural head posture and upper cervical flexor muscle performance. Cephalgia 13:272–282, 1993
269. Waylonis GW, Perkins RH: Posttraumatic fibromyalgia: A long-term follow up. Am J Phys Med Rehab 73:403–412, 1994
270. Weinberg S, Lapointe H: Cervical extension-flexion injury (whiplash) and internal derangement of the temporomandibular joint. J Oral Maxillofac Surg 45:653–656, 1987
271. Westerhaus P: Cervicogenic headache: A clinician's perspective. In: von Piekartz H, Bryden L, eds: Craniofacial Dysfunction & Pain. Oxford, Butterworth-Heinemann, 2001:85–99
272. Westerhaus P: Cervicogenic headache: Physical examination and management. In: von Piekartz H, Bryden L, eds: Craniofacial Dysfunction & Pain. Oxford, Butterworth-Heinemann, 2001:100–115
273. Whittingham W, Ellis WB, Molyneux TP: The effect of manipulation (toggle recoil technique) for headaches with upper cervical dysfunction: A pilot study. J Manip Physiol Ther 17:369–375, 1994
274. Wilke HJ, Wolf S, Caes LE, et al: Stability increase in the lumbar spine with different muscle groups. Spine 20:192–198, 1995
275. Wyke B: Cervical articular contributions to posture and gait: Their relation to senile disequilibrium. Age Ageing 8(4):251–258, 1979
276. Wyke B: Neurology of the cervical spine joints. Physiotherapy 65(3):72–76, 1979
277. Yu YL, Woo E, Huang CY: Cervical spondylitic myelopathy and radiculopathy. Acta Neurol Scand 75: 367–373, 1987
278. Zimmermann M: Pathophysiological mechanisms of fibromyalgia. Clin J Pain 7(S1):S8–S15, 1991
279. Zonn DA, Mennell J McM: Modalities of physical treatment. In: Zonn DA, Mennell J McM, eds: Musculoskeletal Pain: Diagnosis and Physical Treatment. Boston, Little, Brown and Co., 1976:115–152

RECOMMENDED READINGS

Beeton K, Jull G: Effectiveness of manipulative physiotherapy in the management cervicogenic headache: A single case study. Physiotherapy 80:417–423, 1994

Bisbee, LA, Hartsell HD: Physiotherapy management of whiplash. Spine: State of the Art Review 7: 501–516, 1993

Bogduk N: Cervical causes of headache and dizziness. In: Grieve G, ed: Modern Manual Therapy. Edinburgh, Churchill Livingstone, 1986:289–302

Butler D: Mobilization of the Nervous System. Edinburgh, Churchill Livingstone, 1991

Cassidy JD, Lopes AA, Yong-Hing K: The immediate effect of manipulation versus mobilization on pain and range of motion of the cervical spine: A randomized controlled trial. J Manip Physiol Ther 15:570–575, 1992

Dalton M, Coutts A: The effect of age on cervical posture in a normal population. In: Boyling J, Palastanga N, eds: Grieve's Modern Manual Therapy of the Vertebral Column. Edinburgh, Churchill Livingstone, 1994.

Derrick L, Chesworth B: Post-motor-vehicle-accident alar ligament laxity. J Orthop Sport Phys Ther 16:6–11, 1992

Dvorak J: Soft tissue injury to the cervical spine: New possibilities of diagnosis with computed tomography. J Man Med 4:17–21, 1989

Dvorak J, Janssen B, Grob D: The neurologic work-up in patients with cervical spine disorders. Spine 15:1017–1022, 1990

Edward BC: Manual of Combined Movements. Edinburgh, Churchill Livingstone, 1992

Gargan MF, Bannister GC: Long-term prognosis of soft-tissue injuries of the neck. J Bone Joint Surg Br 72:901–903, 1989

Greenman PE: Manual and manipulative therapy in whiplash injuries. Spine: State of the Art Review 7:517–530, 1993

Grant R, ed: Physical Therapy of the Cervical and Thoracic Spine, 2nd ed. Edinburgh, Churchill Livingstone, 1994

Koe B, Bouter L, van Mameren H, et al: The effectiveness of manual therapy, physiotherapy and treatment by the general practitioner for nonspecific back and neck complaints: A randomized clinical trial. Spine 17:28–35, 1992

Labon M: Whiplash: Its evaluation and treatment. Phys Med Rehabil 4:293–307, 1990

Maitland GD: Vertebral Manipulations, 5th ed. London, Butterworths, 1986

Olesen J, Tfelt-Hansen P, Welch KMA, eds: The Headache. New York, Raven Press, 1993

Rocabado M, Iglarsh ZA: The Musculoskeletal Approach to Maxillofacial Pain. Philadelphia, JB Lippincott, 1991

Sjaastad O: Cervicogenic headache: The controversial headache. Clin Neurol Neurosurg 94 (Suppl):147–149, 1990

Sjaastad O, Freriksen TA, Pfaffenrath V: Cervicogenic headache: Diagnostic criteria. Headache 30:725–726, 1991

Sweeny T: Neck school: Cervicothoracic stabilization training. Spine: State of the Art Review 5:367–378, 1992

Teasell R: The whiplash patient: A sympathetic approach. In: Hachinski J, ed: Challenges in Neurology. Philadelphia, FA Davis, 1992:29–52

Teasell R, McCain G: Clinical spectrum and management of whiplash injuries. In: Tollison CD, ed: Painful Cervical Trauma: Diagnosis and Rehabilitative Treatment of Neuromusculoskeletal Injuries. Baltimore, Williams & Wilkins, 1992:2292–2318

Vernon H, Mior S: The neck disability index: A study of reliability and validity. J Manip Physiol 14:409–415, 1991

Vitti M, Fujiwara M, Basmajian JV, et al: The integrated roles of longus colli and sternocleidomastoid muscles: an electromyography study. Anat Rec 177:471–784, 1998

Watson D, Trott P: Cervical headache: An investigation of natural head posture and upper cervical flexor muscle performance. Cephalagia 13:272–284, 1993

Winters JM, Peles JD: Neck muscle activity and 3D head kinematics during quasi-static and dynamic tracking movements. In: Winters JM, Woo SLY, eds: Multiple Muscle Systems; Biomechanics and Movement Organization. New York, Springer-Verlag, 1990

Thoracic Spine

DARLENE HERTLING

EPIDEMIOLOGY AND PATHOPHYSIOLOGY

Few people have a normal thoracic spine, according to Grieve.[101] The diseases that commonly affect the cervical and lumbar spine also occur in the thoracic spine. Degenerative disease changes in the thoracic spine occur as frequently as they do in the cervical and lumbar spine; the peak incidence of involvement is at C7–T1 and T4–T5. However, symptoms and signs from this region are rare because of the anatomy and biomechanics of this area of the spine.[158]

Degenerative joint disease is common in the thoracic spine, but disk lesions are rare. Thoracic involvement occurs in only about 2% of all causes of disk problems. De Palma and Rothman[62] reported that of 1,000 disk operations, only one involved the thoracic spine.

According to Cyriax,[59] unlike the cervical and lumbar regions in which muscle lesions are rare, the muscles of the thorax and abdomen can suffer strain, leading to posttraumatic scarring and persistent symptoms. A pectoral or intercostal muscle may be affected in this way, as may the latissimus dorsi, the rectus abdominis, or the oblique abdominals. Maigne[175] points out that involvement of the rib cage in pathologic processes is often neglected. However, costal sprain is common and is expressed by thoracic or upper lumbar pain. Most rib lesions are accompanied, if not caused, by spasms of the intercostal muscles. A sneeze or cough with a violent contraction of the muscles of the thoracic cage may leave a persistent contraction of one intercostal muscle, leading to approximation of two adjacent ribs, and this may persist. The effect of sustained contraction in one intercostal muscle is to elevate the lower rib (an *inspiratory-type* lesion). *Expiratory-type* lesions, in which the lower rib is held downward, occur only in the lower ribs (mainly the eleventh and twelfth) because of the attachment of the quadratus lumborum.

The thoracic spine is frequently the source of pain of postural origin, particularly in adolescence. McKenzie[187] suggested that although it is not a pathologic entity in itself, poor posture may be a significant factor contributing to the development of Scheuermann's disease in the young and osteoporosis in the aged. Perhaps the most common disease affecting the skeletal thoracic spine is osteoporosis. In the treatment of this disorder, the value of physical therapy has gone largely unrecognized.[187]

FUNCTIONAL ANATOMY

The thoracic vertebrae are characterized primarily by two features: the presence of articular facets on the vertebral bodies (for articulation with the ribs) and the long, thin spinous processes that angle downward in relation to the motion segment (see Fig. 18-4). Unlike the spinous processes in the cervical and lumbar spine, where the tip of the spinous process is found directly posterior to the body of the vertebrae, the tip of the spinous process in the thoracic area lies posterior and inferior to the body of the vertebra. It therefore can be used as a lever to rotate the vertebral body, resulting in a gliding of the facet articulations that is associated with forward and backward bending in the thoracic spine.[71] The spinous processes are quite long and overlap each other, particularly in the middle to lower region (see Fig. 18-1C).

Mitchell and colleagues[197] divide the thoracic vertebrae into groups of three for the purpose of examination. The spinous processes of the first three thoracic vertebrae (T1, T2, T3) project directly backward: the tip of the spinous process is on the same line as the transverse process. The spinous processes of T4 to T6 project half a vertebra below the one to which they are attached. The spinous processes of T7 to T9 are located a full vertebra lower than the vertebra to which they are attached. The spinous processes of T10 to T12 return to being palpable at the same level as the vertebral body to which they are attached (Fig. 20-1).

The typical thoracic vertebra has a body roughly equal in its transverse and anteroposterior diameter. The apophyseal joints are vertical in orientation (at an angle of about 60° from the horizontal plane; see Fig. 18-4). The superior facet faces upward and back, and the inferior facet faces downward and forward, making them particularly well suited for rotation.

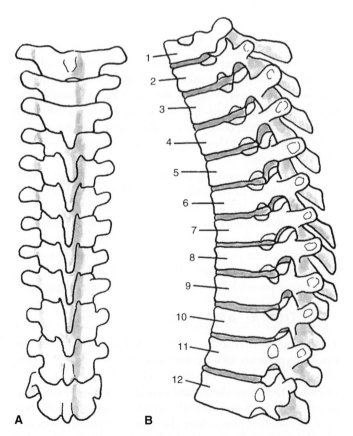

■ **FIG. 20-1.** Thoracic vertebrae—"rule of three." (Adapted with permission from Greenman PE: Principles of Manual Medicine. Baltimore, Williams & Wilkins, 1989:52.)

The *atypical thoracic vertebrae* (T1 and T12) are those that are transitional between the cervical and thoracic spine and the thoracic and lumbar spine. T1 has the longest transverse process in the thoracic spine. The inferior apophyseal joint surface orientation (facing) is typically thoracic, but the superior apophyseal joint is transitional from the cervical spine and may have typical cervical characteristics. T1 is also the junction for the change in the anteroposterior curve between the cervical and thoracic spine. Dysfunction of T1 profoundly affects the functional capacity of the thoracic outlet and related structures.

T12 is the location of transition to the lumbar spine. The superior apophyseal joint facing is usually typically thoracic, but the inferior apophyseal joint facing tends toward lumbar characteristics. T12 is the location for the change in the anteroposterior curve between the thoracic kyphosis and the lumbar lordosis, a location of change in mobility to two areas of the spine, and a point of frequent dysfunction.[99] T12 acts as a bridge between the lumbar–thoracic spine and is essentially a mortise joint.

T3 is the transitional zone between the cervical lordosis and thoracic kyphosis and also serves as the axis of motion for the shoulder girdle complex. T6 is considered the axis of motion for the entire thoracic spine.

The *thoracic kyphosis* is normally a smooth posterior convexity, without severe areas of increased convexity or flattening. The observation of flat spots without the thoracic kyphosis should alert the examiner to evaluate this area carefully for vertebral dysfunction.

Thoracic disks are narrower and flatter than those in the cervical and lumbar spine. They gradually increase in height and width from superior to inferior.

The spinal canal is narrow, with only a small epidural space between the cord and its osseous environment (see Fig. 18-4C).[285] The narrowest region is between T4 and T5.[158] Besides the vertebral joints, there are also the costotransverse joints (see Fig. 18-10B): they are adjacent to the lower portion of the intervertebral foramina and leave the spinal nerve free in the superior portion. The vertebral foramina are quite large, so there is seldom any osseous constriction.

Clinically, the thoracic spine begins at the third vertebra. The upper two thoracic joints and their nerve roots are best examined with the cervical segments.[59]

One must always consider the ribs and their attachments in the evaluation and treatment of the thoracic spine. The ribs move with a complex combination of:

1. Pump-handle motions (similar to flexion and extension; see Fig. 18-11A)
2. Bucket-handle motions (similar to abduction and adduction; see Fig. 18-11B)
3. Caliper-like motions (analogous to internal and external rotation; see Fig. 18-11C)

The upper ribs move mainly in a combined pump-handle and bucket-handle type of motion; middle rib motion is primarily of the bucket-handle type. The lower ribs move much like calipers. However, all ribs move with a complex combination of these motions. Ribs two, three, and four have a somewhat greater proportion of pump-handle movement as they rise and fall with the sternum. Rib one, moving with about half pump-handle and half bucket-handle motions, is acted on during inhalation by the anterior, medial, and posterior scalene muscles. In quieter respiration they may move by the tilting manubrium, or they may not move much at all. Ribs eight to ten have a greater proportion of bucket-handle motion as they increase and decrease the transverse diameter of the chest. The floating ribs have a greater proportion of caliper-type motions.

There are three costovertebral joints for each rib. Except for ribs one and ten to twelve, the head of each rib articulates with two adjacent vertebrae and with one transverse process. The exceptions articulate with one vertebral body (costovertebral joint) and its transverse process. In addition, ribs one to seven articulate anteriorly with the sternum via synovial joints (see Fig. 18-10A). Rib movements are small and gliding to enable pump-handle, bucket-handle, and caliper movements to occur.

Because of the convexity of the thoracic spine, the anterior parts become subjected to considerable load. The intradiskal pressure is high in this region because the load is taken up entirely by the vertebrae and disks. Because of this, compression fractures most often appear anteriorly, and there is an invasion of disk tissue through the end plates into the vertebral bodies.[158] Because of the continuous high intradiskal pressures, degenerative changes develop quite early in the middle and lower sections of the thoracic spine. According to Kramer,[158] disk disease with symptoms from the thoracic spine is not as common as it is in the cervical and lumbar spine. This is because:

1. The intervertebral foramina are not posterior to the disks, as is the case in the cervical and lumbar spine, but are rather on the same level as the vertebral bodies. Nerve root involvement thus requires a large prolapse of disk tissue, and this is uncommon.
2. The movements of the thoracic spine are much more restricted than those of the cervical and lumbar spine. The position of the nerve in relation to the osseous structures is fairly constant and is not subjected to a continuous change of position, as is the case in the cervical and lumbar spine.

Biomechanical Regions

The thoracic spine is intimately related to the rib cage, and they work essentially as a single unit. Alterations in thoracic cage function alter the thoracic spine. Hence, from the respiratory–circulatory model of manual medicine, the thoracic spine assumes major importance in providing optimal functional capacity to the thoracic cage for respiration and circulation.[99]

The thorax can be divided into regions according to their respective anatomic and biomechanical differences.[161,164,165]

• Vertebromanubrial region (C7–T2)
• Vertebrosternal region (T3–T7)
• Vertebrochondral region (T8–T10)
• Thoracolumbar region (T11–T12)

VERTEBROMANUBRIAL REGION

The cervicothoracic junction shares some biomechanical and anatomic features with the cervical and thoracic spine. The C7–T3 segments are a transitional zone between the cervical lordosis and thoracic kyphosis, with all ranges being diminished, although flexion and extension are freer than in the lower thoracic spine. The zygapophyseal facets of the superior articular process lie in the coronal body plane, whereas those of the inferior articular process present a gentle curve in both the transverse and sagittal planes. The first two ribs are always less mobile than T1 or T2, and the movement pattern for flexion and extension is consistent with the stiff thoracic pattern described in the vertebrosternal joints described below.

Lateral Bending. In the mobile thorax, side flexion at this region consists of[162]:

• The same pattern as the midcervical spine region, which is side flexion coupled with ipsilateral rotation. The head of the first rib does not articulate with C7 so the superior-inferior glide of the ribs and the conjunct rotation cannot influence the coupling between C7 and T1 and between T1 and T2.
• An inferior glide of the transverse process relative to the rib on the right, and superiorly relative to the rib on the left, during right side flexion of the head and neck.

Rotation. In the mobile thorax, rotation at this region consists of the same pattern as the midcervical region. During unilateral elevation of the upper limb, the zygapophyseal joints side flex and slightly extend to the same side as the elevated upper limb, producing a rotation of the T1 and T2 vertebrae to the same side.

VERTEBROSTERNAL REGION

Flexion. In the mobile thorax joints, flexion[165] of this region appears to vary among individuals, and can be either a combination of anterior rotation and superior glide or, more commonly, a combination of superior glide of the rib neck and tubercle (T3–T7) and a conjoint anterior rotation. In the stiff thorax the ribs are less mobile than the vertebral column when the stiffer thorax is flexed. The anterior aspect of the ribs travels inferiorly, whereas the posterior aspect travels superiorly. Once the range of motion of the ribs is exhausted, the thoracic vertebrae continue to forward flex on the now stationary ribs.

The third movement pattern occurs when the relative flexibility of the spinal column and the rib cage are the same. During flexion the quantity of movement is reduced, and there is no apparent movement between the ribs and the thoracic vertebrae. Some anterosuperior gliding occurs at the thoracic facet joints; however very little, if any, costotransverse joint motion can be felt.

Extension. Extension[165] occurs during bilateral elevation of the arms and backward bending of the trunk. In the mobile thorax a variety of motion patterns may occur among individuals that can be either a combination of superior glide and a posterior rotation or, more commonly, a combination of a posterior rotation of the rib neck and an inferior glide of the tubercle at the costotransverse joint. An inferior glide of the tubercle results in a posterior rotation of the neck of the rib. Posterior translation is coupled with backward sagittal rotation.

During extension of the stiff thorax the ribs are less flexible than the spinal column. Initially, the anterior ribs travels superiorly while the posterior aspect travels inferiorly. Once the range of motion of the rib cage is exhausted, the thoracic vertebrae continue to extend on the now stationary ribs.

Third Movement Pattern. The third movement pattern occurs when the relative flexibility between the rib cage and the spinal column is the same. During extension of the thorax, the quantity of movement is reduced, and there is no apparent movement between the thoracic vertebrae and the ribs. Some posteroinferior gliding occurs at the zygapophyseal joints. Very little, if any, costotransverse joint motion can be felt.

These are the common patterns noted during flexion and extension; other patterns may be present.

Rotation. According to Lee,[165] in the midthoracic spine, rotation around the y axis has been found to be coupled with ipsilateral rotation around the z axis and contralateral translation along the x axis (see Appendix, Fig. A-1). In the mobile thorax, rotation to the right at this region consists of right rotation and left translation of the superior facet. The right rotation of the superior vertebra produces a "pulling" of the superior aspect of the left rib head forward at the costosternal joint. This in turn produces an anterior rotation of the left rib neck and a superior glide at the left costotransverse joint. At the limits of this horizontal translation both the costovertebral and the costotransverse joint are tensed. If this region is stable, further rotation of the superior costovertebral joint to the right occurs when the superior vertebral body tilts to the right, producing a right side flexion of the superior vertebra during right rotation.

Lateral Bending. Side flexion of the thoracic vertebrae occurs during lateral bending of the trunk. In the mobile thorax, side flexion to the right at this region consists of a left convex curve. As the thorax side flexes to the right, the ribs on the right approximate and the ribs on the left separate at their lateral margins. The costal motion stops first; the thoracic vertebrae then continue to side flex slightly to the right. In both the mobile thorax and the stiff thorax, the ribs appear to stop moving before the thoracic vertebrae. The thoracic vertebrae then continue to side flex to the right.

VERTEBROCHONDRAL REGION

This region consists of T8–T10.[165]

Flexion–Extension. Clinically, during flexion of the thoracic vertebrae in this region it appears that the associated ribs follow the sagittal motion although minimal articular motion is necessary at the costovertebral joints of ribs nine and ten. The zygapophyseal joints glide superiorly during flexion and inferiorly in extension. In the mobile thorax, flexion at the region consists of a superior-medial-posterior (SMP) glide of the rib tubercle but does not induce an anterior rotation of the neck of the rib to the same degree as the middle and upper ribs. In the stiff thorax, at the vertebrochondral and costotransverse joints of the T8–T10, an inferior-lateral-anterior (ILA) glide occurs with flexion. During extension the facets of the costotransverse joints are planar, and the relative glide of the ribs is thus SMP.

Lateral Bending. The biomechanics of the vertebrochondral region during lateral bending of the trunk depends on the apex of the curve produced in side flexion. When the apex of the curve is at the level of the greater trochanter, the ribs do not appear to direct the superior vertebra into contralateral rotation as they do in the vertebrosternal region. The vertebrae are freer to follow the rotation that is congruent with the levels above and below. When the apex of the curve is within the thorax, then the osteokinematics of the lower thoracic vertebrae appear to be very different. The rib cage remains compressed on the right and separated on the left, however the thoracic vertebrae side flex to the left below the apex of the right side flexion curve. The ribs do not appear to direct the superior vertebra to rotate in a sense incongruent to the levels above and below.

Rotation. The same flexibility of motion coupling is apparent in the vertebrochondral region when rotation is considered. The coupled movement pattern for rotation here can be ipsilateral side flexion or contralateral side flexion. This region appears to be designed to rotate with minimal restriction from the costal elements.

THORACOLUMBAR REGION

The T11–L1 segment area[165] is a transitional zone between the thoracic kyphosis and the lumbar lordosis. The last thoracic vertebra (T12), acting as a bridge between the thoracic and lumbar regions, has its inferior zygapophyseal facets in the sagittal plane to match those of L1. The joints in this region are designed to rotate with minimal restriction.[162] Actively, the coupled movement patterns for rotation in this region can be contralateral side flexion or ipsilateral side flexion.

Details of the osteokinematics and arthrokinematic motions during sagittal plane motions of the thorax as well as lateral bending and rotation are described extensively in the works of Lee.[161,164,165] The known biomechanics of the thorax continues to be far from complete.

Innervation

The intercostal nerves (the anterior branches of the thoracic spinal nerves) supply the chest wall, the intercostal muscles, the costotransverse joints, the parietal pleura, and the skin.

When any of these nerves becomes irritated, an intercostal neuralgia develops.

The thoracic spine takes on additional importance from the neurologic perspective because of its relation with the sympathetic division of the autonomic nervous system. The neurovascular supply to the upper limb passes over the first rib, and the sympathetic nervous system has its origin throughout the entire thoracic spine and upper lumbar region. In this way, the thoracic spine becomes an integrated control center for the whole body.

Deformities such as scoliosis and Scheuermann's disease generally develop slowly, and the nerve roots adapt to the change of position. Because of the anterior loading of the disks, dislocation of disk fragments may occur in a posterior direction, with rupture and perforation of the annulus fibrosus. The disk fragment can be as large as a cherry and will in time adhere to the dura.[20] There are also central, anterolateral, and lateral dislocations of fragments, which ultimately protrude posteriorly.[62] The region most involved is T7 to T12.[20,159,170]

COMMON LESIONS AND THEIR MANAGEMENT

Pain in the thoracic spine with referral to various parts of the chest wall and upper abdomen is common in people of all ages and can closely mimic the symptoms of visceral disease such as angina pectoris and biliary colic.[144] Cloward,[53] Maigne,[175] and Cyriax[59] have demonstrated that much of the pain experienced in the upper thoracic region to the level of T7 originates in the cervical spine.

According to Kenna and Murtagh,[144] the significant features to consider with respect to the thoracic region are:

1. People of all ages can experience thoracic problems. They are surprisingly common in young people, including children.
2. Thoracic pain is more common in patients with abnormalities such as thoracic kyphosis and Scheuermann's disease.
3. Trauma to the chest wall (including falls on the chest), such as those experienced in contact sports, commonly leads to disorders in the thoracic spine.
4. Patients recovering from open-heart surgery, when a longitudinal sternal incision is made and the chest wall is stretched out, commonly experience thoracic pain.
5. Unlike the lumbar spine, the joints are quite superficial, and it is relatively easy to find the affected painful segment.

Mechanical causes of thoracic and rib cage dysfunction include disk lesions, facet lesions, costovertebral and costochondral lesions, and spondylosis.

Thoracic Disk Herniations

Disk lesions are relatively rare in the thoracic spine but are of concern because of their possible impingement on the spinal cord.

Disk Prolapse and Pain Patterns

Of the total number of disk problems, thoracic presentations represent 1 to 6 patients per 1,000.[61] This problem appears predominantly in men, and the highest incidence is in the fifth decade. T11 and T12 are most commonly involved.

The clinical history often reveals an axial compression of the trunk, as occurs in a fall on the hindquarter or when lifting a heavy object in the forward-bent position. Localized pain corresponds to the segment involved. Coughing or increasing intrathoracic pressure increases the pain. The cord may be involved and radicular signs may develop, although the only symptom may be localized pain. Evidence of cord compression, with resultant sensory loss, upper motor neuron lesions, and bladder symptoms, is common.[170] A medial prolapse may produce cord symptoms; a disk prolapse that is more posterolateral is more likely to involve the nerve roots.

DISK BULGING AGAINST POSTERIOR LIGAMENT AND DURA

When a prolapsed disk exerts pressure on the posterior ligament and the dura, the result is spondylogenic referred pain, usually experienced in the upper back (if of thoracic origin) or the low back (lumbar origin). The pain, however, can be referred over a wider area. According to Cyriax and Cyriax,[60] as at other spinal levels, involvement of the dura mater, with a central disk protrusion, produces unilateral extrasegmental dural reference of pain. Interference with the dura mater at thoracic levels may produce posterior pain, spreading to the base of the neck or down to the midlumbar region and often pervading several dermatomal levels (Fig. 20-2). Symptoms are usually central or unilateral. Coughing or deep breathing increases the pain.[59,60] The pain is usually dull, deep, and poorly localized.

DISK BULGING POSTEROLATERALLY AGAINST NERVE ROOT

This is a natural route because the annulus fibrosus is no longer reinforced by the posterior longitudinal ligament. According to Cyriax and Cyriax[60] and Cailliet,[41] if the disk exerts pressure on the dural sleeve of the nerve root only, the radicular pain is experienced along the course of the nerve root. Pain can be experienced, therefore, in any part of the dermatome of the affected nerve root.

At T1 and T2 (both rare), symptoms may be felt in the arm. Root pain of lower levels causes symptoms in the side or front of the trunk. A cervical disk lesion is the routine cause of pain felt at upper thoracic levels.[60,177] According to Cyriax and Cyriax,[60] discomfort below the sixth thoracic dermatome may arise from a thoracic disk lesion.

With further pressure on the nerve parenchyma, there is usually no pain. Because conduction down the nerve is affected, paresthesia or anesthesia in the distal end of the dermatome, absent or sluggish reflexes, and motor weakness result.

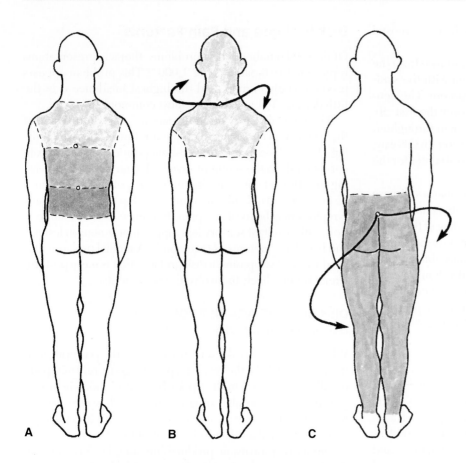

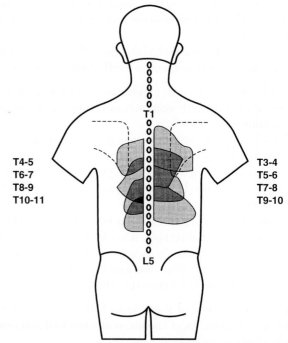

■ **FIG. 20-2.** Extrasegmental reference of pain from the dura mater according to Cyriax and Cyriax.[60] **(A)** Thoracic dural pain could produce pain up to the base of the neck and down to the waist. **(B)** Cervical dura could refer pain to the head and midthoracic spine. **(C)** Low lumbar dural pain could spread to the legs (infrequently to the abdomen and to the midthoracic area). Note that the feet are excluded. (Adapted with permission from Cyriax JH, Cyriax PJ: Illustrated Manual of Orthopaedic Medicine, 2nd ed. London, Butterworths, 1993:245.)

The most common site of prolapse is between T11 and T12. Symptoms include local back pain and radicular pain. Pain refers to the lumbar region, especially the iliac crest.

According to D'Ambrosia,[61] thoracic disk protrusion is difficult to diagnose and more often than not will have a long, puzzling history. It can be confused with ankylosing spondylitis, metastatic tumor, chronic duodenal ulcer disease, intercostal neuralgia, disk space infection, intramedullary spinal cord tumors, or neurofibromas.

Minor Intervertebral Derangement Theory of Maigne

Maigne[177] proposes the existence in the involved segment of a *minor intervertebral derangement* (MID), which is usually reversed by mobilization or manipulation. It is defined as "isolated pain in one intervertebral segment, of a mild character, and due to a minor mechanical cause."[177] Most commonly, a vertebral level is found to be painful and yet has a normal static and radiologic appearance.

The MID always involves one of the two apophyseal joints in the mobile segment, thus initiating nociceptive activity in the posterior primary dermatome and myotome. The overlying skin is tender to pinching and rolling, and the muscles are painful to palpation and feel cordlike.

Referral patterns based on stimulation of the apophyseal joints have been reported by Dreyfuss and associates[67] (Fig. 20-3). This study provides preliminary confirmation that the

■ **FIG. 20-3.** Referral patterns from the T3–T4 to T10–T11 thoracic apophyseal joints: a composite map from asymptomatic volunteers. (Reprinted with permission from Dreyfuss P, Tibiletti C, Dreyer SJ: Thoracic zygapophyseal joint pain patterns: A study in normal volunteers. Spine 19:807–811, 1994.)

thoracic apophyseal joints can cause both local and referred pain. Significant overlap in the referral patterns was reported.

According to Maigne,[177] the functional ability of the mobile segment depends closely on the condition of the intervertebral disk—thus, if the disk is injured, other elements of the segment will be affected. Even a minimal disk lesion can produce apophyseal joint dysfunction, which is a reflex cause of protective muscle spasm and pain in the corresponding segment with loss of function. The result is avoidance of painful pressure or movement of the involved segment. This becomes fixed, and the condition tends to become self-perpetuating.

Thoracic Pain of Lower Cervical Origin

The clinical association between injury to the lower cervical region and upper thoracic pain is well known, especially with whiplash injuries. According to Maigne,[175] 70% of common thoracic pain is of lower cervical origin and is predominant in the intercellular region. These cases represent almost entirely postural thoracic pain, such as that manifested by typists and secretaries.

The examination reveals the same signs in all cases: thoracic signs with a particular localized area of tenderness called the *cervical point of the back* or the interscapular point (ISP) near T5 or T6 (2 cm from the line of the spinous process) and inferior cervical MID (C5–C6, C6–C7, or C6–T1), with the tender facet on the same side as the back pain and the thoracic signs.

An interesting sign that demonstrates the connection between cervical spine involvement and back pain is the anterior cervical doorbell or "push-button" sign.[175,178] Pressure with the thumb over the anterolateral portion of the lower cervical spine, maintained for a few seconds at the responsible vertebral level, triggers the thoracic pain. Another sign is an area of skin more or less thickened and extremely sensitive to the pinch-roll maneuver, which includes all or part of the cutaneous territory of the posterior branch of the second thoracic nerve.[177] This extends from the middle thoracic region (T5–T6) to the acromion.

In addition to these findings, a therapeutic trial of cervical mobilization is important. Disappearance of the cervical MID and ISP with diminished sensitivity in the pinch-roll maneuver of the medial thoracic zone should occur.

Pain from the lower cervical spine can also be referred to the anterior chest and mimic coronary ischemic pain. The associated autonomic nervous system disturbance can cause considerable confusion in making the diagnosis.[144]

Thoracic Pain of Thoracic Origin (According to Maigne[177])

Thoracic pain of thoracic origin is rarer than the preceding. Postural thoracic pain resembles thoracic pain of cervical origin, but the pain is not always localized in the T5 and T6 segments. Clinical examination reveals an MID of a thoracic segment with:

1. Tenderness of the corresponding supraspinous ligament
2. Tenderness of the neighboring skin (infiltrating cellulitis) tested by the skin-rolling maneuver
3. Pain after lateral pressure on one side of the spinous process
4. Elective pain elicited by "resisted" pressure of the spinal processes in one direction

Mobilization and a few sessions of skin-rolling massage involving the tender skin may be used if tenderness persists after the MID is corrected. Muscle reeducation and postural exercises should be prescribed, and static deficiencies should be corrected.

Thoracic Hypomobility Syndromes

The most common cause of disease arising from the apophyseal joints is capsular fibrosis. Most dysfunction is that of hypomobility. Hypermobility is uncommon, but as in the cervical spine, it is equally significant and more difficult to treat. Within their own segment, stiff apophyseal joints may result in reduction of nutrition to the disk. In neighboring segments, they may produce ligamentous and joint instability.

According to McKenzie,[187] the extension dysfunction develops in patients with both Scheuermann's disease and osteoporosis. The loss of movement that characterizes this dysfunction syndrome is caused by adaptive shortening resulting from poor postural habits for a sustained period, or from adaptive shortening as a result of derangement or trauma and the healing process. The dysfunction syndrome is presumed to be caused by a disturbance of some structure within a joint causing mechanical deformation of pain-sensitive structures.[160,187] Many patients lose mobility in extension and rotation as a result of poor postural habits. Treatment is directed at maintaining correct posture and performing extension exercises on a lifelong basis. Management of rotation dysfunction is directed at rotation exercises in sitting and extension in lying.

Mayo Clinic research in postmenopausal spinal osteoporosis has demonstrated that extension exercises performed regularly significantly reduced the number of compression fractures, and that levels of physical activity and back muscle strength may contribute to the bone mineral density of vertebral bodies.[261,262]

A primary cause of thoracic hypomobility in neurologically involved children and adults (e.g., cerebral palsy, traumatic head injury, multiple sclerosis) is the lack of active thoracic extension, leading to immobility of the spine and rib cage. Common problems seen in these patients include:

1. Forward head and increased thoracic kyphosis
2. Decreased thoracolumbar mobility
3. Limited spinal extension with associated hip flexion contractures or excessive lumbar lordosis with increased thoracic kyphosis and genu recurvatum on weight bearing
4. Hypomobility of the rib cage resulting from lack of mobility and postural and muscular imbalances
5. Altered breathing patterns, usually avoiding diaphragmatic breathing (diaphragm is restricted)

6. In the neurologically involved child, retention of the neonatal thoracolumbar kyphosis (thoracolumbar flexion) with posterior tilt of the pelvis (sacral sitting)
7. Spasticity (resulting in hyperactivity of spinal gamma motor neurons) and static postural reflexes. These are often present and interfere with voluntary movement.

Treatment aimed at reducing tone and abnormal movement patterns may be successful using various physical therapy approaches: therapeutic exercise, positioning, and modalities. Joint articulations using long-lever articulations, thoracic stretching, and soft tissue manipulations are useful.

Developmental activities and exercises, as well as joint articulations aimed at reducing tone and restoring motions, should concentrate on trunk and proximal movements, as many patterns of hypertonus seem to arise from these key areas.[26] Trunk activities should include segmental rolling, in addition to upper and lower trunk rotation and counterrotation.[214] Activities, exercise, and articulation techniques that stress extension with trunk rotation are generally most effective. When extensor tone seems to predominate, flexion activities and articulations with trunk rotation should be considered.

Upper Thoracic Spinal Syndromes

The upper thoracic spine is considered the stiffest part of the thoracic spine. Pain is usually well localized but may cause distal symptoms, probably via the autonomic nervous system.[144] A specific syndrome in this region is known as the T4 syndrome.[184] This condition is associated with a hypomobility lesion at the T4 level and has the following features:

1. Arm pain or vague discomfort in the arm associated with paresthesias that do not follow any dermatome pattern, with the hand always involved
2. Diffuse posterior head and neck pain in some patients
3. Hypomobility at one or more levels (T3–T4, T4–T5, or T5–T6); T4 is invariably involved.
4. Tenderness and stiffness, especially at T3–T4 and T4–T5

The mechanism is unknown, but an associated disturbance of autonomic nerve control has been postulated. Predisposing factors have been attributed to unaccustomed lifting, stretching, pushing activities, or trauma (e.g., a motor vehicle accident, a fall). A relaxed posture, with a forward head, accentuated thoracic kyphosis, and protracted shoulder girdle, may predispose the patient to this syndrome.

Butler[38] has explained the symptom distribution and the apparent epiphenomenon of symptomatic involvement based on the clinical observation made by many manual therapists during the past few years that patients with the symptom complex have a positive upper limb tension test and some have a positive slump test. The T4 to T9 segment of the spinal canal is a narrow zone in which minimal reduction in the size of the canal will result in possible compromise of the neuraxis and the meninges.[65] With injury to surrounding joints, a site of adverse tension may be initiated. Other structures such as the

thoracic sympathetic trunk and ganglia, dura mater, nerve roots, and even the preganglionic neurons in the cord may eventually be irritated.

TREATMENT

Articulations or manipulation of this involved area almost always relieve symptoms after three or four treatments, according to Corrigan and Maitland.[57] McGuckin[184] endorsed this and emphasized Klapp's quadripedal exercises.[154,175] If the relaxed posture is considered a predisposing factor, postural correction exercises can be useful.

Butler[38] recommends using both upper limb tension tests 1 and 2 and also the slump test, with combinations of thoracic rotation and lateral flexion in evaluation and treatment if needed. A technique in which the costotransverse joint is mobilized in the slump long-sitting and thoracic rotation positions may be used. For a complete description of the evaluation process and illustrations of these valuable techniques, refer to his textbook.

Midthoracic and Costovertebral Disorders

The T5 to T7 segments are the most common sites for apophyseal joint pain; the T8 to T10 segments are the most common sites for rib articulation problems (costovertebral disorders) and the most common site for referred pain mimicking visceral pain.[144]

Localized degenerative disk lesions are relatively uncommon. There is a higher incidence in people whose occupations involve repeated thoracic rotation (e.g., professional golfers).[57] Nerve root involvement may occur with pain radiating around the chest wall following the line of the rib; this is sometimes associated with paresthesias or numbness over the same distribution. Pain is aggravated by movement and is often worse on lying down. Treatment is difficult: traction, some form of back support, and gentle mobilization techniques may help.

The costovertebral joint may be involved in inflammatory or degenerative joint disease. Complaints of pain in this region are common early in ankylosing spondylitis as a result of synovitis, and examination reveals local tenderness and reduced chest expansion. Chest measurements can also be used to assess disease progress.

Dysfunction of the costovertebral joint commonly causes localized pain about 3 to 4 cm from the midline, where the rib articulates with the transverse process and the vertebral body.[144] The costovertebral joint is frequently responsible for referred pain ranging from the midline, posterior to the lateral chest wall, and even to the anterior chest wall. Diagnosis is confirmed only when movement of the rib provokes pain at the costovertebral joint.

Degenerative changes may occur, although they are usually asymptomatic. They begin in the fourth decade, but symptoms such as tenderness and localized pain usually result only after some form of localized trauma. Nathan and associates[206] found the inferior rather than the superior joint facet to be the usual site of involvement. They also found that the joints with a single facet (one, eleven, and twelve) have a much higher incidence of degenerative changes than those which have two hemifacets.

Treatment with mobilization techniques is usually successful. Local anesthetic injections are often beneficial.

Lower Thoracic Spine and Thoracolumbar Junction Dysfunction

Lower thoracic and thoracolumbar junction pain is common and is the most common level for thoracic disk lesions. Pain is referred to the lumbar region, especially the iliac crest and often the buttock (see Fig. 20-7). There is sometimes pain in the inguinal or apparently in the abdominal areas and occasionally pain in the trochanteric region. The initial impression is that the symptoms are arising from the lower lumbar spine. The pain in these cases is low, lumbar, deep, or sacroiliac, or at the level of the iliac crest.

The skin over the iliac crest and upper outer buttock areas is supplied by the posterior primary rami of nerves arising from the thoracolumbar region.[177] Similarly, anterior groin pain can arise from this region as the nerve supply is from the anterior rami of spinal nerves T12 and L1. The dermatomal symptoms can be present in either the posterior or anterior branches of the dorsal rami. Consequently, with anterior abdominal symptoms, and in some cases of hip pain in which the radiologic examination of the hip is normal, irritation of the twelfth thoracic or first lumbar nerve should be considered.

According to Maigne,[177] in these cases an iliac crest ("crestal") point is found at the gluteal level, usually 8 or 10 cm from the median line, more lateral or more medial. Pressure and friction over the iliac crest will reveal this well-localized and actually painful point. Examination of the thoracolumbar region will also reveal the signs of an MID between T10 and L2. The gluteal pinch-roll maneuver is likely to be painful on the involved side (see Fig. 7-42C). The two most characteristic signs are pain to lateral pressure over the spinous process and posterior articular sensitivity on the same side as the crestal point.

Pain may be acute or chronic. Acute lumbago or dorsalgia of thoracolumbar junction origin or higher can be seen at all ages, but is most common in those older than 40. Typically the patient does not assume an antalgic posture as in the lumbar spine with a lateral shift (lumbar scoliosis). There is, however, marked local contracture, stiffness, vertebral tenderness to pressure, and signs of an acute intervertebral disturbance, probably of diskogenic nature.[66] During attempted active motions there is severe pain on lateral flexion of the trunk and rotation to one side.[175]

Management is similar to that of the lumbar spine (see Chapter 22, Lumbar Spine). Chronic involvement is most common. Treatment with mobilization techniques is usually successful. Therapeutic exercise is usually of little value and may frequently be irritating in this form of low back pain.

Lower thoracic syndromes will involve some aspect of the diaphragm. Because of the relationship of the crura to the quadratus lumborum, symptoms also may occur in the lumbar distribution. Restriction in the lower thorax may increase the load on the lumbar region. Treatment of the lower thorax can help lumbar conditions. Diaphragmatic involvement also may affect the low-pressure lymphatic and venous system.[111]

Thoracic Derangement Syndrome of McKenzie

According to McKenzie,[187] the derangement syndrome is by far the most common cause of pain in those who seek treatment for neck and thoracic pain. The pain of derangement is thought to be produced by displacement or altered position of joint structures, resulting in mechanical deformation of pain-sensitive tissues. Change within the joint may prevent the joint surfaces from moving normally, resulting in altered movement patterns.

McKenzie argues that the derangement syndrome is usually caused by a mechanical disturbance of the intervertebral disk.[187] He has divided these into posterior disk and anterior disk derangements because the clinical presentations suggest that one or the other part of the disk is involved. Anterior derangement is rare in the thoracic spine, with perhaps one case having been identified.[229] The mechanism of posterior derangement may be similar to that demonstrated by Adams and Hutton.[1]

The following derangement patterns are seen in the thoracic spine, but there are many variations and not all patients fit precisely into this listing. The classification is simplified to give a clear explanation of the principles.

- Derangement 1: Central or symmetrical pain between T1 and T12; rapidly reversible
- Derangement 2: Acute kyphosis; rare, usually the result of trauma or serious disease
- Derangement 3: Unilateral or asymmetrical pain across the thoracic region, with or without radiation around the chest wall; rapidly reversible

Diagnosis involves assessing the effect of posture and movement on the symptoms. Each problem is manifested differently, and more than one problem may be present in the same patient. On physical examination, repeated movements or sustained positions can increase or decrease, produce or abolish, or centralize the patient's symptoms. Pain is felt during movement, at end range, or both, and the physical obstruction to movement will increase or decrease in tandem with the symptoms.

With respect to treatment, the patient with a derangement should be taught the postures and movements that will reduce the mechanical deformation of involved structures. In the thoracic spine, this typically involves static thoracic extension (in supine or prone lying) and thoracic rotation in sitting. Such exercises should be expected to reduce the severity or the extent of symptoms. The course of treatment must follow the normal physiologic healing process. Full range of motion without the production of symptoms is the goal.

McKenzie[187] has also classified nonspecific thoracic spine pain into the postural and dysfunction syndrome. Described simply, postural pain appears eventually by the overstretching of normal tissue. Usually the postural syndrome is of insidious onset. Symptoms are time dependent, and range of motion is within normal limits. The postural patient is taught how to maintain optimal alignment of spinal segments to avoid pain.

The pain of the dysfunction syndrome is thought to be caused by the stretching of adaptively shortened pain-sensitive soft tissues.[212] The pain of dysfunction is probably caused by specific shortening or scarring of tissue rather than a general age-related loss of movement. The onset may be acute or insidious; symptoms may or may not be time dependent. The patient usually complains of intermittent pain with increased pain on movement. Range of motion is limited in one or more directions. The patient with dysfunction syndrome should be given exercises to elongate shortened tissues. Such exercises will be expected to produce end-range pain. The principles of treatment for this syndrome are based on the mechanism of tissue healing and the response of soft tissue to the application of controlled forces.[3,4,79,91,221,295]

Back conditions related to mechanical deformation of soft tissue structures do not respond to palliative treatment only. A comprehensive program, including posture and body mechanics instruction and specific individualized exercises, is vital to success. The reader should refer to McKenzie's textbook to plan a treatment program.[187] It is critical to determine the classification or syndrome.

Thoracic Hypermobility Problems

Hypermobility is fairly uncommon but is as significant as hypomobility and more difficult to treat. Hypermobility of the thoracic segments usually results from postural and muscle imbalances, often at levels above restricted segment(s), or from trauma such as pulling, lifting, or reaching, resulting in ligament and capsular sprain.[181] Another common cause of excessive thoracic spine motion is lack of thoracic and hip rotation combined with excessive shoulder girdle protraction.[241] The prevalent movement pattern is to reach with excessive scapular abduction and thoracic flexion.

Several signs and symptoms may alert the examiner to the presence of hypermobility and instability. If the cause is impairment in habitual posture or repetitive movement the clinician must consider the integrated relationship among the upper limbs, the lumbar–pelvic–hip complex, and the foot and ankle in developing a plan of intervention.

HISTORY

Typically the patient reports back pain on assuming a static position (such as sitting) and fatigue of the muscles as a result of their protective role. Movement brings temporary relief, signifying the presence of ligamentous insufficiency.[181,219] Paris[219]

defines hypermobility as a range of motion somewhat in excess of expected for that particular segment given the patient's age, body type, and activity status. Hypermobile joints are generally considered normal. However, complaints of "giving away" or "slipping out" and being able to "twist it back into position" are caused by *instability*. The differences between hypermobility and instability should be detected during the physical examination.

ALIGNMENT

Efficient alignment allows for equal weight-bearing distribution throughout the spine. Functional tasks such as lifting and carrying objects reveal the position and use of the cervical, thoracic, and lumbar spine. Assess the segmental relation of these three areas and any changes that occur during functional activity.

An important objective assessment of the vertical alignment of the thoracic and lumbar spine is the *vertical compression test*.[42,252,253] This test, described by Johnson and Saliba,[130] provides kinesthetic feedback as to how weight is transferred through the spine to the base of support. With the patient standing in a comfortable, natural stance, the therapist applies vertical compression through the shoulders, feeling for any giving away or buckling in the spine (Fig. 20-4). The idea is to test

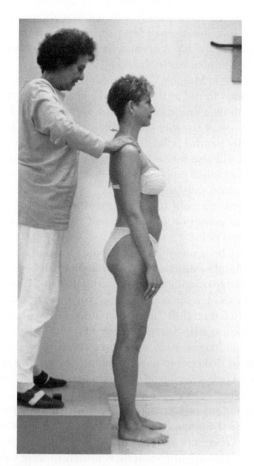

▪ **FIG. 20-4.** Compression testing of the spine.

the amount of "spring" the spine has under direct compression.[42] The patient should relate any increase or reproduction of symptoms. The examiner usually feels and may observe instability at the level of dysfunction, and the patient often reports pressure or pain from the vertical compression in the same area.

Deviations such as an increased posterior angulation of the thoracic spine, increased lumbar lordosis, or anterior shear of the pelvis suggest instability and the prevention of efficient weight transfer through the spine.[83,120,219] According to Saliba and Johnson,[253] when the natural segmental relation of the three spinal curves is interrupted, the spine no longer efficiently transfers the weight to the pelvis, but concentrates the force of the vertical loading at the biomechanically altered segment. This concentration of force appears to facilitate a progressive breakdown of the structural and neuromuscular stability at those segments.[219,243]

Wadsworth[282] describes another test for segmental vertebral instability particularly suited for the lower thoracolumbar spine. In this test the patient lies prone with the legs over the edge of the table and feet resting on the floor. If vertebral posterior–anterior glide applied by the therapist produces pain when the feet are supported by the floor and the paraspinal muscles are relaxed, but not when the legs are actively extended from the hips (bilateral hip extension) and the paraspinal muscles are contracted, the test is positive, implicating segmental instability.

During the objective examination, other signs that suggest hypermobility or instability of the lumbar spine, according to Paris,[219] and that would seem applicable to the middle and lower thoracic spine include:

1. During active forward bending, one may observe (when standing at the patient's side) a sharply angulated segment suggesting hypermobility. If one also observes a "shake," "catch," or "hitch," then there is instability.
2. When examining the patient from behind during forward bending, if the apophyseal joint is hypermobile, the vertebra will slide up more freely on that side, producing a sidebending to the opposite side at that level. Simultaneous uncoordinated muscle contraction or spasm suggests instability.
3. During standing, a hypertrophied band or hypertonic band of muscle may be evident. When palpated, it will show an increased tone or firmness to touch. If the tone is substantially reduced in prone lying, an instability exists, not a simpler hypermobility, according to Paris.[219]
4. Palpation for mobility using passive intervertebral motion has a satisfactory interrater reliability.[96] When performing these tests (forward bending, sidebending, and rotation), the clinician may notice that movements feel "too free" or that there is a forward step or slip in forward bending.

CONSERVATIVE TREATMENT

Treatment should be directed at decreasing the stresses on the unstable segment. The desired outcomes are to prevent worsening of instability and to reduce pain. The most harmful motion appears to be rotation, which produces both compression and shear.[83]

Therapy should include a program of stabilization techniques: isometric, abdominal, and back exercises, as well as localized techniques (segmental stabilization) for the erector spinae muscles, with particular focus on the multifidi (see Thoracic Spine Techniques below). The multifidi are the most influential in extension of small segments and in stabilizing the spine. Work should stress exercises done in midrange or beginning range and those directed at increasing endurance, strength, dynamic control, and sensitivity to stretch. One should also include correction of neighboring hypomobility, support of the involved segment, postural reeducation to reduce the strain, and diaphragmatic breathing exercises.

Rib Conditions

Some painful thoracic or lumbar conditions are associated with small derangements of the costovertebral or costotransverse articulations. Typically they are caused by trauma or an unguarded movement in rotation, such as turning too rapidly, or minimal motions such as reaching back to roll up the back window in a car. There are also anterior chondrocostal sprains, which are usually posttraumatic. According to Maigne,[175] costal sprains are common during judo, particularly at the level of the false ribs. Postural and muscle imbalances may also be a source of pain.

COSTAL SPRAINS

Most rib lesions are related to intercostal muscle spasms that diminish the normal expansion and contraction between the two ribs.[266–268] The most common cause is a sneeze or unexpected cough. These simple dysfunctions consist of restriction of excursion in either inhalation or exhalation and are commonly known as respiratory rib dysfunctions.[29,99] They are associated with hypertonus in the intercostal muscles above and below, and although they may not cause pain, the restriction of motion may cause a predisposition to recurrence of the spinal joint problem if not treated.

Costal sprains are expressed by thoracic or upper lumbar pain. Clinical examination does not reveal tenderness of the spine, but pain is produced by pressure on one rib only. The false ribs are usually involved.[175] The patient complains of a continuous soreness at the costovertebral angle that is aggravated by certain movements or positions. It may vary from a simple feeling of discomfort to pronounced chronic lumbar pain when the false ribs are involved.

A key test in the evaluation of costal sprain is the rib maneuver described by Maigne[175] (see Fig. 20-27). Whenever a rib lesion is suspected, the corresponding apophyseal joint must also be evaluated. Also, because ribs one to seven articulate anteriorly with the sternum, the sternoclavicular and costochondral joints may also need to be assessed.

The course of costal sprain is good, with relief of pain in a few days. If not, the lesion responds very well to a few sessions of deep transverse frictions (see Fig. 8-30).[213] However, a costal sprain may become chronic, resulting in thoracic and lumbar pain, and this may be responsible for diagnostic error. Rib articulations are described later in this chapter. Mobilization is performed by articulating the rib in the nonpainful direction.[175]

HYPOMOBILITY AND HYPERMOBILITY DYSFUNCTIONS

The intercostal muscle may be irritated from a central source—that is, an intervertebral joint lesion may cause nerve irritation and muscle contraction, which leads to restricted rib mobility. This type of dysfunction is sometimes called a structural rib deformity.[29] Positional alterations become evident on palpation and may consist of alterations in *eversion* (the lower rib margin becomes more prominent) or *inversion* (reverse findings), lateral flexion, anteroposterior compression, lateral compression, and subluxation.[29,99,197,266]

FIRST RIB SYNDROME

Often considered a compression syndrome, this condition is characterized by local unilateral pain or tenderness over the supraspinous fossa and by constant referred pain, aching, or paresthesia in the C8 or T1 dermatomal distribution of the arm, forearm, or hand.[189] With involvement of the first rib only, the costotransverse joint may be subluxed superiorly by the pull of the scaleni. This is not uncommon and is often associated with dysfunction of either C7–T1 or T1–T2.[29] The vertebral joints should always be checked and treated first if they are dysfunctional. On palpation, unilateral posteroanterior pressure on the costotransverse joint and on the first rib (caudally) readily reproduces some or all of the symptoms. Functionally there may be hypertrophy or adaptive shortening of the scalenus anticus or medius muscles, with associated elevation, hypomobility, or subluxation of the first rib.

Other signs may include a forward head and protracted shoulders and restriction of the acromioclavicular and sternoclavicular joints. In addition to restricted myofascia of the scalenus anticus and medius, there may also be restriction in the pectoralis minor and major, trapezius, levator scapulae, and sternoclavicular muscles.[181]

Initially the palpation technique that elicits the symptoms is the method used for treatment. Manipulations of restricted joints, soft tissue manipulation for tight muscles, and postural reeducation are all beneficial. There is often associated cervical joint dysfunction, and this must be treated to avoid recurrence from tightness in the scalene muscles.

HYPOMOBILITY

In hypomobility dysfunctions of the ribs the patient often presents with a forward head and increased thoracic kyphosis. Pain is usually posterior at the costovertebral or costotransverse joint, with occasional reference of pain laterally into the chest wall. Diaphragmatic breathing and movements requiring rib cage excursion may be uncomfortable. Signs that may be present during evaluation include[181]:

1. An altered breathing pattern, avoiding diaphragmatic breathing
2. With an *inhalation restriction*, no upward movement of the rib during inspiration; with an *exhalation restriction*, no descent of the rib during expiration
3. On palpation, tenderness involving the costovertebral joint as well as an altered position of the rib
4. Restriction of motion on testing

Treatment includes mobilization of the restricted segments, soft tissue mobilizations, and stretching of the involved intercostal muscles; self-mobilization and stretching to increase rib cage excursion; and postural reeducation.

HYPERMOBILITY

With hypermobility of the ribs, the patient complains of pain localized to the involved costal margin or costochondral area.[181] The pain is usually a dull ache, but there may be sharp episodes. Pain may be intermittent, aggravated by activities involving rotation, such as twisting while bending forward. Clicking sounds may be present. Signs include:

1. Protective posture and shallow breathing
2. Tenderness to palpation of the costochondral junction
3. Excessive joint-play motion or passive motion with spring tests
4. Tenderness of the costochondral junction

Treatment includes gentle stretching to the intercostal area to minimize soft tissue changes resulting from protective postures, correction of any hypomobilities, and advice on body mechanics to decrease the strain to the area.

Kyphosis

Kyphosis is most prevalent in the thoracic spine. There are four types of kyphotic deformities[80]:

1. Localized, sharp, posterior angulation that is called a *gibbous* (or hump back)
2. Dowager's hump, which results from postmenopausal osteoporosis
3. Decreased pelvic inclination (20°) with a mobile spine (flat back)
4. Decrease pelvic inclination (20°) with a thoracolumbar or thoracic kyphosis (round back)

The normal pelvic angle is 30° (Fig. 20-5).

Faulty posture, with excessive thoracic kyphosis and the protracted shoulder position that accompanies this, prevents the shoulder girdle joints from functioning normally. The internal rotators and serratus anterior shorten; the rhomboids and the lower trapezius lengthen. Adaptive anterior shortening of the glenohumeral capsule can result. Consequently, these patients develop restriction of movement of both shoulders as well as the upper thoracic spine.

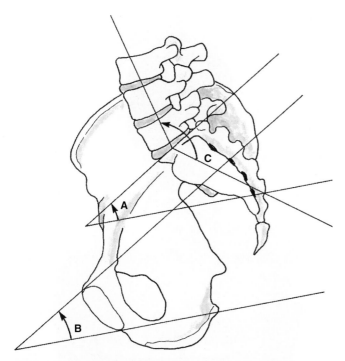

■ **FIG. 20-5.** Angles of the pelvic joint: **(A)** sacral angle (normal 30°); **(B)** pelvic angle (normal 30°); **(C)** lumbosacral angle (normal 140°). (Adapted with permission from Magee DJ: Orthopaedic Physical Assessment, 2nd ed. Philadelphia, WB Saunders, 1992:312.)

Thoracolumbar kyphosis, caused by a postural deficit, is classified as a *round back type I* or *type II*.[80] Patients with type I round back are not round-shouldered but are round-backed. Type I results from postural habits, type II from structural abnormalities. Often this is the presentation seen as a consequence of Scheuermann's disease (osteochondrosis in adolescence) and vertebra plana.[25,80] Scheuermann's disease frequently leads to an anterior wedging of the vertebra. This growth disorder affects about 10% of the population, and several vertebrae are usually affected. The most common area is between T10 and L2.[174] Regularly, with the dramatic and adverse changes of thoracic kyphosis, there is a parallel development of scoliosis.

There are many causes of kyphosis. If the cause is disease such as osteoporosis (see below) or Scheuermann's, exercise intervention cannot reverse the disorder, but it may be able to retard or prevent further exaggeration of the kyphosis.

Few conditions produce decreased kyphosis. Decrease or a reversal of the kyphosis of the interscapular thoracic spine involves the T2 to T6 vertebra. The origin of this flattened spine may be a congenital fixation of the thoracic spine.[80]

Senile Kyphosis

This common condition is responsible for the round shoulders and forward carriage of the head associated with advancing age. It occurs in older patients of either sex and is associated with severe degeneration of the midthoracic intervertebral disks. The principal radiologic changes involve the anterior part of these disks, with loss of disk space.[57]

Upper thoracic kyphosis (dowager's hump), with accompanying fluid retention, is common in postmenopausal women, men with heavy shoulders, and persons with poor postural sense. According to May,[181] the result is a loss of movement in the upper thoracic region, forcing hypermobility in the lower cervical spine, with tenderness and discomfort in the lower cervical spine aggravated by motion or sustained positions. Patients with dowager's hump at the cervicothoracic junction typically present with compensatory increased cervical lordosis and a forward head. They may also have an abnormally flat interscapular region, which is either very stiff or exceptionally irritable on palpation.[25] When this exists, the patient presents with various symptoms including localized upper thoracic, shoulder, cervical, and arm pain.

Senile kyphosis and upper thoracic kyphosis are usually asymptomatic, but some patients present with severe, aching pain that has been present for many years, is worse after activity, disturbs sleep, and tends to be episodic and difficult to control effectively with analgesics.[57]

Pain relief is difficult. Use of a brace, analgesics, exercise, postural control, stretching to the intercostal area, and mobilization techniques may provide temporary or partial relief of symptoms.

Osteoporosis

Osteoporosis frequently is associated with senile kyphosis or upper thoracic kyphosis in postmenopausal women. As a consequence of calcium deficiency, bones weaken; in the spine this causes thinning and wedging of the vertebral bodies, placing the person at risk for fractures. Mayo Clinic research has demonstrated that extension exercises, performed regularly, significantly reduce the number of compression fractures in persons with this disorder (see Figs. 22-21 and 22-68).[261,262] These studies demonstrated a significant correlation of the bone mineral density of the spine and the strength of back extensors with the patient's level of physical activity.

According to McKenzie,[187] the muscles strengthened by performing the exercises recommended by these Mayo Clinic studies are also the muscles responsible for maintaining upright posture. Maintaining good posture may assist in the strengthening process and reduce the likelihood of small compression fractures.

Use caution when prescribing an exercise program for the patient with spinal osteoporosis. Not all types of exercise are appropriate for these patients because of the fragility of their vertebrae. Exercises that place flexion forces on the vertebrae tend to cause vertebral fractures in these patients. Isometric abdominal strengthening exercises seem more appropriate than flexion exercises.[261,262]

McKenzie[187] recommends that extension exercises should be performed from perhaps the age of 40 for the rest of the patient's life. He recommends prone extension with pillows under the abdomen and the hands clasped behind the back. The patient lifts the head, shoulders, and legs simultaneously as high as possible. This position is held for a second, then the patient relaxes. The exercise is repeated as many times as possible; repetitions are increased until at least 15 to 20 are done in each session. In patients with severe osteoporosis the Mayo Clinic recommends extension exercises in sitting to minimize pain.[262]

Postural Disorders

Muscle pain may be felt without any underlying lesion of the cervical or thoracic joints and is related to postural changes. The patient is typically a woman who complains of stiffness and tenderness of the muscle groups related to the shoulder girdle and thorax. Frequently the patient has a sedentary occupation and in general lacks physical fitness. In addition to upper back pain, the patient often describes pain in the cervical and lumbar region. The pain usually worsens as the day goes on, and the patient is often conscious that it may be related to postural activities such as sitting for prolonged periods, typing, or other forms of continuous use. Writers, musicians, dentists, and computer programmers are all common victims. Pain may be aggravated by fatigue or stress or sometimes by changes in the weather.[57] This same pain pattern has been described in women with a postural sagging of the shoulder girdles or in those with large, pendulous breasts.

Treatment of these postural disorders involves simple measures such as reassurance, prophylactic advice, correction of sitting, standing, and sleeping postures, muscle-bracing exercises, relief positions (i.e., upper back stretch, Brugger's relief positions; see Fig. 19-71),[33,34] and special chairs (i.e., chairs with the seat tilted forward and a knee rest; a proper chair enforces lumbar lordosis and thus automatically achieves positional relief), as well as advice regarding problems peculiar to his or her occupation.[43] Changing posture or position is a form of exercise; proprioceptive neural circuits are directly involved.[186,223]

Numerous clinicians have written extensively on exercise programs for postural correction. The principles proposed by Kendall and coworkers[143] and Sahrmann[246–250] are most beneficial. The number of soft tissue treatment options is almost infinite. Muscle length can be restored with stretching techniques. Stretching can be specific for certain muscles or for certain directions, and can be facilitated by activating the antagonist, then activating the agonist.[2,81,157,260]

Assistive devices such as specialized taping procedures can be used to apply external tension (Fig. 20-6).[183,195,248] This tension can be corrective, guiding the soft tissues into a new position and thereby relieving stress on overloaded or overstretched tissues or applying a low-level stretch to restricted tissues, or both.[195] Tension can also serve as a simple behavior reminder, regularly cuing the patient to assume a better position. Other assistive devices include posture-correction

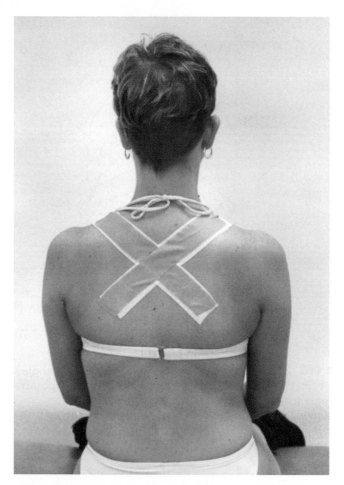

■ FIG. 20-6. Taping for postural correction and reeducation.

braces or a good support bra with criss-cross back straps or large back and shoulder straps.[143,248]

Posture should be addressed from a static viewpoint and more importantly from a dynamic one. Most of these clients, as well as others with thoracic dysfunction, especially with thoracic osteoporosis, will benefit from movement therapies intended to correct inefficient movement patterns (e.g., the Alexander technique,[6,19,94,131] the Feldenkrais method,[84–86,242] Aston patterning,[14,171,194,234] Klein-Vogelbach's functional kinetics,[45,155,156] and Trager's Mentastics,[23,134,135,274,275,284,292–294] which take the form of neuromuscular reeducation).

Other Clinical Syndromes and Differential Diagnosis

Apart from vertebral dysfunction, there are many other causes of thoracic pain. Differential diagnosis between rib and thoracic pain involvement is an important starting point. The first rib may have radiating pain to the upper limb. Neck pain and headache pain also can be associated with upper thoracic dysfunction.[111]

Frozen shoulder or restricted range of motion of the shoulder may be related to dysfunction of the first and second rib, especially the second rib.[111] Upper rib dysfunctions give the chief complaint of a painful shoulder with numbness and tingling into the arm and hand by involvement of the neurovascular bundle near the axilla.[264] Much pain in the first, second, and third rib may refer to the shoulder and must be differentiated from shoulder entrapment-type involvement. Costosternal tenderness with restriction of motion and shoulder restriction frequently is associated with a torsion lesion of the T3 rib.

Other syndromes that may benefit from manual therapy of the thorax include:

- Patient with chronic obstructive lung disease who can be treated with manual therapy and have their subjective complaints eased[111]
- Much attention needs to be placed on the thoracotomy and coronary artery bypass sternotomy patients in whom there has been a mechanical disruption of the normal movement of the thorax. These patients benefit greatly from normalizing the movement of the rib cage and vertebral area.
- Patients with compression deformities in the thoracic spine in the population that is osteoporosis-prone or has posttraumatic vertebral compression deformities respond well to structural evaluation and treatment once the bone has healed. These patients respond well to gentle muscle energy, strain counterstrain, and stretching techniques.

Note: for a discussion of thoracic outlet syndrome, see Chapter 11, Shoulder and Shoulder Girdle.

THORACIC SPINE EVALUATION

Clinical Considerations

Dysfunction of the joints of the thoracic spine is common in people with stresses and strains caused by poor posture and heavy lifting. The costovertebral joints are unique to the thoracic spine. Together with the apophyseal joints, they can present with well-localized pain close to the midline or with referred pain often quite distal to the spine. The major symptoms may appear to have no relation to the thoracic spine.

Clinical features to be considered in the evaluation include the following[144,204,205]:

1. Pain of lower cervical origin (C4 to C7) may be referred to the upper thoracic region. The lower cervical spine must be included in the evaluation of the upper thoracic spine, because the movement of one occurs in conjunction with the other.
2. The upper thoracic spine (T1 to T4) is the stiffest part of the spine. Pain is usually well localized.
3. The midthoracic spine (T5 to T7) is the most common site for apophyseal joint pain. T8 to T10 is the most common site for rib cage articulation problems and for referred pain mimicking visceral pain.

4. Pain of the thoracolumbar region (T11 to L1) is common. Pain can be referred to the lumbar region, especially the iliac crests. T11–T12 is the most common level for thoracic disk lesions.

THORACIC DISK LESIONS

Thoracic disk lesions in this region are less common than those of the cervical and lumbar spine. The clinical history often reveals an axial compression of the trunk, as occurs in a fall on the hindquarter or lifting a heavy object in the forward-bent position. The mode of onset is various: it can be sudden, or a posterior thoracic backache can come on slowly. As at other spinal levels, the mechanism of dural pain may be present, giving rise to unilateral extrasegmental reference of pain in the presence of a central protrusion (Fig. 20-2). Alternatively, a posterolateral displacement produces root pain referred anteriorly. At T1 and T2 symptoms may be felt in the arm; at lower levels symptoms are experienced at the side or front of the trunk (see Fig. 5-6). The dermatomal pain pattern should act as a guide only, because dermatomes overlap and there are variations between patients.

THORACIC PAIN OF LOWER CERVICAL ORIGIN

The clinical association between injury to the lower cervical region and upper thoracic pain is well known.[177] The T2 dermatome, which is in close proximity to the C4 dermatome, appears to represent the cutaneous areas of the lower cervical segments, as the posterior primary rami of C5 to C8. This is why patients present with interscapular pain after cervical spine injury. Such pain may have no connection with dysfunction of the thoracic spine, but instead represents injury to the lower cervical spine (which because of an apparent anomalous dermatome pattern refers pain to the interscapular region, usually corresponding to the T5 and T6 region). The scapula originates as part of the developing limb bud. As the limb develops, the scapula migrates to become folded back on the posterior thoracic wall. This is why the scapula, although it lies level with the thoracic segments, is innervated primarily by cervical segments. Thus, pain of cervical origin is often referred to the scapulae, as well as to the arms. The pain from the lower cervical spine can also refer to the anterior chest and mimic coronary ischemic pain.

COSTOTRANSVERSE JOINTS

So-called costotransverse joint syndrome is caused by arthrosis of these joints. Symptoms develop either spontaneously or when there has been an extenuation of these joints, as after a rib fracture. According to Hohmann,[116] the clinical symptoms include pain on forced and deep breathing that radiates along the ribs, a "whooping" feeling, and a sudden lightening-like pain that makes breathing difficult and may give a feeling of constriction.

Dysfunction of this joint commonly causes localized pain about 3 to 4 cm from the midline, where the ribs articulate.[144]

It may also be responsible for referred pain ranging from the midline, posterior to the lateral chest wall, and even the anterior chest wall. Diagnosis may be confirmed when movement of the rib provokes the pain at the costovertebral joint.

LOWER THORACIC SPINE AND THORACOLUMBAR JUNCTION

Dysfunction of joints in the thoracolumbar region can cause pain presenting primarily as iliac crest or buttock pain.[177] The skin over the iliac crest and upper outer buttock area is supplied by the posterior primary rami of nerves arising from the thoracolumbar junction (T12 and L1; Fig. 20-7). Similarly, anterior groin pain can arise from this region, as the nerve supply is from the anterior rami of the spinal nerves T12 and L1 (Fig. 20-7).[177] Because dermatomal symptoms can be present in either the posterior or anterior branches of the dorsal rami, with anterior abdominal symptoms the thoracic spine must be palpated.

MUSCLE PAIN

Muscle pain may also be experienced with no underlying lesion of the cervical or thoracic joints, and this is often related to postural changes of the thoracic spine.[57] Muscle injury occurs more often in the thoracic region than the cervical or lumbar regions.[60] The strong paravertebral muscles do not

appear to be a cause of chest pain, but strains of the intercostal, pectoral, and latissimus dorsi muscles, as well as the musculotendinous origins of the abdominals, can cause pain. Injuries to these muscles can be provoked by overstrains or attacks of violent coughing or sneezing.

OTHER CAUSES OF THORACIC PAIN

Apart from vertebral dysfunction, there are many causes of thoracic pain. Although posterior pain is often caused by vertebral dysfunction, there are several important visceral (e.g., biliary disorders, ischemic heart disease, penetrating peptic disorders) and vascular origins of this type of pain, some of which can be life threatening. Special problems to consider in the elderly are:

- Malignant disease, e.g., multiple myeloma, lung, prostrate
- Vertebral pathologic fractures
- Polymyalgia rheumatica
- Paget's disease

Features of the history that indicate the pain is arising from thoracic spine dysfunction include the following[144]:

1. Visceral disorders are not influenced by thoracic movements.
2. Aggravation and relief of pain on trunk rotation: the pain may be increased by rotating toward the side of pain but is eased by rotating in the opposite direction.

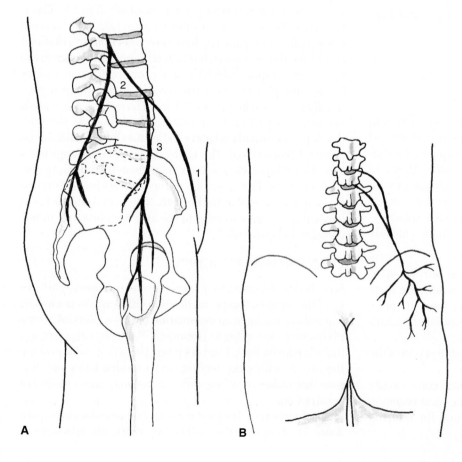

A **B**

■ **FIG. 20-7.** **(A)** Spinal nerves T12 and L1: 1, anterior branch; 2, posterior branch; 3, lateral branch. **(B)** Cutaneous innervation of the upper portion of the gluteal area (T11–T12 to L1) according to Maigne (1980). (Adapted with permission from Rogoff JB, ed: Manipulation, Traction and Massage, 2nd ed. Baltimore, Williams & Wilkins, 1980:100.)

3. Aggravation and relief of pain on trunk side flexion: typically flexion away from the painful side does not hurt, but flexion toward the painful side increases the pain. A neuroma on one side of the spine will painfully limit side flexion away from that side.
4. Aggravation of pain by coughing, sneezing, or deep inspiration tends to implicate the costovertebral joint.
5. Pain is relieved by firm pressure over the back.

Subjective Examination

A general approach to history taking and the subjective examination is described in Chapter 5, Assessment of Musculoskeletal Disorders and Concepts of Management. The concepts there and in Chapter 22, Lumbar Spine, all apply to the evaluation of the thoracic spine. One item peculiar to this area is the effect of breathing on the symptoms. Inspiration frequently causes pain; expiration does so far less commonly.[179] The history should include the chief complaints and a pain drawing (see Fig. 22-5). As with the lumbar spine, the Oswestry function test and McGill Pain Questionnaire are helpful in trying to objectify the quality of pain and its effect on function.[182,191]

When listening to the patient's history of pain, bear in mind the cervical spine, the costochondral articulations, and the scapulothoracic movement, as well as the obvious costovertebral and intervertebral joints. When the patient's symptoms refer to the legs, arms, head, or neck, assess these areas as well. Patience and care with assessment is extremely important, particularly when symptoms have both visceral and vertebral components.

Physical Examination

OBSERVATION

Observe the patient's posture, body type (i.e., ectomorphic, mesomorphic, endomorphic, or mixed), gait, and ability to move freely. A good time to observe the patient's general sitting posture is during the subjective examination. The patient will automatically choose the posture that he or she habitually assumes.

FUNCTIONAL ACTIVITIES

Assess whether spinal movements are free or restricted by watching the patient get in or out of a chair. Observe the position that he or she adopts while sitting and undressing. This can be done before undertaking a more formal inspection of bony structure and alignment. Functional movements that reproduce the patient's symptoms should be part of the objective examination. This information provides reassessment measures that are relevant to the patient and clinician. The functional activities that are likely to aggravate thoracic problems are rotational movements, a combination of flexion and rotation, or sustained unsupported sitting.[129] The lower extremity functional profile is an excellent tool that allows a firm starting

point for objective measurement of the thoracic spine and lower quadrant (see Chapter 10, Functional Exercise).

GAIT

Observe the patient's gait. The typical gait patterns that might be expected in patients with thoracic or lumbar spine are the short-leg gait, Trendelenburg's gait, and the gluteus maximus gait. See Tables 24-1 and 24-2 for an overview of the primary gait abnormalities associated with various common lower thoracic–lumbar or lower limb disorders or structural deviations.

INSPECTION

With the patient standing with the back, shoulders, and legs exposed, observe features such as the level of the pelvis and any disturbance of spinal curves. View the patient from the front, back, and sides. Record specific alterations in bony structure or alignment, soft tissue configurations, and skin status.

Bony Structure and Alignment. Refer to the section on assessment of structural alignment in Chapter 24, Lumbosacral–Lower Limb Scan Examination, for a complete discussion of this part of the examination with respect to the lower thoracic spine. Observe the total body posture from the head to the toes and look for any deviations. Typical postures include the following and are described in more detail in Chapter 7, Myofascial Considerations and Evaluation in Somatic Dysfunction:

- Proximal or shoulder crossed syndrome[125]
- Pelvic or distal crossed syndrome[137] or the kyphosis–lordosis posture (see Fig. 7-23)[143]
- Flat back posture (see Fig. 7-24)[143]
- Sway back posture (see Fig. 7-25)[143]
- Handedness posture (see Fig. 7-26)[143]
- Layer syndrome

The examiner should passively correct any asymmetry to determine its relevance to the patient's problem. Alterations in overall spinal posture may lead to problems in the thoracic spine. Look for kyphosis and scoliosis. Younger patients in particular should be screened for scoliosis.

I. Posterior Alignment (the patient is viewed from behind in the standing position)
  A. Shoulder level: Posteriorly the spine of the scapula should be level with the T3 spinous process. The inferior angle of the scapula is level with the T7 spinous process. The medial borders of the scapulae are parallel to the spine and about 5 cm lateral to the spinous processes.[174] A common sign of scoliosis is unequal shoulder levels and apparent winging of a scapula.
  B. Spinal posture: Look for scoliosis and the presence of a lateral shift.
    1. Lateral shift: This is present if the shoulders and trunk have moved laterally in relation to the pelvis. It is described in terms of the direction of the shift of the

shoulders and the upper trunk—that is, if they have moved to the left it is described as a left lateral shift. When it is present and symptomatic it often indicates a derangement, usually of the lumbar spine.[75,185]

2. Scoliosis: In this deformity there are one or more lateral curves of the lumbar or thoracic spine (Fig. 20-8). It is gauged from the line of the spinous processes and described with respect to the convexity of the curve. Scoliosis may be structural or nonstructural and compensated (Fig. 20-8A) or uncompensated (Fig. 20-8B). A structural scoliosis does not straighten during forward bending or sidebending into the convexity of the spine. Because lateral bending is always accompanied by rotation, there will be a lumbar bulge or rib hump (gibbous) with forward bending if a structural scoliosis is present (Fig. 20-8C). The criteria for screening, evaluation, and diagnosis and a review of nonoperative methods of treatment are covered extensively in the literature.[15,16,40,56,82,89,90,142,143,149,152,199,240,276,286,287,289]

    a. A *functional scoliosis* can be caused by muscle imbalance, poor posture, or a leg-length discrepancy. This type of scoliosis generally straightens on forward bending and sidebending into the convexity, except in the presence of muscle spasm or guarding.

    b. *Acute scoliosis:* Facet joint impingement may cause an acute scoliosis in any area of the spine. This disorder involves the entrapment of soft tissue within the facet joint.[200,255] If this happens, the patient may shift to the opposite side of impingement to take the weight off the painful structure. A more common type of lateral curve is the lateral shift or protective scoliosis (see above).[185]

3. Rib cage: Have the patient cross the forearms in front of the body. Posteriorly, inspect for rib asymmetry and carriage of the scapulae. Palpate for rib prominence by a flat-handed sweep over the posterolateral surface of the hemithorax.

4. Sacral base and leg length: Inspect for the presence of segmental vertical asymmetries. See Chapter 24, Lumbosacral–Lower Limb Scan Examination.

II. Anterior Alignment (the patient is viewed from the front)
    A. Shoulders: Common faults include dropped or elevated shoulders. Note any clavicular, sternoclavicular, or acromioclavicular joint asymmetry.
    B. Rib cage: Inspect for rib cage deformities such as pigeon chest (pectus carinatum), funnel chest (pectus excavatum), or barrel chest (Fig. 20-9). Note any increase or decrease in the infrasternal angle (more or less than 90°). See the section on soft tissue inspection below.

III. Sagittal Alignment (the patient is viewed from the side; obvious abnormalities or asymmetries of the extremities and spine are noted)
    A. Cervical spine: Does the head deviate from the optimal posture (4 to 8 cm) from the apex of the thoracic kyphosis to the deepest point in the cervical lordosis (see Fig. 17-20)?[238]

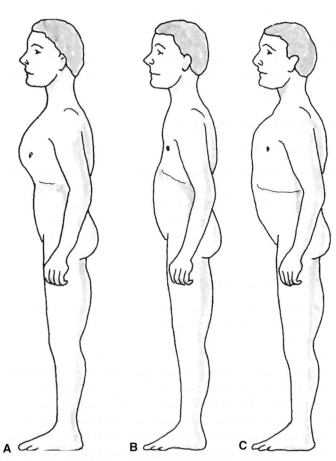

■ **FIG. 20-9.** Chest deformities: **(A)** pectus carinatum, **(B)** pectus excavatum, and **(C)** barrel chest.

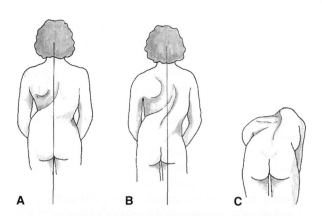

A   B   C

■ **FIG. 20-8.** Scoliosis: To distinguish between a compensated and an uncompensated deviation of the posture, a plumb line is dropped from the first thoracic spinal process. **(A)** Compensated right thoracic–lumbar curve. **(B)** Uncompensated right thoracic curve with a right list. **(C)** When viewed from behind, minor degrees of structural scoliosis can be detected in forward bending. A rotatory component produces a rib deformity or hump.

B. Shoulders: The acromion process often lies anterior to the plumb line; the scapulae are abducted and are associated with excessive kyphosis and forward head. Tightness of the pectoralis major and minor, serratus anterior, and intercostal muscles is most often found.

C. Thoracic spine: Note increased anteroposterior curves (e.g., localized or generalized dowager's hump [osteoporosis causing excessive kyphosis in the C7 to T1 area]). Kyphosis may be generalized, with the back having a smooth, uniform contour, or it may be localized if it is caused by a collapsed vertebra, as occurs in an older person with osteoporosis. Increased posterior convexity (generalized kyphosis) may be caused by tightness of the anterior longitudinal ligament and the upper abdominal and anterior chest muscles. Other muscle findings include stretched thoracic extensors, middle and lower trapezius, and posterior ligaments.

D. The angle of minimum kyphosis can be obtained by a two-inclinometer measurement. Standing and sitting techniques, with the inclinometer at T1 and T12 and with the subject in the erect "military brace" posture, are used to obtain the angle of minimum kyphosis.[9]

E. Chest and rib cage: Note any depression of the anterior thorax and sternum (funnel chest), increased overall anteroposterior diameter of the rib cage (barrel chest), or projection of the sternum anteriorly and downward (pigeon chest).

F. Lumbar spine: Observe for an accentuated or reduced lordosis. Note whether the sacrovertebral or lumbosacral angle is normal (Fig. 20-5).

IV. Transverse Rotary Alignment (the patient is viewed from the front and from behind). The stance width should be normal and the feet slightly (5 to 10°) pointed outward. Assess segmental rotatory alignment, working upward from the feet. See Chapter 24, Lumbosacral–Lower Limb Scan Examination, for assessment of the lower limbs.

A. Anterosuperior iliac spines: These should be positioned in a frontal plane. If the pelvis is rotated (one iliac spine is more anterior then the other) the common causes to be considered are:
   1. A fixed (structural) spinal scoliosis, the rotatory component of which is transmitted to the pelvis through the sacrum via the lumbar spine
   2. Torsional asymmetry of the sacroiliac joints

B. Rib cage: Note whether the ribs are symmetrical and whether the rib contours are normal and equal on both sides. The contours should both be positioned in a frontal plane. In scoliosis the ribs are pushed posteriorly and the thoracic cage is narrowed on the convex side of the curve; the ribs on the concave side move anteriorly.

Soft Tissue Inspection. Note obvious asymmetries in muscle bulk and prominence of the trapezius on one side. Seek regions of muscle tightness and muscle tone, comparing one side with the other. One side of the erector spinae may be tighter than the other, with subsequent listing of the torso. Some muscles are felt to shorten under stress while other muscles weaken, producing muscle imbalance (see Table 5-6). Patterns of muscle imbalance are thought to be one of the causes of altered postures mentioned above. Note abdominal muscle length (i.e., rectus abdominis, internal and external obliques). According to Sahrmann,[248] shortness of the rectus abdominis results in anterior rib cage depression, shortness of the internal oblique results in an increase in the infrasternal angle, and shortness of the external oblique results in a decreased angle. If the internal and external obliques are short, one may find a long lumbar lordosis with paraspinal atrophy and a narrow infrasternal angle, or thoracic kyphosis with a depressed chest and a narrow infrasternal angle.

Observe the skin for any abnormality or scars. If there are scars, what were the causes? Look for any local swelling or cutaneous lesions, such as café-au-lait spots, patches of hair, or areas of pigmentation, or any abnormal depressions. A tuft of hair may indicate a spina bifida occulta or diastematomyelia.[180]

JOINT TESTS: SELECTIVE TISSUE TENSION

Joint tests include integrity tests and active and passive physiologic movements of the thoracic spine and other relevant joints. Segmental mobility (accessory or joint-play movements) completes the joint tests.

I. Joint Integrity Tests
   Nonspecific stability testing of this area involves the use of testing thoracic resilience by the use of vertical pressure to the spinous processes in a rhythmic or springing fashion via pisiform contact.[211] This test gives the examiner an idea of the resilience in the thoracic spine or stiffness of the back. Vertical compression, traction, and spinal translation tests of arthrokinetic function are more specific.[69,162,172] Vertical traction and compression tests stress the anatomic structures that resist vertical forces.

A. Vertical compression is applied to the middle and lower thoracic region by applying a vertical force through the top of the patient's shoulders with the patient in sitting. Compression is applied to the upper thoracic by applying a vertical force through the cranium (see Fig. 19-17).

B. Vertical traction is applied to the upper thorax by applying a vertical force through the cranium (see Fig. 19-18). Traction is applied to the middle and lower thoracic by applying a vertical force through the patient's crossed arms (Fig. 20-10). If the test reproduces the patient's symptoms, injury of the longitudinal ligaments may be present or, in an acutely painful patient, an inflammation of the articular facet joints.[69]

C. Specific passive translation test. A variety of passive translation tests of a segmental spinal unit may be performed.[162,172] Lateral stability (rotation) test for the midthoracic spine (T3–T7) is carried out with the patient sitting with the arms across the chest. The examiner first

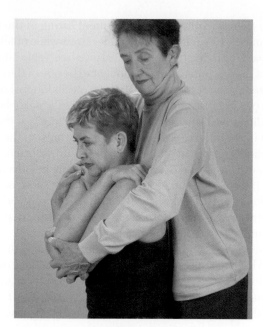

■ **FIG. 20-10.** Vertical traction test.

examines the available range of lateral translation by translating the sixth rib (T5) while stabilizing the spinous processes and transverse process of T6 (Fig. 20-11). The range and end feel of this level are compared with the levels above and below. Stability is then tested by translating the fifth rib (and T5) in the transverse plane while stabilizing the transverse processes and spinous process of T6 and the sixth rib. If there is instability at the T5–T6 level, the clinician will feel movement during the test.[163]

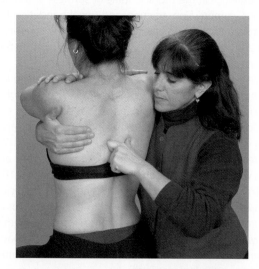

■ **FIG. 20-11.** Examination of available range of lateral translation at the T5–T6 level. The patient is sitting with the arms across the chest. The thumb and index finger of the stabilizing hand stabilize the spinous process and transverse process of T6, while the other hand translates the sixth ribs (and T5) laterally.

II. Active Physiologic Joint Movements of the Spine

   Because the lumbar and thoracic spine form part of a continuous coordinated motion pattern, they are assessed together. With all movements, determine the range, rhythm, and quality of active movement. Note any localized restriction of movement and any protective deformity, muscle guarding, or painful arc of motion. Note whether the patient's symptoms are reproduced. Not every movement listed below is needed for every patient.

   First test the patient while standing. Have him or her extend and laterally flex the spine. This is followed by flexion and rotation.

   A. Standing tests

      1. Extension (backward bending). After observing the global range of motion from the side, kneel behind the patient and while supporting his or her pelvis ask the patient to extend again while observing the thoracic extension. Ask the patient to bend the head, shoulders, middle back, and lower back sequentially.

         a. The thoracic curve should flow backward or at least straighten in a smooth, even manner. If the patient shows excessive kyphosis, this curvature will remain on extension.

         b. Thoracic spine extension is normally 25 to 45°. A tape measure may be used to measure the distance between two points (the C7 and T12 spinous processes). A 2.5-cm difference between standing and extension is normal.[80,174] Inclinometry and spondylometry may also be used to measure spinal extension, either in standing or the sphinx position (Fig. 20-12).[68,95] The values found in the sphinx position may be compared with values in minimal kyphosis or the military posture (in standing). This method (Fig. 20-12) can also be used for measuring extension of the lumbar spine by placing the inclinometer at the sacrum and T12.

      2. Lateral flexion (sidebending; see Fig. 7-31): Have the patient sidebend the head, shoulders, middle back, and lower back, first to one side and then to the other. Symmetry of movement may be judged by comparing the distance from the fingertip to the fibular head on either side and by observing the degree of spinal curvature with movement in either direction. Assess the continuity of segmental movement and look for any tightness or hypermobility at a specific segment when the movement is performed. Lateral flexion is the best movement with which to test the hypomobile lesion.

         a. Bilateral limitation in a young person suggests serious disease but in the elderly person may be attributed to no more than decreased mobility with the passage of time.[60]

         b. With multisegmental capsular restriction, sidebending is restricted in both directions.

         c. Lateral flexion is about 20 to 40°. Some observers measure lateral flexion by measuring the distance between the fingers and knee, or between the fin-

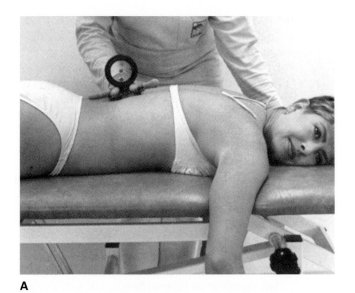
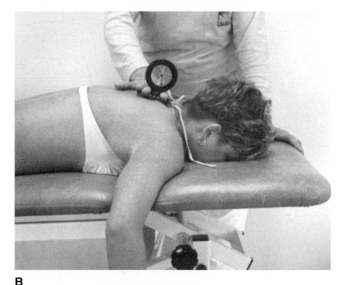

A

B

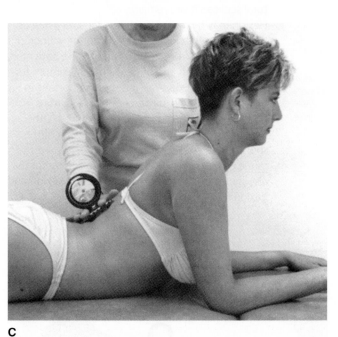
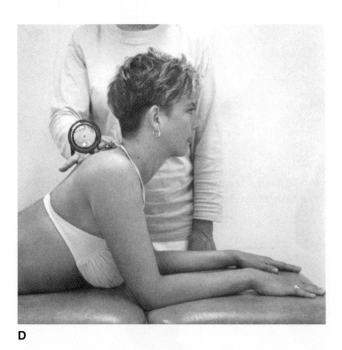

C

D

■ **FIG. 20-12.** Measuring extension of the thoracic spine in the sphinx position. In prone (**A**), the inclinometer is placed over T12 and set at zero. (**B**) The inclinometer is then moved to T1 and the degrees of neutral kyphosis are read. The patient then assumes the sphinx position (**C**), and the inclinometer is moved to T12 and set at zero. (**D**) The inclinometer is then moved to T1, and the degrees are read on the dial. The values taken in the sphinx position are subtracted from the values in neutral kyphosis to determine true extension motion.

gers and the floor. A more objective method devised by Moll and Wright[198] (Fig. 20-13) involves placing two ink marks on the skin of the lateral trunk. The upper mark is placed at a point where a horizontal line through the xiphisternum crosses the coronal line. The lower mark is drawn at the highest point on the iliac crest. The distance between the two marks is measured in centimeters using a tape measure first with the patient standing erect, and again after full lateral flexion. The new distance between the two marks is measured and subtracted from the first measurement. The remainder is taken as an index of lateral spinal mobility. Distraction on the contralateral trunk or approximation of the marks on the homolateral trunk may be used. Lateral spinal movement may also be measured with an inclinometer.[9,95,169]

3. Flexion (forward bending; see Fig. 7-27): Have the patient bend the head and cervical spine forward, then

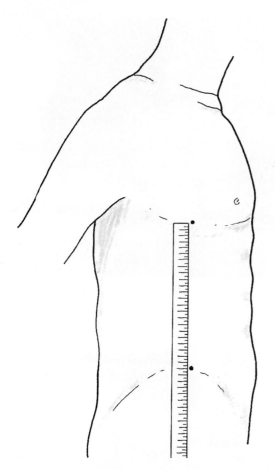

■ FIG. 20-13. Measuring thoracolumbar lateral flexion with a tape measure.

the thoracic spine, and finally the lumbar spine. Have the patient repeat the motion with the eyes closed. Assess the general and specific mobility of the spine. Ask the patient if he or she is experiencing any pain, stiffness, or other symptoms with the movement.

a. Note whether the patient drifts to the left or right instead of bending straight forward. If this is found, it indicates unilateral hypomobility of the apophyseal joint(s), unilateral muscular tightness, or a posterolateral disk protrusion. Drift can often be more readily seen when patients close their eyes, because it is natural for patients to fix their eyes to the floor and guide themselves straight down, thus overriding the tendency to drift laterally.

b. Note whether the thoracic spine shows increased kyphosis or any evidence of a structural scoliosis. With a nonstructural scoliosis, the scoliotic curve will disappear on forward flexion, but with a structural scoliosis it will remain.

c. Flexion may be measured with a tape measure as the distance the fingertips reach from the floor or as the distance from C7 to T12, with the patient in the erect position and then again in maximum forward bending. However, it is more important to observe the relative movement of the spinous processes and to record any loss of range. Other objective clinical methods include the use of the spondylometer and inclinometer.[9,13,95] The normal range of motion is 20 to 45°. The inclinometer may also be used to assess segmental lateral flexion and flexion (Fig. 20-14) of the spine.[95]

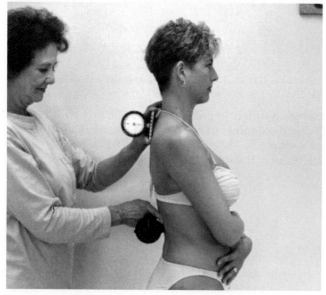
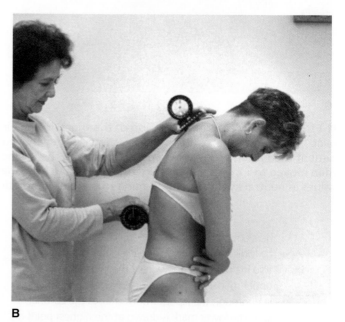

A **B**

■ FIG. 20-14. Testing flexion with an inclinometer. **(A)** One inclinometer is placed in the sagittal plane at the T1 level and the other at the T12 level. Both instruments are zeroed. **(B)** The thoracic spine is flexed forward so as not to involve the lumbar spine. Both instruments' readings are recorded. The T12 value is subtracted from the T1 value to arrive at the thoracic flexion angle.

4. Rotation in standing: Have the patient bend forward to 45° with the hands folded across the chest and the feet together. The patient then rotates fully to the right and left while the examiner observes the amount of rotation and compares one side with the other. When the two-inclinometer method is used, one inclinometer is placed at the T1 level in the coronal plane and the other at the T12 level. Restrained active rotation of the thoracic spine of 20° or less is an impairment of the function of the thoracic spine in the activities of daily living.[80] Rotation in standing can also be tested in the fully erect position with or without the help of outstretched arms or folded arms. Such rotation is more likely to include detectable movement of the lower thoracic spine.

Rotation should be further tested with the patient seated and the trunk alternatively in flexion and then extension (see below).

B. Sitting tests. Overpressure can easily be applied in this position and may be necessary to reproduce the pain. Note the range of each of these movements, whether symptoms are reproduced, any disturbance in normal synchronous rhythm, and the presence of muscle spasm. Correct any movement deviation to determine its relevance to the patient's symptoms.

1. Upper thorax.[69] The patient is asked to raise both arms over the head while keeping the palms together. The patient is asked to move into flexion, lateral flexion, extension, and rotation. During these movements the examiner grasps one of the patient's arms and with the other arm monitors the spinous and transverse processes at specific levels (Fig. 20-15). During these movements the examiner observes the pattern of restriction, taking particular note of restriction of the articular facets during opening and closing and restriction of the costotransverse joint demonstrated by decreased in superior or inferior glide during flexion, extension, side flexion, and rotation.

2. Mid–low thorax. The patient is sitting with the arms across the chest.

a. Flexion. The patient is asked to flex forward as though trying to place the forehead on the knees. Observe areas of segmental restriction and for any paravertebral fullness that might indicate hypertonus. Overpressures may be applied by pushing down on top of the shoulders to increase thoracic flexion.

b. Extension. The patient actively extends. Both hands of the examiner push down on top of the shoulders to increase extension.

c. Lateral flexion. Using a hand placed against the patient's side, the patient is asked to laterally flex over the examiner's hand. One hand on the opposite shoulder applies a force to increase thoracic lateral flexion.

d. Rotation of the thoracic spine is the key movement that requires scrutiny on examination. According to Cyriax and Cyriax,[60] the movement most likely to

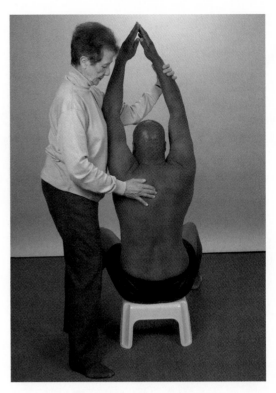

■ **FIG. 20-15.** Upper thoracic mobility test.

hurt with a disk lesion is the extreme of passive rotation. In a minor protrusion this may be the only painful movement.

i. With the patient's arms folded across the chest, active rotation can be tested in the erect or extended position. This can then be compared with the same rotation in the flexed position. In the erect position the patient can usually rotate about 60 to 70°. von Pavelka[220] devised a simple objective clinical method to measure thoracolumbar rotation with a tape measure (Fig. 20-16).

ii. Rotation with passive overpressure (Fig. 20-17). Fix the patient's pelvis by stabilizing his or her knees with your own knees. Have the patient cross the arms with the hands resting on opposite shoulders and actively rotate, or the examiner may move the trunk passively toward end range (patient's arms at side). Apply gentle overpressure by placing a hand on each shoulder and applying further pressure or small oscillatory movements at the end of the painless range in each direction. Note not only the end range but also the end feel of the movement. A normal end feel is springy or elastic; an abnormal end feel is usually that of a firm, hard stop.

If all movements are full and symptom-free on overpressure, and the pressures are aggravated by certain postures, the condition is categorized as a postural syndrome.[222]

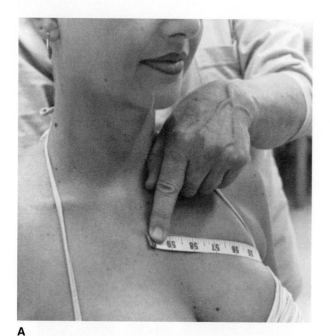

A

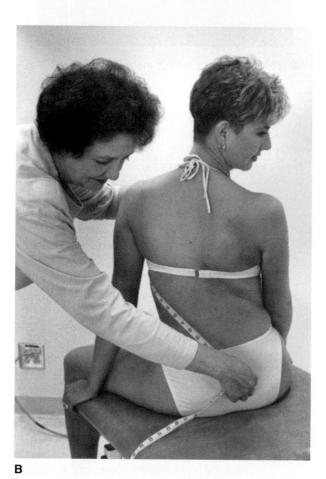

B

■ **FIG. 20-16.** Measurements of thoracolumbar rotation in sitting with a tape measure are made over the spinous process of L5 and over the jugular notch. Using a tape measure, the distance between these two points is recorded before (**A**) and after (**B**) full trunk rotation.

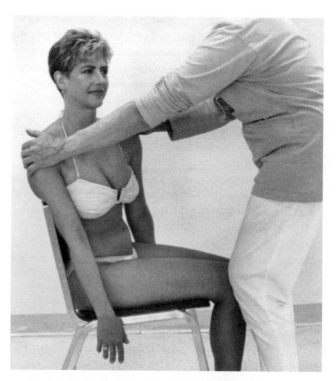

■ **FIG. 20-17.** Thoracic rotation with passive overpressure.

3. Active physiologic (segmental) mobility testing: A useful test of vertebral motion and restriction is to monitor changes in the relation of individual segments during active forward and backward bending (Fig. 20-18).[99,166] Standing behind the seated patient, palpate the transverse processes (with the thumbs and index fingers) at individual levels while having the patient either flex forward or extend. Note the quantity of motion, as well as the cranial and caudal displacement of the transverse processes. Asymmetry indicates dysfunction.

4. Auxiliary tests: If the above movements do not reproduce the patient's pain, auxiliary tests that may do so include:
   • Quadrant tests. This movement is a combination of extension, rotation, and lateral flexion (to the same side). Both hands are placed on top of the shoulders, the patient actively extends, and the clinician then passively rotates and laterally flexes the thoracic spine to one side.[222] Correct any movement deviations to determine its relevance to the patient's symptoms.
   • Performing the test movements repeatedly and at increasing speeds in erect sitting (i.e., flexion, extension, and rotation). Speeds of movement can be altered.
   • Applying sustained pressure at the limit of the range of relevant movements
   • Combined movement tests involving many sequences of combined movements, as well as

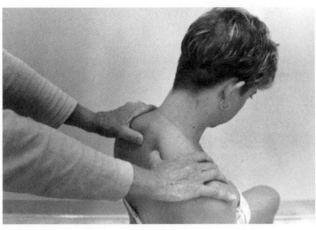

A

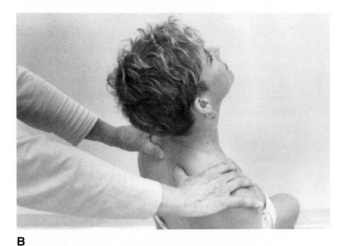

B

■ **FIG. 20-18.** Active (segmental) physiologic mobility testing of forward (**A**) and backward (**B**) bending.

combined motions with compression, can be used, but they are beyond the scope of this text (see Figs. 22-9 to 22-12). See the works of Edwards,[72–74] Lee,[162] and Maitland.[179] When combined motions are performed it should be remembered that coupling is determined in this region by the initiating movement. Rotexion, that is, a motion initiated with rotation, produces the coupling of ipsilateral side flexion and rotation, where as latexion, a motion initiated with side flexion, produces contralateral side flexion and rotation.[162]

- Cervical spine movements should always be tested to exclude pain referred from the lower cervical spine. Cervical flexion may exacerbate any thoracic pain, even if pain arises from the thoracic spine.[57] It helps to keep the thoracic spine immobile to determine whether the cervical spine is responsible for the pain. One way to achieve this, according to McKenzie,[187] is to have the patient sit unsupported in the slump position while active cervical motions

are carried out. If the patient's thoracic symptoms are altered in this position, they probably arise from the cervical spine.

- The upper limbs should also be included. With the patient sitting, examine the upper limbs in a cursory fashion to determine whether they are free of symptoms. Elevating the arms extends the thoracic spine. Try to clarify the effect of neck and arm movements on the thoracic spine. Tightness of the latissimus dorsi muscles and the thoracolumbar fascia will prevent full shoulder joint flexion and flatten the lumbar lordosis.

C. Rib motion and thoracic excursion. Observe breathing pattern and general mobility of the ribs by watching the respiratory range anteriorly and posteriorly with the patient sitting. Note whether expansion is mainly costal or diaphragmatic and if there is a painful phase of inspiration. Assess diaphragmatic breathing also in supine.

1. Evaluation of thoracic excursion during inspiration and exhalation: Have the patient maximally inhale and exhale. Excursion of both the upper and lower halves of the thorax is evaluated by placing the thumbs along the midline of the trunk (posterior and anterior aspect) with the hands embracing the thoracic cage. Note the amount of excursion and asymmetrical movements. Possible findings include decreased thoracic excursion in the presence of various pulmonary diseases, such as ankylosing spondylitis and scoliosis, or pronounced abdominal breathing, which is almost always associated with decreased thoracic excursion.[70]

2. Active physiologic mobility testing (specific articular mobility [individual rib motion testing during respiration])

   a. With the patient prone, palpate the ribs just lateral to the tubercle and medial to the rib angle during full inspiration and expiration. Note the quantity and quality of motion. Repeat this test for each rib. Compare the sides.

   b. With the patient supine, starting on the cranial aspect of the ribs at the sternocostal junction, palpate for rib excursion during full inspiration and expiration. Note the quantity and quality of motion. Repeat this test for each rib. Compare the sides and note any asymmetry.

   c. With the patient supine and during full inspiration and expiration, palpate (with the index fingers) the lateral aspect of the ribs in the midaxillary line. Possible findings include decreased rib motion, either regionally or segmentally, or asymmetry, indicating possible dysfunction.

D. Chest expansion (costovertebral expansion). Rigidity of the thoracic cage is characteristic of spinal and chest disorders and of the late stages of ankylosing spondylitis. An expansion of 3 cm at the T4 level is considered within the lower limits of normal.[198] The patient should be sitting with the hands on the head and the arms flexed in the sagittal plane to prevent maximum contraction of the shoulder adductors. Measure the circumference at rest and during maximum expiration and inspiration at the fourth rib level. Measurements may also be taken at the ninth rib level (three fingers widths below the xiphoid) and subcostally (level of the umbilicus). Record measurements taken at rest, during inspiration, and during expiration. Subtract the smaller figure (expiration) from the larger (inspiration). When the subcostal measurement is greater on expiration and less on inspiration, the results should be recorded as minus.

Determine the affects of inspiration and expiration in flexion and extension. Inspiration and expiration tests in flexion and extension are used to assess spinal contribution to symptoms.[257]

- If full inspiration (which extends the spine) is painful in extension but not in flexion, the spine is implicated.
- If it is painful in both full flexion and extension, a costal problem is implied.

III. Passive Joint Movements

The passive movements that should be tested include the compression test of the spine,[42,197] positional tests,[123] static postures,[186] and passive physiologic movements including segmental palpation (feeling movement between the adjacent spinous processes or ribs) and segmental mobility (accessory movements) of the spine.

A. Passive physiologic joint movements. Passive physiologic intervertebral movements (PPIVMs), which examine the movement at each segmental level, are done with palpation to appreciate the movement of each segment. Palpate between the spinous processes and compare the movement obtained at each level. The chief movements of the T4 to T12 region are forward and backward bending. Sidebending and rotation are limited by the ribs. Rotation occurs mostly at the lower thoracic and upper lumbar spine.

1. C7 to T4 passive motion of flexion (forward bending), extension (backward bending), lateral flexion (sidebending), and rotation at individual segments. Standing at the side of the seated patient, place your middle finger over the spinous process of the vertebra being tested and the index and ring fingers between the spinous processes of the two adjacent vertebrae. Place your other hand on the patient's head or forehead, and introduce flexion and extension (passive movement) to this area (Fig. 20-19A, B). Then introduce passive lateral flexion and rotation (Fig. 20-19C, D). With each motion component introduced, evaluate the movement by assessing its quality, paying particular attention to the coupled movements and determining whether the movement is hypermobile or hypomobile relative to the adjacent vertebrae.

Findings: Asymmetrical movement, abnormal coupling patterns, and hypomobility or hypermobility may indicate disease. Pain with movement, especially in the cervicothoracic junction and during extension, may be caused by a segmental somatic dysfunction—that is, impaired or altered function of related components of the somatic system, such as skeletal, arthrodial, and myofascial structures, as well as related vascular, lymphatic, and neural elements.[29,70]

2. T4 to T12 passive motion testing of flexion and extension. The patient sits with the fingers clasped behind the neck and the elbows together in front. Via the patient's hands or arms, introduce passive flexion and extension (Fig. 20-20) while palpating over the spinous processes as previously described. Pay attention to the gliding motion of the thoracic spinous processes in relation to each other.

Findings: The spinous processes do not separate during flexion, do not approximate during extension, or both. Two or more segments are usually involved. Typically this is caused by joint dysfunction secondary to degenerative joint disease. In young people it may be related to Scheuermann's disease.

3. T4 to T12 passive motion testing of lateral flexion (sidebending). The patient sits with the hands clasped behind the neck and the elbows together in front. Reach across the front of the patient and place the stabilizing hand over the patient's shoulder. Use the fingers of the monitoring hand to palpate the spinous processes (Fig. 20-21). Use your chest to introduce sidebending movement or force against the patient's shoulder girdle, against which the patient rests. During normal passive sidebending, the spinous processes rotate to the same side (toward the side of the convexity of the thoracic spine).[70] Compare movement at the various levels.

Findings: A segmental dysfunction may be suspected when the spinous processes do not exhibit coupled rotation with induced lateral flexion.[70]

4. T4 to T12 motion testing of rotation. The patient sits astride the plinth with arms clasped behind the neck. Standing at the patient's side, reach across the patient from below or thread your arm through the patient's flexed arms and grasp the opposite shoulder. With the patient stabilized against your trunk, move your whole body to effect rotation. Use the fingers of the free hand, placed on the spinous processes as previously described, to palpate the coupled rotatory movement (Fig. 20-22). Evaluate the amount and quality of movement of each segment, as well as that of adjacent segments and any pain induced.

Findings: If the spinous processes do not rotate with passive rotation, a segmental or regional joint or somatic dysfunction is suggested.

B. Passive accessory intervertebral movements (PAIVMs). These passive movements (except for the springing test) are produced by pressure of the thumbs on the spinous process and the transverse process. Spinous processes are

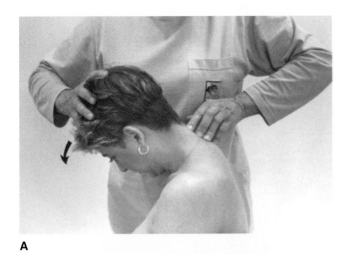

A

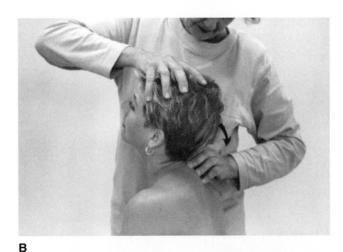

B

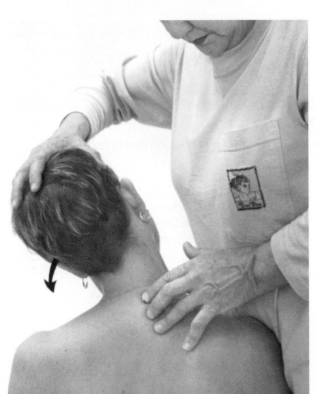

C

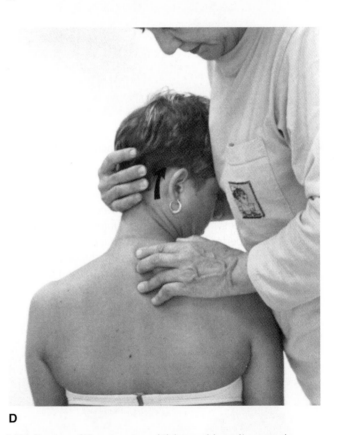

D

■ **FIG. 20-19.** Upper thoracic (C7–T4) passive motion testing of (**A**) flexion, (**B**) extension, (**C**) lateral bending, and (**D**) rotation.

tested using posteroanterior (central) and transverse pressures (on the side of spinous processes); these may be varied by angling the direction of the pressure toward the head or the feet, or diagonally. This is followed by posteroanterior pressures against the transverse processes, over the costotransverse junctions (unilateral), and over the ribs (unilateral).

Passive movement is the key to examination and treatment. It helps identify the site and origin of the pain and is the basis of specific mobilization techniques.

The preferred position for examining the lower thoracic spine is with the patient lying prone across the table (see Fig. 22-14), with a cushion or pillow under the abdomen to place the lower thoracic spine in neutral (resting position). A fully prone position is used for the middle and upper thoracic spine, but ideally the spine should be in slight flexion. This position can be obtained by putting a wedge under the chest or by lowering the top of the table. The head is supported by the palms or with a towel roll.

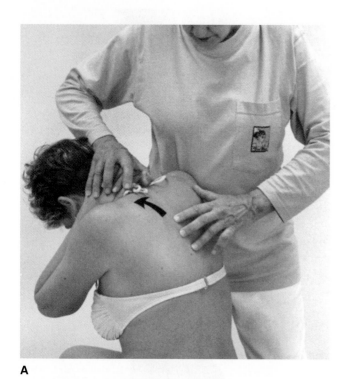

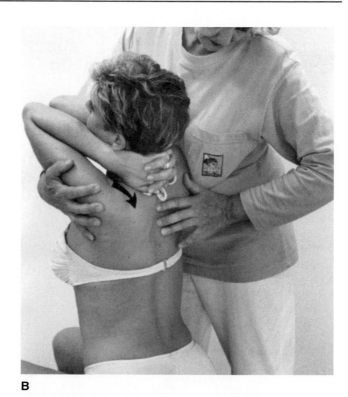

A   **B**

■ **FIG. 20-20.** Middle and lower thoracic spine (T4–T12) passive motion testing of (**A**) flexion and (**B**) extension.

Throughout springing and vertebral and rib pressures, ask the patient to report when and where he or she feels pain or other symptoms; relate this information to the test being performed. Knowing that upper thoracic pain is often cervical in origin, when testing the cervicothoracic junction and upper thoracic region, central and unilateral pressures from C4 to C7 must be done before proceeding to the upper thoracic region.

1. Thoracic vertebrae (springing and vertebral pressures)
   a. Springing tests over the articular processes (transverse processes) of individual segments of the thoracic spine. First, examine for tenderness by palpating

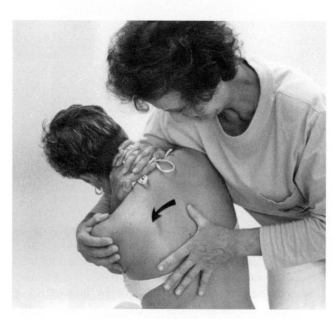

■ **FIG. 20-21.** Middle and lower thoracic spine (T4–T12) passive motion testing of lateral flexion.

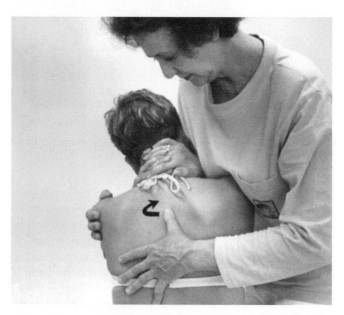

■ **FIG. 20-22.** Middle and lower thoracic (T4–T12) passive motion testing of rotation.

the spinous processes with the fingertips. Then perform the springing test, which examines resistance and tenderness of the deep structures of the spinal segment (i.e., the disk and apophyseal joints).

Stand at the side of the table facing the head of the table (Fig. 20-23) Use the index and middle fingers of the examining hand to palpate the area over the articular processes. With the hypothenar eminence of the other hand, produce a springlike (up and down) motion. Then place the palpating fingers over the costotransverse joint and apply a springing force.

Findings: Pain, either localized or referred, induced by this maneuver indicates segmental instability (with little or no resistance) or articular blockage with increased resistance.[70,168] Additional specific mobility tests must be used to localize the segment precisely.

b. Central postero-anterior pressures against the spinous process. Using the tips of the thumbs applied to the spinous process, direct rhythmic pressure anteriorly (Fig. 20-24A). At first the pressure is applied gently in a rhythmic fashion and then more firmly to reproduce pain if it is present. Pressures over the spinous process may be inclined in a cephalic, caudal, or diagonal direction.

Findings: Dysfunction of a level is characterized by reproduction of local pain or symptoms and restriction of motion. This test may be performed

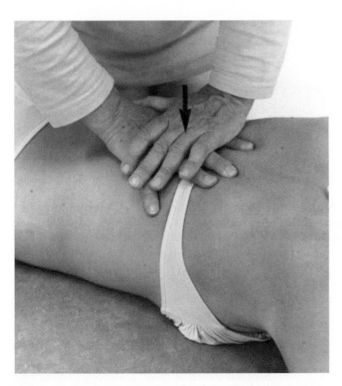

■ **FIG. 20-23.** Springing tests to the articular processes.

several times to determine the quality of motion. Pain may be felt at any stage in the range.

c. Postero-anterior unilateral pressure over the apophyseal joints. Move your thumbs laterally so that they rest on the transverse process of the thoracic vertebra, 2 to 3 cm from the midline to elicit symptoms from the apophyseal facet joints and 4 to 5 cm from the midline to provoke the costovertebral joints (Fig. 20-24B). Pressure may be varied by directing it in a cephalic, caudal, medial, or lateral direction. Again, start gently with rhythmic oscillations and assess the segments immediately above, below, and on the opposite side.

Findings: Same as 1b above, but unlike central palpation this method can determine quite localized symptoms.[144] Remember that the transverse process is not necessarily at the same level as the spinous process (Fig. 20-1).

d. Transverse vertebral pressure. Transverse pressure is the definitive procedure for localizing segmental dysfunction in the thoracic spine.[144,175,177] Place your thumbs along the side of the spinous process, lying flat across the curvature of the thoracic wall (Fig. 20-24C). Apply oscillatory pressure along the side of the spinous process. A rotatory movement (very small in range) is being reproduced, rather than a transverse glide. When the slack is taken up, gently push the spinous process toward the opposite side. Repeat this at each level until the painful segment is located.

Findings: Same as above. The side on which the thumbs are applied to the transverse process is the side responsible for the pain. For example, if pressure from the left toward the right elicits pain, but palpation from the right is painless, the painful lesion is left-sided.

2. Ribs and costovertebral joints. Methods to elicit symptoms at the costovertebral joint include direct pressures over the costovertebral joint and springing of the ribs, thus producing an indirect stretching of the joint and the rib maneuver described by Maigne.[175]

a. Postero-anterior unilateral pressures over the costovertebral joints. The costovertebral joints and intercostal movements are tested by using posteroanterior pressure of the thumbs over the angle of the rib unilaterally, about 4 to 5 cm from the midline. Vary the pressure by directing it in a posterior–anterior direction or in a cranial–caudal direction to attempt to reproduce the symptoms.

Findings: If affected, the costovertebral joint will be very sensitive to pressure because it is relatively superficial and also produces soft tissue irritation in its vicinity.[144] A comparison of the costovertebral joints and thoracic vertebrae should be made. See section on biomechanical regions above.

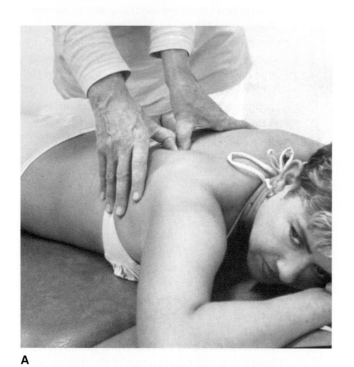

A

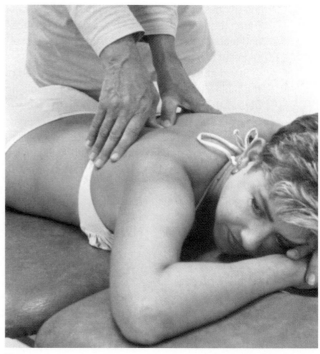

B

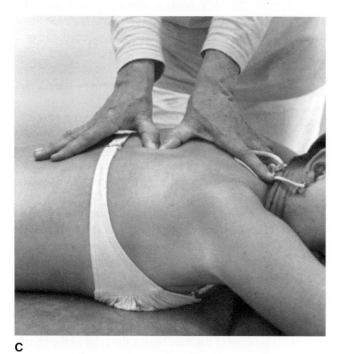

C

■ **FIG. 20-24.** Segmental testing for joint-play movements: **(A)** posteroanterior central pressures, **(B)** posteroanterior unilateral pressures, and **(C)** transverse vertebral pressures.

b. First rib. Palpate the first rib for position and tenderness. Palpation on the superior aspect of the first rib just anterior to the rhomboid muscle commonly shows that a dysfunctional rib is elevated in relation to the contralateral side or that it is hypomobile (Fig. 20-25). To assess mobility, passively flex the cervical spine of the supine patient, and rotate it away from and laterally flex it toward the side to be examined.[99]

Using the thumb of your free hand, after making contact with that rib, introduce an oscillatory or springlike force in the caudal direction while evaluating the mobility and ease of displacement.

Caudal pressures of the first rib with the thumbs should be repeated in prone. The bulk of the trapezius should be raised posteriorly to allow easy access to the rib angle.

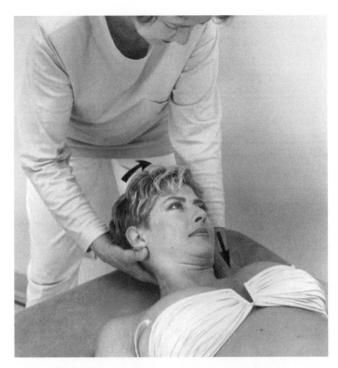

■ **FIG. 20-25.** First rib passive motion testing: Caudal glide.

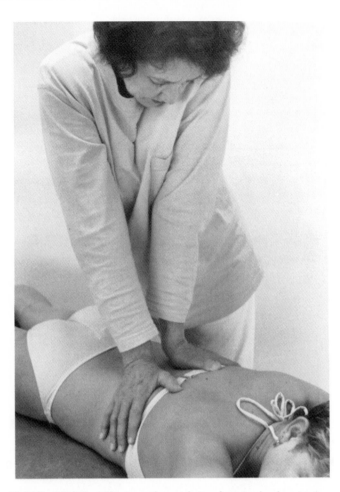

■ **FIG. 20-26.** Ribs two through twelve: Springing tests for joint-play movements.

Findings: Immediate localized pain, arm pain, or both. Pain may be elicited in the cervical region as well with this maneuver, suggesting the presence of the scalenus anticus syndrome.[70,168] Hypertonicity of scalene muscles may also be noted on the ipsilateral side. There may be an absence of springlike movement because of motion restriction.

c. Ribs three to twelve—rib springing. With the patient lying prone, stand at the side or head of the table. Place your hands around the posterolateral aspect of the rib cage so that the heel of each hand rests on the angles of the ribs (Fig. 20-26). Keep your elbows fully extended as you gently spring the ribs, starting at the top of the rib cage and progressing caudally along the whole length of the thoracic spine. Note the amount and quality of movement. This general springing test is especially valuable in providing a good general impression of regional restrictions. If one rib appears hypermobile or hypomobile relative to another, it can be tested individually by applying unilateral posterior rib pressures with the ulnar border of the hand over the rib as it curves around the posterior wall.

Findings: Provocation of the costovertebral symptoms produced by indirect stretching of the joint, and absence of springlike movement because of dysfunction with motion restriction.

d. Rib maneuver for costal sprain.[175] With the patient sitting and the examiner standing behind, move the patient's trunk in lateral flexion to the side opposite the painful side. The arm on the painful side is raised over the head and held there while the ribs are examined. Perform a caudal glide with the tip of the thumb on the upper border of the rib (Fig. 20-27A). Apply the same maneuver with the tips of the fingers pulling upward (cranial glide; Fig. 20-27B). With a costal sprain, one of these maneuvers will increase the pain but the other will be painless. Assessment should include anteroposterior pressures (joint play) and palpation of the ribs at their costochondral junctions. With upper thoracic dysfunction, palpate the sternoclavicular, acromioclavicular, and xiphoid joints and assess them for increase or loss of joint play. Screening tests of the sacroiliac joint should be considered when there is lower thoracic involvement, as joint abnormalities here can refer pain to areas that also receive a thoracic supply. For instance, T12 supplies the lateral aspect of the buttock.[25]

C. Compression testing. In deviations, such as increased lordosis, posterior angulation of the thoracic spine, or anterior shear of the pelvis, or in regions of instability, efficient

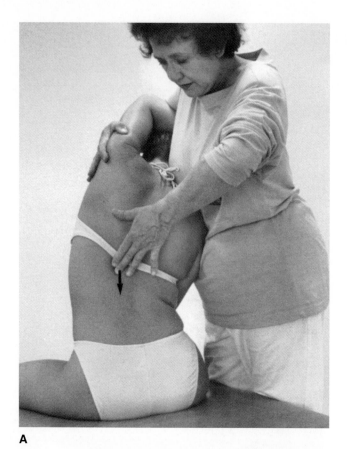
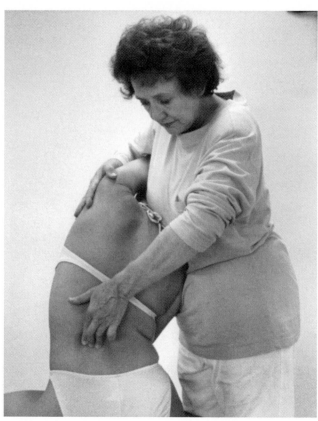

A   B

■ **FIG. 20-27.** Rib maneuver for costal sprain: **(A)** caudal glide and **(B)** cranial glide.

weight transfer through the spine is prevented. A useful objective assessment of the patient's vertical alignment and determination of a biomechanically altered segment is the vertical compression test.[42,130,252] Have the patient stand in a comfortable, natural stance. Apply vertical compression through the shoulders, feeling and observing for any give or buckling in the spine (Fig. 20-4). Generally, patients with accentuated curvatures have an increased springiness, indicating decreased lever arms for the effects of gravity and increased stress on the myofascial structures.[42] The spines of patients with decreased curvatures do not have enough spring, leading to decreased shock attenuation. Have the patient relate any increase or reproduction of symptoms. In the presence of postural deviations, the examiner usually feels instability at the level of the dysfunction, and the patient may report an increase in symptoms.

D. Static postures. When thoracic pain is of postural origin, many of the auxiliary tests above will not provoke pain. In such cases, according to McKenzie,[187] the structures must be loaded for a prolonged time before deformation is sufficient to reproduce the pain. Each position is held for no more than 3 minutes, and the effects are recorded. The test postures include:
1. Static flexion in sitting (slouched with the back totally rounded). The totally flexed position is most

often responsible for the production of mechanical thoracic pain.
2. Lying prone, with the lower thoracic spine fully extended and the weight supported on the hands (Fig. 20-28). The patient allows the lower thoracic spine and pelvic girdle to sag into the treatment table. This position extends the thoracic spine from about T4–T5 to L1.
3. Lying supine in extension, which extends the thoracic spine from about T1 to T4–T5. The patient lies supine over the end of the table so that the head, neck, and shoulders are unsupported down to the level of T4. With the support of one hand the head is lowered until the neck and upper back are fully extended (Fig. 20-29). If the test is impossible in supine, it can be performed in prone on the elbows with cervical extension.

Other Joints as Applicable. To have a lasting treatment effect the clinician has to observe above and below the problem area of the thoracic spine—how movement continues and what avoidance mechanism may be present. Joints likely to be examined are the cervical spine and upper limb joints or the lumbar spine, lower limb, and sacroiliac joints. Thoracic asymmetry (malalignment) may be related to rotational malalignment of the innominate in the sagittal plane or to sacral iliac dysfunction in the vertical plane (i.e., upslip, outflare, inflare).[256]

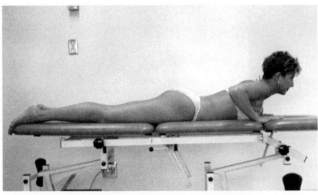

A

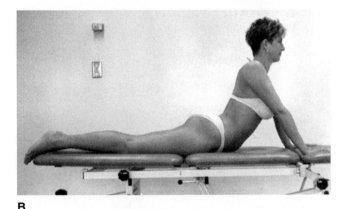

B

■ **FIG. 20-28.** Prone lying thoracolumbar extension: **(A)** starting position; **(B)** end position.

MUSCLE TESTS

The muscles that need to be tested will depend on the area of signs and symptoms and may include the cervical spine and upper quadrant or the lumbar spine and lower quadrant musculature. Many authors have noted patterns of global muscle hyperactivity and dominance.[55,107,123,124,248–250] In the

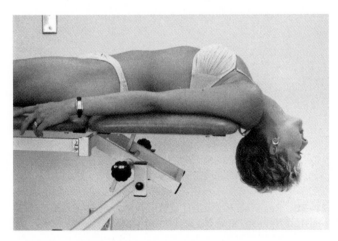

■ **FIG. 20-29.** Supine lying upper thoracic extension.

thoracic spine, the dominant global muscles include the external and internal obliques, rectus abdominus, latissimus dorsi, thoracic erector spinae, and some of the scapular muscles (rhomboids, levator scapulae, and trapezius [lower part]).[165] Other scapular muscles prone to weakness include subscapularis, serratus anterior, and pectoralis major (abdominal part; see Table 5-1).[124,137] Clinically, it has been noted that the deep localized stabilizers become atrophied and weak subsequent to injury to the thorax.[165]

Muscle tests include examining muscle isometric contraction (resisted isometrics), muscle strength, control, and length.

I. Resisted Isometrics

Unlike the cervical and lumbar spine, the muscles of the thorax and abdomen suffer strain more frequently, so that resisted isometric testing has a significant role in the evaluation of the thoracic spine.[60] According to Cyriax and Cyriax,[60] the thorax should be in a neutral position and the most painful movements should be performed last. Grimsby[103] suggests performing resisted tests not only in the midrange but also in the inner and outer ranges to open or close the joint spaces; this helps determine the effect of compression on pain production. The following motions are tested.

A. Side flexion (standing or sitting in a chair with the feet supported). Side flexions (left and right) are resisted by the patient bending outward against the examiner's unyielding resistance. Stabilize the patient's trunk with your trunk and resist the motion with your upper limb(s), which embraces the patient's opposite shoulder. Have the patient match your resistance so that the movement is truly isometric (Fig. 20-30A).

B. Forward flexion (sitting in a chair with the spine in a neutral position). Stabilize the patient's knees. Prevent movement at the sternum and knees as the patient attempts to flex forward (Fig. 20-30B).

C. Rotation (sitting in a chair, spine in a neutral position). Stand in front of the patient and stabilize the lower limbs. Prevent movement of the pelvis by clamping the patient's knees between your knees. Resist the patient by using your hands (which are placed on the shoulders) as he or she tries to rotate right and then left (Fig. 20-30C). Pain on resisted rotation implicates the oblique muscles or inferior posterior serratus.[59]

D. Extension (prone lying). Have the patient try to extend his or her back while you offer unyielding resistance to upper thoracic extension with the cranial hand. The caudal hand stabilizes the pelvic girdle.

II. Muscle Strength

The examiner should test the trunk flexors, extensors, lateral flexors, rotators, and the relevant groups as indicated. For details of these general tests the reader is directed to Clarkson and Gilewich,[52] Cole et al.,[54] Hislop and Montgomery,[115] Kendall et al.,[143] and Palmer and Epler.[216]

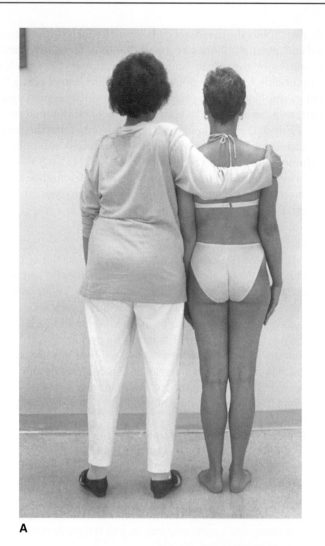

A

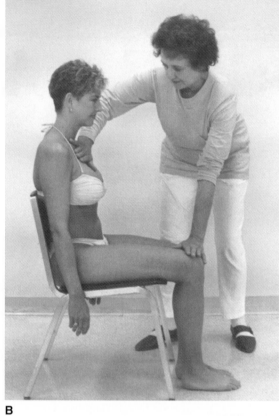

B

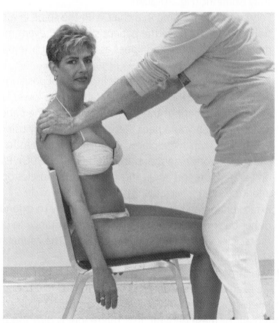

C

■ **FIG. 20-30.** Resisted isometric testing: (**A**) resisted sidebending, (**B**) resisted flexion, and (**C**) resisted rotation.

III. Muscle Control

The relative strength of muscles is considered to be more important than the overall strength of a muscle group.[125] Relative strength of a muscle group is assessed indirectly by observing posture, the quality of movement, noting any changes in muscle recruitment patterns, and coordination, and by palpating muscle activity in various positions.[222] Muscle imbalances of the cervical spine, shoulder girdle, and around the scapulae have been described by a number of workers[106,125,136,148,150,217,249] and can be assessed by observation of upper limb movements. See Chapters 11, Shoulder and Shoulder Girdle, and 19, Cervical Spine.

A. Local stabilizers of the thoracic spine (deep fibers of the multifidi, rotatores breves, levator costarum, and the intercostals). Clinically, it as been noted that atrophy of these deep small stabilizers occurs subsequent to injury to the thoracic spine.[165] A useful clinical method of testing the multifidi and local stabilizers as screening procedures is recommended by Richardson et al.[231] and Lee.[165] This test relies on palpation and comparison of the contraction on each side. With the patient in the prone lying with the head in neutral position and the arms resting comfortably over the edge of the treatment table, the examiner palpates adjacent to the spinous process and asks the patient, "Gently swell out your muscles under my fingers without moving your spine or pelvis." The clinician assesses the ability for the muscles to perform this action.

An alternative method of testing the multifidi of the lower thoracic and lumbar spine is shown in Figure 20-31.[141] The thoracolumbar spine is flexed up to the level of the involved segment; an attempted lateral displacement of the femur will be poorly resisted in the presence of weak multifidi. The pressure should be light. The multifidi primarily functions as contralateral rotators, but because the force is applied through the pelvis, the side on which the pressure is applied is the side providing resistance. These methods of testing can also be used as a training tool for isolated multifidus contraction.

B. Thoracoabdominal diaphragm and intercostals. Assess the strength of the diaphragm and intercostals during quite inspiration and forced expiration.[115,143] Assessment of the diaphragm can be assessed by observation and manual resistance. There is no method of direct assessment of the strength of the intercostal muscles. Indirect methods include observation and measuring the difference in magnitude of chest excursion between maximum inspiration and the girth of the chest at the end of full expiration (pneumograph may be used for the same purpose if one is available).[115] Optimal diaphragmatic breathing involves both abdominal and lower rib cage expansions. The most common component lost in patients with thoracic dysfunction is lateral costal expansion.[165]

C. Abdominals. The abdominal wall muscles work synergistically with the scapula retractors, thoracoabdominal diaphragm, and pelvic diaphragm muscles to align the abdomen and thorax as well as with the relationship of the scapula to the thorax.[225] (See Chapter 7, Myofascial Considerations and Evaluation in Somatic Dysfunction, section on postural musculofascial systems.) Weakness of the abdominal muscles results in the sternum and chest being carried more caudally and may contribute to the rounded shoulder posture. A comprehensive treatment approach for the forward-head rounded shoulder posture should therefore include scapular retractor strengthening, anterior shoulder girdle lengthening, scapulothoracic positioning, and abdominal wall training.

A relatively new method of measuring isolated muscle contraction for the abdominal muscle group has been described by Jull and Richardson[138] and Richardson et al.[231] A pressure sensor (set at a baseline of 40 mm Hg) is placed between the lumbar spine and the table with the patient in prone (Fig. 20-32), sitting, or crook lie position. Abdominal hollowing, i.e., drawing in the stomach and tightening the waist is then attempted by the patient, which normally would cause an increase in pressure of about 10 mm Hg.[143] This is owing to slight flattening of the lumbar spine caused by concentric contraction of the transversus abdominus and internal and external obliques. A greater

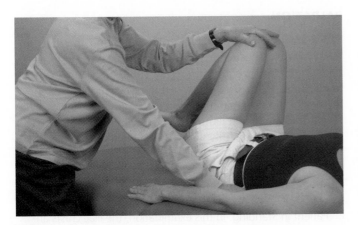

■ **FIG. 20-31.** Segmental multifidus muscle testing.

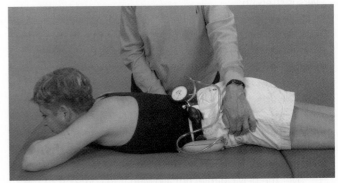

■ **FIG. 20-32.** Abdominal drawing-in test in prone.

increase in pressure (of the order of 20 mm Hg) indicates the incorrect contraction of the rectus abdominus. The time during which the correct activation can be sustained gives an indication of muscle endurance. The abdominal drawing-in test measures a level of motor skill competence, i.e., it measures the ability of the patient to use the correct muscles by drawing the abdominal wall in without moving the spine or pelvis and holding it for 10 seconds while breathing normally.[230,231] Normal function is achieved if the patient is able to sustain the correct contraction for 10 seconds and repeat the contraction 10 times. To palpate transversus abdominis contraction, place your fingers just medial and inferior to the anterior inferior iliac spine. Normal contraction creates a feeling of tightness under the fingers. Overactivity of the internal oblique creates bulging under the fingers. Overactive external obliques appear as a swelling over the lateral lower ribs and an increased lateral abdominal (oblique) line.[113] Overactivity of the rectus abdominus appears as abdominal protuberance.

According to Richardson and associates[231] and others,[58,207,254] the diaphragm and muscles of the pelvic floor are activated with the transverse abdominus and lumbar multifidi during the action of drawing in the abdominal wall. This coactivation of the transversus abdominus and the muscles of the pelvic and diaphragm is likely to act to maintain the intra-abdominal pressure at critical level, thus allowing co-contraction of the transversus abdominis to affect spinal support. Emerging literature suggests that differentiation rather than isolation of the pelvic floor muscles and abdominals of the inner unit are appropriate for treatment of pelvic floor muscles and appears to be indicated.[108] Coactivation-based strengthening of the muscles of the inner unit are appropriate for the treatment of pelvic floor muscle dysfunction, as well as other disorders of the lumbopelvic cylinder.[132,231,232] Assessment and treatment of the pelvic diaphragm muscles and related muscles are described in numerous texts and articles.[10,18,45,46,224,258,259,283]

IV. Muscle Endurance. Testing endurance of the torso flexors (see Fig. 22-19), lateral trunk musculature (see Fig. 22-20), and extensors (see Fig. 22-21) should also be considered. See Chapter 22, Lumbar Spine, for a discussion of torso endurance versus strength.

V. Muscle Length. The examiner checks the length of individual muscles, in particular those muscles prone to become short in the region of the shoulder girdle and cervicothoracic region. See Box 11-1 and Figures 7-34 through 7-37.

Muscle of the anterior trunk that may become tight and have an effect on the thoracic spine and rib cage include the following:

A. Rectus abdominus. Tightness contributes to thoracic kyphosis and a depressed chest. Assessment is made with the patient lying prone. The examiner stabilizes the pelvis over the pelvic girdle, not allowing it to come off of the table as the patient attempts to fully extend the thoracic spine with weight supported on the hands (Fig. 20-28).[17] The patient allows the lower thoracic and pelvic girdle to sag into the treatment table. Full range of motion is the ability to fully extend the elbows. This method tests the length of the abdominal wall, especially the rectus abdominus and obliques.

B. Oblique muscles (internal obliques [IO] and external obliques [EO]). See muscle length testing of the obliques in Chapter 7, Myofascial Considerations and Evaluation in Somatic Dysfunction (see Fig. 7-33). Shortness of the anterior fibers of the IO results in a wide infrasternal angle (greater than 90°) whereas shortness of the anterior fibers of the EO results in a narrow infrasternal angle (less than 90°).[250] Bilateral shortness of the anterior fibers of the EO and IO muscles causes the thorax to be depressed anteriorly, contributing to flexion of the vertebral column.[143] In standing, this will be seen as a tendency to kyphosis and a depressed chest. In a kyphosis–lordosis posture (see Fig. 7-23), the lateral portions of the IO are shortened, and the lateral portions of the EO are elongated.[143] These same findings occur in a swayback posture (see Fig. 7-25). A stiff or short left EO and right IO can limit left thoracic rotation.

C. Latissimus dorsi. Shortness tends to depress the shoulder girdle down and forward. Arm elevation in flexion and abduction will be limited. In a right C-curve of the spine, the lateral fibers of the left latissimus dorsi are usually shortened.[143] The anterior fibers are shortened bilaterally in marked kyphosis. Assessment of forward bending in the standing position should be carried out with stabilization of the patient's pelvis. The client is asked to stop at the point when the sacrum begins to move. Note any thoracic rotation or sidebending and how the arms hang (see Box 11-1). If the arms are held back the latissimus dorsi is most probably tight. Also note the spinal curve and length and tone of the erector spinae.

Cervical spine, lumbar spine, and hip mobility should be tested for mobility impairment in associated regions that may affect thoracic function.

PALPATION

The thoracic spine is palpated for any alteration in bony alignment, muscle spasms or guarding, muscle and skin consistency, temperature alterations, swelling, and any localized tenderness that may be felt over the supraspinous ligament or the side of the interspinous ligament. Tapping sharply with the finger or a percussion hammer on the spinous processes, with the patient standing fully flexed, often elicits local tenderness over the affected level.[57] Palpate for relevant acupressure points, trigger points, strain and counterstrain points, and tender points of fibromyalgia.

I. Patient in Standing. In this examination, the iliac crests are palpated for height and symmetry. The lower ribs and quadratus lumborum may be associated with a painful lower thoracic spine, so both of these areas are assessed. The acromioclavicular joint is palpated for height and symmetry, as well as the position of the head related to midline.

II. Patient in Supine Lying
A. Palpation of the costochondral articulations of the ribs often identifies one or more rib articulations that are exquisitely tender to palpation. This is frequently described as osteochondritis (Tietze's syndrome) but may be associated with dysfunction of that rib.[101,102]
B. Palpate for symmetry of ribs and intercostal spaces.
   • Palpate for positional alterations, such as eversion of the rib. A widened intercostal space above and a narrowed intercostal space below suggest a rib fault. Place the index fingers into corresponding anterior interspaces and feel for approximation or separation. In theory, a rib can be blocked both in the expiration and inspiration positions. From this it follows that the rib is more prominent if blocked in inhalation and less so if blocked in exhalation.
   • Palpate for anteroposterior rib dysfunction. The ribs may shift anteriorly or posteriorly along the axis of rotation that lies between the rib head and transverse process of the vertebra, causing an anterior or posterior dysfunction.[140] An anterior rib dysfunction will feel prominent on the anterior chest wall at the level of the rib, and there will be corresponding depression on the posterior wall.
C. Palpate for rib mobility and dysfunction.[111]
   • Checking individual levels of rib pairs on inhalation and exhalation may reveal a rib that quits moving before its contralateral pair. The rib that quits moving first at the end of inhalation is termed an inhalation restriction on that side. The rib that quits moving first at the end of exhalation is termed an exhalation restriction on the side. The restriction may be anterior or posterior and lateral in direction.
   • If a rib has an inhalation restriction, it has failed to lift fully and will block the ribs below from rising. This top rib is the key rib to be treated in a group of ribs with inhalation restriction.
   • If a rib has an exhalation restriction, it has failed to descend fully and will block the ribs above from descending. This lower rib is the key rib to be treated in a group of ribs with exhalation restriction.
      Rotation of the back occurs mainly in the thoracic spine because of the plane of the apophyseal facets. Rib cage dysfunction can restrict rotation markedly, and correction of rib dysfunction can improve spine rotation dramatically.
D. Search for the presence of tissue texture abnormality, primarily hypertonicity and tenderness of a muscle attachment to a rib.
E. When indicated, palpate the abdomen for tenderness or other signs suggestive of disease.

III. Prone Lying (arms to the side, head to one side)
A. General palpation
   1. Sweep the flat of the hand paravertebrally to assess the state of the skin, texture, and moisture.
   2. Use the skin-rolling technique (pinch while rolling) for painful subcutaneous tissue and regions with loss of mobility—for instance, painful subcutaneous regions in the gluteal area with low back pain may originate in the thoracolumbar junction (see Fig. 7-42C).[175,177] Normally the skin can be rolled over the spine and gluteal regions freely and painlessly.
   3. Palpate the anterior aspect of the medial, lateral, and superior borders of the scapula for any tenderness or swelling. Palpate the posterior aspect of the scapula and the rotator cuff muscles as well.
   4. Palpate the three divisions of the erector spinal group. The intermediate division is the one most useful diagnostically and is felt just lateral to the spinous process in a "gutter" overlying the lamina of the vertebrae with its most lateral border the transverse process.[296]
B. Segmental palpation
   1. Seek abnormalities such as thickening or undue tenderness and bony prominences.
   2. Palpate the spinous processes for tenderness and abnormalities. By placing the fingers in the paravertebral sulcus, note any malalignment of the spinous process, as well as the prominences and depressions of the transverse process.
   3. Apply pressure over the supraspinous ligament with the edge of a coin held lightly between two adjacent spinous processes. Such pressure on the normal ligament is painless; on the involved vertebral area it is usually more painful than over the others.[175,177]
   4. Again, palpate the ribs and intercostal spaces for positional faults and symmetry.
   5. Palpate along the iliac crest for signs such as Maigne's syndrome (Fig. 20-7B).[176,177]

Static Positions (Position Tests)—Middle to Lower Thoracic Spine (Three Positions)[99]. The anteroposterior relationship of the transverse processes to the coronal plane is noted and compared with the level above and below. The position tests are screening tests that, like all screening tests, are valuable in focusing the attention of the examiner on one segment concerning the movement status of the segment, but are not appropriate for making a definitive statement concerning the movement status of the segment.[69] Three positions are commonly tested for symmetry and offer information that will direct the forces used in the treatment approach.

• Forward bent in sitting (Fig. 20-33A)
• Prone (Fig. 20-33B)
• Backward bent (prone propped on elbows; Fig. 20-33C)

To determine the position of the superior vertebra, the anteroposterior relationship of the transverse processes to

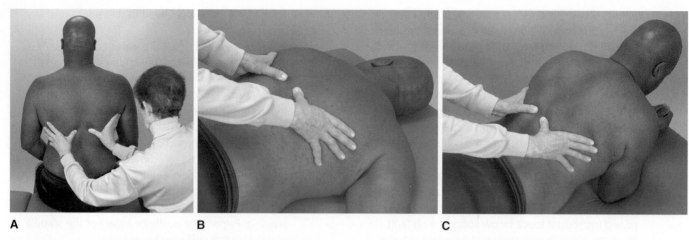

■ **FIG. 20-33.** Position testing: **(A)** flexion (starting position), **(B)** neutral, and **(C)** extension.

the coronal plane is noted and compared with the level above and below in all three positions. When combined with the results of passive movement testing and other tests, positional diagnosis gives the examiner a positional description of the possible restriction and direction to which forces should be applied to restore motion in the segment.

NEUROLOGIC TESTS

Neurologic examination involves examining the integrity and mobility of the nervous system and specific diagnostic tests. Occasionally patients presenting with thoracic pain complain of weakness, pain, and paresthesias in both lower limbs at rest as well as while walking. This should alert the examiner to the possibility of spinal cord involvement. If a tumor is developing, ankle clonus may be present, lower limb reflexes may be exaggerated, and the plantar reflex may be positive. Sensation and power in the lower limbs may be deficient. Neurologic testing should include a full neurologic assessment of the upper and lower limbs. If you suspect a problem with movement of the spinal cord, any of the tests that stretch the cord may be performed: these include the straight-leg raising test, the slump test, and others.

I. Integrity of Nervous System
   A. Dermatomes and myotomes. Gross sensory testing may be performed. Within the thoracic spine there is a great deal of overlap in the dermatomes (see Fig. 5-6). The dermatomes tend to follow the ribs. The absence of only one dermatome may not result in loss of sensation. Remember that sensory changes occur two segments *lower* than the location of a pathologic thoracic spine condition. Like the myotomes, dermatomes of the trunk are arranged in regular bands from T2 to L1. T2, however, includes a Y-shaped area that stretches from the inner condyle of the humerus up the arm and then divides into two areas, reaching the sternum anteriorly and the vertebral border of the scapula behind.[59] T9, T10, and T11 encircle the

trunk at the level of the umbilicus. T12 remains uncertain. L1 is in the region of the groin.
   B. Reflex testing. Although there are no deep tendon reflexes to test in conjunction with the thoracic spine, assess the lumbar reflexes because disease in the thoracic spine can affect them. Other reflexes in this area, which depend on the integrity of the appropriate sensory and motor peripheral nerves and spinal cord segment, as well as on intact suprasegmental input to the spinal reflex center, include the so-called superficial abdominal reflexes.[239] The abdominal reflex in the upper quadrant depends on segments T7 to T9 and in the lower quadrant on segments T10 to T12. Unlike deep tendon reflexes, superficial reflexes are abolished by upper motor neuron lesions. Scratching the skin some distance away from the umbilicus in any one quadrant of the anterior abdominal wall causes contraction of the underlying abdominal muscles. The umbilicus is drawn toward the side of the contraction.

II. Mobility of Nervous System. If you suspect a problem with movement of the spinal cord, any of the tests that stretch the cord may be performed. These include the dural mobility test for the sciatic nerve and the femoral nerve traction test (see Chapter 22, Lumbar Spine). The following tests may also be considered.
   A. Passive neck flexion. Passive neck flexion is done in the supine position. The test should be painless outside of a mild pulling sensation at the cervicothoracic junction. Passive neck flexion stresses neural and nonneural tissue in the neck, and moves and tensions neural tissues in the thorax and lumbar spine.[30,145,271] The test loads thoracic neuromeningeal structures and moves them in relationship to the surrounding spinal canal.
   B. First thoracic nerve root stretch.[59] Have the patient abduct the arms to 90° and flex the pronated forearms to 90°. This should not alter the symptoms. The patient then fully flexes the elbow and puts the hands behind the neck.

This stretches the ulnar nerve, which in turn pulls the T1 nerve root. Pain in the scapular area or arm indicates a positive test.

C. Upper limb neural tension tests.[38,76–78,100,102,139,145] Upper limb tension tests are recommended for all patients with symptoms in the arm, head, neck, and thoracic spine (see Chapter11, Shoulder and Shoulder Girdle).

D. Slump test (see Chapter 22, Lumbar Spine).[179] This test is used to assess the movement of the pain-sensitive structures in the vertebral canal and intervertebral foremen. According to Maitland,[179] this test should be part of the examination of the thoracic spine, but remember that this test causes pain at roughly the T8–T9 area in at least 90% of all subjects. The most commonly useful variation of the test for the cervical and thoracic spine involves performing it in long-sitting position.[39] The suggested base sequence for examination of a nonirritable condition is long sitting with the arms behind the back, plus lumbar flexion and thoracic flexion, plus cervical flexion (Fig. 20-34). The dura is released by then having the patient extend the head and neck. The change in symptom response is noted. If the thoracic pain is brought on by full slump and relieved with extension of the head and neck, involvement of the dura is suggested. Useful variations include:

- Thoracic lateral flexion–rotation and cervical flexion–lateral flexion or rotation can be added to the base test (Fig. 20-34D).
- Neurodynamic sequencing can be altered.

It has also been postulated that the slump test can be refined so as to put more tension onto the sympathetic trunk (sympathetic trunk test).[39,263]

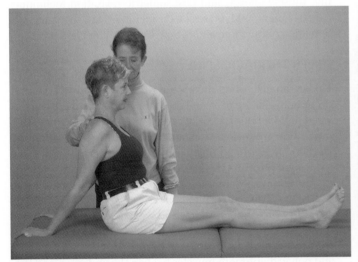

A

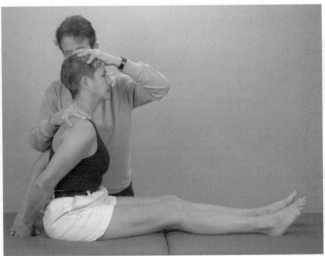

B

C

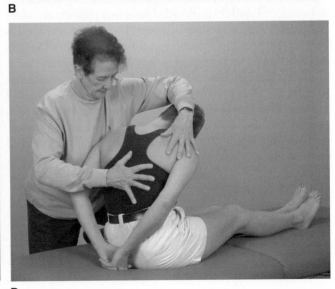

D

■ **FIG. 20-34.** Long sitting slump test: **(A)** starting position, **(B)** addition of thoracic and lumbar flexion, and **(C)** neck flexion. **(D)** Modification for the detection of segmental neural dysfunction within the thoracic spine.

III. Chief Physical Signs. Physical signs that may be helpful in distinguishing the compression or interruption of neighboring spinal nerves include[239]:

A. T1. Intrinsic muscles of the hand are severely affected but more proximal muscles are spared. All reflexes are normal.

B. T2 to T12. Isolated spinal nerve lesions are difficult to detect. The distribution of pain, tenderness, muscle spasm, and careful evaluation of sensory changes are the chief factors in diagnosis. Lesions of upper thoracic nerves may abolish the sympathetic input to the upper limb and head and neck. Abdominal reflexes are absent usually only if more than one of T6 to T12 spinal nerves are blocked.

GENERAL PHYSICAL EXAMINATION

The mechanisms causing pain originating in or from the thoracic spine are numerous.[27] They occur primarily from stimulation of nociceptive endings in the periosteum, ligaments, and joints of the thoracic spine. Fracture, dislocation, arthritis variants, metabolic disorders, infection, or tumors may elicit thoracic pain. Myofascial pain frequently manifests in the thoracic spine muscles as does pain referred from the shoulder.[41] Neuropathic pain from the thoracic cord must always be suspected, for instance from intrinsic and extramedullary spinal cord lesions.[41] About 50% of spinal cord tumors originate in the thoracic area of the cord.[228]

A general physical examination, including the abdomen and chest, may be necessary. Chest pains include those of cardiac origin and those of pulmonary origin involving the pleura, lungs, trachea, and bronchi. The esophagus is a common site and source of chest pain.[41] Chest pain can also occur because of diseases of the mediastinum, the diaphragm, the pancreas, and various visceral organs.[60,133,144,251]

It is important to be able to differentiate between chest pain caused by vertebral dysfunction and that caused by myocardial ischemia.[144] Typically myocardial ischemia patients are older and present with no history of injury. The pain is described as constricting or at times burning in nature. The site of the pain and radiation is epigastric, retrosternal, parasternal, jaw, neck, inside the arm (left more common than right), and interscapular. Exercise, heavy meals, cold, or stress aggravates the pain of myocardial ischemia. The typical elements that increase pain in dysfunction of the thoracic spine include deep inspiration, postural movement of the thorax, slumping, bending, and activities such as lifting.

OTHER STUDIES

See Chapter 22, Lumbar Spine, for a discussion of roentgenograms and other imaging studies.

THORACIC SPINE TECHNIQUES

Numerous manual therapy techniques are available to the clinician. These techniques can be used for hypomobility, hypermobility, instability, and soft tissue dysfunction.

Soft Tissue Manipulation

When hypomobility in the thoracic spine results from osteokinematic restriction, the cause may be articular, myofascial, or both. Patients with longstanding joint restriction are likely to develop myofascial restrictions, requiring concurrent types of intervention. Altered muscle length has implications for strength training (because of length–tension relationships) as well as for mobility. Assessment of the underlying cause of altered myofascial length is crucial for correcting dysfunction in the myofascial system. Functional movement patterns should be taught to reinforce the mobility gained with soft tissue manipulations, joint mobilization, and specific self-management exercises.

Myofascial restrictions commonly found in thoracic spine dysfunction include thoracic kyphosis, hypomobility syndromes, osteoporosis, and postural disorders (see above). These conditions respond well to soft tissue manipulations, stretching, muscle energy, and postisometric relaxation techniques (see Chapters 7, Myofascial Considerations and Evaluation in Somatic Dysfunction, and 8, Soft Tissue Manipulations).

UPPER THORACIC SPINE

Upper thoracic spine myofascial restrictions most commonly occur between the neck and shoulder girdle, producing an elevated shoulder posture, or between the neck and the upper thoracic spine producing a forward head posture (see Fig. 17-19). In the forward-head posture with protracted shoulder and a slumped position, the anterior elements collapse, reducing diaphragmatic excursion and lateral–posterolateral costal expansion. This can lead to increase activity in the secondary accessory breathing muscles and weakness of the abdominal muscles. The abdominal wall muscles work synergistically with the scapular retractors, thoracoabdominal diaphragm, and pelvic diaphragm muscles to align the abdomen and thorax as well as the relationship of the scapula to the thorax.[225] A comprehensive treatment approach for the forward-head rounded shoulder posture should include scapular retractor strengthening, anterior shoulder girdle and rib cage lengthening (see Figs. 8-1, 8-14A, 8-16, 8-38, 8-50, 8-52, 8-53, and 8-56 through 8-58, and Box 8-8), scapulothoracic positioning, and abdominal wall training.

In extreme cases of upper thoracic lordosis, a significant loss of segmental flexion mobility is noted throughout this area. There is usually winging of the scapula associated with weakness of the rhomboids and serratus anterior.[143] Treatment should consist of myofascial manipulation, stretching the extensor musculature (see Figs. 8-2, 8-7, and 8-10), and facilitation and strengthening of the serratus anterior and rhomboids. Prone and wall push-offs (see Figs. 11-71 and 11-76) are excellent ways to self-mobilize this region of the thoracic spine and facilitate the serratus anterior. Quadruped flexion–extension exercises (see Fig. 22-8) can be modified with some specificity by varying the hand position. The closer the hands are to the knees, the higher the apex of flexion motion induced in the spine.[28]

INCREASED THORACIC KYPHOSIS

Below the straight upper thoracic spine is often an accentuated thoracic kyphosis with a significant loss of mobility noted for extension, typically occurring from approximately T6 through T10. Associated with this increased thoracic kyphosis is adaptive shortening of the latissimus dorsi and abducted and internally rotated scapula.[28] Treatment consists of myofascial manipulations and stretching of the latissimus dorsi (see Box 8-8), mobilizing the thoracic kyphosis into extension (see Figs. 20-45, 20-46, and 20-59), and then reeducating lower trapezius activation. According to Bookhout,[28] weakness of the lower trapezius will continue to be perpetuated in the presence of latissimus dorsi tightness and an increased thoracic kyphosis.

The diaphragm is often involved in postural dysfunction and tends to be a flexor of the thorax when it is hypertonic. The diaphragm has been observed to produce a lordosis at the thoracolumbar junction and can lead to overuse of the midthoracic spinal extensors, causing a midthoracic lordosis.[162] For the patient to perform postural reeducation techniques successfully the contracted area of the anterior chest and abdomen (diaphragm and rectus abdominus) must be supple and mobile. Soft tissue manipulations for the diaphragm are illustrated and described in Chapter 8, Soft Tissue Manipulations (see Fig. 8-51), ranging from the least aggressive to most aggressive myofascial manipulations.[42] Techniques for encouraging diaphragmatic breathing are described below.

Joint Mobilization Techniques

As defined earlier, joint mobilization or *articulation* is the gradual application of passive movements in a smooth and rhythmic fashion to stretch contracted muscles, fascia, ligaments, and joint capsules. Direct techniques (on spinous or transverse processes to effect a small range of passive movement between two adjacent vertebrae) or indirect techniques (using a lever system) may be used. Indirect techniques tend to be more effective for the patient with multisegmental restriction.

An important part of treatment deals with active mobility and stability. The goal is to restore normal painless joint range of motion, including the stabilization of unstable segments, correction of muscle weakness or imbalance, restoration of soft tissue pliability and extensibility, relief of pain and reduction of muscle spasms, postural correction, and return to normal activity.

The following are representative passive movement techniques. For complete descriptions and illustrations of the great variety of mobilization, manipulation, and passive movements available for the thoracic spine, consult other texts.[24,29,57,60,64,70,71,74,88,93,99–103,112,139,144,165,166,168,175,177,179,181,187,189,193.197,202,205,218,255,266,267,270]

(For simplicity, the patient is referred to as a female, the operator as a male. P—patient; O—operator; L—localization or fixation; M—movement; WB—weight bearing; NWB—non–weight bearing.)

CERVICOTHORACIC REGION

First and Second Rib Techniques

I. Caudal Glide (Elevated First Rib). WB (Fig. 20-35)
    P—Sitting
    L—The scalene muscles may be placed on slack by sidebending the head to the side of restriction, or by using sufficient sidebending of the head to the side of the restriction with extension and rotation of the head and neck in the opposite direction to lock the cervical column. The examiner maintains the head position by placing the stabilizing hand on top of the head or over the vertex of the skull.
    O—Stand behind the patient. With the mobilizing hand, contact the first rib posteriorly and laterally on the transverse process of the T1 vertebra with the metacarpophalangeal joint of the index finger.
    M—The elbow of the mobilizing hand must be high enough so that the operator can direct downward and forward motion through the hand to the costovertebral joint. Apply mobilization pressure in an inferior, medial, and anterior direction to the first rib. Time movement with exhalation. Follow with stretching of the scalene muscles (see Figs. 7-34, 8-52, and 8-53).

II. Caudal Glide (Elevated First and Second Ribs). NWB, supine (Fig. 20-36)
    P—Supine
    O—Stand at the end of the treatment table by the patient's head.
    L—Place the head in sidebending to the side of the restriction to place the scaleni on slack. By adding rotation away

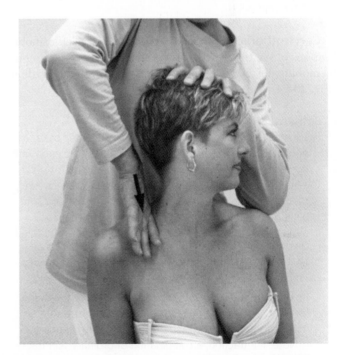

■ **FIG. 20-35.** Technique for the first rib: caudal glide (weight bearing [WB]).

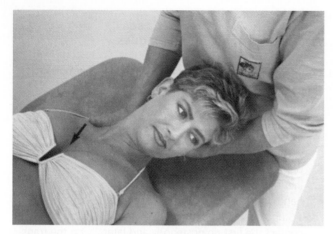

■ **FIG. 20-36.** Technique for the first and second rib: caudal glide (non–weight bearing [NWB]).

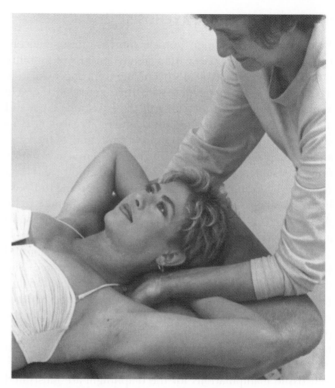

■ **FIG. 20-37.** Backward bending or traction (NWB).

from the restriction, one can lock the cervicothoracic spine. The fixating hand supports the cranium and cervical spine in this position.

M—Using the mobilizing hand, place the radial side of the index finger on the superior aspect of the first rib just posterior to the clavicle. With the mobilizing hand and body, move the first rib in a caudal and ventral direction. To facilitate movement, apply pressure during exhalation. Repeat two or three times, taking up the slack with each exhalation. To modify for the second rib, contact the second rib just lateral to its articulation with the sternum. Follow with stretching of the scaleni muscles (see Fig. 7-34, 8-52, and 8-53).

Cervicothoracic Spinal Articulations. Oscillatory mobilizations of the thoracic spine are extensions of the segmental mobility testing, with the addition of appropriate grading (Fig. 20-24).

I. Backward Bending or Traction. NWB (Fig. 20-37)
   P—Supine with hands behind neck (arms abducted as far as possible), hips flexed, and feet resting on the table, or with the legs positioned over a wedge
   O—Stand behind the patient with the arms laced between the patient's arms by going over the patient's forearm and behind the patient's back so that your fingers can reach underneath to the upper thoracic vertebrae to be mobilized.
   L—Place the fingers on either side of the transverse processes on the cephalic vertebra of the segment to be treated.
   M—By pulling longitudinally toward you and at the same time gently lifting up with the fingers and down with the forearms against the patient's arms, you can strongly mobilize the thoracic vertebrae into backward bending.
      Note: For traction, a combination of ordinary skin traction and of gently lifting the patient toward you can be used. Traction is effected upward and backward by using

body weight and gravity to result in distraction. Do not pull with the fingers; use the body.

II. Forward Bending and Backward Bending. NWB (Fig. 20-38)
   P—Lying on the side; the upper arm is adducted so that the forearm rests on the table in front of the patient.
   O—Facing the patient's head, support the patient's head and cervical spine with the hand and forearm.
   L—The caudal hand grasps the spinous process with the finger and thumb to control or localize the movement on the caudal vertebra of the segment to be treated.
   M—Support the patient's upper shoulder girdle with the trunk. The cephalic or mobilizing hand is then used to produce flexion or extension of the segment to be treated.
      Note: For an alternative NWB forward bending technique for the middle and lower segment see Figure 20-44. WB techniques may also be used (Fig. 20-19A, B).

III. Sidebending and Rotation Techniques. NWB (Fig. 20-39)
   P—Lying on the side
   O—Facing the patient, support the patient's head and cervical spine with the hand and forearm.
   L—The caudal hand stabilizes the segment by stabilizing the lateral aspect of the spinous process (with the finger or thumb) of the caudal vertebra of the segment to be treated to mobilize in either direction (i.e., on the near side of the spinous process when mobilizing in your direction).
   M—With the caudal segment stabilized, the mobilizing (cephalic) hand is used to sidebend or rotate the neck to the limit of range.

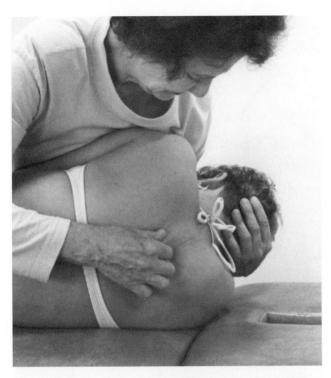

■ **FIG. 20-38.** Forward and backward bending (NWB).

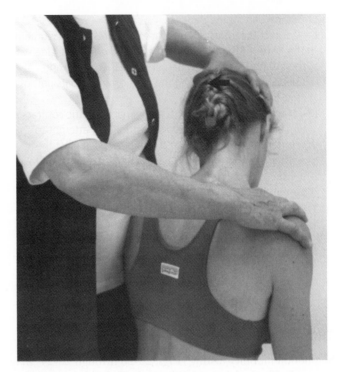

■ **FIG. 20-40.** Sidebending (WB).

Coupled movement in flexion or extension with sidebending and rotation to the same side may also be used.

IV. Sidebending. WB (Fig. 20-40)

    P—Sitting

    O—Stand at the side of the patient to which sidebending is to occur.

    L—With one hand, palpate on the far side of the interspace with the thumb. With the other hand on the vertex of the patient's skull, gently sidebend the head

toward you until motion arrives at the level of the palpating thumb.

    M—Transverse mobilizing pressure is applied to the lateral aspect of the caudal spinous process in the direction of the restriction or the operator.

      Note: This technique can be used effectively for levels C7 to T3.

V. Flexion, Sidebending, and Rotation. Active mobilization in WB (Fig. 20-41)

    P—Sitting

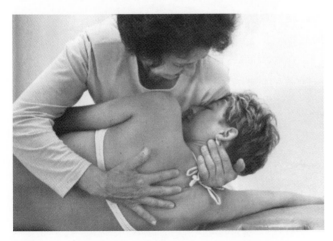

■ **FIG. 20-39.** Sidebending and rotation (NWB).

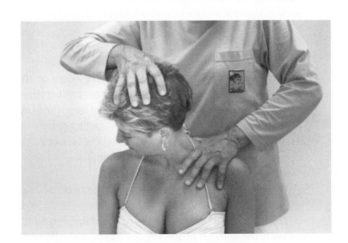

■ **FIG. 20-41.** Flexion, sidebending, and rotation.

O—Stand behind the patient.

L—Contact the interspinous space of the restricted segment. The lower of the two vertebrae is fixed on the far side with the thumb. The motion barrier is localized by flexing, sidebending, and rotating the joint complex to its pathologic limit.

M—Have the patient perform a minimal isometric contraction away from the pathologic barrier (i.e., attempt to extend, backward bend, and rotate away) against the resistance of your hand. Have the patient relax, then take up the slack in forward bending and rotation in the direction of the restricted barrier. Repeat two or three times.

Note: The indication for this technique is combined motion restriction of flexion sidebending and rotation to the same side. Similar combined techniques may be used for the cervical and lower thoracic spine. Many of the techniques described earlier for cervical spine stabilization and articulations can also be effective for C7 and T1–T2, as well as the midthoracic spine techniques described below.

THORACIC SPINE (MIDDLE AND LOWER SEGMENTS)

Segmental mobility testing (Figs. 20-20 through 20-24) may be used effectively for mobilization of the thoracic spine. Graded oscillatory movements (from grade I to IV) should be used appropriately. Many of the segmental spinal movements described in Chapter 22, Lumbar Spine, are appropriate for the thoracic spine (see Figs. 22-33 through 22-37). The long-lever extension (see Fig. 22-38) and rotational mobilization (see Figs. 22-39B and 22-41) are particularly well suited for the lower thoracic spine.

I. Vertical Intermittent Traction. Nonspecific (Fig. 20-42)
    P—Sitting with arms folded across the chest, with hands on the shoulders or with both arms folded across the waist
    O—Stand behind the patient and cup your hands under the patient's elbows, or lace your arms under the patient's arms and secure the patient's forearms.
    M—Crouch behind the patient by bending the legs and flattening the lumbar spine. Both the therapist and the patient lean back slightly, and traction is applied upward by straightening the legs.
       Note: Some degree of localization can be obtained by using the following positions: upper thoracic—position the patient in forward bending; midthoracic—position the patient with the back straight; entire spine—position the patient in backward bending. For a specific level, forward bend the patient to the level with body contact or by using a wedge to fixate the cranial or caudal vertebra between your chest and the patient's body.
II. Forward Bending. WB (Fig. 20-43)
    P—Sitting with the hands clasped behind the neck
    O—Stand at the patient's side.
    L—The pad of the thumb or fingers of the stabilizing hand contacts the spinous process of the caudal vertebra of the segment to be mobilized.

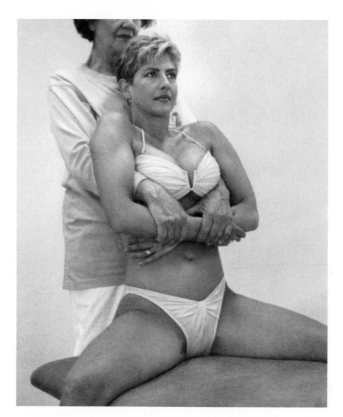

■ **FIG. 20-42.** Vertical intermittent traction: nonspecific.

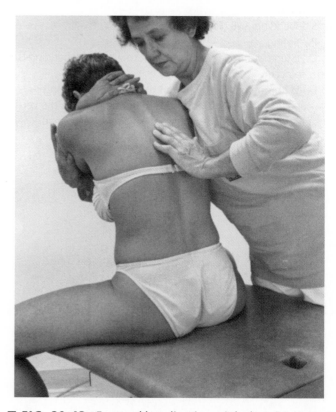

■ **FIG. 20-43.** Forward bending in weight bearing.

M—Using the patient's elbows held close together as a lever, flex the thoracic spine to the segment to be mobilized while fixating the spinous process of the lower vertebra.

Note: If shoulder range is limited, the patient's forearms can be crossed over the chest with hands on the opposite shoulders. Position your mobilizing arm across the patient's forearms with the hand grasping the opposite shoulder. One arm controls the weight of the upper torso and imparts forward bending while the finger or thumb of the opposite hand palpates motions between the segment, or the thumb stabilizes the spinous process to be mobilized.

III. Forward Bending. NWB (Fig. 20-44)

P—Prone with the trunk over a therapy wedge or resting on the forearms, thoracic spine extended

O—Stand at the patient's side. The mobilizing hand supports the top of the patient's head or forehead.

L—With the index finger or thumb, palpate the spinous process of the caudal vertebra of the involved segment. The head is flexed down to the level with your cranial hand.

M—Counterpressure of the thumb or the heel of the hand is applied against the spinous process below the segment to be mobilized. Slow alternating movements of slight pressure and release are applied, thus mobilizing into flexion via the head. In this position the head can be used as a lever for mobilizing into extension, sidebending, or rotation as well as flexion.

Note: An alternative technique in this position is to use one hand to maintain the anterior flexion of the head while the other hand exerts caudal glide (with the heel of the mobilizing hand) on the spinous process of the caudal vertebra of the involved segment.

IV. Backward Bending. WB (Fig. 20-45)

P—Sitting with arms folded across the waist or crossed to opposite shoulders

O—Stand at the patient's side.

L—With the index finger of the dorsal hand, palpate the interspinous space of the restricted segment. Place the ventral hand on the patient's contralateral elbow or shoulder.

M—The ventral hand mobilizes the patient's thoracic spine backward into extension.

V. Backward Bending. WB (middle and lower thoracic region; Fig. 20-46A)[175]

P—Sitting, with arms flexed and supported on the operator's ventral forearm and femur of the supporting leg

O—Stand at the patient's side with one foot on a stool and the ventral forearm supporting the patient's outstretched arms.

M—The dorsal hand exerts pressure on the thoracic region to be mobilized. While accentuating this pressure, move your knee laterally, thus effecting traction of the dorsal spine in extension. Then, as traction is released, perform a series of slow, alternating, rhythmic elastic movements.

Note: For a similar and equally effective technique for the midthoracic region (Fig. 20-46B), stand in front of

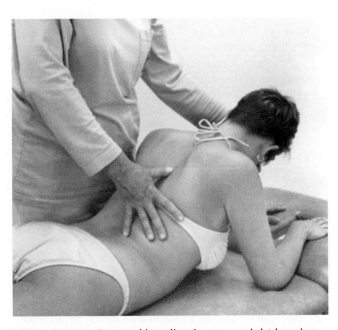

■ **FIG. 20-44.** Forward bending in non–weight bearing.

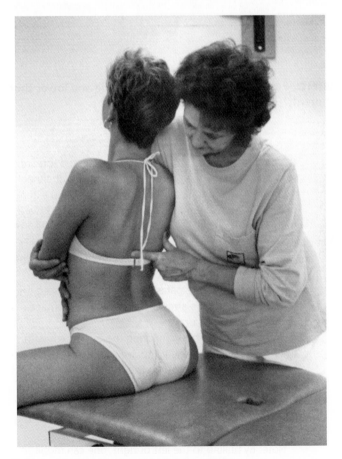

■ **FIG. 20-45.** Backward bending (WB).

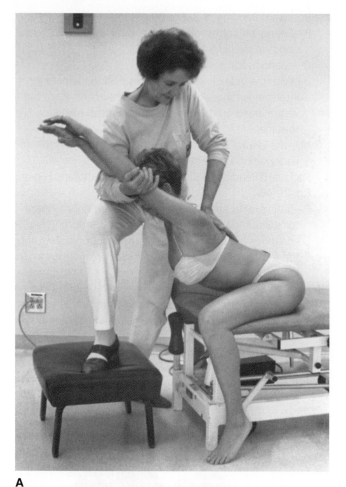

A

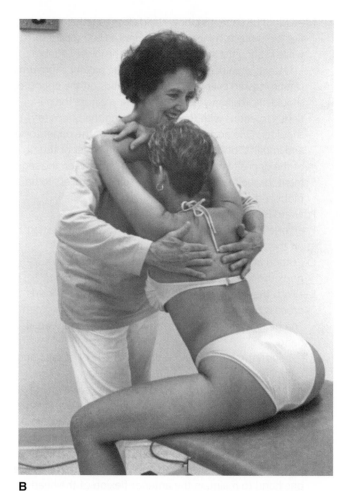

B

■ **FIG. 20-46.** Backward bending, middle and lower thoracic spine: **(A)** operator at side of patient or **(B)** in front of patient.

the patient with the patient resting her crossed forearms on your chest or upper arms. Place your hand at either side of the region to be mobilized. To mobilize in extension, draw the patient toward you by leaning backward, then release the pull by moving forward.

VI. Backward Bending. WB (upper thoracic spine; Fig. 20-47)

P—Sitting with the hands clasped behind the neck and the arms resting on the thorax or on the operator's arms

O—Stand in front of the patient, with your arms laced through the patient's arms with the hands in contact with the patient's thorax.

M—While palpating and monitoring the movement with the fingers, pull the patient toward you by slightly elevating the elbows and extending the trunk backward. Thus a lever is formed that acts on the upper thoracic spine, which is mobilized into extension. The pull is released by moving the trunk forward and lowering the elbows. The movement is repeated several times slowly.

Note: By pulling to the left or right, one can mobilize in combined extension and lateral flexion.

VII. Rotation. WB (Fig. 20-48)

P—Sitting astride the plinth with hands placed on opposite shoulders, clasped across the chest, or behind the neck

O—Stand at the patient's side and grasp the patient's far shoulder with the ventral hand. When the alternative position is used (patient's hands behind the neck), first thread your arm through the patient's flexed arms before grasping the far shoulder.

L—With the thumb or finger of the dorsal hand, palpate the interspinous space of the restricted segment.

M—Rotation of the spine is effected by rotating your whole body and at the same time augmenting and localizing the movement with the dorsal hand.

Note: In a variation of this technique, the restricted segment can be rotated to its pathologic barrier. Steadily increase the pressure over the side of the spinous process of the inferior vertebra of the restricted spinal segment, thereby effecting passive mobilization. Active mobilization can be used by localizing the rotation to its pathologic barrier, and having the patient hold the trunk still

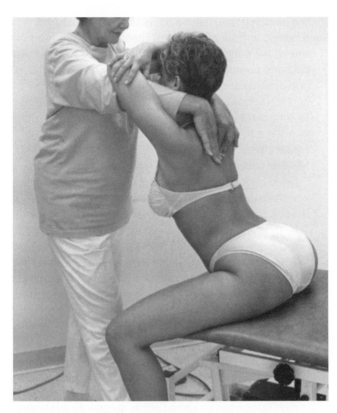

■ **FIG. 20-47.** Backward bending: upper thoracic spine.

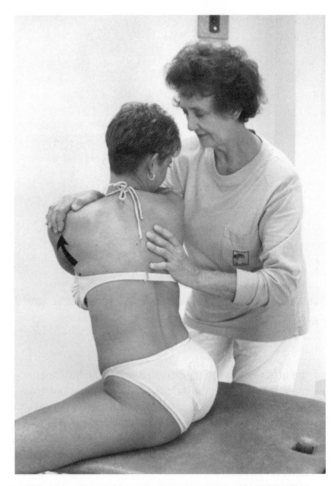

■ **FIG. 20-48.** Rotation: patient with arms across the chest.

while you apply a minimal force toward the midline with the ventral hand. Coupled motions of flexion–rotation–sidebending or extension–rotation–sidebending by localizing to the segment can also be used with active or passive mobilization.[73,74,139,166,197]

VIII. Sidebending. WB (Fig. 20-49)

P—Sitting astride the treatment table with legs over one side and arms clasped across the chest

O—Stand at the patient's side and support the patient's arms and trunk.

L—The thumb or fingers of the dorsal hand are used to palpate laterally between the two spinous processes of the segment to be treated to ensure that movement occurs at that level. For the upper thoracic spine, the ventral hand is wound through the patient's crossed arm to grasp the contralateral shoulder. For the lower thoracic spine, the ventral hand is placed on the contralateral scapula or elbow. The patient's near shoulder is positioned under the operator's axilla.

M—The patient's trunk is sidebent by means of the operator's near axilla, which exerts a downward pressure through the axilla over the near shoulder. An upward lift is given to the patient's contralateral shoulder with the ventral hand on the far shoulder, scapula, or elbow while the dorsal hand palpates the gapping or approximation of the spinous process.

Note: The same NWB technique (see Fig. 22-42) for the lumbar spine, using the patient's thigh as a lever and applying leg abduction until motion arrives at the level of the stabilizing thumb or hand, can be used effectively for the lower thoracic spine.

IX. Posteroanterior Indirect Techniques. Symmetrical techniques to increase flexion.

One of the most effective manipulative techniques for the thoracic spine, especially the central spine, is an indirect (or reverse) technique, whereby the patient lies supine and the operator works from above.[205] A firm base is essential. Because the operator must be able to lean well over the patient a low treatment table or elevation of the operator on a stool is necessary.

Hand grip: A key factor for these techniques is the position and grip of the operator's lower hand. Several grip positions are recommended. The grip position illustrated below uses an extended thumb and index finger to make a V while the third, fourth, and fifth fingers are flexed (Fig. 20-50A).[205] The hand is placed on the spine so that the vertical line of the spinous processes bisects the V and runs in

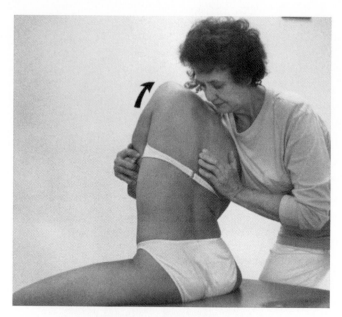

■ FIG. 20-49. Sidebending (WB).

the groove between the clenched fingers and the thenar muscles of the thumb. The position is such that one transverse process lies across the thumb and the transverse process of the level below lies over the flexed middle or ring finger. This serves as a block whereby the movements of the vertebrae are restricted so that when a mobilization (grades I to IV) or a manipulation (grade V) is applied, movement will occur between these two levels. The hand can be cushioned with a small towel roll or cotton bandage to allow greater comfort.

Initial position of the P and O: The patient is sidelying, and with her arms crossed to the opposite shoulders (or

the hands clasped behind the neck and both elbows touching in front of the chin). The operator stands on the side of the patient facing the patient's head with the caudal hand positioned on the segments to be blocked (see grip position above; Fig. 20-50*A*). The other hand and arm lies across and on top of the patient's crossed arms to control the thorax. The operator now brings the thorax into some flexion, which accumulates at the site of the contact hand.

M—The patient is requested to relax, and the patient is rolled back onto the operator's caudal hand. The operator's cephalic arm and body move the patient's upper trunk back (or lets it fall back) over the fulcrum formed by the hand under the patient's back (Fig. 20-50*B*). This technique can be graded from I to V.

To apply a grade V, further increase flexion so as to take up the slack, telling the patient to breathe in and out (this can be repeated as a preparatory mobilization), then apply overpressure along the axis of the humerus, thus compressing the thorax into the caudal hand. It is essential that the overpressure (or thrust) is synchronized with expiration. Instead of delivering a thrust technique, the operator may simply gently increase his pressure, springing the joint while the patient breathes out.[168] This type of mobilization can be carried out as nonspecific treatment, in the rhythm of respiration, mobilizing one segment after the other, rather like a soft tissue manipulation.

An active mobilization assist (muscle energy technique) may be used to effect a change in the muscle tone segmentally.[69] When the motion barrier has been localized, the patient is instructed to gently elevate the crossed arms. The operator resists the motion and the isometric contraction is held up to 5 seconds followed by a period of complete relaxation. The joint is then taken to a new motion

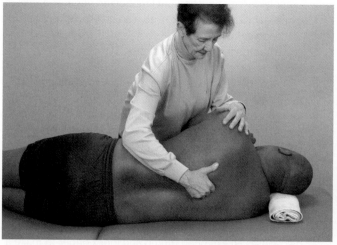

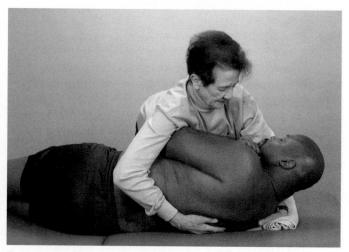

A   B

■ FIG. 20-50. Posteroanterior indirect technique. **(A)** Placement of the hand on the spine. **(B)** Position of patient and operator immediately before indirect technique.

barrier. This may be repeated several times and is followed by reexamination of function.

Other supine indirect techniques can be used both for mobilization (grades 1 to 4) and for a high-velocity thrust, producing either extension or flexion with some degree of sidebending and/or rotation as well.[24,88,139,168,175,205,267]

Thoracic Cage: Articular Techniques of Ribs— Hypomobility of Ribs

Rib dysfunction is indicated if the rib will not move upward during inspiration (inhalation restriction); if the rib will not descend (exhalation restriction); or if there is restriction of motion or position of the rib.

MIDDLE AND LOWER RIB CAGE TECHNIQUES (RIBS TWO TO TWLEVE)

I. Posterior Articulation. NWB (exhalation restriction; Fig. 20-51)
    P—Prone, head facing toward the side to be mobilized
    O—Stand at the patient's head, take hold of the patient's arm just proximal to the elbow, and position the arm into abduction. With the opposite hand, fix each rib involved in turn with the thumb and thenar eminence at the angle of the lower rib.
    M—The ribs are mobilized by stretching the arm into full abduction, achieving quite a powerful stretch of each intercostal space using the leverage of the latissimus dorsi.
        Note: One can also stabilize the arm and mobilize the rib in a caudal direction by contacting the superior angle of the rib with the thumb or the heel of the hand.

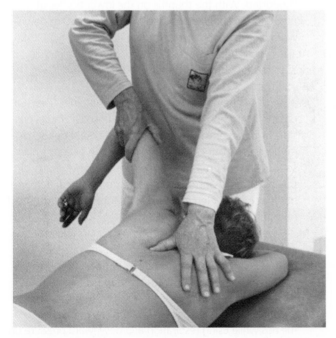

■ **FIG. 20-51.** Posterior articulations.

II. Posterior Articulation. NWB (rib restriction when the arm cannot be used as a lever; Fig. 20-52A)
     P—Prone, head facing toward the side to be mobilized. When working with the upper rib cage, the arm can be abducted or placed behind the patient's back so that the scapula is drawn away from the chest wall to allow easy access to the angle of the rib to be mobilized.
     O—Stand at the patient's head.
     M—For the upper ribs, contact the angle of the rib with pisiform contact and take up the slack in a caudal and lateral or a caudal and central direction. As the patient breathes out toward the limit of expiration, give a series of oscillations. For the middle and lower ribs the contact is with both the pisiform and the base of the metacarpal. Pressure is again applied in a caudal–central or caudal–lateral direction.
         Note: The opposite rib can be stabilized with the other hand. The operator than stands opposite the side to be mobilized (Fig. 20-52B).

III. Anterior Articulation (exhalation restriction; Fig. 20-53)
     P—Supine
     O—Stand on the side to be mobilized, facing the foot of the table. Grasp the forearm above the wrist with the inner hand and stretch the arm upward while fixing the anterior ends of the rib with the outer hand. The operator may use the radial border of the hand or the thumb and thenar eminence to fix the lower of the two ribs.
     M—Quite a powerful stretch of the involved segments can be achieved by using the leverage of the pectoral muscles. To reinforce the stretch and separation of the ribs, muscle energy or proprioceptive neuromuscular facilitation (PNF) techniques may be used, or have the patient inspire deeply as you synchronize the stretch with full inspiration.
         Note: Either a caudal glide may be performed with the right hand as the arm is maintained at its end range, or the right hand may maintain the caudal glide of the rib as the arm is moved into its end range.

IV. Anterior Articulation (exhalation restriction when the arm cannot be used as a lever; Fig. 20-54)
    P—Supine with arms at side
    O—Stand at the patient's head. The stabilizing hand supports the neck, and the mobilizing thumb (reinforced by the hand) contacts the superior edge of the rib to be mobilized.
    M—With the supporting hand, sidebend and forward bend the patient's neck until you feel tension under the mobilizing thumb. During exhalation, apply pressure to the rib in a caudal direction.

V. Cranial–Caudal Glide. WB (lower ribs; Fig. 20-27).[175]
    P—Sitting astradle the table
    O—Stand behind the patient and on the side opposite that to be mobilized.
    M—Move the patient's trunk in lateral flexion to the side 'gers, hook onto the inferior border of the rib and pull

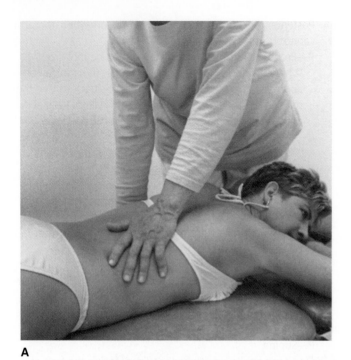
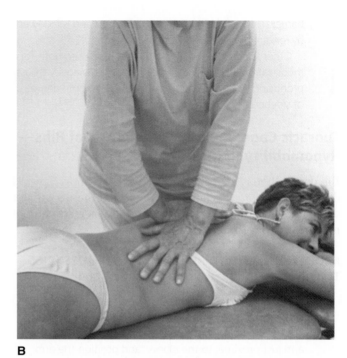

A   **B**

■ **FIG. 20-52.** Posterior articulations: **(A)** without stabilization and **(B)** with stabilization.

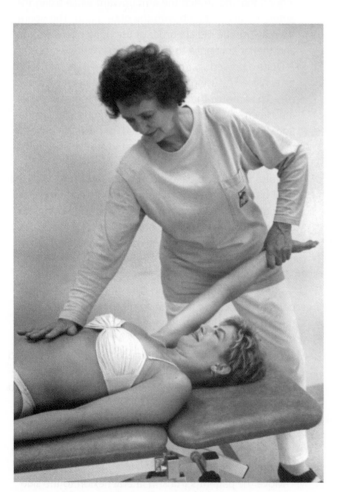

■ **FIG. 20-53.** Anterior articulations using the arm as a lever.

upward (cranial glide) during the end of expiration (Fig. 20-27B). The reverse technique, caudal glide or downward pressure can be used by directing thumb pressure to the superior border of the involved rib (Fig. 20-27A).

Note: This maneuver can also be done in supine (NWB) with both arms of the patient elevated (for a bilateral technique); if a unilateral technique is used, the arm on the side to be mobilized can be maximally elevated and supported. With the thumbs on the lower border of the ribs, glide the rib(s) upward (during expiration) or downward on the upper border (during inspiration; Fig. 20-55).

VI. Active Mobilization (inhalation restriction of the middle ribs, to raise the front of the ribs; Fig. 20-56).[166,197]

P—Supine

O—Stand on the noninvolved side (or same side). The patient's arm on the involved side is flexed as far as possible by your cephalic hand and maintained at end range. Insert your caudal hand under the patient's back so that the fingertips can hook over the inner shafts of the lower ribs. Four ribs can be treated at once. Remember that in restricted inhalation, the uppermost-restricted rib is the key.

M—Have the patient inhale and bring the arm down against your unyielding resistance, if using an isometric contraction. At the same time pull caudally and laterally on the angles of the ribs with the opposite hand.

Note: An isotonic contraction of the serratus anterior and pectoralis major can also be used to raise the front of the ribs while using respiration and downward pressure on the rib angles to assist. To use these muscles, the arm is elevated near its end range with the elbow bent so the

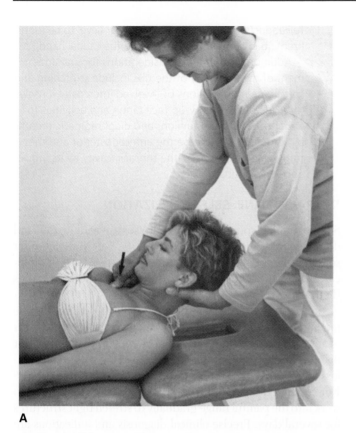

A

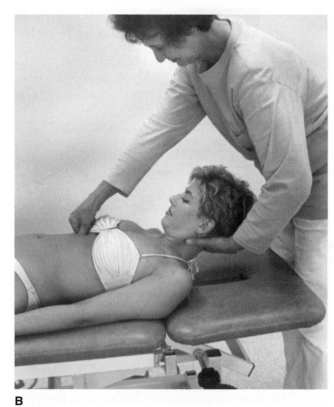

B

■ **FIG. 20-54.** Anterior articulations (alternative technique) when the arm cannot be used as a lever: **(A)** upper ribs and **(B)** lower ribs.

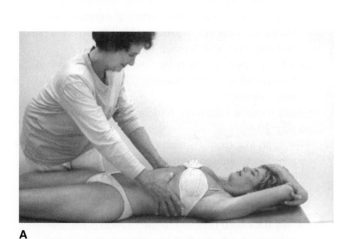

A

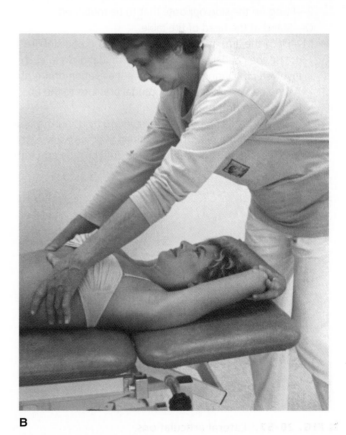

B

■ **FIG. 20-55.** Cephalic and caudal glides (NWB): **(A)** cephalic glide and **(B)** caudal glide.

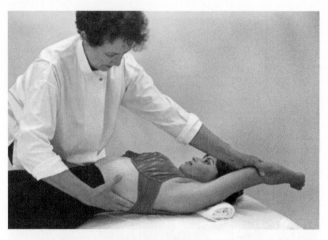

■ FIG. 20-56. Elevation technique using muscle energy or proprioceptive neuromuscular facilitation.

forearm lies above the patient's head (or end range). While resisting at the patient's arm, have the patient inhale deeply and pull the arm down to the side as you resist the arm, and pull caudally and laterally on the angles of the ribs with the opposite hand. Have the patient relax and take up the slack. Repeat three times or more.

There are many variations of PNF or muscle energy approaches. They are extremely effective when the client can isolate movement.

VII. Lateral Articulation (intercostal stretch; Fig. 20-57)

P—Lying on the side opposite that to be mobilized

O—Stand at the head of the table.

M—Place the arm at end range of abduction and stabilize it. Use the caudal hand to impart a caudal glide to each involved rib. During inhalation, resist elevation of the rib. As the patient relaxes, apply caudal pressure to the rib. Repeat two or three times.

Note: This technique can be reversed by using the caudal hand (thumb and thenar eminence or web space) to stabilize the ribs. The cephalic arm stretches the arm into

full abduction, while fixating the lower (level to be mobilized) rib in the midaxillary line with the caudal hand.

Additional treatment considerations for management of hypomobility of the ribs include stretching and soft tissue mobilizations of involved intercostal muscles (see Fig. 8-50); follow-up facilitation and activities to enhance rib cage excursion; and diaphragmatic breathing exercises to increase the anteroposterior and the transverse diameters of the thoracic cavity by its influence on the ribs.

THORACIC SPINE: SELF-MOBILIZATION

Self-segmental spinal mobility exercises are widely used and discussed in the literature.[36,37,102,104,105,117–119,168] Motivation for self-treatment is currently being encouraged, and the logical trend is to teach patients to deal with their problems themselves.

Self-mobilization should be as specific as possible. These techniques should be gentle, deliberate, coaxing movements of small range to induce, at the most, only mild distress. For painful conditions, repetitive motion working within the painless limits provides the proprioceptive input for inhibition.[192] For restricted movement, the patient should be advised to work into the painful range gradually to stretch tight structures for several days. Precise clinical diagnosis and indications are mandatory. The examples presented here correlate with the articulation techniques described above.

I. Extension of the Upper Thoracic Spine (Fig. 20-58)

P—Sitting, back supported by the chair at the level of the lower vertebra (spinous process) of the upper segment to be treated

M—The patient shifts the head and cervicothoracic spine backward to the point of taking up the slack at the segment to be mobilized. This is repeated in a slow, rhythmic fashion.

Note: Use a higher-back chair for upper thoracic levels and the cervical thoracic junction.

II. Flexion–Extension. Middle and lower thoracic spine (Fig. 20-59)

P—Forearm and knees position. The more cranial the mobilization required, the further the elbows are placed forward. For the thoracolumbar region, a hands and knees position is assumed.

M—The patient actively moves the thoracic spine into flexion and extension, breathing in with flexion and out with extension.

III. Localized Thoracic Extension. Middle and lower thoracic spine (Fig. 20-60A)

P—Sitting in a chair. Fixation can be assisted with a pillow adjusted to the segmental level required. By using pillows at various heights and by assuming various erect or slumped sitting positions, almost any level of the thoracic spine can be mobilized.

M—By backward bending to the fixation point, the patient can actively mobilize into extension. Small

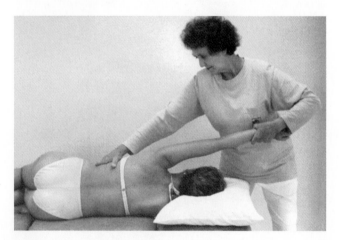

■ FIG. 20-57. Lateral articulations.

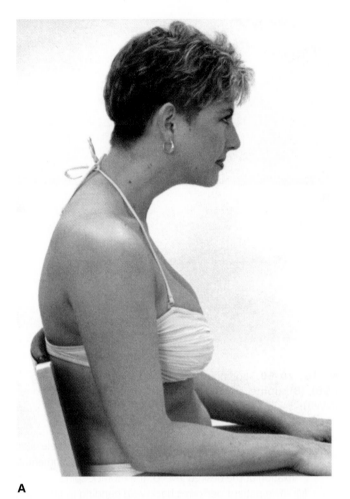

A

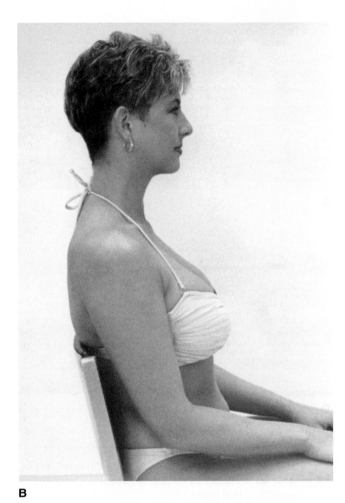

B

■ **FIG. 20-58.** Extension, upper thoracic spine: **(A)** starting position and **(B)** end position.

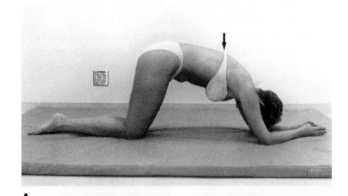

A

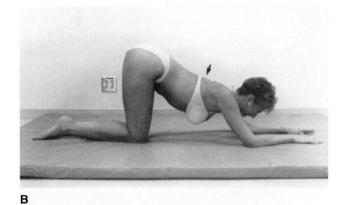

B

■ **FIG. 20-59.** Flexion–extension, middle and lower thoracic spine: **(A)** flexion and **(B)** extension.

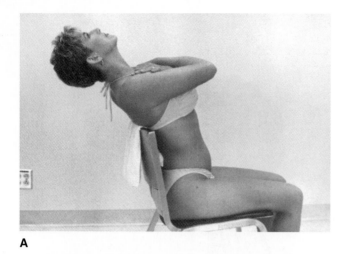

A

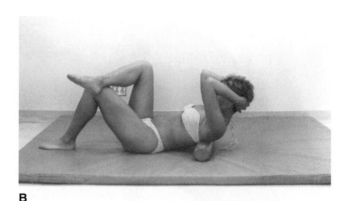

B

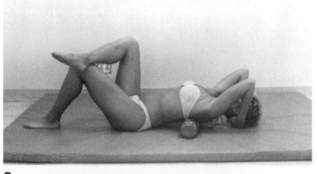

C

■ **FIG. 20-60.** Localized thoracic extension: **(A)** sitting (WB); **(B)** supine, starting position; and (C) end position (NWB).

repetitive oscillatory movements are performed at the end range. With fixation either at a spinous process or a rib, movement can be directed at either the spinal or costovertebral joints.

Note: This self-mobilization technique may also be performed in the supine position over a roll. The level of the axis of motion is determined by the placement of the roll (Fig. 20-60B, C). With this technique the upper ribs are mobilized as well.

IV. Upper Rib–Thoracic Spine Mobilization (Fig. 20-61)

P—Supine with one leg supported by the flexed knee of the opposite side (to flatten the lumbar spine) and with hands clasped behind the neck or with the arms elevated. A foam roll or firm cushion is used to provide segmental fixation at the desired level of the thoracic spine.

M—The patient performs backward bending in time with breathing. The end position should be held as the patient exhales and relaxes.

V. Lower Rib Mobilization (Fig. 20-62)

P—Lying on the side with a hard roll positioned for fixation of the desired thoracic level. The upper leg is extended with the lower leg flexed for stabilization.

M—The patient actively sidebends and reaches with the arm overhead. This technique can be used to effectively mobilize the lower ribs as well as the thoracic spine.

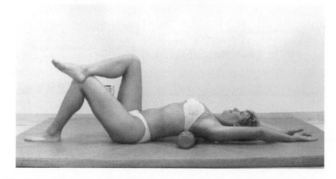

■ **FIG. 20-61.** Upper thoracic spine and rib mobilizations.

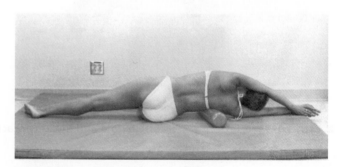

■ **FIG. 20-62.** Lower rib mobilization.

FUNCTIONAL EXERCISES, SENSORIMOTOR TRAINING, AND SPINAL STABILIZATION

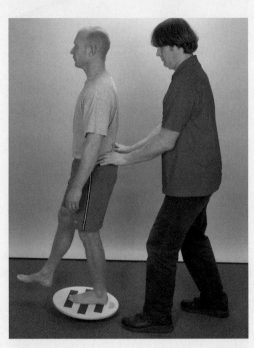

■ **FIG. 20-63.** Applying perturbations to facilitate stabilization response in the deep abdominal muscles.

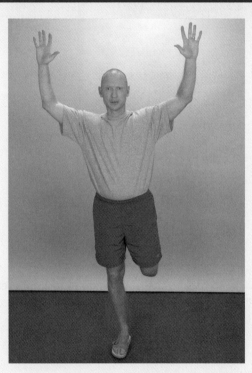

■ **FIG. 20-64.** Internal perturbation with the use of arm movements and balance shoes.

Combining functional exercises (see Chapter 10, Functional Exercises),[7,32,44,45,47,48,49,97,98,150] dynamic stabilization exercises,[51,121,127,201,209,210,237,244,245] reactive neuromuscular training,[277–280] sensorimotor stimulation,[126,203] and other exercise models (i.e., aerobic conditioning,[21] aquatic therapy,[12,31,50] plyometrics–stretch-shortening drills,[114,153,280,291] concentric and eccentric isotonics,[5,153] therapeutic exercise in functional kinetics,[45,155,156] Pilate's method of body conditioning,[11,12,208,236] medical exercise training,[104,105,110,117–119,272,273] movement impairment exercises,[107,246–250] proprioceptive neuromuscular facilitation exercises,[2,109,190,215,265,269,281] and open and closed kinetic chain exercises[150,167,226,290]) will greatly augment the rehabilitation of patients with dysfunction of the thorax, cervicothoracic, and thoracolumbar spine. Many of the functional and dynamic stabilization exercises described in earlier chapters are appropriate for the thoracic spine. See Chapter 10, Functional Exercises (see Figs. 10-1 to 10-5 and 10-7 and 10-9), Chapter 11, Shoulder and Shoulder Girdle (see Figs. 11-71 and 11-73 to 11-89), and Chapter 19, Cervical Spine (see Figs. 19-65, 19-66, and 19-68 to 19-71) for a variety of exercises that can be used to challenge proprioception, range of motion, strength, or endurance of the thoracic spine and lower quadrant.

SENSORIMOTOR TRAINING

Sensorimotor training exercises appropriate for the thoracic spine are described in Chapter 19, Cervical Spine (see Fig.

19-72), Chapter 14, Hip (see Figs. 14-44 and 14-45), Chapter 16, Lower Leg, Ankle, and Foot (see Fig. 16-65) and Chapter 22, Lumbar Spine (see Figs. 22-60 and 22-61). The deep abdominal stabilizers are facilitated by applying the perturbations to the lumbosacral area (Fig. 20-63). Perturbations can be introduced while the patient is kneeling, standing, or marching with the balance shoes via the use of pushes (external perturbations) to the trunk and arm movements (internal perturbations; Fig. 20-64). Both internal and external perturbations can be stimulated by in sequence by throwing an object such as a basketball to and from the patient (see Fig. 16-65). This can also be done with the use of a body blade, which the patient shakes while maintaining stability on a rocker or wobble board.[203] The body blade can be used to place facilitatory focus on the serratus anterior (Fig. 20-65), middle trapezius (Fig. 20-66), lower trapezius (Fig. 20-67), and abdominal stabilizers and deep cervical flexors (Fig. 20-68).[203] Close inspection of the external abdominal oblique reveals that it interdigitates and is typically fused with the serratus anterior.[225] Linkages between shoulder girdle muscles and the abdominal muscles should be appreciated when analyzing or designing exercises to train the abdominal mechanism.

DYNAMIC STABILIZATION

Restoration of dynamic thoracic and lumbar stabilization is part of a more general approach to rehabilitation that follows

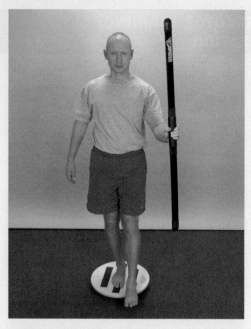

■ **FIG. 20-65.** Using the body blade to facilitate serratus anterior and trunk stabilization.

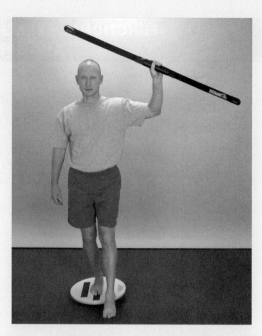

■ **FIG. 20-67.** Using the body blade to facilitate the lower trapezius as well as trunk stabilization responses.

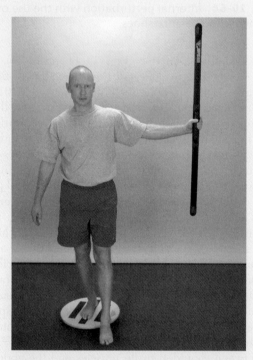

■ **FIG. 20-66.** Using the body blade to facilitate the middle trapezius as well as trunk stabilization responses.

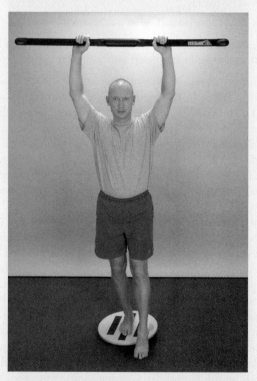

■ **FIG. 20-68.** Using the body blade to facilitate the abdominal stabilizers as well as the deep cervical flexors and trunk stabilization responses.

a sensorimotor format.[126] In this approach, after assessment, tight muscles are stretched, and inhibited (weak) muscles are stimulated and restrengthened. The final and essential stage in the rehabilitation process is to convert movements to an unconscious level. This is achieved by giving an improved activation of the subcortical regulatory systems and increasing sensorimotor stimulation. Subcortical control of stabilization can be achieved by proprioceptive exercise on a labile surface such as therapeutic ball (see Figs. 11-75B, 11-76, 11-78C, 11-82, 22-59, 22-63C, 22-67, and 22-71), wobble board (see Figs. 14-45B and 22-60), rocker board (see Fig. 14-45C), balance shoes (see Fig. 14-45E), a small trampoline (see Figs. 12-32, 14-45A, and 16-68), or foam padding (see Fig. 14-45D).[35,126]

Like the lumbar spine, the dynamic trunk stabilization program for the thoracic spine may be divided into three or four overlapping stages[138,209,210]:

• Stage 1: Reeducation of stabilizing muscles
• Stage 2: Exercise progression for static stabilization
• Stage 3: Exercise progression for dynamic stabilization
• Stage 4: Functional exercise (occupational- or activity-specific stabilization)

The stabilization program starts by identifying the training or functional range in which movement can be performed in a biomechanically correct and painless manner. Normal movement depends not only on active stability but also on passive joint and myofascial mobility. For this reason the practitioner must deal with both myofascial length and muscle strength, and be able to identify and correct faulty movement patterns that affect the thorax, cervicothoracic, thoracic, and thoracolumbar spine. It is quality of a movement rather than simply strength alone that is important to muscle balance. Staying within this range may initially require performing isometric stabilization exercise by co-contracting stability synergists (i.e., gluteus maximus and the transverse abdominus).[230,233] In the case of the trunk, the stability synergists are the transversus abdominus, multifidus, and internal and external obliques. Other stability synergists include the iliopsoas, gluteus maximus, gluteus medius, vastus medialis oblique, soleus, and deep cervical flexors. Muscles such as the rectus abdominus and superficial neck flexors are considered movement synergists. The movement synergists are often a single-joint muscle aligned to oppose gravity and approximate a joint. These muscles and the lateral fibers of the external oblique are not as important to spinal stability because they are prime movers of trunk flexion rather than spinal stabilizers. The ability of a stability synergist to maintain an isometric contraction at low load for a period of time is vital to antigravity function.[233] Facilitating co-contraction of the muscles surrounding the spine can enhance spinal stability. The transversus abdominus and oblique abdominals are particularly important in this respect because of their involvement in the thoracolumbar fascia (TLF) mechanism and in enhancing abdominal pressure.[209,210] Two other muscle groups are activated in synergy with the transversus abdominus and multifidus during the action of drawing in the abdominal wall. These are the diaphragm and pelvic floor musculature. Conceptually, the transversus abdo-

minus forms the walls of a cylinder and the muscles of the pelvic floor and diaphragm form its base and lid, respectively.[231]

STAGE 1: REEDUCATION OF STABILITY MUSCLES

It is critical to isolate contraction of the transversus abdominus and the oblique abdominals from the rectus abdominus, which is often dominant. Action of the multifidus will normally be poor at the level of spinal disease, so facilitation of this muscle segment is important (see muscle control above) as well. Other muscles include the thoracoabdominal diaphragm and the pelvic floor muscles.

Thoracoabdominal Diaphragm. The most common component lost in patients with thoracic dysfunction is lateral costal expansion.[165] Optimal diaphragmatic breathing involves both abdominal and lower rib cage expansions.[63] When lateral costal expansion is absent, excessive excursion occurs in the abdomen (making it difficult to attain a functional transversus abdominus contraction) or in the upper chest. Teaching the client to use diaphragmatic breathing and neutral spine position is the first step in preparing the motor system to learn new stabilization strategies. The patient should be instructed in nasodiaphragmatic breathing, which is best learned in supine followed by sitting, standing, and finally during activity. Proper diaphragmatic breathing is also important for normal temporomandibular function and decreases excessive accessory respiratory muscle activity in the upper chest (see Chapter 17, Temporomandibular Joint).[8,19,43,87,92,128,151,173,188] Breathing exercises exist in many different programs, including the Alexander technique,[6] the Feldenkrais method,[85] Pilates,[236] yoga,[227] meditation schools, and relaxation training.

Abdominal Muscle Training. Both dynamic abdominal bracing and abdominal hollowing have been shown to give muscle activity suitable for lumbar stabilization[231] as well as the thoracic spine.[164] Dynamic abdominal bracing[146,147] is a technique in which the patient is encouraged to expand the abdominal muscles laterally. The patient places his or her hands over the transversus abdominus and oblique abdominals just superior to the iliac spine crests. The action is to contract this abdominal muscle group and to press the hands apart, rather than cause the abdomen to protrude by contracting the rectus abdominus alone.

Abdominal hollowing is achieved by patients pulling the abdomen in, without allowing significant lumbar flexion (neutral spine). Ideally, a neutral lumbar spine should be attained because the neutral lumbar spine is known to facilitate isolation of the transversus abdominus.[254] Abdominal hollowing is facilitated by instructing the patient to pull the umbilicus "in and up" while breathing normally. The initial position chosen to teach this exercise will depend on which position encourages relaxation of the global muscles while providing some stretch on the abdominal wall for proprioceptive feedback.[165] The best position for each patient will vary depending on his or her substitution strategies. Often the quadruped position eases learning by giving stretch facilitation. This position also allows the muscles to contract against gravity.[210] Once the correct contraction is achieved, the exercise is progressed for endurance rather than strength. Restoration of the abdominal hollowing mechanism

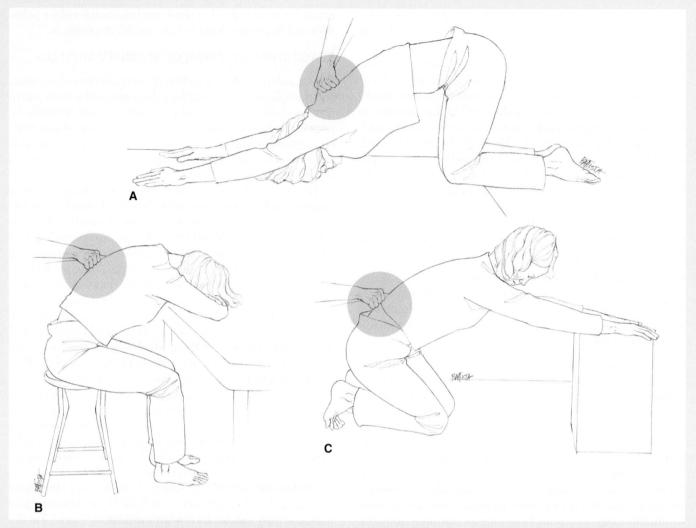

■ **FIG. 20-69.** Segmental flexion–extension stabilization techniques using manual resistance and positioning **(A)** for the upper thoracic spine **(B)** midthoracic spine, and **(C)** lower thoracolumbar spine.

can be enhanced by the use of pressure biofeedback (Fig. 20-32) and multisensory cues (e.g., auditory cues, visual cues, tactile cues, and kinesthetic cueing) to enhance muscle contraction and motor control.[196] There should be a slow development of gentle tension. Only a 15 to 20% contraction of this muscle is required. There should be no pelvic tilt or spinal movements, and little movement in the upper abdomen.

Multifidus Facilitation. Restoration of multifidus activity begins by facilitating the muscle at the level of spinal disorder, as localized dysfunction of this muscle is common. See muscle control testing (above) for assessment and treatment of the deep stabilizers. Low-load rotatory resistance is applied to the affected segment as though testing for PPIVM (Fig. 20-24C).[179] The patient is encouraged to maintain the submaximal contraction against the resistance to rotation applied to the spinous processes of the spine.

As with the abdominal muscles above, multisensory clues can be used to enhance muscle control and muscle contraction. Haynes[113] theoretically suggests that imitating infant rolling

movements can initiate the reflex reactive muscular contraction of the deep spinal muscles. Facilitation can be done in any position; generally it is easiest to minimize excessive global activity in a more supported position. More upright and functional positions can be used as progression occurs (Fig. 20-69). In all of theses segmental methods and more global dynamic stabilization exercises (described below), the clinician should check for normal activation of the transversus abdominus and avoid overactivity of the obliques and rectus abdominus.

STAGE 2: EXERCISE PROGRESSION FOR STATIC STABILIZATION

The aim of the second stage of stabilization is to impose load onto the trunk while maintaining a statically stabilized posture. The patient must recognize when the spine is losing stability. Maintaining the neutral position by muscle bracing is known as static stabilization and is held through all stage 2 exercise progression.[210] In cases in which exercising in the midrange position is not desirable, the spine may be prepositioned to avoid the unwanted range of motion.[201] Active prepositioning is achieved by placing the spine in the desired position and instructing the patient to hold this position with muscle activity only.

Positions used for abdominal hollowing such as the quadruped (see Fig. 11-78A), front bridge (see Fig. 11-79), prone, or the supine position are progressed by using arms and leg loading (Fig. 20-70; also see Figs. 19-65, 19-70D, E, and 22-71 to 22-73) to impose load on to the trunk while maintaining the neutral position.

Work emphasizing the multifidus and obliques may be achieved by using rhythmic stabilization (RS) techniques in various starting positions such as the sidelying crook position (Fig. 20-71). In the sidelying crook position the operator pushes forward on the subject's pelvis and backward on his or her shoulder while the patient resists the action. The movement is then reversed.

In the supine crook position, RS techniques may be applied to the patient's bent knees or to an upper limb arm pattern or to the entire trunk with one manual contact on the knees and the other on an upper trunk pattern (Fig. 20-72) starting in the inner range. The challenge can be increased by applying RS to various arm patterns and moving out of the inner range, altering the lever arm and further challenging the abdominals and extensors of the thoracic spine. Patients

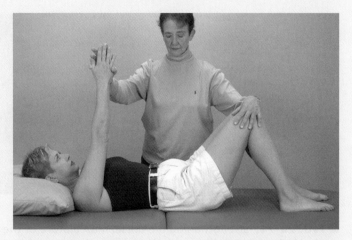

■ **FIG. 20-72.** Supine crook position with an upper limb trunk pattern using rhythmic stabilization to challenge the extensors of the thoracic spine and abdominals.

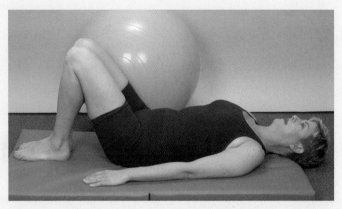

■ **FIG. 20-73.** Home exercises, emphasizing trunk rotation.

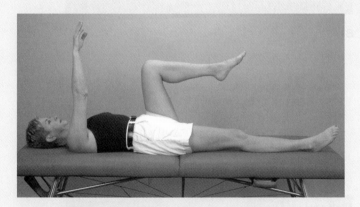

■ **FIG. 20-70.** Dead-bug exercise in supine.

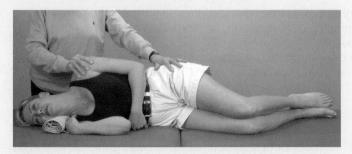

■ **FIG. 20-71.** Rhythmic stabilization applied in the side-lying crook position emphasizing the multifidus and oblique musculature.

may continue these activities at home by pushing into a therapeutic ball secured against a wall with the arms or the legs (Fig. 20-73).

Static work on extension mobility of the thoracic spine and the power of the spinal extensors to develop endurance may begin by sitting on one's heels on the floor and bending forward to rest the forehead on the floor in front of the knees.[102] The forearms are pronated so that the dorsum of the hands rests alongside the legs. Without altering the flexed position of the lumbar spine, the thoracic spine is extended, the arms laterally rotated, and the scapulae approximated, as the head and shoulders are raised to flatten the thoracic spine (Fig. 20-74). The position is held for an increasing number of seconds, as the patient becomes familiar with the purpose and technique of the exercise. The exercise may progress by abducting the arms to 90° while maintaining the neutral spinal position. Often in this position and others an unstable segment remains kyphotic when the rest of the vertebral column extends. Specific extension exercises over a ball (see Fig. 20-78B) together with a 50-Hz stimulating current over the involved segment can help to restore the appropriate motion.[162]

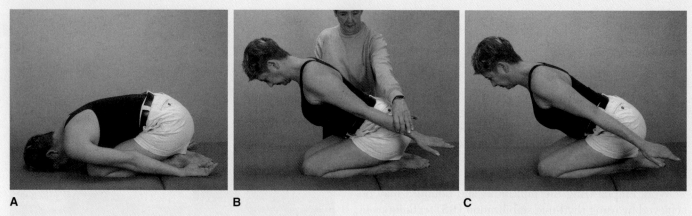

■ **FIG. 20-74.** Strengthening the dorsal musculature of the thoracic spine and shoulder retractors in sitting posture on heels. **(A)** Starting position with the arms resting alongside the legs (forearms pronated). **(B)** Thoracic extension and scapulae approximation with the arms externally rotated. **(C)** Progression to upper limb abduction to 90°.

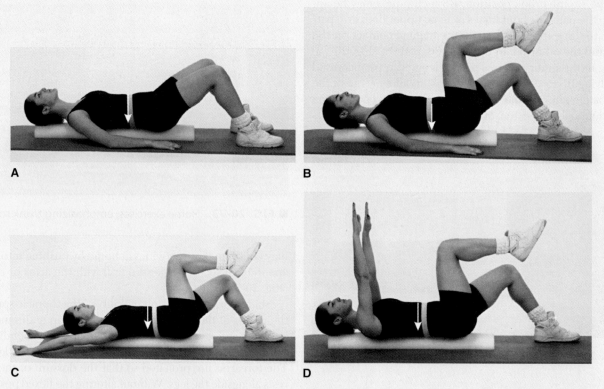

■ **FIG. 20-75.** Trunk bracing in supine. **(A)** The patient is taught to co-contract the anterior and posterior trunk muscles isometrically without excessive posterior tilting. While maintaining the co-contraction, **(B)** alternately lift one foot slightly off the floor and progress to 90° hip flexion, **(C)** repeat with arms over head, and progress **(D)** with both hands above chest without losing trunk control. Note: These movements are more difficult on circular-tubular foam. (Reprinted with permission from Liebenson C: Rehabilitation of the Spine: A Practical Manual. Philadelphia, Lippincott Williams & Wilkins, 1996:306.)

Trunk bracing in supine (Fig. 20-75), trunk control in quadruped (Fig. 20-76; also see Fig. 22-72), back bridge (Fig. 20-77; also see Figs. 22-66 and 22-67), and front bridge activities (see Figs. 11-79, 20-79A, and 22-73) elicit co-contraction between the abdominal muscles, the spinal extensors, and the hip extensors, flexors, and adductors. These activities achieve muscle activity patterns or strategies associated with spinal stabilization. Static stabilization may be combined with stretching exercises for tight muscles identified during the assessment on muscle imbalances. Active stretching of the pectoralis major, latissimus dorsi, and iliopsoas may all be performed while maintaining a neutral position of the spine.

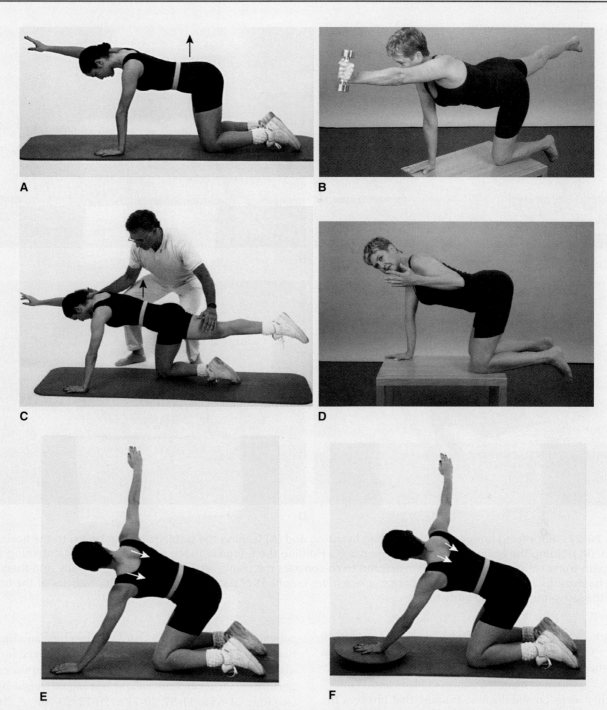

■ **FIG. 20-76.** Quadruped activities might include trunk control **(A)** with independent arm movement, **(B)** independent arm and leg movement on a bench (narrow base of support), **(C)** independent arm and leg movement with manual resistance, **(D)** with lateral flexion of the spine through countermovement of the ipsilateral arm and leg, **(E)** with trunk rotation, and **(F)** with trunk rotation on a balance board. (A, C, E, and F reprinted with permission from Liebenson C: Rehabilitation of the Spine: A Practical Manual. Philadelphia, Lippincott Williams & Wilkins, 1996:302.)

STAGE 3: EXERCISES FOR DYNAMIC STABILIZATION

Dynamic stabilization exercises use many of the starting positions and progressions of stage 2.

Essentially, the patient is taught to specifically recruit the trunk muscles and then maintain this brace as they move the upper and lower limbs independently. Initially the base of support is very stable. The program is progressed by increasing the degree of difficulty by reducing the base of support and by increasing the load, which must be controlled. Figures 20-78 and 20-79 illustrate dynamic upper and lower limb activities over a therapeutic ball to challenge the spinal

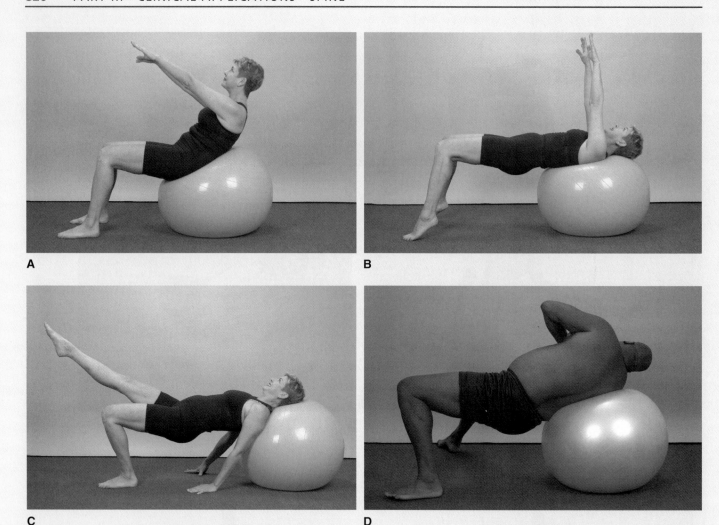

■ FIG. 20-77. Back-lying bridge activities starting in sitting and (**A**) leaning the stable trunk backward to the horizontal position. (**B**) Holding the bridge with arm movements. (**C**) Holding the bridge with leg movements. (**D**) Maintaining the bridge with trunk rotation. The patient is instructed to co-contract the trunk, recruit the gluteus maximus, and then to use the hamstrings. In general back-lying bridges place more emphasis or demand on the posterior muscles of the body such as the latissimus dorsi and gluteals.

extensors, flexors, and rotators. The reader is referred to Biondi,[22] Carriere,[44–46] Clark,[51] Grieve,[102] Hardin,[110] Hyman and Liebenson,[121] Irion,[122] Jemmett,[127] Keely,[141] Lee,[162,164] Morgan,[201] Norris,[210] Saal,[245] Sullivan et al.,[269] and White[288] for further ideas on stabilization training that involves the total musculoskeletal system.

STAGE 4: FUNCTIONAL EXERCISES (OCCUPATIONAL- AND ACTIVITY-SPECIFIC STABILIZATION)

It becomes clear that spinal stabilization patterns produced during rehabilitation must closely match tasks that will be performed in patients' daily living (see Chapter 10, Functional Exercises).[47] To encourage this, actions are chosen that resemble as closely as possible the functional activities the patient uses daily. These are then used as exercises in the rehabilitation program. The program is directed by the patient's needs and is limited only by the clinician's imagination. Like the lumbar spine, the exercise of choice for stimulating disk repair is spinal rotation.[235] Rotation can be performed either in non–weight bearing or weight bearing (see Figs. 11-83 to 11-87, 20-71 to 20-73, 20-76E, F, 20-77D, 20-79C, D, 22-57B, 22-58A, and 22-75 to 22-77).

The current level of quality research in this area gives the clinician scientific evidence to support a program of developing motor control and muscle function for rehabilitation of spinal injuries. In this process, the client should develop freedom of movement, without rigid spinal holding patterns. Efficiency in functional movement should be enhanced through improved proprioceptive abilities, strength, postural endurance, appropriate muscular balance and joint arthrokinematics, and improved neuromuscular efficiency throughout the entire kinetic chain.

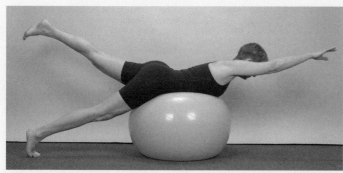

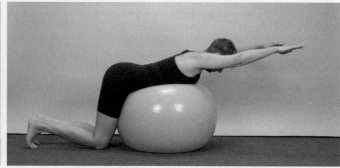

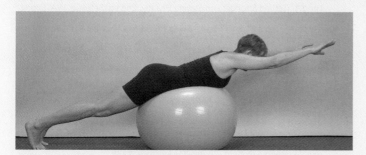

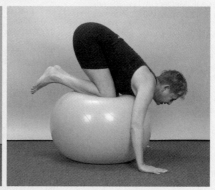

■ **FIG. 20-78.** Upper and lower limb activities over a therapeutic ball to challenge stability, emphasizing spinal extensors. Exercises may include (**A**) trunk control with upper and lower limb lifts, (**B**) scapular retraction with knees flexed, and (**C**) scapular retraction with knees extended. To increase the challenge the patient may perform swimming, reciprocal flexion–extension arm movements. Resistance is optional. These exercises are helpful in strengthening the middle and lower trapezius, the suboccipital muscles, and back extensor muscles.

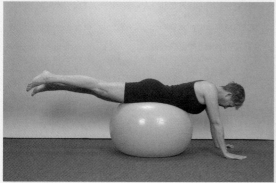

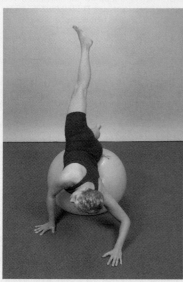

■ **FIG. 20-79.** Trunk activities over a ball to challenge stability of the trunk. (**A**) Front bridge walkouts on a ball. (**B**) Total flexion of the spine and hips on the ball. (**C**) Rotation of the thoracic spine under the shoulder girdle (the weight of the legs has to be stabilized by the trunk). (**D**) Rotation with flexion of the spine. In general prone-lying activities over a ball place more emphasis or demand on the shoulder girdle stabilizers and the anterior muscles such as the abdominals, hip flexors, and adductors.

REFERENCES

1. Adams MA, Hutton WC: Gradual disc prolapse. Spine 10:524–531, 1985
2. Adler SS, Beckers D, Buck M: PNF in Practice: An Illustrated Guide. Berlin, Springer-Verlag, 1993
3. Akeson WH, Amiel D, LaViolette D, et al: The connective tissue response to immobility: An accelerated aging response. Exp Gerontol 3:289–301, 1968
4. Akeson WH, Amiel D, Woo S: Immobility effects of synovial joints: The pathomechanics of joint contracture. Biorheology 17:95–110, 1980
5. Albert M: Eccentric Muscle Training in Sports and Orthopaedics. New York, Churchill Livingstone, 1991
6. Alexander FM: The Alexander Technique. New York, New York University Books, 1967
7. Alfiera RMG: Functional Training: Everyone's Guide to New Fitness Revolution. New York, Hatherliegh Press, 2001
8. Allen RJ, Leischow SJ: The effect of diaphragmatic and thoracic breathing on cardiovascular arousal. In: Proceedings of the VIIth International Respiratory Psychophysiology Symposium. Stockholm, The Nobel Institute for Neurophysiology, 1987
9. American Medical Association: A Guide to the Evaluation of Permanent Impairment, 4th ed. Chicago, American Medical Association, 1993
10. American Physical Therapy Association: Women's Health Gynecological Physical Therapy Manual. LaCrosse, WI, 1997
11. Anderson B: Pilates power. Adv Directors Rehabil 12: 27–30, 76, 2003
12. Anthony A: Pilates takes the plunge. Adv Directors Rehabil 12:53–56, 2003
13. Asmussen E, Heebooll-Nielsen K: Posture, mobility and strength of the back in boys 7 to 16 years old. Acta Orthop Scand 28:174–189, 1959
14. Aston J: Your ideal body: A new paradigm for movement. Phys Ther Today, Summer 1991
15. Axelgaard J, Brown JC: Lateral electrical surface stimulation for the treatment of progressive idiopathic scoliosis. Spine 8:242–260, 1983
16. Axelgaard J, Nordwall A, Brown JC: Correction of spinal curvature by transcutaneous electrical muscle stimulation. Spine 8:463–481, 1983
17. Bajelis D: The Biomechanical Assessment of the Myofascial System. A Practical Manual for Body Therapists. Mount Shasta, CA, Hellerwork, 1995
18. Baker PK: Musculoskeletal problems. In: Steege JF, Metzer DA, Levy BS, eds: Chronic Pelvic Pain: An Integrated Approach. Philadelphia, WB Saunders, 1998:215–240
19. Barlow W: The Alexander Technique. New York, Warner Books, 1980
20. Benson MDK, Byrnes DP: The clinical syndromes and surgical treatment of thoracic intervertebral disk prolapse. J Bone Joint Surg Br 57:471–477, 1975
21. Bezner J: Principles of aerobic conditioning. In: Bandy WD, Sanders B, eds: Therapeutic Exercise: Techniques for Intervention. Philadelphia, Lippincott Williams & Wilkins, 2001:213–238
22. Biondi B: Lumbar functional stabilization program. In: Goldstein TS, ed: Functional Rehabilitation in Orthopedics. Gaithersburg, MD, Aspen, 1995:133–142
23. Blackburn J: Trager psychophysical integration—an overview. J Bodywork Movement Ther 7:233–239, 2003
24. Blackman J, Prip K: Mobilization Techniques, 2nd ed. Edinburgh, Churchill Livingstone, 1988
25. Blair JM: Examination of the thoracic spine. In: Grieves GP, ed: Modern Manual Therapy of the Vertebral Column. New York, Churchill Livingstone, 1986:534–537
26. Bobath B: The treatment of neuromuscular disorders by improving patterns of co-ordination. Physiotherapy 55:18–22, 1969
27. Bonica JJ, Sola AF: Chest pain caused by other disorders. In: Bonica JJ, ed: The Management of Pain, vol. 2, 2nd ed. Philadelphia, Lea & Febiger, 1990:1114–1145
28. Bookhout MR: Exercise and somatic dysfunction. Phys Med Rehabil Clin North Am 7:845–962, 1996
29. Bourdillon JF, Day EA, Bookhut MR: Spinal Manipulation, 5th ed. Oxford, Butterworth-Heinemann, 1992
30. Breig A, Marions O: Biomechanics of the lumbosacral nerve root. Acta Radiol 4:1141–1160, 1963
31. Brody LT: Aquatic physical therapy. In: Hall CM, Brody LT, eds: Therapeutic Exercise: Moving Towards Function. Philadelphia, Lippincott Williams & Wilkins, 1999:286–302
32. Brownstein B, Bronner S, eds: Evaluation, Treatment and Outcomes. Functional Movement in Orthopaedic and Sports Physical Therapy. New York, Churchill Livingstone, 1997
33. Brugger A: Das Sternale Syndrom. Bern, Huper, 1971
34. Brugger A: Die Funktionskrankheiten des Bewegungsapparates. Funktionskrankheiten des Bewegungsapparates 1:69–129, 1986
35. Bullock-Saxton JE, Janda V, Bullock MI: Reflex activation of gluteal muscles in walking. Spine 18:704–708, 1993
36. Buswell J: A Manual of Home Exercises for the Spinal Column. Auckland, NZ, Manipulative Therapy Association, 1978
37. Buswell J: Exercises in the treatment of vertebral dysfunction. In: Grieve GP, ed: Modern Manual Therapy of the Vertebral Column. New York, Churchill Livingstone, 1986:834–838
38. Butler DS: Mobilisation of the Nervous System. Melbourne, Churchill Livingstone, 1991
39. Butler DS, Slater H: Neural injury in the thoracic spine: A conceptual basis for manual therapy. In: Grant R, ed: Physical Therapy of the Cervical and Thoracic Spine. New York, Churchill Livingstone, 1994
40. Cailliet R: Scoliosis. Philadelphia, FA Davis, 1975
41. Cailliet R: Pain: Mechanisms and Management. Philadelphia, FA Davis, 1993
42. Cantu RI, Gordin AJ: Myofascial Manipulations: Theory and Clinical Application. Gaithersburg, MD, Aspen Publications, 1992
43. Caplan D: Back Trouble: A New Approach to Prevention and Recovery. Gainesville, FL, Triad Publishing Co, 1987
44. Carriere B: Therapeutic exercise and self-correction programs. In: Flynn TW, ed: The Thoracic Spine and Rib Cage: Musculoskeletal and Evaluation and Treatment. Boston, Butterworth-Heinemann, 1996
45. Carriere B: The Swiss Ball: Theory, Basic Exercise and Clinical Application. Berlin, Springer-Verlag, 1998
46. Carriere B: Fitness for the Pelvic Floor. Stuttgart, Thieme, 2002
47. Chason N: The Swing Reaction System. Seattle, Biomechanical Golf Exercise Video, 1996
48. Chason N: Total Conditioning for Golfers: Your Definitive Guide to Hitting Longer, Getting Stronger and Staying Healthy, 2nd ed. Bellevue, WA, Sports Reaction Prod, 2002
49. Chason N, Kane M: Functional training for the low back patient. Orthop Phys Ther Clin North Am 8:451–477, 1999
50. Cirullo JA: Aquatic physical therapy approaches in the spine. Orthop Phys Ther Clin North Am 3:179–208, 1994
51. Clark MA: Core stabilization training in rehabilitation. In: Prentice WE, Voight ML, eds: Techniques in Musculoskeletal Rehabilitation. New York, McGraw-Hill, 2001:259–278
52. Clarkson HM, Gilewich GB: Musculoskeletal Assessment: Joint Range of Motion and Muscle Strength. Baltimore, Williams & Wilkins, 1989
53. Cloward RB: Cervical diskography: A contribution to the etiology and mechanism of neck, shoulder, and arm pain. Ann Surg 150:1052–1064, 1959
54. Cole JH, Furness AL, Twomey LT: Muscles in action, an approach to manual muscle testing. Edinburg, Churchill Livingstone, 1988
55. Comerford MJ, Mottram SL: Movement and stability dysfunction—contemporary developments. Man Ther 6:15–20, 2001
56. Connolly BH, Michael BT: Early detection of scoliosis: A neurological approach using the asymmetrical tonic neck reflex. Phys Ther 64:304–307, 1984
57. Corrigan B, Maitland GD: Practical Orthopedic Medicine. Boston, Butterworths, 1983
58. Critchley D: Instructing pelvic floor contractions facilitates transverse abdominus thickness during low-abdominal hollowing. Physiother Res Int 7:65–75, 2002
59. Cyriax JH: Textbook of Orthopaedic Medicine, Diagnosis of Soft-Tissue Lesions, vol. 1, 8th ed. London, Bailliere Tindall, 1982
60. Cyriax JH, Cyriax PJ: Illustrated Manual of Orthopaedic Medicine, 2nd ed. Boston, Butterworths, 1993
61. D'Ambrosia RD, ed: Musculoskeletal Disorders: Regional Examination and Differential Diagnosis, 2nd ed. Philadelphia, JB Lippincott, 1986
62. De Palma A, Rothman RH: The Intervertebral Disc. Philadelphia, WB Saunders, 1970
63. DeTroyer AD: The mechanism of the inspiratory expansion of the rib cage. J Lab Clin Med 114:97–104, 1989
64. DiGiovanna EI, Sahiowitz S, eds: An Osteopathic Approach to Diagnosis and Treatment. Philadelphia, JB Lippincott, 1991
65. Dommisse GF: The blood supply of the spinal cord: A critical vascular zone in spinal surgery. J Bone Joint Surg Br 56:223–235, 1974
66. Dreyfuss P, Levernieux J: Les hernies discales dorsales. In: L'actualite Rheumatologique. Paris, Expansion Scientifique, 1966
67. Dreyfuss P, Tibiletti C, Dreyer SJ: Thoracic zygapophyseal joint pain patterns: A study in normal volunteers. Spine 19:807–811, 1994
68. Dunham WF: Ankylosing spondylitis: Measurement of the hip and spinal movements. Br J Phys Med 12:126–129, 1949
69. Dutton M: The thoracic spine. In: Dutton M: Manual Therapy of the Spine: An Integrated Approach. New York, McGraw, 2002:408–445
70. Dvorák J, Dvorák V: Manual Medicine, Diagnostics. New York, Georg Thieme Verlag, Thieme Medical Publishers, 1990
71. Edmond SL: Manipulation and Mobilization: Extremity and Spinal Techniques. St. Louis, CV Mosby, 1993
72. Edwards BC: Combined movements of the lumbar spine: Examination and clinical significance. Aust J Physiother 25:147–152, 1979
73. Edwards BC: Combined movements in the cervical spine (C2–7): Their value in examination and technique choice. Aust J Physiother 26:165–171, 1980
74. Edwards BC: Manual of Combined Movements, 2nd ed. Oxford, Butterworth-Heinemann, 1999
75. Edwardson B: Musculoskeletal Assessment: An Integrated Approach. San Diego, Singular Publishing Group, 1992
76. Elvey RL: Painful restriction of shoulder movement: A clinical observation study. In: Proceedings, Disorders of the Knee, Ankle and Shoulder. Perth, Western Australian Institute of Technology, 1979
77. Elvey RL: Treatment of arm pain associated with abnormal brachial plexus tension. Aust J Physiother 32:224–229, 1986
78. Elvey RL, Quintner JL, Thomas AN: A clinical study of RSI. Aust Fam Phys 15:1314–1322, 1986

79. Evans P: The healing process at a cellular level. Physiotherapy 66:256–259, 1980

80. Evans RC: Illustrated Essentials in Orthopedic Physical Assessment. St. Louis, CV Mosby, 1994

81. Evjenth O, Hamberg J: Muscle Stretching in Manual Therapy: A Clinical Manual, vol. 2: The Spinal Column and the TMJ. Alfta, Sweden, Alfta Rehab Forlag, 1984

82. Farady JA: Current principles in the nonoperative management of structural adolescent scoliosis. Phys Ther 63:512–523, 1983

83. Farfan H, Gracovetsky S: The nature of instability. Spine 9:714–719, 1984

84. Feldenkrais M: Body and Mature Behavior: A Study of Anxiety, Sex, Gravity and Learning. New York, International Universities Press, 1949

85. Feldenkrais M: Awareness Through Movement—Health Exercises for Personal Growth. New York, Harper & Row, 1972

86. Feldenkrais M: The Potential Self: The Dynamics of Body and the Mind. San Francisco, Harper & Row, 1985

87. Fielding M: Physical therapy in chronic airway limitation. In: Peat M, ed: Current Physical Therapy, Toronto, BC Decker, 1988:12–14

88. Flynn TW: The Thoracic Spine and Rib Cage: Musculoskeletal Evaluation and Treatment. Boston, Butterworth-Heinemann, 1996

89. Ford DM, Bagnall KM, Clements CA, et al: Muscle spindles in the paraspinal musculature of patients with adolescent idiopathic scoliosis. Spine 13:461–465, 1988

90. Ford DM, Bagnall KM, McFadden, KD, et al: Paraspinal muscle imbalance in adolescent idiopathic scoliosis. Spine 9:373–376, 1984

91. Frank C, Akeson WH, Woo S, et al: Physiology and therapeutic value of passive joint motion. Clin Orthop 185:113–125, 1984

92. Frownfelter DL: Chest Physical Therapy and Pulmonary Rehabilitation, 2nd ed. Chicago, Year Book Medical Publishers, 1987

93. Fryette HH: Principles of Osteopathic Technique. Carmel, CA, Academy of Applied Osteopathy, 1954

94. Gelb M: An Introduction to the Alexander Technique. New York, Henry Holt & Company, 1987

95. Gerhardt JJ: Documentation of Joint Motion: International Standard Neutral-Zero Measuring S.F.T.R. Recording and Application of Goniometers, Inclinometers and Calipers. Portland, OR, ISOMED Inc, 1992

96. Gonnella C, Paris S, Kutner M: Reliability in evaluating passive intervertebral motion. Phys Ther 62:437–444, 1982

97. Gray G: Chain Reaction: Successful Strategies for Closed Chain Testing and Rehabilitation. Adrian MI, Wynn Marketing, 1989

98. Gray G: Lower Extremity Functional Profile, Adrian, MI, Wynn Marketing, 1995

99. Greenman PE: Principles of Manual Medicine, 2nd ed. Baltimore, Williams & Wilkins, 1996

100. Grieve GP: Mobilisation of the Spine: Notes on Examination, Assessment and Clinical Method, 4th ed. Edinburgh, Churchill Livingstone, 1984

101. Grieve GP: Thoracic joint problems and simulated visceral disease. In: Grieve GP, ed: Modern Manual Therapy of the Vertebral Column. New York, Churchill Livingstone, 1986:377–395

102. Grieve GP: Mobilization of the Spine: A Primary Handbook of Clinical Method, 5th ed. Edinburgh, Churchill Livingstone, 1991

103. Grimsby O: Lumbar-Thoracic Spine. Continuing Education Course. Nashville, TN, Institute of Graduate Health Sciences, 1976

104. Gustavsen R: Fra aktiv avspenning til trening. Oslo, Norlis, 1977

105. Gustavsen R: Training Therapy: Prophylaxis and Rehabilitation. New York, Thieme, 1993

106. Hall CM: The shoulder girdle. In: Hall CM, Brody LT, eds: Therapeutic Exercise: Moving Toward Function. Philadelphia, Lippincott Williams & Wilkins, 1998:575–625

107. Hall CM, Brody LT: Therapeutic Exercise: Moving Toward Function. Philadelphia, Lippincott Williams & Wilkins, 1998

108. Hampton E: The relationship between pelvic floor and abdominal musculature: Clinical recommendations for rehabilitation based on emerging literature. J Section Womens Health 27:22–25, 2003

109. Hanson C: Proprioceptive neuromuscular facilitation. In: Hall CM, Brody TL, eds: Therapeutic Exercise: Moving Toward Function. Lippincott Williams & Wilkins, 1998:233–251

110. Hardin JA: Medical exercise training. In: Bandy WD, Sanders B, eds: Therapeutic Exercise: Techniques for Intervention. Philadelphia, Lippincott Williams & Wilkins, 2001:121–178

111. Harris JD, Holmes JD: Rib cage and thoracic spine. Phys Med Rehabil Clin North Am 7:761–771, 1996

112. Hartman L: Classification and application of osteopathic manipulative techniques. In: Glasgow EF, Twomey LT, Scull ER, et al, eds: Aspects of Manipulative Therapy, 2nd ed. Edinburgh, Churchill Livingstone, 1985

113. Haynes W: Rolling exercises designed to train the deep spinal muscles. J Bodywork Movement Ther 7:153–164, 2003

114. Helgeson K, Gojdosik RL: The stretch-shortening cycle of the quadriceps femoris muscle group measured by isokinetic dynamometry. J Orthop Sports Phys Ther 17:17–23, 1993

115. Hislop HJ, Montgomery J: Daniel's and Worthingham's Muscle Testing, Techniques of Manual Examination, 6th ed. Philadelphia, WB Saunders, 1995

116. Hohmann G: Orthopadische Technik Bandagen and Apparate. Stuttgart, Ihre Anzeige und ihr Bau, 1968

117. Holten O: Medisinski Treningsterapi. Oslo, Holten Institutt, 1967

118. Holten O: Medical training therapy. Fysiterapueten 11:9–14, 1976

119. Holten O, Torstensen TA: Medical exercise therapy: The basic principles. Fysiterapueten 58:27–32, 1991

120. Howes RG, Isdale IC: The loose back: An unrecognized syndrome. Rheumatol Phys Med 11:72–77, 1971

121. Hyman J, Liebenson C: Spinal stabilization exercise program. In: Liebenson C, ed: Rehabilitation of the Spine. Philadelphia, Lippincott Williams & Wilkins, 1996:293–314

122. Irion JM: Use of the gym ball in rehabilitation of spinal dysfunction. Orthop Phy Ther Clin North Am 1:375–398, 1992

123. Janda V: Muscles, central nervous motor regulation and back problems. In: Korr IM, ed: The Neurobiologic Mechanisms in Manipulative Therapy. New York, Plenum Press, 1978

124. Janda V: Muscle Function Testing. London, Butterworth, 1983

125. Janda V: Muscles and motor control in cervicogenic disorders: Assessment and management. In: Grant R, ed: Physical Therapy of the Cervical and Thoracic Spine, 2nd ed. New York, Churchill Livingstone. 1994:195–216

126. Janda V, Va Vorva M: Sensory motor stimulation. In: Liebenson C, ed: Rehabilitation of the Spine. Philadelphia, Lippincott Williams & Wilkins, 1996

127. Jemmett R: Spinal Stabilization: The New Science of Back Pain. Minneapolis, MN, Orthopedic Physical Therapy Products, 2001

128. Jenks B: Your Body: Biofeedback at Its Best. Chicago, Nelson Hall, 1977

129. Jensen G: Musculoskeletal analysis: Thoracic spine. In: Scully RM, Barnes MR, eds: Physical Therapy. Philadelphia, JB Lippincott, 1989:429–437

130. Johnson GS, Saliba VL: Functional Orthopedics I, Course Outline. San Anselmo, CA: Institute of Physical Arts, 1984

131. Jones FP: The Alexander Technique: Body Awareness in Action. New York, Schocken Books, 1976

132. Jones R: Current concepts of pelvic floor muscle rehabilitation. Orthopedic Division Review of the Canadian Physiotherapy Association. January/February 2002

133. Judge RD, Zuidema GD, Fitzgerald FT: Clinical Diagnosis: A Physiologic Approach. Boston, Little Brown & Co, 1982

134. Juhan D: The Trager approach: Psychophysical integration and Mentastics. In: Drury N, ed: The Body Book. Burbank, CA, Prism Alpha, 1984

135. Juhan D: The Trager approach: The feeling that is healing. Positive Health (March) 26:55–60, 1998

136. Jull GA: Management of cervicogenic headaches. In: Grant R, ed: Physical Therapy of the Cervical and Thoracic Spine, 3rd ed. St. Louis MO, Churchill Livingstone, 2002:239–266

137. Jull GA, Janda V: Muscles and motor control in low back pain: Assessment and management. In: Twoney LT, Taylor JR, eds: Physical Therapy of the Low Back. New York, Churchill Livingstone, 1987:253–278

138. Jull GA, Richardson CA: Rehabilitation of the active stabilization of the lumbar spine. In: Twoney LT, Taylor JR, eds: Physical Therapy of the Low Back, 2nd ed. Churchill Livingstone, New York, 1994:251–273

139. Kaltenborn F: The Spine: Basic Evaluation and Mobilization Techniques. Oslo, Olaf Norlis Bokhandel, 1993

140. Kapandji IA: The Physiology of Joints: The Trunk and Vertebral Column, vol. 3. Edinburgh, Churchill Livingstone, 1974

141. Keely G: Posture, body mechanics, and spinal stabilization. In: Brandy WD, Sanders B, eds: Therapeutic Exercise: Techniques for Intervention. Philadelphia, Lippincott Williams & Wilkins, 2001:263–294

142. Keim HA: Scoliosis. Clin Symp 24:1–30, 1978

143. Kendall FP, McCreary EK, Provance PG: Muscles: Testing and Function, 4th ed. Baltimore, Williams & Wilkins, 1993

144. Kenna C, Murtagh J: Back Pain and Spinal Manipulation: A Practical Guide. Boston, Butterworths, 1989

145. Kenneally M, Rubenach H, Elvey R: The upper limb tension test: The SLR test of the arm. In: Grant R, ed: Physical Therapy of the Cervical and Thoracic Spine. Edinburgh, Churchill Livingstone, 1988

146. Kennedy B: A muscle bracing technique utilizing intra-abdominal pressure to stabilize the lumbar spine. Aust J Physiother 11:102–106, 1965

147. Kennedy B: An Australian programme for management of back problems. Physiotherapy 66:108–111, 1980

148. Kennedy CN: The cervical spine. In: Hall CM, Brody LT, eds: Therapeutic Exercise: Moving Toward Function. Philadelphia, Lippincott Williams & Wilkins, 1999:525–548

149. Kennelly KP, Stokes MJ: Pattern of asymmetry of paraspinal muscle size in adolescent idiopathic scoliosis examined by real-time ultrasound imaging: A preliminary study. Spine 18:913–917, 1993

150. Kibler WB, Herring: Functional Rehabilitation of Sports and Musculoskeletal Injuries. Gaithersburg, MD., 1998

151. Kisner C, Colby LA: Chest therapy. In: Kisner C, Colby LA: Therapeutic Exercise: Foundations and Techniques, 2nd ed. Philadelphia, FA Davis, 1990a:577–616

152. Kisner C, Colby LA: Scoliosis. In: Kisner C, Colby LA: Therapeutic Exercise: Foundations and Techniques, 2nd ed. Philadelphia, FA Davis, 1990b:519–543

153. Kisner C, Colby LA: Therapeutic Exercise: Foundations and Techniques, 2nd ed. Philadelphia, FA Davis, 1990c
154. Klapp B: Das Klappishe Kreichverfahren. Stuttgart, B Thieme, 1955
155. Klein-Vogelbach S: Functional Kinetics: Observing, Analyzing and Teaching Human Movement. Berlin, Springer-Verlag, 1990
156. Klein-Vogelbach S: Therapeutic Exercises in Functional Kinetics: Analysis and Instruction of Individually Adaptable Exercises. Berlin, Springer-Verlag, 1991
157. Knott M, Voss DE: Proprioceptive Neuromuscular Facilitation: Patterns and Techniques, 2nd ed. New York, Harper & Row, 1968
158. Kramer J: Intervertebral Disk Disease: Causes, Diagnosis, Treatment and Prophylaxis. Chicago, Year Book, 1981
159. Kroll F, Reiss E: Der Thoracle Bandscheibeprolaps. Dtsch Med Wschr 76:600–603, 1951
160. Laslett M: The role of physical therapy in soft-tissue rheumatism. Patient Manage 15:57–68, 1986
161. Lee D: Biomechanics of thorax: a clinical model of in vivo function. J Man Manipulative Ther 1:13–24, 1993
162. Lee D: Manual Therapy for the Thorax: A Biomechanical Approach. Delta, BC, Canada, DOPC, 1994
163. Lee D: Rotational instability of the mid-thoracic spine: assessment and management. Man Ther 1:234–238, 1996
164. Lee D: Biomechanics of the thorax. In: Grant R, ed: Physical Therapy of the Cervical Spine and Thoracic Spine, 3rd ed. New York, Churchill Livingstone, 2002:45–60
165. Lee D: The Thoracic: An Integrated Approach, 2nd ed. White Rock, BC, Canada, Lee Physiotherapist Corp, 2003
166. Lee D, Walsh M: A Workbook of Manual Therapy Techniques for the Vertebral Column and Pelvic Girdle. Delta, BC, Canada, Nascent Publishers, 1985
167. Lefever-Button S: Closed kinetic chain training. In: Hall CM, Brody LT, eds: Therapeutic Exercise: Moving Toward Function. Philadelphia, Lippincott Williams & Wilkins, 1999
168. Lewit K: Manipulative Therapy in Rehabilitation of the Motor System, 2nd ed. Boston, Butterworths, 1991
169. Loebl WY: Measurement of spinal posture and range of spinal movement. Ann Phys Med 9:103–110, 1967
170. Love JG, Schorn VG: Thoracic-disk protrusions. JAMA 191:627–631, 1965
171. Low J: The modern body therapies, part 4: Aston patterning. Massage Magazine 1988
172. Lowcock J: Thoracic Joint Stability and Clinical Stress Tests. Proceedings of the Canadian Orthopedic Manipulative Physiotherapists, Orthopaedic Division of the Canadian Physiotherapy Association Newsletter, November/December 1991:15–19
173. MacDonald G, MacDonald G: The Complete Illustrated Guide to the Alexander Technique: A Practical Guide for Health, Poise and Fitness. Rockport, MA, Element Books, 1998
174. Magee DJ: Orthopedic Physical Assessment, 2nd ed. Philadelphia, WB Saunders, 1992
175. Maigne R: Orthopaedic Medicine. Springfield, IL, Charles C. Thomas, 1972a
176. Maigne R: Semeiologie clinique des derangements intervertebraux mineurs. Ann Med Phys 15:275–292, 1972b
177. Maigne R: Manipulation of the spine. In: Basmajian JV, ed: Manipulation, Traction and Massage. Baltimore, Williams & Wilkins, 1986
178. Maigne R, Le Corre F: Sur l'origine cervicale de certaines dorsalgies rebelles et benignes. Ann Med Phys 1:1–18, 1964
179. Maitland GD: Vertebral Manipulation, 5th ed. London, Butterworths, 1986
180. Matson DD, Wood RP, Campbell JB, et al: Diastematomyelia (congenital clefts of the spinal cord). Pediatrics 6:98–112, 1950
181. May P: Thoracic spine. In: Payton OD, Difabio RP, Paris SV, et al, eds: Manual of Physical Therapy. New York, Churchill Livingstone, 1989
182. McCarthy RE: Coping with low back pain through behavioral change. Orthop Nurs 3:30–35, 1983
183. McConnell J: McConnell patellofemoral treatment plan. Course notes, McConnell Seminars, 1990
184. McGuckin N: The T4 syndrome. In: Grieve GP, ed: Modern Manual Therapy of the Vertebral Column. Edinburgh, Churchill Livingstone, 1986:370–376
185. McKenzie RA: The Lumbar Spine: Mechanical Diagnosis and Therapy. Waikanae, New Zealand, Spinal Publications Ltd, 1981
186. McKenzie RA: Care of the Neck. Waikanae, New Zealand, Spinal Publications Ltd, 1983
187. McKenzie RA: The Cervical and Thoracic Spine: Mechanical Diagnosis and Therapy. Waikanae, New Zealand, Spinal Publications Ltd, 1990
188. McManus CA: Group Wellness Programs for Chronic Pain and Disease Management. St. Louis, Butterworth Heinemann, 2003
189. McNair JFS, Maitland GD: Manipulative therapy techniques in the management of some thoracic syndromes. In: Grant R, ed: Physical Therapy of the Cervical and Thoracic Spine. New York, Churchill Livingstone, 1988
190. Meisser L: Proprioceptive neuromuscular facilitation. PNF complex motions. In: Kuprian W, ed: Physical Therapy in Sports, 2nd ed. Philadelphia, WB Saunders, 1995:99–120
191. Melzack R: The McGill pain questionnaire: Major properties and scoring methods. Pain 1:277–299, 1975
192. Melzack R, Wall PD: Pain mechanisms: A new theory. Science 150:971–979, 1965
193. Mennell JM: Back Pain. Boston, Little Brown & Co, 1960
194. Miller B: Alternative somatic therapies. In: White A, Anderson R, eds: Conservative Care of Low Back Pain. Baltimore, Williams & Wilkins, 1991:120–136
195. Miller B: Manual therapy treatment of myofascial pain and dysfunction. In: Rachlin ES, ed: Myofascial Pain and Fibromyalgia. St. Louis, CV Mosby, 1994:415–454
196. Miller MI, Mederios JM: Recruitment of internal oblique and transversus abdominis muscles during the eccentric phase of the curl-up exercise. Phys Ther 67:1213–1217, 1987
197. Mitchell FL, Moran PS, Pruzzo NA: An Evaluation and Treatment Manual of Osteopathic Muscle Energy Procedures. Valley Park, MO, Mitchell, Moran, Pruzzo Associates, 1979
198. Moll JMH, Wright V: Measurement of spinal movement. In: Jayson M, ed: The Lumbar Spine and Back Pain. New York, Grune & Stratton, 1981:93–112
199. Montgomery F, Willner S: Screening for idiopathic scoliosis. Acta Orthop Scand 64:456–458, 1993
200. Mooney V, Robertson J: The facet syndrome. Clin Orthop 115:149–156, 1976
201. Morgan D: Concepts in functional training and postural stabilization for the low-back injured. Top Acute Care Trauma Rehabil 2:8–12, 1988
202. Mulligan BR: Manual Therapy: "Nags," "Snags," "Pops," etc. Wellington, New Zealand, Plane View Services Ltd, 1989
203. Murphy JE: Sensorimotor training and cervical stabilization. In: Murphy JE: Management of Cervical Spine Syndromes. New York, McGraw-Hill, 2000:607–640
204. Murtagh J, Findlay D, Kenna C: Low back pain. Aust Fam Physician 14:1214–1224, 1985
205. Murtagh JE, Kenna CJ: Back Pain and Spinal Manipulation, 2nd ed. Oxford, Butterworth Heinemann, 1997
206. Nathan H, Weinberg H, Robin GC, et al: Costovertebral joints: Anatomico-clinical observation in arthritis. Arthritis Rheum 7:228–240, 1964
207. Neuman P, Gill V: Pelvic floor and abdominal interaction: EMG activity and intra-abdominal pressure. Int Urogynecol J Pelvic Floor Dysfunct 13:125–132, 2002
208. Nickenig T: Stabilizing the Core. Adv Directors Rehabil 11:39–42, 2002
209. Norris CM: Spinal stabilization. Muscle imbalance and the low back. Physiotherapy 3:127–138, 1995a
210. Norris CM: Spinal stabilization. An exercise programe to ehance lumbar stabilization. Physiotherapy 3:138–146, 1995b
211. Nwuga VC: Manipulation of the Spine. Baltimore, Williams & Wilkins, 1976
212. Oliver MJ, Lynn JW, Lynn JM: An interpretation of the McKenzie approach to low back pain. In: Twomey LT, Taylor JR, eds: Physical Therapy of the Low Back. New York, Churchill Livingstone, 1987:250–251
213. Ombergt L, Bisschop P, ter Veer HJ, et al: Disorders of the thoracic cage and abdomen. In: Ombert I, Bisschop T, terVeer HJ, et al, eds: A System of Orthopaedic Medicine, London, WB Saunders, 1995:470–480
214. O'Sullivan SB: Multiple sclerosis. In: O'Sullivan SB, Schmitz, eds: Physical Rehabilitation: Assessment and Treatment. Philadelphia, FA Davis, 1988
215. O'Sullivan DB, Schmitz TJ: Physical Rehabilitation Laboratory Manual: Focus on Functional Training. Philadelphia, FA Davis, 1999
216. Palmer ML, Epler ME: Fundamentals of Musculoskeletal Assessment Techniques, 2nd ed. Philadelphia, Lippincott Williams & Wilkins, 1998
217. Pappas AM, Zaacki RM, McCarthy CF: Rehabilitation of the pitching shoulder. Am J Sports Med 13: 223–235, 1985
218. Paris SV: The Spinal Lesion. New Zealand, Degasus Press, 1965
219. Paris SV: Physical signs of instability. Spine 10:277–279, 1985
220. Pavelka K von: Rotationsmessung der wirbelsaule. A Rheumaforschg 29:366, 1970
221. Peacock E, Van Winkle: Wound Repair. Philadelphia, WB Saunders, 1976
222. Petty NJ, Moore AP: Neuromusculoskeletal Examination and Assessment. A Handbook for Therapists. Edinburgh, Churchill Livingstone, 1998
223. Pickering SG: Exercises for the Autonomic Nervous System. Springfield, IL, Charles C. Thomas, 1981
224. Polden M: Physiotherapy in Obstetrics and Gynecology. Stoneham, MA, Butterworth-Heinemann Publishers, 1990
225. Porterfield JA, DeRosa C: Mechanical Neck Pain: Perspective in Functional Anatomy. Philadelphia, WB Saunders, 1995
226. Prentice WE: Open-versus closed-kinetic chain exercises in rehabilitation. In: Prentice WE, Voight ML, eds: Techniques in Musculoskeletal Rehabilitation. New York, McGraw-Hill, 2001:179–196
227. Pulling Schatz M: Back Care Basics: A Doctor's Gentle Yoga Program for Back and Neck Pain Relief. Berkeley, CA, Rodmell Press, 1992
228. Rasmussen TB, Kernohan JW, Adson AW: Pathologic classification with surgical consideration of intraspinal tumors. Ann Surg 111:513–530, 1940
229. Rath WW, Rath JND, Duffy CG: A Comparison of Pain Location and Duration with Treatment Outcome and Frequency. Presented at the International McKenzie Conference, Newport Beach, CA, 1989
230. Richardson CA: Muscle imbalance: Principles of treatment and assessment. Proceedings of the New Zealand Society of Physiotherapists Challenges Conference, Christchurch, New Zealand, 1992

231. Richardson C, Jull G, Hodges P, et al: Therapeutic Exercise for Spinal Segmental Stabilization in Low Back Pain: Scientific Basis and Clinical Approach. Edinburgh, Churchill Livingstone, 1999
232. Richardson CA, Snidjers CJ, Hides JA et al: The relation between the transverse abdominis muscle and sacroiliac joint mechanics and low back pain. Spine 27:399–405, 2002
233. Richardson C, Toppengerg R, Jull G: An initial evaluation of eight abdominal exercises for their ability to provide stabilization for the lumbar spine. Aust J Physiother 38:105–112, 1992
234. Richardson N: Aston patterning. Phys Ther Forum 6:1–3, 1987
235. Ritzy S, Loren T, Simpson S, et al: Rehabilitation of degenerative disease of the spine. In: Hochschuler SH, Colter HV, Guyer RD, eds: Rehabilitation of the Spine: Science and Practice. St. Louis, CV Mosby, 1993:457–481
236. Robinson L, Fisher H, Knox J, et al: The Official Body Control Pilates Manual, 2nd ed. New York, Barnes & Noble Books, 2001
237. Robinson R: The new back school prescription: Stabilization. Occup Med 7:17–31, 1992
238. Rocabado M: Advanced Upper Quarter. Continuing Education Course. San Francisco, Rocabado Institute, 1984
239. Rosse C: Segmental innervation. In: Rosse C, Clawson DK, eds: The Musculoskeletal System in Health and Disease. Philadelphia, Harper & Row, 1980:169–177
240. Ruggerone M, Austin JHM: Moire topography in scoliosis: Correlations with vertebral lateral curvature as determined by radiography. Phys Ther 66:1072–1076, 1986
241. Rusnak-Smith S, Moffit M: The thoracic spine. In: Hall CM, Brody LT, eds: Therapeutic Exercise. Moving Toward Function. Philadelphia, Lippincott Wiliams & Wilkins 1998:549–574
242. Rywerant Y: The Feldenkrais Method: Teaching by Handling. San Francisco, Harper & Row, 1983
243. Saal JA: Rehabilitation of sports-related lumbar injuries. Phys Med Rehabil 4:613–638, 1987
244. Saal JA: Nonoperative treatment of herniated disc. An outcome study. Spine 14:431–437, 1989
245. Saal JA: The new back prescription: Stabilization training. Part II. Occup Med 7:33–42, 1992
246. Sahrmann S: A program for correction of muscular imbalances and mechanical imbalances. Clin Manage 3:23–28, 1983
247. Sahrmann S: Adult posturing. In: Kraus S, ed: TMJ Disorders: Management of the Craniomandibular Complex. New York, Churchill Livingstone, 1988
248. Sahrmann S: Diagnosis and treatment of muscle imbalances and associated regional pain syndromes: Course notes. Seattle, Team Physical Therapy, 1993
249. Sahrmann S: Diagnosis and Treatment of Movement Impairment. St. Louis, Mosby, 2002
250. Sahrmann S, Hall CM: Diagnosis and Treatment of Muscle Imbalances and Musculoskeletal Pain Syndromes. Continuing Education Course. Seattle, Washington State Physical Therapy Association, 1995
251. Saibil FB, Edmeades J: Chest pain arising from extrathoracic structures. In: Levene DL, ed: Chest Pain: An Integrated Diagnostic Approach. Philadelphia, Lea & Febiger, 1977:130
252. Saliba VL, Johnson GS: Back education and training: Course outline. San Anselmo, CA: The Institute of Physical Arts, 1988
253. Saliba VL, Johnson GS: Lumbar protective mechanism. In: White AH, Anderson R, eds: Conservative Care of Low Back Pain. Baltimore, Williams & Wilkins, 1991
254. Sapsford RR, Hodges PW: Contraction of the pelvic floor muscles during abdominal maneuvers. Arch Phys Med Rehabil 82:1081–1088, 2001
255. Saunders HD: Evaluation, Treatment and Prevention of Musculoskeletal Disorders. Minneapolis, Viking, 1985
256. Schamberger W: The Malalignment Syndrome. Implications for Medicine and Sport. Edinburgh, Churchill Livingstone, 2002
257. Schunk C, Reed K, eds: Therapeutic Associates Rehabilitation Guidelines: Student Volume. Beverton, OR, Tai Publishing, 1995
258. Schussler B, Laycock J, Nortin P, et al, eds: Pelvic Floor Re-education Principles and Practice. New York, Spinger-Verlag, 1994
259. Shelly B: The pelvic floor. In: Hall CM, Brody LT, eds: Therapeutic Exercise: Moving Toward Function. Philadelphia, Lippincott Williams & Wilkins, 1998:353–386
260. Sherrington C: The Integrated Action of the Nervous System, 2nd ed. New Haven, Yale University Press, 1947
261. Sinaki M, Kenneth P, Offord MS: Physical activity in postmenopausal women: Effect on back muscle strength and bone mineral density of the spine. Arch Phys Med Rehabil 69:277–280, 1988
262. Sinaki M, Mikkelsen BA: Postmenopausal spinal osteoporosis: Flexion versus extension exercises. Arch Phys Med Rehabil 65:593–596, 1984
263. Slater H: Adverse neural tension in the sympathetic trunk and sympathetically maintained pain syndromes. Proceedings of the Seventh Biennial Conference of the Manipulative Physiotherapy Association of Australia, Sydney, 1991
264. Stallworth JM, Horne JB: Diagnosis and management of thoracic outlet syndrome. Arch Surg 119:1149–1151, 1984
265. Stalvey MH: Proprioceptive neuromuscular facilitation. In: Bandy WD, Sanders B, eds: Therapeutic Exercise: Techniques for Intervention. Philadelphia, Lippincott Williams & Wilkins, 2001:145–178
266. Stoddard A: Manual of Osteopathic Practice. London, Hutchinson, 1969
267. Stoddard A: Manual of Osteopathic Technique, 8th ed. London, Hutchinson, 1974
268. Stoddard A: The Back—Relief from Pain. London, Dunitz, 1979
269. Sullivan PE, Markos PD, Minor MA: Clinical Decision Making in Therapeutic Exercise. Norwalk, CT, Appleton & Lange, 1994
270. Sydenham RW: Manual therapy techniques for the thoracolumbar spine. In: Donatelli R, Wooden MJ, eds: Orthopedic Physical Therapy. Edinburgh, Churchill Livingstone, 1989:359–401
271. Tencer AF, Allen BL, Ferguson RL: A biomechanical study of thoracic spine fractures with bone in the canal. Part III. Spine 10:741–747, 1985
272. Torstensen TA: The physical therapy approach. In: JW Frymoyer JW, Ducker TB, Hadler NM, et al, eds: The Adult Spine. Philadelphia, Lippincott-Raven 1997:1797–1805
273. Torstensen TA, Ljunggren AE, Meen HD, et al: Efficiency and costs of medical exercise therapy, conventional physiotherapy and self-exercise in patients with chronic low back pain. Spine 23:2616–2624, 1998
274. Trager M: Psychophysical integration and Mentastics. J Holistic Health 7:15–25, 1982
275. Trager M, Guadagno C: Trager Mentastics: Movement as a Way to Agelessness. Barry, NY, Stanton Hill Press, 1987
276. Veldhuizen AG, Sholten PJM: Kinematics of the scoliotic spine as related to the normal spine. Spine 12:852–858, 1987
277. Voight ML: Stretch strengthening: An introduction to plyometrics. Orthop Phys Ther Clin North Am, 1:243–252, 1992
278. Voight ML, Cook G: Clinical applications of closed kinetic chain exercise. J Sport Rehabil 5:25–44, 1996
279. Voight ML, Cook G: Impaired neuromuscular control. Reactive neuromuscular training. In: Prentice W, Voight MI, eds: Techniques in Musculoskeletal Rehabilitation. New York, McGraw-Hill, 2001:93–124
280. Voight ML, Dravitch P: Plyometrics. In: Prentice W, Voight MI, eds: Techniques in Musculoskeletal Rehabilitation. New York, McGraw-Hill, 2001:167–178
281. Voss DE, Ionta MK, Myers BJ: Proprioceptive Neuromuscular Facilitation Patterns and Techniques, 3rd ed. Philadelphia, Harper & Row, 1985
282. Wadsworth CT: Manual Examination and Treatment of the Spine and Extremities. Baltimore, Williams & Wilkins, 1988
283. Wallace K: Female pelvic floor functions, dysfunctions and behavioral approaches to health. Athl Woman 13:459–481, 1994
284. Waltrous I: The Trager approach: An effective tool for physical therapy. Phys Ther Forum 72:22–25, 1992
285. Warwick R, Williams PL, eds: Gray's Anatomy, 35th British ed. Philadelphia, WB Saunders, 1973
286. Weiss HR: The effect of an exercise program on vital capacity and rib mobility in patients with idiopathic scoliosis. Spine 16:88–93, 1991
287. Weiss HR: Influence of an inpatient exercise program on scoliotic curve. Ital J Orthop Trauma 18:395–406, 1993
288. White A: Back school: State of the art. In: Weistein JN, Wiesel SW, eds: The Lumbar Spine. The International Society for the Study of the Lumbar Spine. Philadelphia, WB Saunders, 1990
289. Wilbourn AJ: The thoracic outlet syndrome is overdiagnosed. Arch Neurol 47:328–330, 1990
290. Wilk KE, Reinold MM: Closed-kinetic-chain exercise and plyometric activities. In: Bandy WD, Sanders B, eds: Therapeutic Exercise: Techniques for Intervention. Baltimore, Lippincott Williams & Wilkins, 2001:179–212
291. Wilk KE, Voight ML, Kerins MA, et al: Stretch-shortening drills for the upper extremity; Theory and clinical application. J Orthop Sports Phys Ther 17:225–239, 1993
292. Witt PL: Trager psychophysical integration: An additional tool in treatment of chronic spinal pain and dysfunction. Whirlpool 9:24–26, 1986
293. Witt PL, MacKinnon J: Trager psychophysical integration: A method to improve chest mobility of patients with chronic lung disease. Phys Ther 66:214–217, 1986
294. Witt PL, Parr C: Effectiveness of Trager psychophysical integration in promoting trunk mobility in a child with cerebral palsy: A case report. Phys Occup Ther Pediatr 8:75–94, 1988
295. Woo S, Matthews JV, Akeson WH, et al: Connective tissue response to immobility: Correlative study of biomechanical and biochemical measurements of normal and immobilized rabbit knees. Arthritis Rheum 18:257–264, 1975
296. Zuniga L: Management of thoracic dysfunction. In: Canavan PK, ed: Rehabilitation in Sports Medicine: A Comprehensive Guide. Stamford, CT, Appleton & Lange, 1998:93–108

Cervicothoracic–Upper Limb Scan Examination

21

DARLENE HERTLING

- COMMON DISORDERS OF CERVICOTHORACIC SPINE, TEMPOROMANDIBULAR JOINT, AND UPPER LIMB
- FORMAT OF CERVICOTHORACIC–UPPER LIMB SCAN EXAMINATION

- SUMMARY OF STEPS TO CERVICOTHORACIC–UPPER LIMB SCAN EXAMINATION

The limbs are derived from spinal segments: the myotomes, dermatomes, and sclerotomes. Those corresponding to C4 through T1 extend into the arms, whereas those from L2 through S2 extend into the legs. The clinical significance of this is that symptoms and signs related to pathologic spinal processes are often referred to the limbs, and, conversely, symptoms from common limb lesions are often referred to the spine (or other parts of the involved limb). In the case of deep somatic lesions, referred symptoms and signs are the rule rather than the exception. This is most significant with respect to pain because pain is the most frequent clinical manifestation of deep somatic disorders. Thus, the patient with a cervical problem is very likely to experience scapular, shoulder, or arm pain, perhaps even more so than cervical pain. In addition, paresthesias, weakness, or sensory changes may affect the related segment in the arm or hand. Similarly, it is not unusual for patients with common extremity disorders to experience pain that is referred in a retrograde direction to the proximal aspect of the limb or the related spinal region. Indeed, patients with carpal tunnel syndrome often experience pain up the forearm and arm into the scapular region and neck.

The clinical problem encountered when dealing with the common phenomenon of referred symptoms is that information elicited from the history does not always reliably narrow the source of the problem to a particular region. When this is the case, the clinician may have trouble knowing in which area to direct the physical, or objective, examination. The situation may be compounded by the fact that many patients present with symptoms that occur as the result of summation of afferent input from two separate disorders affecting tissues innervated by the same segment. This is especially true for middle-aged and older people because degenerative joint changes in the cervical spine are common by middle age and may cause "hyperexcitability" of the involved segments.

The purpose of performing a spinal–limb scan examination is to help identify the major area of involvement so that the physical examination can be directed accordingly. It is most useful in cases in which the history or the referring diagnosis does not provide adequate information to indicate the area to be examined. It should be used with most middle-aged

or older patients presenting with chronic musculoskeletal complaints because it will often reveal disorders, other than those identified by the referral or by the history, that are the primary cause. For example, a scan examination often reveals that the patient who describes symptoms suggestive of a C6 radiculopathy actually has carpal tunnel syndrome, that the patient with carpal tunnel syndrome may have symptoms that are enhanced by lower cervical facet joint tightness, that a person with some lower cervical problem is also developing a frozen shoulder, or that someone who describes what sounds like pain referred distally into the C7 segment from the neck actually has pain referred proximally from a tennis elbow condition. Such situations are surprisingly common and can be a frequent source of error in evaluation and treatment planning unless recognized.

The tests that make up the scan examination include those that can be considered *key tests* for the common musculoskeletal lesions affecting the cervical spine and upper limb, or the lumbar spine and lower limb. The basic sequence of testing is geared to patient convenience, to prevent unnecessary movement of the patient. The examiner will also decide the order of testing based on the history and observation. Testing of the vertebral artery and transverse and alar ligaments should be considered if the observation and subjective examination reveal any of the signs and symptoms that have been linked, directly or indirectly, to vertebral artery insufficiency or ligamentous laxity. Listed below are the key tests and positive findings for some the common disorders for which the scan examination is intended to be sensitive.

COMMON DISORDERS OF CERVICOTHORACIC SPINE, TEMPOROMANDIBULAR JOINT, AND UPPER LIMB

I. Temporomandibular Joint
   A. Dysfunction syndrome
      1. Typical subjective complaints include the following:
         a. Often associated with an insidious onset of emotional stress or overload such as bruxism, for a long period of time

b. The presenting complaint is usually pain, which is either in the jaw or ear but which often radiates widely into the face, temporal region, or around the neck. Jaw pain or difficulty in chewing, or worse, after meals and at end of day.

c. Early incoordination associated with clicking, popping, subluxation, and recurrent dislocation. Often reversible but may lead to limitation phase.

d. The patient is often a woman, usually of 20 to 40 years.

2. Key objective findings (incoordination phase): Active motions

a. Excessive joint mobility often characterized by excessive anterior translation during opening. Patient may be able insert three knuckles between the incisors.

b. Clicking, popping, or cracking with mandibular depression or elevation

c. Abnormality of movement: mandibular deviations (protrusively as well as laterally)

d. Tenderness and thickening around the joint with the mouth both closed and open

B. Internal derangement such as a disk or degenerative joint disease

1. Typical subjective complaints include the following:

a. May occur at any age, usually middle or old age, associated with the aging process and repeated minor trauma

b. Pain is present at rest or during movements such as chewing or yawning and is often described as a deep-seated, dull aching type of pain felt in the preauricular region. There may be facial pain that is obscure in character and location.

c. Morning stiffness that subsides with jaw use

d. Jaw pain that is associated with clicking or crepitus

2. Key objective findings

a. Limitation in a capsular pattern of restriction; in unilateral conditions, contralateral excursions and opening are the most restricted.

b. Accessory movements are limited and reproduce temporomandibular joint pain.

II. Cervical Spine

A. Localized cervical facet joint restriction

1. Typical subjective complaints include the following:

a. Aching in the scapular region, perhaps into the arm, usually unilaterally; occasional headaches

b. Gradual onset with perhaps a history of cervical trauma or intermittent acute episodes of neck pain

c. Worse at the end of the day and during periods of prolonged muscular tension such as during emotional stress and long periods of holding the head against gravity (e.g., typing or reading)

d. Patient age is usually 25 to 50 years.

2. Key objective findings

a. Active cervical movements with passive overpressure

i. Pain at the extremes of sidebending and rotation to the involved side

ii. Possible pain on extension

b. Quadrant test (passive rotation, sidebending, and extension to one side). Pain when performed toward the side of involvement.

B. Generalized cervical degenerative changes—Bilateral, multisegmental facet joint capsular tightness

1. Typical subjective complaints include the following:

a. Gradual onset of neck stiffness with associated pain into shoulder girdles and perhaps the arms. Pain and stiffness may be bilateral, although they are usually worse on one side. Frequent headaches (cervicogenic headaches) originate from the occiput and radiate to the frontal region.

b. History of intermittent cervical problems over many years

c. Stiffness and headaches noted in the morning, easing somewhat during midday, with increased neck and shoulder pain by evening

d. The patient is usually 50 years old or older.

2. Key objective findings: Active cervical movements with passive overpressure

a. Marked restriction of extension, moderate restriction of sidebending, mild to moderate restriction of rotations and flexion

b. Pain at the extremes of some movements

C. Cervical nerve root impingements (see Chapter 19, Cervical Spine)

1. Typical subjective complaints include the following:

a. Gradual or sudden onset of unilateral neck, scapular, or arm pain. Often paresthesias into fingers are described. Arm pain may be sharp or aching.

b. Pain may be intense, relieved somewhat with recumbency, and worse with weight bearing.

c. The patient is usually 35 to 60 years old.

2. Key objective findings

a. Quadrant test (foraminal compression); reproduction of *arm* pain

b. Upper limb sensory (see Figs. 5-4 to 5-6), motor (see Fig. 5-9), and reflex tests. Neurologic deficit is confined to the involved segment.

• C5—Weak shoulder abduction or lateral rotation
  • Sensory changes over the radial aspect of the forearm
  • Diminished biceps or brachioradialis jerk
• C6—Weak elbow flexion or wrist extension
  • Sensory changes over the thumb or index finger
  • Diminished biceps or brachioradialis jerk
• C7—Weak elbow pronation, extension, or wrist flexion
  • Sensory changes over the index, middle, and ring fingers
  • Diminished triceps jerk
• C8—Weak thumb abduction, small finger abduction, or wrist ulnar deviation
  • Sensory changes over the little or ring fingers

- T1—Weak adduction of the extended fingers (interossei muscles)
  - Sensory changes over the inner side of the forearm

III. Thoracic Spine
A. Thoracic outlet syndrome
1. Typical subjective complaints include the following:
   a. Defuse arm and shoulder pain, especially when the arm is elevated beyond 90°.
   b. Potential symptoms include pain localized in the neck, face, head, upper limb, chest, shoulder, or axilla; and upper limb paresthesias, numbness, weakness, heaviness, fatigability, swelling, discoloration, ulceration, or Raynaud's phenomenon.[3]
   c. Middle-aged women are more commonly affected, with the typical clinical picture consisting of a rounded-shoulder posture displaying a dowager's hump between C7 and T1.[2]
2. Key objective tests
   a. Thoracic kyphosis is usually stiff, showing tight pectoral tissues and limited shoulder movements. The scapulae are descended.
   b. Reduced movement in the upper and midthoracic regions (dowager's hump).
   c. Tenderness to palpation of upper and midthoracic segments and costal joints. Thoracic segments and rib angles are often exquisitely tender.
   d. The following tests may be positive: overhead test, nerve tension tests, Allen test, elevation test, cervical rotation lateral flexion test, and the Adson's maneuver (see Box 11-2).
B. Thoracic Hypomobility Syndromes
1. Typical subjective complaints include the following:
   a. Dull, aching, occasionally sharp pain; severity related to activity, site, and posture.
   b. Site and radiation: Spinal and paraspinal, e.g., interscapular, arms, lateral chest, anterior chest, substernal, iliac crests
   c. Aggravation: Deep inspiration, postural movement of the thorax, slumping or bending, walking upstairs, and activities—sleeping or sitting for long periods of time, lifting, making a bed, bed too hard or too soft
   d. Associations: Chronic poor posture
2. Key objective findings
   a. Decreased thoracolumbar mobility
   b. Limited spinal extension with associated hip flexion contracture or excessive lumbar lordosis with increased thoracic kyphosis
   c. Hypomobility of the rib cage resulting from lack of mobility and postural and muscle imbalances. In the stiff thorax the ribs are less flexible than the spinal column.[1]
   d. Forward head posture and increased thoracic kyphosis
   e. Altered breathing pattern, usually avoiding diaphragmatic breathing (diaphragm is restricted)
   f. Chest expansion is limited.

IV. Shoulder
A. Frozen shoulder (adhesive capsulitis)
1. Typical subjective complaints include the following:
   a. Gradual onset of shoulder pain and stiffness, noted especially when combing hair, fastening buttons, bras, and such, behind the back, or reaching into the hip pocket.
   b. Frequently there are problems with being awakened at night when rolling onto the painful side.
   c. The patient is more often a woman, usually 40 years old or older.
2. Key objective findings: Active shoulder movements with passive overpressure
   a. Considerable loss of external rotation and abduction, mild to moderate loss of flexion and internal rotation
   b. Pain at the extremes of shoulder movements, especially external rotation and abduction, with a capsular or muscle-spasm end feel
B. Shoulder tendinitis (rotator cuff or biceps)
1. Typical subjective complaints include the following:
   a. Gradual onset of lateral brachial pain, occasionally radiating into arm and forearm.
   b. The onset may be associated with increased use of the arm, such as in athletics.
   c. Painful twinges are felt with specific movements, such as putting on a jacket and reaching behind the back.
   d. The patient is likely to be 20 to 50 years old.
2. Key objective findings: Resisted shoulder, elbow, and forearm movements and pain on contraction of the involved muscle–tendon complex
   a. Supraspinatus: Pain on resisted shoulder abduction
   b. Infraspinatus: Pain on resisted external rotation
   c. Subscapularis: Pain on resisted internal rotation
   d. Biceps (long head): Pain on resisted elbow flexion or forearm supination
C. Shoulder tendon rupture (rotator cuff or biceps)
1. Typical subjective complaints include the following:
   a. Gradual onset of inability to use the arm normally, especially above shoulder level if a rotator cuff tendon is involved. The onset may be sudden, especially in the case of a biceps rupture.
   b. History of intermittent shoulder pain over many years
   c. Possible history of repeated local corticosteroid injections
   d. Pain may or may not be a problem.
   e. The patient is usually 50 years old or older.
2. Key objective findings
   a. Resisted movement tests
      i. Supraspinatus: Resisted abduction is weak and painless
      ii. Infraspinatus: Resisted external rotation is weak and painless.
      iii. Biceps: Resisted elbow flexion and forearm supination are weak and painless.
   b. Observable muscular atrophy

D. Shoulder atraumatic instability
  1. Typical subjective complaints include the following:
    a. Presence of mechanism likely to tear the ligaments or capsule. Typically instability often begins with some minor event or series of events that leads to progressive decompensation of the glenohumeral stability mechanism.
    b. The patient may notice that the shoulder slips out and "clunks" back in with different activities. Patients with multidirectional glenohumeral instabilities may have difficulty sleeping, lifting overhead, and throwing.
    c. Pain may or may not be a problem.
    d. Patients are predominantly younger than 30 years of age.
  2. Key objective findings
    a. Diminished resistance to translation or increased joint-play motions in multiple directions as compared with normal
    b. Duplication of the patient's symptoms with certain motions or position of the arm
E. Acute subdeltoid bursitis
  1. Typical subjective complaints include the following:
    a. Gradual development of relatively intense, constant lateral brachial pain during a 48- to 72-hour period. Pain may radiate down the entire arm.
    b. Often a history of more minor, intermittent shoulder problems suggestive of preexisting tendinitis
    c. Difficulty sleeping or using the arm at all because of intense pain
    d. The patient is likely to be 30 to 50 years old.
  2. Key objective findings: Active shoulder movements with passive overpressure. Marked restriction of active flexion and abduction, with an empty end feel to passive overpressure. Mild to moderate restriction of internal and external rotation with the arm to the side.
V. Elbow
  A. Elbow tendinitis
    1. Typical subjective complaints include the following:
      a. Gradual onset of medial or lateral elbow pain that may radiate into the ulnar aspect of the forearm (medial tennis elbow) or into the dorsum of the forearm and hand and into the posterior brachial region (lateral tennis elbow).
      b. Onset may be associated with some activity such as playing tennis or golf or pruning shrubs.
      c. Pain is aggravated by grasping activities, such as hammering or carrying a suitcase, and by prolonged fine finger activities such as knitting or sewing.
      d. The patient is usually 35 to 60 years old.
    2. Key objective findings
      a. Resisted wrist movements, performed with elbow extended
        i. Lateral tennis elbow (tendinitis at origin of extensor carpi radialis brevis): pain on resisted wrist extension

        ii. Medial tennis elbow (tendinitis at common flexor–pronator origin): pain on resisted wrist flexion
      b. Active wrist movements with passive overpressure, performed with elbow extended
        i. Lateral tennis elbow: pain on full wrist flexion with the elbow extended and forearm pronated
        ii. Medial tennis elbow: pain on full wrist extension with the elbow extended and forearm supinated
V. Wrist and Hand Complex
  A. Carpal tunnel syndrome (pressure on the median nerve in the carpal tunnel)
    1. Typical subjective complaints include the following:
      a. Gradual onset of paresthesias into any or all of the median nerve distribution of hand (thumb and middle three fingers). An aching sensation may be referred up the forearm and arm to the scapula and neck.
      b. Symptoms often awaken the patient at night and are aggravated by activities involving the finger flexors, such as writing, sewing, or knitting.
      c. Women are affected more often than men. The patient is usually 40 years old or older.
    2. Key objective findings: Three-jaw-chuck pinch with wrist held in sustained flexion (modification of Phalen's test). Reproduction of paresthesias into median nerve distribution of the hand (see Fig. 13-31).
  B. De Quervain's disease (tenosynovitis of the abductor pollicis longus and extensor pollicis brevis at the wrist)
    1. Typical subjective complaints include the following:
      a. Gradual onset of pain over the radial aspect of the distal radius that may radiate distally into the thumb or proximally up the radial aspect of the forearm.
      b. Pain is worse with activities involving thumb movements or wrist ulnar deviation.
      c. The patient is usually 40 years old or older.
    2. Key objective findings
      a. Resisted finger movements. Pain occurs over the radial styloid region on resisted thumb extension.
      b. Active wrist movements with passive overpressure. Pain occurs over the radial styloid region on full ulnar deviation with thumb held in patient's clenched fist.
  C. Carpal ligament sprain
    1. Typical subjective complaints include the following:
      a. History of acute trauma, usually a fall on the dorsiflexed or palmarly flexed hand, followed by chronic wrist pain. The patient often has trouble localizing the pain to a particular aspect of the wrist.
      b. Pain is often felt only with specific activities, such as those requiring repeated wrist or weight movements or weight bearing through the hand and wrist.
      c. The patient is usually a young or active person.

2. Key objective findings
   a. Active wrist movements with passive overpressure
      i. Dorsal radiocarpal, dorsal lunocapitate, or capitate–third metacarpal ligament: pain on full wrist flexion
      ii. Palmar radiocarpal or palmar lunocapitate ligament: pain on full wrist extension
   b. Upper limb weight bearing (through dorsiflexed wrist and straight arm). Pain is noted with either dorsal or palmar ligament sprains.

FORMAT OF CERVICOTHORACIC–UPPER LIMB SCAN EXAMINATION

The patient sits at the edge of the plinth with the neck, arm, and shoulder girdles exposed. The examiner briefly inspects the upper spine, shoulder girdles, and arms for obvious muscular atrophy or deformity (see Figs. 19-15 and 19-16).

I. Temporomandibular Joint

This joint is checked by palpation by the patient actively opening and closing the mouth, and by tests of provocation.

A. Active opening and closing of mouth. While the examiner is palpating the temporomandibular joints, the patient is asked to carry out active opening and closing of the mouth to demonstrate the following:
   1. Any localized swelling or tenderness
   2. Abnormal dynamics of the joint or changes in range of motion
   3. Clicking and pain during active motion or on closure

B. Provocation tests. If active movement exhibits a full range of pain-free motion, then provocation tests may be applied to stress the noncontractile structures of the temporomandibular joints by applying loading by forced biting or forced retrusion.

II. Cervicothoracic Tests

Problems in the cervical spine can be ruled out by applying a series of joint-clearing tests.

A. Active cervical movements (see Fig. 19-23). The patient is asked to perform each of the six cervical movements (flexion, extension, right and left lateral flexion, and right and left rotation), or the joints can be passively cleared by spring testing each cervicothoracic segment. If each active movement exhibits a full range of pain-free motion, then some passive overpressure is applied at the extreme of each movement.
   1. Tests for cervicothoracic joint restriction
   2. Overpressure to stress the noncontractile structures

B. Isometrically resisted movements. Isometrically resisted movements at mid range are performed in each direction to stress the contractile units. Test neck flexors, extensors, lateral flexors, and rotator for lesions of the cervical muscles.

C. Quadrant test. Position the patient's head in combined rotation, sidebending, and extension to one side. With the patient's head in this position, a gentle axial compression is applied through the neck by downward pressure to the top of the head.
   1. Tests for localized capsular facet-joint tightness
   2. Tests for interforaminal nerve root impingement

D. Neuromuscular tests
   1. Key sensory areas (C5–C8)—stroking test along dermatomes and sensibility to pin prick (see Fig. 5-5)
   2. Resisted isometric (myotomal) tests (C5–T1). Compare both sides (see Fig. 5-9).
   3. Neural tension tests (brachial tension or upper limb tension tests; see Figs. 11-25 to 11-28)
   4. Reflexes (see Fig. 11-24)
      a. Biceps—C6 (C5)
      b. Wrist extension (brachioradialis)—C5–C6
      c. Triceps—C7

III. Acromioclavicular Joint

A. Inspection and palpation. Inspection may show swelling and elevation of the clavicular end of this joint as a result of sprain. There will be a step deformity in the presence of a third-degree sprain or dislocation. Palpation is performed for normal positioning, tenderness, and crepitation (see Fig. 19-39H).

B. Active and passive movements. Active ranges of depression, elevation, abduction, adduction, protraction, retraction, and circumduction are requested of the patient, followed by passive motion by the examiner through these same ranges. The joint is palpated during active motion for crepitus and abnormal excursions. The patient is instructed to horizontally adduct the arm across the chest. If horizontal flexion exhibits a full range of pain-free motion, then passive overpressure is applied at the end of range to reproduce pain.
   1. Tests for pain. If pain is elicited in any of these movements, the patient should be asked whether it is the same type of pain that brought him or her to the clinician for examination.
   2. Tests for range and symmetry of motion

IV. Sternoclavicular Joint

A. Inspection and palpation. Synovitis is usually evident as a rounded soft tissue swelling localized over the joint. Subluxation of the joint usually occurs in an anterosuperior direction and is best appreciated by looking down onto both joints. With anterior subluxation the clinician should be able to momentarily reduce the subluxation. On palpation there may be tenderness (see Fig. 19-39G).

B. Active and passive movements. The same seven ranges as for the acromioclavicular joint are performed.
   1. Tests for pain
   2. Tests for restriction of motion. The sternoclavicular joint moves with movement of the shoulder girdle, but it is not practical to measure exact range. The examiner should observe range and note symmetry.
   3. Tests for crepitus and abnormal excursions during motion

V. Costosternal Joints and Ribs
   A. Inspection and palpation. Adjacent to the sternum the examiner should palpate the sternocostal and costochondral articulations, noting any swelling or tenderness. Swelling may indicate an inflammation or subluxation of the costosternal joint (costochondritis or Tietze's syndrome). The first rib on both sides is palpated for position and tenderness. Any differences on caudal pressure are noted.
   B. Active and passive motion. There is normally little motion of these joints. Raising and lowering the arms and breathing deeply may elicit a click and produce pain if there is a subluxation. If manual compression of the ribs causes pain, the individual joint or joints should be palpated to determine which ones have abnormal motion.
      1. Tests for abnormal motion
      2. Tests for pain
VI. Scapulothoracic Joint
   A. Inspection. Inspection may reveal winging of the scapula if the long thoracic nerve has been injured.
   B. Active and passive motion. Active motions are observed from behind: elevation, forward, sideways, horizontal abduction–adduction, and lateral and medial rotation. Of particular importance is notation of scapular rotation for bilateral asymmetry and scapulohumeral rhythm. Passive motion testing (retraction, protraction, elevation, depression, and mediolateral rotation [in sidelying]) is included with palpation.
      1. Tests for excessive or reduced movement
      2. Tests for contracture
      3. Tests for pain or tenderness
VII. Costovertebral and Costotransverse Joints
   Palpation may reveal tenderness if there is joint involvement. Deep breathing may induce pain and refer it to the shoulder or arm.
VIII. Upper Thoracic Spine
   A. Inspection and palpation. Inspection may reveal a sharp kyphosis at the site of an injured vertebra or a flat back or reversal of the curve in a mobile spine. Injured vertebrae will usually be tender on compression of the spinous process.
   B. Active and passive movements. Active range of flexion, extension, rotation, and lateral bending should be observed. If active motions are full and painless, overpressure is given to clear the joint.
      1. Tests for limitation and asymmetrical movement
      2. Tests for pain and muscle spasm
IX. Glenohumeral Joint
   A. Active shoulder movements with passive overpressure. The patient is asked to perform flexion of the arm (in the sagittal plane), abduction (in the frontal plane), and horizontal adduction (reaching across to behind the opposite shoulder); to touch the palm to the back of the neck and retract the elbow; and to crawl the thumb up the back as far as possible. If range of motion is full

and painless, gentle passive overpressure is applied at the end point of each movement. Both arms are tested simultaneously for comparison, noting the presence of pain, muscle spasm, or loss of movement.
      1. Tests for shoulder tendinitis: Typically full range of motion with pain at the extremes of elevation and movements that stretch the involved tendon. A painful arc on abduction suggests rotator cuff tendinitis.
      2. Tests for capsular restriction of the glenohumeral joint: Considerable pain and restriction on external rotation and abduction, moderate restriction of flexion and internal rotation
      3. Tests for acute bursitis: Marked pain and restriction of elevation of the arm in any plane
   B. Resisted isometric shoulder movements. The patient sits with the elbows close to the sides, the elbows bent to 90°, and the fingers pointed forward. Abduction is resisted with the arms held at about 30° abduction. Lateral rotation and medial rotation are resisted with the elbows held tight against the sides, applying counterpressure just proximal to the wrist. All movements are resisted bilaterally and simultaneously for easy comparison of one side with the other and for most efficient stabilization against trunk movements. Maximal contractions should be encouraged. Any joint movement should be prevented, and the presence of pain or weakness noted.
      1. Tests for the presence of tendinitis: the contraction of the involved muscle and tendon will be strong and painful.
      2. Tests for the presence of a tendon rupture: the contraction will be weak and painless.
      3. Tests the integrity of the C5 and C6 myotomes
   C. Quadrant test and locking position of the shoulder if applicable. Compare findings with those of the opposite side (see Chapter 11, Shoulder and Shoulder Girdle).
   D. Neurologic test of reflexes, sensation, and distal muscle (C8–T1)
X. Elbow Joint
   A. Active movements with passive overpressure. The patient is asked to fully flex and extend both elbows together. If this exercise is full and painless, passive overpressure is applied at the extremes of each movement, and the patient is observed for pain, spasm, or restricted movement. These tests may be performed with the shoulder extended, in neutral, or flexed to test for involvement of the long head of the biceps or triceps.
      1. Tests for capsular restrictions: Flexion is limited to about 90 to 100°, extension is lacking by 20 to 30°.
      2. Tests for extracapsular pain or restrictions
         a. Loose body—Extension is restricted; flexion is relatively free. Often there are painful twinges or crepitus noted during movement.

    b. Brachialis tightness—Extension is limited; flexion is free. Tightness is felt anteriorly by the patient on forced extension. The restriction is unaffected by the position of the shoulder.

    c. Biceps tendinitis—Pain may be reproduced with elbow extension performed with the shoulder extended.

B. Resisted isometric contractions. The trunk is stabilized by placing a hand over the top of the patient's shoulder and resisting isometric flexion and extension of the elbow. Pronation and supination are resisted with the elbow bent to 90°. Pain or weakness is noted.

    1. Tests the integrity of the C6 and C7 myotomes (biceps [C6], triceps [C7], and pronator teres [C7])

    2. Tests for biceps tendinitis: Resisted elbow flexion and forearm supination will be strong and painful.

    3. Tests for biceps tendon rupture: Flexion and supination will be weak and painless.

XI. Wrist Joint

The patient's elbow is maintained in extension. The patient's arm is held snugly between the examiner's elbow and side, and the patient's forearm is cradled in the examiner's forearm and hand.

A. Active movements with passive overpressure

    1. With the forearm pronated, the wrist is moved into full flexion and ulnar deviation. If movement is full and painless, passive overpressure is applied, once with the patient's fingers flexed, once with them relaxed. Pain or restricted motion is noted.

    2. With the forearm supinated, the wrist is brought into full extension and radial deviation. If movement is full and painless, overpressure is applied, once with the fingers extended, once with them relaxed. Pain or restricted motion is noted.

      a. Tests for lateral tennis elbow: Elbow pain is reproduced on full wrist flexion and ulnar deviation with the forearm pronated and the fingers flexed.

      b. Tests for medial tennis elbow: Elbow pain is reproduced with full wrist extension with the fingers extended and forearm supinated.

      c. Tests for carpal ligament sprain: Pain on movement that stretches the involved ligament.

      d. Tests for de Quervain's tenosynovitis: Pain over the radial styloid region when the wrist is ulnarly deviated while the thumb is held flexed

      e. Tests for capsular restriction of wrist movements: All wrist movements are limited.

B. Resisted isometric wrist movements. With the patient's arm held as described above and the patient's fist clenched, wrist flexion, extension, ulnar deviation, and radial deviation are resisted, and pain or weakness is noted.

    1. Tests the C6 (extension), C7 (flexion), and C8 (ulnar deviation) myotomes

    2. Tests for tennis elbow: Pain on resisted wrist extension

    3. Tests for golfer's elbow: Pain on resisted wrist flexion

C. Modified Phalen's test (see Fig. 13-31). The patient is asked to perform a "three-jaw-chuck" pinch with both hands and to maintain both wrists in extreme flexion by pressing the dorsum of the hands against one another. This position is held for 30 to 60 seconds. The production of pain or paresthesias is noted.

    1. Tests for carpal tunnel syndrome: Paresthesias into the thumb or index, middle, and ring fingers are reproduced on the involved side.

    2. Tests for dorsal carpal ligament sprain: Wrist pain is reproduced on full wrist flexion.

D. Upper extremity weight bearing

    1. While still seated, the patient is asked to place both hands to the side on the plinth and to attempt to raise the body off the plinth by pressing down with the hands.

    2. Tests for carpal ligament sprain: This is often the only maneuver that will reproduce the wrist pain.

XII. Hand Complex

A. Grasp–release. The patient is asked to squeeze two of the examiner's fingers simultaneously with both hands, as hard as possible, and then to open the hands as wide possible. Pain, weakness, or joint restriction is noted.

    1. Tests for the integrity of the T1 myotome: Weakness will be noted on grasp.

    2. Tests for tennis elbow: Strong grasp may reproduce the elbow pain because the wrist extensors must contract to stabilize.

    3. Tests for restriction of finger movement

B. Resisted isometric abduction–adduction. The patient attempts to keep the fingers spread apart as the examiner adducts the small finger and thumb simultaneously. Both hands are tested at the same time for comparison. Then the examiner interlaces his fingers between the patient's extended fingers and asks the patient to adduct the fingers. Pain or weakness is noted.

    1. Tests the C8 myotome (thumb and small finger abduction) and the T1 myotome (finger adduction)

    2. Tests for de Quervain's tenosynovitis: Pain is produced with resisted thumb abduction.

XIII. Sensory Tests

The patient sits with the forearms resting on the thighs, palms facing upward. Using a sharp pin or pinwheel, the examiner assesses sensation by applying the stimulus to a small area on one extremity and asking the patient whether it feels sharp, and then he repeats the test on the same area on the opposite extremity. Then the patient is asked whether it feels the same on both sides. The key sensory areas in the hand are checked first, then various aspects of the forearms, arms, and shoulder girdles, using the procedure described above. Asymmetries and reduction of sensation are noted. For subtler testing, a wisp of cotton or tuning fork may be used.

A. Tests the integrity of the C4 through T1 dermatomes. Rarely is a deficit noted proximal to the distal forearm in the case of nerve root lesions because of the extensive overlapping of dermatomes in all but the wrist and hand (see Figs. 5-5 and 19-37).

C4—Trapezial ridge to tip of shoulder

C5—Upper scapula, lateral brachial region, and radial aspect of forearm

C6—Upper scapula, lateral brachial region, and radial–volar aspect of forearm, thumb, and index finger

C7—Middle scapula, posterior brachial region, dorsum of forearm and hand, and palmar surface of index, middle, and ring fingers

C8—Middle to lower scapula, ulnar aspect of forearm, and palmar surface of ring and little fingers

T1—Ulnar–volar aspect of forearm

B. Tests sensory integrity of upper extremity peripheral nerves

XIV. Deep Tendon Reflex Tests

The patient sits with forearms resting on thighs.

A. Jaw jerk (cranial nerve V; see Fig. 17-30). With the mandible in the physiologic rest position, place the thumb over the mental area of the patient's chin. The examiner then taps the thumbnail with the reflex hammer; the reflex elicited will close the mouth. A brisk reflex may be caused by an upper motor neuron lesion.

B. Biceps (C5, C6; see Fig. 11-24A). As the patient maintains relaxation of the arm, the examiner places his thumb firmly over the patient's biceps tendon at the antecubital fossa and strikes the dorsum of the thumb with the reflex hammer to elicit the reflex. One should feel for tensing of the tendon and observe for contraction of the muscle and slight flexion of the elbow. Asymmetries in responses and clonic responses are noted.

C. Triceps (C7; see Fig. 11-24B). As the patient maintains relaxation of the arm, the examiner grasps the patient's upper arm (near elbow) and, while supporting the forearm at 90° elbow flexion, strikes the distal triceps tendon just above the olecranon. One should observe for triceps contraction and feel for slight elbow extension. Asymmetrical or clonic responses are noted.

D. Brachioradialis (C5, C6). Alternative test: As the patient maintains relaxation of both arms, the examiner supports both forearms at about 90° elbow flexion by grasping both of the patient's thumbs in one hand (or the thumb of one hand). The brachioradialis tendon is struck just above the radial styloid process, slightly volarly. The brachioradialis muscle belly is observed for contraction and felt for slight elbow flexion and forearm pronation. Asymmetrical or clonic responses are noted. The integrity of the C5, C6, and C7 segments is tested.

XV. Referred and Related Tissues

As much as any clinical examination can, the scanning examination attempts to generate a working hypothesis as to the patient's diagnosis by generating a number of signs and symptoms that, taken together, form a pattern distinct enough on which to base an effective intervention. Such diagnosis that the scan can elicit include the possibility of:

A. Visceral conditions. Pain may be referred to the upper quadrant from irritation of the diaphragm or peritoneum because of infection, the presence of free air or blood, an inflamed gallbladder, distended or inflamed stomach, or an injury to the liver or spleen. Cardiac ischemia may also cause shoulder pain.

B. Neoplastic disease

C. Fracture

D. Arthritis

E. Ankylosing spondylitis

SUMMARY OF STEPS TO CERVICOTHORACIC–UPPER LIMB SCAN EXAMINATION

For the scan examination to be of practical use, it must be performed within a very short period of time—5 minutes or less. Otherwise, one of its primary purposes, that of saving time in the clinic, is defeated. To perform the scan examination within a reasonable period of time, the clinician must sequence the tests so that they are performed as efficiently as possible. In doing so, care must be taken to avoid undue haste, which might lead to poor evaluative technique and inaccurate findings. The scan examination condenses a number of tests within a short period; to avoid confusion or the possibility of omitting crucial steps, the clinician must drill himself or herself on the sequencing of steps and the rationale for each step to be able to use the scan examination effectively in the clinic.

The steps to the scan examination are listed below in the order that they can be most efficiently performed.

I. Active Cervical Movements with Passive Overpressure

II. Cervical Resisted Movements

III. Quadrant Test, Left and Right

IV. Active Shoulder Movements with Passive Overpressure
A. Flexion
B. Abduction
C. Hand to opposite shoulder
D. Hand to back of neck, wing elbow back
E. Hand behind and up back

V. Resisted Shoulder Movements
A. Abduction (C5)
B. Internal rotation
C. External rotation

VI. Active Elbow and Forearm Movements with Passive Overpressure, Resisted Elbow and Forearm Movements
A. Flexion (C6): passive overpressure, resist flexion
B. Neutral: resist extension (C7), pronation (C7), and supination

C. Extension: passive overpressure

VII. Active Forearm and Wrist Movements with Passive Over-pressure

   A. Combined wrist flexion and ulnar deviation with the forearm pronated and elbow extended: (1) passive overpressure with fingers flexed; (2) passive overpressure with fingers relaxed

   B. Combined wrist extension and radial deviation with the forearm supinated and elbow extended: (1) passive overpressure with fingers extended; (2) passive overpressure with fingers relaxed

VIII. Resisted Wrist Movements

   A. Flexion (C7)

   B. Extension (C6)

   C. Radial deviation

   D. Ulnar deviation

IX. Modified Phalen's Test

X. Active and Resisted Finger Movements

   A. Grasp–release

   B. Finger abduction (C8)

   C. Finger adduction (T1)

XI. Upper Extremity Weight Bearing

XII. Sensory Tests

   A. C4–T1

XIII. Reflex Testing

   A. Jaw jerk (cranial nerve V)

   B. Biceps (C5, C6)

   C. Triceps (C7, C8)

   D. Brachioradialis (C5–C6)

REFERENCES

1. Lee D: The Thoracic: An Integrated Approach, 2nd ed. White Rock BC, Canada, Lee Physiotherapist Corporation, 2003
2. Norris CM: The thorax. In: Norris CM: Sports Injuries: Diagnosis and Management for Physiotherapists. Oxford, Butterworth-Heinemann, 1993
3. Thompson JF, Jannsen F: Thoracic outlet syndromes. Br J Surg 8:435–436, 1996

RECOMMENDED READING

Altchek DW, Andrews JR: The Athlete's Elbow. Philadelphia, Lippincott Williams & Wilkins, 2001

American Society for Surgery of the Hand: The Hand: Examination and Diagnosis. New York, Churchill Livingstone, 1983

Butler DS: Mobilization of the Nervous System. Melbourne, Churchill Livingstone, 1991

Corrigan B, Maitland GD: Practical Orthopaedic Medicine. London, Butterworths, 1985

Cyriax JH, Cyriax PJ: Illustrated Manual of Orthopaedic Medicine, 2nd ed. London, Butterworths, 1993

Dutton M: Manual Therapy of the Spine: An Integrated Approach. New York, McGraw-Hill, 2002

Dvorak J, Dvorak V: Manual Medicine: Diagnostics. New York, Thieme Medical, 1990

Grant R, ed: Physical Therapy of the Cervical and Thoracic Spine. New York, Churchill Livingstone, 1988

Grant R, ed: Physical Therapy of the Cervical and Thoracic Spine, 3rd ed. New York, Churchill Livingstone, 2002

Grieve GP: Mobilisation of the Spine: A Primary Handbook of Clinical Method, 5th ed. Edinburgh, Churchill Livingstone, 1991

Magee DJ: Orthopedic Physical Assessment, 3rd ed. Philadelphia, WB Saunders, 1997

Maitland GD: Vertebral Manipulations, 6th ed. Boston, Butterworths, 2001

McKenzie RA: The Cervical and Thoracic Spine: Mechanical Diagnosis and Therapy. Waikanae, New Zealand, Spinal Publications, 1990

Petty NJ, Moore AP: Neuromusculoskeletal Examination and Assessment. A Handbook for Therapist. Edinburgh, Churchill Livingstone, 1998

Rocabado M, Iglarsh ZA: Musculoskeletal Approach to Maxillofacial Pain. Philadelphia, JB Lippincott, 1991

Rockwood CA, Matsen FA: The Shoulder, vol. 1. Philadelphia, WB Saunders, 1990

Wadsworth CT: Wrist and hand examination and interpretation. J Orthop Sports Phys Ther 5:108–120, 1983

VI. Extension, passive overpressure

VII. Active Forearm and Wrist Movements with Passive Over-pressure

A. Combined Wrist Flexion and Ulnar deviation with the forearm pronated and elbow extended; (1) passive overpressure with fingers flexed; (2) passive overpressure with forearm flexed

B. Combined wrist extension and radial deviation with the forearm supinated and elbow extended; (1) passive overpressure with fingers extended; (2) passive overpressure with fingers flexed

VIII. Resisted Wrist Movements

A. Flexion (C7)

B. Extension (C6)

C. Radial deviation

D. Ulnar deviation

IX. Modified Phalen's test

X. Active and Resisted Finger Movements

A. Grasp or fist

B. Finger abduction (T1)

C. Finger adduction (T1)

XI. Thumb Extremity Weight Bearing

XII. Sensory Tests

A. C4–T1

XII. Reflex Testing

A. Jaw jerk (Cranial nerve V)

B. Biceps (C5, C6)

C. Triceps (C7)

D. Brachioradialis (C5-C6)

REFERENCES

RECOMMENDED READING

Lumbar Spine

DARLENE HERTLING

EPIDEMIOLOGY

Backache ranks high as a cause of lost working days in the United States. Second only to the common cold as a reason for outpatient visits, it represents the single most common and most expensive industrial and occupational health problem.[149] Each year approximately 500,000 workers in the United States sustain back injuries, leading to lost time from work and financial compensation. Healthcare costs, disability payments, and lost productivity related to low back pain syndromes are estimated at some $20 billion annually. An estimated 8 million Americans suffer from chronic low back pain. Each year more than 200,000 Americans undergo some sort of back surgery. Approximately 30% of workers at some time miss work because of a back ailment; 2 to 4% actually change jobs at least once because of this problem, in addition to the ones who become disabled.[776] According to Kelsey and White,[383] workers who are off the job more than 6 months with back pain have only a 50% chance of returning to work; this decreases to 25% after 1 year.

Nachemson's 1976 report may be the most quoted paper in the field.[555] It states that 80% of citizens will suffer back pain "to some extent," men as often as women, "white collar as often as blue collar workers." About 50 in 100 workers are significantly affected each year, leading to 1,400 to 2,600 lost workdays per 1,000 workers each year. Thus, back pain is the most expensive ailment in the 30- to 60-year-old age group.

The patient with acute low back pain presents different problems owing to the self-limiting nature of the first episode: 88% will be asymptomatic in 6 weeks, 98% in 24 weeks, and 99% in 52 weeks; 97% of causes are unknown, 2% are attributed to disk problems, and 1% to apophyseal joint disorders. No more than 29% require conservative measures, 1% surgery, and the rest recover spontaneously.[416]

According to Dagi and Beary,[149] approximately 80% of all back cases can be attributed to soft tissue conditions (i.e., muscle or ligament sprain, postural abnormalities, poor muscle tone, or neuromuscular disease) and 10% to intervertebral disk disease with or without radiculopathy. The annual incidence of diagnosed disk prolapse is about 5% per year in 20- to 40-year-olds. These lesions occur most often at L4–L5 and L5–S1 segments. Thirty percent of all those who have back pain have a syndrome consistent with radiculopathy at some time in their life.[776] Those who undergo surgery for disk herniation are usually 30 to 39 years old, tending to confirm the theory that partly degenerated disks are the most likely to herniate in such a way as to lead to surgery.

Roentgenographic evidence of disk space narrowing or osteophytosis is found in 70% of men and 50% of women aged 55 to 64 years. Autopsy studies show that disk degeneration begins at 20 to 25 years of age.[383] With respect to facet joint disease, Kelsey and White state that disk and facet joint diseases are closely and most inevitably linked.[383] About 90% of autopsies in patients older than 45 years reveal lumbar facet osteoarthrosis, and more joints are affected as age increases. Most studies have found that symptomatology is not significantly related to such findings.

The epidemiology of other specific diagnoses is not discussed thoroughly in the literature. For example, Shealy suggests that 20% of chronic unoperated back pain patients had sacroiliac joint symptoms as their major complaint, but did not further specify how this was demonstrated.[689] Travel and Simons[763] make only scant reference to the epidemiology of myofascial pain and quote Kraft and Levinthal[409] as stating that the affected patients were most likely aged 31 to 50 years. A large number of soft tissue-related anatomic or clinical syndromes (i.e., iliolumbar ligament strains, piriformis syndrome, lumbodorsal fascia tears, iliac crest syndrome) are described in the literature, but few research studies or controlled tests have been conducted. Many of the more accepted terms used to describe these conditions, as Flor and Turk[218] point out, are more descriptive than etiologic or useful, especially with respect to the treatment of individual patients.

Recently, a considerable amount of work has been done concerning risk factors, individual characteristics, and the natural history of low back pain. Low back pain in general, and disk herniation specifically, are influenced by many factors, including age and gender.[46,52,81,329,332,382,462,463,718,744,776] Low back pain in general is as common in females as in males, but the pattern changes when the work situation is taken into account.[329,744,628] Magora[462,463] found that 35% of women in physically heavy jobs had low back pain, compared with 19.1% of males. Strength factors could be a reason, or a mismatch between the worker's physical strength and the job requirements.[20]

Repeated lifting of heavy loads is often considered a risk factor for back pain,[46,331–333,335,465,466,555] although others deny this.[331,332,508,776] Magora[464] found sudden unexpected maximal efforts to be particularly harmful. Glover,[244] Tichauer,[759] and Troup et al.[770] expressed the same opinion about lifting in combination with lateral bending and twisting. Magora[463,464] found no relation to heavy lifting while standing, but he did find that workers who handled materials while seated and bent over had a high incidence of back pain.

In general, postural deformities, scoliosis/kyphosis, hypolordosis or hyperlordosis, and leg-length discrepancy do not seem to predispose to low back pain.[53,331,332,466,654,718] Although there is considerable disagreement, studies of static work postures indicate an increased risk of low back pain in subjects with predominantly sitting working postures.[332,333,412,426,464] Sitting with a bent-over working posture seems to carry a significant increased risk factor. Kelsey[381] and Kelsey and Hardy[382] found that men who spend more than half their workday in a car have a threefold increased risk of disk herniation. This could be because of the combined effects of sitting and vibration.

Andersson[19] reviewed the industrial epidemiology over a 30-year period and stated that physically heavy, static work postures, frequent bending and twisting, lifting and forceful movements, and repetitive work and vibration were vocational factors in back pain. He and others noted as well that tallness provides an increased risk of injury[19,381,426,751] and that sciatica is more common in the obese.[335]

Physical fitness and conditioning have significant preventive effects on back injuries. Weak trunk muscles and decreased endurance are significant risk factors in the development of back problems.[366] Cady and associates[90] showed that among fire-fighters, muscle strength was an accurate prognostic indicator for the development of low back pain. Chaffin[105] and Keyserling and associates,[390] using pre-employment strength testing, found that the risk of back injury increases threefold when the job requirements exceed the worker's capabilities on an isometric simulation of the job.

Clinical observations led Rowe[654] and Berguist-Ullman and Larsson[46] to conclude that abdominal and spinal extensor muscle strength was decreased in patients with low back pain. Many other investigators have established that patients with low back pain have lower mean trunk strength than do healthy subjects.[5,10,48,294,350,358,514,582,590,622,681] Some investigators have found the extensors to be more influenced (weaker) than the flexors,[575,681] whereas others have identified relatively greater extensor strength.[53–55] Biering-Sorenson found that patients with recurrent back pain had weaker trunk muscles and diminished flexibility (particularly flexion) when compared with asymptomatic persons.[54] Conversely, good isometric endurance in men appears to prevent low back problems. Very little data concerning the endurance capacity of the back muscles are found in the literature.[318,575] The most striking finding of Nicolaisen and Jorgensen[575] in persons with early, serious low back trouble was decreased endurance capacity of the trunk extensors rather than muscle strength, when compared with normal subjects.

Other factors significantly associated with low back pain include smoking and coughing.[236,744] Svensson[744] speculated that coughing led to increased intradiskal pressure and thus to increased loading and low back pain. Disk degeneration, osteoporosis, and spondylolisthesis are all associated with increased low back pain. The major risk for an episode of back pain is a previous history of back pain.[315]

Several reports give a fairly clear picture of how patients with acute back pain fare.[22,46,172,769] Horal[329] documented that 90% of acute symptoms resolve in the 2 months after the first episode. It is often suggested that little can be done in the way of treatment to alter this course. Some evidence exists, however, that short periods of bed rest (2 days), back school, and early and comprehensive care of the patient can speed the return to work.[46,166] Thus, when the initial history and physical examination suggest limited injury or abnormality, without significant neurologic deficit, an initial trial of empirically based conservative treatment and early mobilization is warranted.[166] Nachemson[556] has summarized a variety of data suggesting that motion, rather than rest, may be beneficial in healing soft tissues and joints. For the patient who appears to have a herniated disk with a motor deficit, there is a good biologic rationale for recommending longer periods of bed rest (i.e., reduction of intradiskal pressure).[553]

The risk that the typical patient with acute low back pain will suffer a recurrence over the next few years is about 60%.[46,767] The next attack, however, may be shorter and have a more benign course. According to Troup and associates, attacks of accident-related pain take longer to subside, both during the first attack and with recurrence.[769] Other factors influencing recurrence include sciatic pain, alcoholism, specific job situations, sociopsychologic stigma, and general insurance benefits.[559]

Social problems are greatest in chronic low back pain. Nachemson lists just as many social or psychologic findings as mechanical or occupational ones in considering the correlates of back pain.[555] He mentions abnormal profiles on the Minnesota Multiphasic Personality Inventory (MMPI), the most widely used psychologic test, as well as alcoholism, history of divorce, educational level, and depression as some of the factors that may affect the relation between acute injury or pain and chronic back pain. Severe mental problems are no more common in low back patients, but changes in the MMPI are seen.[20]

Many different diseases can present as low back pain. The purpose of this chapter is not to classify the numerous known causes for low back pain, but rather to deal with the more common types of back pain, including so-called "idiopathic" low back pain.[801] Other sources offer an exhaustive classification of the etiology of low back pain.[12,458,510,559,631]

Musculoskeletal disorders are of primary importance because they are the largest group of complaints most often seen by physical therapists and other healthcare practitioners. However, systemic and visceral problems may mimic low back pain.[73,262,701,811] Thus, a thorough abdominal examination may direct attention away from the spine to a source of viscerogenic pain. Here, we are interested only in minor mechanical derangements; this excludes fractures, dislocations, inflammatory disorders, and tumors.

APPLIED ANATOMY

Three-Joint Segment

At any one level, the motion segment is composed of three distinct parts: the two facet (zygapophyseal) joints and the intervertebral joint (the disk) (Fig. 22-1). In a normal motion

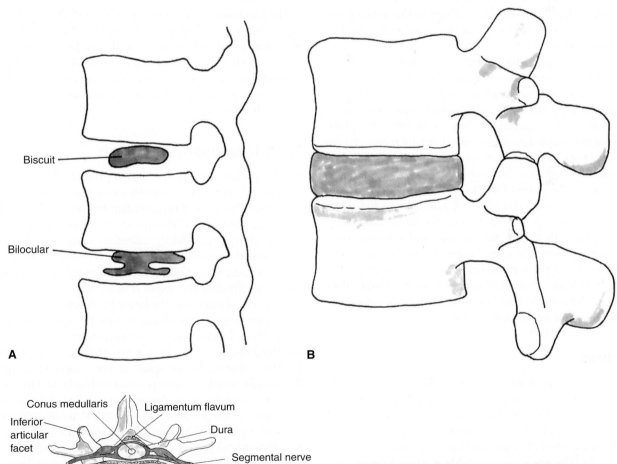

■ FIG. 22-1. (A) Some normal diskogram configurations. (B) A properly spaced lumbar vertebra. (C) Superior view of a normal intervertebral disk. (Part A adapted with permission from Finneson BE: Low Back Pain, 2nd ed. Philadelphia, JB Lippincott, 1980:104.)

segment, these three joints are anatomically linked and mechanically balanced. With age or as a result of various pathologic processes, degeneration may affect the motion segment. The segment as a whole may be somehow programmed to fail, with the chondrocytes of the disk nucleus involuting at the same time that the subchondral bone fractures; or, by attrition, each component structure may succumb to stress in turn. Narrowing of the disk space, spondylolisthesis, and transitional vertebrae tend to apply abnormal stress to the posterior structures.[198,199] Conversely, dysplasia of the lumbosacral facet structures or degenerative changes in the facet joints can cause spondylolisthesis.[571] The two major sites of pathologic change—the intervertebral disks and facet joints—must not be considered independently of one another: dysfunction of one, if allowed to progress, ultimately leads to dysfunction of the other.

The disk depends on normal movement (and therefore adequate mobility at the facet joints) for its nutrition and for an even distribution of force to the annulus over time. On the other hand, normal arthrokinematics at the facet joints depend, in part, on a healthy disk. An inelastic disk at a given level tends to alter the normal centroid of movement for the respective facet joints, a factor likely to contribute to the initiation of a degenerative cycle of events, as discussed in Chapter 3, Arthrology.[205,206,546,803]

In considering joint dysfunction of the spine, as with the peripheral joints, our conceptual model must include all the anatomic and physiologic structures of the joint. Only by looking at the whole picture can we judge which tissues seem to be primarily affected in a particular disorder, as well as the probable or possible secondary effects on other joint tissues. In the spine, it is best to think more in terms of segmental dysfunction rather than joint dysfunction, because of the intimate dependency of the paired facet joints and the intervertebral joint. Therefore, always consider that a segment includes two vertebrae with their paired facet joints, the intervening intervertebral joint with its disk, the muscles and ligaments controlling the segment, the nerves supplying the segment, the nerve tissue within the vertebral canal at the segment, and the spinal nerves leading from the segment and the tissues they innervate.[126] This is why spinal dysfunction is much more complex than peripheral joint dysfunction.

Vertebrae

One of the more important aspects of the skeletal aging process is bone loss. A gradual decrease in cortical bone of 3% per decade can be expected for both genders. In postmenopausal women, a 9% rate of decrease in cortical bone per decade has been demonstrated. Trabecular bone (see Fig. 18-6) also decreases, but the rate is more variable. A 6 to 8% decrease in trabecular bone per decade can be expected to begin between 20 and 40 years of age in both genders.[495]

These changes modify the load-bearing capacity of the vertebrae. After age 40, the load-bearing capacity of cortical cancellous bone changes dramatically.[648] Before age 40, about 55% of load-bearing capacity is attributed to cancellous bone; after age 40, this decreases to about 35%. Bone strength decreases more rapidly than bone quantity.[40] This decrease in strength accounts for the end-plates bending away from the disk, wedge fractures of vertebral bodies, and the end-plate fractures common in osteoporotic spines.[179]

The cartilaginous end-plate of the vertebral body is the weak point of the disk (see Fig. 18-12). It is the site of failure when compressive loads become excessive. Between age 23 and 40, there is a gradual demineralization of end-plate cartilage. By age 60, only a thin layer of bone separates the disk from the vascular channels. These nutrient channels are slowly obliterated and the arterioles and venules progressively thicken.[49] Such changes can have a significant role in the pathogenesis of lumbar disk disease. Because the adult disk has no blood supply, it must rely on diffusion for nutrition.[555]

In the upper lumbar spine, degeneration seems to start early with end-plate fractures and nuclear herniations (Schmorl's nodes) related to the essentially vertical loading of those segments (Fig. 22-2).[205] Facet disease also starts first in the upper lumbar spine. In the lower lumbar spine, disk changes begin in the late teens, facet changes in the mid-20s. Both lesions typically are seen first at L5–S1, then at L4–L5. Degenerative changes of both synovial and vertebral joints seem to occur together, most often at the lumbosacral articulation.[262] Spondylitic and arthrotic changes involving the whole segment are age-related and occur in approximately 60% of persons older than age 45.[434]

Facet (Zygapophyseal) Joints

All the pathologic considerations presented in Chapter 3, Arthrology, apply to the posterior elements and the spinal facet joints (see Fig. 18-9). Primary inflammatory conditions affecting spinal joints are relatively rare; the two major exceptions are ankylosing spondylitis, affecting most often the young male, and rheumatoid arthritis, which primarily involves the upper cervical spine. Osteoarthrosis is probably the major joint condition affecting the spine. It most frequently involves the lower cervical spine and the lower lumbar levels. In the lumbar region, degenerative changes of the facet joints are the rule rather than the exception in virtually everyone living beyond the third decade or so. This fact is attributable in part to the likelihood that the human spine has not completely adapted to the upright, weight-bearing position and to the fact that human life expectancy has been drastically extended. Normal degeneration generally progresses so gradually that only minor symptoms, if any, result. The person may develop a "stiff spine" but usually not until an age at which the normal activity level does not require much mobility anyway. Again, because the process proceeds gradually, the joint tissues gradually adapt by means of fibrosis, bony hypertrophy, or even spontaneous ankylosis; thus, little if any inflammation or pain results. For this reason it is not unusual to see very marked joint narrowing with hypertrophic bony changes on roentgenograms in a person with

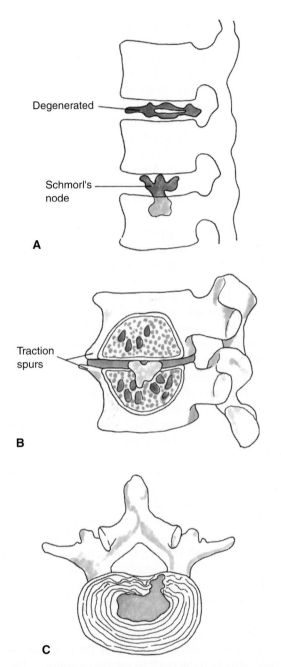

■ **FIG. 22-2.** Some abnormal diskogram configurations. **(A)** Chronic lumbar degenerative joint disease. **(B)** Narrowing of the disk and foramina and hypertrophic changes at the vertebral margins. **(B, C)** Internal disruption of the disk. (Part **A** adapted with permission from Finneson BE: Low Back Pain, 2nd. Philadelphia, JB Lippincott, 1980:104.)

marked restriction of spinal mobility, even if the person denies significant back pain or dysfunction over the years.

Conversely, some persons suffer an acceleration of the normal degenerative processes of the spinal joints. The reasons may include a genetic predisposition, such as asymmetry of facet planes in the lower lumbar spine; an occupational predisposition, such as a job involving abnormal compression of

joint surfaces; or some other factor resulting in considerable alteration in normal joint mechanics, such as excessive muscle tension or sudden changes in disk mechanics. These persons eventually complain of spinal pain; the origin of their pain is the facet joint capsule, which undergoes abnormal stress from the alteration in normal mechanics. In such cases, the altered joint mechanics occur suddenly enough, or to such a degree, that the joint tissues do not have time to adapt through fibrosis and bony hypertrophy. The painful condition continues unless joint stresses sufficient to cause pain are prevented through restoration of normal mechanics and avoidance of certain activities, or until the condition runs its course; that is, over the years, the joint tissues will gradually adapt to the abnormal stresses placed on them. Symptoms are likely to appear before significant radiographic changes; conversely, roentgenographic "degenerative" changes cannot be reliably correlated with symptoms.[467]

Spinal joints, like any synovial joint, can refer pain into the relevant segments, or sclerotomes.[146,148] Pain of spinal joint origin tends to be a deep aching pain felt in an area that often does not correlate well to the skin overlying the site of the lesion; this is characteristic of pain of deep somatic origin.

Posterior element changes proceed from early degenerative joint disease with articular erosion of the facet surfaces to fibrous dysplasia, loss of normal anatomical relations of the facets, osteophyte formation (in an attempt to heal capsular injuries), synovial proliferations, and eventually hypermobility or hypomobility of the joint.[206] Associated with this process are changes in the subchondral bone similar to those seen in degenerative joint disease in other joints, but in the lumbar spine there is also frequently a fatty infiltration of the joint, revealing the "abnormal widening" and the lack of mechanical function of a fully degenerated joint.

The ligamentum flavum (see Fig. 18-8) becomes less elastic and thicker, although the thickness may result from shortening secondary to lost disk height rather than the commonly implied "hypertrophy."[825] Thus, the ligament plays only a passive role in neural entrapment problems. Although the intimate association of the ligamentum flavum with the medial aspect of the facet joint capsule should retract the capsule and synovium when the capsule is slack, this system may not work well because the ligamentum flavum shortens with age and the loss of disk height.[30] Several works refer to the possibility of joint dysfunction and pain secondary to entrapment of the synovium, meniscoid bodies (or meniscoid inclusions), or capsule, or loose joint bodies, especially during re-extension after forward-flexion.[409,605,606]

In quick, poorly controlled movements, or, for example, in the case of a relatively lax ligamentum flavum from segmental narrowing, a meniscoid may become entrapped with a resulting pinching of the innervated portion and a pulling on the capsule to which they attach. This results in a reflex, segmental muscle spasm that tends to prevent the spontaneous release of the entrapped structure. Clinically, the patient presents with a history of a sudden onset of localized pain and "spasm," usually accompanying a combined rotation and extension movement. The pain is immediate, persistent, and associated with rather marked spinal deformity in a direction of flexion, rotation, and sidebending away from the involved side. This must be distinguished from the patient who, while bent forward, feels an immediate pain in the back, which quickly subsides for the most part, then gradually builds to a constant, intense pain over a period of 8 to 12 hours; this is invariably an acute disk protrusion.

This dysfunction concept is highly theoretical. Many believe that it is based on sound anatomical, physiologic, and biomechanical principles. A review and anatomic study by Bogduk and Engel describes three types of meniscoid structures (connective tissue rim, adipose tissue pad, and fibroadipose meniscoid), which are in fact found in various percentages of lumbar facet joints.[62] A histologic study of the fibroadipose meniscoid (the only one long enough to be trapped between the articular surfaces) suggested that it is not strong enough to provide painful traction on the joint capsule in such circumstances.[62] There is a possibility of detachment of the meniscoid with resultant effusion but that would not be relieved with manipulation, which has been considered effective in the facet joint meniscal syndrome. The authors concluded that it would be appropriate to consider other causes of "acute locked back" outside the lumbar facet joint.

Studies of intervention in the form of surgical fusion or surgical, chemical, or thermal denervation of the facets indicate that many cases of back pain may be of facet origin.[98,99,444,611,686] That impression is supported by the experiment of Mooney and Robertson,[540] who produced typical sciatica (sometimes bilaterally) by facet joint injections with hypertonic saline in patients.

Other proponents of the facet joint as a cause of pain have concentrated on root impingement caused by inflammatory hypertrophy of the joint margin, with resulting root compression or irritation. Vertical subluxation of the superior facet occurs with loss of disk space, leading to superior articular facet syndrome and root impingement in the intervertebral foramen by the subluxated process.[198,652]

Damage to the facet joint has always been considered secondary to disk failure. However, according to Farfan,[205,206] Grieve,[262] and others, autopsy evidence clearly shows that facet damage of varying degrees can and frequently does occur in the absence of disk failure. Helfet and Gruebel Lee[300] maintain that lesions of the posterior element always have an effect on the disk and that disk lesions always have an effect on the posterior joints.

Intervertebral Disk

In a manner and at a rate not unlike those of the facet joints, human intervertebral disks (Fig. 22-2) undergo a normal process of degeneration.[628,644] Early changes in the lumbar intervertebral disks are common as early as the second decade, when vascular channels begin to become obliterated. With the developing lumbar lordosis, the posterior lamellae of the annulus become compressed vertically and also horizontally, with an associated tendency toward posterior bulging of the annular fibers. The compaction of the posterior lamellae gives the posterior annulus the appearance of being thinner than the anterior annulus, although the number of lamellae remains the same. The nucleus remains a viscous, incompressible gel with a few collagen fibers embedded.[747]

The nucleus gradually changes from a gel to more of a viscous, fibrous structure. Associated with this process is early breakdown of mucopolysaccharide (with a net loss of chondroitin sulfate); there is a resultant decrease in water-binding capacity and a slight increase in collagen content (from 15% in the first decade to approximately 20% in the remaining years).[88,304,565–567] The original water content decreases from 88 to about 70%.[565] Beginning at the third decade, there is a 55% decrease in the glycosaminoglycan content of the nucleus pulposus.[290] There is a gradual increase in glycoprotein (noncollagen), particularly in the cross-beta form.[456] The posterior annulus gradually becomes more weight bearing, probably due in part to some loss in the preload condition of the nucleus and its ability to withstand vertical compression, but also because of the increasing lumbar lordosis. The posterior lamellae continue to compress posteriorly with an associated posterior bulging. The anterior annular lamellae, which have greater vertical height, remain comparatively loose but also begin bulging posteriorly. The posterolateral annulus becomes dog-eared—it tends to compact and bulge considerably in the posterolateral direction. Between the lamellae of the posterolateral annulus, clefts or gaps appear perhaps secondary to pressure atrophy from the combined vertical forces of weight bearing and the horizontal pressure from the nucleus pulposus. Vascular channels have been shut off and have filled with fibrous scarring.

During the fourth decade, transformation of the nucleus from nearly a pure gel to a largely fibrous mass becomes complete. The nucleus gradually becomes less distinguishable from the surrounding annulus. A considerable portion of the nucleus, in addition to the invading collagen fibers, consists of pulpy debris left from the breakdown of the original protein-polysaccharide material. The water content continues to decrease, although the nucleus retains its volume. The cartilaginous end-plate begins to thin, and some of the scarred vascular channels tend to coalesce to form larger pits. It has been proposed that these weaker, pitted areas are often the site of Schmorl's nodes or invasion of the nucleus into the vertebral body (Fig. 22-2A). Clefting of the posterolateral annulus continues, spreading into the posterior annulus. Some of the clefts meet, forming even larger gaps in the posterolateral annulus. A few radial tears may begin to form across adjacent lamellae, especially in the inner layers of the posterolateral annulus.

Over the next 20 years, roughly from age 40 to 60, similar processes continue. With continued loss of nuclear water content and collapse of the annular lamellae, the disk space begins to narrow. The nucleus is now a pulpy, fibrous mass that is largely adhered to adjacent vertebral bodies (Fig. 22-2C).

Clefts in the annulus continue to increase in number and distribution and to coalesce to form larger clefts. Radial tearing, especially posterolaterally, increases, often with rather large tears extending horizontally across the entire annulus, allowing the nucleus to protrude into the annular space. The annular fibers are correspondingly weaker and have lost their normal elasticity. With gradual narrowing, increased weight bearing peripherally, and increased tension on the outer annular fibers attaching to the vertebral bodies at the periphery, the added stresses to the margins of the vertebral body result in a hypertrophic bony reaction with the development of spurs and osteophytes. These occur both anteriorly and posteriorly (Fig. 22-2B).

After age 60, the disk space is essentially filled with a mass of relatively unorganized fibrous material connecting adjacent vertebral bodies. The area once occupied by the nucleus is virtually indistinguishable from the annular regions. The spaces are narrowed, and bony changes at the periphery of the superior and inferior vertebral bodies are considerable.

Again, this is normal process that occurs in virtually every human spine. So long as the process continues gradually over the years, the involved tissues can be expected to adapt to the altered mechanics so that although considerable changes occur, the person suffers little pain or disability. For example, although the annulus weakens considerably, the nucleus, at the same time, becomes more fibrous and loses volume and therefore exerts less pressure on the annulus, so that the annulus need not be as strong. Although the fibrosis of the disk space results in a very immobile segment, the person, at the age at which this occurs, simply does not require much spinal mobility for activities of daily living.

As with the facet joints, pathologic disk changes are those that occur prematurely or at an accelerated rate, in such a fashion that either the person or the related tissues cannot adapt to the change, resulting in pain or disability. Such pathologic disk changes may result from several factors.[155,188,389,531] Hypermobility or hypomobility at the related facet joints may certainly cause changes in the normal stresses to the intervertebral disk, resulting in accelerated tissue change. For instance, at a segment in which a facet on one side lacks mobility but its mate moves freely, asymmetrical movement will result in increased pressure from the nucleus on an isolated portion of the annulus. This portion of the annulus would tend to degenerate and possibly tear prematurely, resulting in a herniation or protrusion of the nucleus into the torn portion of the annulus (Fig. 22-3). If an entire segment lacks mobility, the segment above or below might tend to become hypermobile, with added stresses on the disk at the hypermobile segment. Again, the annulus at this segment may be unable to withstand the increased horizontal forces applied to it by the nucleus and may give way prematurely, allowing the nucleus to bulge into the space and applying pressure to the sensitive outer annular layers, posterior longitudinal ligament, or nerve root. Occupational factors may also play an important role. The person who must perform continual forward-bending and lifting

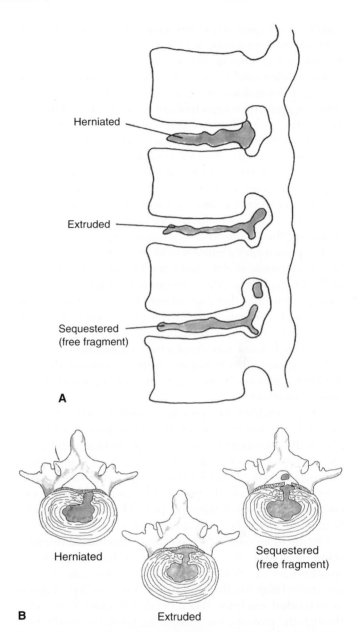

■ **FIG. 22-3.** Abnormal diskograms, with contained and noncontained disks. **(A)** Lateral and **(B)** superior views. (Adapted with permission from Finneson BE: Low Back Pain, 2nd ed. Philadelphia, JB Lippincott, 1980:104.)

activities places heavier, more frequent horizontal stresses on the inner layers of the posterior annulus than the more sedentary person. Conversely, the sedentary person is likely to lose normal annular elasticity and movement between annular lamellae earlier. The annulus is then less able to yield to the relatively higher demand placed on it during more strenuous activities (e.g., occasional sports participation), with an increased likelihood of tearing.

No matter what factors predispose to early disk lesions, persons aged 30 to 50 are much more susceptible to suffering an acute, symptomatic disk injury. At this age, a person usually is still quite active, has a nucleus pulposus that is of good volume, can imbibe fluid, can exert horizontal forces on the annulus, and has an annulus that is beginning to weaken and form clefts and is therefore more likely to tear. Before this age, the annulus is strong and elastic and capable of withstanding pressures transmitted to it by the nucleus. After this period, the nucleus loses volume, narrows, and no longer can bulge posteriorly into sensitive tissues. The nucleus pulposus in the middle-aged person has been invaded by collagen tissue, which may be denser in some areas of the nucleus than in others. Because of this, the nucleus no longer exerts an even distribution of pressure on the posterior annulus; rather, areas of relatively high concentration of forces may result, again increasing the likelihood of an annular tear.

The posterolateral annulus tends to weaken first, with earlier development of clefts and tears. This is perhaps because in the lumbar region, the posterior longitudinal ligament is stronger centrally, thinning out over the posterolateral disk in its characteristic hourglass shape. The central portion of the posterior annulus is, then, better reinforced by this ligament. Also, because functional movements of the trunk tend to be diagonal rather than pure sagittal or coronal, the posterolateral annulus receives more pressure transmitted to it from the nucleus.

The person likely to experience symptoms of disk disease, then, is one in whom the inner layers of the posterior annulus tear in the presence of a nucleus pulposus that is still capable of bulging into the space left by the tear. If the tear is extensive enough, the nucleus may bulge sufficiently to cause increased pressure to the posterior longitudinal ligament or outer annular fibers, resulting in pain. This type of disk protrusion, in which the outer annulus or posterior longitudinal ligament remains intact, is called a **herniated nucleus (contained disk)**. If the outer annular and ligamentous fibers (posterior longitudinal ligament) also give way, allowing the nucleus to bulge into the neural canal, it is called a **prolapsed** or **extruded nucleus.** When the diskal material extrudes through the posterior longitudinal ligament, the condition is known as a **noncontained disk.** As long as the nuclear herniation is connected to the disk itself, a free protrusion is present. If the nuclear material has actually separated from the remaining nucleus, allowing it to be free in the neural canal, it is called a **sequestration of nuclear material** (Fig. 22-3). The term **disk protrusion** is used in a general sense.

A herniation is likely to result in a deep, somatic type of pain or scleratogenous pain, which is deeply, poorly localized and perhaps referred to part or the entire relevant sclerotomal segment. Because the nucleus is still contained, the patient is likely to experience more pain in the morning after the nucleus has imbibed more fluid, because the added volume increases pressure on sensitive structures. A disk prolapse or sequestration (Figs. 22-3 and 22-4) is more likely to impinge on nerve tissue, resulting in "neurogenic" pain and perhaps a progressive nerve root impingement syndrome, in which the symptoms change with prolonged pressure. Central prolapses, although relatively rare, may cause upper motor neuron disturbances if they occur in the cervical spine, with perhaps a plantar-flexion reflex response, lower extremity spasticity, and paresthesias into all four extremities. If the central prolapse occurs in the lumbar region, the lower sacral nerve roots may be compressed, resulting in bowel or bladder dysfunction.

Phases of Degeneration

Generally, three conditions are considered degenerative: spondylosis, osteoarthritis, and herniated (or "slipped") disk (degenerative disk disease).[203,231,732] Alone, or more often together, they can lead to spinal stenosis and nerve root entrapment. Degenerative changes in general are the body's attempt to heal itself. Thus, the body tends to stabilize an unstable joint by immobilizing it, by the natural splintage of muscle spasms or by increasing the surface area of the joint.[178]

To define this process more clearly, Kirkaldy-Willis[391] has proposed a reasonable system based on our current understanding of the degenerating motion segment. The spectrum of degenerative change in the motion segment can be divided into three phases of deterioration.

The first level is the **early dysfunction phase,** with minor pathologic processes resulting in abnormal function of the posterior element and disk. Damage has occurred in the motion segment but is reversible. Changes that occur in the facet joint during this phase are the same as those that occur in any other synovial joint. The pathologic changes usually begin with synovitis. Chronic synovitis and joint effusion can stretch a joint capsule. The inflamed synovium may in turn project folds, which can become entrapped in the joint between the cartilage surfaces and initiate cartilage damage. Most often, this early dysfunction phase involves the capsule and synovium, but it can also involve the cartilage surface or supporting bone. Disk dysfunction during this phase is less clear but probably involves the appearance of several circumferential tears in the annulus fibrosis. If these tears are in the outer layer, healing is possible because there is some vascular supply. In the deeper layers, this is less likely because no blood supply is available. Slowly, there is progressive enlargement of the circumferential tears, which coalesce into radial tears. The nucleus begins to exhibit changes by losing proteoglycan content.

Next, an **intermediate instability phase** results in laxity of the posterior joint capsule and annulus. Permanent changes of instability may develop because of the chronicity and persistence of the dysfunction in earlier years. Restabilization of the posterior segment takes the form of subperiosteal bone formation or bone formation along ligaments and capsular fibers, resulting in perifacetal osteophytes and traction spurs.[178] Finally, the disk is anchored by peripheral osteophytes that pass around its circumference, producing a stable motion segment.

The **final stabilization phase** results in fibrosis of the posterior joints and capsule, the loss of disk material, and the formation of osteophytes.[391,796] Osteophytes form in response to abnormal motion to stabilize the affected motion segment.[572]

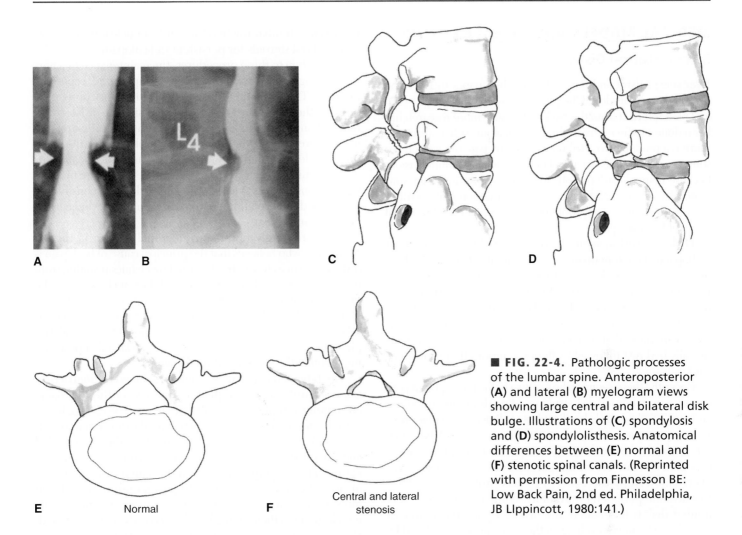

■ **FIG. 22-4.** Pathologic processes of the lumbar spine. Anteroposterior (**A**) and lateral (**B**) myelogram views showing large central and bilateral disk bulge. Illustrations of (**C**) spondylosis and (**D**) spondylolisthesis. Anatomical differences between (**E**) normal and (**F**) stenotic spinal canals. (Reprinted with permission from Finnesson BE: Low Back Pain, 2nd ed. Philadelphia, JB LIppincott, 1980:141.)

Osteophyte formation around the three joints increases the load-bearing surface and decreases motion, resulting in a stiff, less painful motion segment.

Each of these categories defines a pattern of symptoms that may require varied treatment approaches.

Incidental Complications

Although degenerative changes in either the facet joint or the disk may in themselves produce painful syndromes, the pathologic interaction when both parts of the three-joint system are affected is most significant. The three-joint complex can go through these changes with very few symptoms. Pain is only a signal of impending or actual tissue damage and becomes manifest only if the tissue-failure threshold is reached. Thus, patients with minimal degenerative changes may present with chronic recurrent symptoms; others with severe roentgenographic changes present with few or no symptoms.

Each phase carries a specific set of incidental complications that may result in painful clinical syndromes. In the first phase, facet lesions may become manifest as painful facet syndrome. With increased formation of radial tears in the annulus, a disk herniation may occur, often caused by minor trauma. Disk herniations most commonly occur at the end of the dysfunction phase or the beginning of the instability phase, but may occur during the stabilization phase.[391]

During the instability phase, dynamic degenerative spondylolisthesis (Fig. 22-4D) may occur when laxity predominates in the posterior restraining structures, or dynamic degenerative retrolisthesis when laxity predominates in the disk.[179] Both can produce dynamic lateral or central nerve entrapment.[626,777]

In the restabilization phase, narrowing of the central spinal canal at one level may be produced by osteophytic enlargement of the facet joints and circumferential osteophytes around the disk space, which can produce symptomatic central or lateral stenosis (Fig. 22-4F). Later, the degeneration process may spread to involve several levels.

An attempt should be made to correlate this spectrum of degenerative changes and symptoms with diagnosis and treatment. Knowing the natural history of the disease enables the therapist to gain insight into the disease process, to make a more complete assessment, and to formulate a more rational regimen of treatment. An understanding of which forms of treatment are more likely to meet with success is important.

MEDICAL MODELS AND DISEASE ENTITIES

Intervertebral Disks

Ever since Mixter and Barr delivered their paper in 1934, the disk has been considered the principal cause of all low back pain and pain referred from the back.[532] Because more research has been done on the intervertebral disk than any other structure, there is a tendency to attribute almost any type of backache to some type of disk disorder.[559] This often leads to tunnel vision, because many disorders, both spinal and extraspinal, may simulate disk disease. Although a disk dysfunction may result in more serious low back problems, it is rarely if ever the initial cause of low back pain.

Disk protrusion seems to be regarded by most current orthopaedists and neurosurgeons as the most probable diagnosis in cases of back pain with sciatica and evidence of nerve root involvement suggested by physical examination, electromyography, myelography, and other tests.[211,652,722,803] Cases not meeting these criteria are usually designated "mechanical" back pain; those that do meet them are treated conservatively (usually bed rest followed by flexion exercises if improved) or surgically.

Recently, there seems to be a return to the concept that pain can arise from injured disk structures directly in cases of "annular tears."[205,391] Several classifications of clinical syndromes now include pain due to disk degeneration itself.[537,589,803] Although it was established more than 35 years ago, the concept of primary disk pain is relatively unfamiliar to clinicians because it was overshadowed by the concept of disk prolapse.[439–441,649,808] Because the peripheral third of the annulus fibrosis of every lumbar disk is innervated, the disk is a potential source of pain.[60,342] The nerve endings in the disk can be stimulated by involvement of the innervated perimeter of the annulus by the autoimmune inflammatory processes of disk degeneration, by torsional strains of the annulus, or by a bulging nucleus straining the overlying annulus. In each case, the pain is mediated by the nerves that supply the disk.

There is a wide variety of conservative and surgical means of treating intervertebral disk disorders, including immobilization, manipulation, traction, therapeutic exercises, laminectomy, and spinal fusion, to name but a few.[93,102,143,148,201,258,317,318,359,385,457,507,584,651] A frequently mentioned disk-based treatment approach was that of Cyriax,[146] who believed that most back pain (95%) was secondary to disk disease and herniation. The diagnosis is mostly based on physical findings. According to the Cyriax approach, back pain without sciatica is secondary to the blocking effect of a disk protrusion on the motion in the involved segment; back pain with local or buttock-referred symptoms is related to dural "involvement" or irritation by a protrusion that is not affecting a specific root. Muscular pain, sacral joint pain, and buttock pain are referral patterns and are not treated except by treating the disk lesion. Back pain with sciatica or sciatica alone is secondary to root compression or irritation by a disk fragment. Treatment recommended by Cyriax[146] is manipulation for the so-called "hard" or annular

protrusions, lumbar traction for "soft" or nuclear protrusions, and epidural steroids for persistent radiculopathy.

In addition to these procedures, the maintenance of a normal or exaggerated lumbar lordosis is emphasized, especially in sitting. This is thought to prevent or reduce disk protrusion of either the soft or hard type by compressing the disk forward rather than backward. Exercise, stretching, acupressure, and massage are not used for back pain, but prolotherapy (the injection of sclerosants into connective tissue) is advocated for cases in which repeated attacks of pain are thought to indicate ligamentous laxity associated with and perhaps responsible for recurrent disk herniation. Patients are taught to avoid certain positions and stresses.

An increasingly popular conceptual system is that of McKenzie, who believes that the principal cause of back pain is disk disease manifested by abnormal mechanics resulting from the consequences of migration of the intact nucleus within the disk, not frank herniation.[510,511,688] Herniation is seen as a result of untreated, poorly treated, or unusually severe acute nuclear migration. A special case of nuclear migration is the "lateral shift phenomenon," a sciatic scoliosis caused by a lateral or posterior migration of the nucleus within the annulus.

The type of nucleus disk lesion is deduced through a program of prolonged or repeated stresses on the low back, attempting to reproduce painful situations. The change in the pain during such procedures as repeated extension in standing, trunk extension in lying, and lateral bending is recorded and classified according to its peripheralizing or centralizing nature. The geographic pattern of the pain response (central or near the spine as opposed to peripheral) is considered more important than its intensity. A series of positional self-mobilizations is then prescribed, based on the patterns found. Usually, these self-mobilizations are in extension. When a lateral shift is found, it is first reduced by mobilizations (and self-mobilizations) before extension is done to prevent possible peripheralization of symptoms. More conventional spinal manipulations are recommended only for certain situations.

McKenzie also describes a postural syndrome characterized by mechanical deformation of the soft tissue as the result of prolonged postural stress that can lead to pain and a dysfunction syndrome that features pathologically involved muscles, ligaments, fascia, facet joints, and the intervertebral disk.[510] The major factor is adaptive soft tissue shortening (fixation) of the motion segment, causing chronic mechanical deformation and loss of joint play. The precipitating causes are usually by-products of disk migration (derangement syndrome), spondylosis, or poor posture (postural syndrome). Based on the type of motion loss (flexion or extension), mobilization and home exercises are used. For example, when flexion loss is present, a static supine position is used, progressing to sustained and active lumbar stretching into flexion.

In this approach, home therapy is key to maintaining the corrective influences of therapy. McKenzie places a heavy emphasis on prevention of future attacks, usually by the use of lumbar rolls or special seating to maintain lordosis while sitting, and by instruction in body mechanics for daily activities and a daily program of exercise. McKenzie's text is valuable and must be understood in depth. We cannot cover this field adequately here, but other sources should be reviewed.[170,171,424,425,480,481,586,780,782]

Facet Joints

The lumbar facet joints can be a source of both low back pain and referred pain.[59,202,497,540] Pathologically, the lumbar facet joints can be affected by a variety of disorders, but most commonly they undergo degeneration, usually secondary to some form of injury or disk disease.[59] Facet joint pain can be referred to any part of the limb, but most commonly it is the gluteal and proximal thigh or groin region.[59,202,497,540]

Some clinicians place great emphasis on the pathologic processes of the facet joints in the genesis of back pain. Many manual therapists have tended to embrace views propounded by osteopaths,[255,530,551,731] orthopedists,[59,61,108,468,469,523–524] and physical therapists.[368–370,471,472,610]

Mennell[524,525] proposed the theory of joint play (see Chapter 6, Introduction to Manual Therapy), a type of freedom or "slack" considered necessary for the painless function of synovial joints in the spine and extremities. Lack of joint play reduces motion at the joint and produces secondary effects, including referred pain and the myofascial trigger point phenomenon. Treatment is by mobilization of the restricted joints and procedures to break up the cycle of epiphenomena (cryotherapy, heat, electrotherapy, trigger-point injections, and contract–relax programs). Manipulations are often recommended. Determination of the level of the spine to be treated is by observation of gross and segmental movement abnormalities, and oscillations of the vertebral spine, looking for hypersensitive levels ("facilitated segments").[37,222,223,404–406,474] Treatment is directed at an area of the spine that contains one or more symptomatic facet joints, in the expectation that joint mobilization will restore joint play.

Kaltenborn[368–370] and Paris[606,607,610] describe detailed evaluation systems for locating individual hypo- or hypermobile joints. Mobilizations are usually in the direction in which motion is blocked on examination, so that the facet motion is normalized.[607] Maitland (a physical therapist) and Maigne[468,469] (an orthopaedic surgeon) are other well-known manual therapists who operate relatively empirically, attempting to avoid the argument about underlying lesions while using mobilization techniques similar to those of the osteopaths and the "facet school." Maitland's evaluation system[471] is closely linked to treatment and incorporates a widely used graphic record of range of motion and its restrictions. He uses gentle, graded (I to IV), oscillating motions within or at the limit of the available range of motion of the joint, concentrating on end feel and tissue characteristics (see Chapter 6, Introduction to Manual Therapy).

Maigne uses specific mobilizations and manipulation techniques. Based on the evaluation, he implements therapy based on two major rules: no painful manipulations should be performed, because they are unlikely to be successful; and mobi-

lizations or manipulations should be done initially in the direction of greatest mobility found on the examination. The latter rule seems contradictory to other treatment systems (see Chapter 20, Thoracic Spine).[468,469]

Great importance has also been attached to the facets by clinicians that do not necessarily advocate manual therapy.[202,458,540,652,689] Following the works by Kirkaldy-Willis[394] and others, the role of the facet joint in radiculopathies is again becoming prominent, with a re-emergence of the facet joint syndrome theory popular between 1930 and 1945.

Some authors believe that pathologic processes of the facet joints occur after and perhaps because of disk degeneration; others believe they occur with disk degeneration. Asymmetry of the facet joints is well documented and has been given particular significance by Farfan and Sullivan[206] as a contributing factor to pathologic problems in the lower lumbar region. These authors suggest that facet asymmetry (by producing a cam-like effect) may contribute to early degeneration of the L5–S1 intervertebral joint.[206]

Segmental Intervertebral Instability

Instability is a loss of integrity of soft tissue intersegmental control that causes potential weakness and liability to yield under stress.[573] Lumbar instability, where a degenerating segment is functionally incompetent because of insufficient control (whether muscle, ligament, disk, or all three), can be an intractable problem.[189,190,258,259,395,431,542,557,570,572,592,603,604,609,641, 733,734,752] According to Grieve[258] and Paris,[609] segmental hypermobility and ligamentous or disk insufficiency are not necessarily the same thing. Paris defines hypermobility as a range of motion somewhat in excess of that expected for the particular segment, given the subject's age, body type, and activity status.[609] Simple hypermobility may be insignificant and need not result in instability. According to Paris,[609] instability exists when, during active motion, there is a sudden aberrant motion such as a visible slip or shaking of the section. Instability may be the result of postural problems, congenital defects, severe trauma, disk degeneration, traumatic ruptures of ligaments with or without fractures, unsatisfactory results following disk surgery, overtreatment by manipulation, or excessive stretching related to certain sports.[391,393] In spondylolisthesis, the spine sometimes is hypermobile. Hypermobility can also develop in areas adjacent to a hypomobile segment.

Panjabi[602] redefined spinal instability in terms of a region of laxity around the neutral position of a spinal segment called the "neutral zone." This neutral zone is shown to be increased with intersegmental injury and intervertebral disk degeneration[367,529,603] and decrease with simulated muscle forces across a motion segment.[367,603,810] The size of the neutral zone is considered to be an important measure of spinal stability. It is influenced by the interaction between what Panjabi[602] described as the active, neural control and passive systems:

- The active system constituting the muscles and tendons surrounding and acting on the spinal column.

- The neural system constituting the nerves and central control system which direct and control the active system in providing dynamic stability
- The passive system constituting the vertebrae, zygapophyseal joints, intervertebral disks and ligaments.

In light of this, Panjabi[602] defined spinal instability as a significant decrease in the capacity of the stabilizing system to maintain intervertebral neutral zones within the physiologic limits so there is no major deformity, neurologic deficit, or incapacitating pain.

A lumbar segment is considered unstable when it exhibits abnormal movement in quality (abnormal coupling patterns) or in quantity (abnormal increased motion).[179] This instability can be asymptomatic or symptomatic, depending on the demands made on the motion segment. Instability (secondary) is seen in all ages—in the young, in spondylolisthesis or following trauma; and in middle-aged or older patients, in degenerative conditions.[300]

With disk degeneration, vertebral motion becomes irregular, allowing rocking, gliding, and rotation of the adjacent vertebrae with excessive posterior excursion of facet joints. In degenerative spondylolisthesis or retrospondylolisthesis, degenerative subluxation of the facet joint allows posterior or anterior displacement of the vertebral body. The symptoms are those of instability and spinal and intervertebral canal stenosis consequent to secondary changes. Anterior displacement of a vertebral body on the one below causes nerve root traction and compression. These patients (often elderly) may require decompression by laminectomy and stabilization by fusion.

Primary instability occurs chiefly in men in their 30s and 40s, when they are vulnerable to such strains as heavy lifting, falls, and rotational injuries.[300,542] Moran and King[542] found "primary instability" of lumbar vertebrae to be the most common cause of low back pain. Jungham[364,365] labeled this form of lumbar instability "pseudospondylolisthesis" because there is no neural arch defect.

The disk may not be an unstable element in spondylolisthesis or after a ligamentous rupture, despite the fact that it is always involved. In some cases, a deranged disk is part of the complex of instability; in others, it is the only unstable element.

Instability may be present in extension, flexion, lateral tilt, lateral displacement, or rotation.[300,592,752] The main effect of rotational injuries is on the intervertebral disk itself.[300] Hyperextension strains are the most common cause of back pain resulting from segmental instability. This disruption in the normal mechanism of the joint causes a constant position of hyperextension at the posterior facet joint. In this case, there is no free play in the joint; it is held at its physiologic limit constantly, so that even a slight hyperextension strain causes irritation and pain.

Dynamic roentgenograms in flexion-extension and side-bending are a simple, reliable way to determine if motion segment laxity is present.[179] The mobility examination reveals increased active and passive movement at the involved level. Some patients describe a "slipping" or catching sensation or a feeling of instability associated with movement, but this is far from being a reliable or consistent finding. The segment involved is tender to palpation.

Typically, the low back pain of patients with segmental instability is aggravated by both activity and inactivity. Prolonged sitting or standing causes aching, morning stiffness is common, and minor injury causes acute pain with diffuse radiation to the buttocks. The classic sign is lumbar insufficiency (reversal of the normal motion): when extending from the flexed position, rather than extending the upper trunk over the buttocks, the patient brings the buttocks and legs forward beneath the upper trunk in a ducking, irregular movement. Other events observed during active movement tests include pushing up from the thighs for support when returning from flexion; a tendency to maintain a lumbar lordosis during flexion; hinging or fulcruming at one or more spinal levels; a momentary catch during flexion, causing a directional change; and guarded motion performance.[583]

In the classic instability syndrome of spondylosis with a definable skeletal defect (common in adolescents), hamstring tightness (in defense of the instability) is the classical sign.[538] Transient neurologic signs, such as those arising from a spondylolisthesis and causing neurogenic claudication, indicate instability.[609] For example, a runner who clinically has an unstable spondylolisthesis may develop pain and neurologic deficit after 5 to 10 miles. Conservative treatment consists of postural training, muscle strengthening to improve the power of the trunk both regionally and segmentally, lumbosacral supports (corsets or braces), and prophylactic guidance and adherence to good body mechanics. See disorders of movement and spinal stabilization below for additional consideration in assessment and treatment of segmental intervertebral instability.

Effects of Aging

SPINAL STENOSIS

Spinal stenosis includes narrowing of the spinal canal (Fig. 22-4F), nerve root canals, and intervertebral foramina, all of which cause nerve root entrapment.[68] Patients with spinal stenosis experience back pain, transient motor deficits, tingling, and intermittent pain in one or both legs; this is worsened by standing or walking (neurogenic claudication) and somewhat relieved by sitting.[639] Pain of neurogenic claudication, unlike claudication of vascular origin (which disappears quickly with rest), does not ease very readily with rest and may persist for several hours. Clinically, the bicycle test of van Genderen[182] and the stoop test (see below) may be used.

In some patients, symptoms may be relieved by surgical correction.[7,11,27,677] Physical therapy is directed at increasing mobility (flexion–distraction mobilizations, manual stretching, exercises, or traction) and improving the posture to reduce lordosis.[688] Lordosis tends to decrease the size of the intervertebral foramen and increase the symptoms.[608]

Liyang and associates[447] demonstrated that lumbar spinal canal capacity, specifically the dural sac, was enlarged during flexion and decreased with extension. Modification of activities of daily living, achieving ideal lumbar posture through the principles of dynamic lumbar stabilization, endurance exercise, back school, stretching, techniques for unloading the spine, regaining neural mobility, and side-posture spinal manipulations (for lateral recess stenosis and central canal stenosis) are useful in the conservative management of spinal stenosis.[178,392,632,650]

DEGENERATIVE SPONDYLOLISTHESIS

Degenerative spondylolisthesis (Fig. 22-4D) is common in the elderly. Women are more commonly affected than men.[374] Pain includes a neurogenic claudication type with unilateral leg pain. Slip rarely progresses beyond 33%. Foot drop may occur but sciatic tension signs are usually absent. Most patients can be treated nonoperatively (see below) but refractory symptoms may respond to surgery.

DEGENERATIVE LUMBAR SCOLIOSIS

Degenerative lumbar scoliosis is a lateral deviation of the spine that typically develops after age 50.[764] Degenerative scoliosis is associated with loss of lordosis, axial rotation, lateral listhesis, and spondylolisthesis. Although the etiology is unclear, degenerative scoliosis is associated with facet incompetence, degenerative disk disease, and hypertrophy of the ligamentum flavum, leading to back pain and possible neurogenic claudication. Indications for treatment include pain, radiculopathy or myelopathy, and progressive deformity.

Nonsurgical care focuses on exercise, patient education, kinesthetic sense of good alignment, and nonnarcotic medication. Correction of lateral pelvic tilt associated with a lumbar curve can be helped by a proper lift on the side of the low iliac crest. Unilateral pronation may also contribute to the asymmetry and muscle imbalances found in degenerative lumbar scoliosis. The use of a foot orthotic may be indicated. Asymmetrical exercises should be designed to stretch out muscle groups that are too short. Longer and weaker antagonist or synergist should be strengthened and supported to provide balance to the region.

OSTEOPOROSIS

Osteoporosis is the most common metabolic bone disease in adults.[212] Although loss of bone itself does not normally cause symptoms, associated fractures or collapse of vertebrae can cause considerable pain. The pain produced is thought to be secondary to pressure on nerve roots or on sensory fibers in the periosteum. Women are more commonly affected than men; more than half of women age 45 and older have roentgenographic evidence of osteoporosis in the lumbar spine.[339] The cause is unknown, but many theories have been proposed, including lack of estrogen and longstanding calcium deficiency.

The most prominent manifestations of osteoporosis in terms of vertebral collapse are usually localized to the thoracic and upper lumbar region, with pain referred diffusely to the low back (see Chapter 20, Thoracic Spine).[564,683]

Treatment is concentrated on pain-reduction measures and increasing exercise and functional activities. With anterior compression fractures, active and passive exercises are emphasized. All positions and activities involving flexion should be avoided.[669]

Exercise may be an effective strategy, either by improving the peak bone mass attained in young adulthood or by reducing the rate of bone loss in later life.[591] Goals for those with established osteoporosis should include the maintenance of bone mass, strength training, increased coordination, aerobic activity, and sensory integration of balance, postural training, and reduction of pain.[43] Sinaki[702–705] and Bennell and associates[43] have reviewed exercises that are safe and effective for osteoporotic subjects. Isometrics and extension exercises are probably the most useful.[702]

Participation in a variety of high-impact activities should be encouraged to maximize peak bone mass in children and adolescents. In the middle adult years, small increases in bone mass may be achieved by structured weight-training and weight-bearing exercise. In the older adult years, the aim is to conserve bone mass (particularly if osteopenia or osteoporosis is present), reduce the risk of falls, promote good posture and improve mobility and function.[43,692]

KISSING LUMBAR SPINAL PROCESSES

Increased lordosis with disk collapse may lead eventually to "kissing spines" (Baastrup's syndrome).[29] This condition may develop because of degenerative changes in many segments and lordotic postural stresses. The resulting chronic impaction of the spinous processes is accompanied by ligamentous changes and interferes considerably with vertebral mechanics. The flattening of the ligamentous system and disk may create instability of the intervertebral joint and, in some cases, hypermobility of the joint.[364] Of the lumbar movements, extension is the most limited and painful in the low back.[262] Relief is gained by bending forward or by putting the knees to the chest.

The goal of treatment is to reduce the pressure and lordosis. According to Paris, the best method is to lessen the lordosis by stretching the tight myofascia, and strengthening exercises for the abdominal muscles.[608]

Other Tissues and Structures

The most common diagnoses in patients with acute low back pain of 0 to 3 months' duration are nonspecific (e.g., lumbosacral or ligamentous strains, muscular sprains, lumbar dorsal syndromes); only 10 to 20% can be given a precise pathologic diagnosis.[558] Many of the acute temporary painful episodes of low back pain are caused by acute muscular, ligamentous, or capsular strains.[50,130,285,374,455,468,587] Practically all anatomical structures in the region of the motion segment have been cited as a source of pain and have had their proponents in the etiologic discussion. For the most part, conditions involving the soft tissues await further clinical attention and research. There is no clear way to ascribe low back pain to fasciitis, fibrositis, myositis, ruptured or degenerative ligaments, strains or sprains, synovitis of the facet joints, or hypertrophy of the ligamentum flavum.[279,280] It is clear, however, that many of these structures do have sensory innervation and are potential sources of pain.[209,379] Hirsch and associates have documented fine and complex encapsulated nerve endings in the lumbosacral fascia, supraspinous and interspinous ligaments, and vertebral periosteum.[312,314] The facet (apophyseal) joint capsules and the outer third of the annulus are also innervated.

Most cases of uncomplicated acute low back pain can be expected to subside within 3 weeks. Management should be directed at excluding other pathologic processes and providing relief of symptoms and localized therapy. Treatment may progress to graduated activity with a maintenance exercise program and education in the care of the low back in working and recreational life.

LIGAMENTS

Ligaments have been cited as a source of low back pain.[83,587, 634,825] Referred pain from specific spinal ligamentous structures follow no known neurologic pattern.[60,63] Based on clinical experience, Maitland[471] reported that ligamentous pain is felt maximally over the ligament and that the pain may spread into the lower limb. Movements that stretch the ligament/capsule may produce sharp local pain or a stretched sensation at the symptomatic site.[766] Both the supraspinatus and interspinous ligaments have an extensive net work of free nerve endings (type IV receptors) together with Ruffini corpuscles and Pacinian corpuscles. It has been suggested that the proprioceptive role for the ligaments is to prevent excessive strain in fully flexed postures and possibly under excessive shear forces. The iliolumbar ligament, an extremely important structure that stabilizes the lumbar spine on the sacrum, is commonly injured with a mechanism of forward bending combined with twisting.[455]

Postural strain will affect the nociceptors in the capsules of the facet joints and the ligaments of the posterior arch, which happens when prolonged or increased postural pressure falls on the normal tissues, or when abnormal (traumatized, inflamed or deformed) ligaments are subject to normal postural stress.[587] Ligamentous pain is thought to arise from a weakened ligament, which, when stretched, produces pain and perhaps trigger muscle guarding. The postural syndrome, described by Van Wijmen,[782] appears when normal ligaments are subject to abnormal mechanical stress. This happens with inappropriate spinal loading; poor sitting posture or prolonged bent positions. With the aging spine, abnormal mechanical stresses can originate as result of decreasing vertebral height with increased loads applied posteriorly to the spine. Characteristic of the postural syndrome includes intermittent vague lumbar pain, induced by the maintenance of positions

for a prolonged time and abolished by posture correction or movement.[631] Time factor is important in differentiation from dysfunction pain. Some time must pass before pain becomes apparent: the longer the posture is held the more pain. Spinal movements during the examination are full range and usually painless since the stress applied is not maintained long enough to induce pain. Classically, self-treatment and prophylaxis are recommended.[587] The patient should be informed about the pain mechanism and taught how to avoid static postures. Sclerosing and prolotherapy injections are often beneficial.[175,276,277,278,529,587,589,673,822]

Traumatic ligamentous strains include flexion strains that exceed the limits of the interspinous and supraspinous ligaments.[59,83,139,262,276,587] Torn spinal ligaments (interspinous and supraspinous ligaments) appear to be the result of ballistic loading (particularly slips and falls) or traumatic sporting activity with the spine at its end range of motion.[503] Those with recently developing spine symptoms and accompany spine instability can often recount prior incidents in which ligaments could have been damaged. A typical patient with this type of lesion is a middle-aged person who complains of sudden onset (after twisting) of one-sided back pain localized to the fourth or fifth level in the lumbar spine.[550] Pain sometimes radiates down over the gluteal region. Symptoms are increased by certain movements and relieved by rest. The patient particularly resists extension of the affected level, as this movement compresses an already acutely tender and edematous interspinous ligament between the spinous process of the sacrum and that of L5. The intervertebral space is acutely tender, but flexion of the lumbar spine in the supine position gives temporary relief because the injured ligament is no longer compressed.[130]

Ligamentous strains need time to heal. During the subacute stage, if mild mobilization and range of motion are used, normal mobility is likely to be achieved by the time complete healing has occurred. If the joint capsule or ligamentous structures are actually torn or overstretched during injury, the joints may be hypermobile (unstable) when healing is complete. Because ligamentous pain arises from weakened ligaments, it makes sense to reduce the stress on these ligaments by correct or neutral postures supported by adequate muscle action and positions. In time, the ligaments should regain some of their integrity with less movement present on examination.

MUSCLES AND MYOFASCIAL STRUCTURES

Myofascial restrictions may occur from overuse or overstrain and also accompany any other type of injury in low back pain. These restrictions limit function and may lead to adverse changes in other structures, such as the disk or facet joints.

Acute muscle strains, producing partial tears of muscle tissue attachments, typically are a young man's injury, where strong muscles are guarding a healthy spine.[301,378,458,524] Primary muscle disorders will probably heal no matter what care is given, but stiffness, weakness, and postural changes may occur during healing. To avoid loss of function and adaptive postural changes, the activity level and mobilization treatment should be increased as the patient progresses.

Despite the widespread use of exercises, there is little scientific information about their effectiveness in the management of acute low back pain. Kendall and Jenkins[385] compared a variety of exercise regimens and concluded that isometric exercises were most effective.

According to Wyke,[820] myofascial pain is one of the common causes of primary backache resulting from irritation of the nociceptive system that is distributed through the muscle masses of the low back, their fascial sheaths, intramuscular septa, and the tendons that attach them to the vertebral column and pelvis. Contrary to traditional opinions, inflammatory disorders of the back muscles and their related connective tissues are seldom the cause of low back pain. More often, backache of myofascial origin is the result of muscle fatigue, reflex muscle spasm, or trauma. According to Rovere[653] and Keene and Drummond,[378] the most common cause of low back pain in the athlete is overuse, with resultant strains or sprains of the paravertebral muscles and ligaments.

Several muscle pain syndromes are reported in the literature—for instance, the tenderness at motor points described by Gunn and Milbrandt,[270,271] which seem to fall within the myofascial pain and dysfunction group discussed by Travel and Simons.[763] A report by Gunn and Milbrandt and suggestions by others imply that sympathetic phenomena such as trophic changes, cutaneous and myalgic hyperalgesia, increased muscle tone, and piloerection can be seen early and late in patients with "secondary" back pain caused by some degree of injury to the dorsal root ganglion or peripheral nerve.[270,271,695,696] Skin, connective tissue, and muscle may share in sensory disorders, and these detectable changes may be confusing: their typical or unexpected distribution conforms more to a vasal rather than a neural topography. They are ascribed to early and reversible neuropathy rather than late and severe denervation.

Treatment of muscular back pain currently is the cause of some confusion, but major approaches include acupuncture, acupressure, spray and stretch, contract–relax techniques, soft tissue mobilizations, dry needling, and anesthetic injections. Procaine may be the least mycotoxic agent; steroids are not indicated for muscle use.[763]

Spinal disorders primarily of muscle origin are uncommon. Although muscle guarding or intrinsic muscle spasm usually accompanies spinal pain regardless of the underlying cause, there is no neurophysiologic reason for a normal muscle to spontaneously go into spasm. According to Wyke,[818] type IV joint receptors in joint capsules, fat pads, and ligaments, when subjected to sufficient irritation, provoke intense nonadapting motor unit responses simultaneously in all muscles related to the joint, as well in more remote muscles elsewhere in the body.

Dysfunction may lead to nociception (noxious stimulus) that will lead to a state of prolonged involuntary holding. Prolonged muscle guarding leads to circulatory stasis and the retention of metabolites. The muscle then becomes inflamed (myositis) and localized tenderness develops. This intrinsic muscle spasm adds additional pain. Prolonged intrinsic muscle spasm tends to generate up and down the spine and may aggravate areas of degenerative joint and disk disease. During examination, muscle guarding and intrinsic muscle spasm may be noted during palpation or observation, and a positive weight-shift sign may be noted.

According to Nachemson and Bigos,[559] although available data do not support the incrimination of muscle injury as a source of low back disorders, there is indirect evidence to warrant muscle rehabilitation. Even if the musculature was not injured at the time of onset of low back pain symptoms, the subsequent decrease in activity would affect endurance, stamina, and fitness. They advocate aerobic exercise, which also is a means of treating depression, a common finding with at least chronic low back pain.[9,219,341,709] An increase in endorphins has been demonstrated in the cerebrospinal fluid (CSF)[24] and in the bloodstream[207] with aerobic training. Other benefits include positive effects of increased mental alertness,[184,824] sleep,[219,709] stamina,[375] improved self-image, and reversal of activity level compatible with chronic pain.[220,223]

SACROILIAC JOINT

It is impossible to discuss management of the lumbar spine without mentioning the sacroiliac joint. The pain felt at this joint is usually referred from the lumbosacral junction secondary to disk degeneration. However, subluxation (sprains) and dislocations do occur, especially in persons younger than 45. Typical presenting symptoms are pain on resistive hip abduction and weight bearing, as well as tenderness of the symphysis pubis.

Osteopaths, followed by specialists in physical medicine and orthopaedists and others, have suggested that sacroiliac subluxations may be responsible for low back pain and even sciatica.[67,73,160,174,257,530,619,623,730] Involvement of this region must be ruled out when evaluating the lumbar spine. Treatment of this region and even the entire lower quadrant often must be included in the total management of lumbar spine conditions (see Chapter 23, Sacroiliac Joint and Lumbar–Pelvic–Hip Complex).

Combined States

One of the greatest frustrations in the management of spinal pain is that the patient rarely has a single defined abnormality. The nature of degenerative or traumatic spinal disease is such that multiple joints in one or more segments can be involved, and the patient can suffer pain from each component of the disease at different times. In cases of chronic spinal pain with little improvement, the patient usually presents with more than one syndrome.

Degenerative disk disease might not produce any symptoms, but the patient can have pain from secondarily affected facet joints or can suffer from disk pain, complicating the dilemma. Any of these causes of pain can be superimposed on nerve root compression. All the elements of this lesion complex may require treatment.

Other conditions to be considered by the physician include viscerogenic pathologic processes, vascular lesions, ankylosing spondylitis, Scheuermann's disease, and rheumatoid arthritis of the spinal joints, extraspinal lesions, and intraspinal lesions.[746]

EVALUATION

An accurate history is the key component for successful treatment of the low back. The examination entails subjective questions regarding the onset of symptoms and their present status, and the physical examination, which consists of tests and measurements of the symptomatic area. Evaluation of the soft tissues and a scan examination of the lumbar spine and lower extremity are covered in Chapter 5, Assessment of Musculoskeletal Disorders and Concepts of Management, and Chapter 24, Lumbosacral–Lower Limb Scan Examination. The scan examination of the lumbar spine and lower limb is oriented toward detecting gross or subtle biomechanical abnormalities and determining the presence of common lumbar or lower extremity disorders.

Because of the strategic location of the lumbar spine, this structure should be included in any examination of the spine in terms of posture or in any examination of the lower limb joints, particularly the hip and sacroiliac joints. Unless there is a definitive history of trauma, it is difficult to know to which area to direct physical examination procedures after completing the history. Thus, the lumbar spine, sacroiliac joints, and lower extremity joints should be examined sequentially.

History

A general approach to history-taking is described in Chapter 5, Assessment of Musculoskeletal Disorders and Concepts of Management. The concepts presented there apply to the evaluation of the lumbar spine. History-taking of the lumbar spine is probably best done using a combination of a written questionnaire and an interview to assess reliability and to guarantee a thorough review.[336,337,721,788] All aspects of the history are important, because different conditions may be related to the patient's age, gender, occupation, and family history. Previous history of trauma, accidents, or other episodes is considered with respect to recent history. The frequency and duration of each attack and knowledge of the exact mechanism of injury is often helpful and may give clues as to which tissues may have been stressed. For example, disk lesions usually have an insidious onset caused by repeated activities related to slump sitting, lifting, and forward-bending; joint locking is often caused by a sudden, unguarded movement. Inflammatory and systemic disorders usually present with a subtle onset; sprains and strains involve aggravation or trauma.

The history should include the chief complaints and a pain drawing. When using a body chart (Fig. 22-5), the area, type, depth, and intensity of pain are ascertained, and the areas and

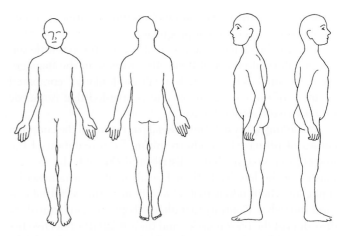

■ **FIG. 22-5.** Body chart for recording subjective and objective information.

types of sensory disturbance are recorded. The pictorial record of information may, by reference to sclerotomes, myotomes, and dermatomes, indicate which nerve root, if any, is involved. It also helps to distinguish organic pain from psychologic pain fairly well.[104,539,636,793] If pain has been present for a significant time, other tests should be used for functional overlay.[569,721,801] The Oswestry function test and the McGill Pain Questionnaire are helpful in objectifying the patient's perception of the quality of pain and its effect on function.[506,520]

Taking each symptomatic area separately, establish by questioning the severity and irritability of the symptoms, and check the level of activity necessary to bring on the pain or other symptoms. Ascertain how the patient eases the symptoms and how long this takes. Determine if there are any reliable historical clues to disease by reviewing the following points:

I. Signs and Symptoms
    A. Are there any postures or actions that specifically increase or decrease the symptoms or cause difficulty? Patients with mechanical problems affecting the low back (i.e., herniated disks, osteoarthritic facet joints, or spondylolisthesis) know precisely which factors aggravate and which relieve their symptoms. For example, pain arising from the facet joints is often relieved by sitting and forward-bending, but walking is likely to be painful.

    According to White,[800] the diagnosis of annular tear is suggested by pain that is aggravated by sitting, relieved by extension, and not stimulated by standing and walking (except prolonged standing).

    Classic radiculopathy causes radicular pain radiating into a specific dermatomal pattern with paresis, loss of sensation, and reflex loss. The classic history for radiculopathy resulting from disk herniation is back pain that progresses to predominantly leg pain. It is worsened by increases in intraspinal pressure such as coughing, sneezing, and sitting. Leg pain predominates over back pain and mechanical factors increase the pain.[686] Physical examination shows positive nerve-stretch signs. A dermatomal distribution of leg pain that is made worse by straight-leg raising, sitting, or supine foot dorsiflexion, neck flexion, jugular compression, and direct palpation of the popliteal nerve is characteristic of radiculopathy.

Patients with mechanical problems do not complain of symptoms being aggravated by "everything" they do. The person who develops spontaneous low back pain initially noted at night but later presenting constantly must be investigated for organic disease (e.g., tumor, abdominal or pelvic disease). The possibility of any nonmechanical pathologic process may be exposed here, perhaps in the way of constant, unremitting pain that is worse at night; the patient regularly must get out of bed to find relief.

B. Establish whether there is any diurnal or nocturnal variation. Is the pain worse in the morning or evening? As the day goes on? For example, in chronic degenerative lumbar disk disease, the history is of sudden catching pain in the back, morning stiffness that wears off to allow activity with minimal pain, and a prolonged (many hours) increase in pain after heavy use or abusive positioning. This is too much like the history given by White for facet arthropathy (transient pain reproduced with certain motions and positions, including rotation, with "catching" pains and relief in neutral) to allow a diagnosis to be made from historical information alone.[800]

C. Which movements hurt? Which movements are stiff? Postural or static muscles tend to respond to pathologic processes by tightness in the form of spasm or adaptive shortening; dynamic or phasic muscles tend to respond by atrophy.[345,346] Tightness of hamstrings or trunk erectors frequently develops in various back syndromes and similar postural defects, whereas abdominal and gluteal muscles show weakness. Janda[345] suggests that just as we have a capsular pattern of joint restriction, so may we have a typical muscle pattern.

1. Does the patient describe a painful arc of movement on forward- or side-flexion? If so, it may indicate a disk protrusion with a nerve root riding over the bulge.[146,731] The phenomenon of a painful arc throws light on intra-articular mechanics (see Chapter 18, Spine), in which the nucleus tends to move backward during trunk flexion (see Fig. 18-13). According to Cyriax,[146] as trunk flexion proceeds, the movement comes to the half-flexed position when the surfaces have moved enough to reverse the tilt. At this point, a mobile fragment of disk moves sharply backward, jarring the dura by pressure transmitted through the posterior longitudinal ligament. Pain may reappear at the extreme of trunk flexion if the loose part is squeezed even further backward.[146]

   Pain associated with an acute injury or inflammation often presents if the joint is moved in any direction. Pain while resting suggests an inflammatory process.

2. In what position does the patient sleep? Prone-lying for a person with restricted extension compresses the posterior tissues and causes ischemia.

3. Is there a change in symptoms in rising from a sitting position? Change may indicate possible ligamentous instability. The action of changing position is painful, but when an upright position is acquired the pain is diminished.

D. Does the patient describe a slipping, popping, or clicking sensation that is associated with certain movements? Popping that cannot be repeated every time is thought to be related to the vacuum effect that is experienced if the joint surfaces are separated suddenly.[131,670] This is a normal phenomenon, and if a joint seems to pop quite easily it indicates a hypermobile joint.

II. Special Considerations for the Lumbar Spine

A. Does the patient experience tingling and numbness in the limbs or the perineal (saddle) or pelvic regions? The adult spinal cord ends at the bottom of the L1 vertebra and becomes the cauda equina. The nerve roots extend in such a way that it is rare for the disk to pinch the nerve root of the same level (except when the protrusion is more lateral). For example, a herniated disk between L4 and L5 usually compresses the fifth lumbar nerve root.

B. Has there been any change in micturition habits associated with back trouble or sphincter disturbance (particularly urinary retention)? If so, proceed with caution; this condition may involve more than the lumbar spine or may result from spinal stenosis or a disk problem. A disk derangement may cause total urinary retention, vesicular irritability, or loss of desire or awareness of the necessity to void.[459]

C. Is the patient taking any medications? Are anticoagulants or steroids being taken, or have they been taken in the past? Long-term steroid therapy can lead to osteoporosis.

D. Is there any increase in pain with coughing, deep-breathing, laughing, or the Valsalva maneuver? All of these actions increase the intrathecal pressure and suggest a pathologic process pressing on the theca (wrapping of the spinal cord).[328]

E. How is the patient's general health? Is body weight stable?

F. Has the patient had a roentgenographic examination? If so, x-ray overexposure must be avoided; if not, roentgenograms may aid in the diagnosis.

G. Has the patient undergone any major surgery? If so, when was the surgery performed, what condition was being treated, and what was the site of surgery?

H. Is there any history (or family history) of rheumatoid arthritis or ankylosing spondylitis, diabetes, or vascular disease? Previous treatment for malignant disease or osteoporosis may be a clue to the current problem. Likewise, a brief systemic history might provide important information.

III. History. The history section completes the impression of the severity, irritability, and particularly the nature of the presenting condition. Putting the history at the end of the subjective examination facilitates constructive questioning.[104]

A. Recent history. A good way to take a current pain history is to ask the patient to describe a typical 24-hour period.

Some points in the recent history of the pain that may help to provide a clue to diagnosis include:

1. When? Sudden or gradual onset?
2. Cause, if any? If there is any obvious cause, obtain the direction, amount, and duration of any forces involved.
3. If there is no obvious cause, were there any predisposing factors?
4. Where was the pain first felt? Did it spread to the leg? Did any sensory disturbances develop?
5. How have the symptoms varied? What has been the effect of any treatment?
6. If the condition is improving or worsening, does the patient know why? Has a different activity or posture been used?

   Often using a pain or symptom scale improves communication. The scale is rated from 0 to 10; 0 is no pain at all and 10 is the worst pain that the patient has ever experienced. Patients may be asked to grade their pain on a graph throughout the day. Pain that does not go below a 3 with rest may be related to a psychologic problem, cancer, or a disease process originating in a location other than a degenerative spinal segment.[804]

B. Past history. Elicit the patient's general history, especially of any past spinal symptoms or injury. When was the first episode? Gradual or sudden? Cause? Site of pain? Any referral? Duration of first attack? What treatment was received, and what was its effect? Did the patient completely recover after the attack?

C. From past to present. How many episodes, and with what frequency? Local or local and referred symptoms? How long do the attacks usually last? Is treatment usually necessary? If so, what treatment is used, and what is the effect? Is the patient symptom-free between episodes?

Dilemma of Diagnosis

According to DeRosa and Porterfield[163] and others, therapists must accept the fact that it is usually impossible to identify the tissues that are causing pain. The Quebec Task Force on Spinal Disorders recognized this dilemma of diagnosis and recommended 11 classifications of activity-related spinal disorders.[723] DeRosa and Porterfield[163] have proposed a modified version of these categories that are more relevant to a scheme for manual therapy diagnosis (Box 22-1).

Physical Examination

OBSERVATION

Observe the patient's posture, body type (i.e., ectomorphic, mesomorphic, endomorphic, or mixed), and ability to move freely. (See Chapter 24, Lumbosacral–Lower Limb Scan Examination, for common gait abnormalities and possible causes.)

BOX 22-1   **SPINAL DISORDERS CLASSIFICATION**

1. Back pain without radiation
2. Back pain with referral to extremity, proximally
3. Back pain with referral to extremity, distally
4. Limb pain greater than back pain
5. Back pain with radiation and neurological signs
6. Postsurgical status (<6 months or >6 months)
7. Chronic pain syndrome

Reprinted with permission from DeRosa CP, Porterfield JA: A physical therapy model for treatment of low back pain. Phys Ther 72:261–269, 1992.

FUNCTIONAL ACTIVITIES

Assess whether spinal movements are free or restricted by watching the patient getting into or out of a chair and observing the position he or she adopts while sitting and while undressing. Then undertake a more formal inspection of bony structures and alignment.

INSPECTION

Have the patient stand with the back, shoulders, and legs exposed for inspection. Features such as pelvic level, disturbances of spinal curves, or other deformities may be observed; view the patient from the front, back, and sides. Record specific alterations in bony structure or alignment, soft tissue configuration, and skin status.

I. Bony Structure and Alignment

   See the section on assessment of structural alignment in Chapter 24, Lumbosacral–Lower Limb Scan Examination, for a discussion of this part of the examination.

II. Soft Tissue Inspection

   A. Muscle contour. Note obvious asymmetries in muscle bulk. The calves or hamstrings on one side may be atrophied in the presence of a chronic S1–S2 radiculopathy. Seek regions of muscle tightness and muscle spasm. Muscle spasm is noted as tautness, particularly in the low back, where the erector spinae is held in a sustained contraction. One side may be tighter than the other, with subsequent listing of the torso.

III. Skin and Markings

   Observe the skin for any local swelling or cutaneous lesions such as café-au-lait spots, patches of hair, areas of pigmentation, or any abnormal depression. A tuft of hair may indicate a spina bifida occulta or diastematomyelia.[482]

IV. Joint Tests

   Joint tests include joint integrity, active and passive physiologic movements of the lumbar spine and other relevant joints. Joint play (accessory) movements complete the joint tests.

A. Joint integrity tests (lumbar stability tests).[180,428,471,617,682] It is recommended that these tests be performed on all patients with a lumbar diagnosis especially in the presence of trauma, subjective reports of cauda equina signs or symptoms, or when treatment will include any manual therapy techniques which approach end range of motion. The key to these tests is to take up the slack of angular motion first, before attempting to gain a further linear glide.[180] A positive test produces excessive motion, shifting, and/or pain.

1. Anterior Shear (Fig. 22-6)
   a. Patient position. Sidelying, knee and hips drawn up into flexion, the examiner resting his or her thighs against the patient's knees.
   b. Fixation. The upper spinous process is fixed, using the index finger and middle finger of the cranial hand and is stabilized by placing the other hand over it. The caudal hand palpates the inferior interspinous space.
   c. Stress. The examiner applies a force through his or her thighs, through the patient's femurs, with the lumbar spine in neutral (~45° flexion). If the test is positive for laxity at 45° of hip flexion, repeat test with lumbosacral spine in flexion (~ 90° hip flexion). Testing in flexion reveals integrity of the thoracolumbar fascia and determines the position of stability.[682]

2. Posterior shear (Fig. 22-7)
   a. Patient position. Sitting in a position of lumbar lordosis with forearms pronated and resting on the examiner's arms or shoulders. Starting at the lower thoracic spine, the examiner moves caudally applying an anterior force to the lower segment as the lumbar spine is extended thus locking the joint.
   b. Fixation. The spinous process of the inferior vertebra is fixed.

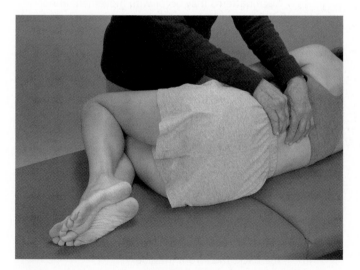

■ **FIG. 22-6.** Anterior stability test position. Knees and hips are drawn into further flexion to rest against the examiner's thighs.

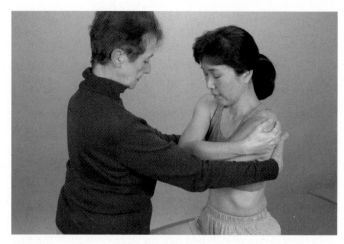

■ **FIG. 22-7.** Posterior stability test position. Hands may be resting on examiner's shoulders.

   c. Stress. While maintaining the lordosis, the patient pushes away from the examiner while the examiner palpates the interspinous space above the stabilized segment.

3. Torsion test (see Fig. 22-39*B*)
   a. Patient position: Prone.
   b. Fixation: The examiner stabilizes the superior lumbar vertebrae.
   c. Stress: the examiner applies spinal rotation by lifting the contralateral innominate bone dorsally. Note the quantity and quality of motion.

B. Active physiologic movements of the spine. With all movements, determine the range, rhythm, and quality of active movement. Watch the body contours and spinous processes carefully to observe whether the spinal joints move smoothly and evenly or whether there is any localized restriction of movement in the spinous processes between two or three vertebrae. Note disturbances of rhythm and the presence or absence of any protective deformity. Note any muscle guarding, a painful arc of motion, and whether the patient's symptoms are reproduced. The patient must actively extend the movement as far as possible. In general, facet joint restrictions are more noticeable during sidebending; conversely, restrictions caused by muscle tightness are proportionately more noticeable in forward-bending.

   With the patient standing (feet a little apart and parallel), assess:

1. Extension (backward-bending). Kneeling behind the patient, support the patient's pelvis or shoulders for stability while observing lumbar extension. Ask the patient to sequentially bend the head, shoulders, middle back, and lower back backward. The lumbar lordosis should increase from the resting position as the patient extends. Note the movement in relation to the painful site and any deviations toward one side. Observe the point on the spine at which extension originates.

a. In an acute spinal derangement, lumbar extension is negligible, with most of the observable backward-bending occurring at higher levels.

b. With multisegmental capsular restriction, lumbar extension is also markedly limited owing to premature close-packing of the facet joints.

c. The spine may deviate away from the side of a localized unilateral capsular restriction.

    The normal range is approximately 20 to 35°. Extension is often the stiffest and most painful movement with lumbar problems. Suitable methods for measuring extension externally include the use of a kyphometer,[542] goniometer (spondylometer or hydrogoniometer),[176,226,449] inclinometer,[200,241] Flexirule,[85,760] and tape measure.[216,459,534,535] The first two methods are based on a mathematical theory of angles outlined by Loebl and are expressed in degrees.[449]

2. Lateral flexion (sidebending). Have the patient sidebend the head, shoulders, middle back, and lower back, first to one side and then to the other (see Fig. 7-31). Symmetry of movement may be judged by comparing the distance from the fingertip to the fibular head on either side and by observing the degree of spinal curvature with movements in either direction. Symmetry of movement, however, is significant only with respect to the starting position; if the resting position of the spine involves a right sidebending curve, then "normal" movement would be a greater degree of sidebending to the right than to the left. Also assess the continuity of segmental movement. Reproduction of pain on passive overpressure is most likely to occur when a capsular restriction exists on the side to which the movement is performed.

a. In acute spinal derangements, such as a posterolateral disk protrusion or unilateral facet joint derangement, lumbar sidebending may be absent on one side (usually toward the involved side), especially if a functional spinal deviation exists in the erect position.

b. With multisegmental capsular restriction, sidebending is moderately restricted in both directions. All serious diseases of the lumbar spine (e.g., malignancy, ankylosing spondylitis) result in equal limitation of both left and right sidebending.[148]

c. With localized unilateral capsular restrictions, sidebending is usually only slightly limited toward the involved side. Unilateral restrictions are often difficult to detect.

    Lateral flexion is about 15° to 20°. Suitable methods for measuring lateral flexion include the use of two gravity-dependent, pendulum goniometers, one or two inclinometers,[200,241] Flexirule,[85,760] and a tape measure, using either distraction or approximation (see Fig. 20-13).[250,533,679]

3. Flexion (forward-bending). Forward flexion is an important movement and the one most likely to be limited by a disk lesion. Have the patient bend the head forward, then the middle back, and finally the low back (see Figs. 7-27 and 7-28). A painful arc may be noted. Observe the level at which lumbar flexion originates. Reversal of normal spinal rhythm on attempting to regain the erect posture after forward flexion is characteristic of disk degeneration associated with a posterior joint lesion.[458] "Hitching" is sometimes seen in patients with osteoarthritis of the facet joints; the patient first extends the lumbar spine, fixing it in lordosis, and then extends at the hips until the erect position is regained.[686] An instability problem may be present if there is a reversal of the normal pelvic rhythm, an arc or listing to one side through the range, or sharp catches of pain, or if the patient exhibits cogwheeling while he or she attempts to rise from the forward-bent position.[391,458,686]

a. If the patient has a relatively acute back problem and this movement is extremely difficult to perform—the patient may support his body weight by placing the hands on the thighs or a nearby plinth—suspect a posterior disk prolapse.

b. If the patient has a relatively acute back problem but can bend forward reasonably well, with only mild discomfort and restriction, an acute facet joint dysfunction or less severe disk prolapse might be considered. It is not unusual to see variations in lateral deviations of the spine as the patient bends forward in either instance. For example, the spine may start out deviated in the upright position and the deviations may disappear during forward-bending, or the spine may be erect on standing and deviate as forward-bending proceeds; the deviation may or may not resolve by the end point of the movement. Such patterns may occur with movement abnormalities resulting from either disk or facet joint derangements.

    If a facet is limited on one side because of meniscoid locking, muscle guarding, or capsular restriction, it will not glide forward on that side. This results in a sudden shift toward the restricted side, followed by a rapid shift back.[606] Conversely, ongoing deviations with forward-bending are typically associated with disk involvement. The patient tends to shift laterally as a unit to move the protrusion away from the irritated nerve root—away from the involved side if the prolapse is lateral to the nerve root and toward the same side if the protrusion is medial to the nerve root.[388]

c. Observe the spine during forward-bending from the back, then from the side.

    When viewing from behind, look for lateral deviation of the spine during movement. A deviated arc of movement is more likely to be secondary to an alteration of intervertebral disk mechanics; a deviation that exists up to the end point of movement is more likely to be the result of a unilateral or asymmetrical capsular restriction or a fixed scoliosis. If a fixed scoliosis exists, a rotary component is present; the side of the convexity appears higher than the side of the concavity in the forward-bent position.

When viewing from the side, assess the continuity of movement at the various spinal segments. The overall spinal curve should be relatively smooth; flattened areas may reflect segmental hypomobility, whereas angular areas may be associated with segmental hypermobility. These flattened areas or sharp angulation of the spinal curvature may also be identified during active sidebending and extension.

With full forward-bending of the lumbar spine, the normal lumbar lordosis should be straightened but is usually not reversed. Inadequate straightening of the lordosis may occur with localized or generalized capsular restriction. Reversal of the lumbar lordosis suggests hypermobility.

The maximum range of motion is 40 to 60°. Suitable methods for measuring flexion include the kyphometer,[176,664] the goniometer (the spondylometer or hydrogoniometer), the inclinometer, and the tape measure (including the Schober test to detect and follow the loss of spinal motions in ankylosing spondylitis). Segmental measurements of flexion of the spine (T12, L3, S1) can also be determined.[200,216,241,459,494,633,679]

4. Lateral shift (side-gliding). Side-gliding movements are performed when a lateral shift is present. Lateral displacement of the pelvis on the thorax is an important test movement, especially for the lower lumbar spine. McKenzie[510] described its application fully. Have the patient move the pelvis and shoulder simultaneously in opposite directions while keeping the shoulders parallel to the ground. Watch for unilateral restriction or blocking. When the patient has a lateral shift, movement is restricted in the opposite direction.

While maintaining a stabilized upper thoracic area, ask the patient to allow the hips and pelvis to slide laterally in the horizontal plane to the left and right.[510]

With the patient sitting, knees together, compare the sitting posture to the standing posture. Note any changes in bony structure and alignment.

5. Rotation. With the arms held straight out in front and the hands together, have the patient turn toward the left and then the right. As rotation occurs in one direction, sidebending occurs in the opposite direction. The spinous processes move in the opposite direction of rotation. Assess symmetry of movement by observing the lateral curvature of the lower spine. The same considerations apply to the assessment of rotation as discussed under sidebending. There is no significant rotation of the lumbar spine (3° to 18°), but it is a useful test for the patient with nonorganic back pain.[550] Structural stresses could include torsional and shear stresses of the disk and neural arch. The contralateral facet is compressed, and the ipsilateral joint is stretched. Suitable methods for measuring lumbar spine rotation externally include the use of a tape measure and application of the rotometer developed by Twomey and Taylor.[535,773]

6. Quadruped tests. With the patient in quadriped:
    a. Observe any asymmetry in the lumbar region. Have the patient cycle through full lumbar flexion and extension (cat/camel exercise) with slow smooth motions (Fig. 22-8).[502,627] Observe segmental mobility and note any excessive segmental hinging at a

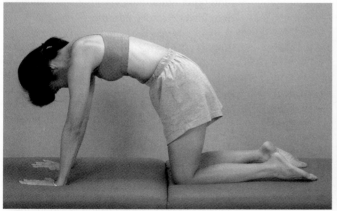
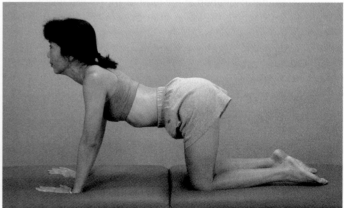

A   **B**

■ **FIG. 22-8.** Quadriped flexion–extension exercises are performed by slowly cycling through **(A)** full spine flexion to **(B)** full extension. Spinal mobility is emphasized.

particular level. Determine whether flexion or extension of the back worsens or lessons symptoms. This may help in deciding which form of exercise (flexion versus extension) should be prescribed.[627]

b. Also assess backward and forward rocking.

c. Rocking backward. Symptoms of the lumbar spine usually decrease because of the slight increase in flexion.[661] Rotation of the primary lumbar segment with instability may increase. Observe for differences in stiffness or range of motion between the two hips that may contribute to lateral tilt or rotation of the pelvis and effect the lumbar spine. If rocking backward causes symptoms, a possible extension syndrome is suggested (see segmental instability below).

d. Rocking forward. Symptoms are often increased with rocking forward motion. Symptoms may decrease (compared with corrected starting position) in the lumbar extension syndrome.[661]

7. Anterior and posterior tilt.

With the patient in a hook-lying position, determine the patient's functional position (SFP).

Morgan[543] describes the spinal functional position as "the most stable and asymptomatic position of the spine for the task at hand." Exploration of posterior and anterior tilting will indicate whether the patient's symptoms are increased, or eliminated at any point between flexion and extension. The most comfortable position is by definition the SFP. Some practitioners also refer to this position as spinal neutral.[658] The position may vary depending on the posture or activity performed by the patient (e.g., standing, supine or sitting). Identifying the SFP assists the practitioner in determining the positions and the ROM in which the patient may safely begin to exercise while controlling pain.

C. Chest expansion and active peripheral joint tests

1. Measure chest expansion from normal expiration to maximal inspiration at the level of T4. An expansion of 3 cm is within the lower limits of normal.[535] Loss of chest expansion is usually a late finding in ankylosing spondylitis. Another late sign is decreased ability to extend the neck.

2. Squatting on the heels from the standing position and returning to the erect position puts the peripheral joints through a full active range of motion. The ability to squat normally reflects the state of the hip joints as well as the power of the quadriceps and gluteal muscles. A patient who complains of low back pain radiating down the anterior aspect of the thigh and who has difficulty squatting may have a midlumbar disk lesion.[686] Changes in symptoms should be noted, as well as where in the range they occur.

D. Auxiliary tests. In most patients with symptoms arising from the lumbar spine, the active tests described above

reproduce the symptoms. If not, the following additional maneuvers may be used:

1. Passive overpressure at the end range of the active physiologic motions described above. The overpressure should be applied with care because the upper body weight is already being applied by virtue of gravity.

2. Repeated motions. It may be helpful to do repeated physiologic movements at various speeds.

3. Sustained pressure. This is applied for about 10 seconds with the lumbar spine first in extension and then in lateral flexion, when necessary to reproduce the pain.

4. Effect of active limb movements on symptoms (i.e., knee extension in sitting, hip abduction with lateral rotation in supine, hip extension and rotation in prone, shoulder flexion in quadriped).[661,778]

5. Combined motions.[79,191–193,586] These passive movement tests are designed to position the joint under maximum stress. The combining of routine physiologic movements to form test movements either opens or closes one side of the intervertebral segment. In this way, a pattern of painful movement may be found or a combination that relieves or increases symptoms. If pain is reproduced, determine whether the pain is felt in the midline or the same or opposite side, and if it radiates down the leg. Determine if the patterns are regular or irregular. These motions may be applied with and without passive overpressure.

a. Active motions without overpressure include:
   i. Lateral flexion combined with extension to the left and right
   ii. Lateral flexion combined with flexion to the right and left

b. Combined movements with passive overpressure. Securely stabilize and maintain the patient's pelvis. Once end range is reached, apply passive overpressure.
   i. Combined movements in flexion
      A. Combined movement of forward-flexion and right lateral flexion (Fig. 22-9). While maintaining a fully flexed position, the patient laterally flexes to the right. At the end of range, the therapist applies passive overpressure. Repeat to the left.
      B. Combined forward-flexion with rotation (Fig. 22-10). The patient bends forward in a fully flexed position. The patient's trunk is rotated to the right. Repeat the sequence with rotation to the left.
   ii. Combined movements in extension.
      A. Extension with lateral flexion to the right (Fig. 22-11). The patient first extends, and lateral flexion is added to this position (the patient is now in a quadrant position). The examiner stands to the side (right) and places one arm across the chest so the hand

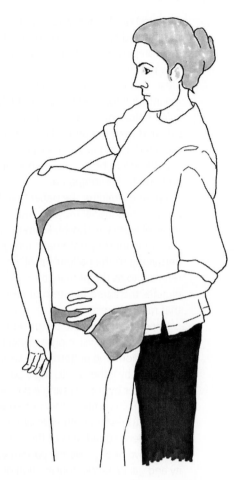

■ **FIG. 22-9.** Combined movement examination: lateral flexion in forward flexion.

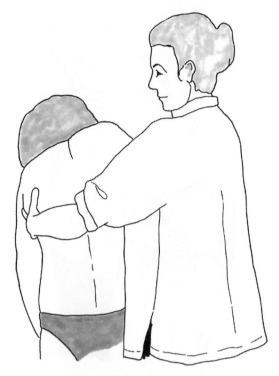

■ **FIG. 22-10.** Combined movement examination: flexion and rotation.

grasps the patient's opposite shoulder, to which extension and lateral flexion will occur. The thumb and index finger of the examiner's opposite hand are placed over the transverse process at the level of the lumbar spine to be examined. Following active extension, the thumb provides counterpressure while the upper arm is used to bring the patient's trunk into lateral flexion. Repeat this sequence on the left side.

B. Extension and rotation to the right (Fig. 22-12). The examiner places one arm across the chest so the hand grasps the opposite shoulder (left). The thumb and index finger of the opposite hand are placed over the transverse process at the level of the lumbar spine to be examined. The patient is encouraged to actively extend to the limit of the range. Using the upper hand (on the patient's shoulder), the examiner guides the trunk into rotation as the thumb applies counterpressure. Repeat this sequence on the left side.

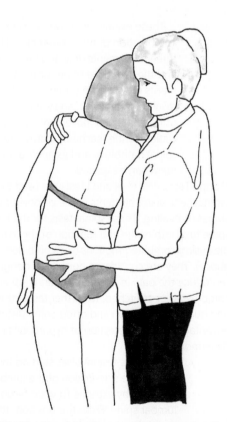

■ **FIG. 22-11.** Combined movement examination: lateral flexion in extension.

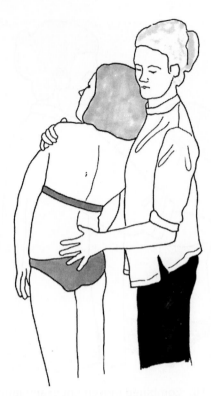

■ **FIG. 22-12.** Combined movement examination: extension and rotation.

These examining movements involve the combination of two movements. However, three movements may also be combined, and the sequence of performing movements may also be varied.[79,191–193,686] As a result of examining, analyzing, and treating using combined movements, a better appreciation of the mechanical presentation of spinal pathology and its application to treatment can be gained.

6. H and I Tests.[79,180,260] H and I tests are used to detect biomechanical impairments in the chronic or subacute stages of healing. These spinal tests for the lumbar spine test both range and function of the joint complex using combined motions (see combined motions above). They are considered quick tests designed to reproduce the pain in a structure that is either being compressed or stretched, to further test active quality and quantity of motion and offers some distinct advantages for the detection of hypomobilities and hypermobilities.

   A. H test. This test involves starting the patient with active side-flexion of the lumbar spine, followed by extreme forward flexion of the lumbar spine. From this position, the patient maintains the side flexion and moves into extension. This sequence of motions is then repeated on the opposite side. Range of motion and end feel is compared. Look for any compensatory motions and the curvature of the spine.

   B. I test. This test starts with the patient moving into full forward flexion of the lumbar spine before moving into side-flexion to one side and then the other. The test is then repeated during extreme extension and side-flexion to both sides. Range of motion and end feel is compared.

   When examining the patient we first look at the conventional movements in their three planes (see above). From them find the single most symptomatic movement pertaining to the patient's problem. This is referred to as the primary movement and dictates the altered pattern of movement that may be present.

   Depending on where the patient's symptoms prevail this will imply a stretching- or compression-type pattern, (i.e., symptoms produced by either stretching a pain-sensitive structure or by compressing a pain sensitive structure). By combing two movements or more, thus testing both sides of the anterior and posterior quadrants of the spine, we can now prove or disprove the pattern's regularity and gain a better appreciation of the mechanical presentation of spinal pathology and greater insight into the possible biomechanical causes of the spinal condition.

   These tests may be repeated in sitting to confirm the findings in standing weight bearing.

7. Positive heel-drop test. Have the patient stand on tiptoes, then drop heavily onto the heels. This causes a jarring of the spine that may be sufficient to reproduce the symptoms.[686]

E. Active segmental mobility. With the patient standing, assess:

   1. Upper lumbar spine lateral flexion. Have the patient stride-stand so that motion is directed at the upper lumbar segments. With the weight transferred to the same side (right), the patient actively sidebends to the right. Repeat to the left.

   2. L5–S1 lateral flexion. Have the patient stride-stand with weight transferred to the opposite side (left). The patient actively sidebends to the right. Repeat to the left.

   3. L5–S1 region. The patient actively tilts the pelvis forward (symphysis up) and then extends it.

F. Passive movement. Movements may include the following:

   1. Vertical compression test (see Chapter 20, Thoracic Spine, and Fig. 20-4).

   2. Posture correction. Posture correction is done to determine if a return to normal posture is possible and if

the symptoms are altered. This may help determine which structures are at fault and to what extent the postural deformity is involved in the current complaints. When an acute lumbar scoliosis is seen during an examination, attempt to correct it. If the scoliosis is caused by a moderate or mild disk protrusion (lateral shift), the correction procedure often causes centralization of the pain in the lumbar region but no increase in peripheral symptoms.[510] If the scoliosis is a protective scoliosis, as described by Finneson,[210] any attempt at correction increases pain and other symptoms in the lower extremities.

The patient stands with the elbow of the arm on the side of the lumbar convexity bent to 90°. The examiner contacts the lateral aspect of the patient's thorax with his clavicular region. The arms encircle the patient and the hands interlock to contact the lateral aspect of the patient's pelvis. The sidebending deformity is very slowly reduced with a mild lateral pressure against the pelvis, toward the therapist. (See Fig. 22-31 for the proper positioning of the therapist and the patient.)

3. Quadrant testing.[471] The quadrant test is a provocative test for a localized capsular restriction that may not cause an obvious restriction of motion or pain on active movement tests. The examiner stands to the patient's side and places one arm across the patient's chest to grasp the opposite shoulder. The other hand is placed over the lower back, with the thumb over the region of the mammillary process of about L2 on the side closest to the examiner (see Fig. 22-12). Use the upper arm to bring the patient's trunk around into sidebending, rotation, and extension, while applying counterpressure forward and inward with the other thumb. When the limit of range is reached, hold the position for 20 seconds to allow for a delayed response. This maneuver localizes a close-packed movement to the facet joint immediately superior to the examiner's thumb, therefore localizing stress to the capsule of that joint. The remaining joints, caudal to the first segment tested, are examined in the same manner in an attempt to reproduce the symptoms. The opposite side of the spine is then tested. This test is less likely to reproduce nerve root symptoms by reducing the size of the intervertebral foramen, as it may in the cervical spine, because the lumbar intervertebral foramina are larger in diameter than the exiting nerve roots.

4. Passive physiologic movements of the spine. Physiologic spinal movements of flexion, extension, rotation, and lateral flexion are tested by passive movements and compared with active motions.
   a. Flexion (forward-bending). The patient lies in supine with the knees bent. Forward-bending is done by having the therapist or patient pull the knees to the chest or by approximating the patient's knees to the axillae (see Fig. 22-25). Make

a general assessment of flexion; compare it with standing forward-bending. Repeated motions may be used to determine if the symptoms change.
   b. Extension (backward-bending). Passive backward bending is checked with the patient lying prone. Have the patient press up with the arms while letting the back sag (see Fig. 22-52). Observe range, changes in pain (centralization or peripheralization), or other symptoms. Measure the distance of the anterior-superior iliac spine from the table; about 2″ is considered within normal limits.[670] Passive backward-bending (press-ups) may also be repeated several times to determine if symptoms change with repeated motion.
   c. Lateral flexion (sidebending). The patient lies supine with the knees bent. The examiner holds the patient's legs together with hips and knees bent to 90°. Spinal sidebending is produced by rotating the patient's pelvis about a vertical axis, using the patient's leg as a lever (see Fig. 22-29).

4. Rotation. The patient lies supine with the knees bent; the thorax is stabilized by placing the arm across the rib cage. The leg furthest from the examiner is grasped behind the knee and the hip is brought to about 90° flexion. This leg is then pulled toward the operator, across the near leg. Repeat on the other side, and compare the two sides (see Fig. 22-27).

5. Passive physiologic joint movements with segmental palpation. This takes the form of passive physiologic intervertebral movements (PPIVM), which examines each segmental level to appreciate the movement of the segment. This is achieved by palpating between the spinous processes and comparing the movement obtained at each level. PPIVMs may be a useful adjunct to passive accessory intervertebral movements to identify segmental hypomobility (see below).

Note the end feels. Determine if tissue tension limits movement before the end of range. Abnormal end feel encountered may be boggy with greater than the expected movement (hypermobility), a rubbery rebound type of resistance, a fairly hard end feel (chondro-osteophyte contact), or a block.[263] Seek abnormalities such as irritability. Does movement elicit spasm, pain, or paresthesias locally or distally?
   a. Flexion–extension. (forward and backward bending; Fig. 22-13A, B). These movements may be tested by the operator flexing one or both of the patient's legs, but it is generally easier to use one leg. The patient lies on the side with the underneath leg slightly flexed at the hip and knee (a small, flat pillow under the waist keeps the lumbar spine in a neutral position). The examiner stands in front of the patient. The index or middle finger of the cranial hand rests between adjunct spinous processes, while the patient's upper leg is grasped

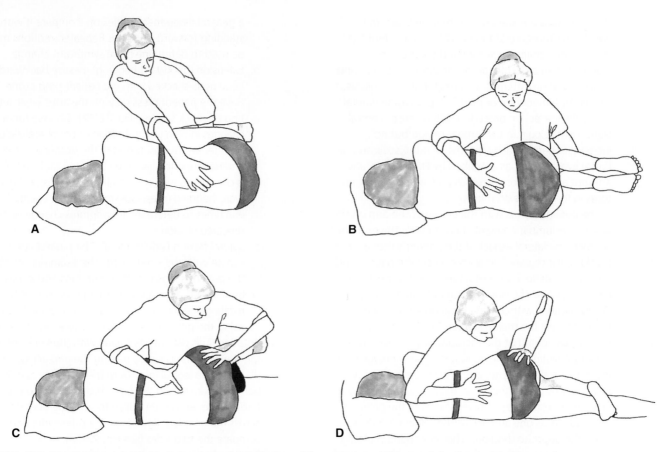

■ **FIG. 22-13.** Passive physiologic testing of **(A)** flexion, **(B)** extension, **(C)** lateral flexion, and **(D)** rotation.

at the knee (with the caudal hand) and passively flexed and released at the hip (extension). The movements of flexion and extension should be stretched to their limits. The amount of movement, noted as an opening and closing of the interspinous gap, is compared to other levels.

b. Lateral flexion (sidebending) (Fig. 22-13C). The patient lies on the side with the knees and hips bent so that the lumbar spine is relaxed midway between flexion and extension. The examiner (facing the patient) applies the caudal arm around the patient's upper pelvis and under the patient's ischial tuberosity. The examiner's cranial hand palpates between the interspinous spaces of the adjacent vertebrae (the pad of the palpating finger is placed facing upward in the underside of the interspinous space). The examiner firmly grasps the patient's pelvis and upper thigh with the caudal hand, then uses a rhythmical side-sway of the trunk toward the patient's head to produce a side-flexion movement from below upward by rocking the pelvis. Movement can be appreciated either as a gapping or approximation by the finger of the cranial hand. Repeat on the opposite side.

c. Rotation (Fig. 22-13D). The positions of the examiner and patient are similar to those used for assessing lateral flexion or sidebending but with a flat pillow placed under the patient's waist to keep the lumbar spine in neutral. The examiner leans across the patient and places the cranial forearm along the lower thoracic spine, with a reinforced finger resting against adjacent spinous processes from underneath. The caudal hand is placed over the patient's greater trochanter. As the examiner stabilizes the thorax with the cranial forearm, the patient's pelvis is rocked backward and forward so the pelvis and lumbar spine rotate. Repeat on the opposite side.

   Note: These three examinations can be modified and used as mobility techniques, using appropriate grades of movement based on the findings found on the evaluation.[370,607]

6. Passive accessory intervertebral movements (PAIVMs) (T10–L5). The examiner should note the following:
   a. The quality of movement.
   b. The range of movement.
   c. The resistance through the range of motion and at the end range of movement.

d. Any provocation of muscle spasm and the behavior of pain through the range.

The patient is in prone-lying across the table, if necessary with a cushion under the abdomen to place the lumbar spine in neutral (resting position; Fig. 22-14). The lower legs are supported on a stool (hips and knees in 90° flexion). The correct movements are achieved by moving the joint by thumb-tip pressure or with pisiform contact against the vertebral prominences. Apply the pressure slowly and carefully so that the "feel" of movement can be recognized. This springing test may be repeated several times to determine the quality of the movement. The basic maneuvers include:

i. Posteroanterior pressure against the spinous processes (using the thumb or pisiform contact).

ii. Transverse pressure against the lateral surface of the spinous process. Pressure should be applied to both sides of the spinous processes to compare the quality of movement.

iii. Posteroanterior unilateral pressures over the mammillary process of the joint to be examined. The same anterior springing pressure is applied as in central pressure evaluation. Both sides are evaluated and compared. For additional information:

A. Alter the direction of posteroanterior pressure movements: cephalad (toward the head), caudally (toward the feet), and diagonally.

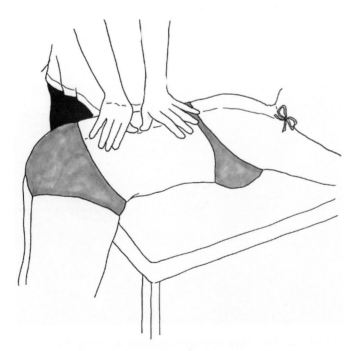

■ **FIG. 22-14.** Position of the patient for palpation and segmental mobility testing of the lumbar spine.

B. Exert counterpressure to the transverse process of the spinal process just below and over the spinous process above a tender segment to determine more precisely the location of the painful or involved segment.[468]

These procedures may elicit pain, restricted movement, or spasm. If the range of movement is limited, assess the type of resistance—caused by either a sense of tightness or muscle spasm. The direction of restriction or painful movement determines the type of mobilization therapy to be used.

7. Passive sacroiliac and peripheral joint tests. Painful joint conditions that may originate from the lumbosacral spine must be assessed. Pain from the spine can be referred to the hip, knee, and sacroiliac joints; pain originating in the hip or sacroiliac joint may be referred to the lumbar spine. Clearing tests of the peripheral joints include:

a. Sacroiliac provocation/mobility tests. These may reproduce pain from a sacroiliac disorder, and a snap might be elicited if the joint is abnormally mobile. Little movement should occur at this joint.

i. Posterior rotation. The patient lies on the side with the side to be tested on top. The examiner flexes the upper knee toward the patient's abdomen, then holds it flexed with the upper thigh or pelvis to free the hands. One hand is placed over the patient's anterior-superior iliac spine, the forearm directed diagonally in the posterocaudal direction with respect to the patient. The opposite hand is placed over the patient's ischial tuberosity, the forearm directed in an anterocephalad direction. The examiner then produces a force-couple movement to rotate the ilium backward on the sacrum while simultaneously moving the patient's hip and knee into more flexion with the examiner's pelvis or anterior thigh (see Fig. 22-46).

ii. Anterior rotation. The patient lies prone. The examiner stands at the side to be tested. The more cephalad hand is placed over the sacrum. With the opposite hand, the examiner grasps around medially to the anterior aspect of the patient's knee. The examiner pushes down on the inferior aspect of the sacrum while simultaneously lifting the patient's leg into extension to move the ilium, by way of the hip joint capsule, into a forward position on the sacrum (see Fig. 22-47).

iii. Tests to demonstrate sacroiliac fixation as described by Kirkaldy-Willis[394] is often included (see Fig. 23-15).

b. Hip joint. A test that may be used to clear the hip joint and also to assess the sacroiliac joint is the hip flexion–adduction test. This test uses the femur as a lever to stretch the posterolateral and inferior portions of the inferior capsule and to compress the superior and medial portions of the capsule. With the patient in supine, the examiner flexes the patient's knee and hip fully and then adducts the femur. As the knee is moved fully toward the patient's opposite shoulder, the examiner compresses the hip joint.

   c. Knee joint. To clear the knee, the anterior drawer test (Lachman test) performed at 25° of knee flexion, and the valgus–varus stress test at 30° of knee flexion is used (see Chapter 15, Knee).

V. Muscle Tests

   Muscle tests include resistive isometric contractions, muscle strength, control and length.

   A. Resisted isometric tests. Resisted trunk isometrics are performed in midrange, the inner and outer ranges to open and close the joint spaces to determine the effect of compression on pain production.[267] With the patient in sitting, legs abducted and feet supported, resists isometrically the trunk in all cardinal planes (forward bending, backward bending, sidebending and rotation) as well as three-dimensional motions. Pain provocated in the middle range is most suggestive of mechanical dysfunction.

   B. Muscle strength. When indicated, the examiner tests the trunk flexors, extensors, lateral flexors and rotators and any other muscles groups indicated. For details of theses tests, the reader is directed to Clarkston and Gilewich,[123] Cole et al.,[127] Hislop and Montgomery,[319] Kendall and McCreary,[384] and Palmer and Epler,[601] to determine exactly which muscles are at fault.

   C. Muscle control and stability. The relative strength of muscles is considered to be more important than the overall strength of a muscle group.[807] Relative strength is assessed by observing posture, quality of movement; and muscle recruitment patterns. Muscle imbalances and arthrokinematic deficits can cause abnormal movement patterns to develop throughout the entire kinetic chain. It is recommended that the interested reader use the reference list to explore a comprehensive muscle imbalance assessment.[64,77,82,108,122,173,323,348,354,384,435,500,659–661]

    1. Multifidi and local stabilizer of the lumbar spine. Lumbar multifidus have been found to atrophy in patients with low back pain and so should be tested.[309] The patient lies prone and the examiner applies deep pressure on either side of the lumbar spinous processes (Fig. 22-15). The patient attempts to contract the muscle fibers under the examiner's hands. Normal function is when the contraction can be held for 10 seconds and repeated 10 times.[617] An alternate method of testing the multifidi of the lower thoracic and lumbar spine is shown in Figure 20-31.[377]

    2. Abdominals. Methods of measuring isolated isometric muscle contraction for the lateral abdominal muscles has

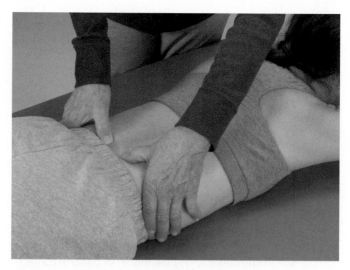

■ FIG. 22-15. Palpation for contraction of the right and left muscles at each lumbar segment of the lumbar multifidus.

been described by Jull and Richardson[362] and Richardson et al.[642] using a pressure sensor (see Fig. 20-32).

   a. Core control and lower abdominal strength can be further assessed using the straight leg-lowering test (Fig. 22-16).[26,122,322,333,363,593,660,661] A pressure sensor (set at a baseline of 40-mm HG) is place under the lumbar spine at approximately at L4-L5. The patient is instructed to perform abdominal hollowing and flatten the back maximally into the pressure cuff and table. The patient is instructed to lower the legs toward the table while maintaining a flat back. The test is over when the pressure in the cuff decreases. The hip angle is then measured.

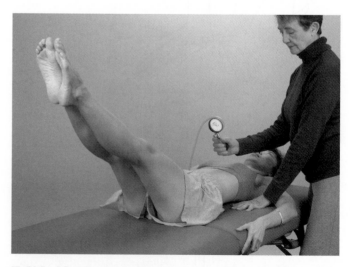

■ FIG. 22-16. Core strength assessed by using the straight leg-lowering test. A pressure sensor is placed at the lumbar spine at L4–L5.

b. Lower abdominal neuromuscular control is assessed in a similar fashion (Fig. 22-17).[26,122,322,323] The knees and hips are flexed to 90° with the pressure sensor under the lumbar spine (L4–L4) with the pressure sensor set at 40 mm Hg. The patient is again instructed in abdominal hollowing to stabilize the lumbar spine. The patient is instructed to slowly lower the legs until the pressure cuff decreases. This test indicates the ability of the lower abdominals to preferentially stabilize the lumbo–pelvic–hip complex. When the lumbar spine begins to move into extension, the hip flexors begin to work as stabilizers. This increases anterior compression and shear forces at the lumbar spine and inhibits the multifidus, internal oblique and transverse abdominus.[122]

c. Active lumbar stabilization can be test further by determining the ability of the patient to control the same position of the lumbar spine (using abdominal hollowing) while it is indirectly loaded via the upper or lower limbs and in more functional postures such as sitting or standing or during exercise or stretching.[617]

d. Torsional trunk control. With the patient in a hooklying position determine the patient's torsional truncal strength control to activate truncal cocontraction (Fig. 22-18) by applying alternating torsional forces to the pelvis.

D. Muscle endurance. Recent work has suggested that endurance has a more protective value than strength and that the balance of endurance among the torso flexors, lateral trunk musculature and extensors better discriminates those who have had back troubles from those who have not.[54,502] Tests proposed by McGill and associates[503,504] include the following:

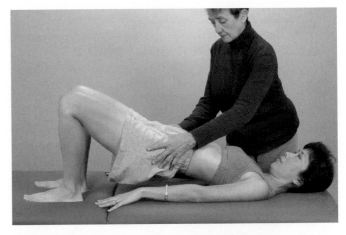

■ **FIG. 22-18.** Bridge position with resistive torsional forces applied to the pelvis to assess truncal cocontraction of back extension.

1. Testing endurance of the abdominals (rectus). (Fig. 22-19)
   a. Position of patient. Patient sitting with back resting on a 60° incline with the arms crossed over the chest and legs in the hooklying position.
   b. Fixation. Examiner provides stabilization of the feet.
   c. Test. Patient holds the isometric position (incline pulled back 10 cm [4 in]) as long as possible. Failure is determined to occur when any part of the client's back touches the incline.

2. Testing endurance of lateral musculature (quadratus lumborum, obliques) (Fig. 22-20)
   a. Position of patient. Patient lying in the full side-bridge position. Patient supports themselves on one elbow and the extended feet (top foot placed in front of lower foot). The top arm is held across the chest or at the side.
   b. Test. Patient supports themselves on the elbow and on their feet while lifting their hips off the plinth to create a straight line over their body length. Failure occurs when the subject loses the side bridge position.

3. Testing endurance of the back extensors (Fig. 22-21).
   a. Position of patient. Prone lying with pelvic girdle and lower limbs supported with a strap. The upper limbs are held across the chest or side of the body with the upper body unsupported once the test begins.
   b. Test. The trunk is raised to the horizontal position (neutral spine) and sustained in this position. Failure occurs when the upper body drops from the horizontal position.

E. Muscle length. Check the length of individual muscles, in particular theses prone to become short i.e., the erector spinae, piriformis, hamstrings, quadratus lumborum (see Fig. 23-32), iliopsoas, rectus femoris,

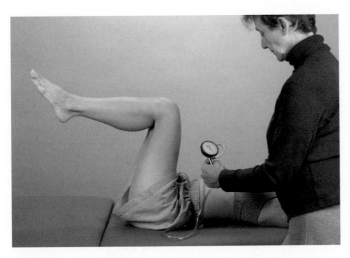

■ **FIG. 22-17.** Lower abdominal neuromuscular assessment. A pressure sensor is placed at the lumbar spine at L4–L5.

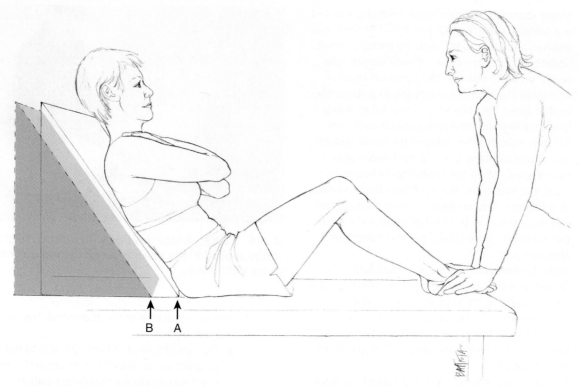

■ **FIG. 22-19.** Trunk flexor endurance test. Begin with person sitting with the trunk supported at 60°, **(A)** knee in the hook position with stabilization of the feet. The back support is pulled back **(B)** and the patient instructed to holds the isometric posture as long as possible without support.

tensor fascia latae and two-joint adductors (see Fig. 23-33).

VI. Palpation

This underused but important examination should be incorporated into the assessment of every patient with back pain. The aims of palpation are to detect abnormalities in bone structure (e.g., spondylolisthesis), to identify the level of the lesion, and to determine the nature of the problem (e.g., muscle spasm, stiffness, pain).

Posterior Aspect

A useful test to assess muscle guarding in the lumbar spine is the weight-shift test.[670] With the patient standing, the examiner places the thumbs on the patient's lumbar paraspinals. The patient is then asked to shift the weight

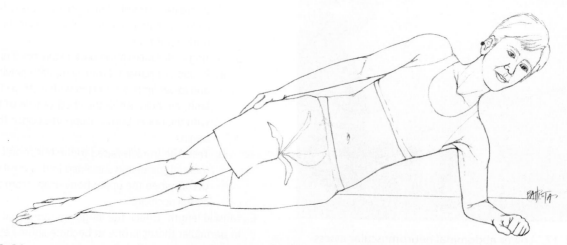

■ **FIG. 22-20.** Lateral trunk endurance test. The subject assumes the full-side bridge position with support on one elbow and on their feet while lifting their hips off the table to create a straight line over their body length.

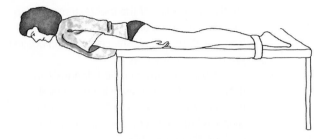

■ **FIG. 22-21.** Back extensor endurance test. The subject is positioned in prone with the pelvis and lower limbs supported on the table with the ankles secured. The upper body is held in a neutral position out over the end of the treatment table. Failure occurs when the upper body drops from the horizontal position.

from one side to the other. Normally, the paraspinals on the side of the stance foot relax, but if muscle guarding or spasm is present, the muscle is not felt to relax. For further palpation of the posterior aspect of the spine, the patient is placed in a relaxed prone position. This is best achieved in the 90–90 position of the hips and knees (Fig. 22-14). Standing behind the patient, the examiner places the fingers on the top of the iliac crests and the thumbs at the same level on the midline of the back (the level of the fourth and fifth lumbar disk interspaces). This reference point is marked and the following are palpated:

A. Ligaments. The supraspinous ligaments are palpated for tenderness and consistency; the supraspinous ligament is normally springy and supple. If it is thick and hardened, the segment may be hypomobile. Tenderness is usually apparent over the involved intervertebral joint. Usually, the interspinous ligament is also tender. This is found by applying exquisitely localized pressure with a key ring or the edge of a coin between the spinous processes.[468]

B. Position of the transverse and spinous processes. Note any alterations in the bony alignment, such as spondylolistheses and evidence of tenderness. Specific pain elicited in one segment is particularly helpful in patients with suspected instability.[559] If each spinous process is tapped sharply with a reflex hammer or fingertip, pain may be reproduced over the painful joint.

C. Sacrum, sulcus, sacral hiatus, and coccyx. Palpate over the pelvis, including the sacrum, sacroiliac joints, sacral hiatus, coccyx (see Fig. 23-11), and any other relevant areas. If indicated, a rectal examination of the coccyx may be performed. The sacroiliac joint is palpated at its inferior extent in the region of the posteroinferior iliac spine. Acute unilateral tenderness is common in painful sacroiliac conditions and when well localized is a useful confirmatory sign.[257]

A comprehensive examination of this joint should be regarded as an expanded section of the lumbar spine. Details of a comprehensive examination of this joint are found in Chapter 23, Sacroiliac Joint and Lumbar–Pelvic–Hip Complex and other sources.[67,131,146–148,198,238,243,394,461,467, 471,530,582,670,799])

D. Iliac crest, ischial tuberosity, and hip joint. Beginning at the posterosuperior iliac spine, the examiner moves along the iliac crest, palpating for signs of pathologic processes such as Maigne's syndrome (see Chapter 20, Thoracic Spine).[394] Pressure and friction over the iliac crest often reveal a well-localized, acutely painful point (crestal point) at the gluteal level (8 to 10 cm from the midline). Pinching and rolling of the skin in the gluteal area (see Fig. 7-42C) will be painful as will lateral pressure over the spinous processes (T11–L1). According to Maigne, referred pain may be mediated by the cluneal nerves, the posterior rami of the T12 or L1 spinal nerves.[469] These nerves pass downward and outward on each side to supply the skin at the level of the iliac crest (Fig. 20-7B). The referred pain is experienced at this level. Irritation of these nerves may be responsible for low back pain, pseudovisceral pain, and pseudohip pain. Because attention is usually directed to the site of referred pain, the source is frequently overlooked.[469] When Maigne's syndrome is suspected, the diagnosis is confirmed when pain is alleviated following manipulation or injections to the symptomatic posterior joints.[394]

The ischial tuberosities are palpated on both sides for any abnormalities, including the hip and greater trochanteric bursa, which sometimes mimics sciatica. It is often difficult to differentiate between hip and spine problems, because the symptoms are often similar.

E. Muscles of the gluteal region and sciatic nerve. Observe for apparent muscle atrophy, particularly of the gluteus maximus on one side. During palpation, one or several of the muscles often have hard, infiltrated fascicles that are sometimes cord-like and may be very sensitive to pressure. According to Maigne, the gluteal muscle pain is responsible for many instances of lumbar pain.[468] Deep pétrissage gives excellent results in this type of chronic pain.[469] Palpating midway between the ischial tuberosity and the greater trochanter, the examiner may be able to palpate the sciatic nerve. Deep to the gluteal muscles, the piriformis muscle should be palpated for potential pathologic processes.

F. Skin and subcutaneous tissue. Palpate the skin for tenderness, moisture, texture, and temperature changes. A quick wipe over the area with the back of the hand is used to register any apparent local changes in temperature or sweating. Examine any moles on the skin to determine whether they are deep or superficial. Normally, the skin can be rolled over the spine and gluteal region freely and painlessly. If there are subcutaneous pathologic changes, there will be tightness and pain with skin-rolling.

Anterior Aspect

A. Abdominal wall, iliac crest, and symphysis pubis. Palpate the abdominal wall including the psoas, iliacus muscles, the iliac crest, and symphysis pubis for tenderness. Palpate the symphysis pubis bilaterally, over the superior aspect, to ensure that the two pubic bones are level and asymptomatic.

B. Inguinal area and femoral triangle. Probe the general area within the triangle for enlarged lymph nodes (infections), symptoms of hernia, abscess, or other pathologic conditions.

C. Arterial pulses. Assess the arterial supply to the legs by palpating the arterial pulses in the inguinal, popliteal, and dorsalis sites.

VI. Neuromuscular Tests

Neurologic examination involves examining the integrity and mobility of the nervous system. The neurologic part of the musculoskeletal evaluation consists of a series of tests to determine if there is segmental interference of neural conduction. The most common cause of such findings is a disk extrusion in the lumbar spine. Other causes of neurologic deficits in the legs are rare but are usually more serious. Any multisegmental deficit should be viewed with some suspicion, because nerve root impingement from a disk protrusion rarely involves more than one root; the occasional exception is an L5–S1 protrusion, which may affect the L5 and S1 roots.

A. Integrity of the nervous system

1. Dermatomes/peripheral nerves. A knowledge of the cutaneous distribution of peripheral nerves and cutaneous distribution of the nerve roots (dermatomes) enables the examiner to distinguish sensory loss owing to a root lesion from that owing to a peripheral nerve lesion (see Fig. 5-8 and Table 5-8).

2. Myotomes/peripheral nerves. A working knowledge of muscular distribution of nerve roots (myotomes) and peripheral nerves enables the examiner to distinguish motor loss owing to root lesions from that owing to peripheral nerve lesion (see Table 5-7). (See Table 5-8 and Fig. 5-10 for myotomal testing of the lumbar and sacral nerve roots.) The following myotomes are tested.

a. Tests with patient in supine

i. L2—Hip flexion (iliopsoas). The patient holds the flexed hip and knee at 90° while resistance is applied just above the knee.

ii. L3—Knee extension (quadriceps). The examiner supports the thigh with one arm underneath it, with the examiner's hand supported on top of the opposite thigh. Resistance is applied to the lower leg while the patient holds the leg just short of full knee extension.

iii. L4—Ankle dorsiflexion and inversion (tibialis anterior). Test bilaterally. The patient holds the feet in dorsiflexion and inversion as resistance is applied against the dorsal-medial aspect of great toe.

iv. L5—Great toe extension (extensor hallucis longus). Toe extension is tested bilaterally. The patient holds the foot and toes dorsiflexed as resistance is applied against the dorsal aspect of great toe.

v. L5–S1—Extension of the toes (extensor digitorum longus). The patient holds the foot and toes dorsiflexed as resistance is applied against the dorsum of the toes.

vi. S1—Ankle eversion (peroneus longus and brevis). The patient tries to keep the heels together with the feet everted as resistance is applied to the lateral borders of the feet, pushing them together.

b. Tests with patient in prone

i. S2—Knee flexion (hamstrings). The hamstrings are tested bilaterally as the patient holds the knees flexed to 90° as resistance is applied behind the heels.

ii. S1—Hip extension (gluteus maximus). The patient holds the hip extended with the knee bent while the examiner applies resistance just above the knee with one hand while palpating the gluteal mass with the other hand to assess firmness.

c. Tests with patient standing

i. S1—Plantar-flexion (gastrocnemius). The patient stands on one leg and plantar-flexes by rising on the toes through a full range of motion. Repeat 6 to 10 times per side. Having the patient walk on the toes can also test plantar-flexion.

ii. L3—Knee flexion (quadriceps). Unilateral half-squats; repeat 6 to 10 times. The girth of the limbs above and below the knee is measured to document any muscle-wasting.

3. Sensory testing

When testing dermatomes and myotomes, subtle sensory deficits are best detected by assessing vibratory perception with a tuning fork. This is because pressure tends to affect the large, myelinated fibers that mediate vibratory and proprioceptive sensation first. Gross sensory testing may be done using a wisp of cotton or a pin.

The key sensory areas to test are in the distal part of the limb, because these are the areas where there is relatively little overlap of segmental innervation. These include L4, the medial aspect of the big toe; L5, the web space between the first and second toes; S1, below the lateral malleolus; and S2, the distal Achilles tendon region. Test these areas first, then the various aspects of the leg and thigh. If a significant deficit is detected proximal to the foot, ensure that more serious pathologic processes have been ruled out.

When performing sensory tests, test a small area of one limb. Ask the patient if the expected sensation is felt (e.g., vibration, touch, or pinprick). Then test the corresponding area on the opposite limb and ask the patient again if it is felt. Ask if the intensity of the stimulus felt is about the same on both sides. Proceed in this fashion for all the areas to be tested.

Sensory tests are most easily done with the patient supine.

4. Reflex testing. The following deep tendon reflexes are tested.
   a. L3/4–knee jerk
   b. S1—ankle jerk
   c. Great toe reflex—L5[754]

   Segmented neurologic deficits may result in diminution of deep tendon reflexes on the involved side. When examining deep tendon reflexes, primarily observe for asymmetry of responses from one side to the other. Difficulty eliciting reflexes on both sides does not necessarily indicate a pathologic process, so long as there is no asymmetry in response. Look for unusual fatigue. Elicit the reflex at least six times, and always compare sides.

   The medial (L5, S1) and the lateral (S1) hamstring reflexes are not routinely tested but may assist in decisions about involvement of those roots.

   Superficial reflex (upper motor neuron) testing may be indicated and includes the abdominal, cremasteric, and anal reflexes.[328,461]

B. Mobility of the nervous system. Neurodynamic tests may be performed to ascertain the degree to which neural tension is responsible for the production of the patient's symptoms. Tests may include passive neck flexion, straight leg raise, passive knee bend, and slump test.

1. Neck flexion. Passive neck flexion is done in supine. The test should be painless outside of a mild pulling sensation of the cervicothoracic junction. This indicative for all possible spinal disorders. It is often positive for low back pain.[768] The neural structures tested are the pons, spinal cord, and meninges. If this test produces lumbar pain, then the cause of the pain lies within the nervous system.

2. Straight leg raise (dural mobility tests). The dura, nerve root sleeves, and nerve roots are sensitive to pain. Their irritants are many, as are the pathologic processes that induce them. Included are disk prolapse,[72,740,774] adhesions (e.g., posttraumatic or postsurgical epidural fibrosis, subarachnoid adhesions),[774,775] hypertrophic changes in the facet joints and margins of the vertebral bodies,[198,540,742] and indirect compressions from ischemic changes secondary to chronic progressive compression (e.g., enlarged masses, thickening of the ligamentum flavum, apophyseal joint swelling).[471]

   Dural mobility tests (sciatic nerve, straight-leg raising) may reproduce symptoms (usually pain) in the case of a disk prolapse, in which a bulging disk may approximate the anterolateral aspect of the dural sac of the cauda equina, or in the case of a disk extrusion, in which the protruded disk material may be adjacent to some part of the dural investment of a nerve root. The dura can be moved in a cephalad direction by flexing the neck, or in a caudal direction by applying tension to the femoral or sciatic nerves. The femoral nerve and its contributing nerve roots are stretched by sidelying or prone knee flexion and hip extension, the sciatic nerve and its roots by straight-leg raising. Additional tension is applied to the sciatic nerve by dorsiflexing the ankle.

   Dural mobility tests for the sciatic nerve roots may be done sitting or supine. It is often best to perform them in both positions and to compare the results. Sitting increases the likelihood of obtaining a positive test in the case of a minor prolapse, because it is a position of relatively high intradiskal pressure. However, to judge improvement, the tests are best performed in the supine position, measuring the distance from the lateral malleolus to the plinth at which pain is produced on straight-leg raising.

   A true-positive dural mobility test will reproduce back pain, hip girdle pain, leg pain, or some combination thereof, and pain should be felt somewhere between 30° and 60° of straight-leg raising. At angles less than 30°, there is very little movement of the nerve roots, and by 60° the dura will have already moved sufficiently to have reproduced pain. Also, above 60°, movement of the spinal column as the pelvis tilts backward may cause the reproduction of pain. Differentiate between pulling on tight hamstrings and reproduction of leg pain from dural impingement. Possible mechanical effects from movement of the spine or sacroiliac joint can be ruled out by seeing if ankle dorsiflexion further accentuates the pain produced; if so, it is likely to be a true-positive dural sign.

   a. The sitting tests are done with the patient sitting at the edge of the plinth. First move one knee toward extension, noting any guarding of the movement and asking whether symptoms are reproduced. If pain is produced, hold the leg just up to the painful point and assess the effects of ankle dorsiflexion and neck flexion. Test the opposite leg similarly.

   b. The supine tests are done in a similar manner by moving first one leg and then the other into flexion with the knee straight. Again, assess the effects of ankle dorsiflexion and neck flexion. Test straight-leg raising with the hip in neutral rotation and slightly adducted during straight-leg raising of the asymptomatic leg. Positive straight-leg raising of the opposite leg can be more important than ipsilateral straight-leg raising. A discussion of this sciatic traction test would be incomplete without mentioning what is called the "well leg of Fajersztan," the crossed straight-leg raising test or crossover sign, a prostrate leg raising test, Lhermitte's sign or sciatic phenomenon.[330,618,758] These tests have a high correlation with large central disk protrusions that impale on the root in its axilla.[183,330,672,817] The pattern of positive results yields clues as to the relation between the protrusion and the pain-sensitive structure (e.g., dura or dural covering of a nerve root).

   i. If prolapsed or extruded material is anterior to the pain-sensitive tissue, ipsilateral leg raising, contralateral leg raising, and neck flexion may all hurt.

   ii. If the protruded material is medial to the nerve root as it exits from the dural sac (rare), leg raising may hurt bilaterally but neck flexion may be painless.

   iii. If the protrusion is lateral to the existing nerve root, ipsilateral leg raising may reproduce symptoms, neck flexion may be painful, and contralateral leg raising is painless.

     Intradiskal pressure increases when the patient sits or stands compared with lying.[561] This may cause a discrepancy in the degree of limitation of straight-leg raising performed in the standing and lying positions, so performing tests in both positions can be valuable.[471]

3. Femoral nerve traction test.[183] The patient lies on the unaffected side with the lower limb flexed at both the hip and knee joints to stabilize the trunk. The head is flexed slightly to increase tension on the cauda equina. The test has two components:

   a. The uppermost part of the thigh is first passively extended just short of provoking lumbar spine extension to create tension in the iliopsoas, and hence traction on the upper lumbar nerve root.

   b. Next, the knee is progressively flexed to increase femoral nerve tension by stretching the quadriceps femoris muscle.

     In the presence of an L3 radiculitis, pain radiates down the medial thigh to the knee. When the L4 root is involved, the pain is more anterior on the thigh and extends to the midtibial portion of the leg.[183]

4. The slump test is an excellent test for a disk lesion and dural tethering; it is performed on the patient who has low back pain with or without leg pain.[68,471,550] Maximum tension can be exerted on the canal structures with the patient's chin on the chest.[471] The following is a description of the slump test for a patient with a nonirritable disorder. Symptoms need to be monitored throughout the test, and the range of motion is estimated after each segment. With the patient sitting erect on the table and the hands behind the back and linked together, have patient do the following:

a. Let the back slump through its full range of thoracic lumbar spine flexion The examiner maintains the cervical spine in neutral (Fig. 22-22A). Overpressure may be applied to encourage maximum thoracic and lumbar flexion.

b. Having established full range of the hip and spine from T1 to the sacrum, actively flex the head and neck fully. The examiner can apply over pressure. In the uninjured patient, pain will be felt 50% of the time in the area of T8 and T9.

   i. Straighten first the unaffected leg and actively dorsiflex the ankle and then the affected leg (Fig. 22-22B). Pain in the hamstrings and popliteal area is common, and a limitation of knee extension is seen frequently.

   ii. The final step is to release cervical flexion and carefully assess the response. With the release of cervical flexion, there is a decrease of symptoms and an increase in knee extension.

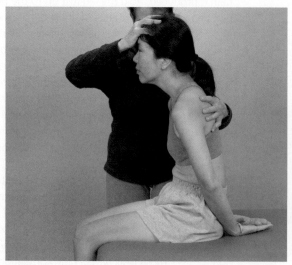

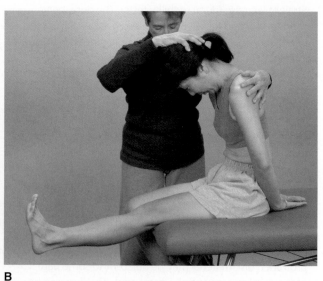

A   **B**

■ **FIG. 22-22.** Slump test. **(A)** Slouch position, maintaining cervical spine in neutral. **(B)** Slump test with full cervical flexion, knee extension, and dorsiflexion.

Note and record the pain response after each step. There are many variations of this test, including passive and sustained overpressure of the head and neck while in the slump position, releasing the neck-flexion component, raising the head to neutral, extending the neck in the slump position, and performing the test in long-sitting. According to Maitland, when assessing the findings of this test, the pain response, particularly in relation to releasing the neck-flexion component, is most important.[470,471]

C. Other neural diagnostic tests

1. Plantar response to test for an upper motor neurone lesion. With the patient's leg extended, stimulate the lateral border of the sole with a blunt object. The stroke begins on the lateral aspect of the heel and moves distally, then across the metatarsals just proximal to the toes. Plantar-flexion is a normal response; dorsiflexion (a positive Babinski response) is pathologic and indicates spinal cord injury (upper motor neuron lesion).

2. Stoop test for intermittent cauda equina compression. The patient is asked to walk briskly for approximately 50 m. The test will produce the patient's buttock and leg pain, and causes lower limb muscle weakness. The test is considered positive—indicating cauda equina compression—if these symptoms are then eased by lumbar spine flexion.[181]

3. Test for ankle clonus. A test to determine if the patient has clonus may be included here. A hyperactive stretch reflex is the mechanism that supports clonus. Ankle clonus is elicited by quickly stretching the gastroc-soleus muscle group by dorsiflexing the foot and then maintaining moderate stretch to the plantar flexors. The clonus response is alternating plantar-flexion and dorsiflexion of the foot.

4. Balance testing. Balance testing is conducted to appraise the receptor integrity in the joints of the lower extremities and lumbar spine.[194,806,819,820] The Romberg test, "stork-standing," or digital balance boards can be used to assess balance. If a mechanical lesion of the low back is suspected, the above tests are generally sufficient. However, if neurologic disease is suspected (e.g., diabetic neuropathy), motor performance, temperature, and proprioception should be tested as well.

TESTS FOR INTERMITTENT CLAUDICATION

Peripheral vascular disease with claudication can be confused with neurogenic claudication and spinal stenosis.[249] The major difference in the clinical features is the response of pain to the rest position of the spine. Peripheral vascular disease pain is not relieved by trunk flexion or aggravated with sustained trunk extension as in neurogenic claudication and spinal stenosis. Tests for intermittent neurogenic claudication include the following.

1. Bicycle test of van Gelden.[182] The patient is seated on an exercise bicycle and is asked to pedal against resistance. The patient starts pedaling while leaning backward to accentuate the lumbar lordosis. If pain into the buttock and posterior thigh occurs, followed by tingling in the affected lower limb, the first part of the test is positive. The patient is then asked to learn forward while continuing to pedal. If the pain subsides over a short period, the second part of the test is positive; if the patient sits up again, the pain returns.

2. Stoop test.[181] The patient with neurogenic claudication is asked to walk briskly, pain ensues in the buttock and lower limb within a distance of 165 ft. To relieve the pain, the patient flexes forward. Symptoms are also relieved by sitting and forward flexion. If flexion does not relieve the symptoms, the test is negative.

The two conditions, neurogenic claudication from lumbar spinal stenosis and vascular claudication from arterial stenosis, commonly coexist in older people.[635] Vascular studies and myelography may be necessary to help determine the source.

GENERAL PHYSICAL EXAMINATION

A general physical examination, including the abdomen and chest, may be necessary. In cases of suspected pelvic lesions, a rectal examination is necessary. These tests help determine the severity of the back pain, the level of the lesion, the presence of nerve root pressure, and the authenticity of the pain. A history and physical examination are usually sufficient to identify most patients for whom specific therapy is required.[631] Other studies may include the following.

I. Roentgenograms and Other Imaging Studies

   The majority of cases of low back pain of less than 4 weeks' duration do not require imaging studies; a thorough history and physical examination are sufficient.[627] In acute injuries in which there is a possibility of spinal fracture or subluxation, or when red flags suggest an increased risk of neoplasm or infections roentgenograms should be obtained. The examiner may review any imaging studies that have been done.[167,357,528] In addition to basic roentgenograms, other special techniques may be used.

A. Magnetic resonance imaging (MRI) has become an invaluable tool in evaluating the spine and is the best test to assess the disks, the soft tissues, and some spinal cord tumors. It should be noted that in asymptomatic adults, up to 25% show degenerative changes on plain film of the spine, and 30% are found to have a major abnormality on MRI. Therefore, correlation between physical and radiographic findings is crucial.[58]

B. Computed tomography (CT) testing. Tomography, which has become a common technique, involves a computerized display that recreates a three-dimensional image of the spine.[726] CT testing reveals most fractures, joint disease, and spinal masses. Herniated disks are also well-visualized as well as structural spinal deformities such as lumbar canal stenosis, abnormalities in the facet joints, and vertebral disease.[99]

C. Other studies that may prove helpful include electromyography (EMG),[131,196] bone scan, venography, and diskography. EMG can diagnose and often localize radiculopathy. It gives information about the actual state of the nerves as opposed to MRI, which simply shows anatomy, regardless of the clinical significance. Myelography gives information about the spinal cord and roots, and is typically combined with CT for better accuracy; however it is seldom used today.[627] Diskography involves the injection of saline or radiopaque contrast into the disk to see if there is leakage of contrast out of a damaged disk or if the injection reproduces pain (Fig. 22-4).

II. Real-Time Ultrasound Imaging and Use for Feedback in Rehabilitation

A review of the application of ultrasonography in medicine is beyond the scope of this chapter. The usefulness of ultrasound of the musculoskeletal has been shown.[119,224,291,373,417,781] Tissues that can be imaged include muscle, tendons, joints, ligaments and bursae. One of the most useful features of real-time ultrasound is that movement of anatomic structures can be observed as it actually occurs. These techniques have been successfully applied to the abdominals and multifidus muscles in LBP patients for assessment and feedback.[305,307,308,310] The results of integration of this modality with assessment and treatment techniques are very encouraging. The use of ultrasound imaging in deep muscle assessment and facilitation are yet to be fully explored and realized.

III. Laboratory Tests

A complete blood count is among the laboratory tests used to investigate spinal disease, and urinalysis should be performed routinely.

TESTS FOR NONORGANIC BACK PAIN

Several tests are useful in the differentiation of organic and nonorganic back pain (e.g., as seen in patients suffering from depression, emotional disturbance, or anxiety).[131,386,652,654,662] It is difficult to assess a patient who has an organic back lesion but whose symptoms are exacerbated or prolonged by psychologic factors. In these patients, the symptoms are usually out of proportion to the signs (e.g., inconsistent joint findings; abnormal postures or gait). Tests include the following:

I. Distraction Test (Leg Test or Flip Test)[386,787,788]

A positive physical finding is demonstrated in a routine manner; this finding is then checked while the patient's attention is distracted. For example, after performing the usual straight-leg raising test in supine, ask the patient to sit up, swing the legs over the end of the table, and repeat leg raising in sitting. If marked improvement is noted, the patient's response is inconsistent. Leg raising is a useful distraction test.

II. Stimulation Tests

These tests should not be uncomfortable: if pain is reported, a nonorganic influence is suggested.

A. Axial loading uses manual pressure through the standing patient's head. Few patients whose lumbar pain is organic will suffer discomfort on this test.[386,787,788]

B. Hip and shoulder rotation.[386] With the patient standing, examine for pain by passively rotating the patient's hips or shoulders while the feet are kept on the ground. This maneuver is usually painless for patients with organic back disorders.

C. Kneeling on a stool (Burns test).[131,386] The patient kneels on a stool or chair and is asked to bend over and try to touch the floor. Even with a severely herniated disk, most patients attempt the task to some degree. Persons with nonorganic pain often refuse on the grounds that it would cause great pain or would tend to overbalance them on the chair.

III. Other Methods

Other tools for assessing nonorganic physical signs include regional disturbances, which involve a divergence from the accepted neuroanatomy (i.e., atypical motor and sensory disturbances), overreaction during examination (i.e., disproportionate verbalization, muscle tension, and tremor), and tenderness.[789,792] Tenderness, when related to physical disease, is usually localized to a particular skeletal or neuromuscular structure. Nonorganic tenderness is nonspecific and diffuse. Further verification is possible by the use of pain drawings, as recommended by Ransford and associates (Fig. 22-5).[636]

Several other psychopathic signs and observations have been described.[458,520,539,618,720] If found, further psychologic evaluation is indicated, and the therapist must guard against potential overtreatment.[618,724,809]

Other types of investigation, such as the MMPI and other psychologic tests, have been used for lumbar spine problems (see other sources).[38,53,71,84,141,150,151,161,220,239,302,403,512,519–522,721,728,771,814] Since its development in 1940 by Hathaway and McKinley,[295] the MMPI has become one of the most widely used personality screening tests.

ACTIVITIES OF DAILY LIVING

A formal exercise obstacle course may be used to evaluate the patient's ability to perform activities of daily living.[804] Activities to be assessed include sitting, standing, walking, bending, lifting, pushing, pulling, climbing, and reaching. Endurance may be evaluated while the patient is walking or riding a stationary bicycle. Quantitative functional capacity measurements can give objective evidence of the patient's physical abilities and degree of effort, and can be useful in designing and administering an effective treatment program.[490] The lower extremity functional profile is an excellent tool that allows a firm starting point for objective measurement of the lumbar spine and lower quadrant (see Chapter 10, Functional Exercise).

COMPUTERIZED TESTS

Isokinetic forms of resisted muscle testing are the most effective and yield reliable measurements of muscular strength, power (at slow and fast speeds), and endurance. These measures can be recorded in graphic form for comparison later in rehabilitation.[179] The potential value of objective measurement of spinal function has been recognized for some time, although practical and clinically useful technology has not been generally available.[53,217,553,743] The increasing understanding of disuse and deconditioning syndromes as a factor in long-term disability and recent developments in the qualification of true spinal range of motion,[491,492,494,748] trunk muscle strength,[156,422,477,560,615,710,757,758] endurance, and lifting capacity bring a new dimension to the management of low back pain.[299,397,493,577,625]

COMMON LESIONS AND MANAGEMENT

Intervertebral Disk Lesions

Sciatica is caused by many intraspinal abnormalities other than disk prolapse.[4,120,256,260,320,436,616,622,711,719,720] For example, a decrease in size of the lateral bony nerve root canal can result from degenerative hypertrophy of the lumbar facets or a trefoil canal (a congenital variant in cross-sectional geometry).[25,393] Other less common causes of sciatica include congenital anomalies of the lumbar nerve roots, "hip-pocket" sciatica, the piriformis syndrome, and even viral infections.[484,725] Space does not permit a full discussion of all the causes of acute spinal dysfunction.

Despite the extensive differential diagnosis, intervertebral disk prolapse is the most common diagnosis of sciatica. Ninety-eight percent of intervertebral disk prolapse cases involve the L4–L5 or L5–S1 lumbar disk space.[719] Older patients have a relatively increased risk of disk prolapse at the L3–L4 and L2–L3 levels.[233,234]

The sensitive spinal cord has an elaborate protective mechanism, including a most pain-sensitive anterior dural sheath and the posterior longitudinal ligament. The following can occur with a prolapsed disk:

1. The disk bulges against the ligament and the dura. This produces a dull, deep, poorly localized pain in the back and over the sacroiliac region because the dura does not have specific dermatomal localization.
2. The disk bulges posterolaterally against the nerve root. This is a natural route because the annulus fibrosus is no longer reinforced by the posterior ligament. The result is sharp nerve root pain (e.g., sciatica).
3. The disk ruptures and the thick gelatinous fluid of the nucleus pulposus flows around the dura and nerve roots. This is an extremely irritating substance and it causes a reaction around the nerve-sensitive tissue. It is the most likely cause of agonizing, persistent back pain. When the disk ruptures, fragments of the harder annulus fibrosus may protrude into the spinal canal; this usually requires surgical intervention.

In experiments using human volunteers by Nachemson and Morris in 1964, the intradiskal pressures in the lumbar spine were measured with a diskogram, and subsequent studies have enhanced our understanding of the intervertebral disk (Figs. 22-23 and 22-24).[555,561] Obviously, bending forward while lifting increases the pressure. The situation is aggravated by sitting and leaning forward with a reduction of the lumbar lordosis.

DISK PROLAPSE

Some clinical features associated with disk prolapse include:

1. Age—The peak age is 20 to 45 years. A prolonged work posture of lumbar flexion is a frequent factor in the history.
2. Gender—Males are more commonly affected than females by about 3:2.
3. Site—In 1,000 lumbar disk operations, Armstrong[24] found that 46.9% occurred at the lumbosacral disk, 40.4% at the L4–L5 disk, and 2.1% at the upper three disks; in 10.7% of the cases, double lesions were present.

History. Back pain may occur for no apparent reason—rather, it may be caused by the cumulative effects of months or even years of forward-bending, lifting, or sitting in a slumped, forward-bent position.[106,157,162,510,576,611,716,719,801] There may be a history of attacks of back pain, sometimes associated with a sensation of back locking. Many patients tend to relate it to some minor traumatic incident or after a strain, such as bending, lifting, or twisting, which may be associated with a tearing sensation.[131]

In the early stages, the patient complains of pain, usually in the lower back but sometimes in the posterior buttocks or thigh. As a rule, leg pain indicates a larger protrusion than does back pain alone.[510] Pain may be described as a dull ache or knife-like. The onset of pain may be sudden and severe or may develop more gradually. Pain at first may be intermittent and relieved by rest, standing, lying, or changing position. Spinal pain tends to be greater on one side than the other. Bilateral spinal pain is probably secondary to a connecting branch of the sinuvertebral nerve, which joins the right and left portions of that nerve.[212] Pain is aggravated by straining, stooping, sneezing, coughing, car travel, and sitting. The patient also often reports that prolonged sitting causes the pain to move from the lower back into the leg. Difficulty in assuming an erect posture after lying down or sitting may also be described. Ultimately, pain usually becomes severe and may disturb sleep.

Back pain may be followed by leg pain, which is almost always unilateral and usually is severe. The back pain may disappear when the leg pain begins. The distribution of the leg pain varies according to the nerve root involved.

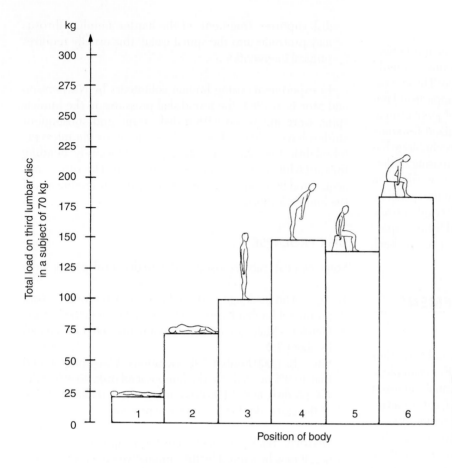

■ **FIG. 22-23.** Intradiskal pressures (relative) as they relate to body positions. (Reprinted with permission from Finneson BE: Low Back Pain, 2nd ed. Philadelphia, JB Lippincott, 1980:41.)

Clinical Examination. Signs consist of varying combinations and degrees of mechanical derangement of the lumbar spinal joints and evidence of nerve root involvement. Mechanical derangement is evidenced by alterations in posture, muscle spasms, disturbance of movements, and alterations in the spinal contours.

Gait and movement are guarded and restricted. Gait may also be antalgic, with as little weight as possible being transferred to the painful side. Transfer activities, such as rising from a sitting position and moving about on the plinth, are performed guardedly; the lumbar spine is reflexively protected from compressive loading or movement.

The patient sits in a slumped posture or insists on standing in the waiting room because of increased intradiskal pressure caused by sitting. In erect standing, patients may be unable to bear any weight on the painful leg, so they stand with the hips and knees flexed and the back held rigid. The patient may have loss of the normal lordosis and flattening of the thoracic

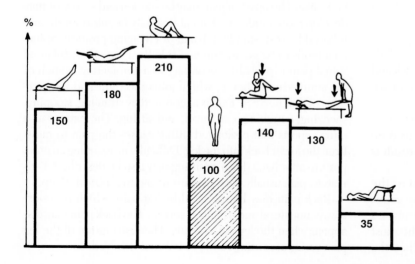

■ **FIG. 22-24.** Intradiskal pressures (relative) as they relate to activities. (Adapted with permission from Nachemson AL: The lumbar spine: An orthopedic challenge. Spine 1:59–71, 1976.)

spine and shoulder girdle retraction as well.[131,146,510,790] The patient may have a lateral shift (lumbar scoliosis) away from the side of pain (contralateral, 85% of cases), but occasionally toward the painful side (ipsilateral, 15% of cases).

Inspection. To evaluate active movement, the physiologic movements of the spine are tested to determine their range, whether pain is reproduced, the behavior of the pain with movement, whether an arc of pain is present, and the presence of any deformity.

Lumbar forward-bending (flexion) is sometimes limited because of the severity of the pain, and the degree of its loss usually reflects the severity of the disk prolapse. The patient often tends to compensate by bending at the hips and knees and may guard the spine against excessive compression by placing the hands on the thighs. In less severe cases, where forward-bending is possible, bending may be associated with a deviated arc of movement in which the spine shifts out of and back toward the midline as movement proceeds. When tested in the standing position, flexion may cause the pain to move peripherally, especially if forward-flexion is repeated several times.[510]

Movement into lateral flexion varies. There may be full and painless range to each side, or there may be painful limitation to one side. This is more common toward the side of pain; lateral flexion to the other side is then usually full. If a lateral shift is present, it should be corrected before testing extension.

Loss of backward-bending (extension) is not as common as loss of flexion. In patients with a loss of the normal lordosis, extension or backward-bending (after the lateral shift has been corrected) is almost always restricted and causes increased pain. The patient usually compensates by extending the thoracic spine and retracting the shoulder girdle. Note whether the increase in pain centralizes or becomes peripheral from the center of the spine into the leg.

The spine is reflexively splinted in a position that compromises between minimizing intradiskal pressure, reducing tension on the dural material, and preventing impingement of the protruded materials. Lordosis is lost because the posteriorly protruded disk material forces the segment toward forward-bending, and backward-bending would tend to compromise the prolapse. Forward-bending is difficult because the marked increase in intradiskal pressure it causes tends to increase the pressure against the pain-sensitive structures.[17,553] Lateral bending is restricted because of increased intradiskal pressure and because of impingement of the protrusion when performed to the involved side. McKenzie[510] maintains that 50% of patients with this disorder have a lateral shift because of the tendency of the nuclear gel to shift posterolaterally. As the gel moves posteriorly, the patient tends to shift the body weight in an anterior direction, flattening the lumbar spine. When the patient shifts the shoulder away from the side of the nuclear movement, a lateral shift occurs.[131,204,212,388,585] Usually, the protrusion is lateral to the existing nerve root, in which case a lateral shift away from the defect minimizes the dural impingement. Less often, the bulge is located at the

axilla formed by the root stemming from the dural sac. The spine is shifted toward the ipsilateral side or painful side (15% of cases). The presence of a lateral shift may be noted while the patient is standing or flexing or extending the lumbar spine. It is not rare for a patient with only unilateral pain and a contralateral list to have this change under treatment to an ipsilateral list, or vice versa.[262]

Passive movements—both physiologic and accessory—are limited because of spasms, stiffness, and pain. Passive physiologic restriction is usually less, because of reduced compression imposed on the spine, in a reclining position. Accessory movements are usually compromised by protective muscle guarding.

Nerve root involvement is indicated by the loss of freedom of movement of the nerve root in the spinal canal or its intervertebral foramen. True neurologic signs and symptoms are produced. The patient has all the signs and symptoms previously discussed, with the addition of positive neurologic signs such as strength loss, decreased muscle stretch reflexes, loss of sensation, and positive dural mobility signs. Tests should include straight-leg raising and the femoral nerve traction test. Neurologic assessment to determine the nerve root involved and the degree of compression is essential. The most important clinical features are the localization of pain to an affected nerve root and the reproduction of the pain by a positive nerve root tension sign.[672]

Palpation. The affected spinal level is usually tender to palpation in the midline or in the paravertebral area on the same side as the disk prolapse. The sciatic nerve may also be tender. If the patient has had pain for more than 1 or 2 days, the muscles may be tender from guarding and muscle spasm. Positional changes can occasionally be felt by palpating the spinous processes. For example, if the segment is locked in rotation and sidebending, the superior spinous process will not be in alignment with the adjacent inferior spinous process.

Clinical Variations. Many clinical variations of the pain pattern and neurologic involvement are possible. The most common pain pattern is back pain followed by leg pain, but the patient may present with back pain alone, sciatic pain alone, or simultaneous back and leg pain. Pain may radiate into both legs simultaneously and consecutively. A large posterior prolapse may implicate two nerve roots on either side at the same level or at different levels.[131]

Acute nerve root compression is a severe back problem usually caused by an advanced disk protrusion. It must be handled with care. The disorder has a protracted course of 6 to 12 weeks; more than 50% of patients recover in 6 weeks.[21] Rarely is surgical treatment required, so delaying surgery is appropriate in most cases.

Conservative Treatment. In the acute stage, the nonsurgical treatment of acute symptomatic disk prolapse includes bed rest, medications, epidural steroids, and minimizing the lesion by reducing intradiskal pressure. The therapist must be aware of the positions and activities that increase intradiskal pressure and must carefully instruct the patient to avoid situations that may cause the protrusion to progress (Figs. 22-23 and 22-24).[16,17,135,136,553,556]

The optimal amount of bed rest remains to be established, but Deyo and associates[166] observed no difference in outcome between patients with 2 days of bed rest versus those with 1 week of bed rest. In patients with a demonstrated radicular compression, bed rest is efficacious, as shown in Weber's study of 2 weeks of bed rest.[794] This does not mean absolute bed rest, however, because with prolonged recumbency, the disk tends to imbibe fluid from the adjacent vertebral bodies. Activities related to feeding and personal hygiene may actually be more difficult to achieve in bed than out of bed.

Epidural infiltrations of cortisone and local anesthetics have been the topic of several clinical studies, and results have been variable; their utility remains controversial.[68,140,588,715] Epidural steroids reduced pain and increased function in one randomized study.[169] However, a recent comparison of epidural steroid therapy and placebo (saline) demonstrated no differences 24 hours after the injections.

Traction can be applied by means of inversion traction, gravity reduction, 90–90 traction, and motorized techniques, including three-dimensional lumbar traction (see other sources).[86,87,133,142,164,327,432,478–481,548,581,597,614,662,668,670,719,772,795] Some clinical studies have compared the effects of different types of traction, but no controlled study has demonstrated their relative efficacy.[432,631,672,708,833] At least 60% of the body weight must be applied for dimensional changes in the lumbar disk to occur.[234] Claims that disk prolapse can be reduced are unproven. Gravity axial traction and positional traction have a short-lived benefit in acute low back pain and sciatica.[86,606]

When treating an acute disk protrusion with spinal traction, the treatment time should be short. The patient may feel less pain while the distractive force is applied, but as the traction is released a marked increase in pain often is experienced.[672] Such an effect is probably secondary to absorption of additional fluid by the nucleus while the traction is applied, and the development of a high intradiskal pressure as the distractive force is relaxed. This adverse reaction has not been observed if treatment times are kept under 10 minutes for intermittent traction and under 8 minutes for sustained traction.[668]

Braces and lumbar corsets remain controversial. Morris et al.[545] and Nachemson and Morris[561] have shown that when a garment such as a lumbosacral corset that compresses the abdomen is worn, intradiskal pressure is diminished by approximately 25%. Significant unloading of the disk occurs in both the standing and sitting positions.

The first step in any treatment program for acute low back pain should be education. The following points should be considered with respect to the reduction of intradiskal pressure:

1. Sitting (Fig. 22-23), especially with the lumbar part of the spine in a forward-bent position, causes high intradiskal pressure.[555] Sitting with the knees and hips flexed is especially contraindicated. The patient must be taught to sit and rise to standing without bending forward at the lumbar part of the spine. Sitting for a bowel movement may cause a significant increase in intradiskal pressure because of the Valsalva maneuver. The patient must be taught to sit leaning back, with a wide base of support, with one or both legs outstretched. Use of a raised toilet seat and a laxative may be advisable.

2. Most patients are more comfortable while standing than sitting, which confirms Nachemson and Morris's findings that on standing intradiskal pressure is decreased by 29%.[561] The normal lumbar curve should be maintained. If the patient is fixed in some degree of forward-bending, walking should be allowed only with the aid of crutches to reduce weight-bearing compressive forces to the disk.[651]

3. Isometric abdominal contractions and pelvic-tilt exercises that increase intradiskal pressure should not be instituted in the early acute stage.

Physical Therapy. Oscillatory techniques may relieve pain by increasing large-fiber proprioceptive input, which in turn relieves some of the protective muscle spasm. Physical programs (e.g., ultrasound, hot packs, cold packs, and diathermy) have no impact on the disease process but provide temporary pain relief.[131,555]

Perhaps the most controversial form of treatment is **manipulative therapy,** which Haldeman has divided into manipulation, mobilization, manual traction, soft tissue massage, and pressure-point massage.[283,284] Others have evaluated multiple critical trials that have compared manipulative therapy with other treatments such as medications and sham therapy; they concluded that short-term manipulative treatment might temporarily decrease pain and improve function.[74,165,282,283,595] Although sciatica is not considered a contraindication to manipulation by its proponents, there are reports that forceful manipulations may cause new or increased neurologic deficits.[152]

Total management often involves passive exercises as soon as they can be done without increasing peripheral signs and symptoms. An organized form of exercise, "the McKenzie program," has been found to be effective for both chronic and acute low back pain.[780] This program uses a series of individualized progressive exercises to localize and ultimately to eliminate the pain. A comparative study found the McKenzie protocol twice as effective in alleviating low back pain as traction and back schools.[170,780] More than 40 different exercise regimens are available. The appropriate exercise regimen must be individualized, incorporating only those movements (done in the proper sequence and with or without the effects of gravity) that bring about symptom centralization.[170]

Typically, McKenzie advocates correction of any lateral shift and passive extension exercises to move the nucleus of the disk centrally.[510] He also advocates constant maintenance of the correction to allow healing of the annular fibers. Healing of the disk can occur.[205,230,293,313,445] The key is to reduce the bulge and then to maintain the posterior aspect of the disk in close approximation so the scar formed will protect it from further protrusion.[142,510,614] The patient must avoid positions and activities that increase the intradiskal pressure or cause a posterior force on the nucleus (e.g., slump sitting, forward-bending, and flexion exercises). The restoration of full mobility is a necessary component of treatment as soon as the protrusion is stable. Passive exercises and joint mobilization are indicated if mobility is restricted. Finally, a full fitness program should be implemented.

Disorders of Movement

Disorders of spinal movement may be classified as acute mechanical derangement, hypomobility, and hypermobility lesions.

ACUTE MECHANICAL DERANGEMENT

The **acute locked back, sudden backache, facet syndrome, facet blockage, subluxation or fixation,** and **acute lumbago** are all terms used to describe sudden pain in the back. This condition may be regarded as an acute form of mechanical derangement and locking of the intervertebral joint complex. Several theories have been proposed to explain its occurrence: ligamentous tears,[50,83,503] a primary muscle lesion,[158,285,374,458,737] apophyseal joint (facet) lesions (including subluxation, an overriding or shifting of the facet joint out of its normal congruous relation),[587,685] synovitis, an impacted synovial fringe or intra-articular structure such as a meniscoid body,[407,409] acute nuclear prolapse of the disk, acute hydrops of the disk,[114] and an annular tear.

In this form of acute backache (lumbago), more than one condition can produce a typical attack.[263] The term **lumbago** is used here to describe a lumbar spinal syndrome characterized by the sudden onset of severe persistent pain, marked restriction of lumbar movements, and a sensation of locking in the back. Attacks may vary in severity from severe and incapacitating to more minor discomfort. During an attack, it is impossible to know the exact mechanism; one can only speculate.

Lumbago can occur at any age but is most common between ages 20 and 45 years.[685] The mechanism of injury is usually a sudden, unguarded movement involving backward-bending, forward-bending, sidebending, or rotation. If the attack is severe, the patient presents with an onset of sudden, intense lower lumbar pain. It may be bilateral but typically is unilateral. The pain and sensation of back locking may render the patient immobile, with the back stuck in one position. The patient may even fall down or may have had to crawl on hands and knees off a tennis court or into bed from the bathroom. Not all attacks are severe: the patient may be aware only of a mild discomfort in the low back after the triggering movement. Symptoms are initially mild but within a few hours or after having gone to bed, the patient awakens to find that he or she cannot get out of bed because of agonizing pain in the low back. Some examples of sudden back pain, which may serve as a guide when planning initial treatment, are described below.

Impacted Synovial Meniscoid[263]**.** The patient with a sudden backache caused by a presumed locking of a facet joint by an impacted synovial meniscoid is often a young person with a degree of hypermobility. Lumbar synovial joint locking typically occurs during some activity involving reaching up (e.g., to open a window) or after a forward-flexion movement, which may have been slight (e.g., picking up a piece of paper or a tennis ball), in which a hypermobile segment undergoes additional distraction.

Examination reveals:

1. Significant paraspinal muscle spasm, more prominent on one side than the other. A spinal deformity is present.
2. Physiologic movements. Extension and lateral flexion toward the painful side may be nearly full, with pain near the extremes of range; lateral flexion toward the painless side is restricted early in the range and is more painful. Flexion is cautious and limited.
3. Straight-leg raising is limited by pain, with movement of the contralateral (painless) leg equally restricted. Straight-leg raising usually provokes acute discomfort in the region of the posterosuperior iliac spine.
4. Negative neurologic signs.

Locking of Arthrotic Facet Joint[261]**.** The typical patient is a middle-aged or older person, with a degree of presupposed degenerative joint disease, who complains of sudden onset (after twisting) of one-sided back pain localized to the fourth or fifth level in the lumbar spine. The history is that of a simple, nonstressful daily activity such as getting out of a bathtub, bending over to tie a shoe, leaning over a bathroom sink, coughing, sneezing, or lifting a weight. Sudden pain to one side fixes the patient in a flexed posture, and a vertical position can be regained only with some difficulty. The patient may present with a kyphosis or a reversal of the normal lumbar curve.

Examination reveals:

1. Pain is unilateral; extension and lateral flexion away from the side of pain are the most painful.
2. Flexion may not appear to be limited and may be painless, but is performed with the lumbar spine fixed in lordosis. Passive overpressure may provoke localized lumbosacral pain.
3. There are no neurologic signs. Straight-leg raising is usually negative; there may be localized pain at the extreme of leg raising on the painful side.

Most cases of acute mechanical derangement subside within 3 weeks; spinal mobilizations shorten that time. One mobilization technique useful in early treatment is gentle, rhythmic manual traction applied to the patient's legs (see Fig. 22-43). As the patient improves, other mobilization techniques may be added. Specific and nonspecific rotational manipulations are appropriate. Vertebral manipulation is probably the therapeutic modality most frequently studied in controlled trials. A few studies have shown that short-term manipulative treatment may temporarily decrease pain and improve function.[74,134,165,168,254,279,283,324,352,372,469, 481,595,631,637]

Traction can be applied by manual, gravity reduction, and motorized methods. It is often wise to precede mobilization or traction with ice or heat and massage to relieve the muscle guarding and spasm that may accompany acute mechanical derangement. Finally, the restoration of normal mobility of the lumbar spine, particularly in patients who have had several attacks, is facilitated by appropriate therapeutic exercise.

This condition cures itself in most cases when enough time is allowed to pass and when rest (relative) is prescribed. Nevertheless, mobilizations shorten the duration of pain, often dramatically.

HYPOMOBILITY LESIONS

Localized Restriction. Facet joint capsular tightness or degenerative changes in the disk result in localized hypomobility lesions. The chronic form of a mechanical derangement, usually of the intervertebral joint complex, is the result of prolonged immobilization secondary to injury or poor posture. Often there is a history of acute low back dysfunction. The onset of pain may be gradual or sudden; the patient may relate it to bending, twisting, or trauma. Pain varies in degree from minor to severe and is usually described as a dull aching in the lumbosacral region or referred into the buttocks, leg, or abdomen. Symptoms are aggravated by long periods of standing, walking, or activity involving prolonged or repetitive lumbar extension. Symptoms are worse in the evening than in the morning.

When evaluating a patient, it is often difficult, if not impossible, to determine if pain is coming from the disk or the facet joints. Determining the mechanism of aggravation and analyzing the most painful position may give reliable clues. If extension (standing and walking) is the most aggravating, the facets are probably involved. If the pain is diskogenic in nature, it may be because of mechanical irritation or inflammation of the outer wall of the annulus.[670] In this case, flexion (sitting and forward-bending) is the most painful movement or is the mechanism of aggravation.

Consider the following points and tests in evaluating the patient:

1. Possible subtle predisposing biomechanical factors, such as leg-length discrepancy
2. Physiologic motions may appear normal but usually show some evidence of restricted motion only in certain directions (e.g., minor restriction of sidebending to the involved side; deviation of the spine toward the involved side on forward-bending and away from the involved side on extension). When motions are restricted, they should also reproduce the patient's pain. The normal, rhythmic pattern of lumbar movement may also be disturbed. This is best appreciated by standing behind the patient to observe spinal movement.

3. There is usually loss of the normal passive joint-play movements that reproduce the pain. However, because degenerative joint or disk disease can develop because of hypermobility or instability of the joint, accessory movements are sometimes excessive. Pain may occur within the limited range, but most often it occurs at the limits of the range. The examination consists of direct pressure over the spinous process, lateral pressure over the spinous process, pressure over the facet joints, and pressure over the interspinous and supraspinous ligaments. Pain may be referred and is usually unilateral.
4. Special tests may be indicated if the above tests fail to reproduce symptoms. The quadrant test, combined movements or H and I tests are used in attempt to reproduce the symptoms at the appropriate level. Examination using combined movements and recognition of regular (or irregular) patterns of movement can be most helpful in the selection of treatment techniques.[191]
5. The involved level is tender to palpation. Often, a thickened supraspinous ligament can be palpated.
6. Roentgenograms should be normal for the patient's age.

Manipulations, segmental distraction techniques, and mobilizations (including muscle energy techniques and combined movements) are the manual treatments of choice. On the whole, mobilization techniques are most effective because of the variety of joint responses that can be facilitated.[419] A vast array of mobilization techniques can be used.

With hypermobility, localized stabilization techniques should be used instead. Sometimes both mobilization and stabilization techniques are indicated. Mobilizing exercises are indicated if the condition has been present for a long time. Based on the evaluation, the home program should include localized segmental self-mobilization or stabilization techniques (see Figs. 22-62 and 22-63). Prolonged rest and use of supports are contraindicated, because they tend to increase the restrictions.

Multisegmental Bilateral Capsular Restriction. Degenerative joint or disk disease, osteoarthritis, lumbar spondylosis, and facet arthritis are included in this category. Various terms, including spondylosis, are used to describe the osteoarthritic changes in the spine that may lead to back pain, which is more common in middle-aged or older persons. Although degenerative joint or disk disease is a natural process of aging and is often asymptomatic, symptoms sometimes develop as the result of hypomobility and repeated trauma. Hypermobility can also contribute to the development of degenerative joint or disk disease. Patients with symptomatic degenerative joint disease often have difficulty bending because of stiffness and aching in the low back. On stooping over a wash basin, they usually lean on one arm to support the body weight. After simple loosening-up exercises or a hot shower, the discomfort eases tremendously. As the condition progresses, the patient tends to get worse as the day goes on, but at times the pain may be more pronounced after a night of rest and then ease as the patient becomes more mobile. Patients also may note discomfort with increasing sports activities and may even cut down on sports as they become aware that pain and stiffness tend to be more pronounced the following day.

A striking symptom relates to many patients' avocations or occupational activities—they do not like to hold their backs in a flexed position.[685] Homemakers, carpenters, plumbers, and others who must frequently work in a stooped position find their symptoms increased. They do not like standing for lengthy periods because this increases the lumbar lordosis. Aching is relieved if one foot is placed on a stool or step while standing. If facet arthrosis is more advanced, turning over in bed becomes increasingly difficult because of movement imposed on the facet joints.

Because degenerative changes involve both the anterior and posterior portions of the intervertebral joint complex, it is impossible to determine the exact mechanism of symptom production. The most likely basis for attacks of mechanical derangement is recurrent episodes of synovitis in the facet joints after overuse, such as excessive bending (as in gardening), stressful unaccustomed activity, or abrasive positioning with resultant strain of the joints. After several hours of heavy use, pain develops that can last for hours. Pain is typically at the lower lumbar midline but may radiate out to the groin or buttock. Degenerative joint or disk disease may also occur with neurologic complications (i.e., lateral spinal stenosis). Pain may be experienced in one or both legs, and three mechanisms may be involved: pain may be referred with stimulation of the sinuvertebral nerve; sciatica may result from nerve root pressure, or leg pain may be caused by the pressure of a spinal canal stenosis.[131]

Consider the following in evaluating a patient:

1. Activities that aggravate and relieve symptoms. Some loss of normal lordosis may be noted. The pain may increase if the patient tries to sit up straight or slumps. Symptoms are decreased with the back in a neutral or functional position. Pain is increased when upright (standing and walking). One test that Seimons[685] found positive in almost all of these patients is to have the patient stand semi-stooped and to maintain this position for 1 to 2 minutes. This increases the tension in the disks and also strains the capsular ligaments of the facet joints.
2. Physiologic movements. Early on, spinal motions may appear normal. Most of the discomfort and stiffness occurs early in the day and may have subsided by the time of the assessment. With advanced chronic degeneration, restriction of active and passive motions occurs in a generalized capsular pattern: marked restriction and equal limitation of side flexion, and moderate restriction of rotation, forward-bending, and backward-bending.
3. Moderate to significant restriction of all accessory motions may be noted.
4. The neurologic findings in uncomplicated degenerative disease are normal. Patients who complain of pain on coughing, sneezing, jarring movements, or turning over in bed often have a positive heel-drop test.
5. Degenerative changes are observed on roentgenograms, affecting the disk and facet joints. The severity of pain is out of proportion to the roentgenographic findings.[685]

With advanced degenerative joint or disk disease, movements are stiff in all directions, so treatment requires several techniques in different directions, including intermittent variable lumbar traction, mobilization, and a program of exercises. There may also be attacks of mechanical derangement. First, settle any localized single joint signs superimposed on an otherwise stiff spine by local treatment, as these will be worsened by a generalized regimen. The facet joints are more vulnerable to facet impingement, sprains, and inflammation when degenerative joint disease is present.

Nonsteroidal anti-inflammatory drugs are used in patients with more severe degrees of degenerative joint disease in an attempt to reduce any associated synovitis.[550]

Passive movements (i.e., flexion, extension, and sidebending) play a major role in the management of patients with multisegmental involvement. Starting in the direction opposite that of pain aggravation, exercises are progressed to include motions in all directions. Manual and mechanical lumbar traction and spinal mobilization techniques increase mobility and relieve pain. Use joint mobilization and exercise cautiously in the presence of nerve root irritation, because they may increase symptoms. Postural training and carefully instituted isometric exercises to strengthen the abdominal and back muscles may be indicated. Patients may be overweight, and their type of work may aggravate the disorder. The overweight patient should be encouraged to lose weight and to exercise by walking or swimming within the limits of pain. Brisk walking (in patients who are bothered by standing) often relieves pain.

SEGMENTAL INTERVERTEBRAL INSTABILITY

The reader is referred to the earlier discussion of segmental instabilities under Medical Models and Disease Entities in this chapter. When the ligaments of the spinal segment, including the outer annulus of the intervertebral disk, the iliolumbar ligament, the sacroiliac ligaments as well as the muscles of the low back and abdominal region, become weakened or lose their normal tone, the result is spinal instability Ligamentous conditions can either start as a traumatic spondylolisthesis or lead to a degenerative spondylolisthesis (see below). The principle risk is a disk rupture. Factors that can be responsible for the development of a hypermobile segment include trauma, pathology (e.g., degenerative joint changes), anatomic impairment (e.g., spondylolisthesis, asymmetric tropic changes in the zygapophyseal joint, herniated nucleus pulposus) or repetitive movement patterns. With repetitive movement, segmental hypermobility can develop within the lumbopelvic region in response to a relatively less mobile segment or region. Abnormal or excessive movement is imposed on segments with the least amount of stiffness. With repeated movements over time, the more stiff segments decrease in mobility, and the least stiff segments increase in mobility.

Clinical Variations. Clinical classifications have been developed from clinical observation and are based on the mechanism of injury to the spine, resultant tissue damage, the reported and observed aggravating activities and movement problems relating to specific movement quadrant or quadrants.[592,661] Common to all the patient presentations is the repeated vulnerability and observed lack of movement control and related symptoms within the neutral zone. Instabilities may be present in extension, flexion, rotation, or lateral displacement. As the motion within the lumbar spine is three-dimensional and involves coupled movement, tissue damage is likely to result in movement dysfunction in more than one direction (e.g., rotation with flexion syndrome, rotation with extension and multi-direction patterns).[592,661]

Flexion Pattern or Flexion Syndrome. The flexion pattern appears to be the most common. These patients may relate their injury to either a single flexion/rotational injury or to repetitive strains relating to flexion/rotational activities.[592] Symptoms are present or increase with positions or movements associated with lumbar flexion (e.g., sitting, forward bending, driving).[661] They predominantly report aggravation of their symptoms during flexion/rotational movements, with an inability to sustain semiflexed postures.[592,752] Movements into forward bending are associated with a tendency to flex more at the symptomatic level than at the adjacent levels. This movement may be associated with a painful arc and an inability to return from flexion to neutral without the use of hands to assist the movement.[592]

Specific muscle tests reveal an inability to activate lumbar multifidus in co-contraction with the deep abdominal muscle at the unstable motion segment within a neutral lordosis. Many patients are unable to assume a neutral lordotic posture, particularly in four point kneeling or sitting. The preferred alignment is a flexed lumbar spine in both sitting and quadriped. Symptoms are present or increased, relative to sitting with the lumbar spine in neutral or slightly arched inward.

According to Sahrmann,[661] the primary dysfunction of the flexion syndrome is that lumbar flexion motion is more flexible than hip flexion motion. Most often, the back extensors are elongated and flexible while the hip extensors are short and stiff.

Extension Pattern and Lumbar Extension Syndrome. The primary dysfunction in this pattern or syndrome is that the position of stress that aggravates their symptoms is extension and extension/rotation.[592,752] Activities such as standing, fast walking, and carrying out overhead activities, sitting in lumbar extension, or back lying with their legs straight also aggravate their symptoms.[752] Patients find walking with a stoop posture is more comfortable.[300] They typically relate their injury to an extension rotation incident or repetitive movement patterns frequently associated with sporting activities involving extension.[592,752]

Examination elicits tenderness between the spinous processes of the involved joint. In the quadriped position, rocking backward increases the symptoms compared with rocking forward.[661] Extension activities usually reveal hinging at the affected segment with a loss of segmental lordosis above this level. In the standing position, younger individual may exhibit an increase in lumbar lordosis. Sometimes there is segmental lordosis at the unstable segment with an increased level of segmental muscle activity. Muscle findings reveal difficulty or inability to cocontract segmental lumbar multifidus and the deep abdominal muscles in the neutral position.[752] There may be weakness, excessive length, or inadequate stiffness of the external oblique.[661]

Sahrmann[661] indicates the primary dysfunction in the extension syndrome is that the lumbar spine extends more readily than the hip extensors and the hip flexors exert an anterior shear forces on the spine. The hip flexors and lumbar paraspinals are short or stiff.

Lumbar Rotation Syndrome. The primary dysfunction in this syndrome is that a segment of the lumbar spine rotates, sidebends, glides and translates more easily than the other segments.[661] Symptoms are often unilateral or greater on one side and increase with rotation. It is not common to find a patient that has a pure lumbar rotation syndrome because of coupled movements of sidebending and rotation. Patients may experience increase symptoms with sidebending or rotation, activities requiring repeated movements into rotation (e.g., tennis, golf). Symptoms are often transient and occur with change in position. There may be increase in symptoms with extension of the hip and knees in supine. One may observe loss of lumbopelvic rotation control in supine with hip and knee flexion, and hip abduction and lateral rotation. Preventing excessive lumbopelvic rotation by controlling the abdominals is more important than muscular strength. Weakness, excessive length or poor control of oblique abdominals muscles maybe a contributing factor (internal oblique on one side and external oblique on the opposite side). Many patients however have strong abdominals but can not control lumbopelvic rotation associated with movement of the lower limbs.

As described earlier the main effect of rotational injuries is on the intervertebral disk itself. Associated diagnosis includes spinal stenosis, facet syndrome, scoliosis, spondylolysis and osteoporosis. Differential movement patterns include the lumbar rotation-flexion and lumbar rotation-extension syndrome. See the works of Sahrmann[661] and Van Dillen and associates[778,779] for details of these rotation movement impairment syndromes.

Lateral Shift Pattern. The lateral shift pattern is usually unidirectional and is associated with unilateral low back pain. Patients present with a loss of lumbar segmental lordosis at the affected level and usually with an associated lateral shift in the lower lumbar spine.[752] Sidebending in the direction of the shift commonly reveals a lateral translatory movement rather than sidebending.

Muscle findings reveals an inability to bilaterally activate segmental lumbar multifidi and co-contraction with the deep abdominal muscles, with dominance of activation of the lumbar erector spinae, the quadratus lumborum and superficial multifidi on the side ipsilateral to the shift. Palpation of the lumbar multifidi muscle in standing commonly reveals atrophy and low tone on the contralateral side. There is an inability to activate segmental lumbar multifidi on the contralateral side.

Multidirectional Pattern. This is the most serious and debilitating of the clinical presentations.[592,752] Usually all weight-bearing activities are painful and excessive segmental shifting and hinging patterns may be observed in all movement directions. These patients have the poorest prognosis for conservative treatment particularly, if they present with an inability to tolerate compression loading and a high degree of irritability.

Management of Lumbar Intervertebral Instability. The findings of the physical examination dictate the treatment approach to be taken. The aim of the examination is to identify the symptomatic hypermobile motion segment,[592] the local muscle system dysfunction and faulty movement patterns of global muscle system substitutions,[640] and the neuromuscular control strategy utilized by the patient to stabilize the spine during functional movement and limb loading tasks.[659] Special tests to identify the symptomatic hypermobile segment may include joint integrity testing (e.g., anterior shear, posterior shear, torsion tests), PPIVMs, PAIVMs, the vertical compression test (see Fig. 20-4) and quadriped tests (e.g., flexion, extension, forward and backward rocking). Once the aim has been achieved, the specific exercise intervention can be used to retrain appropriate motor control strategies with integration in a functional manner. See Functional Exercise, Sensorimotor Training and Spinal Stabilization below.

LUMBAR SPONDYLOLYSIS AND SPONDYLOLISTHESIS

Lumbar spondylosis, a bilateral defect in the pars interarticularis, occurs in 58% of adults.[13] The etiology of spondylolysis is multifactorial with genetic predisposition, developmental defects, and repetitive microtrauma all contributing as a risk factor.[240,460,729] In athletes, repetitive flexion and extension stresses cause an initial stress reaction in pars articularis. With repetitive activity, low back pain gradually occurs. Typically the pain is reproduced by back extension. A positive one-legged hyperextension test is especially indicative of ipsilateral spondylolysis.[823] Pain on the support leg is suspicious for an ipsilateral spondylolysis. Patients may also have hamstring tightness or spasm.[460,729]

Approximately 50% of spondylolysis never progress to any of degree of spondylolisthesis, a condition of forward slippage of a cephalad vertebra onto a caudal vertebra (Fig. 22-4D).[7] There are different types of lumbar spondylolisthesis. These types are described in a classic article by Wiltse et al.[813] in 1976. The two most common forms of spondylolisthesis are isthmic and degenerative spondylolisthesis.[380] Degenerative spondylolisthesis refers to the anterior slippage of a vertebrae related to degenerative changes within the facet joint and has been discussed earlier (see section on effect of aging). Isthmic spondylolisthesis occurs in relation to a defect in the pars interarticularis that may be caused by a fracture. The defect itself is known as a **spondylolytic defect.** It may occur at any level but is most common at L5–S1 segmental level, primarily because of the angulation of the L5 segment with respect to vertical. The slip or spondylolisthesis generally occurs during adolescence. The majority of isthmic spondylolisthesis that become symptomatic do so during the adult years, generally in the four and fifth decades of life.[380]

EXAMINATION AND EVALUATION FINDINGS

The patient may complain of backache, localized lumbosacral discomfort, gluteal pain, lower limb pain, paraesthesia in the legs, and stiffness after exercise. Increase symptoms are more commonly provoked with activities of repetitive flexion, extension and rotation. Pain is described as a dull ache, episodic, depending on the activity. Onset usually is mid-morning after standing. Symptoms worsen on extension and return from forward bending. Significant physical findings include[550]:

- Stiff waddling gait
- Increased lumbar lordosis
- Flexed knee stance
- A depression at the listhesis level
- Tender prominent spinous process of "slipped" vertebra
- Limited flexion
- Hamstring tightness or spasm
- Percussion over the segment may elicit pain

Neurologic examination is usually negative. Radiologic confirmation can be made by a lateral view of the lumbosacral region.

Although 5% of the population have spondylolisthesis, not all are symptomatic.[550] The pain is usually caused by extreme stretching of the interspinous ligaments or of the nerve root. The onset of back pain in many of these patients is caused by concurrent disk degeneration rather than a mechanical problem.

TREATMENT

Treatment initially consists of modification of activity and control of pain (e.g., cryotherapy or heat, grades I and II joint mobilizations at level of instability, strain–counterstrain). If the patient has a hot bone scan, the use of a rigid lumbosacral brace in neutral or slight flexion has been advocated as a means to increase speed of recovery.[197,460,526,527,638] Unilateral pars defects have a greater chance of healing than do bilateral defects. The presence of a bilateral pars defect shown on x-ray may significantly decrease the chance of bony healing, even with immobilization.[372] If back pain persists despite bracing and rehabilitation, surgery may be considered.

Most patients with isthmic spondylolysis will benefit from initial nonsurgical treatment. Stabilization exercises aimed at the lumbosacral area by combining realignment with a muscle-strengthening program, activity modification, and movement re-education is the cornerstones of rehabilitation.[594] As for patients with lumbar stenosis, extension and shearing forces should be avoided initially. If anterior shear is positive in neutral and flexion, patients should exercise and perform body mechanic in neutral.[682] If anterior shear is positive in neutral and negative in flexion, patient should perform body mechanics with a posterior pelvic tilt.[682]

Other methods of stabilization include sclerosant injections, prolotherapy injections (to strengthen the ligaments by stimulating collagen formation),[276,399,400,562,589,629,673] and surgical fusion. Indications for surgical intervention include lack of response to conservative measures, significant restriction of the patient's activities, and neurologic findings that are progressing, or in spondylolisthesis progression of the slip itself.[69]

Chronic Low Back Pain

After 3 months of low back pain, only 5 to 10% of patients have persisting symptoms,[234,559] but these patients account for 85% of the costs in terms of compensation and loss of work related to low back pain.[235,717] In these patients, the presence of a treatable active disease has been carefully eliminated. Pain has become the patient's preoccupation, limiting daily activity.[631] It is important to reach a definitive diagnosis if possible, and to rule out any of the causes for back pain for which specific treatment exists. No study demonstrates a specific method of treatment for chronic idiopathic low back pain.[559]

The differential diagnosis of chronic low back pain includes all the conditions previously discussed, which may be overlooked or neglected during the acute and subacute phases. Lumbar segmental instability, in the absence of defects of the bony architecture of the lumbar spine, has been sited as a significant cause of chronic low back pain.[450] A number of studies have reported increased and abnormal intersegmental motion in subjects with chronic low back pain, often in the absence of other radiologic findings.[242,442,693] Additional diagnostic possibilities include various degenerative conditions, spondyloarthropathies, and ill-defined syndromes of fibrositis or fibromyalgia. Some psychologists[220] maintain that this pain represents a behavior reaction, whereas neurophysiologists lean toward the hypothesis that nervous structures irritated for a prolonged period generate new mechanisms of pain generation. Chronic pain has also been described as a variant of depression. In a study of patients with chronic low back pain, a structured diagnosis was possible in 50%; no diagnosis could be determined in the remainder.[621]

Included in this diagnostic category are degenerative spondylolisthesis[776] and degenerative lumbar stenosis,[25,394] affecting either the central canal or the lateral recesses, or consisting of isolated disk resorption.[138] Also included are several degenerative conditions with less certain criteria such as facet syndromes,[540] disk disruption syndrome,[139] segmental instability,[237,258,396,542,557,736] idiopathic vertebral sclerosis,[802] diffuse idiopathic skeletal hyperostosis,[237] inflammatory spondyloarthropathy,[94] myofascial syndromes,[736]

fibrositis,[2,95,315,408,448,712–714,762,617,815,816] and primary fibromyalgia[45,95,96,109,371,762,816,826–831] (also see other sources[28,44,96,213,214,245,281,318,475,496,598,691,695–700,763,816,828]).

According to Maigne,[468] in many cases of chronic distal lumbago and sciatica, a cellulomyalgic syndrome is often present, revealed by the presence of myalgic cordlike structures in the muscles of the external iliac fossa (i.e., the gluteus medius, tensor fasciae latae, gluteus maximus, or piriformis). In the syndromes of sciatica, in addition to the muscles of the iliac fossa, the distal portion of the biceps femoris, the lateral gastrocnemius (S1), and the anterior lateral aspect of the leg (L5) may be involved. With joint manipulation, tenderness often disappears, but in some cases pain remains. In addition to procaine injections of trigger points, treatment by slow, deep massage and long, continued stretching may be helpful.

EVALUATION

A definitive diagnosis requires a careful history to identify the distribution of back and leg pain as well as such aggravators of pain as poor posture, mechanical loads, and walking.[187] The physical examination should include observation of gait, trunk mobility, deformities, leg-length inequalities, and assessment of coordination, endurance, and function. The examination should also include a careful search for neurosensory and motor loss and signs of nerve root tension. The neurologic examination may be confusing and show no anatomical sensory losses in patients with spinal stenosis.[251] In addition to a detailed neuromuscular examination, abdominal and vascular evaluations should be included, particularly in the elderly and those with symptoms suggesting neurogenic claudication. The degenerative conditions that may be causing the pain can be classified according to the clinical history, roentgenographic findings, diagnostic blocks, and imaging studies. Psychologic testing should be used to determine the patient's psychologic status and to explore the relations between pain behavior and reinforcing consequences.

The results of a physical examination in such patients are often nonspecific, except for demonstration of restricted motion and muscle spasm. However, many degenerative conditions can be strongly suggested by roentgenographic studies. When segmental instability is suspected, flexion and extension films may demonstrate abnormal displacements.[237,391,542] If nerve root symptoms or claudication is present, myelography is the most sensitive study for identifying the level of neural encroachment, followed by CT scanning. CT and MRI are rapidly surpassing myelography as the imaging technique of choice in most patients with radiculopathies. Electromyography may also be used to provide additional confirmation of the levels of nerve root involvement.[195] In patients with suspected facet syndrome, a CT scan may reveal degeneration, but a definitive diagnosis is based on the relief of symptoms by the injection of local anesthetics into the affected joints.[202,536,539]

TREATMENT CONSIDERATIONS

Most patients with chronic low back pain can be treated with anti-inflammatory medications and exercise programs.[234] As in other nonmalignant chronic pain syndromes, narcotic analgesics are avoided. Alternative therapeutic modalities have been used, including biofeedback, acupuncture, transcutaneous nerve stimulation, implanted neurostimulators, and ablative neurosurgical procedures.[521] These methods have varying degrees of success; all have methodologic problems.[165] For selected patients, trigger-point injections may be beneficial.[639]

Soft Tissue Manipulation, Massage, and Relaxation. Soft tissue manipulations, with the specific purpose of improving the vascularity and extensibility of the soft tissues, are another approach to pain management (see Chapters 7 and 8). Massage and myofascial manipulations are being used now more than ever before.[32,42,111,113,144,147,185,186,303,356,414,415,468,469,517,547,588,599,588,791,798] These techniques are beneficial, although research has been lacking in this area for hundreds of years.[262,263] Recent studies have found massage to be effective for persistent back pain and may reduce the cost of care after an initial course of therapy.[110,118] Effectiveness is attributed in part to increased circulation to the area, release of muscle spasm, stretching of abnormal fibrous tissue (connective tissue), increased proprioception, and extensibility of the soft tissues. An increase in extensibility may also allow a secondary increase in circulation.[124] Acupressure massage presumably produces some of the same beneficial effects as acupuncture and acupuncture-like transcutaneous electrical nerve stimulation.[112,749,821] Rocking-chair therapy and mechanical vibration are other forms of sensory stimulation that reportedly relieve both chronic and acute pain.[146,288,289,451–453,522,596,819] Relaxation techniques can affect the pain cycle by eliciting relaxation, increasing circulation, and decreasing pain (see Chapter 9, Relaxation and Related Techniques). Stress and tension influence strongly the perception of pain and pain tolerance.

Anterior Element Pain. **Anterior element pain** is pain that is made worse by sustained flexion of the lumbar spine.[694] Characteristically, anterior element pain is made worse by sitting and is relieved by standing. Patients assume the hyperlordotic posture to relieve pain. Fracture of the vertebral body and prolapsed intervertebral disks produce anterior element symptoms. In young patients, in whom anterior element pain is the most common presentation, extension exercises and press-ups are more likely to produce remission than flexion exercises.[385] This is borne out by the tendency of many flexion exercises to increase intradiskal pressure; extension exercises unload the disk.[341] Therefore, the hyperextension principles advocated by Cyriax[146] and McKenzie[510,511] are logical for patients with anterior element pain.[425] Lesions resulting in chronic anterior pain are obscure; it is tempting to assume that anterior element pain is diskogenic in origin, but there is no evidence for this. Unlike the acute group, patients with chronic anterior element pain may respond to manipulative techniques.[424,649]

Posterior Element Pain. In posterior element pain, pain is worsened by increasing the lumbar lordosis, standing, and walking. It is eased by maintained forward-flexion, sitting, and hip flexion (with or without the knees extended). Patients with structural or postural hyperlordosis, facet arthropathy, or foraminal stenosis show features of posterior element pain.[676,694] Pain from extension and rotation is usually of facet origin.[804] Flexion treatment frequently improves facet disease, spondylolysis, flexion dysfunction, and certain types of derangement.[170,171,510,804] Hyperextension exercises may make the condition worse.[385]

Movement-Related Pain. Patients with movement-related pain are most comfortable at rest; pain is precipitated only by activity or jarring. Heavy manual work, repeated twisting, fast walking or running (especially on hard surfaces), and traveling in cars over rough ground all precipitate pain. Movement-related pain occurs in association with traumatic fracture/dislocations, in symptomatic spondylolysis or spondylolisthesis, and as a result of chronic degenerative segmental instability. Diagnosis may be confirmed by obtaining lateral flexion and extension roentgenograms of the lumbar spine and noting abnormal translational movements. A basic scheme of progressive stabilization by strengthening regional and segmental muscles isometrically should be considered.[258,259,266] According to Grieve,[266] mature patients and those in most pain may need to start abdominal exercises with their knees bent, and progress more slowly. Sidelying stabilization techniques and dynamic abdominal bracing also may be used (see spinal stabilization and dynamic functional exercises below).[387] Home exercises must be efficiently monitored, and the patient must be taught to avoid aggravating postures and activities.[678]

Mechanical Pain without Postural or Movement Exacerbation. Patients with static-sensitive low back pain cannot maintain any one position (other than lying) for a normal length of time and obtain relief by changing position and moving. Many of these patients appear to have discrete structural disease, such as scoliosis.[76]

Altered Pattern of Muscle Recruitment. Janda has delineated the altered patterns of muscle recruitment in chronic low back pain (see Table 6-1).[345–350,360,361] One of the most common is the overuse and early recruitment of the low back muscles.[516] Another common pattern associated with low back pain is overuse of the hip flexors (psoas) and weakness of the abdominals. Often the gluteal muscles must be retrained and the overuse of lumbar extension inhibited, a common maladaptive pattern.

Numerous clinicians have written on exercise programs for the treatment of muscle imbalances and programs for postural correction, with or without mechanical or manual resistance or assistance (see sensorimotor and neuromuscular training below). (See other sources.[64,92,173,238,265,272–275,294,384,443,541,612,613,656–661,663,741])

Spinal Bracing. Several lumbar supports have been advocated. Spinal bracing seems justified in patients with osteoporotic compression fractures, spondylolisthesis, or segmental instability, and in some patients with spinal stenosis, although no controlled studies have demonstrated its efficacy. Approximately 80 to 90% of patients wearing a simple support find it of benefit.[559] It prevents excessive motion and reminds the wearer not to exaggerate the lumbar load.

EDUCATIONAL PROGRAMS

Educational programs are an essential part of the care of patients with chronic low back pain.[94,103,125,145,201,215,228,296, 398,412,413,430,437,487,489,508,509,669,671,680,685,727,736,738,739,741,784,786,804] All patients must be educated in how to live with their discomfort. Advice regarding everyday activities must be individualized; in many instances this is the most important aspect of treatment.

Functional Training. These structured programs include the identification of routine daily living and work postures and activities, and advice on re-education exercises and instructions.[631] Mayer and associates[487,489] have devised a functional program that emphasizes restoration of muscle strength and aerobic capacity, vocational assessment, and short-term psychologic intervention, with careful qualification of progress. One year after this 3-week intervention, 85% of patients had returned to work (see Chapter 10, Functional Exercise).

Back Schools. These structured intervention programs are aimed at groups of patients and include general information on the spine, recommended posture and physical activities, preventive measures, and exercises for the back.[3,46, 215,225,286,297,398,423,443,446,483,509,804,812,832] The main objective is to transmit information on anatomy and disorders of the spine and to teach the principles underlying healthy posture, daily activities, and sports. The content of the programs varies considerably. Overall patient satisfaction with back schools is 75 to 96%. According to White,[804] 70 to 90% of patients find their pain is at an acceptable level after attending back school.

Acute back schools and education can often keep patients out of the hospital and return many of them to a normal life in just days.[804] Back schools in the home and at work, and athletic back schools for chronic patients have also been described.

Work-hardening or work-capacity training are the "Super Bowl" of back schools. A high rate of recurrent low back injury and poor work tolerance may be owing to underlying pathologic processes and incomplete rehabilitation before return to work. With the work-endurance program, there has been a significant improvement in work tolerance and a decreased rate of recurrent injury.[427,430,437,438,489,805]

Specialized Centers. Exercises and therapeutic activities may be prescribed, directed, and supervised by a health professional.[238,325,387,543,544] Generally, exercises are done in a specialized center for a limited time only, mainly to instruct the patient, and then are continued at home by the patient. Sometimes specific rehabilitation demands prolonged therapy in a specialized environment.

Most of these programs emphasize the functional position of the spine, defined by Morgan and Vollowitz as "the optimal position in which the spine functions."[544] These positions vary depending on the physical condition of the spine and the

stresses it must withstand. There is no one position for all functional tasks, and the best functional position varies from person to person. It is often near the midrange of all available movement. The functional position should not be confused with the theoretical "neutral" position of the spine.

The spinal control method (stabilization) is a form of body mechanics that trains and uses any or all of the muscles associated with body alignment to place a given spinal segment in its functional balanced position and hold it there while other joints and muscle groups accomplish a specific task. Thus, the involved spinal segment is stabilized to whatever degree is necessary to allow pain-free activity.[544]

PAIN CLINICS

Pain clinics focus on behavioral adaptation to help patients withstand and control their condition.[498,631] This form of intervention is recommended to evaluate the factors that modify the patient's perception of pain and to support the patient. Improved understanding of the relation between pain and activity has resulted in a change in management from a negative philosophy of treatment for pain to more active restoration of function. Fordyce and colleagues[222] and other behavioral psychologists have investigated the relation between chronic pain and physical activity, and suggest that pain behaviors are influenced and modified by their consequences.[221,223,443,690]

Ergonomics. Knowledge of the patient's work environment and a functional evaluation can help ensure a better balance between job assignments and capabilities.[631] For chronic conditions, ergonomic interventions are an integral component of therapy. Ergonomists seek to create a harmonious balance between workers and their equipment, work patterns, and the working environment, both at work and at home. Manual handling and lifting has received more attention from ergonomists[106,107,159,235,236,464,465,745] than virtually any other topic. Since Brackett[70] first identified the possible dangers of lifting a heavy load from the ground with the back in a fully flexed position. Many ergonomists have sought to identify safer lifting techniques and load limits.[157,296–298,553,554,438,439]

Another aspect of back pain that has interested ergonomists is work postures, particularly the seated work posture. Several epidemiologic studies point to the relation between sitting and back pain, and clinicians use the increase of pain in sitting as a diagnostic indicator.[381,382] Many authors—as early as Staffel in 1884[724]—have made recommendations about seating design.[65,80,296,473,784] The importance of the design of the back rest was underlined by Akerblom in 1948.[8,376] Andersson and associates[15–17] measured changes in intradiskal pressure at the L3–L4 disk in different sitting positions and for different configurations of the backrest and lumbar support. To reduce intradiskal pressure, they recommended a positive lumbar support maintaining the lumbar spine in lordosis.

Reports about seating and driving positions have demonstrated a confusing lack of agreement. Until recently, concepts of correct design have been based more on aesthetics, ethics, and wishful thinking than on science, but that is beginning to change. The chair is a principal adjunct in industrialized labor, and seating design must be integrated into the whole of the workspace and also the job design. It is hoped that car manufacturers will propose alternative seating designs to substantially reduce stresses on the spine.

Exercise. Currently, aerobic exercise is a popular form of treatment. The bases for these exercise programs have been extensively reviewed with respect to their effects on disk nutrition, pain modulation, and spinal mechanics.[152,341,558] Knowledge of the body's endogenous chemical pain-modulating capability, the endorphin system, continues to increase.[9,563,684,755,824] Activity in large muscle groups yields an increased amount of endorphins in both the bloodstream and the CSF.[9,207] This, in turn, lessens the pain sensitivity.[486,563,684,824] Johansson and associates[355] demonstrated in 10 patients with chronic back pain a significantly lower amount of endorphins in the CSF, a finding corroborated by Pug and coworkers.[630] Aerobic exercise also relieves depression,[219,709] a common finding with at least chronic low back pain. Other benefits include increased mental alertness,[184,824] sleep,[219,709] and stamina[375]; improved self-image; and an increase in the activity level compatible with chronic pain.[220,709]

Walking and jogging on soft, even ground are recommended. Indoor cross-country skiing machines are preferable to stationary bikes, and water aerobics are preferable to swimming. High levels of physical fitness reduce the risk of further injury and speed rehabilitation. The more physically fit a person is, the more pain he or she can tolerate.[129,227,684] However, there is little agreement about what form the exercise should take. Any exercises selected must be based on a thorough clinical evaluation.[341]

TREATMENT TECHNIQUES

Assessment continues throughout the treatment period, and the patient's response guides the next step in treatment. Do not overtreat; when signs and symptoms are cleared, stop. Treatment should be adapted according to presenting signs and symptoms; as these changes, so should the treatment.

Soft Tissue Manipulations

When hypomobility of the lumbopelvic region results from osteokinematic restrictions, the cause may be articular, myofascial or both. Muscle contraction is often a primary source of lumbopelvic dysfunction.[393] In low back pain or dysfunction, it is typical for the erector spinae to be held in a sustained contraction.[303] The hypertonicity limits the movement in the joints, creating a fixation of the facets. This stimulates the joint mechanoreceptors, which have neurologic reflexes to the surrounding muscles. Some muscles increase their tension, and others become inhibited, such as the multifidus. Janda,[346,349] has discovered predictable patterns of muscle imbalances. Jull and Janda[361] called this muscle imbalance the pelvic or distal crossed syndrome (see Chapter 8, Soft Tissue Manipulations). These imbalances alter movement

patterns and therefore add a continuing stress to the joint system. Muscles that tend to be tight include the iliopsoas, lumbar portion of erector spinae, the piriformis, iliotibial band and tensor fascia lata, the adductors, hamstrings and quadratus lumborum.

Box 8-9 illustrates self-stretches for the muscles prone to tightness in the pelvic or distal crossed syndrome. Manual stretches are also described in Figures 8-3 through 8-6, 8-13, 8-15, 8-17, 8-19, 8-34 through 8-37, 8-66, and 8-68 through 8-75. It is important to remember that not all tight structures should be stretched or release by soft tissue manipulations. Oftentimes, tightness is a protective guarding mechanism designed to control loads to the injured tissue. Porterfield and DeRosa[624] have proposed the following useful guideline. "If the forces of tightness generate unwanted forces and loads into the injured area—stretch the tight structures. If the forces of generate unwanted loads away from the injured area—avoid stretching of those specific tight structures." Assessment of the underlying cause of altered myofascial length and the forces generated is crucial for correcting dysfunction in the myofascial system. Muscles that tend to be inhibited and weak include the multifidi, gluteus maximus, minimus and the abdominals. Clinically, it is more effective to release the hypertonicity in a muscle and to lengthen a short muscle and its connective tissue before trying to strengthen a weak or inhibited muscle.[347,350]

Neural Tension Techniques

According to Grieve,[264] the development of neural tension techniques of the lumbar spine has been encouraged by the success of including hamstring stretching techniques in the treatment plan,[31,343] progressive stretching of nonirritable (presumed) lumbar root adhesions,[264] and the slump test.[89,471,766] Maitland[471] described the "slump test," which maximally stresses the dural sheath and the nerve roots (see Fig. 22-22). This test exerts a cephalad and caudally directed force on the dura mater and additionally places a tensile stress on the nerve roots of the lower limbs.

Localized segmental changes should generally be treated first when tethering lesions are suspected. If this does not relieve the so-called canal signs, neural tension techniques should be considered. Any of the slump tests may be used in treatment as a mobilization technique. Clinicians have prescribed straight-leg raising stretches for many years not only to stretch the hamstrings but also, in some situations, to stretch the sciatic nerve. Butler[89] recommends that to turn a hamstring stretch into a neural system stretch, it should be done with the hip in medial rotation; this allows better access to the neural tissue. Several variations of straight-leg raising techniques and prone knee bends to stretch the upper part of the femoral nerve are described in the literature.[89,471,687] Neural tension techniques are beyond the scope of this text, but manipulative and clinical reasoning courses are available that include the concepts and practice of mobilization of the nervous system.

Joint Mobilization Techniques

The following are examples of spinal movement techniques that should be useful in treating properly selected patients when applied according to the guidelines below. For complete descriptions and illustrations of the great variety of mobilization techniques, other texts should be consulted.[148,255,264,370,392,468,469,471,510,523–525,606,731] For mobilization to be effective, a sense of "feel" of movement is required. The movements occurring are often not seen but sensed.[131]

Many passive movements have been described for the lumbar spine, but only a few of the more common techniques are presented here. Although some of McKenzie's techniques[510] are briefly described here, refer to his textbook to plan a treatment program. Determination of the tissue type involved is critical.

NONSPECIFIC SPINAL MOBILIZATIONS

Note: P—patient, O—operator, M—movement.

1. Flexion (Fig. 22-25)
   P—Supine with knees bent.
   O—Grasps across the anterior aspect of both proximal tibias and approximates the patient's knees to the axillae.
   M—Traction may be used by passing the left arm behind the knees and the right arm in front of the thighs. The hands are interlocked; by lifting and pulling with the arms, the knees are flexed toward the chest. Some traction is carried out along the line of the femurs by lifting the pelvis with the left arm as the knees are flexed.

   Global stretching into flexion is used for patients with a generally tight back (particularly with loss of flexion), or for apprehensive patients beginning a home stretching program. Large-amplitude oscillations can increase general mobility, stimulate joint motion, or reduce active muscle guarding. Gentle, small-amplitude oscillations can relieve pain.

2. Extension (Fig. 22-26)
   P—Lies prone.
   O—Grasps across the anterior aspect of the patient's distal femurs.
   M—The spine is extended by extending the patient's legs and pelvic girdle.

   This technique is used as in flexion above and to prepare the patient for more specific techniques. Sometimes this method is better tolerated than specific, more vigorous techniques.

3. Rotation (Fig. 22-27)
   P—Supine with knees bent.
   O—Stabilizes the patient's thorax by placing an arm across the lower rib cage. The leg further from the operator is grasped at the knee and the hip is brought to about 90° flexion.
   M—This leg is then pulled toward the operator, across the near leg. Maintain some knee and hip flexion of the near leg to prevent overextension of the spine.

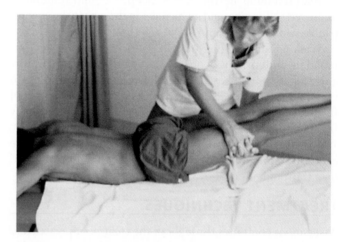

■ FIG. 22-26. Nonspecific long-lever extension mobilization of the lumbar spine.

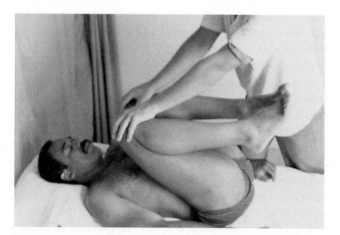

■ FIG. 22-25. Nonspecific long-lever flexion mobilization of the lumbar spine.

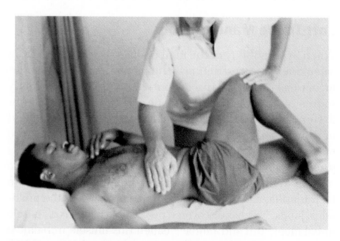

■ FIG. 22-27. Nonspecific long-lever rotation mobilization of the lumbar spine.

4. Rotation (Fig. 22-28)

P—Sidelying, hips and knees slightly flexed. This movement is localized to one area by the positioning of the patient's pelvis and thorax. For the lower lumbar spine, rotation is used with the spine toward flexion; for the upper lumbar spine, rotation is used with the spine in minimal extension.

O—Stands behind patient. Simultaneously rotate the patient's top shoulder toward and the hip away until all slack is taken up. Then, positioned directly over the patient with both elbows straight, apply firm pressure down and cranially against the shoulder, and down and caudally against the greater trochanter, taking up additional slack.

M—An oscillation movement is produced by the therapist's caudal hand, which rotates the pelvis while the cranial hand stabilizes the thorax (grade III). Additional stretch or thrust (given through the shoulder and hip) may be performed (grade IV).

This is a useful technique for unilateral back or leg pain. Gentle, small-amplitude oscillations can relieve pain, and large-amplitude oscillations can increase general mobility or reduce active guarding.

5. Lateral Flexion (sidebending; Fig. 22-29)

P—Supine with knees bent.

O—Holds the patient's legs together with the hips and knees bent to 90°.

M—Spinal sidebending is produced by rotating the patient's pelvis about a vertical axis, using the patient's legs as a lever.

6. Lateral Flexion (sidebending; Fig. 22-30)

P—Lies on the side toward which sidebending is to occur. A small, soft roll may be placed under the lumbar spine to create a greater excursion of movement. The hips and knees are comfortably flexed.

O—Contacts the lateral aspects of the patient's hip girdle and shoulder girdle with the forearms. The fingertips contact the far sides of the spinous processes.

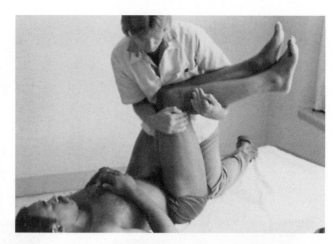

■ FIG. 22-29. Nonspecific long-lever lateral flexion mobilization of the lumbar spine.

M—Movement is produced by pressing outward, then down, with the forearms and pulling up on the spinous processes. Additional leverage is gained by caudal pressure of the operator's chest on the patient's top hip and thigh.

This technique is useful for global stretching and pain relief. Its potential for separating vertebral bodies and opening intervertebral foramina may be valuable in relieving nerve root entrapment.

7. Correction of Acute Lateral Deviation (Fig. 22-31)

P—Standing, with the elbow bent to 90° and resting on the side to which the thorax deviates (see Fig. 20-31A).

O—Contacts the patient's thorax and arm with the shoulder or chest. The operator's arms encircle the patient and the hands interlock to contact the lateral aspect of the patient's pelvis.

M—The lateral deviation is *slowly* (may take several minutes or attempts) reduced with simultaneous pressure

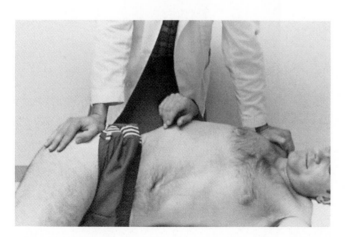

■ FIG. 22-28. Alternative method for nonspecific long-lever rotational mobilization of the lumbar spine.

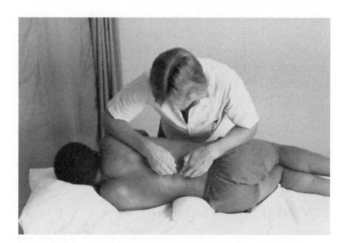

■ FIG. 22-30. Alternative method for nonspecific long-lever lateral flexion mobilization of the lumbar spine.

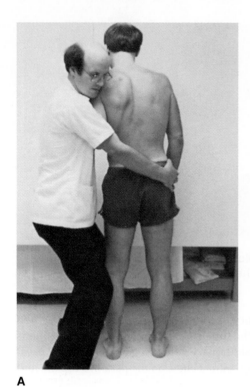
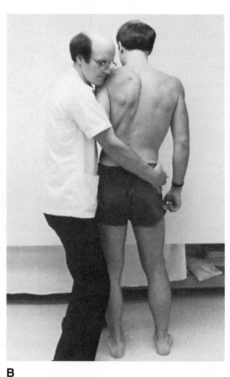

A   **B**

■ **FIG. 22-31.** Correction pressure to the patient's trunk for lateral deviation. **(A)** The initial contact and **(B)** with slight "overcorrection" at the end.

against the thorax and the hips. Small-amplitude oscillations may be superimposed on slow pressure, for patient comfort. The original deviation should be slightly overcorrected (Fig. 22-31*B*).

Note: The patient may be taught to perform this maneuver at home (see Fig. 22-53). In performing this technique, original or more central back discomfort is acceptable; more distal pain is not. This technique is useful for acute disk prolapse and is more successful if radicular signs or symptoms are not present.[507,510] This procedure is usually followed by the next technique.

8. Correction of Flexion Deformity in Standing (Fig. 22-32)
   P—Standing, as relaxed as possible.
   O—Contacts the low lumbar spine with the thenar eminence of one hand (if the level at which the blockage occurs can be identified, the thenar eminence should contact the spinous process *below* that level). The opposite arm reaches across the front of the patient's thorax to grasp the shoulder on the opposite side.
   M—Extension is slowly and gradually produced with a mild forward pressure of the contacting hand, while the thorax is gently moved backward.
   Note: The patient may be taught to perform this maneuver at home (see Fig. 22-51).

SEGMENTAL SPINAL MOVEMENTS

1. Posteroanterior Central Vertebral Pressure (Fig. 22-33)
   P—Prone. The spine may be positioned in the desired degree of extension by placing a pillow under the abdo-

men (for more flexion) or the chest or thighs (for more extension).
O—Contacts the spinous process of the vertebra to be mobilized with the thumb pads of both hands. The fingertips or knuckles are used to stabilize the handhold by placing them along the spine on both sides.

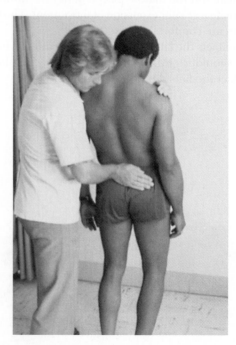

■ **FIG. 22-32.** Correction pressure to the patient's trunk for flexion deformity.

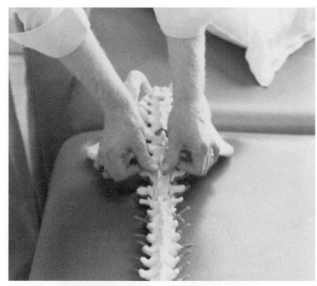

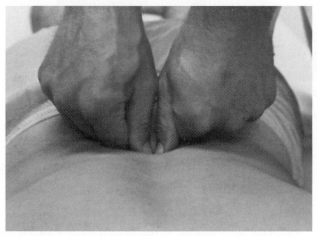

A

B

■ **FIG. 22-33.** Posteroanterior central vertebral pressure on the spinous process.

M—Segmental movement is localized by downward pressure through the arms, forearms, and thumbs. Graded oscillations are used.

2. Posteroanterior Central Vertebral Pressure (Fig. 22-34)
   P—Prone; may be positioned as described in the previous technique.
   O—Contacts the spinous process of the vertebra to be mobilized with the ulnar border of the hand closest to the patient's head (Fig. 22-34A). The other hand is used for support, as shown in Figure 22-34B.
   M—Same as for the previous technique. If the patient is positioned in flexion, overpressure may be applied cranially into more flexion.

   This is a technique of choice for pain reduction or gentle, specific mobilization, for stretching stiff segments, and for helping patients with disk prolapse to achieve greater extension.

3. Posteroanterior Unilateral Vertebral Pressure (Fig. 22-35)
   P—Prone, with the spine positioned in the desired degree of initial extension.
   O—Places both thumb pads over the mammillary process of the joint to be mobilized; these are roughly level with the spaces between the spinous processes and perhaps one to the side.
   M—Movement is produced with a downward pressure in an oscillatory manner through the arms, forearms, and thumbs, in a direction perpendicular to the contour of the spine.

4. Transverse Vertebral Pressures (rotational gliding; Fig. 22-36)
   P—Prone.
   O—The thumbs are applied against the side of the spinous process at the painful level or the level to be mobilized.
   M—The thumbs apply a rhythmic oscillatory force directed toward the opposite side (the painful side or the side of restriction). It is often useful to overlap the thumbs to generate reinforcement.

   This technique achieves a rotational mobilization by means of localized direct pressure to the side of the spinous process of the affected vertebral level. Its greatest value is in conditions in which the symptoms have a unilateral distribution.

5. Flexion (Fig. 22-37A)
   P—Sidelying, with the hips and knees comfortably flexed, arms resting in front of the body.
   O—Rest the patient's upper arm across the lateral aspect of the thorax. Grasp the lower arm at the distal humerus, gaining a purchase on the humeral epicondyles. Pull the shoulder forward until the restricted segment is localized and engaged by rotating the thoracic and lumbar vertebrae above the restricted segment (slack is taken up to the restricted segment). The hip is flexed to prevent further motion in that joint. The patient's lower leg rests against the operator's body.
   The operator's cranial forearm stabilizes along the patient's upper shoulder and rib cage with the fingers placed on the transverse processes or the spinous process of the cranial vertebra of the targeted segment to provide fixation.
   The caudal arm and forearm encircle the sacrum, and the fingers are placed on the spinous or transverse processes of the caudal vertebra of the targeted segment.
   M—Flexion is introduced by the operator's caudal hand and body moving as a unit, stabilizing with the cranial hand. The pelvis is moved in a caudal–ventral direction.

   This technique involves locking the cranial segments in extension and rotation. If this position is not tolerated well, locking from above (via rotation) may be achieved by rotating the thoracic and lumbar spine forward (Fig. 22-37B). Active mobilization (muscle energy or postisometric relaxation techniques) is often effective. The operator introduces traction to the spinous process of the

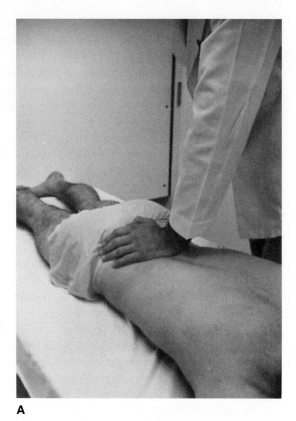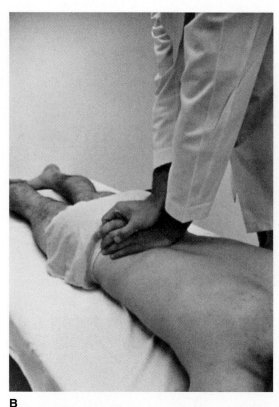

A   **B**

■ **FIG. 22-34.** Alternative method for posteroanterior central vertebral pressure on the spinous processes, with **(A)** ulnar border contact and **(B)** support of the other hand.

caudal segment, thereby effecting passive mobilization and flexing the spinal segments. The hips are concurrently flexed as well.

The restricted segment is brought up to the pathologic barrier. Isometric extension is effected away from the barrier during inhalation. During the relaxation phase, the

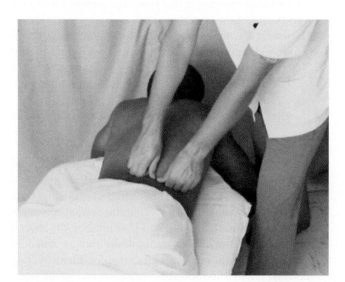

■ **FIG. 22-35.** Posteroanterior unilateral vertebral pressure.

segment is mobilized beyond the pathologic barrier while the patient exhales.

6. Extension (Fig. 22-38)
    P—Prone.
    O—The ulnar border of the cranial hand contacts the spinous process of the segment to be mobilized (Fig. 20-38A). The other hand grasps firmly around the patient's near thigh, just above the knee, and raises (extends) that leg until motion occurs at the desired segment. Alternatively, the thumb pad contacts the mammillary process on the near side for unilateral extension (Fig. 22-38B).
    M—Movement is produced by pressing down on the spinous process or mammillary process, or extending the leg.
    Because of the long lever arm (the patient's leg), a significant amount of force can be applied with this technique, so it is a technique of choice for patients with chronic lumbar stiffness. It may be too vigorous for patients with more acute disorders and should be used with caution.

7. Rotation (Fig. 22-39)
    P—Prone.
    O—Grasp across to the opposite anterosuperior iliac spine with the more caudal hand. Contact the far side of the spine over the mammillary process of the upper vertebra of the segment to be mobilized with the ulnar border or the pisiform of the opposite hand (Fig. 22-

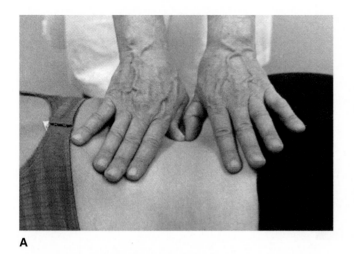

A

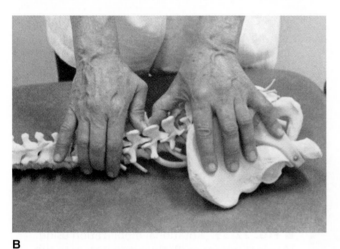

B

■ **FIG. 22-36.** Transverse vertebral pressures. (**A**) Transverse directed rotational gliding using the thumbs. (**B**) Position of the thumbs on the spinous processes for transverse gliding.

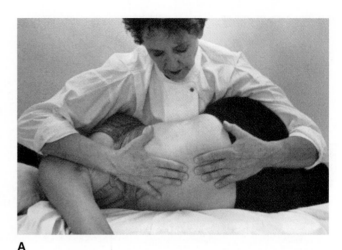

A

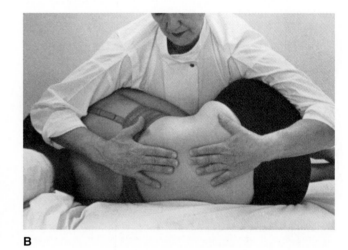

B

■ **FIG. 22-37.** (**A**) Segmental flexion mobilization and (**B**) alternative method for flexion mobilization.

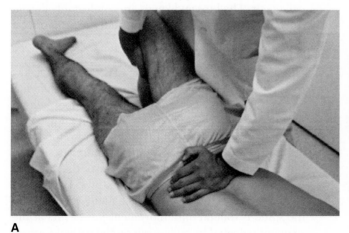

A

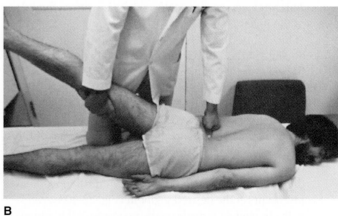

B

■ **FIG. 22-38.** Long-lever extension mobilization of the lumbar spine with (**A**) ulnar border contact or (**B**) thumb contact with the stabilizing hand.

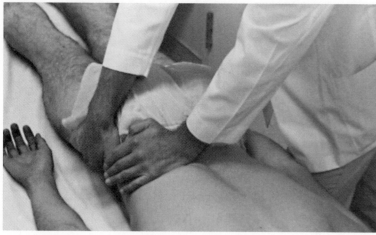

A

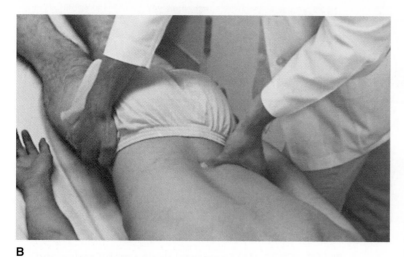

B

■ **FIG. 22-39.** Rotational mobilization using **(A)** ulnar border or **(B)** thumb contact with the lumbar spine.

39A). Alternatively, the thumb or pisiform can contact near the side of the spinous process of the upper vertebra of the segment to be mobilized (Fig. 22-39B).

M—Movement is performed by simultaneously lifting the pelvis and pressing down with the contacting hand. This produces rotation (of the spine) away from the side of the pelvis contacted.

This is an effective stretching (grade IV) and pain-reducing (grades I to III) technique and is also useful for disk prolapse (without neurologic deficit), usually with the painful side toward the operator.

8. Rotation (Fig. 22-40)

P—Prone, knees flexed to 90°.

O—The cranial hand contacts the upper vertebra of the segment to be mobilized at the far side (mammillary process), using pisiform contact. The other hand grasps the patient's ankles and lowers them until movement just occurs at the desired segment (Fig. 22-40A). Alternatively, contact is made on the near side of the spinous process of the upper vertebra with the pisiform or thumb (Fig. 22-40B).

M—Movement is produced by lowering the ankles or pressing down and laterally with the contacting hand.

9. Rotation (Fig. 22-41)

P—Lying on the side opposite that to which movement will occur. The hips and knees are comfortably flexed, the head and neck slightly flexed, and the arms at rest in front of the patient.

O—Flexes the upper hip, keeping the knee level with the plinth, until movement just occurs at the segment below that to be moved (palpate motion with the middle finger). Position the dorsum of the patient's foot behind the opposite knee or thigh. Rest the patient's upper arm across the lateral aspect of the thorax. Grasp the lower arm at the distal humerus, gaining a purchase on the humeral epicondyles. The third finger of the opposite hand palpates between the spinous processes at the level above that to be moved. The patient relaxes and the spine is rotated until movement just occurs at the segment palpated by pulling out on the patient's arm. The forearm is placed across the posterolateral aspect of the patient's pelvis, the opposite forearm across the

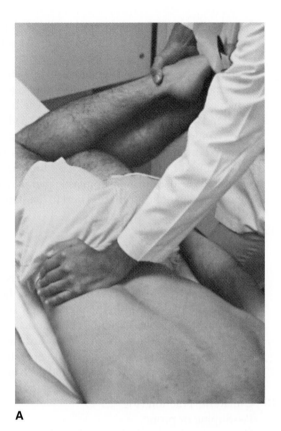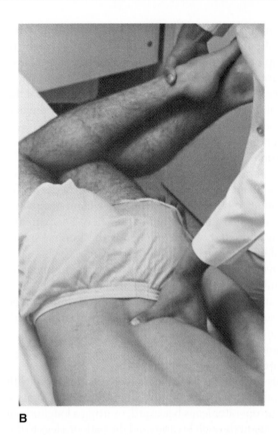

A   B

■ **FIG. 22-40.** Alternative method for rotational mobilization using **(A)** pisiform contact on the far side or **(B)** thumb contact on the near side of the lumbar spine.

deltopectoral groove. The middle finger of the caudal hand hooks underneath to the opposite side of the spinous process of the more caudal vertebra of the segment to be moved. The opposite middle finger or thumb contacts the near side of the spinous process of the more cranial vertebra.

Slack is taken up in the shoulder girdle by pushing down and away with the forearm, and in the hip girdle by pulling down and toward the operator.

M—Movement is produced by pulling up on the caudal spinous process while continuing to move the pelvic girdle (as above), and simultaneously pushing

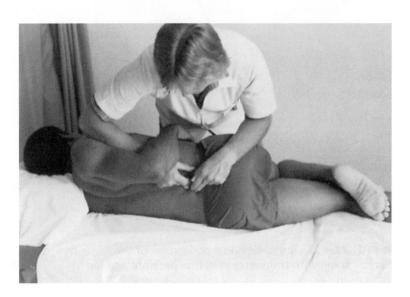

■ **FIG. 22-41.** Alternative method for rotational mobilization of the lumbar spine.

down on the cranial spinous process while moving the shoulder girdle (as above). Use body weight to complete end-range distraction. Oscillations can also be used.

Note: A contract–relax technique or gentle thrust at the end point of movement may be used to facilitate maximum range of motion.

10. Sidebending (Fig. 22-42)

P—Prone.

O—The cranial hand makes thumb or pisiform contact at the near side of the upper spinous process of the segment to be mobilized. The other hand grasps the patient's near thigh just above the knee. The patient's leg is abducted, which sidebends the lumbar spine, until motion reaches the desired level.

M—Overpressure is applied at the spine through the thumb or at the leg (into more abduction).

Because of the long lever arm, significant force can be used, so this is a technique of choice for patients with chronic joint stiffness.

11. Traction (Fig. 22-43)

P—Supine, knees and hips flexed.

O—Sits or stands at the patient's feet, securing them with the buttocks or thighs. Grasps behind the patient's knees.

M—The operator leans backward, exerting a longitudinal movement through his arms and the patient's legs to the

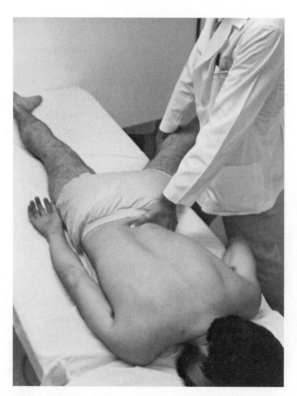

■ **FIG. 22-42.** Lateral flexion mobilization of the lumbar spine with transverse vertebral pressure and leg abduction.

patient's spine. Movement can be graded, depending on patient tolerance and desired result. This technique provides gentle traction to relieve pressure on the disk and also comfortable stimulation and movement to pain segments that may not tolerate more vigorous techniques. Belt traction may be used.[548] The belt is placed around the patient's upper calves, with a pad interposed for comfort. The clasped loop of the adjustable belt is placed around the therapist's upper back. By leaning the trunk in the desired direction, lumbar traction is applied. A foam or nonslip plastic pad may be placed under the patient's trunk and next to the skin to prevent slipping.

12. Traction (Fig. 22-44)

P—Supine, at the end of the plinth.

O—Assumes a walk-standing position at the foot of the table, facing the patient. The patient's crossed legs are placed over the operator's shoulder, and the operator clasps the hands around the patient's proximal thighs, keeping the elbows in tight to the chest.

M—The patient's hips are drawn toward the operator, thus distracting the spine, when the operator's body is simultaneously rocked backward and the trunk is tucked (flexed).

13. Unilateral Traction (Fig. 22-45)

P—Supine or prone.

O—Grasps the distal tibia on the side to be distracted, gaining a purchase on the malleoli. The patient's leg is flexed and adducted just until movement occurs at the spinal level below that at which movement is desired.

M—Movement is produced by a longitudinal pull through the leg, leaning backward with body weight. Countermovement is provided against the sole of the patient's opposite foot with the anterior aspect of the operator's thigh. The opposite leg may be placed in a hook position (hip and knee flexed, feet flat on the plinth) or held in the Thomas position, to flatten out the lumbar spine.

14. Sacroiliac Backward Rotation (Fig. 22-46)

P—Lying on the side opposite the joint to be moved.

O—Flexes the patient's hip and knee as far as possible and holds the leg in that position by contacting the anterior aspect of the leg around the operator's waist. The patient's other leg is extended, and the dorsum of the foot is secured at the far edge of the plinth. The operator's more cranial hand contacts the patient's anterosuperior iliac spine, and the opposite hand contacts the ischial tuberosity. The forearms are parallel to each other in a direction to create a force-couple around the joint axis.

M—Movement is produced by a force-couple, pushing the anterosuperior iliac spine backward and the ischial tuberosity forward. Further pressure is placed against the patient's leg with the operator's abdomen.

This is an effective technique for correcting anterior sacroiliac dysfunction. Contract–relax or muscle-energy techniques may be used.

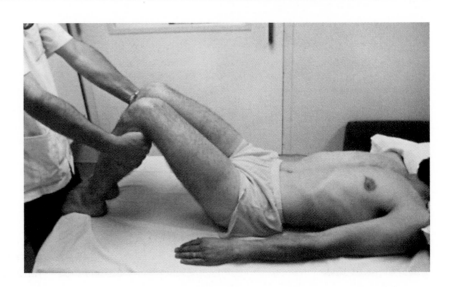

■ **FIG. 22-43.** Traction mobilization of the lumbar spine, using the legs.

15. Sacroiliac Anterior Rotation (Fig. 22-47)
    P—Prone.
    O—Places the cranial hand directly over the patient's sacrum. The opposite hand reaches around to grasp the anterior aspect of the distal thigh of the near leg.
    M—Movement is produced by simultaneously pressing on the distal sacrum with the heel of the hand and lifting the leg, thus rotating the proximal ilium forward (anteriorly).

This is an effective technique for correcting posterior sacroiliac dysfunction.

Note: This technique may be used with an isometric relaxation or muscle-energy technique.[50,67,108,422,429,435,530] The leg is elevated in extension and usually slight abduction and rotation to loose-pack the sacroiliac joint (the operator monitors the sulcus with the fingers). Pressure is exerted on the iliac crest slightly above the posterior iliac spine. The leg is elevated in extension until the re-

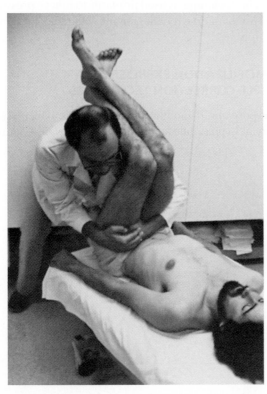

■ **FIG. 22-44.** Alternative method for traction mobilization of the lumbar spine, using the hips.

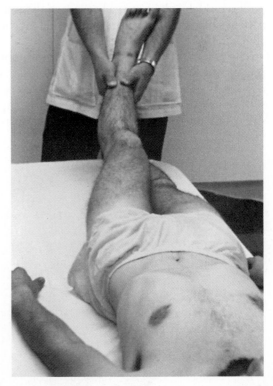

■ **FIG. 22-45.** Unilateral traction mobilization of the lumbar spine, using the leg.

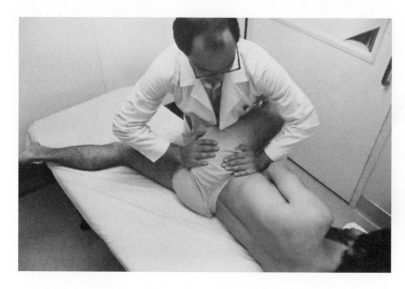

■ **FIG. 22-46.** Posterior rotation of the innominate on the sacrum.

strictive barrier at the limit of passive range of motion is engaged. The patient then pulls the leg down toward the table against the resistance of the therapist's hand. The patient relaxes and additional slack in the joint motion is taken up until a new restrictive barrier is engaged. This process is repeated three or four times.

16. Positional Distraction (Fig. 22-48)

   P—Sitting on the side of the plinth, with a soft roll placed at the side, between the pelvic crest and the chest wall (Fig. 22-48A).

   O—The patient is carefully assisted into the sidelying position; sidebending occurs because of the roll. The patient's hips and knees are slightly flexed for comfort (Fig. 22-48B).

   M—The operator palpates between the spinous processes at the level where maximal positional traction is desired. Grasping the patient's top knee, the operator slides it up the edge of the plinth, flexing the hip and spine until movement just occurs at the level palpated.

The dorsum of the patient's foot is secured behind the other knee or thigh (Fig. 22-48C).

The operator then palpates at the next highest level, with the third finger of the other hand. The opposite hand grasps the patient's distal humerus and pulls up and out, rotating the upper spine, until motion just occurs at the level palpated (Fig. 22-48D).

The patient's arm is placed across the chest. This position is maintained as long as tolerated (usually 5 to 25 minutes).

This technique is used primarily to relieve pressure on the lumbar nerve root in patients with radicular signs and symptoms.

SELF-MOBILIZATION EXERCISES AND SELF-CORRECTION TECHNIQUES

The purpose of self-mobilization exercises is to increase joint mobility at hypomobile segments. Specificity of motion may

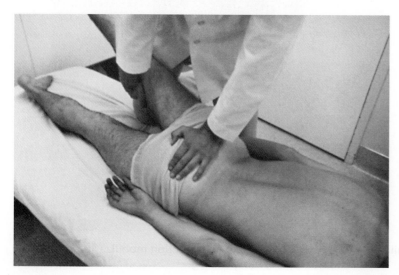

■ **FIG. 22-47.** Anterior rotation of the innominate on the sacrum.

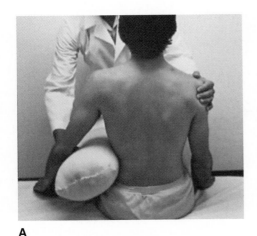

A

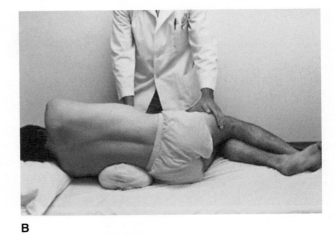

B

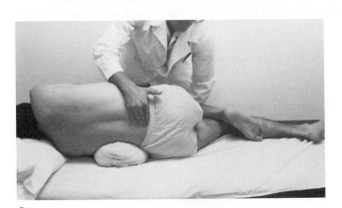

C

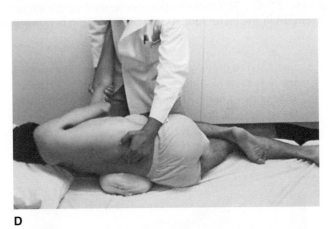

D

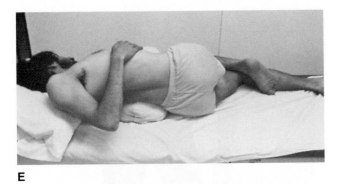

E

■ **FIG. 22-48.** Positional distraction technique. Beginning with the patient (**A**) sitting on the side of the plinth, (**B**) assist him into sidelying. While palpating the level where maximal positional traction is desired, the hip and spine are flexed (**C**), the upper spine is rotated (**D**), and the position is maintained (**E**).

be accomplished through ligamentous or facet-locking techniques, by the use of the patient's hands, or by a device (e.g., a roll or the back of the chair) to allow motion to occur at a particular segment without creating unwanted extension at other areas (see Fig. 20-60).

I. Quadriped Flexion–Extension
  A. In quadriped, flexion-extension is performed by slowly cycling through full spine flexion to full extension (Fig. 22-8).
  B. Extension can be localized to different areas of the spine by allowing the spine to sag and then rocking forward or backward.[64] When maintaining the sag, rocking forward promotes extension lower in the spine (Fig. 22-49*A*); rocking backward promotes extension higher in the spine (Fig. 22-49*B*).

  Note: These flexion-extension exercises emphasize spine mobility rather than "pressing" at the end range of motion. This exercise provides motion for the spine with very low loading of the intervertebral joints and reduces viscous stresses for subsequent exercises.[502]

II. Sidebending (Fig. 22-50)
  A. Standing, arms behind neck. Positioning of the lower limbs is critical to localize motion to the targeted seg-

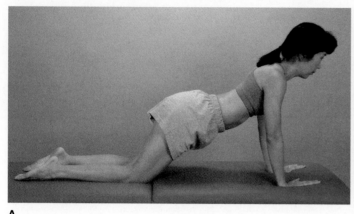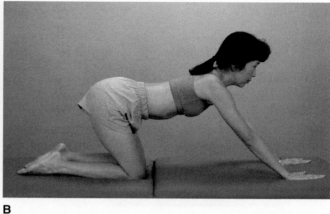

A   **B**

■ **FIG. 22-49.** Self-mobilization—extension of the spine in the quadriped position. **(A)** Rocking forward to increases extension in the lower lumbar spine. **(B)** Rocking backward increases extension in the lower thoracic and upper lumbar spine.

ment and to prevent sagging of the pelvis. By moving the legs apart or abducting the ipsilateral leg to the level of the targeted segment, active mobilization can be localized to the hypomobile segment while avoiding hypermobile segments that may be present distal to the segment.

   B. The patient actively sidebends the upper trunk.
      Note: Combined motions may be done (i.e., extension, right sidebending and left rotation).
III. Standing Extension (Fig. 22-51)
   A. General. Place hands on hips, thumbs forward. Keeping the knees straight, bend back over the hips,

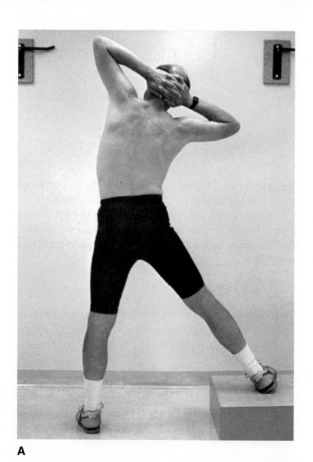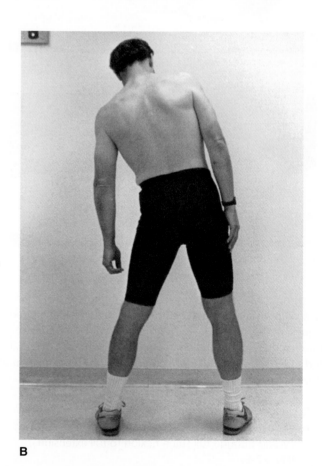

A   **B**

■ **FIG. 22-50.** Self-mobilization—sidebending using the lower limbs for localization. **(A)** Ipsilateral leg abduction and **(B)** legs apart.

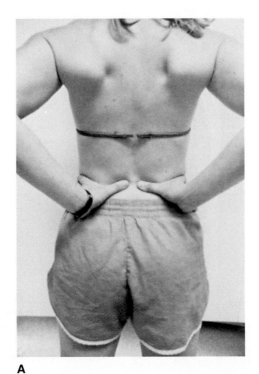 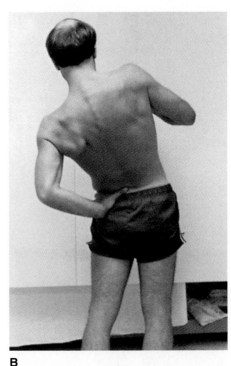

A   **B**

■ **FIG. 22-51.** Self-mobilization. **(A)** Specific bilateral and **(B)** unilateral extension techniques for localized acute back pain with some loss of normal lumbar lordosis.

extending the lumbar spine. Keep the cervical spine neutral.

B. Specific. Place hands on hips, thumbs making contact with the lower spinous process of the segment to be mobilized. Extend the lumbar spine, maintaining pressure with the thumbs and localizing the force at the desired level (Fig. 22-51A).

C. Unilateral. As above, with single general or specific contact (thumb just lateral to the spinous process) only. Bend back and to the side of hand contact (Fig. 22-51B).

IV. Prone Extension (Fig. 22-52)

A. Prolonged. Lie prone with elbows and shoulders flexed about 90°, cervical spine neutral. Relax the back and abdomen, allowing the spine to stretch into extension (see Fig. 22-52A).

B. Intermittent. Lie prone with hands at shoulder level. Push the shoulders up until motion is halted by stiffness or discomfort. The back and abdomen remain completely relaxed (see Fig. 22-52B).

Prolonged or intermittent, vigorous stretching into extension is used to relieve stiffness, or to allow the patient with acute disk prolapse to achieve desired extension.

V. Self-Correction of Lateral Deviations (Fig. 22-53)[509]

A. Standing, the hands contact the protruding hip and chest (lateral chest wall to the same side as trunk deviation, and the pelvic crest on the opposite side). Hand pressure slowly forces the spine into straight, then slightly overcorrected, position (Fig. 22-53A).

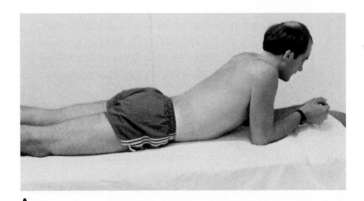

A

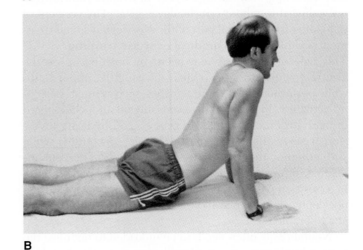

B

■ **FIG. 22-52.** **(A)** Prolonged and **(B)** intermittent prone extension.

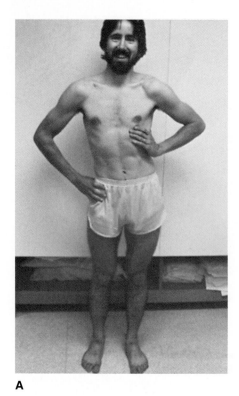

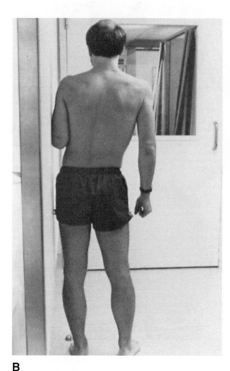

A   **B**

■ **FIG. 22-53.** Self-correction of lateral deviation using **(A)** hand pressure and **(B)** wall contact. (Note: In both A and B, a left lateral deviation has been slightly overcorrected so that the patient is shown in a slight right lateral deviation.)

B. Alternatively, the elbow to the side of deviation is held at 90° against the lateral chest wall. Contact the wall with that arm and shoulder. Slowly move hips toward the wall, eventually assuming a slightly overcorrected position (Fig. 22-53B).

Unloading Techniques

Many spinal patients are sensitive to axial loading during exercise and activities of daily living. When this is the case, an attempt should be made to control the axial load that that spine may bear during exercise or to allow intermittent unloading throughout out the day.[208,325,499] The concept of unloading is an integral part of the Norwegian spinal treatment technique called **medical exercise training.**[292,325,761] This type of unloading may occur by pushing up on the arm rest while sitting in a chair or using the upper limbs while performing lower limb activities, such as squats or step-up activities (Fig. 22-54), by exercising on an incline board or over a therapeutic ball (in prone), and by using inversion traction (hanging from the lower extremities) while strengthening the trunk muscles (Fig. 22-55).[91,92] Axial unloading improves the body's ability to control and stabilize in a position with reduced body weight and decreases the nociceptive input, while allowing the affected tissues to adapt at a tolerable level.

Neural tissue often needs to be unloaded to optimize the treatment outcome in patients with chronic low back and leg pain who lack extension and external rotation during gait. This can be achieved by taping the buttock and down the leg, following the dermatome to shorten the inflamed tis-

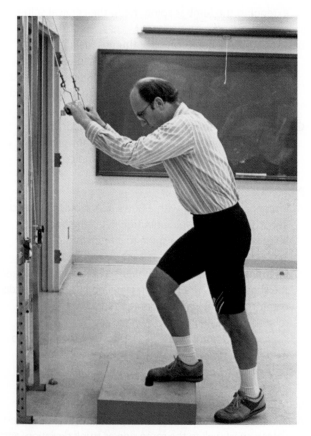

■ **FIG. 22-54.** Unloading a patient (so-called minus weight exercise) performed by utilizing a wall pulley with weights to assist with stair climbing. This exercise might be used with patients who can bear only partial weight on one limb.

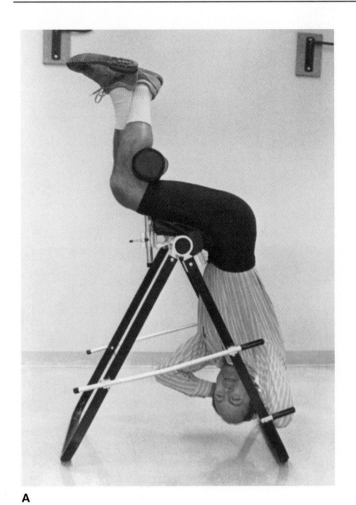
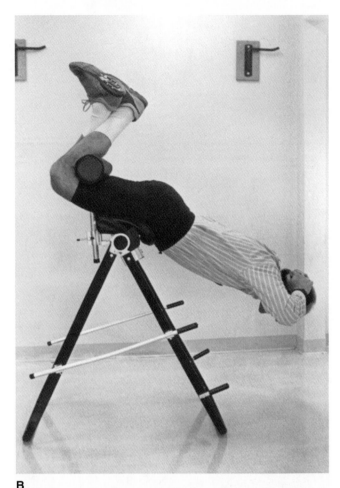

A   **B**

■ **FIG. 22-55.** Inversion machine. **(A)** Gravity-assisted traction and **(B)** gravity-assisted traction with active exercise (extension).

sue so that symptoms are not increased when there is an attempt, in treatment, to gain range.[499] Typically, flexibility needs to be gained in the anterior hip structures (see Figs. 8-42 and 14-10) and the thoracic spine, while stability is required at the mobile lumbar/s and often pelvis. Refer to McConnail[499] for a detailed discussion of this taping and treatment method.

Unloading or "de-weighting" the spine with the use of manual (Figs. 22-43 through 22-45),[138,264] positional (Fig. 22-48), suspended, or gravity-assisted traction (see Fig. 22-55) is often used to bring temporary pain relief when an irritable tissue (i.e., nerve root) is provoked by an exercise program or activities of daily living. These mild forms of traction should not be confused with other forms of traction in which a body part's gravitational weight is exceeded by the distraction force. Self-traction (Fig. 22-56),[674,675] positional traction,[606,610] Cottrell 90–90 traction,[132,133] inversion traction,[91,92,229,243,421,666] and the development of various forms of gravity traction,[87,246,597,665,756] in which gravity is applied to the body, are useful home traction methods for the lumbar spine. The principle of gravity traction is that the weight of the upper or lower body stretches all the tissues of the low back—the

muscles, fascia, ligaments, and possibly the disk.[91,92,675] Traction may exert some of its beneficial effects by stretching the mechanoreceptors of the apophyseal joints, disk, and ligaments.[750]

One of the more common methods of unloading the spine is through hydrotherapy or aquatic therapy.[1,39,121,338,513,707,765,797] Although a fair amount has been written regarding the benefits of water exercises for people with orthopaedic problems of the spine and extremities, Cirullo[121] was one of the first to address specific low back diagnoses. A land-based program is integrated with an aquatic program of basic lumbar stabilization training. Before engaging in multiple stabilization training activities, full understanding of what lumbopelvic motion is at both ends of the available range, training in cocontraction techniques, and demonstration of the concept of midrange or pelvic neutral[656] is stressed. As with land programs, early emphasis is placed on lengthening the "guy wires" of the spine (iliopsoas, quadriceps, hamstrings, and hip rotators) if needed, and strengthening the key stabilizing muscles (abdominals and latissimus dorsi).[656] All four abdominals are strengthened separately at first, and then together for more advanced work. The program also includes strengthening of

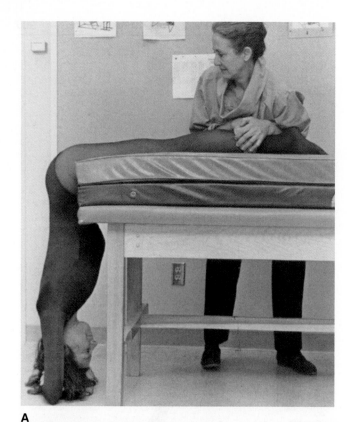

A

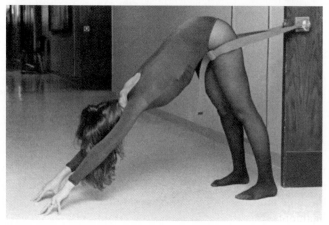

B

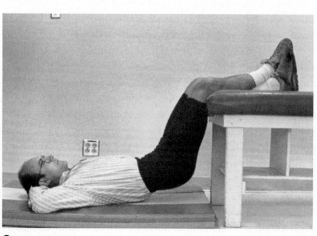

C

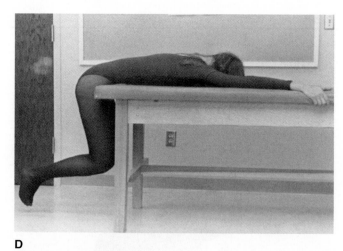

D

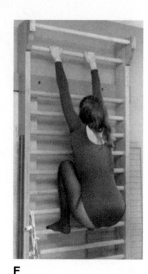

E

F

■ **FIG. 22-56.** Self tractions. Traction methods include **(A)** torso hang over a table or **(B)** via a belt around the pelvis; **(C)** leg hang over a table in supine or **(D)** prone position; and **(E)** arm hang in either an extended or **(F)** flexed position.

the gluteus maximus, spinal extensors, and multifidi. Also included is a general program for cervicothoracic stabilization training.

Unloading is recommended for most spinal dysfunction patients with radicular syndromes, disk derangement, hypomobility, strains, sprains, and degenerative disk disease. Unloading with activity offers great benefits because it allows patients to engage in activity at a reduced percentage of body weight.

CONSIDERATIONS

Joint structures and the optimal stimulus for regeneration that should always be considered:

1. Vertebrae. The optimal stimulus for regeneration of bone is biomechanical energy in the line of stress (longitudinal axis of bone). This biomechanical energy is transmitted to the bone through intermittent compression and distraction by way of antigravity muscle contraction and through the forces of gravity and body weight in upright postures (see Chapter 3, Arthrology). Exercises involving repeated high-force movements in weight-bearing positions produce greater bone densities.[735]

2. Zygapophyseal joints. The optimal stimulus for regeneration of articular cartilage is intermittent compression and decompression and gliding, which can be achieved through specific active movements of the lumbar spine while avoiding static loading.[269]

3. Ligaments. Joint immobilization results in reduced synthesis of proteoglycan and plasticity of ligaments over time. Ligamentous laxity tends to be prominent in the lumbar spine secondary to chronic improper postural loading or traumatic ligamentous strain.[645] When ligaments are torn or overstretched, they may remain lax, in which case neutral postures and muscle stabilization is required. According to

Grimsby,[269] ligaments respond well to modified tension in the line of stress. This modified tension may be applied to the ligaments through selected exercises designed to target the specific ligament. Tension to the posterior longitudinal, interspinous, and supraspinous ligaments, for example, may be applied by flexion of the lumbar spine at the end range (Fig. 22-25), either by the therapist or the patient.

4. The disk. The annulus, like ligaments, contains mainly type I collagen fibers, which are highly organized and resist tension. The nucleus pulposus contains mainly type II collagen fibers, which respond to pressure. The nucleus pulposus has a greater concentration of water and proteoglycans than the annulus. The exercise of choice for stimulating disk repair is lumbar rotation. Modified tension in the line of stress stimulates protein synthesis of type I collagen of the annulus; intermittent compression and distraction promotes regeneration of type II collagen and proteoglycans.[645] Rotations can be performed either in non-weight bearing (supine or prone; Fig. 22-57) or in weight bearing (Fig. 22-58), with (Fig. 22-59) or without weights. Producing mechanoreceptor activity theoretically reduces pain. Strengthening and segmental coordination of the deep rotators may also be improved. In sitting, because of the ability to produce end-range stretch, this may be useful in restoring function.

5. Muscles. Phasic muscles, such as the erector spinae, act as movers of the spine; tonic muscles, such as the multifidi, act as stabilizers. The lumbar multifidus, considered to be particularly important for stability,[434] is prone to atrophy.[311] The optimal stimulus for the regeneration of tonic fibers is high-repetition, low-resistance exercise to improve capillarization to the muscle. Because tonic muscles atrophy first, muscle endurance exercises should be performed initially, followed by strengthening exercises.[269]

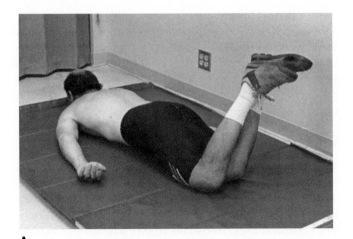

A

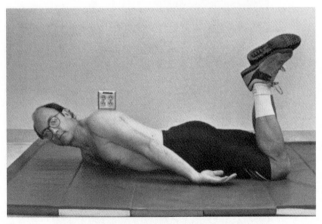

B

■ **FIG. 22-57.** Prone rotations (**A**) performed caudad-to-cephalad with knee flexion. The patient is instructed to slowly lift the pelvis and anterior thigh with the rotator muscles. (**B**) Cephalad-to-caudad. The patient is instructed to roll slowly while lifting one shoulder and stabilizing the pelvis.

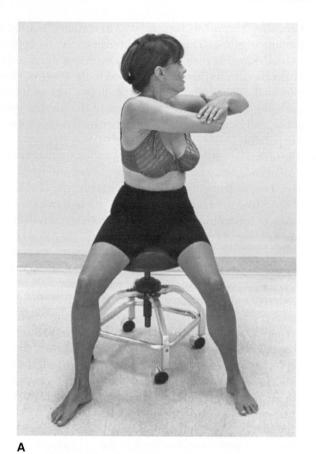

A

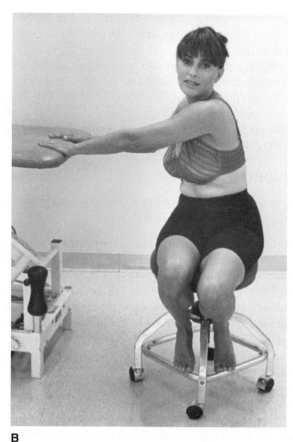

B

■ **FIG. 22-58.** Sitting rotations. **(A)** Cephalad-to-caudad with active upper trunk rotation performed with a neutral lumbar spine and a fixed pelvis, and **(B)** caudad-to-cephalad performed with a fixed upper torso. The patient is rotating the pelvis (while sitting on a swivel stool).

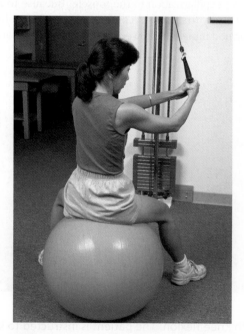

■ **FIG. 22-59.** Pulley resisted trunk rotation on a therapeutic ball.

The optimal stimulus for regeneration of phasic fibers is low-repetition, high-resistance exercise without increasing speed.[645]

Based on Holten's medicine training theory, muscle endurance is enhanced by performing about 30 repetitions at 60% of one resistance maximal (1 resistance maximum [RM]).[274,294,325] Pure strength is achieved by performing 8 to 12 or fewer repetitions at 80 to 100% of 1 RM. For a combination of strength and endurance, Holten proposed performing 20 to 25 repetitions at 70% of 1 RM.

Sensorimotor and Neuromuscular Training

Many sensorimotor training exercises appropriate for the lumbar spine are described in Chapter 20, Thoracic Spine (see Figs. 20-63 through 20-68), Chapter 14, Hip (see Figs. 14-44 through 14-46), and Chapter 16, Lower Leg, Ankle, and Foot (see Figs. 16-64 and 16-65). The uses of twisters, rollers, balance shoes, wobble boards, rocker boards, mini trampolines and therapeutic balance balls in the treatment of back pain have gain popularity. One of the advantages of balance balls is that they are safe and help to activate proprioception, balance and equilibrium control. An incredible variety of balance exercises can be used to establish improved kinesthetic awareness, spinal stability and new movement patterns.

The mini trampoline is a particularly useful devise.[348] Jogging or jumping activities activates proprioceptors more effectively than a similar exercise performed on a firm floor (see Fig. 16-68).[348] In addition, it protects the joints because if functions as a shock absorber. Exercises on the trampoline are not limited to upright positions but can be performed in sitting (a particularly effective method for strengthening the abdominals) and quadriped.

An endless variety of exercises may be performed on balance boards with the use of perturbation to facilitate differ-

ent muscles groups.[549] Applying the perturbation to the lumbosacral area (see Fig. 20-63) may facilitate the deep abdominal stabilizers. This causes a tendency for increased lumbar lordosis and anterior tilt. The stabilizers of the trunk have to counteract this tendency by maintaining neutral posture. Applying the perturbations to the anterior aspect of the hip joint (Fig. 22-60) while balance is challenged on a wobble board facilitates the gluteus maximus. Applying perturbations in a lateral to medial direction (Fig. 22-61) facilitates the gluteus medius. Both internal and external perturbations can be stimulated by weight bearing activities such as throwing a ball (see Fig. 16-65) or using a body blade to facilitate stabilization responses (see Figs. 20-65 through 20-68).[549]

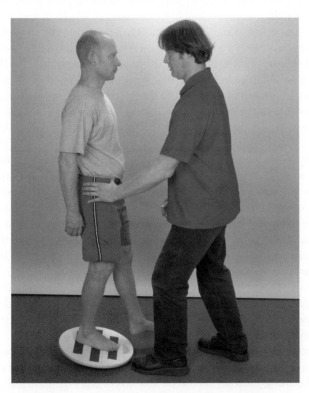

■ **FIG. 22-60.** Applying peturbations to facilitate stabilization responses in the gluteus maximus.

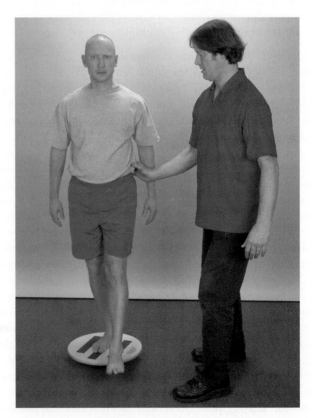

■ **FIG. 22-61.** Applying perturbations to facilitate stabilization responses in the gluteus medius.

SPINAL STABILIZATION AND DYNAMIC FUNCTIONAL EXERCISES

Bergmark[47] proposed the concept of different trunk muscles playing different roles in the provision of dynamic stability of the spine. He hypothesized the presence of two muscle systems in the maintenance of spinal stability.

1. The "global muscle system," which consists of large torque producing muscles that act on the trunk and spine without directly attaching to it. These muscles include the thoracic part of lumbar iliocostalis, obliquus abdominis externus, and rectus abdominis.
2. The local muscle system, which consist of muscles directly attach to the lumbar vertebrae spine, and are responsible for providing segmental stability and controlling the lumbar segment. This local system consists of the thoracoabdominal diaphragm, psoas major, quadratus lumborum, the lumbar part of the iliocostalis and longissimus, transversus abdominis, posterior fibers of the obliquus abdominus internus, and lumbar multifidus.

There is growing evidence that the deep abdominal and lumbar multifidus muscles are preferentially adversely affected in the presence of acute low back pain,[306,309] chronic low back pain,[51,153,154,321–323,655] and lumbar instability.[442,592,639,752] (See Chapter 20, Thoracic Spine, for further discussion of abdominal muscle training and multifidus facilitation.)

Grieve[258,263,266] proposed a basic scheme of progressive stabilization techniques for strengthening regional and segmental muscles. Abdominal exercises and dynamic abdominal bracing may also be used.[360] Exercises are selected that avoid extreme positions (flexion, extension, or rotation) liable to exacerbate the condition. For example, a potent cause of aggravation of low back pain, owing to hypermobility, is that of active forced extension in the neutral starting position of prone-lying.

Mobilizations are used to relieve the pain of the hypermobile segments within the normal range of accessory movement and to mobilize stiff segments as part of the treatment for lumbar instability (i.e., where neighboring osteochondrotic segments have slowly induced hypermobility at the L5–S1 segment). If the spinal extensor muscles are weak or need extra strengthening, exercises to strengthen them should avoid outer-range hyperextension movements. Therefore, the starting position should be such that the resisted movement occurs in middle range and the excursion ceases when the normal postural length of the muscle is reached.[458] A segment held in hyperextension has no safety margin, so painful capsular lesions result.

Batson[34–36] Bronner,[77] Carriere,[100,101] Chason,[116,117] Clark,[122] Comerford,[128] Dominguez,[173] Fritz and Hicks,[232] Jemmett,[353] Gunnari,[272] Gustavsen,[273,274] Harden,[292] Holten,[325] Hyman,[334] Keely,[373] Kolster,[402] May,[485] McGill,[501–504] Morgan,[543,544] Norris,[578–580] O'Sullivan,[592] Richardson et al.,[642] Robinson,[647] Saal,[657,658] Sahrmann,[661] Taylor and O'Sullivan,[752] and White,[806] use similar schemes of progressive stabilization for strengthening regional and segmental muscles when the joints are hypermobile or painful. Self-stabilization exercises, with the patient's active participation, and training in synergies are useful prophylaxis. The prime importance of soft tissues, particularly muscles, as opposed to the skeletal elements of joint structures is underscored by selected exercises that not only emphasize pure strength training but also improve speed and endurance.[325]

Many other approaches used in clinical practice have some potential to assist the integration of local and global stability retraining once the basic motor control correction has been made. Alternative approaches include Tai Chi,[66,247,326,333,340,344,420] yoga,[33,78,137,351,410,674,753] the Feldenkrais technique[287,418,476,613,620] and Pilates programs.[14,23,515,552,574,646] In Pilates programs, clients are taught to stabilize the core before each movement. When performed correctly, Pilates workouts develop trunk muscle endurance and tone, an importune factor in preventing low back pain.

Examples of stabilization exercises involving the strengthening of regional and segmental muscles are shown in Figures 22-62 and 22-63. Isometric exercises for strengthening the segmental muscles related to a hypermobile joint may be performed in a similar fashion to the preceding segmental spinal movements (Figs. 22-33 to 22-36). The patient is taught to prevent displacement of the spinous or mammillary process at the level of the hypermobile segment. The direction of the applied sustained pressures may be altered (diagonally, transversely, posteroanteriorly, caudally, and cephalad) to recruit the appropriate muscles. Increasing the pressure being sustained and the duration of the hold allows progression. These are just a few of the exercises often necessary to complement passive movement techniques, and at times they make up the main form of treatment. When attempting to stabilize the unstable segment and to avoid further stress, there are two goals. The first is to encourage the patient to recognize and maintain functional back positions during all activities and to teach the patient to avoid postures and activities that aggravates the back dysfunction. The second goal is to improve the strength and endurance of the trunk musculature and its function specific to the task demanded and the directional intent. The trunk muscles should be able to contract (isometrically), contract and shorten (concentrically), contract and lengthen (eccentrically), stretch, and—most importantly—rest, ideally at their resting length.

Hypermobile joints should be trained initially with many repetitions, at low speed, and with minimal resistance at the beginning or midrange.[267] This is followed by increasing (isometric) contractions in the inner range of motion to facilitate increased sensitivity to stretch, particularly of the deep rotators such as the multifidi (Figs. 22-62 and 22-63). Finally, the patient is trained with submaximal resistance (isometric contractions) in any range except the outer range.

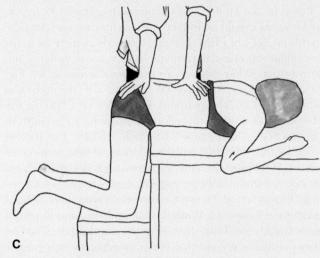

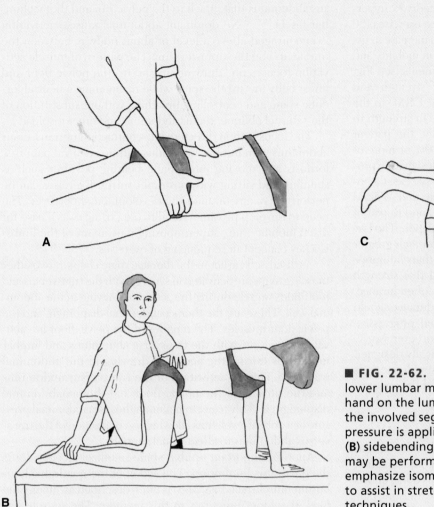

■ FIG. 22-62. Segmental stabilization exercises of the lower lumbar musculature. The therapist may use one hand on the lumbar region immediately above or below the involved segment. Moderate but increasing sustained pressure is applied to the patient's pelvis. **(A)** Rotation, **(B)** sidebending, and **(C)** flexion–extension techniques may be performed. Techniques may be modified to emphasize isometric, concentric, and eccentric control and to assist in stretching shortened tissue by using hold–relax techniques.

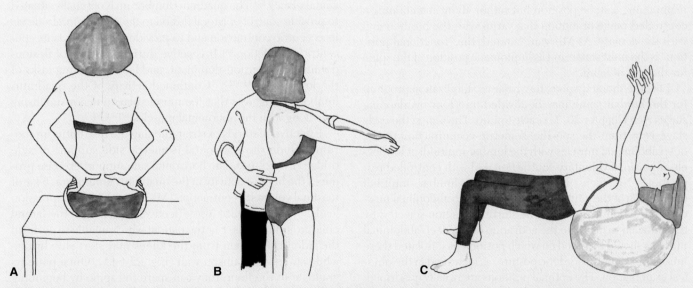

■ FIG. 22-63. Exercises for stabilization and strengthening. **(A)** Self-resistance may be applied using posteroanterior or lateral pressures for strengthening the segmental musculature. Regional strengthening may be achieved through **(B)** standing exercises and **(C)** assuming the bridging position while maintaining a functional back position.

Based on the Holten's medicine training theory,[325] hypermobile joints should be trained with endurance exercises (30 repetitions, 60% of 1 RM) initially to provide an increase in tissue capillarization and to promote an increase in mobility and control through low-intensity repetitive movements (see Fig. 11-34).[274] This is followed by training for strength and endurance (15 to 30 repetitions, 60 to 75% of 1 RM) in the outer range of motion; this allows an increase in strength to maintain the gained range of motion. Finally, the patient should be trained with 8 to 12 repetitions at 80% or more of their 1 RM for pure strength. Such training is designed to provide optimal stimulus for the regeneration of tissue (see Chapter 1, Properties of Dense Connective Tissue and Wound Healing and Chapter 2, Wound Healing: Injury and Repair of Dense Connective Tissue) as well as pain modulation. The few studies available suggest that endurance has a much greater value than strength.[454] McGill[501–503,505] indicates that endurance has more protective value than strength and that strength should not be overemphasized at the expense of endurance. Furthermore, it appears emphasis placed on endurance should precede specific strengthening in a graduated progressive exercise program (i.e., long duration, lower-effort exercise).[502]

Stabilization training uses exercises specifically designed to provide a "muscle corset,"[656] limiting undesirable motions and allowing healing to occur. Saal[656] described the anatomical basis for this method of control, stating that the "abdominal mechanism, which couples the midline ligaments as well as the thoracolumbar fascia, combined with a slight reduction in lumbar lordosis, can eliminate shear stresses to the lumbar intervertebral segments." He argued that the coupled action of this musculature, together with the latissimus dorsi, allows a muscle "fusion" for spinal protection. Spinal extensors, particularly the multifidi, are essential for balancing the stress to the intervertebral segments.

Contrary to some beliefs, spinal stabilization is not about maintaining a static position but rather about maintaining a controlled range of motion that varies with the position and with the activity. As Morgan[543] stated, the "functional position" is the most stable and asymptomatic position of the spine for the task at hand.

Like the thoracic spine, the dynamic stabilization program for the lumbar spine may be divided into four overlapping stages (see Chapter 20, Thoracic Spine). The aim in the early stage is to train the specific isometric cocontraction of the deep abdominal muscles with the lumbar multifidi at low levels of maximal voluntary contraction and with controlled respiration. No focus is placed on the lumbar multifidi contraction at the very early stage until deep abdominal muscle contraction is isolated. The starting position selected by the clinician to facilitate the activation of the deep abdominal muscles should be based on which position best isolated these muscles in a neutral lordotic posture, as identified in the physical examination. The optimal positions are usually quadriped, prone lying or the supine crook position.

For the lumbar spine there should be focused contraction of the muscles of the lower and middle fibers of the transversus abdominus that attach to the pelvic rim and thoracolumbar fascia.[592,752] No dominant abdominal muscle activation is encouraged above a level of about midway between the umbilicus and the xiphisternum. The pattern of muscle activation focuses on "drawing up and in" the pelvic floor and lower belly toward the spine while maintaining a neutral lordotic spine and controlling breathing without substitution of the external oblique, rectus abdominis and erector spinae.

The focus is then directed at cocontraction of transversus abdominis with lumbar multifidus within a neutral pain free lordosis and moving into weight bearing postures such as standing and sitting with postural control. Exercises can be performed in any or all of the developmental postures. The need to develop proximal stability (i.e., truncal) as a base for distal mobility (i.e., superimposing movement of the limbs) is a key concept in sequencing of exercises.[6,401,543,741,785]

As discussed earlier in the thoracic spine chapter, two other muscle groups are activated in synergy with the transversus and multifidus muscle during the action of drawing in the abdominal wall. These are the thoracoabdominal diaphragm and the pelvic floor muscles. The muscles of the pelvic floor are activated in synergy with the transverse abdominus and lumbar multifidus during the action of drawing in the abdominal wall.[642,667] This co-activation of the transversus abdominus and the muscle of the pelvic floor and thoracoabdominal diaphragm is likely to act to maintain the intraabdominal pressure at a critical level, thus allowing co-contraction of the transversus abdominus to affect spinal support.

Another important lumbar spine stabilizer to consider is the quadratus lumborum. The action of the quadratus lumborum muscle (see Fig. 23-8) is often described as "hiking the hip." It seldom functions in this manner. The muscle has perhaps a more important function relative to moving and stabilizing the pelvis and lumbar spine in the frontal and horizontal planes.[624] The quadratus lumborum is optimally situated to provide control of lateral flexion to the contralateral side via its eccentric contraction and to provide the return via its concentric contraction.[661] It is active during a variety of flexion-dominant; extension-dominant, and lateral bending tasks of the lower back.[18,502,505] Continued activity of the quadratus lumborum suggests that the muscle plays a major stabilizing role along with the abdominal muscles.[501,502,505]

Effective methods of strengthening the quadratus lumborum include the horizontal isometric side support or side bridge (Fig. 22-64). The horizontal side support exercise produces the highest activity in the quadratus lumborum (54% of maximal voluntary contraction [MVC]) with low compression loads.[232] This exercise also effectively challenges the lateral oblique abdominals. For the patient who is unable to perform the side bridge even from the knees may start side bridge while standing against a wall (Fig. 22-64A). Once patients graduate to the floor, they can spare the spine by beginning with the knees on the floor (Fig. 22-64B). Supporting the body with the feet increases the challenge, but also the spine load (Fig. 22-20). This exercise can be done for a sustained iso-

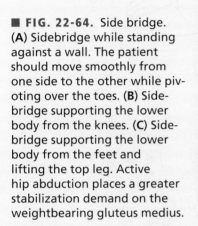

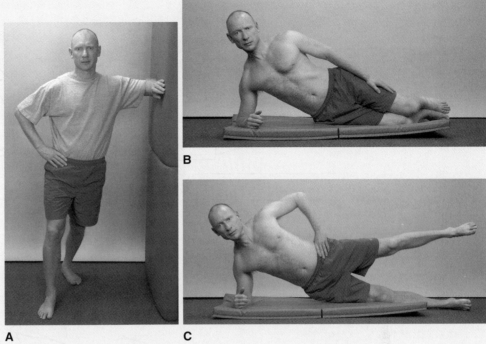

■ **FIG. 22-64.** Side bridge. **(A)** Sidebridge while standing against a wall. The patient should move smoothly from one side to the other while pivoting over the toes. **(B)** Side-bridge supporting the lower body from the knees. **(C)** Side-bridge supporting the lower body from the feet and lifting the top leg. Active hip abduction places a greater stabilization demand on the weightbearing gluteus medius. **A**   **C**

metric hold or in a more dynamic fashion with lowering and raising repetitions of the body. An even greater challenge is to add hip abduction of the upper hip (Fig. 22-64*C*).[353] As the upper hip is abducted, a greater stabilization demand is placed on the weightbearing gluteus medius. Patients who present with painful shoulder that cannot tolerate shoulder load can perform a side bridge by lying on the floor and attempting to raise the legs laterally (Fig. 22-65*A*) or by attempting to take the weight off the legs. Another option for patients with shoulders that can not tolerate load through the humerus because of pain or weakness (some elderly women) is to stand, with the side of the body supported on a tilt table or 45° bench (with the feet anchored) and the arms folded across the chest.[503] The torso can either be elevated from the table or bridged from the shoulder girdle.

Basic lateral sidebends can be performed by raising the torso laterally with the lower limbs secured (Fig. 22-65*B*). Progression of sidebends calls for a difference of where the hands are placed. The hands may be placed behind the head. It is important that both side bridges and sidebends movement be performed under control—with a slow, steady, sustained effort; with a static end point; and with a return in the same manner.[173] Lateral sidebends may reveal an imbalance in the oblique muscles.[384] A forward twist of the thorax denotes a stronger pull by external obliques, while a backward twist denotes a stronger pull by the internal obliques Further progression of sidebend exercises include positioning the arms straight above the head, adding combined trunk rotation (Fig. 22-65*C*), and adding weight.

The second and third stages of trunk stabilization and motor learning are the associated stages, where the focus is on refining particular movement patterns. Once the pattern of cocontraction of the multifidus and transversus abdominus is achieved it is immediately incorporated into dynamic tasks or static hold postures as determined by the patient's individual complaints. The program is progressed by increasing the difficulty by reducing the base of support, by increasing the load that must be controlled, and by using arm and leg loading to impose load on the trunk while maintaining the neutral position (see Figs. 11-78, 11-79, 11-82 through 11-87, 11-89, 14-45, 15-58 through 15-61, 16-65, 20-68, 20-70 through 20-73, and 20-75 through 20-79).

It has been found that general stabilization exercises and dynamic intensive resistive training have no significant effect on the cross sectional area of the lumbar spine in patients with chronic low back pain.[153,154] However, stabilization training combined with dynamic-static resistive training (static holding between concentric and eccentric phase with a five-second static contraction) was found to be critical in inducing muscle hypertrophy and an appropriate method of restoring the size of the multifidus muscle. Exercises included leg extension in quadriped (see Fig. 20-76*B,C*), trunk lifting from the prone position with straps over the calves (Fig. 22-21) and leg lifting from the prone position (see Fig. 20-78*A*).

The often-performed exercise of lying prone on the floor and raising the upper body and legs off the floor (hyperextension) is contraindicated for anyone at risk of low back injury or reinjury.[503,555] The bridging position can be used to begin exercising the spinal extensors, gluteals and hamstrings (Fig. 22-63*C*). Richardson et al.[643] examined EMG activity during eight exercises to determine which reflected the optimal stabilizing pattern. Recruitment of the obliques and back extensor was

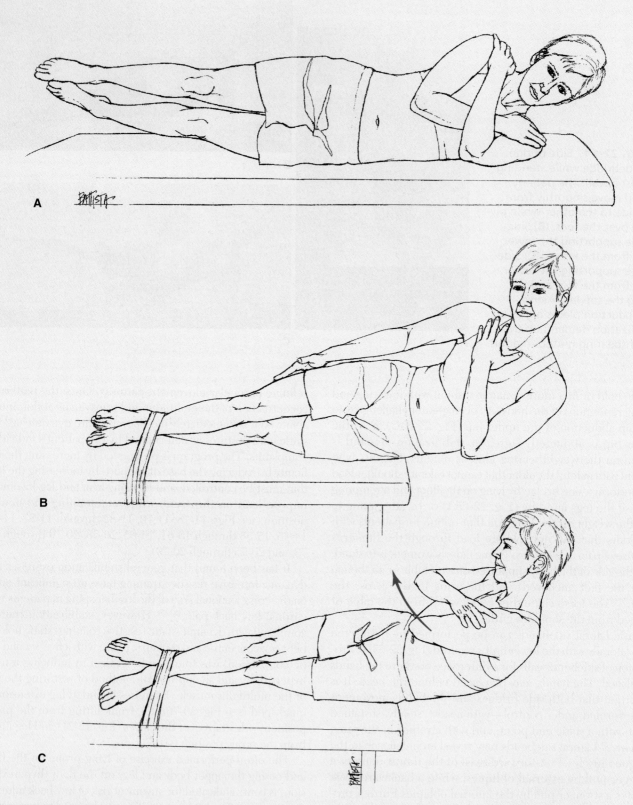

■ **FIG. 22-65.** Sidebends (lateral spine flexion). **(A)** Modified sidebend by attempting to raise the legs laterally. **(B)** Basic sidebend with top arm at the side and bottom arm across the chest. **(C)** High-performance lateral flexion with rotation.

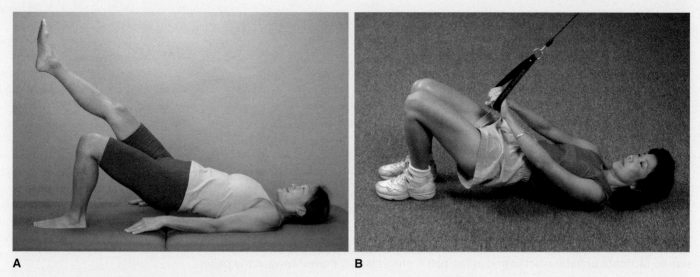

■ **FIG. 22-66.** Bridge position. **(A)** Maintaining the bridge position while extending one leg. **(B)** Maintaining the bridge position with pulley resistance of the upper limbs.

considered a goal of stabilization. Exercises that involved trunk stabilization during isometric resisted trunk rotation were judged one of the most optimal patterns; the most effective bridging with isometric resisted rotation (Fig. 22-18) Other effective bridging activities include superimposing arm or leg movements while maintaining the bridge (Fig. 22-66). To further facilitate bridging, a therapeutic ball can be used to challenge balance and proprioception as well (Fig. 22-67).

Endurance and strength for the back extensors can be facilitated by performing the extension motion on a tilt table or over

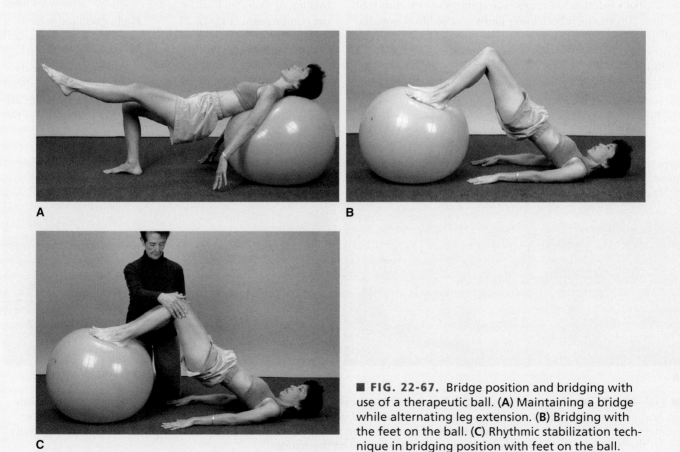

■ **FIG. 22-67.** Bridge position and bridging with use of a therapeutic ball. **(A)** Maintaining a bridge while alternating leg extension. **(B)** Bridging with the feet on the ball. **(C)** Rhythmic stabilization technique in bridging position with feet on the ball.

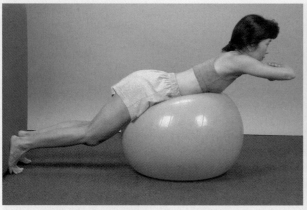
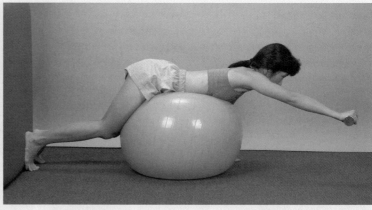

A   **B**

■ **FIG. 22-68.** (A) Spinal extension exercises over a therapeutic ball (feet secured). (B) A dumbbell can be added on one side to facilitate unilateral activation as the ball is progressively moved toward the pelvis.

a therapeutic ball where the feet are secured (Fig. 22-68A). When the objective is focus on activation on one side of the extensors, a hand weight can be added to one side and the exercise repeated as the ball is moved progressively toward the pelvis with each set (Fig. 22-68B).[504] Moving the ball toward the pelvis allow a greater portion of the torso to be cantilevered. McGill and associates[504] discovered that more motor units are recruited with active extensor motion as compared to isometric back extensor exercises. The spine never extends past neutral. Alternatively both lower limbs may be lifted from the ball as the patient maintains neutral spine position (with the arms secured).

Similar to attempts at strengthening the back extensor, strengthening of the rectus abdominis (part of the global muscle system) should only be considered after the patient learned the limits of the SFP in hook lying, sidelying, quadriped.

Graduated abdominal strengthening of the rectus should simultaneously include drawing in the umbilicus and tightening of the muscles of the rectum to ensure strengthening of not only rectus abdominis, but also the transversus abdominis and the pelvic floor muscles. The patient may begin with abdominal wall bracing using isometric "hold" positions as a basis for progression (Fig. 22-69).[75,265,387] There seems to be some obsession in our society with doing vertical sit-ups or curl ups with a twisting motion. Such curl-ups are expensive in terms of lumbar compression (Fig. 22-21).[503,555] Higher oblique activation with lower spine load may be accomplished with the side bridge (Fig. 22-64). The preferred progression of the curl-up should begin with tightening up the muscles of the pelvic floor and contraction of the transversus abdominus. Only the head is raised with the shoulders clearing the plinth (Fig. 22-70). The back should not be flattened to the floor which takes the

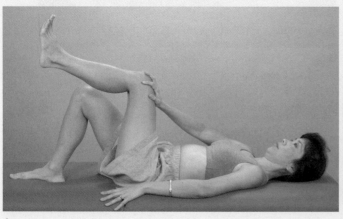
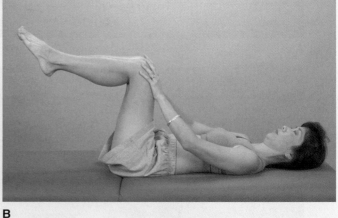

A   **B**

■ **FIG. 22-69.** Abdominal bracing. (A) While breathing freely, one leg is lifted and resisted by opposite hand to initiate an isometric contraction of the obliques and the abdominal wall. (B) Both legs are resisted with the hands to initiate an isometric contraction of the abdominal wall. Progression can be made with the hips more flexed, as the patient attempts to lift the buttock from the table, against manual resistance of the hands.

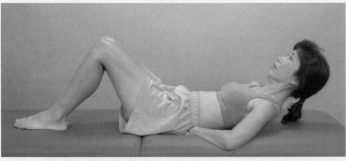
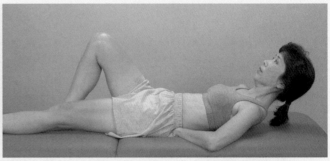

A   **B**

■ **FIG. 22-70.** Curl-up. **(A)** The beginners curl-up is performed by lifting the head and shoulders off the ground with the hands under the lumbar spine region to help stabilize the spine and support the neutral spine. **(B)** A variation of the curl-up; the straight leg assists in pelvic stabilization and maintenance of a "neutral" lumbar curve.

spine out of the elastic equilibrium and raises the stresses in the passive tissues.[503] An intermediate curl-up is to raise the elbows a couple of centimeters, off of the table thus shifting more load to the rectus while an advanced curl up requires using the arms in different positions (i.e., placing fingers lightly on the forehead) as long as the lumbar posture is controlled.

Progression of abdominal control exercises can be performed in any or all of the developmental positions, supine with arm and leg movements (Fig. 22-71), quadriped (Fig. 22-72),[128,402] front bridge (Fig. 22-73) (also see Fig. 11-79),[122,353] sitting (Fig. 22-74),[402,741] and standing with a body blade (see Fig. 20-68) or hand held weight (Fig. 22-75).[116,252,253] All exercises should begin with a contraction of the transversus abdominus and pelvic floor. Wobble boards, therapeutic balls, foam rolls and balance cushions can be used to further challenge balance and proprioception and to facilitate recruitment of the spinal stabilizers.

It is clear from what is known about normal gait that transverse plane motion is critical to the spine and that transverse plane forces are in inevitable. The lumbar spine is a system that must react to forces created from the ground up as the pelvis rotates in the transverse plane during ambulation. Lumbopelvic rotation control (transverse plane) becomes critical during the rehabilitation of the lumbar spine (Figs. 22-57 and 22-59). Early on lumbo pelvic rotational and oblique abdominal load control can be facilitated by supine limb loading first on a stable base with progression on unstable base with increased proprioceptive challenges (Fig. 22-76; also see Figs. 23-67, 23-68, 23-70, and 23-71).[128] Progression must ultimately include dynamic functional control to reproduce the movements, loads and forces encountered at all the joints of the lower limbs in the foot to the spine (Fig. 22-75).[116,252]

The gluteus maximus through it attachment of the raphe of the thoracolumbar fascia is coupled with the contralateral latissimus dorsi muscle. This coupling establishes it function

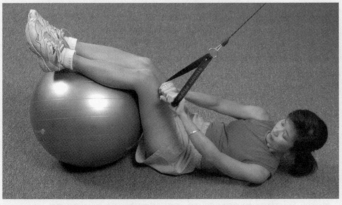
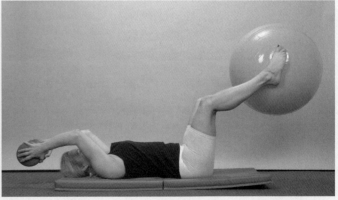

A   **B**

■ **FIG. 22-71.** Exercises to challenge the abdominals in supine. **(A)** Diagonal pull of the upper limbs using resistive cords. **(B)** Moving the upper and lower limbs in opposite directions using weight held in the hands and a therapeutic ball between the legs.

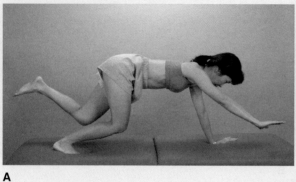
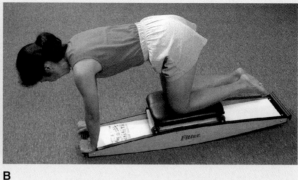

A   **B**

■ **FIG. 22-72.** Exercises to challenge abdominal flexion control in quadriped. **(A)** One leg is raised from the floor while the patient is standing on tiptoe. In this position one hand at a time and the opposite leg is raised simultaneously. **(B)** Backward rocking with independent hip flexion on a Fitter (or Pilates Reformer), but only as far as the neutral lumbopelvic position can be maintained.

creating a self-bracing mechanism for the sacroiliac joints and allows the muscle to help transmit forces from the lower limbs to the spine and trunk.[783] Figure 22-77 demonstrates a dynamic exercise in which cross-coupling of the pelvis and trunk is facilitated.

Conditioning program initially focuses on mobility, followed by endurance and progressive resistive exercise training for strength, including both resistive and repetitive low-load exercises. Endurance is can be further improved through aerobic exercise, followed by protocols to improve whole-body coordination and agility.[488] It becomes clear that spinal stabilization patterns produced during rehabilitation must closely match tasks that the patient will perform in patient's daily living (see Chapter 10, Functional Exercise).[116,117]

For the athlete, plyometrics is useful in late-stage rehabilitation and functional precompetitive testing after injury (see Chapter 12, Hip).[578] Although plyometric activity is primarily used for lower limb training, it is also important in training the upper limb and trunk. Throwing and catching from a bent-knee position is only one example (Fig. 11-89*B*,*C*).

Active exercise programs are a critical element in the successful rehabilitation of patients with low back pain. The selection of a specific exercise routine should be based on the presentation of the individual patient.

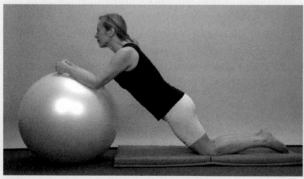
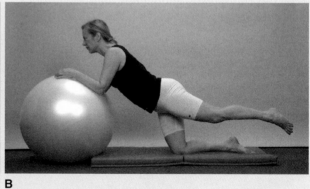

A   **B**

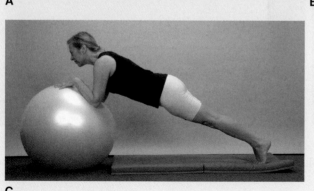

C

■ **FIG. 22-73.** High performance exercise to challenge abdominal flexion control and stabilization of the shoulder girdle in the front bridge. **(A)** Front bridge on a ball with two knees on the floor. **(B)** Front bridge on a ball with one knee on the floor. **(C)** Front bridge on a ball with two feet on the floor. Further progression includes front bridge on the ball with one foot on the floor. These exercises are difficult in terms of balance and strength; a lack of shoulder girdle and trunk strength often limit patient's ability to do these exercises.

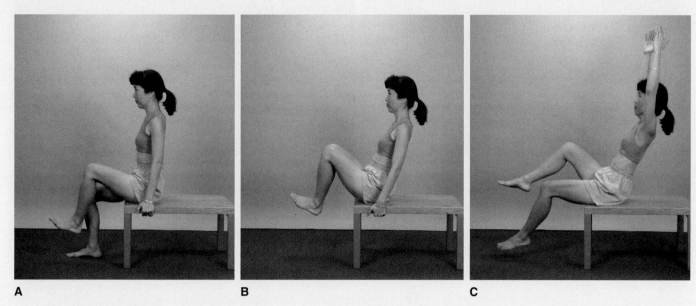

A   **B**   **C**

■ **FIG. 22-74.** Exercises to challenge the abdominals control in sitting. (**A**) Sitting on a table, one knee is raised toward the chest. (**B**) While maintaining abdominal control, the other leg is brought toward the chest. (**C**) Sitting on the edge of a table where the feet are flat on the floor, the trunk is moved into a backward lean. While maintaining a neutral spine the arms are elevated above the head in a continuation of the trunk line. With the trunk in a backward lean, the legs are raised a little alternately, like riding a bicycle.

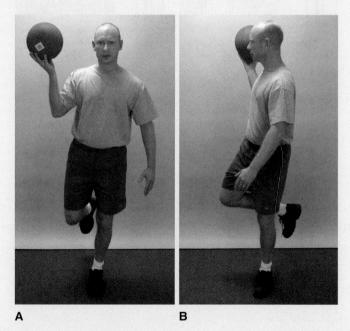

A   **B**

■ **FIG. 22-75.** Functional abdominal strengthening. The subject is challenged to balance on one leg with toe-touch support of the opposite foot. A weight is held on the contralateral hand and placed near the side of the head just above the shoulder. The patient stands with a wall or door behind that is used as a target. While squatting on the stance leg, the trunk is rotated posteriorly and extended with a goal of touching the right elbow and posterior aspect of the shoulder to the wall. Once the touch is made, the patient returns to the erect position by extending the knee and derotating the trunk.

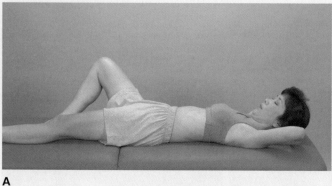
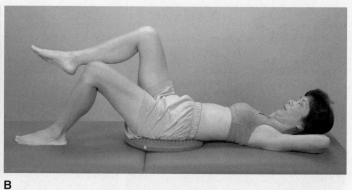

A   B

■ **FIG. 22-76.** Lumbopelvic rotational control. (**A**) With one leg in the hook position beside the straight, the leg is lowered out slowly as far as no rotation of the pelvis occurs. The stabilizing abdominal muscles must coordinate with the adductor control muscles. (**B**) Oblique abdominal control can be facilitated by alternately lifting and lowing one foot at a time off the floor slowly. A further progression would be to perform the exercise on an unstable base with a balance cushion or wobble board and increasing the proprioceptive challenge.

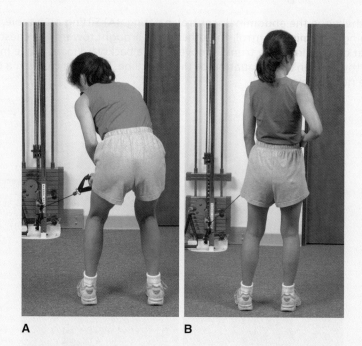

A   B

■ **FIG. 22-77.** Diagonal rotational squat which creates optimal coupling of the gluteal muscles and contralateral latissimus dorsi.

REFERENCES

1. Abboudi SY: The aquatic solution. Rehabil Manage 6:77–79, 1993
2. Abel OJR, Siebert WJ: Fibrositis. J Missouri Med Assoc 36:43–437, 1939
3. Aberg J: Evaluation of an advanced back pain rehabilitation program. Spine 7:317–318, 1982
4. Adams MA, Hutton WC: Gradual disc prolapse. Spine 10:524–531, 1985
5. Addison R, Schultz A: Trunk strength in patients seeking hospitalization for chronic low back disorders. Spine 5:539–544, 1980
6. Adler SS, Beckers D, Buck M: PNF in Practice. An Illustrated Guide. Berlin, Springer-Verlag, 1993
7. Admundson GM, Wenger DR: Spondylolisthesis: Natural history and treatment. Spine 1:323–328, 1987
8. Akerblom B: Standing and Sitting Posture with Special Reference to the Construction of Chairs. Thesis. Stockholm, Nordiska Bockhandeln, 1948
9. Almay BG, Johansson F, Von Knorring L, et al: Endorphins in chronic pain: I. Differences in CSF endorphin levels between organic and psychogenic pain syndromes. Pain 5:153–162, 1978
10. Alston W, Carlson KE, Feldman DJ, et al: A quantitative study of muscle factors in chronic low back syndrome. J Am Geriatr Soc 14(10):1041–1047, 1966
11. Alvarez JA, Hardy RH Jr: Lumbar spine stenosis: A common cause of back and leg pain. Am Fam Phys 57:1825–1834, 1999
12. American Academy of Orthopaedic Surgeons: A Glossary on Spinal Terminology. Chicago, American Academy of Orthopaedic Surgeons, 1981
13. Amundsen T, Weber H, Nordal HJ et al: Lumbar spinal stenosis: Conservative or surgical management? Prospective 10-year study. Spine 25:1424–1436, 2000
14. Anderson B: Pilates power. Adv Dir Rehabil 12:27–30, 2003
15. Andersson BJ, Murphy RW, Ortengren R, et al: The influence of back-rest inclination and lumbar support on lumbar lordosis. Spine 4:52–58, 1979
16. Andersson BJ, Ortengren R, Nachemson A, et al: Lumbar disc pressure and myoelectric back muscle activity during sitting: 1. Studies on an experimental chair. Scand J Rehabil Med 6:104–114, 1974
17. Andersson BJ, Ortengren R, Nachemson A, et al: The sitting posture: An electromyographic and discometric study. Orthop Clin North Am 6:105–120, 1975
18. Andersson EA, Oddsson Lie, Grundstrom H, et al: EMG activities of the quadratus lumborum and erector spinae muscles during flexion-relaxation and other motor tasks. Clin Biomech 11:392–400, 1996
19. Andersson GBJ: Epidemiologic aspects on low back pain in industry. Spine 6:53–60, 1981
20. Andersson GBJ, Pope MH: The patient. In: Pope MH, Frymoyer JW, Andersson G, eds: Occupational Low Back Pain. New York, Praeger, 1984:137–156
21. Andersson GBJ, Sevensson HO, Oden A: The intensity of work recovery in low back pain. Spine 8:880–884, 1983
22. Andersson JAD: Back pain and occupation. In: Jayson M, ed: The Lumbar Spine and Back Pain. London, Pittman Medical, 1980:57–82
23. Anthony A Pilates takes the plunge. Adv Dir Rehabil 12:53–56, 2003
24. Armstrong JR: Lumbar Disc Lesions. London, Livingstone, 1967
25. Arnoldi CC, Brodsky AE, Cauchoix J, et al: Lumbar spinal stenosis and nerve root entrapment syndromes: Definitions and classification. Clin Orthop 115:4–5, 1976
26. Ashmen KJ, Swanik CB, Lephart SM: Strength and flexibility characteristics of athletes with chronic low back pain. J Sports Rehab 5:275–286, 1996
27. Atlas SJ, Keller RB, Robinson D, et al: Surgical and nonsurgical management of lumbar spinal stenosis four-year outcomes from the main lumbar spine study. Spine 25:556–562, 2000
28. Awad EA: Interstitial myofibrositis: Hypothesis of mechanism. Arch Phys Med Rehabil 54:449–453, 1975
29. Baarstrup C: On the spinous processes of the lumbar vertebrae and soft tissues between them and on pathological changes in that region. Acta Radiol 14:52, 1933
30. Badgley CE: The articular facets in relation to low-back pain and sciatica radiation. J Bone Joint Surg 23:481–496, 1941
31. Baer WS: Sacroiliac strain. Bull Johns Hopkins Hosp 28:159, 1917
32. Bajelus D: Hellerwork: The ultimate. International J Altern Complement Med 12:26–38, 1994
33. Bastille JV, Gill-Body KM: A yoga-based exercise program for people with chronic poststroke hemiparesis. Phys Ther 84:33–48, 2004
34. Batson G: Balancing mobility with stability for dynamic spine function: Part I. Mobility. Kinesiol Dance 9(3):8–10, 1987
35. Batson G: Balancing mobility with stability for dynamic spine function: Part II. Stability. Kinesiol Dance 9(4):12–15, 1987
36. Batson G: Balancing mobility with stability for dynamic spine function: Part III. Strengthening the trunk. Kinesiol Dance 10(1):12–16, 1987
37. Beal M: Palpatory testing of somatic dysfunction in patients with cardiovascular disease. J Am Osteopath Assoc 82:822–831, 1983
38. Beals RK, Hickman NW: Industrial injuries of the back and extremities. J Bone Joint Surg Am 54:1593–1611, 1972
39. Becker BE: Aquatic exercise therapy. In: Liemohn W, ed: Exercise Prescription and the Back. New York, McGraw, 2001:197–213
40. Bell GH, Dunbar O, Beck SJ, et al: Variation in strength of vertebrae with age and their relation to osteoporosis. Calcif Tissue Res 1:75–86, 1967
41. Bell GR, Rothman RH: The conservative treatment of sciatica. Spine 9:54–56, 1984
42. Benjamin BE: Are You Tense? The Benjamin System of Muscular Therapy: Tension Relief Through Deep Massage and Body Care. New York, Pantheon Books, 1978
43. Bennell K, Khan K, McKay H: The role of physiotherapy in the prevention and treatment of osteoporosis. Man Ther 5:198–213, 2000
44. Bennet RM: Fibrositis: Misnomer for a common rheumatic disorder. West J Med 134:405–413, 1981
45. Bennett K: Therapeutic exercise for fibromyalgia syndrome and chronic fatigue syndrome. In: Hall CM, Brody LT, eds: Therapeutic Exercise: Moving Toward Function. Philadelphia, Lippincott Williams & Wilkins, 1999:200–212
46. Berguist-Ullman M, Larsson U: Acute low back pain in industry: A controlled prospective study with specific reference to therapy and vocational factors. Acta Orthop Scand (Suppl) 170:1–117, 1977
47. Bergmark A: Stability of the lumbar spine. A study in mechanical engineering. Acta Orthop Scand (Suppl) 230(60):20–24, 1989
48. Berkson M, Schultz A, Nachemson A, et al: Voluntary strengths of male adults with acute low back syndromes. Clin Orthop 129:84–95, 1977
49. Bernick S, Cailliet R: Vertebral end-plate changes with aging of human vertebrae. Spine 7:97–102, 1982
50. Bianco AJ: Low back pain and sciatica: Diagnosis/indications for treatment. J Bone Joint Surg Am 50:170–181, 1968
51. Biedermann HJ, Shanks GL, Forrest W, et al: Power spectrum analysis of electromyographic activity: Discriminators in the differential assessment of patients with chronic back pain. Spine 16:1179–1185, 1991
52. Biering-Sorensen F: Low back trouble in a general population of 30-, 40-, 50- and 60-year-old men and women: Study design, representativeness and basic results. Dan Med Bull 29(6):289–299, 1982
53. Biering-Sorensen F: A prospective study of low back pain in a general population: I. Occurrence, recurrence and aetiology. Scand J Rehabil Med 15(2):71–78, 1983
54. Biering-Sorensen F: Physical measurement as risk indication for low back trouble over a 1-year period. Spine 9:106–118, 1984
55. Biering-Sorensen F, Hilden J: Reproducibility of the history of low-back trouble. Spine 9:280–286, 1984
56. Blades K: Hydrotherapy in orthopedics. In: Champion MR, ed: Adult Hydrotherapy. London, Heinemann, 1990
57. Blumett AE, Modesti LM: Psychological predictions of success or failure of surgical intervention for intractable back pain. In: Bonica JJ, Albefessard D, eds: Advances in Pain Research and Therapy, vol. I. New York, Raven Press, 1976:323–326
58. Boden SD, Davis DO, Dina TS, et al: Abnormal magnetic-response scans of the lumbar spine in asymptomatic subjects. J Bone Joint Surg Am 74:403–408, 1990
59. Bogduk N: Lumbar dorsal ramus syndrome. Med J Aust 2:537–541, 1980
60. Bogduk N: The innervation of the lumbar spine. Spine 8:286–293, 1983
61. Bogduk N: Lumbar dorsal ramus syndrome. In: Grieve GP, ed: Modern Manual Therapy of the Vertebral Column. New York, Churchill Livingstone, 1986
62. Bogduk N, Engel R: The menisci of the lumbar zyapophyseal joints. Spine 9:454–460, 1984
63. Bogduk N, Tynan W, Wilson AS: The nerve supply to the human intervertebral disk. J Anat 132:39–56, 1981
64. Bookhout MR: Examination and treatment of muscle imbalances. In: Bourdillon JF, Day EA, Bookhout MR, eds: Spinal Manipulation, 5th ed. Oxford, Butterworth Heinemann, 1992:313–333
65. Boothby B: Seating by design. Physiotherapy 70:44–47, 1984
66. Bottomley JM: Tai Chi: Choreography of Body & Mind. In: Davis CM, ed: Complementary Therapies in Rehabilitation, Thorofare, Slack, 1997
67. Bourdillon JF, Day EA, Bookhout MR: Spinal Manipulations, 5th ed. Oxford, Butterworth Heinemann, 1992
68. Bourne IHJ: Treatment of chronic back pain comparing corticosteroid-lignocaine injections with lignocaine alone. Practitioner 228:333–338, 1984
69. Boxall D, Bradford DS, Winter RB, et al: Management of severe spondylolisthesis in children and adolescents. J Bone Joint Surg Am 61:479–495, 1979
70. Brackett EG: Low back strain with particular reference to industrial accident. JAMA 83:1068–1075, 1924
71. Bradley LA, Prokop CK, Margolis R, et al: Multivariate analyses of the MMPI profiles of low back pain patients. J Behav Med I(3):235–272, 1978
72. Braunarski DT: Clinical trails of spinal manipulations: A critical appraisal and review of the literature. J Manip Physiol Ther 7:243–249, 1984
73. Breig A, Troup JDG: Biomechanical consideration in straight leg-raising test. Spine 4:242–250, 1979
74. Brewerton DA: The doctor's role in diagnosis and prescribing vertebral manipulations. In: Maitland GD, ed: Vertebral Manipulations, 5th ed. London, Butterworths, 1986:14–17
75. Brill PW: The Core Program. Fifteen Minutes a Day that can Change Your Life. New York, Bantam Books, 2001
76. Brinckmann P: Injury of the annulus fibrosus and disc protrusions: An in vitro investigation on human lumbar disc. Spine 11:149–153, 1986

77. Bronner S: Functional rehabilitation of the spine: The lumbopelvis as a key of control. In: Brownstein B, Bronner S, eds: Evaluation, Treatment and Outcomes: Functional Movement in Orthopaedic and Sports Medicine. New York, Churchill Livingstone, 1995:141–190

78. Bronson KM: The therapeutic benefits of yoga. Orthop Phys Ther Pract 14:11–15, 2002

79. Brown L: An introduction to the treatment and examination of the spine by combined movements. Physiotherapy 74:347–353, 1988

80. Brunswic M: Ergonomics of seat design. Physiotherapy 70:40–43, 1984

81. Buckle PW, Kember PA, Wood AD, et al: Factors influencing occupational back pain in Bedfordshire. Spine 5:254–258, 1980

82. Bullock-Saxton JE: Muscles and joint: Inter-relationships with pain and movement dysfunction. Course manual, 1997

83. Burnell A: Injection techniques in low back pain. In: Twomey LT, ed: Symposium: Low Back Pain. Perth, Western Australia Institute of Technology, 1974:111

84. Buros OK: Eighth Mental Measurements. Lincoln, University of Nebraska Press, Year Book, 1978

85. Burton AK: Regional lumbar sagittal mobility: Measurement by flexicurves. Clin Biomech 1:20–26, 1986

86. Burton CV: Conservative management of low back pain. Postgrad Med 70(5):168–183, 1981

87. Burton CV, Nida G: Gravity Lumbar Reduction Therapy. Rehabilitation Publication No. 731. Minneapolis, Sister Kenny Institute, 1976

88. Bush HD, Horton WG, Smare DL, et al: Fluid content of the nucleus pulposus as a factor in the disk syndrome. Br Med J 2:831–832, 1956

89. Butler DS: Mobilization of the Nervous System. Melbourne, Churchill Livingstone, 1991

90. Cady LD, Bischoff DP, O'Connell ER, et al: Strength and fitness and subsequent back injuries in firefighters. J Occup Med 21:269–272, 1979

91. Cailliet R: Low Back Pain Syndrome, 4th ed. Philadelphia, FA Davis, 1988

92. Cailliet R: Soft Tissue Pain and Disability, 2nd ed. Philadelphia, FA Davis, 1988

93. Cairns D, Thomas L, Mooney V, et al: A comprehensive treatment approach to chronic low back pain. Pain 2:301–308, 1976

94. Calin A, Porta J, Fries JF, Schurman DJ: Clinical history as a screening test for ankylosing spondylitis. JAMA 237:2613–2614, 1977

95. Campbell SM, Clark S, Tindall EA, et al: Clinical characteristics of fibrositis: I. A "blinded" controlled study of symptoms and points. Arthritis Rheum 26:817–824, 1983

96. Caro XJ: Immunofluorescent studies of skin in primary fibrositis syndrome. Am J Med [Suppl 3A] 81:43–48, 1986

97. Caro XJ, Wolfe F, Johnston WH, et al: Controlled and blinded study of immunoreactant deposition at dermal/epidermal junction of patients with primary fibrositis syndrome. J Rheumatol 13:1086–1092, 1986

98. Carrera GF: Lumbar facet arthrography and injection in low back pain. Wisc Med J 78:35–37, 1979

99. Carrera GF, Haughton VM, Syversten A, et al: Computerized tomography of the lumbar facet joints. Radiology 134:145–148, 1980

100. Carriere B. The Swiss Ball: Theory, Basic Exercise and Clinical Applications. Berlin, Springer-Verlag, 1998

101. Carriere B: Fitness for the Pelvic Floor. Stuttgart, Thieme, 2002

102. Carvin PJ, Jennings RB, Stern IJ: Enzymatic digestion of the nucleus pulposus: A review of experimental studies with chymopapain. Orthop Clin 8:27–35, 1977

103. Chadwick PR: Advising patients on back care. Physiotherapy 65:277–278, 1979

104. Chadwick PR: Examination, assessment and treatment of the lumbar spine. Physiotherapy 70:2–7, 1984

105. Chaffin DB: Human strength capacity and low back pain. J Occup Med 16:248–253, 1974

106. Chaffin DB: Manual materials handling: The case of overexertion injury and illness in industry. J Environ Pathol Toxicol 2:31–36, 1979

107. Chaffin DB, Herrin GD, Keyserling WM: Pre-employment strength testing—An updated position. J Occup Med 20:403–408, 1978

108. Chaitow L: Muscle Energy Techniques. New York, Churchill Livingstone, 1996

109. Chaitow L: Fibromyalgia Syndrome: A Practitioner's Guide to Treatment. Edinburg, Churchill Livingstone, 2000

110. Chaitow L, Comeaux Z, Dommerholt J, et al: Efficacy of manipulation in low back pain treatment: The validity of meta-analysis conclusions. J Bodywork Move Ther 8:25–31, 2004

111. Chamberlain GJ: Cyriax's friction massage: A review. J Orthop Sports Phys Ther 4:16–22, 1982

112. Chan PC: Finger Acupressure. Los Angeles, Price/Stern/Sloan, 1982

113. Cantu R, Grodin A: Myofascial Manipulations. Gaithersburg, Aspen, 1992

114. Charnley J: Orthopaedic signs in the diagnosis of disc protrusion with specific reference to straight leg-raising test. Lancet 1:186–192, 1951

115. Chason N: The Swing Reaction System. Seattle, Biomechanical Golf Exercise Video, 1996

116. Chason N, Kane M: Functional training for the low back patient. Ortho Phys Ther Clin North Am 8:451–477, 1999

117. Chason N: Total Conditioning for Golfers: Your Definitive Guide to Hitting Longer, Getting Stronger and Staying Healthy, 2nd ed. Bellevue, WA, Sports Reaction Productions, 2002

118. Cherkin DC, Sherman KJ, Deyo RA, et al: A review of the evidence for the effectiveness, safety, and cost of acupuncture, massage therapy, and spinal manipulations for back pain. Ann Intern Med 138:898–906, 2003

119. Chhem RK, Kaplan PA, Dussault RG: Ultrasonography of the musculoskeletal system. Radiol Clin North Am 32:275–289, 1994

120. Chrisman DO, Mittnacht A, Snook GA: A study of the results following rotatory manipulation in the lumbar intervertebral disc syndrome. J Bone Joint Surg Am 46:517–524, 1964

121. Cirullo JA: Aquatic physical therapy approaches for the spine. Orthop Phys Ther Clin North Am 3:179–208, 1994

122. Clark MA: Core stabilization training in rehabilitation. In: Prentice WE, Voight ML, eds: Techniques in Musculoskeletal Rehabilitation. New York, McGraw-Hill, 2001:259–278

123. Clarkston HM, Gilewish GB: Musculoskeletal Assessment, Joint Range of Motion and Manual Muscle Strength. Baltimore, Williams & Wilkins, 1989

124. Clelland J, Savinar E, Shepard KF: The role of the physical therapist in chronic pain management. In: Burrows GD, Elton D, Stanley GV, eds: Handbook of Chronic Pain Management. New York, Elsevier, 1987:243–258

125. Clements L, Dixon M: A model role of occupational therapy in back education. Can J Occup Ther 46:161–163, 1979

126. Cloward RB: The clinical significance of the sinuvertebral nerve of the cervical spine in relation to the cervical disc syndrome. J Neurol Neurosurg Psychiatry 23:321–326, 1960

127. Cole JH, Furness AL, Twoney LT: Muscles in Action, an Approach to Manual Muscle Testing. Edinburg, Churchill Livingstone, 1988

128. Comerford MJ, Mottrom SL: Functional stability retraining: Principles and strategies for managing mechanical dysfunction. Man Ther 6:3–14, 2001

129. Colt EWD, Wardlaw SL, Frantz AG: The effect of running on plasma B-endorphin. Life Sci 28:1637–1640, 1981

130. Coplans CW: The conservative treatment of low back pain. In: Helfet AJ, Gruebel LDM, eds: Disorders of the Lumbar Spine. Philadelphia, JB Lippincott, 1978:135–183

131. Corrigan B, Maitland GD: Practical Orthopaedic Medicine. Boston, Butterworths, 1985

132. Cottrell GW: 90/90 traction in the treatment of low back pain. Orthop Trans/J Bone Joint Surg 4:80, 1981

133. Cottrell GW: New, conservative and exceptionally effective treatment for low back pain. Compr Ther 11:59–65, 1985

134. Coulehan JL: Chiropractic and the clinical art. Soc Sci Med 21:383–390, 1985

135. Coventry MB, Ghormley RK, Kernohan JW: The intervertebral disc: Its microscopic anatomy and pathology: 2. Changes in the intervertebral disc concomitant with age. J Bone Joint Surg 27:233–247, 1945

136. Coventry MB, Ghormley RK, Kernohan JW: The intervertebral disc: Its microscopic anatomy and pathology: 3. Pathological changes in the intervertebral disc. J Bone Joint Surg 27:460–474, 1945

137. Craig C: Pilates on the Ball. Rochester, VT, Healing Arts Press, 2001

138. Crock HV: Isolated lumbar disk resorption as a cause of nerve root canal stenosis. Clin Orthop 115:109–115, 1976

139. Crock HV: Internal disc disruption: A challenge to disc prolapse 50 years on. Spine 11:650–653, 1986

140. Cuckler JM, Bernini PA, Wiesel SW, et al: The use of epidural steroids in the treatment of lumbar radicular pain: A prospective, randomized, double-blind study. J Bone Joint Surg 67:63–66, 1985

141. Cummings GS, Routon JL: Validity of unassisted pain drawings by patients with chronic pain [abstract]. Phys Ther 5:668, 1985

142. Cyriax J: Treatment of lumbar disk lesions. Br Med J 2:1434–1438, 1950

143. Cyriax J: Conservative treatment of lumbar disc lesions. Physiotherapy 50:300–303, 1964

144. Cyriax J: Deep friction. Physiotherapy 63:60–61, 1977

145. Cyriax J: The Slipped Disc. New York, Charles Scribner's Sons, 1980

146. Cyriax J: Textbook of Orthopaedic Medicine, 8th ed, vol. I: Diagnosis of Soft-Tissue Lesions. London, Bailliere-Tindall, 1982

147. Cyriax JC, Coldham M: Textbook of Orthopaedic Medicine, 11th ed, vol. 2: Treatment by Manipulation, Massage and Injection. Philadelphia, Bailliere-Tindall, 1984

148. Cyriax J, Cyriax P: Illustrated Manual of Orthopedic Medicine. Boston, Butterworths, 1983

149. Dagi FT, Beary JF: Low back pain. In: Beary JF, ed: Rheumatology and Outpatient Orthopedic Disorders: Diagnosis and Therapy, 2nd ed. Boston, Little, Brown, 1987:97–103

150. Dahlstrom WG, Welsh GS, Dahlstrom LE: MMPI Handbook, vol. 1. Minneapolis, University of Minnesota Press, 1975

151. Dahlstrom WG, Welsh GS, Dahlstrom LE: MMPI Handbook, vol. 2. Minneapolis, University of Minnesota Press, 1975

152. Dan NG, Saccason PA: Serious complications of lumbar spine manipulations. Med J Aust 2:672–673, 1983

153. Danneels LA, Coorevits PL, Cools AM et al: Differences in electromyographic activity in the multifidus muscle and iliocostalis lumborum between healthy

subjects and patients with sub-acute and chronic low back pain. Eur Spine J 11:13–19, 2002

154. Danneels LA, Vanderstraeten GG, Camber DC et al: Effects of three different training modalities on the cross sectional area of lumbar multifidus muscle in patients with chronic low back pain. Br J Sports Med 35:186–191, 2001

155. Davidson EA, Woodhall B: Biochemical alterations in herniated intervertebral disks. J Biol Chem 234:2951–2954, 1959

156. Davies G, Gould J: Trunk testing using a prototype Cybex II isokinetic stabilization system. J Orthop Sports Phys Ther 3:164–170, 1982

157. Davis P: Reducing the risk of industrial bad backs. Occup Health Safety 48:45–47, 1979

158. DeFazio FA, Barth RA, Frymoyer JW et al: Acute lumbar paraspinal compartment syndrome. J Bone Joint Surg Am 73:1101–1103, 1991

159. Dehlin O, Lindberg B: Lifting burden for a nursing aide during patient care in a geriatric ward. Scand J Rehabil Med 7:65–72, 1975

160. Delmas A: Fonction sacro-iliaque et statique du corps. Rev Rhuna 17:475–481, 1950

161. Dennis MD, Greene RL, Farr SP, et al: The Minnesota Multiphasic Personality Inventory: General guidelines to its use and interpretation in orthopaedics. Clin Orthop 150:125–130, 1980

162. DePalma A, Rothman RH: The Intervertebral Disc. Philadelphia, WB Saunders, 1970

163. DeRosa CP, Porterfield JA: A physical therapy model for the treatment of low back pain. Phys Ther 72:261–269, 1992

164. deVries HA, Cailliet R: Vagotonic effect of inversion therapy upon resting neuromuscular tension. Am J Phys Med 64(3):119–129, 1984

165. Deyo RA: Conservative therapy for low back pain: Distinguishing useful from useless therapy. JAMA 250:1057–1062, 1983

166. Deyo RA, Diehl A, Rosenthal M: How many days of bed rest for acute low back pain? N Engl J Med 315:1065–1070, 1986

167. Deyo RA, Diehl AK: Lumbar spine films in primary care: Current use and the effects of selective ordering criteria. J Gen Intern Med 1:20–25, 1986

168. DiFabio RP: Clinical assessment of manipulation and mobilization of the lumbar spine: A critical review of the literature. Phys Ther 66:51–54, 1986

169. Dike TFW, Burry HC, Grahame R: Extradural corticosteroid injection in management of lumbar nerve root compression. Br Med J 2:635–637, 1973

170. Dimaggio A, Mooney V: Conservative care of low back pain: What works? J Musculoskel Med 4(4):27–34, 1987

171. Dimaggio A, Mooney V: The McKenzie program: Exercise effective against back pain. J Musculoskel Med 4(12):63–74, 1987

172. Dixon ASJ: Progress and problems in back pain research. Rheumat Rehabil 12(4):165–175, 1973

173. Dominguez RH, Gajda R: Total Body Training. New York, Warner Books, 1982

174. Dontigny RL: Function and pathomechanics of the sacroiliac joint: A review. Phys Ther 65:35–44, 1985

175. Dorman TA: Prolotherapy: A survey. J Orthop Med 15:2–3, 1993

176. Dunham WF: Ankylosing spondylitis measurement of hip and spine movements. Br J Phys Med 12:126, 1949

177. DuPriest CM: Nonoperative management of lumbar spinal stenosis. J Manip Physiol Ther 16:411–414, 1993

178. Dupuis PR: The natural history of degenerative changes in the lumbar spine. In: Watkins RG, Collis JS, eds: Principles and Techniques in Spine Surgery. Rockville, Aspen, 1987

179. Dupuis PR, Yong-Ling K, Cassidy JD, et al: Radiologic diagnosis of degenerative lumbar spinal instability. Spine 10:262–276, 1985

180. Dutton M: The lumbar spine. In: Dutton M, ed: Manual Therapy of the Spine: An Integrated Approach. New York, Mc Graw, 2002:272–341

181. Dyck P: The stoop-test in lumbar entrapment radiculopathy. Spine 4:89–92, 1979

182. Dyck P, Doyle JB: "Bicycle test" of van Gelderen in diagnosis of intermittent cauda equina compression syndrome. J Neurosurg 46:667–670, 1977

183. Dyck P: Sciatic pain. In: Watkins C, ed: Lumbar Discectomy and Laminectomy. Rockville, Aspen, 1987

184. Eastmond CJ, Woodrow JC: The HLA system and the arthropathies associated with psoriasis. Ann Rheum Dis 36:112, 1977

185. Ebner M: Connective tissue massage. Physiotherapy 64:208–212, 1978

186. Ebner M: Connective Tissue Manipulations, Therapy and Therapeutic Application. Malabar, FL, Robert Kreiger, 1985

187. Echternach JL: Evaluation of pain in the clinical environment. In: Echternach JL, ed: Pain. New York, Churchill Livingstone, 1987:39–72

188. Eckert C, Decker A: Pathological studies of intervertebral discs. J Bone Joint Surg 29:447–454, 1947

189. Edgar MA: Backache. Br J Hosp Med 32:290–301, 1984

190. Edgar MA, Park WM: Induced pain patterns on passive straight leg-raising in lower disc protrusion. J Bone Joint Surg Br 56:658–667, 1974

191. Edwards BC: Combined movements of the lumbar spine: Examination and significance. Aust J Physiother 25:147–152, 1979

192. Edwards BC: Combined movements in the lumbar spine: Examination and treatment. In: Grieve GP, ed: Modern Manual Therapy of the Vertebral Column. New York, Churchill Livingstone, 1986:561–566

193. Edwards BC: Clinical assessment: The use of combined movements in assessment and treatment. In: Twomey LT, Taylor JR, eds: Physiotherapy of the Low Back. New York, Churchill Livingstone, 1987:81–109

194. Eggart JS, Leigh D, Vergamini G: Preseason athletic physical evaluations. In: Gould JA, Davies GJ, eds: Orthopaedic and Sports Physical Therapy. St. Louis, CV Mosby, 1985:605–642

195. Ehard R, Blowling R: The recognition and management of the pelvic component of low back and sciatic pain. Presented at the Annual Meeting of the American Physical Therapy Association (Orthopaedic Section), Miami, 1967

196. Eisen A, Hoirch M: The electrodiagnostic evaluation of spinal root lesions. Spine 8:98–106, 1983

197. Eismont FJ, Kitchel SH: Thoracolumbar spine. In: DeLee JC, Drez D, eds: Orthopaedic Sports Medicine: Principles and Practice. Philadelphia, Saunders, 1994:1018–1062

198. Epstein JA, Epstein BS, Lavine LS, et al: Lumbar nerve root compression at the intervertebral foramina caused by arthritis of the posterior facets. J Neurosurg 39:362–369, 1973

199. Epstein JA, Epstein BS, Lavine LS, et al: Surgical treatment of nerve root compression caused by scoliosis of the lumbar spine. J Neurosurg 41:449–454, 1974

200. Evans RC: The lumbar spine. In Evans RC (ed): Illustrated Essentials in Orthopedic Physical Assessment. St. Louis, Mosby, 1994:249–343

201. Fahrni WH: Conservative treatment of lumbar disc degeneration: Our primary responsibility. Orthop Clin North Am 6:93–103, 1975

202. Fairbanks JCT, Park WN, Mc Call JW, et al: Apophyseal injection of local anesthetic as a diagnostic aid in primary low back syndromes. Spine 6:598–605, 1981

203. Fajersztajn J: Ueber das gekreuzte ischiasphanomen. Wien Klin Wochenschr 14:41–47, 1901

204. Falconer MA, McGeorge M, Begg AC: Observation on the cause and mechanism of symptom production and low back pain. J Neurosurg Psychiatry 11:13–26, 1948

205. Farfan HF: Mechanical Disorders of the Low Back. Philadelphia, Lea & Febiger, 1973

206. Farfan HF, Sullivan JD: The relation of facet orientation to intervertebral disc failure. Can Surg 10:179–185, 1967

207. Farrell PA, Gates WK, Maksud MG: Plasma beta-endorphin/beta-lipotropin immunoreactivity increases after treadmill exercise in man [abstract]. Med Sci Sports 13(2):134, 1981

208. Farrell PA, Koury M, DryeTaylor C: Therapeutic exercise for back pain. In: Twomey LT, Taylor JT, eds: Physical Therapy of the Low Back, 3rd ed. New York, Churchill Livingstone, 2000

209. Feinstein B, Langton J, Jameson R: Experiments on pain referred from deep skeletal structures. J Bone Joint Surg Am 36:981–997, 1954

210. Finneson B: Low Back Pain. Philadelphia, JB Lippincott, 1973

211. Finneson BE: A lumbar disc surgery predictive score-card: A retrospective evaluation. Spine 4:141–144, 1979

212. Finneson BE: Low Back Pain, 2nd ed. Philadelphia, JB Lippincott, 1980

213. Fischer AA: Documentation of myofascial trigger points. Arch Phys Med Rehabil 69:286–291, 1988

214. Fischer AA, Chang CH: Temperature and pressure threshold measurements in trigger points. Thermology 1:212–215, 1986

215. Fisk J, Dimonte P, Courington S: Back schools. Clin Orthop 179:18–23, 1983

216. Fitzgerald KG, Wynveen KJ, Rhealt W, et al: Objective assessment with establishment of normal values for lumbar spinal range of movement. Phys Ther 63:1776–1781, 1982

217. Flint M: Effect of increasing back and abdominal strength on low-back pain. Res Q 29:160–171, 1955

218. Flor H, Turk DC: Etiological theories and treatments for chronic back pain: Somatic models and interventions. Pain 19:105–121, 1984

219. Folkins CH, Sime WE: Physical fitness training and mental health. Am Psychol 36(4):373–389, 1981

220. Fordyce WE: Behavioral Methods for Chronic Back Pain and Illness. St. Louis, CV Mosby, 1976

221. Fordyce WE, Fowler RS, Lehmann JF, et al: Some implications of learning in problems of chronic pain. J Chron Dis 21:179–190, 1968

222. Fordyce WE, Mc Mahon R, Rainwater G, et al: Pain compliant/exercise performance relationship in chronic pain. Pain 10:311–321, 1981

223. Fordyce WE, Shelton JL, Dundore DE: The modification of avoidance learning pain behaviors. J Behav Med 5:405–414, 1982

224. Fornage BD, Rifkin MD: Ultrasound examination of tendons. Radiologic Clinics of North America 22: 87–107, 1990

225. Forssell MZ: The back school. Spine 6:104–106, 1981

226. Fox RF, Van Breemer J: Chronic Rheumatism: Causation and Treatment. London, Churchill, 1934

227. Fraioli F, Moretti C, Paulucci D, et al: Physical exercise stimulates marked concomitant release of B-endorphins and adrenocorticotrophic hormones (ACTH) in peripheral blood in man. Experientia 36:987–989, 1980

228. Fredrickson BE, Trief PM, Van Beveren P, et al: Rehabilitation of the patient with chronic back pain. Spine 13:351–353, 1987

229. Friberg RR, Weinreb RN: Ocular manifestation of gravity inversion. JAMA 253:1755–1757, 1985

230. Friberg S, Hirsch C: Anatomical and clinical studies on lumbar disc degeneration. Acta Orthop Scand 19:222–242, 1949
231. Fries JF, Mitchell DM: Joint pain or arthritis. JAMA 233:199–204, 1976
232. Fritz JM, Hicks GE: Exercise protocol for low back pain. In: Liemohn W, ed: Exercise Prescription and the Back. New York, McGraw-Hill, 2001:167–181
233. Frymoyer JW: Basics for all [abstract]. Challenge of the Lumbar Spine: Ninth Annual Meeting, New York City, 1987
234. Frymoyer JW: Back pain and sciatica. N Engl J Med 318:291–300, 1988
235. Frymoyer JW, Pope MH, Clements JH, et al: Risk factors in low back pain: An epidemiological survey. J Bone Joint Surg 65A:213–218, 1983
236. Frymoyer JW, Pope MH, Clostanza MC, et al: Epidemiologic studies of low-back pain. Spine 5:419–423, 1980
237. Frymoyer JW, Selby DK: Segmental instability: Rationale for treatment. Spine 10:280–286, 1985
238. Garrett R: Back strength and fitness programme using Norsk and sequence training. Physiotherapy 73:573–575, 1987
239. Gatchel RJ, Mayer TG, Capra P, et al: Qualification of lumbar function: VI. The use of psychological measures in guiding physical functional restoration. Spine 11:36–42, 1986
240. Gerbino PGI, Micheli IJ: Back injuries in the young athlete. Clin Sports Med 14:571–590, 1995
241. Gerhardt JJ: Documentation of Joint Motion. International Standard Neutral-Zero Measuring SFTR. Recording and Application of Goniometers, Inclinometers and Calipers. Portland, Isomed Inc., 1992
242. Gertzbein S: Segmental instability of the lumbar spine. Semin Spinal Surg 3:130–135, 1991
243. Gianakopoulos G, Waylonis GW, Grant PA, et al: Inversion devices: Their role in producing lumbar distraction. Arch Phys Med Rehabil 66:100–102, 1985
244. Glover JR: Back pain and hyperaesthesia. Lancet 1:1165–1169, 1960
245. Goldenberg DL: Psychologic studies in fibrositis. Am J Med 81(Suppl 3A):67–81, 1986
246. Goldish GD: Lumbar traction. In: Tollison CD, Kriefel ML, eds: Interdisciplinary Rehabilitation of Low Back Pain. Baltimore, Williams & Wilkins, 1989:305–321
247. Goldstein TS: Tai Chi for Rehabilitation. Physical Therapy Association of Washington, Seattle, WA, 2000
248. Gonnella C, Paris S, Kutner M: Reliability in evaluating passive intervertebral motion. Phys Ther 62:437–444, 1982
249. Goodman CC, Synder TE: Differential Diagnosis in Physical Therapy, 2nd ed. Philadelphia, WB Saunders, 1995
250. Gorman HO, Gwendolen J: Thoracic kyphosis and mobility: The effect of age. Physiother Pract 3:154–162, 1987
251. Grabias S: The treatment of spinal stenosis. J Bone Joint Surg Am 60:308–313, 1980
252. Gray G: Chain Reaction: Successful Strategies for Closed Chain Testing and Rehabilitation. Adrain, MI, Wynn Marketing, 1989
253. Gray G: Lower Extremity Functional Profile. Adrain MI, Wynn Marketing, 1995
254. Greenland S, Reisbord LS, Haldeman S, et al: Controlled clinical trials of manipulation: A review and proposal. J Occup Med 22:670–676, 1980
255. Greenman, PE: Principles of Manual Medicine, 3rd ed. Philadelphia, Lippincott Williams & Wilkins, 2003
256. Grieve GP: Sciatica and the straight leg-raising test in manipulative treatment. Physiotherapy 58:337–346, 1970
257. Grieve GP: The sacroiliac joint. Physiotherapy 62:384–400, 1976
258. Grieve GP: Lumbar instability. Physiotherapy 68:2–9, 1982
259. Grieve GP: Lumbar instability. In: Grieve GP, ed: Modern Manual Therapy of the Vertebral Column. New York, Churchill Livingstone, 1986:416–441
260. Grieve GP: Diagnosis. Physiotherapy Practice 4:73–77, 1988
261. Grieve GP: Pathological changes: Combined regional. In: Grieve GP, ed: Common Vertebral Joint Problems, 2nd ed. New York, Churchill Livingstone, 1988:249–298
262. Grieve GP: Clinical features. In: Grieve GP, ed: Common Vertebral Joint Problems, 2nd ed. New York, Churchill Livingstone, 1988:299–353
263. Grieve GP: Common patterns of clinical presentation. In Grieve GP: ed: Common Vertebral Joint Problems, 2nd ed. New York, Churchill Livingstone, 1988:355–458
264. Grieve GP: Passive movements. In: Grieve GP, ed: Mobilisation of the Spine: A Primary Handbook of Clinical Methods, 5th ed. Edinburgh, Churchill Livingstone, 1991:177–285
265. Grieve GP: Manually assisted or manually resisted movements. In: Grieve GP, ed: Mobilisation of the Spine: A Primary Handbook of Clinical Methods, 5th ed. Edinburgh, Churchill Livingstone, 1991:305–318
266. Grieve GP: Active movements. In: Grieve GP, ed: Mobilisation of the Spine: A Primary Handbook of Clinical Methods, 5th ed. Edinburgh, Churchill Livingstone, 1991:319–358
267. Grimsby O: Advanced Course: Lumbar—Thoracic Spine. Continuing Education Course, Institute of Graduate Health Sciences, Nashville, 1976
268. Grimsby O: Advanced Extremity Mobilizations. Continuing Education Course, Sorlandet Institute, Portland, OR, 1979
269. Grimsby O: Fundamentals of Manual Therapy: A Course Workbook, 3rd ed. Norway, Sorlandet Fusikalske Institutt, 1981
270. Gunn CC, Milbrandt WE: Tenderness at motor points: A diagnostic and prognostic aid for low back injury. J Bone Joint Surg Am 58:815–825, 1976
271. Gunn CC, Milbrandt WE: Early and subtle signs in low back sprain. Spine 3:267–281, 1978
272. Gunnari H, Evjenth O, Brady MM: Sequence Exercise. Oslo, Breyers Forlag, 1983
273. Gustavsen R: Fra aktiv avspenning. Oslo, Olaf Norlis Bokhandel, 1977
274. Gustavsen R, Streeck R: Training Therapy: Prophylaxis and Rehabilitation, 2nd ed. Stuttgart, Georg Thieme Verlag, 1993
275. Guymer AJ: Proprioceptive neuromuscular facilitation for vertebral joint conditions. In: Grieve GP, ed: Modern Manual Therapy of the Vertebral Column. New York, Churchill Livingstone, 1986:622–634
276. Hackett GS: Referred pain from low back ligament disabilities. AMA Arch Surg 73:878–883, 1956
277. Hackett GS, Hemwall GA, Montgomery GA: Ligament and Tendon Relaxation Treated by Prolotherapy, 5th ed. Oak Par, IL, Gustav A. Hemwall, 1991
278. Hackett GS, Henderson DG: Joint stabilization: An experimental, histological study with comments on the clinical application in ligament proliferation. Am J Surg 89:968–973, 1955
279. Hadler NM: Legal ramifications of the medical definition of back disease. Ann Intern Med 89:992–999, 1978
280. Hadler NM: A critical reappraisal of the fibrositis concept. Am J Med 81A:26–30, 1986
281. Hadler NM: Regional back pain. N Engl J Med 315:1090–1092, 1986
282. Hadler NM: A benefit of spinal manipulations as adjunctive therapy for acute low back pain: A stratified controlled trail. Spine 12:703–706, 1987
283. Haldeman S: Spinal manipulative therapy as a status report. Clin Orthop 179:62–70, 1983
284. Haldeman S: Soft-Tissue Techniques. Challenge of the Lumbar Spine, Ninth Annual Meeting, New York, 1987
285. Hall C: Therapeutic exercise for lumbopelvic region. In: Hall CM, Brody LT, eds: Therapeutic Exercise, Moving Towards Function. Philadelphia, Lippincott Williams & Wilkins, 1999:303–352
286. Hall H, Iceton JA: Back school: An overview with specific reference to the Canadian Back Education Units. Clin Orthop 179:10–17, 1983
287. Haller C: Alternative movement related therapies. In: Hall C, Brody LT, eds: Therapeutic Exerrcise, Moving Towards Function. Philadelphia, Lippincott Williams & Wilkins, 1999:274–285
288. Hansson P, Ekblom A: Acute pain relieved by vibratory stimulation [letter]. Br Dent J 151:213, 1981
289. Hansson P, Ekblom A: Transcutaneous electrical nerve stimulation (TENS) as compared to placebo: TENS for the relief of acute orofacial pain. Pain 15:157–165, 1983
290. Happey T, Pearson CH, Palframan J, et al: Proteoglycans and glycoproteins associated with collagen in the human intervertebral disc. Z Klin Chem 9:79, 1971
291. Harcke HT, Grissom LE, Finkelstein MS: Evaluation of the musculoskeletal system with sonography. AJR 150:1253–1261, 1988
292. Hardin JA: Medical exercise training. In: Bandy WD, Sanders B, eds: Therapeutic Exercise: Techniques for Intervention. Philadelphia, Lippincott Williams and Wilkins, 2001:121–144
293. Harris RI, MacNab I: Structural changes in the lumbar intervertebral disc: Their relationship to low back pain and sciatica. J Bone Joint Surg 36B:304–322, 1954
294. Hasue M, Fujiwara M, Kikuchi S: A new method of quantitative measurement of abdominal and back muscle strength. Spine 5(2):143–148, 1980
295. Hathaway SR, McKinley JC: A multiphasic personality schedule (Minnesota): I. Construction of the schedule. J Psychol 10:249, 1940
296. Hayne CR: Ergonomics and back pain. Physiotherapy 70:9–13, 1984
297. Hayne CR: Back schools and total care programs. Physiotherapy 70:14–17, 1984
298. Hayne CR: Prophylaxis and ergonomic considerations. In: Grieve GP, ed: Modern Manual Therapy of the Vertebral Column. New York, Churchill Livingstone, 1986:860–872
299. Hazard RG, Reid S, Fenwick J, et al: Isokinetic trunk and lifting strength measurements: Variability as an indicator of effort. Spine 13:54–57, 1988
300. Helfet AJ, Gruebel Lee DM: Disorders of the Lumbar Spine. Philadelphia, JB Lippincott, 1978
301. Henderson I: Low back pain and sciatica: Evaluation and surgical management. Aust Fam Phys 14:1149–1159, 1985
302. Hendler N: Psychological tests for chronic pain. In: Hendler N, ed: Diagnosis and Nonsurgical Management of Chronic Pain. New York, Raven Press, 1981:101–120
303. Hendrickson T: Massage for Orthopedic Conditions. Philadelphia, Lippincott Williams & Wilkins, 2003
304. Hendry NGS: The hydration of the nucleus pulposus and its relation to intervertebral disc derangement. J Bone Joint Surg Br 40:132–144, 1958
305. Hides JA, Cooper DH, Stokes MJ: Diagnostic ultrasound imaging for measurement of the lumbar multifidus muscle in normal young adults. Physiother Theory Pract 8:19–26, 1992
306. Hides JA, Jull GA, Richardson CA: Long-term effect of specific stabilizing exercises for first-episode low back pain. Spine 26:243–248, 2001

307. Hides JA, Richardson CA, Jull GA: Magnetic resonance imaging and ultrasonography of the lumbar multifuds muscle: Comparison of two different modalities. Spine 20:54–58, 1995

308. Hides JA, Richardson CA, Jull GA, et al: Ultrasound imaging in rehabilitation. Physiotherapy 41:187–193, 1995

309. Hides JA, Richarson CA, Jull G: Multifidus recovery is not automatic following resolution of acute first episode of low back pain. Spine 21:2763–2769, 1996

310. Hides JA, Richarson CA, Jull GA: Use of real-time ultrasound imaging for feedback in rehabilitation. Manual Therapy 3:125–131, 1998

311. Hides JA, Stokes MJ, Saide M, et al: Evidence of lumbar multifidus muscle-wasting ipsilateral to symptoms in patients with acute/subacute low back pain. Spine 19:165–172, 1993

312. Hirsch C: Studies on the mechanism of low back pain. Acta Orthop Scand 20:261–273, 1951

313. Hirsch C: The reaction of the intervertebral discs to compressive forces. J Bone Joint Surg Am 37:1188–1196, 1955

314. Hirsch C, Ingelmark BE, Miller M: The anatomical basis for low back pain: Studies on the presence of sensory nerve endings in ligamentous, capsular and intervertebral disc structures in the human lumbar spine. Acta Orthop Scand 33:1–17, 1963

315. Hirsch C, Jonsson B, Lewin T: Low-back symptoms in a Swedish female population. Clin Orthop 63:171–176, 1969

316. Hirsch C, Nachemson A: The reliability of lumbar disc surgery. Clin Orthop 29:189–195, 1963

317. Hirschberg GG: Treating lumbar disc lesions by prolonged continuous reduction of intradiscal pressure. Tex Med 70:58–68, 1974

318. Hirschberg GG, Froetscher L, Naem F: Iliolumbar syndrome as a common cause of low back pain: Diagnosis and prognosis. Arch Phys Med Rehabil 60:415–419, 1979

319. Hislop HJ, Montgomery J: Daniels and Worthingham's Muscle Testing Techniques, 6th ed. Philadelphia, WB Saunders, 1995

320. Hitselberger WE, Witten RM: Abnormal myelograms in asymptomatic patients. J Neurosurg 28:204–206, 1968

321. Hodges PW: Core stability exercise in chronic low back pain. Orthop Clin N Am 34:245–254, 2003

322. Hodges PW, Richardson C: Inefficient muscular stabilization of the lumbar spine associated with low back pain: A motor control evaluation of transversus abdominis. Spine 21:2640–2650, 1996

323. Hodges PW, Richardson CA, Jull G: Evaluation of the relationship between laboratory and clinical tests of transverse abdominus function. Physiother Res Int 1:30–40, 1996

324. Hoehler FK, Tobin JS, Buerger AA: Spinal manipulations for low back pain. JAMA 245:1835–1838, 1981

325. Holten O: Medisinsk Trenigsterapi Trykk. Fugseth and Lorentzen, Medical Training Course, Salt Lake City, 1984

326. Hong YL, Li JX, Robinson PD: Balance control, flexibility, and cardiorespiratory fitness among older Tai Chi practitioners. Sports Sci Med 34:29–34, 2000

327. Hood LB, Chrisman D: Intermittent pelvic traction in the treatment of the ruptured disc. Phys Ther 48:21–30, 1968

328. Hoppenfeld S: Physical Examination of the Spine and Extremities. New York, Appleton-Century-Crofts, 1976

329. Horal J: The clinical appearance of low back pain disorders in the city of Goteborg, Sweden: Comparison of incapacitated probands and matched controls. Acta Orthop Scand (suppl 118):1–109, 1969

330. Hudgins WR: The crossed straight leg-raising test. N Engl J Med 297:1127, 1977

331. Hult L: The Munfors investigation: A study of the frequency and causes of the stiff-neck brachalgia and lumbago-sciatica syndromes as well as observation on certain signs and symptoms from the dorsal spine and the joints of the extremities in industrial and forest workers. Acta Orthop Scand (suppl 16):1–76, 1954

332. Hult L: Cervical, dorsal and lumbar spinal syndromes: A field investigation of a nonselected material of 1200 workers in different occupations with special reference to disc degeneration and so-called muscular rheumatism. Acta Orthop Scand (suppl 17):1–102, 1954

333. Husted C, Pham L, Hekking A, Niederman R: Improving quality of life for people with chronic conditions: The example of T'ai Chi and multiple sclerosis. Alten Therap 5:70–74, 1999

334. Hyman J, Liebenson C: Spinal stabilization exercise program. In: Liebenson C, ed: Rehabilitation of the Spine: A Practitioner's Manual. Philadelphia, Lippincott Williams & Wilkins, 1996:293–328

335. Ikata T: Statistical and dynamic studies of lesions due to overloading spine. Shikoku Acta Med 40:262–286, 1965

336. Ingham JG: A method of observing symptoms and attitudes. Br J Soc Clin Psychol 4:131–140, 1965

337. Ingham JG: Quantitative evaluation of subjective symptoms. Proc R Soc Med 62:492–494, 1969

338. Irion JM: Aquatic therapy. In: Brandy WD, Sanders B, eds: Therapeutic Exercise: Technique for Intervention. Philadelphia, Lippincott Williams & Wilkins, 2001:295–331

339. Iskrant AP, Smith RW: Osteoporosis in women 45 years and over related to subsequent fracture. Public Health Rep 84:33–38, 1969

340. Ives JC, Sosnoff J: Beyond the mind-body exercise hype. Phys Sportsmed 28:67–81, 2000

341. Jackson CP, Brown MD: Is there a role for exercise in the treatment of patients with low back pain? Clin Orthop 179:39–45, 1983

342. Jackson HC, Winkelmann RK, Bichel WH: Nerve endings in ligamentous, capsular and intervertebral disc structures in the human lumbar spine. J Bone Joint Surg Am 48:1272–1281, 1966

343. Jackson RH: Chronic sacroiliac sprain with attendant sciatica. Am J Surg 24:456–477, 1934

344. Jacobson BH, Chen HC, Cashel C, et al: The effect of tai chi chuan training on balance, kinesthetic sense, and strength. Percept Motor Skills 84:27–33, 1997

345. Janda V: Muscles, central nervous motor regulation and back problems. In: Korr I, ed: The Neurobiologic Mechanisms in Manipulative Therapy. London, Plenum Press, 1978:27–42

346. Janda V: Muscle Function Testing. Boston, Butterworths, 1983

347. Janda V: Muscle weakness and inhibition (pseudoparesis) in back pain syndromes. In: Grieve GP, ed: Modern Manual Therapy of the Vertebral Column. New York, Churchill Livingstone, 1986:197–201

348. Janda V: Evaluation of muscular imbalance. In: Liebenson C, ed: Rehabilitation of the Spine: A Practitioner's Manual. Philadelphia, Lippincott Williams & Wilkins, 1996:97–112

349. Janda V, Va Vrova M: Sensory motor stimulation. In: Liebenson C, ed: Rehabilitation of the Spine: A Practitioner's Manual. Philadelphia, Lippincott Williams & Wilkins, 1996:319–328

350. Janda V, Schmid HJA: Muscles as a pathogenic factor in back pain. Proceedings of the 4th Conference of International Federation of Orthopaedic Manipulative Therapists, Christchurch, New Zealand, 1980

351. Janisse M: Therapeutic use of yoga. Orthop Phys Ther Practice 12:15–20, 2002

352. Jayson MIV, Sim-Williams H, Young S, et al: Mobilization and manipulations for low back pain. Spine 6:409–416, 1981

353. Jemmett R: Spinal Stabilization: The New Science of Back Pain. Minneapolis, OPTP, 2001

354. Jesse J: Hidden Causes of Injury, Prevention, and Correction for Running Athletes. Pasadena, Athletic Press, 1997

355. Johansson F, Almay BG, von Knorring L, et al: Predictors for the outcome of treatment with high-frequency transcutaneous electrical nerve stimulation in patients with chronic pain. Pain 9:55–61, 1980

356. Johnson GS: Soft tissue mobilization. In: Donatelli RA, Wooden MJ, eds: Orthopaedic Physical Therapy, 3rd ed. New York, Churchill Livingstone, 2001:578–617

357. Jones MD: Basic Diagnostic Radiology. St. Louis, CV Mosby, 1969

358. Jorgensen K: Back muscle strength and body weight as limiting factors for work in the standing slightly stooped position. Scand J Rehabil Med 2:149–153, 1970

359. Judovich B, Nobel GP: Lumbar traction therapy: A study of resistive forces. Am J Surg 93:108–114, 1957

360. Jull GA: Examination of the lumbar spine. In: Grieve GP, ed: Modern Manual Therapy of the Vertebral Column. New York, Churchill Livingstone, 1986:547–560

361. Jull GA, Janda V: Muscles and motor control in low back pain: Assessment and management. In: Twomey LT, Taylor JR, eds: Physical Therapy of the Low Back. New York, Churchill Livingstone, 1987:253–278

362. Jull GA, Richardson CA: Rehabilitation of the active stabilization of the lumbar spine. In: Twoney LT, Taylor JR, eds: Physical Therapy of the Low Back, 2nd ed. Churchill Livingstone, New York, 1994:251–283

363. Jull G, Richardson CA, Hamilton C, et al: Towards the validation of a clinical test for the deep abdominal muscles in back pain patients. Sydney, Manipulative Physiotherapists Association of Australia, 1995

364. Jungham H: Spondylolisthesen ohne Spalt im Zwischengelenkstuck (pseudospondylolisthesen). Arch Orthop Unfall-chir, 29:118–123, 1930

365. Jungham H: Die wirbelsaule in der Arbeitmedizin. Wirbel saule Forch Praxis 79:1–395 Teil II, 1979

366. Kahanovitz N, Nordin M, Verderame R, et al: Normal trunk muscle strength and endurance in women and the effect of exercises and electrical stimulation: Part 2. Comparative analysis of electrical stimulation and exercise to increase trunk muscle strength and endurance. Spine 12(2):112–118, 1987

367. Kaigle A, Holm S, Hansson T: Experimental instability in the lumbar spine. Spine 20:421–430, 1995

368. Kaltenborn FM: Manual Therapy for the Extremity Joints. Oslo, Olaf Norlis Bokhandel, 1976

369. Kaltenborn FM: Manual Mobilizations of the Extremity Joints, vol. II. Advanced Treatment Techniques. Oslo, Olaf Norlis Bokhandel, 1986

370. Kaltenborn FM: The Spine: Basic Evaluation and Mobilization Techniques, 2nd ed. Oslo, Olaf Norlis Bokhandel, 1993

371. Kalyan-Raman UP, Kalyan-Raman K, Yunus MB, et al: Muscle pathology in primary fibromyalgia syndrome: Light microscopic, histochemical and ultrastructural study. J Rheumatol 11:808–813, 1984

372. Kane RL, Craig L, Olsen D, et al: Manipulating the patient: A comparison of the effectiveness of physician and chiropractor care. Lancet 1:1333–1336, 1974

373. Kaplan PA, Matamoros A, Anderson JC: Sonograpy of the musculoskeletal system. AJR 155:237–245, 1990

374. Kaul M, Herring SA: Rehabilitation of lumbar spine injuries. In: Kibler WB, Herring SA, Press JM, eds: Functional Rehabilitation of Sports and Musculoskeletal Injuries. Gaithersburg, Aspen, 1998:188–215

375. Kavanagh T: Exercise: The modern panacea. Ir Med J 72:24–27, 1979

376. Keegan JJ: Alterations to the lumbar curve related to posture and seating. J Bone Joint Surg 35:589–603, 1953

377. Keely G: Posture, body mechanics, and spinal stabilization. In: Brandy WD, Sanders B, eds: Therapeutic Exercise: Techniques for Intervention. Philadelphia, Lippincott Williams & Wilkins, 2001:263–294

378. Keene JS, Drummond DS: Mechanical back pain in the athlete. Compr Ther 11:7–14, 1985

379. Kellgren JH: On the distribution of pain arising from deep somatic structures with charts of segmental pain areas. Clin Sci 4:35, 1939

380. Kelly LA: New advances in lumbar spine surgery. In Donatelli RA, Wooden MJ: Orthopaedic Physical Therapy, 3rd ed. New York, Churchill Livingstone, 2001:324–334

381. Kelsey JL: An epidemiological study of the relationship between occupations and acute herniated lumbar intervertebral discs. Int J Epidemiol 4:1997–204, 1975

382. Kelsey JL, Hardy RJ: Driving a motor vehicle as a risk factor for acute herniated lumbar intervertebral disc. Am J Epidemiol 102:63–67, 1975

383. Kelsey JL, White AA: Epidemiology and impact of low-back pain. Spine 5:133–142, 1980

384. Kendall FP, Mc Creary EK, Provance PG: Muscles: Testing and Function, 4th ed. Baltimore, Williams & Wilkins, 1993

385. Kendall PH, Jenkins JM: Exercises for backache: A double-blind controlled study. Physiotherapy 54:154–157, 1968

386. Kenna O, Murtagh A: The physical examination of the back. Aust Fam Physician 14:1244–1256, 1985

387. Kennedy B: An Australian programme for management of back problems. Physiotherapy 66:108–111, 1980

388. Kessler RM: Acute symptomatic disc prolapse: Clinical manifestations and therapeutic considerations. Phys Ther 59:978–987, 1979

389. Keyes DC, Compere EL: The normal and pathological physiology of the nucleus pulposus of the intervertebral disc. J Bone Joint Surg 14:897–938, 1932

390. Keyserling WM, Herrin GD, Chaffin DB: Isometric strength testing as a means of controlling medical incidents on strenuous jobs. J Occup Med 22:332–336, 1980

391. Kirkaldy-Willis WH: The three phases of the spectrum of degenerative disease. In: Kirkaldy-Willis WH, ed: Managing Low Back Pain. New York, Churchill Livingstone, 1983:75–90

392. Kirkaldy-Willis WH: Manipulation. In: Kirkaldy-Willis WH, ed: Managing Low Back Pain. New York, Churchill Livingstone, 1983:175–183

393. Kirkaldy-Willis WH: The relationship of structural pathology to the nerve root. Spine 9:49–52, 1984

394. Kirkaldy-Willis WH, ed: Managing Low Back Pain, 4th ed. New York, Churchill Livingstone, 1999

395. Kirkalady-Willis WH, Farfan HF: Instability of the lumbar spine. Clin Orthop 165:110–123, 1982

396. Kirkaldy-Willis WH, Wedge JH, Yong-Hing K, et al: Lumbar spinal nerve entrapment. Clin Orthop 169:171–178, 1982

397. Kishino ND, Mayer TG, Gatchel J, et al: Qualification of lumbar function IV: Isometric and isotonic lifting simulation in normal subjects and low-back dysfunction patients. Spine 10:921–927, 1985

398. Klaber Moffett JA, Chase SM, Portek I, et al: A controlled prospective study to evaluate the effectiveness of a back school in low back pain. Spine 11:120–122, 1986

399. Klein RG, Dorman TA, Johnson CE: Proliferant injections for low back pain: histological changes of injected ligaments and objective measurements of lumbar spine mobility before and after treatment. J Neurolog Orthop Med Surg 10:123–126, 1989

400. Klein RG, Eek BC, Delong WB, et al: A randomized double-blind trail of dextrose-glycerine-phenol injections for chronic, low back pain. J Spinal Disord 6:23–33, 1993

401. Knott M, Voss DE: Proprioceptive Neuromuscular Facilitation, 2nd ed. New York, Harper & Row, 1968

402. Kolster B, Frank A: Look after Your Back. Cologne, Konemann Verlagsgesellschaft, 1998

403. Kopala B, Matassarin-Jacobs E: Sensory-perceptual pain assessment. In: Bellack J, Banford PA, eds: Nursing Assessment: A Multidimensional Approach. Belmont, CA, Wadsworth, 1984

404. Korr IM: The emerging concept of the osteopathic lesion. J Am Osteopath Assoc 48:127–138, 1948

405. Korr IM: Proprioceptive and somatic dysfunction. J Am Osteopath Assoc 74:123–135, 1975

406. Korr IM: Sustained sympatheticotonia as a factor in disease. In: Korr I, ed. The Neurobiological Mechanism in Manipulative Therapy. New York, Plenum Press, 1978

407. Kos J, Wolf J: Intervertebral menisci and their possible role in intervertebral blockage. Bull Orthop Sect Am Phys Ther Assoc 1:8, 1976

408. Kraft GL, Johnson EW, LaBan MM: Fibrositis syndrome. Arch Phys Med Rehabil 49:155–162, 1968

409. Kraft GL, Levinthal DH: Facet synovial impingement. Surg Gynecol Obstet 93:439–443, 1951

410. Kraftsow G: Yoga for Wellness. New York, Penguin, 1999

411. Kramer J: Intervertebral Disc Disease. Chicago, Year Book, 1987

412. Kroemer KHE, Robinette JC: Ergonomics in the design of office furniture. Industr Med Surg 38:115–125, 1969

413. Kvien TK, Nilsen H, Vik P: Education and self-care of patients with low back pain. Scand J Rheumatol 10:318–320, 1981

414. La Freniere JG: The Low-Back Patient: Procedures for Treatment by Physical Therapy. New York, Masson, 1979

415. La Freniere JG: La Freniere Body Techniques. Chicago, Year Book, 1984

416. Lageard P, Robinson M: Back pain: Current concepts and recent advances. Physiotherapy 72:105, 1986

417. Laine HR, Peltokallo P: Ultrasonography possibilities and findings in most common sports injuries. Annales Cirugiae et Gynaecologiae 80: 127–133, 1991

418. Lake B: Treatment by the application of Feldenkrais principles. Aust Fam Phys 11:1175–1178, 1985

419. Lamb DW: A review of manual therapy for spinal pain with reference to the lumbar spine. In: Grieve GP, ed: Modern Manual Therapy of the Vertebral Column. New York, Churchill Livingstone, 1986:605–621

420. Lan C, Chen SY, Lai JS, et al: Cardiorespiratory function, flexibility, and body-composition among geriatric tai chi chuan practitioners, Arch Phys Med Rehabil 77:612–616, 1996

421. Lancourt JE: Traction technique for low back pain. J Musculoskel Med 3:44–50, 1986

422. Langrana N, Lee C, Alexander H, et al: Quantitative assessment of back strength using isokinetic testing. Spine 9:287–290, 1984

423. Lankhorst GL, Vanderstadt RJ, Vogelaar JW, et al: The effect of the Swedish back school in chronic idiopathic low back pain. Scand J Rehabil Med 15:141–145, 1983

424. Laslett M: The role of physical therapy in soft tissue rheumatism. Patient Man 15:57–68, 1986

425. Laslett M: Use of manipulative therapy for mechanical pain of spinal origin. Orthop Rev 16:65–73, 1987

426. Lawrence JS: Rheumatism in coal miners: Part III. Occupational factors. Br J Industr Med 12:249–261, 1955

427. Lee CL: Work hardening: Return to work and work hardening [abstract]. Challenge of the Lumbar Spine: 9th Annual Meeting, New York, 1987

428. Lee DG: The Pelvic Girdle: An Approach to the Examination of the Lumbo-Pelvic-Hip Region, 2nd ed. Edinburgh, Churchill Livingstone, 1999

429. Lee D: A Workbook of Manual Therapy Techniques for the Verebral Column and Pelvic Girdle. Delta BC, Canada, Nascent Publishers, 1985

430. Lee SLK, Wesers B, McInnis S, et al: Analysing risk factors for preventive back education approaches: A review. Physiother Can 40:88–98, 1988

431. Lettin AWF: Diagnosis and treatment of lumbar instability. J Bone Joint Surg Br 49:520–529, 1967

432. Levernieux J: Traction Vertebrale. Paris, Expansion Scientifique, 1960

433. Lewin T: Osteoarthrosis in lumbar synovial joints. Gottesborg, Orstadius Bokryckeri Aktiebolag, 1964

434. Lewin T, Moffett B, Viidik A: The morphology of the lumbar synovial intervertebral joints. Acta Morph Neder Scand 4:299–319, 1962

435. Lewit K: Manipulative Therapy in Rehabilitation of the Locomotor System, 2nd ed. London, Butterworth, 1991

436. Leyshon A, Kirwan E, Wynn-Parry GB: Is it nerve root pain? J Bone Joint Surg Br 62:119, 1980

437. Lichter R: Work hardening: Simulated job training using work performances for worker rehabilitation and testing [abstract]. Challenge of the Lumbar Spine: 9th Annual Meeting, New York, 1987

438. Lichter RL, Hewson JK, Radke S, et al: Treatment of chronic low-back pain. Clin Orthop 190:115–123, 1984

439. Lindblom K: Technique and results in myelography and disc puncture. Acta Radiol 34:321–330, 1950

440. Lindblom K: Technique and result of diagnostic disc puncture and injection (discography) in the lumbar region. Acta Orthop Scand 20:316–326, 1951

441. Lindblom K: Intervertebral disc degeneration considered as a pressure atrophy. J Bone Joint Surg Am 39:933–945, 1957

442. Lindgren K, Sihovonen T, Leino E, et al: Exercise therapy effects on functional radiographic findings and segmental electromyographic activity in lumbar spine instability. Arch Phys Med Rehabil 74: 993–939, 1993

443. Linton SJ: The relationship between activity and chronic pain. Pain 21:289–294, 1985

444. Lippit AB: The facet joint and its role in spine pain management with facet joint injections. Spine 9:746–750, 1984

445. Lipson SJ, Muir H: Proteoglycans in experimental intervertebral disc degeneration. Spine 6:194–210, 1981

446. Liston CB: Back schools and ergonomics. In: Twomey LT, Taylor JR, eds: Physical Therapy of the Low Back. New York, Churchill Livingstone, 1987:279–303

447. Liyang D, Yinkan X, Wenming Z, et al: The effect of flexion–extension motion of the lumbar spine on the capacity of the spinal canal. Spine 14:523–525, 1989

448. Llewellyn RLJ, Jones AB: Fibrositis. London, Heinemann, 1915

449. Loebl WY: Measurement of spinal posture and range of spinal movement. Ann Phys Med 7:103–110, 1967

450. Long D, BenDebba M, Torgenson W: Persistent back pain and sciatica in the United States: Patient characteristics. J Spinal Disord 9:40–58, 1996

451. Lundeberg T: Vibratory stimulation for alleviation of chronic pain. Acta Physiol Scand [Suppl] 523:8–51, 1983

452. Lundeberg T: Long-term results of vibratory stimulation as a pain-relieving measure for chronic pain. Pain 20:13–23, 1984

453. Lundeberg T, Nordemar R, Ottoson D: Pain alleviation by vibratory stimulation. Pain 20:25–44, 1984

454. Luoto S, Heliovaara M, Hurri H, et al: Static back endurance and the risk of low back pain. Clin Biomech 10:323–324, 1995

455. Lux KDK, Ho HC, Leong JCY: The iliolumbar ligament. A study of its anatomy, development and clinical significance. J Bone Joint Surg Br 68:197–200, 1986

456. Lyon HE, Jones FE, Quinn FE, et al: Changes in the protein-polysaccharide fraction of the nucleus pulposus from human intervertebral disc with age and disc herniation. J Lab Clin Med 68:930, 1966

457. MacNab I: Chemonucleolysis. Clin Neurosurg 20:183–191, 1973

458. MacNab I: Backache, 2nd ed. Baltimore, Williams & Wilkins, 1990

459. MacRae IF, Wright V: Measurement of back movement. Ann Rheum Dis 28:584–589, 1969

460. Madelbaumn BR, Gross ML: Spondylolysis and spondylolisthesis. In: Reider B, ed: Sports Medicine in the School-age Athlete, 2nd ed. Philadelphia, Saunders, 1996:44–156

461. Magee DJ: Orthopedic Physical Assessment, 3rd ed. Philadelphia, WB Saunders, 1997

462. Magora A: Investigation of the relation between low back pain and occupation: Age, sex, community, education and other factors. Industr Med Surg 39:465–471, 1970

463. Magora A: Investigation of the relation between low back pain and occupation: 2. Work history. Industr Med Surg 39:504–510, 1970

464. Magora A: Investigation of the relation between low back pain and occupation: 3. Physical requirements: Sitting, standing and weight-lifting. Industr Med Surg 41:5–9, 1972

465. Magora A: Investigation of the relation between low back pain and occupation: 4. Physical requirements: Bending, rotation, reaching, and sudden maximal effort. Scand J Rehabil Med 5:186–190, 1973

466. Magora A: Investigation of the relation between low back pain and occupation: 7. Neurologic and orthopedic conditions. Scand Rehabil Med 7(4):146–151, 1975

467. Magora A, Schwartz A: Relation between the low back pain syndrome and X-ray findings: I. Degenerative osteoarthritis. Scand J Rehabil Med 8:115–125, 1976

468. Maigne R: Orthopaedic Medicine. Springfield, Charles C. Thomas, 1976

469. Maigne R: Manipulation of the spine. In: Rogoff JB, ed: Manipulations, Traction and Massage, 2nd ed. Baltimore, Williams & Wilkins, 1980:59–120

470. Maitland GD: Movement of pain-sensitive structures in the vertebral canal in a group of physiotherapy students. S Afr J Physiother 36:4–12, 1980

471. Maitland GD: Maitland's Vertebral Manipulation, 6th ed. Oxford, Buttersworth Heineman, 2001

472. Maitland GD: The Maitland concept: Assessment, examination and treatment by passive movements. In Twomey LT, Taylor JR (eds): Physical Therapy of the Low Back. New York, Churchill Livingstone, 1987:135–156

473. Mandal AC: The correct height of school furniture. Physiotherapy 70:48–53, 1984

474. Mannheimer JS, Lampe GN: Clinical Transcutaneous Electrical Nerve Stimulation. Philadelphia, FA Davis, 1984

475. Masi AT, Muhammad B, Yunus MD: Concepts of illness in populations as applied to fibromyalgia syndromes. Am J Med [Suppl 3A]81:19–25, 1986

476. Master R, Houston J: Listening to the Body: The Psychophysical Way to Health and Awareness. New York, Dell, 1982

477. Matheson L, Ogden L: Work Tolerance Screening. Trabues Canyon, CA, Rehabilitation Institute of Southern California, 1983

478. Mathews J: Dynamic discography: A study of lumbar traction. Ann Phys Med 9:275–279, 1968

479. Mathews J: The effects of spinal traction. Physiotherapy 58:64–66, 1972

480. Mathews JA, Hickling J: Lumbar traction: A double-blind controlled study for sciatica. Rheumatol Rehabil 14:222–225, 1975

481. Mathews JA, Mills SB, Jenkins VM, et al: Back pain and sciatica: Controlled trials of manipulation, traction, sclerosant and epidural injections. Br J Rheumatol 26:416–423, 1987

482. Matson DD, Woods RP, Campbell JB, et al: Diastematomyelia (congenital clefts of the spinal cord). Pediatrics 6:98–112, 1950

483. Mattmiller AW: The California back school. Physiotherapy 66:118–121, 1986

484. Maxwell TD: The piriformis muscle and its relation to the long-legged syndrome. J Can Chiro Assoc 51:10–24, 1978

485. May P: Exercise and training for spinal patients: Part A. Movement awareness and stabilization training. In: Basmajian JV, Nyberg R, eds: Rational Manual Therapies. Baltimore, Williams & Wilkins, 1993:347–359

486. Mayer DJ, Price DD: CNS mechanisms of analgesia. Pain 2:379–404, 1976

487. Mayer H, Mayer TG: Functional restoration: New concepts in spinal rehabilitation. In: Kirkaldy-Willis, ed: Managing Low Back Pain. New York, Churchill Livingstone, 1988

488. Mayer TG: Rehabilitation of the patient with spinal pain. Orthop Clin North Am 14:623–637, 1983

489. Mayer TG, Gatchel RJ: Functional Restoration for Spinal Disorders: The Sports Medicine Approach. Philadelphia, Lea & Febiger, 1988

490. Mayer TG, Gatchel RJ, Kishino N, et al: Objective assessment of spine function following industrial injury: A prospective study with comparison and 1-year follow-up. Spine 10:482–493, 1985

491. Mayer TG, Kishino N, Kedy J, et al: Using physical measurements to assess low back pain. J Muscoloskel Med 2:44–51, 1985

492. Mayer TG, Smith SS, Keeley J, Mooney V: Qualification of lumbar function: II. Sagittal plane trunk strength in chronic low-back pain patients. Spine 10:765–772, 1985

493. Mayer TG, Smith SS, Tencer A, et al: Measurement of Isometric and Multispeed Isokinetic Strength of Lumbar Spine Musculature Using a Prototype Cybex Testing Device on Normal Subjects and Patients with Chronic Low Back Pain. Proceedings of the International Society for Study of the Lumbar Spine, Montreal, 1983

494. Mayer TG, Tencer AF, Kristoferson S, et al: Use of noninvasive techniques for qualification of spinal range-of-motion in normal subjects and chronic low-back dysfunction patients. Spine 9:588–595, 1984

495. Mazess RB: On aging bone loss. Clin Orthop 165:237–252, 1983

496. McCain GA: Role of physical fitness training in the fibrositis/fibromyalgia syndrome. Am J Med [Suppl 3A]81:73–77, 1986

497. McCall IW, Park WM, O'Brien JP: Induced pain referral from posterior lumbar elements in normal subjects. Spine 4:441–448, 1979

498. McCarthy RE: Coping with low back pain through behavioral change. Orthop Nurs 3:30–35, 1983

499. McConnell J: Recalcitrant chronic low back and leg pain: A new theory and different approach to management. Man Ther 7:183–192, 2002

500. McDonnell MK, Sahrmann S: Movement-impairment syndromes of the thoracic and cervical spine. In: Grant R, eds: Physical Therapy of the Cervical and Thoracic Spine, 3rd ed. New York, Churchill Livingstone, 2002:335–354

501. McGill SM: Low back exercises: evidence for improving exercise regimens. Phys Ther 78:754–765, 1998

502. McGill SM: Mechanics and pathomechanics of muscles acting on the lumbar spine. In Oatis C: Kinesiology: The Mechanics and Pathomechanics of Human Movement. Philadelphia, Lippincott Williams & Wilkins, 2004:563–575

503. McGill SM: Low Back Disorders: Evidence-Based Prevention and Rehabilitation. Champaign, Human Kinetics, 2002

504. McGill SM, Childs A, Liebenson C: Endurance times for stabilization exercises: Clinical targets for testing and training from a normal database. Arch Phys Med Rehabil 80: 941–944, 1999

505. McGill SM, Juker D, Kropf P: Quantitative intramuscular myoelectric activity of the quadratus lumborum during a wide variety of tasks. Clin Biomech 11:170–172, 1996

506. McKenna O, Murtagh A: The physical examination of the back. Aust Fam Physician 14:1244–1256, 1985

507. McKenzie RA: Manual correction of sciatic scoliosis. NZ Med J 76(484):194–199, 1972

508. McKenzie RA: Prophylaxis in recurrent low back pain. NZ Med J 89:22–23, 1979

509. McKenzie RA: Treat Your Own Back. Waikanae, New Zealand, Spinal Publications Ltd, 1980

510. McKenzie RA: The Lumbar Spine: Mechanical Diagnosis and Therapy. Waikanae, New Zealand, Spinal Publications, 1981

511. McKenzie RA: Mechanical diagnosis and therapy for low back pain: Toward a better understanding. In: Twomey LT, Taylor JR, eds: Physical Therapy of the Low Back. New York, Churchill Livingstone, 1987:157–174

512. McKinley JC, Hathaway SR: The identification and measurement of the neuroses in medical practice. JAMA 23:161–167, 1943

513. McNeal RL: Aquatic therapy for patients with rheumatic disease. Rheum Dis Clin North Am 16:915–929, 1990

514. McNeill T, Warwick D, Andersson G, et al: Trunk strengths in attempted flexion, extension and lateral bending in healthy subjects and patients with low back disorders. Spine 5:529–538, 1980

515. McNergney E: Spine healthy. Adv Dir Rehabil 13:59–62, 2004

516. McQuarrie A: Physical therapy. In: Kirkaldy-Willis WH, ed: Managing Low Back Pain. New York, Churchill Livingstone, 1988:345–354

517. Meagher J, Boughton P: Sports Massage. New York, Doubleday, 1980

518. Meikle JCE: The Minnesota Multiphasic Personality Inventory (MMPI) and back pain. Clin Rehabil 1:143–145, 1987
519. Melzack R: The Puzzle of Pain. New York, Basic Books Inc, 1973
520. Melzack R: The McGill pain questionnaire: Major properties and scoring methods. Pain 1:277–299, 1975
521. Melzack R, Vetere P, Finch L: TENS for low back pain. Phys Ther 63:489–493, 1983
522. Melzack R, Wall PD: The Challenge of Pain. New York, Basic Books, 1983
523. Mennell JB: The Science and Art of Joint Manipulation, vol. 2. London, Churchill, 1952
524. Mennell JMCM: Back Pain. Boston, Little, Brown & Co, 1960
525. Mennell JMCM: Joint Pain. Boston, Little, Brown & Co, 1960
526. Micheli LJ: Back injuries in gymnastics. Clin Sports Med 4:85–94, 1985
527. Micheli LJ, Hall JE, Miller ME: Use of a modified Boston brace for back injuries in athletes. Am J Sports Med 4:85, 1980
528. Miller WT: Introduction to Clinical Radiology. New York, Macmillan, 1982
529. Mimura M, Panjabi M, Oxland T, et al: Disc degeneration affects the multi-directional flexibility of the lumbar spine. Spine 19:1371–1380, 1994
530. Mitchell FL: An Evaluation and Treatment Manual of Osteopathic Muscle Energy Procedures, 1st ed. Valley Park, MO, Mitchell Moran Pruzzo, 1979
531. Mitchell PEG, Hendry MGC, Billewicz WZ: The chemical background of inter-vertebral disc prolapse. J Bone Joint Surg Br 43:141–151, 1961
532. Mixter WJ, Barr JS: Rupture of the intervertebral disc with involvement of the spinal canal. N Engl J Med 211:210–215, 1934
533. Moll JMH, Liyanange SP, Wright V: An objective clinical method to measure lateral spine flexion. Rheum Phys Med 11:225–239, 1972
534. Moll JMH, Liyanange SP, Wright V: An objective clinical method to measure spinal extension. Rheum Phys Med 11:293–312, 1972
535. Moll JMH, Wright V: Measurement of spinal movement. In Jayson M (ed): The Lumbar Spine and Back Pain. New York, Grune & Stratton, 1981:93–112
536. Mooney V: Alternative approaches for the patient beyond the help of surgery. Orthop Clin 6:331–334, 1975
537. Mooney V: The syndromes of low back disease. Orthop Clin North Am 14:505–515, 1983
538. Mooney V: Evaluation and guidelines for nonoperative care of the low back. In Stauffer SE (ed): American Academy of Orthopaedic Surgeons—Instructional Course Lectures. St. Louis, CV Mosby, 1985
539. Mooney V, Cairns D, Robertson JA: A system for evaluating and treating chronic back disability. West J Med 124:370–376, 1976
540. Mooney V, Robertson J: The facet syndrome. Clin Orthop 115:149–156, 1976
541. Moore M: Endorphins and exercise: A puzzling relationship. Phys Sports Med 10:111–114, 1982
542. Moran FP, King T: Primary instability of the lumbar vertebrae as a common cause of low back pain. J Bone Joint Surg Br 39:6–22, 1957
543. Morgan D: Concepts in functional training and postural stabilization for low-back-injured. Topics in Acute Care and Trauma Rehabilitation: Part II. Clinical Applications. Aspen, Aspen Publishers, 1988
544. Morgan D, Vollowitz E: Training the Patient with Low Back Dysfunction. Folsom, Folsom Physical Therapy Education Division, 1988
545. Morris JM, Lucus DB, Besler B: The role of the trunk in the stability of the spine. J Bone Joint Surg Am 43:327–351, 1961
546. Morris JM, Markoff KL: Biomechanics of the lumbar spine. In American Academy of Orthopaedic Surgeons: Atlas of Orthotics. St. Louis, CV Mosby, 1975:312–331
547. Mottice M, Goldberg D, Bennr EK, et al: Soft-Tissue Mobilization. Monroe Falls, Ohio, JEMD Publications, 1986
548. Mulligan BR: Belt techniques. In: Grieve GP, ed: Modern Manual Therapy of the Vertebral Column. New York, Churchill Livingstone, 1986
549. Murphy JE: Sensorimotor training and cervical stabilization. In: Murphy JE, ed: Management of Cervical Spine Syndromes. New York, McGraw-Hill, 2000:607–640
550. Murtagh J, Findlay D, Kenna C: Low back pain. Aust Fam Physician 14:1214–1224, 1985
551. Murtagh JE, McKenna OJ: Muscle energy therapy. Aust Fam Physician 15:756–765, 1987
552. Muscolino JE, Ciprini S: Pilates and the "powerhouse"—I. Journal of Bodywork and Movement Therapies, 8: 15–24, 2004
553. Nachemson AL: The load on lumbar discs in different positions of the body. Clin Orthop 45:107–122, 1966
554. Nachemson AL: Towards a better understanding of low back pain: A review of the mechanics of the lumbar disc. Rheum Rehabil 14:129–143, 1975
555. Nachemson AL: The lumbar spine: An orthopedic challenge. Spine 1:59–71, 1976
556. Nachemson AL: Work for all: For those with low back pain as well. Clin Orthop 179:77–85, 1983
557. Nachemson AL: Lumbar instability: A critical update and symposium summary. Spine 10:290–291, 1985
558. Nachemson AL: Recent advances in the treatment of low back pain. Intern Orthop 9:1–10, 1985
559. Nachemson A, Bigos SJ: The low back. In: Cruess RL, Rennie WRJ, eds: Adult Orthopedics, Vol. 2. New York, Churchill Livingstone, 1984:843–938
560. Nachemson A, Lindh M: Measurement of abdominal and back muscle strength with and without low back pain. Scand J Rehabil Med 1:60–65, 1965
561. Nachemson A, Morris JM: In vivo measurement of intradiskal pressures. J Bone Joint Surg 46A:1077–1092, 1964
562. Nacim F, Froetscher L, Hirshberg GG: Treatment of the chronic iliolumbar syndrome by infiltration of the iliolumbar ligament. West J Med 136:372–374, 1982
563. Nagi SZ, Riley LE, Newby LG: A social epidemiology of back pain in a general population. J Chronic Dis 26:769–779, 1973
564. Nassim R, Burrows HJ, eds: Modern Trends in Diseases of Vertebral Column. London, Butterworths, 1959
565. Naylor A: The biophysical and biochemical aspects of intervertebral disc herniation and degeneration. Ann R Coll Surg 31:91–114, 1962
566. Naylor A: Intervertebral disc prolapse and degeneration. Spine 1:108–114, 1976
567. Naylor A, Happey F, MacRae T: The collagenous changes in the intervertebral disc with age and their effect on its elasticity. Br Med J 2:570–573, 1954
568. Nelson J: The Feldenkrais and Alexander techniques. In Liemohn W: Exercise Prescription and the Back. New York, McGraw-Hill, 2001:157–166
569. Nelson MA, Allen P, Clamp SE, et al: Reliability and reproducibility of clinical findings in low back pain. Spine 4:97–101, 1979
570. Newman PH: Sprung back. J Bone Joint Surg Br 34:30–37, 1952
571. Newman PH: The etiology of spondylolisthesis. J Bone Joint Surg Br 45:39–59, 1963
572. Newman PH: The spine, the wood and the trees. Proc R Soc Med 61:35–41, 1968
573. Newman PH: Surgical treatment for derangement of the lumbar spine. J Bone Joint Surg Br 55:7–19, 1973
574. Nickening T: Stabilizing the core. Adv Dir Rehabil 11:39–42, 2002
575. Nicolaisen T, Jorgensen K: Trunk strength, back muscle endurance and low-back trouble. Scand J Rehabil Med 17:121–127, 1985
576. Norby E: Epidemiology and diagnosis in low back injury. Occup Health Safety 50:38–42, 1981
577. Nordin M, Kahanovitz N, Verderame R, et al: Normal trunk muscle strength and endurance in women and the effect of exercise and electrical stimulation Part I: Normal endurance and trunk muscle strength in 101 women. Spine 12(2):105–111, 1987
578. Norris CM: Physical training and injury. In Norris CM (ed): Sports Injuries: Diagnosis and Management for Physiotherapists. Oxford, Butterworths-Heinemann, 1993:89–116
579. Norris CM: Spinal stabilization. Muscle imbalances and low back pain. Physiotherapy 3:127–138, 1995
580. Norris CM: Spinal stabilization. An exercise programe to enhance lumbar stabilization. Physiotherapy 3:138–146, 1995
581. Nosse LJ: Inverted spinal traction. Arch Phys Med Rehabil 59:367–370, 1978
582. Nummi J, Jarvinen T, Stambej U, et al: Diminished dynamic performance capacity of back and abdominal muscles in concrete-reinforcement workers. Scand J Work Environ Health 4 (Suppl 1):39–46, 1985
583. Nyberg R: Clinical assessment of the low back: Active movement and palpation testing. In: Basmajian JV, Nyberg R, eds: Rational Manual Therapies. Baltimore, Williams & Wilkins, 1993:97–140
584. O'Brian JP: The role of fusion for chronic low back pain. Orthop Clin North Am 14:639–647, 1983
585. O'Connell JEA: Protrusion of lumbar intervertebral discs: A clinical review based on 500 cases treated by excision of the protrusion. J Bone Joint Surg Br 33:8–30, 1951
586. Oliver JO, Lynn JW, Lynn JM: An interpretation of the McKenzie approach to low back pain. In: Twomey LT, Taylor JR, eds: Physical Therapy of the Low Back. New York, Churchill Livingstone, 1987:225–251
587. Ombergt L, Bisschop P, ter Veer HJ, et al: The ligamentous concept. In: Ombergt L, Bisschop P, ter Veer HJ, et al., eds: A System of Orthopaedic Medicine. London, WB Saunders, 1995:560–568
588. Ombergt L, Bisschop, P, ter Veer HJ, et al: Principles of treatment. In: Ombergt L, Bisschop P, ter Veer HJ, et al., eds: A System of Orthopaedic Medicine, London, WB Saunders, 1995:71–100
589. Ongley MJ, Klein RG, Dorman TA, et al: A new approach to the treatment of chronic low back pain. Lancet 2:143–146, 1987
590. Onishi N, Nomara H: Low back pain in relation to physical work capacity and local tenderness. J Human Ergo 2:119–132, 1973
591. Orwoll ES: The influence of exercise on osteoporosis and skeletal health. In: Goldberg L, Elliot DL, eds: Exercise for Prevention and Treatment of Illness. Philadelphia, FA Davis, 1994:228–244
592. O'Sullivan PB: Lumbar segmental "instability": Clinical presentation and specific stabilizing exercise management. Man Ther 5:2–12, 2000
593. O'Sullivan P, Twomey L, Allison G, et al: Altered patterns of abdominal muscle activation in patients with chronic back pain. Austral J Physiother 43:9198, 1997
594. O'Sullivan PB, Twoney L, Allison G: Evaluation of specific stabilizing exercises in the treatment of chronic low back pain with radiological diagnosis of spondylolisthesis. Spine 22:2959–2967, 1997

595. Ottenbacker K, Defabio RP: Efficacy of spinal manipulations/mobilization therapy: A meta-analysis. Spine 10:833–837, 1985

596. Ottoson D, Ekblom A, Hansson P: Vibratory stimulation for the relief of pain of dental origin. Pain 10:37–45, 1981

597. Oudenhoven RC: Gravitational lumbar traction. Arch Phys Med Rehabil 59:510–512, 1978

598. Pace JB, Nagle D: Piriformis syndrome. West J Med 124:435–439, 1976

599. Palastanga N: The use of transverse frictions of the soft tissue. In: Grieve GP, ed: Modern Manual Therapy of the Vertebral Column. New York, Churchill Livingstone, 1986:819–826

600. Palastanga N: Connective tissue massage. In: Grieve GP, ed: Modern Manual Therapy of the Vertebral Column. New York, Churchill Livingstone, 1986:827–833

601. Palmer ML, Epler ME: Fundamental of Musculoskeletal Assessment and Techniques, 2nd ed. Philadelphia, Lippincott Williams & Wilkins, 1998

602. Panjabi M: The stabilizing system of the spine. Part 1 and Part 2. J Spinal Disord 5:383–397, 1992

603. Panjabi M, Abumi K, Duranceau J, et al: Spinal stability and intersegmental muscle forces: A biomechanical model. Spine 14:194–199, 1989

604. Panjabi M, Lydon C, Vasavada A, et al: On the understanding of clinical instability. Spine 19:2642–2650, 1994

605. Paris SV: The theory and technique of specific spinal manipulations. NZ Med J 62:320–321, 1963

606. Paris SV: The Spinal Lesion. New Zealand, Pegasus Press, 1965

607. Paris SV: Mobilization of the spine. Phys Ther 59:988–995, 1979

608. Paris SV: Clinical decision: Orthopaedic physical therapy. In: Wolf SL, ed: Clinical Decision-Making in Physical Therapy. Philadelphia, FA Davis, 1985:215–254

609. Paris SV: Physical signs of instability. Spine 10:277–279, 1985

610. Paris SV: The lumbar spine. In Payton OD (ed): Manual of Physical Therapy. New York, Churchill Livingstone, 1989: 349–361

611. Park WM: Radiological investigation of the intervertebral disc. In: Jayson MIV, ed: The Lumbar Spine and Back Pain, 2nd ed. Kent, England, Pittman, 1980:185–230

612. Parker I: Beyond conventional exercise. Forum July 24:4–7, 1992

613. Parker I: Integrated Feldenkrais for Stabilization Approach to Exercise: The Connecting Link Between the Neurological and Musculoskeletal System. Continuing education course. Seattle, 1993

614. Parson W, Cummings J: Mechanical traction in the lumbar disc syndrome. Can Med Assoc J 77:7–11, 1957

615. Pederson OF, Peterson R, Staffeldt ES: Back pain and isometric back muscle strength of workers in a Danish factory. Scand J Rehabil Med 7(3):125–128, 1975

616. Peltier LF: The classic back strain and sciatica. Clin Orthop 219(6):4–6, 1987

617. Petty NJ, Moore AP: Neuromuscular Examination and Assessment: A Handbook for Therapists. Edinburgh, Churchill Livingstone, 1998

618. Pheasant HC: Sources of failure in laminectomies. Orthop Clin North Am 6:319–329, 1975

619. Piedalla P: Problemes sacroiliaques. Home Sain II. Bordeaux, Biere, 1952

620. Plotke RJ: The power of the center. Phys Ther Forum 9:1–5, 1994

621. Pope MH: Rosen JD, Wilder DG, et al: The relation between biomechanical and psychological factors in patients with low back pain. Spine 5:173–178, 1980

622. Porter RW, Hibbert C, Evans C: The natural history of the root entrapment syndrome. Spine 9:418–421, 1984

623. Porterfield JA: The sacro-iliac joint. In: Gould JA, Davies GJ, eds: Orthopaedic and Sports Physical Therapy. St. Louis, CV Mosby, 1985:550–580

624. Porterfield JA, DeRosa C: Mechanical Low Back Pain: Perspective in Functional Anatomy, 2nd ed. Philadelphia, WB Saunders, 1998

625. Porterfield JA, Mostardi RA, King S, et al: Simulated lift testing using computerized isokinetics. Spine 12:683–687, 1987

626. Posner I, White AA, Edwards WT, et al: A biomechanical analysis of the clinical stability of the lumbar and lumbosacral spine. Spine 7:374–389, 1982

627. Prahlow ND, Buschbacher RM, Conti AR: Back. In Buachbacher RM: Practical Guide to Musculoskeletal Disorders: Diagnosis and Rehabilitation, 2nd ed. Boston, Butterworth-Heinemann, 2002:87–112

628. Pritzker KPH: Aging and degeneration in the lumbar intervertebral discs. Orthop Clin North Am 8:65–75, 1977

629. Proulx WR: Comparison of efficacy of prolotherapy versus steroid injection in the treatment of low back pain. Presented at the annual meeting of the American Association of Orthopedic Medicine, Denver, CO, 1990

630. Pug MM, Laorden ML, Miralles FS, et al: Endorphin levels in cerebrospinal fluid of patients with postoperative and chronic pain. Anesthesiology 57:1–4, 1982

631. Quebec Task Force on Spinal Disorders: Report. Spine [Suppl] 12:S1–S54, 1987

632. Rademeyer I: Manual therapy for lumbar spinal stenosis: a comprehensive physical therapy approach. Phys Med Rehabil Clin North Am 14:103–110, 2003

633. Rae PS, Waddell B, Verner RM: A simple technique for measuring lumbar flexion. J R Coll Surg Edinb 29:281–284, 1984

634. Ramani PS, Perry RH, Tomlinson BE: Role of ligamentum flavum in the symptomatology of prolapsed lumbar intervertebral disc. J Neurol Neurosurg Psychiatry 38:550–557, 1975

635. Randall T, McMahon K: Screening for musculoskeletal system disease. In: Boissonnault WG, ed: Examination in Physical Therapy Practice. Screening for Medical Disease, 2nd ed. New York, Churchill Livingstone,1995:223–256

636. Ransford AO, Cairns D, Mooney V: The pain drawing as an aid to the psychologic evaluation of patients with low back pain. Spine 1:127–134, 1976

637. Rasmussen GG: Manipulation in the treatment of low back pain: A randomized clinical trial [abstract]. Man Med 1:8–21, 1979

638. Reid DC: Injuries and conditions of the neck and spine. In Reid DC (ed). Sports Injury Assessment and Rehabilitation. New York, Churchill Livingstone, 1992:784–837

639. Reuler JB: Low back pain. West J Med 143:259–265, 1985

640. Richarson C, Jull GA: Muscle control—pain control. What Exercise would you prescribe? Man Therapy.1:2- 10, 1995

641. Richardson C, Jull G, Hides J: A new clinical model of the muscle dysfunction linked to the disturbance of spinal stability: Implications for treatment of low back pain. In: Twomey LT, Taylor JR, eds: Physical Therapy of Low Back, 3rd ed. New York, Churchill Livingstone, 2000: 249–267

642. Richardson C, Jull G, Hodges P, Hides J: Therapeutic Exercise for Spinal Segmental Stabilization in Low Back Pain: Scientific Basis and Clinical Approach. Edinburgh, Churchill Livingstone, 1999

643. Richardson C, Toppenberg R, Jull G: An initial evaluation of eight abdominal exercises for their ability to provide stabilization for the lumbar spine. Aust J Physio 36:6–11, 1990

644. Ritchie JH, Faharni WH: Age changes in intervertebral discs. Can J Surg 13:65–71, 1970

645. Ritzy S, Lorren T, Simpson S, et al: Rehabilitation of degenerative disease of the spine. In: Hochschuler SH, Colter HB, Guyer RD, eds: Rehabilitation of the Spine: Science and Practice. St. Louis, CV Mosby, 1993:457–481

646. Robinson L, Fisher H, Knox J, et al: The Official Body Control Pilates Manual, 2nd ed. New York, Barnes and Nobles, 2001

647. Robinson R: The new back school prescription: Stabilization training: Part I. Occupational Medicine: State of the Art Review. Philadelphia, Hanley & Belfus, 1992:17–31

648. Rockoff SD, Sweet E, Bluestein J: The relative contribution of trabecular and cortical bone to the strength of human lumbar vertebrae. Calcif Tissue Res 3:163–175, 1969

649. Roofe PG: Innervation of annulus fibrosis and posterior longitudinal ligaments: Fourth and fifth lumbar level. Arch Neurol Psych 44:100–103, 1940

650. Rosomoff HL, Rosomoff RS: Nonsurgical aggressive treatment of lumbar spinal stenosis. Spine: State of the Art Review 1:383–400, 1987

651. Rothman RH: Indications for lumbar fusion. Clin Neurosurg 20:215–219, 1973

652. Rothman RH, Simeone FA: The Spine. Philadelphia, WB Saunders, 1982

653. Rovere GD: Low back pain in athletes. Phys Sports Med 15:105–117, 1987

654. Rowe ML: Low back pain in industry: A position paper. J Occup Med 11(4):161–169, 1969

655. Roy S Deluca C, Casavant D: Lumbar muscle fatigue and chronic low back pain. Spine 14:992–1001, 1989

656. Saal JA: Rehabilitation of sports-related lumbar spine injuries. In Saal JA (ed): Physical Medicine and Rehabilitation: State of the Art Reviews. Philadelphia, Hanley & Belfus, 1987:613–637

657. Saal JA: The new back school prescription: Stabilization training: Part II. Occupational Medicine: State of the Art Review. Philadelphia, Hanley & Belfus, 1992:33–42

658. Saal JA, Saal JS: Nonoperative treatment of herniated lumbar inteveterbral disk with radiculopathy: An outcome study. Spine 14: 431–437,1989

659. Sahrmann S: A program for correction of muscular imbalance and mechanical imbalance. Clin Manag 3:23–28, 1983

660. Sahrmann S: Posture and muscle imbalance: Faulty lumbo-pelvic alignment and associated musculoskeletal pain syndromes. Orthop Div Rev—Can Phys Ther 12:13–20, 1992

661. Sahrmann S: Diagnosis and Treatment of Movement Impairment Syndromes. St. Louis, Mosby, 2001

662. Salib R: Gravity lumbar reduction traction: The results for documented lumbar disc herniation. Presented at the meeting of the Society for the Study of the Lumbar Spine, Sydney, Australia, 1985

663. Saliba V, Johnson G: Lumbar protective mechanism. In: White AH, Anderson R, eds: Conservative Care of Low Back Pain. Baltimore, Williams & Wilkins, 1991:112–119

664. Salisbury PJ, Porter RW: Measurement of lumbar saggital mobility: A comparison of methods. Spine 12(2):190–193, 1987

665. Sallade J: Variation on Robin McKenzie's technique for correction of lateral shift. J Orthop Sports Phys Ther 8:417–420, 1987

666. Sanborn GE, Friberg TE, Allen R: Optic nerve dysfunction during gravity inversion: Visual field abnormalities. Arch Ophthalmol 105:774–776, 1987

667. Sapsford RR, Hodges PW: Contraction of the pelvic floor muscles during abdominal maneuvers. Arch Phys Med Rehabil 82:1081–1088, 2001

668. Saunders DH: Use of spinal traction in the treatment of neck and back conditions. Clin Orthop 179:31–37, 1983

669. Saunders DH: Educational back care programs. In: Saunders DH, ed: Evaluation, Treatment and Prevention of Musculoskeletal Disorders. Minneapolis, Viking Press, 1985:297–324

670. Saunders DH: Evaluation, Treatment and Prevention of Musculoskeletal Disorders. Minneapolis, Viking Press, 1985

671. Sawyer WM: The role of the physical therapist before and after lumbar spine surgery. Orthop Clin North Am 14:649–659, 1983

672. Scham SM, Taylor TKF: Tension signs in lumbar disc prolapse. Clin Orthop 75:195–204, 1971

673. Schamberger W: A comprehensive treatment approach. In: Schamberger W, ed: The Malalignment Syndrome: Implications for Medicine and Sports. Edinburgh, Churchill Livingstone, 2002:319–387

674. Schatz MP: Living with your lower back. Yoga J July/August:316–345, 1984

675. Schatz MP: Back Care Basics. Berkeley, Rodmell Press, 1992

676. Schatzker J, Pennal GF: Spinal stenosis: A cause of cauda equina compression. J Bone Joint Surg Br 50:606–608, 1968

677. Schillberg B, Nystrom B: Quality of life before and after microsurgical decompression in lumbar spinal stenosis. J Spinal Disord 13:237–241, 2000

678. Schmorl G, Jungham H: The Human Spine in Health and Disease, 2nd ed. New York, Grune & Stratton, 1971

679. Schned ES: Ankylosing spondylitis. In: Beary JF, Christian CL, Johanson MA, eds: Manual of Rheumatology and Outpatient Orthopedic Disorders: Diagnosis and Therapy. Boston, Little, Brown & Co., 1987

680. Schuchmann JA: Low back pain: A comprehensive approach. Compr Ther 14:14–18, 1987

681. Schultz A, Andersson G, Ortengren R, et al: Loads on the lumbar spine: Validation and biomechanical analysis by measurements of intradiscal pressures and myoelectric signals. J Bone Joint Surg Br 64:713–720, 1982

682. Schunk C, Reed K, ed: Therapeutic Associates Rehabilitation Guidelines: Student Volume. Beverton, OR. Tai Publishing, 1995

683. Scott ME: Spinal osteoporosis in the aged. Aust Fam Phys 3:281, 1974

684. Scott V, Gijsbers K: Pain perception in competitive swimmers. Br Med J 283:91–93, 1981

685. Seimons LP: Low Back Pain: Clinical Diagnosis and Management. Norwalk, CT, Appleton-Century-Crofts, 1983

686. Selby DK, Paris SV: Anatomy of facet joints and its correlation with low back pain. Contemp Orthop 31:1097–1103, 1981

687. Shacklock M: Mobilization of the nervous system. Initial course notes, Part of a neuro-orthopedic approach. Seattle, WA, 1997

688. Shah JS: Structure, morphology and mechanics of the lumbar spine. In Jayson M (ed): The Lumbar Spine and Low Back Pain. London, Pittman Medical, 1980:359–406

689. Shealy CN: Facet denervation in the management of back and sciatic pain. Clin Orthop 115:159–164, 1976

690. Shealy CN, Shealy M: Behavioral techniques in control of pain: A case for health maintenance vs. disease treatment. In: Weisenberg M, Tursky B, eds: Pain: New Perspectives in Therapy and Research. New York, Plenum Press, 1976:21–34

691. Sheon RP: Regional myofascial pain and the fibrositis syndrome (fibromyalgia). Compr Ther 12(a):42–52, 1986

692. Shumway-Cook N, Woollacott M: Motor Control: Theory and Practical Applications, 2nd ed. Philadelphia, Lippincott Williams, & Wilkins, 2001.

693. Sihvonen T, Partanen J: Segmental hypermobility in lumbar spine and entrapment of dorsa rami. Electromyogr Clin Neurophysiol 3:175–180, 1990

694. Sikorski JM: A rationalized approach to physiotherapy for low-back pain. Spine 10:571–579, 1985

695. Simons DG: Muscle pain syndromes: Part I. Am J Phys Med 54:289–311, 1975

696. Simons DG: Muscle pain syndromes: Part II. Am J Phys Med 55:15–42, 1976

697. Simons DG, Travell JG: Myofascial origins of low back pain: 1. Principles of diagnosis and treatment. Postgrad Med 73:66–77, 1983

698. Simons DG, Travell JG: Myofascial origins of low back pain: 2. Torso muscles. Postgrad Med 73:81–92, 1983

699. Simons DG, Travell JG: Myofascial origins of low back pain: 3. Pelvic and lower extremity muscles. Postgrad Med 73:99–108, 1983

700. Simons DG, Travell JG: Myofascial pain syndromes. In Wall PD, Melzack R (eds): Textbook of Pain. New York, Churchill Livingstone, 1984:263–276

701. Sims FH, Dahlin DC: Primary bone tumors simulating lumbar disc syndrome. Spine 2:65–74, 1977

702. Sinaki M: Postmenopausal spinal osteoporosis: Physical therapy and rehabilitation principles. Mayo Clin Proc 57:699–703, 1982

703. Sinaki M: Beneficial musculoskeletal effects of physical activity in the older woman. Geriatr Med Today 8:53–72, 1989

704. Sinaki M: Osteoporosis. In: Delisa JA, Gans BM, Currie DM, et al., eds: Rehabilitation Medicine: Principles and Practice, 2nd ed. Philadelphia, JB Lippincott, 1993:1018–1035

705. Sinaki M, Mikkelsen BA: Postmenopausal spinal osteoporosis: Flexion versus extension exercises. Arch Phys Med Rehabil 65:593–703, 1984

706. Sinaki M, Ito E, Rogers JW et al: Correlation of back extensor strength with thoracic kyphosis and lumbar lordosis in estrogen-deficient women. Am J Phys Med Rehabil 75:370–374, 1996

707. Skinner AT, Thompson AM, eds: Duffield's Exercise in Water. London, Bailliere Tindall, 1983

708. Smidt G: Inversion traction: Effects on spinal column, heart rate and blood pressure [abstract]. Presented at the meeting of the International Society for the Study of the Lumbar Spine, Sydney, Australia, 1985

709. Smith AE: Physical activity: A tool in promoting mental health. J Psychiatr Nurs 11:24–25, 1979

710. Smith SS, TG Mayer, Gatchel RJ, et al: Qualification of lumbar function: I. Isometric and multispeed isokinetic trunk strength measures in saggittal and axial planes in normal subjects. Spine 10:757–764, 1985

711. Smyth MJ, Wright V: Sciatica and intervertebral disc: An experimental study. J Bone Joint Surg Am 40:1401–1418, 1958

712. Smythe HA: Nonarticular rheumatism and the fibrositis syndrome. In Hollander JL, McCarty DJ (eds): Arthritis and Allied Conditions, 8th ed. Philadelphia, Lea & Febiger, 1972:874–884

713. Smythe HA: Nonarticular rheumatism and psychogenic musculoskeletal syndromes. In: McCarty DJ, ed: Arthritis and Allied Conditions: Textbook of Rheumatology, 9th ed. Philadelphia, Lea & Febiger, 1979:1083–1094

714. Smythe HA: Referred pain and tender points. Am J Med (Suppl 3A) 81:90–98, 1986

715. Snoek W, Weber H, Jorgensen B: Double-blind evaluation of extradural methylprednisolone for herniated lumbar disc. Acta Orthop Scand 48:635–641, 1977

716. Snook SH: The design of manual handling tasks. Ergonomics 21:963–641, 1978

717. Snook SH: Low back pain in industry. In: White AA, Gordon SL, eds: American Academy of Orthopaedic Surgeons Symposium on Idiopathic Low Back Pain. St. Louis, CV Mosby, 1982:23–48

718. Sorensen KH: Scheuermann's Juvenile Kyphosis. Thesis. Copenhagen, Munksgaard, 1964

719. Spangfort EV: The lumbar disc herniation: A computer-aided analysis of 2504 operations. Acta Orthop Scand (Suppl 142):1–95, 1972

720. Spencer DL, Irwin GS, Millar JAA: Anatomy and significance of fixation of the lumbosacral nerve roots in sciatica. Spine 8:672–679, 1983

721. Spengler DM, Freeman CW: Patient selection for lumbar discectomy: An objective approach. Spine 4:129–134, 1979

722. Spengler DM, Freeman CW: Low Back Pain: Assessment and Management. New York, Grune & Stratton, 1982

723. Spitzer WO: Quebec task force on spinal disorders: Scientific approach to the assessment and management of activity-related spinal disorders. Spine 12:S1–S58, 1987

724. Staffel F: Zur Hygiene des Sitzens. Gesundheitspflege 3:403–421, 1983

725. Steiner C, Staubs C, Ganon M, et al: Piriformis syndrome: Pathogenesis, diagnosis, and treatment. J Am Osteopathic Assoc 87:318–323, 1987

726. Steinmetz ND: MRI of the Lumbar Spine: A Practical Approach to Image Interpretation. Thorofare, Slack, 1987

727. Sternbach RA: Pain Patients: Traits and Treatment. New York, Academic Press, 1974

728. Stewart ML: Measurement of clinical pain. In: Jacox AK, ed: Pain: A Source Book for Nurses and Other Health Professionals. Boston, Little, Brown & Co., 1977

729. Stinson JT: Spondylolysis and spondylolishtesis in the athlete. Clin Sports Med 12:517–528, 1993

730. Stoddard A: Conditions of the sacro-iliac joints and their treatment. Physiotherapy 44(4):97, 1958

731. Stoddard A: Manual of Osteopathic Technique. London, Hutchinson, 1959

732. Stoddard A: Cervical spondylosis and cervical osteoarthritis. Man Med 2:31, 1970

733. Stokes I, Frymoyer J: Segmental motion and instability. Spine 12:688–691, 1987

734. Stokes IAF, Frymoyer JM, Lunn RA: Segmental motion and segmental instability [abstr]. Orthop Trans 10:517–518, 1986

735. Stone MH: Implications of connective tissue and bone alterations resulting from resistance exercise training. Med Sci Sports Exerc 20(suppl):162–168, 1988

736. Strachan A: Back care in industry. Physiotherapy 65:249–251, 1949

737. Strange FG: Debunking the disc. Proc R Soc Med 9:952–956, 1966

738. Stubbs DA, Buckle PW, Hudson MP, et al: Back pain in the nursing profession: I. Epidemiology and pilot methodology. Ergonomics 26:755–765, 1983

739. Stubbs DA, Buckle PW, Hudson MP, et al: Back pain in the nursing profession: II. The effectiveness of training. Ergonomics 26:767–779, 1983

740. Sugiura K, Yoshida T, Mimatsu T: A study of tension signs in lumbar disc hernia. Int Orthop 3:225–228, 1979

741. Sullivan PE, Markos PD: Low back. Clinical Decision Making in Therapeutic Exercise. Norwalk, Appleton &Lange, 1994, 159–193

742. Sunderland S: The anatomy of the intervertebral foramen and mechanism of compression and stretch of nerve roots. In: Haldeman S, ed: Modern Developments in Principles and Practice of Chiropractic. New York, Appleton-Century-Crofts, 1980:297–299

743. Suzuki N, Endo S: A quantitative study of trunk muscle strength and fatigability in low-back syndrome. Spine 8:69–74, 1983

744. Svensson HL, Andersson GBJ: Low back pain in 40- to 47-year-old men: I. Frequency of occurrence and impact on medical services. Scand J Rehabil Med 14(2):47–53, 1982
745. Svensson HL, Andersson GBJ: Low back pain in 40- to 47-year-old men. Spine 8:272–276, 1983
746. Svensson HL, Vedin A, Wihelmsson C, et al: Low back pain in relation to other diseases and cardiovascular risk factors. Spine 8(3):277–285, 1983
747. Sylven B: On the biology of nucleus pulposus. Acta Orthop Scand 20:275–279, 1951
748. Tanigawa M: Comparison of the hold/relax procedure and passive mobilization in increasing muscle length. Phys Ther 52:725–735, 1972
749. Tappan FM: Healing Massage Techniques: Holistic, Classic and Emerging Methods. Norwalk, Appleton & Lange, 1988
750. Tasuma T, Makina E, Saito S, et al: Histological development of intervertebral disc herniation. J Bone Joint Surg 68A:1066–1072, 1986
751. Tauber J: An unorthodox look at backaches. J Occup Med 12:128–130, 1970
752. Taylor JR, O'Sullivan PB: Lumbar segmental instability: Pathology, diagnosis, and conservative management. In: Twomey LT, Taylor JR, eds: Physical Therapy of the Low Back, 3rd ed. New York, Churchill Livingstone, 2000:201–247
753. Taylor MJ: Putting movement system back in the patient: An example of holistic physical therapy. Orthop Phys Ther Pract 12:15–20, 2000
754. Taylor TKF, Weiner M: Great-toe extensor reflexes in the diagnosis of lumbar disc disorder. Br Med J 2:487, 1969
755. Terenius L: Endorphins and pain. Front Horm Res 8:162–171, 1981
756. Thery Y, Bonjean P, Calen S, et al: Anatomical and roentgenological basis for the study of lumbar spine with the body in suspended position. Anat Clin 7:161–169, 1985
757. Thompson NN, Gould JA, Davies GJ, et al: Descriptive measures of isokinetic trunk testing. J Orthop Sports Phys Ther 7:43–49,1985
758. Thorsteinsson A, Nilsson J: Trunk muscle strength during constant and velocity movements. Scand J Rehabil Med 14:61–68, 1982
759. Tichauer ER: The Biomedical Basis of Ergonomics: Anatomy Applied to the Design of the Work Station. New York, Wiley Inter-Sciences, 1978
760. Tillotson LM, Burton AK: Noninvasive measurement of lumbar saggital mobility, an assessment by Flexicurves technique. Spine 16:29–33, 1991
761. Torstensen TA, Ljunggren AE, Meen HD et al: Efficiency and costs of medical exercise therapy, conventional physiotherapy, and self-exercise in patients with low back pain. Spine 23:2616–2624, 1998
762. Traut FF: Fibrositis. J Am Geriatr Soc 16:531–538, 1968
763. Travel JG, Simons DG: Myofascial Pain and Dysfunction: The Trigger Point Manual: The Lower Extremities, vol. 2. Baltimore, William & Wilkins, 1992
764. Tribus CB: Degenerative lumbar scoliosis: evaluation and management. J Am Acad Othrop Surg 11: 174–183, 2003
765. Triggs M: Orthopedic aquatic therapy. Clinical Management 11:30–31, 1991
766. Trott PH, Grant R: Manipulative physical therapy in the management of selected low lumbar syndromes. In: Twomey LT, Taylor JR, eds: Physical Therapy of the Low Back. New York, Churchill Livingstone, 2000:167–234
767. Troup JDG: Causes, prediction and prevention of back pain at work. Scand J Work Environ Health 10:419–428, 1984
768. Troup JDG: Biomechanics of the lumbar spinal canal. Clinical Biomechanics 1:31–43, 1986
769. Troup JDG, Martin JW, Lloyd DCEF: Back pain in industry: A prospective survey. Spine 6:61–69, 1981
770. Troup JDG, Roantree WB, Archibald RM: Survey of cases of lumbar spinal disability: A methodological study. Medical Officers' Broadsheet, National Coal Board, 1970
771. Tursky B: The development of a pain perception profile: A psychophysical approach. In: Weisenberg M, Tursky B, eds: Pain: New Perspectives in Therapy and Research. New York, Plenum Press, 1976:171–194
772. Twomey LT: Sustained lumbar traction: An experimental study of long spine segments. Spine 10(2):167–169, 1985
773. Twomey LT, Taylor JR: A description of two new instruments measuring the ranges of sagittal and horizontal plane motions in the lumbar region. Aust J Physiother 31:106–112, 1985
774. Urban LM: The straight-leg raising test: A review. J Orthop Sports Phys Ther 2:117–133, 1981
775. Urban LM: The straight-leg raising test: A review. In: Grieve GP, ed: Modern Manual Therapy of the Vertebral Column. New York, Churchill Livingstone, 1986:567–575
776. Valkenberg HA, Haanen HCM: The epidemiology of low back pain. In: White AA, Gordon SL, ed: American Academy of Orthopaedic Surgeons, Symposium on Idiopathic Low Back Pain. St. Louis, CV Mosby, 1982:9–22
777. Van Akkerveeken PF, O'Brien JP, Park WM: Experimentally induced hypermobility in the lumbar spine. Spine 4:236–241, 1979
778. Van Dillen FR, Sharmann SA, Nortin BJ, et al: Effect of active limb movement on symptoms in patients with low back pain. J Othrop Sports Phys Ther 31:402–418, 2001
779. Van Dillen LR, Sahrmann SA, Nortin BJ et al: Movement system impairment-based categories for low back pain: Stage 1 Validation. J Orthop Sports Phys Ther 33:126–142, 2003
780. Vanharanta H, Videman T, Mooney V: McKenzie exercise, back traction and back school in lumbar syndrome [abstract]. Orthop Trans. 10:533, 1986
781. van Holsbeeck M, Introcaso JH: Musculoskeletal ultrasonography. Radiol Clin North Am 30:907–925, 1992
782. Van Wijmen PM: The management of recurrent low back pain. In: Grieve GP, ed: Modern Manual Therapy of the Vertebral Column. New York, Churchill Livingstone, 1986:756–776
783. Vleeming A, Pool-Goudzwaard AL, Stoechart R, et al: The posterior layer of the thoracolumbar fascia: its function in load transfer from spine to legs. Spine 20:753–758, 1995
784. Vollowitz E: Furniture prescription for the conservative management of low back pain. In Topics in Acute Care and Trauma Rehabilitation, Industrial Back Injury, Part II: Clinical Applications. Aspen, CO, Aspen Publications, 1988
785. Voss DE, Ionta MK, Myer BJ: Proprioceptive Neuromuscular Facilitation, 3rd ed. Philadelphia, Harper & Row, 1985
786. Waddell G: A new clinical model for treatment of low back pain. Spine 12:632–644, 1987
787. Waddell G, Main CJ, Morris EW, et al: Normality and reliability in the clinical assessment of backache. Br Med J 284:1519–1523, 1982
788. Waddell G, Main CJ, Morris EW, et al: Chronic low back pain, psychological distress and illness behavior. Spine 9:209–213, 1984
789. Waddell G, McCulloch JA, Kummel EG, et al: Nonorganic physical signs in low back pain. Spine 5:117–125, 1980
790. Waitz E: The lateral bending sign. Spine 6:388–397, 1981
791. Walker JM: Deep transverse frictions in ligament healing. J Orthop Sports Phys Ther 6:89–94, 1984
792. Walters A: Psychogenic regional pain alias hysterical pain. Brain 84:1–18, 1961
793. Watkins R, O'Brien J, Drauglis R, et al: Comparison of preoperative and postoperative MMPI data in chronic back patients. Spine 11:385–390, 1986
794. Weber H: Lumbar disc herniation: A controlled prospective study with 10 years of observation. Spine 8:131–140, 1983
795. Weber H, Ljunggren AI, Walker L: Traction therapy in patients with herniated lumbar intervertebral disc. J Oslo City Hosp 34:61–70, 1984
796. Wedge JH: The natural history of spinal degeneration. In Kirkaldy-Willis WH (ed): Managing Low Back Pain. New York, Churchill Livingstone, 1983:3–8
797. Weider DL: Jumping in with both feet: Water therapy in sports. Rehabil Management June/July:135, 1993
798. Weintraube A: Soft-tissue mobilization of the lumbar spine. In: Grieve GP, ed: Modern Manual Therapy of the Vertebral Column. New York, Churchill Livingstone, 1986:750–755
799. Wells PE: The examination of the pelvic joints. In: Grieve GP, ed: Modern Manual Therapy of the Vertebral Column. New York, Churchill Livingstone, 1986:590–602
800. White AA: Injection technique for the diagnosis and treatment of low back pain. Orthop Clin North Am 14:553–567, 1983
801. White AA, Gordon SL: Synopsis workshop on idiopathic low-back pain. Spine 7:141–149, 1982
802. White AA, McBride ME, Wiltse LL, et al: The management of patients with back pain and idiopathic vertebral sclerosis. Spine 11:607–616, 1986
803. White AA, Panjabi MM: Clinical Biomechanics of the Spine, 2nd ed. Philadelphia, JB Lippincott, 1990
804. White AH: Back Schools and Other Conservative Approaches to Low Back Pain. St. Louis, CV Mosby, 1983
805. White AH: Work hardening: General conditioning [abstr 91]. Challenge of the Lumbar Spine: 9th annual meeting, New York, 1987
806. White AH: Stabilization of the lumbar spine. In White AH, Anderson R (ed): Conservative Care of Low Back Pain. Baltimore, Williams & Wilkins, 1991:106–111
807. White SG, Sahrmann SA: A movement system balance approach to musculoskeletal pain. In Grant R (ed): Physical Therapy of the Cervical and Thoracic Spine, 2nd ed. Edinburgh, Churchill Livingstone, 1994: 339
808. Wiberg G: Back pain in relation to the nerve supply of the intervertebral disc. Acta Orthop Scand 19:211–221, 1949
809. Wiesel SW, Bernini P, Rothman RM, et al: Effectiveness of epidural steroids in the treatment of sciatica: A double-blind clinical trial. Presented at the meeting of the International Society for the Study of the Lumbar Spine, Toronto, 1982
810. Wilke H, Wolf S, Claes L, Arand M, Wiesend A: Stability increase of the lumbar spine with different muscle groups. Spine 20:192–198, 1995
811. Wilkinson M: A neurological perspective. Rheum Rehabil 14:162–163, 1975
812. Williams SJ: The back school. Physiotherapy 63:90, 1977
813. Wiltse LL, Newman PH, McNab I: Classification of spondylolysis and spondylolisthesis. Clin Orthop 117:23–24, 1976
814. Wiltse LL, Rocchio PD: Preoperative psychological tests as predictors of the success of chemonucleolysis in treatment of low back syndrome. J Bone Joint Surg Am 57:478–483, 1975
815. Wolfe F: The clinical syndrome of fibrositis. Am J Med (Suppl 3A)81:99–104, 1986
816. Wolfe F, Hawley DJ, Cathey MA, et al: Fibrositis: Symptom frequency and criteria for diagnosis: Evaluation of 291 rheumatic disease patients and 58 normal individuals. J Rheumatol 12:1159–1163, 1985

817. Woodhall B, Hayes GJ: The well leg-raising test of Fajersztajn in the diagnosis of ruptured intervertebral disc. J Bone Joint Surg Am 32:786–792, 1950
818. Wyke B: The neurological basis of thoracic spinal pain. Rheumatol Phys Med 10:356–367, 1970
819. Wyke B: Articular neurology and manipulative therapy. In: Idezak RM, ed: Aspects of Manipulative Therapy. Carlton, Victoria, Australia, Lincoln Institute of Health Sciences, 1980
820. Wyke B: The neurology of low back pain. In: Jayson MIV, ed: The Lumbar Spine and Back Pain, 2nd ed. London, Pittman Medical, 1980:265–340
821. Yao J: Acutherapy: Acupuncture, TENS and Acupressure. Libertyville, IL, Acutherapy Postgraduate, 1984
822. Yelland MJ, Glasziou PP, Bogduk N et al: Prolotherapy injections, saline injections, and exercises for chronic low-back pain: a randomized trial. Spine 29: 9–16, 2004
823. Young C, Riley LH, Lachacz JG: The lumbar spine, ilium, and sacrum. In Canavan PK: Rehabilitation in Sports Medicine. Stamford, Conn. Appleton & Lange, 1998
824. Young RJ: The effect of regular exercise on cognitive functioning and personality. Br J Sports Med 3:110–117, 1979
825. Young-Hing K, Reilly J, Kirkaldy-Willis WH: The ligamentum flavum. Spine 1:226–234, 1976
826. Yunus MB: Primary fibromyalgia syndrome: Current concepts. Compr Ther 10:21–28, 1984
827. Yunus MB, Kalgan-Raman UP, Kalyan-Raman K: Primary fibromyalgia syndrome and myofascial pain syndrome: Clinical features and muscle pathology. Arch Phys Med Rehabil 69:451–454, 1988
828. Yunus MB, Kalgan-Raman UP, Kalyan-Raman K, et al: Pathologic changes in muscle in primary fibromyalgia syndrome. Am J Med 81(suppl 3a):38–42, 1986
829. Yunus MB, Masi AT: Association of primary fibromyalgia syndrome with stress-related syndrome. Clin Res 33:923A, 1985
830. Yunus MB, Masi AT, Aldag JC: Criteria studies of primary fibromyalgia syndrome. Arthritis Rheum 30(Suppl):S50, 1987
831. Yunus MB, Masi AT, Calabro JJ, et al: Primary fibromyalgia (fibrositis)—Clinical study of 50 patients with matched normal controls. Semin Arthritis Rheum 11:151–171, 1981
832. Zachrisson-Fossell M, Forssell M: The back school. Spine 6:104–106, 1981
833. Zylbergold RS, Piper MC: Cervical spine disorders: A comparison of three types of traction. Spine 10:867–871, 1985

RECOMMEND READINGS

Hides J, Richardson C: Exercise and Pain. In: Strong J, Unruh AM, Wright A, et al., eds: Pain: A Textbook for Therapists. New York, Churchill Livingstone, 2002:245–266
Hubley-Kozey CL, McCulloch TA, McFarland DH: Chronic low back pain: A critical review of specific therapeutic exercise protocols on musculoskeletal and neuromuscular parameters. J Man Manip Ther 11:78–87, 2003
Maher C, Latimer J, Refshauge K: Prescription of activity for low back pain. What works? Aust J Physiol 45:121–132, 1999
McAuley JA: Exercise for patients with chronic low back pain. Orthop Phys Ther Practice 16:19–22, 2004
McGill S: Low Back Disorders: Evidence-Based Prevention and Rehabilitation. Champaign, Human Kinetics, 2002
McGill S: Analysis of the forces on the lumbar spine during activity. In: Oatis CA, ed: Kinesiology: The Mechanics & Pathomechanics of Human Movement. Philadelphia, Lippincott Williams & Wikins, 2004:576–593
Moseley GL: Joining forces—Combing cognition-targeted motor control training with group or individual pain physiology education: A successful treatment for chronic low back pain. J Man Manip Ther 1:8–94, 2003
O'Sullivan PB, Phyty GD, Twomey LT, et al: Evaluation of specific stabilizing exercise in the treatment of chronic low back pain with radiologic diagnosis of spondylolyisis or spondylolisthesis. Spine 22:2959–2967, 1997
Richardson CA, Jull GA, Hodges P, et al: Therapeutic Exercise for Spinal Stabilization in Low Back Pain. 2nd ed. New York, Churchill Livingstone, 2004

Sacroiliac Joint and Lumbar–Pelvic–Hip Complex

DARLENE HERTLING

The sacroiliac joint (SIJ) is probably the most controversial in the human body. In the early years of the 20th century, disorders of the SIJ were considered responsible for a large percentage of patients presenting with low back pain.[29] It was not until the 1930s, when the role of the nucleus pulposus became an established entity in low back pain, that the SIJ tended to be overlooked. There is a constant debate regarding the type and amount of movement and the location of the axes. Medical students are often taught that the SIJ is immobile and therefore cannot be a cause of low back pain. More recently attention has been paid to the SIJ and its involvement in low back pain.[11,13,29,43.45,51,57,58,63,80,145,156,161,232,233,270,296,313]

FUNCTIONAL ANATOMY

Arthrokinematics and Osteokinematics

When discussing the pelvic girdle, we must always consider the interrelatedness of the lumbar–pelvic–hip complex (Fig. 23-1). We can think of the lumbar–pelvic–hip complex as consisting of the fourth and fifth lumbar joints (four apophyseal joints), the sacrum (two synovial joints), the two hip joints, and the pubic symphysis (amphiarthrodial joint). This complex should always be considered as a mechanical unit; do not attempt to isolate it. Involvement of any one structure affects the positioning and movement of the others. The sacrum is mechanically associated with the spine, whereas the innominate is aligned with and affected by movement of the femur. Any frontal plane asymmetry, leg-length discrepancy, or loss of motion in one joint of the complex that might alter the forces (from the spine above or the lower limbs below) can affect the lumbar–pelvic–hip complex, resulting in abnormal mechanical

stresses and symptoms of overuse.[86,154,231,232] For example, fusion of the lower lumbar vertebrae can cause a compensatory increase in motion at the SIJ.[103] Cibulka and Delitto[44] compared two different treatments for hip joint pain in runners who had primary hip and SIJ dysfunction and found that a manipulative technique designed to reduce SIJ dysfunction effectively reduced hip pain. They concluded that the therapist should evaluate the SIJ in patients with hip pain.

By establishing the relation among these functional components of the kinetic chain, the clinician can better evaluate the patient and formulate more-effective treatment programs. Keep in mind the possible effect and influences of other components of the kinetic chain, such as the foot, ankle, and knee, to complete the picture of dysfunction.

The center of activity in the human body for static weight bearing, normal biomechanics, and posture is the lumbar–pelvic–hip region. Kendall and colleagues[140,141] regard the position of the pelvis as the keynote in postural alignment. The two SIJs form an integral part of this region. During ambulation the SIJs decrease the effort of ambulation and absorb shear forces to protect the disks and to decrease the effects of impact loading on the femoral heads.[65]

The pelvis (meaning basin) is a bony ring formed by the two innominate bones, the sacrum, and the cavity of this arrangement. It is interposed between the fifth lumbar vertebra and the femoral heads (Fig. 23-1). The ancient phallic worshipers named the base of the spine the *sacred bone*. The sacrum is the seat of the transverse center of gravity, the keystone of the pelvis, and the foundation for the spine. The most important mechanical function of the pelvic girdle is to transmit the weight of the head, upper limbs, and trunk to the lower limbs and to transmit in the opposite direction the contact forces

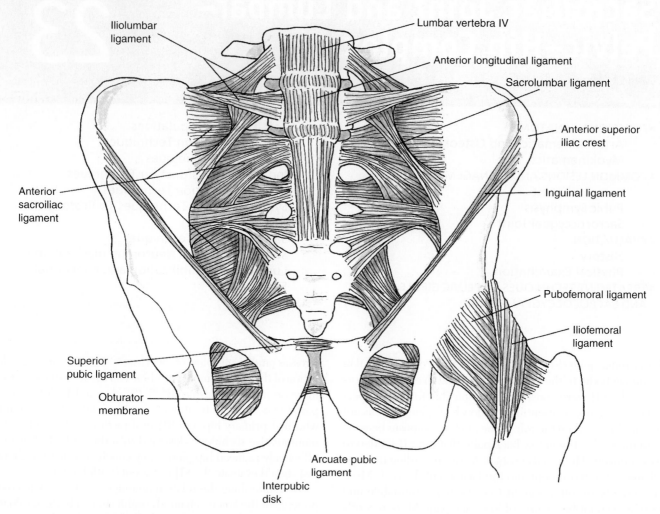

■ **FIG. 23-1.** The lumbar–pelvic–hip complex.

from the ground, through the leg, up into the trunk.[139] When trunk and ground forces exceed the normal physiologic adaptive capacity of its tissues, a chronic painful condition can result.[53,182,190]

The pelvis also plays a role in energy absorption.[190] Weight is transmitted to the sacrum via the lumbosacral junction (fifth lumbar vertebra and lumbosacral disk to the first sacral segment), distributed equally along the alae of the sacrum, and transmitted through the SIJs to the acetabulum and hence to the lower limbs. The force of the body weight tends to separate the sacrum from the ilia and tends to push the first sacral segment into flexion (nutation).

SACROILIAC JOINTS

The SIJ is a synovial joint formed between the medial surface of the ilium and the lateral aspect of the upper sacral vertebrae. The articular surface on the iliac side of the joint, however, is fibrocartilage. The cartilage covering the opposing joint surface (sacral) is hyaline cartilage 1.7 to 5 times thicker than the fibrocartilage of the iliac component.[8,28] The surfaces

of the sacroiliac articulation exhibit irregular elevations and depressions that fit into one another, restrict movement, and contribute to the strength of the joint.

The SIJ changes as we age. In early childhood the joint surfaces are smooth and flat: gliding motions are possible in all directions.[28,128,171,264,303,304] After puberty the joint surfaces change their configuration, and motion is restricted to anteroposterior movement of the sacrum on the ilium or the ilium on the sacrum (flexion or rotation and extension or counter-rotation).[211] Most investigators describe a decrease in motion with age.[8,28,222,254,263,264,297] Sturesson and colleagues,[281] however, noted no decrease in mobility in a sample of persons aged 19 to 45 years, and reported 0.08 mm of translation. In the elderly, the joint cavity is at least partly obliterated by fibrous adhesions and synovitis (osseous union may occur). Mobility is lower in men than in women, and the joint usually becomes ankylosed in elderly men.[99,305]

The articular surface of the sacrum is shaped like a letter L lying on its side, with its upper, more-vertical limb being shorter than its lower, more-horizontal limb (Fig. 23-2).[5,28,305]

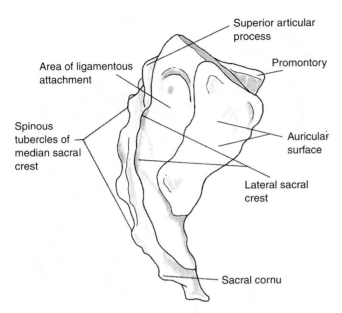

■ FIG. 23-2. Articular surface of the sacrum.

The sacral surface is slightly concave, the iliac surface convex.[8,28] The size, shape, roughness, and complexity of the articular surfaces vary greatly among individuals; this contributes to the unique stability of the joint.[62,276]

Besides the bony architecture, SIJ stability depends primarily on the anterior and posterior ligaments (see Fig. 18-19). The stronger posterior ligaments are necessary to provide stability and prevent the tendency for the upper sacrum to be driven forward during weight bearing. All adjacent muscles (i.e., the quadratus lumborum, gluteus maximus, gluteus minimus, iliacus, latissimus dorsi, and piriformis) have fibrous expansions that blend with the anterior and posterior SIJ ligaments and contribute to the strength of the joint capsule and ligaments, and thus to the joint's stability.[299]

In addition there are the accessory ligaments. The most important is the *iliolumbar ligament*, which extends from the transverse process of the fifth lumbar vertebra (although it can reach as far superiorly as the fourth lumbar vertebra) to the posterior iliac crest (Fig. 23-1). The multidirectional aspect of the iliolumbar bands of this ligament allows the ligament to check various motions of the L5 vertebra on the sacrum and is important in squaring the L5 vertebra on the sacrum. This ligament is frequently painful when there is true sacroiliac dysfunction.

The pelvis can move in all three body planes: in the sagittal plane during forward and backward bending, in the coronal plane during sidebending (lateral flexion), and in the axial plane during twisting of the trunk. During these movements, motion also occurs within the pelvis. Experiments using several different techniques (i.e., gross examination, roentgenography, tomography) to demonstrate sacroiliac movement have been described.[26,32,40,45,48,50,64,72,77,89,95,101,102,139,147,154,167,177,192,197,214,228,229,241,254,261,281,291,295,305,309,310] Although there has been considerable con-

troversy and speculation about the role and type of movements that occur in this joint, there seems no doubt that the normal range of SIJ movement (although only a few millimeters) is important.[103] Recent studies seem to have confirmed the rotatory movement described by Brooke,[32] but it is generally considered minimal.[254,276] Motion is often described as a nodding type of movement of the sacrum, in that the sacral promontory can move forward and backward between the iliac bones. Flexion or *nutation* involves movement of the anterior tip of the sacral promontory anteriorly and inferiorly while the coccyx moves posteriorly in relation to the ilium (Fig. 23-3A). Extension or *counternutation* refers to the opposite movement: the anterior tip of the sacral promontory moves posteriorly and superiorly while the coccyx moves anteriorly in relation to the ilium (Fig. 23-3B).[139] The arthrokinematics of the sacrum during rotation have not been studied, although several theories have been proposed.[85,185,198,234]

When a human stands erect, the line of gravity is posterior to the acetabula, causing a posterior rotation of the innominate bones around the acetabula. At heel-strike there is a posterior rotational force on the innominate (Fig. 23-4).[199,280] As the lower extremity proceeds through the stance phase and approaches push-off, a resultant anterior rotational force creates a flexion force on the sacrum around a horizontal axis. Most agree that the axis occurs at the intersection of the cranial and caudal portions of the sacroiliac articular surfaces. However, Lavignolle and colleagues[154] calculated that the horizontal axis of the SIJ was just posterior to the pubic symphysis.

Wilder[310] reported, that Farabeuf described sacral flexion about an extra-articular axis lying posterior to the center of the articular facet while Bonnaire argued that the axis was intra-articular at the convergence of the facetal limbs allowing pure spin. Weisl[305] rejected the idea of a transverse axis and theorized pure linear motion, with sacral flexion being a straight displacement of the sacrum along the caudal facet anterosuperiorly. Wilder and associates[310] used topography and theoretical modeling with best-fit axes of rotation for each contour to calculate the optimal axes of rotation. They concluded that motion did not occur exclusively around axes proposed by Weisl, Bonnaire, or Farabeuf, or in optimized axes in the median or frontal planes. They argued that translation motion occurred about a "rough axis" if some separation of the surfaces was present.

Osteopathic theory demands at least three transverse and two diagonal axes to accommodate sacroiliac and iliosacral motions and sacral torsion. It is likely that all of these axes are operative during some phase of motion, depending on the load being carried through the articulations and the age and stage of degeneration of the joint. Mitchell and associates[198,199] have described the following axes and movements:

1. *Superior transverse axis* (runs through the second sacral segment). This is often referred to as the respiratory axis. This axis is actually a fulcrum formed by the attachments of the posterior sacroiliac ligaments and the thoracodorsal

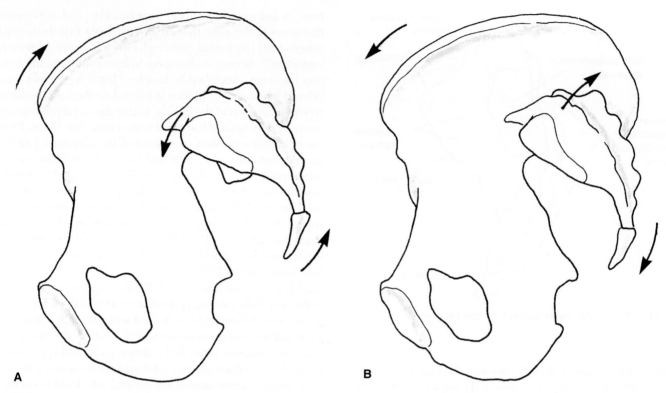

■ **FIG. 23-3.** Nutation (**A**) and counternutation (**B**) of the sacrum.

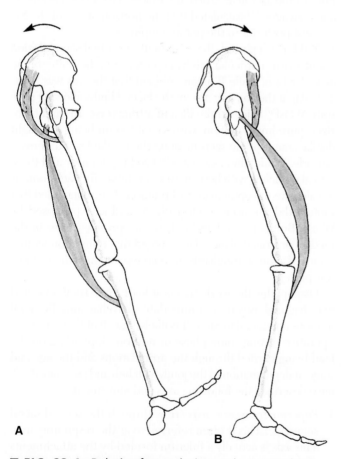

■ **FIG. 23-4.** Relative forces during early stance phase (**A**) and swing phase of gait (**B**).

fascia. As one inhales, the sacrum counternutates; as one exhales, the sacrum nutates (Fig. 23-5A).
2. *Middle transverse axis* (located at the second sacral body). This is the principal axis of normal sacroiliac flexion and extension (nutation and counternutation; Fig. 23-5A).
3. *Inferior transverse axis* (runs transversely through the inferior pole of the sacral articulations). This is the principal axis of normal iliosacral motion (anterior and posterior rotation of the innominates; Fig. 23-5A).
4. *Right and left oblique axes* (run from the superior end of the articular surface of the sacrum obliquely to the opposite inferior lateral angle). Iliosacral motion occurring about the inferior transverse axis is consorted with rotation at the pubis and through the sacrum at the contralateral oblique axis (Fig. 23-5B).

In osteopathic medicine, the SIJ is often described as two joints: the iliosacral and the SIJ.[313] The term *iliosacral* implies the innominates moving on the sacrum; conversely, the term *sacroiliac* implies the sacrum moving within the innominates. Functionally these designations hold true because they are based on the recruitment of motion and transmission of forces from the spine or lower limbs through the pelvis, although it is one and the same joint. The sacrum is mechanically associated with the spine, whereas the ilium is aligned with and affected by the lower limbs. As the lumbar spine goes, so goes the sacrum; similarly, as the lower extremity goes, so goes the ilium.[231]

It is generally agreed that the innominate bones are capable of anteroposterior rotation, but the quantity of movement and

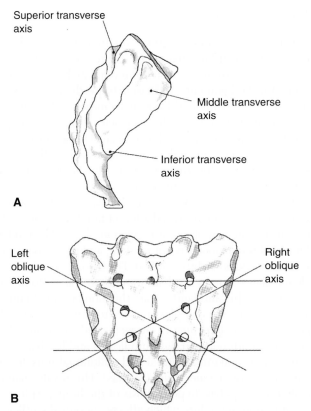

A

B

■ **FIG. 23-5.** Principal axes (about which motion of the sacrum or innominate bones moves) that have been proposed (Mitchell 1965, 1968). **(A)** Superior, middle, and inferior transverse axes. **(B)** Left and right oblique axes. (Adapted with permission from Saunders D: Evaluation, Treatment and Prevention of Musculoskeletal Disorder. Minneapolis, Viking Press, 1985.)

the specific axes remain controversial.[292,293] The axis of innominate rotation is not thought to lie in the coronal plane but rather is thought to run obliquely in the posterolateral direction. The craniocaudal orientation of this axis varies during anteroposterior rotation. Anterior translation (arthrokinematic) of the innominate bone (6 to 8 mm) conjoined with both anterior and posterior rotation (osteokinematic) has been confirmed, although the quantity of this translation is disputed (0.5 to 1.6 mm).[154,281]

During spinal flexion or standing up from lying down, the sacral promontory moves ventrally so that the anteroposterior diameter of the pelvic inlet is reduced and the apex of the sacrum moves dorsally. At the same time, a movement occurs in the iliac bones, in which the iliac crests and the posterosuperior iliac spines (PSIS) become approximated, and the anterosuperior iliac spines (ASIS) and the ischial tuberosities move apart (Fig. 23-6).[139] Flexion increases tension in the iliolumbar ligaments, the short posterior SIJ ligament, the interosseous ligaments, and the sacrotuberous ligaments, which then dynamically return the SIJs to their normal resting position.[65] In studies of functional movements, motion of the sacrum has been found to peak in the act of rising from a supine to a standing or long-sitting position.[48,50,259,281]

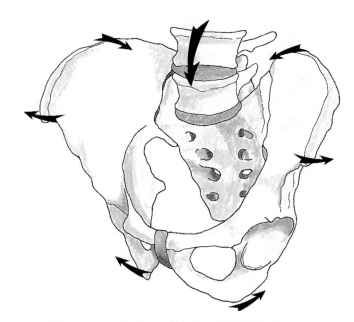

■ **FIG. 23-6.** Osteokinematic motion of the pelvic girdle during trunk flexion.

Alternatively, on spinal extension or on lying down, opposite movements occur so that the base of the sacrum moves dorsally and the apex of the sacrum moves ventrally, increasing the anteroposterior diameter of the pelvic inlet. At the same time, the iliac crests and the PSIS separate and the ASIS and the ischial tuberosities approximate (Fig. 23-7).[139] Tension is increased mostly in the anterior sacroiliac ligaments, causing a relative unloading of the posterior ligaments.[63]

Other movements of the ilia on the sacrum are possible, but do not normally occur except in dysfunctional states. These

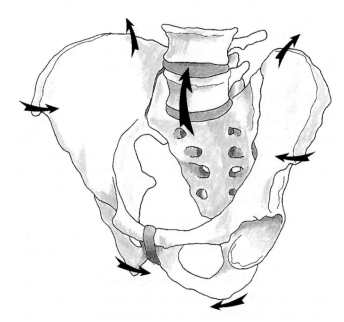

■ **FIG. 23-7.** Osteokinematic motion of the pelvic girdle during trunk extension.

uncommon movements are described as up or down slips and in or out flares of the ilia.[63,85,100,158,199,214,306,313] Sacroiliac dysfunction is also termed *subluxation* or *posterior* or, more frequently, *anterior fixed innominate.* There are numerous tests for SIJ dysfunction, basically of two types: palpation of bony landmarks with or without measurement, and pain provocation tests.[51,63,102,103,158,299]

Several investigators have reported the presence of "supernumerary articular facets"[263] or "axial"[60] or accessory SIJs that may contribute to, or be responsible for, sacroiliac dysfunction.[5,60,78,110,111,288] According to Walker,[298] the fact that higher frequencies are observed in adult samples with increasing age, with no reports in fetuses or children, supports the theory that the accessory SIJs may be acquired as a result of the stress of weight bearing.

SACROCOCCYGEAL JOINT

The coccyx is formed by fusion of four rudimentary vertebrae. The first coccygeal joint has a base for articulation with the apex of the sacrum and two cornu. The apex of the sacrum and base of coccyx are united by a thin fibrocartilaginous intervertebral disk. The sacrococcygeal joint is a true joint with a joint capsule and ligaments (see Fig. 8-28).[215] Other ligaments covering the posterior aspect of the coccyx are the posterior intercoccygeal ligaments. The gluteus maximus partly inserts at the posterolateral aspect of the coccyx via its coccygeal fibers. To the ventral surface of its inferior two segments attaches the ischiococcygeal portions of the levator ani muscle (see Fig. 7-18*B, C*). The coccyx is innervated by S1–S4 and may refer pain throughout the pelvic floor.[4]

In persons up to middle age, there is slight movement of the coccyx posteriorly on defecation, and during childbirth. Movements are restricted to flexion and extension. Flexion movements are performed by the levator ani and the sphincter ani externus muscle (see Fig. 7-18*C*).[174] Extension is caused by relaxation of these muscles. In elderly persons the first coccygeal vertebra is frequently fused to the apex of the sacrum, thereby eliminating the sacrococcygeal joint.[202]

PUBIC SYMPHYSIS

The symphysis pubis, a cartilaginous joint, should not be overlooked as a source of symptoms or dysfunction.[55,161] The symphysis pubis permits limited mobility between the two oval articular surfaces of the bones and can be affected by excessive mobility in the SIJs.[164] Stability of this articulation is vital to both the kinetic and kinematic functions of the pelvic girdle. The joint is supported superiorly by the pubic ligament, which extends to connect the pubic tubercles, and inferiorly by a strong fibrous band, the arcuate pubic ligament (Fig. 23-1). A fibrocartilaginous disk separates the articular surfaces of the two pubic bones. Many forces act on this joint, especially those exerted by the muscles of the lower limbs, some of which cross the pubic symphysis, adding significantly to pelvic stability.

Myokinematics

Specific balanced muscle groups are fundamental to balancing the pelvis and lumbar spine. There are 35 muscles that attach directly to the sacrum or innominate bones and function with the ligaments and fascia to produce synchronous motion of the trunk and lower extremities.[158] Decreases in the length or strength of these muscles, caused by adaptive shortening or neuromuscular imbalances, can alter normal pelvic mechanics. Several authors have stressed that soft tissue evaluation is the crucial factor in the diagnosis of lumbar spine and sacroiliac dysfunction.

Certain muscles respond in a typical way to a given situation, whether this is pain, impaired afferent input from the joint, or impairment in central motor regulation.[132,138,226] The tendency for muscles to respond is not random, and typical patterns of muscle reactions can be identified. The two regions where muscle imbalance is more evident or in which it starts to develop, according to Jull and Janda,[138] are the shoulder–neck complex and the pelvic–hip complex (pelvic crossed syndrome). The *pelvic crossed syndrome* is characterized by an imbalance between shortened and tight hip flexors and lumbar erector spinae and weakened gluteal and abdominal muscles (see Chapter 8, Soft Tissue Manipulations). This results in anteversion of the pelvis, hyperlordosis of the lumbar spine, and slight flexion of the hip, which affects not only the efficiency of the static postural base but also dynamics such as gait.[226] In dysfunction, tonic muscles tend to shorten and hypertrophy; phasic muscles tend to become weak and atrophy.[130–132,134,138] The clinical significance is that it is essential to stretch or lengthen the tight, short tonic muscle groups before trying to reeducate the weak, dysfunctional phasic muscle groups. The main muscles and muscle groups of the pelvic–hip complex that illustrate the characteristic differences between tonic and phasic muscles are listed in Table 23-1.

According to Chapman and Nihls,[41] elsewhere in the body multijoint muscles affect the joints they traverse, and the pelvis is no exception. Pelvic articulations may also be affected by the

TABLE 23-1   FUNCTIONAL DIVISION OF MUSCLE GROUPS

MUSCLES PRONE TO TIGHTNESS	MUSCLES PRONE TO WEAKNESS
Erector spinae	Gluteus maximus
Quadratus lumborum	Gluteus medius
Rectus femoris	Gluteus minimus
Iliopsoas	Rectus abdominis
Tensor fasciae latae	Vastus medialis
Piriformis	Vastus lateralis
Short hip adductors	
Hamstrings	

transarticular and swing component of the muscle forces, as well as osteokinematics affecting tension, compression, and shear.

Consider the *quadratus lumborum* (Fig. 23-8), a multijoint muscle. The quadratus lumborum has three portions (iliocostal, iliotransverse, costotransverse) that produce lateral guy wire forces to the lumbar spine. Working with such structures as the iliolumbar ligament and the deep portion of the erector spinae muscles, the quadratus lumborum helps maintain the stability of the lumbar spine. Bilateral contraction may produce an anterior flexion of the sacrum through its attachments onto the base and ala. By the law of approximation, contraction of this muscle brings bony attachments together. This could produce a lateral tilt of the pelvic girdle and maintain a cranial displacement of the ipsilateral ilium on the sacrum.[41]

According to Travell and Simons,[286] the quadratus lumborum is one of the most commonly overlooked muscular sources of low back pain. Mechanical perpetuation of quadratus lumborum trigger points may depend on skeletal asymmetries, particularly inequality in leg length, or a small hemipelvis. Many authors have identified the quadratus lumborum as a source of back pain.[97,107,210,272,274,312] More specifically, they have identified it as referring pain to the sacroiliac region,[138,142,242,267,273,285] to the hip or buttock,[96,267,273,285] and to the greater trochanter.[267,285]

The abdominal muscles are also longitudinal, multijoint muscles. The abdominal muscles, including the two obliques,

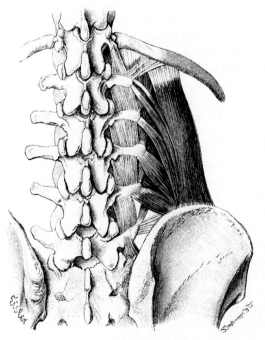

the transversus abdominis, and the rectus abdominis (see Fig. 7-13), insert on the superior aspect of the pelvic girdle and are joined by the quadratus lumborum, the lumbodorsal fascia, and the erector spinae. A key point with respect to the abdominal muscles is their contribution to the stability of the symphysis pubis.[139,302] They retain the viscera and act in respiration and maintenance of the lumbosacral angle. The abdominal wall contributes to the attenuation of trunk and ground forces as they converge into the lumbopelvic region.[284] A weak abdominal wall promotes a forward pelvic tilt (increases the lumbosacral angle), creating an anterior migration of the center of gravity. To counter the anterior migration and maintain postural equilibrium, the person must increase the extension of the lumbar spine with a posterior movement of the weight line.[232]

The first sacral segment, which is inclined slightly anteriorly and inferiorly, forms an angle with the horizontal called the *lumbosacral angle* (see Fig. 20-5). The size of the angle varies with the position of the pelvis and affects the lumbar curvature. An increase in this angle increases the anterior convexity of the lumbar curve and increases the amount of shear stress at the lumbosacral joint.[211] The greater the sacral angle, the greater the shear forces and, therefore, the greater the weight carried by the soft tissues and articular processes, as opposed to the sacrum itself.[168] Added weight bearing must be taken on by the apophyseal joints and may become an important source of both low back pain and referred pain.[20,21,81,167,179,201,223]

Lower limb rotation is directly related to pelvic inclination and thus to the lumbosacral angle. External hip rotation facilitates posterior pelvic tilt and so may decrease the lumbosacral angle. One of the external rotators, the piriformis (see Figs. 7-18A and 7-21B), primarily a tonic muscle, is considered responsible for restricting SIJ motion or producing local pain and symptoms of the piriformis syndrome (see Chapter 8, Soft Tissue Manipulations).[36,115,198,207,218,219,267,279,287] Imbalance in piriformis length and strength appears to strongly influence movement of the sacrum between the innominates.[100]

The gluteus maximus has considerable mechanical advantage in humans as compared with other primates, given the increased anteroposterior depth of the human pelvis. More than half of this muscle inserts into the iliotibial band (see Fig. 7-2).[83] It is a short, multipennate muscle designed for power. Its bony attachments are close to both hip joints and SIJs, so its action involves a large transarticular force. It can posteriorly rotate the ilium. Because the gluteus maximus, medius, and minimus are phasic muscles, in a weakened and dysfunctional state they reduce the dynamic stability of the pelvic girdle, thus predisposing to recurrent articular strains of the lumbosacral junction and the SIJ.[158] Weakness of the gluteus medius results in limited hip abduction and loss of lateral stabilization of the ilium (see gluteus medius syndrome, Chapter 8, Soft Tissue Manipulations).

The hamstrings (multijoint muscles; see Fig. 7-21), with their distal attachments further from the pelvic joint, help reduce the lumbosacral angle, and with unilateral action there is the potential for posterior torsion of one ilium.[41] Along with the deep rotators of the hip and the gluteus maximus, the force of these posterior thigh muscles is readily transmitted to the pelvis when the femur or foot becomes fixed and a closed kinetic chain is established.

The multifidus (see Fig. 18-16*A*, *C*), along with the rotatores (transversospinalis group), is considered primarily a tonic or postural muscle and stabilizes the lumbar spine.[268] The extensive attachment of the multifidus muscle to the dorsal surface of the sacrum makes it a major mass filling the deep sulcus formed by the overlapping ilium and sacrum. The attachment of the multifidus to the spinous processes results in an effective lever arm for extension of the lumbovertebral segments.[20,21] A unilateral contraction may produce a posterior rotation of the vertebrae on that side. A bilateral contraction may produce a posterior force on the pelvis through its attachments with the erector spinae, the PSIS, and the posterior sacroiliac ligaments. Contraction also exerts a compressive force between each lumbar vertebra and between L5 and the sacrum. Stability of the lumbar spine increases when compressive forces are placed on it. Also, because of its greater tonic or stabilizing function, functional training of the multifidus may offer treatment for segmental instability. Evidence of lumbar multifidus muscle-wasting ipsilateral to symptoms in patients with acute and subacute low back pain indicate that wasting may be attributable to inhibition from perceived pain via a long-loop reflex pathway.[123]

The psoas (see Fig. 7-16), a longitudinal, multijoint muscle, does not directly attach to either the innominate bone or the sacrum but does have a significant biomechanical influence because of its potential to increase lumbar lordosis and produce hip flexion. Thoracolumbar lordosis effects a compensatory change in the lumbosacral angle and can produce a unilateral anterior iliac torsion and anterior movement of the sacrum on that side. Simultaneously, it may produce torsion of the sacrum on the opposite side.[313] The force of the multifidus muscle is opposite that of the psoas muscle, and they may function together to "square" the vertebral unit in the sagittal plane.[232]

Other muscles to consider are:

1. Tensor fasciae latae (see Fig. 7-2*B*). Unilateral tightness produces a lateral pelvic tilt. Tightness may be one of the causes if an iliac downslip.[213] Bilateral tightness produces an anterior pelvic tilt.
2. Sartorius (see Fig. 7-19). The sartorius may exert an anterior influence on the innominate when the knee is fixed in some flexion and the hip is extended.
3. Rectus femoris (see Fig. 7-19; multijoint) muscles can act as potential anterior rotators of the ipsilateral innominate.
4. The muscles of the adductor group (see Fig. 7-20) have a direct effect on superior and inferior motions of the pubic rami. The short adductors and obturator externus, functioning as a unit, could produce a distracting force at the pubic ramus. Tightness or weakness of the adductors may influence hip position, which in turn influences the SIJ.

5. The pelvic floor muscles play an important supporting role (see Fig. 7-18 and Chapter 7, Myofascial Considerations and Evaluation in Somatic Dysfunction). If the lumbosacral angle is increased, the stretched urogenital diaphragm becomes inefficient in its action.[41] Imbalance is highly significant in patients with rectal, gynecologic, and urologic problems.[100] Spasms or tight pelvic diaphragm musculature can cause symphysis compression.[213]

Always consider the influence of the thoracolumbar fascia, which represents not only fascial tissue but also the fused aponeurosis of several muscles (see Figs. 7-9 through 7-12 and Chapter 7, Myofascial Considerations and Evaluation in Somatic Dysfunction).[125] It serves as an attachment for the transversus abdominis, the internal oblique, and the latissimus dorsi muscles. The thoracolumbar fascia can influence and be influenced by the lumbar spine and pelvic positions and their surrounding muscles. Motions of the pelvis directly influence the thoracolumbar fascia: anterior pelvic movements tighten it and posterior pelvic movements loosen it.

COMMON LESIONS AND MANAGEMENT

Sacroiliac Joint

SIJ pain is normally described as a dull ache and is characteristically experienced over the back of the SIJ and buttock.[51] It may also refer to the groin, over the greater trochanter, down the back of the thigh to the knee, and occasionally down the lateral or posterior calf to the ankle, foot, and toes.[144] Pain may also be referred to the lower abdomen; pain is then felt in the iliac fossa and is usually associated with a localized area of deep tenderness over the iliacus muscle (see Fig. 7-16) known as Baer's sacroiliac point.[51,188] This point is located about 20 cm from the umbilicus on an imaginary line drawn from the ASIS to the umbilicus. Because the pelvis is a bony ring, pain may also be experienced anteriorly over the pubic symphysis or the adductor tendon origin.[51]

Clinical signs of sacroiliac dysfunction are pain and local tenderness, with increased pain on position changes such as ascending or descending stairs or slopes or rising from sitting or lying to standing. Pain may also increase with prolonged postures in standing or sitting. Pain may be initially transient but becomes deep and boring. Typically there is early-morning stiffness that eases after a period of weight bearing.

Abnormal or asymmetric forces reaching the lumbar or hip area are ultimately translated to the pelvis and render the weight-bearing joints vulnerable to injury.[80] Mechanical lesions may be caused by hypomobility (with or without pain), hypermobility (with or without pain), or normal mobility with pain of the SIJ.[51,158]

HYPOMOBILITY LESIONS

Hypomobility lesions usually occur in young people and may be associated with movements that place a rotational stress on the SIJ, such as ballet or golfing.[51] It may also develop after pregnancy or trauma. It can also occur insidiously and may be associated with certain structural faults such as asymmetric development of the pelvis or unequal leg length. Pain may result from sustained contraction of the muscle overlying the joint[143] or from a muscle-pain disorder.[286] This hypertonicity may accompany dysfunction of the SIJ or the lumbar spine.

Disparity in leg lengths, functional or structural, and pelvic muscle length asymmetries are considered prime factors in detecting sacroiliac dysfunction.[46,103] According to Grieve,[103] the pelvis can become stuck or blocked at the SIJ, not necessarily in a position of torsion but sometimes so in people with unequal leg length. Bourdillon and Day[27] wrote, "In patients with leg inequality there is a natural tendency for the pelvis to adopt the twisted position which most nearly levels the anterior-superior surface of the sacrum." When there is frontal plane asymmetry or a leg-length discrepancy, the pelvis must drop a distance equal to the amount of the discrepancy with every step. Ground forces reach the lumbopelvic tissues in an abnormal, asymmetric manner, resulting in comparatively more compression forces applied to the shorter side and more shear forces to the opposite sacroiliac side. The tilted position of the sacrum also results in alteration at the hip (see Chapter 14, Hip), lumbar spine, and knee. The most serious complication is osteoarthritis of the hip on the longer side.[92,93] With respect to the lumbar spine, there is sidebending motion away from the short side, with compressive forces placed on the concave side and tensile forces on the convex side.[231] Osteophytes may develop on the lumbar vertebrae on the side of the concavity produced by leg-length inequality.[86,87,91,204] Giles and Taylor[91] illustrated wedging of the lumbar vertebrae in a manner that would represent the conversion of a functional scoliosis to a fixed scoliosis.

Conversely, when innominate torsion is present (in the absence of structural leg-length discrepancy); this gives an appearance of unequal leg length, when measured from the ASIS or by noting the relation of the medial malleoli bilaterally when using a functional sit-up test.[199,231,255,296,313] Fisk[84] illustrated how anterior rotation of an innominate bone elevates the side of the sacrum. Thus, compensatory anterior rotation of the innominate is associated with a short lower limb, compensatory posterior rotation with a long lower limb. One would expect this functional compensation to become increasingly fixed with time.[287] Denslow and associates[59] also noted the likelihood of a compensatory horizontal rotation of the pelvis toward the longer side. Studies have also shown a relation between the SIJ and limited hip mobility[73,152] and between low back pain and asymmetric hip rotation.[43,79,82,187]

HYPERMOBILITY LESIONS

Hypermobility lesions, like those in which hypomobility is the causative factor, occur in one of two situations.[51] According to Corrigan and Maitland,[51] the first situation is secondary to instability of the symphysis pubis, which occurs predominantly in athletes.[117] This condition may be complicated by a mechanical lesion of the lumbar spine or one or both SIJs, and may be

associated with an osteitis condensans ilii. The second occurs in young women, usually during or soon after pregnancy. Ligaments may remain lax for 6 to 12 weeks after delivery or longer. Occasionally the symphysis may become a truly mobile joint, with pelvic instability as a result.[258] Movement abnormalities of the sacroiliac, the pubic joints, and the lumbar spine may be a cause of persistent postpartum pain.

Sacroiliac pain appears to be an accepted problem during pregnancy. Berg and colleagues[11] found that of 862 women who experienced low back pain during pregnancy, 79 could not continue work because of very severe low back pain. The most common cause was dysfunction of the SIJs. Under the influence of the hormone relaxin, there is a physiologic pelvic girdle relaxation that may produce symptoms.[281] Dietrichs and Kogstad[61] have suggested the terms *physiologic pelvic girdle relaxation* for normal ligament relaxation during pregnancy and *symptom-giving pelvic girdle relaxation* for that which results in pain or pelvic instability. When pain in one or more pelvic joints is experienced outside pregnancy and the puerperium, the authors propose the term *pelvic joint syndrome*.[298] This term reflects their findings that pain, and not mechanical dysfunction, was the common symptom. There is clinical and radiologic evidence to support the presence of increased SIJ mobility near the end of pregnancy.[112,149,170,186]

Simple mobilizing techniques localized to the SIJ structures are very effective after careful exclusion of problems from the intervertebral joints.[103] Passive stabilization for SIJ hypermobility may involve sacroiliac supports or belts, as advocated by Cyriax,[54] Grieve,[103] Lee,[158] Macnab,[172] Mennell,[189] and Porterfield and DeRosa,[231] taping, or compression shorts. Use of sacroiliac belts appears to be justified in theory, but outcome data are not yet available.[158,232,299] Possible mechanisms by which the belt exerts its effect include:

- It brings the adjoining sacral and iliac surfaces of the SIJ together.[291]
- It enhances a self-bracing mechanism that normally ensures stability of the SIJ and allows for transfer of the lumbosacral load to the legs while minimizing the shear between the iliac and sacral surfaces.[271]
- It decreases the amount of anterior rotation of the innominates and posterior tilting of the lower part of the sacrum by exerting a direct pressure against these structures.[257]

A sacroiliac belt is often used prepartum, postpartum, and after trauma; it is especially helpful for women just before delivery. The belt is worn when the patient is most active and is removed when sitting or lying. During the initial phase after trauma, a support is used to help stabilize the area, to enhance soft tissue healing and minimize reinjury. The patient must be instructed thoroughly about the nature of the condition and how to prevent recurrence. Doran and Newell[67] found that the response to a corrective corset was slow, but the long-term effects were as good as those of other treatments. The support should be put on after a correction has been made to help prevent recurrence.[63]

A loose joint can become overridden and stuck so that it may appear hypomobile. Grieve,[101] in a study on lumbopelvic rhythm during simple knee-raising, found that some patients present a paradox: the joint does not move in the moving phase and is hypermobile in the stance phase.

Prolotherapy[68,70,108,109,124,148,235] may be the treatment of choice if the sacroiliac dysfunction has been corrected but the ligaments continue to be an ongoing source of pain, or if the dysfunction keeps reoccurring and laxity of the supporting tissue is evident or suspected. The principal concept is to inject material that stimulates proliferation of collagen in ligament, to strengthen the ligament (particularly its attachment to bone), and to reduce the ligamentous-related pain.[100] The most popular current solution is that advocated by Ongley and associates[216] and consists of hypertonic glucose, glycerin, and phenol, diluted with water and then combined with lidocaine hydrochloride for injection. Remember that muscles, in particular the iliopsoas, coccygeus, and piriformis, may be chronically contracted and stabilizing what otherwise prove to be an unstable joint.[257]

Hypermobility in any joint is the result of overstretching the elastic tissue in the ligaments and joint capsule. Normal tone in ligaments depends on the natural stimulus of intermittent gentle stretching. Therefore, controlled gentle joint mobilization techniques are useful in reducing pain and serve as a natural stimulus to the elastic tissue.

Unless otherwise specified, strengthening and stabilization exercises should be carried out with a focus on the pelvic core muscles for strengthening in particular:

- The elements of the inner unit (multifidus, transversus abdominis, thoracic diaphragm, and pelvic floor). Work by Richardson et al.[243] and others suggests that contraction of specific abdominal muscles is coupled with contraction of specific pelvic floor muscles (e.g., contraction of transversus abdominis and pubococcygeus, the oblique abdominals and the iliococcygeus or ischiococcygeus, and rectus and puborectalis). The simultaneous contraction of some muscles of the inner core may be able to set up a force couple capable of affecting the stability of the SIJ and the lumbosacral junction.
- The outer units consist of the posterior oblique system (the continuum of latissimus dorsi connected, by way of the thoracolumbar fascia, to the contralateral gluteus medius), which will on contraction compress the SIJ on the side of the gluteus maximus and contribute to load transfer through the pelvic region with rotational activities and during gait.[98,100,200]
- The anterior oblique system (the external and internal abdominal obliques on one side connected by way of the anterior abdominal fascia to the contralateral adductors of the thigh). The lower horizontal fibers of the internal abdominal oblique may augment the transversus abdominis in its role of supporting the SIJ.[243]
- The deep longitudinal system (the continuum of the erector spinae muscle connected by way of the deep lamina of the thoracolumbar fascia to the contralateral sacrotuerous ligament and the biceps femoris), which will on contraction enhance the ability of the fascia to contribute to an SIJ force closure mechanisms acting across it.[98,290,311]
- The lateral system, which includes the gluteus medius and minimus, and the contralateral adductors of the thigh, which are more involved with the proper function of the pelvic girdle in standing and walking rather with force closure. SIJ instability is said to result in a reflex inhibition of these muscles and may account for the feeling of the hip giving away.[69,71,159,289]

For further discussion of form and force closure (a self-locking mechanism) and its contribution to the sacroiliac joint, see Chapter 18, Spine—General Structure and Biomechanical Considerations.

DEGENERATIVE CHANGES

Degenerative changes are increasingly common with advancing age and may occur secondary to disorders in which movement is decreased.[51] SIJ degeneration is often associated with chronic neurologic conditions such as paraplegia and hemiplegia. Degenerative changes are also associated with chronic structural abnormalities such as leg-length discrepancies, scoliosis, or pelvic asymmetries, or hip disease (osteoarthritis).[297,298] In patients with unilateral hip disease, degenerative changes are usually found in the contralateral SIJ.[51]

Degenerative changes first involve the iliac surface, where the cartilage is thinner than on the sacral surface. The cartilage changes are similar to those in peripheral joints with, ultimately, a fibrous ankylosis of the joint cavity.[239,240] Vleeming and associates[291,292] consider the noninflammatory fibrous or chondroid ankylosis and radiologically visible hyaline cartilage-covered ridges to be physiologic, not pathologic, a response to joint stress and an adaptation for greater stability.

OSTEITIS CONDENSANS ILII

Osteitis condensans ilii (a noninflammatory condition) is characterized by a condensation of bone on the iliac side of the SIJ. Its nature is uncertain, but it probably represents a bony reaction to unequal stress in this joint. It is usually bilateral and occurs mostly in young adults, more commonly in postpartum women. It disappears with menopause, and is important medically as it mimics inflammatory disease.[299] Treatment consists of reassurance, analgesics, correction of any postural problems present, and if necessary the use of a sacroiliac belt.[51]

INFLAMMATORY DISEASE AND INFECTIONS

Other conditions to be considered in the differential diagnosis of sacroiliac dysfunction include infections and metabolic conditions. Infections usually involve only one SIJ and may be a staphylococcal or tubercular infection, a sexually acquired infection, or one related to intravenous drug abuse, among many other sources.[299] Inflammatory sacroiliitis conditions are either infectious or seronegative spondyloarthropathies. Of the latter, the major ones are ankylosing spondylitis, Reiter's syndrome, and psoriasis.[299] Ankylosing spondylitis is usually bilateral and symmetric; involvement of the SIJs is the hallmark.

Pubic Symphysis

Dysfunction of the symphysis pubis is very common and frequently overlooked. Pubic shears are probably the most commonly overlooked pubic dysfunction.[313] However, their recognition and proper treatment are mandatory for success in treating pelvic dysfunction. The unleveling of the pubic symphysis could also be called a subluxation.[100]

INFERIOR AND POSTERIOR PUBIC SHEARS

Unleveling of the pubic symphysis is either superior or inferior (superior pubic shear and inferior pubic shear). Muscle imbalances between the abdominals above and the adductors below are major contributors. Strain or adaptive shortening of the adductors in either acute trauma or long-term adaptive shortening may produce abnormal superior or inferior separation of the pubis via their action at the pubis.[4] Pubic shears very frequently occur with innominate rotations or upslips and are often the cause of groin pain as a presenting symptom. Causes of superior, posterior pubic dysfunction include abnormal upward force through an extended leg, a fall on an ischial tuberosity, hip hyperflexion, and weak hip abductor (middle and anterior abductors fibers especially), whereas causes of inferior, anterior dysfunction include an upward lift of the body with the foot fixed, tight hip adductors, and hip hyperflexion.[213] A palpable difference in the comparative superior and inferior heights of the pubis right to left in conjunction with tenderness and edema in the suprapubic area are usually indicative of dysfunction in this articulation.

PUBIC SEPARATION

An increase in separation at the pubic symphysis may occur during labor and delivery and if unresolved in the postpartum period may lead to chronic lower abdominal discomfort and perhaps tension myalgia in the pelvic floor and hips.[4] More severe cases are likely to be accompanied by painful alteration in gait and possibly a posture of external rotation and iliac outflare.[23] The three bones and three joints of the pelvis work in unison; dysfunction of one joint leads to instability the entire structure. Anterior or posterior rotation of an innominate bone cannot occur without causing the rotation of one pubic bone relative to the other. An upslip or downslip causes simultaneous upward and downward translation respectively on both SIJs and the symphysis pubis. The displacement is usually 3 to 5 mm and easily discernable.[257] The impairment generally shows up on x-rays taken in a one-legged weight-bearing stance and often requires surgical intervention to stabilize the symphysis.

PUBIC SYMPHYSIS COMPRESSION

Causes of symphysis compression include spasm or tight pelvic diaphragm musculature, trauma (to lateral aspect of ASIS), and hip hyperadduction or internal stress.[213] The patient typically complains of symphyseal, medial hip, and thigh pain. Pain is increased with stair climbing and walking. Management includes soft tissue manipulations (inhibition-stretch) to the pelvic diaphragm and pubic decompression or distraction (see Fig. 23-40). Movement within pain tolerance is encouraged to promote pubic motion.

OSTEITIS PUBIS SYNDROME

Osteitis pubis is a painful, chronic syndrome that affects the symphysis pubis, adductor and abdominal muscles, and the surrounding fascia. It may affect either joint mobility or the musculotendinous attachments of the abdominal muscles and adductors. The abdominal and adductor muscles act antagonistically to each other, predisposing the symphysis to mechanical traction microtrauma and resulting in osteitis pubis.[246] It may be mistaken for adductor strain, which is characterized by tenderness to direct pressure about the symphysis. Osteitis pubis usually appears during the third and fourth decade of life and occurs most commonly in men.[88] This is most likely to occur in participants involved in any active sport, particularly kicking sports such as soccer or football, and in activities that create continual shearing forces at the pubic symphysis, as with unilateral leg support, or acceleration–deceleration forces required during multidirectional activities (e.g., tennis, race walking, distance runners, and basketball).[74,166,183,246,294]

Many theories have been put forward concerning the origin and progression of the disease. Overuse is the most likely cause of the inflammation.[196] Muscle imbalances between the abdominal muscles and hip adductors have been also suggested as an etiologic factor. Because of their attachment to the thoracic cage proximally and the pubis distally, the abdominal muscles act synergistically with the paravertebral muscles to stabilize the symphysis, allowing single-leg stance while maintaining balance during many sporting activities. Imbalances of these muscle groups disrupt the equilibrium of forces around the symphysis pubis, predisposing the athlete to subacute periostitis cause by chronic microtrauma. This microtrauma exceeds the dynamic capacity of tissue for hypertrophic remodeling, resulting in tissue degeneration.[35,116] Shear stress at the symphysis pubis can also cause sacroiliac dysfunction if hip internal rotation is limited in either flexion or extension.[246]

The pain or discomfort can be located at the pubic area, one or both groins, and in the lower rectus abdominus. Pain may radiate to the hip, testis, or perineum and may also cause low back pain when it is associated with a lesion of the SIJ.[51] Pain is usually made worse by exercise, straining, coughing and sneezing, walking up stairs, or thrusting the leg forward. An audible or palpable click over the symphysis might be detected on certain movements.[51,196]

During the physical examination, pain can be elicited by having the patient squeeze a fist between the knees with resisted isometric adductor contraction (pubic symphysis gap test; see Fig. 23-26).[246] Pain may also be reproduced by passively abducting the hip, and by resisting the patient's attempt to sit up. The inguinal ligament is usually tender to palpation on the side of the impairment. Diagnosis is confirmed by radiographic (x-ray and bone scan) findings. It is common to find the pubic symphysis held in one of the four following positions[74]:

- Anterior-inferior
- Posterior-superior
- Anterior-superior
- Posterior-inferior

Management includes rest as pain is exacerbated by most weight-bearing activities. All sporting activities that involve running or walking must be avoided for several months, although swimming is usually possible.[51] Conservative management includes:

- Pharmacologic management and therapeutic modalities (e.g., cryomassage, laser, and ultrasound or electrical stimulation) as indicated.
- Gentle joint mobilization techniques. If mobilization is used, only one direction needs to be chosen for correction, because of the osteokinematic motion (see Figs. 23-59 through 23-62).[74] Improvement of position (see superior and inferior pubic shears above) and decreased pain on palpation of the inguinal ligament and symphysis pubis should be found if the technique has been successful. Alternatively, isometric contraction of the hip abductors and adductors (see Fig. 23-40) can be used for impairments that do not respond to the mobilization techniques. The short adductors when recruited bring the joint into a level position. Tests for sacroiliac fixation (see Fig. 23-15) and positional tests should be evaluated. If there is no improvement, a sacroiliac dysfunction is a probable cause.
- Progressive rehabilitation program, including stretching exercises to the hip (particularly the adductors and the muscles of internal rotation), pelvic stabilization and abdominal (particularly the transversus abdominis) exercises, and correction of biomechanical problems (e.g., agonist–antagonist muscle imbalances). The return to sports needs to be gradual.

Corticosteroid injections, wedge resection of the symphysis, curettage, arthrodesis, and surgical treatment of the sheath of the rectus abdominus together with an epimysial adductor release have all been used with variable success.[14,137]

Sacrococcygeal Joint

Coccygeal pain is a fairly common occurrence. The causes can be muscle scarring or trauma (i.e., a fall or childbirth injury). Injury to the sacrococcygeal joint (see Fig. 8-28) may occur as a sprain, subluxation, fractures, luxation, or hypermobility. The patient will be unable to sit on both buttocks at the same time. External and internal examination will reveal tenderness to palpation of the coccyx, and mobility of the coccyx may be very limited or absent.

The coccyx is a vital link between the bony pelvis and the soft tissue of the pelvic region. Tension myalgia may occur as a secondary response to the inflammation of traumatic coccyx injury in both acute and chronic states.[4] Length and tone of the pelvic floor muscles may be altered by coccyx displacements caused by sprain or fracture. Reproduction of pelvic floor pain with resisted hip extension is indicative of coccyx dysfunction owing to this relationship.[4] Pelvic pain arising from the coccyx may be reported to worsen with stair climbing and hip extension. Irritation of the coccygeal fibers of the gluteus maximus (which has tendinous attachments in the sacrococcygeal joint) may result in unilateral pain to one buttock.[215]

The normal coccyx flexes while sitting and extends when standing.[255] When the coccyx is injured or subluxed it may heal in the more extended position. The coccyx can also be dislocated or fractured and heal in a flexed position, often with an accompanying deviation, or become fragmented or unstable in a flexed position. These disorders can be diagnosed by palpating the position of the coccyx and testing the passive mobility of the sacrococcygeal joint, or it may be diagnosed by lateral dynamic x-rays and coccygeal discography.[174] Palpation may reveal four types of coccygodynia[54]:

- Contusions of the tip of the coccyx and the immediate tissue around it. This is the most common type.
- Sprain of the posterior intercoccygeal ligament
- Sprain of the sacrococcygeal joint
- Irritation of the coccygeal fibers of the gluteus maximus

From clinical findings as well as from the therapeutic results it can be assumed that tension in the gluteus maximus and the levator ani is a main cause of a tender coccyx.[161] Several of the conditions causing pelvic pain are specifically identified with the levator ani muscle: pelvic floor syndromes,[165] levator ani spasm syndrome,[163,314] levator spasm syndrome,[269] and levator syndrome.[252]

In addition, evaluate the gross range of motion of the whole spine as well as sacroiliac mobility. Evaluate the spinal dural system for irritability using the slump test (see Fig. 22-22), noting the range of motion in the lower limbs and spine as the dural barrier is engaged. Patrick's signs may be positive as well as straight-leg raising; the iliacus may be in spasm.[161]

The manual therapist can expect good results with ultrasound, passive joint mobilization, soft tissue manipulations including friction massage (see the section on pelvic floor disorders in Chapter 8, Soft Tissue Manipulations, and Box 8-3), and postisometric muscle relaxation (PIR) along with other conservative treatment, such as a coccyx pillow that transfers weight to the ischia, if the joint is hypomobile or subluxed and positioned in extension. A treatment of choice is often strain and counterstrain (see Fig. 23-63),[151] or PIR of the gluteus maximus (including self-treatment; see Fig. 8-65) and some-times the piriformis (see Fig. 8-66). Strain and counterstrain techniques of the obturator internus, levator ani, or pubococcygeus are also effective.[151] Surgical removal of the coccyx may be indicated if it is unstable or dislocated in a flexed position.[237] Other treatment for unstable coccyges includes local intradiskal corticosteroid injections and prolotherapy.[174,215]

It should be noted that the coccyx is directly attached to the sacrotuberous ligament[6,7] and to the dural sac by the filum terminales. Mechanical dysfunction of this small bone can impact directly on the axial skeleton by way of the dura.[238] It can create visceral dysfunctions by straining all the muscles and ligamentous structures of the pelvic floor. Somatic joint dysfunction can create symptoms that include low back pain, headaches, and even incontinence in women.[238] Conversely, visceral pain can also cause pelvic floor hypertonicity, which may deform the sacrococcygeal joint and cause back pain.

In the absence of a history of trauma to the sacrococcygeal region, a concerted effort must be made to exclude any underlying visceral disease effecting the bowel, rectum, or urogenital system. If tests are negative, the problem may simply be related to coexisting malalignment. In particular, distortion of the pelvic ring and L5 vertebral and sacrococcygeal rotation should be sought and addressed.[257] Further investigation and treatment (e.g., biofeedback and pelvic floor exercises) may be in order if the symptoms fail to respond to realignment alone.[52,300]

EVALUATION

History

A general approach to history-taking is described in Chapter 5, Assessment of Musculoskeletal Disorders and Concepts of Management; the concepts there as well as in Chapter 14, Hip, and Chapter 22, Lumbar Spine, all apply to the evaluation of the lumbar–pelvic–hip complex.

In the history, certain traumatic incidents might point to involvement of the joints of the pelvis, such as a fall on the buttock, an unexpected heel-strike, a golf swing, or abnormal stresses occurring in such activities as punting a football. Chronic pain commencing after giving birth or starting oral contraceptives is another consideration. Most patients present with the typical history of acute or chronic back pain.

The history of the patient with SIJ pain typically includes:

1. Unilateral pain, most often local to the joint (sulcus) itself, but possibly referring down the leg (usually posterolaterally and not below the knee) because of innervation from the L2 through S2 segments. It may occasionally refer into the hip, groin, or abdomen.
2. The absence of lumbar articular signs or symptoms (although patients may have lesions at both areas)
3. Pain aggravated by walking, rolling over in bed, and climbing stairs, especially when leading with the involved side
4. Increased pain with prolonged postures or with standing or sitting on the affected side ("twisted-sitting" posture)
5. Morning stiffness that eases after a short period of weight bearing

Additional considerations are whether the patient has a past history of conditions that can involve the SIJ, such as ankylosing spondylitis,[96,259] Reiter's disease,[10,90] or rheumatoid arthritis.[220]

Finally, this area is a common site for secondary malignant deposits or Paget's disease (osteitis deformans). Paget's disease is characteristically aggravated by exercise and is more severe during sleep.[56,119]

Physical Examination

When assessing patients with sacroiliac pain, remember that pain felt in this area may be referred from either the lower lumbar spine or the hip joint. The SIJ should not be examined comprehensively until after the lumbar spine and hip joint examinations, including neurologic tests. The goal of assessment is to determine what force(s) reproduces the patient's symptoms.

OBSERVATION

Observe the patient's posture, body type, and ability to move freely. Refer to Chapter 24, Lumbosacral–Lower Limb Scan Examination, for a discussion of common gait abnormalities and possible causes.

GAIT

Careful observation of the patient's gait pattern can be informative, as formal bipedal striding requires optimal lumbar–pelvic–hip function. Sacroiliac dysfunction may originate from a leg-length discrepancy and the accompanying excessive increase or decrease in lordosis. A painful SIJ may cause reflex inhibition of the gluteus medius, leading to a Trendelenburg gait or lurch.[173] The patient may sidebend the trunk away from the painful side or walk with difficulty.

POSTURE

Postural asymmetry does not necessarily indicate pelvic girdle dysfunction, but pelvic girdle dysfunction is often reflected through postural asymmetry. Observe the patient's standing posture, sitting posture (sitting on a stool or bench without back support), and long sitting. In the coronal and sagittal planes, observe the head, shoulder alignment, spinal curves, and level of the pelvis. In particular, carefully observe the distribution of body weight through the lower quadrant. In weight bearing, note whether the patient stands with equal weight on both feet or has a lateral pelvic tilt, suggesting an apparent or real leg-length discrepancy. Patients tend to bear weight on the unaffected side in standing and sitting and to step up with the unaffected side. Note the posture of the feet (pronation or supination) and the knees (hyperextension, varus, valgus). Variations in the resting position of these joints can be the result of compensation for a longstanding leg-length discrepancy. The lower limbs are also an important link in the transference of ground forces to the pelvis. In anterior dysfunction of the innominate, the lower limb may be medially rotated. With spasm of the piriformis muscle, the limb may be laterally rotated on the affected side.

In integrating the myofascial system, look for muscle asymmetry, connective tissue asymmetry, and increased muscle activity that may correlate with abnormal structural deviations. For example, muscle asymmetry may be a result of prolonged shortening or lengthening of a muscle group as a result of pelvic obliquity or a leg-length discrepancy. Although asymmetry is important, remember that the human body is by nature's design asymmetric; the critical factor in determining whether the asymmetry is significant is its correlation to other relevant evaluation findings.

INSPECTION

Bony Structure and Alignment. Refer to the section on assessment of structural alignment in Chapter 24, Lumbosacral–Lower Limb Scan Examination, for a complete discussion of this part of the examination.

I. In the standing position, compare the levels of the PSIS, the iliac crests, and the ASIS. The most common finding is the posterior innominate in which the PSIS is lower than the opposite side. The reverse is found with the anterior innominate.
   A. Palpate the summit of the greater trochanter for levelness as an indicator of apparent or structural leg-length discrepancy. See Chapter 14, Hip, for measurement of functional leg length.
   B. The depth caliper or meter stick method may be used clinically for detecting pelvic movement (Fig. 23-9).[2] Measurement of PSIS displacement is used. By this method Alviso and colleagues[2] determined an average total pelvic tilt range of 14.3°, with a standard deviation of 5.2°. Anterior pelvic tilt averaged 7.9°; posterior tilt range of motion was an average of 6.5°.
II. In sitting (erect on a level surface), repeat palpation of the bony landmarks of the innominate. Determine whether lateral pelvic tilt is still present or whether the previous lateral tilt in standing is now eradicated.
III. In hyperflexion (sitting, feet supported, knees at a right angle and apart, sufficient to allow the shoulders to come between them and the lumbar spine to be fully flexed), determine the position of the sacrum for possible sacral dysfunction (Fig. 23-10). To determine the position of the sacrum, compare the posteroanterior relation of the sacral base or the depth of the two sacral sulci and the inferior lateral angles (Fig. 23-11).[27,158]
   A. The level of the sacral base is often called the *depth of the sacral sulcus*.[100] The sacral base can be described as anterior or posterior if it is not level against the coronal

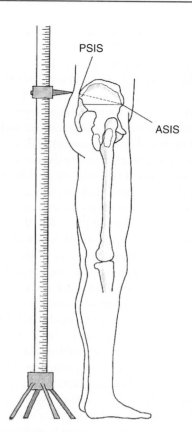

■ **FIG. 23-9.** Measurement of pelvic inclination: measuring the distance from the posterosuperior iliac spine (PSIS) to the floor. ASIS, anterosuperior iliac spine. (Adapted with permission from Basmajian JV, Nyberg R: Rational Manual Therapies. Baltimore, Williams & Wilkins, 1993:103.)

plane; if one sacral base is more anterior than the other, the sacral sulcus is said to be deep on that side. Using the thumbs, palpate the sacral depth (dorsal ventral distance) between the PSIS and the base of the sacrum, medially from the caudal aspect of the PSIS bilaterally.

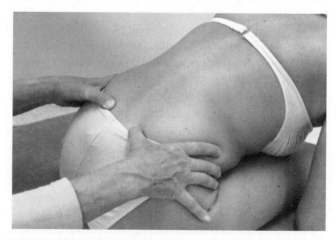

■ **FIG. 23-10.** Positional testing in hyperflexion of the lumbosacral junction.

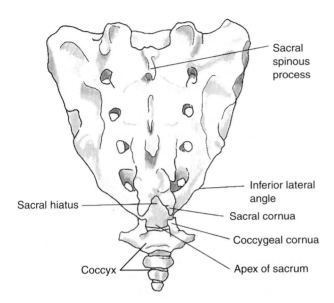

■ **FIG. 23-11.** The posterior aspect of the sacrum: anatomic landmarks used in palpation of the posterior aspect of the sacrum.

B. The *inferior lateral angle* is the transverse process of S5 and is found by placing one finger in the sacral hiatus and the index and middle fingers of the other hand on either side at the same level about 2 cm away (Fig. 23-11).[27] An anterior right sacral base or a deep (anterior) sacral sulcus, together with a left inferior lateral angle, suggests a left-rotated sacrum.[158,213] This is the most common sacral torsion dysfunction. When palpating the inferior lateral angle, one is also palpating the superior attachment of the sacrotuberous ligament. Note any tissue texture abnormality (see Fig. 18-19*B*).

As these positional findings may be manifested only in one position of the vertebral column, it is necessary to evaluate in neutral (prone) and finally in hyperextension.[158] For other types of sacral torsion lesions, refer to the works of Bourdillon and Day,[27] Greenman,[100] Lee,[158] Maitland,[178] Mitchell and colleagues,[198,199] and Woerman.[313]

IV. With the patient in supine and the crook position, have him or her lift the buttock and drop it down to the mat or treatment table, or do it for the patient. Bring the knees to the chest and slowly bring the legs down with the knees extended.

A. Check the iliac crests for asymmetry. With the radial border of the index fingers, palpate the highest point of the iliac crest bilaterally. Compare the craniocaudal relation of the two sides.

B. Check the set of the pelvis. Determine whether either ilium is inflared (one ilium ASIS is closer to the midline than the opposite ASIS) or outflared (one ilium ASIS is further from the midline than the opposite ASIS). Use an imaginary line from the tip of the xiphoid to the pubis; ignore the navel, which is often off to one side. Over time an inflared or outflared ilium will lead to muscle imbalance.

C. Palpate bilaterally the caudal aspect of the ASIS. Check for rotation (craniocaudal relation) and the anteroposterior relation (deep or higher).

D. Determine whether both pubic bones are level at the symphysis pubis. Test for levelness (craniocaudal position) by placing the thumbs on the superior aspect of each pubic bone and comparing the height (Fig. 23-12). This can be correlated with anterior or posterior dysfunction and the relation of the ASIS. In posterior dysfunction, one would expect the pubic bone also to be higher.

E. Assess leg-length equality (non–weight bearing). See Chapter 14, Hip.

V. In prone, determine the following:

A. Palpate the coccyx, noting its anteroposterior angulation, any deviations to one side, and any tenderness around its tip and any thickening or hypertrophy of the soft tissue inserting into it.

B. Determine whether the ischial tuberosities are level (superoinferior position). Using the thumbs, palpate the most caudal aspect of the ischial tuberosity bilaterally (Fig. 23-13). Compare the craniocaudal relation. If one tuberosity is higher, it may indicate an upslip of the ilium on the sacrum on that side.[313]

C. The position of the sacrum (see above). If one sacral sulcus is deeper than the other, this could indicate a possible sacral torsion or an innominate rotation. Compare the inferior lateral angles for their relative caudad–cephalad and anteroposterior positions (Fig. 23-11). If the angles are level and a deep sacral sulcus is found, it suggests a dysfunction of the innominates.[313]

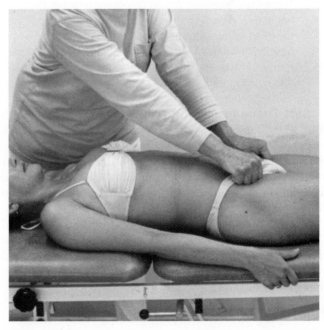

■ **FIG. 23-12.** Determining the level of the pubic tubercles.

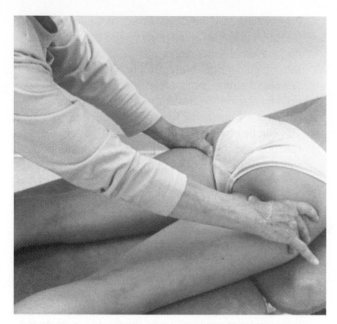

■ FIG. 23-13. Determining the position of the ischial tuberosities.

VI. In the press-up or backward-bending position (prone on elbows with the patient's chin resting in the hands and the lumbar spine in hyperextension), determine the position of the sacrum by palpating the position of the:
  A. Sacral sulci, to determine whether there has been a change in the relative depth of the sacral sulci from that noted in the neutral prone position. In sacroiliac dysfunction, the side that is blocked will remain shallow and the side that is free to move will go deeper.[100,313]
  B. The inferior lateral angles, to determine whether there has been a change in their position. If the angle opposite the deep sacral sulcus becomes more posterior in this position, it suggests a forward sacral torsion. If the angle is more inferior on the same side as the deep sacral sulcus, it suggests unilateral sacral flexion.[313]

Soft Tissue Inspection and Muscle Contour. With the patient standing, it is not unusual to observe a loss of bulk of the gluteal muscles of one side coexisting with sacroiliac dysfunction. View the abdominal outline and the lumbar region from the side. A weak protruding abdominal wall and a marked lumbar lordosis may be a source of stress falling on the pelvic joints.

With the patient prone, look for pelvic asymmetry and flattening of the buttock. Decreased tone in the glutei of the affected side may cause the hip to fall into more medial rotation compared with the opposite side.[307] Note a swollen appearance over either joint.

JOINT TESTS: SELECTIVE TISSUE–TENSION

Active Movements. See Chapter 24, Lumbosacral–Lower Limb Scan Examination, for a complete discussion of this part of the examination. Perform active physiologic movements of the spine and peripheral joints of the lower extremity. Note the quantity and quality of motion achieved. Look for loss of movement or hypermobility, the patient's willingness to move, and the presence and location of evoked symptoms.

I. Forward Flexion (standing and seated)
  A. Lumbosacral junction (flexion). While palpating the transverse processes of the L5 vertebra, determine whether any abnormal coupling (i.e., two or more types of motion occurring simultaneously, such as rotation or side flexion) manifests with flexion or extension. The transverse processes of the L5 vertebra should travel an equal distance in a superior direction. Monitor the lower thoracic and lumbar spine for segmental dysrhythmia or a compensatory scoliotic curvature.
  B. Pelvic girdle. Active physiologic mobility testing of the pelvis is a useful preliminary test of pelvic girdle function, as asymmetry of motion is present in all unilateral hypomobility disorders.[27,100,158,199,306]
  C. Standing flexion test
    1. Palpate the inferior slope of the PSIS bilaterally (following the excursion of motion), as the patient actively forward bends, for any innominate distortion (Fig. 23-14A). The PSIS should travel an equal distance in a superior direction.
    2. Repeat while palpating the sacral base or inferior lateral angles for sacral distortion (Fig. 23-14B). The angles of the sacrum should travel an equal distance in a superior direction without deviating in the anteroposterior plane. The test for innominate excursion is positive on the side in which the PSIS appears to move more cephalically and ventrally.[100] It is thought that the downward and backward glide of the two limbs of the SIJ has been lost, so the sacrum and the innominate move as a unit on the positive side.
  D. Seated flexion test. Repeat the test in sitting to rule out extrinsic influences on the pelvis from below, such as leg-length discrepancy or the effect of a tight hamstring.
    1. Position the patient seated with the feet flat on the floor and knees at right angles and apart, sufficient to allow the shoulders to come between them in forward bending. Note the spinal movements and correlate them with standing forward bending. If they have changed, the problem may be in the lower extremity.
    2. Have the patient repeat forward bending and follow the excursion of the bony processes as in standing. This assesses the movement of the sacrum with the ilium stabilized. If the PSIS moves in the same manner as in standing (more cephalically and ventrally on one side), it suggests a sacroiliac problem (as opposed to iliosacral).[306]
II. Lateral Bending (standing). Note the ability of the pelvic girdle to translate laterally to the opposite side without deviation. See Chapter 18, Spine, for the specific osteokinematics required during this test.

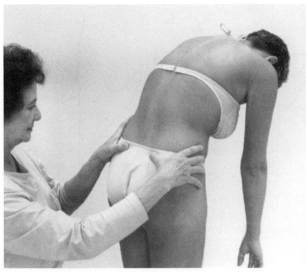

A

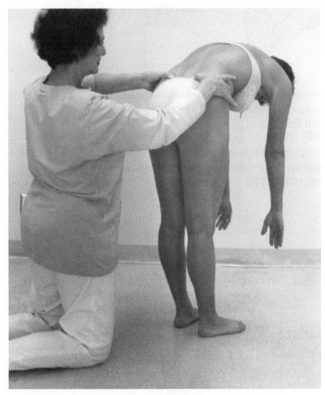

B

■ **FIG. 23-14.** Active physiologic mobility tests: **(A)** forward bending of innominate bones and **(B)** forward bending of the sacrum.

III. Auxiliary Tests. In most patients with symptoms arising from the SIJ, the active tests described above are sufficient to reproduce the patient's symptoms. If not, consider applying passive overpressure at the end range of the active physiologic motions described above or using repeated motions, sustained pressure, and combined motions of the

active physiologic motions of the spine as well as combined motions with overpressure (see Chapter 22, Lumbar Spine). When applying passive overpressure, consider whether the overpressure is increasing compressive or tensile forces to the area.

IV. Hip Mobility (weight-bearing flexion). Have the patient perform a bilateral or unilateral squat. Functionally, the dynamic stabilization of the hip joint and its ability to bear full weight during flexion and standing is of paramount importance.

V. Sacroiliac Fixation Tests.[144,145] Several tests have been devised to demonstrate sacroiliac fixation. This signifies ipsilateral locking, in which the sacrum and ilium move as a whole owing to muscular contraction that prevents motion of the sacrum on the ilium (intrapelvic torsion). These tests include the one-legged stork test,[27,100] the ipsilateral kinetic test,[85,158,160] Gillet's test,[313] and Piedallu's sign.[101,227,256]

A. With the patient standing and using one hand for support on a table or the back of a chair, palpate the inferior aspect of the PSIS with one thumb while using the other to palpate the median sacral crest directly parallel (spinous process of S2). Have the patient flex the ipsilateral femur at the hip joint and knee to 90°. Observe the displacement of the PSIS relative to the sacrum (Fig. 23-15A–C). This test examines the ability of the innominate bone to laterally flex and laterally rotate, as well as the ability of the sacrum to rotate.[158]

B. In a similar manner, place one thumb over the last sacral spinous process and the other thumb over the ischial tuberosity. Have the patient repeat hip flexion as above, and observe the displacement of the thumb on the ischial tuberosity (Fig. 23-15D–F). Repeat both tests on the opposite side and compare the results.

C. A third test is required to examine the ability of the innominate bone to extend and medially rotate.[158] With the patient prone, palpate the PSIS with one thumb while the other palpates the median sacral crest directly opposite. Have the patient extend the ipsilateral femur at the hip joint. Note the superolateral displacement of the PSIS relative to the sacrum.

Passive Movements

I. Lumbosacral Junction (L5 vertebra and the sacral base). Osteokinematic tests of physiologic mobility and arthrokinematic tests of accessory motion should be performed as described in Chapter 22, Lumbar Spine.

II. Pelvic Girdle: Osteokinematic Tests of Physiologic Mobility
   A. Pelvic rock test (Fig. 23-16). The pelvic rock test involves getting a sense of the mobility of the joint and the end feel for the relative ease or resistance to passive overpressure for each innominate. With the subject in supine, place the palms on the ASIS and gently glide and then spring or shear the innominates alternately in a medial anteroposterior direction (in the plane of the joint). While maintaining light pressure on the opposite side, press more firmly on first one side and then the other to detect

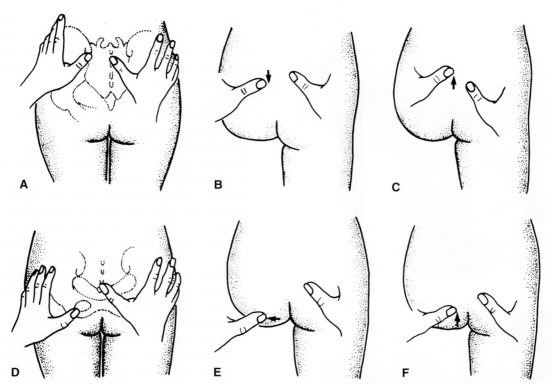

■ FIG. 23-15. Test for sacroiliac joint fixation. The patient is examined in standing and is instructed to flex the hip and knee to 90° during each test. To test the upper part of joint (left side): **(A)** Place one thumb over the spinous process of S2 and the other hand over the PSIS. **(B)** In the normal joint the thumb will move caudally. **(C)** In the abnormally fixed joint the thumb will move cephalad. To assess the lower part of the joint: **(D)** Place one thumb over the last sacral spinous process and the other thumb over the ischial tuberosity. **(E)** In the normal joint the thumb will move laterally. **(F)** In the abnormally fixed joint the thumb will remain stationary. (Reprinted with permission from Kirkalday-Willis WH, ed: Managing Low Back Pain, 2nd ed. New York, Churchill Livingstone, 1988:137.)

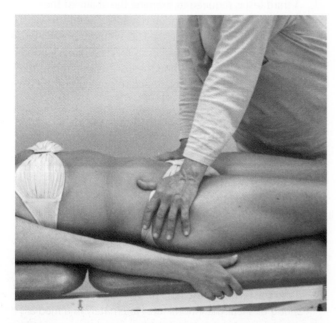

■ FIG. 23-16. Pelvic rock test (anteroposterior glide of the innominate). Alternately glide the innominate bone in an anterior–posterior direction.

resilience. A harder end feel on one side indicates a probable restriction of movement on that side.

B. Flexion–extension of the innominate bone (Fig. 23-17). With the patient sidelying, hips and knees comfortably flexed, contact the ASIS with one hand while the other contacts the ipsilateral ischial tuberosity. The innominate bone is passively flexed and extended (posteriorly and anteriorly rotated) on the sacrum; note the quantity of motion.

III. Pelvic Girdle: Arthrokinematic Tests of Accessory Joint Mobility

A. Anteroposterior iliac glide (Fig. 23-18).[75,307] With the patient lying prone, palpate the sacral base with the fingertips of the cranial hand, placing them over the joint in question (over the short posterior sacral ligaments). The ilium, held by hooking the fingers under the ASIS with the caudal hand, is gently and repeatedly lifted in an anteroposterior direction. If the amplitude of movement is too large it will merely rotate the lumbar spine and override the small but detectable joint play. The palpating fingers register the relative displacement between the iliac bone and the sacrum, which should be about 2 to 3 mm.[75]

B. Sacrococcygeal region. Posteroanterior central coccygeal pressures (see Fig. 23-66), anteroposterior coccygeal pres-

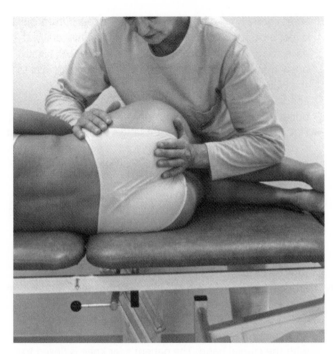

■ **FIG. 23-17.** Passive flexion–extension (posteroanterior rotation) of the innominate bone.

sures (see Fig. 23-64), and transverse coccygeal pressures described in the treatment section are used as examination techniques in the presence of sacrococcygeal and intercoccygeal dysfunction. This area is quite commonly the site of pain, and it is not always easy to determine whether the pain is a referred phenomenon from the lumbosacral area or whether it is a local pain from a joint disorder.

Arthrokinematic Tests of Stability. Movement of the SIJ is produced by a series of passive movements designed to stress the joint or ligaments and to reproduce the patient's pain. That numerous tests have been devised is proof of their inadequacy. The stress tests also stress other structures, so false-positive and false-negative results are common.[51]

I. Sacral Apex Pressure Test or Tripod Test.[51,75,103,307] The patient lies prone. Apply vertical pressure to the sacrum with the heel of the caudal hand. Rock the sacrum by repetitive pressure to its apex. Because the three-point contact of the pubis and the anterior ends of the ilium with the surface of the treatment table will stabilize the pelvis, repetitive downward pressures on the sacral apex will induce a small degree of movement of the sacrum on the ilium. This may be detected with the palpating fingers of the cephalad hand in the sulcus; compare it with the opposite side. If reproduction of symptoms is sought (stress test), the pressure is carefully but increasingly firmly applied with one hand reinforcing the other; the arms are kept fully extended (Fig. 23-19). This produces a shearing movement across the SIJs as well as movement of the lumbosacral joint. Incline the hand medially or laterally, or in a cephalad or caudad direction, to amplify the findings.

   Note: In manual therapy practice, testing procedures are often used as subsequent treatment techniques. The sacral apex pressure test is a good example. As a technique it is considered a sacral counternutation manipulation to increase joint play and range of motion into sacral counternutation or to reduce a sacral nutation positional fault. Bilateral sacral flexion dysfunction may be thought of as a failure to return from a fully nutated position; bilateral sacral extension dysfunction may be thought of as a failure to return from the fully counternutated position.

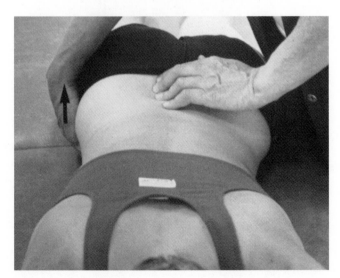

■ **FIG. 23-18.** Anteroposterior gliding of the innominate to detect movement of the sacroiliac joint.

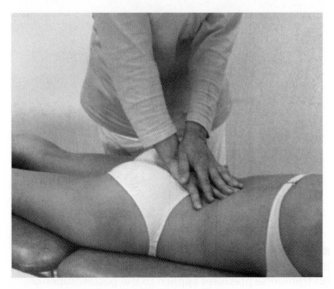

■ **FIG. 23-19.** Sacral apex pressure test.

II. Posteroanterior and Transverse Oscillatory Pressure (Fig. 23-20).[177,307] Unlike pressures applied to the spinal joints to explore the characteristics of accessory motion, these pressures, when applied to the sacroiliac region, are used to determine whether they provoke or relieve the patient's symptoms. Such pressures may also be used as treatment. Thumb pressures are directed over the sacrum and adjacent ilium in an attempt to reproduce the patient's symptoms.

This useful routine was suggested by Wells.[307] With the patient in prone, first direct posteroanterior thumb pres-

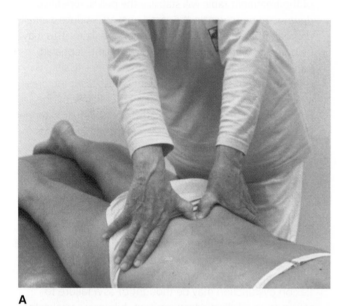

A

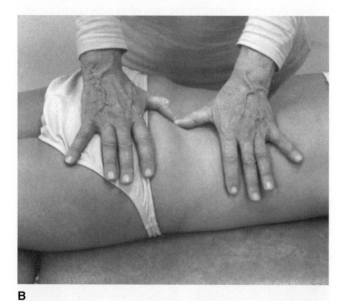

B

▪ **FIG. 23-20.** Oscillatory pressures: **(A)** posteroanterior pressures applied unilaterally at each sacral level and **(B)** transverse pressures applied to the posterosuperior iliac spine.

sures centrally on each sacral spinous process in turn. Next, direct posteroanterior oscillatory pressures unilaterally at each sacral level and over each PSIS (Fig. 23-20A). Finally, apply transverse pressures directed laterally just medial to the PSIS (Fig. 23-20B).

III. Longitudinal Stress of the Sacrum (craniocaudal and caudocranial pressures or caudocephalad shearing procedures; Fig. 23-21).[51,103,104,307] To test these two motions, the patient is placed in the prone position. Place the heel of one hand near the apex of the sacrum and apply pressure in a cephalad direction while the heel of the other hand stabilizes the posterior third of the iliac crest. Next, apply pressure near the base of the sacrum in a caudad direction while the ilium is stabilized at the ischial tuberosity.

Note: These tests may be useful as gentle treatment techniques, applied to areas of pain noted when used as tests of sacroiliac strain.

IV. Prone Gapping Test (Fig. 23-22).[104,307] This test can be done only if the hip is normal and full internal rotation is painless. With the patient prone, stabilize the pelvis with your thigh or abdomen while palpating the sacroiliac sulcus with the cranial hand. The patient's far knee is flexed to 90° and the hip placed in end range medial rotation while small-range oscillatory stresses are placed on the hip by the caudal hand and forearm. A small amount of sacroiliac gapping can be appreciated by the palpating fingers. Repeat the test on the opposite side, comparing the degree of opening and the quality of movement.

Note: This test is another that can be used as a treatment procedure.[101] Gentle repetitive movements can be

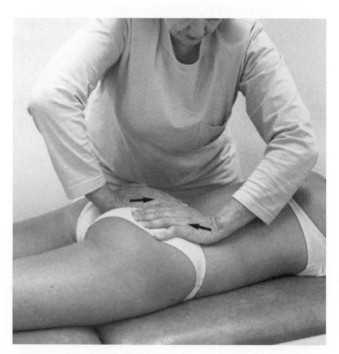

▪ **FIG. 23-21.** Longitudinal stress applied to the sacrum (in a cephalad direction) and the ilium (in a caudad direction).

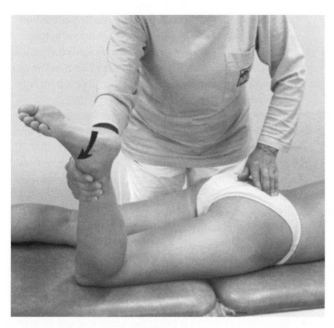

■ **FIG. 23-22.** Prone gapping test.

very precisely graded when used as a treatment procedure.

V. Torsional Stress (Fig. 23-23).[307] With the patient in the prone position, stabilize the sacrum at its apex with the caudad hand while the cephalad hand simultaneously applies vertical downward pressure over the PSIS on the far side. According to Wells,[307] this maneuver is particularly informative when examining a chronically hypomobile and nonirritable joint problem. Repeated

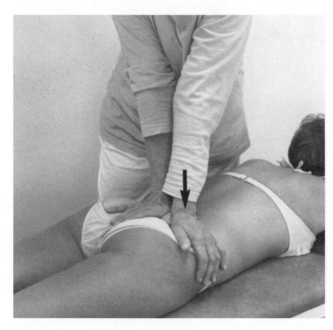

■ **FIG. 23-23.** Torsional stress test.

oscillatory pressures reveal a markedly unyielding response in this case.

Note: This evaluation procedure can also be used either as an effective mobilization or manipulation technique for posterior dysfunction of the innominate.[103]

VI. Compression–Distraction Tests (transverse anterior stress test and gapping test; Fig. 23-24).[51,126,173,255,313] Compression–distraction tests are used to ascertain a serious disease or the presence of hypermobility and to stress the ligaments and joint. The subject lies supine while the examiner applies crossed-arm pressure to the ASIS with the heels of the hands (Fig. 23-24A). The slack is taken up and a posterolateral spring is given. This action compresses the SIJs posteriorly and gaps them anteriorly, stressing the anterior sacroiliac ligaments and the transverse pubic ligament. Then move the hands to the lateral iliac wings and compress the pelvis toward the midline of the body (Fig. 23-24B). Doing

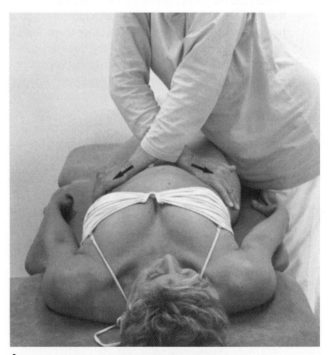

A

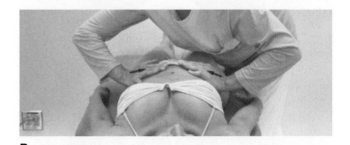

B

■ **FIG. 23-24.** Compression–distraction test using the crossed hand method (**A**) and (**B**) from the lateral aspect of the innominate.

so compresses the anterior and distracts the posterior SIJs and ligaments. Some authors suggest applying a slow, steady force through the pelvic girdle (maintained for 20 seconds) rather than a springlike force.[158]

VII. Isometric Contraction of Hip Abductors and Adductors (Fig. 23-25)[51,85,199]

A. Hip abduction (Fig. 23-25A). The patient is supine with knees bent, feet flat on the treatment table, hips slightly abducted. The pelvis is in a neutral position. Place each hand on the lateral aspect of each of the patient's knees. Have the patient resist a force provided by the examiner into hip abduction, thus distracting the iliac joint surfaces away from the sacrum as the abductors contract and pull on their attachment to the iliac crest.

B. Hip adduction (Fig. 23-25B). With the patient in the same position as above, the adductors of the hip are isometrically contracted by attempting to maximally adduct the hip joints against the examiner's hands, thereby recruiting the patient's short adductors. Adduction stresses the symphysis pubis because these short muscles cross the inferior aspect of the pubic articulation in a cruciate manner; when recruited, they strongly bring the joint into a balanced level position.[85] A slight popping noise is often elicited; this is thought to bring the joint strongly into a level position.[85,199]

After this test, the fixation and positioning tests are reevaluated. If no change has occurred, a sacroiliac or iliosacral dysfunction is the probable cause.

Pain experienced over the SIJ on resisted abduction (in the absence of hip joint disease) in sidelying (positional test with the knee extended) is highly suggestive of an SIJ lesion. According to Macnab,[172] when the gluteus maximus contracts to abduct the hip, it pulls the ilium away from the sacrum.

VIII. Pubic Symphysis Gap Test with Isometric Adduction Contraction (Fig. 23-26).[246] The patient is in a 90°/90° hip and knee position with the legs supported by the examiner. The patient then performs an isometric adductor muscle contraction against the examiner's fist; painful isometric muscle action is considered a positive test result.

IX. Active Straight-Leg Test (Fig. 23-27).[162,193–195] This test can be used to verify which SIJ is unstable and as a posttreatment check to determine whether a trail test is of value. The patient lies supine and actively lifts (knee straight) one leg at a time 20 cm off the table. The test is positive if:
- The leg cannot be raised off the table.
- Significant heaviness of the leg is reported.
- Decreased strength is exhibited when manual resistance is added.
- Significant ipsilateral trunk rotation occurs.

It has been shown that altered kinematics of the diaphragm and pelvic floor muscles are present in those with a positive active straight-leg test.[217]

X. Sacrotuberous Ligament Stress Test (Fig. 23-28).[157,158,173,232] With the patient in a supine position, the contralateral hip and knee are fully flexed and then adducted. The innominate bone is flexed and medially rotated until tension of

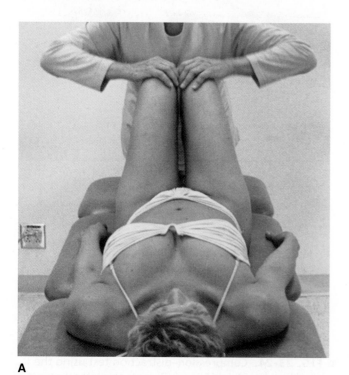
A

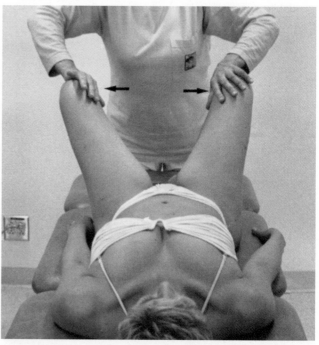
B

■ FIG. 23-25. Isometric contractions: (A) hip abduction and (B) hip adduction.

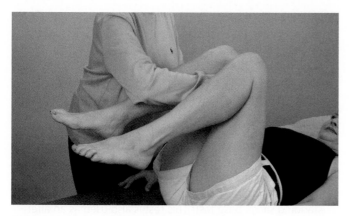

■ **FIG. 23-26.** Pubic symphysis gap test.

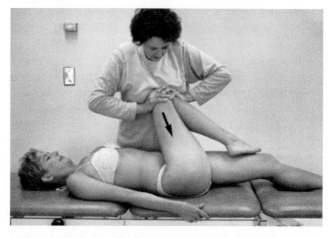

■ **FIG. 23-28.** Sacrotuberous ligament stress test.

the sacrotuberous ligament is perceived. From this position, a slow, steady, longitudinal (axial-loading) force is applied with both hands through the femur in an obliquely lateral direction to stress the posterior sacroiliac ligament further. The force is maintained for 20 seconds; note whether local pain is provoked.[158] Another example of using the femur as a lever is to rock the SIJ by flexion and adduction of the hip, moving the knee toward the patient's opposite shoulder.[173] A long-axis force is then applied down through the femur until all the tissues have become taut, and then a small adduction force is imparted through the shaft of the femur, which compresses the anterior aspect of the SIJ and results in a significant gapping at the posterior aspect.[232] These tests induce ligamentous stretch pain, indicating a functionally shortened or stressed (overloaded) posterior sacroiliac ligament.[75]

XI. Femoral Shear Test (Fig. 23-29).[173,232] With the patient in the supine position, the leg is flexed, abducted, and laterally rotated until the thigh is at about 45°, so as to line up the force with the plane of the ipsilateral SIJ. Apply a graded force through the long axis of the femur, causing an anteroposterior shear to the SIJ.

Note: There are many other tests commonly used to stress the SIJ, including the Patrick or Fabere test,[75,118,126,313] the Gaenslen test,[118,126,173] Gillet's (sacral fixation) test,[313]

the flamingo test or single-leg stand,[156,173] Yeoman's test,[47,173,256] and Goldthwait's test.[47,173,256]

Tests To Determine Functional Leg-Length Difference

I. Supine-to-Sit Test (long-sitting test).[8,9,75,228,255,296,313] This test is used to assess the ability of the SIJs to move in response

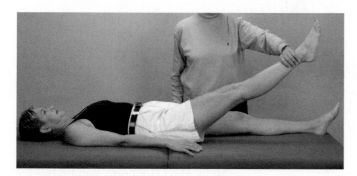

■ **FIG. 23-27.** Active straight-leg raise test.

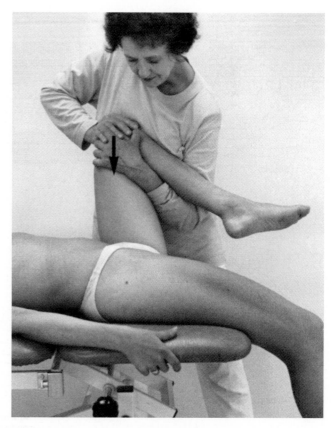

■ **FIG. 23-29.** Femoral shear test.

to external forces that passively rotate the innominates (Fig. 23-30). To ensure a neutral alignment of the pelvis on the table, the patient performs a bridging technique, which consists of flexing the knees to place the feet flat on the table, extending the hips to lift the buttocks from the surface, and then relaxing to allow the buttocks to return to the table. With the subject in the supine position, compare the positions of the medial malleoli using the borders of the thumbs. Have the patient sit with the knees extended and recheck the malleoli for symmetry. Caudad positioning of one malleolus may indicate posterior rotation of the ilium. If the standing flexion test is positive on the same side, then this test is considered positive. Conversely, a cephalad malleolus indicates an anteriorly rotated ilium. This phenomenon (short to long or equal to long) is thought to occur because in the posterior innominate, posterior rotation of the innominate moves the acetabulum in a superior direction and carries the leg along with it; the opposite occurs in anterior rotation. A difference of less than 2 cm is probably not clinically significant.[75]

Note: A study by Bemis and Daniel[9] suggests that this test is an accurate method of predicting iliosacral dysfunction. As with other tests, however, it should not be used alone but in conjunction with other conformational data for accurate diagnosis.

II. Wilson–Barlow Test of Pelvic Motion Symmetry.[199,255,313] The patient lies supine and flexes the knees and hips. Grasp the ankles with the thumbs under the medial malleoli. To equalize the patient's position on the table, have the patient then lift the buttocks from the table, then return to the resting position. Next, passively extend the patient's legs toward yourself, maintaining good alignment. Compare the positions of the malleoli using the borders of the thumbs. A difference in leg length should agree with the standing sacral base test. This test is also used as an alternative test for the standing and seated flexion tests. Additional steps include:

A. Passive flexion of one leg on the abdomen and then abduction, external rotation, and extension of the leg. Then compare the malleoli for levelness. The leg should appear longer.

B. Flexion of the same leg on the abdomen, internal rotation, and then extension. The leg should appear shorter.

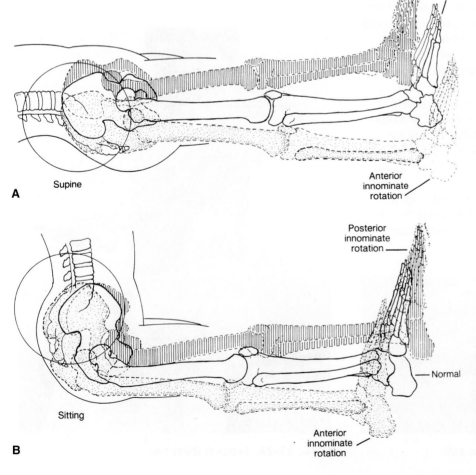

■ **FIG. 23-30.** Supine-to-sit test. Leg-length reversal: supine (**A**) versus sitting (**B**). (Reprinted with permission from Wadsworth CT, ed: Manual Examination and Treatment of the Spine and Extremities. Baltimore, Williams & Wilkins, 1988:82.)

Failure of the leg to shorten or lengthen may indicate pelvic dysfunction.

III. Testing for Leg Length (prone).[100,198] The patient is prone with the dorsum of the foot free at the edge of the table. Both legs are pulled toward the operator to ensure good alignment. Palpate the medial malleoli to determine any differences in length. This test is used to evaluate the position of the sacrum between the two innominates (which are triangulated on the examination table by the symphysis pubis and the two ASIS). It is also used to evaluate sacroiliac dysfunction. Whether functional leg shortness will develop depends on the ability of the lumbar curvature to adapt to the tilted sacral base.

In all these examinations, observer error is possible. Also, these non–weight-bearing tests for the most part disregard the neuromuscular control of movement. Gravity-eliminated body mechanics are very different from the body mechanics in antigravity standing, and standing assessment is thought to yield more clinically relevant information.

MUSCLE TESTS

Myokinematic Tests for Muscle Function. The entire lumbar and hip regions should be evaluated or screened because sacroiliac dysfunction occurs in combination with tissue injury to other lumbopelvic tissues. The pelvic girdle is the link between the lower limbs and the spine. Ligaments and fascia connect the lumbar spine, pelvis, and femur and should be tested when this area is being assessed. Important ligaments and fascia include the thoracolumbar (lumbodorsal) fascia, iliolumbar ligament, lateral fascia of the thigh, sacroiliac ligament, sacrotuberous ligament, sacrospinous ligament, and iliotibial band. The ligamentous structures (iliofemoral, ischiofemoral, and pubofemoral ligaments) and the hip joint's fibrous capsule also influence the lower limb kinetic chain. Restrictions, contractures, or laxity of the capsule can result in hip and lower quadrant mechanical dysfunction.

If the pelvis is not symmetrically balanced, then muscle imbalances occur, and with time some muscles will develop tightness while their antagonists will develop stretch weakness. Several muscles link the lumbar spine, sacrum, pelvis, and lower limbs into one kinetic chain, so any muscle imbalance or injury can influence the whole kinetic chain. A common finding in the examination of sacroiliac dysfunction is decreased passive range of motion on the side of the lesion. Hip capsule tightness or muscle shortness creates a biomechanical alteration that makes the SIJ vulnerable to overuse and sprain from what would otherwise be activities within normal tolerance.

I. Sagittal Plane Alignment
  A. Anterior or posterior rotation dysfunction. If a unilateral posterior innominate rotation exists, the gluteus maximus, hamstrings, and adductor magnus on that side tend to become shortened and tight while the hip flexors, sartorius, and remaining adductors become stretched and weak on the affected side.[118] Conversely, if unilateral anterior rotation dysfunction exists, the hip flexors,

adductors, and tensor fasciae latae become tight on that side while the hamstrings, glutei, and abdominals become stretched and weak. Anterior or posterior dysfunction can cause these muscle imbalances, or these rotations can result from muscle imbalances. These rotations can cause SIJ dysfunction and eventual hip and lumbar spine problems.

  B. Anterior or posterior tilt. Excessive anterior or posterior tilt of the whole pelvis can lead to muscle imbalances and can also subject the SIJ, the lumbar spine, and the hip joint to abnormal forces and loads.
  1. If there is an anterior pelvic tilt, the lumbar spine moves into excessive lordosis and the lumbosacral angle increases. The hip flexors (chiefly the iliopsoas) and erector spinae shorten and become tight, and the abdominals, glutei, and hamstrings become stretched and weakened.[118] The anterior longitudinal ligaments in the lumbar spine and the sacrotuberous, sacroiliac, and sacrospinous ligaments are stretched.[221] There is increased compression of the lumbar spine posteriorly on the vertebrae and the articulating facets.[141]
  2. If there is a posterior pelvic tilt, the lumbar spine moves into a flat-back posture, characterized by a decreased lumbosacral angle (see Fig. 7-24). In the flat-back posture (rigid), the lumbar paraspinals become lengthened, and perhaps the hip flexors, while the hamstrings and adductor magnus become tight.[118] There is compression of the lumbar vertebrae anteriorly, stretching of the hip capsule,[221] and stress to the posterior longitudinal ligament. Kendall and associates[141] describe the flexible flat-back posture in which the low back muscles are usually normal and the abdominal muscles, especially the lower abdominals, tend to be stronger than normal. The hip extensors are usually strong and the hamstrings are short.

II. Frontal Plane Alignment. A unilateral change in limb length in the closed kinetic chain position in the presence of tight muscles can alter mechanics and cause pain anywhere in the body.[301] If the leg is longer, the ilium on that side is higher, which causes imbalances of forces through the SIJ, hip joint, pubic symphysis, sacrum, lumbar spine, and whole lower limb.[118] Altered weight-bearing forces also go through the opposite side. On the long side the quadratus lumborum, iliocostalis lumborum, iliopsoas, obliques, and rectus abdominis become tight, while the hamstrings, adductors, rectus femoris, sartorius, and tensor fasciae latae become stretched and weak.[118] The opposite muscle imbalances occur on the side of the shorter leg. Subjects with leg-length differences are generally weaker on the short side.[22,301]

Any alteration of the joints or muscles in the lower quadrant can result in a functional leg-length difference—that is, a foot with pronation that produces a shortening effect, or the knee in recurvatum with a weak quadriceps and gastrocnemius, which generally has a lengthening effect.[301] Anterior rotation dysfunction (ASIS low) causes a functional lengthening; posterior rotation causes a functional shortening. It is easy to miss a small right–left difference if the patient is evaluated only in a non–weight-bearing position.

With lateral pelvic tilt (a sideways tilt of the pelvis from neutral position, often associated with handedness pattern), the posterior lateral trunk muscles and thoracolumbar fascia are tighter on the high side of the pelvis, and the leg abductors and tensor fasciae latae are tighter on the low side of the pelvis.[141]

III. Transverse Plane Alignment[118]
A. On the outflare side, the adductors, obliques, and sartorius become tight; the gluteus medius, minimus, and tensor fasciae latae become stretched and weak.
B. On the inflare side, the gluteus medius, minimus, and tensor fasciae latae become tight; the adductors, obliques, and sartorius become stretched and weak. These muscle imbalances twist the pelvic girdle and cause excessive rotational forces through the lumbar spine and the whole lower limb on the involved side. The hip joint becomes rotated, and the symphysis pubis, SIJ, or lumbar spine may develop dysfunction.

Muscle Tests: Examination of Lower Quadrant Movement Patterns and Muscle Strength.

Muscle tests are the same as those of the lumbar spine and hip joint (see Chapters 14, Hip, and 22, Lumbar Spine). If indicated, muscle testing should include a detailed examination of the contractile tissue function of all the muscles attaching to the lumbar–pelvic–hip complex. This may involve:

- Resisted isometrics for the presence of pain. It should be noted that resisted isometric contraction of the gluteus medius pulls the ilium away from the sacrum. In the absence of hip joint disease, pain experienced over the SIJ is highly suggestive of a sacroiliac lesion.[55]
- Muscle strength. Relative to the pelvic girdle, the phasic muscles that tend to weaken (the abdominals, gluteus maximus, medius, and minimus) should be specifically assessed for strength. Also observe for sequencing, quality, and coordination of muscle activity during movement. Muscle strength testing of the pelvic floor muscles can provide pertinent information about factors that may contribute to lumbopelvic dysfunction.
- Positional strength can be used to determine the length–tension properties of the relevant muscle. If a muscle tests weak in the short range, it most likely is an elongated muscle.[141] Positional strength combined with mobility tests and functional movement tests can determine the length, strength, and function about the SIJ and hip joint.[113,114]
- Muscle endurance. Evidence indicates that endurance has more protective value than strength; strength gains should not be overemphasized at the expense of endurance.[169,180,181] See endurance tests of the trunk muscles in Chapter 22, Lumbar Spine, and Figures 22-19 through 22-21.

- Muscle control and stability. Tests for muscle control and stability include:

A. Neutral lordosis or heel slide (abdominals; Fig. 23-31).[283] With the patient lying supine with the hip joints flexed to at least 60° and the soles of the feet flat on the table, have the patient pull in their abdominals by pulling the navel to the spine. While maintaining a neutral spine, with co-contraction of the transversus abdominis and the lumbar multifidus, have the patient slide one foot along the table; if this is performed easily, have him or her slide both feet. This test assesses the ability of the lower abdominals to maintain a neutral spine while the iliopsoas muscles are activated. It is important to note the activation of the low and middle fibers of the transversus abdominus that attach to the pelvic rim. No dominant abdominal muscle activation should occur above the level of midway between the umbilicus and the xiphisternum.

B. Hip extension (gluteus maximus).[24,131,138] The patient is prone with the knees extended. Three muscle groups are principally involved when the patient extends the leg actively: the gluteus maximus and hamstrings acting as prime movers, and the erector spinae, which stabilize the lumbar spine and pelvis. The correct order of patterning is ipsilateral hamstrings first, then gluteus maximus, contralateral erector spinae, and ipsilateral erector spinae. Signs of altered patterning may include the following:

1. The hamstrings and erector spinae are readily activated during the contraction, with delayed or minimal contraction of the gluteus maximus. This action may be strong enough to produce active hip extension, with little weakness noted on manual muscle testing.

2. The poorest pattern occurs when the erector spinae initiate the movement, and the activity of the gluteus maximus is again delayed or weak. Little hip extension occurs, and the leg lift is achieved through forward pelvic tilt and hyperextension of the lumbar spine.

According to Bookhout,[24] chronic hamstring tightness may be a response to the substitution pattern for gluteus maximus weakness and will continue unless this muscle imbalance is corrected.

Hip extension also tests the ability of the ilium to extended and medially rotate and the ability of the

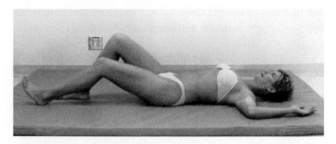

■ FIG. 23-31. Pelvic tilt or heel slide test for the ability of the lower abdominals to maintain a posterior pelvic tilt.

sacrum to rotate. Lack of superolateral movement of the PSIS while palpating the sacrum and PSIS on the side of active hip extension suggests hypomobility of the SIJ on that side.[159]

C. Hip abduction (gluteus medius and minimus).[131,138] The patient lies on the side with the lower leg flexed and the upper leg extended. When abducting the leg, the gluteus medius and minimus and the tensor fasciae latae act as prime movers, while the quadratus lumborum stabilizes the pelvis. Signs of an altered pattern of movement can be observed (as well as palpated) when:

1. The patient's leg laterally rotates during upward movement, indicating that the tensor fasciae latae has initiated and even dominated the movement performance.

2. The patient compensates for weakness of the glutei by allowing flexion and lateral rotation, indicating substitution of hip flexors and iliopsoas activity for true abduction movement.

3. The quadratus lumborum acts not only to stabilize the pelvis but also to initiate the movement through lateral pelvic tilt. This pattern of movement can cause excessive stress to the lumbosacral segments and lumbar spine during walking.

D. Pelvic clocks and pelvic diagonal patterns. Pelvic clocks[25,30] (see Fig. 23-67) and proprioceptive neuromuscular facilitation (PNF) diagonal pelvic patterns of motion (Box 23-1)[1,251] can be used to assess general coordination and kinesthetic awareness of this area and ability to isolate movement, as well as tolerance and control of small combined movements. Pain or inability to perform a specific portion of the pelvic clock or diagonal pattern can often be correlated to segmental vertebral or sacral motion restrictions. Bookhout[25] suggests that type II extended–rotated–sidebent (ERS) and flexed–rotated–sidebent (FRS) dysfunctions can be correlated to pelvic clock quadrant dysfunction. Osteopathic type II lesions are named for their osteoarticular positional diagnosis (see Appendix Table A-1). The actual dysfunction is in the opposite direction and may be caused by articular or neuromuscular elements, or by elements of both.

Examination of Lower Quadrant Muscle Length. Relative to the pelvic girdle, the postural muscles that tend to tighten should be assessed for their extensibility and influence on the mobility of the lumbar–pelvic–hip complex.[130–132] The postural muscles include:

A. Erector spinae and quadratus lumborum. Tightness of the erector spinae and quadratus lumborum is revealed in the seated forward bending position. Note the quantity of the available motion, the symmetry or asymmetry of the paravertebral muscles, and the presence or absence of a multisegmental spinal curve at the limit of range. Multisegmental rotoscoliosis may indicate unilateral tightness of the erector spinae or the quadratus lumborum.[158]

An insight into quadratus lumborum tightness can be gained by positioning the patient in a half-sidelying position (Fig. 23-32).[131] Note any changes in the shape of the lumbar curve. Normally there is a smooth, symmetrical lateral curve; when the quadratus lumborum is tight, the lumbar spine remains straight or the curve reverses itself. Simultaneously, abnormal tension can be felt on deep palpation.

B. Hamstrings. The hamstring muscles may be assessed in the conventional straight-leg raise in supine with the knee extended. Monitor any subsequent flexion of the innominate bone via the anterior aspect of the iliac crest. A straight-leg raise with the hip in lateral rotation and abduction tests the length of the medial hamstrings. A straight-leg raise with the hip in medial rotation and adduction tests the length of the lateral hamstrings.[24]

The knee extension test in the sitting position offers a significant insight into restrictive hamstring length, in the presence of excessive flexibility of the lumbar spine rather than the hip extensors (flexion syndrome according to Sahrmann[249,250]). Typical findings in this syndrome are short abdominal muscles and associated paraspinal atrophy (multifidi).[249] While sitting in 90° of hip flexion with the lumbar spine neutral, have the patient extend the knee. Monitor the lumbar spine and pelvic girdle to assess the motion of the lumbar spine during knee extension. The patient should be able to extend the knees within 10° of complete extension without lumbar flexion or rotation and without eliciting pain.[249]

C. Iliopsoas, rectus femoris, tensor fasciae latae, and the adductors. With the patient lying at the end of the firm treatment table, one leg is flexed toward the chest and maintained in this position by the examiner or by the patient holding onto the knee, allowing the pelvis to tilt back and the lumbar spine to assume a flattened or neutral position. Monitor the low back position. If the knee is pulled too far forward and the back is allowed to assume a kyphotic position, the result is that the one-joint hip flexors, which may be normal in length, will appear short. The flexed leg may be supported against the examiner's trunk (Fig. 23-33A). The leg to be tested must hang free of the table.

1. Initially observe the position of the leg to assess the length of the iliopsoas and the relative length of the rectus femoris. A tight iliopsoas muscle will restrict extension of the femur; a tight rectus will restrict knee flexion. End feel is noted, and passive overpressure is applied to hip extension and knee flexion.

2. If the anterior band of the tensor fasciae latae is tight, full femoral extension and knee flexion will occur; however, knee flexion will be possible only in conjunction with lateral tibial torsion.[158] If tibial rotation is passively blocked during the test, knee flexion will be restricted. Passive overpressure should also be applied to adductions. Hip adduction of less than 15 to 20°

BOX 23-1　PELVIC PATTERNS

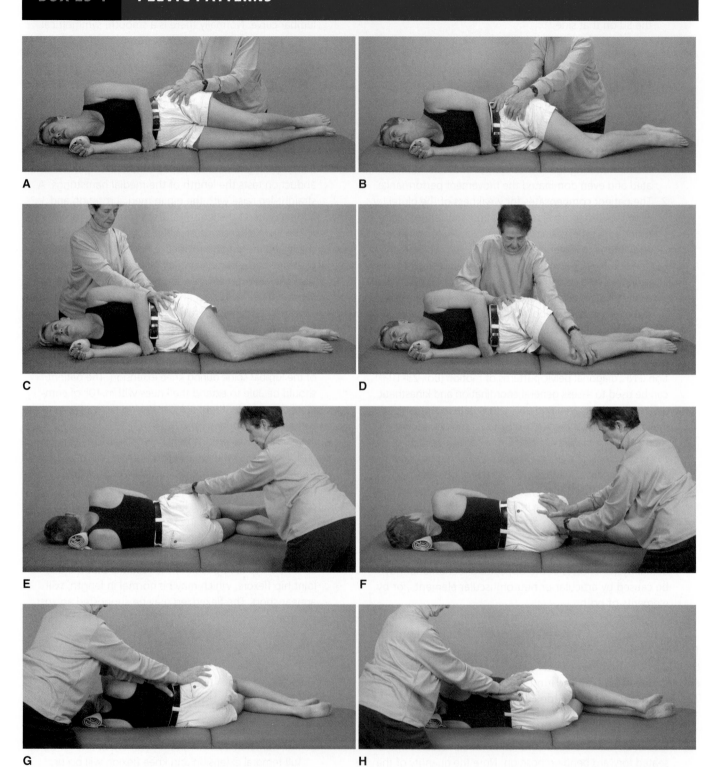

Anterior elevation: (**A**) elongation position and (**B**) end position. Anterior depression: (**C**) elongated position and (**D**) end position with alternative grip on patient's knee. Posterior depression: (**E**) elongated position and (**F**) end position. Posterior elevation: (**G**) elongated position with grip on the greater trochanter and (**H**) end position.

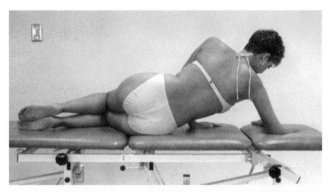

■ **FIG. 23-32.** Muscle length test of the quadratus lumborum.

indicates tightness of the tensor fasciae and iliotibial band.[138] There will be an associated increased deepening on the outside of the thigh over the iliotibial tract.

3. To isolate the two-joint hip adductors from the one-joint adductors, the leg is abducted with the knee in extension (Fig. 23-33*B*), and the test is repeated with the knee flexed to 90°. A decreased range of abduction with the knee straight is a sign of shortness of the long adductors (two-joint adductors); a decreased range and compensatory flexion of the hip joint are signs of shortness of the one-joint thigh adductors.[131]

D. Piriformis. The patient lies supine with the hip flexed to 90° on the side where the muscle is being examined. At this point, the piriformis muscle acts as a pure abductor of the femur. Before 60° it also laterally rotates the femur, but after 60° it medially rotates the femur.[158] Adduct the patient's hip and at the same time provide an axial force to the femur to prevent the pelvis from lifting off the table. If there is shortening of the piriformis, adduction and medial rotation are decreased and may be accompanied by stretch pain. This test does not differentiate between shortening of the piriformis muscle and a painful iliolumbar ligament. According to Janda,[131] palpation of the piriformis usually gives better results than the stretch test.

PALPATION

For bony palpation and position see the section on bony structure and alignment above. The SIJ can be palpated in one locality only—at its inferior extent in the region of the posteroinferior iliac spine. Acute unilateral tenderness and thickening are common in painful sacroiliac conditions, and when well localized serve as a useful confirmatory sign.[101] Tenderness here often represents a referred area of tenderness from disorders of the lower lumbar spine.

Soft tissue palpation in prone should include the skin, subcutaneous tissues (using a skin-rolling test) (see Fig. 7-42*C*), gluteus maximus and medius, piriformis, and erector spinae. The lateral aspect of the erector spinae muscle is the anatomic location of the lateral raphe. At the inferior aspect of the raphe,

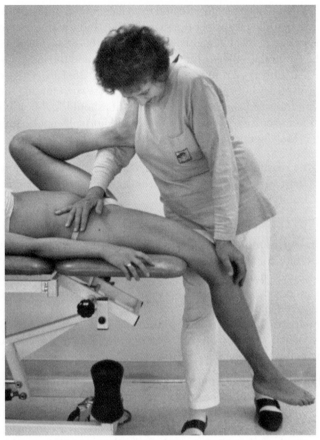

A

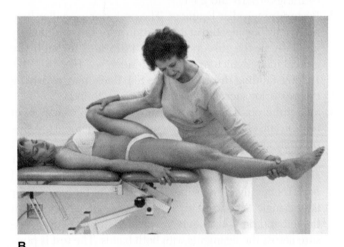

B

■ **FIG. 23-33.** Muscle length: **(A)** iliopsoas, rectus femoris, tensor fascia latae, and **(B)** two-joint hip adductors.

corresponding to the level of the iliac crest, is an important connective tissue junction where the thoracolumbar fascia, the lateral aspect of the iliocostalis lumborum tendon, the deep erector spinae muscle, the quadratus lumborum, and the lateral third of the iliolumbar ligament converge to attach to the iliac crest.[232] This region is frequently tender to palpation.

Ligaments typically affected by malalignment (and upslip) most consistently affect the sacrospinous and the four major posterior pelvic ligaments on each side: the sacrotuberous, the iliolumbar, the posterior SIJ ligaments, and the long posterior (dorsal sacroiliac) ligament (see Fig. 18-19B).[257] Also involved are interosseus ligaments and those surrounding the symphysis pubis (Fig. 23-1). Ligaments should feel neither lax nor excessively taut, and they should normally not be tender. Malalignment can increase tension by:

1. Increasing the distance between the origin and insertion
2. Increasing tension in a muscle that attaches to, or is in continuity with the ligament

Persistent increase in tension in a ligament has four undesirable consequences.[257] The ligament ultimately lengthens and fails to provide adequate support. Second, the ligament becomes painful. Third, an elongated, irritated, and inflamed ligament can become a source of aberrant proprioceptive referred-pain symptoms, and finally, pain from the ligaments results in a reflex splinting of muscles, which may eventually result in chronic tension myalgia and myofascial pain. Routinely palpate the following ligamentous structures:

1. Iliolumbar ligaments. The iliolumbar ligaments lie deep and in a small space. The fibers arising from L4 are accessible to palpation. From a laterosuperior direction, the origin at the transverse process is palpated, whereas the insertion is palpated mediosuperiorly at the iliac crest, if accessible (see Figs. 18-19 and 23-1).[75]
2. Posterior sacroiliac ligament. The posterior sacroiliac ligament may be palpated at its insertion inferiorly and slightly medially in the direction of the PSIS and through the gluteal mass (which may also be tender; see Fig. 18-19B). In longstanding disorders of the SIJ, thickening overlying the posterior sacroiliac ligament may be found.
3. Sacrotuberous ligament. According to Grieve,[101] changes in tension and elasticity of the sacrotuberous ligament are surprisingly easy to feel through the gluteal mass (Fig. 23-34). Using the index finger or thumb, proceed from the inferior aspect of the ischial tuberosity medially, then superiorly and posterolaterally to the superior attachment on the inferior lateral angle. A contrast in tension can be detected between the left and right ligaments by applying simultaneous pressure across the ligaments with both hands. The test is positive if one sacrotuberous ligament is more lax or tense than the normal or opposite side.[100] If the sacrum is dysfunctional in a position that places the ligament in tension; it will be tense and usually tender.
4. Anteriorly, palpate the abdominal wall, inguinal area, femoral triangle, and Baer's sacroiliac point for tenderness, muscle spasms, or other signs that may indicate the source of disease. Note any ganglions, nodules, and lymph nodes in the femoral triangle. Also palpate the trochanteric bursae and psoas bursa (palpable if swollen) and nerve. Palpate ligaments spanning the pubic symphysis (Fig. 23-1). A dis-

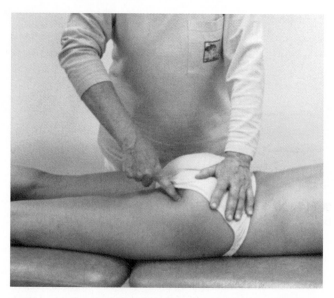

■ **FIG. 23-34.** Palpation of the sacrotuberous ligament.

placement or torsion of one pubic bone relative to the other creates stress on the ligaments and the disk.

Also palpate for relevant trigger points and tender points of fibromyalgia.

Neurologic Testing. Neurologic testing at this point has been completed as part of the earlier lumbar spine and hip examination, which should always precede the SIJ examination. A sacroiliac condition can coexist in the presence of lumbosacral nerve root or cauda equina involvement. Patients with sacroiliac problems may report paresthesias in the absence of neurologic signs; these appear to simulate lumbosacral involvement.[315]

Radiographic Evaluation. SIJ dysfunction is diagnosed by clinical examination; radiographs rarely add any useful information but do help exclude other conditions, such as early ankylosing spondylitis.[12,144,145] The presence of degenerative changes usually bears no correlation with symptoms because 24.5% of patients older than 50 years of age have abnormal-appearing SIJs on plain radiographs.[49,129,144,212,247] Radionuclide scanning of the SIJ is the procedure of choice for demonstrating infection, inflammation, stress fracture, or neoplasm involving the SIJ.[12]

TREATMENT TECHNIQUES OF PELVIC GIRDLE AND SACROCOCCYGEAL REGION

Treatment of the pelvic girdle follows the same guidelines as for other areas of the body. Acutely, when pain is present, rest becomes an important consideration. Ice, massage, or other modalities at the disposal of the clinician may be helpful to deal effectively with the pain. If the pain is acute or severe, a scultetus binder or sacroiliac belt is recommended.[224] Relief by either the belt or binder is generally confirmatory of the diagnosis. Heel-lifts may be a valuable adjunct while tissue heals if they are used under the foot of the short side to minimize ground forces.[86,231] Pelvic traction may be helpful in the presence of a neurologic deficit and may help correct compromised sacroiliac dysfunction by pulling the innominates caudally on the sacrum.[63]

At the appropriate time, nondestructive passive and active movements should be started to stimulate the tissue to adapt to the proper lines of stress, to modulate pain, and to provide proprioceptive input. Education, in the form of ergonomic counseling, is the most important aspect of treatment. Habitual working stresses and sitting postures should be corrected. Exercises should proceed with the goal of normalizing stresses by balancing muscle length and strength and ground and trunk forces.

Soft Tissue Manipulations

Janda[131] has identified the common pattern of muscle imbalances that occur in the lower quadrant with hypertonic postural muscles and muscles showing a tendency toward inhibition and reflex muscle weakness (see Table 5-6). Tightness of the hip flexors and spinal extensors and inhibition and weakness of the gluteal and abdominal muscles characterize the pelvic or distal crossed syndrome (see Chapter 8, Soft Tissue Manipulations).[133,138] Clinical consequences of the lower crossed syndrome include increased thoracolumbar facet and SIJ strain, altered hip mechanics, and overstress of the lumbosacral junction.[42,133,138] Many other overuse syndromes of the lower quadrant may contribute to sacroiliac dysfunction, including the tensor fascia lata overuse syndrome, the piriformis muscle syndrome, and the gluteus medius syndrome (see Chapter 8, Soft Tissue Manipulations).

Soft tissues manipulations to consider include myofascial manipulations of the thoracolumbar fascia and lumbar mass (see Figs. 8-1B, 8-13, 8-15, 8-17B, C, and 8-34A through 8-37) and postisometric relaxation and stretching of the hip adductors (see Fig 8-76 and Box 8-9E), piriformis (see Figs. 8-3, 8-66, and 8-75), hamstrings (see Figs. 7-32, 7-45B, 7-46B, and 8-19A, and Box 8-9H), quadratus lumborum (see Figs. 8-15C, 8-35, and 8-37), iliopsoas (see Fig. 8-4 and Box 8-9F), latissimus dorsi (see Box 8-8F–H), erector spinae (see Figs. 8-5, 8-10, 8-35, and 8-37), or tensor fascia lata (see Figs. 8-14B, and 8-68 through 8-72). Soft tissue manipulation should always be carried out in conjunction with a home program of self-stretch of the myofascial structures of the pelvic girdle and the lower quadrant (see Box 8-9) and correction of biomechanical problems (e.g., agonist–antagonist muscle imbalances of the spine and lower limbs; see sensorimotor training, neuromuscular reeducation, lumbopelvic stabilization, and functional exercises below).

It is often necessary and productive to mobilize the connective tissue of the sacral borders and sacral pad before attempting to mobilize the sacrum out of various positional faults or movement dysfunctions.[38] The latissimus dorsi, thoracolumbar fascia, and heavy fascial sheet of the erector spinae

blend into a heavy connective pad on the sacrum and coccyx.[262] At its lower edge the gluteus maximus attaches to it above the tailbone. This area may also be restricted in conjunction with iliac crest restrictions at the PSIP, lateral border of the iliac crest, and lateral border of the sacrum, coccyx, and sacrotuberous ligament. To fully mobilize this area the insertion of the tensor fascia lata (see Fig. 8-71) and lateral border of the sacrum should also be mobilized. Release of the sacral borders may be executed by using the same hand position as the iliac crease release described earlier (see Fig. 8-11) by a reinforced thumb technique or a leverage-distraction technique with the fingertips (see Fig. 8-35B). Similar techniques may used to release the thoracolumbar fascia and erector spinae aponeurosis in this area (see Figs. 8-35A, 8-36, and 8-37).

SOFT TISSUE MANIPULATIONS FOR RELEASING THE SACRAL PAD AND SACRUM

1. Patient lying prone. Using a supported hand technique, place one hand over the sacrum with the heel over the base and fingertips techniques over the apex including the lateral angles. The other hand is placed on top (Fig. 23-35). The operator's hand pressure is applied anteriorly and inferiorly with a rocking motion from side to side, forward and backward, and across the oblique axis.[100]

2. Patient lying prone. The operator places his or her partially flexed elbow in the sacral sulcus. With his or her elbow in the sacral sulcus, the operator applies slow sustained pressure in an anterior inferior direction to cover the entire length of the sacrum. Using this same technique the iliac crest can be treated as well (see Fig. 8-11).[209] Starting superficially with light pressure, the elbow is pushed along the iliac crest to approximately the midaxillary line. When restrictions to mobility are palpated, the specific restrictions can be determined using the imaginary clock. After the restriction is treated, the examination and treatment of this area continues at deeper tissue levels.

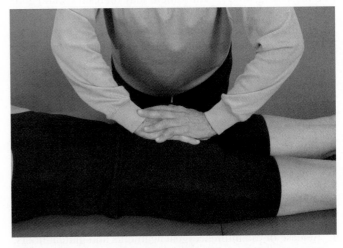

■ **FIG. 23-35.** Soft tissue manipulation of the sacrum.

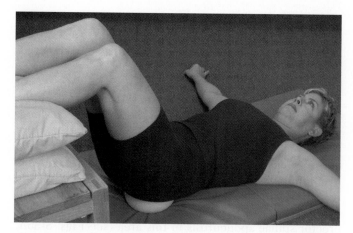

■ **FIG. 23-36.** Self-treatment to release the thoracolumbar fascia, erector spinae, and sacral pad with the use of a ball.

More superficial strokes to the sacrum affect the superficial layer of the thoracolumbar and erector spinae aponeurosis. Deeper strokes affect the deeper laminal layers of the thoracolumbar fascia and multifidi and iliolumbar ligaments (see Figs 7-9 through 7-11, 18-16, and 23-1). A number of other soft tissue manipulations may be used to release the sacral pad, such as J-stroking (see Fig. 8-8) and S myofascial pressure release (see Fig. 8-12).

Self-treatment for increasing the extensibility of the sacral pad, erector spinae aponeurosis, and the L4–L5 segments can be done with the use of a small ball to apply slow, prolonged stresses to this region, creating both a stretch of the elastic tissue and relaxation of the collagen.[225,275] Self-stretching in this way allows for release of the tight shortened back muscles at the lumbosacral junction as well as the sacral pad and surrounding ligamentous and muscular attachments of the sacrum. The ball can either be rolled across the region into the areas of restriction (in supine or sitting) or the patient may simply rest on the ball (positioned under the apex of the sacrum) for a period of time, allowing the surrounding tissues to release (Fig. 23-36). The patient may then slowly and gently press into the ball to engage more of the low back with lengthening of the abdominals in the same process.[225] Slow gentle repetitions for 10 to 15 minutes is recommended.

Release of the restricted ligaments of the coccyx and the origin of the gluteus maximus (see Fig. 8-28) may be indicated as well (see Box 8-3*E*).

COCCYGEAL SOFT TISSUE MANIPULATIONS

Mobilization of the sacrococcygeal joint and the surrounding soft tissues can be used to free up sacral extension so that the sacral base can tip anteriorly (which is the physiologic movement of the sacrum that occurs with lumbar extension)[257] and enhance the mobility of the coccyx.

1. Release of the intercoccygeal ligaments and gluteal fibers. The patient lies prone with a pillow under the pelvis. The operator sits next to the patient and places one thumb on the restricted area. To release the intercoccygeal ligaments, impart alternating small adduction–abduction movement of the thumb and work the posterior aspect of the coccyx. To release the gluteal fibers the thumb contacts the area between the muscle and the lateral border of the coccyx. Apply up and down movements along the edge of the bone.

2. Release of the coccygeus muscle (see Fig. 7-18) to enhance mobility of the coccyx.[120] The patient is sitting near the end of the treatment table, with arms crossed holding the elbows. The operator stands to the side of the patient and grasps under the patient's arms, the other hand with the index finger on the coccygeus muscle besides the coccyx. Have the patient slump sit and shift weight onto the operator's finger ("sit on finger"), thus increasing the ischemic pressure and releasing the muscle.

Myofascial manipulations of the coccygeus muscle, sacrotuberous ligament, and gluteal muscle fibers can be performed in sidelying, prone, or sitting (as above).

Pelvic floor muscle (see Fig. 7-18) contractions can be used to mobilize the coccyx into flexion.[120] Bo et al.[19] found via dynamic magnetic resonance imaging of the pelvic floor that in the upright sitting position the coccyx moves with pelvic floor contractions (15° flexion with contraction and 13° with extension). To mobilize coccyx flexion (with the patient in the same sitting position as above), ask the patient to slump sit, while holding the coccyx in flexion. Have the patient contract the pelvic floor muscles, and take up the slack into flexion. This is usually repeated with a coccyx hold into flexion three times.

MYOFASCIAL MANIPULATION OF SACROTUBEROUS LIGAMENT

Myofascial manipulation of the sacrotuberous ligament may be used to balance the sacrotuberous ligaments and urogenital diaphragm (see Fig. 7-18*C*). The sacrotuberous ligament origin is particularly vulnerable to weakness in that[257]:

- Anterior rotation of the innominate, sacral nutation, sacral torsions, and coccygeal rotation not only increase the distance between its origin and insertion, but can also separate its points of origin and insertion and innominate from each other.

- An upslip can similarly increase tension in the long dorsal sacrotuberous ligament, the part of the ligament that originates from the sacrum, by moving the PSIS upward and away from the sacrum.

- Tension in the ligament will be increased by active contraction of the hamstrings, gluteus maximus, or piriformis. The ligament is also put at increased risk of injury by any passive increase in tension of these muscles, such as occurs with straight-leg raising, stretching, and jumping.

It is not surprising that the sacrotuberous ligament is tender to palpation in 70 to 80% of those presenting with malalignment.[257] The referred pain pattern overlies primarily the poste-

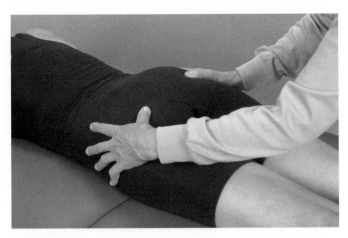

■ **FIG. 23-37.** Myofascial manipulation of the sacro-tuberous ligament.

rior thigh and calf and an area around the heel–calcaneal scle-rotome and overlaps to a large extent that of the sacrospinous ligament.[108] A side to side difference in tension is usually appar-ent on palpating the ligament with the patient lying prone.

Technique: Manipulation of Sacrotuberous Liga-ment (Fig. 23-37).[100] Patient is in prone position. The oper-ator at the side of the table places his or her hands over the buttock in contact with the sacrotuberous ligament at the infe-rior lateral angles of the sacrum. Tension in the sacrotuberous ligament is tested for symmetric balance. The hands are twisted in counterclockwise and clockwise directions, sensing for tight-ness and looseness. The operator then applies load to balance the tension in the sacrotuberous ligament while the patient performs enhancing maneuvers (e.g., respiration, contraction of the gluteals).

Myofascial manipulations, as an approach, encompass ele-ments from many other techniques. The primary motive is to achieve a biomechanical release of the myofascia.

Joint Mobilization Techniques

PHYSICAL FINDINGS OF COMMON PELVIC GIRDLE DYSFUNCTION

The following physical findings characterize some of the more common pelvic girdle dysfunctions. There are, how-ever, numerous rare pelvic girdle dysfunctions; for complete coverage of these conditions, refer to the works of Bookhout,[24] Bourdillon and Day,[27] Greenman,[100] Mitchell,[198] Nyberg,[213] Schamberger,[257] and Woerman.[313] In all dysfunctions of the pelvic girdle, correction of habitual postural stresses and sit-ting postures should receive primary attention. Shoe-lifts or a buttock-lift when sitting may be needed. Functional integra-tion, neuromuscular reeducation, and ergonomic measures should be emphasized.

I. Signs and Symptoms of Innominate Lesions. With respect to the pelvis, displacement of the innominate on the sacrum

determines the direction of the dysfunction. The following pos-itive findings are the most common innominate dysfunctions:

A. Anterior dysfunction (anterior innominate rotation). When unilateral anterior dysfunction is present, the PSIS is higher and more anterior on the affected side compared with the contralateral side when standing—that is, the ASIS is lower and more posterior. This indicates a poste-rior torsion (counternutation) of the sacrum on that side.[175,176,199] The ischial tuberosity is posterior on the involved side, and the lower limb is usually medially rotated. Traumatically, anterior rotation dysfunction occurs most frequently in any forced anterior diagonal pattern, such as a golf or baseball swing, or in a posterior horizontal thrust of the femur (dashboard injury).[313]

1. In the supine-to-sit test in supine, an anterior dysfunc-tion can cause the leg to appear longer than the contra-lateral limb because it brings the acetabulum closer to the plane of the table and reduces the angulation at the hip. In sitting, with unilateral anterior dysfunction, the leg may appear shorter because the acetabulum moves posteriorly relative to the SIJ (Fig. 23-30).

2. On the involved side, the PSIS moves first and farther superiorly during the standing trunk flexion test.

3. Muscle findings include weak abdominals, weak gluteus maximus and medius, and tight hip flexors (particularly the psoas and iliotibial band) on the involved side.[191,213]

B. Posterior dysfunction (posterior innominate rotation). Just the opposite will occur in posterior dysfunction of the innominate. This torsion may result in a spinal scoliosis and an altered functional leg length (shorter on the involved side). The posterior dysfunctions are usually the result of falling on an ischial tuberosity, lifting when for-ward flexed with the knees straight, repeated or pro-longed standing on one leg, vertical thrusting onto an extended leg, or sustaining hyperflexion and abduction of the hips.[173]

1. In standing, the ASIS is higher and the PSIS is lower on that side; this indicates an anterior rotation of the sacrum (nutation).[176] In the standing flexion test, the PSIS on the involved side moves first or farther superi-orly. In the supine-to-sit test, the malleolus moves from short to long (Fig. 23-30). The sulcus is deep on the involved side.

2. Muscle findings include hamstring and adductor mag-nus tightness, tightness or tenderness of the tensor fas-ciae latae or piriformis, and gluteus medius weakness.

C. Innominate outflare (external rotation) The pelvis on the involved side opens up so that the SIJ moves outward and opens the SIJ anteriorly while closing it posteriorly. Poste-rior landmarks, such as the PSIS, move medially, whereas anterior landmarks, such as the ASIS, move laterally. The shift results in increased tension in the ipsilateral anterior SIJ capsule and ligaments, the deep iliolumbar ligaments, and across the symphysis pubis, whereas tension is decreased in the sacrospinous ligament, the ipsilateral posterior SIJ ligaments, interosseous ligaments, and long sacrotuberous and long posterior sacroiliac ligaments.[257] Causes of a right iliac outflare include right hip internal rotation or adduction restrictions, tight hip abductors or internal rotators on the right, or a fall on the lateral aspect of the right PSIS.[213]

D. Innominate inflare. The front of the innominate moves inward, opening up the SIJ posteriorly while closing it anteriorly. Posterior landmarks move laterally, anterior ones medially. Tension decreases in the ipsilateral anterior SIJ capsule and ligaments, the deep iliolumbar ligaments, and across the symphysis pubis, whereas tension increases in the sacrotuberous ligament, long sacrotuberous and ipsilateral long posterior sacroiliac ligaments, interosseous ligaments, and posterior SIJ ligaments.[257] Cause of a left iliac inflare includes left hip restriction, left posterior sacroiliac weakness, or a fall onto the lateral aspect of the ASIS.[213]

In palpating for inflares and outflares, find the ASIS with your client in a supine position. Place the pad of your thumbs on the medial inferior edge of each ASIS. Next draw an imaginary line down the center of your client's body to represent the midsagittal axis. Then compare how far each thumb is from this centerline. If the thumb on the right ASIS seems closer to the midline than the left, then you are probably looking at a unilateral inflare or outflare. If the standing flexion test (Fig. 23-14) or the test for SIJ fixation (Fig. 23-15) reveals a fixation on the right, then you are dealing with a right inflare; if fixation is on the left, then you are dealing with a left inflare.[178]

E. Innominate upslip (superior innominate shear). Vertical shear lesions of an entire innominate occur more frequently than originally thought.[100] Upslips are usually the result of jumping or falling suddenly on an extended leg.[214]

1. In standing, with unilateral anterior or posterior dysfunction, there are differences in the relation of the ASIS and PSIS. With a unilateral upslip of the innominate, the ASIS and PSIS are higher than the ASIS and PSIS on the opposite side.[199,313]

2. The quadratus lumborum may be in muscle spasm; there may be a tight hip adductor on that side.

II. Signs of a Sacral Lesion

A. Sacral torsion (left-on-left anterior torsion). The left-on-left forward torsion is the most common sacroiliac lesion.[100,214,313] The primary axis of dysfunction is the left oblique axis. A left-on-left sacral torsion signifies flexion movement at the right sacral base and inferior movement of the left side of the sacrum. As a result, the sacrum is positioned in left rotation and left sidebending.[213] Usually there is a history of a pelvic twist injury.

1. The right sacral sulcus is deep; the left is shallow. The inferior angle is inferior and posterior on the left. Lumbar lordosis is usually increased, with a convex scoliosis on the right.[100] In prone, the left malleolus is short.

2. The piriformis, tensor fasciae latae, and posterior sacroiliac ligaments are tender on the right. The gluteus medius is usually weak (especially on the right) and the left piriformis tight.

B. Unilateral sacral flexion. A unilateral sacral flexion exists when the sacrum rotates in one direction and sidebends. It may be thought of as failure of one side of the sacrum to counternutate from a fully nutated position.[313] Some of the findings for a right unilateral sacral flexion are the following:

1. The seated flexion test is positive: the blocked side (right) moves first. In prone the medial malleolus is long on the right. On the right side, the base of the sacrum (sulcus) is anterior and the inferior angle is posterior.

2. The left tensor fasciae latae is tight. Increased right piriformis and psoas tone and tenderness over the right sacroiliac ligaments are usually found.

JOINT MOBILIZATION AND MUSCLE ENERGY TECHNIQUES

The role of mobilization is limited to passive mobility, but the most important part of treatment deals with active mobility and patient self-treatment or mobilization on an ongoing basis outside the clinical setting. Joint mobilization (or stabilization) is just part of the treatment of chronic dysfunction in one or both SIJs, which is most often associated with dysfunction of the hip and lumbosacral joints. Treatment will not bring the expected relief of symptoms unless soft tissue dysfunctions are addressed in addition to the loss of muscle strength and flexibility. Active mobilization and corrective exercises play an integral role; passive mobilization is useless if it is not followed by active specific mobilization. When patients with hypermobility are treated symptomatically, the dysfunction will reappear, leading to repeated symptoms. Recurrence can be prevented only by stabilizing the hypermobile joint or vertebral segment.

Many joint mobilization and muscle energy techniques have been described for the pelvic girdle complex, but only a few of the more common ones are presented here. (See the following references for more techniques.[27,45,51,63–66,70, 76,80,85,100,103–105,121,122,157–160,176,177,178,199,213,223,231,232,257,260,280,306,307,313])

Osteopathic muscle energy techniques are very useful in treating pelvic and sacral positional faults. Direct manipulation with graded thrust techniques is also appropriate when hypomobility or positional faults are encountered. Muscle energy direct techniques, which are safer and very effective, often obviate the need for manual manipulation and can be performed by the patient to maximize correction maintenance. Although controversial, many osteopaths suggest first treatment and correction of lower limb muscles, next the pubis, then the sacral deformity followed by the ilia, and finally L5–S1 altered mechanics. All of these areas must be assessed and treated to effectively correct the mechanical system. Correction of biomechanical problems (e.g., agonist–antagonist muscle imbalances) is key for resetting the joints' neutral position, both mechanically and neurologically with stretching, soft tissue manipulations, toning, and strengthening of flaccid muscles.

Several of the evaluation maneuvers are useful as treatment techniques for pelvic dysfunction. The following maneuvers were described and illustrated in the section on passive movement above.

I. Osteokinematic Tests of Physiologic Mobility
    A. Pelvic rock test—Anterior–posterior glide of the innominate (Fig. 23-16). When used as a technique in the presence of asymmetric dysfunction (i.e., when gliding the innominate bones in an anteroposterior direction in the plane of the sacroiliac articular surfaces), emphasis is placed on the more hypomobile innominate.
    B. Flexion–extension of the innominate (Fig. 23-17). According to Maitland and colleagues,[177] the test movement that reproduces the pain should be used first as a treatment technique. At the onset it should be performed using a grade that produces only minimal discomfort.
II. Arthrokinetic Tests of Stability
    A. Posteroanterior and transverse pressures around the SIJ (Fig. 23-20). If such pressures consistently yield a response to the same pressure and direction at certain points, they may be used not only for assessment but also for treatment.[177,307]
    B. Prone gapping test (Fig. 23-22). This technique can be used as regional mobilization with a gentle gapping and

gliding for the SIJ, with the near ilium stabilized. It can also be used to stretch the piriformis passively or to improve its extensibility by hold–relax or isometric techniques.[102,103]

    C. Torsional stress of the SIJ (Fig. 23-23). This technique can be used as a downward, outward, and caudal mobilization of the innominate while the sacrum is stabilized, or as an outward manipulation of the SIJ.[103,104]
    D. Compression–distraction tests of the innominates (Fig. 23-24). These techniques can be used to reduce a positional fault (pubic compression) or to promote motions (pubic di traction) at the pubic symphysis.[213]
        Note: Other evaluation maneuvers useful in treatment techniques (not described below) include the sacral apex pressure test (Fig. 23-19) and the longitudinal stress test of the sacrum (Fig. 23-21).

Nonspecific Techniques

(For simplicity, the operator is referred to as the male, the patient as the female. (P—patient; O—operator; M—movement.)

I. Pelvic Shift. Forward and backward, sitting (Fig. 23-38)
    P—Sitting on the treatment table or bolster, or straddling a large therapy roll, with the legs abducted. Arms may

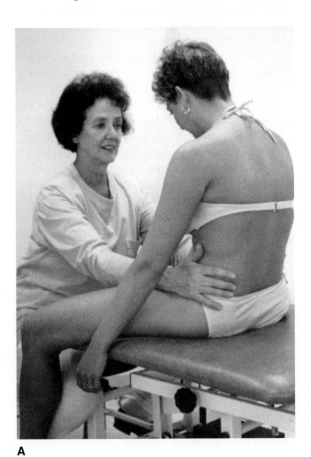
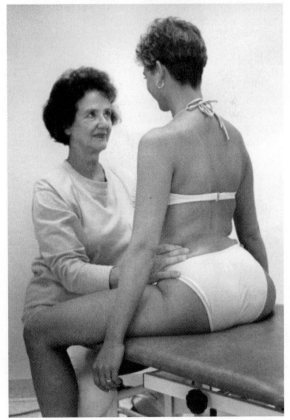

A   **B**

■ **FIG. 23-38.** Pelvic shift forward (**A**) and backward (**B**).

be positioned on the operator's head or shoulders to facilitate upper thoracic flexion with lumbar spine extension.

O—Sits on the floor or on a mat or stool in front of the patient

M—With his hands on the posterior aspect of the pelvic girdle, the operator shifts the pelvis forward and backward into its end range or barrier.

Note: This a useful technique for general mobilization of the pelvic girdle as well as for increasing the extensibility of the inferior hip joint capsule. It is particularly valuable in the management of pelvic dysfunction in the neurologically involved adult and child. Active pelvic shift is an excellent lead-up exercise in preparation for standing and walking.

II. Self-Mobilization of the SIJ (Fig. 23-39)[106,161]

With this technique, sidebending and rotation of the lower lumbar spine are mobilized as well.

P—Kneeling on a table, close to the edge, with the trunk supported on the hands (elbows extended) or on the

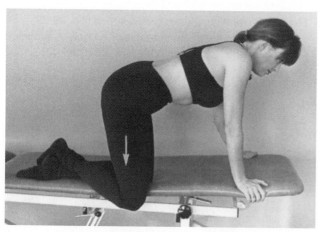

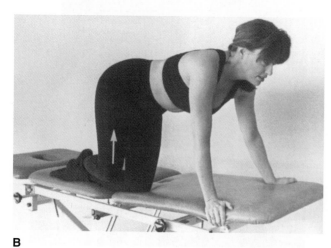

■ **FIG. 23-39.** Self-mobilization of the sacroiliac joint: **(A)** starting position and **(B)** end position.

elbows. One leg is shifted to hang the flexed knee over the edge of the table, with the foot supported over the heel of the other leg.

M—The patient relaxes so the pelvis slopes obliquely down from the ilium. The slack is taken up at the SIJ of the supported side on the table. Once the patient senses tension in the joint, very small downward vertical springing motions are performed with the knee over the edge of the table, thus mobilizing the SIJ on the supported side.

III. Distraction of Pubic Symphysis: Muscle Energy Technique (MET; "shotgun technique;" Fig. 23-40).[27,76,100,199,232,313]

A. Distraction of SIJ pubic symphysis (Fig. 23-40A)

P—Supine with knees bent, feet resting on the table, knees together

O—Stands at the end of the table facing the patient

M—With patient's knees held together to resist abduction, have the patient try to spread the legs apart (abduct the legs). This is done with a maximum isometric contraction for 7 to 10 seconds. After relaxation, repeat this procedure but with the legs abducted 30 to 45°. Repeat three times and proceed to the next phase (below).

The resisted force provided by the operator into hip abduction results in distraction of the iliac joint surfaces away from the sacrum because the abductors contract and pull on their attachments to the iliac crest.[76]

B. Distraction of pubic symphysis (Fig. 23-40B)

P—Same position as above

O—Same position as above

M—Place the hands or one forearm (used as a brace to keep the knees apart) on the medial aspects of the patient's knees to resist adduction. Have the patient try to bring the knees together as you oppose the adduction motion, thus distracting the pubic symphysis joint surfaces away from one another as the adductors contract and pull on their attachments to the pubic rami. After a maximum isometric hold for 7 to 10 seconds, have the patient relax. Repeat several times. Retest and repeat if indicated.

Note: These two techniques can be used separately or in combination. Often by releasing the pubis or changing the forces in the pelvis, the sacrum is likely to correct its position as well as a left-on-left sacral torsion.[232]

Self-treatment using contraction–relaxation of the hip abductors and adductors can be carried out by using the same position as above with a belt around the thighs and a cushion or ball between the knees to resist hip abduction and adduction (Fig. 23-41). Self-treatment can also be done in sitting using the hands or a belt to resist abduction and a forearm to resist adduction.

Innominate Dysfunction Techniques

I. Forward Rotation. Prone position

This is a basic technique for a posterior innominate rotation dysfunction (see Fig. 22-47). Signs on the involved side

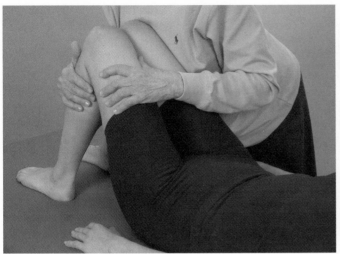

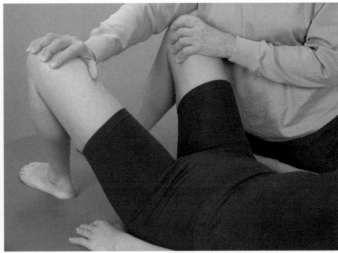

A   **B**

■ **FIG. 23-40.** Muscle energy technique (MET): Distraction of pubic symphysis. **(A)** Resisted abduction effort of the knees. **(B)** Resisted adduction of the knees.

include an inferior and posterior PSIS, a superior and anterior ASIS, a positive standing flexion test, and an apparent short leg in the supine position. Hypermobility or restriction in innominate anterior rotation is apparent. The hip and pelvic girdle muscles should be checked for asymmetry.

II. Forward Rotation. Supine position (Fig. 23-42)

For posterior innominate rotation dysfunction, signs on the involved side are the same as above.

P—Supine, with the leg on the side to be mobilized extended over the edge of the table

O—Stands opposite of the side to be mobilized. The patient or operator flexes and stabilizes the opposite leg.

M—Place the caudal hand over the thigh and use it to push the hip into further extension; the cephalic hand can be applied to the patient's PSIS, pushing upward to increase the forward rotation of the innominate on the sacrum.

Note: This technique can be modified to use muscle correction, which can place an anterior rotatory moment on the innominate (muscle energy) using the iliopsoas as the desired force.[231,313] Have the patient push the freely hanging leg up against your hand with a submaximal force while you give unyielding resistance to the contraction

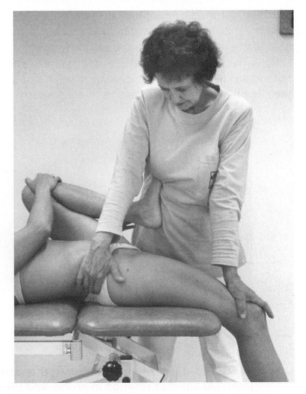

■ **FIG. 23-42.** Forward rotation for posterior iliac dysfunction.

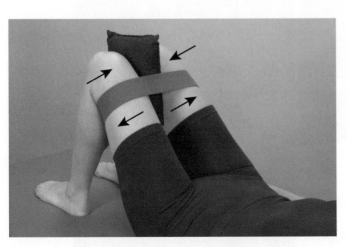

■ **FIG. 23-41.** MET: Self-treatment of pubic symphysis dysfunction.

for 7 to 10 seconds. This procedure is repeated three or four times or until all the slack is taken up.

Management for posterior innominate rotation dysfunction should include soft tissue inhibition and stretching to the involved muscles (hamstrings and piriformis and occasionally the tensor fasciae latae, according to Mennell[191]); promotion of hip extension activities, such as prone press-ups or pushing the head and shoulders up while the pelvis remains on the floor or table; functional integration and strengthening of involved muscles (gluteus medius, hip rotators, hip flexors); and functional activity requiring this range (i.e., coming-to-sit over the hip joint). Rolling and assuming the half-kneeling position are other activities that can improve sacroiliac mobility while gaining functional strength. Increase non–weight-bearing rest time if unstable (consider a pelvic corset or belt if necessary).[213]

Self-treatment techniques to counteract posterior iliac rotation may consist of passive hip extension (Fig. 23-43A) in prone or supine (Fig. 23-43B). In the supine correction technique it is important that the (left) leg is off the table. The hip is should be maximally adducted and literally be suspended above the horizontal by the hip capsule and soft tissue.[121,122] This position should be held for about 2 minutes.

III. Backward Rotation

This is the basic technique for anterior innominate dysfunction (see Fig. 22-46). Signs on the involved side include a superior and anterior PSIS, an inferior and posterior ASIS, a positive flexion test, an apparent long leg in the supine position, and innominate posterior rotation. The hip and pelvic girdle muscles should be checked for symmetry.

Note: The same maneuver can be used to produce anterior rotation (for a posterior innominate rotation dysfunction), but the operator produces a force–couple pushing the ASIS forward and the ischial tuberosity backward. Contract–relax or muscle-energy techniques may be used effectively in either of these techniques.

IV. Backward Rotation. Supine position (Fig. 23-44)

This technique is useful for anterior innominate rotation dysfunction. The cephalic hand cups the ASIS in the palm while the caudal hand grasps the ischial tuberosity. Transfer your weight toward the patient's head; this results in a backward rotation of the innominate on the sacrum.

Muscle correction (muscle energy) of this positional fault uses muscles that can rotate the innominate in a posterior direction, mainly the gluteus maximus.[76,313] Have the patient resist a force provided by your trunk (or against the patient's own hands, which fixates the knee) with a sustained submaximal contraction for 7 to 10 seconds. This is repeated three or four times, not allowing the hip to move into extension, only flexion.

This treatment may be given to the patient to do as a home program in sitting, supine (Fig. 23-45A), or standing.[63,64] In standing, the patient places the foot on a table or bench, leans toward the knee, and stretches it into the axilla (Fig. 23-45B). DonTigny[63] recommends repeating this exercise several times a day, and always making a correction when going to bed to relieve the strain on the involved ligaments. An alternative method can be created by using a lever effect by letting the trunk hang down in forward flexion (Fig. 23-45C).[122,257] These techniques are powerful rotators of the innominate and can be overdone unless specific guidelines are given.[313]

Management for anterior iliac rotation dysfunction should include soft tissue mobilization techniques and stretching of tight hip flexors (particularly the psoas and tensor fasciae latae); strengthening of the abdominal and gluteal muscles; and exercise and functional activities to promote hip flexion, abduction, and external rotation.

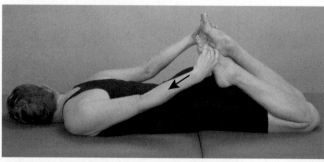

A

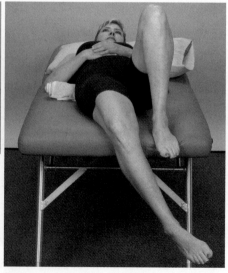

B

■ **FIG. 23-43.** Self-mobilization of the sacroiliac joint: **(A)** anterior rotation in prone, and **(B)** anterior rotation in supine to counteract posterior rotation of the innominate.

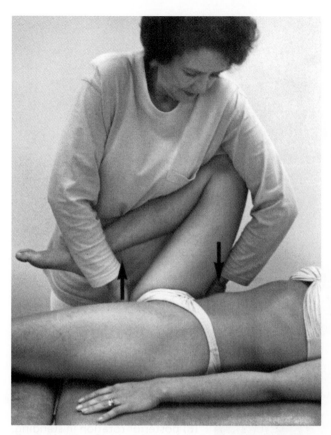

■ **FIG. 23-44.** Backward rotation for anterior innominate dysfunction.

V. Mobilization Techniques for Innominate Outflare
   A. Passive prone technique (left side; Fig. 23-46)[213]
      P—Prone
      O—Stands on the left side. The caudad hand contacts the left ankle and the cephalad hand the right side of the sacral base.
      M—The cephalad hand applies posteroanterior pressure to the right side of the sacral base. The caudad hand internally rotates the left hip to inflare and internally rotates the left innominate.
   B. Muscle energy supine technique (Fig. 23-47)[100]
      P—Supine
      O—Flexes the patient's hip and knee, rolling the pelvis to the opposite side. The operator's fingers of the cephalad hand contact the medial aspect of the PSIS, and the patient's pelvis is returned to neutral.
      M—The caudad hand adducts the femur to the internal rotation barrier while maintaining lateral traction on the PSIS with the cephalad hand. The patient is instructed to abduct and externally rotate the leg against the resistance of the operator's hand three to five times. The operator engages a new internal rotational barrier after each patient relaxation. The operator should maintain pressure through the femur toward the table to prevent the

pelvis from rotating to the opposite side during muscle contraction.
   C. Self-treatment (Fig. 23-48).[121] The patient lies on her back and bends the involved hip to 90°. With her hand, she pushes the thigh to the opposite side. A cushion or folded pillow under the foot and lower leg may be necessary to maintain 90° of hip flexion. The stretch is maintained for 2 minutes.
   D. Management. Based on the findings consider soft tissue inhibition and stretch to the piriformis, hip abductors, and external rotators on the involved side and exercises to promote hip internal rotation or adduction when tolerated.[213]
VI. Innominate Inflare Techniques
   A. Prone technique (left side; Fig. 23-49)[213]
      P—Prone with the left leg externally rotated
      O—Stands on the left side. The cephalad hand contacts the medial aspect of the left ASIS. The caudad hand contacts the area just lateral to the PSIS.
      M—The cephalad hand pulls the ASIS laterally and inferiorly while the caudad hand applies medial and superior force to the PSIS.
   B. Muscle energy supine technique (Fig. 23-50)[100]
      P—Supine
      O—Stands on the involved side. The operator flexes the patient's hip and knee, placing the foot on the opposite knee, and contacts the medial aspect of the knee of the involved side. The cephalad hand contacts the ASIS on the opposite side and stabilizes the pelvis.
      M—The hip is externally rotated until the first barrier is engaged. The patient performs three to five muscle contractions for 3 to 5 seconds, attempting to internally rotate the leg against the resistance of the operator. The operator engages a new external rotation barrier after each patient contraction.
   C. Self-treatment. Muscle energy technique (Fig. 23-51).[257] The patient anchors the foot of the involved side on thigh of the opposite leg, which is positioned with the hip in flexion and the foot resting on the table. The patient resists internal rotation three to five times, engaging a new external barrier after each contraction.
   D. Management. Consider soft tissue inhibition to the piriformis and functional integration and strengthening of the gluteus medius on the involved side. Include postural reeducation of the involved hip to reduce hip internal rotation stress loads on the sacroiliac joint. The use of a sacroiliac binder or corset may be indicated.
VII. Innominate Upslip. Inferior glide (Fig. 23-52)
   An upslip is a superior subluxation of the innominate on the sacrum at the SIJ. The dysfunction is primarily articular with secondary muscle imbalances (as opposed to anterior and posterior innominate rotations, which primarily result from muscle imbalances that secondarily restrict SIJ motion).[85] Possible muscle findings include quadratus lumborum spasm and tight hip adductors. Causes include

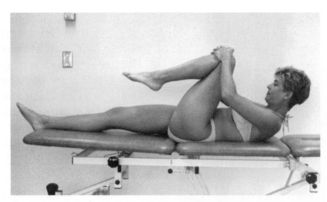

A

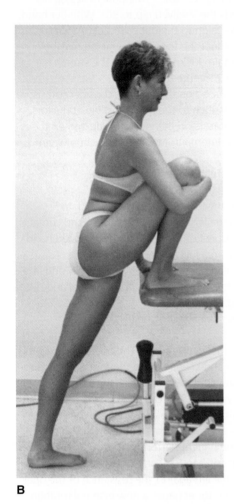

B

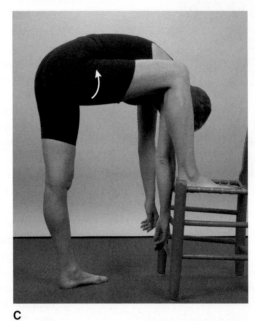

C

■ **FIG. 23-45.** Self-mobilization of the sacroiliac joint: **(A)** posterior rotation in supine and **(B)** posterior rotation in standing. **(C)** Alternative method to correct right anterior rotation: a right posterior lever effect can be created by resting right foot on a high stool (hip flexed 90° and abducted 45°), and then letting the trunk hang down in forward flexion as far as feels comfortable.

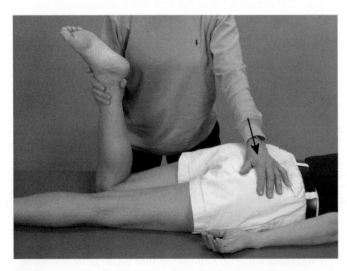

■ **FIG. 23-46.** Passive mobilization for innominate outflare in prone.

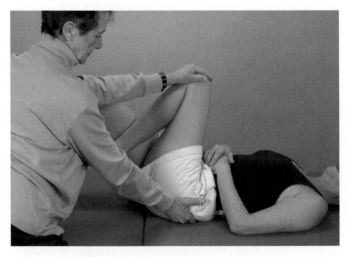

■ **FIG. 23-47.** MET for innominate outflare in supine.

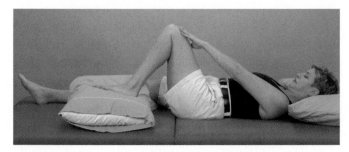

■ **FIG. 23-48.** Self-treatment to counteract an innominate outflare.

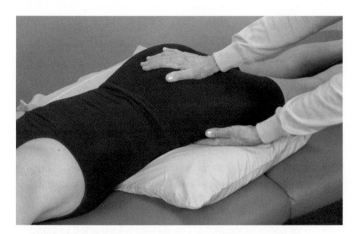

■ **FIG. 23-49.** Passive mobilization for innominate inflare in prone.

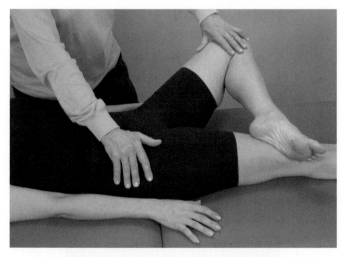

■ **FIG. 23-50.** MET for innominate inflare in supine.

jumping or falling suddenly on an extended leg or, more commonly, from a fall on the ischial tuberosity.[85,213] Signs on the involved side include superior positioning of the ASIS, PSIS, iliac crest, pubic tubercle, and ischial tuberosity. Inferior glide of the ilium is restricted.

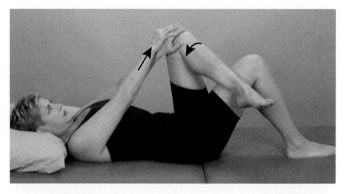

■ **FIG. 23-51.** Self-treatment to counteract an innominate inflare: resisting internal rotation.

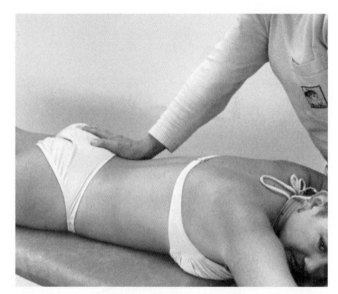

■ **FIG. 23-52.** Inferior glide of the innominate for an upslip.

P—Prone
O—Stands to the involved side at the head
M—The outer hand contacts the superior aspect of the iliac crest and applies an inferior and slightly medial force in the plane of the joint.

VIII. Innominate Upslip. Distraction

Simple longitudinal distraction of one lower limb tends to induce a combined downward and forward movement of the innominate on that side.[101] Distraction may be applied in either supine or prone.

A. Distraction in supine (Fig. 23-53A). The signs are the same as in the iliac upslip, except that the innominate is also in anterior rotation so that the PSIS is superior and the ASIS is inferior on the involved side (iliac upslip with an anterior rotation).

P—Supine with both legs extended
O—Stands at the foot of the table and grasps the

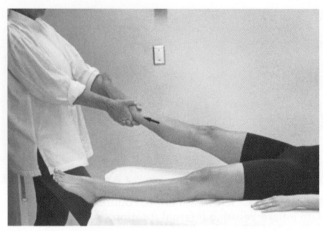

A

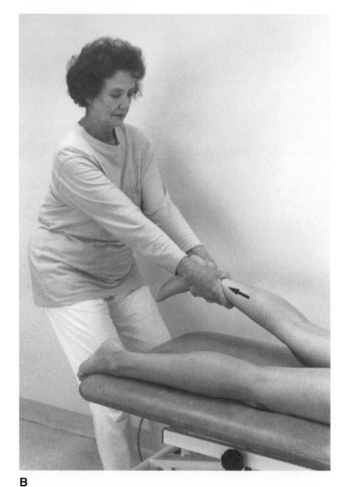

B

■ **FIG. 23-53.** Distraction in **(A)** supine and **(B)** in prone for an innominate upslip.

patient's ankle on one side just proximal to the malleolus. A belt may be used around the patient's trunk, or you may support the opposite foot with your thigh to stabilize the patient.

M—Apply a gentle, caudal distraction force through the lower leg until the exact position of the leg that

will localize the force to the SIJ is attained. Distraction is then applied by pulling the leg, leaning backward with the trunk, and twisting the pelvis, while pushing against the other (outstretched) leg with the thigh.

B. Distraction in prone (Fig. 23-53*B*)

The signs are the same as in the iliac upslip, except that the PSIS is inferior and the ASIS is superior (iliac upslip with posterior rotation). This procedure can be performed in the prone position (Fig. 23-53*B*). Distraction can also be performed in prone with the leg in a neutral position and the knee extended or bent to 90°. In this case the mobilizing hand applies distraction via the uppermost region of the calf; this increases the tension of the rectus femoris.

Manipulation is particularly helpful for correcting an SIJ upslip, which can usually be corrected with quick downward traction on the leg. The exact position of the innominate needs to be determined to know how the maneuver should be carried out. Sudden traction is applied during the exhalation on the second or third cycle. The reader is referred to Lee,[159] Lee and Walsh,[160] and Vleeming et al.[290] for further reading on this topic.

Management of an upslip should include soft tissue inhibition and stretch to the quadratus lumborum and hip adductor muscle and soft tissue mobilization and stretch to tight hip flexors. Self-traction, as proposed by Schamberger,[257] can be used if an upslip fails to correct or keeps reoccurring. The patient is instructed to stand with one leg on a stool and hang the affected leg down over the side with a weight attached (e.g., ankle weights, heavy boot; Fig. 23-54). Traction is applied for 15 to

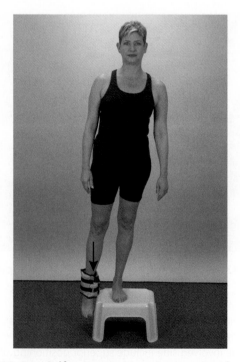

■ **FIG. 23-54.** Self-treatment to counteract an innominate upslip.

30 minutes. The patient should be encouraged to move the leg gently through a limited range of motion at the hip to help relax the muscles and stretch out any structures in the hip and pelvic girdle region. Alternatively hip long axis extension in supine can be used (see Fig. 14-35).

Sacral Dysfunction Techniques

I. Sacral Nutation Technique (Fig. 23-55)

This is used to reduce a sacral counternutation positional fault, commonly caused by a postural flat back, or flexed sitting or standing postures and coccygeal muscle spasm.[213] Signs include lumbar spine hyperflexion, shallow (posterior) sacral sulci, deep (anterior) inferior lateral angles, less prominent PSIS, sacral flexion restriction, and L5 to S1 (and possibly generalized) restriction in lumbar extension.

   P—Prone with a pillow under the abdomen and the legs externally rotated

   O—Stands at the level of the pelvis on the involved side, facing the foot of the table

   M—The base of the inner hand contacts the sacral base, with the arm directed at a right angle to the base. The mobilizing hand glides the cranial surface of the sacrum ventrally, directing the sacrum into nutation. Incline the pressure toward the patient's feet.

   Management of sacral extension dysfunction includes postural reeducation to avoid flexed sitting and standing positions, functional activities to promote lumbar extension mobility, and possibly a home exercise program of prone press-ups. Also consider soft tissue inhibition and stretch to the pelvic diaphragm.[213]

II. Sacral Counternutation Technique (Fig. 23-56)

This is used for sacral nutation dysfunction, commonly caused by an increase in the lumbosacral angle because of structure or poor abdominal tone combined with lumbar

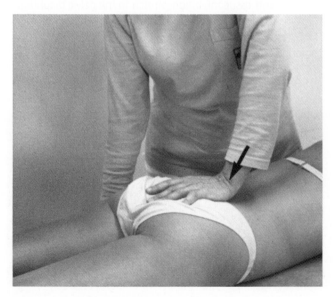

■ **FIG. 23-55.** Sacral nutation.

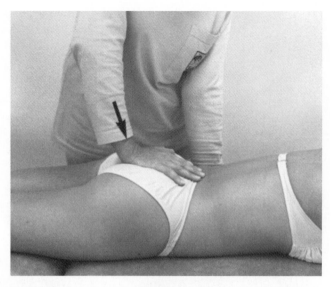

■ **FIG. 23-56.** Sacral counternutation.

spine hyperextension and a weak gluteus medius and maximus.[213] Signs include deep (anterior) sacral sulci and shallow (posterior) inferior lateral angles, increased piriformis and psoas tone, sacral flexion hypermobility or sacral extension restriction,[213] and possibly tenderness and tightness bilaterally in the tensor fasciae latae.[313]

   P—Prone with the legs internally rotated

   O—To one side of the pelvis, facing the head

   M—With thenar or ulnar contact of the inner hand on the sacral apex, apply a posteroanterior force on the apex of the sacrum when the sacrum is felt to extend.

   Management of sacral flexion dysfunction includes promotion of lumbar flexion activities and postures, soft tissue mobilization and stretch for tight structures (piriformis, psoas, and possibly the tensor fasciae latae), and strengthening of the gluteus medius and maximus, as well as the abdominal muscles.

III. Sacral Right Sidebending Technique. Left-on-left sacral torsion dysfunction[213]

   The most common sacral torsion dysfunction, the left-on-left sacral condition, is presented here. By definition, a sacral torsion occurs as a result of sacral rotation and tilt (sidebending) to the same side. Three other types of sacral torsion lesions exist: (1) left-on-right sacral torsion, (2) right-on-right sacral torsion, and (3) right-on-left sacral torsion. The causes, signs, and symptoms will vary somewhat; however, the concept in evaluation and treatment of one type will carry over to the other types. Causes of the left-on-left sacral torsion include right-sided posterior sacroiliac ligamentous weakness, tight left piriformis, weak gluteus medius (especially on the right), a short left leg, spinal left rotation force, hip hyperflexion (left), or hip hyperextension (right). Two techniques are used: sacral right sidebending and right rotation.

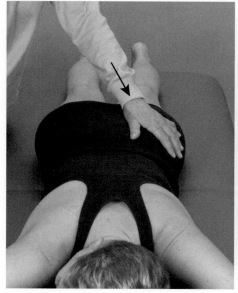

A

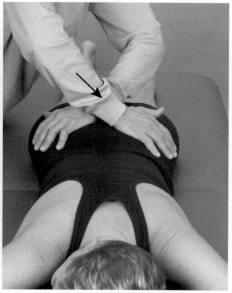

B

■ **FIG. 23-57.** Techniques for a left-on-left sacral torsion dysfunction: **(A)** sacral right sidebending and **(B)** sacral right rotation.

A. Sacral right sidebending (Fig. 23-57A)
   P—Prone
   O—On the right side of the patient facing the feet. The ulnar aspect of the left hand contacts the posterior aspect of the left side of the sacrum with the fingers pointed toward the feet.
   M—An inferior, slightly medial force is applied onto the left side of the sacrum by taking up tissue tension on the posterior aspect.
B. Sacral right rotation (Fig. 23-57B)
   P—Prone
   O—Stands on the right side of the patient with the ulnar aspect of the right hand on the posterior aspect of the left inferior lateral angle. The left hand contacts over the PSIS of the right ilium.
   M—The right hand applies posteroanterior force to the posterior aspect of the left inferior lateral angle, and the left hand applies anterolateral force to the right ilium for stabilization.

   Management should include functional integration and strengthening of the abdominal, gluteus maximus, and gluteus medius, soft tissue manipulation of the piriformis or psoas, and postural reeducation to reduce hip hyperflexion (right) or hyperextension (left) and left-sided rotation stresses of the L5–S1 facets. Other considerations include a decrease in weight-bearing activities with a pelvic belt or corset if unstable, and a shoe lift for correction of a short leg.[213] Also consider distraction of the pubic symphysis (isometric contraction of hip adductors and abductors; Fig. 23-40).

IV. Self-Treatment of Left Sacral Rotation (Fig. 23-58)[122]
   The patient lies supine with the hips and knees flexed. A padded dowel (2/5 cm × 10 cm) is placed vertically on the left side of the sacrum to encompass L5–S1 and S1–S3. The patient maintains this position for 2 minutes. After treatment, retest mobility.

   Other patterns of sacral dysfunction and methods of treatment are described in detail elsewhere.[27,100,122,158,177,257,313]

Symphysis Pubis Techniques To Restore Joint Dysfunction

I. Pubic Decompression Technique (Fig. 23-24A)[213]
   P—Supine with legs externally rotated
   O—Stands on one side of the patient facing the patient
   M—Crossed-armed lateral pressure is applied to the medial aspect of the ASIS with the heels of the hands to decompress.

   Soft tissue inhibition–stretch to the pelvic diaphragm is usually indicated. Encourage movement within pain tolerance to promote pubic motion.

II. Inferior–Superior Pubic Glide Technique (Fig. 23-59)
   P—Supine

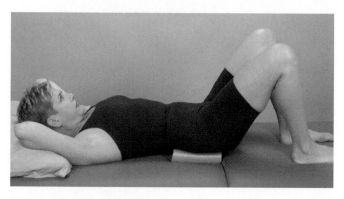

■ **FIG. 23-58.** Self-treatment of left sacral rotation.

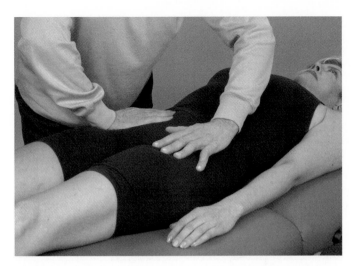

■ **FIG. 23-59.** Inferosuperior pubis glide technique via the ASIS.

O—Stands to the side of the patient, the heel of one hand is placed against the ASIS from above on the far side so the direction of movement is caudad on the ASIS. The heel of the opposite hand is placed against the underside of the other ASIS so the direction of movement of this hand is cephalad on the ASIS.

M—The ASIS are moved in the opposite caudad and cephalad directions.

More localized accessory movements can be performed directly on the pubic ramus. Figure 23-60 illustrates a technique for a superior, posterior dysfunction. The base of the left hand contacts the superior aspect of the pubic ramus on the involved side (left side). The arm applies a gentle inferior and anterior force to move the pubis down and forward.

III. Muscle Energy Technique. Superior pubic symphyseal joint (Fig. 23-61)[27,100,133]

Findings: The standing forward flexion test is positive on the left. The left pubic tubercle is superior to the right and there may be tissue texture changes at the insertion of the inguinal ligament.

   P—Supine, near the left side of the table

   O—Stands on the involved side, toward the foot of the table facing the patient, and supporting the leg over the edge of the table with one hand while stabilizing the patient's right ASIS with the other hand

   M—Slowly glide the leg toward the floor while also slightly abducting it, until the motion barrier is reached. From this position, the patient is asked to lift her knee "up and in" against the operator's hand. The contraction is held for 3 to 5 seconds. After each patient effort, the operator engages new barriers by additional leg extension. About three repetitions are usually required for a correction.

   Reevaluate. Management may include rest from function if unstable and the use of a pelvic girdle binder or corset if necessary. Promote hip extension or lumbar extension when tolerated. Correct any biomechanical problems. Strengthening of the gluteus medius is usually indicated.

IV. Muscle Energy Technique. Inferior pubic symphyseal joint (Fig. 23-62)[27,100,133]

Findings: The pubic tubercle is further inferior on the right with tissue texture changes at the insertion of the inguinal ligament and sensitivity of the hip adductors.

   P—Supine with the right knee and hip flexed, adducted, and slightly medially rotated

   O—Stands on the left side of the patient and stabilizes the patient's left ASIS, while placing the palm of the left hand under the patient's right ischial tuberosity and returns P's pelvis to table.

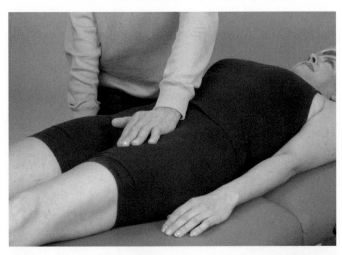

■ **FIG. 23-60.** Inferior and anterior pubis glide via the pubic ramus.

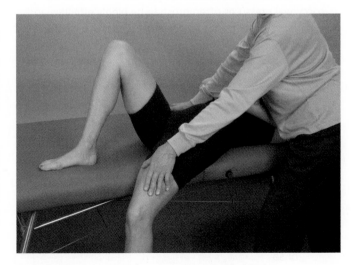

■ **FIG. 23-61.** MET for superior symphysis.

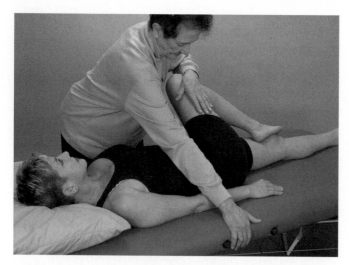

■ **FIG. 23-62.** MET for inferior symphysis (starting position). Hip is flexed further and stabilized under O's shoulder.

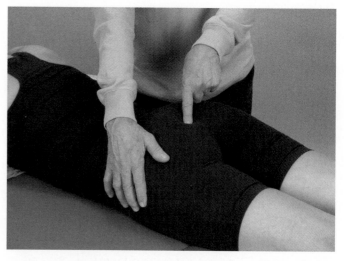

■ **FIG. 23-63.** Strain–counterstrain technique for coccygeal dysfunction.

M—From this position the patient is asked to attempt to straighten her leg in the caudad direction. The operator resists three to four efforts of three to five contractions. After each effort, the operator engages a new barrier by more hip flexion and compression against the ischial tuberosity. Retest.

Also see nonspecific technique for distraction of pubic symphysis and SIJ using muscle energy (Fig. 23-40).

Sacrococcygeal Techniques

I. Anterior Restrictions

These dysfunctions are seen in both women and men and are typically sequelae of falls or direct trauma. Before attempting an invasive technique, using the rectal route, postisometric muscle relaxation (see Fig. 8-65), friction massage (see Box 8-3), strain and counterstrain techniques, and Maitland's anteroposterior pressure and transverse coccygeal pressures often prove to be highly effective and eliminate the need for coccygeal manipulations via the anal passage.

A. Strain and counterstrain correction, coccyx dysfunction (Fig. 23-63).[151] Palpate both sides of the coccyx for tenderness.

P—Lies prone

O—Stands at the side of the patient. One hand is place over the sacrum, the opposite hand monitors the tender point on the coccyx.

M—Place the coccyx in the position of ease by caudally gliding the sacrum. Rotation or lateral flexion of the sacrum, usually toward the tender point side, may be added to fine tune the position. Once the ideal position is achieved, it is held for a period of 90 seconds or so.

B. Anteroposterior coccygeal pressure (Fig. 23-64)[177]

P—Lies prone

O—Places as much of the pad of the tip of the thumbs as possible deeply alongside the coccyx to reach the anterolateral margin of the coccyx

M—When performed unilaterally the therapist directs his thumb pads to the coccyx so that an angulated anteroposterior movement is achieved.

C. Transverse coccygeal pressure[177]

P—Lies prone

O—Places the thumb pads to one side of the coccyx. It is necessary with this technique to maintain a very deep position of the thumbs if the whole lateral aspect is to be reached.

M—Vary the point of contact and pressure (e.g., cephalad, caudad) so that pain produced by bone-to-bone contact is avoided. The thumbs apply an oscillatory force directed toward the opposite side.

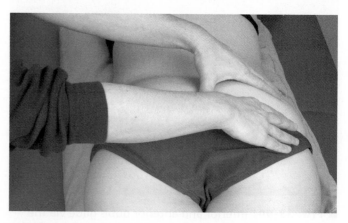

■ **FIG. 23-64.** Anteroposterior coccygeal pressure.

II. Posterior Restrictions[7]

These are seen almost exclusively in women. During childbirth, the head of the fetus pushes the coccyx posteriorly. The anterior sacrococcygeal ligament is stretched, whereas the posterior sacrococcygeal ligament gradually shortens, fibroses, and keeps the coccyx extended.[6,7]

A. Posteroanterior glide (Fig. 23-65)[7]

P—Seated

O—Stands at the side of the patient and places the palm of the mobilizing hand over the sacrum and fingers on the coccyx

M—Move the coccyx anterosuperiorly. The mobilization may be easier if the other hand places slight compression on the skull.

Alternatively this technique may be performed in supine. Many times just performing the evaluation in sitting will free the coccyx and put it back in place.

B. Posteroanterior central pressure (Fig. 23-66)[177]

P—Lies prone

O—Places as much of the tip of the thumb pad as possible over the mid-coccyx

M—Gentle posteroanterior central pressures are applied at first. Grades should only be increased if the pain response permits it. The point of contact as well as the angle of pressure can be varied for a more effective technique.

Posteroanterior central, anteroposterior, and transverse coccygeal pressures are also used as examination techniques.[177] The examination technique that produces the predicted pain response is used as the treatment technique. It is advisable to use these techniques as grade II or III techniques until it is known that there will not be any unfavorable reaction to firmer techniques.

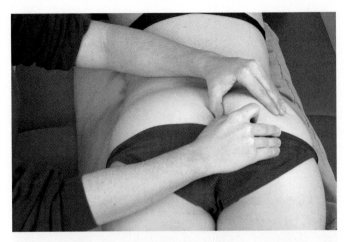

■ **FIG. 23-66.** Posteroanterior central coccygeal pressure.

Sensorimotor and Neuromuscular Training

Understanding the full nature of SI disturbance requires understanding the interdependence concept of the pelvic girdle system. The lower lumbar spine, hips, and SIJs are virtually inseparable components of the pelvis. Involvement of any one structure will directly affect the positioning and movement of the other. Correction of biomechanical problems (e.g., agonist–antagonist muscle imbalance) of the spine and lower limbs is key. The sacrum is mechanically associated with the spine, whereas the ilium is aligned with and affected by the lower limbs. Management of the SIJ complex takes considerable vigilance.

Sensorimotor activities are the same as those suggested in Chapter 22, Lumbar Spine. Sensorimotor stimulation is beneficial when used as part of any exercise program in that it helps improve muscle coordination and motor programming and increases the speed of activation of a muscle.[133,135] Chronic lumbopelvic pain represents one of the most important indications. Better control of the trunk, improved activation of the gluteal muscles, and thus better stability of the pelvis is achieved by sensorimotor training.

The neuromuscular system is under the control of the sensorimotor loop. With people in chronic pain, the functioning of this feedback loop has been distorted as a result of the deleterious effect of habituation. These patients' perception must be dishabituated; that is to say, they must learn to sense their movements and must refine that sensitivity.[94] Strengthening exercises can often be counterproductive if a patient performs the movements in such a way that they have the opposite effect. Janda[130] has demonstrated experimentally that people with chronic back pain can perform so-called abdominal muscle strengthening and end up strengthening the spinal extensors instead.

Particularly useful pelvic girdle techniques for neuromuscular reeducation in the sensorimotor dimension are the pelvic clock or compass (Fig. 23-67)[30,33,34,94,100,244] and PNF using

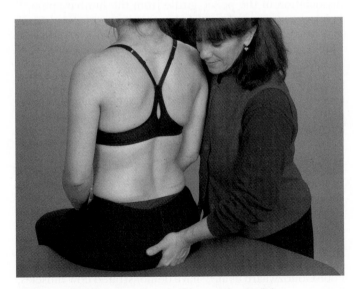

■ **FIG. 23-65.** Posteroanterior coccygeal glide.

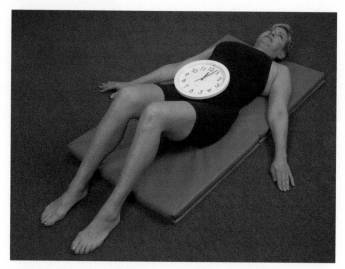

■ FIG. 23-67. Pelvic clock exercise for integration of the lumbopelvic musculature.

pelvic diagonal patterns of movement.[1,282] Pelvic clocks, used by Feldenkrais practitioners, are not only useful in diagnosis but can be used for self-mobilization and for neuromuscular reeducation of the pelvic and lumbar musculature. There are numerous variations of the pelvic clock in the supine position. Progression of pelvic motions in hooklying on a rocker board, half roll, or inflatable air cushion is even more challenging (Fig. 23-68). Once the patient has good control in these relaxed positions, pelvic clocks can be performed on all fours, standing with bent knees, and in a sitting position on a therapeutic ball to assist in establishing a kinesthetic awareness of this region.

The use of PNF pelvic diagonals like the pelvic clock allows the therapist to move quickly and effectively to evaluate neuromuscular control and range of motion within synergistic muscle groups. When dysfunctions are identified, specific PNF techniques can be applied to enhance the desired functional

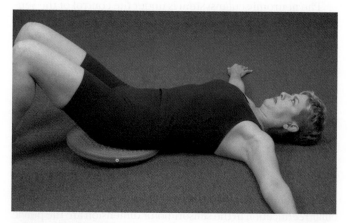

■ FIG. 23-68. Pelvic motions on an inflatable cushion.

movement through facilitation, inhibition, strengthening, and relaxation of muscle groups. The techniques use concentric, eccentric, and static muscle contractions combined with properly graded resistance and suitable facilitatory procedures and are combined and adjusted to fit the needs of each patient. Patterns can be done with the patient lying, sitting, or standing. Sidelying allows free motion of the pelvis and easy reinforcement of the trunk and lower limbs (Box 23-1). The movements and muscle components mainly involved are as follows[141]:

Anterior elevation	Internal and external oblique abdominal muscles
Posterior depression	Contralateral quadratus lumborum, iliocostalis lumborum, iliocostalis lumborum, and longissimus thoracis
Posterior elevation	Ipsilateral quadratus lumborum, ipsilateral latissimus dorsi, iliocostalis lumborum, and longissimus thoracis
Anterior depression	Contralateral internal and external oblique abdominal muscles

For anterior elevation patterns to occur efficiently, the lower abdominals (transversus abdominus and internal obliques), trunk extensors, body of the psoas, and quadratus lumborum must perform in a coordinated sequence of contraction and elongation.[251] The posterior depression pattern occurs along the same track of motion but requires efficient antagonistic muscle function to develop coordination of pelvic and hip motions and dissociation of pelvic and lumbar motions. The primary tools for treating dysfunction in the patterns are contract or hold-relax to increase mobility and a combination of isotonics to improve the proper sequencing of muscle recruitment and dissociation of the pelvic girdle from the lumbar spine.[251] Pelvic patterns can be carried out with scapular and trunk patterns allowing unlimited variety of patterns and techniques and activation of the pelvic sling muscles. As motion becomes integrated, lower limb motions can be resisted to develop synergistic lumbopelvic–lower limb control. The success achieved through PNF is derived from the therapist's ability to appropriately identify faulty characteristics of neuromuscular control and analyze and select the appropriate technique. Details of these PNF techniques are beyond the scope of this text. The reader is referred to the works of Adler et al.,[1] Saliba et al.,[251] Stalvey,[277] and Sullivan and Markos.[282]

Lumbopelvic Stabilization and Functional Exercises

Pool-Goudzwaard et al.[230] have demonstrated how muscles, ligaments, and the thoracolumbar fascia aid in stabilizing the pelvis, thus achieving force closure. Force closure is necessary during gait when unilateral loading of the legs introduces shear forces, and the muscle–ligament–fascia system is required to stabilize by compressing the SIJ. The sacrotuberous and long dorsal sacroiliac ligaments are responsible for limiting nutation and counternutation, respectively. Insufficient ligamentous tension will decrease force closure. Three muscle slings—anterior oblique, posterior oblique, and longitudinal slings—are the active components in the pelvic sling system. The muscular slings and other core muscles of the inner unit and the lateral system have been described earlier.

Stabilization programs advocated for the lumbar spine and thoracic spine are also useful for problems of the SIJs.[106,203,245,248,308] After a detailed evaluation, exercises should focus on reactivating the deep intrinsic stabilizers such as the transverse abdominals, internal oblique abdominal, and multifidus (see Figs. 20-31, 20-32, 20-70, 20-71 through 20-73, 20-75, 22-16, 22-17, and 22-68 through 22-75) and possible endurance training of the quadratus lumborum (see Figs. 22-20, 22-64, and 22-65), gluteus medius (see Figs. 14-38*B* and 14-39), gluteus maximus (see Fig. 14-38*A*), and latissimus dorsi (see Figs. 11-75 and 11-85). Both Pilates core exercises[184,205,206,244] and yoga strengthening exercises[31,136,150,153,236] have been found useful. One of the best yoga methods recommend by Lasater[153] is simple backbends, such as the bow pose (Dhanurasana; Fig. 23-69), in which the pelvis moves forward and contraction of the posterior muscles is required. This helps to move the sacroiliac joint into place and also strengthens the muscles of the lower back and hip that can help hold it in place.

To facilitate the pelvic stabilizers it is often necessary to balance the left and right transversus abdominus in coordination with gross pelvic movements. Figures 23-70 and 23-71 illustrate two such exercises proposed by Browne.[34]

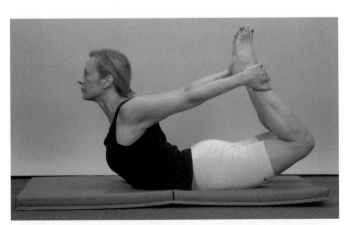

■ **FIG. 23-69.** Bow pose. The knees are lifted straight up off the floor as the chest lifts simultaneously and the shoulders retract. Strong engagement of the buttock muscles is required.

In Figure 23-70 the patient assumes supine position on the floor with the pelvis on a small to medium ball—feet off the floor allowing the pelvis to fall to the left and right until a neutral position is found. In this position the patient attempts to reach alternately with the feet toward the ceiling while straightening the knees, then with the knees and feet wide apart. It is important for the patient to differentiate the upper abdominals from the lower abdominals while maintaining lumbopelvic control. Figure 23-71 introduces some lumbar thoracic differentiation by crossover movements to the left and right while maintaining the pelvis in neutral. The head moves in one direction and the knees in the opposite. The aim is to achieve rotation of the spine with controlled stability. Also see Figure 22-76 for lumbopelvic rotational control.

Use of the pelvic floor muscles (PFM) is one of the most effective ways of achieving contraction of the transversus abdominus to contribute to stabilization of the spine and also plays an important supporting role in sacroiliac dysfunction. Hypomobility or hypermobility of the sacroiliac, pubic symphysis, or sacrococcygeal joint may cause the secondary impairment of the altered tone of the PFM. Pain from joint dysfunction may lead to tonic holding of the PFMs, and sacroiliac mobility impairments may also cause pain-induced PFM muscle weakness. Discussion of specific strengthening programs of the PFM is beyond the scope of this chapter, and the reader is referred to the current literature.[3,15–18,27,37,39,120,127,155,208,253,265,266,278,300]

Stabilization must also include training in functional core exercises using stability patterns in movements and positions similar to those of daily living, recreation, and sport demands. For instance, lunges and diagonal rotational squats (see Fig. 22-77) create optimal coupling of the gluteal muscles and contralateral latissimus dorsi and pushing and pulling movements.

SUMMARY

Dysfunctions of the pelvic girdle are often complex and not easily understood. All of the areas—the lumbar spine, pelvis, and hips—are anatomically and functionally related, and all should be examined in detail so that treatment can be applied based on these findings. The treatment goal is to normalize stresses in the lumbar–pelvic–hip complex by balancing muscle length and strength, ground and trunk forces, and afferent–efferent neural pathways. The myokinetics and arthrokinematics of the region are in their infancy as far as research is concerned; investigations have shown that motion exists at the SIJ, but it is variable and limited. Restoring pelvic girdle function within the walking cycle is a major therapeutic goal from the biomechanical, postural, and structural point of view. The most powerful healer is often not to create the torque of sacrum and ilium moving apart in functional activities and everyday life.

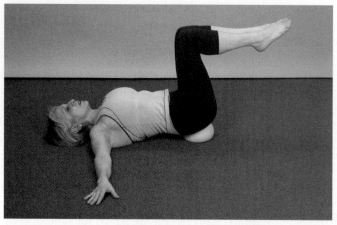

A

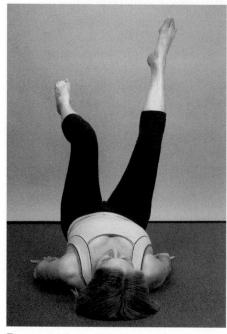

B

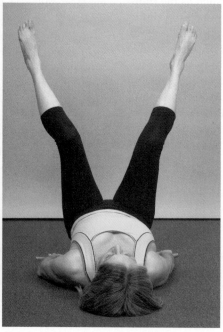

C

■ **FIG. 23-70.** Balancing the pelvis on a ball (medium size) to help balance the left and right transversus abdominus. With the feet off the floor, the pelvis is allowed to fall left and right a small amount off the ball to find neutral and train the transversus abdominus (**A**). A variety of leg patterns can be added such as reaching to the ceiling with straightening of the knees (**B**) and performing movements with the legs wide apart (**C**).

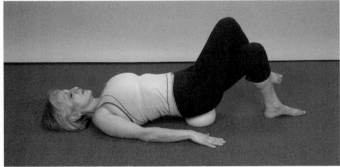

A

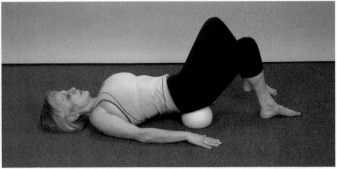

B

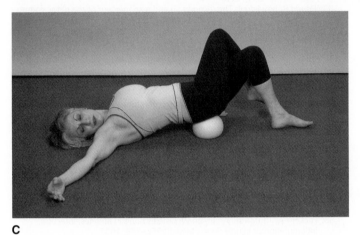

C

■ **FIG. 23-71.** Balancing the pelvis on a ball to help balance left and right transversus abdominus with some lumbar and thoracic differentiation. With the ball under one side of the pelvis, one leg is crossed over the other (**A**). As the lower trunk rotates to the opposite side (**B**), the head and trunk rotate to the same side with control (**C**).

REFERENCES

1. Adler SS, Beckers D, Buck M: PNF in Practice. An Illustrated Guide. Berlin, Springer-Verlag, 1993
2. Alviso DJ, Dong GT, Lentell GL: Intertester reliability for measuring pelvic tilt in standing. Phys Ther 68:1347–1351, 1988
3. Appell RA, Bourcier AP, Torre FL: Pelvic Floor Dysfunction-Investigations and Conservative Treatment. Rome, Casa Editrice Scientifica Internazionale, 1999
4. Baker PK: Musculoskeletal problems. In: Steege E, ed: Chronic Pelvic Pain. Philadelphia, WB Saunders, 1998:215–240
5. Bakland O, Hansen JH: The axial SIJ. Anat Clin 6:29–36, 1984
6. Barral JP: Visceral Manipulation. Seattle, Eastland Press, 1988
7. Barral JP: Urogenital Manipulations. Seattle, Eastland Press, 1993
8. Beal MC: The sacroiliac problem: Review of anatomy, mechanics and diagnosis. J Am Osteopath Assoc 81:667–679, 1982
9. Bemis T, Daniel M: Validation of the long-sit test on subjects with iliosacral dysfunction. J Orthop Sports Phys Ther 8:336–345, 1987
10. Benson DR: The back: Thoracic and lumbar spine. In: D'Ambrosia RD, ed: Musculoskeletal Disorders: Regional Examination and Differential Diagnosis, 2nd ed. Philadelphia, JB Lippincott, 1986:287–366
11. Berg G, Hammer M, Moller-Nielsen J, et al: Low back pain during pregnancy. Obstet Gynecol 71:71–75, 1979
12. Bernard TN, Cassidy JD: The SIJ syndrome: Pathophysiology, diagnosis and management. In: Frymoyer JW, ed: The Adult Spine: Principles and Practice. New York, Raven Press, 1991:2107–2130
13. Bernard TN, Kirkalday-Willis WH: Recognizing specific characteristics of non-specific low back pain. Clin Orthop 217:266–280, 1987
14. Biedert RM, Warnke K, Meyer S: Symphysis syndrome in athletes: surgical treatment for chronic lower abdominal, groin, and adductor pain in athletes. Clin J Sports Med 13:278–284, 2003
15. Bo K: Pelvic floor muscle exercise for the treatment of stress urinary incontinence: An exercise physiology perspective. Int Urogynecol 6:282–291, 1995
16. Bo K: Single blind, randomised controlled trial of pelvic floor exercises, electrical stimulation, vaginal cones, and no treatment in management of genuine stress incontinence in women. J Section Women's Health 26:17–23, 2002
17. Bo K, Hagen RH, Kvarstein B, et al: Pelvic floor muscle exercise for the treatment of female stress urinary incontinence. III: Effects of two different degrees of pelvic floor muscle exercise. Neurourol Urodyn 9:489–502, 1990
18. Bo K, Kvarstein B, Larsen S: Pelvic floor muscle exercise for the treatment of female stress urinary incontinence. II: Validity of vaginal pressure measurements of pelvic floor muscle strength and the necessity of supplementary methods for control of correct contraction. Neurourol Urodyn 9:479–487, 1990
19. Bo K, Lilleas F, Talseth T, et al: Dynamic MRI of the pelvic floor muscle in an upright sitting position. Neurourol Urodyam 20: 167–174, 2001
20. Bogduk N: Lumbar dorsal ramus syndrome. Med J Aust 2:537–541, 1980
21. Bogduk N, Twomey LT: Clinical Anatomy of the Lumbar Spine and Sacrum, 3rd ed. London, Churchill Livingstone, 1997
22. Boltz S, Davies GJ: Leg-length differences and correlation with total leg strength. J Orthop Sports Phys Ther 6:123–129, 1984
23. Bookhout MM, Boissonnault JS: Musculoskeletal dysfunction in the female pelvis. Orthop Phys Ther Clin North Am 5: 23–45, 1996
24. Bookhout MR: Examination and treatment of muscle imbalances. In: Bourdillon JF, Day EA, Bookhout MR, eds: Spinal Manipulation, 5th ed. Oxford, Butterworth-Heinemann, 1992a:313–333
25. Bookhout MR: Exercise as a compliment to manual therapy. In: Bourdillon JF, Day EA, Bookhout MR, eds: Spinal Manipulation, 5th ed. Oxford, Butterworth-Heinemann, 1992b:335–355
26. Borel U, Fernstrom I: The movements of the SIJs and their importance to changes on pelvic dimensions during parturition. Acta Obstet Gynecol Scand 36:42–57, 1957
27. Bourdillon JF, Day EA, Bookhout MR, eds: Spinal Manipulation, 5th ed. Oxford, Butterworth-Heinemann, 1992
28. Bowen V, Cassidy JD: Macroscopic and microscopic anatomy of the SIJ from embryonic life until the eighth decade. Spine 6:620–627, 1981
29. Broadhurst NA: Sacroiliac dysfunction as a cause of low back pain. Aust Fam Phys 18:623–628, 1989
30. Bronner S: Functional rehabilitation of the spine: The lumbopelvis as a key point of control. In: Brownstein B, Bronner S, eds: Evaluation Treatment and Outcomes: Functional Movement in Orthopaedic and Sports Physical Therapy. New York, Churchill Livingstone, 1995:141–190
31. Bronson KM: The therapeutic benefits of yoga. Orthop Phys Ther Pract 14:3:11–15, 2002
32. Brooke R: The SIJ. J Anat 58:299–305, 1924
33. Browne G: A Manual Therapist's Guide to Movement. Edinburg, Elsevier, In press.
34. Browne G: Outsmarting Lower Back Pain. Facilitating Lumbopelvic Stability. Seattle, Motor Learning Seminars, 2003
35. Cabot J, Marin M, Cisa J: Pubialgia del deportista. Rev Orthop Trauma 291B:255–258, 1985

36. Cailliet R: Miscellaneous low back conditions relating to pain. In: Cailliet R, ed: Low Back Pain Syndrome, 4th ed. Philadelphia, FA Davis, 1988:252–270
37. Calais-Germain B: The Female Pelvis Anatomy and Exercise. Seattle, Eastland Press, 2003
38. Cantu R, Grodin A; Myofascial Manipulations. Gaithersburg, MD, Aspen Publishing, 1992
39. Carriere B: Fitness for the Pelvic Floor. Stuttgart, Thieme, 2002
40. Chamberlin WE: The symphysis pubis in the roentgen examination of the SIJ. J Bone Joint Surg Am 23:621–625, 1930
41. Chapman L, Nihls M: Myokinematics of the pelvis. Proceedings of the 5th Conference of International Federations of Orthopaedic Manipulative Therapists. Vancouver, British Columbia, 1984
42. Chapman SA, DeFranca CL: Rehabilitation of the low back. In: Cox JM, ed: Low Back Pain: Mechanism, Diagnosis, and Treatment. Baltimore, 6th ed. Baltimore, Williams & Wilkins 1999:653–678
43. Cibulka M: The treatment of the SIJ component to low back pain. Phys Ther 72:917–922, 1992
44. Cibulka M, Delitto A: A comparison of two different methods to treat hip pain in runners. J Orthop Sports Phys Ther 17:172–176, 1993
45. Cibulka MT, Delitto A, Koldehoff RM: Changes in innominate tilt after manipulation of the SIJ in patients with low back pain: An experimental study. Phys Ther 68:1359–1363, 1988
46. Cibulka MT, Koldehoff RM: Leg-length disparity and its effect on SIJ dysfunction. Clin Manage 6:10–11, 1986
47. Cipriano JJ: Photographic Manual of Regional Orthopedic Tests. Baltimore, Williams & Wilkins, 1985
48. Clayson SJ, Newton IM, Debeucc DF, et al: Evaluation of mobility of hip and lumbar vertebrae in normal young women. Arch Phys Med Rehabil 43:1–8, 1962
49. Cohen AS, McNeill JM, Calkins E, et al: The "normal" SIJ: Analysis of 88 sacroiliac roentgenograms. Am J Roent Radium Ther 100:559–563, 1967
50. Colachis SD, Warden RE, Bechtol CO: Movement of the SIJ in the adult male: A preliminary report. Arch Phys Med Rehabil 44:490–498, 1963
51. Corrigan B, Maitland GD: Practical Orthopaedic Medicine. London, Butterworths, 1983
52. Costello K: Myofascial syndromes. In: Steege JF, Metztger DA, Levey BS, eds: Chronic Pelvic Pain. An Integrated Approach. Philadelphia, WB Saunders, 1998:251–266
53. Coventry MB, Tapper EM: Pelvic instability. J Bone Joint Surg Am 54:83–101, 1972
54. Cyriax JH: Textbook of Orthopaedic Medicine: Diagnosis of Soft-Tissue Lesions, vol. 1, 8th ed. London, Bailliere Tindall, 1982
55. Cyriax JH, Coldham M: Textbook of Orthopaedic Medicine: Treatment by Manipulation, Massage, and Injection, vol. 2, 11th ed. Philadelphia, Bailliere Tindall, 1984
56. D'Ambrosia RD: The hip. In: D'Ambrosia RD, ed: Musculoskeletal Disorders: Regional Examination and Differential Diagnosis, 2nd ed. Philadelphia, JB Lippincott, 1986:447–490
57. Daly JM, Frame PS, Rapoza PA: Sacroiliac subluxation: A common, treatable cause of low-back pain in pregnancy. Fam Pract Res J 11:149–159, 1991
58. Davis P, Lentle BC: Evidence of sacroiliac disease a common cause of low backache in women. Lancet 2:496–497, 1978
59. Denslow JS, Chance JA, Gardner DL, et al: Mechanical stresses in the human lumbar spine and pelvis. J Am Osteopath Assoc 61:705–712, 1962
60. Derry DE: Note on accessory articular facets between the sacrum and ilium, and their significance. J Anat Physiol 45:202–211, 1911
61. Dietrichs E, Kogstad O: "Pelvic girdle relaxation"—Suggested new nomenclature. Scand J Rheumatol Suppl 88:3, 1991
62. Dijkstra PF, Vleeming A, Stoeckart R: Complex motion tomography of the SIJ: An anatomical and roentgenological study. Rofo Forstschr Geb Rontgenstr Neuen Bildgeh Verfahr 150:635–642, 1989
63. DonTigny RL: Functions and pathomechanics of the SIJ: A review. Phys Ther 65:35–44, 1985
64. DonTigny RL: Dialogue on SIJ [letter]. Phys Ther 69:164–165, 1989
65. DonTigny RL: Pathomechanics and treatment of SIJ dysfunction. In: International Federation of Orthopaedic Manipulative Therapists, 5th International Conference, Vail, 1992
66. DonTigny RL: Mechanic and treatment of the sacroiliac joint. In: Vleeming A, Mooney V, Doraman T, et al, eds: Movement, Stability, and Low Back Pain: The Essential Role of the Pelvis. New York, Churchill Livingstone, 1997:461–476
67. Doran DMI, Newell DJ: Manipulation in treatment of low back pain: A multicentre study. BMJ 2:161–164, 1975
68. Dorman TA: Prolotherapy: A survey. J Orthop Med 15:2–3, 1993
69. Dorman TA: Failure of self-bracing at the sacroiliac joint: The slipping clutch syndrome. J Orthop Med 16:49–51, 1994
70. Dorman TA: Pelvic mechanics and prolotherapy. In: Vleeming A, Mooney V, Dorman T, et al, eds: Movement, Stability, and Low Back Pain: The Essential Role of the Pelvis. New York, Churchill Livingstone, 1997:501–522
71. Dorman TA, Brierly S, Fray J, et al: Muscles and pelvic clutch; hip abductor inhibition in anterior rotation of the ilium. In: Vleeming A, Mooney V, Tischler H, et al, eds: Proceedings of the Third Interdisciplinary World Congress on Low Back and Pelvic Pain. Vienna, November 19–21, 1998:140–148

72. Drerup B, Hierholzer E: Movement of the human pelvis and displacement of related anatomical landmarks on the body surface. J Biomech 20:971–977, 1987
73. Dunn EJ, Bryon DM, Nugent JT, et al: Pyogenic infections of the hip joint. Clin Orthop 118:113–117, 1976
74. Dutton M: The sacroiliac joint. In: Dutton M: Manual Therapy of the Spine, An Integrated Approach. New York, McGraw-Hill, 2002:446–493
75. Dvorák J, Dvorák V: Manual Medicine: Diagnostics, 2nd ed. Stuttgart, Georg Thieme Verlag/Thieme Medical Publisher, 1990
76. Edmond SL: Manipulation and Mobilization: Extremity and Spinal Techniques. St. Louis, Mosby, 1993
77. Egund N, Olsson TH, Schmid H: Movement in the SIJs demonstrated with roentgen stereophotogrammetry. Acta Radiol (Stockh) 19:833–846, 1978
78. Ehara S, El-Koury GY, Bergman RA: The accessory SIJ: A common anatomic variant. AJR Am J Roentgenol 150:857–859, 1988
79. Ellison JB, Rose SJ, Sahrmann SA: Patterns of hip rotation range of motion: Comparison between healthy subjects and patients with low back pain. Phys Ther 70:537–541, 1990
80. Erhard R, Bowling R: The recognition and management of the pelvic components of low back pain and sciatic pain. Bulletin of the Orthopaedics Section, APTA 2:4–15, 1977
81. Fairbanks JCT, Park WN, McCall JW, et al: Apophyseal injection of local anesthetic as a diagnostic aid in primary low back syndromes. Spine 6:598–605, 1981
82. Fairbanks JCT, Pysant PB, Van Poortvliet JA, el al: Influence of anthropometric factors and joint laxity in the incidence of adolescent back pain. Spine 9:461–464, 1984
83. Farfan C: The biomechanical advantage of lordosis and hip extension for upright activity. Spine 3:336–342, 1978
84. Fisk JW: Medical Treatment of Neck and Back Pain. Springfield, IL, Charles C Thomas, 1987
85. Fowler C: Muscle energy techniques for pelvic dysfunction. In: Grieve GP, ed: Modern Manual Therapy of the Vertebral Column. Edinburgh, Churchill Livingstone, 1986
86. Friberg O: Clinical symptoms and biomechanics of lumbar spine hip joint in leg-length inequality. Spine 8:643–650, 1983
87. Friberg O: The statics of postural pelvic tilt scoliosis: A radiographic study on 288 consecutive chronic LBP patients. Clin Biomech 2:211–219, 1987
88. Fricker PA, Tauton JE, Ammann W: Osteitis pubis in athletes. Infection, inflammation or injury? Sports Med 12:266–279, 1991
89. Frigerio NA, Stowe RR, Howe JW: Movement of the SIJ. Clin Orthop 100:370–377, 1974
90. Gibofsky A: Reiter syndrome. In: Beary JF, Christian CL, Johanson NA, eds: Manual of Rheumatology and Outpatient Orthopedic Disorders: Diagnosis and Therapy, 2nd ed. Boston, Little, Brown and Co, 1987
91. Giles LGF, Taylor JR: Lumbar spine structural changes associated with leg-length inequality. Spine 7:159–162, 1982
92. Goften JP: Studies in osteoarthritis of the hip: Part IV. Biomechanics and clinical considerations. Can Med Assoc J 104:1007–1011, 1971
93. Goften JP, Trureman GE: Studies in osteoarthritis of the hip: Part II. Osteoarthritis of the hip and leg-length disparity. Can Med Assoc J 104:791–799, 1971
94. Goldfarb LW: The Feldenkrais Method for Moving Smarter. Tucson, AZ, Therapy Skill Builders, 1994
95. Goldthwait JE: The pelvic articulations: A consideration of their anatomic, physiologic, obstetric and general surgical importance. JAMA 49:768–774, 1907
96. Good MB: Diagnosis and treatment of sciatic pain. Lancet 2:597–598, 1942
97. Good MB: What is "fibrositis"? Rheumatism 5:117–123, 1949
98. Gracovetsky SA: Linking the spinal engine with the legs: A theory of human gait. In: Vleeming A, Mooney V, Dorman T, et al, eds: Movement, Stability and Low Back Pain: The Essential Role of the Pelvis, New York, Churchill Livingstone, 1997
99. Gray H: SIJ pain, Part II. Mobility and axes of rotation. Int Clin 11:65–76, 1938
100. Greenman PE: Principles of Manual Medicine, 3rd ed. Philadelphia, Lippincott Williams & Wilkins, 2003
101. Grieve E: Lumbopelvic rhythm and mechanical dysfunction of the SIJ. Physiotherapy 67:171–173, 1981
102. Grieve EFM. Mechanical dysfunction of the SIJ. Int Rehabil Med 5:46–52, 1983
103. Grieve GP: The SIJ. Physiotherapy 62:384–400, 1976
104. Grieve GP: Mobilization of the Spine: Notes on Examination, Assessment and Clinical Method, 4th ed. Edinburgh, Churchill Livingstone, 1984
105. Grieve GP: Common Vertebral Problems. Edinburgh, Churchill Livingstone, 1988
106. Gustavsen R, Streeck R: Training Therapy: Prophylaxis and Rehabilitation, 2nd ed. Stuttgart, Georg Thieme Verlag, 1993
107. Gutstein-Good M: Idiopathic myalgia simulating visceral and other diseases. Lancet 2:326–328, 1940
108. Hackett GS: Ligament and Tendon Relaxation (Skeletal Disability) Treated by Protherapy (Fibro-Osseous Proliferation), 3rd ed. Springfield, IL, Charles C Thomas, 1958
109. Hackett GS, Hemwall GA, Montgomery GA: Ligament and Tendons Relaxation Treated by Proliferation, 5th ed. Oak Park, IL, Gustav A Hemwell, 1991
110. Hadley LA: Accessory sacroiliac articulations with arthritic changes. Radiology 55:403–409, 1950

111. Hadley LA: Accessory sacroiliac articulations. J Bone Joint Surg Am 34:149–155, 1952

112. Hagen R: Pelvic girdle relaxation from an orthopaedic point of view. Acta Orthop Scand 45:550–563, 1974

113. Hall C: Diagnosis and Treatment of Movement System Imbalances and Musculoskeletal Pain as Taught by Shirley Sahrmann. Continuing education course, Seattle, 1993

114. Hall C, Brody LT: Impairment in muscle performance. In: Hall C, Brody LT: Therapeutic Exercise Moving Toward Function. Baltimore, Lippincott Williams & Wilkins, 1999:43–69

115. Hallin RP: Sciatic pain and the piriformis muscle. Postgrad Med 74:69–72, 1983

116. Hanson PG, Angevine M, Juhl J: Osteitis pubis in sports activities. Physician Sportsmed 7:111–114, 1978

117. Harris NH, Murry RO: Lesions of the symphysis pubis in athletes. BMJ 4:211–214, 1974

118. Hartley A: Practical Joint Assessment: A Sports Medicine Manual. St. Louis, Mosby Year Book, 1990

119. Healy JH: Paget disease of bone. In: Beary JF, Christian CL, Johanson NA, eds: Manual of Rheumatology and Outpatient Orthopedic Disorders: Diagnosis and Therapy, 2nd ed. Boston, Little, Brown and Co, 1987

120. Herman H, Shelly B: Intermediate pelvic floor dysfunction. Continuing education course. Sponsored by The Section on Women's Health, APTA, Seattle, 2003

121. Hesch J: Course workbook—The Hesch method of treating sacroiliac joint dysfunction: an integrated approach. Albuquerque, 1996

122. Hesch J: Evaluation and treatment of the most common patterns of sacroiliac joint dysfunction. In: Vleeming A, Mooney V, Dorman T, et al, eds: Movement, Stability, and Low Back Pain: The Essential Role of the Pelvis. New York, Churchill Livingstone, 1997:535–545

123. Hides JA, Stokes MJ, Saide M, et al: Evidence of lumbar multifidus muscle wasting ipsilateral to symptoms in patients with acute/subacute low back pain. Spine 19:165–172, 1994

124. Hirschberg GG: Sclerosant solution in low back pain. West J Med 143:682–686, 1985

125. Hollinshead WH, Jenkins DB: Functional Anatomy of the Limbs and Back. Philadelphia, WB Saunders, 1981

126. Hoppenfeld S: Physical Examination of the Spine and Extremities. New York, Appleton-Century-Crofts, 1976

127. Hume JA: Beyond Kegels: Fabulous Four Exercises and More to Prevent and Treat Incontinence. Missoula, MT, Phoenix Publishing, 1997

128. Ishimino T: Histopathological study of the aging process in the human SIJ [in Japanese]. Nippon Seikeigeka Gakkai Zasshi 63;1070–1084, 1989

129. Jajic I, Jajic Z: The prevalence of osteoarthrosis of the SIJs in an urban population. Clin Rheumatol 6:39–41, 1987

130. Janda V: Muscles, central nervous motor regulation and back problems. In: Korr I, ed: The Neurobiologic Mechanisms in Manipulative Therapy. London, Plenum Press, 1978:27–42

131. Janda V: Muscle Function Testing. Boston, Butterworths, 1983

132. Janda V: Muscle weakness and inhibition (pseudoparesis) in back pain syndromes. In: Grieve GP, ed: Modern Manual Therapy of the Vertebral Column. New York, Churchill Livingstone, 1986:197–201

133. Janda V: Evaluation of muscle imbalance. In: Liebensen C, ed: Rehabilitation of the Spine: A Practitioner's Manual. Philadelphia, Lippincott Williams & Wilkins, 1996:97–112

134. Janda V, Schmid H: Muscles as a pathogenic factor in back pain. Proceedings, 4th Conference of International Federation of Orthopaedic Manipulative Therapist. Christchurch, New Zealand, 1980

135. Janda V, Vavrova M: Sensory motor stimulation. In: Liebenson C, ed: Rehabilitation of the Spine. Philadelphia, Lippincott Williams & Wilkins, 1996:319–328

136. Janisse M: The therapeutic use of yoga. Orthop Phys Ther Pract 14:7–12, 2002

137. Johnson R: Osteitis pubis. Curr Sports Med Rep 2:98–102, 2003

138. Jull GA, Janda V: Muscles and motor control in low back pain: Assessment and management. In: Twomey LT, Taylor JR, eds: Physical Therapy of the Low Back. New York, Churchill Livingstone, 1987:253–278

139. Kapandji IA: Physiology of the Joints. The Trunk and the Vertebral Column, vol. 3, 2nd ed. Edinburgh, Churchill Livingstone, 1974

140. Kendall HO, Kendall FP, Boynton DA: Posture and Pain. Baltimore, Williams & Wilkins, 1952. Reprinted Melbourne, FL, Robert E Krieger, 1971

141. Kendall HO, McCreary EK, Provance PG: Muscle Testing and Function, 4th ed. Baltimore, Williams & Wilkins, 1993

142. Kidd R: Pain localization with the innominate upslip dysfunction. Man Med 3:103–105, 1988

143. Kirkaldy-Willis WH, ed: Managing Low Back Pain, 2nd ed. New York, Churchill Livingstone, 1988a

144. Kirkaldy-Willis WH: The site and nature of the lesion. In: Kirkaldy-Willis WH, ed: Managing Low Back Pain, 2nd ed. New York, Churchill Livingstone, 1988b:133–154

145. Kirkaldy-Willis WH, Hill RJ: A more precise diagnosis for low back pain. Spine 4:102–109, 1979

146. Kirkaldy-Willis WH, Wedge JH, Yong-Hing K, et al: Pathology and pathogenesis of lumbar spondylosis and stenosis. Spine 3:319–128, 1978

147. Kissling R, Brunner C, Jacob HA: Mobility of the SIJ in vitro [in German]. Y Orthop 128:282–288, 1990

148. Klein RG, Eek BC, DeLong WB, et al: A randomized double-bind trail of dextrose-glycerine-prenol injections in chronic, low back pain. J Spinal Disord 6:23–33, 1993

149. Kogstad D, Birnstad N: Pelvic girdle relaxation: Pathogenesis, etiology, definition, epidemiology [in Norwegian]. Tidssk Nor Laegeforen 110:2209–2211, 1990 [English abstract]

150. Kraftsow G: Yoga for Wellness. New York, 1999

151. Kusunose RS: Strain and Counterstrain III: Cranial with Advanced Techniques. Continuing Education Course, Jones Institute, Seattle, 2003

152. LaBan MM, Meerschaert JR, Taylor RS, et al: Symphyseal and sacroiliac pain associated with pubic symphysis instability. Arch Phys Med Rehabil 59:470–472, 1978

153. Lasater JH: Out of joint. Yoga J 162:109–115, 2001

154. Lavignolle B, Vital JM, Senegas J, et al: An approach to the functional anatomy of the SIJs in vivo. Anat Clin 5:169–176, 1983

155. Laycock J, Haslam J, eds: Therapeutic Management of Incontinence and Pelvic Pain. London, Springer-Verlag, 2002

156. Leblanc KE: Sacroiliac sprain: An overlooked cause of back pain. Am Fam Physician 46:1459–1463, 1992

157. Lee D: Principles and practice of muscle energy and functional techniques. In: Grieve GP, ed: Modern Manual Therapy of the Vertebral Column. Edinburgh, Churchill Livingstone, 1986

158. Lee D: The Pelvic Girdle: An Approach to the Examination and Treatment of the Lumbopelvic region. Edinburgh, Churchill Livingstone, 1989

159. Lee D: Treatment of pelvic instability. In: Vleeming A, Mooney V, Dorman A, et al, eds: Movement, Stability, and Low Back Pain: The Essential Role of the Pelvis. New York, Churchill Livingstone, 1997:445–459

160. Lee DG, Walsh MC: A Workbook of Manual Therapy Techniques for the Vertebral Column and Pelvic Girdle. Delta, British Columbia, Nascent, 1986

161. Lewit K: Manipulative Therapy in Rehabilitation of the Locomotor System, 2nd ed. Oxford, Butterworth-Heinemann, 1991

162. Liebenson C: The relationship of the sacroiliac joint, stabilization musculature, and lumbo-pelvic instability. J Bodywork Movement Ther 8:43–45, 2004

163. Lilius HG, Valtonen EJ: The levator ani spasm syndrome: A clinical analysis of 31 cases. Ann Chir Gynaecol Fenn 62:93–97, 1973

164. Linder HH: Clinical Anatomy. Norwalk, CT, Appleton & Lange, 1989

165. Long C II: Myofascial pain syndromes: Part III. Some syndromes of trunk and thigh. Henry Ford Hosp Med Bull 4:102–106, 1956

166. Lovell G: The diagnosis of chronic groin pain in athletes: A review of 189 cases. Aust J Sci Med Sport 1:76–69, 1995

167. Lumsden RM, Morris JM: An in vivo study of axial rotation and immobilization at the lumbosacral joint. J Bone Joint Surg Am 50:1591–1602, 1968

168. Lundgren B: Osteokinematics of the pelvis. Proceedings of the International Federation of Orthopedic Manipulative Therapists, 5th International Conference, Vancouver, 1984

169. Luoto S, Heliovaara M, Hurri H, et al: Static back endurance and the risk of low back pain. Clin Biomech 10:184–192, 1995

170. Lynch FW: The pelvic articulations during pregnancy, labor and puerperium: A x-ray study. Surg Gynecol Obstet 30:575–580, 1920

171. MacDonald GR, Hunt TE: SIJs: Observations on the gross and histological changes in the various age groups. Can Med Assoc J 66:157–162, 1952

172. Macnab I: Lesions of the SIJs. In: Macnab I, McCulloch J, eds: Backache, 2nd ed. Baltimore, Williams & Wilkins, 1990

173. Magee DJ: Orthopedic Physical Assessment, 3rd ed. Philadelphia, WB Saunders, 1997

174. Maigne JY: Lateral dynamic X-rays in the sitting position and coccygeal discography in common coccygodynia. In: Vleeming A, Mooney V, Dorman T, et al: Movement, Stability, and Low Back Pain: The Essential Role of the Pelvis. New York, Churchill Livingstone, 1997:385–391

175. Maigne R: The concept of painless and opposite motion in spinal manipulations. Am J Phys Med 44:55–69, 1965

176. Maigne R: Orthopedic Medicine. Springfield, Ill., Charles C. Thomas, 1972

177. Maitland GD, Banks K, English K, et al: Vertebral Manipulations, 6th ed. Oxford, Butterworths-Heinemann, 2001

178. Maitland J: Spinal Manipulation Made Simple: A Manual of Soft Tissue Techniques. Berkley, CA, North Atlantic Books, 2001

179. McCall IW, Park WM, O'Brien JP: Induced pain referral from posterior lumbar elements in normal subjects. Spine 4:441–448, 1979

180. McGill SM: Low Back Disorders: Evidence-Based Prevention and Rehabilitation. Champaign, IL, Human Kinetics, 2002

181. McGill SM: Mechanics and pathomechanics of muscles acting on the lumbar spine. In: Oatis C, ed: Kinesiology: The Mechanics and Pathomechanics of Human Motion. Philadelphia, Lippincott Williams & Wilkins, 2004

182. McKenzie RA: Mechanical Diagnosis and Therapy of the Lumbar Spine. Waikanae, New Zealand, Spinal Publications, 1981

183. McMurty CT, Avioli LV: Osteitis pubis in an athlete. Calcif Tissue Int 38:76–77, 1986

184. McNerney E: Spine healthy. Adv Directors Rehabil 13: 59–62, 2004

185. Meadows J: Pelvic arthrokinematics. Proceedings of the International Federation of Orthopaedic Manipulative Therapists, 5th International Conference, Vancouver, 1985

186. Meisenbach RO: Sacroiliac relaxation: With analysis of 84 cases. Surg Gynecol Obstet 12:411–434, 1911

187. Mellin G: Correlations of hip mobility with degree of back pain and lumbar spinal mobility in chronic low-back pain patients. Spine 13:668–670, 1990
188. Mennell JB: Physical Treatment, Movement, Manipulation, and Massage. Philadelphia, Blakiston, 1947
189. Mennell JB: The Science and Art of Joint Manipulation, vols. 1 and 2. London, Churchill, 1952
190. Mennell JB: The Science and Art of Joint Manipulation, vol. 2: The Spinal Column. London, Churchill, 1962
191. Mennell J McM: Back Pain. Boston, Little, Brown & Co, 1960
192. Mennell J McM: Diagnosis and Treatment Using Manipulative Techniques: Joint Pain. Boston, Little, Brown & Co, 1964
193. Mens JMA, Vleeming A, Snijder CJ, et al: The active straight leg raising test and mobility of the pelvic joints. Eur Spine J 8:468–473, 1999
194. Mens JMA, Vleeming A, Snijder CJ, et al: Reliability and validity of active straight leg raise test in posterior pelvic pain since pregnancy. Spine 26:1167–1171, 2001
195. Mens JMA, Vleeming A, Stoeckart R, et al: Understanding peripartum pelvic pain; implications of a patient survey. Spine 21:1363–1370, 1996
196. Middleton R, Carlisle R: The spectrum of osteitis pubis. Compr Ther 19:99–105, 1993
197. Miller JAA, Schultz AB, Andersson GBJ: Load-displacement behavior of SIJs. J Orthop Res 5:92–101, 1987
198. Mitchell F: Structural Pelvic Function. Carmel, CA, Academy of Applied Osteopathy, 1965
199. Mitchell FL, Moran PS, Pruzzo NA: An Evaluation and Treatment Manual of Osteopathic Muscle Energy Procedures. Valley Park, MO, Mitchell, Moran and Pruzzo Associates, 1979
200. Mooney V, Pozos R, Vleeming A et al: Coupled motion of contralateral latissimus dorsi and gluteus maximus: Its role in sacroiliac stabilization. In: Vleeming A, Mooney V, Dorman T, et al, eds: Movement, Stability, and Low Back Pain: The Essential Role of the Pelvis. New York, Churchill Livingstone, 1997:115–122
201. Mooney V, Robertson J: The face syndrome. Clin Orthop 115:149–156, 1976
202. Moore KL: Clinically Oriented Anatomy, 2nd ed. Baltimore, Williams & Wilkins, 1985
203. Morgan D: Concepts in functional training and postural stabilization for low-back-injured. Top Acute Care Trauma Rehabil 2:8–17, 1988
204. Morscher E: Etiology and pathophysiology of leg-length discrepancies. Progr Orthop Surg 1:9–19, 1977
205. Muscolino JE, Cipriani S: Rehabilitation and core stability. Pilates and the powerhouse—I. J Bodywork Movement Ther 8:15–24, 2004a
206. Musculino JE, Cipriani S: Rehabilitation and core stability. Pilates and the "power house"–II. J Bodywork Movement Ther 8:122–130, 2004b
207. Namey TC, An HS: Emergency diagnosis and management of sciatica: Differentiating the nondiskogenic causes. Emerg Med Rep 6:101–109, 1985
208. Neumann P, Gill V: Pelvic floor and abdominal muscle interaction: EMG activity and intraabdominal pressure. Int Urolgynecol J Pelvic Floor Dysfunct 3:124–132, 2002
209. Nicholson GG, Clendaniel RA: Manual techniques. In: Schully RM, Barnes MR, eds: Physical Therapy. Philadelphia, JB Lippincott, 1989:926–985
210. Nielsen AJ: Spray and stretch for myofascial pain. Phys Ther 58:567–569, 1978
211. Norkin CC, Levangie PK: Joint Structure and Function, 2nd ed. Philadelphia, FA Davis, 1992
212. Norman GF: Sacroiliac disease and its relationship to lower abdominal pain. Am J Surg 116:54–56, 1968
213. Nyberg R: Pelvic girdle. In: Donatelli R, Wooden MJ, eds: Orthopaedic Physical Therapy. New York, Churchill Livingstone, 1989
214. Nyberg R: Clinical studies of sacroiliac movement. In: International Federation of Orthopedic Manipulative Therapists, 5th International Conference, Vail, 1992
215. Ombergt L, ter Veer HJ: Anatomy and disorders of the coccyx. In: Ombergt L, Bisschop P, ter Veer HJ, et al, eds: A System of Orthopaedic Medicine, London, WB Saunders, 1995: 709–711
216. Ongley MJ, Klein RG, Dorman TA, et al: A new approach to the treatment of chronic back pain. Lancet 2:243–246, 1987
217. O'Sullivan PB, Beales DJ, Beetham JA, et al: Altered motor control strategies in subjects with sacroiliac joint pain during the active straight-leg-test. Spine 27:E1–E8, 2002
218. Pace JB: Commonly overlooked pain syndromes responsive to simple therapy. Postgrad Med 58:107–113, 1975
219. Pace JB, Nagle D: Piriformis syndrome. West J Med 124:435–439, 1976
220. Paget S, Bryan W: Reiter syndrome. In: Beary JF, Christian CL, Johanson NA, eds: Manual of Rheumatology and Outpatient Orthopedic Disorders: Diagnosis and Therapy, 2nd ed. Boston, Little, Brown & Co, 1987
221. Palmer LM, Epler M: Fundamentals of Musculoskeletal Assessment Techniques, 2nd ed. Philadelphia, Lippincott Williams & Wilkins, 1998
222. Paquin JD, Rest M, Marie PJ, et al: Biochemical and morphologic studies of cartilage from the adult human SIJ. Arthritis Rheum 26:887–895, 1983
223. Paris SV: The Spinal Lesion. New Zealand, Degasus Press, 1965
224. Paris SV: Differential diagnosis of lumbar and pelvic pain. In: Vleeming A, Mooney V, Dorman T, et al, eds: Movement, Stability, and Low Back Pain: The Essential Role of the Pelvis. New York, Churchill Livingstone, 1997:319–330
225. Petrone E: The Miracle Ball Method. New York, Workman Publishing, 2003
226. Phillips M: Myokinetic of the pelvis. Proceedings, 5th Conference of International Federation of Orthopaedic Manipulative Therapists, Vancouver, 1984
227. Piedallu P: Problemes Sacro-iliaque. Bordeaux Biere, Homme Sain No. 2, 1952
228. Pierrynowski MR, Schroeder BC, Garrity CB, et al: Three-dimensional sacroiliac motion during locomotion in asymptomatic male and female subjects. In: Cotton CE, Lamontagne M, Roberson DGE, et al, eds: Proceedings of the 5th Biennial Conference and Human Locomotion Symposium of the Canadian Society for Biomechanics, London, Ontario, 1988
229. Pitkin HD, Pheasant HC: Sacro-arthrogenetic telalgia. J Bone Joint Surg Am 18:365–374, 1936
230. Pool-Goudzwaard A, Vleeming A, Stoeckart C, et al: Insufficient lumbopelvic approach to a clinical, anatomical and biomechanical approach to "a specific" low back pain. Man Ther 3:31–37, 1998
231. Porterfield JA, DeRosa CP: The SIJ. In: Gould J, ed: Orthopaedic and Sports Physical Therapy, 2nd ed. St. Louis, CV Mosby, 1990
232. Porterfield JA, DeRosa CP: Mechanical Low Back Pain: Perspectives in Functional Anatomy. Philadelphia, WB Saunders, 1991
233. Potter NA, Rothstein JM. Intertester reliability for selected clinical tests of the SIJ. Phys Ther 65:1671–1675, 1985
234. Pratt WA: The lumbopelvic torsion syndrome. J Am Osteopath Assoc 51:335–343, 1952
235. Proulx WR: Comparison of efficacy of prolotherapy versus steroid injection in the treatment of low back pain. Presented at the annual meeting of the American Association of Orthopedic Medicine, Denver, CO, 1990
236. Pulling Schatz M: Back Care Basics: A Doctor's Gentle Yoga Program for Back and Neck Pain Relief. Berkeley, CA: Rodmell Press, 1992
237. Pyper JB: Excision of the coccyx for idiopathic coccygodynia. J Bone Joint Surg Br 39:733–737, 1957
238. Ravin T: Visualization of pelvic biomechanical dysfunction. In: Vleeming A, Mooney V, Dorman T, et al, eds: Movement, Stability, and Low Back Pain: The Essential Role of the Pelvis. New York, Churchill Livingstone. 1997:369–383
239. Resnick D, Niwayama G, Georgen TG: Degenerative disease of the SIJ. Invest Radiol 10:608–621, 1975
240. Resnick D, Niwayama G, Georgen TG: Clinical, radiographic and pathologic abnormalities in calcium, pyrophosphate dihydrate deposition disease (CPPD): An analysis of 85 patients. Radiology 122:1–15, 1977
241. Reynolds HH: Three-dimensional kinematics in the pelvic girdle. J Am Osteopath Assoc 80:277–280, 1980
242. Reynolds MD: Myofascial trigger point syndromes in the practice of rheumatology. Arch Phys Med Rehabil 62:111–114, 1981
243. Richardson C, Jull G, Hodges P, et al: Therapeutic Exercise for Spinal Segmental Stabilization in Low Back Pain: Scientific Basis and Clinical Approach. Edinburgh, Churchill Livingstone, 1999
244. Robinson L, Fisher H, Knox J, et al: The Official Body Control Pilates Manual, New York, Barnes & Noble, 2000
245. Robinson R: The new back school prescription: Stabilization training, part I. Occup Med State of the Art Rev 7:17–31, 1992
246. Rodriguez C, Miguel A, Lima H, et al: Osteitis pubis syndrome in the professional soccer athlete: A case report. J Athl Train 36:437–440, 2001
247. Ryan LM, Carrera GF, Lightfoot RW, et al: The radiographic diagnosis of sacroiliitis—A comparison of different views with computed tomograms of the SIJ. Arthritis Rheum 26:760–763, 1983
248. Saal JA: The new back school prescription: Stabilization training, part II. Occup Med–State of the Art Rev 7:33–42, 1992
249. Sahrmann S: Diagnosis and Treatment of Muscle Imbalances and Associated Regional Pain Syndromes, Level II course notes. Seattle, 1993
250. Sahrmann S: Diagnosis and Treatment of Movement Impairment. St. Louis, Mosby, 2002
251. Saliba V, Johnson GS, Wardlaw C: Proprioceptive neuromuscular facilitation. In: Basmajian JV, Nyberg R, eds: Rational Manual Therapies. Baltimore, Williams & Wilkins, 1993:243–284
252. Salvati E: The levator syndrome and its variant. Gastroenterol Clin North Am 16:71–78, 1987
253. Sapsford RR, Hodges PW, Richardson CA et al: Co-activation of the abdominal and pelvic floor muscles during voluntary exercise. Neurourol Urodyn 20:31–42, 2001
254. Sashin O: A critical analysis of the anatomy and the pathological changes of the SI joints. J Bone Joint Surg Am 12:891–910, 1930
255. Saunders HD, Saunders R: Evaluation, Treatment and Prevention of Musculoskeletal Disorders, 3rd ed. Minneapolis, H Duane Saunders, 1993
256. Schafer RC: Clinical Biomechanics, Musculoskeletal Action and Reactions. Baltimore, Williams & Wilkins, 1987
257. Schamberger W: The Malalignment Syndrome: Implications for Medicine and Sport. Edinburgh, Churchill Livingstone, 2002
258. Schmorl G, Junghanns H: The Human Spine in Health and Disease. New York, Grune & Stratton, 1971
259. Schned ES: Ankylosing spondylitis. In: Beary JF, Christian CL, Johanson NA, eds: Manual of Rheumatology and Outpatient Orthopedics: Diagnosis and Therapy, 2nd ed. Boston, Little Brown & Co, 1987:133–141
260. Schneider W, Dvorak J, Dvorák T: Manual Medicine Therapy. New York, Georg Thieme Verlag Stuttgart/Thieme Medical Publisher, 1988
261. Scholten PJM, Schultz AB, Luchico CW, et al: Motions and loads within the human pelvis: A biomechanical model study. J Orthop Res 6:840–850, 1988
262. Schultz RL, Feitz R: The Endless Web: Fascial Anatomy and Physical Reality. Berkeley, CA, North Atlanta Books, 1996

263. Schunke GB: The anatomy and development of the sacroiliac joint in man. Anat Rec 72:313–331, 1938
264. Schunke GB: The anatomy and the development of the SIJ and their relation to the movements of the sacrum. Acta Anat 23:80–91, 1955
265. Schussler B, Laycock J, Nortin P, et al, eds: Pelvic Floor Re-education Principle and Practice. New York, Springer-Verlag, 1994
266. Shelly B: The pelvic floor. In: Hall CM, Brody LT, eds: Therapeutic Exercise: Moving toward Function. Philadelphia, Lippincott Williams & Wilkins, 1999
267. Simons DG, Travell JG: Myofascial origins of low back pain, torso muscles. Postgrad Med 73:81–92, 1983
268. Sirca A, Kostevc V: The fibre type composition of the thoracic and lumbar paravertebral muscles in man. J Anat 141:131–137, 1985
269. Smith WT: Levator spasm syndrome. Minn Med 42:1076–1079, 1959
270. Snaith ML, Galvin SEJ, Short MD: The value of quantitative radioisotope scanning in the differential diagnosis of low back pain and sacroiliac disease. J Rheumatol 9:435–440, 1982
271. Snijders CJ, Vleeming A, Stoeckart R: Transfer of lumbosacral load to iliac bones and legs. I. Biomechanics of self-bracing of the sacroiliac joints and its significance for treatment and exercise. Clin Biomech 8:285–294, 1992
272. Sola AE: Trigger point therapy. In: Roberts JR, Hedges WB, eds: Clinical Procedures in Emergency Medicine. Philadelphia, WB Saunders, 1985:674–686
273. Sola AE, Kuitert JH: Quadratus lumborum myofasciitis. Northwest Med 53:1003–1005, 1954
274. Sola AE, Williams RL: Myofascial pain syndromes. Neurology 6:91–95, 1956
275. Soleway C: Small Ball Release Program: Basic Back and Body Routine. Longmount, CO, Ball Dynamics International, 2001
276. Solonen VA: The SIJ in the light of anatomical roentgenological and clinical studies. Acta Orthop Scand Suppl 27:1–127, 1957
277. Stalvey MH: Proprioceptive neuromuscular facilitation. In: Bandy WD, Sanders B, eds: Therapeutic Exercise: Techniques for Intervention. Baltimore, Lippincott Williams & Wilkins, 2001:145–177
278. Steege JF, Metzger DA, Levy B: Chronic Pelvic Pain: An Integrated Approach. Philadelphia, WB Saunders, 1998
279. Stein JM, Warfield CA: Two entrapment neuropathies. Hosp Pract:100A–100P, 1983
280. Stoddard A: Manual of Osteopathic Technique. London, Hutchinson and Co, 1959
281. Sturesson B, Selvik G, Uden A: Movement of the SIJs: A roentgen stereophotogrammetric analysis. Spine 14:162–165, 1989
282. Sullivan P, Markos PD: Low back. In: Sullivan P, Markos PD: Clinical Decision Making in Therapeutic Exercise. Norwalk, CT, 1994:159–193
283. Taylor JR, O'Sullivan PO: Lumbar segmental instability: pathology, diagnosis, and conservative treatment. In: Twomney LT, Taylor JR, eds: Physical Therapy of the Low Back, 3rd ed. New York, Churchill Livingstone, 2000:201–247
284. Tesh KM, Dunn JS, Evans JH: The abdominal muscles and vertebral stability. Spine 12:501–508, 1987
285. Travell JG, Simons DG: Quadratus lumborum muscle. In: Travell JG, Simons DG: Myofascial Pain and Dysfunction, The Trigger Point Manual, Volume 2: The Lower Extremities. II, Baltimore, MD, Williams & Wilkins, 1992
286. Travell JG, Simons DG: Quadratus lumborum muscle. In: Travell JG, Simons DG, eds: Myofascial Pain and Dysfunction: The Trigger Point Manual, vol. 2. Baltimore, Williams & Wilkins, 1992a:28–88
287. Travell JG, Simons DG: Piriformis and other short lateral rotators. In: Travell JG, Simons DG, eds: Myofascial Pain and Dysfunction: The Trigger Point Manual, vol. 2. Baltimore, Williams & Wilkins, 1992b:186–213
288. Trotter M: A common anatomical variation in the sacroiliac region. J Bone Joint Surg 22:293–299, 1940
289. Vleeming A, Pool-Goudzwaard AI, Stoeckart R, et al: The posterior layer of the thoracolumbar fascia; its function in load transfer from spine to legs. Spine 20:753–758, 1995
290. Vleeming A, Snijders CJ, Stoeckart R, et al: The role of the sacroiliac joint in coupling between spine, pelvic, legs and arms. In: Vleeming A, Mooney V, Dorman T, et al, eds: Movement, Stability, and Low Back Pain: The Essential Role of the Pelvis. New York, Churchill Livingstone, 1997:53–71
291. Vleeming A, Stoeckart R, Snijder CJ, et al: The SIJ—anatomical, biomechanical and radiological aspects. Man Med 5:100–102, 1990
292. Vleeming A, Stoeckart R, Volkers ACW, et al: Relation between form and function in the sacroiliac, part I: Clinical anatomical aspects. Spine 13:133–135, 1990
293. Vleeming A, Volkers ACW, Snijders CJ, et al: Relation between form and function in the sacroiliac joint II. Biomechanical aspects. Spine 15:133–136, 1990
294. Volpi P, Melegati G: La pubalgia del calciatore: Aspetti eziopatogenetici e classificcativi. Ital J Sports Traumatol 8:271–274, 1985
295. Vukicevic S, Plitz W, Vukicevic D, et al: Holographic study of the stresses in the normal pelvis with particular reference to the movement of the sacrum. In: Huiskes R, Van Campen D, Dewijn J, eds: Biomechanics: Principles and Applications. Dordrecht, The Netherlands, Marinus Nijhoff, W Junk Publisher, 1982:223–239
296. Wadsworth CT: Manual Examination and Treatment of the Spine and Extremities. Baltimore, Williams & Wilkins, 1988
297. Walker JM: Age-related differences in the human SIJ—A histological study: Implications for therapy. J Orthop Sports Phys Ther 7:325–331, 1986
298. Walker JM: Pathology of the SIJ. In: Proceedings, International Federation of Orthopaedic Manipulative Therapists 5th International Conference, Vail, 1992a
299. Walker JM: The SIJ: A critical review. Phys Ther 72:903–916, 1992b
300. Wallace KA: Pelvic floor muscle dysfunction and its behavioral treatment. In: Agostini R, ed: Medical and Orthopedic Issues of Active and Athletic Women. Philadelphia, Hanley & Belfus, 1994:200–212
301. Wallace LA: Limb-length difference and back pain. In: Grieve GP, ed: Modern Manual Therapy of the Vertebral Column. Edinburgh, Churchill Livingstone, 1986
302. Warwick R, Williams P: Gray's Anatomy, 36th ed. Philadelphia, JB Lippincott, 1980
303. Weisl H: The relation of movement to structure in the SIJ. Thesis, University of Manchester, 1953
304. Weisl H: The articular surfaces of the SIJ and their relation to movement of the sacrum. Acta Anat (Basel) 22:10–14, 1954
305. Weisl H: The movements of the SIJ. Acta Anat (Basel) 23:80–91, 1955
306. Weismantel A: Evaluation and treatment of SIJ problems. Bull Orthop Section, Am Phys Ther Assoc 3:5–9, 1978
307. Wells PE: The examination of the pelvic joints. In: Grieve GP, ed: Modern Manual Therapy of Vertebral Column. Edinburgh, Churchill Livingstone, 1986
308. White A: Stabilization of the lumbar spine. In: White A, Anderson R, eds: Conservative Care of Low Back Pain. Baltimore, Williams & Wilkins, 1991
309. Wicks T: Motion in the SIJ scanned with ultrasonography. Proceedings of the International Federation of Orthopedic Manipulative Therapists, 5th International Conference, Vancouver, 1984
310. Wilder DG, Pope MH, Frymoyer JW: The functional topography of the SIJ. Spine 5:575–579, 1980
311. Wingerden JP van, Vleeming A, Snijders CJ, et al: Functional anatomical approach to the spine-pelvis mechanism interaction between the biceps femoris muscle and the sacrotuberous ligament. Eur Spine J 2:140–144, 1993
312. Winter Z: Referred pain in fibrositis. Med Rec 157:34–37, 1944
313. Woerman AL: Evaluation and treatment of dysfunction in the lumbo-pelvic-hip complex. In: Donatelli R, Wooden MJ, eds: Orthopaedic Physical Therapy. New York, 3rd ed. Churchill Livingstone, 2001:378–436
314. Wright RR: The levator ani spasm syndrome. Am J Proctol 6:477, 1969
315. Young HH: Non-neurological lesions simulating protruded intervertebral disc. JAMA 148:1101–1105, 1952

RECOMMENDED READINGS

Fortin JD, Aprill CN, Ponthieux B, et al: SIJ: Pain referral maps upon applying a new injection/arthrography technique. Part II: Clinical evaluation. Spine 19:1483–1489, 1994

Fortin JD, Dwyer MD, West S, et al: SIJ: Pain referral maps upon applying a new injection/arthrography technique. Part I: Asymptomatic volunteers. Spine 19:1475–1482, 1994

Hungerford B, Gilleard W, Hodges P: Evidence of altered lumbopelvic muscle recruitment in the presence of sacroiliac joint pain. Spine 28:1593–1600, 2003

Laslett M, Young SB, Aprill CN, et al: Diagnosing painful sacroiliac joints: A validity study of McKenzie evaluation and sacroiliac provocation tests. Aust J Physiother 49:89–97, 2003

O'Sullivan PB, Beales DJ, Beetham JA, et al: Altered motor control strategies in subjects with sacroiliac joint pain during active straight-leg-raise test. Spine 27:E1–E8, 2002

Pool-Goudzwaard A, Hoek van Dijke G, et al: The iliolumbar ligament: its influence on stability of the sacroiliac joint. Clin Biomech 18:99–105, 2003

Richardson CA Snijders CJ, Hides JA, et al: The relation between the transversus abdominus muscles, sacroiliac joint mechanics, and low back pain. Spine 27:399–405, 2002

Van Wingerden JP, Vleeming A, Buyruk HM, et al: Stabilization of the sacroiliac joint in vivo: verification of muscular contribution to force closure of the pelvis. Eur Spine J, in press, 2004

Lumbosacral–Lower Limb Scan Examination

24

DARLENE HERTLING

- COMMON LESIONS OF LUMBOSACRAL REGION AND LOWER LIMBS AND THEIR PRIMARY CLINICAL MANIFESTATIONS
    - Lumbosacral Region
    - Hip
    - Knee
    - Lower Leg, Ankle, and Foot
- SCAN EXAMINATION TESTS
    - Gait Analysis
    - Assessment of Structural Alignment
    - Regional Tests
- CLINICAL IMPLEMENTATION OF LUMBOSACRAL–LOWER LIMB SCAN EXAMINATION

A common problem in the clinical examination of patients presenting with chronic, insidious musculoskeletal problems of the low back and lower extremities is not knowing in which area to direct physical examination procedures after completing the history portion of the examination. The reason is twofold:

1. Chronic musculoskeletal disorders affecting the low back and the various regions of the lower limbs often present with similar pain patterns.
2. Biomechanical disorders affecting the back and various lower extremity regions often coexist.

The former is a result of the common phenomenon of referred pain that is characteristic of most common musculoskeletal disorders; localized pain arising from deep somatic tissues is usually perceived in an area not corresponding well to the exact pathologic site. Thus, patients with low back pain usually feel discomfort primarily in the upper buttock or sacroiliac region, patients with trochanteric bursitis often have significant pain in the posterior hip and lateral thigh areas, and those with chondromalacia patellae frequently feel pain over the medial aspect of the distal thigh and upper leg. Also, as the severity of the pathologic process increases, there is greater likelihood that pain may be perceived throughout a distribution corresponding to any or all of the relevant sclerotome. Thus, if a relatively acute disorder affects a tissue innervated primarily by the L5 segment, the patient may feel pain in any or all of those regions also innervated by L5.

A typical example would be the patient with moderate to advanced degenerative hip disease who invariably experiences pain in the groin, which spreads into the anterior thigh and to the knee—the L3 sclerotome. This occurs because the anterior aspect of the hip joint capsule, from which the pain primarily arises, is innervated largely by the L3 segment. Similarly, the patient with involvement of the L3 segment of the spine from, for example, the facet joint or disk, may feel pain that spreads in the same distribution as that described for hip joint disease. It may not be obvious from subjective informa-

tion alone whether the hip, the low back, or both are involved. Likewise, it is often difficult to determine on the basis of subjective information alone whether a patient has trochanteric bursitis, an L5 spinal disorder, or both. The trochanteric region is innervated primarily by L5, and pain arising in conjunction with trochanteric bursitis is often felt down the lateral aspect of the thigh and dorsum of the leg (the L5 sclerotome), as may be the case with pain originating at the L5 spinal level.

Another classic example of localization of pain to distant regions of a relevant sclerotome occurs in the child with a hip joint disorder, such as a slipped capital femoral epiphysis, who feels pain primarily in the knee; both the hip and the knee joints are innervated largely by L3. Because delocalization and reference of pain are common phenomena, the subjective account of pain distribution does not provide a reliable indication of the true site of the pathologic process. Additional objective information is often required.

The prevalence of coexistent disorders or abnormalities of the low back and lower extremity regions is largely a result of the biomechanical interdependency of the weight-bearing joints in the closed kinetic chain. Normal attenuation of the energy introduced to the weight-bearing joints by the vertical displacement of the center of gravity requires that the overall displacement of the center of gravity be minimized, which, in turn, requires normal movement of the weight-bearing joints during stance phase of gait. Loss of critical movement at any of the weight-bearing joints will cause increased energy input to the entire weight-bearing skeleton from the force of the body weight acting over a greater distance, with the result being added vertical compressive loading during stance phase. Similarly, energy input to the weight-bearing joints in a horizontal plane is normally attenuated by joint movements. With the foot fixed to the ground, for the body to be normally moved through space in the presence of reduced critical movement at any joint, compensation is required at some other joint. Such an alteration in function is likely to result in added stresses to the compensating joint. Thus, the patient with loss of hip extension tends to walk with greater extension of the lower lumbar joints, and the person with loss of ankle dorsiflexion undergoes greater-than-normal extension movements at the knee. Because the close-packed positions of the spine and knee are extended, these abnormalities are likely to cause increased subchondral compressive stresses and increased capsular tensile stresses to the knee and spinal joints.

Less obvious are the results of abnormalities in transverse rotation of the weight-bearing joints during stance phase of gait. From heel-strike to foot-flat the pelvis, thigh, and leg normally undergo internal rotatory movements, the distal segments more so than their supra-adjacent neighbors. The segments of the leg similarly undergo external rotation during foot-flat to toe-off. Because the foot is relatively fixed to the ground, however, it does not rotate. This means that the ankle–foot complex must absorb the rotatory movements imposed from above; internal rotation is absorbed by pronation of the foot, and external rotation is transmitted to the foot as a supinatory movement. One should observe the result of rotating the leg over the foot that is fixed to the ground; internal rotation causes the calcaneus to shift into valgus position and the medial arch to lower (pronation of the hindfoot), whereas external rotation brings the heel into varus position and raises the arch (supination of the hindfoot). It should also be noted that internal rotation of the thigh with the knee slightly bent causes an increased valgus angulation at the knee. This is of practical significance because the knee remains slightly bent during all phases of the gait cycle.

Again, because attenuation of the forces of the body weight moving over the fixed foot requires a normal contribution of movement from all weight-bearing joints, abnormalities of function at any one joint may affect the function of one or more of the others in the chain. A common example occurs in the person with increased femoral antetorsion, who tends to walk with excessive internal rotation during stance phase of gait. This results in abnormal valgus angulation at the knee and increased foot pronation. The former may predispose to patellar tracking problems, whereas the latter may lead to a variety of problems, including plantar fasciitis, heel spurs, hallux valgus, metatarsalgia, and fatigue of the intrinsic foot musculature (see Chapter 16, Lower Leg, Ankle, and Foot). On the other hand, a primary problem of abnormal foot pronation may lead to excessive internal rotatory and valgus stresses to the knee and increased internal rotation of the hip during gait. It should be clear that the best approach to management of pathologic lesions resulting from such biomechanical derangements would be one that takes into consideration primary causative factors. This often requires that evaluating procedures be directed to areas other than simply the primary region of involvement.

The above considerations should help emphasize the need to evaluate all of the weight-bearing joint regions in many, if not most, chronic musculoskeletal disorders affecting the low back or lower limb. A further factor to consider in this regard is the common phenomenon of summation of otherwise subliminal afferent input from coexistent minor disorders involving tissues innervated by the same or adjacent spinal segments. A common example is the person who stresses the joint capsules of the low back excessively throughout the day and who also has some low-grade inflammation of the trochanteric bursa. Noxious input from both areas may summate at the dorsal horn of the spinal cord and other central neural connections to cause more low back pain as well as more lateral thigh pain than would be present if either disorder existed by itself. In this particular example, the clinician must differentiate between the possibility of one lesion referring pain into another part of the relevant segment and two distinct pathologic processes within the same segment. This cannot be determined without evaluating both the low back and the hip regions. Pain arising from the summation of input from different sites of the same segment will, of course, be more likely to occur in the patient with multisegmental restrictions of motion of the lower spine, inasmuch as with daily activities the soft tissues (joint capsules and ligaments) of the spine will be stressed more, causing an increase in afferent input to the relevant spinal levels. In such cases, the threshold of pain arising from minor disorders affecting tissue in the lower limbs innervated by the corresponding spinal segments is probably reduced. Any back pain is likely to be enhanced by such segmentally related pathologic processes. Most persons, by middle age or later, develop some lower lumbar facet-joint capsular restriction secondary to disk narrowing or other causes. Thus, middle-aged or older persons with chronic low back or lower limb pain should always be examined for coexistent segmental disorders that may be contributing to the amount of pain the person experiences.

In summary, the low back–lower extremity scan examination may be used to:

- Determine the area of involvement in cases in which relatively vague subjective information fails to suggest the site of the pathologic process. This is not an uncommon occurrence and is related to the fact that pain of deep somatic origin may be referred to any or all of the relevant sclerotome.
- Examine for the presence of some distant biomechanical derangement that may be related, in cause or effect, to the patient's primary physical lesion that causes his or her pain.
- Rule out the possibility of some segmentally related disorder that may, by the mechanism of summation of segmentally related afferent input, contribute to the patient's pain perception.

The scan examination is oriented, then, toward detecting gross or subtle biomechanical abnormalities and toward determining the presence of common lumbar or lower extremity musculoskeletal disorders. Essential to the detection of significant biomechanical derangements are careful assessment of function (gait analysis), evaluation of bony structure and alignment, and examination of joint mobility. These examination procedures are combined with the key objective tests for the common chronic disorders affecting the lower back and lower limbs, to constitute the lumbosacral–lower limb scan examination. A discussion of the common pathologic processes and their primary clinical manifestations will facilitate understanding and interpretation of the examination procedures involved in the scan examination.

COMMON LESIONS OF LUMBOSACRAL REGION AND LOWER LIMBS AND THEIR PRIMARY CLINICAL MANIFESTATIONS

Lumbosacral Region

I. Acute (Severe) Posterolateral Disk Prolapse (Outer Annulus or Posterior Longitudinal Ligament Still Intact)
    A. Subjective complaints
       1. Sudden onset of unilateral lumbosacral pain, often with gradual buildup of pain intensity. Occasionally the patient denies a sudden onset and notes first experiencing pain on rising in the morning. There may be some aching in the leg.
       2. Worse with sitting and on rising after a long period of recumbency; somewhat relieved with recumbency
    B. Key objective signs
       1. Functional lumbar deformity, with a loss of lordosis and usually a lumbar scoliosis with the convexity to the involved side
       2. Marked, painful restriction of spinal movement, especially forward and backward bending
       3. Positive dural mobility tests
II. Acute Facet Joint Derangement
    A. Subjective complaints
       1. Sudden onset of lumbosacral pain and deformity; little or no leg discomfort
       2. Pain is aggravated by being up and about and is relieved by sitting or recumbency.
    B. Key objective findings
       1. Marked lumbar deformity; loss of lordosis and lumbar scoliosis with convexity to side of involvement
       2. Lumbar extension and sidebending to the side of involvement are painfully restricted. Forward bending and contralateral sidebending are slightly restricted.
       3. Negative dural signs
III. Localized, Unilateral, Facet Joint Capsular Tightness
    A. Subjective complaints
       1. Often a history of past episodes of acute low back dysfunction
       2. Aching in the lumbosacral region, aggravated by long periods of standing, walking, or activities involving prolonged or repetitive lumbar extension; also worse with increased muscular tension, such as during periods of emotional stress, and worse in the evening than in the morning
    B. Key objective findings
       1. Possible subtle predisposing biomechanical factors such as a leg-length disparity

       2. Possible minor restriction of sidebending to the involved side and deviation of spine toward the involved side on forward bending and away from the involved side on extension
       3. Discomfort on quadrant tests when localized to the involved segment
IV. Multisegmental Bilateral Capsular Restriction of Lumbar Facet Joints—Degenerative Joint Disease
    A. Subjective complaints
       1. The patient is middle-aged or older.
       2. Often there is a long history of intermittent back problems.
       3. Aching across the lower back and hip girdle is made worse with long periods of standing or walking. The back is stiff in the morning, somewhat better at midday, and aching again by evening. Some intermittent aching in one or both legs may occur.
    B. Key objective findings
       1. Some loss of the normal lumbar lordosis
       2. Restriction of spinal motion in a generalized capsular pattern of limitation: marked restriction of spinal extension, moderate restriction of sidebending bilaterally, and mild to moderate restriction of rotations and forward bending
V. Lower Lumbar Disk Extrusion with Nerve Root Impingement
    A. Subjective complaints
       1. Sudden or gradual onset of lumbosacral pain and unilateral leg pain. The patient may describe an onset suggestive of an acute posterolateral prolapse (see earlier) with progressive loss of back pain and increase in leg pain.
       2. The leg pain may be relatively sharp and is usually felt down the posterolateral thigh and into the anterolateral or posterior aspect of the lower leg. The leg pain may be aggravated by sitting or by being up and about and is relatively relieved by rest.
    B. Key objective findings
       1. Mild to moderate loss of lumbar movement, usually toward extension and in movements toward the side of involvement; it occasionally occurs away from the involved side.
       2. Mild segmental neurologic deficit
       3. Positive dural mobility signs
VI. Acute Sacroiliac Dysfunction
    A. Subjective complaints
       1. Sudden onset of unilateral sacroiliac pain, often associated with some twisting motion
       2. Occasional spread of pain to the posterior thigh
       3. Pain is usually aggravated by activities involving combined hip and spine extension, such as standing erect (posterior torsional displacement). Less often it is aggravated by combined hip and spine flexion, such as sitting (anterior torsional displacement).

B. Key objective findings
1. Posterior torsional displacement (most common)
   a. Tendency to stand with the hip, knee, and low back slightly flexed on the involved side. If so, the knee landmarks and the greater trochanter will be lower on the involved side than on the uninvolved side. The posterosuperior iliac spine and iliac crest will also be lower on the involved side, more so than the knee landmarks and trochanter. The anterosuperior iliac spine will not be as low on the involved side as the knee and trochanteric landmarks. The pelvis will be shifted away from the involved side.

   If the patient stands with the legs straight, all of the landmarks up to and including the trochanters will be level. The posterosuperior iliac spine and iliac crest will be lower on the involved side than on the uninvolved side, but the anterosuperior iliac spine will be higher. The pelvis will appear to be rotated forward on the involved side.
   b. The anterior rotation test will be quite painful; the posterior rotation test will be less painful.
   c. Contralateral straight-leg raising may cause some pain, which is relieved when the involved leg is raised.
2. Anterior torsional displacement (rare)
   a. Tendency to stand with the hip and knee in more extension on the involved side than on the uninvolved side. The pelvis may be shifted toward and inclined away from the involved side. If the patient stands in this manner, the knee landmarks and trochanter will be lower on the uninvolved side. The posterosuperior iliac spine and iliac crest will also be lower on the uninvolved side, more so than the knee landmarks and trochanter. The anterosuperior iliac spine will not be as low on the uninvolved side as the other landmarks.

   If the patient can stand erect, the trochanters and landmarks below will be level. The posterosuperior iliac spine and iliac crest will be higher on the involved side; the anterosuperior iliac spine will be lower on the involved side.
   b. Posterior rotation test will be quite painful; anterior rotation test will be less painful.
   c. Ipsilateral straight-leg raising test may cause some pain, which is relieved when the opposite leg is raised.
VII. Chronic Sacroiliac Hypermobility
A. Subjective complaints
1. History suggestive of intermittent acute sacroiliac dysfunction with gradual progression to more chronic sacroiliac and posterior thigh pain. Development may be associated with past pregnancy.
2. Pain is aggravated by prolonged or repetitive activities involving:

a. Combined hip and spine extension or hip extension with contralateral hip flexion
b. Combined hip and spine flexion or hip flexion with contralateral hip extension
B. Key objective findings
1. Possible signs of sacroiliac asymmetry on assessment of structural alignment (see earlier under Acute Sacroiliac Dysfunction)
2. Pain or crepitus on one or more sacroiliac stress tests

Hip

I. Degenerative Joint Disease
A. Subjective complaints
1. Gradual, progressive onset of hip pain and dysfunction
2. Pain is felt first and most in the groin region. With progression, pain may spread to the anterior thigh, posterior hip, and lateral hip regions.
3. Pain is first noticed after long periods of weight-bearing activities. Later, pain and stiffness are noted on rising in the morning, easing somewhat by midday, and then increased again by evening.
B. Key objective findings
1. Tendency to stand with hip and knee flexed and lumbar spine hyperextended; pelvis is shifted toward the involved side
2. Gait abnormality characterized by tendency to incline the trunk toward the involved side during stance phase
3. Painful limitation of hip motions in a capsular pattern of restriction; marked limitation of internal rotation and abduction; moderate restriction of flexion and extension; mild to moderate restriction of abduction and external rotation
II. Trochanteric Bursitis
A. Subjective complaints
1. Insidious onset of lateral hip pain, often spreading into the lateral thigh, aggravated most by climbing stairs or, occasionally, by sitting with the involved leg crossed over the uninvolved leg
2. Occasionally an acute onset is described, associated with a "snap" felt in the hip region (the iliotibial band snapping over the greater trochanter).
B. Key objective findings
1. Pain on resisted hip abduction
2. Pain on approximation of the knee on the involved side to the opposite axilla
3. Possible pain on stretch of the iliotibial band
4. Possible pain on full passive hip abduction
III. Iliopectineal Bursitis
A. Subjective complaint: Gradual, usually nontraumatic, onset of anterior hip pain, made worse by activities involving extreme or repetitive hip extension
B. Key objective findings
1. Pain on resisted hip flexion
2. Pain on full passive hip extension
3. Possible pain on full hip flexion

Knee

I. Acute Medial Ligamentous Injury
   A. Subjective complaints
      1. Sudden onset of knee pain usually associated with some athletic activity. There may or may not have been some external force acting on the knee at the time of injury in the case of a partial tear.
      2. Gradual buildup of swelling during several hours in the case of a partial tear; there is little swelling in the case of a complete rupture.
      3. The patient often attempts to continue the activity in which he or she was engaged in the case of a complete rupture, but much less so in the case of a partial tear.
   B. Key objective findings
      1. Antalgic, toe-touch gait in the acute phase of a partial tear; less severe gait disturbance or no gait disturbance in a complete rupture
      2. Effusion with limitation of motion in a capsular pattern in the case of a partial tear; little swelling and relatively free range of motion if a complete rupture
      3. Pain and spasm on valgus and external rotary stress if a partial tear; painless hypermobility in the case of a complete rupture
II. Acute Meniscus Tear
   A. Subjective complaint: Essentially the same as for a partial ligamentous tear. The patient is very hesitant to continue to engage in the activity.
   B. Key objective findings
      1. The same as for a partial ligament tear except no pain on stress tests
      2. Point tenderness over the anteromedial joint line
      3. Disproportionate loss of extension (e.g., locked knee) if a mechanical block to movement is created by a displaced piece of the meniscus
III. Lateral Patellar Tracking Dysfunction (Chondromalacia Patellae)
   A. Subjective complaints
      1. Gradual onset of medial knee pain aggravated especially by descending stairs and sitting for long periods of time
      2. The onset may be associated with an increase in some activity involving repeated loaded knee extension.
   B. Key objective findings
      1. There may be some predisposing structural factor such as anteversion of the hip, genu valgum, a small patella, a high-riding patella, or a diminution in the prominence of the anterior aspect of the lateral femoral condyle.
      2. There may be some atrophy of the vastus medialis.
      3. Lateral glide of the patella may cause some medial discomfort.
      4. Palpation of the medial aspect of the backside of patella may cause discomfort.
      5. Femoropatellar crepitus may be noted on weight-bearing knee flexion–extension.

IV. Chronic Coronary Ligament Sprain (Adhesion)
   A. Subjective complaint: Sudden medial knee pain associated with some weight-bearing twisting movement, followed by persistent aching or twinging of pain over the medial knee region. There is usually no significant disability.
   B. Key objective findings
      1. Point tenderness over the anteromedial joint line
      2. Pain on passive external rotation of the tibia on the femur; no pain on valgus stress
V. Tendinitis—Biceps, Iliotibial, or Pes Anserinus
   A. Subjective complaint: Gradual onset of pain, almost always associated with long-distance running or some other athletic activity. The pain is lateral for biceps or iliotibial tendinitis and medial for pes anserinus tendinitis. There is little that reproduces the pain except the activity that caused the problem.
   B. Key objective findings
      1. Pain on resisted knee flexion and external tibial rotation in the case of biceps tendinitis
      2. Pain on resisted knee extension and external tibial rotation in the case of iliotibial tendinitis
      3. Pain on resisted knee flexion and internal rotation for pes anserinus tendinitis
      4. Pain on straight-leg raising for biceps tendinitis
      5. Point tenderness over the site of the lesion, usually at the tenoperiosteal junction
      6. Pain on iliotibial band extensibility test for iliotibial tendinitis

Lower Leg, Ankle, and Foot

I. Overuse Syndromes of the Leg
   A. Subjective complaints
      1. The term *shin splint* is often used as a blanket description of any persistent pain occurring between the knee and ankle usually associated with some increased athletic activity, such as jumping or running on a hard surface.
      2. When overuse is a contributing factor, there will be a characteristic history of gradual onset of pain that may be accentuated by excessive pronation or supination. Pain is aggravated by activity and relieved by rest.
   B. Key objective findings
      1. There may be some predisposing structural factors such as excessive pronation or supination, tibial varum, or the coxa varum–genu valgum combination.
      2. Pain and tenderness over the involved soft tissue (tendinitis or compartment syndromes) or in an area devoid of muscles such as the tibial shaft (tibial stress reaction and stress fracture).
      3. Pain is increased by stressing the involved muscles (compartment syndromes and tendinitis) actively or with manual resistance.
      4. In tibial stress reaction, percussion of the tibia increases the pain. Tuning fork vibration may or may not be positive.

II. Acute Ankle Sprain
  A. Subjective complaints
    1. Sudden onset of lateral ankle pain, associated with plantar flexion–inversion strain, usually during some athletic activity. Continued participation in the activity, at the time of injury, is usually not possible.
    2. Gradual development of lateral ankle swelling over the subsequent several hours with continued difficulty in weight bearing.
  B. Key objective signs
    1. Obvious limp associated with traumatic arthritis of the ankle mortise joint (Table 24-1)
    2. Swelling and often marked ecchymosis over the lateral aspect of the ankle
    3. Pain is reproduced on:
      a. Plantar flexion–inversion stress
      b. Anterior glide of the talus in the mortise
III. Chronic Recurrent Ankle Sprains
  A. Subjective complaint: History of acute ankle sprain (see earlier) followed by one or more episodes of the ankle giving way during activities involving jumping or quick lateral movements. Pain, swelling, and dysfunction associated with subsequent episodes are usually not as severe as that occurring with the original injury.
  B. Key objective findings: These are variable, depending on the causative factors. Consider the following possible causes and the related clinical manifestations.
    1. True structural instability (rare)—Hypermobility of anterior glide of the talus in the mortise
    2. Residual ligamentous adhesion—Hypomobility or pain on anterior glide of the talus in the mortise
    3. Alteration in proprioceptive neuromuscular protective response—Poor balance reactions on one-legged standing
IV. Achilles Tendinitis and Bursitis
  A. Subjective complaint: Usually a gradual onset of posterior ankle pain that may be associated with some increase in activity level. The pain is made worse when wearing lower-heeled shoes and is improved with wearing higher heels.
  B. Key objective findings
    1. Pain on strong resisted or repetitive resisted ankle plantar flexion
    2. Pain on extreme hindfoot dorsiflexion
    3. Tenderness to palpation over the distal Achilles region
V. Medial Metatarsalgia
  A. Subjective complaint: Pain over the first two metatarsal heads after long periods of weight bearing. The onset is usually insidious, occasionally associated with a change in footwear.
  B. Key objective findings
    1. Pressure metatarsalgia
      a. Often associated with a pronated or pronating foot
      b. The first metatarsal may be abnormally short.
      c. The medial metatarsal heads may be tender to deep palpation.

    2. Tension metatarsalgia (from increased tension on the distal insertion of the plantar fascia)
      a. Usually associated with a pronating foot
      b. The pain may be reproduced by everting the hindfoot while supinating the forefoot and dorsiflexing the toes.
VI. Plantar Fasciitis
  A. Subjective complaints
    1. Pain and tenderness localized to plantar aspect of foot. Pain may be localized to the heel or may present as a burning pain over the arch.
    2. Pain is made worse by activity, such as climbing stairs, walking, or running, and relieved by rest.
  B. Key objective findings
    1. There may be some predisposing factors such as a high-arched cavus foot, a tight plantar fascia or Achilles tendon, weak peronei or chronic irritation from excessive pronation, or a variety of malalignment faults.
    2. Localized tenderness at the plantar fascial attachment into the calcaneus, just distal to this attachment and over the medial band of the plantar fascia. A tight plantar band can be palpated.
    3. Pain may be increased on actively and passively dorsiflexing the foot, especially if the big toe is also dorsiflexed.

SCAN EXAMINATION TESTS

Gait Analysis

The reader should refer to Tables 24-1 and 24-2 for an overview of the primary gait abnormalities associated with various common lumbar or lower limb disorders or structural deviations. These tables emphasize the biomechanical interplay among the weight-bearing regions. A careful assessment of gait is an essential component of the evaluation of chronic low back and lower limb disorders because it is, of course, the most important functional requirement of these regions and also because many biomechanical abnormalities will not be evident on other parts of the examination.

When evaluating chronic disorders, most of which are the result of stress overloads, it is important to realize which functional abnormalities are present and to appreciate that these are not always manifested as obvious static deviations or deformities. For example, a person's foot may undergo excessive pronation while walking but the foot may not necessarily appear pronated on assessment of bony structure and alignment during standing. Experience in gait analysis is invaluable in understanding the pathomechanics and, in some instances, the causes of many common chronic disorders. For this reason it also leads to greater sophistication in devising and implementing treatment strategies because many chronic disorders are temporarily relieved by symptomatic treatment but will inevitably recur unless the underlying causes are addressed.

Tables 24-1 and 24-2 are organized to serve as a guide to the clinical assessment of gait abnormalities associated with

TABLE 24-1 EFFECTS OF COMMON PATHOLOGIC CONDITIONS ON GAIT: SAGITTAL PLANE (PATIENT VIEWED FROM THE SIDE)

	PAINFUL OR RESTRICTED ANKLE PLANTAR FLEXION	PAINFUL OR RESTRICTED ANKLE DORSIFLEXION	PAINFUL OR RESTRICTED KNEE EXTENSION	PAINFUL OR RESTRICTED HIP EXTENSION	PAINFUL OR RESTRICTED LOW BACK EXTENSION
Nature of Gait Disturbance					
	1. Capsular restriction (e.g., postimmobilization) 2. Traumatic arthritis (e.g., post-ankle sprain)	1. Capsular restriction (e.g., postimmobilization) 2. Heel-cord tightness (e.g., postimmobilization) 3. Traumatic arthritis (e.g., post-ankle sprain)	1. Capsular restriction (e.g., DJD or postimmobilization) 2. Traumatic arthritis (e.g., post-sprain) 3. Locked knee (e.g., bucket-handle meniscus tear)	1. Capsular restriction (e.g., DJD) 2. Iliopectineal bursitis	1. Multisegmental capsular restriction (e.g., DJD) 2. Posterior disk prolapse 3. Acute facet joint dysfunction
Pattern of Gait Disturbance					
Loss of heel-strike a. Toe-touch gait			X (if painful or locked)		
b. Flatfooted gait	X		X (if stiff)		
Loss of plantar flexion after heel-strike with accelerated stance phase	X		X (if stiff)		
Loss of dorsiflexion during foot-flat stage of stance → premature heel-rise, exaggerated hip and knee flexion during early swing phase		X	X (if stiff)		
Loss of push-off and heel-rise	X		X	X	
Shortened stance phase on involved side	X	X	X	X	X (stance shortened bilaterally)
Tendency toward increased knee extension during stance		X (if stiff)			

(continued)

TABLE 24-1 EFFECTS OF COMMON PATHOLOGIC CONDITIONS ON GAIT: SAGITTAL PLANE (PATIENT VIEWED FROM THE SIDE) (Continued)

	PAINFUL OR RESTRICTED ANKLE PLANTAR FLEXION	PAINFUL OR RESTRICTED ANKLE DORSIFLEXION	PAINFUL OR RESTRICTED KNEE EXTENSION	PAINFUL OR RESTRICTED HIP EXTENSION	PAINFUL OR RESTRICTED LOW BACK EXTENSION
Trunk lurch forward during stance		X	X	X (if painful)	
Knee held in increased flexion during stance	X (early and late stance)		X	X	X
Loss of hip extension during stance		X	X	X	X
Loss of low back extension during stance; trunk held in forward position				X (if painful)	X
Tendency toward increased low back extension during stance				X (if stiff)	

DJD, degenerative joint disease.

the common disorders affecting the low back and lower limbs. After having documented the salient features of some abnormal gait pattern, the clinician may consult the tables to estimate what the underlying physical dysfunction may be and to see what the common causes are. This information should then be correlated with findings from the remainder of the physical examination.

Assessment of Structural Alignment

Static alterations in skeletal alignment are significant if they are relatively pronounced or if they are acquired. In either case, they affect a considerable reduction in the stresses that may be imposed on related tissues without pain or degenerative changes. Congenital skeletal deviations, as long as they fall within relatively normal limits, are usually insignificant under normal activity levels because the related tissues automatically adapt to the various stresses they must withstand as the musculoskeletal system develops. However, such normal deviations may make the patient more susceptible to certain stress-overload disorders under conditions of increased activity, such as recreational or competitive athletics. To avoid omitting crucial assessments, the examination of structural alignment may be organized into the following three components: (1) frontal alignment, (2) sagittal alignment, and (3) transverse (rotary) alignment.

The patient's unstructured stance is noted. In this habitual stance the patient may be compensating for a number of postural asymmetries. It may be easier to detect these problems if the stance is structured by asking the patient to stand with the feet hip-width apart and the feet pointed slightly (about 5 to 10°) outward. The primary assessments of each position are carried out with the patient in relaxed standing position, with the low back and lower extremities well exposed. The patient is instructed to look straight ahead and to keep arms to the side.

TESTS IN STANDING

I. Frontal Alignment. Patient viewed from behind
   A. Horizontal asymmetry is best detected by use of a plumb bob. The plumb bob is hung so that it barely clears the ground; the patient is positioned as close as possible to the plumb line, without touching it, and with the plumb bob bisecting the heels.
      1. It should be noted, first, whether the plumb line bisects the legs, pelvis, and lower spine. If there is a lateral shift of the pelvis with respect to the plumb line, consider the following possibilities:
         a. A shorter leg on the side of the shift; this will be checked for later during assessment of vertical symmetry.

b. Tight hip abductors (almost always the iliotibial band) on the side opposite the shift. This is often associated with a valgus deviation of the knee on the tight side. Iliotibial band extensibility should be checked later.

c. Loss of hip abduction on the side of the shift. The most common cause is a capsular restriction secondary to degenerative hip disease. Hip range of motion should be assessed later to determine whether a capsular pattern of restriction exists.

2. Note obvious valgus or varus deviations or asymmetries of the knee

a. Bilateral genu valgum (knock knees) is often associated with femoral antetorsion, foot pronation, or both.

b. Unilateral genu valgum is often associated with iliotibial band tightness, lateral compartment degenerative joint disease of the knee, unilateral femoral antetorsion, or unilateral foot pronation.

c. Bilateral genu varum (bowed legs) is often associated with femoral retrotorsion.

d. Unilateral genu varum is often associated with medial degenerative knee disease or unilateral femoral retrotorsion.

e. Tibial varum or valgum should be differentiated from genu varum or valgum.

f. Calcaneal valgum is usually associated with foot pronation, genu valgum, femoral antetorsion, or some combination thereof. It is evidenced by inward bowing of the Achilles tendon.

g. Calcaneal varum may be present with foot supination, femoral retrotorsion, genu varum, or some combination and is seen as outward bowing of the Achilles tendon.

3. Note obvious asymmetries in muscle bulk. The calves or hamstrings on one side may be atrophied in the presence of a chronic S1 or S2 radiculopathy.

4. Note lateral spinal curvatures. A lumbar scoliosis may be associated with:

a. A lateral pelvic inclination. The lumbar convexity will be toward the side on which the pelvis is lower.

b. A lateral pelvic shift. The convexity will be on the side toward which the pelvis is shifted.

c. Acute spinal derangements (disk prolapse or facet joint dysfunction). The lumbar convexity is usually toward the side of the problem, except in some prolapses in which protruding disk material is medial to the sensitive structure (e.g., the nerve root).

d. Asymmetric lumber degenerative changes, with asymmetric disk narrowing and facet joint tightness. The convexity is usually away from the side of the degeneration.

e. A structural thoracolumbar scoliosis. The patient is asked to bend forward to observe for a fixed rotary component, typical of structural curves. The lumbar convexity is usually to the left, with a left rotary component; the thoracic convexity is to the right, with a right rotary component (see Fig. 20-8C). These curves, unless severe, are generally asymptomatic.

B. Sacral base and leg length. The presence of segmental vertical asymmetries (leg-length disparities) is best determined by comparing the heights of the key bony landmarks listed below. This is usually done by palpating similar prominences or contours with the same finger of both hands, then assessing the relative heights of the palpating fingers. For each of the landmarks, it is not so important that the examiner feel some precise point as it is that he or she feels the same prominence or contour with both palpating fingers.

1. Medial malleoli. The most common cause of one being lower than the other is a foot that is more pronated on the lower side. The examiner should check transverse alignment later and correlate this with the position of the calcaneus, because with foot pronation the calcaneus will tend to be in a valgus position.

2. Fibular heads and popliteal folds. If the malleoli are level and these are not level, disparity in tibial length should be suspected. One should inquire about a previous fracture or other possible causative factors.

3. Greater trochanters. If the ankle and knee landmarks are level but the trochanters are not level, the shaft of one femur is probably shortened, barring severe degenerative changes of the knee. Again, one should inquire about previous fractures.

4. Posterosuperior iliac spines. If the ankle and knee landmarks as well as the trochanters are level, but the posterosuperior iliac spines are not, the following are possible: (1) torsional asymmetry in the sacroiliac joints, (2) valgus–varus asymmetry in the proximal femur, and (3) advanced degenerative changes of one hip joint.

a. The most common torsional displacement at the sacroiliac joint is a backward torsion of the ilium on the sacrum, in which the posterosuperior iliac spine on the involved side is lower than the one on the opposite side; however, the anterosuperior iliac spine on the involved side is higher. In this case, one should check the relative heights of the anterosuperior iliac spines.

b. In the case of femoral valgus or varus asymmetry, both the posterosuperior and anterosuperior iliac spines are higher on the side that is in relative valgus position. Nélaton's line may be used to confirm the existence of valgus–varus asymmetry. The position of the greater trochanter is assessed with respect to a line formed from the anterosuperior iliac spine to the ischial tuberosity; with a valgus femur the trochanter will fall more inferiorly with respect to Nélaton's line compared with a varus femur. It should be realized that valgus angulation of the femur is usually associated with increased

TABLE 24-2 EFFECTS OF COMMON PATHOLOGIC CONDITIONS ON GAIT: FRONTAL PLANE AND TRANSVERSE PLANES (PATIENT VIEWED FROM THE FRONT OR BACK)

	PRONATION DEFORMITY OR FUNCTIONAL PRONATION DEVIATION OF HINDFOOT	PAINFUL OR RESTRICTED ANKLE OR KNEE FLEXION OR EXTENSION	VARUS DEFORMITY OR VALGUS DEFORMITY DEVIATION OF KNEE	VARUS DEFORMITY OR DEVIATION OF KNEE	EXTERNAL TIBIAL TORSION
Nature of Gait Disturbance					
	1. Congenital hypermobility of foot (flexible deformity) 2. Tarsal coalition (fixed deformity) 3. Increased femoral anteversion (functional) 4. Genu valgum (functional) 5. Loss of hindfoot dorsiflexion (e.g., tight heel cord)	See Table 24-1	1. DJD of lateral knee (deformity) 2. Increased femoral antetorsion (function→ structural) 3. Increased foot pronation (functional) 4. Tight iliotibial band (functional)	1. DJD of medial knee (deformity) 2. Increased femoral retrotorsion (functional)	1. Congenital (structural) 2. Acquired compensation for femoral antetorsion
Pattern of Gait Disturbance					
Toeing inward					
Lowered navicular (flatfoot)	X				
Valgus deviation of heel	X		X		
Toeing outward		X			X (uncompensated)
Patella facing outward during swing phase				X (if 2° retroversion)	
Patella facing inward during swing phase					
Patella facing inward during stance	X		X (if 2° anteversion)		X (if compensated)
Patella facing outward during stance					
Pelvis rotates excessively externally (contralateral side forward) during stance					
Pelvis shifted ipsilaterally					
Pelvis shifted contralaterally					
Trunk inclined ipsilaterally during stance					
Trunk inclined contralaterally during stance					

DJD, degenerative joint disease.

TABLE 24-2 EFFECTS OF COMMON PATHOLOGIC CONDITIONS ON GAIT: FRONTAL PLANE AND TRANSVERSE PLANES (PATIENT VIEWED FROM THE FRONT OR BACK) (Continued)

INTERNAL TIBIAL TORSION	INCREASED FEMORAL ANTETORSION OR FUNCTIONAL INTERNAL ROTATORY DEVIATION OF FEMUR	INCREASED FEMORAL RETROTORSION OR FUNCTIONAL EXTERNAL ROTATORY DEVIATION OF FEMUR	PAINFUL OR RESTRICTED HIP ABDUCTION AND INTERNAL ROTATION	RESTRICTED HIP ADDUCTION	PAINFUL OR RESTRICTED LUMBAR LATERAL DEVIATION
Nature of Gait Disturbance					
1. Congenital (structural) 2. Acquired compensation for for femoral retrotorsion	1. Congenital (structural) 2. Increased foot pronation (functional) 3. External tibial torsion (compensatory)	1. Congenital (structural) 2. Internal tibial torsion (compensatory)	Capsular restriction (e.g., hip DJD)	Tight iliotibial band	1. Posterolateral disk protrusion 2. Acute facet joint dysfunction (unilateral)
Pattern of Gait Disturbance					
X (uncompensated)	X (uncompensated)				
	X (if compensated for by external torsion)				
	X (if compensated for by external torsion)				
		X (uncompensated)	X		
		X			
	X				
	X				
X (uncompensated)		X			
	X				
			X		
				X	
			X		X (rare)
					X

antetorsion and a relatively mobile hip joint, whereas a varus femur is usually associated with retrotorsion and a more stable hip joint.

c. Advanced degenerative changes of a hip joint, sufficient to cause noticeable lowering of the pelvis on the involved side, will invariably be associated with a capsular restriction of motion at the hip. Internal rotation and abduction are markedly restricted, flexion and extension are moderately restricted, and adduction and external rotation are somewhat limited.

5. Iliac crests. If these are not level, the cause of asymmetry should be looked for at some lower segment (see earlier). Note: Asymmetry in the height of landmarks at any level should result in a corresponding asymmetry of all landmarks situated more superiorly. If not, combined segmental asymmetries must be suspected (one asymmetry compensating for, or adding to, another).

II. Sagittal Alignment. Patient viewed from the side

Obvious abnormalities or asymmetries in flexion–extension positioning of the lower extremity joints and spine are noted. It should be realized that a fairly broad range of normal variation exists in sagittal alignment. For some persons, it is normal to stand with the ankles, hips, and knees slightly flexed and the spinal curves somewhat flattened. For others it might be normal to stand with the lower extremity joints well extended and with more accentuation of the spinal curves. Any deviation must be considered in light of other findings. Asymmetries can be considered to be more reliably significant.

A. Hip, pelvic, and lumbar region. In general, the front of the pelvis and thigh are in a straight line. All the muscles that control the pelvis are balanced so the angle of the top of the sacrum to a horizontal line does not exceed 50° (30° optimal; see Fig. 20-5). The buttocks do not look prominent but slope slightly downward. Common faults include:

1. The low back arches forward too much (lordosis; see Fig. 7-23). The pelvis tilts forward excessively and the front of the thigh forms an angle with the pelvis when this tilt is present. The anterosuperior iliac spines lie anterior to the pubic symphysis. The amount of lordotic curve is determined not only by the slope of the sacrum but the wedge shape of L5 and the wedge shape of the L5–S1 intervertebral disk, the surrounding musculature, and the stabilizing lumbar ligament.

2. The normal forward curve in the low back has straightened out. The symphysis pubis lies anterior to the anterosuperior iliac spines. The lumbosacral angle is decreased and hip extension is characteristic.

3. The entire pelvic segment shifts anteriorly, resulting in hip extension, and shift of the thoracic segment posteriorly results in flexion of the thorax on the upper lumbar spine (swayback posture; see Fig. 7-25).[5] A compensatory increased thoracic kyphosis and forward head placement is also seen. This results in an increased lor-

dosis in the lower lumbar region and increased kyphosis in the lower thoracic region.

4. The most common unilateral finding of the pelvis is posterior iliac torsion: the posterosuperior spine is lower than the opposite side. The reverse is found with anterior iliac torsion.

B. Knees and Legs. Looking at the knees from the side, the knees are straight (i.e., neither bent forward nor locked backward). The plumb line passes slightly anterior to the midline of the knee, creating an extension moment. Abnormal considerations include:

1. Abnormal hyperextension (genu recurvatum). The knee is hyperextended, and the gravitational stress lies far forward of the joint. Abnormal hyperextension of the knees is often seen with an anterior pelvic tilt and the resulting excessive lumbar lordosis. Abnormal extension is often the result of restricted ankle dorsiflexion, as from a tight heel cord or capsular ankle restriction. A less common and more serious cause of severe "back" knee is neuropathic arthropathy such as may occur with tertiary syphilis.

2. Abnormal flexion (flexed knees or antecurvatum). The plumb line falls posterior to the joint axis. Abnormal flexion of the knees occurs with a greater variety of disorders, including the following:

a. Restricted ankle plantar flexion (rare), the most common cause of which is capsular restriction after immobilization

b. An internal derangement, such as a bucket-handle meniscus tear, causing a mechanical block to knee extension

c. An acute spinal derangement, such as a disk herniation or facet joint lesion

d. Multisegmental capsular restriction, which occurs with significant degenerative changes (e.g., ankylosing spondylosis)[3]

C. Ankles. The plumb line lies slightly anterior to the lateral malleolus aligned with the tuberosity of the fifth metatarsal. In the forward posture (anterior deviation of the body), the plumb line is posterior to the body; body weight is carried on the metatarsal heads of the feet.[5,6] The ankles are in dorsiflexion because of the forward inclination of the leg and overstretched posterior musculature. The posterior muscles of the trunk and lower extremities tend to remain in a state of constant contraction.

III. Transverse Rotary Alignment. Patient viewed from the front

The stance width should be normal and the feet slightly (5 to 10°) pointed outward. Obvious foot deformities, such as hallux valgus (see Fig. 16-33D), should be noted. Hallux valgus is often associated with abnormal foot pronation, which, in turn, often occurs in conjunction with transverse rotary abnormalities of more proximal segments. Assessment of segmental rotary alignment is performed, working upward from the feet, by examining the positioning and symmetry of the following landmarks:

A. Navicular tubercles. The positions of the navicular tubercles are assessed compared with a line from the medial malleolus to the point at which the first metatarsal contacts the ground. The tubercle should fall just on, or below, this line. The person with a static (i.e., resting) pronation deviation of the foot will have a navicular tubercle that falls well below the line. This is a true flatfoot and will invariably be associated with a valgus heel. Abnormality in bony alignment must be confirmed because many persons have considerable bulk of the medial soft tissues of the foot, which gives the foot a flattened appearance. When a true flatfoot is detected, one must determine whether it is structural (fixed) or functional (mobile). To do so, the patient is asked to raise up on the balls of the feet or to attempt to externally rotate the legs over the stationary foot; in both cases, the arch will be seen to rise significantly if the pronated position of the foot is functional. The common cause of a structurally pronated foot is tarsal coalition. The common causes of a mobile flatfoot are congenital ligamentous laxity and femoral antetorsion. It must be appreciated that a person who does not have static pronation deviation of the foot, as evidenced on examination of structural alignment, may still have a problem from abnormal foot pronation during gait. On the other hand, a person with a static pronation deviation of the foot does not necessarily have a pronation problem, especially if the deviation has existed since childhood. The tissues of the foot will have adapted to the increased pronatory stresses during development.

B. Intermalleolar line. A line passing through the tips of the medial and lateral malleoli should make an angle, opening laterally, of about 25° with the frontal plane when the knee axis is situated in the frontal plane (i.e., when the patellae are facing straight forward).

   Note: Twenty-five degrees corresponds to the lateral malleolus being about 4 cm posterior to the medial malleolus when the intermalleolar distance is 10 cm, about 3.5 cm posterior for a 9-cm intermalleolar width, or about 3 cm posterior for an 8-cm width.

   1. If the angle is excessive, the examiner must suspect increased external tibial torsion or increased femoral antetorsion. It is not unusual for these to coexist, the two having a mutual compensatory effect to cancel abnormal toeing inward (from femoral antetorsion) or toeing outward (from external tibial torsion). Compensation would occur during development. The presence of femoral antetorsion is best determined clinically by femoral torsion tests (Craig's test or Ryder's method) (Fig. 14-25) and by assessing hip rotational range of motion in the prone position. The hip with medial femoral torsion is a very mobile hip that appears to have an increase in internal rotation at the expense of a loss of external rotation.

   2. Similarly, if the angle the intermalleolar line makes with the frontal plane is diminished when the patellae

face straight forward, there may be an increase in femoral retrotorsion or abnormal internal tibial torsion. A hip with lateral femoral torsion is a less mobile hip that will appear to have a loss of internal rotation, with external rotation perhaps somewhat increased.

C. Patellae. With the feet pointed slightly outward the patellae should face straight forward.

   1. If the patellae face inward, the examiner should suspect increased femoral antetorsion, increased external tibial torsion, or both (see earlier).

   2. If the patellae face outward when the feet are in a normal position, the cause may be femoral retrotorsion, internal tibial torsion, or both (see earlier).

D. Anterosuperior iliac spines. These should be positioned in a frontal plane. If the pelvis is rotated (one iliac spine more anterior than the other), there are two common causes to be considered:

   1. A fixed (structural) spinal scoliosis, the rotary component of which is transmitted to the pelvis through the sacrum by way of the lumbar spine

   2. Torsional asymmetry of the sacroiliac joints. The pelvis will appear to be rotated forward on the side on which the ilium is in more anterior torsion with respect to the sacrum.

IV. Vertical Compression Test (see Fig. 20-4).[1,8] The concept behind compressive testing is to test the amount of "spring" that the spine has when a direct compression force is applied. Spines of patients with decreased curvatures (decreased lordosis or axially extended spines) will not have enough spring, which leads to decreased shock attenuation.[1] Deviations such as an increased lumbar lordosis, posterior angulation of the thoracic spine, or regions of instability preventing sufficient weight transfer through the spine may be revealed during this test.[2,4,7]

V. Tests in Sitting. Observe posture with the patient seated with the back unsupported and feet on the ground. Note any changes in posture. As in the standing position, this observation is carried out for frontal, sagittal, and transverse rotatory alignment. Note any changes in the spinal curvatures. If scoliosis is observed when the client is standing and disappears in sitting, then the asymmetry is caused by the lower limbs and is therefore functional.

Regional Tests

I. Lumbosacral Tests

A. With the patient standing, the examiner demonstrates the movement to be performed as verbal instructions are given. The examiner is looking for the patient's willingness to do the movements and for limitation of motion and its possible causes, such as pain, stiffness, or spasm. When viewing from behind, the movements are observed for asymmetry and for the levels affected. The examiner can determine whether any deviations are painful or painless when corrected. When viewing the patient from the side, the examiner should assess the continuity of movement at the various spinal segments and look for reversal of the lumbar lordosis. The most painful movements should be done last. The following active movements are carried out in the lumbosacral spine:

1. Extension (backward bending): When viewing from behind stabilize the crest of the pelvis. The pelvis should not tilt nor should the hips extend. Areas of the spine that appear to bend easier (hypermobile) and areas that seem restricted (hypomobility) should be noted.

2. Lateral flexion (sidebending; left and right): Normally the lumbar curve should form a smooth curve on side flexion, and there should be no obvious angulations. If angulation does occur, it may indicate hypomobility or hypermobility at one level of the lumbar spine. A localized capsular restriction will limit sidebending slightly toward the involved side, but a multisegmental capsular restriction can cause restriction to both sides.

3. Flexion (forward bending): The examiner must ensure that the movement is occurring in the lumbar spine and not in the hips. It should be determined whether iliosacral movement is blocked or hypomobile during palpation.

4. Active return from forward bending: The lumbosacral rhythm should be a smooth transition during lumbar reversal and pelvic return.

5. Active flexion (forward bending) in sitting position: Observe for sacroiliac motion.

6. Lateral shift (side glide): Observe unilateral restriction.

7. Rotation (patient seated, knees together, with the arms folded or held in 90° flexion and hands together; left and right). Observe for asymmetry.

B. Active auxiliary tests. If the patient's symptoms have not been reproduced, the following additional maneuvers may be conducted (patient standing):

1. Passive overpressure at end range of active physiologic spinal motions
2. Repeated physiologic motions at various speeds
3. Sustained pressure at end range of extension and lateral flexion
4. Active combined motions without overpressure (left and right)
   a. Flexion (forward bending) with rotation
   b. Lateral flexion with flexion (forward bending)
5. Passive combined motions with passive overpressure (left and right)
   a. Flexion (forward bending) and lateral flexion
   b. Flexion (forward bending) with rotation
   c. Extension (backward bending) with lateral flexion
   d. Extension with rotation

C. Active segmental mobility. With the patient in stride-standing position, the examiner can assess the following:

1. Upper lumbar spine for lateral flexion
2. L5–S1 for lateral flexion
3. Active pelvic tilt (L5–S1 for whether painful or painless)

D. Passive movements

1. Whether posture correction is painful or painless
2. Quadrant test (patient standing); passive auxiliary test for segmental involvement
3. Passive physiologic movements (non–weight bearing).
   a. Flexion (forward bending)
   b. Extension (backward bending)
   c. Lateral flexion (sidebending; left and right)
   d. Rotation (left and right)
4. Passive physiologic movements with segmental palpation. Note type of end feel and seek abnormalities.
   a. Flexion–extension (forward and backward bending)
   b. Lateral flexion (sidebending; left and right)
   c. Rotation (left and right)
5. Segmental mobility
   a. Posteroanterior central pressures for T10–L5
   b. Transverse pressures for T10–L5
   c. Posteroanterior unilateral pressures for T10–L5
      For the fullest information, one should alter the direction of posteroanterior pressure; counterpressures are exerted to the spinous process of the segment above and below, and posteroanterior pressures may be applied diagonally in caudal and cephalad directions—T10–L5.

E. Passive movements of the sacroiliac and peripheral joints

1. Sacroiliac auxiliary (provocation) and mobility tests
   a. Posterior rotation test
   b. Anterior rotation test
2. Hip joint: Hip flexion–adduction test
3. Knee joint
   a. Anterior drawer (Lachman) test
   b. Valgus–varus stress test at 30° knee flexion

F. Neuromuscular tests

1. Key sensory areas (L4–S2); stroking test and sensibility to pin prick, if applicable
2. Resisted isometric (myotomal) tests (L2–S2; see Fig. 5-10). Compare both sides.
3. Dural mobility testing
   a. Straight-leg raising (sciatic nerve); sitting and supine, with and without cervical spine flexion
   b. Slump test (sciatic nerve)
   c. Femoral nerve traction test
4. Reflexes
   a. Knee jerk (L3) and plantar response
   b. Ankle jerk (S1)
   c. Great toe jerk (L5)
   d. Posterior tibial reflex (L5)
   e. Test for ankle clonus

II. Pelvic Joint and Sacroiliac Joint Tests

A. Active movements. Active movements of the spine puts a stress on the sacroiliac joints as well as the lumbar and lumbosacral joints. Forward flexion movement while standing tests the movement of the ilium on the sacrum. The hip movements are also affected by sacroiliac lesions.

1. Standing and sitting active trunk flexion tests for possible locking of the ilium on the sacrum or restriction

2. Sacroiliac fixation test (active hip flexion) for fixation or restriction
B. Passive movements. Special tests include:
   1. Posterior rotation test
   2. Anterior rotation test
   3. Anterior ligament distraction test
   4. Posterior ligament distraction test
C. Functional leg difference caused by pelvis imbalance: Supine-to-sit test

III. Hip Tests
A. Active movements. The emphasis is on assessing functional activities involving the use of the hip. If the patient is able to do active flexion (knee to chest), extension in standing, and abduction and rotation in non–weight bearing with little difficulty, the examiner may use a series of functional tests to see whether increased intensity of activity produces pain or other symptoms (e.g., squatting, going up and down stairs, running, and jumping).
B. Passive movements. Passive movements should be performed to determine the end feel and the degree of passive range of motion.
   1. Perform passive hip flexion–extension, abduction–adduction, internal–external rotation, and combined flexion, adduction, and rotation.
   2. If indicated, the assessment of muscle lengths is included: the Thomas test to detect a hip flexion contracture, Ely's test for the iliopsoas and rectus femoris, knee extension with the hip in 90°, straight-leg raising for hamstrings, and the Ober test for the iliotibial band.
C. Resisted isometric movements
   1. Resisted hip flexion–extension, adduction, and internal–external rotation are tested isometrically in the supine position to determine which muscles may be at fault or for the presence of a possible bursitis. Resisted hip flexion is also done as a test for the integrity of the L2 myotome.
   2. Resisted hip abduction is tested with the patient in the prone position for the presence of possible trochanteric bursitis or gluteus medius tendinitis.

IV. Knee Tests
A. Active movements. Flexion–extension can be assessed at the same time as hip flexion and extension and, in a weight-bearing situation, while testing the L3 myotome.
   1. During weight-bearing movements, the examiner should palpate at the femoropatellar joint and at the femorotibial joint for crepitus that may indicate degenerative changes. Snapping and popping during movement is common, but a continuous grinding, suggestive of sand in the joint, is more significant.
   2. During non–weight bearing, the knee is assessed for loss of dynamic tibial function and for any evidence of quadriceps lag. These tests allow the examiner to detect subtle abnormalities that may predispose to

chronic knee pain and perhaps progressive degeneration. These patients often respond well to manual therapy techniques.
   3. Functional tests. If the preceding tests are performed with little difficulty, the examiner may put the patient through a series of functional tests to see whether these activities reproduce the patient's symptoms or pain.
B. Passive physiologic movement with passive overpressure. More information may be derived by testing passive ranges of extension, flexion, and axial rotation in cardinal planes and combined motions.
C. Patellar glide. The patella is moved passively, posteriorly, medially, and laterally. At the extremes of medial movement, the underside of the medial patella is palpated for tenderness.
D. Resisted isometric movements
   1. Internal–external rotation with the knee bent. Resisted internal rotation will reproduce pain from pes anserinus; resisted external rotation may reproduce pain from iliotibial band tendinitis.
   2. Knee flexion (also tests for the S2 myotome). This may reproduce pain from pes anserinus tendinitis or biceps tendinitis.
   3. Knee extension (L3). Pain may be reproduced in patellar tendinitis.

V. Ankle and Foot Tests
A. Active motion and passive movements
   1. Flexion–extension. The patient lies prone with the feet over the edge of the table. With the foot in subtalar neutral, active and passive dorsiflexion are assessed and then repeated with the knee bent to 90°. Pain from Achilles tendinitis may be reproduced at the extremes of dorsiflexion. Pain from an anterior talofibular ligament sprain or adhesion may be reproduced on plantar flexion–inversion with passive overpressure.
   2. Hindfoot inversion–eversion. With the patient sitting, the range of passive calcaneal inversion–eversion is assessed.
   3. Forefoot supination–pronation. With the subtalar joint maintained with the calcaneus in subtalar neutral, the examiner should maximally supinate (untwist) and pronate (twist) the forefoot. With the foot held untwisted, the toes are moved into sustained dorsiflexion. Untwisting of the foot may reproduce pain from a calcaneocuboid ligament sprain; sustained toe dorsiflexion may reproduce pain from plantar fasciitis or calcaneal periostitis because this stretches the plantar fascia.
   4. Anterior glide of the talus in the mortise. Hypermobility will be present in the case of chronic anterior talofibular ligament rupture. Pain will be reproduced from a talofibular ligament sprain or adhesion.
   5. Functional tests. If the patient is able to do the preceding activities with little difficulty, functional tests may be performed to see whether these

activities reproduce the symptoms or pain (e.g., standing and walking on the toes, standing on one foot at a time, running, and jumping). These activities should be selected and geared to the individual patient.

B. Resisted isometrics. With the patient in the supine position, the presence of pain and weakness is assessed. Movements tested isometrically include the following:
1. Knee flexion (S2)
2. Tibialis anterior (L4; dorsiflexion–inversion)
3. Tibialis posterior (L5; plantar flexion–inversion)
4. Peroneus tertius (dorsiflexion–eversion)
5. Peroneus longus and brevis (S1; plantar flexion–eversion)
6. Toe flexion–extension: extensor digitorum (L5–S1) and hallucis longus (L5)

CLINICAL IMPLEMENTATION OF LUMBOSACRAL–LOWER LIMB SCAN EXAMINATION

Gait analysis and a comprehensive assessment of structural alignment should be included in the assessment of virtually all chronic disorders of the low back and lower extremities. It is rare, however, to include all of the regional tests discussed during any one examination; tests are chosen as indicated by subjective information and findings on gait analysis and inspection of structural alignment. The clinician must be prepared to judge which tests might be relevant in a particular case—a judgment that is facilitated by experience.

For the scan examination to be of practical use in a busy clinical setting, the clinician must be able to perform the examination within a reasonable time, for example, 15 minutes or less. This requires knowledge of which tests are to be performed, understanding of the rationale for each test, skill in appropriately carrying out each test, and ability to interpret the results.

Clinically, the tests of the scan examination must be carried out according to the patient's position to minimize time requirements and to prevent omission of crucial tests. The following is a summary of the tests included in a complete lumbosacral–lower limb scan examination, according to the position of the patient. This format should be followed in the clinical implementation of the scan examination.

I. Standing
   A. Gait analysis
      1. Sagittal
      2. Frontal
      3. Transverse
      4. Equilibrium. The patient stands on one leg with the eyes closed. Check stabilization efficiency of each hip.
   B. Inspection of structural alignment and soft tissue
      1. Frontal—from behind
      2. Sagittal—from the side
      3. Transverse (rotatory)—from the front
      4. Posture correction
      5. Vertical compression
   C. Functional tests
      1. Active lumbar (physiologic) movements
         a. Extension (backward bending)
         b. Lateral flexion (sidebending)
         c. Flexion (forward bending)
         d. Lateral shift (side gliding)
      2. Active lumbar segmental movements
         a. Upper lumbar
         b. L5–S1
         c. Active pelvic tilt
      3. Active peripheral joint movements
         a. Hip flexion–extension
         b. Standing unilateral half squats (L3)
         c. Standing unilateral toe raises (S1–S2)
      4. Auxiliary tests (if indicated) to clear joints
II. Sitting
   A. Alignment
      1. Sitting posture compared with standing
      2. Position of the patellae
      3. Rotatory position of the tibia
   B. Function
      1. Active lumbar spine rotation
      2. Resisted isometrics—hip flexion (L2)
      3. Tibial rotatory mechanics
      4. Dural mobility
   C. Resisted isometrics
      1. Resisted hip flexion (L2)
      2. Resisted knee extension (L3)
III. Supine
   A. Functional tests
      1. Active lumbar movements: Effect on symptoms
         a. Flexion
         b. Repeated flexion
      2. Passive tests—Hip, knee, ankle, and foot ranges compared with other limbs, with assessment of end feel and overpressure if applicable. Regions of muscle tightness are sought: hamstrings, hip adductors, and gastrocnemius and soleus muscles.
         a. Hip and knee flexion–extension range
         b. Hip adduction–abduction range
         c. Knee internal-external rotation
         d. Patellar glide, medially and laterally
         e. Ankle dorsiflexion–plantar flexion
         f. Hindfoot inversion–eversion and forefoot twisting and untwisting; dorsiflex toes when untwisted
   B. Resisted isometrics
      1. Resisted hip abduction
      2. Resisted dorsiflexion (L4)–plantar flexion; tibialis posterior (L5)
      3. Resisted large toe extension (L5)
   C. Sensation: Include vibratory perception, stroking test, and sensibility to pin prick, if applicable

D. Dural mobility

E. Reflexes

  1. Knee jerk (L3–L4)

  2. Great toe jerk (L5)

  3. Test for ankle clonus

  4. Plantar response

IV. Sidelying. Function

A. Passive physiologic movements with segmental palpation; lumbar spine

  1. Flexion–extension (forward and backward bending)

  2. Lateral flexion (sidebending)

  3. Rotation

B. Sacroiliac posterior rotation

C. Iliotibial band extensibility

V. Prone

A. Active movements: Effect on symptoms

  1. Lumbar spine extension

  2. Lumbar spine; repeated extension

  3. Lateral shift; correction

B. Passive movements: Effect on symptoms

  1. Sacroiliac anterior rotation

  2. Hip internal–external rotation range of motion and femoral torsion tests

  3. Lumbar spine

    a. Sidebending

    b. Rotation

C. Accessory movements

  1. Sacral springing

  2. Posteroanterior gliding and rotation; lumbar spine

D. Resisted isometrics

  1. Resisted hip extension (S1)

  2. Resisted knee rotations

  3. Resisted knee flexion

    a. Assess strength; S1, S2, myotomes

    b. Assess irritability; biceps or pes anserinus tendonitis

E. Reflexes: Ankle jerk (S1, S2)

REFERENCES

1. Cantu RI, Grodin AJ: Myofascial Manipulation: Theory and Clinical Application. Gaithersburg, MD, Aspen, 1992
2. Farfan H, Gracovetsky S: The nature of instability. Spine 9:714–719, 1984
3. Hartley A: Practical Joint Assessment: A Sports Medicine Manual. St. Louis, Mosby Year Book, 1990
4. Howes RG, Isdale IC: The loose back: An unrecognized syndrome. Rheumatol Phys Med 11:72–77, 1971
5. Kendall FP, McCreary EK, Provance PG: Muscles: Testing and Function, 4th ed. Baltimore, Williams & Wilkins, 1993
6. Palmer ML, Epler M: Clinical Assessment Procedures in Physical Therapy 2nd ed. Philadelphia, Lippincott Williams & Wilkins, 1998
7. Paris SV: Physical signs of instability. Spine 10:277–279, 1985
8. Saliba VL, Johnson G: Lumbar protective mechanism. In: White A, Anderson R, eds: Conservative Care of Low Back Pain. Baltimore, Williams & Wilkins, 1991:112–119

RECOMMENDED READINGS

Boyling J, Palastanga N, eds: Grieve's Modern Manual Therapy of the Vertebral Column. Edinburgh, Churchill Livingstone, 1994

Butler D: Mobilisation of the Nervous System. Melbourne, Churchill Livingstone, 1991

Corrigan B, Maitland GD: Practical Orthopaedic Medicine. London, Butterworths, 1985

Cyriax JF, Cyriax PJ: Illustrated Manual of Orthopaedic Medicine, 2nd ed. Boston, Butterworths, 1993

Dutton M: The scanning examination. In: Dutton M: Manual Therapy of the Spine: An Integrated Approach. New York, McGraw-Hill, 2002:171–224

Dvorák J, Dvorák V: Manual Medicine: Diagnostics. New York, Thieme Medical, 1990

Edwards BC: Combined movements in the lumbar spine: Their use in examination and treatment. In: Grieve GP, ed: Modern Manual Therapy of the Vertebral Column. New York, Churchill Livingstone, 1986:561–566

Edwards BC: Manual of Combined Movements, 2nd ed. Oxford, Butterworth-Heinemann, 1999

Evans RC: Illustrated Essentials in Orthopedic Physical Assessment. St. Louis, CV Mosby, 1994

Grant R: Physical Therapy of the Cervical and Thoracic Spine. 3rd ed. New York, Churchill Livingstone, 2002

Greenfield BH: Rehabilitation of the Knee: A Problem Solving Approach. Philadelphia, FA Davis, 1993

Greenman PE: Principles of Manual Medicine 3rd ed. Philadelphia, Lippincott Williams & Wilkins, 2003

Grieve P: Mobilisation of the Spine: A Primary Handbook of Clinical Methods, 5th ed. Edinburgh, Churchill Livingstone, 1991

Kaltenborn FM: The Spine: Basic Evaluation and Mobilization Techniques, 2nd ed. Oslo, Olaf Norlis Bokhandel, 1993

Kenna C, Murtagh J: Back Pain and Spinal Manipulation. Sydney, Butterworths, 1989

Kibler WB, Herring SA: Functional Rehabilitation of Sports and Musculoskeletal Injuries. Gaithersburg, MD, Aspen Publications, 1998

Lee D: The Pelvic Girdle. Edinburgh, Churchill Livingstone, 1989

Lee D: The Thorax: An Integrated Approach. White Rock, BC, Canada, Lee Physiotherapist Corporation, 2003

Magee DJ: Orthopedic Physical Assessment, 3rd ed. Philadelphia, WB Saunders, 1997

Maigne R: Orthopedic Medicine. Springfield, IL, Charles C Thomas, 1976

Maitland GD, Banks K, English K, et al: Vertebral Manipulations, 6th ed. Oxford, Butterworths-Heinemann, 2001

McKenzie R: The Lumbar Spine: Mechanical Diagnosis and Therapy. Waikanae, New Zealand, Spinal Publications, 1981

Nicholas JA, Hershmann EB, eds: The Lower Extremity and Spine in Sports Medicine. St. Louis, CV Mosby, 1986

Porterfield JA, DeRosa C: Mechanical Low Back Pain: Perspectives in Functional Anatomy. Philadelphia, WB Saunders, 1991

Wells PE: The examination of the pelvic joints. In: Grieve GP, ed: Modern Manual Therapy of the Vertebral Column. Edinburgh, Churchill Livingstone, 1986:590–602

Woermann AL: Evaluation and treatment of dysfunction in the lumbar-pelvic-hip complex. In: Donateli R, Wooden MJ, eds: Orthopaedic Physical Therapy, 3rd ed, New York, Churchill Livingstone, 2001:387–436

Case Histories and Management Problems

KAREN SHRADER DASILVA, RPT

25

- OTHER FORMS OF THERAPEUTIC EXCHANGE BETWEEN PATIENT AND PRACTITIONER
- NONCLINICAL MANAGEMENT CHALLENGES
- CASE STUDY FORMAT
- CASE STUDY OUTLINE
- DEFINITIONS OF CASE STUDY FORMAT
- CASE STUDIES
    - Mark
    - Elizabeth
    - Kathy
    - Mary
    - Larry
    - Sally
- CONCLUSION

It is important to remember when treating patients that they are more than a simple diagnosis. The most effective treatment of a patient often comes when one considers not only the objective findings of their dysfunction, but also the subjective aspects of the patient as well. The practitioner needs to consider the entire person, and not just their injured body part. Many management challenges can arise from the objective problems of the patient. However, additional management challenges arise from the less quantifiable subjective roadblocks to a successful rehabilitation. Such factors range from the patient's psychological health, their socioeconomic situation, language barriers, transportation issues, insurance limitations, and other factors. The goal of this chapter is to present an overview of other forms of therapeutic exchange between patients and practitioners, in addition to a variety of case studies, beginning with initial subjective complaints through objective findings, leading to treatment plans, therapeutic procedures, management problems, and actual outcomes.

OTHER FORMS OF THERAPEUTIC EXCHANGE BETWEEN PATIENT AND PRACTITIONER

The therapeutic relationship between patient and practitioner begins the first moment that you make contact with your patient. A great deal is communicated to the patient by your professionalism, tone, nonverbal behavior, responses, and mood. These factors need to be considered as setting the stage for the patient's successful therapeutic outcome. A primary goal is to instill a sense of trust and confidence in you by your patient. Once this is established, there is a much stronger base on which to build your treatment.

On first meeting your patient it is helpful to call the patient by their name, introduce yourself, and make eye contact with a pleasant look on your face. You are trying to communicate that you enjoy what you are doing, you are sincerely pleased

to have the opportunity to treat a new patient, and you are committed to helping them. Although it can be difficult with a high patient load, try to keep in mind how you would like to be treated if you were the patient in this situation. This may seem trivial, but you are telling the patient that you respect them and have genuine concern for them. Without this basis, patients are much less likely to be compliant with their home exercise programs, be honest with you about their complaints, or integrate your instructions into their daily lives.

Once you begin to take their subjective history, strive to practice active listening. Acknowledge patients' concerns and complaints as they tell you about their situation. For example, if a patient is telling you that they have had to quit their job and go on part-time disability because of their back problems, rather than keeping your eyes focused on what you are writing, you might try looking up, making eye contact and saying something like, "Oh I am sorry to hear that, that must be difficult for you." This type of acknowledgment is not necessarily *feeling sorry for the patient,* but rather an empathetic statement letting the patient know you are really listening to them and care. This type of interaction validates the patient's situation. If patients perceive that their therapist values and understands their situation, they may be less likely to exaggerate their complaints or feel it is necessary to be overly verbose in their communications to you (Box 25-1, Active Listening Guidelines).

It is important for practitioners to have genuine compassion for their patients. This is especially true with a difficult or combative patient. It can be helpful if a patient feels that they have some sort of common ground with you. For example, try to find a brief conversation topic that relates to their life. If they are telling you about their frustrations of not being able to play tennis because of their elbow pain, you might make a comment like, "I would be frustrated too if I could not play for that long. I've been playing tennis for years myself." Your goal is to find some sort of common ground. When even this approach seems challenging and you simply cannot find anything in common

BOX 25-1	ACTIVE LISTENING GUIDELINES

- Look at the patient, observe their reactions, and generally maintain eye contact when possible. Show that you're interested in what he or she is saying. Encourage the patient by unobtrusive use of "yes" and "I see."
- Use positive body cues at appropriate points—nods, smiles, note taking, sympathetic glances, and so forth.
- Engage the patient by looking for opportunities to subtly mirror his or her cues. Do not mimic, but do look for ways to be congruent. For example, if he or she speaks slowly, match his or her cadence.
- Don't say much yourself. You can't listen while you're talking. Be careful not to interrupt the patient's flow.

BOX 25-2	OTHER FORMS OF THERAPEUTIC TREATMENT

- Instill trust and confidence in the practitioner
- Communicate respect and genuine concern
- Practice active listening
- Acknowledge patients' concerns, feelings, and fears
- Find common ground and genuine compassion
- Try to get patients to acknowledge their progress through functional gains

with your patient, it may be helpful to simply comment on something situational that day. For instance, "That is a beautiful ring. I had not noticed it before and I really admire jewelry." This is not meant to suggest that you are going to get into an in-depth personal conversation with each patient, but a few brief comments can make a difference for both the patient and you.

Yet another way you can connect better with your patients is the way you choose to explain things. Choose analogies that relate to the patient's reality and background. For example, if you know that your patient is a construction worker you might be more successful explaining his disk disease with an example like, "The disk and vertebrae are like a washer and a bolt. The washer is there to protect the bolt, but after years of rubbing back and forth, the washer begins to wear thin." Even the words you choose can be important, you may go into greater technical detail about the benefits of ultrasound to an electrical engineer, or more about the anatomy of their problem to a massage therapist, or you may keep your language very simple and use more visual aids to a 11-year-old patient or the non–English-speaking patient. Whatever your approach, do your best to understand your audience.

Try to get patients to see their own progress. There is a certain type of patient that no matter how things have gone since their last visit will answer the question "How are you today?" with "About the same." As a practitioner, you can tell by the way patients are walking or holding themselves that they appear better to you. At this point you might try asking them what they have done since your last visit. They may report something like "Well, I mowed the lawn over the weekend and watched a ball game, but I still hurt." You could then take the opportunity to point out that they were previously unable to push or pull anything greater than 5 pounds and they also could not sit for more than 15 minutes without increased pain. The fact that they can do so much more indicates that they are improving. This type of functional quantification of progress is not only helpful to your patient, but also to insurance compa-

nies. In summary, effective treatment extends beyond clinical assessment and implementation of your treatment plan. The successful practitioner will also take care to address the less objective aspects of treatment. No matter what the therapeutic setting, patients will respond more favorably if they feel that they are being treated with respect and dignity and if they believe that their practitioner has a genuine investment in their care (Box 25-2, Other Forms of Therapeutic Treatment).

NONCLINICAL MANAGEMENT CHALLENGES

In addition to clinical challenges in treatment, today's practitioner will be faced with many other nonclinical management challenges. Such factors range from the patient's psychological health, family circumstances, socioeconomic situations, language barriers, transportation issues, insurance limitations, and other factors.

A patient's psychological health may impact their ability to understand and follow your directions. There may also be some secondary gain issues involved. If a patient is experiencing secondary gains, this can be a substantial roadblock to rehabilitation. Secondary gain is a psychiatric term meaning that a person has a hidden reason for holding on to an undesirable condition. Frequently this reason is unconscious. It is obviously unconscious because the loss of holding on to the condition is often far greater than the perceived gain. For example, this term is often used in chronic pain management. Chronic pain is pain that continues on past the time of an injury being healed, often having no apparent cause in the present. Identifying and addressing the perception of secondary gain, such as the attention one receives, monetary compensation for disability, or just the need to deny the original cause of the pain, can greatly contribute to healing. A patient also may be in a depressed state, which can interfere with many aspects of care. In this situation it may be best to contact their referral source or case manager and see whether you can get them referred for additional mental health intervention.

Family circumstances can also present challenges to care. Although not always in the best interest for a patient's rehabilitation, it may be necessary to stop treatment or have inconsistent care for your patient to address issues within their family. Sometimes this is in the form of caring for sick children, parents, or spouse; other times it is divorce or other family tragedies that demand the full attention of the patient. Other times, care is interrupted because other family members are having difficulty caring for the patient. Whatever the circumstances, it might be necessary to adapt your treatment plan. If care is greatly interrupted, it likely will also be necessary to contact the patient's referral source or case manager and let them know the current situation.

There also may be socioeconomic issues that present challenges. For example, not speaking the patient's language may mean that they must come with an interpreter. Scheduling with the interpreter can be problematic, as all parties need to be present for treatment. Sometimes the patient cannot drive and has to rely on family, friends, or the bus for transportation. Attending timely scheduled appointments can be difficult for patients in these situations. With insurance plans paying smaller percentages, often the patient cannot afford to pay for their portion of care. It might be necessary to develop a plan of care that is limited by a number of visits for financial reasons. These are some examples of socioeconomic issues that need to be considered when treating patients.

Unfortunately in current times, medical insurance coverage needs to be seriously considered as part of the treatment plan. Most insurance plans now have a maximum number of rehabilitation visits per year or maximum dollar amount limitations. As practitioners we must be aware of these sorts of financial limitations. If a patient can only afford six sessions of care or their insurance only allows 10 sessions a year, then you must design the best treatment plan you can with the current limitations. Often practitioners must act as an advocate for their patients, working with claims adjustors, case managers, or insurance companies to try to maximize quality of care for their patients.

Whether it is psychological health, family circumstances, socioeconomic situations, language barriers, transportation issues, insurance limitations, and other factors, many other nonclinical challenges need to be considered when treating patients. Overall, it is the practitioner's responsibility to be aware of all of these nonclinical factors and to consider them in the treatment of their patients.

CASE STUDY FORMAT

Six case studies will be presented in this chapter. The case studies presented are about real patients and actual outcomes. The variety of cases presented is meant to demonstrate realistic challenges and obstacles that one can experience as a practitioner and possible ways to overcome those obstacles. Each case study will be presented in the following format: the subjective complaints and history of the patient, a table of their significant clinical findings, a table of their management challenges, the working assessment, the treatment plan and goals, what therapeutic procedures were performed, the clinical outcome, and lastly a summary of key points.

CASE STUDY OUTLINE

1. Subjective Narrative
2. Significant Clinical Findings
3. Treatment Challenges
4. Assessment
5. Treatment Plan and Goals
6. Therapeutic Procedures Performed
7. Outcome
8. Case Summary

DEFINITIONS OF CASE STUDY FORMAT

The subjective narrative section will present a brief summary of the patient's complaints and history. Further description will include the onset of their pain, the quality of their pain including the location, the nature of the pain, and what increases or decreases their pain. The patient's functional limitations will be noted. The patient's goals will also be presented.

The table of significant clinical findings requires the greatest clarification. This table will be based on the physical examination format presented in earlier chapters of this book. One should assume that any finding not noted was unremarkable or within normal limits. It is the physical examination that leads the practitioner to the significant clinical findings. The format of the physical examination is detailed in Box 25-3.

The presentation of the clinical and management challenges will include what restrictions were placed on treatment as well as how to compensate or accommodate for those challenges. The challenges can be varied from physical or other medical complications, cognitive limitations of the patient, socioeconomic difficulties, cultural considerations, insurance limitations, and other such challenges.

The description of the assessment is somewhat self-explanatory. However, it must be noted that all assessments are working assessments and should be updated every time the patient is seen. New information and data gathered during treatment can more clearly refine the assessment and focus the treatment plan. Often updates in the assessment will slightly or

BOX 25-3	**PHYSICAL EXAMINATION FORMAT**

1. Observation, including posture and functional use
2. Inspection, including structure and soft tissue
3. Selective tissue tension, including:
   a. Active range of motion
   b. Passive range of motion
   c. Resisted isometric movement
   d. Joint play and osteomechanics
   e. Neuromuscular tests
   f. Palpation
4. Other special tests

even dramatically alter the treatment plan. Sometimes new information is presented by the patient that they withheld or forgot to mention during your initial examination; other times additional special tests have been performed by the practitioner, and further outside tests such as a magnetic resonance imaging report or electromyographic findings also may be presented. Additionally, as treatment progresses the patient's response to treatment must be considered. An effective practitioner is like a good detective, always gathering clues and information that lead to the further clarification of the problem.

The treatment plan and goals are based on the most current significant objective findings. As the objective findings are being refined, so must the treatment plan. The plan may need to be updated as further clinical information is presented. Although what is presented in the following case studies appears stagnant in its presentation, the plans were refined during the course of treatment.

The therapeutic procedures performed will include a variety of procedures and techniques. Many of these techniques are learned in continuing education courses and may not be immediately familiar to the reader and are beyond the scope of this chapter to illustrate. This section will cover therapeutic procedures ranging from soft tissue techniques, modality applications, joint and neural or dural mobilization techniques, stabilization exercises, taping and bracing techniques, neuromuscular reeducation techniques, other exercise approaches, and more. No specific treatment style or technique is universally applied to every patient. A skilled practitioner will have many different tools in their toolbox to be used as needed. Remember, if all you have is a hammer, every patient will look like a nail. As such, this section will be broad in its representation of techniques and procedures.

Lastly, the actual therapeutic outcome for each patient will be described. This section will focus primarily on functional outcomes and the patient's reports. The outcome for some cases may not be full recovery, but rather the highest level of recovery possible within the given set of challenges.

CASE STUDIES

Mark

SUBJECTIVE

Mark is a 14-year-old boy who comes to the clinic with complaints of left knee pain. Mark plays basketball up to 15 hours a week. His knee pain has been slowly increasing during the last 4 months, but he cannot recall any specific incident that started it. He reports that he has pain at the inferior patella with deep knee bends, kneeling, and landing and taking off from jumps. The pain is sharp during movement, but can remain achy after he has stopped. He denies any locking or giving way of the knee. Currently Mark is unable to effectively push off for his jump shots or land without pain. Mark has a very busy basketball schedule, and he is preparing for the junior high championships. He would like to know how he can most quickly begin to manage his problem and still be able to play.

PAST MEDICAL HISTORY (PMH)

Mark has grown more than 2 inches in the last year; otherwise unremarkable and not taking any medications (Tables 25-1 and 25-2).

TABLE 25-1 MARK—SIGNIFICANT CLINICAL FINDINGS

	SIGNIFICANT CLINICAL FINDINGS
Observation	Slight anterior pelvic tilt with hyperextended knees in standing. Left foot pronation in standing. Left patella alta.
Inspection	Swelling and tenderness over left tibial tubercle.
Selective tissue tension	
Range of motion	Knee flexion right 130°, left 119°. Mild pain with overpressure of full flexion. Ankle dorsiflexion right 20°, left 14°.
Resisted isometrics	Pain with resisted left knee extension and squatting.
Joint play	Decreased left patellar inferior glide and medial glide.
Neuromuscular tests	Overuse of the left proximal quadriceps and substitution by the hamstring with active knee extension from 15 to 20° of knee flexion. Poor left eccentric control of quadriceps, hamstring, and gastrocnemius on landing from small jump.
Palpation	Tender at inferior patella, patellar odd facet, and tibial tubercle.
Special tests	Positive provocation tests of resisted quadriceps contraction with the knee held at 30 to 40° flexion.
Other	Poor proximal stabilization of pelvis and low back with closed kinetic chain movements of the left lower extremity.

TABLE 25-2 MARK—TREATMENT CHALLENGES

SPECIFIC TREATMENT CHALLENGE	HOW IT AFFECTS TREATMENT
Needs to continue to play up to 15 hours of basketball a week	Difficult to control inflammation at tibial tubercle.
14-year-old boy	Need to emphasize importance of compliance with exercise program and wearing neoprene sleeve. Modalities may be contraindicated secondary to age and growth plate issues.
Hard for him to find time in schedule for physical therapy appointments	Need to work with parent for optimum schedule.
Grew 2 inches in last year	Soft tissue in lower extremity may not have been able to keep up with growth of bony skeleton and hence greater soft tissue restrictions.

ASSESSMENT

Mark presents with signs and symptoms consistent with left patellofemoral dysfunction and associated Osgood-Schlatter disease. With his growth in the last year and many hours of basketball, it is likely that the adaptive shortening and extensor inefficiencies of his quadriceps are strong contributing factors. In addition, his postural habit of standing in hyperextension with the gravity line anterior to the knee, his moderate left foot pronation, and his decreased left ankle dorsiflexion on landing from jumps may be contributing biomechanical factors to increased pressure on the patella.

TREATMENT GOALS

- Bilateral symmetrical range of motion of the knees and ankles and associated peripheral joints
- Compliance with therapeutic home exercise program as prescribed
- Obtain and trial use of foot arch support and knee neoprene sleeve
- Demonstration of appropriate standing postures with neutral pelvis and knees in neutral
- Continue playing basketball up to 10 hours a week with significantly decreased or absent symptoms (may need a brief rest before returning to playing to allow for inflammation to resolve)

TREATMENT PLAN

- Normalize left patellar mobility
- Reduce inflammation at left tibial tubercle with rest and ice
- Increase left knee flexion to 130°
- Increase left ankle dorsiflexion to 20°
- Increase length of left quadriceps, iliotibial band, and gastrocnemius
- Appropriate rehabilitative exercises to correct inefficiencies of the left extensor mechanism and left hamstrings, and include core stabilization exercises for proximal control

- Trial of over-the-counter arch supports, consider possible custom orthotics
- Trial of patellar support, such as a neoprene rubber knee sleeve and McConnell taping

THERAPEUTIC PROCEDURES

Decreased inflammation using ice and rest. Increased knee and ankle range of motion using myofascial soft tissue techniques on the quadriceps and lateral leg including the iliotibial band, and the gastrocnemius and soleus complex. Performed gentle joint mobilization techniques to the left patellar femoral joint and ankle, including medial and inferior patellar glide mobilizations and dorsiflexion mobilization to the ankle mortise joint. Applied McConnell taping techniques to improve osteomechanics and tracking of the patella. Instructed patient in quadriceps and hamstring stretching, closed kinetic chain exercises for the extensor mechanism, core stabilization exercises for the trunk and pelvis, and proximal hip stabilization and ankle dorsiflexion strategies for improved eccentric control. Assisted patient in obtaining medial arch support shoe inserts and neoprene sleeve for the knee.

OUTCOME

Mark had to take 10 days off from playing basketball to allow for some resolution of the inflammation in his knee. During that time he took nonsteroidal anti-inflammatory medication as prescribed by his doctor, and he began a gentle home exercise program. He later was able to progress to a more aggressive program. Mark responded well to over-the-counter shoe inserts and his neoprene sleeve with a cutout for the patella to improve tracking. Mark reported that he found the taping to be too restrictive, and he did not feel comfortable doing it on his own. Mark also purchased more supportive shoes for basketball that provided better shock absorption as well as pronation control. He iced his knee for 15 minutes both before and after every game or practice. Mark made time in his schedule to attend physical therapy one time a week and was compliant with his home exercise program. After 6 weeks of treatment, he was playing basketball 15 hours a week and reported feeling "almost back to normal, as long as I do all the stuff that I am supposed to."

CASE SUMMARY

Mark had primarily biomechanical factors contributing to his knee pain with an acute inflammatory problem. His poor eccentric control in landing from jumps, as well as his extensor weakness, did not support the knee or patellar tracking well. His postural habits of anterior pelvic tilt, knee hyperextension, and foot pronation placed greater forces through the medial aspect of the patellar femoral joint and altered patellar femoral tracking. Partly because of his growth spurt, Mark also had a shortened quadriceps, iliotibial band, and gastrocnemius–soleus complex that affected the patellar tracking as well as range of motion of knee and ankle. By improving and normalizing the underlying biomechanical issues, Mark was able to manage his knee problems and return to playing basketball.

Elizabeth

SUBJECTIVE

Elizabeth is a 34-year-old woman who is 24 weeks pregnant with her second child. She comes to the clinic with complaints of left hip and low back pain that have been slowly increasing during the last few weeks. She describes her hip pain as a constant, deep, dull ache at the lateral aspect of her hip. She says it is much worse with standing or with anything that com-

presses it, such as lying on that side or wearing tight clothes. She has also had some radiating pain into the lateral aspect of her left leg and a little anterior thigh pain when it has been at its worst. Elizabeth reports that she notices the hip pain even more when her back is bothering her. She denies any numbness, tingling, or sense of weakness. Her back pain is also dull and achy; however, it can be sharp with certain forward bending or twisting movements. She says that ice on her hip and back is helpful, as is sitting down. She finds that it wakes her up a great deal at night and is particularly sore first thing in the morning and again at the end of the day, especially if she has been on her feet a lot. Climbing stairs is particularly painful for her at the hip and low back. Elizabeth's goal is to be able to sleep for at least 4 hours before the pain awakens her.

PHM

First pregnancy was normal and uncomplicated; baby was delivered by cesarean section (Tables 25-3 and 25-4).

ASSESSMENT

Elizabeth presents with signs and symptoms consistent with left trochanteric bursitis and associated left sacroiliac dysfunction. It is likely that she has an upslip of her left innominate that is contributing to the altered resting length of the iliotibial band, the iliopsoas, the gluteals, and the piriformis. The increased muscle tension is adding compressive forces to the trochanteric bursa. The osteomechanical dysfunction at the sacrum and L5 is also likely contributing to increased muscle tension of the surrounding musculature. As the pregnancy progresses, Elizabeth's increasing anterior tilt is also

TABLE 25-3 ELIZABETH—SIGNIFICANT CLINICAL FINDINGS

	SIGNIFICANT CLINICAL FINDINGS
Observation	Slight antalgic gait on the left, considerable anterior pelvic tilt with hyperextended knees and bilateral foot pronation.
Inspection	Left iliac landmarks high, both posterior and anterior iliac spine. Left shoulder elevated at scapula. Warmth over left greater trochanter.
Selective tissue tension	
Range of motion	Left hip internal rotation reduced with soft tissue end feel. Full passive left hip abduction painful. Lumbar spine full ROM, but painful arc with forward flexion and left side bending.
Resisted isometrics	Pain in left hip with resisted abduction, external rotation, and extension.
Joint play	Altered osteomechanics of the left L5–S1 facet and left sacral iliac joint with lumbar forward flexion; loss of sacral extension with lumbar flexion on the left. Restrictions on the left with pelvic rocking test.
Neuromuscular tests	Within normal limits
Palpation	Discrete tenderness over greater trochanter. Moderately tender over left sacroiliac joint. Tender to palpation of the left piriformis, gluteals, iliotibial band, paraspinals, iliopsoas, and quadratus lumborum. Palpation to left sacrotuberous ligament was slack compared with right.
Special tests	Positive left: Ober's test, one-legged stork test, and compression–distraction test.
Other	Difficulty stabilizing right side in standing single-leg stork test on the left.

TABLE 25-4 ELIZABETH—TREATMENT CHALLENGES

SPECIFIC TREATMENT CHALLENGE	HOW IT AFFECTS TREATMENT
Modalities and oral anti-inflammatories are contraindicated secondary to pregnancy.	Difficult to resolve local hip inflammation without ultrasound, electrical stimulation or oral anti-inflammatories.
Patient cannot lie prone on normal treatment table.	Assessment and treatment of lumbar spine and sacrum difficult.
Patient cannot exercise supine or bridge as contraindicated for her stage of pregnancy.	Find alternative ways for some therapeutic exercise.
Generalized hypermobility owing to pregnancy.	Challenging to stabilize hypermobile joints.
Patient needs to sleep on sides, primarily the left for appropriate blood flow during pregnancy.	Cannot alter sleeping postures to unload the left hip.
History of cesarean section, likely deconditioned abdominal muscles.	Cannot address abdominal strengthening effectively during pregnancy.

placing strain on the ligamentous system of the pelvis and all the way down the closed kinetic chain.

TREATMENT GOALS

- Reduce or resolve inflammation of the left trochanteric bursa
- Normalize positional faults of the boney pelvis
- Tolerate sleeping on left side for more than 3 hours
- Tolerate standing for more than 1 hour without increased pain in the left hip
- Be compliant with use of sacroiliac belt, shoe inserts, and foam sleeping pad as appropriate
- Demonstrate neutral spine postures at least 75% of the time
- Be compliant with gentle home exercise program as prescribed including self-mobilization techniques

TREATMENT PLAN

- Ice massage over trochanteric bursa (may be a candidate for a local cortisone injection to bursa if inflammation cannot be reduced within four visits)
- Soft tissue massage and myofascial release of the quadratus lumborum and surrounding left hip musculature with emphasis on the gluteals, piriformis, and iliotibial band
- Mobilization to correct positional faults of the left sacroiliac joint, innominate, and lumbar spine
- Trial of maternity sacroiliac stabilization belt
- Trial of over-the-counter shoe inserts to decrease pronation
- Trial of custom foam pad with hole cut out to release pressure off the bursa when in left sidelying
- Neuromuscular reeducation of neutral spine in pregnancy
- Instruction in home mobilization techniques for the pelvis
- Appropriate home exercise program to stretch tight hip and lumbar musculature as well as a gentle stabilization program for the low back and hips

THERAPEUTIC PROCEDURES

Performed ice massage over left trochanteric bursa to reduce inflammation in bursa. Used soft tissue, myofascial release, and strain–counterstrain techniques to left quadratus lumborum, gluteals, piriformis, quadriceps, and iliotibial band to reduce resting tone and improve fascial mobility. Mobilized L4, L5, left innominate, and sacrum to correct positional faults using primarily muscle energy techniques owing to stage of pregnancy. Performed varied manual mobilization techniques to improve osteomechanics of the facets from L4 through S1. Provided patient with information on over-the-counter orthotics, assisted patient in ordering sacroiliac stabilization belt that included a sacral stabilization pad, assisted patient in creating foam pad with cutout for relief to the trochanteric bursa. Instructed patient in neutral spine postures and provided written information about postural changes during pregnancy. Taught patient home exercise program that included abdominal bracing in sitting and standing (patient unable to be supine), modified piriformis and gluteal stretch for the hip in sidelying, quadruped lumbar range of motion and stabilization activities, and self-mobilization and self-stabilization techniques to maintain correction of left sacroiliac joint.

OUTCOME

Elizabeth responded well to therapy and was treated for eight visits. After her fourth visit, her back pain and radiating leg pain were greatly improved, but she was still awakening with hip pain after prolonged compression of the bursa. After the therapist consulted with her physician, she had a cortisone injection to the left trochanteric bursa, which resolved the inflammation and discrete trochanteric tenderness. Elizabeth found great relief with use of her sacroiliac stabilization belt, foam cut-away pad, and over-the-counter orthotics. She tolerated her home program well and enjoyed working quadruped.

By discharge Elizabeth had met all of her long-term goals and was on her way to a more comfortable pregnancy.

CASE SUMMARY

Elizabeth had many challenges to her treatment because of her pregnancy. By avoiding any modalities, using a prone pregnancy pillow, and using gentle joint mobilization techniques, Elizabeth's care was safe and effective. Elizabeth's trochanteric bursitis was likely a secondary problem related to the altered osteomechanics and positional faults of her low back and pelvis. Because of the increased ligamentous laxity during pregnancy, the increased forces on the pelvis from the growing baby, and the abdominal muscle weaknesses perhaps from the first pregnancy and cesarean section, it was challenging to stabilize Elizabeth's low back and pelvic girdle. Safely working in quadruped, she was able to increase her core stability and strength. By using orthotics and a sacroiliac stabilization belt, Elizabeth was better able to maintain a neutral spine and pelvis. Addressing the acute bursitis as well as the entire closed kinetic chain, Elizabeth had a positive therapeutic outcome.

Kathy

SUBJECTIVE

Kathy is a 44-year-old female interior designer who comes to the clinic with complaints of bilateral hand pain and tingling. Kathy began to notice her hands about 2 years ago, but has had a significant increase in her symptoms in the last 2 weeks after a weekend of heavy yard work. She describes the feeling in her hands as dull and achy, but with certain movements she feels an "electric shock" sort of pain from her wrist to her hands. When it is at its worst, Kathy reports that both arms feel achy and heavy. She also describes a sense of increased weakness in her hands, right more than left, and an increased incidence of dropping objects. After activities like writing, using scissors, blow-drying her hair, or driving more than 20 minutes, she gets pins and needles in her thumb and first two digits that will progress to numbness if she does not stop the activity. She finds herself awakening with her thumb and first two digits numb and then needing to "shake them out" to regain feeling. Kathy also complained today of increased neck pain with a sense of stiffness. Currently, Kathy has found it difficult to do many of her work activities because of the numbness and pain in her hands. She would like to be able to return to cutting, writing, and sewing-type activities as well as not be awakened by numbness.

PMH

History of C5–C6 disk injury in motor vehicle accident 5 years ago; congenital palmar keratoses (Tables 25-5 and 25-6).

ASSESSMENT

Kathy presents with signs and symptoms consistent with bilateral carpal tunnel with an overlay of postural dysfunction and possible C6 nerve root facilitation. The hypermobility of both the carpal bones and midcervical spine may be contributing factors to the irritation of the median nerve. The soft tissue restrictions in the scalenes and pectoralis minor proximally and the pronator teres and long flexors distally may also be adding to the compression of the median nerve resulting in a double crush presentation.

TABLE 25-5 KATHY—SIGNIFICANT CLINICAL FINDINGS

	SIGNIFICANT CLINICAL FINDINGS
Observation	Rounded shoulders with forward head. Protracted scapula. Very thick palmar skin secondary to keratoses.
Inspection	Slight warmth and edema at the carpal tunnel, right greater than left.
Selective tissue tension	
Range of motion	Wrist: flexion right 67°, left 74°; extension right 52°, left 64°; supination right 72°, left 76°. Neck: flexion 40°; right rotation 63°, left rotation 69°.
Resisted isometrics	Pain with resisted wrist flexion and pronation bilaterally and right neck sidebending.
Joint play	Generalized hypermobility in carpal joints bilaterally. Restricted segmental movements of C2–C3, C3–C4, and T1–T3. Excessive segmental movements at C5–C6, C6–C7, and T4–T5. Decreased mobility in scapular retraction and depression.
Neuromuscular tests	Slightly decreased sensation to light touch in median nerve dermatome, right greater than left. Grip strength using dynamometer, right 17 kg and left 20 kg.
Palpation	Tender to palpation over carpal tunnel, in belly of pronator teres and long wrist flexors bilaterally, levator scapula, upper trapezius, rhomboids, scalenes, and pectoralis minor bilaterally with right greater than left.
Special tests	Positive bilateral modified Phalen's and Tinel's signs.
Other	Positive upper limb tension test with median nerve bias bilaterally, right greater than left.

TABLE 25-6 KATHY—TREATMENT CHALLENGES

SPECIFIC TREATMENT CHALLENGE	HOW IT AFFECTS TREATMENT
Palmar keratoses	Thickening of palmar tissues makes application of modalities less effective and palpation more difficult.
Past history of cervical injury	Cervical spine dysfunction may be playing role in wrists, may need additional treatment to cervical spine.
Self-employed as interior designer	Patient is not able to easily take time off from repetitive hand activities. Job requires a lot of driving.

TREATMENT GOALS

- Reduce local inflammation at carpal tunnel
- Full range of motion of wrist and cervical spine
- Normalize soft tissue in forearms and cervical spine
- Normalize neural mobility in upper extremities
- Demonstrates appropriate posture and biomechanics at least 75% of the time
- Compliant with progressive home exercise program
- Not be awakened by hand tingling, numbness, or pain
- Tolerate 2 hours of driving or more without increased symptoms in hands
- Tolerate cutting and writing activities for 30-minute periods without increased symptoms in hands

TREATMENT PLAN

- Reduce or resolve inflammation in the carpal tunnel bilaterally with trial of ultrasound, electrical stimulation, and ice. If there are no changes after three visits, discontinue modalities.
- Education on the anatomy of wrist and carpal tunnel including activities and positions of aggravation
- Ergonomic and biomechanical information on ways to reduce compression on the carpal tunnel
- Soft tissue mobilization with emphasis on myofascial release of the forearm, scalenes, and pectoralis minor
- Mobilization of hypomobile segments of the cervical and thoracic spine
- Neural mobilization with emphasis on median nerve
- Stabilization of wrists through night bracing
- Postural education and neuromuscular reeducation to correct forward head
- Progressive home exercise program with emphasis on forearm stretching, wrist stabilization, and proximal scapular stabilization program

THERAPEUTIC PROCEDURES

Ultrasound, interferential electrical stimulation, and ice were applied to reduce inflammation. Various soft tissue techniques including manual lymph drainage to upper extremity, soft tissue massage and myofascial release to the forearm, scapular gir-dle, and cervical spine musculature, and strain–counterstrain to the pronator teres were performed. Mobilized upper cervical and upper thoracic spine using direct manual techniques as well as muscle energy techniques. Neural mobilization techniques to the upper extremity with a median nerve bias were applied. Educated and instructed in appropriate posture, biomechanics, and ergonomics, and provided written information and illustrations. Assisted patient in obtaining appropriate night splints for her wrists. Taught progressive home exercise program including range of motion activities for the cervical spine, scapula, and wrists, especially to increase wrist extension and supination. Program also emphasized inner range stabilization for the carpals, proximal stabilization for the scapulothoracic complex, and cervical spine stabilization.

OUTCOME

Kathy was able to continue her work activities throughout her care and was seen for a total of 14 visits. To control her symptoms, she did need to wear her wrist braces during the day as well as the night for a period of 4 weeks; after that she was able to use only night bracing. Modalities other than ice were discontinued after three visits, as they did not seem to change her symptoms or swelling. Kathy had some difficulty with compliance in doing her exercise program in the first few weeks of treatment, which may have contributed to the longer time in the braces. Kathy does experience intermittent tingling in her hands if she "overdoes repetitive activities" like cutting or painting for more than 3 consecutive hours. She reported that she had not realized the discomfort her neck was causing her until the symptoms were relieved. She states that she now understands the anatomy and other factors of carpal tunnel and has been able to modify both her activities and ergonomic setup at work and home.

CASE SUMMARY

Kathy's carpal tunnel may have had contributing origins in postural dysfunction, decreased scapular stability, and cervical spine hypermobility. Her increased neural tension in the median nerve pathway and the excessive tension in the pronator teres also added to compressive forces on the median nerve before it even passed through the carpal tunnel. Beyond traditional treatment for carpal tunnel, it was necessary in treating Kathy to address her cervical and thoracic hypomobilities to improve her cervical lordosis and thoracic spine extension, to correct her scapular osteomechanics, and to decrease forces on hypermobile segments, especially at C5–C7 to calm down any segmental facilitation adding to her nerve root irritation. Imagine Kathy's median nerve as a garden hose: the more kinks in the hose, the less the water can flow, until by the end there is very little water coming out. It was necessary to eliminate multiple kinks that individually were not significant, but their aggregate was.

Mary

SUBJECTIVE

Mary is a pleasant 70-year-old, obese woman who comes to the clinic with multiple areas of concern. Mary's primary complaint today is of right leg pain. She describes this pain as intense with a "pulling sensation in the tendons behind my knee." The leg pain began more than 2 weeks ago. She has used a cane to walk when it is at its worst. She has also had the sensation that her right knee was "going to give out." She denies any changes to her bowel or bladder function. She reports experiencing new problems in the right low back as well as intermittent tingling in her right foot. Her leg seems to bother her more after standing or prolonged walking. Mary also reports pain at the top of both of her feet with the left being worse than the right. The left foot hurts most sig-

nificantly on the lateral aspect on the fourth and fifth rays and metatarsal heads. She received a cortisone injection into the left foot that has brought her some relief, but not significant. Mary has difficulty making her bed, dressing, and walking any further than 100 yards. She would like to be able to return to her normal activities of daily living as well as tolerate up to 20 minutes of walking to maintain her general conditioning.

PMH

Bilateral vein legation in lower extremities; Doppler tests reveal good circulation at present. Left total knee replacement in 1998. Rare form of glaucoma treated with high doses of steroids; bone scan reveals good density. Severe osteoarthritis in feet revealed by x-ray. Children were less than 1 year apart; both by cesarean section (Tables 25-7 and 25-8).

ASSESSMENT

Patient presents signs and symptoms consistent with lumbar facet dysfunction, osteoarthritis of bilateral metatarsals, lack of core strength, and deconditioning. Mary is expected to respond well to conservative treatment of her low back, but if her symptoms change or worsen after three visits, she may need further diagnostic evaluation of her spine. With Mary's knees and feet, as well as her size, I would be concerned about the outcome of a fall. At this time the focus of her treatment will be on her back and leg, but her feet will be addressed with some gentle home exercise to maintain range of motion in

TABLE 25-7 MARY—SIGNIFICANT CLINICAL FINDINGS

	SIGNIFICANT CLINICAL FINDINGS
Observation	Antalgic gait with Trendelenburg lurch to the left, slight right lateral shift and trunk flexion, appears in distress.
Inspection	Warmth over dorsal aspects of bilateral feet with mild edema noted in legs.
Selective tissue tension	
Range of motion	Lumbar Spine: flexion 60°; extension 15°; rotation right 20°, left 30°. Hip: within normal limits. Knee: flexion right 125°, left 119°. Ankle: plantar flexion right 31°, left 29°.
Resisted isometrics	Pain with resisted lumbar extension and right rotation, ankle and tarsal dorsiflexion bilaterally, and bilateral resisted hip adduction.
Joint play	Significantly decreased passive intervertebral movements of L4 on L5, capsular restriction pattern of right L4–L5 facet joint, unable to test tarsals and metatarsals secondary to pain.
Neuromuscular tests	All deep tendon reflexes normal. Unable to accurately test sensation secondary to paresthesia from vein legation surgery. Unable to test distal strength or functional strength secondary to foot and ankle pain. Patient able reach 3 of 5 grade with abdominal testing, gluteals 4 of 5.
Palpation	Exquisitely tender over L4–L5 facet on the right. Mild tenderness over right sacroiliac joint. Moderate tenderness over dorsal aspects of bilateral feet. Pain on palpation of right piriformis, right iliotibial band, right paraspinals, bilateral gastrocnemius–soleus complex.
Special tests	Pain with combined motion of lumbar extension and right sidebending.
Other	Positive sciatic neural tension tests on the right.

TABLE 25-8 MARY—TREATMENT CHALLENGES

SPECIFIC TREATMENT CHALLENGE	HOW IT AFFECTS TREATMENT
Obesity	Palpating bony landmarks difficult, excessive forces through lower extremities and lumbar spine, low tolerance to exercise.
Decreased sensation in lower legs because of vein legation surgery	Challenging to increase standing proprioception, at greater risk for falls.
Arthritis in feet	Full weight-bearing exercise challenging.
History of total knee replacement	Limitations of kneeling, squatting, and quadruped for exercise.
Glaucoma	Variable pressures in eye make prone or quadruped positioning contraindicated.
History of two cesarean births in 3 years	Very poor abdominal strength, patient believes she is unable to strengthen her abdominals.
Unable to drive independently to therapy	Limited scheduling availability and unable to independently get to public pool.

non–weight bearing. Mary voiced that she would like to lose some weight, but feels frustrated by her inability to exercise secondary to her pain. She does not enjoy swimming. Mary's lack of trunk and abdominal strength needs to be addressed in relation to her back and feet. She has been under the impression that because of the cesarean sections, she will not be able to strengthen her abdominal muscles successfully. This issue will be gently addressed.

TREATMENT GOALS

- Achieve functional range of motion of the lumbar spine and right hip
- Normalize joint mechanics of lumbar spine especially right L4–L5 facet
- Be compliant with home exercise program as prescribed to address trunk and abdominal strength
- Participate in at least two sessions of pool therapy with emphasis on general conditioning as well as core stabilization
- Demonstrate appropriate posture and biomechanics at least 50% of the time
- Return to gentle walking up to 15 minutes daily with significantly decreased or absent symptoms
- Tolerate standing for 1 hour or more without increased leg pain

TREATMENT PLAN

- Decrease pain and inflammation in the low back and feet with ice, ultrasound, and interferential current
- Myofascial release and soft tissue mobilization of the piriformis, tensor fasciae latae, iliotibial band, lumbar paraspinals, and gastrocnemius complex
- Segmental mobilization of the lumbar spine and pelvis, with focus on L4–L5 segment
- Education and instruction in biomechanics particularly for activities of daily living, sit to stand, stairs, and lifting

- Instruction in home exercise program with focus on supine core stabilization with a flexion bias and hip strengthening in sidelying, supine, and closed kinetic chain positions as tolerated by her feet
- Neuromuscular reeducation and proprioception training for neutral spine postures, abdominal control, and lower leg balance strategies

THERAPEUTIC PROCEDURES

Performed ultrasound over right lumbar spine and bilateral dorsal aspect of feet, interferential current, and ice to reduce pain and swelling. Used soft tissue, myofascial release, and trigger point techniques to affected soft tissue to increase circulation, reduce guarding, and improve fascial mobility. Mary was able to achieve a much more upright posture with a significant decrease in her anterior pelvic tilt posture through myofascial release of her iliopsoas, anterior hips, and iliotibial band. Performed segmental mobilization of L4 on L5 with emphasis on capsular mobility of right facet using primarily direct manual techniques. Instructed patient in neutral spine postures, appropriate biomechanics for activities of daily living, stairs, sit to stand, and lifting. Taught patient home exercise program and performed in the clinic, including supine low abdominal series, bridging, hip adduction, and sidelying hip abduction activities as well as stretches for the hip rotators, lumbar paraspinals, and gastrocnemius–soleus complex. Mary's exercise program had a lumbar spine flexion emphasis to avoid irritation of the facet joints. Encouraged Mary to participate in pool exercise and provided schedules of classes in her area.

OUTCOME

Mary responded well to therapy for the first four visits with centralization of her right lower extremity pain and decreased low back pain. She also reported a significant decrease in her foot pain. However, in the next three visits Mary's range of motion and subjective complaints of her low back pain remained unchanged. Her right L4–L5 facet joint was becoming more irritated with therapy and was not displaying a capsular pattern of restriction. Mary was advised to check back with her physician, and the therapist sent a progress note requesting possible additional diagnostic testing for the lumbar spine. A magnetic resonance imaging revealed a golf ball-sized fluid-filled cyst on the anterior aspect of her right L4–L5 facet. The cyst was then aspirated under fluoroscopy, and an epidural injection was given at that level. Mary returned to therapy a week later with reports of significant improvement. She continued therapy for eight more visits. Her facet joint mechanics were restored to within normal limits, and she reported being able to tolerate up to an hour of standing without increased pain. She also tried a pool program and found it enjoyable. The therapist contacted the instructor and helped to transition Mary's exercise program to the pool.

CASE SUMMARY

Mary had many challenges to her treatment, the most significant being limitations in ways she could exercise safely. The therapist had to take care with her exercise program to avoid any positions that were contraindicated by her past medical history as well as by pain. Gentle encouragement was necessary to allow Mary to explore the option of pool therapy. Mary was able to successfully work in the pool, which allowed her greater exercise options that were safe with her contraindications. When her improvement plateaued and then began to regress, it was vital to seek additional medical consultation. Additional intervention was necessary for the treatment of Mary's low back problems. The unusual finding on the magnetic resonance imaging of the lumbar facet cyst demonstrates that practitioners need to take care to listen to the feedback from their patients and compare it with the objective findings.

Larry
SUBJECTIVE

Larry is a 36-year-old man who comes to the clinic with complaints of low back pain and left leg pain. He has been having back problems for more than 6 years, but reports that in the last year "it has gotten really bad." He rates his pain at worst at 8 of 10 and at best at 5 of 10. He reports that he has had a magnetic resonance imaging study but does not know the results yet. He is considering surgery. Larry describes his pain as sharp in his low back with radiating pain into his left knee. He also reports pain in both hips and a great deal of spasms in the back, especially after forward bending activities and Valsalva maneuvers. Larry works as a lead pastry chef, which requires a great deal of bending and stooping, and reports that he is unable to take any time off from work. He reports that he will occasionally "get stuck" when trying to rise from forward bending. He describes mild numbness and tingling in his left lateral lower leg and big toe. He also expresses a sense of weakness in the left leg, but has not had any episodes of his leg giving way or buckling. The morning is the worse time for Larry, but pain will also keep him awake at night. He is frustrated and would like to do more exercise and return to his gym, but is only able to walk at this time because of the pain.

PMH

Smoker, otherwise unremarkable (Tables 25-9 and 25-10).

ASSESSMENT

Larry presents with signs and symptoms consistent with probable lumbar disk injury and nerve root involvement. Larry discussed the plan of his treatment in physical therapy today, and

TABLE 25-9 LARRY—SIGNIFICANT CLINICAL FINDINGS

	SIGNIFICANT CLINICAL FINDINGS
Observation	Left lateral shift and decreased lumbar lordosis in standing. Significant bilateral foot pronation in standing.
Inspection	Slight swelling noted over left low back and paraspinals.
Selective tissue tension	
Range of motion	Lumbar spine: flexion limited to 75° by pain; left sidebending decreased 50 % from the right; right rotation decreased 25% from the left.
Resisted isometrics	Pain with resisted lumbar extension and left hip external rotation.
Joint play	Tenderness to grade II posterior glides of L4 and L5. Generalized hypomobility at L1–L3 and hypermobility at L4–S1. Positional fault of L4 in right rotated and flexed position.
Neuromuscular tests	Decreased sensation in left L4 dermatome, left patellar reflex 1, manual muscle testing of left tibialis anterior 4 of 5 grade.
Palpation	Tender to palpation of bilateral lumbar paraspinals, left quadratus lumborum, and left gluteals.
Special tests	Positive left straight-leg raise at 45° hip flexion and dorsiflexion.
Other	Positive sitting slump test for reproduction of pain at left low back and hip.

TABLE 25-10 LARRY—TREATMENT CHALLENGES

SPECIFIC TREATMENT CHALLENGE	HOW IT AFFECTS TREATMENT
Cannot take time away from work	Difficult to control chronic irritation because of poor body mechanics and tasks of job. Patient may aggravate symptoms and inflammation through work activities.
Insurance restrictions of 30 consecutive days of physical therapy per diagnosis	Timeline for care too short to achieve significant changes in strength and core stabilization. Challenging for patient to tolerate more demanding exercise and neuromuscular reeducation.

he expressed a desire to try physical therapy before considering surgery. He would like to explore the option of an epidural injection if appropriate in the future as well. It should be noted that his insurance plan will only pay for 30 consecutive days of treatment for this problem. This may limit his ability to progress and increase strength. It would be unfortunate if because of insurance limitations Larry felt pushed too quickly into a surgical solution before he was able to fully see the benefits of physical therapy.

TREATMENT GOALS

- Achieve functional range of motion of hips and lumbar spine, including full unrestricted ability to squat and return to neutral
- Normalize left lateral pelvic shift
- Be compliant with home exercise program with an extension bias to increase core trunk stability and endurance, including returning to his gym with a specific exercise program
- Demonstrate appropriate posture and biomechanics at work and home at least 75% of the time
- Tolerate working an 8-hour shift without increased back or leg pain
- Fall asleep easily and sleep through the night without pain

TREATMENT PLAN

- Modalities of ultrasound, interferential electrical stimulation, portable TENS unit, and ice to decrease pain and inflammation in the lumbar spine
- Myofascial release and soft tissue mobilization of the involved musculature of the low back and hips
- Segmental mobilization of the lumbar spine to correct positional fault of L4 and increase general mobility of L1–L3
- Education and instruction in home exercise program and appropriate biomechanics at work and home including McKenzie protocols
- Develop appropriate individual program at patient's gym including aerobic and strengthening components
- Neuromuscular reeducation and proprioception training for neutral spine in sitting and standing including proper foot positioning

- Trial of over-the-counter orthotics to support medial arch; if helpful, consider custom orthotics
- If no significant decrease is reported in pain level of 6 of 10 after three visits, discuss possible epidural injection with referring physician.

THERAPEUTIC PROCEDURES

Performed ultrasound over bilateral lumbar spine paraspinals, administered interferential current, and applied ice to reduce pain and swelling. After a successful trial in the clinic of the TENS unit, the patient was dispensed a unit for home and work use for a month rental period. Applied soft tissue technique to bilateral lumbar paraspinals, left quadratus lumborum, left gluteals, and left iliopsoas. Administered Jones's strain–counterstrain techniques to the left quadratus lumborum. Using the McKenzie approach, instructed patient in home exercises to correct left lateral pelvic shift. Corrected positional fault of L4 using muscle energy techniques. Increased general mobility of L1–L3 using direct mobilizations techniques as well as Mulligan's mobilization with movement techniques. Mobilized left sciatic nerve using Butler's neural gliding techniques, in addition to general dural mobilization. Instructed patient in neutral spine postures, standing lumbar extension activities to reduce pain, abdominal bracing techniques for lifting and transitional movements, and appropriate mechanics for work activities and activities of daily living. Taught patient home exercise program with emphasis on extension activities, trunk and proximal hip stabilization, and general aerobic conditioning. Also addressed weakness of left tibialis anterior with tubing exercises and functional standing exercises. Assisted patient in purchasing over-the-counter orthotics. Encouraged Larry to try to take a 10-minute break at least once every 2 hours when working and ideally ice his low back during these breaks.

OUTCOME

After the first three visits, Larry reported a centralization of his symptoms, with significantly decreased left leg pain. However, he still rated his low back pain at a 6 of 10 and a 4 of 10 with use of the TENS unit. Larry was referred back to his physician for a consultation regarding a lumbar epidural injection. The magnetic resonance imaging study did reveal a moderate lateral left disk bulge at L4–L5. Larry received an L4–L5 epidural injection and returned to therapy a week later. He responded well to the injection, and he now rated his pain as a 3 of 10 with only local low back pain. He was able to tolerate a more aggressive exercise program and demonstrate appropriate body mechanics. Because of his 30-day insurance limitation, it would likely be necessary that he would have to make his own informed decision regarding surgery in the future. Larry was presented with information regarding the current literature on the short-term and long-term outcomes of lumbar disk surgery versus exercise, physical therapy, and time. At the end of his 30 consecutive days of treatment, Larry had reached most of his treatment goals. However, he was still unable to tolerate working an 8-hour shift without increased back pain or return to his previous level of exercise at his gym. On discharge Larry was scheduled for a second epidural injection. Larry was provided a written progression of his exercise program to be carried out independently during the next 8 weeks. He was comfortable with this plan and chose to hold off on surgery for at least 6 months and reevaluate his situation at that time.

CASE SUMMARY

The most significant challenge to Larry's treatment was the 30-day limitation imposed by his insurance company. The therapist had to consider the time limitation when designing and implementing his treatment plan. It was necessary to communicate to Larry the importance of his independent compliance with the progression of his exercise program after physical therapy ended. In this case further medical intervention was necessary to help resolve the local disk inflammation and allow Larry to progress in his home exercise program.

Sally

SUBJECTIVE

Sally is a 34-year-old woman who comes to the clinic with a variety of complaints associated with fibromyalgia and chronic fatigue. During the past 2 years Sally has gone through significant life stresses including the sudden death of her mother, divorce from her husband, and the death of both grandparents. Sally is now a single mom with a 7-year-old daughter. Her primary complaints are of neck and shoulder pain, distal joint pain, headaches, pressure in her ears, stomach problems, and general fatigue. She also has intermittent low back problems. Sally is currently off work on medical leave. She is unable to tolerate more than 3 hours of any one activity because of pain and fatigue. She does not notice any pattern to her symptoms or what might aggravate them. Her stated goal today is to gain strength and endurance and focus on wellness.

PMH

A 1988 rear-ender motor vehicle accident; meningitis in 2001; recent diagnosis of depression (Tables 25-11 and 25-12).

ASSESSMENT

Sally presents with signs and symptoms consistent with fibromyalgia and associated disorders. She has considerable neck and thoracic spine segmental dysfunction as well as associated

TABLE 25-11 SALLY—SIGNIFICANT CLINICAL FINDINGS

	SIGNIFICANT CLINICAL FINDINGS
Observation	Forward head, elevated shoulders, increased thoracic kyphosis, and rounded shoulders. Patient was tearful in much of session, with an unwillingness to make eye contact.
Inspection	Patient looks generally "unwell," slumped postures, pale, and slow moving.
Selective tissue tension	
Range of motion	Cervical spine: flexion full, painful at end range; left rotation 40°, right rotation 48°; extension full, painful at end range.
Resisted isometrics	Pain with resisted cervical spine extension and head retraction.
Joint play	Hypomobility in upper cervical retraction and rotation bilaterally, T1–T3 restricted into extension; C5–C6 tender to anterior glides, right first rib tender to caudal glides, T4 tender to anterior forces with pain at costovertebral junction with caudal–anterior glides of right fourth rib.
Neuromuscular tests	All within normal limits
Palpation	Palpation to upper cervical spine, right first and fourth rib, anterior neck, and anterior chest all very tender and painful. Also tender to palpation: suboccipitals, scalenes, levator scapula, upper and middle trapezius, cervical paraspinals, strap musculature, sternocleidomastoid, pectoralis major and minor, thoracic paraspinals, and rhomboids.
Special tests	Tender to light palpation at 7 of 12 fibromyalgia points; Chapman's points positive; positive slump test for pain at thoracic T4 area and suboccipital area; thoracic rib provocation tests positive.

TABLE 25-12 SALLY—TREATMENT CHALLENGES

SPECIFIC TREATMENT CHALLENGE	HOW IT AFFECTS TREATMENT
The nature of fibromyalgia and chronic fatigue, patient has low endurance and low tolerance of a progressive exercise program.	Challenging to design exercise program to increase conditioning and core stability. Patient is also not able to tolerate more than grade I to II soft tissue techniques and joint mobilizations.
Patient presents with depression.	Depression contributes to low energy, difficulty with compliance of home exercise program, and much of the treatment session being taken up with conversation and reassurance.
Family circumstances.	As a single mother, patient has to cancel treatment often to handle needs of her child.

tender points. She displays a forward head posture that is likely aggravating her headaches and ear problems. Sally also has anterior neck and anterior trunk myofascial restrictions as well as general upper thoracic spine hypomobility that are likely contributing to her postural problems. Sally would gain from therapeutic intervention to improve her myofascial mobility, increase segmental mobility, and assist her with increasing her physical endurance and core stability through gentle exercise, as well as education in pacing herself and setting reasonable goals.

TREATMENT GOALS

- Achieve full range of motion of the neck and thoracic spine, including normalizing upper thoracic kyphotic curve
- Be compliant with a gentle home exercise program, with the goal of some regular form of exercise outside the house like yoga or a pool program
- Demonstrate appropriate head and neck posture and biomechanics
- Return to working at least 4 hours a day with modified duty
- Report one headache or less a week

TREATMENT PLAN

- Myofascial release and soft tissue mobilization of the cervical spine musculature, trunk, anterior neck, and chest
- Segmental mobilization to correct positional faults or hypomobility cervical spine and thoracic spine with an emphasis on restoring upper cervical osteomechanics, upper thoracic spine segmental extension, and rib movement
- Education and instruction in home exercise program and biomechanics; assist with trial of independent outside class such as yoga or pool program
- Neuromuscular reeducation and proprioception training for proper posture and head alignment

THERAPEUTIC PROCEDURES

Performed soft tissue techniques including gentle myofascial release, effleurage, strain–counterstrain, and manual lymph drainage to the neck, thoracic spine, and anterior chest. Mobilized the cervical spine, thoracic spine, and ribs using gentle muscle energy techniques and mobilization with movement. Applied cranial sacral techniques, trigger point release, and Chapman reflex points. Performed manual traction techniques with an emphasis on decompressing the upper cervical spine and stretching suboccipital musculature. Instructed patient in gentle core stabilization exercises including scapular retraction, abdominal series, cervical and thoracic multifidi endurance activities, and general global range of motion activities to open up the thoracic outlet and assist with scapular retraction. Also taught patient independent dural mobilization exercises including upper extremity neural glides and flexion activities of the head and cervical and thoracic spine. Assisted patient with research on yoga and pool classes in her area.

OUTCOME

Sally was able to return to modified work for 4 hours a day after 12 visits during a 3-month period. She reported having headaches less than once a week and much less intense when they did occur. Overall her neck pain reduced to a 4 of 10 at baseline. Sally began taking a therapeutic yoga class two times a week and found this most enjoyable. Sally was compliant with her home exercise program to gently increase core stability and global range of motion. Sally gained insight into the systems of perception of pain and how her emotional reactions may affect her pain. Sally was presented with a great deal of information about fibromyalgia, the importance of pacing herself, the likelihood of flares and remission, and general expectations. She also learned more about the affects of fibromyalgia on other systems of her body such as sleep and irritable bowel and bladder issues. Better understanding this connection she reported, "I feel less like I am completely falling apart . . . understanding that much of my problems are related to the fibromyalgia gives me more of a sense of control and it makes sense to me." At the suggestion of her physical therapist, Sally also talked to her primary care physician about her depression. She began taking an antidepressant as well as seeing a counselor. Sally also now sees a massage therapist monthly as part of her overall wellness plan. Sally is continuing to work toward her goal of returning to work full time.

CASE SUMMARY

The largest challenge for Sally's case was the diagnosis of fibromyalgia itself. The combination of systems that this disorder affects makes it particularly challenging to treat; however, it is that much more rewarding when goals are achieved. Gaining additional intervention for Sally's depression was quite helpful. Getting Sally to be compliant with any form of regular movement was very useful. Finding a therapeutic yoga class was not only appropriate, it was also a nice place for Sally to gain a network of support from people struggling with similar issues. Working within the constraints of her family circumstances also presented challenges to consistent care. Sally became frustrated at times with her slow progress. It was important to bring to her attention that she was capable of improvement; she was not improving because she was inconsistent with her care and her home program. Reframing her perception that she "would never get better" was a critical step in her treatment. It was necessary to address the myofascial and segmental restrictions contributing to Sally's poor posture and forward head. By reducing the compressive forces on her suboccipital region through improved cervical lordosis and trunk extension, Sally found significant improvement in her headaches and neck pain.

CONCLUSION

The most successful treatment of a patient occurs when one considers the subjective aspects of the patient as well as the objective findings. An effective practitioner will also respond creatively to other management challenges. As covered in this chapter it is important to establish a good therapeutic relationship between patient and practitioner. This involves instilling a sense of trust and confidence in the skills of the practitioner, communicating genuine respect and concern for the patient, acknowledging patients' concerns, feelings, and fears, and trying to get patients to see their own progress through functional gains. In addition, today's practitioner will be asked to respond to other obstacles to patient care ranging from the patient's psychological health, family circumstances, socioeconomic situation, language barriers, insurance limitations, and other external factors.

As presented in the case studies, a patient's objective findings and other unique complexities must be considered on an individual basis. It is important to evaluate a particular dysfunction in context and within the entire biomechanical system. Other factors such as the patient's current medical conditions, specific contraindications, age, emotional state, personal goals, motivation, and compliance may also direct your treatment. Every patient is unique even if they present with the same diagnosis; therefore a "cookie-cutter approach" to treatment is generally not as effective. The successful practitioner will evaluate all aspects of a patient's case, synthesize the subjective and objective data, arrive at a working assessment, and continually refine the assessment and treatment plan based on new information and the needs of the patient.

RECOMMENDED READING LIST

Butler D: The Sensitive Nervous System. Adelaide, Australia, Noigroup Publications, 2000

Butler D: Explain Pain. Adelaide, Australia, Noigroup Publications, 2003

Corrigan B, Maitland GD: Practical Orthopedic Medicine. London, Prentice Hall, 1976

Hall C, Brody LT: Therapeutic Exercise: Moving Toward Function. Philadelphia, Lippincott Williams & Wilkins, 1999

Hoppenfeld S: Physical Examination of the Spine and Extremities. London, Prentice Hall, 1976

Jones L: Jones Strain-Counterstrain. Boise, Jones Strain-Counterstrain, Inc, 1995

Kaltenborn F: Manual Mobilization of the Joints: vol. 1 The Extremities. Minneapolis, OPTP, 1999a

Kaltenborn F: The Spine: Basic Evaluation and Mobilization Techniques, 2nd ed. Minneapolis, OPTP, 1999b

Kisner C, Colby LA: Therapeutic Exercise: Foundations and Techniques, 3rd ed. Philadelphia, FA Davis, 1996

Kulund D: The Injured Athlete, 2nd ed. Philadelphia, JB Lippincott, 1988

Loth T, Wadsworth C: Orthopedic Review. St. Louis, Mosby, 1998

Magee D: Orthopedic Physical Assessment, 3rd ed. Philadelphia, WB Saunders, 1997

McKenzie R: Treat Your Own Back, 7th ed. Waikanae, New Zealand, Spinal Publications New Zealand Ltd, 2001a

McKenzie R: Treat Your Own Neck, 3rd ed. Waikanae, New Zealand, Spinal Publications New Zealand Ltd, 2001b

Mulligan B: Manual Therapy "Nags," "Snags," "MWMs," etc., 4th ed. Wellington, New Zealand, Hutcheson Bowman & Stewart Ltd, 1999

Myers T: Anatomy Trains: Myofascial Meridians for Manual and Movement Therapists. Edinburgh, Churchill Livingstone, 2001

Component Motions, Close-Packed Positions, Loose-Packed Positions, Rest Positions, and Capsular Patterns

Component motions are the motions in the joint complex or related joints that accompany, and are necessary for, full active range of motion. An example of a component motion is inferior glide of the head of the humerus into the lower portion of the glenoid fossa during active movement of the shoulder.

The most stable position of a joint is called the close-packed position.[6] In this position the tension on the articular capsule and ligaments is maximal, with the joint surfaces often temporarily locked together. This locking together is frequently performed by a screw-home component. The close-packed configuration usually occurs at a position that is the extreme of the most habitual position of the joint. For example, the close-packed position for the wrist joint is full extension. The other extreme position of the joint that is less commonly assumed is also very congruent and is called the *potential close-packed position*.[1,18,29,37]

In the close-packed position, the joint capsule and major ligaments are twisted, causing the joint surfaces to become firmly approximated. This is a direct result either of the conjunct rotation that necessarily accompanies a diadochal movement into this position, or of the spin that accompanies an impure swing into the position. Movement into or out of a close-packed position is never accomplished by a pure chordate swing alone. Habitual movements of daily activities usually involve motions that move a joint closer to or farther from

a close-packed position. An example would be the motions at the hip when walking.

Consider the relation between the close-packed position at a particular joint and the capsular pattern of restriction, as described by Cyriax,[6] at the same joint. The more intimate the anatomic and functional relation between the joint capsule and major supporting ligaments, the more likely it is that the close-packed position will be the most restricted position of the joint in a capsular pattern of restriction. Thus, in the hip and shoulder joints, in which the major ligaments blend with the joint capsule, movements into the close-packed position are the first to be lost with a capsular pattern of restriction. In the knee, however, in which the ligaments are easily distinguished from the capsule, flexion may be the most limited in a capsular restriction, whereas extension constitutes the close-packed position.

In any position of the joint other than the close-packed position, the articular surfaces are noncongruent, and some part of the joint capsule is lax. In these positions the joint is *loose-packed*. Often there is enough laxity in midrange to allow distraction of the joint surfaces by an externally applied force. The laxity of the capsule in the loose-packed position allows for the elements of spin, glide, and roll, which are present in most joint movements in various degrees. The *resting position* is the maximum loose-packed position and is the ideal position for evaluation and early treatment procedures used in restoring joint play. The resting position is also the position in which the joint capsule has its greatest capacity and in which the joint is under the least stress. Accessory movement must be determined (this is traditionally part of the joint mobilization examination) if the therapist is to restore the normal roll–glide action that occurs during joint movements: joint-play and component motions.

TEMPOROMANDIBULAR JOINT

Both temporomandibular joints (TMJs) are involved in every jaw movement, forming a bicondylar arrangement.

Component Motions

OPENING OF THE MOUTH

1. The head of the mandible first rotates around a horizontal axis (rolls dorsally) in relation to the disk (lower compartment).
2. This movement is then combined with gliding of the head anteriorly (and somewhat downward) in contact with the lower surface of the disk.
3. At the same time, the disk glides anteriorly (and somewhat downward) toward the articular eminence of the glenoid fossa (upper compartment). The forward gliding of the disk ceases when the fibroelastic tissue attaching to the temporal bone posteriorly has been stretched to its limits.
4. Thereafter, there is some further hinging and gliding anteriorly of the head of the mandible until it articulates with the most anterior part of the disk and the mouth is fully opened.

CLOSING OF THE MOUTH

The movements are reversed.

PROTRUSION

The disks glide anteriorly in the upper compartment (simultaneously on both sides). Both condyles glide anteriorly and slightly downward but do not rotate.

RETRACTION

The movements are reversed.

LATERAL MOVEMENTS

Anterior gliding occurs in one joint while rotation around a cranial–caudal axis occurs in the other joint. One condyle glides downward, forward, and inward, while the other condyle in the fossa rotates and glides ipsilaterally. When the jaw is moved from side to side (as in chewing), a movement involving a shuttling of the condylar disk assembly occurs in the concave parts of the fossa.

Resting Position

The mouth is slightly open. The teeth of the mandible and maxilla are not in contact but are slightly apart.

Close-Packed Position

Unlike other joints, both TMJs become nearly close-packed with full occlusion of the dental arches.[12] It remains questionable whether these joints have a truly close-packed position, as the restraining capsule and ligaments are not maximally tightened during the maximum occlusion of the dental arches.[19]

Normally there is 3 to 4 mm of movement from the position of rest to the position of centric relation.[12] According to Rocabado,[33] the TMJ has two close-packed positions: maximal retrusion, where the condyles cannot go farther back and the ligaments are tight, and the maximal anterior position of the condyles with maximal mouth opening (potential close-packed position).

Potential Close-Packed Position

This is full or maximal opening. The ligaments, in particular the temporomandibular ligament and capsular constraints of the craniomandibular articulation, seem particularly tightened during maximum opening.[17]

Capsular Pattern of Restriction

In bilateral restriction, lateral movements are most restricted; opening of the mouth and protrusion are limited; closing of the mouth is most free. In unilateral capsular restrictions, contralateral excursions are most restricted. In mouth opening, the mandible deviates toward the restricted side.

UPPER LIMB

Glenohumeral Joint

COMPONENT MOTIONS

Flexion (Elevation in Sagittal Plane)

1. At full elevation of the humerus, whether accomplished through coronal abduction or sagittal flexion, the humerus always ends up back in the plane of the scapula, as if it had been elevated through a pure swing (i.e., at an angle midway between the sagittal and coronal planes). Because sagittal flexion is an impure swing, the humerus tends to undergo a lateral conjunct rotation on its path to full elevation. If this occurred, however, the humerus would end up with the medial condyle pointed backward, rather than forward, with the capsule of the glenohumeral joint completely twisted. This essentially would involve a premature close-packing that would prevent full elevation. To avoid this, the humerus must rotate medially on its long axis during the complete arc of sagittal flexion. The rotation occurs because the anterior aspect of the joint capsule pulls tight on flexion while the posterior capsule remains relatively lax.
2. Downward (inferior) glide of the head of the humerus on the glenoid

Abduction

1. Lateral rotation of the humerus on its long axis to counter the medial conjunct rotation that tends to occur during this impure swing (see above). In this case, the posterior capsule pulls tight during abduction, effecting a lateral rotation of the humerus.
2. Inferior glide of the humeral head on the glenoid
   External rotation—Anterior glide of the head of the humerus
   Internal rotation—Posterior glide of the head of the humerus
   Horizontal adduction—Posterior glide of the humeral head
   Horizontal abduction—Anterior glide of the humeral head

RESTING POSITION

Semiabduction: 55 to 70° abduction, 30° horizontal adduction, neutral rotation

CLOSE-PACKED POSITION

Maximum abduction and external rotation are combined.

CAPSULAR PATTERN OF RESTRICTION

External rotation is most limited; abduction, quite limited; internal rotation and flexion, somewhat limited (relatively free).

Acromioclavicular Joint

COMPONENT MOTIONS

1. Allows widening and narrowing of the angle (looking from above) between the clavicle and the scapula. Narrowing occurs during protraction; widening occurs during retraction (about 10° total). This occurs about a vertical axis.
2. Allows rotation of the scapula upward, such that the inferior angle of the scapula moves away from the midline; or downward, such that it moves toward the midline. This occurs about a horizontal axis lying in the sagittal plane. Actually, very little acromioclavicular joint motion is involved in this rotation of the scapula. About 30° occurs with elevation of the clavicle at the sternoclavicular joint, but much of the remaining 30° occurs because of axial rotation of the clavicle; because the clavicle is S-shaped anteroposteriorly, an axial rotation converts the S to a superoinferior attitude, the distal end pointing more or less upward. This occurs as a result of tightening of the coracoclavicular ligaments as the scapula begins to rotate upward (the coracoid rotating downward).
3. Allows rotation of the scapula such that the inferior angle swings anteriorly and posteriorly. As the scapula moves upward and forward on the thorax, the inferior angle swings posteriorly. This occurs about an axis lying horizontally in the frontal plane and probably is accompanied by considerable length rotation at the sternoclavicular joint as well.

RESTING POSITION

Arm rests by the side in the normal physiologic position.

CLOSE-PACKED POSITION

Upward rotation of the scapula relative to the clavicle is combined with narrowing of the angle between the scapula and clavicle as seen from above. This occurs during elevation of the arm (arm abducted 90°) and during horizontal adduction (see Fig. 11-3).

CAPSULAR PATTERN

Primarily there is pain into the close-packed position, such as when horizontally adducting the arm, and limitation of full extension.

Sternoclavicular Joint

COMPONENT MOTIONS

1. Allows length rotation of the clavicle, as discussed above; about 50° total. This occurs during elevation of the arm and somewhat during protraction and retraction.
2. Allows upward and downward swing of the clavicle, such as during shoulder shrugging or elevation of the arm. This occurs about an axis passing through the costoclavicular ligament, so that with elevation the clavicular articular surface slides inferiorly on the sternum and, with depression, superiorly; about 30° total.
3. Allows forward and backward swing of the clavicle, such as with protraction and retraction. This occurs about an axis lying somewhat medial to the joint, so that the clavicular articular surface slides forward on protraction; about 45 to 60° total.

RESTING POSITION

Arm rests by the side in the normal physiologic position.

CLOSE-PACKED POSITION

Arm abducted to 90°.

CAPSULAR PATTERN

Pain occurs at the extremes of motion. To emphasize the interplay of all joints involved with shoulder movements, we will review here the components of shoulder abduction in the frontal plane, one of the more complex shoulder movements.

With the arm at the side in the resting position, the glenoid faces almost equally anteriorly and laterally. The humerus rests in the plane of the scapula, or in alignment with the glenoid, such that the medial humeral condyle points about 45° inward and backward (see Fig. 11-2).

During the first 30° or so of abduction, the effects on the scapula are variable, but during this time it becomes set or fixed against the thoracic wall in preparation for movement.

From 30° to full elevation, for every 15° of movement about 10° occurs at the glenohumeral joint and 5° at the scapulothoracic joint. The scapula must rotate upward as well as forward around the chest wall. The early part of this movement occurs as a result of elevation at the sternoclavicular joint, as well as movement at the acromioclavicular joint, such that its angle narrows (looking from above) and the scapula rotates slightly upward on the clavicle. This close-packs the acromioclavicular joint but also draws the coracoclavicular ligaments tight because of the downward movement of the coracoid relative to the clavicle. Thus, between, say, 90 and 120°, motion stops at the acromioclavicular joint. Further elevation from scapular rotation is possible only because the coracoclavicular ligaments pull the clavicle into long-axis rotation.

The S-shape of the clavicle becomes oriented superoinferiorly such that the distal end of the clavicle points somewhat upward, allowing the acromioclavicular joint to maintain apposition as the scapula continues to rotate upward. This clavicular rotation occurs, of course, at the sternoclavicular joint.

Because the convex humeral head is moving in relation to the concave glenoid cavity to allow upward swing of the humerus, it must glide inferiorly in the glenoid. The humerus must move out of the plane of the scapula to be elevated in the frontal plane; it must undergo an impure swing. As with any impure swing, a conjunct rotation occurs, in this case a medial rotation. However, the posterior and inferior capsular fibers cannot allow this amount of rotation, so for the humerus to come back into the plane of the scapula on full elevation, it must rotate laterally on its long axis. This lateral rotation is necessary for clearance of the greater tuberosity under the acromial arch.

The clinically important considerations are that elevation is impossible without appropriate sternoclavicular and acromioclavicular movements, especially rotation of the clavicle on its long axis, without inferior glide of the humeral head, and without lateral rotation of the humerus on its long axis.

Furthermore, we must consider the motions occurring in the thoracic and lower cervical spines on shoulder movement. For example, bilateral elevation of the arms requires considerable thoracic extension; the person with a significant thoracic kyphosis will not be able to perform this movement throughout the full range. On unilateral elevation, the upper thoracic spine must sidebend toward, and the lower thoracic spine must sidebend away from, the side of motion.

Elbow

COMPONENT MOTIONS

Extension
1. Superior glide of ulna on trochlea
2. Pronation of ulna relative to humerus
3. Abduction of ulna relative to humerus
4. Distal movement of radius on ulna
5. Pronation (inward rotation) of radius relative to humerus

Flexion
1. Inferior glide of ulna on trochlea
2. Supination of ulna relative to humerus
3. Adduction of ulna relative to humerus
4. Proximal movement of radius on ulna
5. Supination (outward rotation) of radius on humerus

HUMEROULNAR JOINT

Resting Position. Semiflexion: 70° flexion, 10° supination
Close-Packed Position. Full extension and supination
Capsular Pattern. More limitation of flexion than extension. Pronation and supination are limited only if condition is severe.

HUMERORADIAL JOINT

Resting Position. Full extension and supination
Close-Packed Position. 90° flexion, 5° supination
Capsular Pattern. Flexion and extension are most restricted; supination and pronation are limited only if condition is severe.

Forearm

COMPONENT MOTIONS

Pronation–Supination
Proximal Radioulnar Joint and Radiohumeral Joint. This movement is essentially one of pure spin of the head of the radius on the capitellum and, therefore, one of roll and slide of the radius in the radial notch of the ulna and annular ligament.

Distal Radioulnar Joint. Here the radius is said to rotate around the head of the ulna, being largely a sliding movement. However, functionally the ulna also tends to move backward and laterally during pronation and forward and medially during supination. Therefore, component movements during pronation are as follows:

1. Palmar glide of radius on ulna
2. Inward rotation of radius on ulna (looking palmarly)
3. Dorsal glide of ulna on radius
4. Outward rotation of ulna on radius (looking palmarly)
5. Abduction of ulna on humerus

The reverse would naturally occur on supination.

Proximal Radioulnar Joint
Resting Position. 70° flexion, 35° supination
Close-Packed Position. Supination, full extension
Capsular Pattern. Pronation = supination
Distal Radioulnar Joint
Resting Position. 10° supination, 90° flexion
Close-Packed Position. 5° supination
Capsular Pattern. Involvement of the distal radioulnar joint produces little limitation of movement, but there is pain at the extremes of pronation and supination. Pronation = supination.

Wrist

COMPONENT MOTIONS

Radiocarpal Joint
Palmar Flexion
1. Dorsal movement of proximal carpals (scaphoid and lunate) on radius and disk
2. Distraction of radiocarpal joint

Dorsiflexion
1. Palmar movement of proximal carpals on radius (the scaphoid also spins—supinates—on the radius at full wrist dorsiflexion)
2. Approximation of scaphoid and lunate to radius and disk

Radial Deviation
1. Approximation of scaphoid to radius
2. Ulnar slide of proximal carpals on radius (this movement is quite limited and is somewhat increased by the tendency for the scaphoid to extend [slide palmarly and supinate] on the radius)

Ulnar Deviation
1. Distraction of scaphoid from radius
2. Radial slide of proximal carpals on radius

Ulnomeniscotriquetral Joint. The ulnomeniscotriquetral joint is primarily involved with pronation and supination of the forearm. During pronation and supination, the disk moves with the radius and carpals and must therefore sweep around the distal end of the ulna. During flexion and extension, the disk stays with the radius and ulna and movement occurs between the disk and the carpals. In this situation the disk acts as an ulnar extension of the distal radial joint surface to become, functionally, part of the radiocarpal joint.

During wrist radial deviation, there is considerable distraction of the triquetrum and pisiform from the ulna, with approximation on ulnar deviation.

Radiocarpal and Ulnomeniscotriquetral Joints
Resting Position. Neutral with slight ulnar deviation
Close-Packed Position. Full extension
Potential Close-Packed Position[1,27,37]**.** Full flexion
Capsular Pattern. Limitation is equal in all directions.
Midcarpal Joint
Component Motions
Palmar Flexion
1. Dorsal slide of hamate and capitate on triquetrum and lunate
2. Palmar slide of trapezoid on scaphoid

Dorsiflexion. From full flexion to neutral, the reverse of the above occurs. At neutral, the hamate, capitate, and trapezoid become close-packed on the scaphoid, and these four bones tend to move together in a palmar slide and supinatory spin on the radius, lunate, and triquetrum. The scaphoid acts as a proximal carpal from neutral into palmar flexion and as a distal carpal from neutral into full dorsiflexion. Also note the supination and radial deviation that tend to occur on extreme dorsiflexion of the wrist.

Radial Deviation. There is some ulnar slide of the hamate and capitate on the triquetrum and lunate, with considerable distraction of the base of the hamate from the lunate. The trapezoid slides radially on the scaphoid.

Ulnar Deviation. This is the reverse of radial deviation. The entire carpus might be divided into four functional units: (1) hamate, capitate, and trapezoid, always acting as distal carpals; (2) scaphoid, acting as proximal carpal into flexion and distal carpal into extension; (3) triquetrum and lunate, always acting as proximal carpals; and (4) trapezium, acting primarily in its articulation with the first metacarpal of the thumb, playing little part in movements at the wrist.

Resting Position. Semiflexion: near neutral with slight ulnar deviation
Close-Packed Position. Of the wrist as a whole, extension (dorsiflexion) with radial deviation
Capsular Pattern. Equal limitation of palmar flexion and dorsiflexion

Hand

"INTERMETACARPAL JOINTS"

Although these are not true synovial joints, movement does occur between the heads of the metacarpals on grasp and release.

Grasp. The metacarpals form an arch through the following movements:

1. Palmar movement of second relative to third, fourth relative to third, and fifth relative to fourth metacarpal head
2. Supination of fourth and fifth metacarpals; perhaps slight pronation of the second

Release. The arch is flattened through the reverse of the above movements.

COMPONENT MOTIONS

Metacarpophalangeal Joints
Flexion
1. Palmar glide of base of phalanx on head of metacarpal
2. Supination of phalanx on metacarpal, especially with grasp or pinch
3. Ulnar deviation of phalanx on metacarpal, especially with grasp or pinch
4. Approximation of phalanx and metacarpal
   Extension. Reverse of flexion
   Radial Deviation. Radial slide of base of phalanx on head of metacarpal
   Ulnar Deviation. Ulnar slide of base of phalanx on head of metacarpal

COMPONENT MOTIONS

Interphalangeal Joints
Flexion
1. Palmar glide of base of more distal phalanx on head of more proximal phalanx
2. Distraction of distal phalanx on proximal phalanx

3. Supination of distal phalanx on more proximal phalanx (more at distal interphalangeal than proximal interphalangeal joint)
4. Radial deviation of distal phalanx on more proximal phalanx
   Extension. Reverse of flexion

COMPONENT MOTIONS

Trapeziometacarpal Joint. This is a sellar joint, with the trapezium concave in the plane of the palm and convex perpendicularly.
Extension. With radial deviation, there is ulnar slide of the base of the first metacarpal on the trapezium. A slight amount of lateral rotation (supination) occurs.
Flexion. Opposite of extension
Abduction. With motion away from the plane of the palm, there is palmar slide of the base of the first metacarpal.
Adduction. Dorsal slide of the base of the metacarpal
Opposition. This is a combined movement with considerable conjunct rotation as a consequence of the impure swing. It is easily visible by the rather marked medial rotation that occurs, allowing the thumb pad to oppose the pads of the fingers. It is typical for relatively more conjunct rotation to occur at a sellar joint such as this or at the interphalangeal joints or humeroulnar joint than at ovoid joints.

RESTING POSITION

1. First carpometacarpal: Neutral position
2. Carpometacarpal (2–5): Midway between flexion and extension, with slight ulnar deviation
3. Metacarpophalangeal (2–5): Semiflexion and slight ulnar deviation
4. Metacarpophalangeal (1): Semiflexion
5. Proximal interphalangeal (1–5): 10° flexion
6. Distal interphalangeal (1–5): 30° flexion

CLOSE-PACKED POSITION

1. Most intercarpal joints: Full extension
2. Trapeziometacarpal: Full opposition
3. Metacarpophalangeal (2–5): Full flexion
4. Metacarpophalangeal (1): Full extension
5. Interphalangeal joints: Full extension

CAPSULAR PATTERNS

1. Trapeziometacarpal joint: Abduction and extension limited, flexion free
2. Carpometacarpal (2–5): Equal in all directions
3. Metacarpophalangeal joint: More restricted in flexion than extension
4. Interphalangeal joints: Flexion greater than extension

LOWER LIMB

Sacroiliac and Pubic Symphysis[8]

RESTING POSITION

Not described

CLOSE-PACKED POSITION

Not described

CAPSULAR PATTERNS

For both joints, pain when joints are stressed

Hip

COMPONENT MOTIONS

Flexion. Posterior and inferior glide of femoral head in acetabulum
Abduction. Inferior glide of femoral head in acetabulum
External Rotation. Anterior glide of femoral head
Internal Rotation. Posterior glide of femoral head

RESTING POSITION

The hip is flexed to about 30°, abducted to about 30°, and slightly externally rotated.[14]

CLOSE-PACKED POSITION

Ligamentous: Internal rotation with extension with abduction

POTENTIAL CLOSE-PACKED POSITION

Bony: The hip is flexed to about 90°, abducted and externally rotated slightly.

CAPSULAR PATTERN

Internal rotation and abduction are most restricted; flexion and extension are restricted; external rotation is relatively free.

Knee

COMPONENT MOTIONS

Flexion
1. Medial rotation of tibia on femur during first 15 to 20° flexion from full extension
2. Posterior glide of tibia on femur
3. Inferior movement of patella
4. Inferior movement of fibula
   Extension. Reverse of flexion
   Analysis of Knee Motion. The knee primarily moves about a single axis that lies horizontally in the frontal plane. If the tibia moves on a stationary femur, roll and slide occur in the same direction. If the femur moves on a fixed tibia, roll and slide occur in opposite directions. Toward the last 10 to 20° extension, almost a pure roll occurs, the rolling phase being somewhat longer on the lateral side. Moving into flexion, the rolling motion between the joint surfaces gradually becomes more and more a sliding motion. Thus, the articular contact point on the femur gradually moves backward (while moving into flexion); the articular contact point on the tibia moves backward during the first phase of flexion, then gradually narrows to a point (in the case of the femur moving on the tibia).

A length rotation also occurs between the femur and tibia during flexion and extension at this joint. This rotation is a necessary part of normal joint kinematics and may be lost in certain pathologic conditions, such as a torn meniscus or adhered capsule. Considering the case of the femur moving on the tibia during the last, say, 30° extension, the femur must rotate inward for close-packing and full extension to occur. There are many explanations for this phenomenon. Most include the fact that because the lateral femoral condyle is smaller, it reaches its close-packed congruent position in extension before the medial condyle does. For the medial condyle to continue movement, it must slide backward around an axis passing somewhere through the lateral femoral condyle. The resultant rotation of the lateral condyle forces the anterior segment of the lateral meniscus forward over the convex lateral tibia condyle such that the lateral femoral condyle is no longer congruent and may continue into somewhat more extension. Of course, this all happens simultaneously and continues until the knee becomes locked in its close-packed position of full extension (about 5° hyperextension). In this position, the cruciate ligaments are pulled tight and twisted so as to prevent internal rotation of the tibia on the femur. The collateral ligaments also become twisted relative to each other (the medial ligament passes downward and forward, the lateral ligament passes downward and backward) so as to prevent outward rotation of the tibia on the femur. Both sets of ligaments prevent further extension, with help from the soft tissues posteriorly.

RESTING POSITION

About 25° knee flexion[15]

CLOSE-PACKED POSITION

Full extension with lateral rotation

CAPSULAR PATTERN

Flexion is most restricted; extension is somewhat restricted.

Proximal Tibiofibular Joint

RESTING POSITION

25° knee flexion, 10° plantar flexion[8]

CLOSE-PACKED POSITION

Not described

CAPSULAR PATTERN

Pain when joint stressed

Distal Tibiofibular Joint

RESTING POSITION

10° plantar flexion, 5° inversion[8]

CLOSE-PACKED POSITION

None; not a synovial joint

CAPSULAR PATTERN OF RESTRICTION

None; not a synovial joint

Talocrural

COMPONENT MOTIONS

Dorsiflexion. Backward glide of talus on tibia; spreading of distal tibiofibular joint
Plantar Flexion. Reverse of dorsiflexion

RESTING POSITION

The foot is in about 10° plantar flexion and midway between maximal inversion and eversion.[14]

CLOSE-PACKED POSITION

Full dorsiflexion

CAPSULAR PATTERN

Dorsiflexion and plantar flexion are both limited, plantar flexion slightly more so unless the heel cord is tight.

Subtalar Joint

COMPONENT MOTIONS

The subtalar joint is essentially bicondylar. The posterior facet of the talus on the calcaneus is a concave-on-convex surface; the combined anterior and medial facet forms a convex-on-concave joint. On eversion of the calcaneus on the talus, the posterior joint surface of the calcaneus must glide medially, while the anterior and medial facets must glide laterally.

RESTING POSITION

The foot is midway between maximal inversion and eversion with 10° plantar flexion.

CLOSE-PACKED POSITION

Full inversion

CAPSULAR PATTERN

Inversion (varus) is very restricted; eversion (valgus) is free.

Midtarsal Joints: Talonavicular and Calcaneocuboid

RESTING POSITION

10° plantar flexion, midway between supination and pronation

CLOSE-PACKED POSITION

Full supination

CAPSULAR PATTERN

Supination greater than pronation (limited dorsiflexion, plantar flexion, adduction, and medial rotation)

Tarsometatarsal

RESTING POSITION

Midway between supination and pronation

CLOSE-PACKED POSITION

Full supination

CAPSULAR PATTERN

Not described

Metatarsophalangeal

RESTING POSITION

Neutral (extension 10°)

CLOSE-PACKED POSITION

Full extension

CAPSULAR PATTERN

For the first metatarsophalangeal joint, extension is greater than flexion; for metatarsophalangeal joints two through five, variable, tends toward extension greater than flexion.

Interphalangeal Joints

RESTING POSITION

Slight flexion

CLOSE-PACKED POSITION

Full extension

CAPSULAR PATTERN

Tends toward extension restrictions

Orientation of Joint Axes

In the embryo the lower limb started out abducted and externally rotated so that the sole of the foot faced forward. During development, the leg must rotate medially and adduct. As a result, the femoral condyles are rotated inward (about 10° in the adult) in relation to the neck of the femur, and the shaft of the femur is adducted (forming an angle of about 125° in the adult) with respect to the femoral neck. The shaft of the tibia is rotated about 25° outwardly so the axis of the ankle mortise is 25° outwardly rotated, relative to the knee. The axis of the subtalar joint runs about 20° from back and out to front and in.

SPINE

In three-dimensional space, the spine has six components (degrees of freedom) of the vertebral segments.[38] A vertebral body can move in six different ways (Fig. A-1):

1. Forward and backward in the sagittal plane (anterior and posterior translation)
2. Forward and backward tilting on a frontal axis (i.e., flexion and extension)
3. Laterally, in the frontal plane by a slight translation or gliding motion (i.e., lateral translation)
4. Lateral tilting or rotation around a sagittal axis (movement in the frontal plane) or sidebending
5. Rotation in the horizontal plane, around a vertical axis
6. Compression or distraction in the longitudinal axis of the spine

A vertebra may rotate or translate along any of these axes or move in various combinations of these motions (longitudinal, vertical, and sagittal). Pure movement in any of these three principal planes very seldom occurs. The facet joints act to guide and limit these motions; the plane of the facet joints determines the direction and amount of motion at each segment. The torsional stiffness of the spine is largely determined by the design of the facet joints.

Cervical Spine

LOWER CERVICAL SPINE (C2–T2)

The only pure motions that exist in the cervical spine from C2 through C7 are that of flexion and extension in the sagittal plane, because lateral flexion and rotation are combined motions. The site of maximum motion in flexion and extension occurs between C4 and C6. In the combined movements of lateral flexion and rotation, the spinous processes of the vertebral bodies move toward the convexity of the curve, or opposite to rotation of the vertebral body. The direction of physiologic rotation combined with lateral flexion appears to be the same regardless of whether the cervical spine is in flexion or extension. When we laterally bend to one side, we automatically get some physiologic rotation to that side; when we rotate to one side, we automatically get some lateral flexion to the same side. According to Brown,[5] there are two degrees of coupled axial rotation for every three degrees of lateral bending. Between C2 and C7 there is a gradual cephalocaudal decrease in the amount of axial rotation that is associated.

Although movement rapidly diminishes from above downward, lateral flexion is accompanied by rotation to the same side at the cervicothoracic region (C6–T3).

Resting Position. Slight forward flexion
Close-Packed Position. Full backward bending
Capsular Pattern. Lateral flexion and rotation are equally limited with greater limitation than extension.

OCCIPITAL–ATLANTOAXIAL COMPLEX (OCCIPUT–C1–C2)

The atlantooccipital joint permits primarily a nodding motion of the head (i.e., flexion and extension in the sagittal plane around a coronal axis).[2,19] Although there is dispute as to whether any rotation occurs between the occiput and the atlas, a small amount of rotation may be felt between the mastoid

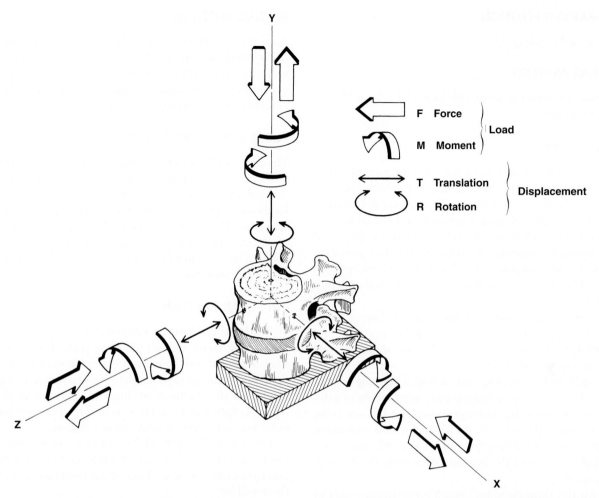

FIG. A-1. Scheme to illustrate the six degrees of freedom of vertebral segments. (Reprinted with permission from White AA, Panjabi MM: Clinical Biomechanics of the Spine, 2nd ed. Philadelphia, JB Lippincott, 1990:132)

process and the transverse process on passive testing. During lateral flexion, the occiput moves in a direction opposite to that in which the head is laterally flexed.[4]

Motion at the atlantoaxial joint includes flexion, extension, lateral flexion, and rotation. About 50% of the total rotation of the cervical region occurs at the median atlantoaxial joint before rotation in the rest of cervical spine. When the atlas pivots around the dens at the median atlantoaxial joint, the skull and atlas move as one unit. The lateral atlantoaxial joint serves to guide the rotation, which is about 45°.

Resting Position. Midway between flexion and extension
Close-Packed Position. Not described
Capsular Pattern. Atlantooccipital joint: extension and sidebending, equally restricted; atlantoaxial joint: restriction with rotation[16]

Thoracic Spine

Motion in the upper thoracic spine most likely mimics the cervical spine, with sidebending and rotation coupled to the same side.[15,36,38] Motion in the midthoracic spine is variable

and inconsistent among individuals.[15,38] Lee[21,22] has proposed that at the T3–T10 levels, the coupling depends on which of the two coupled motions initiates the movement (rotation or sidebending). She proposes that if rotation initiates the motion (rotexion) then ipsilateral sidebending is produced, but if sidebending initiates the motion (laxexion) then the sidebending produces a contralateral rotation.

In the lower thoracic spine (as in the lumbar spine) sidebending is accompanied by rotation to the same side only in flexion.[15] In the neutral and extended position, sidebending is accompanied by rotation to the opposite side.[15]

Vertebral rotation in the thoracic spine produces associated movement of the corresponding ribs. The rib on the side to which the vertebra is rotated moves in a dorsal direction, and the rib on the opposite side to which the vertebra is rotated moves in a ventral direction.[8] If a positional fault of the thoracic spine is detected, an associated positional fault of the ribs should also be investigated.

RESTING POSITION

Not described

CLOSE-PACKED POSITION

Full backward bending

CAPSULAR PATTERN

Side flexion and rotation are equally limited; backward bending is quite limited.

Lumbar Spine

The lumbar region is the pivot point for most general movements of the trunk, with movements of the lower lumbar spine being the freest. The large lumbar intervertebral disks potentially allow free flexion, extension, and lateral flexion. However, these motions are limited in the lumbar spine, and the direction of the movement is controlled by the orientation of the facet joints. Because of the shape of the facets, rotation in the lumbar spine is minimal and is accomplished only by a shearing force.

The lumbar region shows certain cross-coupling of spinal motions. Two types of motion may occur at the same time, and frequently three motions simultaneously occur during normal physiologic movements.[9,10,14,23,33]

Forward bending (flexion) and backward bending (extension) may be considered relatively pure movements to a degree. Some coupling has been proposed but has not been clearly delineated.[20,31,34,36,38] Both flexion and extension reduce the range of sidebending and rotation. Flexion sometimes slightly reverses the lumbar curve from the L3 segment upward.

As with the thoracic spine, much controversy exists in the literature as to the nature of coupling. Because of facet joint orientation, relatively less sidebending and rotation occur at the lower lumbar segments than at the upper lumbar joints.[32,38] In the three upper segments (as in the lower thoracic spine), sidebending and rotation to the opposite side are thought to be coupled weakly.[20,31,32,38] The L4–L5, a transitional segment, appears to exhibit inconsistent behavior but is thought to result in sidebending and rotation to the same side.[32]

Stoddard[35] stated that the direction of axial rotation varies depending on whether the lateral flexion was performed with the lumbar spine in flexion or extension. He suggests that the axial rotation is to the same side when lateral flexion is performed in flexion and to the opposite side when lateral flexion is performed in extension. Fryette[11] stated that axial rotation occurs to the same side if the segments are in full flexion or extension with the facets engaged; in neutral, without locking of the facets (erect standing), rotation is to the opposite side as sidebending. According to Edwards,[9] the direction of axial rotation is in the opposite direction to which the lumbar spine is laterally flexed, regardless of whether the spine is in flexion or extension. Although these combined movement tendencies require further investigation, they offer a useful objective examination tool.

RESTING POSITION

According to MacConaill,[26] flexed spinal joints are loose-packed and movement is limited by soft tissue contact. The anti–close-packed position is extreme flexion with minimal convexity of the lumbar portion of the column and minimal kinking of the lumbosacral junction.

CLOSE-PACKED POSITION

The close-packed position is that of full extension. In this position there is maximum forward convexity of the lumbar and cervical portions of the column and maximum kinking of the lumbosacral junction. At the thoracolumbar junction region, a mortise effect is produced on full extension by engagement of the articular facets. This is one of the few articular mechanisms in the body in which a practically solid lock occurs at the extreme of movement.[7]

CAPSULAR PATTERN

Bilateral Pattern of Restriction. As in many synovial joints, movements toward the close-packed position are the most restricted and the earliest restricted in cases of capsular tightness. Thus, the capsular patterns of restriction in bilateral facet joint involvement are marked. There is marked and equal limitation of lateral flexion and rotation and limitation of flexion and extension (extension > flexion).

Unilateral Pattern of Restriction. In general, motion loss is most noticeable in sidebending opposite to and in rotation to the involved side. Thus, if the right facet is restricted, there will be:

1. Considerable limitation of sidebending left and rotation to the right
2. Moderate restriction of forward bending (swings to the right)
3. Mild to slight restriction of sidebending right and rotation to the left

Spinal Motion Characteristics and Nomenclatures for Vertebral Dysfunction

Osteopathic evaluation and discussion of spinal motions builds on the early work of Lovett[24,25] and Fryette.[11] Although referred to as "laws," these statements are better referred to as concepts as they have undergone review and modification over time. However, the concepts serve as useful guidelines in evaluation and treatment of spinal dysfunction. Spinal sidebending and rotation were found to be coupled motions. This has been confirm by Oxland et al.[30] and Panjabi et al.,[31] who determined that that abnormal patterns of coupled motion are associated with patients with low back pain. Fryette's laws of spinal motions and type I and type II dysfunctions are summarized in Boxes A-1 and A-2.

Law 1 describes the coupling for the lower thoracic (T11–T12) and lumbar spine. Dysfunctions that occur in the neu-

BOX A-1 | **FRYETTE'S LAWS OF SPINAL MOTION**

- Law 1: When the spine is in neutral (facets are idling), sidebending to one side is accompanied by rotation to the other side (contralateral coupling).
- Law 2: When the spine is fully extended or flexed, sidebending to one side is accompanied by rotation to the same side (ipsilateral coupling).
- Law 3: When motion is introduced into a segment in one plane, motion in all other planes is reduced.

BOX A-2 | **TYPES OF SPINAL DYSFUNCTION**

Dysfunctions are named for positional findings, not for movement restrictions.
Type I dysfunction: Neutral group dysfunction
- Three or more vertebral segments
- Principle restriction is sidebending
- Found above or below a type II dysfunction
- Adaptive or accommodating
- Type I neutral, sidebend, rotated are contralateral (abbreviated, NS left or right).
Type II dysfunction: Nonneutral dysfunction
- Single vertebral segment
- Usually traumatic
- Includes a flexion or extension component
- Type II flexed, rotated, sidebend dysfunction is apparent in extension motion (abbreviated, FRS left or right).
- Type II extended, rotated, sidebend dysfunction is apparent in flexion motion (abbreviated, ERS left or right).
- Rotation and sidebending are ipsilateral.

(Data from Bourdillion et al.,[3] Greenman,[13] and Mitchell et al.[28])

tral range are termed, by osteopaths, *type I dysfunctions*. The cervical spine is not included in this law, as the zygapophysial joints of this region are always engaged.

Recent research confirms most of Fryette's work but suggests that law 2 may not be true for lumbar extension. Lumbar extension may in fact revert back to law 1: in normal physiologic motion there is a coupled contralateral sidebending and rotation.[3]

Dysfunction occurring in flexion or extension ranges is described, by osteopaths, as *type II dysfunction*. This law describes the coupling that occurs in C2–T3 areas of the spine.

Although both type I and type II dysfunctions can occur in the thoracic and lumbar regions, in the cervical spine the

picture is not the same. In the typical cervical joints there is only type II motion, and therefore all dysfunctions are of the type II, nonneutral variety. At the atlantoaxial joint the dysfunction is rotation only and at the atlantooccipital joint there is a small amount of rotation in the opposite direction to sidebending.

The osteopathic model names a segmental dysfunction by its position. If while palpating forward bending of L4 on L5, the right transverse process is more prominent or posterior, the positional diagnosis is ERS right L4–L5 (extended, rotated, and sidebending right). The motion restriction is into flexion, rotation, and sidebending left. For a more complete discussion, the reader is referred to Bourdillion et al.,[3] Mitchell et al.,[28] and Lee.[21,22]

It is important to remember during the structural evaluation that asymmetries, even on a segmental level, may be caused by any of the following: articular dysfunction, soft tissue restriction, spasm, or asymmetric neuromuscular dysfunction.

REFERENCES

1. Barnett C, Davies D, MacConaill MA: Synovial Joints—Their Structures and Mechanics. Springfield, IL, Charles C Thomas, 1961
2. Basmajian BE: Primary Anatomy, 7th ed. Baltimore, Williams & Wilkins, 1976
3. Bourdillion JF, Day EA, Boothout MR: Spinal Manipulations, 5th ed. Anatomy and Biomechanics. Oxford, Butterworth-Heinemann, 1992
4. Braakman R, Penning L: Injuries of the Cervical Spine. Amsterdam, Excerpta Medica, 1971
5. Brown L: An introduction to the treatment and examination of the spine by combined movements. Physiotherapy 77:347–353, 1988
6. Cyriax J: Textbook of Orthopedic Medicine, vol. 1: Diagnosis of Soft-Tissue Lesions, 5th ed. Baltimore, Williams & Wilkins, 1969
7. Davis PR: The thoracolumbar mortise joint. J Anat 89:370–377, 1955
8. Edmonds S: Manipulation and Mobilization: Extremity and Spinal Techniques. St. Louis, Mosby, 1993
9. Edwards BC: Clinical assessment: The use of combined movements in assessment and treatment. In: Twomey LT, Taylor JR, eds: Physical Therapy of the Low Back. New York, Churchill Livingstone, 1987
10. Farfan HF: Muscular mechanisms of the lumbar spine and the positions of power and efficiency. Orthop Clin North Am 6:135–145, 1975
11. Fryette HH: The Principles of Osteopathic Technique. Carmel, CA, Academy of Applied Osteopathy, 1954
12. Graber TM: Overbite: The dentist's challenge. J Am Dent Assoc 79:1135–1139, 1969
13. Greenman PE: Principles of Manual Medicine, 3rd ed. Philadelphia, Lippincott Williams & Wilkins, 2003
14. Gregerson GC, Lucas DB: An in vivo study of the axial rotation of the human thoracolumbar spine. J Bone Joint Surg Am 49:247–262, 1967
15. Grieve GP: Vertebral movement. In: Grieve GP, ed: Mobilisation of the Spine, A Primary Handbook of Clinical Method, 5th ed. Edinburgh, Churchill Livingstone, 1991:9–19
16. Hartley A: Practical Joint Assessment: Upper Quarter, 2nd ed. St Louis, Mosby, 1995
17. Hesse JR, Hansson JR: Factors influencing joint mobility in general and in particular respect of craniomandibular articulation: A literature review. J Craniomandibular Disord 2:19–28, 1988
18. Kaltenborn F: Manual Therapy for the Extremity Joints. Oslo, Olaf Norlis Bokhandel, 1986
19. Kent BA: Anatomy of the trunk: A review, part I. Phys Ther 54:722–744, 1976
20. Kulak RF, Schultz AB, Belytschko T, et al: Biomechanical characteristics of vertebral motion segments and intervertebral discs. Orthop Clin North Am 6:121–133, 1975
21. Lee D: Manual Therapy for the Thorax: A Biomechanical Approach. Delta, BC, Canada, DOPC, 1994
22. Lee D: The Thoracic: An Integrated Approach, 2nd ed. White Rock, BC, Canada, Lee Physiotherapist Corporation, 2003
23. Loebl WY: Regional rotation of the lumbar spine. Rheumatol Rehabil 12:223–231, 1973
24. Lovett RW: The mechanics of lateral curvature of the spine. Boston MSJ; 142:622–627, 1902a

25. Lovett RW: The study of the mechanics of the spine. AM J Anat 2:457–462, 1902b

26. MacConaill MA: Joint movement. Physiotherapy 50:359–367, 1964

27. MacConaill MA, Basmajian JV: Muscles and Movements: A Basis for Human Kinesiology, 2nd ed. Hunting, NY, RE Krieger Publisher, 1977

28. Mitchell FL, Moran SP, Pruzzo NA: An Evaluation and Treatment Manual of Osteopathic Muscle Energy Procedures. Valley Park, MO, Mitchell, Moran, and Pruzzo, 1979

29. Osborn JW: The disc of the human temporomandibular joint: Design, function and dysfunction. J Oral Rehabil 12:279–293, 1985

30. Oxland TR, Crisco JJ, Panjabi MM, et al: The effect of injury on rotational coupling at the lumbosacral junction: A biomechanical investigation. Spine 17:17–31, 1992

31. Panjabi M, Yamamoto I, Oxland T, et al: How does posture affect coupling in the lumbar spine? Spine 14:1002–1011, 1989

32. Pearcy MU, Tibrewal SB: Axial rotation and lateral bending in the normal lumbar spine measured by three-dimensional radiography. Spine 9:582–587, 1983

33. Rocabado M: Arthrokinematics of the temporomandibular joints. Dent Clin North Am 27:573–594, 1983

34. Rolander SD: Motion of the lumbar spine with special reference to the stabilising effect of posterior fusion: An experimental study on autopsy specimens. Acta Orthop Scand Suppl 90:1–144, 1966

35. Stoddard A: Manual of Osteopathic Technique. London, Hutchinson, 1962

36. Veldhuizen AG, Scholten PJM: Kinematics of the scoliotic spine. Spine 12:852–858, 1987

37. Warwick R, Williams P, eds: Gray's Anatomy, 36th British ed. Philadelphia, JB Lippincott, 1980

38. White AA, Panjabi MM: Clinical Biomechanics of the Spine, 2nd ed. Philadelphia, JB Lippincott, 1990

Index

Page numbers in *italics* denote figures; those followed by a t denote tables.